IMAGING OF THE DISEASES OF THE CHEST

FOURTH EDITION

To our families

Commissioning Editor: Michael Houston
Project Development Manager: Joanne Scott
Project Manager: Naughton Project Management
Designer: Sarah Russell

IMAGING OF THE DISEASES OF THE CHEST

FOURTH EDITION

David M. Hansell

Professor of Thoracic Imaging, Department of Radiology, Royal Brompton Hospital, London, UK

Peter Armstrong

Professor of Radiology, Academic Department of Radiology, St. Bartholomew's Hospital, London, UK

David A. Lynch

Professor of Radiology and Medicine, Department of Radiology, University of Colorado Health Services Center, Denver, Colorado, USA

H. Page McAdams

Associate Professor of Radiology, Department of Radiology, Duke University Medical Center, Durham, North Carolina, USA

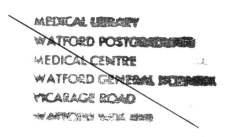
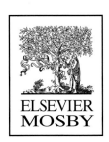

ELSEVIER
MOSBY

Philadelphia   Edinburgh   London   New York   Oxford   St Louis   Sydney   Toronto   2005

ELSEVIER
MOSBY

An imprint of Elsevier Limited

First edition 1990
Second edition 1995
Third edition 2000
Fourth edition 2005
   Reprinted 2005

ISBN 0 3230 3660 0

British Library Cataloguing in Publication Data
A catalogue record for this book is available from the British Library

Library of Congress Cataloguing in Publication Data
A catalogue record for this book is available from the Library of Congress

Notice
Medical knowledge is constantly changing. Standard safety precautions must be followed, but as new research and clinical experience broaden our knowledge, changes in treatment and drug therapy may become necessary r appropriate. Readers are advised to check the most current product information provided by the manufactactureer of each drug to be administered to verify the recommended dose, the method and duration of administration, and contraindications. It is the responsibility of the practitioner, relying on experience and knowledge of the patient, to determine dosages and the best treatment for each individual patient. Neither the Publisher nor the editors assume any liability for any injury and/or damage to persons or property arising from this publication.

The Publisher

ELSEVIER your source for books, journals and multimedia in the health sciences
www.elsevierhealth.com

Working together to grow
libraries in developing countries

www.elsevier.com | www.bookaid.org | www.sabre.org

ELSEVIER   BOOK AID International   Sabre Foundation

The
publisher's
policy is to use
**paper manufactured
from sustainable forests**

Printed in China
Last digit is the print number: 9 8 7 6 5 4 3 2

Contents

Preface

This book has been written to provide radiologists, physicians, and thoracic surgeons with a one-volume account of chest imaging, primarily in the adult patient. An attempt has been made to present an integrated review of the appearances encountered in diseases of the lung, pleura and mediastinum using the various imaging techniques available in a modern imaging department. Our aim has been to provide answers to the many queries that in our experience arise in the day-to-day practice of chest radiology.

From the preface to the first edition (1990)

Despite the advances in thoracic imaging that have occurred since the publication of the first edition, the scope and intention of this fourth edition remain the same.

A major change has come about with the retirement of Alan Wilson and Paul Dee and the stepping aside of Peter Armstrong as senior author. We are delighted that Page McAdams and David Lynch agreed to help with updating the text and renewing many of the illustrations - their expertise and input is readily evident throughout this new edition. The value of the contributions of Alan Wilson and Paul Dee to the preceding editions cannot be overstated. Their legacy is the authoritative bedrock that underpins many of the chapters.

This edition has been completely revised and the references brought up to date. For instance, the ramifications of the latest classification of the idiopathic interstitial pneumonias and the emerging role of PET in lung cancer staging are given particular attention.

In line with the ethos of earlier editions, we have chosen to present the clinical and pathologic features of the differing diseases in varying degrees of detail, based on our perception of the needs of readers. Complicated and rare entities are discussed in much more detail than commoner and well understood conditions. Once again, we hope that our efforts provide a useful resource for anyone who uses thoracic imaging in its many and varied forms.

David M. Hansell
Peter Armstrong
David A. Lynch
H. Page McAdams
2005

Acknowledgements

The number of individuals who have wittingly, or otherwise, helped with the production of this book increases with each succeeding edition, to the extent that it is now impossible to name them all; but that does not diminish our gratitude to them. Buried within some chapters are sections of enduring value from various contributors, who are not individually cited – their reward must be the knowledge that the quality of their contribution has ensured its continued inclusion.

Secretarial help with an endeavour of this size is crucial and we have been ably assisted by Jenni Hillsley, Lisa Bolt, Julie Jessop, Ann Willard and Brenda Baker, all of whom undertook the painstaking process of ensuring that the references were correctly transferred to an electronic database. Mary Anne Hansell sorted and renumbered the surviving figures from previous editions and in so doing spared the authors many hours of vexation.

Most of the numerous new illustrations were acquired in digital format direct from electronic image archives but the skills of medical photographers, notably the Medical Illustration Department of St Bartholomew's Hospital, were still occasionally required. It goes without saying that we have relied on many long-suffering colleagues to supply us with illustrations of some of the rarer conditions and we hope that they spot their prized cases in the following pages. Thanks are due to our publishers, in particular to Joanne Scott who was subjected to many impetuous requests and to Michael Houston for sanctioning most of them. We are also indebted to Nora Naughton and Sam Gear for their flexibility and efficiency at the eleventh hour.

Our wives Mary Anne, Carole, Anne, and Emma, know that we could not have completed this task without their fortitude and support.

David M. Hansell
Peter Armstrong
David A. Lynch
H. Page McAdams

Technical considerations

The chest radiograph remains the prime imaging investigation in respiratory medicine and the basic technique has changed little over the last 100 years. Of all the cross-sectional imaging techniques computed tomography (CT) has had the greatest impact on diagnosis of lung and mediastinal disease, while magnetic resonance imaging, ultrasonography and positron emission tomography have complementary roles in a few situations. Refinements to CT scanning protocols continue as more specific applications are developed. Despite technological advances the radiation burden inherent in CT scanning remains relatively high. The trend towards routine narrow-collimation volumetric acquisition represents a significant radiation burden to the patient and the optimal protocol for each patient should always be considered.

CHEST RADIOGRAPHY

The standard views of the chest are the erect posteroanterior (PA) and lateral projections. The PA chest radiograph is taken at near total lung capacity with the patient positioned so that the medial ends of the clavicle are equidistant from the spinous process of the thoracic vertebra at that level. The scapulae are held as far to the side of the chest as possible by rotating the patient's shoulders forward and placing the backs of the patient's wrists on the iliac crests. A chest radiograph obtained at nearer residual volume (expiratory film) can dramatically change the appearance of the mediastinal contour, as well as giving the misleading impression of diffuse lung disease (Fig. 1.1). Even on a correctly exposed film just under half the area of the lungs is obscured, to a greater or lesser extent, by overlying structures.[1]

Furthermore, many technical factors, notably the kilovoltage and film–screen combination used, determine how well lung detail is seen.

The steep S-shaped dose/response curve of conventional radiographic film–screen combinations (Fig. 1.2) makes it impossible to obtain perfect exposure of the most radiolucent and radiodense parts of the chest in a single radiograph. Methods of overcoming this shortcoming of radiographic film have included the use of high-kilovoltage (above 120 kV) techniques,[2] asymmetric screen–film combinations,[3] "trough" or more complex filters,[4] and sophisticated scanning equalization radiographic units.[5]

High-kilovoltage radiographs have several advantages over low-kilovoltage films. Because the coefficients of x-ray absorption of bone and soft tissue approach each other at high kilovoltage, the bony structures no longer obscure the lungs to the same degree as on low-kilovoltage radiographs (Fig. 1.3). Furthermore, the better penetration of the mediastinum with high-kilovoltage techniques allows greater detail of the large airways to be seen. At high kilovoltage, exposure times are shorter, so that structures within the lung tend to be sharper. Although scattered radiation is greater with high kilovoltage, the use of a grid means that there is a net reduction of image-degrading scattered radiation compared with a low-kilovoltage, nongrid technique. With high-kilovoltage technique an air gap of 15 cm in depth is often used, instead of a grid to disperse the scattered radiation; this is as effective as a grid, and the radiation dose to the patient is similar for the two techniques.[6] To counteract the unwanted magnification and penumbra effects of interposing an air gap, the focus–film (or anode-to-image) distance is increased to approximately 4 m. Although high-kilovoltage radiographs are preferable for

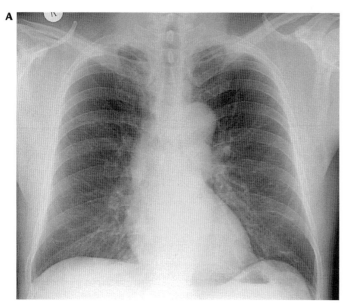 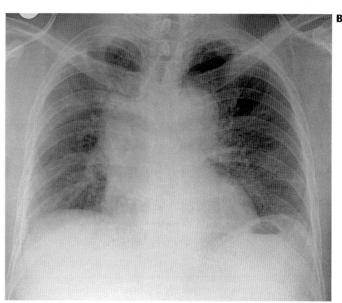

Fig. 1.1 **A**, A normal chest radiograph of an individual breath holding at full inspiration. **B**, By comparison, at full expiration, the mediastinum appears abnormally widened and there is the appearance of diffuse lung shadowing.

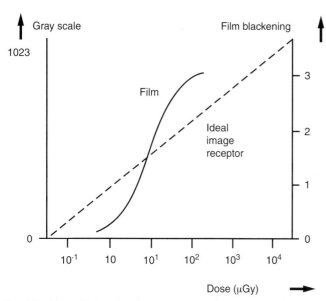

Fig. 1.2 The radiation dose/response curve of a conventional film–screen combination compared with the linear response (dotted line) of an ideal image receptor.

routine examination of the lungs and mediastinum, low-kilovoltage radiographs provide excellent detail of unobscured lung because of the better contrast between lung vessels and surrounding aerated lung. Moreover, calcified lesions, such as pleural plaques, and small pulmonary nodules[7] are particularly well demonstrated on low-kilovoltage films.

A major advance was the introduction of "faster" rare earth phosphor screens and the development of wide-latitude film.

The improved light emission from rare earth phosphors over traditional calcium tungstate crystal screens resulted in shorter exposure times and thus sharper images. A significant improvement for chest imaging came with the development of an asymmetric combination consisting of a thin front screen and high-contrast film emulsion and, on the reverse side of the film base, a thicker back screen and a low-contrast film emulsion. With this combination the two ends of the wide spectrum of transmission of x-rays through the thorax could be accommodated. Such a film–screen combination reveals significantly more detail in the mediastinum and lung obscured by the diaphragm and heart[3,8,9] (Fig. 1.4). However, there may be some loss of detail in the unobscured lung.[10]

Because attenuation of x-rays by the mediastinum is up to 10 times greater than that by the lungs, several devices have been designed to produce a more uniformly exposed chest radiograph. One of the most widely used was the advanced multiple beam equalization radiography (AMBER) system.[5] The AMBER unit comprised a horizontally oriented scanning slit beam effectively divided into 20 segments, each modulated by an electronic feedback loop from 20 corresponding detectors on the far side of the patient. Such a system is particularly good at demonstrating pulmonary lesions behind the heart and diaphragm (Fig. 1.4).[11] Nevertheless, recent advances with digital acquisition technology mean that scanning equalization devices are now largely obsolete.

Extra radiographic views

The frontal and lateral projections suffice for most purposes. Other radiographic views are becoming much less frequently requested because of the ready availability of cross-sectional

A 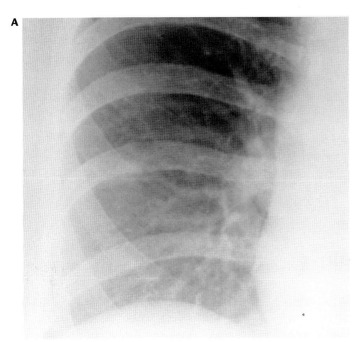 **B**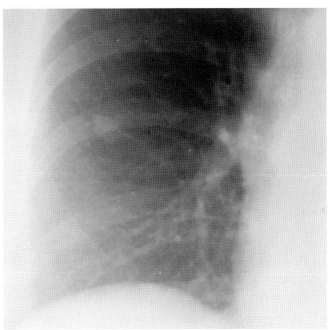

Fig. 1.3 The effect of kilovoltage on chest radiography. **A**, A low-kilovoltage (70 kVp) technique providing good detail of the ribs. A small nodule in the right mid zone is partially obscured by overlying ribs. **B**, By comparison, a high-kilovoltage (140 kVp) technique radiograph diminishes the visibility of the ribs and reveals the small carcinoid tumour in the right mid zone. (Courtesy of Dr MB Rubens, London)

imaging, particularly CT. Nevertheless, an additional view may occasionally solve a particular clinical problem quickly and cheaply.

The lateral decubitus view is not, as its name implies, a lateral view. It is a frontal view taken with a horizontal beam with the patient lying on his or her side. Its main purpose is to demonstrate the movement of fluid in the pleural space. If a pleural effusion is not loculated, it gravitates to the dependent part of the pleural cavity. If the patient lies on his or her side, the fluid layers between the chest wall and the lung edge. Because the ribs, unlike the diaphragm, are always identifiable, comparison of a standard frontal view with a lateral decubitus view is a reliable way of recognizing free pleural fluid. A lateral shoot-through radiograph may be used to advantage to show a small anterior pneumothorax in recumbent patients in intensive care (Fig. 1.5).[12]

A lordotic view is now rarely used, but is included here for completeness. It is performed by angling the x-ray beam 15° craniad, either by positioning the patient upright and angling the beam up or by leaving the beam horizontal and leaning the patient backward. In this way the lung apices are better demonstrated, free from the superimposed clavicle and first rib. The lordotic view may be useful for distinguishing a pulmonary shadow from incidental calcification of the costochondral junctions (Fig. 1.6). With the exception of identifying rib fractures and confirming the presence of a rib lesion, such as a lytic metastasis, oblique views of the thorax are rarely required.

Portable chest radiography

Portable or mobile chest radiography has the obvious advantage that the examination can be performed without moving the patient to the radiology department. In many medical centers the proportion of portable to departmental chest radiographs has gradually increased over the years. However, the many disadvantages of portable radiography should not be forgotten.

The shorter focus–film distance results in undesirable magnification. High-kilovoltage techniques cannot be used because portable machines are unable to deliver high kilovoltage and because accurately aligning the x-ray beam with a grid is difficult. Furthermore, the maximum milliamperage is severely limited, necessitating long exposure times with the risk of significant blurring of the image. Portable lateral radiographs with conventional film radiography are even less likely to be successful because of the extremely long exposure times. Radiation exposure of nearby patients and staff is a further consideration.

Positioning of bed-bound patients is difficult, and the resulting radiographs are often of half-upright or rotated subjects. Even in the so-called "erect position" with the patient sitting up, the chest is rarely as vertical as it is in a standing patient. More important, the patient is unable to take a deep breath when propped up in bed. Many patients cannot be moved to the radiology department and the improved quality of digital portable radiographs, especially phosphor plate computed radiography, represents a significant advance.

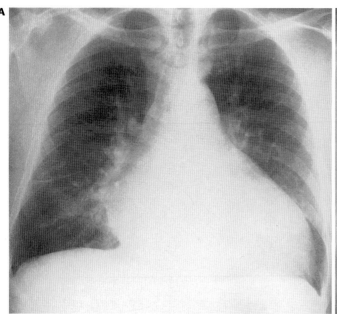

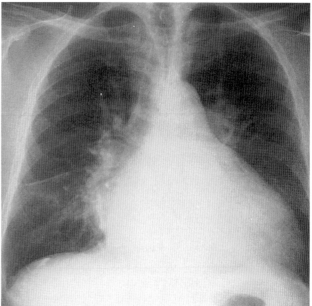

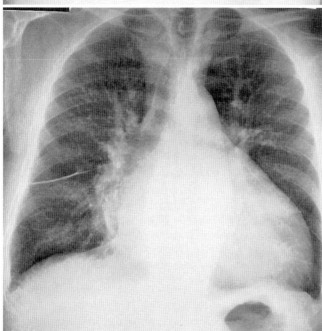

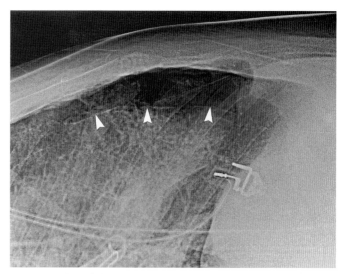

Fig. 1.4 A patient with mitral valve disease. The three chest radiographs were taken at 140 kVp using: **A**, a conventional film and rare earth screen combination; **B**, INSIGHT asymmetric film; C, an AMBER scanning equalization unit. Note the differences in mediastinal detail between the radiographs produced with the three techniques.

Fig. 1.5 A lateral shoot-through computed radiograph of a patient on the intensive care unit. The supine AP radiograph did not reveal a pneumothorax, but on this lateral radiograph an anterior pneumothorax is seen. The visceral pleural edge of the lung (arrowheads) has fallen away from the anterior chest wall.

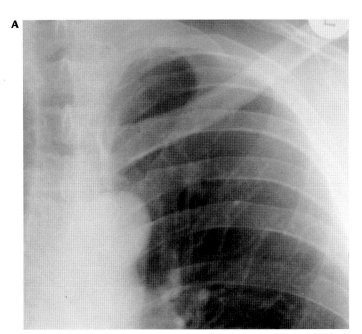
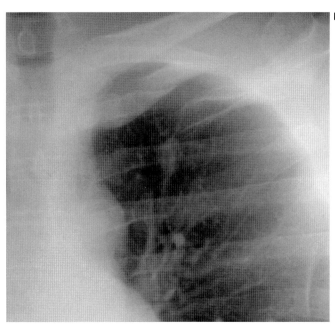

Fig. 1.6   Use of the lordotic view. **A**, A selective view of the left apex showing a small opacity projected over the anterior end of the left first rib. **B**, A lordotic view confirms that the opacity is intrapulmonary, rather than part of a calcified costochondral cartilage.

DIGITAL CHEST RADIOGRAPHY

It has long been recognized that conventional film as a means of image capture, storage, and display represents something of a compromise,[13] and over the years it has become apparent that digital image acquisition, transmission, display, and storage can, with advantage, be applied to projectional chest radiography.[14] The earliest work on digital chest radiography used digitization of conventional film radiographs by means of optical drum scanners or laser scanners. A great deal of useful information that helped to establish the parameters for clinically acceptable digital radiographs derived from observer performance studies of digitized conventional film.[15–17]

A well-established digital system employs conventional radiographic equipment but uses a reusable photostimulable phosphor plate (Europium-doped barium fluorohalide)[18] instead of a conventional film–screen combination. Phosphor plate computed radiography has been used successfully for many years, particularly as a substitute for portable film radiography.[19,20] The phosphor plate is a large-area detector housed in a "filmless" cassette. The phosphor plate stores some of the energy of the incident x-ray photons as a latent image. When the plate is scanned with a focused laser beam, the stored energy is emitted as light that is detected by a photomultiplier and converted to a digital signal (Fig. 1.7). The digital information can then be manipulated, stored and displayed in whatever format is desired (Fig. 1.8). The phosphor plate can be reused once the latent image has been erased by exposure to white light. Most currently available computed radiography systems produce a digital radiograph with a 2 K × 2 K matrix (with a pixel size of 0.2 mm) and a gray scale of up to 1024 discrete levels. The fundamental requirement of segmenting the image into a finite number of pixels entailed much work to determine the relationship between pixel size, which affects spatial resolution, and lesion detectability.[16,21,22] Digital radiography probably cannot match conventional film radiography

for the detection of extremely subtle pneumothoraces[23] and early interstitial lung disease.[24] Although an image composed of pixels of the smallest size possible would seem desirable, there is a direct inverse relationship between the pixel size and the cost and ease of data handling. In fact, there is not always a measurably significant difference in observer performance between 2 K and 4 K formats.[25] In general, pixel size is ultimately a practical compromise between image fidelity and ease of data processing and storage.

Single-shot dual-energy imaging, a technique in which the bony thorax can be removed to reveal a "soft tissue image", can be performed relatively simply with phosphor plate computed radiography by separating two phosphor plates by a thin copper filter.[26,27] The resulting images, which separate the anatomic information into bone and soft tissue components, although remarkable, have not gained widespread clinical acceptance, probably because dual-energy imaging is competing with computed tomography to provide similar information.

There has been much interest in systems using selenium as a broad area detector, particularly the commercially available Thoravision system (Philips Medical Systems).[28] This device consists of a large drum coated with amorphous selenium which, on exposure to x-rays, stores an electrostatic charge on the selenium surface. The charge pattern is then recorded by electrometer probes while the drum is rapidly rotated. Amorphous selenium is an exceedingly efficient x-ray detector which is superior to conventional film–screen and phosphor plate radiography. Phantom and clinical studies have shown that selenium detector radiography is at least as good,[29,30] or superior[31,32] to conventional radiography, or indeed phosphor plate radiography.[33,34] The overall appearance of chest radiographs obtained with a selenium detector system seems to be readily accepted by chest and general radiologists.[35] Considerable dose reduction is possible with selenium detector radiography: in studies of both chest phantoms and patients, there was no significance difference in diagnostic performance

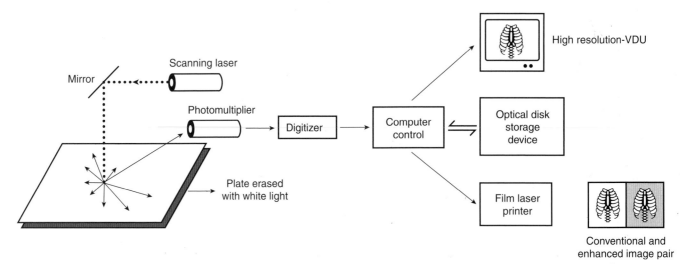

Fig. 1.7 The components of a phosphor plate computed radiography system.

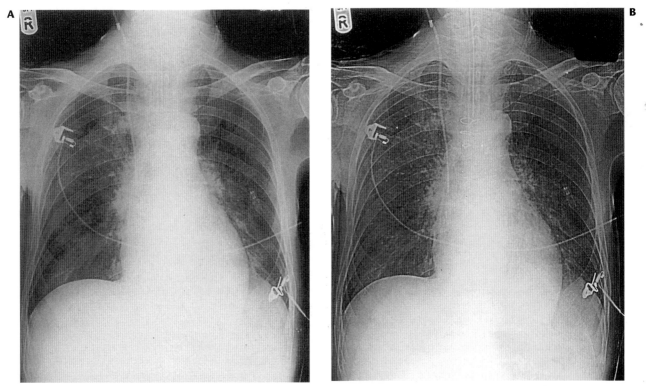

Fig. 1.8 A portable radiograph (phosphor plate) – **A**, manipulated to resemble a conventional radiograph and **B**, digitally processed to give wider latitude and edge enhancement.

between radiographs obtained with conventional exposures and those taken with up to a two-thirds reduction.[36,37] However, if an anti-scatter grid is used the dose needed for optimal images becomes comparable to conventional radiography.[38,39] In contrast to conventional film–screen chest radiography, a high kilovoltage technique may be detrimental and the recommended optimum is in the range 90–110 kVp.[40] Selenium detectors are susceptible to "memory artifact" whereby direct radiation may cause a lingering silhouette on subsequent images, unless sufficient time is given for the artifact to resolve.[41] By the nature of the drum design, selenium detector radiography is currently limited to

departmental use, and the new "direct" digital acquisition devices will probably supplant selenium technology.

There is considerable commercial activity in developing direct digital acquisition of images using new solid-state thin-film transistor flat-panel x-ray detectors.[14,42] An increasing array of "flat-panel radiography detectors" are now being marketed – the term is used to denoted the property of an active matrix with direct readout (integrated into a flat panel).[43] At present, many of these panel detectors are too heavy (and expensive) to be used for portable radiography. Clinical experience with flat-panel detectors for thoracic imaging is relatively limited but early phantom and clinical studies suggest that their favorable quantum efficiency[44–49] and performance compared with phosphor plate computed radiography[50–52] will encourage their further implementation. The report of observer preference for flat-panel chest radiographs, compared to state-of-the-art film–screen and phosphor plate chest radiographs, coupled with an overall decrease in radiation dose of 50% is promising.[53] Whether further technological developments and reduced manufacturing cost of flat-panel detectors will result in the demise of the robust, relatively inexpensive, and now mature phosphor plate technology remains to be seen.

An unequivocal advantage of digital acquisition systems over conventional film radiography is the exactly linear photoluminescence–dose response, which is a full order of magnitude greater than that of conventional film (Fig. 1.2). This extremely wide latitude, coupled with the facility for image processing, produces diagnostically acceptable images over a wide range of exposures. The ability to retrieve an image of diagnostic quality from a suboptimal exposure, which with conventional film would have resulted in an uninterpretable radiograph, has led to the increasing implementation of digital systems. Nevertheless, although overall optical density is maintained on an underexposed computed radiograph, the decreased signal-to-noise ratio may result in a loss of diagnostic content.[54] Early claims by manufacturers of phosphor plate computed radiography systems that a significant radiation dose reduction could be achieved seem to have been exaggerated[55]; indeed, in the intensive care setting the dose may actually be higher than that needed with a flat film–screen combination.[56] In addition, there are several artifacts, peculiar to computed radiography, that may hamper accurate interpretation.[57]

Numerous observer performance studies have shown that computed radiography can equal conventional film–screen radiography in virtually any specific task.[58–61] For this, however, postprocessing of the digital image may have to be used to match the digital radiograph to the task.[62] For example, unsharp masking improves the detection of central lines and other devices on intensive care portable radiographs.[63,64] A problem inherent in all forms of digital manipulation is that enhancement of the image for one purpose degrades it for another.

Many studies suggest that 2 K × 2 K monitors are adequate for making primary diagnoses of digital chest radiographs.[65–67] Indeed, for the interpretation of chest radiographs obtained on a coronary care unit, 1 K × 1 K monitors are probably sufficient.[68] There are many differences between the image appearance, radiation dose, unit cost, and applicability of the various techniques now available for obtaining a chest radiograph. Studies that have attempted to compare, for example, storage phosphor, selenium and film–screen systems[69–71] do not address every one of these factors and the final choice of system depends as much on local circumstances as objective image quality.[72]

COMPUTED TOMOGRAPHY

CT relies on the same physical principles as conventional radiography: the absorption of x-rays by tissues with constituents of differing atomic number. With multiple projections and computed calculations of radiographic density, slight differences in x-ray absorption can be displayed in a cross-sectional format.

The basic components of a CT machine are an x-ray tube and an array of x-ray detectors opposite the tube; the number and geometry of these detectors are variable. The signal from the x-ray detectors is reconstructed by a computer, and the resulting images are either laser-printed or, increasingly, displayed on a workstation. The speed with which a CT scanner acquires a single sectional image depends on the time the anode takes to rotate around the patient. The rotation time of the latest machines can be as fast as 0.42 s, allowing the acquisition of up to 38 images per second. Electron beam ultrafast CT scanning technology dispenses with a rotating mechanical anode: the patient is surrounded by a tungsten target ring, and a focused electron beam sweeps around the tungsten ring at high speed to produce an x-ray beam. Such machines are capable of acquiring an image in 100 ms or less.

Continuous volume (formerly referred to as spiral or helical) scanning has altered routine CT scanning protocols since the 1990s.[73] The basic principle of volumetric CT entails moving the patient into the CT gantry at a constant rate while data are continuously acquired, often within a single breath hold.[74,75] The resulting "corkscrew" of information is then reconstructed, most frequently as a contiguous set of axial images, similar to conventional single-slice CT sections. To achieve this, some interpolation is needed because direct reconstruction results in nonorthogonal images of nonuniform thickness. Continuous volume CT scanning has several advantages over conventional CT of the thorax: (1) rapid scan acquisition in one or two breath holds; (2) reduced volume of contrast needed for optimal opacification of vessels, for example the pulmonary arteries; (3) no misregistration between sections obtained in one acquisition, thus improving nodule detection; and (4) potential for multiplanar or three-dimensional (3D) reconstructions.[76–79] With the advent of multidetector (4–16 detector rings) technology, the possible variation in scanning protocols has become vast, as has the potential number of images generated in a single examination.[80] Multidetector computed tomography (MDCT) not only permits shorter acquisition times and greater coverage and image resolution, but also provides data sets that increasingly exploit multiplanar reformations and sophisticated 3D renditions[81] (Fig. 1.9). The potentially huge number of images generated by some protocols, for example more than 350 contiguous 1 mm sections in CT pulmonary angiography, represents a challenge in terms of efficient interpretation and the logistics of image storage and transmission. The technique of volumetric MDCT scanning of the thorax continues to be refined, and the full potential of acquiring and analyzing data in a truly volumetric form is still to be realized.[82]

General considerations

The CT image is composed of a matrix of picture elements (pixels). There is a fixed number of pixels within the picture matrix so that the size of each pixel varies according to the diameter of the circle to be scanned. The smaller the scan circle size, the smaller the area represented by a pixel and the higher the spatial resolution of the final image. In practical terms the field of view size should be adjusted to the size of area of interest, usually the thoracic diameter of the patient. Depending on the field of view size, the pixel size varies between 0.3 and 1 mm across. By selecting a specific area of interest, the operator can achieve optimal spatial resolution for that region (targeted

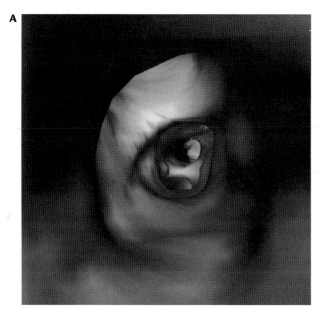
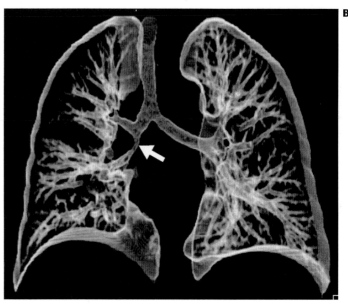

Fig. 1.9 Two examples of three-dimensional reconstructions from continuous volume CT data. **A,** A simulated endobronchial view (virtual bronchoscopy) derived from a routine CT protocol showing two segmental bronchi in the distance. **B,** A volume reduced reconstruction showing narrowing of the bronchus intermedius (arrow) caused by a central lung cancer.

reconstruction of the raw data); extra information is available that is not displayed when the whole body section is viewed at once. Targeted reconstruction is used only when the finest morphologic detail is required.

Sometimes a striking difference is apparent in the characteristics and "look" of the final CT image between different scanners. This is generally the result of differences in the software reconstruction algorithms that "smooth" the image to a greater or lesser extent by averaging the density of neighboring pixels. Smoothing is used to reduce the conspicuity of image noise and improve contrast, but it has the drawback of reducing the definition of fine structures. The lung is a high-contrast environment, and such smoothing is thus less necessary. Higher spatial resolution algorithms (which make image noise more conspicuous) are generally more desirable, and it has been recommended that they should be applied to both standard contiguous and high-resolution CT.[83,84] Because of the inherent high contrast between soft tissue structures and aerated lung, it is possible to reduce the photon flux by up to tenfold (for example, a decrease of 200 to 20 mAs) and preserve the diagnostic yield for the detection of pulmonary nodules,[85] a factor which has been exploited in the context of screening for lung cancer. Theoretically, even lower dose protocols may be practicable for the detection of high-contrast lesions. In one report, 6 mA was achieved with the use of aluminum filtration, and there was no significant difference in the detection rate of artificial focal lesions between this ultralow-dose protocol and a low-dose (50 mA) protocol.[86]

Acquisition parameters

Although a single CT section appears a two-dimensional image, it has a third dimension of depth. Thus each pixel has a volume, and the three-dimensional element is referred to as a voxel. The average radiographic density of tissue within each voxel is calculated, and the final CT image consists of a representation of the numerous voxels in the section. The single attenuation value of a voxel represents the average of the attenuation values of all the various structures within the voxel. The thicker the section, the greater the chance of different structures being included within the voxel and so the greater the averaging that occurs. The most obvious way to reduce this "partial volume" effect is to use thinner sections (Fig. 1.10).

When the whole thorax is examined, contiguous sections are employed. Thinner sections are required to clarify partial volume effects or to study areas of anatomy that are oriented obliquely to the plane of scanning. A specific example of the use of narrow sections (less than 3 mm) to display differential densities (which would otherwise be lost because of the partial volume effect) is the demonstration of small foci of fat or calcium that are sometimes seen within a hamartoma. Thin sections of 1–1.5 mm thickness are used to study the fine morphologic detail of the lung parenchyma (high-resolution CT). Apart from the evaluation of diffuse lung disease, when sampling of a few parts of the lung (traditionally with sections taken at 20 or 30 mm intervals) is adequate, contiguous section scanning is necessary to allow accurate interpretation in most situations.

For volumetric CT scanning, consideration needs to be given to the speed of table travel, volume of interest, duration of scanning (usually within one breath hold) and reconstruction interval. Pitch is defined as the distance travelled by the table per gantry revolution divided by the section thickness (collimation). A potential source of confusion arises from the two definitions of pitch used in the context of multidetector CT: it should be borne in mind that either the section thickness or the total z-axis length of the detector array may be used. The latter definition is most frequently quoted in the literature. It also should be emphasized that definitions of

A

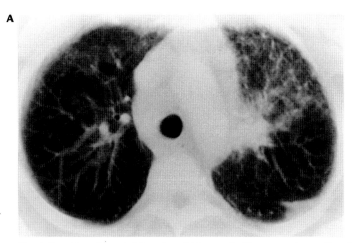

B

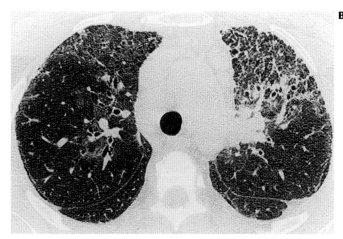

Fig. 1.10   The effect of CT section thickness. **A,** 10 mm section collimation with a standard reconstruction algorithm showing indistinct abnormalities in the lungs of a patient with pulmonary fibrosis and lymphangitis carcinomatosa. **B,** 1.5 mm section with a high spatial resolution reconstruction algorithm at the same anatomic level. Both the normal structures (for example the oblique fissures and airways) and the abnormal features including a reticular pattern and thickened interlobular septa are more clearly seen (courtesy of Dr SR Desai, London).

acquisition parameters and protocols for MDCT may, because of unique detector array designs, be specific to a given manufacturer.

A typical pitch of 1 describes the situation, assuming a gantry revolution in one second, in which the table travels at 10 mm/s with 10 mm collimation. During a 10 second breath hold, 10 cm in longitudinal axis will be covered. If the travel speed is increased to 20 mm/s, the pitch will be increased to 2 and twice the distance will be covered. In general, the useful range of pitch for thoracic work is between 1 and 2.[87] When detection of small pulmonary nodules is the primary aim, a pitch of less than 1.5 is recommended.[88] Conversely, when radiation dose is a major consideration scanning at a higher pitch reduces the radiation burden to the patient.[89] Although the spatial resolution of spiral CT images in the transaxial plane is nearly comparable to conventional CT, there is some image degradation because of broadening of the slice profile, inherent in all spiral CT scanning; this results in additional partial volume averaging in the longitudinal (z-) axis.[90] The faster the table feed, the broader the slice profile. The use of a 180° interpolation algorithm produces a slice profile close to the nominal section thickness, although this causes a slight increase in image noise.[91] Greatly increased z-axis resolution is a feature of MDCT, with isotropic imaging (identical resolution in all planes) being the ultimate goal pursued by manufacturers.

A higher pitch and increased section thickness together enable greater coverage at the expense of increased partial volume effects. However, this can be partly ameliorated by reducing the reconstruction increment, thus producing a larger number of overlapping images.[92,93] The ability retrospectively to reconstruct axial images with considerable overlap by choosing a small reconstruction interval is a major advantage of spiral CT.[94] Nowadays, with the increasing implementation of MDCT, adequate anatomical coverage in a single breath hold is becoming less of an issue.

Intravenous contrast enhancement

The high contrast on CT between vessels and surrounding air in the lung, as well as between vessels and surrounding fat

within the mediastinum, means that intravenous contrast enhancement is needed only in specific instances, for example for the detection of emboli within the pulmonary arteries. The exact timing of the injection of contrast media depends most on the time the CT scanner takes to scan the thorax. With fast spiral CT scanning the circulation time of the patient becomes an important factor. However, general guidance about the time of arrival of contrast medium from the antecubital vein to various structures is possible.[95] In normal individuals arrival time in the superior vena cava is 4 seconds, pulmonary arteries 7 seconds, ascending aorta 11 seconds, descending aorta 12 seconds, and inferior vena cava 16 seconds. Occasionally small bubbles of air, introduced with the contrast medium infusion, will be seen, particularly in the main pulmonary artery.[96]

The contrast medium rapidly diffuses out of the vascular space into the extravascular space, so that opacification of the vasculature following a bolus injection quickly declines and nonvascular structures such as lymph nodes steadily increase in density over time. Because of these dynamics, there is a time at which a solid structure may have exactly the same density as an adjacent vessel. The timing and duration of the contrast medium infusion must therefore be taken into account when interpreting a contrast-enhanced CT examination. Rapid scanning protocols with automated injectors improve contrast enhancement of vascular structures at the expense of enhancement of solid lesions because of the rapidity of scanning. With rapid CT scanning it is possible to achieve good opacification of all the thoracic vascular structures with a total dose of less than 100 ml contrast (iodine content of 150–350 mg/ml) at a rate of about 2 ml/s.[97] Some CT scanners generate streak artifact centered on the high-density bolus of contrast, usually as it passes through the superior vena cava. This beam-hardening artifact may be troublesome if it obscures detail in the adjacent pulmonary arteries, particularly in patients being investigated for pulmonary embolism (Fig. 7.16). One solution is to reduce the iodine concentration and use a high volume of dilute contrast at an increased flow rate.[98] A reduction in both the streak artifact and amount of contrast needed can also be achieved by employing a power injector to "push" a smaller volume of contrast with a following bolus of saline solution.[99] One protocol recommended for general thoracic CT scanning is

100 ml of 150 mg iodine/ml (300 mg iodine/ml diluted 50:50) injected at a rate of 2.5 ml/s after a 25 second delay.[100] However, Loubeyre et al have shown that satisfactory enhancement of the hilar vasculature can be obtained with a relatively modest amount of contrast (60 ml of 250 mgI/ml at 3 ml/s).[101] For the examination of inflammatory lesions it may be necessary to delay scanning by at least 30 seconds to allow contrast to diffuse into the extravascular space. Each CT examination must be carefully tailored to the clinical problem; the protocol needed for the evaluation of an empyema with a single-slice CT is very different to that required for the investigation of pulmonary embolism using MDCT.

Consideration must be given to the consequences of accidental extravasation of contrast medium: the flow rate used, within reason, is not predictive of the likelihood of extravasation,[102] nevertheless large volumes (more than 100 ml) introduced into the soft tissues of the forearm by an automated power injector may be associated with severe complications, including compartment syndrome and tissue necrosis; in the event of extravasation of a large volume of contrast, urgent surgical advice should be sought.[103]

Window settings

The average density of each voxel is measured in Hounsfield units (HU); these units have been arbitrarily chosen so that zero is water density and −1000 is air density. The range of Hounsfield units encountered in the thorax is wider than in any other part of the body, ranging from aerated lung (approximately −800 HU) to ribs (+700 HU). The operator uses two variables to select the range of densities to be viewed: window width and window center or level.

The window width determines the number of Hounsfield units to be displayed. Any densities greater than the upper limit of the window width are displayed as white, and any below the limit of the window are displayed as black. Between these two limits the densities are displayed in shades of gray. The median density of the window chosen is the center or level, and this center can be moved higher or lower at will, thus moving the window up or down through the range (Fig. 1.11). The narrower the window width, the greater the contrast discrimination within the window. No single window setting can depict this wide range of densities on a single image. For this reason, thoracic work requires at least two sets of images, usually to demonstrate the lung parenchyma and the soft tissues of the mediastinum. Furthermore, it may be necessary for the operator to adjust the window settings to improve the demonstration of a particular abnormality. Standard window widths and centers for thoracic CT vary between institutions, but some generalizations can be made: for the soft tissues of the mediastinum and chest wall a window width of 300–500 HU and a center of +40 HU are appropriate. For the lungs a wide window of approximately 1500 HU or more at a center of approximately −600 HU is usually satisfactory.[104] For skeletal structures the widest possible window setting at a center of 30 HU is best. Allowing observers to adjust window settings, compared with images at fixed window settings, does not appear to improve performance in terms of identifying fine lung structures or detecting diffuse lung disease.[105]

Window settings have a profound influence on the visibility and apparent size of normal and abnormal structures. The most accurate representation of an object appears to be achieved if the value of the window level is halfway between the density of the structure to be measured and the density of the surrounding tissue.[106,107] For example, the diameter of a pulmonary nodule, measured on soft tissue settings appropriate for the mediastinum, will be grossly underestimated.[108] It is also important to remember that when inappropriate window settings are used, smaller structures (for example, peripheral pulmonary vessels) are proportionately much more affected than larger structures. The optimal window settings for the postprocessed data, for example minimum intensity projection images or 3D volume rendered images, cannot be prescribed and are largely a matter of observer preference.

In the context of HRCT the window settings have a substantial effect on both the appearance of the lungs and the apparent dimensions of, for example, the thickness of bronchial walls[109,110] (Fig. 1.12). Alterations of the window settings may sometimes make detection of parenchymal abnormalities impossible in cases in which there is a subtle increase or decrease in attenuation of the lung parenchyma. Although no absolute window settings can be given because of machine variation and individual preferences, uniformity of window settings from patient to patient will aid consistent interpretation of the lung images. In general, a window level of −500 to −800 Hounsfield units (HU) and a width of between 900 and 1500 HU is usually satisfactory. Modifying the window settings for particular tasks is often desirable: for example in looking for pleuro-parenchymal abnormalities in asbestos-exposed individuals, a wider window of up to 2000 may be useful. Conversely, a narrower window width of approximately 600 HU may usefully emphasize the subtle density differences encountered in patients with emphysema or small airways disease. There does not appear to be any significant diagnostic gain, or otherwise, in allowing observers to adjust window settings freely.[105]

Indications and protocols

There is no single protocol which can be recommended for every clinical eventuality without being prohibitively excessive in terms of radiation dose, time taken, or data acquired. The optimal protocol is one that makes a difference to patient outcome by providing clinically relevant information at the lowest possible radiation dose. There is a constant tension between the desire for a comprehensive examination and the unnecessary exposure of the patient to ionizing radiation.[111] Despite its obvious benefits, MDCT encourages indiscriminate "catch-all" protocols, a problem exacerbated by unfocused clinical requests, for example: "Dyspnea, Rule out bronchiectasis, Nodule on CXR – ?neoplasm". A combination protocol for a general lung examination using MDCT might include contiguous 5 or 3 mm sections from which thin sections (3 or 1.25 mm respectively) can be extracted. Clearly the radiation dose of contiguous 3 mm sections, compared to a tailored protocol appropriate to the scenario above (e.g. HRCT 1 mm sections interspaced 20 mm and contiguous 3 mm sections through the putative nodule), could be regarded as unacceptably high, especially in a young patient.

Attempts to contain and, wherever possible reduce, the radiation dose of a CT examination should be a constant consideration.[111,112] As a practical and simple example, Wildberger et al found that with a Siemens Volume Zoom MDCT (Siemens,

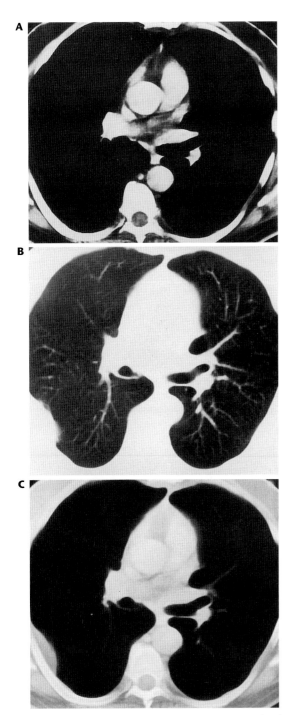

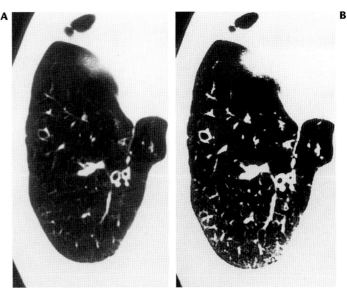

Fig. 1.12   The effect of window settings. **A**, There is cylindrical bronchiectasis in the right lower lobe with wall thickening of the affected bronchi (level –600 HU, width 1300 HU). **B**, Bronchial wall thickening is exaggerated on inappropriately narrow window settings (level –500 HU, width 800 HU).

Fig. 1.11   An illustration of the effects of varying CT window levels and window widths. The section shows an extrapleural lipoma lying against the right chest wall. **A**, Window center 30 HU, window width 350 HU shows mediastinal soft tissue differences to advantage but does not show lung detail, nor is the lipoma easy to see. **B**, Window center 30 HU, window width 1500 HU shows the whole range of densities so that bone detail is well seen, the lipoma is recognizable as a soft tissue mass, and the mediastinal and lung structures are visible but subtle distinctions of contrast are invisible. **C**, Window center –600 HU, window width 1000 HU shows lung detail to advantage but provides no information about the mediastinum other than the outline.

Forchheim, Germany) adaptation of the mAs based on the patient's weight (body weight in kilograms minus 10) produced image quality comparable to the standard dose recommended by the manufacturer (120 mAs).[113] Such a maneuver resulted in an approximate 45% reduction in radiation dose; these findings have been reproduced elsewhere[114] and it is surprising that more centers have not adopted this simple radiation reducing strategy.

Indications for CT can be broadly divided into situations in which CT elucidates an abnormality shown on a plain chest radiograph and those in which the chest radiograph appears normal but cryptic disease is suspected (Box 1.1). Some of the technical modifications, idiosyncracies and artifacts of the more common protocols used for specific clinical indications, notably high-resolution computed tomography, are now considered. Specific aspects of CT technique peculiar to a particular clinical indication (for example, CT pulmonary angiography for pulmonary embolism) appear in the relevant chapters.

High-resolution CT (HRCT) technique for parenchymal disease

Three factors significantly improve the spatial resolution of CT images of the lung: narrow scan collimation, a high spatial resolution reconstruction algorithm, and a small field of view.[115] Other aspects that affect the final image, over which the user has no control, include the x-ray focal spot size, the geometry and array of detectors, and the frequency of data sampling and scan acquisition time.[116] It is worth appreciating that the same imaging parameters (for example, scan collimation and reconstruction algorithm) applied to two different CT scanners can result in images of very different appearance, although such differences in image quality rarely cause diagnostic confusion.

Scan collimation

Narrow collimation of the x-ray beam reduces volume averaging within the section and so increases spatial resolution compared with standard (for example, 8 mm) collimation.[117,118] Collimation of between 0.5 and 1.5 mm can be used.[117,119,120] A section thickness greater than 3 mm does not improve spatial resolution substantially compared with standard section widths. In contrast, reducing the section thickness below 0.5 mm will not yield any significant further improvement in spatial resolution and at the same time significantly reduces the signal-to-noise ratio of the image. Differences between 1.5 mm and 3 mm collimation are probably insignificant for the detection of small structures,[117] but subtle regional variations in the density of the lung parenchyma are more easily appreciated with 1.5 mm collimation images. Narrow section collimation has a marked effect on the appearance of the lungs, notably the vessels and bronchi: the branching vascular pattern seen particularly in the mid zones on standard 10 mm sections has a more nodular appearance on narrow sections, because shorter segments of the obliquely running vessels are included in the plane of section (Fig. 1.10). The resulting "nodular" pattern of the normal lungs can be pronounced on some CT scanners. Another effect of narrow collimation is an apparent increase in the diameter of vessels that run parallel with the plane of section. This is due to the elimination of the partial volume effect of air surrounding the rounded surface of the vessel encountered in standard width sections. The diameter of vessels or bronchi running perpendicular to the plane of section are the same irrespective of the scan collimation.

Interspacing between each section is usually 1 or 2 cm. Studies have shown that wider intervals do not have a deleterious effect on diagnosis in a wide spectrum of interstitial lung diseases[121,122]; a more minimalist approach might entail images being obtained at the level of the arch, tracheal carina, and 2 cm above the right hemidiaphragm. In practice, however, even experienced radiologists need the reassurance that confirmatory or ancillary features are not being missed by keeping the interspace distance to less than 3 cm.

The application of MDCT to high-resolution CT has implications in terms of image quality, novel image presentation (reformations), and radiation burden. Schoepf et al acquired scans with 1 mm collimation with multidetector CT and reconstructed 5 mm contiguous and 1.25 mm high-resolution CT sections from the original data.[123] Image quality (assessed subjectively) of the 5 mm "fused" images was significantly superior to the 5 mm single detector CT images, and the 1.25 mm images were of similar quality to conventional HRCT (1 mm sections acquired at 10 mm increments) using single detector CT. For the patient in whom such a comprehensive examination is required, this may be an appropriate and useful technique. However, for the majority of patients being evaluated for suspected interstitial lung disease, conventional HRCT remains an adequate examination. A standard HRCT examination yields approximately 30 transaxial images; a protocol involving the reconstruction of 5 mm contiguous sections and 1.25 mm sections at 10 mm increments (from a MDCT volumetric set acquired with 1 mm detector collimation) would produce approximately 90 images. In an attempt to reduce the number of images that need to be interrogated using this protocol, Remy-Jardin et al evaluated the diagnostic accuracy of coronal thin sections as an alternative to transaxial HRCT scans. Reconstructions in the coronal plane result in fewer images (owing to the overall conformation of the thorax) and diagnostic accuracy was similar to that of conventional transaxial HRCT.[124] Not surprisingly, coronal reformations produced from "isotropic" data obtained from volumetric 0.5 mm collimation acquisitions can be of high quality.[120] The issue of dose with respect to MDCT is an important one. Volumetric imaging of the chest with 1 mm collimation (performed on a MDCT Somatom Plus 4 Volume Zoom machine) entails an effective dose of between 6.4 and 7.8 mSv even when a relatively low dose (70 mAs) is used. This is considerably higher than the effective dose of a conventional (1.5 mm at 10 mm intervals) HRCT which is approximately 0.98 mSv (140 kVp and 175 mAs).

It has been estimated that the mean skin radiation dose delivered with HRCT using 1.5 mm sections at 20 mm intervals is 6% of that of conventional 10 mm contiguous scanning protocols.[125] A study of the differences of the more meaningful parameter of effective radiation dose has shown that a standard HRCT protocol (1.5 mm sections at 10 mm intervals) delivers approximately 6.5 times less effective dose than a conventional single detector CT (10 mm contiguous sections); the effective dose from a standard HRCT (0.98 mSv) is about 12 times that of a PA and lateral chest radiograph.[126] It is possible to reduce the milliamperage of an HRCT examination by up to tenfold and still obtain comparably diagnostic images.[127] Such low-dose techniques result in a considerable increase in image noise, and subtle parenchymal abnormalities such as early emphysema or ground-glass opacification may be obscured. Lee et al compared relatively low (80 mAs) and high dose (340 mAs) HRCTs and found no difference in diagnostic accuracy in 50 patients with chronic diffuse infiltrative lung disease.[121] Taking these options into account, one approach might be to use 80–90 mAs for the initial HRCT and to use the lower dose (40–50 mAs) for subsequent follow up (Fig. 1.13).

Reconstruction algorithm

The type and characteristics of the software algorithm used to reconstruct the CT image are at least as crucial as the chosen

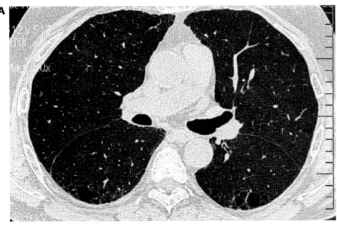
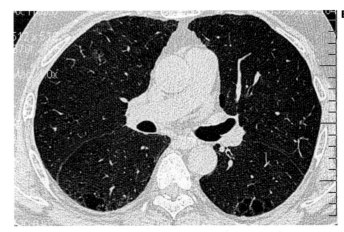

Fig. 1.13 HRCT of a patient with suspected interstitial lung disease. **A**, HRCT obtained at 90 mAs. **B**, HRCT at the same anatomic level at 50 mAs showing no appreciable difference in image quality.

section width. In conventional body CT, images are reconstructed with a medium or relatively low spatial frequency algorithm which is designed to smooth the image and so reduce the visibility of image noise and improve contrast resolution. In HRCT lung work, a high spatial frequency algorithm is used which takes advantage of the inherently high-contrast environment of the lung. The high spatial frequency algorithm (also known as the edge-enhancing, sharp or formerly "bone" algorithm) reduces image smoothing and makes structures visibly sharper but at the same time makes image noise more conspicuous.[115,117] More than any other manipulation in HRCT technique, it is the combination of section thickness and the unique reconstruction algorithm of a particular CT scanner that determines the final appearance of the lung image; occasionally the variations in appearances of images obtained on different CT scanners make comparisons difficult.

Targeted reconstruction

HRCT scanning is usually performed using a field of view which encompasses the whole patient in cross section (approximately 35 cm diameter). After acquiring the image data, it is possible to "target" the reconstruction to a single lung, thus reducing the image pixel size and so increasing spatial resolution. For example, with a matrix of 512 × 512 pixels and a 40 cm field of view the pixel size is 0.78 mm. If the image reconstruction is targeted to a 25 cm diameter field of view (large enough to encompass an average size single lung in cross section) the pixel size is reduced to 0.5 mm and the spatial resolution is correspondingly increased. In practice, targeted reconstruction is now seldomly performed, largely because of the laborious nature of the process and the inability to view both lungs on a single image.

Artifacts

Several artifacts can be consistently identified on HRCT images but they do not usually degrade the diagnostic content. It is useful to be aware of the commonest artifacts, which are caused by patient motion, quantum noise, and aliasing.

Probably the most frequently encountered artifact on HRCT images of the lung is a streaking appearance due to patient motion. When scan acquisition time is less than 3 seconds respiratory motion is rarely responsible for significant motion artifact. However, even with millisecond scan acquisition, movement of the lung due to cardiac motion sometimes causes

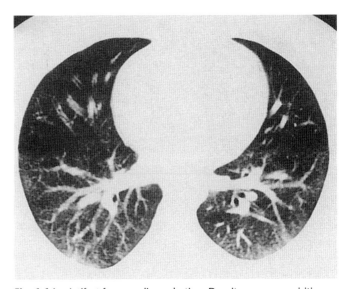

Fig. 1.14 Artifact from cardiac pulsation. Despite a scan acquisition time of 0.2 s, some of the vessels in the right middle lobe are "double-imaged" and so resemble bronchiectatic airways (6 mm collimation section).

degradation of image quality of the adjacent lingula and, to a lesser extent, the right middle lobe. Pulsation artifacts take the form of high-density linear streaks, usually arising from the heart border. Another manifestation of movement is a "star" pattern centered on pulmonary vessels[128] and these vessels may show a superficial resemblance to bronchiectatic airways in cross section.[129] Sometimes the oblique fissure may be seen as two fine lines in parallel.[130] This artifact is due to linear structures being scanned in different positions after the gantry has turned through 180°. Although the double fissure artifact is unlikely to cause misdiagnosis, "double vessels" may occasionally resemble bronchiectasis[129] (Fig. 1.14). Some scanners are capable of prospective ECG gating. Schoepf et al subjectively assessed image quality and the presence of motion artifacts on ECG-gated versus non-ECG-gated HRCT sections.[131] ECG gating clearly reduces artifacts adjacent to the heart but it has not yet been determined whether it actually improves the diagnostic accuracy of HRCT. In theory, at least, it should be

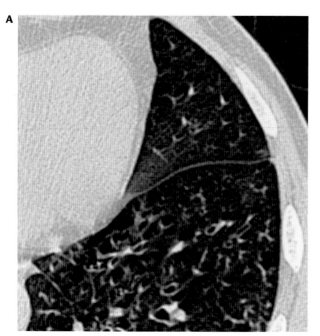 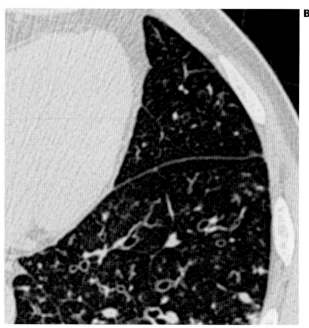

Fig. 1.15 A detail of HRCT of a patient with cylindrical bronchiectasis. **A**, A non-ECG-gated image shows considerable image degradation caused by cardiac motion artifact. **B**, An ECG-gated image provides clearer visualization of the airways in the left lower lobe and lingula.

easier to detect subtle parenchymal and airway abnormalities on images with less artifact (Fig. 1.15).

The size of the patient has a direct effect on the quality of the lung image: the larger the patient, the more conspicuous the noise because of increased x-ray absorption by the patient. Image noise or quantum mottle takes the form of granular streaks arising from high-attenuation structures and is particularly evident in the posterior lung adjacent to the vertebral column (Fig. 1.16). Image noise rarely interferes with diagnosis and while the problem can be counteracted by increasing the kVp and mA settings, the reduction in noise is, except in the largest patients, barely perceptible. The phenomenon of aliasing results in a fine streak-like pattern radiating from sharp, high-contrast interfaces. The severity of the aliasing artifact is related to the geometry of the CT scanner and particularly the spacing of the detectors and scan collimation; unlike quantum mottle, aliasing is independent of the radiation dose. Aliasing and quantum mottle are most prominent in the paravertebral regions and often parallel the pleural surface.[115] These artifacts are exaggerated by the non-smoothing high spatial resolution reconstruction algorithm but do not mimic normal anatomical structures and are rarely severe enough to obscure important detail in the lung parenchyma.

When early interstitial fibrosis is suspected, for example in asbestos-exposed individuals, HRCT scans are often performed in the prone position to prevent any confusion with the increased opacification seen in the dependent posterobasal segments of many normal individuals scanned in the usual supine position. The increased density seen in the posterior dependent lung in the supine position will disappear in normal individuals when the scan is repeated at the same level with the patient in the prone position (Fig. 1.17). The physiological mechanism of the increased opacification in the dependent lung in normal individuals is not fully understood and has been ascribed to gravity dependent perfusion[132] and/or relative

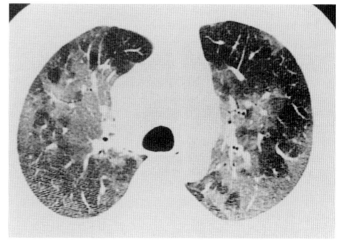

Fig. 1.16 Artifact (quantum mottle) in the paravertebral regions of a large patient. The patchy ground-glass opacity in this case was caused by desquamative interstitial pneumonia.

atelectasis of the dependent lung.[133] Prone sections are mandatory in patients with suspected diffuse lung disease and a normal or near-normal chest radiograph, but are unnecessary if the chest radiograph is clearly abnormal.[134]

Maximum intensity projection (Max IP)

One of the early reported limitations of HRCT for the assessment of diffuse infiltrative lung disease was the perception that micronodules were more reliably distinguished from blood vessels on standard collimation sections.[135,136] The problem of making this distinction has probably been overstated in the past. However, with MDCT it is possible to acquire volumetric data rapidly: the entire thorax can be imaged with a high-

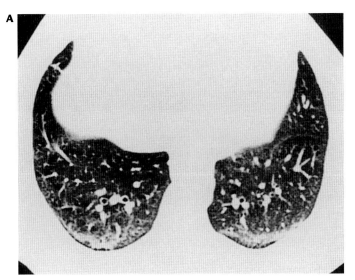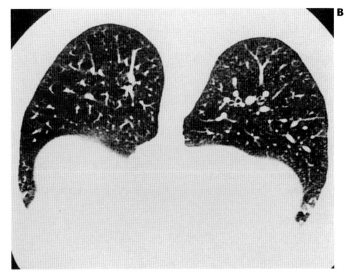

Fig. 1.17 **A**, Increased parenchymal opacity in the dependent lung in a supine patient. **B**, When the patient is turned over into the prone position, the density in the posterolateral segments disappears, confirming that this is a normal gravity-dependent phenomenon rather than fixed pathology.

resolution technique in 17 seconds using a pitch of 6, 1.0 mm detectors, and a rotation time of 0.5 seconds.[137] Maximum intensity projection (Max IP) images have been advocated as an additional tool in the evaluation of diffuse infiltrative lung diseases; the diagnostic benefit of Max IP postprocessing for the detection of larger nodules, for example pulmonary metastases, is unequivocal.[138] Remy-Jardin and colleagues[139] compared conventional CT (1 mm and 8 mm collimation) with Max IP images (sliding slabs of 3 mm, 5 mm, and 8 mm thickness generated from volumetric CT performed at the level of the region of interest) in patients with a suspicion of micronodular infiltration. Max IP images showed micronodular disease involving less than 25% of the lung when conventional CT was inconclusive, and better defined the profusion and distribution of micronodules when they were identified on conventional images. However, in patients with normal 1 mm and 8 mm images, sliding thin-slab Max IP images did not reveal additional lung abnormalities. Bhalla et al[140] used Max IP reconstruction in 20 patients with known diffuse lung disease and found two main advantages over thin-section CT: more precise identification of nodules and more accurate characterization of suspected nodule distribution (perivascular versus centrilobular). The technique is not widely used routinely in the context of diffuse lung disease, largely because volumetric data have to be acquired, and in most cases of suspected interstitial lung disease a standard HRCT technique will have been performed.

CT technique for airways diseases

Bronchiectasis

The simplest and most widely used technique for patients with suspected bronchiectasis remains narrow collimation (1.0–1.5 mm) sections every 10 mm from lung apex to base with images reconstructed using a high spatial frequency reconstruction algorithm.[141,142] Potential advantages of volumetric CT include improved detection of subtle bronchiectasis missed between HRCT sections, reduced motion artifact, and seamless reconstruction of oblique airways.[143,144] In a study that compared HRCT with spiral CT for the detection of bronchiectasis, Lucidarme et al showed that the detection rate of bronchiectasis

with spiral CT (3 mm collimation, pitch of 1.6; 24 s breath hold) was superior to a standard HRCT protocol (1.5 mm collimation at 10 mm intervals).[145] Furthermore, interobserver agreement was superior with the spiral CT protocol. However, the radiation burden to patients using the spiral CT protocol was 3.4 times greater (skin dose) than that of conventional HRCT. In another study that compared HRCT with spiral CT (5 mm collimation, pitch of 1; 40 s breath hold), spiral CT with 5 mm section thickness was not as sensitive as HRCT.[146] More recently Remy-Jardin et al have shown that in terms of diagnostic accuracy there are no important differences between 3 mm and 1 mm reconstructed images acquired with MDCT,[147] the implication being that there could be a modest radiation saving if 3 mm sections were acquired from 4 × 2.5 mm detectors (rather than 4 × 1 mm detectors necessary for 1 mm reformations). Yi et al investigated the effects of radiation dose on volumetric acquisitions and concluded that a tube current of 70 mA or higher provided image quality compatible to standard (170 mA) HRCT images[148]; nevertheless, the radiation dose of the volumetric protocol is considerably higher (five times) than that of HRCT. Nevertheless, whether such volumetric acquisitions are necessary for the majority of patients with suspected bronchiectasis remains open to question, although the ability of these data sets to provide coronal and other reformations has some attractions.[149]

Variations in window settings have a marked effect on the apparent thickness of bronchial walls[109] (Fig. 1.12). Narrow window settings will also alter the apparent bronchial diameter unless the measurement of the diameter is made between points in the "center" of the bronchial walls.[150] In the context of suspected bronchiectasis a window level of between −400 and −950 Hounsfield units (HU) and a width of between 1000 and 1600 HU have been widely recommended.[151–153] A more liberal recommendation about the appropriate window level for the accurate evaluation of bronchial wall thickness has been reported in a study by Bankier et al that correlated thin-section CT with planimetric measurements of inflation-fixed lungs.[110] For the accurate estimation of bronchial wall thickness the authors suggest that, irrespective of the chosen window width, the window center should be between −250 and −700 HU, and that within this range bronchial wall thickness is not appreciably affected. Window width should be greater than 1000 HU (a narrower window width will cause a spurious appearance of bronchial wall thickening); the suggested window width range lies between 1000 and 1400 HU.[110]

Small airways disease

HRCT is currently regarded as the imaging method of choice for the detection of small airways disease. Standard HRCT technique is satisfactory for demonstrating constrictive obliterative bronchiolitis and diffuse panbronchiolitis. The former requires attention to appropriate contrast resolution to demonstrate sometimes subtle regional attenuation differences caused by air-trapping (mosaic attenuation pattern). The latter is more dependent on adequate spatial resolution to depict the small branching structures that characterize exudative panbronchiolitis (tree-in-bud pattern).[154] In this context a suggested HRCT protocol is 1–1.5 mm collimation sections every 10 mm from apices to costophrenic angles with the patient breath-holding at full inspiration.[155] Care should be exercised when choosing window widths as minor differences in lung attenuation may only be visible when narrow (<1000 HU) window widths are used.[156]

Expiratory CT

The necessity of the routine acquisition of expiratory CT sections is controversial. The regional inhomogeneity of the lung density is accentuated and small or subtle areas of air-trapping may be revealed on CT performed at end-expiration[157,158] (Fig. 1.18). Expiratory CT may be helpful in differentiating between the three main causes of a mosaic pattern (infiltrative lung disease, small airways disease, and occlusive pulmonary vascular disease) which may be problematic on inspiratory CT.[159,160] A lesser number of expiratory than inspiratory HRCT sections (e.g. at 30 or 40 mm intervals) are usually obtained. Although expiratory images almost invariably make regional inhomogeneity more conspicuous, and occasionally reveal the presence of air-trapping not suspected on the inspiratory images, in most patients with clinically significant small airways disease the mosaic pattern is apparent on inspiratory images.

Dynamic studies in which sections are obtained in rapid succession at a given level during forced expiration may improve the conspicuity and apparent extent of air-trapping.[161] A recent study that compared low-dose (40 mA) dynamic expiratory CT with the more conventional end-expiratory CT technique demonstrated that the density changes were significantly greater with the dynamic technique.[162] In very specific circumstances, for example the surveillance of lung transplant patients when the early detection of small airways dysfunction may be important, dynamic expiratory low-dose thin-section CT may be indicated. Each dynamic sequence (acquired at the level of the arch, carina, and 2 cm above the right hemidiaphragm) is obtained as a 6-second cine-acquisition with no table movement.

Minimum intensity projection (Min IP)

The contrast between normal and low attenuation lung parenchyma in patients with constrictive obliterative bronchiolitis may be subtle on inspiratory HRCT images, and image processing techniques such as minimum intensity projections (Min IPs) can improve the conspicuity of such regional density differences.[140,163] In a study by Fotheringham et al, Min IP images showed good correlation with pulmonary function tests and had the lowest observer variation when compared with inspiratory and expiratory images.[163] Window settings for the interpretation of Min IP slabs have not been standardized; window widths of 350–500 HU and a window level of –750 to –900 HU have been used in the few studies that have investigated this technique.

Central airways disease

The near-isotropic volume data sets that can be acquired with multidetector CT coupled with advances in volume rendering software have made possible routine 3D airway imaging. Axial imaging currently remains widely used for the evaluation of the central airways despite several limitations including underestimation of subtle bronchial stenoses, difficulties in depicting complex 3D relationships of the airways, and inadequate representation of the airways that lie obliquely to the axial plane.[76,77,164,165] Two-dimensional (2D) multiplanar and

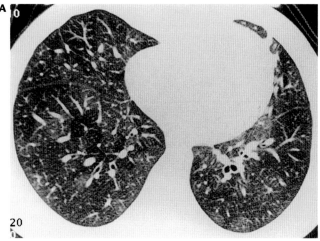 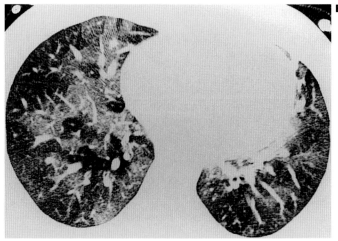

Fig. 1.18 Expiratory CT in a patient with constrictive bronchiolitis following bone marrow transplantation. **A,** A mosaic attenuation pattern, most easily appreciated in the right lower lobe on standard inspiratory HRCT. **B,** Marked enhancement of the mosaic pattern on expiratory HRCT.

3D reconstruction images aid assessment of a wide variety of airway diseases.[166]

Multiplanar reconstructions

Quint et al evaluated CT images from lung transplant patients using 3 mm collimation, pitch of 1, and a 1.5 mm reconstruction interval and found that axial images were 91% accurate in the detection of bronchial stenoses.[167] By comparison, viewing the axial images with multiplanar reconstructions (sagittal and coronal) improved accuracy, marginally, to 94%. However, observers found it easier to identify mild stenoses on the multiplanar images, highlighting the difficulty of accurately assessing luminal caliber on sequential axial images. Multiplanar reconstructions also depict the lengths of stenotic segments more clearly due to the orientation of the section along the long axis of the airway.

Improvements in computing power and speed have led to the replacement of shaded surface display renditions with 3D volume rendering. Volume rendering converts the volume of information acquired by MDCT into a simulated 3D form that surpasses the technique of surface-shaded display[168] which is limited by threshold voxel selection. The volume-rendered 3D image is the computed sum of voxels along a ray projected through the data set in a specific orientation, thus using all the MDCT data to form the final image. The volume rendering technique assigns a continuous range of values to a voxel, allowing the percentage of different tissue types to be reflected in the final image while maintaining 3D spatial relationships. Remy-Jardin et al compared overlapping axial CT images with volume-rendered bronchographic images for the detection of airway abnormalities and identification of lesion morphology.[76] Findings on the volume-rendered images were concordant but added no complementary value to those on the transverse CT images in half of the cases. However volume-rendered images provided supplemental information in a third and could correct potential interpretative errors from viewing only transverse CT images in 5%.

The most alluring technique to be applied to airway imaging is "virtual bronchoscopy" (Fig. 1.9A). These images are obtained using volume rendering techniques that allow internal rendering of the tracheo-bronchial tree producing an appearance similar to that seen by a bronchoscopist. Adequate images can be obtained even with low (50 mA) tube currents.[169] Despite these exciting possibilities, virtual bronchoscopy remains just that, and despite software advances the technique cannot be regarded as an indispensable tool in airway imaging. Studies using this technique have revealed several limitations. Summers et al used virtual bronchoscopy to assess 14 patients with a variety of airway abnormalities.[170] They found that, overall, 90% of segmental bronchi that were measurable at CT could be measured at virtual bronchoscopy. However, of the total bronchi expected to be visible, only 82% could be evaluated at virtual bronchoscopy and only 76% of segmental bronchi were demonstrated compared with 91% and 85% respectively for multiplanar CT images. Axial CT and the "virtual" images were of similar accuracy in estimating the maximal luminal diameter and cross-sectional area of the central airways. These authors used 3 mm sections, pitch of 2, a field of view of 26 cm or less, and 1 mm reconstruction intervals. Virtual bronchoscopy demonstrates stenoses of the central airways (proved with fiberoptic bronchoscopy) in most cases,[171,172] but in the former study[171] all the stenoses demonstrated by virtual bronchoscopy

were also shown on the axial CT images. In addition, evaluation of the length of the stenoses and surrounding tissues required simultaneous display of multiplanar reformations.

The use of airway stents for benign and malignant stenotic disease provides another potential, but limited, use for volume rendering techniques. As stents require frequent follow up, 3D CT of the airway offers an easier way to monitor cases until adjustment requires direct intervention.[173] From experience so far it seems that for many central airways diseases 3D CT does not have a greater sensitivity than conventional transaxial images, but it does confer an advantage in describing spatial relationships of airway disease, particularly in communicating this information to clinicians.[165]

MAGNETIC RESONANCE IMAGING

In thoracic imaging the most significant advantage of magnetic resonance imaging (MRI) over other cross-sectional imaging is its excellent contrast resolution of soft tissues. It also has the benefit of not using ionizing radiation. However, it has taken several years of accumulated published evidence and clinical experience to allow the conclusion that CT, particularly multidetector CT, is the technique of choice for the investigation of most commonly encountered mediastinal and lung diseases. There are, however, specific instances in which MRI is traditionally considered a useful problem-solving technique: these include the identification of mediastinal or chest wall invasion by tumor,[174–177] the differentiation between solid and vascular hilar masses,[178,179] the demonstration of diaphragmatic abnormalities,[180] and the assessment of mediastinal disease in patients with treated lymphoma.[181–183] However, it is notable that most of the studies that describe the application of MRI to these clinical situations are from the 1980s or early 1990s, and nowadays most centers use MDCT for thoracic imaging, including the specific areas thought earlier to be the domain of "problem-solving" MRI. There is continued interest in the role of MR angiography for the diagnosis of pulmonary embolism, either by direct demonstration of intravascular thrombus[184–187] or by decreased signal areas representing underperfused lung on gadolinium-enhanced MRI.[188]

High spatial resolution imaging with MRI is technically possible, but there is a trade-off between resolution on one hand and signal-to-noise ratio and acquisition time on the other. The relatively poor spatial resolution of MRI remains an obstacle to its more widespread use in thoracic imaging. For example, the spurious appearance of small clusters of lymph nodes in the mediastinum, which appear as a single mass, prevents the routine application of MRI to the staging of bronchogenic carcinoma. However, faster spin-echo techniques improve contrast and spatial resolution for the evaluation of the lungs by reducing motion artifact.[189–192] Imaging sequences and protocols have been developed for obtaining an adequate and reproducible signal from lung parenchyma,[193,194] although considerable technical difficulties remain. More recently, various inhaled agents have been investigated for imaging the airspaces of the lung.[195–198] Hyperpolarized noble gases, specifically Helium-3, have been used to demonstrate ventilated parts of the lung.[199,200] In addition, Xenon gas, which rapidly crosses lipid membranes, has the potential to be used for imaging the lung interstitium.[195] Ventilation imaging has been performed using oxygen as a paramagnetic contrast agent with inversion recovery (IR) sequence or multiple IR sequences,[201] and perfusion imaging has been succesfully demonstrated using arterial spin labeling (ASL). Combining oxygen-enhanced and ASL methods yields an MR technique to correlate ventilation and perfusion[202] (Fig. 1.19). Nevertheless, the generation of some contrast agents is complex and so these techniques remain in the experimental domain.

Technical considerations

MRI of the lung poses some unique challenges, particularly the consequences of cardiac and respiratory movement and the

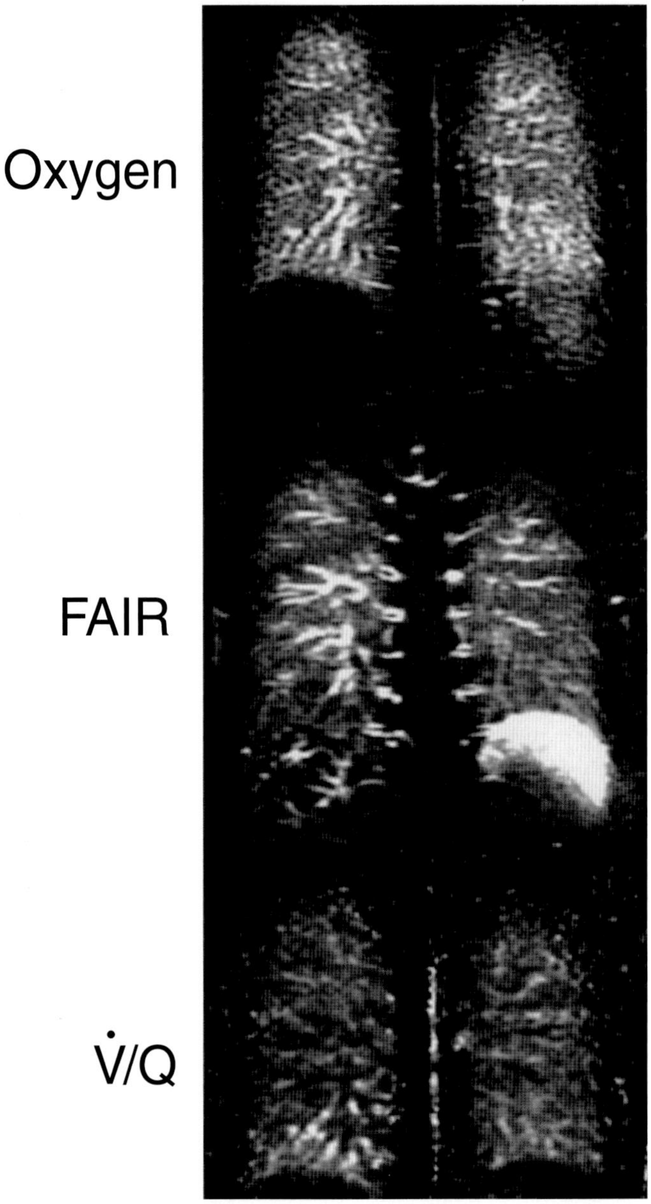

Fig. 1.19 A sophisticated MR depiction of ventilation (oxygen) and perfusion (flow-sensitive alternating inversion recovery [FAIR]) in a healthy individual. The V̇/Q image represents the signal intensity from the combined oxygen and FAIR acquisitions. (With permission from Mai VM, Liu B, Polzin JA, et al. Ventilation-perfusion ratio of signal intensity in human lung using oxygen-enhanced and arterial spin labeling techniques. Magn Reson Med 2002;48:341–350.)

extremely low proton density of normal lung. The large tissue–air interface of the lung induces susceptibility artifacts that affect magnetic field homogeneity and lead to signal loss from intravoxel phase dispersion of spins in lung parenchyma.[203] An experimental technique that circumvents this rapid decay in signal has been reported.[204]

With the numerous imaging sequences, gating techniques, and planes of sections available to the radiologist, no single protocol can be prescribed for a thoracic MRI examination; more than any other imaging investigation in the chest, the protocol needs to be tailored to the clinical question to be answered. For example, the MRI examination of suspected pulmonary embolism will be different in virtually every detail from an examination of the diaphragm.

An appreciation of the factors that affect the signal-to-noise ratio (SNR) is crucial when considering the method of obtaining optimal MR images of the thorax. In MRI, signal intensity is proportional to the volume of tissue within a voxel. Because background noise is constant through the entire tissue volume, the voxel size in MRI needs to be larger than in CT to maintain a tolerable SNR. The same consideration applies to section thickness: section width is directly related to SNR. Sections less than 5 mm wide usually result in an unacceptably low SNR. The signal is further reduced with contiguous sections because of a phenomenon known as "cross-talk". For this reason most protocols include an interspace of approximately 25% of the section thickness between individual sections.[95]

The field of view has a profound effect on SNR. Although the field of view should be equivalent in size to the region of interest, SNR decreases dramatically below a field of view of 30 cm because of the reduction in pixel size inherent in decreasing the field of view (halving the field of view reduces the pixel size fourfold and therefore the SNR by the same factor). The SNR can be increased by increasing the number of radiofrequency excitations and averaging the signal from each pixel. Doubling the number of radiofrequency excitations entails doubling the scanning time for what is only a modest increase in SNR; for this reason it is rarely employed.

MR images are degraded by periodic respiratory and cardio-vascular motion. The result is blurring of the image and superimposition of ghost images. At higher magnetic fields, degradation of the image by motion is more marked and the ghost images are more obvious because of the higher SNR. Artifacts from cardiovascular motion are minimized by synchronizing the acquisition of the images to a certain point in the cardiac cycle by electrocardiographic triggering. Such gating increases the scan time by approximately 15% while significantly improving image quality.[205]

Artifact from the movement of normal breathing cannot be countered by gating simply because the respiratory cycle is too long and a basic gating technique would require extremely long examination times.[206] Many data acquisition and processing techniques, including averaging, rephasing, and reordering of phase encoding (ROPE)[207] and navigator[192] techniques, have been developed to overcome this problem. None is ideal, but fast scan techniques with acquisition within one breath hold have been reported.[208] Rapid breath-hold MRI has been successfully applied to cardiac studies.[209] For lung imaging, however, this technique suffers from the susceptibility artifacts encountered with gradient echo imaging.

Fast spin-echo (FSE), also called turbo spin-echo (TSE) imaging, has been developed.[210] This sequence uses a multiecho spin-echo sequence that changes the phase-encode gradient for each of the echoes, which allows the acquisition of multiple lines of k-space within a given repetition time. This significantly reduces the total imaging time, compared to an ordinary spin-echo sequence. The dominant image contrast is determined by the echo times of the low-order k-space acquisitions (low-order phase encoding steps give global image contrast, high-order phase encoding steps give edge detail). Therefore, by changing the k-space coverage and changing which echo the low k-space acquisitions are acquired over, it is possible to change the effective echo time and produce images with different T1 or T2 weightings. On T2-weighted (long effective echo time) FSE images, fat signal appears bright due to the T1 weighting from signals acquired at shorter echo times. To preempt this, fat saturation is sometimes employed for clinical imaging.

Artifacts sometimes simulate or obscure the presence of thrombus in the major cardiovascular structures. In spin-echo imaging increased signal intensity may be returned from slow-flowing blood because of the second echo of a symmetric double spin-echo sequence (known as even-echo rephasing). On the other hand, immobile thrombus often shows a reduction in signal intensity (with the caveat that the signal intensity of thrombus is affected by its age). Phase display images show either a high or a low signal intensity from moving objects, whereas static structures show contrast signal intensity.[211,212] Perhaps the simplest technique for differentiating slow-flowing blood from a suspected thrombus is the use of gradient echo pulse sequences. The extremely high signal from even relatively slow-flowing blood usually allows the distinction to be made (Fig. 1.20). However, if the vessel runs parallel to the plane of section, the contained blood receives multiple radiofrequency pulses and thus has a reduced signal, so that it potentially mimics thrombus. This can be resolved by imaging the vessel perpendicular to the scan plane.[213]

Imaging of structures located in areas with physiological motion (thorax and abdomen) is commonly performed using rapid imaging during a breath hold (typically 15 s). However, this may be difficult in a patient with lung disease. In addition, as patients are required to breath hold reproducibly at the same diaphragm position, slice misregistration can occur. This refers to imaging artifact caused by imperfect alignment of individual image slices. In addition to the reproducibility problem, the signal-to-noise ratio and spatial resolution are inherently low because of the limited acquisition time of a single breath hold. In recent years, respiratory monitoring has become possible using an MR navigator echo, which tracks the diaphragm position in real time and uses this information to gate image data acquisition. The navigator echo can also be used for sophisticated and intelligent phase-encode ordering.[192]

Tissue characteristics and paramagnetic contrast agents

Differences in MR signal intensity among various tissues are due to a complex relationship between proton density and spin-lattice (T1) and spin-spin (T2) relaxation times.[214] After excitation by a radiofrequency pulse the nuclei return to their resting state. In the process an exchange of energy occurs; if the exchange is inefficient, the T1 time is long. The T1 time is a constant which reflects the rate of energy exchange between protons and the surrounding lattice. Fat has the shortest T1 relaxation time of all human tissues. In contrast, the large collagen macromolecules of fibrous (solid) tissue have much longer T1 relaxation times.

The T2 relaxation time is more complex and is influenced by inhomogeneity of the external (applied) and induced (local) magnetic field. Although the mobile molecules of water and fat generate the most signal, these molecules usually interact with the surrounding macromolecules that constitute the bulk of the soft tissue and thus their relaxation times are altered. It is this fundamental influence on water (and to a lesser extent fat) molecules by the macromolecular components of different tissues that produces the striking contrast differences among various tissues on MRI. Thus an increase in the concentration of freely mobile water molecules and a decrease in the proportion of macromolecules (particularly protein) capable of interacting with water give long T1 and T2 relaxation times. Conversely, tissue with a high protein content shortens T1 relaxation times and at the same time has a less predictable effect on T2 relaxation times. Paramagnetic agents, in the form of blood or gadolinium-complex contrast media, reduce T1 times; this phenomenon is the result of increasing the range of resonant frequency of protein protons by varying the magnetic field in the immediate vicinity of the paramagnetic material. In this way a wider range of proton-bearing molecules are recruited. The net result is a greater signal on T1 images with no substantial effect on T2 images at usual concentrations of gadolinium.

The MR signal intensity of a given tissue is an average of the contribution from each constituent of the tissue. In the same way, different pathologic processes produce different signal intensities depending on the proportions of, for example, fibrosis, edema, and necrosis. Because of the wide overlap in signal intensity resulting from the many components that contribute to the final signal, the signal intensity of a lesion cannot be regarded as specific; different pathologic conditions may produce similar signals. Any change in the various components of a tissue over time is reflected in the MR signal. For this reason, MRI, unlike CT, is more sensitive to serial change in a pathologic lesion; this characteristic has been exploited in monitoring some tumors. The naturally occurring contrast agents in the thorax that provide the most clinically useful information on MRI are fat, flowing blood, and air. The high signal intensity of fat on T1-weighted images is of particular value because of its abundance in the

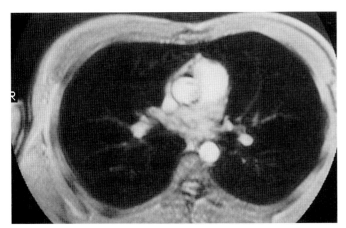

Fig. 1.20 A gradient echo magnetic resonance image showing high signal from flowing blood, particularly in the great vessels running perpendicular to the plane of section.

mediastinum and in the extrapleural region around the chest wall: the detection of local invasion by a tumor relies largely on the striking contrast between its signal and the adjacent fat.

Certain pathologic conditions lend themselves to characterization by MRI because of their distinctive signals; hemorrhagic lesions or hematoma,[215] the proteinaceous contents of some foregut duplication cysts,[216] the high lipid content of lipoid pneumonia,[217] and to a lesser extent alveolar proteinosis, all result in a shortened T1 relaxation time. Differences in relaxation time between reactive mediastinal lymph nodes and those containing metastases are not large enough to be clinically useful.[218,219] Nevertheless, the differences in T2 relaxation time between tumor and established fibrosis are substantial enough to allow clinically useful judgments about tumor recurrence versus postradiation fibrosis, particularly in patients with lymphoma.[181,182] Early studies showed that increased signal on T2-weighted images reflected edema associated with diffuse active alveolitis but this is not generally used for following patients with diffuse interstitial lung disease.[191,194] Although the administration of gadopentetate dimeglumine may increase the conspicuity of honeycomb lung in patients with fibrosing alveolitis, it does not appear to affect the detection of areas of ground-glass opacification as shown on HRCT.[220]

Sequences for thoracic magnetic resonance imaging

Spin-echo sequences that have a short repetition time (TRI) and a short echo time (TE), referred to as T1-weighted, increase the contrast between fat and surrounding tissues. T1-weighted images are therefore suited to anatomic studies. T2-weighted images have long TR and TE times and may allow further characterization of abnormalities detected on the T1-weighted images (Fig. 1.21).[221,222] In general, if no abnormality is found on these T1-weighted sequences, further imaging with T2-weighted sequences is unlikely to reveal additional information that would otherwise be overlooked.[95]

Cardiac and respiratory gating considerably improve image quality by reducing motion artifact, particularly for the areas adjacent to the heart or diaphragm. Relatively static lesions, for example at the lung apex, can be imaged satisfactorily without such gating. When cardiac gating is used, the TR time is equal to the R–R wave interval of the cardiac cycle. At a normal heart rate, cardiac gating produces pulse sequences with a TR of 800–1000 ms. The optimal echo time for lung studies depends on the magnetic field strength, but for most thoracic work the TE should be 20 ms or less. The long TR time of T2-weighted scans must be matched with the heart rate of the patient, and if necessary cardiac gating is adjusted to cover every third or fourth heartbeat. A further consideration with T2-weighted images is that thicker sections are desirable; sections less than 8 mm make tissue characterization difficult because of poor signal-to-noise ratio.

In some circumstances suppressing the signal from fat may be useful; this can be done by choosing an appropriately short inversion time so that the signal from fat can be caught at its null time and thus be eliminated. The technique used for fat suppression is the so-called "STIR (short T1 inversion recovery) sequence". It has the disadvantage that some signal loss from other tissues occurs.

Rapid imaging using TSE sequence imaging, gradient echo sequences (which have numerous acronyms such as FEER, GRASS, FAST, and FLASH), and imaging during steady-state precession (SSFP) have been developed. TSE uses a multiecho spin-echo sequence that changes the phase-encode gradient for each of the echoes, which allows the acquisition of multiple lines of k-space within a given repetition time. In gradient echo sequences magnetic field gradients are used to dephase and then rephase the protons following an excitation pulse, and an echo is produced much more rapidly than by the spin-echo sequence. Reduced flip angles are used for the initial exciting pulse to avoid saturation. An additional maneuver to maintain signal from moving blood is to make use of the "even echo rephasing" phenomenon and to acquire the second echo rather than the first. An extremely fast acquisition version of this sequence enables images to be acquired during a breath hold. The striking property of gradient echo images is the great contrast between the high signal from flowing blood and the surrounding structures. With SSFP sequences, rapid, repetitive excitation pulses induce a state of equilibrium for both longitudinal and transverse magnetization. True-FISP (true fast

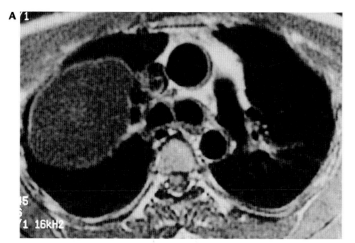
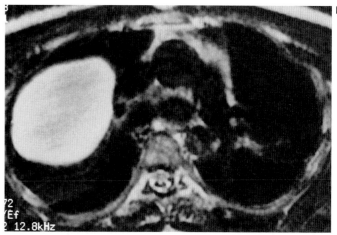

Fig. 1.21 **A**, A T1-weighted MR image of a patient with a hydatid cyst in the right lung. **B**, A T2-weighted image showing increased contrast discrimination and increased noise associated with T2-weighted images.

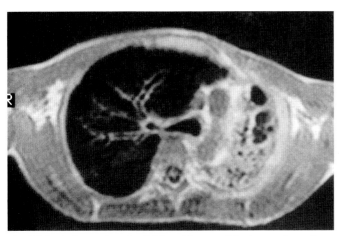

Fig. 1.22 A short spin-echo (TE 8 ms) image of the lungs of a patient with cystic fibrosis, showing bronchiectatic airways in the right lung.

imaging in steady-state precession, also called balanced fast-field echo and FIESTA) is a widely used steady-state sequence that uses fully balanced gradients.[223]

Several studies have shown that extremely short spin-echo sequences improve the demonstration of lung detail[191,193,224] but the images obtained with such techniques do not compare with the high spatial resolution images of computed tomography (Fig. 1.22).

REFERENCES

1. Chotas HG, Ravin CE. Chest radiography: estimated lung volume and projected area obscured by the heart, mediastinum, and diaphragm. Radiology 1994;193:403–404.
2. Revesz G, Shea FJ, Kundel HL. The effects of kilovoltage on diagnostic accuracy in chest radiography. Radiology 1982;142:615–618.
3. Swensen SJ, Gray JE, Brown LR, et al. A new asymmetric screen-film combination for conventional chest radiography: evaluation in 50 patients. AJR Am J Roentgenol 1993;160:483–486.
4. Peppler WW, Zink F, Naimuddin S, et al. Patient-specific beam attenuators. Proceedings of the Chest Imaging Conference. Madison, Wis: 1987: 64–78.
5. Vlasbloem H, Schultze Kool LJ. AMBER: A scanning multiple-beam equalization system for chest radiography. Radiology 1988;169:29–34.
6. Trout ED, Kelley JP, Larson VL. A comparison of an air gap and a grid in roentgenography of the chest. AJR Am J Roentgenol 1975;124:404–411.
7. Kelsey CA, Moseley RD, Mettler FA, et al. Comparison of nodule detection with 70-kVp and 120-kVp chest radiographs. Radiology 1982;143: 609–611.
8. Morishita J, MacMahon H, Doi K, et al. Evaluation of an asymmetric screen-film system for chest radiography. Med Phys 1994;21:1769–1775.
9. Rottenberg GT, Chinn RJS, Allen CM, et al. Portable chest radiography in intensive care: comparison of a new dual characteristic film-screen system (Insight) incorporating a flexible grid with a standard film-screen system. Clin Radiol 1996;51:494–498.
10. Logan PM, Tunney T, McCoy CT, et al. Comparison of a new dual characteristic film-screen system (insight) with a standard film-screen system for chest radiology. Br J Radiol 1994;67:162–165.
11. Schultze Kool LJ, Busscher DLT, Vlasbloem H, et al. Advanced multiple-beam equalization radiography in chest radiology: a simulated nodule detection study. Radiology 1988;169:35–39.
12. Morgan RA, Owens CM, Collins CD, et al. The improved detection of pneumothoraces in critically ill patients with lateral shoot-through digital radiography. Clin Radiol 1993;48: 249–252.
13. Goodman LR, Wilson CR, Foley WD. Digital Radiography of the chest: promises and problems. AJR Am J Roentgenol 1988;150:1241–1252.
14. Schaefer-Prokop C, Uffmann M, Eisenhuber E, et al. Digital radiography of the chest: detector techniques and performance parameters. J Thorac Imaging 2003;18:124–137.
15. Goodman LR, Foley WD, Wilson CR, et al. Digital and conventional chest images: observer performance with film digital radiography system. Radiology 1986;158:27–33.
16. Lams PM, Cocklin ML. Spatial resolution requirements for digital chest radiographs: an ROC study of observer performance in selected cases. Radiology 1986;158:11–19.
17. MacMahon H, Metz CE, Doi K, et al. Digital chest radiography: effect on diagnostic accuracy of hard copy, conventional video, and reversed gray scale video display formats. Radiology 1988;168:669–674.
18. Sonoda M, Takano M, Miyahara J, et al. Computed radiography utilizing scanning laser stimulated luminescence. Radiology 1983;148:833–838.
19. Freedman MT, Artz DS. Digital radiography of the chest. Semin Roentgenol 1997;32:38–44.
20. Niklason LT, Chan HP, Cascade PN, et al. Portable chest imaging: comparison of storage phosphor digital, asymmetric screen-film, and conventional screen-film systems. Radiology 1993;186: 387–393.
21. Foley WD, Wilson CR, Keyes GS, et al. The effect of varying spatial resolution on the detectability of diffuse pulmonary nodules. Radiology 1981;141:25–31.
22. MacMahon H, Vyborny CJ, Metz CE, et al. Digital radiography of subtle pulmonary abnormalities; an ROC study of the effect of pixel size on observer performance. Radiology 1986;158:21–26.
23. Fajardo LL, Hillman BJ, Pond GD, et al. Detection of pneumothorax: comparison of digital and conventional chest imaging. AJR Am J Roentgenol 1989; 152:475–480.
24. Kido S, Ikezoe J, Takeuchi N, et al. Interpretation of subtle interstitial lung abnormalities: conventional versus storage phosphor radiography. Radiology 1993;187:527–533.
25. Miro SP, Leung AN, Rubin GD, et al. Digital storage phosphor chest radiography: an ROC study of the effect of 2K versus 4K matrix size on observer performance. Radiology 2001;218:527–532.
26. Ishigaki T, Sakuma S, Horikawa Y, et al. One-shot dual-energy subtraction imaging. Radiology 1986;161:271–273.
27. Kido S, Ikezoe J, Naito H, et al. Clinical evaluation of pulmonary nodules with single-exposure dual-energy subtraction chest radiography with an iterative

noise-reduction algorithm. Radiology 1995;194:407–412.

28. Chotas HG, Floyd CEJ, Ravin CE. Technical evaluation of a digital chest radiography system that uses a selenium detector. Radiology 1995;195:264–270.

29. van Heesewijk HP, van der Graaf Y, de Valois JC, et al. Chest imaging with a selenium detector versus conventional film radiography: a CT-controlled study. Radiology 1996;200:687–690.

30. Bernhardt TM, Otto D, Reichel G, et al. Detection of simulated interstitial lung disease and catheters with selenium, storage phosphor, and film-based radiography. Radiology 1999;213:445–454.

31. van Heesewijk HP, Neitzel U, van der Graaf Y, et al. Digital chest imaging with a selenium detector: comparison with conventional radiography for visualization of specific anatomic regions of the chest. AJR Am J Roentgenol 1995;165:535–540.

32. Schaefer-Prokop CM, Prokop M, Schmidt A, et al. Selenium radiography versus storage phosphor and conventional radiography in the detection of simulated chest lesions. Radiology 1996;201:45–50.

33. Biemans JM, Van Heesewijk JP, Van Der Graaf Y. Digital chest imaging: selenium radiography versus storage phosphor imaging. Comparison of visualization of specific anatomic regions of the chest. Invest Radiol 2002;37:47–51.

34. Awai K, Komi M, Hori S. Selenium-based digital radiography versus high-resolution storage phosphor radiography in the detection of solitary pulmonary nodules without calcification: receiver operating characteristic curve analysis. AJR Am J Roentgenol 2001;177:1141–1144.

35. Floyd CEJ, Baker JA, Chotas HG, et al. Selenium-based digital radiography of the chest: radiologists' preference compared with film-screen radiographs. AJR Am J Roentgenol 1995;165:1353–1358.

36. van Heesewijk HP, van der Graaf Y, de Valois JC, et al. Effects of dose reduction on digital chest imaging using a selenium detector: a study of detecting simulated diffuse interstitial pulmonary disease. AJR Am J Roentgenol 1996;167:403–408.

37. van Heesewijk HP, Casparie HW, de Valois JC, et al. Effect of dose levels on the diagnostic performance of a selenium-based digital chest system. Invest Radiol 2001;36:455–459.

38. Ravin CE, Chotas HG. Chest radiography. Radiology 1997;204:593–600.

39. Otto D, Ludwig K, Fessel A, et al. Digital selenium radiography: detection of subtle pulmonary lesions on images acquired with and without an additional antiscatter grid. Eur J Radiol 2000;36:108–114.

40. Launders JH, Cowen AR, Bury RF, et al. Towards image quality, beam energy and effective dose optimisation in digital thoracic radiography. Eur Radiol 2001;11:870–875.

41. Chotas HG, Floyd CEJ, Ravin CE. Memory artifact related to selenium-based digital radiography systems. Radiology 1997;203:881–883.

42. Chotas HG, Dobbins JT, Ravin CE. Principles of digital radiography with large-area electronically readable detectors: a review of the basics. Radiology 1999;210:595–599.

43. Kotter E, Langer M. Digital radiography with large-area flat-panel detectors. Eur Radiol 2002;12:2562–2570.

44. Fink C, Hallscheidt PJ, Noeldge G, et al. Clinical comparative study with a large-area amorphous silicon flat-panel detector: image quality and visibility of anatomic structures on chest radiography. AJR Am J Roentgenol 2002;178:481–486.

45. Hosch WP, Fink C, Radeleff B, et al. Radiation dose reduction in chest radiography using a flat-panel amorphous silicon detector. Clin Radiol 2002;57:902–907.

46. Strotzer M, Volk M, Reiser M, et al. Chest radiography with a large-area detector based on cesium-iodide/amorphous-silicon technology: image quality and dose requirement in comparison with an asymmetric screen-film system. J Thorac Imaging 2000;15:157–161.

47. Strotzer M, Volk M, Frund R, et al. Routine chest radiography using a flat-panel detector: image quality at standard detector dose and 33% dose reduction. AJR Am J Roentgenol 2002;178:169–171.

48. Chotas HG, Ravin CE. Digital chest radiography with a solid-state flat-panel x-ray detector: contrast-detail evaluation with processed images printed on film hard copy. Radiology 2001;218:679–682.

49. Hennigs SP, Garmer M, Jaeger HJ, et al. Digital chest radiography with a large-area flat-panel silicon X-ray detector: clinical comparison with conventional radiography. Eur Radiol 2001;11:1688–1696.

50. Goo JM, Im JG, Lee HJ, et al. Detection of simulated chest lesions by using soft-copy reading: comparison of an amorphous silicon flat-panel-detector system and a storage-phosphor system. Radiology 2002;224:242–246.

51. Herrmann A, Bonel H, Stabler A, et al. Chest imaging with flat-panel detector at low and standard doses: comparison with storage phosphor technology in normal patients. Eur Radiol 2002;12:385–390.

52. Floyd CE Jr, Warp RJ, Dobbins JT III, et al. Imaging characteristics of an amorphous silicon flat-panel detector for digital chest radiography. Radiology 2001;218:683–688.

53. Ganten M, Radeleff B, Kampschulte A, et al. Comparing image quality of flat-panel chest radiography with storage phosphor radiography and film-screen radiography. AJR Am J Roentgenol 2003;181:171–176.

54. Kimme-Smith C, Aberle DR, Sayre JW, et al. Effects of reduced exposure on computed radiography: comparison of nodule detection accuracy with conventional and asymmetric screen-film radiographs of a chest phantom. AJR Am J Roentgenol 1995;165:269–273.

55. Heggie JC, Wilkinson LE. Radiation doses from common radiographic procedures: a ten year perspective. Australas Phys Eng Sci Med 2000;23:124–134.

56. Weatherburn GC, Bryan S, Davies JG. Comparison of doses for bedside examinations of the chest with conventional screen-film and computed radiography: results of a randomized controlled trial. Radiology 2000;217:707–712.

57. Volpe JP, Storto ML, Andriole KP, et al. Artifacts in chest radiographs with a third-generation computed radiography system. AJR Am J Roentgenol 1996;166:653–657.

58. Schaefer CM, Greene R, Hall DA, et al. Mediastinal abnormalities: detection with storage phosphor digital radiography. Radiology 1991;178:169–173.

59. Schaefer CM, Greene R, Oestmann JW, et al. Digital storage phosphor imaging versus conventional film radiography in CT-documented chest disease. Radiology 1990;174:207–210.

60. Thompson MJ, Kubicka RA, Smith C. Evaluation of cardiopulmonary devices on chest radiographs: digital vs analog radiographs. AJR Am J Roentgenol 1989;153:1165–1168.

61. Elam EA, Rehm K, Hillman BJ, et al. Efficacy of digital radiography for the detection of pneumothorax: comparison with conventional radiography. AJR Am J Roentgenol 1992;158:509–514.

62. Prokop M, Neitzel U, Schaefer-Prokop C. Principles of image processing in digital chest radiography. J Thorac Imaging 2003;18:148–164.

63. Jennings P, Padley SPG, Hansell DM. Portable chest radiography in intensive care: a comparison of computed and conventional radiography. Br J Radiol 1992;65:852–856.

64. Nodine CF, Liu H, Miller WTJ, et al. Observer performance in the localization of tubes and catheters on digital chest images: the role of expertise and image enhancement. Acad Radiol 1996;3:834–841.

65. Frank MS, Jost RG, Molina PL, et al. High-resolution computer display of portable, digital, chest radiographs of adults: suitability for primary interpretation. AJR Am J Roentgenol 1993;160:473–477.

66. Hayrapetian A, Aberle DR, Huang HK, et al. Comparison of 2048-line digital display formats and conventional radiographs: An ROC study. AJR Am J Roentgenol 1989;152:1113–1118.

67. Razavi M, Sayre JM, Taira RK, et al. Receiver operating characteristic study of chest radiographs in children: digital hard-copy film vs 2K × 2K soft-copy images. AJR Am J Roentgenol 1992; 158:443–448.

68. Steckel RJ, Batra P, Johnson S, et al. Comparison of hard- and soft-copy digital chest images with different matrix sizes for managing coronary care unit patients. AJR Am J Roentgenol 1995;164:837–841.

69. Kehler M, Lyttkens K, Andersson B, et al. Phantom study of chest radiography with storage phosphor, selenium, and film-screen systems. Acta Radiol 1996; 37:332–336.

70. Leppert AG, Prokop M, Schaefer-Prokop CM, et al. Detection of simulated chest lesions: comparison of a conventional screen-film combination, an asymmetric screen-film system, and storage phosphor radiography. Radiology 1995;195:259–263.

71. Woodard PK, Slone RM, Sagel SS, et al. Detection of CT-proved pulmonary nodules: comparison of selenium-based digital and conventional screen-film chest radiographs. Radiology 1998; 209:705–709.

72. MacMahon H. Digital chest radiography: practical issues. J Thorac Imaging 2003;18:138–147.

73. Zeman RK, Baron RL, Jeffrey RB Jr, et al. Helical body CT: evolution of scanning protocols. AJR Am J Roentgenol 1998; 170:1427–1438.

74. Kalender WA, Seissler W, Klotz E, et al. Spiral volumetric CT with single-breath-hold technique, continuous transport, and continuous scanner rotation. Radiology 1990;176:181–183.

75. Vock P, Soucek M, Daepp M, et al. Lung spiral volumetric CT with single breath-hold technique. Radiology 1990;176: 864–867.

76. Remy-Jardin M, Remy J, Artaud D, et al. Volume rendering of the tracheobronchial tree: clinical evaluation of bronchographic images. Radiology 1998;208:761–770.

77. Ravenel JG, McAdams HP, Remy-Jardin M, et al. Multidimensional imaging of the thorax: practical applications. J Thorac Imaging 2001; 16:269–281.

78. Lawler LP, Fishman EK. Multi-detector row CT of thoracic disease with emphasis on 3D volume rendering and CT angiography. Radiographics 2001;21:1257–1273.

79. Salvolini L, Bichi SE, Costarelli L, et al. Clinical applications of 2D and 3D CT imaging of the airways – a review. Eur J Radiol 2000;34:9–25.

80. Rubin GD. Data explosion: the challenge of multidetector-row CT. Eur J Radiol 2000;36:74–80.

81. Prokop M. General principles of MDCT. Eur J Radiol 2003;45 Suppl 1:S4–10.

82. Rubin GD, Napel S, Leung AN. Volumetric analysis of volumetric data: achieving a paradigm shift. Radiology 1996;200:312–317.

83. Zwirewich CV, Terriff B, Müller NL. High-spatial-frequency (bone) algorithm improves quality of standard CT of the thorax. AJR Am J Roentgenol 1989;153: 1169–1173.

84. Hopper KD, Kasales CJ, Mahraj R, et al. Routine use of a higher order interpolator and bone algorithm in thoracic CT. AJR Am J Roentgenol 1996;167:947–949.

85. Rusinek H, Naidich DP, McGuinness G, et al. Pulmonary nodule detection: low-dose versus conventional CT. Radiology 1998;209:243–249.

86. Nitta N, Takahashi M, Murata K, et al. Ultra low-dose helical CT of the chest. AJR Am J Roentgenol 1998;171:383–385.

87. Paranjpe DV, Bergin CJ. Spiral CT of the lungs: optimal technique and resolution compared with conventional CT. AJR Am J Roentgenol 1994;162:561–567.

88. Wright AR, Collie DA, Williams JR, et al. Pulmonary nodules: effect on detection of spiral CT pitch. Radiology 1996;199: 837–841.

89. Rubin GD, Napel S. Increased scan pitch for vascular and thoracic spiral CT. Radiology 1995;197:316–317.

90. Brink JA, Heiken JP, Balfe DM, et al. Spiral CT: decreased spatial resolution in vivo due to broadening of section-sensitivity profile. Radiology 1992;185: 469–474.

91. Polacin A, Kalender WA, Marchal G. Evaluation of section sensitivity profiles and image noise in spiral CT. Radiology 1992;185:29–35.

92. Buckley JA, Scott WWJ, Siegelman SS, et al. Pulmonary nodules: effect of increased data sampling on detection with spiral CT and confidence in diagnosis. Radiology 1995;196:395–400.

93. Kasales CJ, Hopper KD, Ariola DN, et al. Reconstructed helical CT scans: improvement in z-axis resolution compared with overlapped and nonoverlapped conventional CT scans. AJR Am J Roentgenol 1995;164: 1281–1284.

94. Kalender WA, Polacin A, Suss C. A comparison of conventional and spiral CT: an experimental study on the detection of spherical lesions. J Comput Assist Tomogr 1994;18:167–176.

95. Naidich DP, Webb WR, Müller NL, et al. Principles and techniques of thoracic CT and MR. Computed tomography and magnetic resonance of the thorax, 3rd edn. Philadelphia: Lippincott-Raven, 1999:14–15.

96. Groell R, Schaffler GJ, Rienmueller R, et al. Vascular air embolism: location, frequency, and cause on electron-beam CT studies of the chest. Radiology 1997;202:459–462.

97. Loubeyre P, Debard I, Nemoz C, et al. Using thoracic helical CT to assess iodine concentration in a small volume of nonionic contrast medium during vascular opacification: a prospective study. AJR Am J Roentgenol 2000;174: 783–787.

98. Rubin GD, Lane MJ, Bloch DA, et al. Optimization of thoracic spiral CT: effects of iodinated contrast medium concentration. Radiology 1996;201: 785–791.

99. Hopper KD, Mosher TJ, Kasales CJ, et al. Thoracic spiral CT: delivery of contrast material pushed with injectable saline solution in a power injector. Radiology 1997;205:269–271.

100. Leung AN. Spiral CT of the thorax in daily practice: optimization of technique. J Thorac Imaging 1997;12:2–10.

101. Loubeyre P, Debard I, Nemoz C, et al. High opacification of hilar pulmonary vessels with a small amount of nonionic contrast medium for general thoracic CT: a prospective study. AJR Am J Roentgenol 2002;178:1377–1381.

102. Federle MP, Chang PJ, Confer S, et al. Frequency and effects of extravasation of ionic and nonionic CT contrast media during rapid bolus injection. Radiology 1998;206:637–640.

103. Bellin MF, Jakobsen JA, Tomassin I, et al. Contrast medium extravasation injury: guidelines for prevention and management. Eur Radiol 2002;12: 2807–2812.

104. Stern EJ, Frank MS, Godwin JD. Chest computed tomography display preferences. Survey of thoracic radiologists. Invest Radiol 1995;30: 517–521.

105. Maguire WM, Herman PG, Khan A, et al. Comparison of fixed and adjustable window width and level settings in the CT evaluation of diffuse lung disease. J Comput Assist Tomogr 1993;17: 847–852.

106. Baxter BS, Sorenson JA. Factors affecting the measurements of size and CT number in computed tomography. Invest Radiol 1981;16:337–341.

107. Koehler PR, Anderson RE, Baxter B. The effect of computed tomography viewer controls on anatomical measurements. Radiology 1979;130:189–194.

108. Harris KM, Adams H, Lloyd DCF, et al. The effect on apparent size of simulated pulmonary nodules of using three standard CT window settings. Clin Radiol 1993;47:241–244.

109. Webb WR, Gamsu G, Wall SD, et al. CT of a bronchial phantom. Factors affecting appearance and size measurements. Invest Radiol 1984;19:394–398.

110. Bankier AA, Fleischmann D, Mallek R, et al. Bronchial wall thickness: appropriate window settings for thin-section CT and radiologic-anatomic correlation. Radiology 1996;199:831–836.

111. Mayo JR, Aldrich J, Müller NL. Radiation exposure at chest CT: a statement of the Fleischner Society. Radiology 2003;228:15–21.

112. Mayo JR, Hartman TE, Lee KS, et al. CT of the chest: minimal tube current required for good image quality with the least radiation dose. AJR Am J Roentgenol 1995;3:603–607.

113. Wildberger JE, Mahnken AH, Schmitz-Rode T, et al. Individually adapted examination protocols for reduction of radiation exposure in chest CT. Invest Radiol 2001;36:604–611.

114. Prasad SR, Wittram C, Shepard JA, et al. Standard-dose and 50%-reduced-dose chest CT: comparing the effect on image quality. AJR Am J Roentgenol 2002;179:461–465.

115. Mayo JR, Webb WR, Gould R, et al. High-resolution CT of the lungs: An optimal approach. Radiology 1987;163:507–510.

116. Mayo JR. High resolution computed tomography: technical aspects. Radiol Clin North Am 1991;29:1043–1049.

117. Murata K, Khan A, Rojas KA, et al. Optimization of computed tomography technique to demonstrate the fine structure of the lung. Invest Radiol 1988;23:170–175.

118. Murata K, Khan A, Herman PG. Pulmonary parenchymal disease: evaluation with high-resolution CT. Radiology 1989;170:629–635.

119. Webb WR, Müller NL, Naidich DP. Technical aspects of HRCT. High-resolution CT of the lung, 3rd edn. Philadelphia: Lippincott Williams & Wilkins, 2000:1–21.

120. Honda O, Johkoh T, Yamamoto S, et al. Comparison of quality of multiplanar reconstructions and direct coronal multidetector CT scans of the lung. AJR Am J Roentgenol 2002;179:875–879.

121. Lee KS, Primack SL, Staples CA, et al. Chronic infiltrative lung disease: comparison of diagnostic accuracies of radiography and low- and conventional-dose thin-section CT. Radiology 1994; 191:669–673.

122. Leung AN, Staples CA, Müller NL. Chronic diffuse infiltrative lung disease: comparison of diagnostic accuracy of high-resolution and conventional CT. AJR Am J Roentgenol 1991;157:693–696.

123. Schoepf UJ, Bruening RD, Hong C, et al. Multislice helical CT of focal and diffuse lung disease: comprehensive diagnosis with reconstruction of contiguous and high-resolution CT sections from a single thin-collimation scan. AJR Am J Roentgenol 2001;177:179–184.

124. Remy-Jardin M, Campistron P, Amara A, et al. Usefulness of coronal reformations in the diagnostic evaluation of infiltrative lung disease. J Comput Assist Tomogr 2003;27:266–273.

125. Mayo JR, Jackson SA, Müller NL. High-resolution CT of the chest: radiation dose. AJR Am J Roentgenol 1993;160:479–481.

126. van der Bruggen-Bogaarts BA, Broerse JJ, Lammers JW, et al. Radiation exposure in standard and high-resolution chest CT scans. Chest 1995;107:113–115.

127. Zwirewich CV, Mayo JR, Müller NL. Low dose high resolution CT of lung parenchyma. Radiology 1991;180:413–417.

128. Kuhns LR, Borlaza G. The "twinkling star" sign: an aid in differentiating pulmonary vessels from pulmonary nodules on computed tomograms. Radiology 1980;135:763–764.

129. Tarver RD, Conces DJ, Godwin JD. Motion artifacts on CT simulate bronchiectasis. AJR Am J Roentgenol 1988;151:1117–1119.

130. Mayo JR, Müller NL, Henkelman RM. The double-fissure sign: a motion artifact on thin-section CT scans. Radiology 1987;165:580–581.

131. Schoepf UJ, Becker CR, Bruening RD, et al. Electrocardiographically gated thin-section CT of the lung. Radiology 1999;212:649–654.

132. Cailes JB, Du Bois RM, Hansell DM. Density gradient of the lung parenchyma on CT in patients with lone pulmonary hypertension and systemic sclerosis. Acad Radiol 1996;3:724–730.

133. Morimoto S, Takeuchi N, Imanaka H, et al. Gravity-dependent atelectasis: radiologic, physiologic and pathologic correlation in rabbits on high-frequency oscillation ventilation. Invest Radiol 1989;24:522–533.

134. Volpe J, Storto ML, Lee K, et al. High-resolution CT of the lung: determination of the usefulness of CT scans obtained with the patient prone based on plain radiographic findings. AJR Am J Roentgenol 1997;169:369–374.

135. Mathieson JR, Mayo JR, Staples CA, et al. Chronic diffuse infiltrative lung disease: comparison of diagnostic accuracy of CT and chest radiography. Radiology 1989;171:111–116.

136. Remy-Jardin M, Degreef JM, Beuscart R, et al. Coal worker's pneumoconiosis: CT assessment in exposed workers and correlation with radiographic findings. Radiology 1990;177:363–371.

137. Dawn SK, Gotway MB, Webb WR. Multidetector-row spiral computed tomography in the diagnosis of thoracic diseases. Respir Care 2001;46:912–921.

138. Gruden JF, Ouanounou S, Tigges S, et al. Incremental benefit of maximum-intensity-projection images on observer detection of small pulmonary nodules revealed by multidetector CT. AJR Am J Roentgenol 2002;179:149–157.

139. Remy-Jardin M, Remy J, Gosselin B, et al. Sliding thin slab, minimum intensity projection technique in the diagnosis of emphysema: histopathologic-CT correlation. Radiology 1996;200:665–671.

140. Bhalla M, Naidich DP, McGuinness G, et al. Diffuse lung disease: assessment with helical CT – preliminary observations of the role of maximum and minimum intensity projection images. Radiology 1996;200:341–347.

141. Grenier P, Lenoir S, Brauner M. Computed tomographic assessment of bronchiectasis. Semin Ultrasound CT MR 1990;11:430–441.

142. Hansell DM. Bronchiectasis. Radiol Clin North Am 1998;36:107–128.

143. Grenier P, Beigelman C. Spiral CT of the bronchial tree. In: Remy-Jardin M, Remy J, eds. Spiral CT of the chest. Berlin: Springer-Verlag, 2000:185–199.

144. Engeler CE, Tashjian JH, Engeler CM, et al. Volumetric high-resolution CT in the diagnosis of interstitial lung disease and bronchiectasis: diagnostic accuracy and radiation dose. AJR Am J Roentgenol 1994;163:31–35.

145. Lucidarme O, Grenier P, Coche E, et al. Bronchiectasis: comparative assessment with thin-section CT and helical CT. Radiology 1996;200:673–679.

146. van der Bruggen-Bogaarts BAHA, van der Bruggen HMJG, van Waes PFGM, et al. Assessment of bronchiectasis: comparison of HRCT and spiral volumetric CT. J Comput Assist Tomogr 1996;20:15–19.

147. Remy-Jardin M, Amara A, Campistron P, et al. Diagnosis of bronchiectasis with multislice spiral CT: accuracy of 3-mm-thick structured sections. Eur Radiol 2003;13:1165–1171.

148. Yi CA, Lee KS, Kim TS, et al. Multidetector CT of bronchiectasis: effect of radiation dose on image quality. AJR Am J Roentgenol 2003;181:501–505.

149. Sung YM, Lee KS, Yi CA, et al. Additional coronal images using low-milliamperage multidetector-row computed tomography: effectiveness in the diagnosis of bronchiectasis. J Comput Assist Tomogr 2003;27:490–495.

150. Desai SR, Wells AU, Cheah FK, et al. The reproducibility of bronchial

circumference measurements using computed tomography. Br J Radiol 1994;67:257–262.

151. Grenier P, Cordeau MP, Beigelman C. High-resolution computed tomography of the airways. J Thorac Imaging 1993;8:213–229.

152. Seneterre E, Paganin F, Bruel JM, et al. Measurement of the internal size of bronchi using high resolution computed tomography (HRCT). Eur Respir J 1994;7:596–600.

153. Kang EY, Miller RR, Müller NL. Bronchiectasis: comparison of preoperative thin-section CT and pathologic findings in resected specimens. Radiology 1995;195:649–654.

154. Hansell DM. Small airways diseases: detection and insights with computed tomography. Eur Respir J 2001;17: 1294–1313.

155. Miller WT Jr, Kotloff RM, Blumenthal NP, et al. Utility of high resolution computed tomography in predicting bronchiolitis obliterans syndrome following lung transplantation: preliminary findings. J Thorac Imaging 2001;16:76–80.

156. Stern EJ, Frank MS. Small-airways disease of the lungs: findings at expiratory CT. AJR Am J Roentgenol 1994;163:37–41.

157. Arakawa H, Webb WR, McCowin M, et al. Inhomogeneous lung attenuation at thin-section CT: diagnostic value of expiratory scans. Radiology 1998;206: 89–94.

158. Lucidarme O, Coche E, Cluzel P, et al. Expiratory CT scans for chronic airway disease: correlation with pulmonary function test results. AJR Am J Roentgenol 1998;170:301–307.

159. Arakawa H, Niimi H, Kurihara Y, et al. Expiratory high-resolution CT: diagnostic value in diffuse lung diseases. AJR Am J Roentgenol 2000;175: 1537–1543.

160. Stern EJ, Swensen SJ, Hartman TE, et al. CT mosaic pattern of lung attenuation: distinguishing different causes. AJR Am J Roentgenol 1995;165:813–816.

161. Lucidarme O, Grenier PA, Cadi M, et al. Evaluation of air trapping at CT: comparison of continuous- versus suspended-expiration CT techniques. Radiology 2000;216:768–772.

162. Gotway MB, Lee ES, Reddy GP, et al. Low-dose dynamic expiratory thin-section CT of the lungs using a spiral CT scanner. J Thorac Imaging 2000;15: 168–172.

163. Fotheringham T, Chabat F, Hansell DM, et al. A comparison of methods for enhancing the detection of areas of decreased attenuation on CT caused by airways disease. J Comput Assist Tomogr 1999;23:385–389.

164. Remy-Jardin M, Remy J, Artaud D, et al. Tracheobronchial tree: assessment with

volume rendering – technical aspects. Radiology 1998;208:393–398.

165. Naidich DP, Gruden JF, McGuinness G, et al. Volumetric (helical/spiral) CT (VCT) of the airways. J Thorac Imaging 1997;12:11–28.

166. Boiselle PM, Reynolds KF, Ernst A. Multiplanar and three-dimensional imaging of the central airways with multidetector CT. AJR Am J Roentgenol 2002;179:301–308.

167. Quint LE, Whyte RI, Kazerooni EA, et al. Stenosis of the central airways: evaluation by using helical CT with multiplanar reconstructions. Radiology 1995;194:871–877.

168. Kauczor HU, Wolcke B, Fischer B, et al. Three-dimensional helical CT of the tracheobronchial tree: evaluation of imaging protocols and assessment of suspected stenoses with bronchoscopic correlation. AJR Am J Roentgenol 1996;167:419–424.

169. Choi YW, McAdams HP, Jeon SC, et al. Low-dose spiral CT: application to surface-rendered three-dimensional imaging of central airways. J Comput Assist Tomogr 2002;26:335–341.

170. Summers RH, Feng DH, Holland SM, et al. Virtual bronchoscopy: segmentation method for real-time display. Radiology 1996;200:857–862.

171. Ferretti GR, Knoplioch J, Bricault I, et al. Central airway stenoses: preliminary results of spiral-CT-generated virtual bronchoscopy simulations in 29 patients. Eur Radiol 1997;7:854–859.

172. Fleiter T, Merkle EM, Aschoff AJ, et al. Comparison of real-time virtual and fiberoptic bronchoscopy in patients with bronchial carcinoma: opportunities and limitations. AJR Am J Roentgenol 1997;169:1591–1595.

173. Lawler LP, Corl FM, Haponik EF, et al. Multidetector row computed tomography and 3-dimensional volume rendering for adult airway imaging. Curr Probl Diagn Radiol 2002;31: 115–133.

174. Bergin CJ, Healy MV, Zincone GE, et al. MR evaluation of chest wall involvement in malignant lymphoma. J Comput Assist Tomogr 1990;14:928–931.

175. Brown L, Aushenbaugh G. Masses of the anterior mediastinum: CT and MRI findings. AJR Am J Roentgenol 1991; 157:1171–1180.

176. Heelan RT, Demas BE, Caravelli JF, et al. Superior sulcus tumors: CT and MR imaging. Radiology 1989;170: 637–641.

177. Padovani B, Mouroux J, Seksik L, et al. Chest wall invasion by bronchogenic carcinoma: evaluation with MR imaging. Radiology 1993;187:33–38.

178. Glazer GM, Gross BH, Aisen AM, et al. Imaging of the pulmonary hilum: a prospective comparative study in

patients with lung cancer. AJR Am J Roentgenol 1985;145:245–248.

179. Webb WR, Gamsu G, Stark DD, et al. Magnetic resonance imaging of the normal and abnormal pulmonary hila. Radiology 1984;152:89–94.

180. Mirvis SE, Keramati B, Buckman R, et al. MR imaging of traumatic diaphragmatic rupture. J Comput Assist Tomogr 1988;12:147–149.

181. Glazer HS, Lee JKT, Levitt RL, et al. Radiation fibrosis: differentiation from recurrent tumor by MR imaging. Radiology 1985;156:721–726.

182. Nyman R, Rehn S, Glimelius B, et al. Magnetic resonance imaging for assessment of treatment effects in mediastinal Hodgkin's disease. Acta Radiol 1987;28:145–151.

183. Webb WR. MR imaging of treated mediastinal Hodgkin disease. Radiology 1989;170:315–316.

184. Meaney JFM, Weg JG, Chenevert TL, et al. Diagnosis of pulmonary embolism with magnetic resonance angiography. N Engl J Med 1997;336:1422–1427.

185. Gupta A, Frazer CK, Ferguson JM, et al. Acute pulmonary embolism: diagnosis with MR angiography. Radiology 1999;210:353–359.

186. Ley S, Kauczor HU, Heussel CP, et al. Value of contrast-enhanced MR angiography and helical CT angiography in chronic thromboembolic pulmonary hypertension. Eur Radiol 2003;13:2365–2371.

187. Oudkerk M, van Beek EJ, Wielopolski P, et al. Comparison of contrast-enhanced magnetic resonance angiography and conventional pulmonary angiography for the diagnosis of pulmonary embolism: a prospective study. Lancet 2002;359:1643–1647.

188. Amundsen T, Kvaerness J, Jones RA, et al. Pulmonary embolism: detection with MR perfusion imaging of lung – a feasibility study. Radiology 1997;203: 181–185.

189. Bergin CJ, Glover GM, Pauly J. Magnetic resonance imaging of the lung parenchyma. J Thorac Imaging 1993;8:12–17.

190. Bergin CJ, Pauly JM, Macovski A. Lung parenchyma: projection reconstruction MR imaging. Radiology 1991;179:777–781.

191. Müller NL, Mayo JR, Zwirewich CV. Value of MR imaging in the evaluation of chronic infiltrative lung diseases: comparison with CT. AJR Am J Roentgenol 1992;158:1205–1209.

192. Schmidt MA, Yang GZ, Keegan J, et al. Non-breath-hold lung magnetic resonance imaging with real-time navigation. Magma 1997;5:123–128.

193. Mayo JR, MacKay A, Müller NL. MR imaging of the lungs: value of short TE spin-echo pulse sequences. AJR Am J Roentgenol 1992;159:951–956.

194. McFadden RG, Carr TJ, Wood TE. Proton magnetic resonance imaging to stage activity of interstitial lung disease. Chest 1987;92:31–39.

195. Albert MS, Cates GD, Driehuys B, et al. Biological magnetic resonance imaging using laser-polarized 129Xe. Nature 1994;370:199–201.

196. MacFall JR, Charles HC, Black RD, et al. Human lung air spaces: potential for MR imaging with hyperpolarized He-3. Radiology 1996;200:553–558.

197. Edelman RR, Hatabu H, Tadamura E, et al. Noninvasive assessment of regional ventilation in the human lung using oxygen-enhanced magnetic resonance imaging. Nat Med 1996;2: 1236–1239.

198. Thomas SR, Gradon L, Pratsinis SE, et al. Perfluorocarbon compound aerosols for delivery to the lung as potential 19F magnetic resonance reporters of regional pulmonary pO_2. Invest Radiol 1997;32: 29–38.

199. Kauczor HU, Hofmann D, Kreitner KF, et al. Normal and abnormal pulmonary ventilation: visualization at hyperpolarized He-3 MR imaging. Radiology 1996;201:564–568.

200. Salerno M, Altes TA, Brookeman JR, et al. Rapid hyperpolarized 3He diffusion MRI of healthy and emphysematous human lungs using an optimized interleaved-spiral pulse sequence. J Magn Reson Imaging 2003;17:581–588.

201. Mai VM, Chen Q, Bankier AA, et al. Multiple inversion recovery MR subtraction imaging of human ventilation from inhalation of room air and pure oxygen. Magn Reson Med 2000;43: 913–916.

202. Mai VM, Liu B, Polzin JA, et al. Ventilation-perfusion ratio of signal intensity in human lung using oxygen-enhanced and arterial spin labeling techniques. Magn Reson Med 2002; 48:341–350.

203. Bergin CJ, Glover GH, Pauly JM. Lung parenchyma: magnetic susceptibility in MR imaging. Radiology 1991;180: 845–848.

204. Alsop DC, Hatabu H, Bonnet M, et al. Multi-slice, breathhold imaging of the lung with submillisecond echo times. Magn Reson Med 1995;33:678–682.

205. Mark AS, Winkler ML, Peltzer M, et al. Gated acquisition of MR images of the thorax: advantages for the study of the hila and mediastinum. Magn Reson Imaging 1987;5 (1):57–63.

206. Lewis C, Prato FS, Drost DJ, et al. Comparison of respiratory triggering and gating techniques for the removal of respiratory artifacts in MR imaging. Radiology 1986;160:803–810.

207. Bailes DR, Gilderdale DJ, Bydder GM, et al. Respiratory ordered phase-encoding (ROPE): a method for reducing respiratory motion artifacts in MR imaging. J Comput Assist Tomogr 1985;9:835–838.

208. Moody AR, Bolton SC, Horsfield MA. Optimization of a breath-hold magnetic resonance gradient echo technique for the detection of interstitial lung disease. Invest Radiol 1995;30:730–737.

209. Edelman RR, Manning W, Burstein D, et al. Coronary arteries: breath-hold MR angiography. Radiology 1991;181: 641–643.

210. Hennig J, Nauerth A, Friedburg H. RARE imaging: a fast imaging method for clinical MR. Magn Reson Med 1986;3:823–833.

211. Miller SW, Holmvang G. Differentiation of slow flow from thrombus in thoracic magnetic resonance imaging, emphasizing phase images. J Thorac Imaging 1993;8:98–107.

212. White EM, Edelman RR, Wedeen VJ, et al. Intravascular signal in MR imaging: use of phase display for differentiation of blood-flow signal from intraluminal disease. Radiology 1986; 161:245–249.

213. Haase A, Frahm J, Matthaei D, et al. FLASH imaging: rapid NMR imaging using low flip angle pulses. J Magn Reson 1986;67:258–266.

214. Schmidt HC, Tscholakoff D, Hricak H, et al. MR image contrast and relaxation times of solid tumours in the chest, abdomen and pelvis. J Comput Assist Tomogr 1985;9:738–748.

215. Takahashi N, Murakami J, Murayama S, et al. MR evaluation of intrapulmonary hematoma. J Comput Assist Tomogr 1995;19:125–127.

216. Nakata H, Egashira K, Watanabe H, et al. MRI of bronchogenic cysts. J Comput Assist Tomogr 1993;17:267–270.

217. Brechot JM, Buy JN, Laaban JP, et al. Computed tomography and magnetic resonance findings in lipoid pneumonia. Thorax 1991;46:738–739.

218. Glazer GM, Orringer MB, Chenevert TL, et al. Mediastinal lymph nodes: relaxation time/pathologic correlation and implications in staging of lung cancer with MR imaging. Radiology 1988;168:429–431.

219. Webb WR. Magnetic resonance imaging of the hila and mediastinum. Cardiovasc Intervent Radiol 1986;8:306–313.

220. King MA, Bergin CJ, Ghadishah E, et al. Detecting pulmonary abnormalities on magnetic resonance images in patients with usual interstitial pneumonitis: effect of varying window settings and gadopentetate dimeglumine. Acad Radiol 1996;3:300–307.

221. Link KM, Samuels LJ, Reed JC, et al. Magnetic resonance imaging of the mediastinum. J Thorac Imaging 1993;8:34–53.

222. Shioya S, Haida M, Ono Y, et al. Lung cancer: differentiation of tumor, necrosis and atelectasis by means of T1 and T2 values measured in vitro. Radiology 1988;167:105–109.

223. Carr JC, Simonetti O, Bundy J, et al. Cine MR angiography of the heart with segmented true fast imaging with steady-state precession. Radiology 2001;219:828–834.

224. Carr DH, Oades P, Trotman-Dickenson B, et al. Magnetic resonance scanning in cystic fibrosis: comparison with computed tomography. Clin Radiol 1995;50:84–89.

The normal chest

This chapter describes the normal anatomy of the airways, lungs, mediastinum, and diaphragm as demonstrated on plain chest radiographs (Fig. 2.1), computed tomography (CT), and magnetic resonance imaging (MRI).

AIRWAYS AND LUNGS

Central airways

The trachea[1,2] is a tube which, in children and young adults, passes downwards and backwards close to the midline and has sufficient flexibility to adapt to body position. In adults, the aorta may cause a recognizable impression and, in infants and young children, the brachiocephalic artery may indent the trachea. In older individuals, the intrathoracic trachea deviates slightly to the right to accommodate the left-sided arch. With unfolding and ectasia of the aorta, the trachea deviates more to the right as it descends into the chest and may also bow forward. In a CT study of 50 normal individuals, the mid point of the trachea in the thorax lay between 1.6 cm to the right and 0.7 cm to the left of the midline.[3]

The trachea has 16–20 incomplete C, U or horseshoe-shaped cartilage rings which can give the trachea a corrugated outline. Calcification of the cartilage rings is a common normal finding after the age of 40 years, increasing in frequency with the age of

the individual[4]; it was seen on CT in 50% of subjects in their seventh and eighth decades.[5] The prevalence of visible tracheal calcification on chest radiography is very small, less than 1% in a series of 5000 inpatients, most of whom were females over 70 years old.[6]

In cross section, the trachea is usually round, oval, or oval with a flattened posterior margin, the posterior margin being formed by the fibromuscular membrane. It may occasionally show other configurations such as a square or inverted pear shape.[4,7,8] The trachea enters the thorax 1–3 cm above the level of the suprasternal notch and the intrathoracic portion is 6–9 cm in length.[8] The range of tracheal diameters in adults on chest radiography in men is 13–25 mm in coronal plane, and 13–27 mm in sagittal plane; in women the diameters are 10–21 mm in coronal plane, and 10–23 mm in sagittal plane.[9] At CT, which allows precise assessment of diameters and cross-sectional areas without magnification, the mean transverse diameter is 15.2 mm (standard deviation [SD] 1.4) for women and 18.2 mm (SD 1.2) for men, the lower limit of normal being 12.3 mm for women and 15.9 mm for men.[10] The diameters in the growing child and young adult have been documented by Griscom and Wohl.[11] In addition to gender and age differences, it is probable that there are inter-racial differences in the diameter and configuration of the trachea.[12] Cross-sectional areas can also be measured: the mean is 194 mm^2 (SD 35) in women and 272 mm^2 (SD 33) in men. The normal cross-sectional

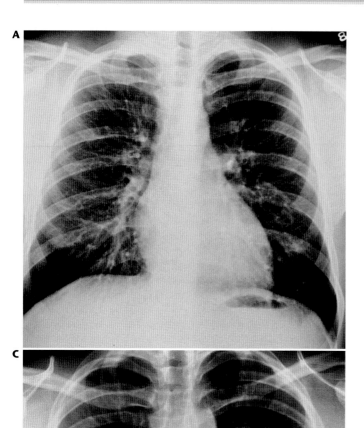

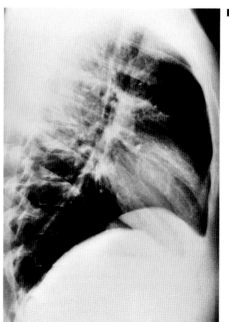

Fig. 2.1 Radiograph of a normal chest: **A**, posteroanterior (PA) view; **B**, lateral view; **C**, PA view on expiration (same patient). Note the differences between appearances on inspiration and expiration, especially widening of the heart and mediastinum on expiration.

area on forced expiration is considerably less than on full inspiration: in 10 normal male volunteers the cross-sectional area dropped from a mean of 280 mm² (SD 50.5) at full inspiration to 178 mm² (SD 40.2) at end-expiration.[13] The major change is forward movement or invagination of the posterior wall of the trachea leading to a significant reduction in the anteroposterior diameter (Fig. 2.2).

The trachea divides into the two mainstem bronchi at the carina at approximately the level of D5. The left main bronchus extends up to twice as far as the right main bronchus before giving off its upper lobe division. (The left main bronchus is

approximately 50 mm long and the right main bronchus is approximately 25 mm in length.) In children the angles are symmetric, but in adults the right mainstem bronchus has a steeper angle than the left. The range of subcarinal angles is wide[14]; in one survey they varied between 35° and 90.5° (mean 60.8°; SD 11.8°).[15] Abnormalities of angle can, therefore, only be diagnosed by right–left comparisons, not by absolute measurement.

The lobar and segmental branching pattern is shown in Figure 2.3 and the branching pattern of the airways beyond the segmental bronchi is shown diagrammatically in Figure 2.4. The

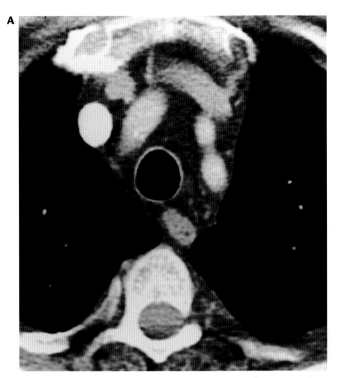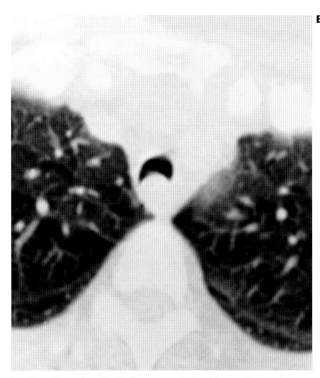

Fig. 2.2   A, Inspiratory CT of the trachea showing an almost round cross-sectional configuration. **B**, Similar anatomic level in another patient obtained at full expiration showing invagination of the posterior membrane.

walls of the segmental bronchi are invisible on chest radiography except when seen end-on as ring shadows. They are, however, clearly seen on CT, particularly if thin (1–5 mm) contiguous sections are taken; some authors recommend 20° angled CT in selected patients.[16] The CT anatomy of central airways has been described in the literature.[8,17–19] The reader is also referred to a number of detailed articles concerning the CT appearance of the segmental and subsegmental airways: upper lobes,[20–23] lower lobes,[24,25] and lingular segments.[20]

Variations in bronchial anatomy,[26–29] particularly those affecting segmental and subsegmental airways, are fairly common but are rarely clinically significant (Fig. 2.5); however, they can be confusing to bronchoscopists searching for landmarks. There are two kinds of anomalous airways: (1) displaced, in which a standard airway arises from an unusual site; and (2) supernumerary. Displaced airways are much more common than supernumerary ones. Ghaye et al have written a detailed, illustrated review including an analysis of their experience of both types of variants on CT examination.[30] Anomalous bronchi can be well shown by thin-section spiral CT with three-dimensional reconstructions or by MR imaging.[28,31] The reported variations are:

1. Tracheal bronchus, also known as bronchus suis, is an anomaly in which either a segment of the right upper lobe or the entire right upper lobe bronchus originates from the trachea rather than the main bronchus (Fig. 2.6). Tracheal bronchus is found in 0.5–3% of bronchoscopies.[32,33] A tracheal bronchus arises from the lateral wall of the trachea,[30,34,35] usually within a few centimeters of the mainstem takeoff. It is much more common on the right side and is usually a displaced apical segmental bronchus, but it may be supernumerary supplying the apical segment, a displaced upper lobe airway, or even a supernumerary upper lobe airway.[36] When a tracheal bronchus is a displaced upper lobe airway, the more distal trachea is narrowed.[37] The anomaly is usually clinically inapparent, but occasionally the orifice is narrow[36,38,39] or the airway bronchiectatic,[36,38] which may lead to recurrent distal pneumonia and abscess formation. Apical cyst formation in the lung supplied by a tracheal bronchus is also described.[40]

2. There may be a common origin of the right upper and middle lobe bronchi.[41]

3. An accessory cardiac bronchus is a supernumerary bronchus arising from the medial aspect of the right main bronchus or intermediate stem bronchus proximal to the origin of the right superior (apical) segmental airway of the lower lobe (Fig. 2.7). It usually passes downward and medially toward the heart, paralleling the intermediate stem bronchus. It is either blind-ending, in which case it may have a nodule of unaerated lung tissue at its tip, or supplies a small ventilated "lobule".[42,43] Most patients are

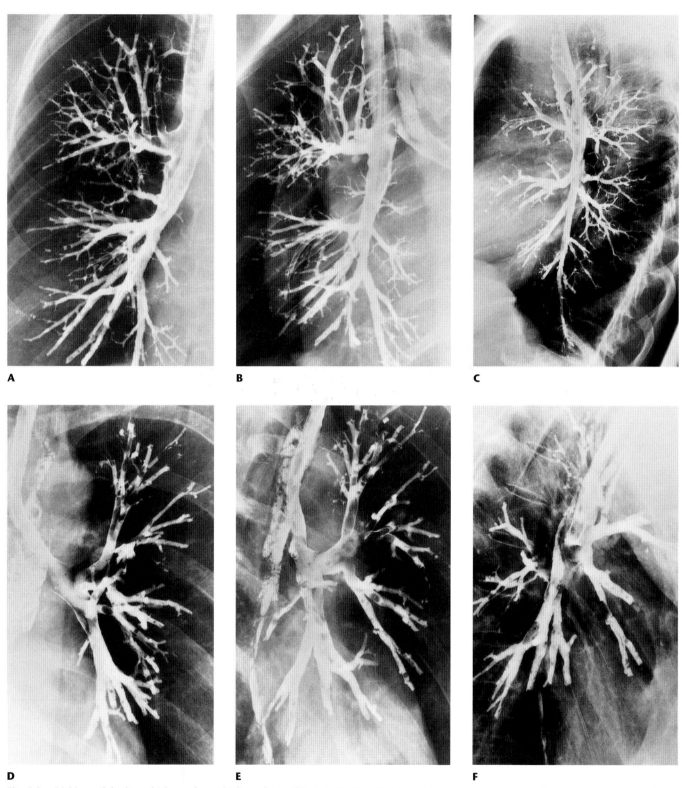

Fig. 2.3 Divisions of the bronchial tree shown by bronchography. **A**, Right bronchial tree, anteroposterior (AP) view. **B**, Right bronchial tree, right posterior oblique view. **C**, Right bronchial tree, lateral view. **D**, Left bronchial tree, AP view. **E**, Left bronchial tree, left posterior oblique view. **F**, Left bronchial tree, lateral view.

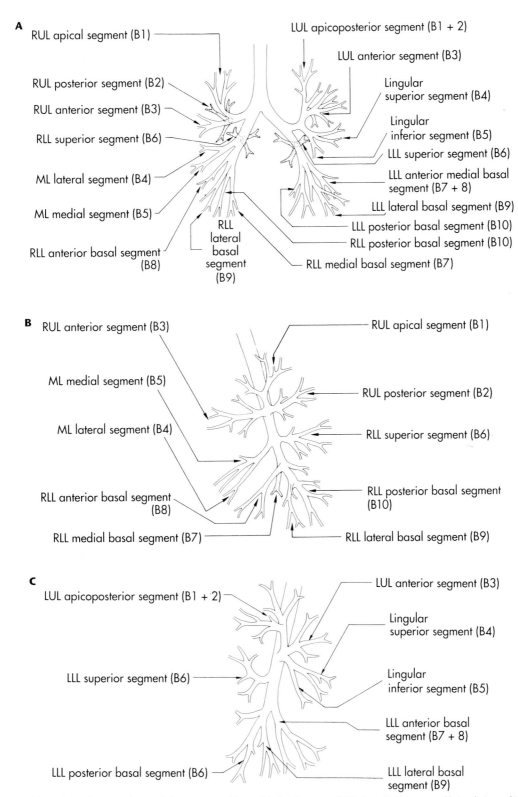

A
RUL apical segment (B1)

LUL apicoposterior segment (B1 + 2)

RUL posterior segment (B2)

LUL anterior segment (B3)

RUL anterior segment (B3)

Lingular superior segment (B4)

RLL superior segment (B6)

Lingular inferior segment (B5)

ML lateral segment (B4)

LLL superior segment (B6)

LLL anterior medial basal segment (B7 + 8)

ML medial segment (B5)

LLL lateral basal segment (B9)

LLL posterior basal segment (B10)

RLL anterior basal segment (B8)

RLL posterior basal segment (B10)

RLL lateral basal segment (B9)

RLL medial basal segment (B7)

B
RUL anterior segment (B3)

RUL apical segment (B1)

ML medial segment (B5)

RUL posterior segment (B2)

ML lateral segment (B4)

RLL superior segment (B6)

RLL anterior basal segment (B8)

RLL posterior basal segment (B10)

RLL medial basal segment (B7)

RLL lateral basal segment (B9)

C
LUL anterior segment (B3)

LUL apicoposterior segment (B1 + 2)

Lingular superior segment (B4)

LLL superior segment (B6)

Lingular inferior segment (B5)

LLL anterior basal segment (B7 + 8)

LLL posterior basal segment (B6)

LLL lateral basal segment (B9)

Fig. 2.4   Diagram of branches of airways beyond the segmental bronchi. **A**, Diagram of AP view. **B**, Diagram of lateral view of L right bronchial tree. **C**, Diagram of lateral view of left bronchial tree.

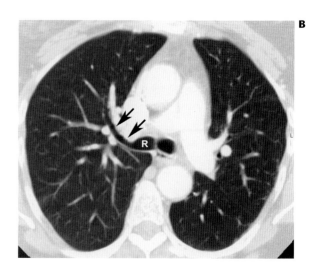

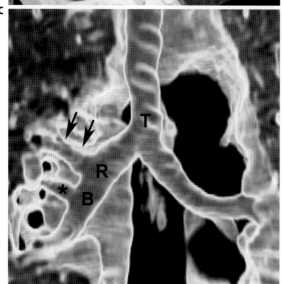

Fig. 2.5 Anomalous bronchial origin in a middle-aged asymptomatic woman. **A**, The posterior segment bronchus (white arrow) originates, anomalously, from bronchus intermedius (B). **B** and **C**, The anterior and apical segmental bronchi (black arrows) originate from the right upper lobe bronchus (R), but the posterior segment bronchus (asterisk) has an anomalous origin. T, trachea.

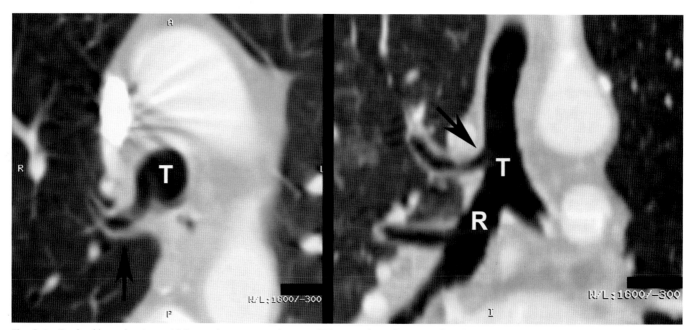

Fig. 2.6 Tracheal bronchus in a middle-aged asymptomatic man. CT images show the anomalous bronchus (black arrows) originating from the distal trachea (T). R, right main bronchus.

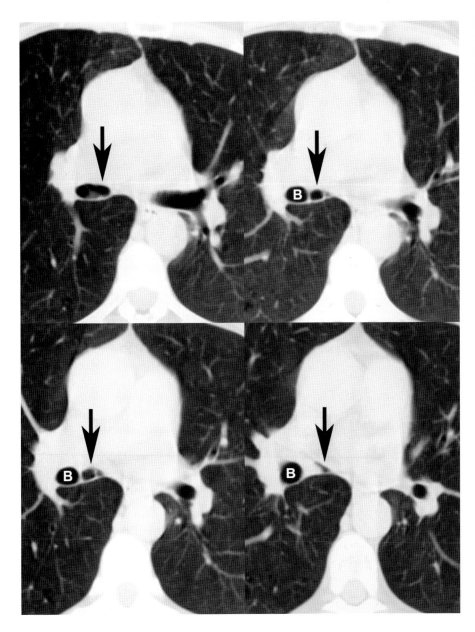

Fig. 2.7 Accessory cardiac bronchus in a 21-year-old man with hemoptysis. CT shows the anomalous bronchus (black arrows) originating from the medial wall of bronchus intermedius (B) and terminating in a distal lung bud.

asymptomatic, however an accessory cardiac bronchus may be associated with local infection[44] or hemoptysis. Ghaye et al[30] found a frequency of accessory cardiac bronchus of 0.08% in 17,500 consecutive patients. The diameter of the accessory bronchus ranged from 4 to 14 mm and the length ranged from 4 to 23 mm. The simultaneous occurrence of an accessory cardiac and tracheal bronchus has been reported.[43,45,46]

4. Lateral inversion of right- and left-sided airways occurs in situs inversus. With situs ambiguus the airway has either a bilateral right-sided or left-sided configuration. Such anomalies are strongly associated with serious congenital heart disease.[47,48]

5. Isolated cases of the so-called "bridging bronchus" have been described.[49] In this condition, the right lower lobe bronchus arises from the left main bronchus and crosses or "bridges" the mediastinum to reach the right lung (Fig. 2.8). This anomaly is exceedingly rare.

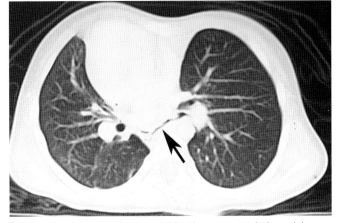

Fig. 2.8 Bridging bronchus in a child with recurrent right lower lobe pneumonia. CT shows the bronchus (black arrow) arising from the left lung and crossing the mediastinum to supply the right lower lobe. (Case courtesy of NL Müller, MD, PhD, Vancouver, BC, CA)

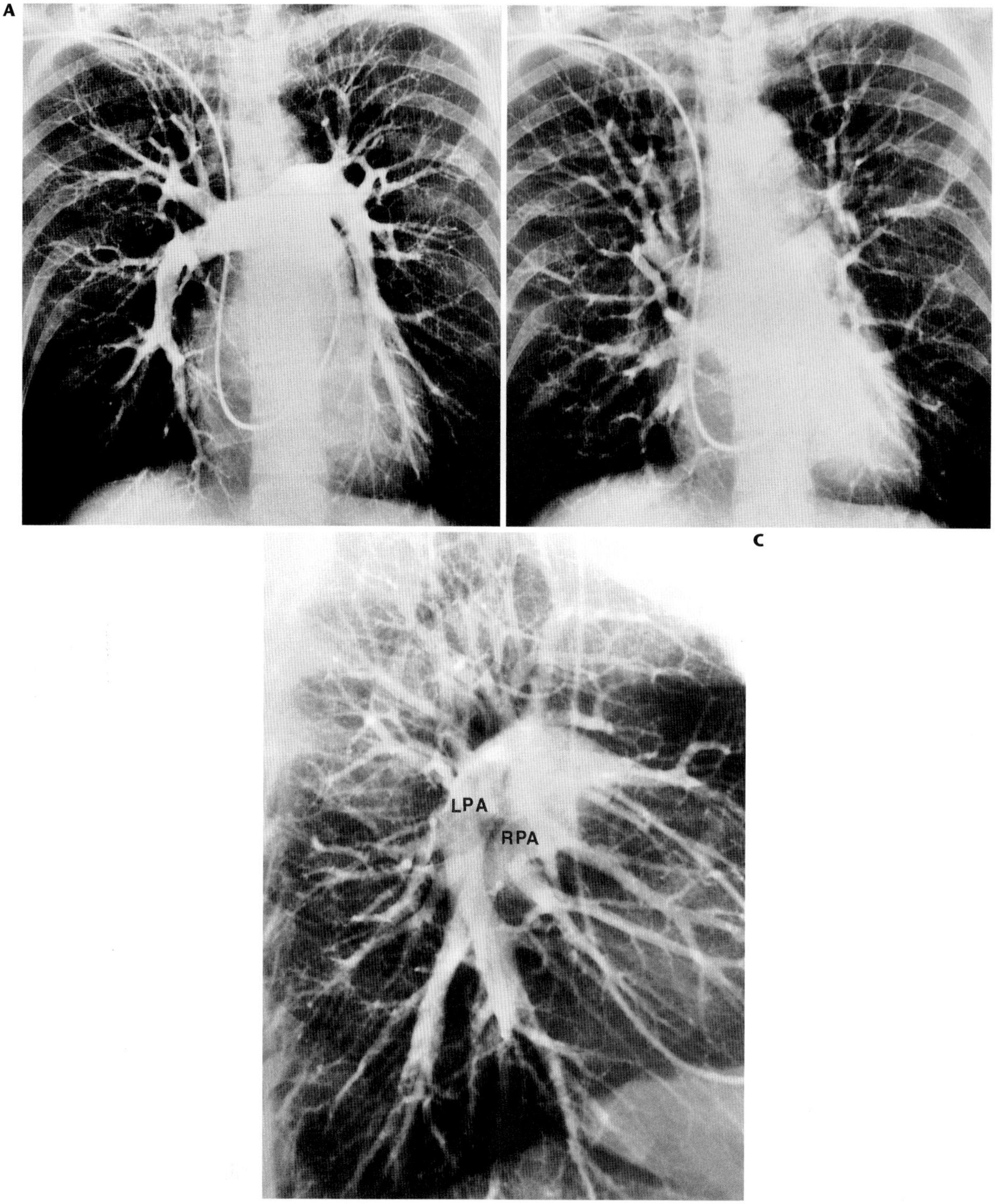

Fig. 2.9 Pulmonary arteries and veins shown by pulmonary angiography. **A**, Anteroposterior (AP) view of pulmonary arteries. **B**, AP view of pulmonary veins in the same patient. **C**, Lateral view of pulmonary arteries (different patient). LPA, Left pulmonary artery; RPA, right pulmonary artery.

Pulmonary hila

Understanding the appearances of the normal hila requires an appreciation of the anatomy of the major bronchi (Fig. 2.3), hilar blood vessels (Figs 2.9 and 2.10),[19,50–52] and hilar lymph nodes,[53,54] because it is these structures that are demonstrated with imaging. Connective tissue does not contribute significantly to the bulk of the hila, and the small amount of fat between the vessels is, for practical purposes, visible only at CT and MRI.

The following points of anatomy should be remembered:

1. The right main bronchus has a more vertical course than the left main bronchus, and the right upper lobe bronchus arises more proximally than the left upper lobe bronchus.

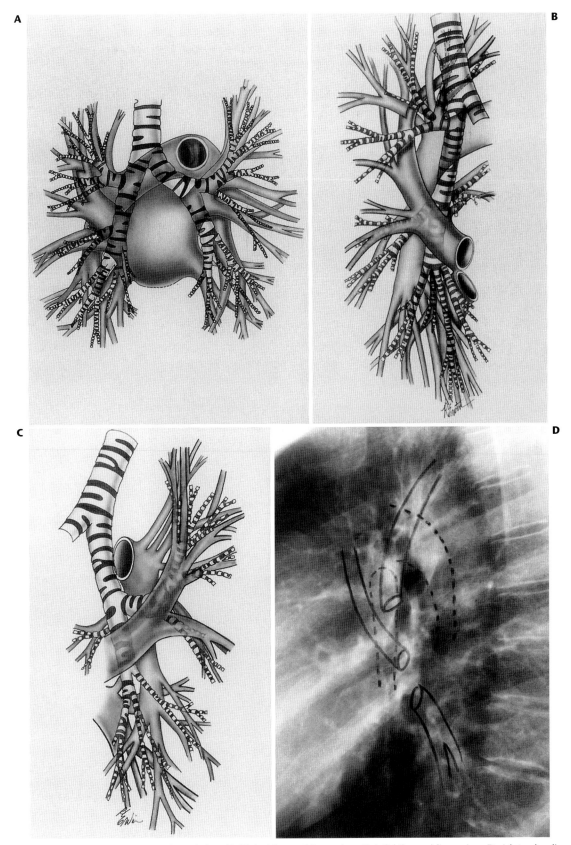

Fig. 2.10 Diagram of the hilar structures. **A**, Frontal view. **B**, Right hilum: oblique view. **C**, Left hilum: oblique view. **D**, A lateral radiograph with the position of the central pulmonary arteries and veins drawn in. The left and right pulmonary arteries are indicated by dotted lines (the left lies posterior to the right). The inferior pulmonary veins are similar on the two sides and are superimposed (only one is drawn in). The right superior pulmonary vein is on a more anterior plane than the left superior pulmonary vein.

2. The right mainstem bronchus and its divisions into the right upper lobe bronchus and bronchus intermedius are outlined posteriorly by lung so that the posterior wall of these portions of the bronchial tree is seen as a thin stripe (Figs 2.11 and 2.12), except for a focal nodule, representing a small draining pulmonary vein in some 5% of normal subjects.[55] This region is, therefore, an important area in which to look for masses, such as lymphadenopathy. On the left side the lower lobe artery intervenes between the lung and the bronchial tree, and only a small tongue of lung can

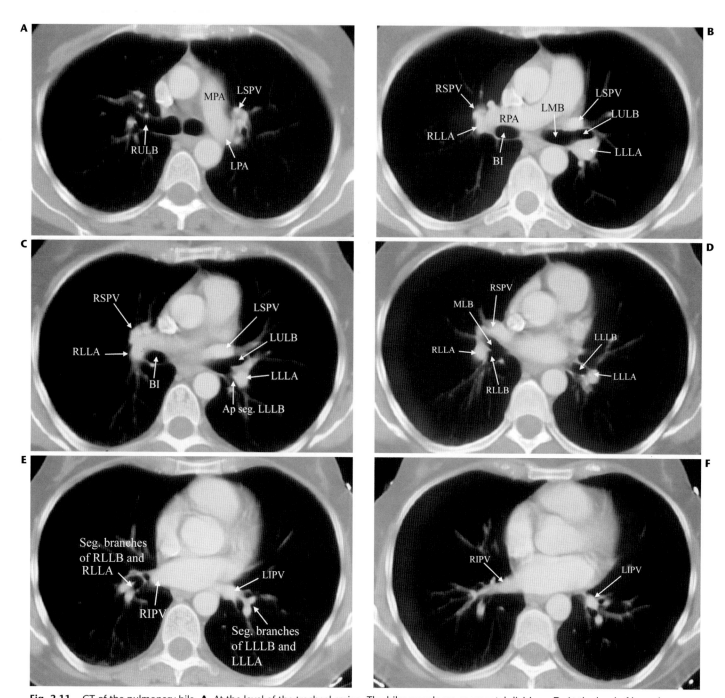

Fig. 2.11   CT of the pulmonary hila. **A,** At the level of the tracheal carina. The hilar vessels are segmental divisions. **B,** At the level of bronchus intermedius. Note the lack of major vessels behind bronchus intermedius and the conglomerate density formed by the right pulmonary artery and right superior pulmonary vein. **C,** At the level of (right) middle lobe bronchus. **D,** At the level of the inferior pulmonary veins. **E** and **F** illustrate the posterior relationships of the left and right bronchial tree. The section shown in **E** is 1 cm higher than that in **F**. BI, Bronchus intermedius; LIPV, left inferior pulmonary vein; LLLA, left lower lobe artery; LLLB, left lower lobe bronchus; LMB, left main bronchus; LPA; left pulmonary artery; LSPV, left superior pulmonary vein; LULB, left upper lobe bronchus; MLB, middle lobe bronchus; MPA, main pulmonary artery; RIPV, right inferior pulmonary vein; RLLA, right lower lobe artery; RLLB, right lower lobe bronchus; RPA, right pulmonary artery; RSPV, right superior pulmonary vein; RULB, right upper lobe bronchus.

A
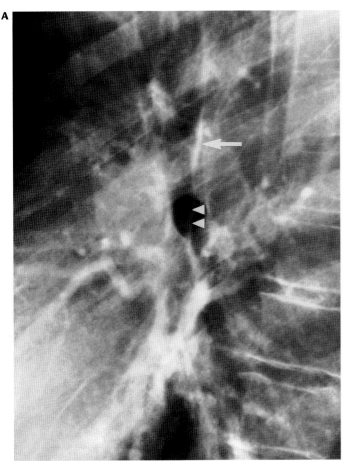

B
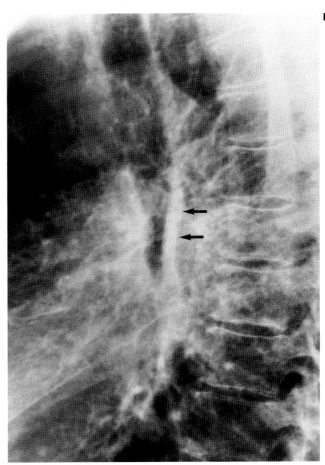

Fig. 2.12 **A**, A lateral radiograph of normal pulmonary hila. The arrow points to the posterior wall of the right main bronchus, and the arrowheads point to the posterior wall of bronchus intermedius. **B**, A lateral view in a patient with lymphangitis carcinomatosa shows thickening of the tissues posterior to bronchus intermedius (arrows).

invaginate between the left lower lobe artery and the descending aorta to contact the posterior wall of the left mainstem bronchus (Fig. 2.11).[56]

3. The right pulmonary artery passes anterior to the major bronchi to reach the lateral aspect of the bronchus intermedius and right lower lobe bronchus, whereas the left pulmonary artery arches over the left main bronchus and left upper lobe bronchus to descend posterolateral to the left lower lobe bronchus.

4. The pulmonary veins are similar on the two sides. The superior pulmonary veins are the anterior structures in the upper and mid hilum on both sides, and the inferior pulmonary veins run obliquely forward beneath the divisions of each lower lobe artery to enter the left atrium. Because the central portions of the pulmonary arteries are so differently organized on the two sides, the relationship between the major veins and arteries differs. On the right the superior pulmonary vein is separated from the central bronchi by the lower division of the right pulmonary artery, whereas on the left the superior pulmonary vein is separated from the lower division of the left pulmonary artery by the bronchial tree.

5. On chest radiographs the transverse diameter of the lower lobe arteries prior to their segmental divisions can be measured with reasonable accuracy. These arteries should normally be 9–16 mm in diameter (Fig. 2.13). The large round shadow seen on lateral and oblique views of the right hilum is a combination of the right pulmonary artery and the superior pulmonary vein. The combined shadows of these two vessels may be sufficiently large to be confused with a mass (Fig. 2.14).

6. Normally there are no large vessels traversing the angle between the middle and the lower lobe bronchi on the right, or the angle between the upper and lower lobe bronchi on the left, on lateral or oblique plain chest radiographs. Therefore a rounded shadow larger than 1 cm in either of these angles is likely to be a mass rather than a normal vessel.[57]

7. Normal hilar lymph nodes are not recognizable on plain chest radiography but are identifiable at high-quality contrast-enhanced spiral CT as triangular or linear soft tissue densities.[53] The normal range of size of hilar lymph nodes has not yet been fully established, but Remy-Jardin et al[53] suggested a short-axis figure of up to 3 mm, except around the left lower lobe artery where the diameter may normally be somewhat larger. The shape of the hila on CT is important when trying to assess the normality of lymph nodes. In normal patients the interfaces with the lungs are concave except at the sites of blood vessels.[54]

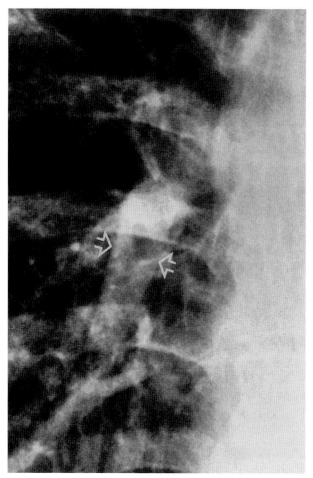

Fig. 2.13 The right lower lobe artery. The diameter indicated by the arrows should be between 9 and 16 mm.

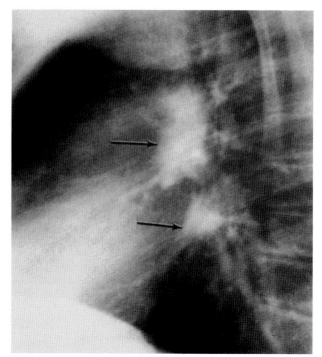

Fig. 2.14 Lateral chest radiograph showing combination shadow of right pulmonary artery and superior pulmonary vein (upper arrow), which can be confused with a hilar mass, and confluence of the lower lobe pulmonary veins (lower arrow) which is sometimes mistaken for a pulmonary nodule.

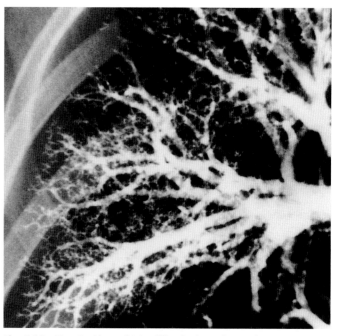

Fig. 2.15 Terminal bronchiolar filling by bronchography.

8. A collection of fat between the bifurcation of the right pulmonary artery as it exits the mediastinum, lying anterolateral to the bronchus intermedius, may be confused with lymphadenopathy if this anatomic variant is not recognized.[58] The major difficulty is that the fat in question may be combined in the same CT section as horizontal portions of the adjacent right pulmonary artery and appear to be of soft tissue rather than fat density due to partial volume artifact.

Lung parenchyma

The segmental bronchi divide into progressively smaller airways until, after six to 20 divisions, they become bronchioles (Fig. 2.4). The bronchioles divide, and the last of the purely conducting airways is known as the terminal bronchiole. Beyond the terminal bronchioles lie the acini, the gas exchange units of the lung. The entire airway down to the terminal bronchiole can be demonstrated on a well-filled bronchogram (Fig. 2.15).

The bronchopulmonary segments are based on the divisions of the bronchi and can be identified with reasonable accuracy at CT.[18,22] The boundaries between segments are complex in shape;

the segments have been likened to the pieces of a three-dimensional jigsaw puzzle. With the rare exception of accessory fissures, the segments are not delimited by septa. Although processes such as atelectasis, pneumonia, or edema may predominate in one segment or another, these processes never conform precisely to the whole of just one segment, since collateral air drift occurs from adjacent segments. In other words, it is very unusual to see visible evidence of precise segmental boundaries.

The pulmonary blood vessels (Fig. 2.9) are responsible for the branching linear markings within the lungs. It is not possible to distinguish arteries from veins in the outer two-thirds of the lungs on chest radiography. More centrally the orientation of the arteries and veins differs: the inferior pulmonary veins draining the lower lobes run more horizontally, and the lower lobe arteries more vertically. In the upper lobes the arteries and veins show a similar gently curving vertical orientation, but the upper lobe veins (when not superimposed on the arteries) lie lateral to the arteries and can sometimes be traced to the main venous trunk, the superior pulmonary vein, even on chest radiographs.

The diameter of the blood vessels beyond the hilum varies according to the patient's position. On films taken with the patient in the upright position, the diameter of both the arteries and veins increases gradually from apex to base; for comparisons of diameter to be valid, the measurements must be made equidistant from the hilum. These changes in vessel size correlate with physiologic studies of perfusion, which show that in an erect subject there is a gradation of blood flow increasing from apex to base, a difference that is less marked when supine. Although general statements regarding differences in regional blood vessel size can be made, meaningful measurements of individual peripheral pulmonary vessels are difficult to make on plain chest radiographs, since it is not possible to know whether the vessel being measured is an artery or a vein or what degree of magnification has been used. Certain measurements are suggested for upright chest films:

1. The artery and bronchus of the anterior segment of either or both upper lobes are frequently seen end on. The diameter of the artery is usually slightly less than the diameter of the bronchus (4–5 mm).[59]
2. Woodring[60] measured the visible bronchi and immediately adjacent arteries in the upper and lower half of the chest in upright patients and found that the artery/bronchus ratio was 0.85 (SD 0.15) for the upper zone and 1.34 (SD 0.25) for the lower zone.
3. Vessels in the first anterior interspace should not exceed 3 mm in diameter.[61]

An acinus, which is 5–6 mm in diameter, comprises respiratory bronchioles, alveolar ducts, and alveoli. Up to 24 acini are grouped together in secondary pulmonary lobules, each 1–3 cm in diameter, which in the lung periphery are separated by interlobular septa. When thickened by disease, these septa form so-called "septal lines" (Kerley B lines). The anatomy of the secondary pulmonary lobule and the appearance of the normal pulmonary parenchyma on HRCT is discussed on page 144 in Chapter 4.

A rich network of lymphatics drains the lung and pleura. The subpleural lymphatic vessels are found just beneath the pleura, at the junction of the interlobular septa and pleura, where they interconnect with one another as well as with the lymphatic vessels in the interlobular septa. The lymph then flows to the hilum by way of lymphatic channels that run peribronchially and in the deep septa. The lymphatic network is radiographically invisible, but in certain conditions, such as when the lung is edematous or when the lymphatic channels are occluded by tumor, the thickened septa containing the dilated lymphatics may become visible.

There are a few intrapulmonary lymph nodes, which are small and are not identifiable on plain chest radiographs. Very occasionally CT shows them as small, peripherally located, often coffee bean-shaped, nodules (Fig. 2.16).[62,63] In one series of 19 cases shown by CT, the intrapulmonary lymph nodes were either abutting the pleura or within 8 mm of the pleura, were round or oval in shape with homogeneous density, and had well-defined borders with the exception of one node that showed an irregular border resembling a small carcinoma. None of the nodes was larger than 12 mm. All were in the lower lobes or middle lobe/lingula.[64] The subpleural, lower lobe predominance of intrapulmonary lymph nodes and the fact that a few have an irregular outline indistinguishable from lung cancer on CT have also been emphasized by others.[65,66] Pathologically, visible intrapulmonary lymph nodes are believed to result from the presence of inorganic dust within the lungs and lymphatic obstruction.[67]

The pleura

The pleural space is lined by a smooth membrane consisting of a single layer of flat, in part cuboidal, mesothelial cells, lubricated by a small amount of fluid. Inferiorly the parietal pleura is tucked into the costophrenic sulcus. The disposition of the sulcus is important in upper abdominal interventional procedures. On the surface of the body the inferior edge of the sulcus crosses the xiphoid and eighth costochondral junction to reach the midaxillary line at the level of the tenth rib.[68,69] It then passes horizontally across the eleventh and twelfth ribs to reach the first lumbar vertebral body. The cephalad part of the sulcus is occupied to a variable extent by lung, whereas caudally the sulcus is empty and the diaphragm and chest wall are separated only by the two layers of parietal pleura. The distance between

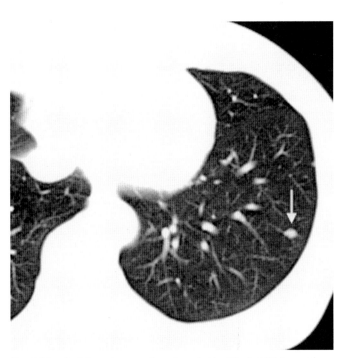

Fig. 2.16 An intrapulmonary lymph node identified at CT (proved following surgical resection, undertaken because the finding was thought to be a possible small lung cancer).

the lowest part of the sulcus and the lung edge depends on the phase of respiration and the segment of sulcus being considered. The right midaxillary intercostal approach is often used for percutaneous introduction of needles into the upper abdomen, and because the pleural reflection reaches the tenth rib in this region, it is common for the pleura to be punctured, for example during percutaneous transhepatic biliary or subphrenic abscess drainage when bile or pus may flow into the pleural space.

The parietal mesothelial cells lie on loose, fat-containing, areolar connective tissue bounded externally by the endothoracic fascia. Five layers can be defined in the visceral pleura[70,71]: (1) a mesothelial layer; (2) a thin layer of connective tissue; (3) a strong layer of connective tissue – the chief layer; (4) a vascular layer; and (5) the limiting lung membrane, connected by collagen and elastic fibers to the chief layer.[70]

The normal pleura cannot be imaged as such by CT, even by HRCT, because it cannot be separated from immediately adjacent structures. The CT appearances of the normal interface between chest wall and pulmonary parenchyma have been reported in detail by Im and co-workers.[72]

In normal subjects, there is a linear opacity of soft tissue density, 1–2 mm thick, overlying an intercostal space, connecting the inner aspects of the ribs (Figs 2.17 and 2.18). This opacity, the intercostal stripe, is produced by two layers of pleura, extrapleural fat, the endothoracic fascia, and the innermost intercostal muscle. It is marginated centrally by air in the lung and peripherally by fat lying between the innermost and internal intercostal muscles. The intercostal stripe disappears on the inner aspect of ribs, since at this point it generally consists only of pleura, extrapleural fat, and endothoracic fascia, which are too thin to resolve. In some circumstances, however, it can be seen:

1. Posteriorly, where the ribs are parallel to the scan plane and the CT section is through the lower tapering edge, the intercostal stripe is then seen on the inner aspect of the rib (Fig. 2.18).

2. When there is significant fat between the parietal pleura and endothoracic fascia; this characteristically occurs laterally at the level of the fourth to eighth ribs and in obese individuals may be conspicuous on the plain chest radiograph.

3. Low in the parasternal and paravertebral region poorly developed muscle slips (anteriorly the sternocostal muscle and posteriorly the subcostal muscle) lie on the inside of the ribs, producing linear, soft tissue opacities 1–2 mm thick (Fig. 2.17). The sternocostal muscle is commonly identified, but the subcostal muscle is seen less often (Fig. 2.19). These muscles are distinguished from pleural thickening by being smooth, uniform, and bilateral.

4. Paravertebrally, intercostal muscles are absent and the lung–soft tissue interface is formed by a very thin line produced by two layers of pleura and the endothoracic fascia (Figs 2.17 and 2.18). Linear soft tissue opacities 2–3 mm thick lying immediately underneath this interface are produced by intercostal veins, which can be positively identified when they join the azygos or hemiazygos vein.

Fissures

The lobes of the lungs are separated by fissures[73] that in the majority of people are incomplete. In other words, lung parenchyma, together with its bronchovascular bundles and draining veins, passes from one lobe to another through holes in the fissures.[21,74,75] The frequency of incomplete fissures in different series ranges from 12.5% to 73% for the major fissures[76] and from 60% to 90% for the minor fissures.[77–79] These defects are important because they allow collateral air drift between lobes, permit disease to "cross" fissures and also limit the accumulation of pleural fluid in the interlobar portions of the pleural cavity.[80–82]

The major fissures on each side are similar. The left major (oblique) fissure divides the left lung into an upper and lower lobe. The right lung has an additional fissure, the minor (horizontal) fissure, which separates the middle from the right

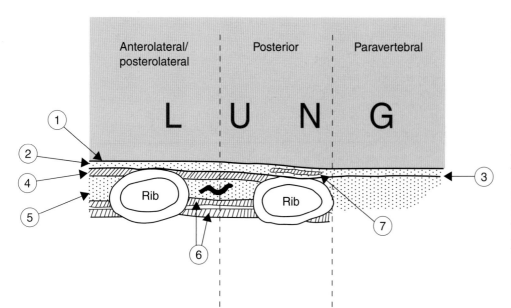

Fig. 2.17 Diagramatic anatomy of the lung–chest wall interface. The component layers vary in different segments. Anatomically identifiable layers (as illustrated) are not necessarily separately demonstrated on images and consist of (1) parietal and visceral pleura, which is too thin to image; (2) subpleural fat, which may be absent or if present is of variable thickness; (3) endothoracic fascia; (4) innermost intercostal muscle (3 and 4 appear as one structure on images); (5) intercostal fat and intercostal vessels; (6) internal and external intercostal muscles; and (7) subcostal muscle (anteriorly the transverse thoracic muscle).

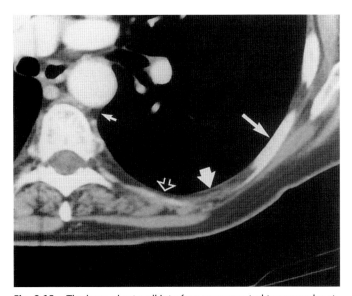

Fig. 2.18 The lung–chest wall interface on computed tomography at 10 mm collimation. Joining the inner rib margins is a soft tissue layer made up of pleura, endothoracic fascia, and innermost intercostal muscle (broad arrow). It lies on intercostal fat, outside which are internal and external intercostal muscles. No soft tissue is seen inside the ribs (large arrow) except where the thinner rib margin is sectioned (open arrow). The paravertebral interface is marginated by a thin or invisible line (small arrow), adjacent to which it is "thickened" by a posterior intercostal vein draining into the hemiazygos vein.

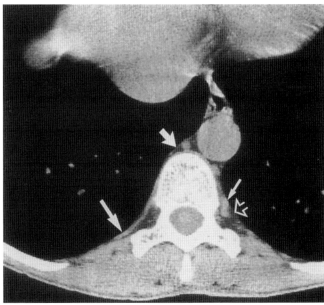

Fig. 2.19 The lung–chest wall interface in the paravertebral region on high-resolution computed tomography. The normal interface is marginated by a layer that is undetectable (open arrow) or very thin (broad arrow). The soft tissue density on the left (small arrow) is a posterior intercostal vein. That on the right (large arrow) is probably also venous but at this low level in the chest could be caused by subcostal muscle.

upper lobe. The major fissures run obliquely forward and downward, passing through the hilum, commencing at approximately the level of the fifth thoracic vertebra to contact the diaphragm up to 3 cm behind the anterior chest wall. Portions of one or both major fissures are frequently seen on the lateral chest radiograph. It is, however, unusual to be able to trace both fissures in their entirety on chest radiographs.

In Proto and Speckman's study of lateral chest radiographs, a part of a right fissure was seen in 22% of the images, a part of the left fissure was seen in 14%, and part of a major fissure of indeterminate side was seen in 62%; in only 2% of radiographs was a complete major fissure identified.[83] When the major fissure is incompletely seen, it is almost always the lower portion that is detected.

Each major fissure follows a gently curving plane somewhat similar to that of a propeller blade, with the upper portion facing forward and laterally and the lower portion facing forward and medially. Below the hila the lateral portions of the major fissures lie further forward than do the medial portions, whereas above the hila this relationship reverses (Fig. 2.20). These undulations cannot be traced on the plain chest radiograph. Therefore, on a lateral view the radiologist cannot be certain what portion of the fissure is being profiled, and it is easy to misinterpret a fissure as displaced when it is in fact in normal position. The inferior few centimeters of either or both major fissures are often wide as a result of fat or pleural thickening between the leaves of the pleura. This thickening may lead to loss of silhouette where the fissure contacts the diaphragm.

The major fissure is not usually seen on a frontal radiograph, but it may be detected under three circumstances. First, the upper edge may become visible where it contacts the posterior chest wall when extrapleural fat enters the lips of the fissure. This generates the "superolateral major fissure" (Fig. 2.21), a curved line or stripe that starts medially above the hilum and curves downward and laterally.[84] Second, the upper aspect of the major fissure can be tangential to the x-ray beam, particularly on lordotic projections,[85] generating a hairline opacity that runs obliquely across the mid zone (Fig. 2.22). Medially, this fissure line often crosses the hilum to end against the spine, allowing it to be distinguished from the minor fissure, which never crosses hilar vessels. Third, reorientation of the lateral aspect of the lower part of the oblique fissure probably accounts for the vertical fissure,[86-88] seen particularly on the right, low down close to the chest wall. It is most often described in babies with lower lobe volume loss and cardiomegaly.[86]

The minor fissure fans out forward and laterally in a horizontal direction from the right hilum. On a standard upright frontal chest radiograph the minor fissure contacts the lateral chest wall at or near the axillary portion of the right sixth rib. The fissure curves gently, usually downward in the anterior and lateral portions. Because of the undulations of the major fissure the posterior portion of the minor fissure may be projected posterior to the right major fissure on a normal lateral view.

On frontal chest radiographs some or all of the minor fissure is seen in approximately 50–60% of patients.[89] The whole fissure is seen in only 7% of individuals. When just a portion is seen, it is much more commonly the lateral than the medial portion. Felson[89] pointed out that on a frontal chest radiograph the fissure ends medially at the interlobar pulmonary artery within about 1 cm of the point at which the superior venous trunk crosses the lower lobe artery (Fig. 2.23). This observation can be helpful in finding and identifying the fissure. On a lateral view,

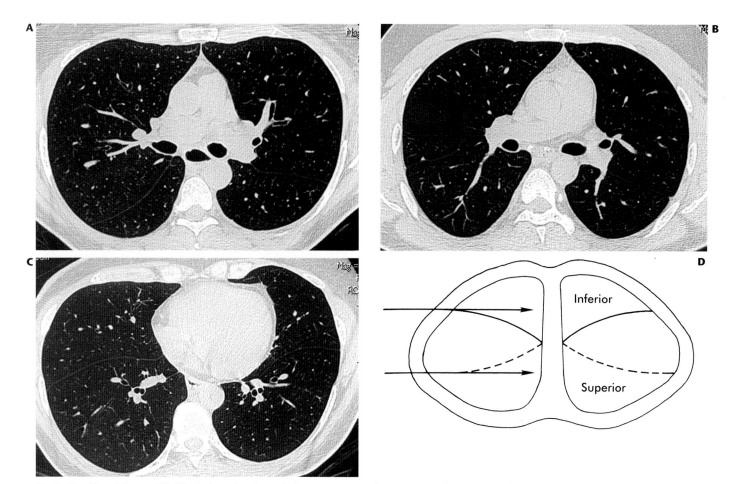

Fig. 2.20 Pleural fissures (HRCT). **A,** A section through the upper zones. The curving major fissures are clearly seen as lines. **B,** The minor fissure is seen as a zone of avascularity radiating out from the right hilum. **C,** A section through the lower zones showing the major fissures. Note the reverse curvature compared to the section through the upper zones. **D,** Diagram showing the common configuration of major fissures oriented as for CT. The arrows indicate the direction of the x-ray beam for lateral chest radiographs.

the minor fissure is seen in about half of chest radiographs: in part in 44% and in total in 6%.[83]

On 5–10 mm CT sections (see Fig. 2.24) the position of the major fissures can usually be predicted by noting the relatively avascular zone that forms the outer cortex of the lobe.[75,90,91] The region of the major fissures is seen as a band of avascularity, or a zone with much smaller vessels, traversing the lung. The major fissures may be seen as lines but, because they run obliquely through the sections, the fissure itself may be invisible or may be seen as a poorly defined band of density.[75,92] With thin-section CT the left major fissure is seen as a line throughout its course in almost all subjects (see Fig. 2.20), but the line may not be visible in upper and middle portions of the right major fissure in up to one-fourth of patients, presumably because the right major fissure is more obliquely oriented to the scanning plane.[75]

The major fissures may be seen as two parallel lines rather than a single line on thin-section CT at least at one level.[93] This so-called "double fissure sign" (Fig. 2.25) is an artifact related to cardiac and respiratory motion when exposure times are long.[75,93]

The minor fissure is in the plane of section of the CT scanner, and therefore when in normal position is not seen as a line on axial sections. Its position can usually be inferred from the large, triangular or oval deficiency of vessels on one or more sections just above the level of the bronchus intermedius (Fig. 2.20).[91,94,95] With HRCT a variety of normal patterns are encountered, depending on the precise shape of the minor fissure.[74] Because the fissure may assume the shape of an upward-arching dome, some portions may run sufficiently obliquely through the section to be seen as a line, an ill-defined band shadow, or even a rounded density (Fig. 2.26).[74,95]

Accessory fissures

Accessory fissures are clefts of varying depth in the outer surface of the lung that separate portions of lung. In one CT study of 50 patients, 22% had some form of accessory fissure,[96] and in another comprising 186 patients, 32% had an accessory fissure.[97] Five accessory fissures are either common or easily recognized:

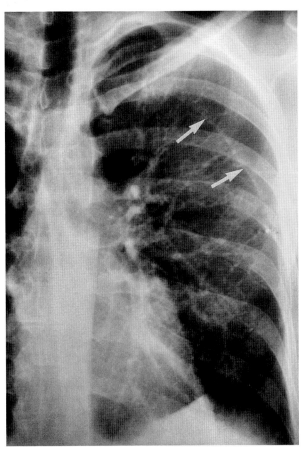

Fig. 2.21 The superolateral major fissure. This curvilinear opacity (arrows) marks the line along which the major fissure contacts the posterior chest wall.

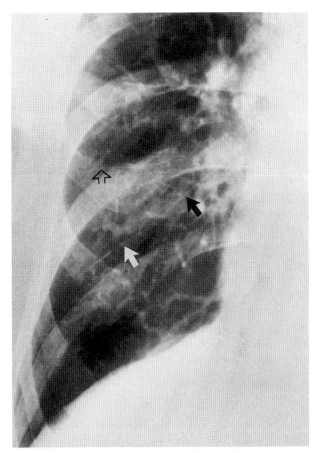

Fig. 2.22 The major fissure on a frontal radiograph. The reoriented major fissure (closed arrows) is visible on a frontal radiograph as an oblique line. It can be distinguished from the minor fissure (open arrow) because it passes more medially, overlying the right hilum and ending at the spine.

1. The best known accessory fissure, seen in up to 1% of the population, is the "azygos lobe fissure" (Fig. 2.27), so called because it contains the azygos vein within its lower margin. The fissure is almost invariably on the right side, although left-sided "azygos" fissures have been described, in which case the vein at the base of the fissure is the superior intercostal vein.[98] The fissure results from failure of normal migration of the azygos vein from the chest wall through the upper lobe to its usual position in the tracheobronchial angle, so that the invaginated visceral and parietal pleurae persist to form a fissure in the lung. The altered course of the azygos vein together with the fissure is readily seen at CT.[99] Since there is no corresponding alteration in the segmental architecture of the lung, the term "lobe" is a misnomer: the portion of the lung is supplied by branches of the apical segment bronchus with or without a contribution from the posterior segmental airway.[100] The "azygos lobe" is not unduly susceptible to disease. A potential diagnostic pitfall is that the "azygos lobe" may occupy less volume than the equivalent normal lung and may therefore appear relatively opaque,[101] even when no disease is present (Fig. 2.28). The right brachiocephalic vein may on rare occasion course through the anterior portion of the azygos fissure.[102]

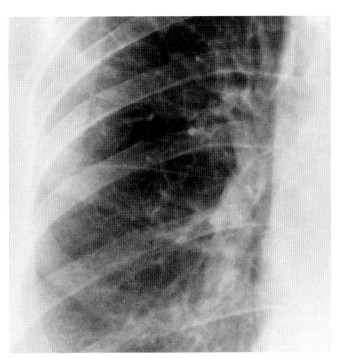

Fig. 2.23 The minor fissure. The fissure stops medially at the lateral margin of the interlobar pulmonary artery at a point approximately 1 cm beyond the Y-point of the hilum where the artery and vein cross. This is a useful identifying feature of the minor fissure.

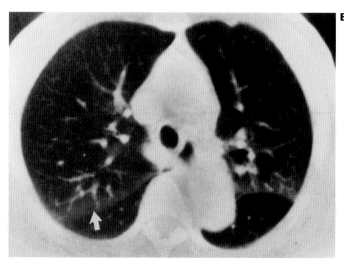

Fig. 2.24   The major fissures (arrows) on conventional CT (10 mm sections). The fissure is seen **A**, as a band of avascularity or, **B**, as a band opacity.

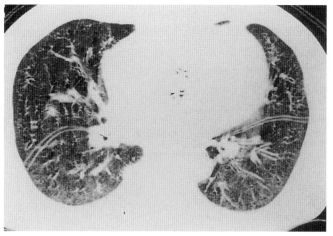

Fig. 2.25   The double fissure sign on CT (HRCT). The major fissures (and vessels) appear doubled because of lung movement during exposure.

2. The "inferior accessory fissure" usually incompletely separates the medial basal segment from the rest of the lower lobe. Because this segment lies anteromedially in the lower lobe, the accessory fissure has components that are oriented both sagittally and coronally (Figs 2.29 and 2.30) and are tangential to frontal and lateral x-ray beams; even so the fissure is rarely seen on lateral radiographs. The frequency of occurrence is difficult to ascertain because the fissure varies greatly in depth and prominence from one examination to the next.[96] The reported prevalence also depends on the method of detection. The fissure is present in 30–50% of anatomic specimens,[89] in 16–21% of CT scans,[96,97] and in 5–10% of plain radiographs.[89,96,103] On the frontal radiograph the fissure is a hairline that arises from the medial aspect of the hemidiaphragm and ascends obliquely toward the hilum (Fig. 2.30). Sometimes there is a small triangular peak at its diaphragmatic end, and this, with a very short fissure line, may be all that is seen. At the other extreme the fissure may be long, reaching all the way

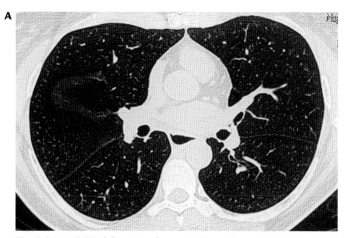

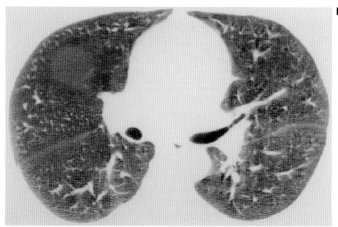

Fig. 2.26   HRCT of the minor fissure. **A**, Sometimes the minor fissure is bounded by a curvilinear band of density because the section is close to the dome of the fissure. **B**, The minor fissure may be seen as a faint homogeneous density when the section is through the apex of the dome of the fissure.

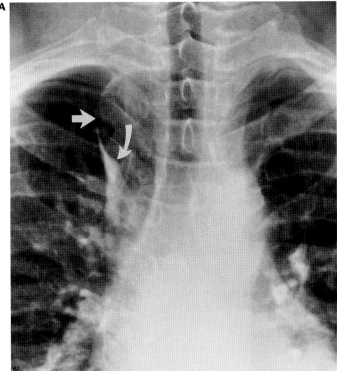

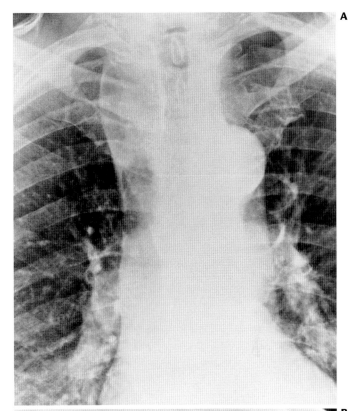

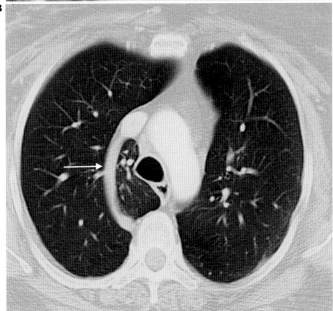

Fig. 2.27 A typical example of the azygos fissure. **A,** The horizontal arrow points to the fissure. The curved arrow points to the azygos vein in the lower margin of the fissure. Note that the azygos vein is not in its usual position in the tracheobronchial angle. **B,** A CT scan (in a different patient) shows the azygos vein coursing through the lung (arrow) and lying adjacent to the spine at a level higher than normal.

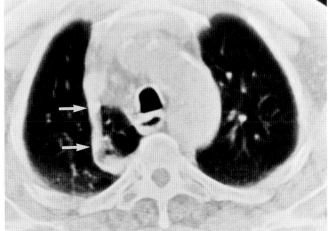

Fig. 2.28 **A,** Opaque lung medial to the azygos fissure. This appearance can be a normal finding. The opacity does not represent disease as proved in **B,** a CT of the same patient (the arrows point to the azygos vein in the lower end of the azygos fissure).

to the hilum.[89] Although the left lower lobe lacks a separate medial basal segment, the anteromedial basal bronchus divides early into two components analogous to the medial and anterior segmental bronchi on the right,[96] and an inferior accessory fissure is about as common on the left as the right. However, it is not detected with equal frequency on radiologic examination: in one series of 500 radiographs 80% of inferior accessory fissures were right-sided, 12% left-sided, and 7% bilateral.[103] On the lateral radiograph the inferior accessory fissure is occasionally seen as a vertical line, often associated with a diaphragmatic peak in the region of the esophagus.[96] The inferior pulmonary ligament is close to the medial portion of the inferior accessory fissure, and some diaphragmatic peaks on the lateral radiograph in this region are really due to the inferior pulmonary ligament and its septum. On CT (Fig. 2.29) the fissure appears on sections near the diaphragm as an arc, concave to the mediastinum, extending from the major fissure back to the mediastinum near the esophagus.[96,97]

3. Should the inferior accessory fissure marginate a pneumonia in the medial basal segment, the triangular opacity has a

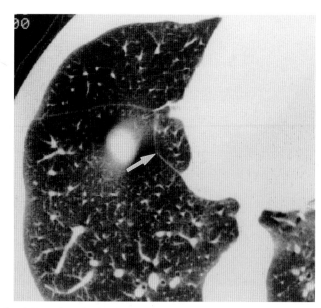

Fig. 2.29 The inferior accessory fissure on CT. The fissure (arrows) separates the medial basal segment from the rest of the lower lobe.

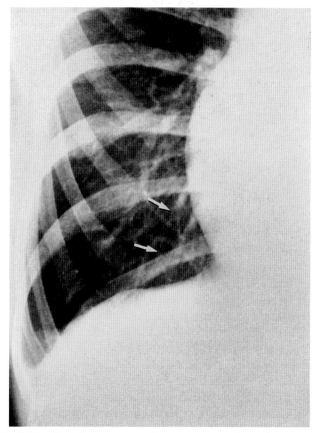

Fig. 2.30 The inferior accessory fissure on chest radiography.

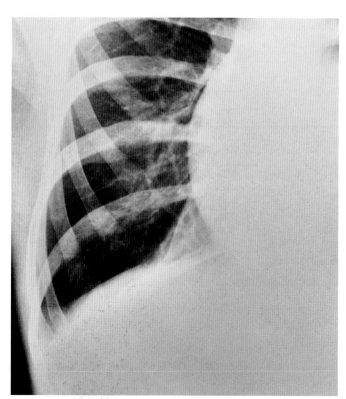

Fig. 2.31 The inferior accessory fissure. Consolidation in the medial basal segment of the right lower lobe is sharply demarcated laterally by the inferior accessory fissure. (Courtesy of Dr CJ Dow, London)

and superficially resembles a minor fissure on a frontal radiograph. It was identified on 6% of lateral radiographs in one series,[83] a figure that seems high when judged by general experience and CT series.[97] The minor fissure lies above the middle lobe bronchus, and the superior accessory fissure lies below the superior segmental bronchus. Because both of these airways arise at approximately the same level, the superior accessory fissure is projected below the minor fissure on frontal radiographs. On the lateral view it differs from the minor fissure in that it extends backward across the vertebral bodies.[83] The original descriptions of the superior accessory fissure suggested it was horizontal in orientation, but a recent evaluation of CT images suggests that it is often oriented obliquely,[105] traveling upward as it sweeps laterally and posteriorly from the hilum. On CT, like the minor fissure, it may appear as an avascular area, which should be distinguished from downward angulation of the upper end of the major fissure, a distinction that depends on identification of the superior segmental bronchus.[96] It may also be seen as a line or a boundary to atelectasis or pleural fluid, similar to the major fissures.[105]

5. The "left minor fissure" is present in 8–18% of people but is only rarely detected on posteroanterior and lateral radiographs, with a reported frequency of 1.6%.[106] It separates the lingula from the rest of the left upper lobe and is analogous to the minor fissure. It is usually arched and located more cephalad than the minor fissure. It slopes medially and downward (Fig. 2.32).

6. Rare accessory fissures include intersegmental fissures between the medial and lateral segments of the right middle

sharp outer border (Fig. 2.31),[104] which may mimic a collapsed lower lobe. Other lesions such as pleural effusion, mediastinal mass, hernia, or fat pad may be simulated.[96]

4. The "superior accessory fissure" separates the superior (apical) segment of a lower lobe from the basal segments

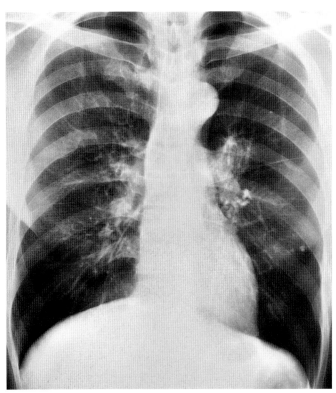

Fig. 2.32 The left minor fissure. This separates the lingula from the rest of the left upper lobe. It characteristically slopes downward and medially.

lobe, the superior and inferior segments of the lingula, and the anterobasal and laterobasal segments of both the right and left lower lobe.[97]

(Inferior) pulmonary ligaments

The (inferior) pulmonary ligaments consist of a double sheet of pleura that hangs down from each hilum like a curtain and joins the lungs to the mediastinum and to the medial part of the hemidiaphragms.[107]

The two layers of pleura contact each other below the inferior pulmonary vein and end in a free border that usually lies over the inner third of the hemidiaphragm but is sometimes displaced toward the hilum. The right inferior pulmonary ligament is short and wide-based and is related on its mediastinal aspect to the azygos vein. On the left the ligament is longer and attaches to the mediastinum close to the esophagus and anterior to the aorta (Fig. 2.33).[107] The ligament overlies a septum within the lung that separates posterior and medial basal segments.[108] The bare area of the ligament contains connective tissue, small systemic vessels, lymphatics, and lymph nodes.[109]

The ligament is not visible on chest radiographs. On CT it is visible in approximately 50–75% of patients (Fig. 2.33).[108,110,111] It is best detected just above the diaphragm as a thin curvilinear line passing outward and slightly backward from the mediastinum at the level of the esophagus. There is strong evidence that this line represents an intrapulmonary septum associated with the ligament rather than the ligament itself.[108,112,113] Often a small, triangular elevation is present at the mediastinal base of the ligament.

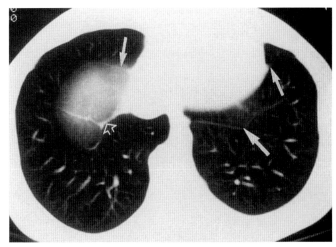

Fig. 2.33 The inferior pulmonary ligament. A CT section just above the diaphragm shows a septum associated with the left inferior pulmonary ligament (large arrow). The linear branching structure (open arrow) arising from the lateral aspect of the inferior vena cava is too anterior to be the inferior pulmonary ligament and is caused by the phrenic nerve or vessels (see Fig. 2.59, p. 63). The small anterior projections from the mediastinum (smaller arrows) are related to the major fissures.

The ligament and variations in its degree of development have been considered important for the following reasons:

1. The ligament determines the shape of a collapsed lower lobe (see Fig. 3.61D, p. 100).
2. The ligament determines the ultimate shape of the collapsed lung in a pneumothorax.[114]
3. Pleural effusion collecting posterior to the ligament tends to produce a triangular opacity, not unlike a lower lobe collapse.[114]
4. The juxtaphrenic peak sign described with volume loss of an upper lobe (see p. 92) may be due to diaphragmatic traction by way of the ligament and septum.
5. The ligament provides a pathway from lung to mediastinum and allows pathologic processes to travel in either direction.

MEDIASTINUM

The mediastinum is divided by anatomists into superior, anterior, middle, and posterior divisions. The exact anatomic boundaries between these divisions are unimportant to the radiologist because they do not provide a clear-cut guide to disease, nor do these boundaries form barriers to the spread of disease. Moreover, almost every writer on the subject seems to have a different definition.[77,109,115,116]

The mediastinal structures and spaces as seen on CT and MRI are described before the appearances on plain film because the complex interfaces between the mediastinum and the lungs are best understood by careful correlation with cross-sectional images.

Normal mediastinum

The normal mediastinal structures always identified at CT and MRI (Figs 2.34 and 2.35) are the heart and blood vessels, which

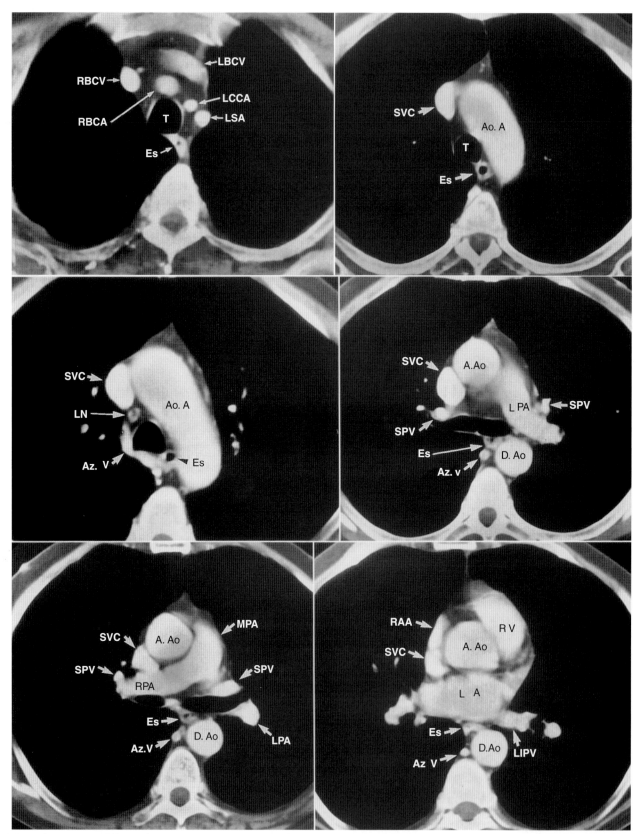

Fig. 2.34 The anatomy of the mediastinum on contrast-enhanced CT. A.Ao, Ascending aorta; Ao.A, aortic arch; Az.V, azygos vein; D.Ao, descending aorta; Es, esophagus; LBCV, left brachiocephalic vein; LCCA, left common carotid artery; LA, left atrium; LIPV, left inferior pulmonary vein; LN, lymph node; LPA, left pulmonary artery; LSA, left subclavian artery; LV, left ventricle; MPA, main pulmonary artery; RA, right atrium; RAA, right atrial appendage; RBCA, right brachiocephalic artery; RBCV, right brachiocephalic vein; RPA, right pulmonary artery; RV, right ventricle; SPV, superior pulmonary vein; SVC, superior vena cava; T, trachea.

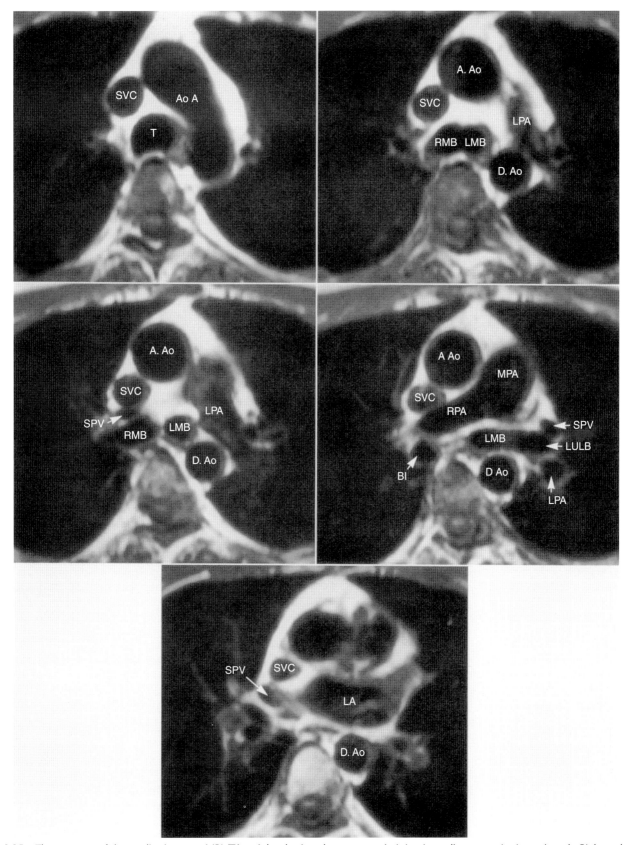

Fig. 2.35 The anatomy of the mediastinum on MRI (T1-weighted spin-echo sequences). A.Ao, Ascending aorta; Ao.A, aortic arch; Bl, bronchus intermedius; D.Ao, descending aorta; LA, left atrium; LMB, left main bronchus; LPA, left pulmonary artery; LULB, left upper lobe bronchus; MPA, main pulmonary artery; RMB, right middle lobe bronchus; RPA, right pulmonary artery; SPV, superior pulnomary vein; SVC, superior vena cava; T, trachea.

make up the bulk of the mediastinum; the major airways; and the esophagus. These structures are surrounded by a variable amount of connective tissue, largely fat, within which lie lymph nodes, the thymus, the thoracic duct, and the phrenic and laryngeal nerves.

Mediastinal blood vessels

On transaxial CT images the vertically oriented ascending and descending portions of the aorta appear round, whereas the arch is seen as a tapering oval that becomes narrower as it gives rise to the arteries to the neck, head, and arms. The average diameter of the ascending aorta is 3.5 cm, and that of the descending aorta is 2.5 cm.[117] Sections above the aortic arch show the three major aortic branches arranged in a curve lying anterior and to the left of the trachea. Their order from right to left is the brachiocephalic (innominate), left common carotid, and left subclavian arteries. The brachiocephalic artery is appreciably larger than the other two vessels. It varies slightly in position: in about half the population it is directly anterior to the trachea, and in the remainder, although still anterior to the trachea, it is either slightly to the right or left of the midline.[118] The left common carotid artery lies to the left of the trachea; the left subclavian artery also lies either to the left of the trachea or posterior to it. It is the most lateral vessel of the three and often contacts the left lung.

In 0.5% of the population the right subclavian artery arises as a separate fourth major branch of the aorta, known as an aberrant right subclavian artery. Instead of arising from the brachiocephalic artery, it runs behind the esophagus from left to right, at or just above the level of the aortic arch, to lie against the right side of the vertebral bodies before entering the root of the neck. In individuals with an aberrant right subclavian artery the brachiocephalic artery (now the right common carotid artery) is smaller than usual and is similar in diameter to the left common carotid artery.

As the descending aorta travels through the chest, it gradually moves from a position to the left of the vertebral bodies to an almost midline position before exiting from the chest through the aortic hiatus in the diaphragm. The diameter should remain nearly constant, but dilatation and tortuosity may develop with increasing age.

The mediastinal venous anatomy[119] is illustrated in Figure 2.36. The superior vena cava (SVC) has an oval or round configuration on transaxial section. Its diameter is one-third to two-thirds the diameter of the ascending aorta.[117] It can, however, be considerably smaller and may appear flattened.

A left SVC is present in 0.3–0.5% of the healthy population, but in 4.4–12.9% of those with congenital heart disease (Fig. 2.37).[120,121] This anomaly results from failure of obliteration of the left common cardinal vein during fetal development. A right SVC and an interconnecting brachiocephalic vein are also present in most cases. A left SVC arises from the junction of the left jugular and subclavian veins and travels vertically through the left mediastinum, passing anterior to the left main bronchus before joining the coronary sinus on the back of the heart. From this point the blood flows into the right atrium through the coronary sinus, which is significantly larger than normal because of the increased blood flow. At unenhanced CT a left SVC may be confused with lymphadenopathy if the full course of the vessel is not appreciated.

The left brachiocephalic vein forms a curved band anterior to the arteries arising from the arch of the aorta. Since it takes an oblique, downward course to join the SVC, its image on axial sections is usually oval rather than tubular. On rare occasions the left brachiocephalic vein descends vertically through the mediastinum before crossing the midline to join the right brachiocephalic vein,[122] and like a left superior vena cava (which it resembles) may mimic lymphadenopathy.

The right brachiocephalic vein, which travels vertically, lies anterolateral to the trachea in line with the three major arteries; it is often oval in configuration, larger than the arteries, and is the farthest right of the vessels.

The azygos vein travels anterior to the spine, either behind or to the right of the esophagus, until at some variable point it arches forward to join the posterior wall of the SVC. Usually it remains within the mediastinum and occupies the right tracheobronchial angle. In the 1% of the population who have an azygos lobe, the azygos vein traverses the lung before entering the SVC, in which case the SVC may appear distorted both on plain film and CT.[99]

The hemiazygos and accessory hemiazygos veins also lie against the vertebral bodies but in a more posterior plane, usually just behind the descending aorta. The accessory hemiazygos vein may cross the midline in the midthoracic level to join the azygos vein, or it may drain into the left superior intercostal vein, which arches around the aorta more or less at the junction of the arch and the descending portion to join the left brachiocephalic vein. The azygos and hemiazygos veins are routinely identifiable at CT, but they are generally not big enough to confuse with lymphadenopathy or other masses.[123] The left superior intercostal vein is much smaller than the azygos vein and is only occasionally identified on plain films or on CT, although in 1–9.5% of normal patients it is seen on plain chest radiography as a small nipple on the lateral margin of the aortic arch (see Fig. 2.47, p. 57).[124–126]

Occasionally the inferior vena cava (IVC) does not develop in the usual fashion and the azygos vein forms the venous conduit draining inferior vena caval blood back to the heart, an arrangement known as azygos continuation of the IVC. The hepatic veins in these cases drain into the right atrium, not into the IVC. The azygos vein is therefore enlarged and is only slightly smaller than the IVC. Its anatomy is otherwise unaltered. Azygos continuation of the IVC may resemble a mediastinal mass or lymphadenopathy.

The main pulmonary artery runs obliquely backward and upward to the left of the ascending aorta. Its average diameter on a study of 100 normal subjects was 2.72 cm (SD = 0.3 cm); in another series the diameter averaged 2.8 cm.[117,127] It divides into right and left branches. The right branch travels more or less horizontally through the mediastinum, between the ascending aorta and SVC anteriorly and the major bronchi posteriorly. The left pulmonary artery arches higher than the right pulmonary artery and passes over the left main bronchus to descend posterior to it. This configuration leads to two important observations: the left pulmonary artery is often seen on a higher CT section than the right pulmonary artery, and the lung abuts the posterior wall of the right airway but is partly or totally excluded from contact with the left airway by the descending limb of the left pulmonary artery. The right pulmonary artery is two-thirds the diameter of the main pulmonary artery.

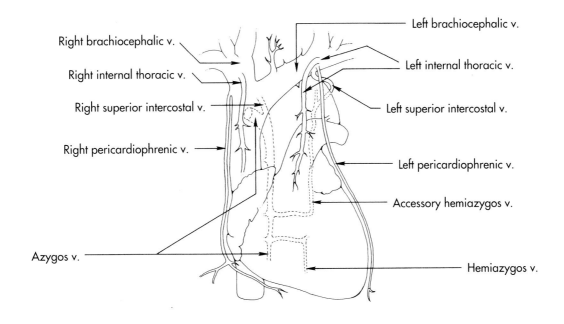

Right brachiocephalic v.
Right internal thoracic v.
Right superior intercostal v.
Right pericardiophrenic v.

Left brachiocephalic v.
Left internal thoracic v.
Left superior intercostal v.
Left pericardiophrenic v.
Accessory hemiazygos v.

Azygos v.
Hemiazygos v.

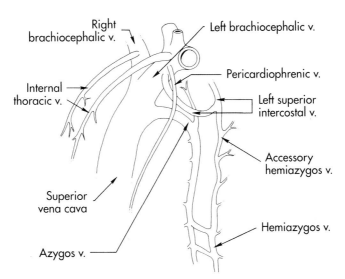

Right brachiocephalic v.
Internal thoracic v.
Superior vena cava
Azygos v.

Left brachiocephalic v.
Pericardiophrenic v.
Left superior intercostal v.
Accessory hemiazygos v.
Hemiazygos v.

Fig. 2.36 Diagrams illustrating mediastinal venous anatomy. (Redrawn from Godwin JD, Chen JTT. Reprinted with permission from the American Journal of Roentgenology)

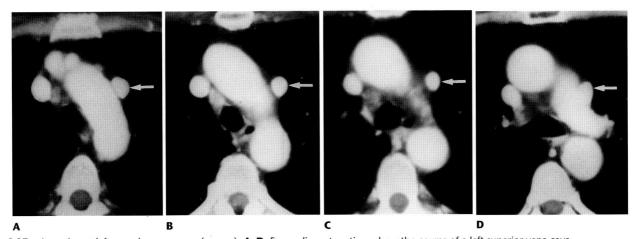

A **B** **C** **D**

Fig. 2.37 A persistent left superior vena cava (arrows). **A–D**, Four adjacent sections show the course of a left superior vena cava.

Esophagus

The esophagus is visible on all CT and MRI axial sections from the root of the neck down to the esophageal hiatus through the diaphragm. In approximately 80% of normal persons the esophagus contains air, sometimes just a small amount. If there is sufficient mediastinal fat, the entire circumference of the esophagus can be identified. If air is present in the lumen, the uniform thickness of the wall can be appreciated. Without air the collapsed esophagus appears either circular or oval and is usually approximately 1 cm in its narrowest diameter. On MRI the signal intensity on T1-weighted images is similar to that of muscle, but on T2-weighted images the esophagus often shows a much higher signal intensity than muscle.

Thymus

Microscopic examination of the thymus shows many lobules, each divided into a medulla, consisting predominantly of epithelial cells, and a cortex containing the major cell of the thymus, the T lymphocyte. Epithelioid cells form a general framework. Hassall's corpuscles are a characteristic feature of the medulla of the thymus; they consist of mature keratinized epithelial cells that layer on each other in concentric fashion. Myoid cells, similar to striated skeletal muscle, are found adjacent to Hassall's corpuscles; they are much more prevalent in children than in adults.

The thymus is anterior to the aorta and the right ventricular outflow tract or pulmonary artery. At CT it is usually found inferior to the left brachiocephalic vein and superior to the level of the horizontal portion of the right pulmonary artery; it is often best appreciated on a section through the aortic arch.[128]

Before puberty,[129] the thymus occupies most of the mediastinum in front of the great vessels (Fig. 2.38). The gland remains fairly constant in weight, enlarging slightly until puberty, after which the thymic follicles atrophy and fatty replacement occurs until eventually little or no residual thymic tissue can be seen. In children the gland varies so greatly in size that measurement is of little value in deciding normality. Shape is a more useful criterion: the thymus is soft and fills in the spaces between the great vessels and the anterior chest wall as if molded by these structures. The lateral margins may be

concave, straight, or bulged outward, but approximate symmetry is the rule. In children under 5 years of age the gland is usually quadrilateral in shape with a convex lateral margin.[130] A sharp angular border equivalent to the sail sign on plain films is occasionally visible at CT.[129] In young children the thymus may extend all the way into the posterior mediastinum[131,132] and may occasionally be confused with a posterior mediastinal mass.[133–136]

The thymus consists of two lobes, each enclosed in its own fibrous sheath.[137] Up to 30% of the population have a fat cleft visible by CT at the junction of the two lobes. The left lobe is usually larger[138] and slightly higher than the right,[139] but these asymmetries are moderate and the two lobes cannot always be clearly defined.[128] A focal swelling, or a large lobe on one side with little or no thymic tissue visible on the other, suggests a mass. At CT the thymus is bilobed, triangular, or shaped like an arrowhead. In one series of normal children, the mean thickness of the right lobe was 9 mm and that of the left lobe was 11 mm.[140] The maximum width and thickness of each lobe decrease with advancing age. Between 20 and 50 years of age the average thickness measured by CT decreases from 8 or 9 mm to 5 or 6 mm, the maximum thickness of one lobe being up to 1.5 cm.[132,141] These diameters are greater at MRI, presumably because MRI demonstrates the thymic tissue even when it is partially replaced by fat.[138] At MRI, sagittal images demonstrate that the gland is 5–7 cm in craniocaudad dimension.[138] It is impractical to measure the craniocaudad dimension at CT, but the gland may be visible over a similar distance.[132,141]

In younger patients the CT density of the thymus is homogeneous and close to, or slightly higher than, muscle. The gland often enhances appreciably with intravenous contrast material.[129] After puberty the density gradually decreases owing to fatty replacement.[142] In patients older than 40 years of age the thymus may have an attenuation value identical to that of fat.[141] In some patients the whole gland shows fat density[141,143] and is therefore indistinguishable from mediastinal fat. In others residual thymic parenchyma is visible as a streaky or nodular density (Fig. 2.39).[128,143]

On T1-weighted MR images (Fig. 2.40) the intensity of the normal thymic tissue is similar to or slightly higher than that of muscle.[130,144] As fatty replacement progresses, the thymus shows higher signal intensity to eventually blend in with the surrounding fat. On T2-weighted images the signal intensity is similar to or sometimes higher than fat[130,144,145] and does not change with age. Proton density images show significantly less signal than the surrounding fat.

Ultrasonography has been used to evaluate the thymus in children.[146–148] Longitudinal ultrasound scans can be obtained by scanning intercostally, to the right and left of the sternum, angling the probe medially to visualize the substernal thymus. Axial images can be obtained by scanning in the suprasternal notch.[146] On longitudinal scans the thymus appears triangular or tear-drop in shape, but may rarely be round in shape. On transverse scans the gland is trapezoid in shape with slight lateral convexity and molds to the shape of the adjacent great vessels. In general the gland is symmetric about the midline.[146,147] Adam and Ignotus gave the following measurements for children aged 2–8 years: mean anteroposterior and longitudinal measurements were 1.4 and 2.5 cm, respectively, for the right lobe, and 1.4 and 2.9 cm, respectively, for the left lobe. The internal echogenicity of the thymus in both infants and children is similar to that of the liver.[146–148]

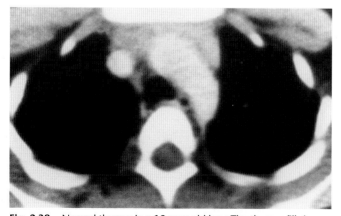

Fig. 2.38 Normal thymus in a 12-year-old boy. The thymus fills in most of the mediastinum and molds to the aorta and superior vena cava.

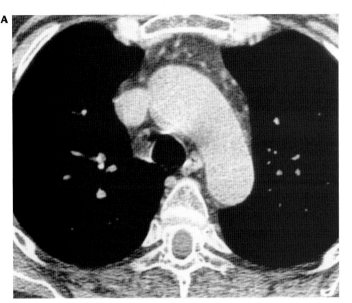

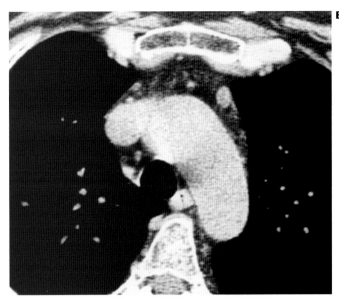

Fig. 2.39 Normal thymic remnants in adulthood. **A,** Typical small nodular and linear remnants. **B,** Large nodular and linear remnants in a 36-year-old man.

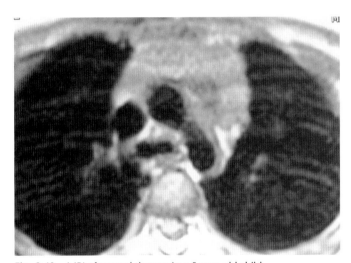

Fig. 2.40 MRI of normal thymus in a 5-year-old child.

The normal thymus may take up various radionuclides, such as fluoro-deoxyglucose (FDG) and iodine-131, and this should not be confused with disease.[149–151]

"Mediastinal spaces"

The nomenclature of the connective tissue spaces within the mediastinum is not standard, and there are no exact definitions for the boundaries between them. Nevertheless, radiologists need to understand the terms in common use. Four named spaces surround the central airways: the pretracheal space, the aortopulmonary window, the subcarinal space, and the right paratracheal space. All four contain lymph nodes that drain the lung and are therefore likely to be involved by bronchial carcinoma. In addition to these central spaces are the junction areas, so called because in these areas the two lungs approximate each other. One lies anterior to the aorta and pulmonary artery

and is variously known as the anterior junction[152] or the prevascular space[118]; the other lies posterior to the trachea and esophagus and is known as the posterior junction.[153] Finally, there are the paraspinal lines on either side of the spine and the junctional area between mediastinum and retroperitoneum known as the retrocrural space.

Pretracheal space

The pretracheal space[154] has no boundary with the lung and is therefore not imaged on plain chest radiographs. It is well known to surgeons because it is the space explored by transcervical mediastinoscopy. The space is triangular in axial cross section; the three boundaries are the trachea or carina posteriorly, either the superior vena cava or the right innominate vein anteriorly to the right, and the ascending aorta with its enveloping superior pericardial sinus anteriorly to the left.[155] The superior pericardial recess is a small pocket of pericardium investing the aorta. When distended, the pericardial configuration is easy to recognize (Fig. 2.41D). In normal individuals, however, a small amount of pericardial fluid in the retroaortic extension of the superior pericardial recess (Fig. 2.41) may mimic lymph-adenopathy on CT. At spin-echo MRI the signal characteristics of fluid permit differentiation from lymphadenopathy or other masses, but on gradient echo MR imaging the high signal intensity of fluid may resemble the signal from flowing blood and the superior pericardial recess may then mimic aortic dissection.[156]

The pretracheal space is continuous with the right paratracheal space, the aortopulmonary window, and the subcarinal space. Consequently, lymph nodes or other masses arising in any of these spaces may grow large enough to encroach on the pretracheal space and vice versa.

Aortopulmonary window

The aortopulmonary window is situated under the aortic arch above the left pulmonary artery. It is bounded medially by the

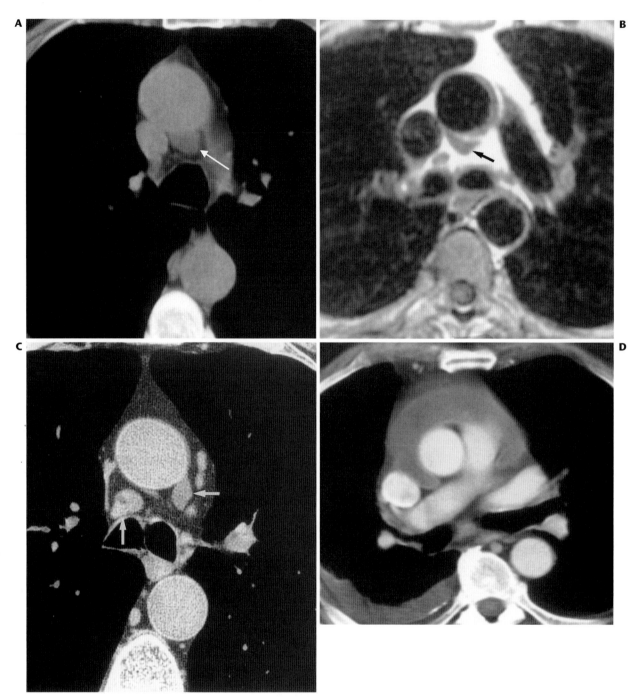

Fig. 2.41 The superior pericardial recess. **A**, CT showing a normal superior pericardial recess posterior to the ascending aorta (arrow). **B**, MRI showing a similar appearance. **C**, HRCT showing a normal superior pericardial recess (horizontal arrow) tucking into the aortopulmonary window. The vertical arrow points to an enlarged mediastinal lymph node. Note that the node is not immediately next to the aorta. **D**, A patient with a large pericardial effusion showing marked distension of the superior pericardial recess on CT.

trachea and esophagus and laterally by the lung.[157] Its fatty density is not always appreciated at CT because so often the sections include either the aortic arch or the left pulmonary artery, and volume averaging results in higher than fat density.

The ligamentum arteriosum and the recurrent laryngeal nerve traverse this space. They are rarely identified with conviction, but in any event they are not likely to be confused with lymphadenopathy or other masses. In older patients, calcification of the ligamentum is common and causes recognizable curvilinear calcification in approximately half of patients

undergoing chest CT.[158] However, it is often confused with atheromatous calcification of the adjacent aortic wall. It is easier to distinguish from atheromatous aortic calcification in younger patients, in whom calcification of the ligamentum was seen in 13% of 53 patients in one series,[159] but none had evidence of a patent ductus arteriosus.

The left pulmonic recess of the pericardium envelops the main pulmonary artery and even normal amounts of pericardial fluid can mimic lymphadenopathy if the anatomic position and shape of this pericardial extension is not recognized (Fig. 2.41C).[160]

Subcarinal space

The subcarinal space, lying beneath the tracheal carina, is bounded on either side by the major bronchi. The azygoesophageal recess of the right lung lies behind the subcarinal space, and distortion of the azygoesophageal recess is a sensitive method of detecting masses, usually lymphadenopathy, in this space. The posterior boundary is partly formed by the esophagus.

Right paratracheal space and posterior tracheal space

These two adjacent spaces (they should more properly be called stripes) are best considered together. Normally the right lung is separated from the trachea only by a thin layer of fat (the only exception being at the tracheobronchial angle where the azygos vein lies between the lung and the airway). The degree to which the lung envelops the posterior wall of the trachea is variable. In up to half the population a substantial portion of the posterior tracheal wall is outlined by lung as it interposes between the spine and the trachea to contact the esophagus.

Anterior junction (prevascular space)

The anterior junction[152] lies anterior to the pulmonary artery, the ascending aorta, and the three major branches of the aortic arch. It lies between the two lungs and is bounded anteriorly by the chest wall. If the two lungs approximate each other closely enough, the intervening mediastinum may consist of little more than four layers of pleura and is then sometimes known as the anterior junction line (see Fig. 2.48, p. 58). Coursing through the prevascular space superiorly is the left brachiocephalic vein. The internal mammary vascular bundles are to be found laterally and are visible at CT only if intravenous contrast material is administered. Embedded within the prevascular space are lymph nodes, the thymus, and the phrenic nerve.

Posterior junction and paraspinal areas

The term "posterior junction" describes the mediastinal region posterior to the trachea and the heart, where the two lungs lie close to each other.[153] The right lung always invaginates behind the right hilar structures and heart to contact the pleura overlying the azygos vein and esophagus, forming the so-called "azygoesophageal recess". Displacement of the lung from the azygoesophageal recess is an important sign of a subcarinal mediastinal mass, particularly lymphadenopathy. Above the level of the azygos arch, the lung contacts the esophagus alone.

On the left, the lung interface is with the aortic arch and descending aorta rather than with the esophagus, but in some individuals the lung below the aortic arch invaginates anterior to the descending aorta to reach almost to the midline.

The paraspinal areas are contiguous with the posterior junction. Normally there is little or no discernible connective tissue between the lateral margins of the spine and the lungs but fat may make these lines more evident (Fig. 2.42). The only structures contained in these areas are intercostal vessels and small lymph nodes.

Retrocrural space

The aorta exits the chest by passing through the aortic hiatus, which is bounded by the diaphragmatic crura and the spine

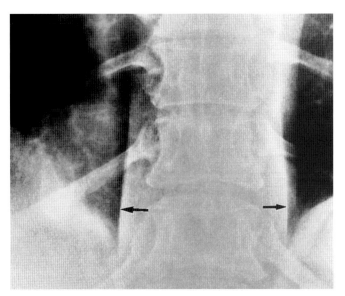

Fig. 2.42 The paraspinal lines (arrows) are made more obvious by fat deposition in this case. (Streiter ML et al: Steroid induced thoracic lipomatosis: paraspinal involvement, AJR 1982;139:679).

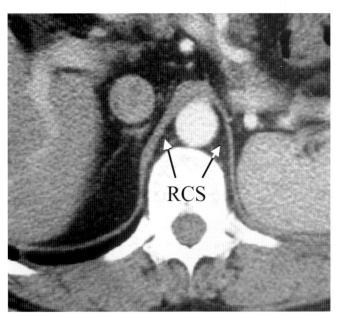

Fig. 2.43 The retrocrural spaces (RCS) behind the diaphragmatic crura.

(Fig. 2.43). The diaphragmatic crura are ligaments that blend with the anterior longitudinal ligament of the spine. Apart from the aorta, the structures that pass through the aortic hiatus are the azygos and hemiazygos veins, intercostal arteries, and splanchnic nerves. All these structures are too small to be mistaken for lymphadenopathy.[161]

Mediastinal and hilar lymph nodes

Lymph nodes are widely distributed through the mediastinum and hila. There have been several classifications over the years. The following description uses terms agreed by the American Joint Committee on Cancer and the Union Internationale Contre

Box 2.1 AJCC–UICC classifications of regional lymph nodes[162]

1. *Highest mediastinal nodes* lie above a horizontal line at the upper rim of the brachiocephalic (left innominate) vein
2. *Upper paratracheal nodes* lie above a horizontal line drawn tangential to the upper margin of the aortic arch and below the inferior boundary of No. 1 nodes
3. *Prevascular and retrotracheal nodes* may be designated 3A and 3P; midline nodes are considered to be ipsilateral
4. *Lower paratracheal nodes* lie to the right or left of the midline of the trachea between a horizontal line drawn tangential to the upper margin of the aortic arch and a line extending across the right or left main bronchus at the upper margin of the ipsilateral upper lobe bronchus. They are contained within the mediastinal pleural envelope. NB: The left lower paratracheal nodes lie medial to the ligamentum arteriosum
5. *Subaortic (aortopulmonary window) nodes* lie lateral to the ligamentum arteriosum or the aorta or left pulmonary artery and proximal to the first branch of the left pulmonary artery and lie within the mediastinal pleural envelope
6. *Paraaortic nodes (ascending aorta or phrenic)* lie anterior and lateral to the ascending aorta and the aortic arch or the innominate artery, beneath a line tangential to the upper margin of the aortic arch
7. *Subcarinal nodes* lie caudal to the carina of the trachea, but not associated with the lower lobe bronchi or arteries within the lung
8. *Paraesophageal nodes (below carina)* lie adjacent to the wall of the esophagus and to the right or left of the midline, excluding subcarinal nodes
9. *Pulmonary ligament nodes* lie within the pulmonary ligament, including those against the posterior wall and lower part of the inferior pulmonary vein
10. *Hilar nodes* lie distal to the mediastinal pleura reflection and the nodes adjacent to the bronchus intermedius on the right
11. *Interlobar nodes* lie between the lobar bronchi
12. *Lobar nodes* lie adjacent to the distal lobar bronchi
13. *Segmental nodes* lie adjacent to the segmental bronchi
14. *Subsegmental nodes* lie around the subsegmental bronchi

NB. Station 1–9 nodes lie within the mediastinal pleural envelope whereas station 10–14 nodes lie outside the mediastinal pleura within the visceral pleura.

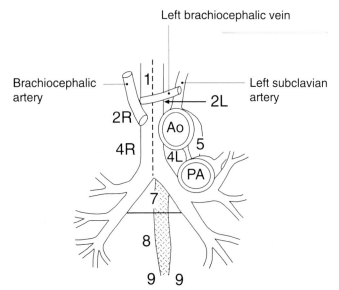

Fig. 2.44 The AJCC–UICC lymph node classification illustrating selected nodal stations. Those included in the diagram are all within the mediastinum. Mediastinal stations not shown are the prevascular (3A) and retrotracheal (3P) and the paraaortic group (6).

le Cancer (AJCC–UICC) designed primarily for the staging of carcinoma of the bronchus (Box 2.1 and Fig. 2.44).[162–164] The nomenclature is similar to that previously used by the American Thoracic Society (ATS),[165] except that all nodes around the main bronchi lying inside the mediastinal pleura are classified as paratracheal, and all hilar nodes lie outside the mediastinal pleura.

The AJCC–UICC classification is based on cross-sectional imaging in that it is directly referable to axial cross-sectional anatomy. The plane tangential to the upper margin of the aortic arch is an important dividing plane with nodes above this level being designated as: "highest mediastinal nodes" (station 1 if they are above the upper rim of the left brachiocephalic vein); "right, left and posterior upper paratracheal" (stations 2R, 2L, and 3P, respectively); and "prevascular" if they lie anterior to the arteries to the head and neck (station 3A).

The nodes below the plane tangential to the upper margin of the aortic arch include the following: right and left lower paratracheal (stations 4R and 4L); subaortic (aortopulmonary window) nodes (station 5); paraaortic nodes which lie anterior and lateral to the ascending aorta, the aortic arch, or the proximal brachiocephalic artery (station 6); subcarinal nodes, which lie beneath the main bronchi within the mediastinal pleura (station 7). Low down in the mediastinum are the paraesophageal (station 8) and pulmonary ligament nodes (station 9). Nodes are also present in the retrocrural areas and cardiophrenic angles.

The nodes outside the mediastinal pleura are hilar (station 10), interlobar (station 11), lobar, segmental and subsegmental (stations 12–14).

Normal lymph node size

The CT series documenting normal mediastinal lymph node size are in general agreement.[154,162,166–168] In these studies 95% of normal mediastinal lymph nodes were less than 10 mm in short-axis diameter, and the remainder, with very few exceptions, were less than 15 mm in short-axis diameter. There is a significant variation in the number and size of lymph nodes seen in different locations within the mediastinum. Nodes in the region of the brachiocephalic veins are generally smaller, with over 90% measuring 5 mm or less, whereas nodes in the aortopulmonary window, the pretracheal and lower paratracheal spaces, and the subcarinal compartment are often 6–10 mm in short-axis diameter. Nodes in the paracardiac areas are rarely visible in normal subjects: their maximum size in a series of 50 persons was 3.5 mm.[169] Nodes in the retrocrural area do not normally exceed 6 mm in diameter.[161]

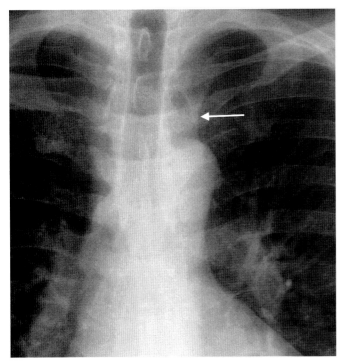

Fig. 2.45 The shadow of the left subclavian artery (arrow) may simulate a pleural or parenchymal density.

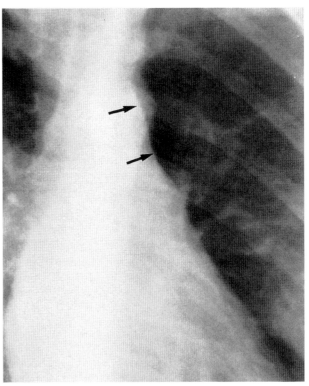

Fig. 2.46 The aortopulmonary stripe, the reflection of mediastinal pleura from aorta to pulmonary artery (arrows). This should not be confused with displacement of mediastinal pleura resulting from adenopathy. (Keats TE: The aortic-pulmonary mediastial stripe, AJR 1972;116:107).

Normal mediastinal contours on plain chest radiographs

For descriptive convenience the frontal and lateral projections are treated separately, although in practice the information from these two views should be integrated. For further details of the normal appearances in the lateral projection, the reader is referred to the excellent accounts by Proto and Speckman.[83,170]

Frontal projection

Left mediastinal border

Above the aortic arch the mediastinal shadow to the left of the trachea is of low density and is due to the left carotid and left subclavian arteries and the jugular veins. The usual appearance in the frontal projection is a gently curving border that fades out where the artery enters the neck (Fig. 2.45). The border is formed by the left subclavian artery or more usually by the adjacent fat[171]; occasionally the interface is with the left carotid artery.[171] A separate interface may be discernible for the left carotid artery. The outer margin of the left tracheal wall is very rarely outlined[172] because the lung is almost invariably separated from the trachea by the aorta and great vessels.

Below the aortic arch the left mediastinal border is formed by the aortopulmonary pleural stripe (Fig. 2.46),[157,173] the main pulmonary artery, and the heart. A small "nipple" may occasionally be seen projecting laterally from the aortic knob. This projection is caused by the left superior intercostal vein arching forward around the aorta just beyond the origin of the left subclavian artery before entering the left brachiocephalic vein (Fig. 2.47).[174] This vein should not be misinterpreted as lymph-

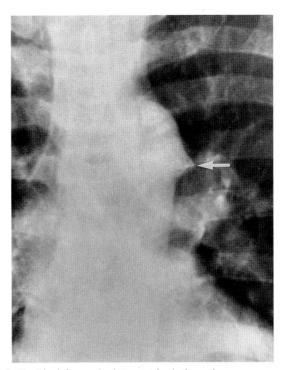

Fig. 2.47 The left superior intercostal vein (arrow) seen as a so-called "aortic nipple".

adenopathy projecting from the aortopulmonary window. Fat can sometimes be identified in the aortopulmonary window beneath the aortic arch.

The left border of the descending aorta can be traced through the shadow of the main pulmonary artery and heart as a continuous border from the aortic arch down to the aortic hiatus in the diaphragm in the great majority of normal patients. In a small proportion, 9% in a series from Japan, a portion of the interface between lung and descending aorta is indistinct due to contact or proximity of the aortic margin branches of the left hilar vessels.[175] In patients with pectus excavatum a small portion of the left wall of the middle descending aorta may appear indistinct because it is in contact with the left atrium and left inferior pulmonary vein.[176]

Right mediastinal border

The right mediastinal border is normally formed by the right brachiocephalic (innominate) vein, the SVC, and the right atrium. The right paratracheal stripe can be seen through the right brachiocephalic vein and SVC because the lung contacts the right tracheal wall from the clavicles down to the arch of the azygos vein (Fig. 2.48). This stripe,[177] which should be of uniform thickness and no greater than 4 mm in width, is visible in approximately two-thirds of healthy subjects. It consists of the wall of the trachea and adjacent mediastinal fat, but there should be no focal bulges caused by individual paratracheal lymph nodes. The azygos vein is outlined by air in the lung at the lower end of this stripe. The diameter of the azygos vein in the tracheobronchial angle is variable; it may be considered normal when 10 mm or less. The nodes immediately beneath the azygos vein, which are sometimes known as azygos nodes, are not recognizable on normal chest radiographs. The right paratracheal stripe has diagnostic value because it excludes space-occupying processes in the area where the stripe is visible and appears normal.

Anterior junction

The two lungs approximate each other above the level of the heart and below the manubrium; the term "anterior junction" has therefore been applied to this area of the mediastinum.[152] When the two lungs are separated only by pleura, the anterior junction forms a visible line, known as the anterior junction line (Fig. 2.48), which is usually straight and diverges to fade out superiorly as it reaches the clavicles. It descends for a variable distance, usually deviating to the left. The anterior junction line sometimes follows a vertical course or, very rarely, deviates to the right. It cannot extend below the point where the two lungs separate to envelop the right ventricle. Since the line is only occasionally seen, failure to identify it is of no significance.

More often the two lungs are separated by fat and thymus, with the result that the borders of the anterior junction are invisible on plain film or that only one of the borders can be identified. Bulging of one or both borders indicates the presence of a mass. In young children the thymus can be a prominent structure and the sail shape is characteristic (Fig. 2.49).

Proto et al[152] used the terms "superior" and "inferior recesses" to describe the lung interfaces above and below the anterior junction region. The interfaces of the superior recesses are concave laterally. They are formed by mediastinal fat anterior to the arteries that supply the head and neck. (The left

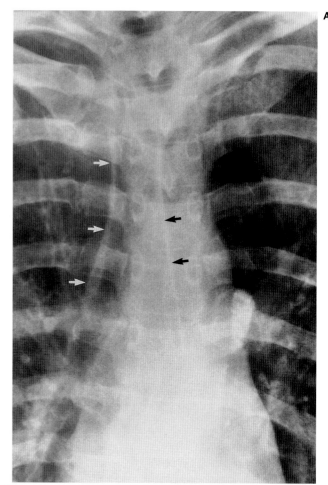

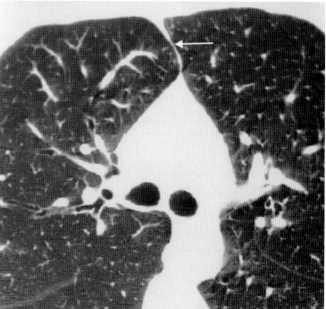

Fig. 2.48 **A**, The anterior junction line (black arrowheads) and right paratracheal stripe (white arrows). The lowest white arrow points to the azygos vein. **B**, CT in another patient shows the anterior junction line (arrow).

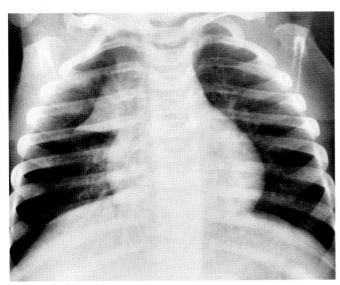

Fig. 2.49 Normal thymus in a 3-year-old child. The sail shape projecting to the right of the mediastinum is characteristic.

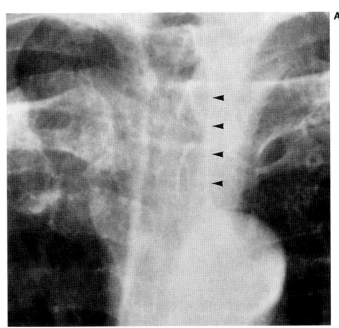

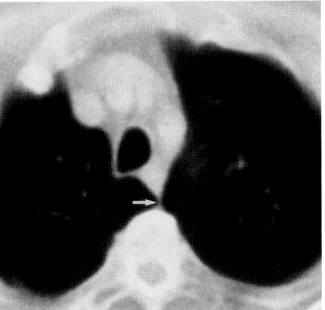

Fig. 2.50 **A,** The posterior junction line (arrowheads). **B,** CT shows the origin of the line (arrow) in the same patient.

and right brachiocephalic veins course through this fat but do not form visible borders on the frontal view.) The inferior recesses are due to divergence of the lungs around fat in the lower mediastinum anterior to the heart.[152]

Posterior junction and azygoesophageal recess

In some individuals the lungs almost touch each other behind the esophagus to form the posterior junction line, a structure that can be thought of as an esophageal mesentery (Fig. 2.50).[77] This line, unlike the anterior junction line, diverges to envelop the aortic and azygos arches. Above the aortic arch the posterior junction line extends to the lung apices, where it diverges and disappears at the root of the neck, well above the level of the clavicles. The differences in the superior extent of the anterior and posterior junction lines are related to the sloping boundary between the thorax and the neck. Once again the width of the line depends on the amount of mediastinal fat. Whether both sides of the line are seen on plain chest radiograph depends on the tangent formed with the adjacent lung. Bulging of the borders of any portion of the posterior junction line or its superior recesses suggests a mass or other space-occupying process. The only normal convexities are those attributable to the azygos vein or aortic arch.

Whether or not there is a visible posterior junction line above the aortic arch, the interface between the lung and the right wall of the esophagus can often be seen as a very shallow S extending from the lung apex down to the azygos arch. If there is air in the esophagus, which there frequently is, the right wall of the esophagus is seen as a stripe, usually 3–5 mm thick.[178] This interface is known as the pleuroesophageal line or stripe (Fig. 2.51).

Below the aortic arch the right lower lobe makes contact with the right wall of the esophagus and the azygos vein as it ascends next to the esophagus. This portion of lung is known as the "azygoesophageal recess", and the interface is known as the azygoesophageal line (Fig. 2.52). The shape of the azygos arch

varies considerably in different subjects, and therefore the shape of the upper portion of the azygoesophageal line varies accordingly. In its upper few centimeters, however, the azygoesophageal line in adults is always straight or concave toward the lung, and a convex shape suggests a subcarinal mass. Before 3 years of age the azygoesophageal line is usually convex and various configurations, including a high proportion showing a convex or straight border, are seen as the child becomes older.[179,180] The azygoesophageal line can be traced down into the posterior costophrenic angle in subjects with normal anatomy.

The left wall of the esophagus (Fig. 2.53) is rarely visible; the near vertical border seen through the heart represents the left

A

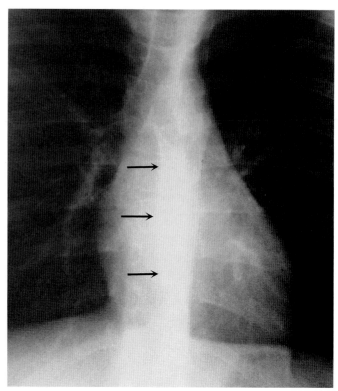

Fig. 2.52 The azygoesophageal line (arrows).

B

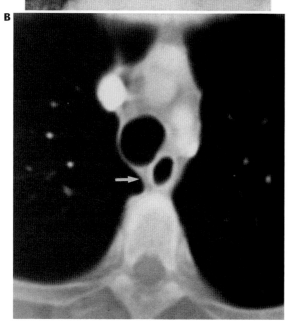

Fig. 2.51 **A**, The pleuroesophageal line (arrowheads). **B**, CT shows the origin of the line (arrow) in the same patient.

wall of the descending aorta. This border can be traced, with virtually no loss of continuity, upward to the aortic arch and downward to the diaphragm. In a few subjects a small segment of aortic outline may be invisible because of contact between the aorta and the descending division of the left pulmonary artery behind the left main bronchus.

Occasionally the lung contacts the left wall of the esophagus, and then the esophagus is outlined both from the right and the left. Because air is frequently present in the esophagus, identifying separately the thickness of the right and left walls may even be possible. The usual site for trapped air within the esophagus is just beneath the aortic arch (Fig. 2.54).[181]

Paraspinal lines

The term "paraspinal line" refers to a stripe of soft tissue density parallel to the left and right margins of the thoracic spine. Although lymph nodes and intercostal veins share this space with mediastinal fat and pleura, these structures cannot normally be recognized individually. With little fat the interface may closely follow the undulations of the lateral spinal ligaments, but with larger quantities of fat these undulations are smoothed out (see Fig. 2.42, p. 55). The left paravertebral space is usually thicker than the right. The paravertebral stripes are usually less than 1 cm wide, although they can be wider in obese persons. Aortic unfolding contributes to the thickness of the left paraspinal line; as the aorta moves posteriorly, it strips the pleura away from its otherwise close contact with the profiled portions of the spine.

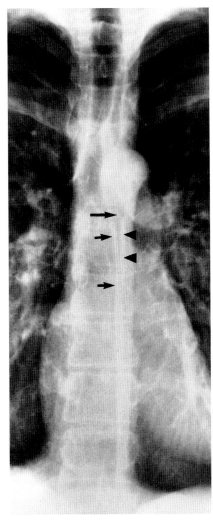

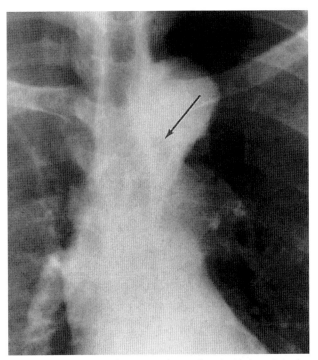

Fig. 2.54 Air in the esophagus may be confused with free air in the mediastinum. In elderly people, the esophagus follows the ectatic descending aorta and air is trapped in the knuckle of the esophagus below the arch (arrow). (Proto AV. Air in the esophagus: a frequent radiologic finding. AJR 1977;129:433).

Fig. 2.53 The right and left walls of the esophagus. The arrowheads point to the left wall. The arrows point to the right wall (azygoesophageal line). The uppermost arrow points to air in the lumen of the esophagus trapped beneath the aortic arch.

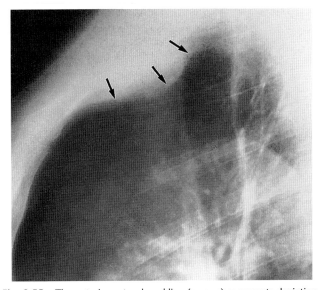

Fig. 2.55 The anterior extrapleural line (arrows) represents deviation of the pleura produced by the innominate artery and vein and the costal cartilage of the first ribs. It should not be mistaken for a lesion of the sternum or a mediastinal mass.

Lateral view

Mediastinum above the aortic arch

A variable portion of the aortic arch and head and neck vessels is visible in the lateral view, depending on the degree of aortic unfolding. The brachiocephalic artery is the only artery recognized with frequency. It arises anterior to the tracheal air column. Unless involved by atheromatous calcification, the origin is usually invisible, but after a variable distance its posterior wall can be seen as a gentle S-shaped interface crossing the tracheal air column. The left and right brachiocephalic veins are also visible in the lateral view. The left brachiocephalic vein often forms an extrapleural bulge behind the manubrium (Fig. 2.55).[182] The posterior border of the right brachiocephalic vein and SVC can occasionally be identified curving downward in much the same position and direction as the brachiocephalic artery, but they are sometimes traceable below the upper margin of the aortic arch.

Trachea and retrotracheal area[183]

The air column in the trachea can be seen throughout its length as it descends obliquely downward and posteriorly. The course of the trachea in the lateral view of adult subjects is straight, or bowed forward in patients with aortic unfolding, with no visible indentation by adjacent vessels. The carina is not visible

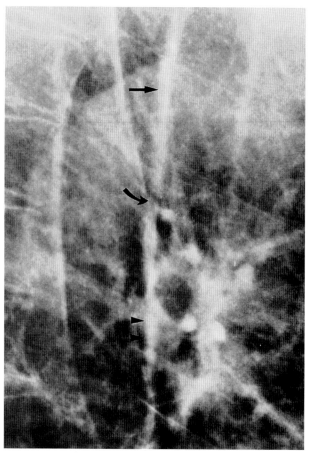

Fig. 2.56 The posterior tracheal band (straight arrow). Note that the posterior walls of the trachea, right main bronchus (curved arrow), and bronchus intermedius (arrowheads) are seen as a continuous thin band.

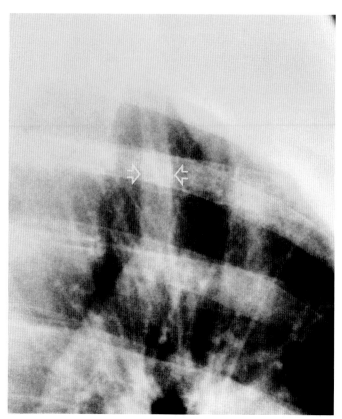

Fig. 2.57 A normal collapsed esophagus appearing as a band shadow (arrows) posterior to the trachea.

on the lateral view. The anterior wall of the trachea is visible in only a minority of patients, but its posterior wall is usually visible because lung often passes behind the trachea, allowing the radiologist to see the "posterior tracheal stripe or band" (Fig. 2.56).[4,172] This stripe is seen in 50–90% of healthy adults.[172,184] It is uniform in width and measures up to 3 mm (rarely, 4 mm). There is, however, a problem in applying this measurement. Because air is frequently present in the esophagus, the anterior wall of the esophagus may contribute to the thickness of the stripe in healthy subjects.[184] Alternatively, the lung may be separated from the trachea by the full width of a collapsed esophagus, leading to a band of density 1 cm or more in thickness (Fig. 2.57). Thus caution is needed in diagnosing abnormalities on the basis of an increase in thickness of the posterior tracheal stripe. A CT study has shown that the visibility of the posterior tracheal stripe is dependent on the degree to which the lung passes behind the trachea.[185] Sometimes the airway is close to the spine and what little space is present is occupied by the esophagus and connective tissue. Clearly the quantity of mediastinal fat is an important factor in determining how much lung invaginates behind the trachea.

Retrosternal line

A bandlike opacity simulating pleural or extrapleural disease is often seen in healthy individuals along the lower half or lowest

third of the anterior chest wall on the lateral view (Fig. 2.58).[186] This density is due to the differing anterior extent of the left and right lungs. The left lung does not contact the most anterior portion of the left thoracic cavity at these levels because the heart and its epicardial fat occupies the space.

Inferior vena cava

In most healthy subjects the posterior wall of the inferior vena cava is visible just before it enters the right atrium. Even patients with azygos continuation of the inferior vena cava may show a similar vessel formed by the continuation of the hepatic veins as they drain into the right atrium. In approximately 5% of healthy people the posterior wall of the inferior vena cava is not visible on the lateral chest radiograph.

DIAPHRAGM

The diaphragm consists of a large, dome-shaped central tendon with a sheet of striated muscle radiating from the central tendon to attach to ribs 7 through 12 and to the xiphisternum.[187–190] The two crura arise from the upper three lumbar vertebrae and arch upward and forward to form the margins of the aortic and esophageal hiatuses. The median arcuate ligament connecting the two crura forms the anterior margin of the aortic hiatus, and the crura themselves form the lateral boundary of the aortic hiatus. Accompanying the aorta through this opening are the azygos and hemiazygos veins and the thoracic duct. Anterior to the aortic hiatus lies the esophageal hiatus, through which run

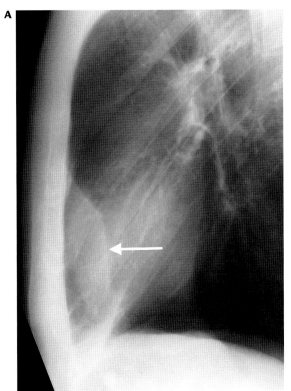

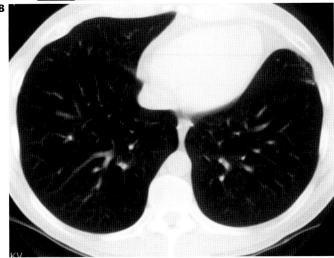

Fig. 2.58 **A**, The retrosternal line (arrows). **B**, CT in the same patient shows that the anterior margin of the left lung lies more posterior than the anterior margin of the right lung, in part because of the heart and in part because of epicardial fat.

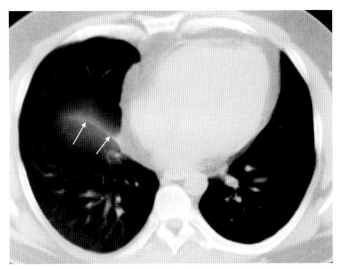

Fig. 2.59 The phrenic nerve (or according to some authors, the phrenic vessels) (arrows) coursing over the surface of the right hemidiaphragm. (See also Fig. 2.33, p. 47.)

the esophagus, the vagus nerve, and the esophageal arteries. The most anterior of the three diaphragmatic hiatuses is the hiatus for the IVC, which is situated within the central tendon immediately beneath the right atrium. The diaphragm has a smooth dome shape in most individuals, but a scalloped outline is also common.

The position of the diaphragm in healthy subjects on upright plain chest radiographs taken at full inspiration was investigated by Lennon and Simon.[191] They used the anterior ribs to describe the position of each hemidiaphragm because the dome's are closer to the anterior chest wall and both the domes and the anterior ribs are closer to the film in the PA projection. The normal right hemidiaphragm is found at about the level of the anterior sixth rib, being slightly higher in women and in individuals over 40 years of age. The range covers approximately one interspace above or below this level. In most people the right hemidiaphragm is 1.5–2.5 cm higher than the left, but the two hemidiaphragms are at the same level in approximately 9% of the population. In a few (3% in the series by Felson[89]) the left hemidiaphragm is higher than the right, but by less than 1 cm. The normal excursion of the domes of the diaphragm as measured by plain chest radiography is usually between 1.5 and 2.5 cm, although greater degrees of movement are sometimes seen. Transabdominal ultrasound, which allows more accurate real-time measurement of movement, shows that the normal range is considerable: between 2 and 8.6 cm, with the mean excursion of the right hemidiaphragm on deep inspiration 53 mm (SD 16.4) and that of the left side 46 mm (SD 12.4).[192]

Incomplete muscularization, known as eventration, is also common. An eventration is composed of a thin membranous sheet replacing what should be muscle. Usually it is partial, involving one-half to one-third of the hemidiaphragm, frequently the anteromedial portion of the right hemidiaphragm. The lack of muscle manifests itself radiographically as elevation of the affected portion of the diaphragm, and the usual pattern is a smooth hump on the contour of the diaphragm. Total eventration of a hemidiaphragm, which is much more common on the left than the right, results in elevation of the whole hemidiaphragm; on fluoroscopy, hemidiaphragm movement is poor, absent, or paradoxic. In severe cases, eventration cannot be distinguished from acquired paralysis of the phrenic nerve.

A linear density arising from the lateral wall of the IVC (Fig. 2.59) is often seen coursing over the superior surface of the right hemidiaphragm. This line represents an envelope of fat with investing pleura surrounding either the phrenic nerve, according to Berkmen and co-workers,[193] or the inferior phrenic artery and vein, according to Ujita and associates.[113]

REFERENCES

1. Holbert JM, Strollo DC. Imaging of the normal trachea. J Thorac Imaging 1995;10:171–179.
2. Dennie CJ, Coblentz CL. The trachea: normal anatomic features, imaging and causes of displacement. Can Assoc Radiol J 1993;44:81–89.
3. Bhalla M, Noble ER, Shepard JA, et al. Normal position of trachea and anterior junction line on CT. J Comput Assist Tomogr 1993;17:714–718.
4. Gamsu G, Webb WR. Computed tomography of the trachea: normal and abnormal. AJR Am J Roentgenol 1982; 139:321–326.
5. Lloyd DC, Taylor PM. Calcification of the intrathoracic trachea demonstrated by computed tomography. Br J Radiol 1990;63:31–32.
6. Bravo JM, Stark P, Jacobson F. Tracheobronchial cartilage calcifications in an inpatient population. J Thorac Imaging 1995;10:220–222.
7. Davis SD, Maldjian C, Perone RW, et al. CT of the airways. Clin Imaging 1990;14:280–300.
8. Gamsu G, Webb WR. Computed tomography of the trachea and mainstem bronchi. Semin Roentgenol 1983;18:51–60.
9. Breatnach E, Abbott GC, Fraser RG. Dimensions of the normal human trachea. AJR Am J Roentgenol 1984;142:903–906.
10. Vock P, Spiegel T, Fram EK, et al. CT assessment of the adult intrathoracic cross section of the trachea. J Comput Assist Tomogr 1984;8:1076–1082.
11. Griscom NT, Wohl ME. Dimensions of the growing trachea related to age and gender. AJR Am J Roentgenol 1986; 146:233–237.
12. Dimopoulos PA, Yarmenitis SD, Nikiforidis G, et al. Anatomical shape of the airways in two different European populations. A radio-anatomical study of the airways. Acta Radiol 1995;36: 448–452.
13. Stern EJ, Graham CM, Webb WR, et al. Normal trachea during forced expiration: dynamic CT measurements. Radiology 1993;187:27–31.
14. Murray JG, Brown AL, Anagnostou EA, et al. Widening of the tracheal bifurcation on chest radiographs: value as a sign of left atrial enlargement. AJR Am J Roentgenol 1995;164:1089–1092.
15. Haskin PH, Goodman LR. Normal tracheal bifurcation angle: a reassessment. AJR Am J Roentgenol 1982;139:879–882.
16. Remy-Jardin M, Remy J. Comparison of vertical and oblique CT in evaluation of bronchial tree. J Comput Assist Tomogr 1988;12:956–962.
17. Naidich DP, Terry PB, Stitik FP, et al. Computed tomography of the bronchi: 1. Normal anatomy. J Comput Assist Tomogr 1980;4:746–753.
18. Osborne D, Vock P, Godwin JD, et al. CT identification of bronchopulmonary segments: 50 normal subjects. AJR Am J Roentgenol 1984;142:47–52.
19. Webb WR, Glazer G, Gamsu G. Computed tomography of the normal pulmonary hilum. J Comput Assist Tomogr 1981;5:476–484.
20. Lee KS, Im JG, Bae WK, et al. CT anatomy of the lingular segmental bronchi. J Comput Assist Tomogr 1991;15:86–91.
21. Otsuji H, Uchida H, Maeda M, et al. Incomplete interlobar fissures: bronchovascular analysis with CT. Radiology 1993;187:541–546.
22. Lee KS, Bae WK, Lee BH, et al. Bronchovascular anatomy of the upper lobes: evaluation with thin-section CT. Radiology 1991;181:765–772.
23. Otsuji H, Hatakeyama M, Kitamura I, et al. Right upper lobe versus right middle lobe: differentiation with thin-section, high-resolution CT. Radiology 1989;172:653–656.
24. Jardin M, Remy J. Segmental bronchovascular anatomy of the lower lobes: CT analysis. AJR Am J Roentgenol 1986;147:457–468.
25. Naidich DP, Zinn WL, Ettenger NA, et al. Basilar segmental bronchi: thin-section CT evaluation. Radiology 1988;169:11–16.
26. Atwell SW. Major anomalies of the tracheobronchial tree: with a list of the minor anomalies. Dis Chest 1967;52: 611–615.
27. Boyden EA. Developmental anomalies of the lungs. Am J Surg 1955;89:79–89.
28. Beigelman C, Howarth NR, Chartrand-Lefebvre C, et al. Congenital anomalies of tracheobronchial branching patterns: spiral CT aspects in adults. Eur Radiol 1998;8:79–85.
29. Wu JW, White CS, Meyer CA, et al. Variant bronchial anatomy: CT appearance and classification. AJR Am J Roentgenol 1999;172:741–744.
30. Ghaye B, Szapiro D, Fanchamps JM, et al. Congenital bronchial abnormalities revisited. RadioGraphics 2001;21: 105–119.
31. Freeman SJ, Harvey JE, Goddard PR. Demonstration of supernumerary tracheal bronchus by computed tomographic scanning and magnetic resonance imaging. Thorax 1995;50:426–427.
32. Doolittle AM, Mair EA. Tracheal bronchus: classification, endoscopic analysis, and airway management. Otolaryngol Head Neck Surg 2002; 126:240–243.
33. Lee KH, Yoon CS, Choe KO, et al. Use of imaging for assessing anatomical relationships of tracheobronchial anomalies associated with left pulmonary artery sling. Pediatr Radiol 2001;31:269–278.
34. Carpenter LM, Merten DF. Radiographic manifestations of congenital anomalies affecting the airway. Radiol Clin North Am 1991;29:219–240.
35. Morrison SC. Demonstration of a tracheal bronchus by computed tomography. Clin Radiol 1988;39: 208–209.
36. McLaughlin FJ, Strieder DJ, Harris GB, et al. Tracheal bronchus: association with respiratory morbidity in childhood. J Pediatr 1985;106:751–755.
37. Hosker HS, Clague HW, Morritt GN. Ectopic right upper lobe bronchus as a cause of breathlessness. Thorax 1987; 42:473–474.
38. Ritsema GH. Ectopic right bronchus: indication for bronchography. AJR Am J Roentgenol 1983;140:671–674.
39. Setty SP, Michaels AJ. Tracheal bronchus: case presentation, literature review, and discussion. J Trauma 2000;49:943–945.
40. Siegel MJ, Shackelford GD, Francis RS, et al. Tracheal bronchus. Radiology 1979;130:353–355.
41. Mannes GP, van der Jagt EJ, Wouters B, et al. Dextrocardia? Chest 1989;96: 391–392.
42. Mangiulea VG, Stinghe RV. The accessory cardiac bronchus. Bronchologic aspect and review of the literature. Dis Chest 1968;54:433–436.
43. McGuinness G, Naidich DP, Garay SM, et al. Accessory cardiac bronchus: CT features and clinical significance. Radiology 1993;189:563–566.
44. Endo S, Saitoh N, Murayama F, et al. Symptomatic accessory cardiac bronchus. Ann Thorac Surg 2000; 69:262–264.
45. Jackson GD, Littleton JT. Simultaneous occurrence of anomalous cardiac and tracheal bronchi: a case study. J Thorac Imaging 1988;3:59–60.
46. Bentala M, Grijm K, van der Zee JH, et al. Cardiac bronchus: a rare cause of hemoptysis. Eur J Cardiothorac Surg 2002;22:643–645.
47. Landay MJ, Chaw C, Bordlee RP. Bilateral left lungs: unusual variation of hilar anatomy. AJR Am J Roentgenol 1982;138:1162–1164.
48. Landing BH, Lawrence TY, Payne VC Jr, et al. Bronchial anatomy in syndromes with abnormal visceral situs, abnormal spleen and congenital heart disease. Am J Cardiol 1971;28:456–462.
49. Starshak RJ, Sty JR, Woods G, et al. Bridging bronchus: a rare airway anomaly. Radiology 1981;140:95–96.

50. Genereux GP. Conventional tomographic hilar anatomy emphasizing the pulmonary veins. AJR Am J Roentgenol 1983;141:1241–1257.

51. Naidich DP, Khouri NF, Scott WW Jr, et al. Computed tomography of the pulmonary hila: 1. normal anatomy. J Comput Assist Tomogr 1981;5:459–467.

52. Vix VA, Klatte EC. The lateral chest radiograph in the diagnosis of hilar and mediastinal masses. Radiology 1970;96:307–316.

53. Remy-Jardin M, Duyck P, Remy J, et al. Hilar lymph nodes: identification with spiral CT and histologic correlation. Radiology 1995;196:387–394.

54. Shimoyama K, Murata K, Takahashi M, et al. Pulmonary hilar lymph node metastases from lung cancer: evaluation based on morphology at thin-section, incremental, dynamic CT. Radiology 1997;203:187–195.

55. Kim JS, Choi D, Lee KS. CT of the bronchus intermedius: frequency and cause of a nodule in the posterior wall on normal scans. AJR Am J Roentgenol 1995;165:1349–1352.

56. Webb WR, Gamsu G. Computed tomography of the left retrobronchial stripe. J Comput Assist Tomogr 1983;7:65–69.

57. Park CK, Webb WR, Klein JS. Inferior hilar window. Radiology 1991;178:163–168.

58. Ashida C, Zerhouni EA, Fishman EK. CT demonstration of prominent right hilar soft tissue collections. J Comput Assist Tomogr 1987;11:57–59.

59. Kim JS, Müller NL, Park CS, et al. Bronchoarterial ratio on thin section CT: comparison between high altitude and sea level. J Comput Assist Tomogr 1997;21:306–311.

60. Woodring JH. Pulmonary artery–bronchus ratios in patients with normal lungs, pulmonary vascular plethora, and congestive heart failure. Radiology 1991;179:115–122.

61. Jefferson K, Rees S. Clinical cardiac radiology. London: Butterworths, 1973.

62. Bankoff MS, McEniff NJ, Bhadelia RA, et al. Prevalence of pathologically proven intrapulmonary lymph nodes and their appearance on CT. AJR Am J Roentgenol 1996;167:629–630.

63. Perez N, Lhoste-Trouilloud A, Boyer L, et al. Computed tomographic appearance of three intrapulmonary lymph nodes. Eur J Radiol 1998;28:147–149.

64. Oshiro Y, Kusumoto M, Moriyama N, et al. Intrapulmonary lymph nodes: thin-section CT features of 19 nodules. J Comput Assist Tomogr 2002;26:553–557.

65. Fujimoto N, Segewa Y, Takigawa N, et al. Two cases of intrapulmonary lymph node presenting as a peripheral nodular shadow: diagnostic differentiation from lung cancer. Lung Cancer 1998;20:203–209.

66. Yokomise H, Mizuno H, Ike O, et al. Importance of intrapulmonary lymph nodes in the differential diagnosis of small pulmonary nodular shadows. Chest 1998;113:703–706.

67. Kradin RL, Mark EJ. Benign lymphoid disorders of the lung, with a theory regarding their development. Hum Pathol 1983;14:857–867.

68. Neff CC, Mueller PR, Ferrucci JT Jr, et al. Serious complications following transgression of the pleural space in drainage procedures. Radiology 1984;152:335–341.

69. Nichols DM, Cooperberg PL, Golding RH, et al. The safe intercostal approach? Pleural complications in abdominal interventional radiology. AJR Am J Roentgenol 1984;142:1013–1018.

70. Light RW. Pleural diseases. Philadelphia: Lippincott Williams and Wilkins, 1995.

71. Wang NS. Anatomy and physiology of the pleural space. Clin Chest Med 1985;6:3–16.

72. Im JG, Webb WR, Rosen A, et al. Costal pleura: appearances at high-resolution CT. Radiology 1989;171:125–131.

73. Hayashi K, Aziz A, Ashizawa K, et al. Radiographic and CT appearances of the major fissures. RadioGraphics 2001;21:861–874.

74. Berkmen YM, Auh YH, Davis SD, et al. Anatomy of the minor fissure: evaluation with thin-section CT. Radiology 1989;170:647–651.

75. Glazer HS, Anderson DJ, DiCroce JJ, et al. Anatomy of the major fissure: evaluation with standard and thin-section CT. Radiology 1991;180:839–844.

76. Raasch BN, Carsky EW, Lane EJ, et al. Radiographic anatomy of the interlobar fissures: a study of 100 specimens. AJR Am J Roentgenol 1982;138:1043–1049.

77. Heitzman ER. The mediastinum: radiologic correlations with anatomy and pathology. Berlin: Springer-Verlag, 1988.

78. Kent EM, Blades B. Surgical anatomy of pulmonary lobes. J Thorac Surg 1942;12:18–30.

79. Medlar EM. Variations in interlobar fissures. AJR Am J Roentgenol 1947;57:723–725.

80. Dandy WE Jr. Incomplete pulmonary interlobar fissure sign. Radiology 1978;128:21–25.

81. Hogg JC, Macklem PT, Thurlbeck WM. The resistance of collateral channels in excised human lungs. J Clin Invest 1969;48:421–431.

82. Scanlon TS, Benumof JL. Demonstration of interlobar collateral ventilation. J Appl Physiol 1979;46:658–661.

83. Proto AV, Speckman JM. The left lateral radiograph of the chest. Part 1. Med Radiogr Photogr 1979;55:29–74.

84. Proto AV, Ball JB Jr. The superolateral major fissures. AJR Am J Roentgenol 1983;140:431–437.

85. Fisher MS. Significance of a visible major fissure on the frontal chest radiograph. AJR Am J Roentgenol 1981;137:577–580.

86. Davis LA. The vertical fissure line. AJR Am J Roentgenol 1960;84:451–453.

87. Friedman E. Further observations on the vertical fissure line. Am J Roentgenol Radium Ther Nucl Med 1966;97:171–173.

88. Webber MM, O'Loughlin BJ. Variations of the pleural vertical fissure line. Radiology 1964;82:461–462.

89. Felson B. Chest roentgenology. Philadelphia: W B Saunders, 1973.

90. Marks BW, Kuhns LR. Identification of the pleural fissures with computed tomography. Radiology 1982;143:139–141.

91. Proto AV, Ball JB Jr. Computed tomography of the major and minor fissures. AJR Am J Roentgenol 1983;140:439–448.

92. Sakai O, Takahashi K, Nakashima N, et al. CT visualization of the major pulmonary fissures: value of 25 degrees cranially tilted axial scans. AJR Am J Roentgenol 1993;161:523–526.

93. Mayo JR, Müller NL, Henkelman RM. The double-fissure sign: a motion artifact on thin-section CT scans. Radiology 1987;165:580–581.

94. Goodman LR, Golkow RS, Steiner RM, et al. The right mid-lung window. Radiology 1982;143:135–138.

95. Frija J, Yana C, Laval-Jeantet M. Anatomy of the minor fissure: evaluation with thin-section CT. Radiology 1989;173:571–572.

96. Godwin JD, Tarver RD. Accessory fissures of the lung. AJR Am J Roentgenol 1985;144:39–47.

97. Ariyurek OM, Gulsun M, Demirkazik FB. Accessory fissures of the lung: evaluation by high-resolution computed tomography. Eur Radiol 2001;11:2449–2453.

98. Takasugi JE, Godwin JD. Left azygos lobe. Radiology 1989;171:133–134.

99. Speckman JM, Gamsu G, Webb WR. Alterations in CT mediastinal anatomy produced by an azygos lobe. AJR Am J Roentgenol 1981;137:47–50.

100. Boyden EA. The distribution of bronchi in gross anomalies of the right upper lobe, particularly lobes subdivided by the azygos vein and those containing pre-parietal bronchi. Radiology 1942;58:797–807.

101. Caceres J, Mata JM, Alegret X, et al. Increased density of the azygos lobe on frontal chest radiographs simulating disease: CT findings in seven patients. AJR Am J Roentgenol 1993;160:245–248.

102. Mata JM, Caceres J, Llauger J, et al. CT demonstration of intrapulmonary right brachiocephalic vein associated with an azygos lobe. J Comput Assist Tomogr 1990;14:305–306.

103. Rigler LG. The inferior accessory lobe of the lung. AJR Am J Roentgenol 1933;29:384–392.

104. Trapnell DH. The differential diagnosis of linear shadows in chest radiographs. Radiol Clin North Am 1973;11:77–92.

105. Davis SD, Yu LS, Hentel KD. Obliquely oriented superior accessory fissure of the lower lobe of the lung: CT evaluation of the normal appearance and effect on the distribution of parenchymal and pleural opacities. Radiology 2000;216:97–106.

106. Austin JH. The left minor fissure. Radiology 1986;161:433–436.

107. Rabinowitz JG, Cohen BA, Mendleson DS. Symposium on Nonpulmonary Aspects in Chest Radiology. The pulmonary ligament. Radiol Clin North Am 1984;22:659–672.

108. Godwin JD, Vock P, Osborne DR. CT of the pulmonary ligament. AJR Am J Roentgenol 1983;141:231–236.

109. Fraser RS, Müller NL, Colman N, et al. Diagnosis of diseases of the chest. Philadelphia: W B Saunders, 1999.

110. Cooper C, Moss AA, Buy JN, et al. CT appearance of the normal inferior pulmonary ligament. AJR Am J Roentgenol 1983;141:237–240.

111. Rost RC Jr, Proto AV. Inferior pulmonary ligament: computed tomographic appearance. Radiology 1983;148:479–483.

112. Berkmen YM, Drossman SR, Marboe CC. Intersegmental (intersublobar) septum of the lower lobe in relation to the pulmonary ligament: anatomic, histologic, and CT correlations. Radiology 1992;185:389–393.

113. Ujita M, Ojiri H, Ariizumi M, et al. Appearance of the inferior phrenic artery and vein on CT scans of the chest: a CT and cadaveric study. AJR Am J Roentgenol 1993;160:745–747.

114. Rabinowitz JG, Wolf BS. Roentgen significance of the pulmonary ligament. Radiology 1966;87:1013–1020.

115. Zylak CJ, Pallie W, Jackson R. Correlative anatomy and computed tomography: a module on the mediastinum. Radiographics 1982;2:255–292.

116. Felson B. The mediastinum. Semin Roentgenol 1969;4:41–58.

117. Guthaner DF, Wexler L, Harell G. CT demonstration of cardiac structures. AJR Am J Roentgenol 1979;133:75–81.

118. Gamsu G. Computed tomography of the mediastinum. Philadelphia: W B Saunders, 1983.

119. Godwin JD, Chen JT. Thoracic venous anatomy. AJR Am J Roentgenol 1986;147:674–684.

120. Buirski G, Jordan SC, Joffe HS, et al. Superior vena caval abnormalities: their occurrence rate, associated cardiac abnormalities and angiographic classification in a paediatric population with congenital heart disease. Clin Radiol 1986;37:131–138.

121. Cha EM, Khoury GH. Persistent left superior vena cava. Radiologic and clinical significance. Radiology 1972;103:375–381.

122. Fujimoto K, Abe T, Kumabe T, et al. Anomalous left brachiocephalic (innominate) vein: MR demonstration. AJR Am J Roentgenol 1992;159:479–480.

123. Takasugi JE, Godwin JD. CT appearance of the retroaortic anastomoses of the azygos system. AJR Am J Roentgenol 1990;154:41–44.

124. Ball JB Jr, Proto AV. The variable appearance of the left superior intercostal vein. Radiology 1982;144:445–452.

125. Friedman AC, Chambers E, Sprayregen S. The normal and abnormal left superior intercostal vein. AJR Am J Roentgenol 1978;131:599–602.

126. McDonald CJ, Castellino RA, Blank N. The aortic "nipple". The left superior intercostal vein. Radiology 1970;96:533–536.

127. Edwards PD, Bull RK, Coulden R. CT measurement of main pulmonary artery diameter. Br J Radiol 1998;71:1018–1020.

128. Moore AV, Korobkin M, Olanow W, et al. Age-related changes in the thymus gland: CT–pathologic correlation. AJR Am J Roentgenol 1983;141:241–246.

129. Heiberg E, Wolverson MK, Sundaram M, et al. Normal thymus: CT characteristics in subjects under age 20. AJR Am J Roentgenol 1982;138:491–494.

130. Siegel MJ, Glazer HS, Wiener JI, et al. Normal and abnormal thymus in childhood: MR imaging. Radiology 1989;172:367–371.

131. Cohen MD, Weber TR, Sequeira FW, et al. The diagnostic dilemma of the posterior mediastinal thymus: CT manifestations. Radiology 1983;146:691–692.

132. Francis IR, Glazer GM, Bookstein FL, et al. The thymus: reexamination of age-related changes in size and shape. AJR Am J Roentgenol 1985;145:249–254.

133. Bach AM, Hilfer CL, Holgersen LO. Left-sided posterior mediastinal thymus – MRI findings. Pediatr Radiol 1991;21:440–441.

134. Meaney JF, Roberts DE, Carty H. Case of the month: pseudo-tumour of the postero-superior mediastinum. Br J Radiol 1993;66:741–742.

135. Rollins NK, Currarino G. MR imaging of posterior mediastinal thymus. J Comput Assist Tomogr 1988;12:518–520.

136. Shackelford GD, McAlister WH. The aberrantly positioned thymus: a cause of mediastinal or neck masses in children. Am J Roentgenol Radium Ther Nucl Med 1974;120:291–296.

137. Rosai J, Levine GD. Normal thymus. Washington, DC: Armed Forces Institute of Pathology,1976.

138. de Geer G, Webb WR, Gamsu G. Normal thymus: assessment with MR and CT. Radiology 1986;158:313–317.

139. Sagel SS, Aronberg DJ. Thoracic anatomy and mediastinum. New York: Raven Press, 1982.

140. St Amour TE, Siegel MJ, Glazer HS, et al. CT appearances of the normal and abnormal thymus in childhood. J Comput Assist Tomogr 1987;11:645–650.

141. Baron RL, Lee JK, Sagel SS, et al. Computed tomography of the normal thymus. Radiology 1982;142:121–125.

142. Siegelman SS, Scott WW, Baker RR, et al. CT of the thymus. New York: Churchill Livingstone, 1984.

143. Dixon AK, Hilton CJ, Williams GT. Computed tomography and histological correlation of the thymic remnant. Clin Radiol 1981;32:255–257.

144. Boothroyd AE, Hall-Craggs MA, Dicks-Mireaux C, et al. The magnetic resonance appearances of the normal thymus in children. Clin Radiol 1992;45:378–381.

145. Molina PL, Siegel MJ, Glazer HS. Thymic masses on MR imaging. AJR Am J Roentgenol 1990;155:495–500.

146. Adam EJ, Ignotus PI. Sonography of the thymus in healthy children: frequency of visualization, size, and appearance. AJR Am J Roentgenol 1993;161:153–155.

147. Han BK, Babcock DS, Oestreich AE. Normal thymus in infancy: sonographic characteristics. Radiology 1989;170:471–474.

148. Hasselbalch H, Nielsen MB, Jeppesen D, et al. Sonographic measurement of the thymus in infants. Eur Radiol 1996;6:700–703.

149. Patel PM, Alibazoglu H, Ali A, et al. Normal thymic uptake of FDG on PET imaging. Clin Nucl Med 1996;21:772–775.

150. Veronikis IE, Simkin P, Braverman LE. Thymic uptake of iodine-131 in the anterior mediastinum. J Nucl Med 1996;37:991–992.

151. Weinblatt ME, Zanzi I, Belakhlef A, et al. False-positive FDG-PET imaging of the thymus of a child with Hodgkin's disease. J Nucl Med 1997;38:888–890.

152. Proto AV, Simmons JD, Zylak CJ. The anterior junction anatomy. Crit Rev Diagn Imaging 1983;19:111–173.

153. Proto AV, Simmons JD, Zylak CJ. The posterior junction anatomy. Crit Rev Diagn Imaging 1984;20:121–173.

154. Schnyder PA, Gamsu G. CT of the pretracheal retrocaval space. AJR Am J Roentgenol 1981;136:303–308.

155. Aronberg DJ, Peterson RR, Glazer HS, et al. The superior sinus of the

pericardium: CT appearance. Radiology 1984;153:489–492.

156. Black CM, Hedges LK, Javitt MC. The superior pericardial sinus: normal appearance on gradient-echo MR images. AJR Am J Roentgenol 1993; 160:749–751.

157. McComb BL. Reflecting upon the left superior mediastinum. J Thorac Imaging 2001;16:56–64.

158. Wimpfheimer O, Haramati LB, Haramati N. Calcification of the ligamentum arteriosum in adults: CT features. J Comput Assist Tomogr 1996;20:34–37.

159. Bisceglia M, Donaldson JS. Calcification of the ligamentum arteriosum in children: a normal finding on CT. AJR Am J Roentgenol 1991;156:351–352.

160. Protopapas Z, Westcott JL. Left pulmonic recess of the pericardium: findings at CT and MR imaging. Radiology 1995;196: 85–88.

161. Callen PW, Korobkin M, Isherwood I. Computed tomographic evaluation of the retrocrural prevertebral space. AJR Am J Roentgenol 1977;129:907–910.

162. Mountain CF, Dresler CM. Regional lymph node classification for lung cancer staging. Chest 1997;111: 1718–1723.

163. Cymbalista M, Waysberg A, Zacharias C, et al. CT demonstration of the 1996 AJCC–UICC regional lymph node classification for lung cancer staging. Radiographics 1999;19:899–900.

164. Mountain CF. Revisions in the International System for Staging Lung Cancer. Chest 1997;111:1710–1717.

165. Glazer GM, Gross BH, Quint LE, et al. Normal mediastinal lymph nodes: number and size according to American Thoracic Society mapping. AJR Am J Roentgenol 1985;144:261–265.

166. Genereux GP, Howie JL. Normal mediastinal lymph node size and number: CT and anatomic study. AJR Am J Roentgenol 1984;142:1095–1100.

167. Ingram CE, Belli AM, Lewars MD, et al. Normal lymph node size in the mediastinum: a retrospective study in two patient groups. Clin Radiol 1989;40:35–39.

168. Murray JG, O'Driscoll M, Curtin JJ. Mediastinal lymph node size in an Asian population. Br J Radiol 1995;68:348–350.

169. Sussman SK, Halvorsen RA Jr, Silverman PM, et al. Paracardiac adenopathy: CT evaluation. AJR Am J Roentgenol 1987; 149:29–34.

170. Proto AV, Speckman JM. The left lateral radiograph of the chest. Med Radiogr Photogr 1980;56:38–64.

171. Proto AV, Corcoran HL, Ball JB Jr. The left paratracheal reflection. Radiology 1989;171:625–628.

172. Bachman AL, Teixidor HS. The posterior tracheal band: a reflector of local superior mediastinal abnormality. Br J Radiol 1975;48:352–359.

173. Keats TE. The aortic-pulmonary mediastinal stripe. Am J Roentgenol Radium Ther Nucl Med 1972;116: 107–109.

174. Lane EJ, Heitzman ER, Dinn WM. The radiology of the superior intercostal veins. Radiology 1976;120:263–267.

175. Takahashi K, Shinozaki T, Hyodo H, et al. Focal obliteration of the descending aortic interface on normal frontal chest radiographs: correlation with CT findings. Radiology 1994; 191:685–690.

176. Takahashi K, Sugimoto H, Ohsawa T. Obliteration of the descending aortic interface in pectus excavatum: correlation with clockwise rotation of the heart. Radiology 1992;182:825–828.

177. Savoca CJ, Austin JH, Goldberg HI. The right paratracheal stripe. Radiology 1977;122:295–301.

178. Cimmino CV. The esophageal-pleural stripe: an update. Radiology 1981;140: 609–613.

179. Fitzgerald SW, Donaldson JS. Azygoesophageal recess: normal CT appearance in children. AJR Am J Roentgenol 1992;158:1101–1104.

180. Miller FH, Fitzgerald SW, Donaldson JS. CT of the azygoesophageal recess in infants and children. RadioGraphics 1993;13:623–634.

181. Proto AV, Lane EJ. Air in the esophagus: a frequent radiographic finding. AJR Am J Roentgenol 1977;129:433–440.

182. Whalen JP, Oliphant M, Evans JA. Anterior extrapleural line: superior extension. Radiology 1975;115:525–531.

183. Raider L, Landry BA, Brogdon BG. The retrotracheal triangle. RadioGraphics 1990;10:1055–1079.

184. Palayew MJ. The tracheo-esophageal stripe and the posterior tracheal band. Radiology 1979;132:11–13.

185. Kormano M, Yrjana J. The posterior tracheal band: correlation between computed tomography and chest radiography. Radiology 1980;136: 689–694.

186. Whalen JP, Meyers MA, Oliphant M, et al. The retrosternal line. A new sign of an anterior mediastinal mass. Am J Roentgenol Radium Ther Nucl Med 1973;117:861–872.

187. Gale ME. Anterior diaphragm: variations in the CT appearance. Radiology 1986;161:635–639.

188. Heitzman ER. Kerley Pergamon lecture: The diaphragm. Radiologic correlations with anatomy and pathology. Clin Radiol 1990;42:15–19.

189. Kleinman PK, Raptopoulos V. The anterior diaphragmatic attachments: an anatomic and radiologic study with clinical correlates. Radiology 1985;155:289–293.

190. Panicek DM, Benson CB, Gottlieb RH, et al. The diaphragm: anatomic, pathologic, and radiologic considerations. Radiographics 1988;8:385–425.

191. Lennon EA, Simon G. The height of the diaphragm in the chest radiograph of normal adults. Br J Radiol 1965;38: 937–943.

192. Houston JG, Morris AD, Howie CA, et al. Technical report: quantitative assessment of diaphragmatic movement – a reproducible method using ultrasound. Clin Radiol 1992;46:405–407.

193. Berkmen YM, Davis SD, Kazam E, et al. Right phrenic nerve: anatomy, CT appearance, and differentiation from the pulmonary ligament. Radiology 1989;173:43–46.

Basic patterns in lung disease

One of the most crucial decisions when viewing chest radiographs is determining the location of any lesion, in particular whether the process is primarily in the lung, the hilum, the mediastinum, the pleura, the chest wall, or the diaphragm. Indeed the distinction is so important that most textbooks, including this one, are organized according to anatomic divisions. In this chapter, and the following one on high-resolution computed tomography (HRCT), the discussion centers on the signs of pulmonary disease on chest radiographs and CT.

Two interrelated plain film signs – the silhouette sign and the air bronchogram – are considered first because they have widespread applicability in the diagnosis of many chest disorders.

SILHOUETTE SIGN

Felson and Felson[1] popularized the term "silhouette sign". They wrote, "An intrathoracic lesion touching a border of the heart, aorta, or diaphragm will obliterate that border on the roentgenogram. An intrathoracic lesion not anatomically contiguous with a border of one of the structures will not obliterate that border". The lesion responsible for obliterating a silhouette (Figs 3.1 and 3.2) does not have to be large, nor does the opacity have to originate within the lung; pleural fluid, extrapleural fat, chest wall deformity, and mediastinal masses may all cause a loss of silhouette.

Felson and Felson[1] believed the sign depended solely on direct contact. It may, however, be due to absorption of x-rays by whatever lies in the path of the beam; the reason the border is lost only in cases of direct contact is that precise anatomic conformity of shape occurs only when intimate contact is present.

The silhouette sign can be used in two ways:

1. To localize a radiographic density (Figs 3.3 and 3.4) because, in practice, the lesion lies immediately adjacent to the structure in question. Thus opacities in the right middle lobe or lingula may obliterate the right and left borders of the heart, respectively (Figs 3.1 and 3.5), whereas opacities in

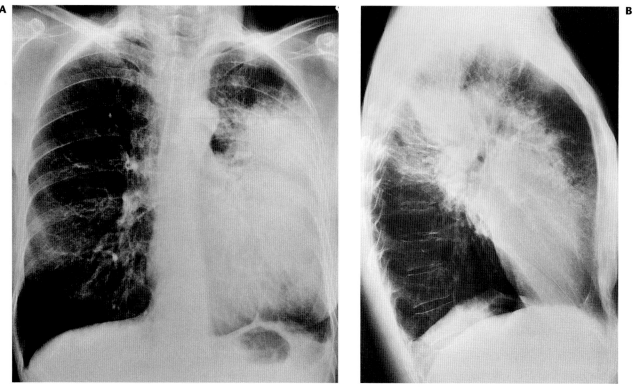

Fig. 3.1 The silhouette sign. The left heart border is invisible because of consolidation in the adjacent left upper lobe. **A**, Posteroanterior view. **B**, Lateral view.

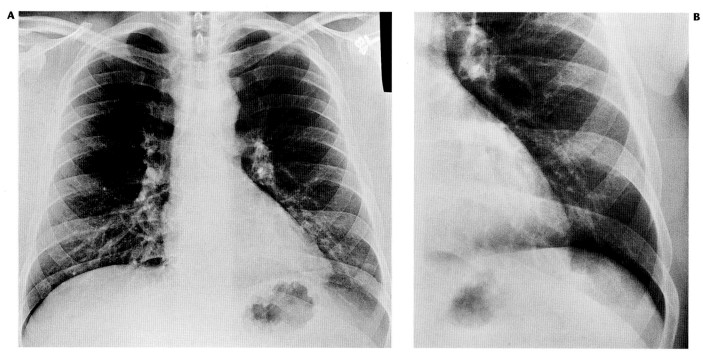

Fig. 3.2 The silhouette sign. **A**, A small patch of pneumonia in the anterior segment of the left lower lobe has resulted in lack of visibility of the outer half of the left hemidiaphragm. (The lateral view in this patient is shown in Fig. 3.14.) **B**, Normal diaphragm outline after the pneumonia has resolved.

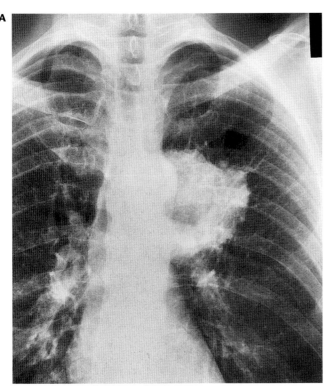
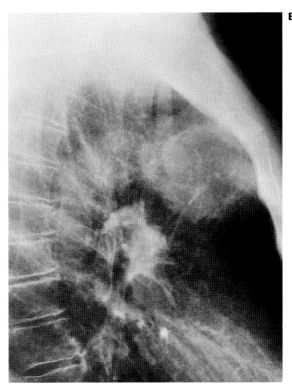

Fig. 3.3 **A**, Preservation of the silhouette of the aortic knob and descending aorta in the posteroanterior view is good evidence that the pulmonary mass does not lie in the superior segment of the lower lobe. **B**, The lateral view shows that the mass, in fact, lies well anteriorly. (It proved to be a squamous cell carcinoma.)

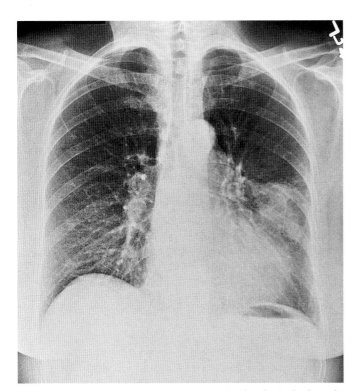

Fig. 3.4 The loss of silhouette of the left cardiac border in the frontal view localizes the pulmonary consolidation to the lingula. It proved to be postobstructive pneumonia beyond a carcinoma in the lingular bronchus.

the lower lobes may partially obliterate the outline of the descending aorta and diaphragm but leave the cardiac outline clearly visible (Fig. 3.6). Similarly, the aortic knob will be rendered invisible if there is no air in the adjacent left upper lobe. A good example of detecting lesions of low radiopacity is collapse of the right middle lobe (Fig. 3.5).

2. To detect lesions of low radiopacity when the loss of silhouette is more obvious than the shadow itself (Fig. 3.2).

Felson and Felson[1] warned that mistakes will be made unless the following points are borne in mind:

- The technical quality of the radiograph must be such that the diseased area is adequately penetrated. Underpenetration may result in loss of visibility of a normal border.
- The outline of a portion of the cardiovascular structure in question must be clearly visible beyond the shadow of the spine. In many healthy individuals the right border of the heart and ascending aorta do not project into the right side of the thorax. In these patients the silhouette sign cannot be applied on the right side.
- In patients with pectus excavatum the right border of the heart is frequently obliterated because the depressed thoracic wall replaces aerated lung alongside the cardiac silhouette (Fig. 3.7).

Felson and Felson also pointed out that there are patients in whom no disease and no satisfactory explanation for the loss of the right heart border is found.[1] These cases are, however, few and far between and do little to reduce the value of the sign.

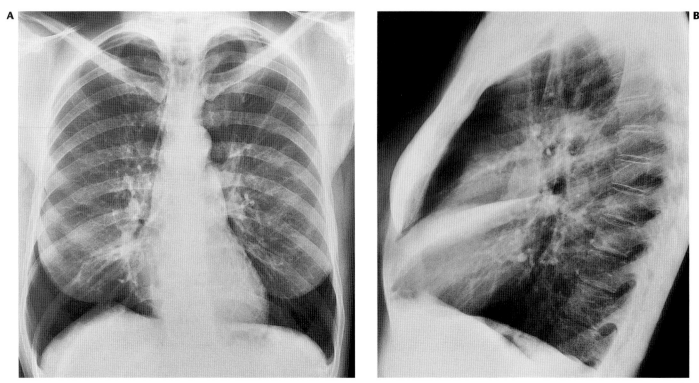

Fig. 3.5 Right middle lobe atelectasis and consolidation obliterating the right heart border. **A**, Posteroanterior view. **B**, Lateral view.

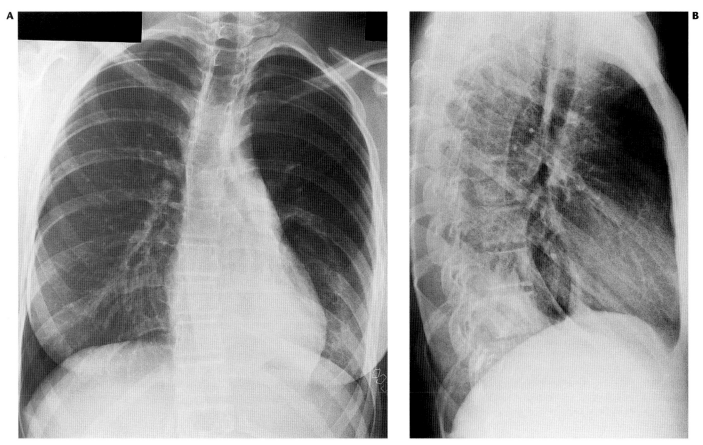

Fig. 3.6 Left lower lobe atelectasis and consolidation obliterating the outline of the adjacent descending aorta and medial left hemidiaphragm. **A**, Posteroanterior view. **B**, Lateral view.

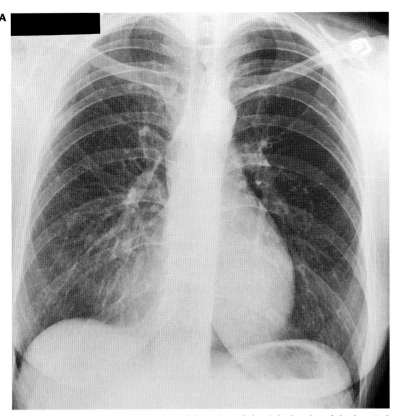

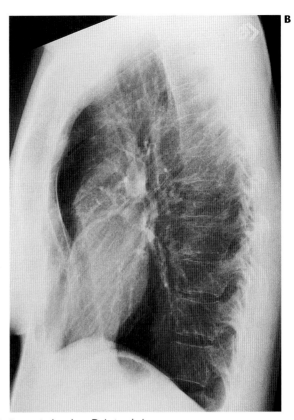

Fig. 3.7   Pectus excavatum causing obliteration of the right border of the heart. **A**, Posteroanterior view. **B**, Lateral view.

AIR BRONCHOGRAM

Normal intrapulmonary airways are invisible on a chest radiograph unless end-on to the x-ray beam, but air within bronchi, or bronchioles, passing through airless parenchyma may be visible as branching linear lucencies: a so-called "air bronchogram" (Fig. 3.8). An air bronchogram within an opacity reliably indicates that the opacity is intrapulmonary, not pleural or mediastinal, in location. The sign is particularly well demonstrated with CT (Fig. 3.9).

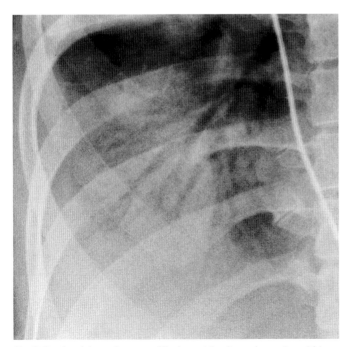

Fig. 3.8   An air bronchogram. The branching linear lucencies within the consolidation in the right lower lobe are particularly well demonstrated in this example of staphylococcal pneumonia.

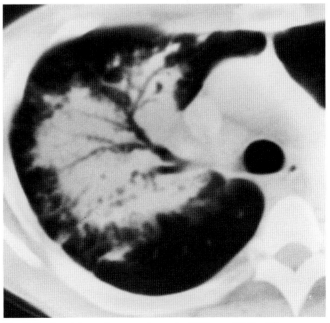

Fig. 3.9   An air bronchogram shown by CT in a patient with pneumonia.

Normal expiratory radiograph
Consolidation
Pulmonary edema
Acute respiratory distress syndrome (in adults) or hyaline membrane disease (in neonates)
Compression atelectasis (e.g. pleural effusion)
Scarring, e.g. radiation fibrosis, bronchiectatic lobe
Severe interstitial disease (e.g. sarcoidosis)
Certain neoplasms (notably bronchioloalveolar carcinoma, lymphoma)

The most common causes of an air bronchogram (Box 3.1) are pneumonia and the various forms of pulmonary edema. Similarly, widespread air bronchograms are seen in hyaline membrane disease. Air bronchograms are also seen in atelectatic lobes on chest radiographs when the airway is patent, notably when atelectasis is caused by pleural effusion, pneumothorax, or bronchiectasis.

There are four less predictable situations in which air bronchograms are seen:

1. Bronchioloalveolar carcinoma (Fig. 3.10) and lymphoma grow around airways without compressing them and, therefore, air bronchograms may be visible even on plain chest radiographs. Air bronchograms in other lung cancers are commonly present but are seen only on CT.[2]
2. Interstitial fibrosis, notably advanced usual interstitial pneumonia and radiation fibrosis, may be so intense that in addition to causing dilatation of the bronchi, which remain patent, it renders the lung parenchyma almost airless, producing an air bronchogram (Fig. 3.11).[3] Air bronchograms may also be seen in areas of dense involvement of the lung by sarcoidosis (Fig. 3.12).
3. Air bronchograms can sometimes be seen in postobstructive pneumonia, particularly on CT (see Fig. 13.13, p. 794), even though replacement of air by secretions beyond the obstruction might have been expected.
4. Air bronchograms can be normal on plain chest radiographs at low lung volumes and in segmental bronchi behind the heart in children.

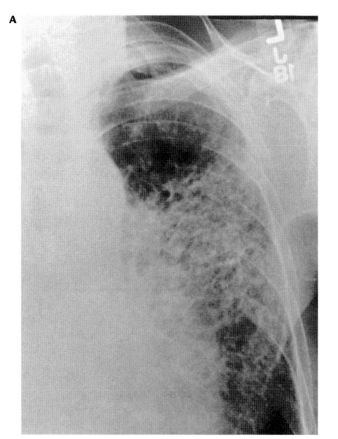

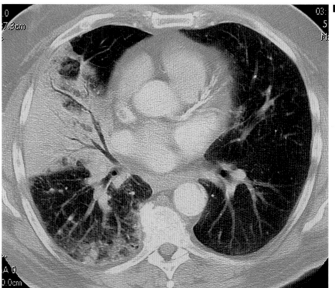

Fig. 3.10 An air bronchogram in bronchioloalveolar cell carcinoma. **A**, Chest radiograph. **B**, CT of a different patient. (See Fig. 3.89 for another example.)

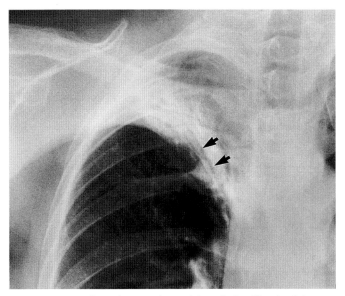

Fig. 3.11   An air bronchogram (arrows) in radiation fibrosis of the right upper lobe following treatment of carcinoma of the breast.

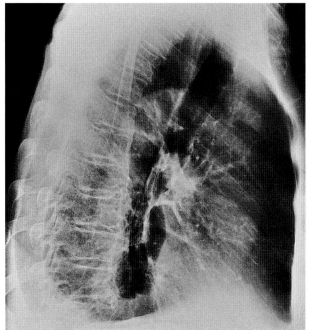

Fig. 3.12   An air bronchogram in severe sarcoidosis of the lung shown by CT.

PULMONARY OPACITY

A focal pulmonary opacity is usually readily detected in the frontal view by comparing one lung with the other. In the lateral view such right/left comparisons are not possible and therefore alternative signs are needed. In the normal lateral view, each thoracic vertebral body appears blacker than the one above it, as the eye travels down the spine, until the diaphragm is reached. Pulmonary opacity projected over the spine alters this con-

tinuum (Fig. 3.13). Another helpful point is that in a healthy subject there is no abrupt change in density across the heart shadow in the lateral projection (Fig. 3.14). The rib shadows are of course an exception, but the observer should mentally subtract the ribs from the image. Also, but less reliably, the high retrosternal area is usually more transradiant than all other areas on the lateral chest radiograph except the region immediately behind the heart.

Although search patterns among experienced viewers are far from orderly it seems wise, particularly for the inexperienced, to adopt a systematic approach. The apices, the hila, the retrocardiac regions, the lung below the domes of the diaphragm and the strip just inside the chest wall should be specifically

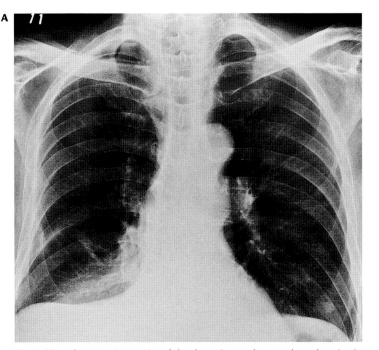

Fig. 3.13   Alteration in opacity of the thoracic vertebrae on lateral projection as a sign of lower lobe density. In this case, increasing opacity of the vertebral bodies as the eye travels down the spine is one of the most obvious signs indicating the presence of right lower lobe atelectasis. **A**, Posteroanterior view. **B**, Lateral view.

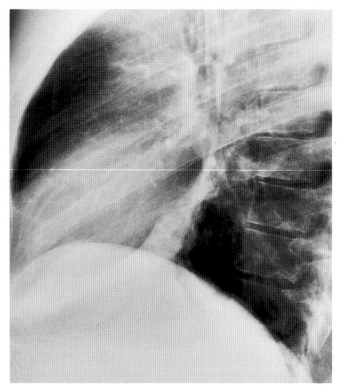

Fig. 3.14 Abrupt change in density overlying the cardiac shadow. A lateral view in a patient with pneumonia in the anterior segment of the left lower lobe. (The posteroanterior view of this patient is shown in Fig. 3.2.)

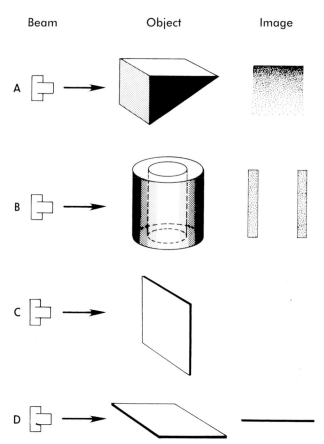

Fig. 3.15 The density characteristics of pulmonary shadows. See text for explanation. (From Wilson AG. The interpretation of shadows on the adult chest radiograph. Br J Hosp Med 1987;37:526–534.)

examined, because experience has shown that opacities in these areas are easily overlooked.

The characteristics of a radiographic shadow depend on the absorptive capacity and geometry of the object. In order of increasing absorptive capacity, the major components of the chest are air, fat, fluid and soft tissues, and bone. For practical purposes, fluid and soft tissues, apart from fat, are isodense on plain film radiography. The following geometric features are worth noting (Fig. 3.15)[4]:

- Interfaces tangential to the x-ray beam are sharp and distinct, whereas oblique interfaces are not seen because they fade off and cannot be identified (Fig. 3.15A).
- Hollow cylinders and hollow spheres are most absorptive at their edges because at the edge the beam has a longer path within the object and is therefore more attenuated. Also, the outside and inside marginal interfaces are sharp and distinct (Fig. 3.15B).
- A thin sheet perpendicular to an x-ray beam usually causes no detectable opacity (Fig. 3.15C), whereas a thin sheet oriented in the direction of the beam casts a definite shadow (Fig. 3.15D).

There are innumerable patterns of pulmonary opacity, with no clear-cut divisions between them. Nevertheless, categorizing patterns is worthwhile; the more certain the observer is of the description of an individual opacity, the shorter the differential diagnostic list will be. The diagnostic considerations for a particular pattern may be further reduced by reviewing serial images and by correlating the radiographic pattern with the clinical findings and laboratory data. The following classification of pulmonary shadows is used in this chapter (pleural shadows are considered separately in Ch. 15):

1. Airspace filling
2. Atelectasis (collapse)
3. Pulmonary mass (nodule)
4. Line shadows and band shadows
5. Ring shadows, cysts, and bullae
6. Widespread nodular, reticulonodular, and honeycomb shadowing.

More than one pattern may be present. Calcification and cavitation should be looked for; their presence will limit the number of diagnostic possibilities.

AIRSPACE FILLING

There is considerable variation in the terms used for describing one or more discrete, ill-defined pulmonary densities.

The expressions "airspace filling" and "airspace shadows" are the best because they imply a radiographic appearance.[5] The term "consolidation" can be confusing because pathologists use it synonymously with exudate, whereas its use by radiologists is less specific. The word "infiltrate" is also used differently by radiologists and pathologists. Some radiologists use the term to describe almost any pulmonary shadow, whereas pathologists restrict its use to processes showing the specific histologic features of infiltration. In this chapter, in accordance with terminology recommended by the Fleishner Society,[5] the phrase "air-space filling/shadowing" is used for a radiographic appearance that implies replacement of air in the distal airways and alveoli by fluid or other material, such as neoplasm or alveolar proteinosis, and no destruction or displacement of the gross morphology of the lung. The fluid can be a transudate, an exudate, pus, or blood. Where it is possible to be certain that the shadow is caused by edema, the expression "pulmonary edema" is used instead. The term "consolidation" is restricted to shadows thought to be due to exudate, pus, blood, or tumor. Thus edema and consolidation are subdivisions of airspace filling.

The features of airspace filling on plain chest radiography are one or more shadows with ill-defined margins, except where the shadow abuts pleura. When multiple, the shadows may coalesce. An air bronchogram may be visible, often as scattered branches or small twigs. On plain chest radiography the normal vascular markings within the shadow are invisible because of the silhouette sign. The lack of clarity of the edge of the shadows results, in part, from the piecemeal spread of the process through the alveoli, the poorly defined margin being analogous to the edge of a three-dimensional jigsaw puzzle. Once the process abuts a fissure, the edge appears sharp. The ease with which it is possible to appreciate this edge on plain chest radiographs depends on how much of the fissure is tangential to the x-ray beam.

Many sublobar processes are vaguely conical, sometimes resembling the shape of a segment. Precise conformity to a segment almost never occurs because, with the rare exception of accessory fissures, there are no anatomic barriers to prevent the spread of fluid or other processes across segmental boundaries. Airspace filling is often peripheral in location, crossing segmental boundaries with impunity. Spherical consolidations are also seen but are unusual.

Ill-defined nodular shadows between 0.5 and 1 cm are sometimes seen within or adjacent to the larger opacities of airspace filling, particularly with pulmonary edema and lung infections, notably varicella or tuberculosis (Fig. 3.16; see also Fig. 3.19). These shadows have been called "acinar shadows", since they are believed to be opaque acini contrasted against aerated lung.[6] They may coalesce as the disease progresses. The converse of the acinar shadow is the air alveologram (Fig. 3.17), a pattern of small rounded lucencies seen when aerated acini are surrounded by opaque lung.

Cavitation may occur within areas of airspace filling. The term "cavitation" implies necrosis and liquefaction of lung tissue. If the necrotic center communicates with the bronchial tree, air enters the cavity (Fig. 3.18) and is seen as a translucency within the shadow, often accompanied by an air–fluid level (Fig. 3.18).

The term "ground glass" has a slightly different meaning depending on whether it is being applied to chest radiographs or to CT images, notably HRCT. When applied to chest radiographs it refers to a homogeneous veiling opacity which often makes the pulmonary vessels indistinct or invisible. Such opacity is seen in a large number of conditions, including airspace filling disorders and interstitial pulmonary diseases. Ground-glass opacity on HRCT (see Ch. 4) refers to an increase in attenuation of the lung parenchyma ("gray lung") without obscuration of the underlying bronchovascular structures.

Computed tomography (the topic of high-resolution CT is discussed in Ch. 4) may on occasion provide additional information about airspace filling. It shows acinar shadows to advantage (Fig. 3.19). The excellent contrast discrimination of CT allows pneumonia in the immunocompromised host, for example, to be diagnosed when plain chest radiographs still have a normal appearance.[7] It can also demonstrate the size,

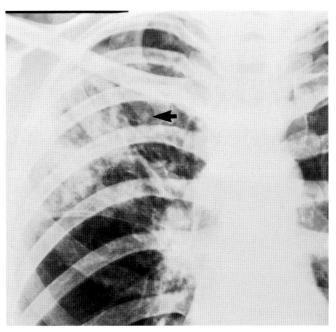

Fig. 3.16 Acinar shadows in pulmonary tuberculosis (arrow). The acinar shadows have become confluent in the lateral portion of the right upper lobe. (The appearance of acinar shadows on CT is shown in Fig. 3.19.)

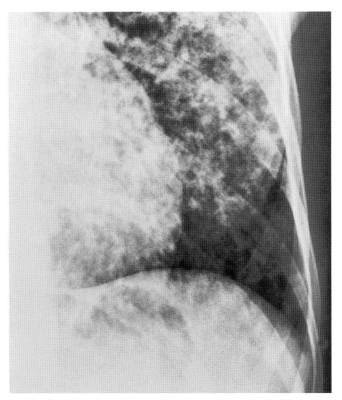

Fig. 3.17 An air alveologram in bronchogenic spread of tuberculosis.

shape, and precise position of any cavities (Fig. 3.20).[8] Better definition of a cavity or the demonstration of more cavities may improve diagnostic accuracy, but if a cavity is clearly demonstrated on plain films, CT usually has little additional information to offer. Other morphologic features of airspace filling that are particularly well demonstrated by CT are air bronchograms

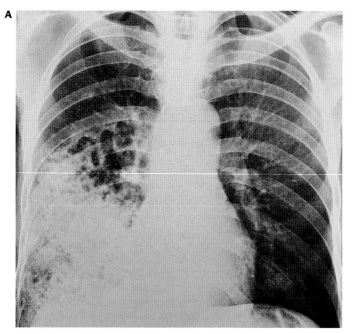
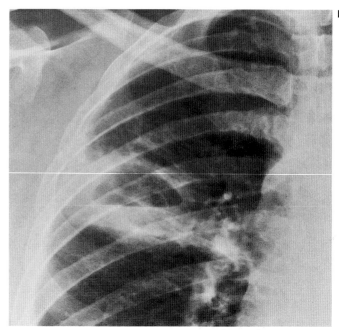

Fig. 3.18 Cavitation. **A,** In this example of staphylococcal pneumonia there are multiple transradiant areas within consolidation but no air–fluid levels. **B,** Another patient, illustrating an air–fluid level in a cavity within an area of pneumonia.

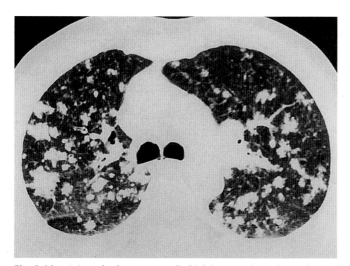

Fig. 3.19 Acinar shadows, some of which have coalesced. CT of bronchogenic spread of tuberculous pneumonia.

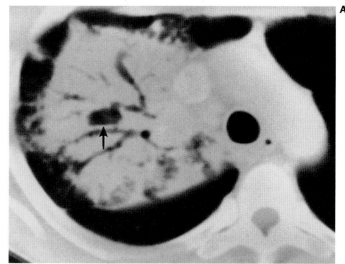
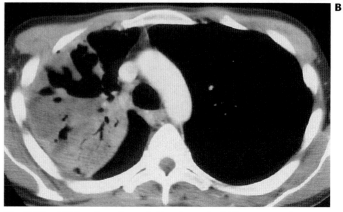

Fig. 3.20 CT showing: **A,** cavitation (arrow) within pneumonia; **B,** complex cavitation with lower density fluid in the dependent portion of a cavity.

(Fig. 3.9), the satellite lesions of infectious inflammation, including a tree-in-bud pattern, and the conformity of radiation fibrosis to the radiation port (Fig. 3.21).

It has been suggested that measuring CT numbers is sometimes helpful in diagnosing the nature of airspace shadowing. The CT density may be high in pulmonary hemorrhage, progressive massive fibrosis, and pulmonary calcinosis, and low in lipoid pneumonia.[9,10] Great care must be taken in accepting a low CT number, however, because part of the volume being measured could be air in aerated alveoli or bronchi.

A CT angiogram sign may be present. The term[11] refers to the presence of visible contrast-enhanced blood vessels coursing through areas of consolidation (Fig. 3.22).[12] The sign was originally described as reasonably specific for bronchiolo-alveolar carcinoma,[12] but with the more rapid rate of contrast medium injection that has become common in the last decade it

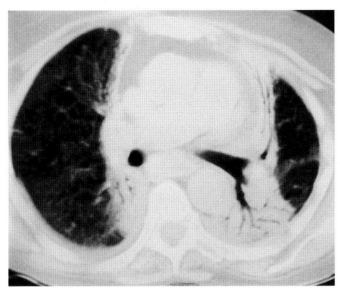

Fig. 3.21 Radiation fibrosis. CT showing conformity of the radiation fibrosis to the radiation portal. Note the obvious air bronchograms in the fibrotic lung.

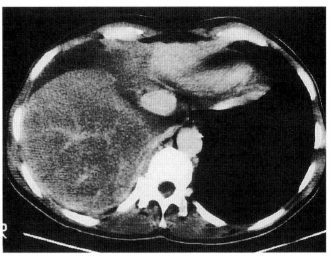

Fig. 3.22 CT angiogram sign. Branching contrast-enhanced pulmonary vessels are seen coursing through low-density pulmonary consolidation. In this instance, the diagnosis was lymphoma. (From Vincent JM, Ng YY, Norton AJ, et al. CT "angiogram sign" in primary pulmonary lymphoma. J Comput Assist Tomogr 1992;16:829–831.)

is apparent that the CT angiogram sign is seen in a variety of causes of consolidation, notably pneumonia, obstructive pneumonitis, pulmonary edema, bronchioloalveolar carcinoma, and lymphoma.[12–16] The CT angiogram sign, however, is useful in the differential diagnosis of atelectatic lung resembling pleural effusion: its presence definitively indicates pulmonary pathology, since the sign cannot occur within pleural pathology.[17]

Differential diagnosis of airspace filling

The differential diagnosis of airspace shadows is long and covers diseases that require quite different forms of management.

Solitary airspace shadowing (Fig. 3.23) is usually the result of pneumonia, atelectasis, infarction (Fig. 3.24), or hemorrhage

A

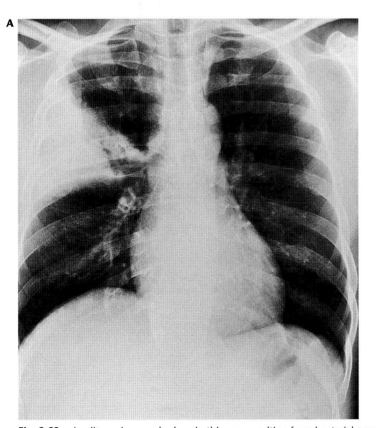

B

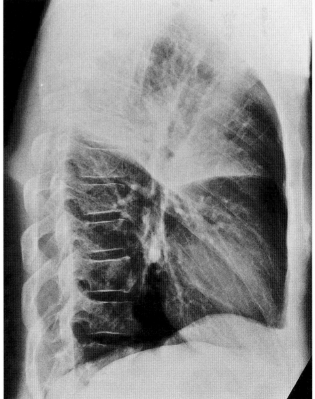

Fig. 3.23 A solitary airspace shadow, in this case resulting from bacterial pneumonia. Note that the pneumonia occupies the gravitationally dependent portions of lobes, rather than being distributed according to segmental anatomy. **A**, Posteroanterior view. **B**, Lateral view.

A

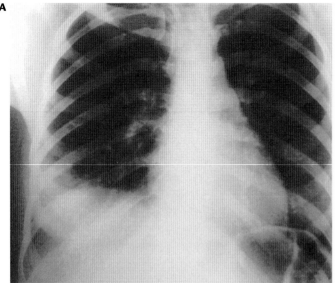

B

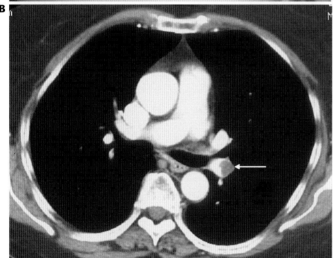

C

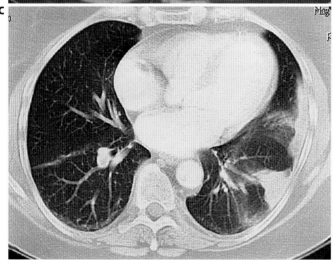

Fig. 3.24   Pulmonary consolidation caused by pulmonary infarction. **A**, A chest radiograph showing an infarct peripherally in the right lower lobe. **B** and **C**, CT showing infarct peripherally in the left lower lobe and the responsible emboli (arrow) on the CT pulmonary angiogram.

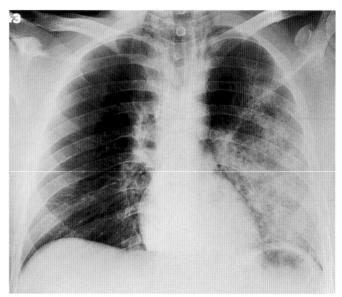

Fig. 3.25   A solitary airspace shadow caused by pulmonary hemorrhage (contusion) following a motor vehicle accident. (A pneumomediastinum is also present.)

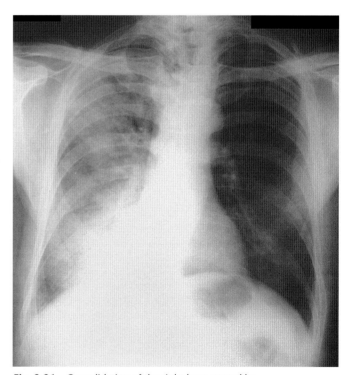

Fig. 3.26   Consolidation of the right lung caused by bronchioloalveolar cell carcinoma.

(Fig. 3.25). Neoplasms, particularly bronchioloalveolar carcinoma (see Figs 3.10, 3.26, and 3.89) and lymphoma (Fig. 3.27), may appear sufficiently ill-defined to be called consolidation. The full list of causes of solitary airspace shadows is given in Table 3.1.

Airspace filling is often multifocal and tends to coalesce as it progresses (Fig. 3.28). The list of causes is given in Boxes 3.2 and 3.3.

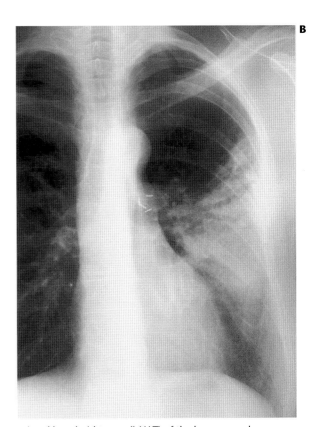

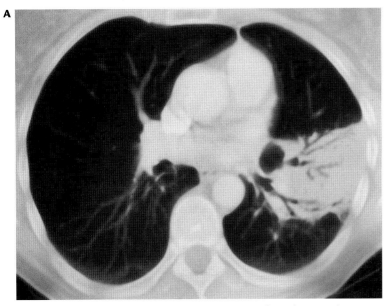

Fig. 3.27 A solitary airspace shadow with obvious air bronchograms in a mucosa-associated lymphoid tumor (MALT) of the lung parenchyma. **A**, Chest radiograph. **B**, CT of the same patient.

Certain generalizations may be helpful when considering airspace shadows:

1. Clinical correlation is essential and is often decisive. A few examples suffice to emphasize this point: (a) in patients with noncardiogenic pulmonary edema, the chest film may not become abnormal until several hours after the onset of symptoms, whereas with cardiogenic pulmonary edema the pulmonary shadowing is almost always evident early on; (b) widespread pneumonia is almost invariably accompanied by cough and fever; (c) aspiration should be suspected as the cause of airspace shadowing in patients who have known predisposing factors such as alcoholism, a recent seizure, or a period of unconsciousness; (d) immunocompromised patients are a special and complicated group (see Ch. 6) and widespread pulmonary shadows in such patients usually indicate infection, often from opportunistic organisms; (e) substantial hemoptysis associated with widespread pulmonary consolidation usually indicates pulmonary hemorrhage.

2. Opacity of over half a lobe with no loss of volume is virtually diagnostic of pneumonia (Fig. 3.29). The common causes in patients living in the community are pneumococcal or *Mycoplasma* pneumonia and pneumonia distal to a bronchial neoplasm. Neoplastic obstruction of a lobar bronchus usually causes some degree of atelectasis, but consolidation without loss of volume due to an obstructing neoplasm is not uncommon. Bronchioloalveolar carcinoma (see Fig. 3.10) and lymphoma may on occasion appear identical to lobar pneumonia

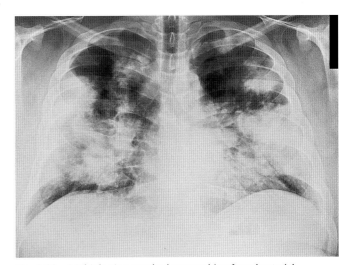

Fig. 3.28 Multiple airspace shadows resulting from bacterial pneumonia.

radiologically. The lobar consolidation in these cases is due to neoplastic tissue spreading through the alveolar spaces without necessarily occluding the central bronchi.

3. Lobar consolidation with expansion of the lobe suggests bacterial pneumonia (particularly due to *Streptococcus pneumoniae, Klebsiella pneumoniae, Pseudomonas aeruginosa*, and *Staphylococcus aureus*) or obstructive pneumonia caused by a centrally positioned carcinoma of the bronchus, the so-called "drowned lung".

Table 3.1 Differential diagnosis of a solitary airspace shadow on chest radiography

Diagnosis	Comments
Pneumonia	Pneumonia is the most common cause of solitary airspace filling. The opacity may be almost any shape from segmental/lobar to round or irregular. Cavitation and accompanying pleural effusion are both distinct features. In adults an associated hilar mass suggests a centrally located neoplasm causing postobstructive pneumonia, whereas in children an associated hilar mass suggests primary tuberculosis.
Organizing pneumonia	Can be responsible for a variety of radiographic patterns, including a focal rounded or segment-shaped area of consolidation.
Atelectasis	The diagnosis of atelectasis is based on its characteristic shape. The appearances and causes are discussed in the section Atelectasis/Collapse later in this chapter. Discoid atelectasis results in a characteristic bandlike shape coursing through the lung, often in a horizontal orientation. Large areas of atelectasis that do not conform to either of these patterns may be indistinguishable from the other causes of airspace shadowing listed in this table.
Infarction or hemorrhage associated with pulmonary embolism	Infarcts are usually segmental in size, rarely larger. Their shape is similar to a truncated cone with the base on the pleura. The apex of the cone, which may be rounded, points toward the hilum. The rounded medial margin, known as Hampton's hump (see Ch. 7), is a well known but infrequent sign suggestive, but not diagnostic, of the condition. Septic infarcts cavitate frequently, whereas bland infarcts rarely cavitate.
Pulmonary contusion	Contusions appear within hours of injury and clear within a few days. They are usually maximal in the general area of injury, although contrecoup damage may be seen at a distance. Pneumatocele formation is a distinct feature. Pulmonary contusion may surround a pulmonary hematoma. Hematomas resemble masses, may liquefy and cavitate, and take much longer to clear than contusions.
Connective tissue disease, vasculitis	These conditions are infrequent causes of solitary airspace shadowing. They need to be considered in patients with appropriate clinical features. The opacity is usually sublobar in size and nonspecific in shape. Cavitation may be seen. Most solitary shadows in patients with connective tissue disease or vasculitis represent pneumonia, organizing pneumonia, or infarction.
Drug reactions and allergic reactions	Airspace shadows in these conditions are rarely solitary. They may be almost any shape except lobar.
Hemorrhage	Solitary airspace shadows caused by hemorrhage are usually due to pulmonary emboli or to pulmonary trauma. When caused by systemic disease, pulmonary hemorrhage is usually multifocal. When single, the opacity can be any shape, even including lobar.
Neoplasm	Postobstructive pneumonia is a common cause of solitary airspace shadowing. Some neoplasms, particularly bronchioloalveolar carcinoma and lymphoma, can closely resemble focal pneumonia and may even contain air bronchograms. The absence of clinical features of pneumonia and the lack of change of the shadow over many weeks point to one of these neoplasms. The longer the opacity persists, particularly if it grows slowly, the more likely it is to be a neoplasm.
Radiation pneumonitis/ fibrosis	Airspace shadowing caused by radiation therapy conforms, usually but not invariably, to the approximate shape of the radiation port, a feature that is particularly evident in CT scans. The shape, and the fact that radiation therapy was given, usually permits a specific diagnosis to be made.
Eosinophilic pneumonia	Airspace shadowing in this condition is almost invariably multifocal; it is very rarely solitary. The opacity is likely to be noticeably peripheral in location.

4. Spherical consolidation is likely to be due to pneumonia (Fig. 3.30). The organisms most likely to cause round (spherical or nodular) pneumonia are *S. pneumoniae, S. aureus, K. pneumoniae, P. aeruginosa, Legionella pneumophila* or *Legionella micdadei, M. tuberculosis* and a variety of fungi. Clearly the major differential diagnosis is from neoplasm. Ground-glass opacity surrounding rounded consolidation on CT is highly suggestive of hemorrhage; the causes of this so-called "CT halo sign" (see Fig. 3.91) are discussed on page 119.

5. Air lucencies within consolidated lung may be due to (a) intervening normal lung, either because those particular portions of lung, often secondary pulmonary lobules, were never involved or because they have cleared prior to the remainder of the pneumonia, (b) preexisting emphysema, (c) necrosis of tissue with cavitation, or (d) pneumatoceles.[18] The development of air–fluid levels within an area of consolidation that is known or presumed to be pneumonia strongly suggests necrotizing pneumonia (true abscess formation). Bacteria are the likely pathogens, notably *S. aureus*, gram-negative bacteria (especially *K. pneumoniae, Proteus* and *P. aeruginosa*), anaerobic bacteria, and tuberculosis. Those few cases of segmental or lobar

Box 3.2   Causes of multifocal airspace shadows on chest radiography

Exudates and transudates
Pneumonia
Organizing pneumonia
Pulmonary emboli causing infarction (bland or septic)
Eosinophilic pneumonia
Connective tissue disease and vasculitis
Pulmonary edema, both circulatory and noncirculatory
(acute respiratory distress syndrome)
Inhalation of noxious gases or liquids
Hydrocarbon ingestion
Drug reactions
Allergic reactions
Alveolar proteinosis

Hemorrhage
Pulmonary contusion and hematoma
Hemorrhage due to pulmonary embolus
Aspiration of blood
Idiopathic hemorrhage, Goodpasture syndrome,
anticoagulant therapy, bleeding tendency

Neoplasm
Bronchioloalveolar carcinoma
Lymphangitis carcinomatosa
Metastases
Lymphoma

Miscellaneous
Sarcoidosis
Silicosis, coal worker's pneumoconiosis
Alveolar microlithiasis
Diffuse pulmonary calcification

Box 3.3   Widespread airspace shadows on chest radiography: likelihood of bat's wing pattern

Common pattern for disease
Pulmonary edema, both circulatory and noncirculatory
(acute respiratory distress syndrome)
Pneumonia, notably pneumonia caused by aspiration or
Pneumocystis carinii
Inhalation of noxious gases or liquids
Alveolar proteinosis
Pulmonary hemorrhage
  • Spontaneous
  • Goodpasture syndrome
  • Anticoagulant therapy
  • Bleeding tendency

Occasional or rare pattern for disease
Aspiration of blood
Bronchioloalveolar carcinoma
Lymphangitis carcinomatosa
Alveolar microlithiasis
Diffuse pulmonary calcification
Lymphoma
Pulmonary emboli causing hemorrhage or infarction (bland
or septic)
Connective tissue disease / vasculitis
Drug reactions
Allergic reactions
Amyloidosis

Extremely rare pattern for disease
Eosinophilic pneumonia
Metastases
Sarcoidosis
Silicosis, coal worker's pneumoconiosis

consolidation with cavitation not caused by infection will be caused by vasculitis or, rarely, lymphoma. A meniscus of air within an area of segmental or lobar consolidation almost always represents resolving invasive fungal infection. (Cavitation in pulmonary masses is a separate subject and is dealt with on p. 118.)

6. The presence of rib or vertebral body destruction in the vicinity of a pulmonary shadow, whatever the shape of the shadow, is virtually diagnostic of invasion by primary carcinoma of the lung. With the rare exception of actinomycosis and the occasional case of pulmonary tuberculosis[19] or fungal disease, neither pulmonary infections nor other non-neoplastic pulmonary processes invade the adjacent bones.

7. Multiple airspace shadows that are clearly lobar or segmental in shape constitute another potentially useful diagnostic subgroup (Fig. 3.31; Box 3.4).

8. It is useful to separate out those cases of multifocal airspace shadowing that show the so-called *bat's wing* or *butterfly pattern*, because the presence of this pattern makes certain diagnoses more or less likely. These fanciful terms are an attempt to describe bilateral perihilar shadowing. The shadowing consists of coalescent densities with ill-defined borders, sometimes with acinar shadows at the periphery. The outer portion of each lobe is less involved than the perihilar area and is often normal (Fig. 3.32). Bat's wing

shadowing may be symmetric, but it is often more severe on one side than the other. Air bronchograms and air alveolograms may be prominent features. By far the most common cause is pulmonary edema (Fig. 3.32), particularly if air bronchograms, air alveolograms, or acinar shadows are present. Cases of bat's wing shadowing not caused by pulmonary edema are likely to be due to pneumonia, inhalation of noxious gases or liquids (including aspiration of gastric contents), multifocal pulmonary hemorrhage (Fig. 3.33), vasculitis, or neoplasm, particularly lymphangitis carcinomatosa. Multifocal pneumonia can be due to a vast array of organisms, but the bat's wing pattern in the immunocompetent patient should suggest particularly aspiration pneumonia, gram-negative bacterial pneumonia, and nonbacterial pneumonias such as mycoplasmal, viral, and rickettsial pneumonia. Pneumonia in the immunocompromised host often results in the bat's wing pattern, most notably in infections with opportunistic organisms such as *Pneumocystis carinii* and various fungi. The coexistence of the bat's wing pattern and thickened interlobular septa (Kerley A and B lines) visible on plain chest radiography, for practical purposes, limits the diagnostic possibilities to pulmonary edema and lymphangitis carcinomatosa.

Bat's wing shadowing that remains unchanged over several weeks and is associated with nonspecific chronic symptoms

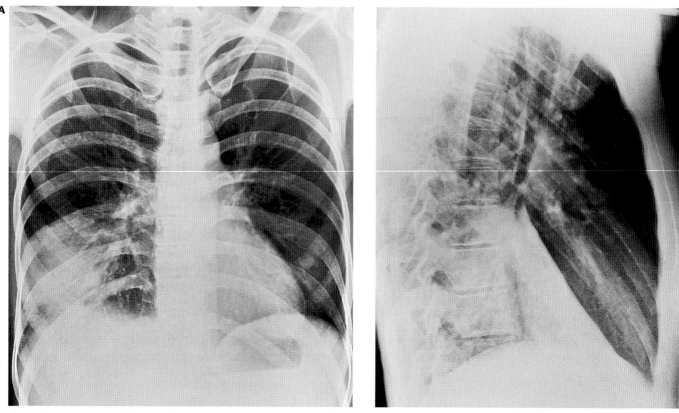

Fig. 3.29 Lobar consolidation resulting from bacterial pneumonia. In this case, the superior segment of the right lower lobe is spared. **A**, Posteroanterior view. **B**, Lateral view.

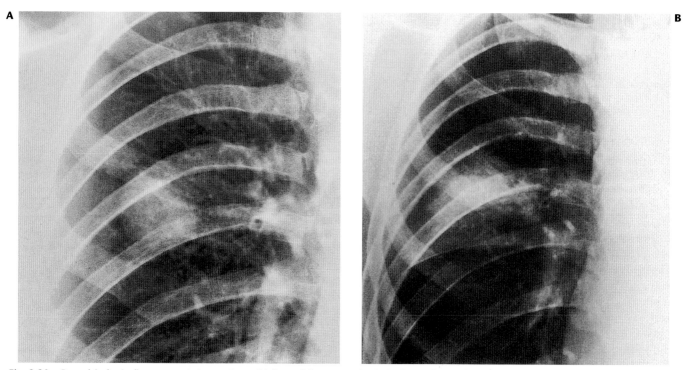

Fig. 3.30 Round (spherical) pneumonia in a patient with bacterial pneumonia. **A**, Radiograph on admission to hospital. **B**, One day later, the pneumonia has spread through the adjacent lung.

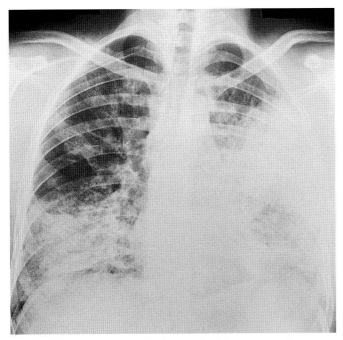

Fig. 3.31 Multiple airspace shadows with a lobar-segmental distribution in a case of bacterial pneumonia.

Box 3.4 Differential diagnosis of multiple airspace shadows on chest radiography when their shape is clearly lobar or segmental

Pneumonia
Infarction or hemorrhage caused by pulmonary emboli
Pulmonary edema*
Neoplasm (bronchioloalveolar carcinoma, lymphangitis carcinomatosa*, malignant lymphoma)

---

*Segmental or lobar shapes are a rare manifestation of the entity.

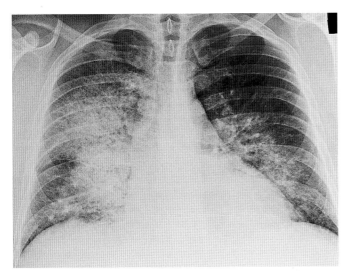

Fig. 3.32 "Bat's wing" pattern caused by pulmonary edema. This example is typical in that it is bilateral, but asymmetric. The shadowing is maximal in the central (perihilar) portions of the lung, and the outer portions of the lungs are relatively clear.

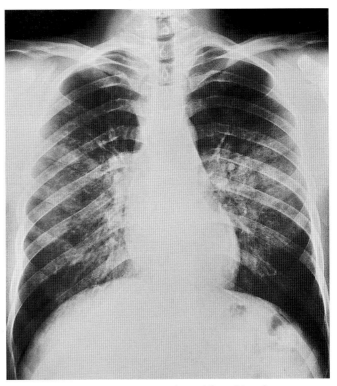

Fig. 3.33 "Bat's wing" shadowing due to idiopathic pulmonary hemorrhage.

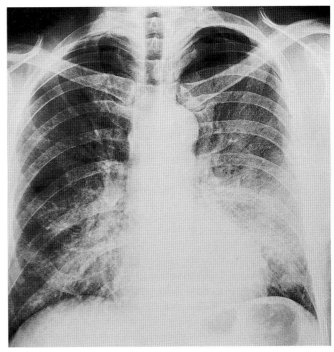

Fig. 3.34 "Bat's wing" shadowing due to alveolar proteinosis.

suggests alveolar proteinosis (Fig. 3.34) or a neoplasm, notably lymphangitis carcinomatosa (Fig. 3.35), bronchioloalveolar carcinoma, or malignant lymphoma. Sarcoidosis and Wegener granulomatosis are extremely rare possibilities for such shadowing.

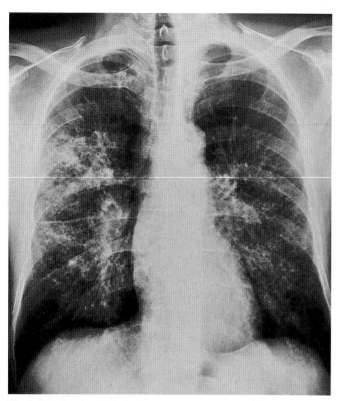

Fig. 3.35 "Bat's wing" shadowing due to lymphangitis carcinomatosa.

9. Nonsegmental airspace shadows that are widespread, yet clearly peripheral in location (sometimes called "the photographic negative of pulmonary edema"), strongly suggest chronic eosinophilic pneumonia when upper zone predominant (Fig. 3.36).[20] The peripheral distribution may be more readily apparent on CT than on plain chest radiography.[21] When there is no upper zone predominance the differential diagnosis widens to include drug reactions and organizing pneumonia (Fig. 3.37).

10. Many of the causes of multiple airspace shadows appear rapidly, but pulmonary edema and hemorrhage are the only ones that clear within hours.

11. Airspace shadowing that resolves only to reappear either in the same area or in some other part of either lung suggests: pulmonary edema; eosinophilic pneumonia, either acute or chronic; or asthma, particularly when associated with bronchopulmonary aspergillosis.

12. Very fine punctate calcification may cause focal or multifocal areas of pulmonary opacity closely resembling consolidation on plain chest radiographs (Fig. 3.38). This phenomenon occurs in patients with hypercalcemia caused by conditions such as hyperparathyroidism, particularly secondary hyperparathyroidism resulting from renal failure, and in children who have had cardiac surgery or liver transplants.[22–26] The calcifications may be so minute that it is not possible to appreciate on plain chest radiographs that the cloudlike shadows are in fact due to a myriad of calcifications. The appearance may then be confused with the other causes of multiple airspace shadows. CT allows the observation of widespread parenchymal calcification to be made with confidence.

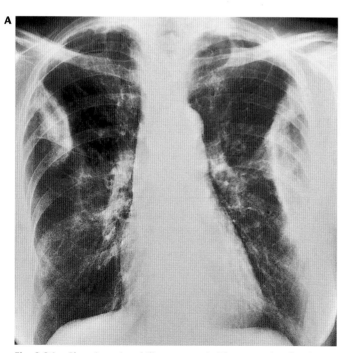

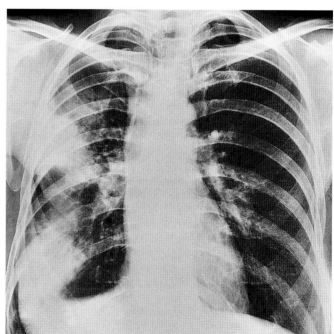

Fig. 3.36 Chronic eosinophilic pneumonia. Two examples showing nonsegmental peripheral distribution of airspace shadowing. **A**, As is more usual, the airspace shadowing is bilateral. **B**, An example with unilateral airspace shadowing.

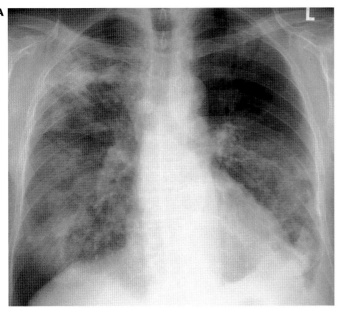

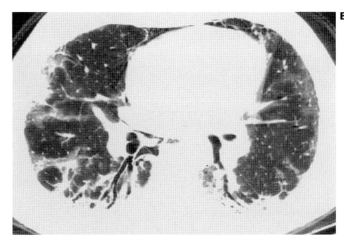

Fig. 3.37   Cryptogenic organizing pneumonia showing patchy, peripherally predominant, airspace shadowing. **A**, Chest radiograph. **B**, CT of a similar case.

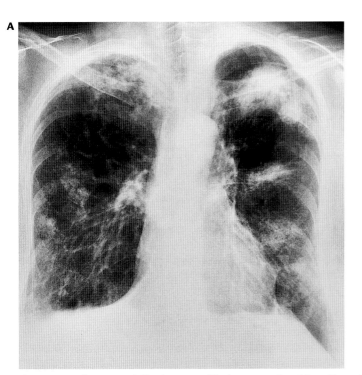

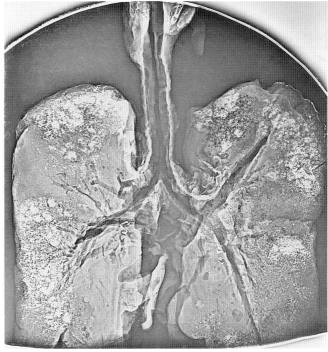

Fig. 3.38   Pulmonary calcification caused by hyperparathyroidism. Fine calcifications are deposited in the lung in a patchy fashion and produce coalescent cloud-like shadows. The patient died despite parathyroidectomy. **A**, Posteroanterior radiograph. **B**, An autopsy radiograph of the same patient shows the pulmonary calcifications to advantage.

13. Acute (formerly known as "adult") respiratory distress syndrome (ARDS) is the most likely diagnosis for uniform opacity of the whole of both lungs without pleural effusion in the immunocompetent patient (Fig. 3.39). Air bronchograms are a noteworthy feature in these patients. The presence of associated pneumothorax or pneumomediastinum increases the likelihood of ARDS.

14. Sarcoidosis occasionally causes patchy shadows in the lungs that tend to be spherical, contain air bronchograms,

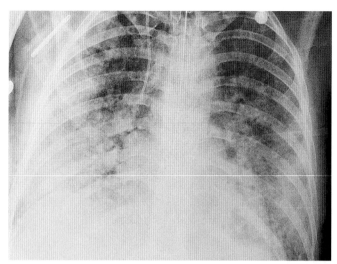

Fig. 3.39 Widespread, uniform airspace shadowing in acute respiratory distress syndrome.

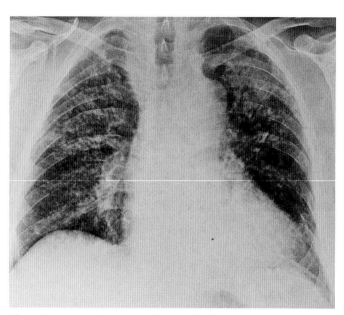

Fig. 3.41 Progressive massive fibrosis (PMF) in a coal miner. The conglomerate PMF shadow in the left upper lobe is ill-defined enough to resemble airspace shadowing, but the typical location and the presence of widespread small nodules in the lungs are characteristic of mineral dust pneumoconiosis.

and are associated with obvious hilar and mediastinal lymph node enlargement. Sometimes these opacities dominate the picture and, when irregular in shape, are radiologically indistinguishable from multifocal pneumonia (Fig. 3.40).

15. Progressive massive fibrosis may, rarely, resemble airspace shadowing (Fig. 3.41). The lesions are, however, characteristic in shape and position, they do not contain air bronchograms, and the other findings of pneumoconiosis are almost invariably visible. So, true diagnostic confusion is most unusual.

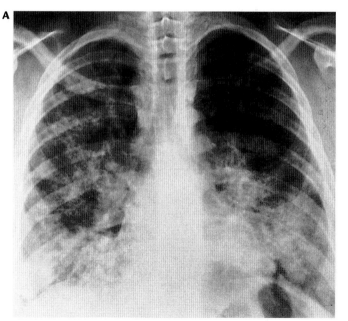

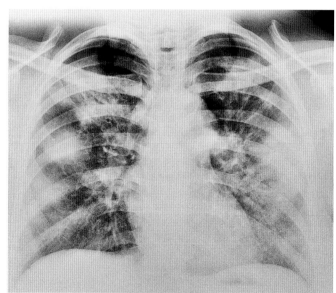

Fig. 3.40 **A**, Sarcoidosis showing multiple, rounded, ill-defined areas of pulmonary shadowing closely resembling pneumonia. **B**, A similar case with bilateral hilar and mediastinal adenopathy.

ATELECTASIS/COLLAPSE

The terms "atelectasis", "loss of lung volume", and "collapse" are often used synonymously, although the term "collapse" is sometimes, particularly in North America, restricted to mean total atelectasis.[5]

Mechanisms of atelectasis

There are several mechanisms for atelectasis, the most frequent being bronchial obstruction.[27]

Bronchial obstruction in adults is usually the result of a bronchial neoplasm or mucus plug. On occasion, it is due to an inhaled foreign body, inflammatory or post-traumatic bronchostenosis, a broncholith, or extrinsic compression by such phenomena as enlarged lymph nodes, aortic aneurysm, or left atrial enlargement.

Because bronchial tumors are uncommon in children, the probable causes of childhood obstructive atelectasis differ significantly from those in adults. In young children the airways are smaller and more vulnerable to obstruction by inflammatory exudate and mucus in pneumonia, or mucus plug obstruction in conditions such as asthma or cystic fibrosis. The other likely cause of lobar atelectasis in children is an inhaled foreign body. Rare causes include inflammatory or post-traumatic bronchostenosis, compression of the bronchial tree by anomalous vessels and, very rarely, neoplastic obstruction.

Any process that occupies increased space within the thorax either compresses the lung (**compressive atelectasis**) or allows it to retract (**passive atelectasis**). With large pleural effusions the lobes surrounded by fluid may show substantial atelectasis. Large intrathoracic masses frequently press on the lung and may therefore acquire an ill-defined margin because of adjacent atelectatic lung. Similarly, emphysematous bullae are often surrounded by atelectatic lung. The best example of passive atelectasis, due to normal elastic recoil, is pneumothorax, which allows retraction of the lung.

Pulmonary fibrosis leads to loss of lung volume owing to a combination of lung destruction and loss of compliance. There are many different patterns, the precise radiographic features depending on the distribution of the primary disease.

Following infection a lobe may lose volume because of destruction, often accompanied by bronchiectasis, and fibrosis. The most common cause in the upper lobes and superior segment of the lower lobes is previous granulomatous infection. If the disease affects the dependent portions of the lung, the patient may have the clinical features of bronchiectasis. The "**middle lobe syndrome**" is a particular example of the phenomenon (see p. 98). The following features, all of which are best seen at CT, may be inferred from plain chest radiographs: no endobronchial mass; dilated, thick-walled bronchi within the atelectatic lobe; and associated extensive pleural thickening.[28] The loss of volume can be very severe and may be greater than is generally observed in lobar collapse caused by endobronchial obstruction.

Widespread pulmonary fibrosis causes generalized loss of lung volume. Reticulonodular shadowing of the lung is then the dominant radiographic feature (see the section Widespread Nodular, Reticulonodular, and Honeycomb Shadowing, p. 127).

Discoid atelectasis (also known as plate or linear atelectasis) is a form of adhesive atelectasis. First described by Fleischner,[29] and formerly known as Fleischner lines, the atelectasis is disk or

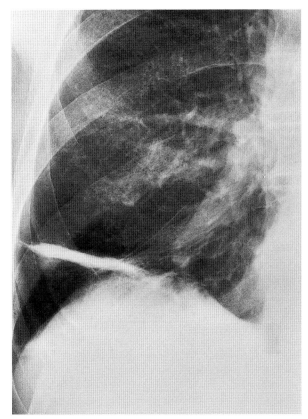

Fig. 3.42 Discoid atelectasis showing a typical bandlike shadow.

plate shaped (Fig. 3.42). Sometimes the disk is so large that it crosses the whole lobe. Discoid atelectasis may be single or multiple. It usually abuts the pleura and is perpendicular to the pleural surface[30] with no predisposition to point toward the hilum. The orientation may be in any plane from horizontal to vertical. The thickness ranges from a few millimeters to a centimeter or more, and the lesions are therefore usually seen as line or band shadows.

Westcott and Cole[30] reviewed the mechanisms that lead to discoid atelectasis. The subject is complex but, put simply, discoid atelectasis is due to hypoventilation, which leads to alveolar collapse. Alveoli lying at the lung bases and those lying posteriorly are most likely to collapse, not only because they have the lowest volume but also because the physiologic mechanisms responsible for keeping the small airways and alveoli open are at their most vulnerable in these sites. In addition, discoid atelectasis may be seen in the lingula in patients with substantial collapse of the left lower lobe, possibly because of kinking of bronchi in the hyperexpanded lingula.[31,32]

Discoid atelectasis is common, particularly in hospitalized patients. Since it reflects hypoventilation, it is seen in a large variety of conditions.[33] Of itself, it is usually of little clinical importance, although the associated conditions may be of great significance. Occasionally, discoid atelectasis is of such magnitude and so widespread that it causes hypoxemia. It should be remembered that plain films may substantially underestimate the extent of the condition. Following general anesthesia, for example, widespread discoid atelectasis can be clinically significant, even in cases that show few signs on plain chest radiograph.

Imaging lobar atelectasis

Chest radiographs are usually sufficient to diagnose the presence of lobar atelectasis. CT can be useful when the plain film findings are ambiguous,[33] for example, when pleural fluid and pulmonary disease processes are both present.

The fundamental signs of lobar atelectasis on both plain films[27,34–36] and CT[35–37] are opacity of the lobe and evidence of loss of volume which they can be divided into (1) direct signs, such as displacement of fissures, pulmonary blood vessels, and major bronchi, and (2) shift of other structures to compensate for the loss of volume. The compensatory shifts are in principle similar for each lobe, and they are therefore discussed before describing the appearance of atelectasis of individual lobes.

Compensatory over-expansion of the adjacent lobe may result in recognizable spreading of the vessels so there are fewer vessels per unit volume. This sign should not be relied upon if it is an isolated finding, since previous lung damage, from infection for example, can lead to a similar appearance. Another sign of compensatory expansion is the shifting granuloma sign as illustrated in Figure 3.43.

The amount of mediastinal shift accompanying lobar atelectasis is variable. In general, it is greatest with lower lobe atelectasis or chronic fibrotic loss of volume of an upper lobe, relatively mild with acute upper lobe atelectasis, and virtually nonexistent with atelectasis of the middle lobe. Its recognition depends on noting displacement of the trachea and mediastinum. Normally, on a correctly centered frontal view, the trachea lies midway, or slightly to the right of the mid point, between the medial ends of the clavicles. Minor obliquity of the chest radiograph does not make much difference because the trachea is only just behind the plane of the medial ends of the clavicles. The normal position of the mediastinum varies so greatly that displacement of the mediastinal contour is an insensitive sign of loss of volume. Normally, one-fifth to one-half of the cardiac shadow lies to the right of the midline. More than one-half or less than one-fifth suggests mediastinal shift.

Hemidiaphragm elevation is another manifestation of compensatory shift. Loss of volume of either lower lobe or of the left upper lobe may lead to obvious elevation of the ipsilateral hemidiaphragm. It is usually unrecognizable in right middle lobe collapse and may be subtle in right upper lobe atelectasis. The sign is, however, of limited value because the position of the normal diaphragm is highly variable, particularly in a hospital population. Diaphragm position depends on many factors, including the amount of gas in the stomach, and can vary from day to day. Therefore great care must be taken before relying on elevation of a hemidiaphragm to support the diagnosis of lobar atelectasis.

Inward movement of the chest wall causes narrowing of the spaces between the affected ribs. This sign, which is only seen with a severely collapsed lobe, can be difficult to evaluate on chest films. It is much easier to recognize on axial CT imaging where the cross-sectional area of each hemithorax can be readily compared. Clearly, confusion with preexisting chest wall deformity, particularly when consequent to scoliosis, may cloud the issue.

Obliteration or narrowing of the bronchial air column at the site of any obstruction is often visible, even on plain film. Opaque foreign bodies or calcified broncholiths may be directly visible. Even though CT demonstrates the size and site of the responsible obstructing lesion in virtually all patients with a lobar collapse[38–41] (Figs 3.44 and 3.45), bronchoscopy is indicated

A 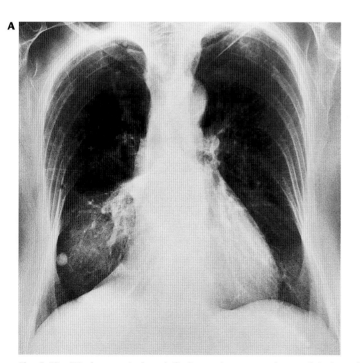 **B**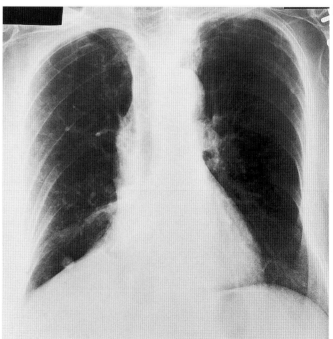

Fig. 3.43 Displacement of a calcified granuloma secondary to right lower lobe atelectasis: **A**, at a time when mild right lower lobe collapse is present; **B**, when complete atelectasis of the right lower lobe is present.

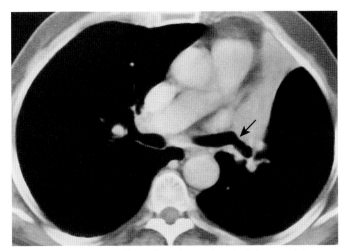

Fig. 3.44 Carcinoma of bronchus obstructing the left upper lobe bronchus and causing left upper lobe atelectasis. Bronchial occlusion by tumor (arrow) is well shown by CT.

to diagnose the nature of the obstruction and where possible, as with foreign body inhalation, mucus plug obstruction and broncholith, to treat the cause.

When the peripheral lung collapses and the central portion is prevented from collapsing by the presence of a mass, the relevant fissures are concave peripherally but convex centrally; the shape of the fissure then resembles an S or a reverse S – hence the name Golden S sign, after Golden's description of cases of lobar collapse caused by carcinoma of the lung.[42] This sign is recognizable both on plain film and at CT (Fig. 3.46).[33,43] On occasion, the fact that there is lobar atelectasis may be overlooked and the patient misdiagnosed as having a mediastinal or hilar mass (see Fig. 3.49). Similarly, bronchi that are massively dilated due to tuberculosis may deform the central portion of the atelectatic lobe, leading to a misdiagnosis of a pulmonary, hilar, or mediastinal mass.[44]

Bronchial dilatation and air bronchograms within atelectatic lobes

Mucus-filled, dilated bronchi are frequently present beyond an obstructing lesion responsible for lobar atelectasis. They cannot be recognized on plain films, although they are readily identified at CT as low-density branching structures (Figs 3.45B and 3.47).[33,45,46] The low density is due to trapped secretions. Finding a so-called "mucoid" or "fluid bronchogram" should prompt a search for a central obstructing lesion.

Air bronchograms within atelectatic lobes are very rarely identified on plain chest radiographs, but may be seen on CT even when the loss of volume is due to central bronchial obstruction, possibly because of collateral air drift or necrosis of the obstructing tumor.[41]

In one series,[47] the MR signal intensity on proton density and T2-weighted images was high in atelectasis due to central obstruction but was low in nonobstructive atelectasis. The authors postulated that the high T2 signal was related to trapped secretions, which were present only when the atelectasis was due to obstruction.

Right upper lobe atelectasis

In right upper lobe atelectasis (Figs 3.46A and 3.48), the major and minor fissures move upward toward each other rather like a half-closed book, the spine of which is represented by the hilum. At the same time these fissures rotate toward the mediastinum, with the result that the right upper lobe packs against the mediastinum and lung apex. The more the loss of volume, the greater is the concavity of the minor fissure. Eventually, with extreme collapse, the minor fissure parallels the mediastinum and thoracic apex and resembles pleural thickening or mediastinal widening. The lobe is attached to the hilum by a conical wedge of collapsed lung, and therefore the curving inferior margin of the lobe always connects to the hilum. The

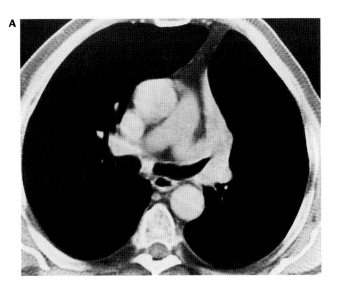

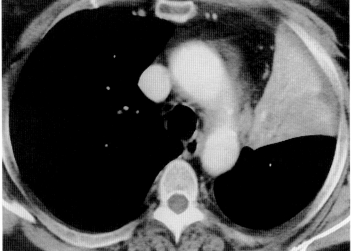

Fig. 3.45 Left upper lobe collapse due to bronchial carcinoma. **A**, Severe collapse. Note that the carcinoma has caused "rat tail" narrowing of the left upper bronchus. **B**, Moderately severe collapse with substantial consolidation. Fluid-filled bronchi are seen within the obstructed lobe.

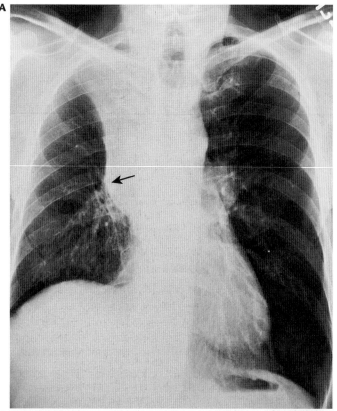

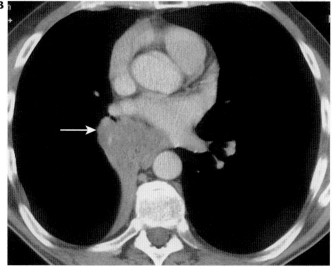

Fig. 3.46 Golden S sign. **A**, Chest radiograph showing right upper lobe atelectasis with the Golden S sign. The outward bulge (arrow) of a displaced minor fissure indicates the underlying mass, which proved to be bronchial carcinoma. **B**, CT in a patient with a large carcinoma obstructing the right lower lobe bronchus causing lobar collapse. The arrow points to the bulge of the major fissure which cannot move more medially because of the underlying tumor.

intrinsic bulk of the central vessels and bronchi means there is a limit to the loss of volume possible at the hilum; hence an outward bulge is discernible at the hilum in examples of extreme collapse even when no hilar mass is present. Because the atelectatic right upper lobe has extensive contact with the mediastinum, the normal superior vena caval border is

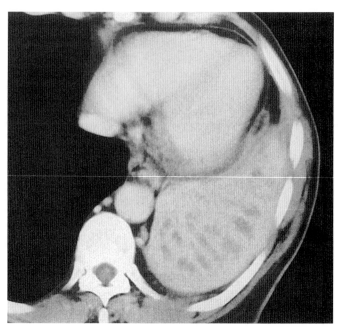

Fig. 3.47 Fluid bronchogram at CT. Fluid-filled bronchi beyond a carcinoma in the atelectatic lower left lobe are clearly visible.

"silhouetted" out on the frontal chest film, as is the ascending aorta on the lateral view.

The middle and lower lobes expand to occupy the vacated space, leading to outward and upward displacement of the right lower lobe artery. This displacement is most readily seen on frontal radiographs. The corresponding upward angulation of the right mainstem and lower lobe bronchi is more difficult to recognize. Over-expansion of the opposite upper lobe is usually minor; for practical purposes it is visible only at CT scanning.

On the lateral view the upward displacement of the major and minor fissures is usually obvious. With severe loss of volume the wedge of collapsed lung radiating out from the hilum may be no more than an indistinct density on lateral views, since neither of the fissures is tangential to the x-ray beam. The elevation of the right pulmonary trunk and the anterior displacement of the right bronchial tree can be identified on the lateral projection,[48] but only with great difficulty.

Occasionally, collapse of the right upper lobe around a large obstructing bronchial tumor closely mimics a mediastinal mass (Fig. 3.49). An error in interpretation can be avoided by carefully analyzing the film for compensatory shift of other intrathoracic structures.

On rare occasions, the normal chest wall contact is maintained even in severe collapse.[49] This appearance (Fig. 3.50) is most frequently reported in neonates and young children,[50] but is also seen in adults.[51] It has been termed peripheral atelectasis[50,52,53] because the atelectatic lobe lies against the lateral chest wall and the over-expanded lower lobe lies centrally.[54] The appearance may mimic loculated pleural effusion.[53]

A juxtaphrenic peak may be visible.[55] This term refers to a small triangular shadow based on the apex of the dome of the hemidiaphragm with loss of silhouette of the adjacent hemidiaphragm (Fig. 3.48), usually caused by traction on an inferior accessory fissure,[56–58] or, on occasions, due to traction on the intrapulmonary septum associated with the inferior pulmonary ligament.[57]

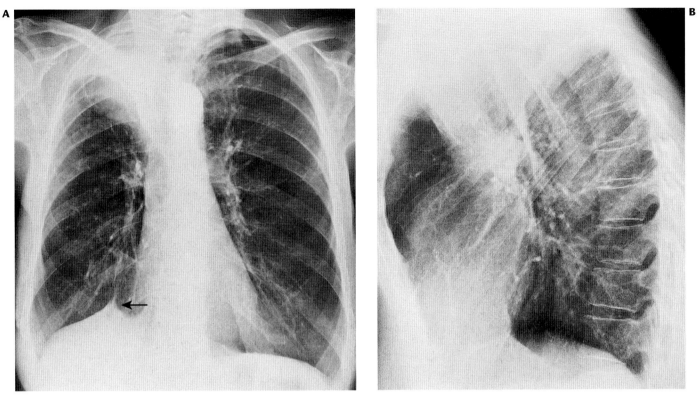

Fig. 3.48 Right upper lobe atelectasis – a typical example. Also note the juxtaphrenic peak (arrow). **A**, Posteroanterior view. **B**, Lateral view.

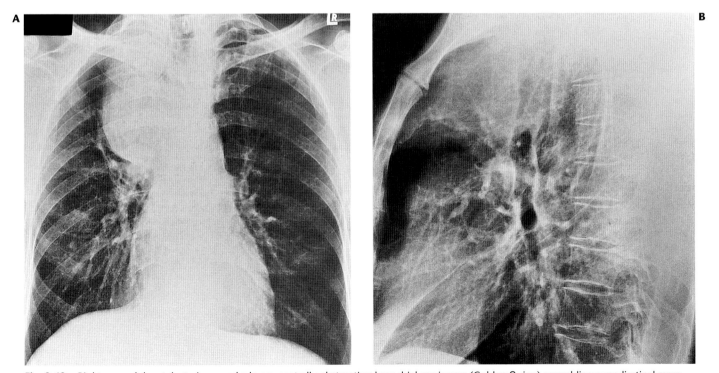

Fig. 3.49 Right upper lobe atelectasis around a large, centrally obstructing bronchial carcinoma (Golden S sign) resembling a mediastinal mass. The best clue to the correct interpretation is elevation of the right lower lobe artery. **A**, Posteroanterior view. **B**, Lateral view.

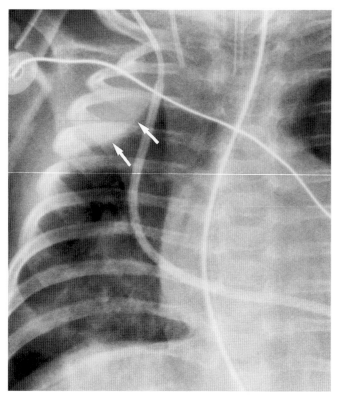

Fig. 3.50 "Peripheral atelectasis" of right upper lobe (arrows) in an infant following cardiac surgery. The lobe has collapsed against the chest wall.

At CT,[28,36,37,39,59] an atelectatic right upper lobe appears as a triangular soft tissue density lying against the mediastinum and the anterior chest wall. The border formed by the major fissure posteriorly and the minor fissure laterally is sharp (Fig. 3.51). In the absence of large intrapulmonary masses, each fissural boundary should be uniformly concave or convex, not a combination of the two. A severely collapsed right upper lobe assumes a bandlike configuration plastered against the mediastinum, an appearance that can be confused with mediastinal disease. Sometimes the hyperexpanded superior segment of the lower lobe insinuates itself between the mediastinum and the medial border of the atelectatic lobe. Elevation of the right upper lobe bronchus may cause the bronchus intermedius to move laterally, and the right middle lobe bronchus may be displaced anteriorly and reoriented in a more horizontal position.

Left upper lobe atelectasis

Because there is no minor fissure on the left, the appearance of atelectasis of the left upper lobe is significantly different from atelectasis of the right upper lobe (Fig. 3.52). The lobe moves predominantly forward, pulling the expanded left lower lobe behind it. Except at the edges the lobe retains much of its original contact with the anterior chest wall and mediastinum.

Since the lobe thins as the fissure is pulled forward, the usual appearance on a frontal radiograph is a hazy density extending out from the left hilum, often reaching the lung apex, and fading laterally and inferiorly. The loss of the left cardiac and mediastinal silhouette is a striking feature on the frontal view. With mild loss of volume – provided the lobe is opaque – the entire cardiac and upper mediastinal border, together with the diaphragm outline adjacent to the cardiac apex, becomes invisible. With increasing loss of volume the upper margin of the aortic knob once again becomes visible because the superior segment of the lower lobe takes the place of the posterior segment of the upper lobe – a sign that has been called the "luftsichel" sign.[60] With further loss of volume the upper border of the pulmonary opacity becomes hazy and its medial border becomes sharp because the apex is now occupied by the greatly over-expanded superior segment of lower lobe (Fig. 3.53). The superior mediastinal and left hemidiaphragm contours then reappear, but with very few exceptions the left border of the heart remains indistinct even in the most severe cases of left upper lobe atelectasis.

The over-expansion of the left lower lobe results in elevation of the left hilum and outward angulation of the left lower lobe artery. The left bronchial tree assumes an S-shaped

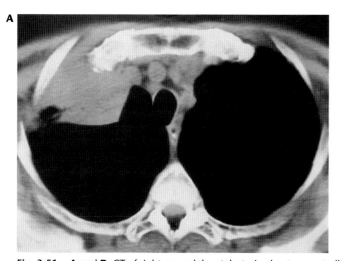
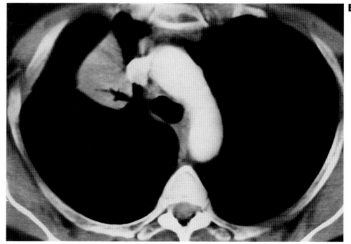

Fig. 3.51 **A** and **B**, CT of right upper lobe atelectasis, due to a centrally located lung cancer, showing a characteristic wedge-shaped density radiating from the right hilum with a broad base against the anterior chest wall. Note the air bronchogram leading into the collapsed lobe on **B**, an example of the "bronchus sign".

A 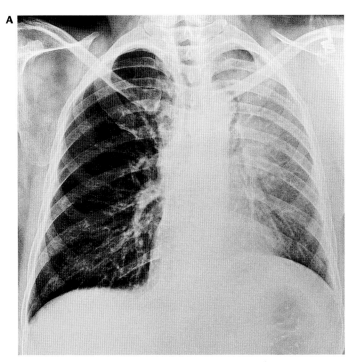 **B**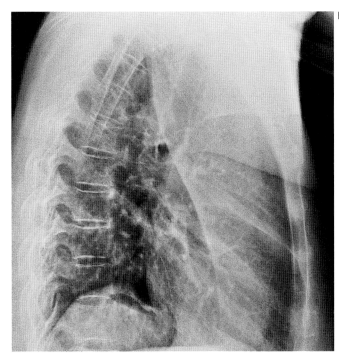

Fig. 3.52 Left upper lobe atelectasis due to bronchial carcinoma. **A**, Posteroanterior view. **B**, Lateral view.

A 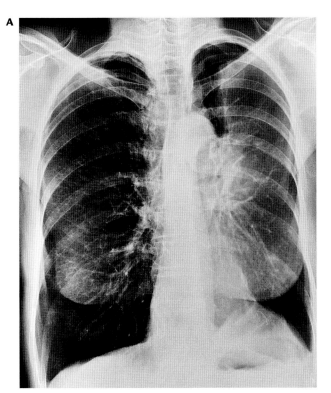 **B**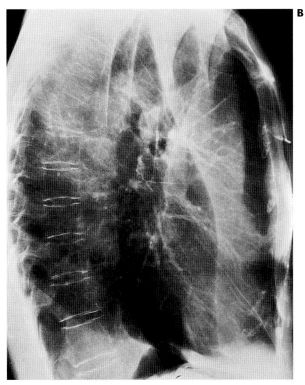

Fig. 3.53 Left upper lobe atelectasis. **A**, Posteroanterior view. In this example, the greatly expanded superior segment of the left lower lobe occupies the apex, and consequently the upper surface of the aortic arch is visible. **B**, Lateral view. The posterior boundary of the collapsed left upper lobe is formed by the displaced major fissure. The anterior boundary is against the anterior chest wall. The ascending aorta is particularly well seen, and should not be mistaken for the anterior boundary of the collapsed lobe.

configuration, the left main bronchus running a near horizontal course and the lower lobe bronchus being more vertical than usual (Fig. 3.54).

On the lateral view the lateral portion of the major fissure is usually seen as a clearly defined concave margin running approximately parallel to the anterior chest wall. The wedge of tissue radiating from the hilum is indistinct on the lateral projection unless there is a hilar mass to alter the tangents. The lingular segment, being thinner to start with, often is no more than a sliver. The whole fissure may be so far forward that a

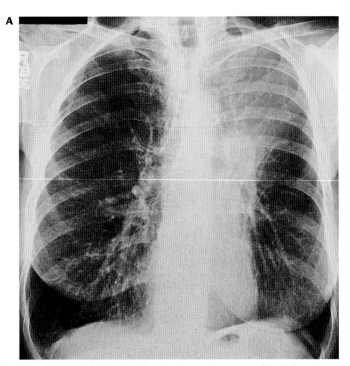 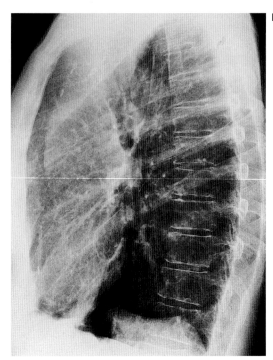

Fig. 3.54 Left upper lobe atelectasis showing reorientation of the left mainstem bronchus and left lower lobe bronchus. Note the near horizontal alignment of the mainstem bronchus and the near vertical alignment of the lower lobe bronchus. **A**, Posteroanterior view. **B**, Lateral view.

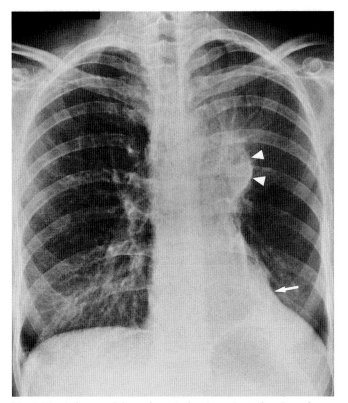

Fig. 3.55 Left upper lobe atelectasis showing a juxtaphrenic peak (arrow) and a Golden S sign (arrowheads). The atelectasis was caused by a centrally obstructing bronchial carcinoma.

collapsed upper lobe can be overlooked or misinterpreted as an anterior mediastinal density. Sometimes the fissure rotates, so that no part of it is tangential to the x-ray beam and, in these cases, the edge of the shadow is ill-defined in the lateral view also.

A striking feature of left upper lobe atelectasis is herniation of the opposite lung into the left hemithorax in front of the aorta (see Fig. 3.44), which leads to increased visibility of the ascending aorta on the lateral chest radiograph (Fig. 3.53), an appearance that should not be misinterpreted as the anterior edge of the collapsed lobe. In rare instances the edge of the herniated lung can be seen projected over the aortic knob on a frontal film. The more usual cause of aerated lung lying medial to the opacity of an atelectatic left upper lobe is over-expansion of the left lower lobe invaginating between the atelectatic lung and the mediastinum (Fig. 3.53).

A juxtaphrenic peak on the hemidiaphragm (Fig. 3.55) and the phenomenon of "peripheral" atelectasis may be seen on the left just as they may with atelectasis of the right upper lobe.

At CT (Figs 3.44, 3.45, and 3.56)[28,36,37,39,59] atelectatic left and right upper lobes appear similar, but with left upper lobe atelectasis the airless lingular segments are identified on sections below the carina as a narrow triangular density based on the heart and anterior chest wall extending almost to the diaphragm. The herniation of the right lung anterior to the aorta is particularly well demonstrated at CT scanning.

Right middle lobe atelectasis

The opacity of an atelectatic middle lobe on the frontal chest radiograph may, in severe cases, be so minimal that middle lobe atelectasis is easy to overlook, because its depth in the plane of the beam may be no more than a few millimeters (Fig. 3.57), but

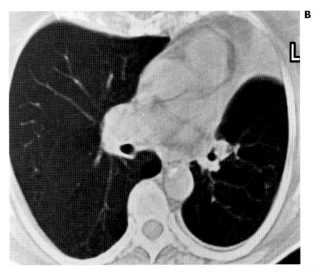
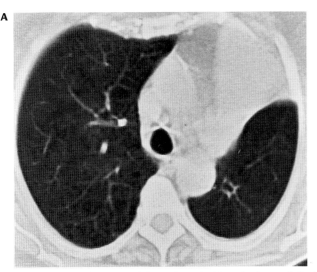

Fig. 3.56 CT showing left upper lobe atelectasis. Note the forward displacement of the major fissure and mediastinal shift to the left. **A**, A section above the level of the left mainstem bronchus showing the atelectatic anterior, posterior, and apical segments. **B**, A section through the collapsed lingular segments.

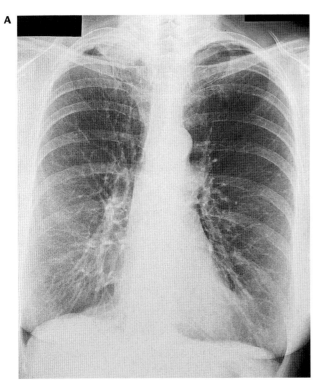
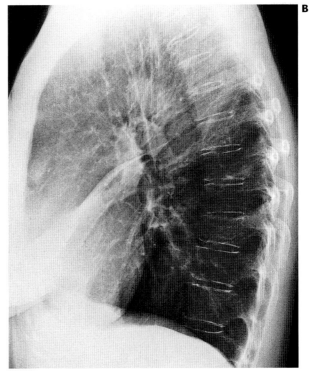

Fig. 3.57 Right middle lobe atelectasis. **A**, The lobe is so severely atelectatic that the opacity is difficult to see in the frontal view. There is, however, loss of the right heart border due to the silhouette sign. **B**, The lateral view shows the atelectatic lobe to advantage. In this case, the atelectasis was chronic and the result of the "middle lobe syndrome".

loss of silhouette of the right border of the heart is almost always a feature. The bronchial and vascular realignments in right middle lobe atelectasis are so slight that there is no recognizable alteration in the appearance of the right hilum. The atelectatic lobe is, however, easily and reliably recognized on the lateral chest radiograph. The major and minor fissures approximate one another and, if the atelectasis is pronounced, the lobe resembles a curved, elongated wedge. The wedge tapers in two directions: medial to lateral, and anterior to posterior.

The collapsed lobe may be so thin that it may be misinterpreted as a thickened fissure. Alternatively, there may occasionally be difficulty in distinguishing between atelectasis of the middle lobe and loculated fluid in the major fissure. With atelectasis the inferior margin of the opacity is concave, whereas with loculated fluid the fissure bulges downward. Also the fissures should not be separately visible in their normal positions, an important point in the differential diagnosis from pleural fluid, pleural thickening, or tumors lying within the fissures.

A 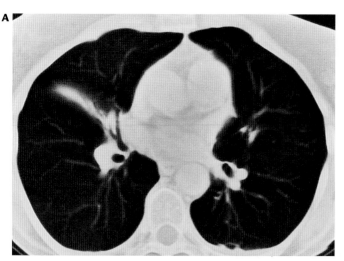 B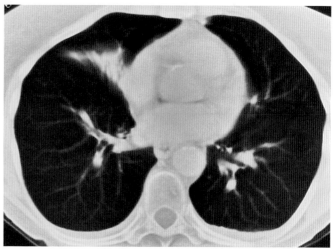

Fig. 3.58 CT of right middle lobe atelectasis in the same patient as in Figure 3.57. Note the patent middle lobe bronchus and air bronchogram. Two adjacent sections are shown: **A**, a section at the level of the right middle lobe bronchus; **B**, a lower section.

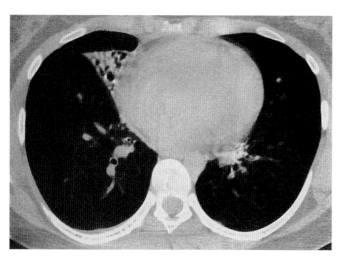

Fig. 3.59 CT of right middle lobe atelectasis showing dilated air-filled bronchi within the atelectatic lobe. This combination is typical of the "right middle lobe syndrome".

At CT (Figs 3.58 and 3.59),[28,36,37,39,59] right middle lobe atelectasis appears as a triangular density bounded posteriorly by the major fissure, medially by the mediastinum at the level of the right atrium, and anteriorly by the minor fissure. The posterior boundary should be well defined. Unless the minor fissure is pulled well down, the anterior margin may be poorly defined on the CT images. The right middle lobe bronchus enters the posteromedial corner of the opacity, an important point in the differential diagnosis from loculated pleural fluid. Because the atelectatic middle lobe is effectively a sheet of tissue running obliquely through the chest, the axial sections of CT are not aligned with the lobe and only small portions of the atelectatic lobe are seen on any one section.

The term "middle lobe syndrome" refers to chronic non-obstructive middle lobe collapse (Figs 3.57, 3.58 and 3.59). The condition was originally thought to be due to tuberculous lymphadenopathy pressing on the middle lobe or lingular bronchus, but it is now believed that the entity is due to chronic inflammatory disease, which clears very slowly because of poor collateral drift.[61] Pathologically, the atelectatic lung may show

bronchiectasis, chronic bronchitis with lymphoid hyperplasia, organizing pneumonia, and abscess formation.[62] In one series of 129 patients with chronic disease in the right middle lobe or lingula, most of whom were middle-aged women, 58 had no evidence of central obstruction, either by endobronchial or extrabronchial masses.[63]

Lower lobe atelectasis

The appearance of atelectasis of the lower lobes is sufficiently similar on the two sides that it is convenient to consider right and left lower atelectasis together. The loss of volume may affect the whole lobe, but the superior segment is frequently spared.

With atelectasis of either lower lobe (Figs 3.60 and 3.61), the major fissure rotates backward and medially, and the upper half of the fissure swings downward. Thus atelectatic lower lobes lie posteromedially in the lower thoracic cavity. The resulting triangular opacity is based on the diaphragm and mediastinum, with the fissure running obliquely through the thorax. On frontal projection the opacity of an atelectatic lower lobe is easier to recognize on the right than on the left because on the left it is often hidden by the heart, especially if the film is under-penetrated. With severe loss of volume the lobe becomes notably thin and appears as a sliver lying against the mediastinum (Fig. 3.61). Sometimes, presumably when the inferior pulmonary ligament does not attach to the diaphragm, the lobe is plastered against the mediastinum but has little if any contact with the diaphragm. In these cases the atelectatic lobe assumes a rounded configuration and may resemble a mediastinal mass (Fig. 3.61). Care should be taken not to confuse a large but normal left cardiophrenic fat pad with left lower lobe collapse (Fig. 3.62).

If the superior segment remains aerated, the upper half of the major fissure will often be identified on the frontal view (Fig. 3.63). In these cases the major fissure may be confused with the minor fissure, a misinterpretation that can be avoided by remembering that the minor fissure does not cross medial to the hilum.

Lower lobe atelectasis is sometimes more obvious in the lateral than the frontal view. Unless the atelectasis is very severe, the density of the posterior thorax, notably the spine, is increased

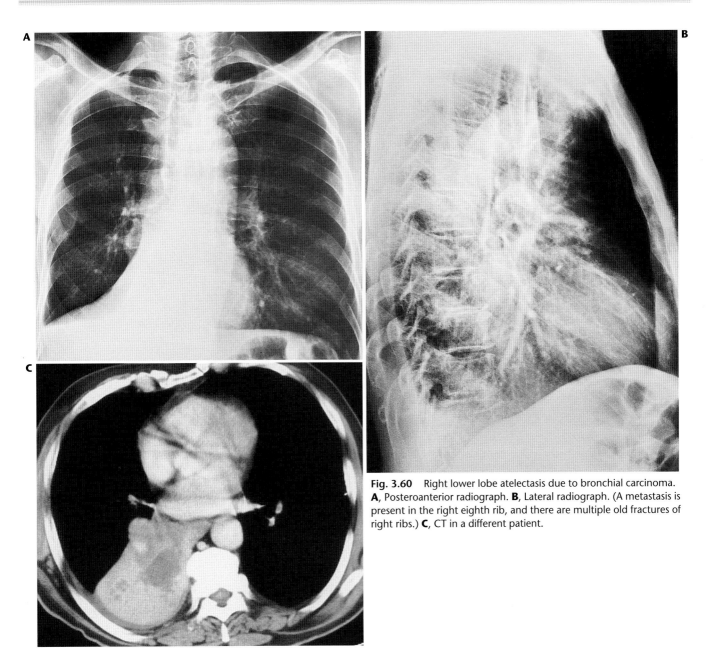

Fig. 3.60 Right lower lobe atelectasis due to bronchial carcinoma. **A**, Posteroanterior radiograph. **B**, Lateral radiograph. (A metastasis is present in the right eighth rib, and there are multiple old fractures of right ribs.) **C**, CT in a different patient.

and the outline of the posterior half of the right or left hemidiaphragm shadow is lost. Normally, on lateral projection each vertebra appears blacker than the one above as the eye descends through the thorax to the diaphragm. In lower lobe atelectasis the lower vertebrae appear whiter than those higher up (Figs 3.60 and 3.61). With very severe collapse the outline of the ipsilateral hemidiaphragm may once again become visible, because compensatory expansion of the upper and middle lobe brings them into contact with the previously effaced diaphragm (Fig. 3.61). The opacity of the collapsed lobe may be difficult to recognize unless the observer is careful to observe the density of the vertebrae.

The major vascular trunks supplying the lobes are displaced but, more importantly from a diagnostic point of view, they are invisible because they are coursing through an opaque lobe. Therefore, with complete lower lobe collapse, the lower lobe artery and its segmental divisions are displaced and invisible. Careful analysis of the hilum may, however, be needed to recognize this difference because displaced middle or upper lobe trunks may resemble the lower lobe arteries. A similar analysis of the bronchi may be more revealing: in most cases air within the bronchus can be identified coursing into the triangular density of the collapsed lobe.

Bronchial displacement can also be recognized on lateral chest films, but the signs are subtle and demand confident knowledge of the normal anatomy.[48] Normally the central bronchi run in the same direction as the trachea and travel obliquely backward as they descend, so that the right and left major airways are virtually superimposed on one another in a true lateral projection. The only difference is the higher origin of the right upper lobe bronchus and the differences inherent in the right lung having a middle lobe. Lower lobe atelectasis leads

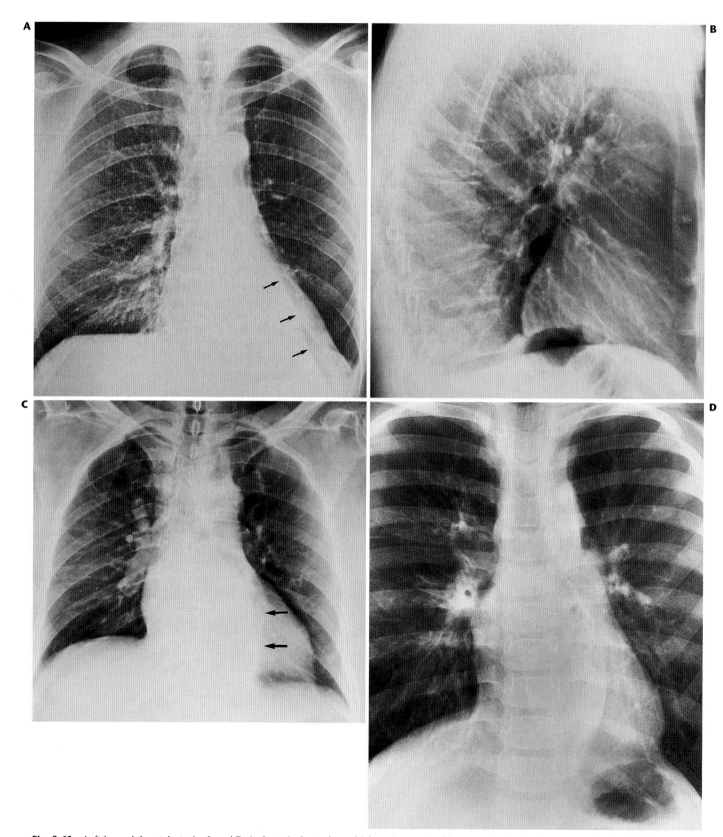

Fig. 3.61   Left lower lobe atelectasis. **A** and **B**, Atelectasis due to bronchial carcinoma. In this example, the displacement of the left hilar vessels is particularly well demonstrated. The left lower lobe artery is invisible because it is within the atelectatic lobe. Note also the splaying of the blood vessels in the over-expanded left upper lobe and the flat waist sign. (Arrows point to the displaced major fissure.) **C**, Very severe atelectasis in which the lobe is no more than a sliver against the mediastinum. The altered configuration of the left hilum is perhaps the most obvious sign. **D**, Atelectasis in a patient with an underdeveloped pulmonary ligament with resultant lack of tethering of the lower lobe to the diaphragm. The collapsed lobe mimics a mediastinal mass. The disposition of the left main bronchus, lack of visibility of left lower lobe artery, and air bronchograms within the opacity indicate the correct diagnosis.

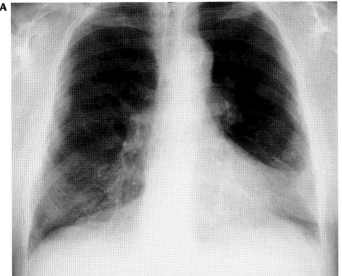

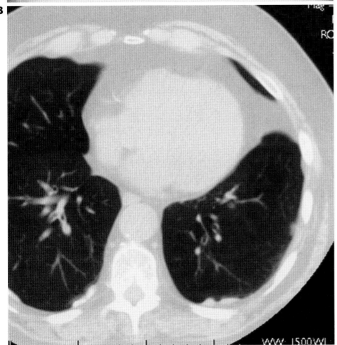

Fig. 3.62 **A,** A large cardiophrenic fat pad, which mimics left lower lobe atelectasis on the posteroanterior chest radiograph. **B,** CT showing the fat pad and the absence of left lower lobe atelectasis.

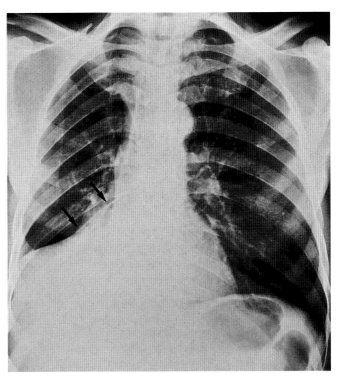

Fig. 3.63 Right lower and right middle lobe atelectasis with partial aeration of the superior segment of the right lower lobe. Arrows point to the displaced major fissures.

to backward displacement of the relevant airways. This displacement is useful in differentiating opacity caused primarily by pleural fluid from that caused by lower lobe collapse. With collapse the bronchi are pulled back, whereas with pleural fluid the bronchi may be pushed forward.[64]

The appearance of the upper mediastinal contours may occasionally be helpful in drawing attention to, or confirming, the possibility of lower lobe atelectasis. Kattan[65] emphasized three signs:

1. The upper triangle sign[66] refers to a low-density, clearly marginated triangular shadow on frontal chest radiographs that resembles right-sided mediastinal widening. It is seen in right lower lobe atelectasis and is caused by

rightward displacement of the anterior junctional tissues of the mediastinum (Fig. 3.64). The appearance superficially resembles right upper lobe atelectasis but should not be confused with it, because the fissural, vascular, and bronchial realignments all point to over-expansion of the right upper lobe rather than to atelectasis.

2. The flat waist sign[67] refers to flattening of the contours of the aortic knob and adjacent main pulmonary artery (Fig. 3.61). It is seen in severe collapse of the left lower lobe and is due to leftward displacement and rotation of the heart. The appearance therefore resembles a shallow right anterior oblique view of the normal mediastinum.

3. The outline of the top of the aortic knob may be obliterated in severe left lower lobe collapse.[65]

At CT,[28,36,37,39,59] an atelectatic lower lobe produces a triangular opacity of soft tissue density in the posterior chest against the spine (Figs 3.60 and 3.65). The major fissure rotates to lie obliquely across the thoracic cavity. The lobe is fixed at the hilum, and the medial basal segment cannot move further back than the attachment of the inferior pulmonary ligament to the mediastinum. In cases where the inferior pulmonary ligament is incomplete, collapse of the basal segments may simulate a mass on CT, just as it may on the plain chest radiograph.[68]

Whole lung atelectasis

Whole lung atelectasis on either side leads to opacity of the whole hemithorax. The signs of compensatory shift are usually

A 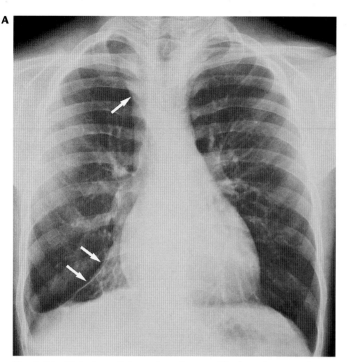 **B**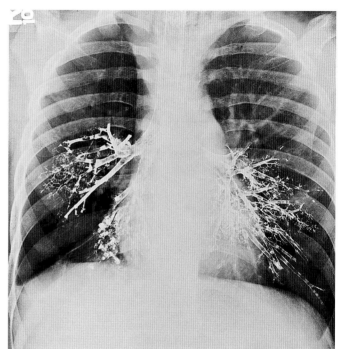

Fig. 3.64 Right lower lobe atelectasis caused by bronchiectasis showing the "upper triangle sign" (upward-pointing arrow). The displaced major fissure (downward-pointing arrows) and the right lower lobe artery entering the atelectatic lobe are well demonstrated. **A**, Posteroanterior radiograph. **B**, Bronchogram showing the arrangement of the bronchi.

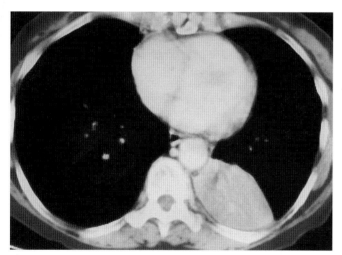

Fig. 3.65 Contrast-enhanced CT of left lower lobe atelectasis.

obvious. Mediastinal shift is invariably present, and herniation of the opposite lung is usually a striking feature (Fig. 3.66).

Combined right upper and middle lobe atelectasis

Because there is no single bronchus to the right upper and middle lobes that does not also supply the right lower lobe, collapse of these two lobes with normal aeration of the lower lobe is unusual. This phenomenon is seen particularly with neoplastic disease, when, for instance, tumor obstructs one bronchus and extends through lung parenchyma or peribronchially to obstruct the other bronchus. The appearances[69,70] are virtually identical to those seen with left upper lobe atelectasis

on both plain chest radiography and CT (Fig. 3.67). Occasionally atelectasis of the right upper lobe alone precisely mimics combined collapse of the right upper and middle lobes.[71]

Combined right lower and middle lobe atelectasis

The combination of right lower and middle lobe atelectasis is seen with obstruction to the bronchus intermedius. The appearances are similar to atelectasis of the right lower lobe alone in both PA and lateral projections except that the abnormal density extends all the way to the lateral costophrenic angle (Fig. 3.68).[34,69] The upper border of the opacity, formed by a combination of the major and minor fissures, can be convex or concave. In either case, the appearances can be confused with subpulmonary pleural effusion. Similarly, on the lateral view the opacity extends from the front to the back of the thorax.[34]

Diagnosing combined middle and lower lobe atelectasis is much easier at CT[36] because the bronchi can be individually identified. It is therefore possible to identify the middle lobe specifically and so diagnose or exclude the presence of combined middle and lower lobe atelectasis.

Distinguishing lower lobe collapse from pleural fluid

Lower lobe atelectasis can be difficult, and sometimes impossible, to distinguish from pleural effusion on conventional PA and lateral radiographs. This diagnostic dilemma is most frequent in postoperative or acutely ill patients and is compounded by the fact that these patients are frequently examined with portable equipment in frontal projection only.

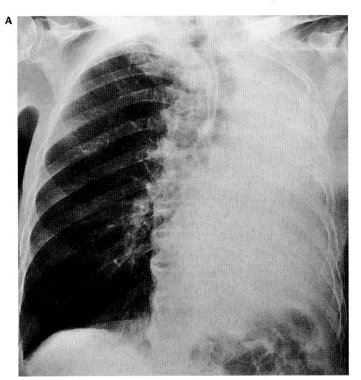

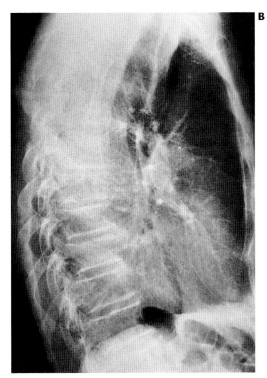

Fig. 3.66   Atelectasis of the left lung. The left lung is opaque, and there is striking shift of the mediastinum. **A**, Posteroanterior view. **B**, Lateral view.

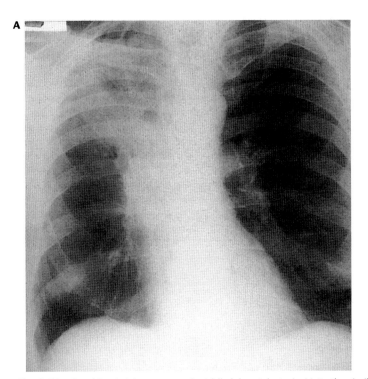

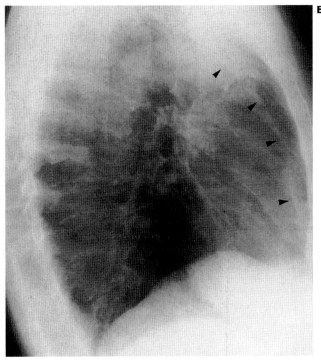

Fig. 3.67   Combined right upper and middle lobe atelectasis. Note the similarity to left upper lobe atelectasis. Arrowheads point to the greatly displaced major fissure. **A**, Posteroanterior view. **B**, Lateral view. (Courtesy of Dr Michael Pearson, London)

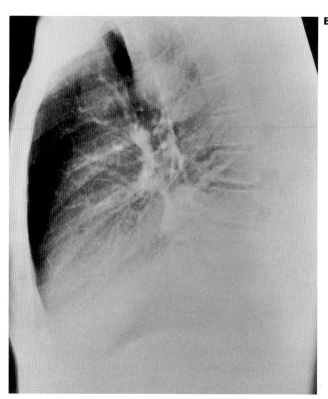

Fig. 3.68 Combined right middle and lower lobe atelectasis. Note the similarity to right lower lobe atelectasis alone, except that the abnormal density extends all the way to the costophrenic angle in the frontal view and from front to back in the lateral view. **A,** Posteroanterior view. **B,** Lateral view.

The diagnosis of lobar atelectasis depends on recognizing shift of structures, particularly the fissures, the hilar blood vessels, and the major bronchi. If the position of the fissures can be confidently established, the diagnosis is easy. If not, attention should be turned to the hila, particularly the position of the lower lobe arteries and bronchi. Two questions should be addressed: (1) do these structures enter the opacity in question, and (2) are they displaced in a direction that suggests collapse? For example, in a patient with basal opacity, if the lower lobe artery is obscured and the lower lobe bronchus runs vertically through the opacity, lower lobe atelectasis should be diagnosed. If, on the other hand, the lower lobe artery is clearly seen lateral to the opacity and the bronchus is not surrounded by the density, the opacity is not the result of lower lobe atelectasis.

Distinguishing between pleural effusion and lobar atelectasis is easy at CT and/or ultrasound (Fig. 3.69). At CT the density of the atelectatic lobe is usually appreciably greater than that of the pleural effusion, particularly if intravenous contrast enhancement is used.[28,39] Also, blood vessels and bronchi can be traced into the compressed lung.

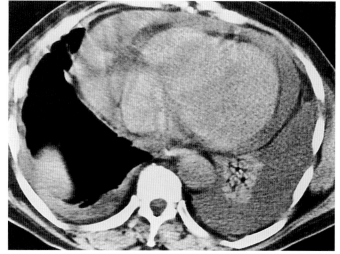

Fig. 3.69 CT of combined pleural effusion and left lower lobe atelectasis. The atelectatic lobe with its air bronchogram is clearly distinguishable from the adjacent left pleural effusion. (The patient, who had small cell carcinoma of the lung, also has extensive mediastinal adenopathy, pericardial effusion, and right pleural effusion.)

Lobar atelectasis due to bronchiectasis

Lobar atelectasis may be the result of bronchiectasis (Fig. 3.70). The loss of volume is due to a combination of multiple occlusions of bronchi beyond subsegmental bronchial divisions. The topic is discussed in more detail on page 89, but the essential feature is lobar atelectasis, the lobe in question often being of strikingly low volume and containing dilated thick-walled bronchi.[28]

Round atelectasis

Round atelectasis, also known as folded lung, Blesovsky syndrome[72] or atelectatic pseudotumor, is a form of chronic atelectasis that resembles a mass, which on plain films can be confused with bronchial carcinoma.[73–75] The process is commonly

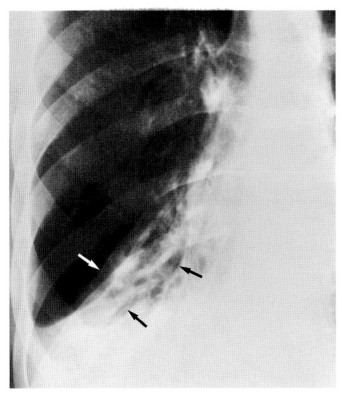

Fig. 3.70 Right lower lobe atelectasis caused by bronchiectasis. Air in the dilated bronchi (black arrows) is an important clue to the cause of the atelectatic lobe. The white arrow points to the displaced major fissure.

encountered in individuals with asbestos-related pleural disease (see p. 456),[76–78] but it has been reported in association with other benign pleural conditions,[79,80] including tuberculosis, other infections, therapeutic pneumothorax, uremic pleuritis,[81] pulmonary infarction, and Dressler syndrome,[82] as well as with idiopathic pleural exudates. It can also be seen in association with malignant mesothelioma.[83]

The mechanism leading to the formation of round atelectasis is uncertain but pleural thickening, usually benign fibrosis, is the common element.[80,84] One suggestion is that a pleural exudate is the initial event and the resulting effusion causes passive atelectasis of the adjacent lung and pleural invagination.[85] The pleural surface of the atelectatic lung may then develop fibrinous adhesions to the adjacent parietal pleura and across any adjacent fissure. As the pleural effusion clears, the atelectatic lung is trapped and folds in on itself. An alternative explanation is that a sheet of pleural fibrosis alone is responsible: as the pleural fibrosis matures, it retracts, causing infolding and atelectasis of the underlying lung.[76,86,87] Probably both mechanisms operate in different patients.[76]

The imaging features on plain films and CT scans are listed in Box 3.5.[78,82,84,88–92] A constant sign is the peripheral location of the opacity based against thickened pleura. Round atelectasis is usually oval or wedge-shaped in configuration and angled with respect to the pleural surface (Fig. 3.71). The top, bottom, and lateral edges of the mass are usually smooth, but the edge pointing to the hilum is often irregular or ill defined and blends with the bronchi and blood vessels that lead into the atelectatic mass. A feature of great diagnostic value, and one that is almost universally present,[82,91] is the distortion and displacement of the blood vessels and bronchi leading to, and immediately adjacent to,

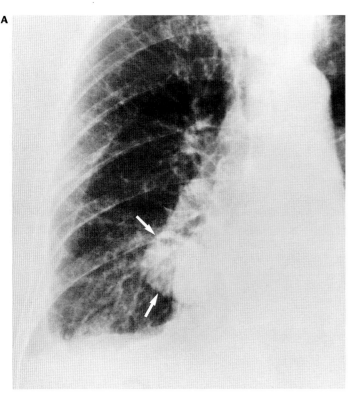
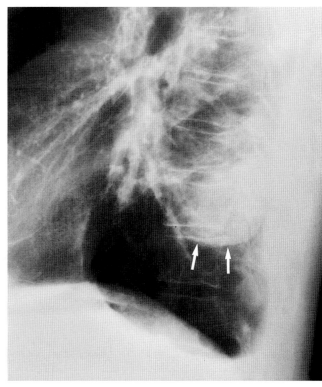

Fig. 3.71 Round atelectasis (arrows) showing the typical features of an oval mass aligned obliquely against pleural thickening along the posterior chest wall. **A**, Posteroanterior radiograph. **B**, Lateral radiograph.

Box 3.5   Imaging features of round atelectasis

Rounded, oval, or wedge-shaped mass
Smooth margin except at site of entry of bronchi and vessels
Convergence of bronchovascular markings
Curvilinear vessels and bronchi entering mass
Subpleural in location
Pleural thickening adjacent to mass
Indistinct margins
Air bronchograms within mass
Loss of volume of affected lobe
Pleural thickening/plaques elsewhere

the area of round atelectasis. The vessels and bronchi appear pulled toward the lesion, are more numerous than normal for that portion of lung, and show a characteristic curvilinear configuration (Fig. 3.72), sometimes referred to as a comet tail sign. Air bronchograms are seen within the opacity at CT in the majority of cases; the thinner the CT section, the more frequently air bronchograms are identified. Calcifications may be seen within the area of rounded atelectasis, and the volume of the affected lobe is reduced. Round atelectasis, like lung cancer and many other

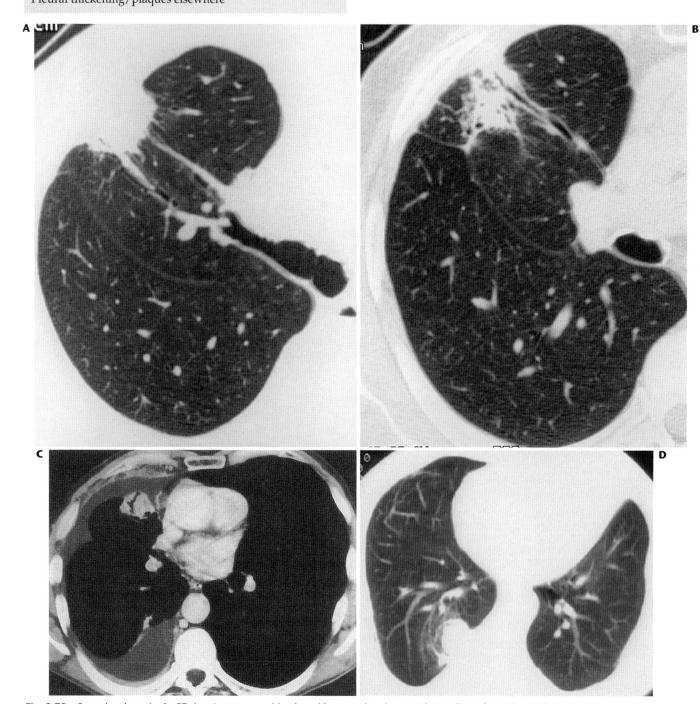

Fig. 3.72   Round atelectasis. **A**, CT showing a mass with a broad base on the pleura and crowding of vessels supplying the lesion. **B**, Adjacent section showing an air bronchogram within the lesion. **C**, Contrast-enhanced CT in another patient showing contrast enhancement and air bronchograms. **D**, CT showing distortion of vessels entering the "mass".

pathologic conditions, enhances after intravenous injection of contrast agent; contrast enhancement is therefore of little diagnostic value.[93] Although usually static, round atelectasis may grow,[94] or shrink,[85] or even on occasion resolve spontaneously.[76,81]

CT (Fig. 3.72) shows all the features to advantage and may show more extensive pleural disease than can be appreciated on plain films. The CT findings may be definitive, so further investigation to exclude carcinoma, the major differential diagnosis, as the cause of the mass is unnecessary.

Ultrasound can show a pleurally based mass with thickening of the adjacent pleura and extrapleural fat. A highly echogenic line extending from the pleural surface into the mass, believed to correspond to scarred invaginated pleura, is a frequent ultrasound feature.[95]

MRI can show the curving vessels to advantage, particularly when a sagittal imaging plane is used, and low-intensity lines can be seen at MRI within the folded lung, thought to be due to thickened invaginated pleura.[84,96,97] Round atelectasis shows signal that is higher than muscle and lower than fat on T1-weighted sequences and similar to or lower than fat on T2-weighted sequences; homogeneous enhancement occurs after intravenous contrast administration.[97] Round atelectasis, unlike most lung carcinomas of similar size, is not metabolically active on ^{18}F-fluoro-deoxyglucose PET scanning.[98]

SOLITARY PULMONARY NODULE/MASS

The term "pulmonary mass" refers to an essentially spherical opacity with a well-defined edge. Although the Fleischner Society[5] and others use the word "nodule" for a lesion of up to 3 cm in diameter and "mass" for a lesion greater than 3 cm in diameter, the two terms are used interchangeably in this book. (The multiple 2–5 mm nodules seen with widespread nodular or miliary shadowing are a separate category and are discussed in the section Widespread Nodular, Reticulonodular, and Honeycomb Shadowing later in this chapter.)

The first step in the work-up of a solitary pulmonary nodule (SPN) is to ensure that the nodule is in fact solitary and truly arises in the lung parenchyma and is not merely callus around a rib fracture, a hypertrophied costochondral junction (Fig. 3.73), an exostosis arising from a rib, a pleural nodule or plaque, or a skin nodule or other extrathoracic opacity projected over the lung on a chest radiograph.

The possible diagnoses of an SPN seen on plain chest radiography or CT are numerous (see Box 3.6 and Fig. 3.74), but over 95% fall into one of three groups:

1. Malignant neoplasm, either primary or metastatic
2. Infectious granulomas, either tuberculous or fungal
3. Benign tumors, notably hamartomas.

The subsequent steps are highly dependent on the size of the nodule, the age of the patient, and certain clinical features, e.g. fever, or a known primary tumor with a propensity to metastasize to the lungs. A solitary nodule larger than 10 mm in diameter is sufficiently likely to be a primary lung cancer that a definitive diagnosis is required without undue delay, whereas a 6 mm nodule discovered incidentally or on screening CT is up to 30 times more likely to be benign than malignant. Since, for practical purposes, the only lung cancers that can be recognized on plain chest radiographs as a discrete SPN are 10 mm or greater in diameter, the diagnostic work-up for SPNs recognized

---

Box 3.6   Differential diagnosis of a solitary pulmonary nodule or mass identified on chest radiography

Neoplastic
Bronchial carcinoma*
Metastasis*
Pulmonary lymphoma*
Pulmonary carcinoid*
Atypical adenomatous hyperplasia
Hamartoma
Connective tissue and neural tumors, e.g. lipoma, fibroma, chondroma, neurofibroma, blastoma,* sarcoma

Inflammatory
Infective
Granuloma,* e.g. tuberculosis, histoplasmosis, cryptococcosis, blastomycosis, coccidioidomycosis, nocardiosis
Round pneumonia, acute or chronic*
Lung abscess*
Septic emboli*
Hydatid cyst*
Dirofilariasis
Noninfective
Rheumatoid arthritis*
Wegener granulomatosis*
Lymphomatoid granulomatosis*
Sarcoidosis*
Necrotizing sarcoidosis*
Lipoid pneumonia
Behçet disease*

Congenital
Arteriovenous malformation
Sequestration*
Lung cyst*
Bronchial atresia with mucoid impaction

Miscellaneous
Organizing pneumonia
Pulmonary infarct*
Round atelectasis
Intrapulmonary lymph node
Progressive massive fibrosis*
Mucoid impaction*
Hematoma*
Amyloidosis*
Pulmonary artery aneurysm or venous varix
First costochondral junction

Mimics of solitary pulmonary nodule
External object (e.g. nipple, skin nodule)
Bone island in rib
Healing rib fracture
Pleural plaque
Loculated pleural fluid

* May cavitate

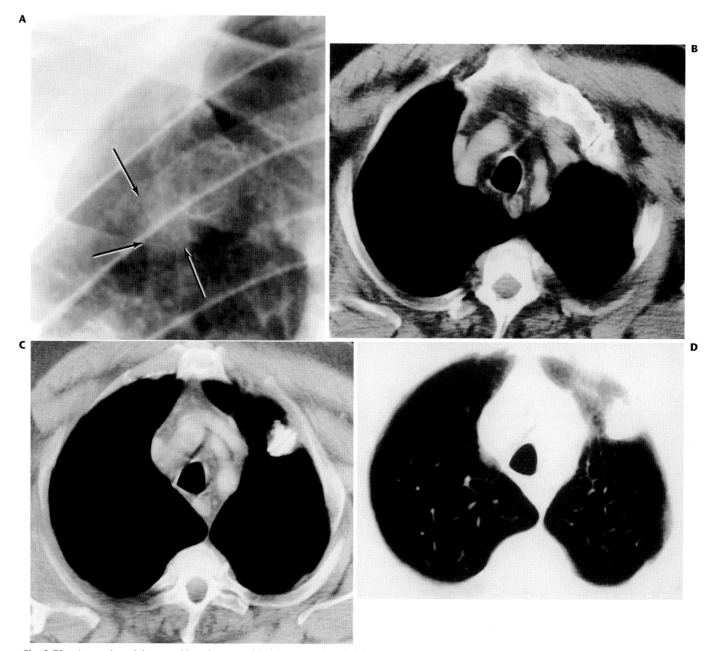

Fig. 3.73 A pseudonodule caused by a hypertrophied first costochondral junction projecting into the lung. **A**, Chest radiograph showing how closely a carcinoma of the lung can be simulated. **B**, CT (in another patient) showing the costochondral junction. **C** and **D**, CT sections show how the downward-projecting costochondral junction simulates a solitary pulmonary nodule.

on plain films is different to that for nodules less than 10 mm found only on CT. (The approach to SPNs detected only on CT is discussed in the section on CT screening for lung cancer in Chapter 13, p. 824.)

Patients with SPN are generally divided into two groups: those in whom malignant neoplasm is either unlikely or impossible; and those in whom malignancy remains a serious consideration.

If there is no known extrathoracic primary tumor, the problem usually centers on deciding whether or not the patient has a primary malignant neoplasm of the lung, notably bronchial carcinoma. In one large multicenter series of chest radiographs,[99] only 3 of 877 resected SPNs were metastases, and in

another study of 705 patients without a known primary tumor,[100] only one nodule was a metastasis. If a patient has a known extrathoracic malignant neoplasm and a solitary pulmonary nodule then the likelihood of a metastasis depends on the patient's age and the site of origin of the extrathoracic neoplasm. In their analysis of 149 patients, Quint et al[101] found that patients with carcinomas of the head and neck, bladder, breast, cervix, bile ducts, esophagus, ovary, prostate, or stomach, in whom a solitary pulmonary nodule was discovered, were more likely to have primary lung carcinoma than metastasis. Patients with carcinomas of the salivary glands, adrenals, colon, kidney, thyroid, thymus or uterus had fairly even odds, and patients with melanoma, sarcoma, or testicular cancer were

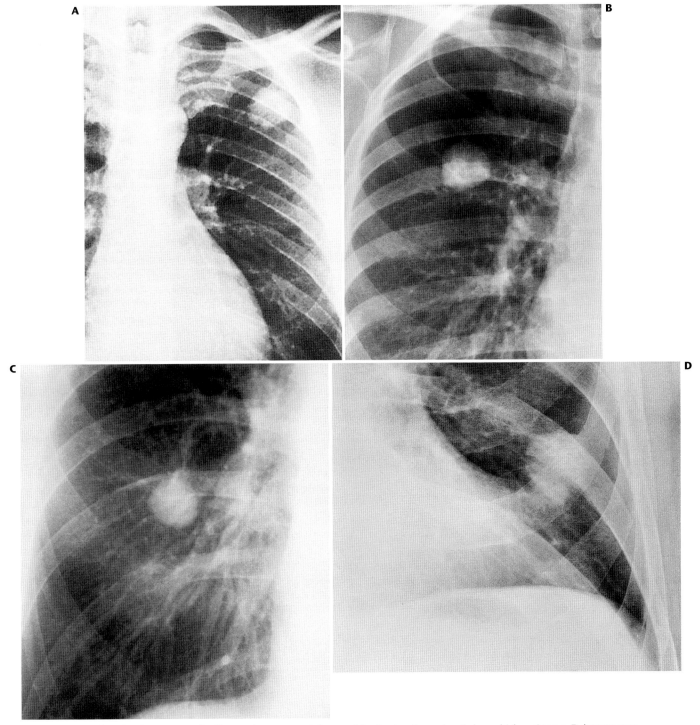

Fig. 3.74 Examples of various causes of solitary pulmonary nodules on plain chest radiography: **A**, bronchial carcinoma; **B**, hamartoma; **C**, bronchial carcinoid; **D**, pulmonary infarct.

more likely to have a solitary metastasis than bronchial carcinoma.

Morphologic features such as size, shape, and cavitation, which can be diagnostically helpful, are discussed later, but it must be emphasized that no radiologic feature is entirely specific for lung carcinoma (or other primary malignant tumors). There are, however, four imaging observations that exclude the diagnosis with reasonable certainty: (1) the detection of a benign pattern of calcification; (2) a rate of growth that is either too slow or too fast for the nodule to be primary lung cancer; (3) a specific shape indicating a benign process; and (4) unequivocal evidence on previous examinations that the nodule is the end stage of a previous benign process such as infarction or granulomatous infection.[102]

Calcification

Various types of calcification may be identified within an SPN: concentric, laminated, punctate, cloud-like, and uniform (homogeneous).

Concentric (laminated) calcification is virtually specific to tuberculous or fungal granulomas (Fig. 3.75) and *popcorn calcifications*, which are randomly distributed, often overlapping, small rings of calcification, are seen only when there is cartilage in the nodule, a feature specific to hamartoma and cartilage tumors (Fig. 3.76). *Punctate calcification* occurs in a variety of benign and malignant lesions: granuloma, hamartoma, amyloidoma, carcinoid, and metastases, particularly osteosarcoma. Punctate calcification is rare in bronchial carcinoma unless the tumor engulfs a preexisting calcified granuloma (Fig. 3.77), in which case the calcification is rarely randomly distributed or at the center of the nodule. The presence of one or more punctate calcifications arranged in an eccentric group and widespread *cloud-like calcification* of a nodule substantially reduces the probability of bronchial carcinoma, particularly if the calcification is present in sufficient quantities to be visible on plain chest radiographs, although, as discussed below, it does not exclude the diagnosis entirely. *Uniform calcification* of an SPN (Fig. 3.78) is virtually diagnostic of a calcified granuloma and excludes the diagnosis of bronchial carcinoma.

Calcification is better seen on plain chest radiographs taken with low kilovoltage than high kilovoltage. Attempts to analyze nodules using single- or dual-energy kilovoltage techniques with chest radiography and CT remain experimental.[103–105]

CT, because of its superb density discrimination, is far superior to plain chest radiography for the detection of calcification in an SPN[106] (Fig. 3.79). Care must, however, be taken not to misdiagnose artifactual high density as calcification at the edge of smaller nodules on high-spatial-frequency reconstruction algorithms (the algorithm used for HRCT).[107]

Siegelman and co-workers[108] were the first to use CT to identify nodules as benign by determining their CT density. They found that SPNs with a representative CT number of above 164 HU were benign. Proto and Thomas,[109] using a different scanner, confirmed this observation but recommended 200 HU as the cut-off point above which the diagnosis of a benign lesion could be made. Assessments of density are made directly on an imaging console. If the high density is either uniformly distributed or clearly lies centrally within the nodule, the nodule is unlikely to be a bronchial carcinoma, but as with plain film and conventional tomographic evaluation, CT scans may show calcification within a bronchial carcinoma if the tumor engulfs a preexisting calcified granulomatous lesion.[109,110] There are also well-documented reports of amorphous calcification in bronchial carcinoma (Fig. 3.80 and see Fig. 13.7, p. 791).[111–117] It has been shown[111,114] that 6–7% of bronchial carcinomas show calcification of some type or another within the tumor mass at CT. To avoid misdiagnosing a benign lesion in those cases of carcinoma that show calcification, the radiologist should consider a high-density lesion benign only if the edge of the nodule is smooth.[110,111] Also, evaluation of a nodule by CT scanning rarely yields a confident diagnosis of benign disease if the nodule is larger than 3 cm. CT densitometry is therefore not recommended for lesions greater than 3 cm in diameter or for nodules with irregular or spiculated borders,[111] nor is it recommended in patients with nodules that are known to be increasing in size at a rate compatible with bronchial carcinoma. Such nodules

should not be automatically regarded as benign just because they show calcification.

Accurate detection of diffuse calcification of a nodule at CT densitometry depends on obtaining a section through the equator of the nodule and ensuring the measurements are not artefactually reduced because air in the adjacent lung is included in the section of the nodule. This is not possible with very small nodules detected at routine 7 or 10 mm section CT. It has been suggested, however, that it is possible to detect diffuse calcification in 3–7 mm nodules lying within thick sections even when the measured CT density is well below 200 HU. Yankelevitz and Henschke[118] showed in a phantom study that 3–7 mm individual nodules that are still visible on routine mediastinal window and level settings on 10 mm thick sections are probably diffusely calcified and therefore benign. How this suggestion translates to clinical practice remains to be seen.

Even with good technique and awareness of pitfalls, however, some malignant nodules will be misdiagnosed as benign based on CT densitometry: in the series of Swensen and associates at least 10 of the 85 nodules diagnosed as benign by nodule densitometry proved to be malignant.[117]

Zerhouni and associates[111,119] designed a reference phantom that simulated the shape, dimensions, and density of the thorax at multiple levels, in order to replicate the conditions under which an SPN was measured, and provide a standard for density regardless of equipment- or patient-related variations. The patient's nodule was considered to be above the critical density level if more than 10% of the voxels in the patient nodule were higher in density than in the phantom nodule. The phantom technique has not, however, remained in general use.

Fat density within a nodule

Unequivocal demonstration of fat within a solitary pulmonary nodule is almost completely specific for hamartoma (Fig. 3.81). Lipoid pneumonia and metastatic liposarcoma are very rare alternatives.[120] When using CT, care must be taken not to include adjacent aerated lung in the section, because the density reading may then be a mixture of air and cancer and lie within the fat range.

Ground-glass opacity

A number of different pathologic processes can give rise to a solitary small round area of pure ground-glass opacity (Fig. 3.82): a small area of focal pulmonary scarring; a patch of pneumonia; atypical adenomatous hyperplasia; bronchioloalveolar carcinoma; and invasive adenocarcinoma. The probability of invasive adenocarcinoma for a lesion composed entirely of ground-glass opacity under 1 cm in diameter is very low.[121] A small nodule of ground-glass opacity with a central area composed of standard soft tissue density is, however, likely to be a lung cancer, sometimes bronchioloalveolar carcinoma but often invasive adenocarcinoma.[122]

Contrast enhancement

Solitary pulmonary nodules caused by malignant neoplasm show a greater degree of contrast enhancement with iodinated

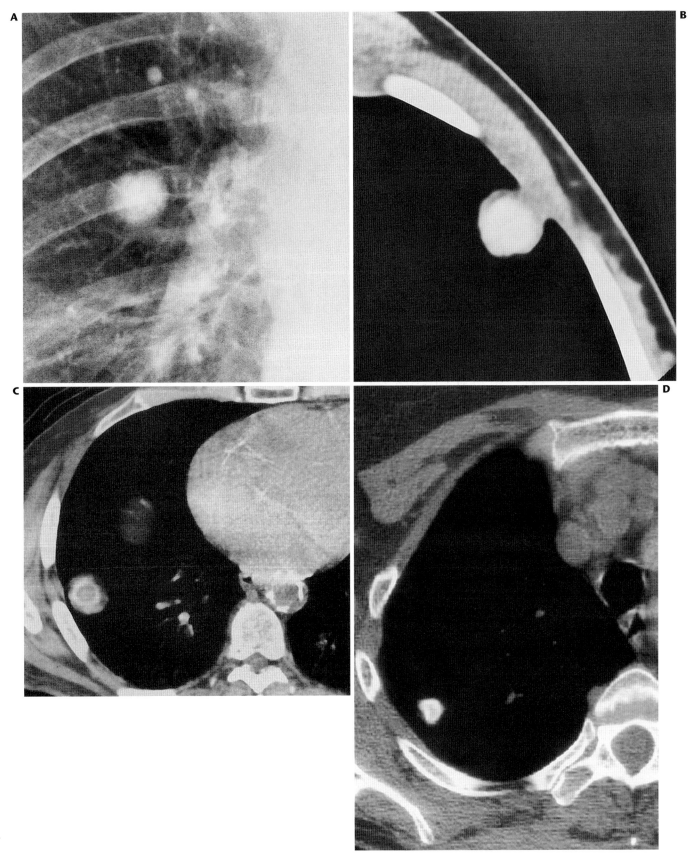

Fig. 3.75 Concentric calcification in fungal and tuberculous granulomas. **A**, A histoplasmoma on chest radiography showing laminated concentric calcification. **B**, A histoplasmoma on CT showing homogeneous concentric calcification. **C**, A histoplasmoma on CT showing laminated concentric calcification. **D**, A tuberculoma on CT showing laminated concentric calcification.

A

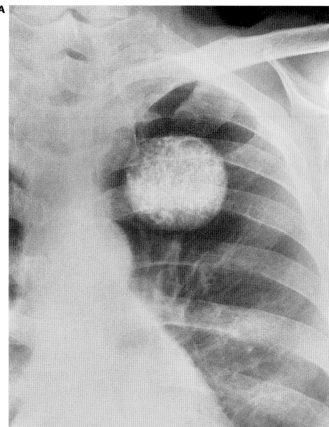

B

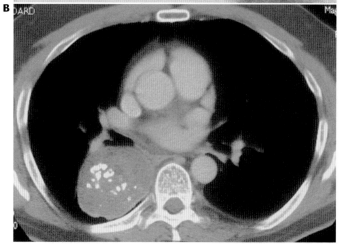

Fig. 3.76 Popcorn calcifications in pulmonary hamartoma: **A**, on chest radiography; **B**, on CT.

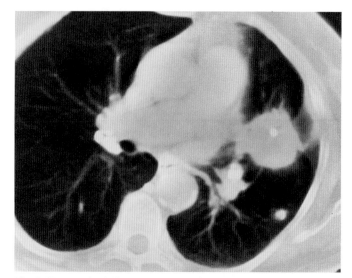

Fig. 3.77 Focal calcification in a granuloma engulfed by a bronchial adenocarcinoma. Note another similar granuloma in the lung behind the tumor and widespread calcification in hilar lymph nodes.

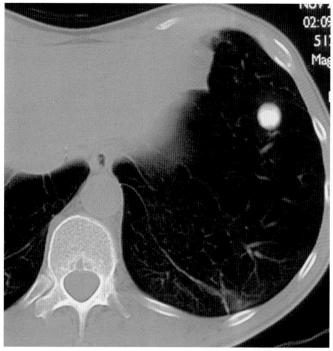

Fig. 3.78 Uniform calcification in a tuberculoma shown by CT.

contrast media than benign nodules. The basis of this enhancement is likely to be the presence of angiogenesis.[123] Littleton and co-workers[124] first demonstrated contrast enhancement using very high-quality conventional tomography together with film densitometry. Swensen et al in a prospective[125] and, subsequently, in a multicenter study[126] of contrast-enhanced CT showed that enhancement of an SPN can be a good predictor of lung carcinoma, and failure to enhance above a certain level can be a good predictor of a benign lesion. However, careful attention to technique and interpretation is required. The prospective study[126] demonstrated that all but one of 44 primary lung

carcinomas showed at least a 20 HU increase in density during dynamic contrast enhancement, whereas 15 of 56 benign lesions failed to enhance to this degree (sensitivity 98%, specificity 73%, positive predictive value 77%, negative predictive value 98%). A multicenter study was designed to test the hypothesis that SPNs that enhance less than 15 HU on all the images obtained at 1, 2, 3, and 4 minutes are benign. It found that only 4 out of 171 malignant SPNs showed less than 15 HU enhancement on all these images (i.e. sensitivity 98%). Sensitivity of 100% for diagnosing malignancy was achieved if the threshold was reduced to <10 HU enhancement. It is important to emphasize

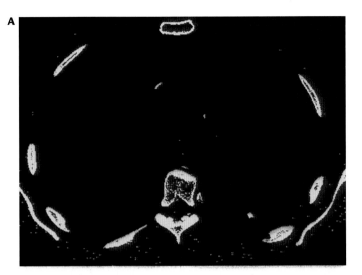

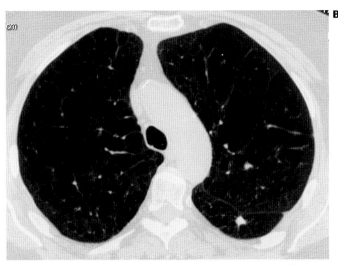

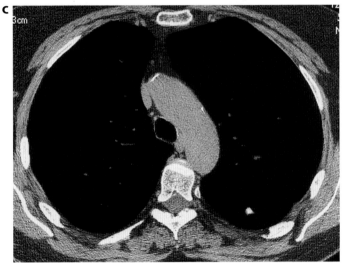

Fig. 3.79   A simple visual method of CT densitometry. **A**, By viewing the nodule at a window width (WW) of 1 HU and a window level (WL) of 200 HU, it is possible to see that over one-third of the area of the nodule on this section is heavily and uniformly calcified, and lung cancer for practical purposes is ruled out. **B**, The same lesion showing a nodule that could be a bronchial carcinoma if viewed only on a standard lung window (WW 1000, WL –700). **C**, The standard mediastinal window (WW 350, WL 35) also shows that on visual grounds the nodule is of calcific density.

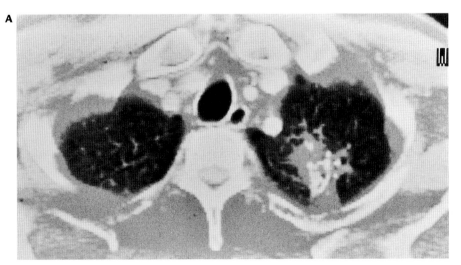

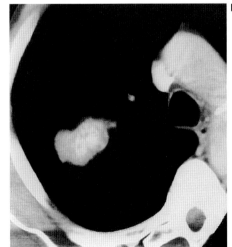

Fig. 3.80   Calcification in a primary carcinoma of lung. **A**, Adenocarcinoma: the punctate, conglomerate calcification in this case proved to be necrotic foci of tumor (courtesy of Dr John Pitman, Williamsburg, Va.). **B**, Small cell carcinoma, showing extensive punctate cloud-like calcification.

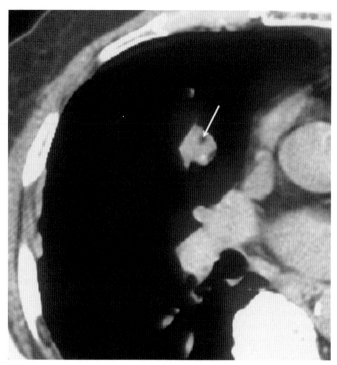

Fig. 3.81   Fat within a hamartoma (arrow).

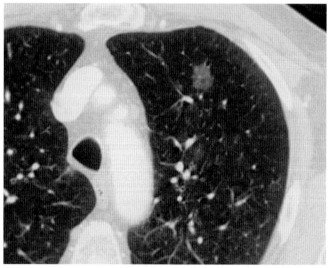

Fig. 3.82   Rounded solitary ground-glass opacity. The nature of this nodule was never confirmed. It did not grow and is assumed to be benign, possibly atypical adenomatous hyperplasia.

that the enhancement must be measured at each of 1, 2, 3, and 4 minutes, and the contrast medium dose must be adequate (the doses used in the multicenter study were adjusted for the weight of the patient with 30 grams of iodine [100 ml] being given for 72 kg patients), because many lung cancers showed enhancement of <10 HU on at least one of these observations. Inevitably, a conservative figure for enhancement (in order to achieve 100% sensitivity) means that benign lesions will also be classified as positive. Only 107 of 185 benign lesions showed <15 HU enhancement (specificity 58%) and 93 showed <10 HU enhancement (specificity 50%).

Zhang et al[127] performed dynamic contrast-enhanced CT in 65 patients with an SPN of less than 3 cm in diameter. In their series, peak enhancement almost always occurred in the first minute (in Swensen's series enhancement was more uniform throughout the 4 minutes of measurement). They showed that inflammatory SPNs have similar enhancement characteristics to malignant tumors, but confirmed Swensen's observation that other benign lesions show significantly slower and less marked enhancement. Other, previous studies have shown sensitivities of 95% to 100% for the diagnosis of malignancy based on contrast enhancement of an SPN.[128,129]

The potential usefulness of this technique now appears to be the 95% or greater predictive value for benignity in nodules, 5 mm or greater in diameter, that fail to enhance by more than 15 HU (Fig. 3.83), with the predictive values at, or approaching, 100% if more conservative criteria for enhancement are used.

Noncalcified tuberculous granulomas may show peripheral ring enhancement or curvilinear central enhancement, a feature that may help diagnostically.[130] The nonenhanced portions of the nodules correspond to caseous necrosis.

Nodules due to lung carcinoma also show enhancement with gadolinium DTPA at MRI. The difference between benign and malignant lesions is best shown by dynamic enhancement during the transit of the bolus of contrast material.[131,132] The number of patients studied so far is too small to draw conclusions about the utility of the technique in clinical practice. Preliminary reports on the use of Gd-DTPA enhanced MRI noted that tuberculomas tend to show ring enhancement of their capsule with slight or no enhancement of the caseous center, whereas lung cancers below 3 cm in diameter show homogeneous enhancement, similar to that observed with contrast-enhanced CT.[133–135]

Radionuclide imaging/PET

[18]F-fluoro-deoxyglucose PET imaging and SPECT imaging using depreotide (a somatostatin analog labeled with technetium-99m)[136,137] can be used to characterize SPNs as either benign or malignant. Lung cancer also concentrates a variety of other radionuclides including gallium-67, thallium-201, ^{99m}Tc-DMSA,[138] MIBI,[139] and sestamibi.[140]

[18]F-fluoro-deoxyglucose (FDG), a glucose analog with ^{18}F substituted for one of the hydroxy groups, is the most widely used PET agent.[141–153] It is a marker for glucose metabolism which, after phosphorylation, is not metabolized further but remains trapped within tumor cells thus making it a suitable imaging agent (Fig. 3.84). FDG uptake is proportional to the metabolic rate of the cells which take up glucose and correlates with tumor aggressiveness and tumor growth rates.[154,155]

The sensitivity and specificity of FDG PET for diagnosing an SPN as a lung cancer depend on the equipment and technique used for imaging and the criteria chosen for a positive result. Dedicated PET scanners can identify lung cancers as small as 5 mm.[153] Gamma camera-based PET systems can produce acceptable sensitivity,[156,157] but do not have quite as good specificity or resolution.[158,159]

The criterion for a positive scan can be based on standardized uptake value (SUV) in which the uptake of tracer by the tumor is quantified and the ratio of the activity per estimated tumor volume is compared to the activity administered to the patient (corrected for lean body mass). Some authors have considered

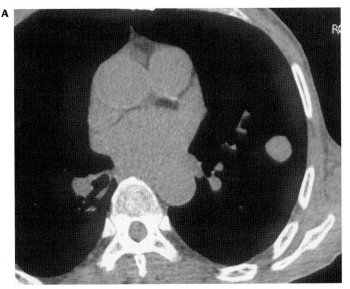
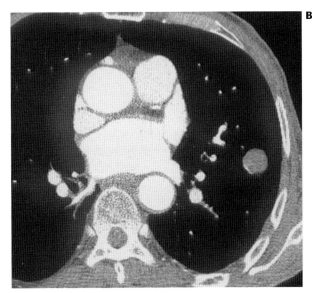

Fig. 3.83 A benign nodule showing less than 15 HU of contrast enhancement. This nodule was stable in size during more than 5 years of observation. **A**, Pre-contrast scan. **B**, Following a 100 ml bolus of intravenous contrast.

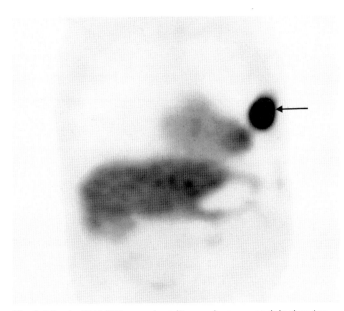

Fig. 3.84 An FDG PET scan of a solitary pulmonary nodule showing intense uptake of the FDG in the nodule (arrow) which was, as expected, a bronchial carcinoma. (Courtesy of Ms Tiba Seear, Alliance Medical, London)

SUVs of 2.5 or greater to indicate malignancy, and others have used slightly different values.[151,160,161] Measuring the SUV at two different times to observe the change in uptake over time increased the accuracy of diagnosis in one report.[150] A visual assessment, whereby the scan is regarded as positive if the activity in the nodule is greater than the activity in the mediastinum, can also be used.[153] A recent comprehensive analysis of the English language literature showed an average sensitivity for diagnosing malignancy of 95.9%, an average specificity of 74.1%, with positive and negative predictive values from pooled data of 92.6% and 87.0% respectively.[161] Virtually identical results were obtained in a meta-analysis of FDG imaging, combining

the results from both dedicated PET scanners and modified gamma cameras in coincidence mode, with a sensitivity of 96.8% and a specificity of 77.8%.[162] Marom et al[153] reviewed the PET images in 192 histologically proven T1 lung cancers (tumors up to 3 cm in diameter): 95% showed increased FDG or PET.

In practice, therefore, when PET is negative, the probability that an SPN is malignant is low. False negative results occur with tumors less than 1 cm in diameter and, rarely, with low-grade malignancies such as slow-growing lung cancers, notably bronchioloalveolar carcinoma,[163] and carcinoid tumors, and it would appear that lung cancers with a negative PET result are less aggressive and have a better survival than the average lung cancer. In the series of T1 lung cancers reported by Marom et al, for instance, of the 9 tumors that were PET negative, 5 were either bronchioloalveolar carcinoma or carcinoid, and the 9 patients who were PET negative had a significantly better 5-year survival.[153] The good survival of PET-negative patients, implying slower growing tumors, led the authors to suggest that it may be acceptable to follow up PET-negative SPNs >5 mm in diameter with conventional imaging. An uncommon cause for false negative FDG PET studies is competitive inhibition from hyperglycemia. Diabetic control should, therefore, be optimized and serum glucose values checked at the time of examination.[164]

Active infections or other inflammatory lesions, notably tuberculous granulomas, coccidioidomycosis, aspergillosis, rheumatoid nodules, and recent surgical wounds can show substantial uptake of FDG[161,164–166] and are responsible for the majority of false positive interpretations of lung cancer for nodules that prove to be benign.

FDG PET is a very expensive technique and availability and access are currently limited, but the test result can have a major impact on the likelihood of an SPN being or not being a lung cancer compared with the standard analyses based on CT and the plain chest radiograph.[167] A number of cost–benefit analyses have been performed. Gambhir et al found that the most cost-effective strategy was a combination of CT and PET for SPNs with a pre-test probability of malignancy between 12% and

69%.[168] Above 69% CT alone was a more cost-effective approach, and below 12% follow up to assess growth was more cost-effective.

Depreotide complexed with ^{99m}Tc can be used as a radio-nuclide to diagnose malignant tumors. Depreotide is a somato-statin analog that binds avidly to lung cancers. It has the advantage that SPECT with standard gamma cameras can be used to image ^{99m}Tc depreotide.[136,169] In a large multicenter study[137] of 114 indeterminate focal lung lesions, 85 of the 88 patients with malignant neoplasms had a positive ^{99m}Tc depreo-tide scintigram (sensitivity 97%), a result that compares reasonably favorably with FDG PET.

Rate of growth

Bronchial carcinomas usually take between 1 and 18 months to double in volume (Fig. 3.85), the average time being 4.2 to 7.3 months, depending on cell type.[170–177] A few take as long as 24 months or very occasionally even longer, and a few double their volume in under a month. Therefore doubling times faster than 1 month or slower than 18 months make bronchial carci-noma unlikely but do not exclude the diagnosis completely (Fig. 3.86). (An increase in diameter of 26% corresponds to a doubling of volume.)

Volume doubling times faster than 1 month suggest infec-tion,[178] infarction,[178] aggressive lymphoma,[179] or a fast-growing metastasis from tumors such as germ cell tumor and certain sarcomas.[180] Doubling times slower than 18 months suggest processes such as granuloma, hamartoma, bronchial carcinoid,

and round atelectasis. A practical guideline in common use is that if a nodule becomes smaller or has remained the same size over a period of 2 years, it is so likely to be benign that follow up is a reasonable course of action. If growth occurs during follow up, the nodule should be resected.[181] One point to bear in mind is that primary lung tumors close to 1 cm are usually invisible on plain chest radiographs, so that it is not possible to calculate an accurate growth rate for small nodules that have developed in a part of the lung that was previously normal on plain films.

Patients whose SPN is 10 mm or greater in diameter with a rate of growth that is either indeterminate or in keeping with bronchial carcinoma, who do not have an extrathoracic primary tumor, and who do not show a benign pattern of calcification in the nodule form a discrete group. Based on several large series,[99,100,182–184] between 25% and 50% of such cases in patients above 35 years of age prove to be bronchial carcinoma, with the remainder composed of the various lesions listed in Box 3.6. The precise incidence varies greatly according to geography. The proportion is higher in Europe than in the United States because of the virtual absence of fungal granulomas. (Nodules less than 10 mm in diameter discovered on CT are considered separately in the section on Screening for Lung Cancer Using Low dose CT, p. 823.)

Size and shape

An SPN due to lung cancer can be any size, but those less than 9 mm in diameter are virtually never visible on plain chest

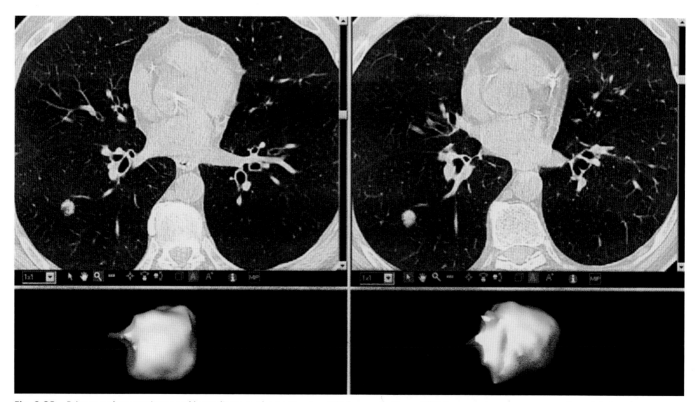

Fig. 3.85 Primary adenocarcinoma of lung discovered on screening CT demonstrating a 33% increase in volume over a 6-week interval, corresponding to a volume doubling time of just under 4 months. (Courtesy of Dr Mary Roddie, Medicsight, London)

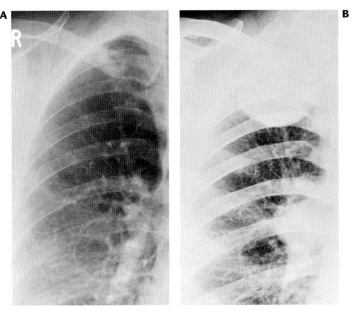

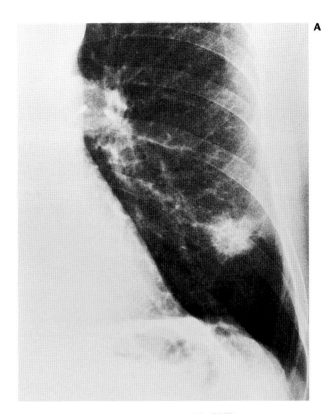

Fig. 3.86 **A** and **B**, Unusually rapid growth of a primary large cell carcinoma of lung. The two views were taken 2 months apart.

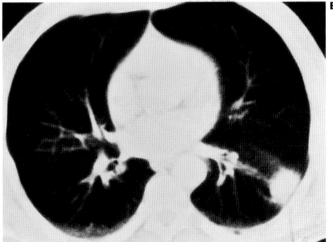

Fig. 3.87 Organizing pneumonia showing **A**, irregular edges on chest radiograph and **B**, nodular shape on CT. The lesion was removed surgically because it was believed to be a bronchial carcinoma preoperatively.

radiographs. A well-defined nodule of smaller size that is clearly seen on plain radiographs is likely to be calcified and is, therefore, likely to be benign. An SPN below 1 cm in size is readily detected at CT (see section on Screening for Lung Cancer Using Low dose CT, p. 823). When the nodule is between 1 cm and 3 cm in diameter, there is no diagnosis in Box 3.6 that can be excluded on the basis of size alone. Above 3 cm the probabilities begin to change dramatically. Most solitary nodules larger than 3 cm in diameter are bronchial carcinoma. With few exceptions, SPNs above this size that are not primary or metastatic carcinoma prove to be lung abscess, Wegener granulomatosis, lymphoma, round pneumonia, round atelectasis or hydatid cyst. The first three resemble one another and may be indistinguishable from bronchial carcinoma. The latter three, however, often show characteristics that permit a specific diagnosis to be made.

There is substantial discussion in the literature over how much attention should be paid to the shape of nodule when trying to determine the nature of an SPN. Good,[185] referring to plain chest radiographs and plain film tomography, believed that calcification and lack of growth were the only important factors, and many authors have subsequently agreed. However, certain shapes, particularly with CT[110] and HRCT, provide important diagnostic information and, in practice, shape is often used to make management decisions.

A very irregular edge makes bronchial carcinoma highly probable,[186] and a corona radiata, the appearance of numerous strands radiating into the surrounding lung, is almost specific for bronchial carcinoma.[182,187] Exceptions do exist, however. For example, infectious granulomas and other chronic inflammatory lesions, notably organizing pneumonia, may occasionally have a very irregular edge (Fig. 3.87) and may even show a corona radiata.[187,188]

Lobulation and notching, signs that indicate uneven growth, are seen with almost all the diagnostic possibilities, but the more pronounced these two signs are, the more likely it is that the lesion is a bronchogenic carcinoma. A well-defined, smooth,

non-lobulated edge is most compatible with hamartoma, granuloma, and metastasis. It is rarely seen in patients with bronchial carcinoma.[187]

If the opacity is composed of one or more narrow linear shadows (Fig. 3.88) without focal nodularity, the chances of bronchial carcinoma are so low that a benign cause can be assumed and follow up is the only recommendation.[182]

The presence of a pleuropulmonary tail associated with a peripherally located nodule is not helpful in the differential diagnosis of an SPN. Much has been written about the "tail" sign because at one time it was believed to be of potential diagnostic value. However, it turns out that the sign is seen with

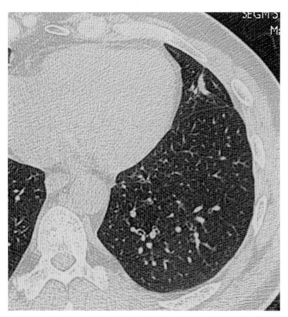

Fig. 3.88 HRCT showing that an abnormal density that looked like a nodule is in fact made up of clear-cut linear components with no nodular elements. The lesion is therefore benign and likely to be a scar or a small area of atelectasis.

a variety of lesions, both malignant and benign, particularly granulomas.[186,187,189–191]

The precise relationship between an SPN and the adjacent pulmonary vessels may prove helpful when deciding the nature of the nodule. The sign known as the "feeding vessel sign" can be used to suggest a diagnosis of hematogenous metastasis.[192] The sign refers to a small pulmonary artery shown by CT to lead directly to a nodule. Similarly, Mori and associates,[193] using multiplanar CT reconstructions, found that involvement of a pulmonary vein was a feature of lung cancer and infrequent in non-neoplastic lesions.

Air bronchograms and bubble-like lucencies

The presence of air bronchograms visible within an SPN on chest radiography makes lung carcinoma (other than bronchioloalveolar carcinoma) or metastasis an unlikely diagnosis. They may be seen in bronchioloalveolar carcinoma and lymphoma, as well as in round pneumonia and round atelectasis. Air bronchograms are, however, seen with some frequency in primary bronchial carcinoma on CT, particularly HRCT.

Bubble-like low-attenuation areas, similar to air bronchograms but more spherical in configuration (Fig. 3.89), are not uncommon in adenocarcinomas on CT and HRCT, particularly bronchioloalveolar carcinomas.[186,194,195] These lucencies are due to patent small bronchi within the nodule or to lepidic growth of tumor around alveolar walls. Another valuable sign is the "positive bronchus sign",[196] originally described to predict the likelihood of obtaining a positive transbronchial biopsy diagnosis of bronchial carcinoma.[197] The sign refers to a patent bronchus entering the nodule – in effect a variation of the air bronchogram sign in which tissue, typically bronchial carcinoma, infiltrates around but does not totally occlude an adjacent bronchus.

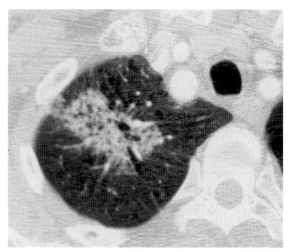

Fig. 3.89 Air bronchograms and bubble-like lucencies in a bronchioloalveolar carcinoma.

Cavities and air crescent sign

A cavity is defined by the Fleischner Society[5] as a gas-filled space within a zone of pulmonary consolidation, a mass, or a nodule. There may or may not be an accompanying fluid level.

As can be seen from Box 3.6, many of the causes of SPN may result in cavitation, so the presence or absence of cavitation is of limited diagnostic value. The morphology of the cavity may, however, be helpful. Lung abscesses and benign lesions in general have a thinner, smoother wall than cavitating malignant neoplasms. Woodring and Fried[198] compared 126 patients with solitary cavities and found that when the maximum wall thickness was 16 mm or more, 35 cases were due to malignant neoplasm whereas only 4 cases were benign. Conversely, with a maximum wall thickness of 4 mm or less, only 2 cases were malignant neoplasm and 30 were benign. Between 4 and 16 mm the cases were almost equally divided, with 33 cases benign and 22 malignant.

In practice, the diagnosis of acute lung abscess usually depends on the clinical features together with the appearance of a cavity evolving in an area of undoubted pneumonia. The more difficult problem is distinguishing between cavitating neoplasm and chronic inflammatory processes. Fungal pneumonia, particularly cryptococcosis and blastomycosis, and various connective tissue diseases, particularly Wegener granulomatosis and rheumatoid arthritis, can appear identical to carcinoma of the lung and may even be indistinguishable clinically.

A cavity may contain a mass within it, the air within the cavity forming a peripheral halo or crescent of air between an intracavitary mass and the cavity wall, giving rise to the so-called "air crescent" or "air meniscus sign". Intracavitary masses are most often due to fungal mycetomas. Other causes include complicated hydatid disease, blood clot (as a result of tuberculosis, laceration with hematoma, or infarct), abscess and necrotizing pneumonias (particularly caused by *Klebsiella* or *Aspergillus fumigatus*), and necrotic neoplasm. Another cause of the air crescent sign is crescentic cavitation – a phenomenon that appears to be unique to invasive fungal infection, notably invasive aspergillosis.

CT is a useful modality for diagnosing or excluding the presence of a cavity within the lung but it has little or no

A 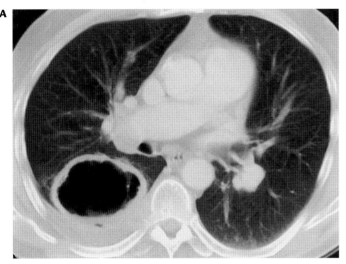 **B**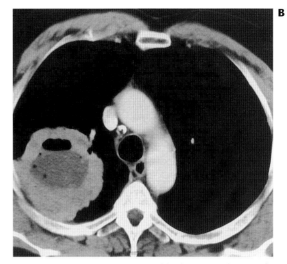

Fig. 3.90 CT of cavitation in bronchial carcinoma. **A**, The more usual thick wall. **B**, The wall can, however, be notably thin, as in this example.

advantage over plain films in diagnosing the nature of the cavity because it rarely limits the differential diagnosis (Fig. 3.90). CT can, however, distinguish with great reliability between lung abscess and empyema when this is a diagnostic problem on plain chest radiographs (see Ch. 5).[199,200]

The CT halo sign

The term "CT halo sign"[201] refers to ground-glass attenuation surrounding a nodule on CT (Fig. 3.91). Apart from malignant neoplasms and hemorrhage following biopsy,[202] the most common cause of a CT halo sign is infection, notably invasive aspergillosis.[203,204] The other causes are candidiasis, coccidioidomycosis, tuberculosis, cytomegalovirus, herpes simplex, Wegener granulomatosis, metastatic angiosarcoma, and Kaposi sarcoma.[204,205] A feature that links many of these conditions is hemorrhage into the lung adjacent to the basic pathology.

It is worth bearing in mind that a CT halo sign surrounding a small asymptomatic nodule in a patient in the lung cancer age range is likely to be a bronchogenic carcinoma and that when a CT halo sign is seen surrounding central consolidation in a patient who is immunocompromised due to leukemia or drug treatment the diagnosis is highly likely to be invasive aspergillosis.

Adjacent bone destruction

Invasion of adjacent bone by a pulmonary mass is almost pathognomonic of bronchogenic carcinoma. Alternative possibilities include actinomycosis and occasionally tuberculosis[19] or fungal disease.

Management of a solitary pulmonary nodule

The management of a patient with an SPN depends on a combination of clinical and radiologic factors.[181,206–213] A clinical evaluation to find evidence of diseases such as rheumatoid arthritis, Wegener granulomatosis, hydatid disease, and extrathoracic primary malignant tumor should be undertaken.

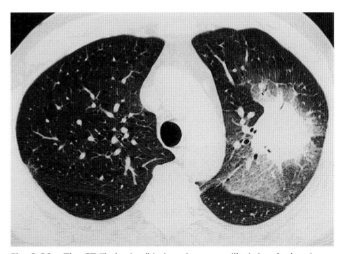

Fig. 3.91 The CT "halo sign" in invasive aspergillosis in a leukemic patient. The central rounded pneumonia is surrounded by a ground-glass halo due to hemorrhagic infection.

Solitary masses larger than 3 cm, unless they show the specific features of round atelectasis or a congenital malformation such as an arteriovenous malformation, are so frequently lung cancers that benign entities should be diagnosed with caution.

The radiological approach for patients in the cancer age group who have an asymptomatic SPN between 1 and 3 cm in diameter is to examine all available images carefully for visible calcification conforming to a definite benign pattern, fat within the nodule, or stability of size on retrospective review of the images for at least 18 months. Any one of these features is sufficient evidence for a benign lesion to obviate surgical resection.

If the nodule does not show any of these features, thin-section CT can be used to assess the morphologic and density characteristics, notably calcification and/or fat[120] (using formal CT density measurements if necessary). The presence of occult calcification must be interpreted with care and is not absolute proof of benignity, but because the probability of cancer becomes very low when more than 10% of a nodule shows calcification, it is prudent to institute a watch and wait program.[102] CT densitometry for calcification is not advised for nodules greater than 3 cm in diameter, because the probability of a benign lesion above this size diminishes greatly. If the presence of fat is used to diagnose a hamartoma, care must be taken to ensure the CT section is at the equator of the nodule and that the section does not include adjacent lung which could, by partial volume effect, lower the density from soft tissue to lie within the range of fat.

A nodule that is still indeterminate after all the preceding considerations have been taken into account may be benign, a solitary metastasis, or a bronchogenic carcinoma. A negative result from FDG PET scanning is an excellent method of determining that lung cancer is highly unlikely, but a positive result is less reliable for predicting malignancy. The same applies to contrast enhancement of the nodule at CT. Fine needle aspiration biopsy can usually prove that a nodule is malignant but is less reliable at excluding malignancy. Resection of the nodule, with appropriate prior staging, is the recommended course of action in many instances unless the likelihood of primary lung cancer is deemed very low, e.g. in a young non-smoker, or in a patient for whom the risk of pulmonary resection outweighs the potential benefit of removal of possible malignant tumor. When follow up is deemed a reasonable course of action, an appropriate scheme is plain chest radiography or CT after 3 months and, if there is no significant growth, at further intervals of 6–12 months until stability at 24 months has been established. If the nodule has not grown over a 2-year period then primary lung cancer is sufficiently unlikely that further follow up can be stopped.

Gurney calculated likelihood ratios for malignancy as the cause of an SPN based on all the published distinguishing features.[208] Gurney et al then used the likelihood ratios to predict malignancy or benignity and found that readers using likelihood ratios performed better than expert observers using more conventional analysis.[214] When using Bayesian analysis for a noncalcified nodule, additional tests beyond the initial chest radiograph or CT are most helpful when the pre-test probability of lung cancer is in the intermediate range.[215]

MULTIPLE PULMONARY NODULES

The differential diagnosis for multiple pulmonary nodules is given in Box 3.7. Once again the list is long, but well over 95% of multiple pulmonary nodules on plain chest radiographs are metastases or tuberculous/fungal granulomas. The larger and more variable the size of the nodules, the more likely they are to be neoplastic. This remark does not apply to nodules too small to be seen on plain chest radiographs and found only by CT; here the probability of multiple metastases is lower and the chance of multiple granulomas is higher. CT can be useful[216] when the morphologic features of the nodules are unclear or when the distinction between multiple nodules and multifocal consolidation is not certain from the plain chest radiographs.

The following points may help limit the diagnostic possibilities:

1. In patients with metastases the presence of an extrathoracic primary tumor is usually known or at least suspected because of clinical findings.
2. A cluster of two or more small (<1 cm) pulmonary nodules within 1 cm of each other in a focal area of the lung is highly likely to be infectious or inflammatory in origin. In a series of 31 adult patients with a cluster of small pulmonary

nodules identified at chest CT, none of the nodules proved to be malignant.[217] Patients with a dominant nodule, i.e. a nodule more than twice the size of the adjacent nodules, were excluded from consideration.
3. Cavitation is seen in many of the disorders listed in Box 3.7. The major diagnostic value of cavitation is that it indicates an active disease process. It is not a feature of incidental lesions such as inactive granulomas.
4. Metastases are usually spherical and have well-defined outlines (Fig. 3.92), although metastases with irregular margins and poorly defined edges are occasionally encountered. Metastases vary considerably in size.
5. Nodules containing calcification are usually infectious granulomas, notably tuberculous or histoplasmal granulomas. On rare occasions, they are multiple hamartomas or even amyloidomas. Thus nodules that are extensively calcified can, with one important exception, be assumed to be benign. The exception is in patients with osteosarcoma or chondrosarcoma, because metastases from these tumors frequently calcify (Fig. 3.93). In the case of

---

Box 3.7 Differential diagnosis of multiple pulmonary nodules/masses

Neoplastic
Malignant
Metastatic carcinoma or sarcoma*
Lymphoma*
Multifocal neoplasms, e.g. Kaposi sarcoma and
    bronchioloalveolar carcinoma
Benign
Hamartomas, chondromas
Laryngeal papillomatosis*
Benign metastasizing leiomyoma

Inflammatory
Infective
Granulomas,* e.g. tuberculosis, histoplasmosis,
    cryptococcosis, coccidioidomycosis, nocardiosis
Round pneumonias, particularly fungal and opportunistic
    infections*
Lung abscesses,* especially septicemic
Septic infarcts*
Atypical measles
Hydatid cysts*
Paragonimiasis*
Noninfective
Rheumatoid arthritis,* Caplan syndrome*
Wegener granulomatosis*
Sarcoidosis*
Drug-induced

Congenital
Arteriovenous malformation

Miscellaneous
Progressive massive fibrosis*
Hematomas*
Amyloidosis*
Pulmonary infarcts*
Mucoid impactions*

*May cavitate

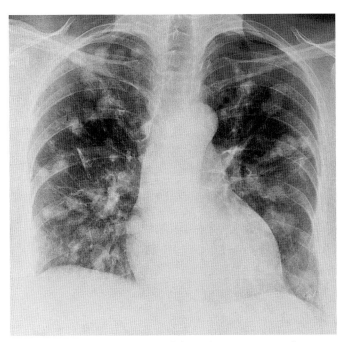

Fig. 3.92 Multiple pulmonary nodules owing to metastases from a squamous cell carcinoma of salivary gland.

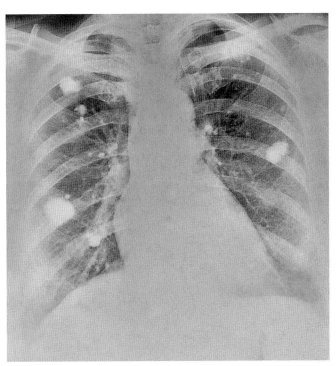

Fig. 3.93 Multiple calcified pulmonary nodules caused by metastases from an extrathoracic osteosarcoma.

metastases from chondrosarcoma, the calcification may be the typical popcorn calcification of cartilage tumors. If calcified and noncalcified nodules coexist, it cannot necessarily be assumed that the noncalcified nodules are also benign.

6. Growth rate can be a useful discriminator between granuloma and metastases. Straus,[174] reviewing the literature on the doubling times of pulmonary metastases, found a wide range, much wider than for primary lung carcinoma: 11–745 days for breast carcinoma; 11–150 days for colorectal carcinomas; 10–205 days for testicular tumors; and 17–253 days for soft tissue and bone sarcomas. Some tumors, for example choriocarcinoma and osteosarcoma, may show explosive growth, doubling their volumes in less than a month.[218] Others, for example thyroid carcinoma, can remain the same size for a very long time.[219]

7. Small pulmonary granulomas are common in the histoplasmosis belt of the United States. Elsewhere in the United States granulomas are less common. In parts of the world where pulmonary fungal disease is uncommon, granulomas are also uncommon and when encountered are usually caused by tuberculosis. Thus the likelihood of pulmonary nodules being granulomas is strongly influenced by where the patient has lived.

8. Multiple arteriovenous malformations can usually be diagnosed with certainty by noting large feeding arteries and draining veins. They are very rare and are usually part of the Osler–Weber–Rendu syndrome.

9. Sarcoidosis can produce multiple nodular shadows in the lung that may resemble metastases or lymphoma. The uniform size, the slightly ill-defined edge, and the accompanying hilar and mediastinal adenopathy are important clues to the diagnosis of sarcoidosis (Fig. 3.94). Also, the relatively young age of the patient and the frequent lack of signs and symptoms of malignant neoplastic disease often help to resolve the diagnostic difficulty.

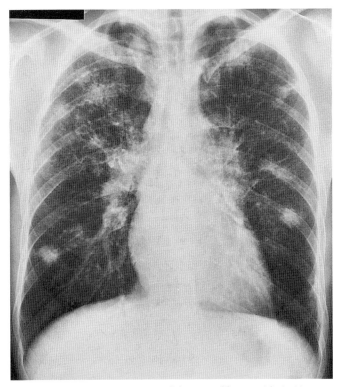

Fig. 3.94 Multiple pulmonary nodules caused by sarcoidosis. Note that there is also hilar and mediastinal adenopathy. As is so often the case in sarcoidosis, the nodules are ill defined in outline and much the same size.

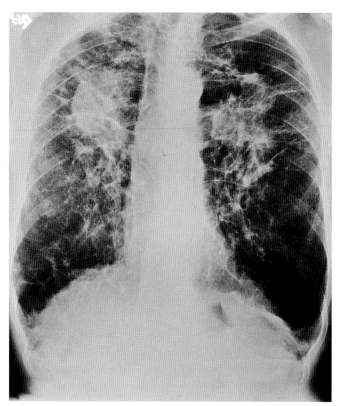

Fig. 3.95 Multiple pulmonary nodules caused by progressive massive fibrosis (PMF). The diagnosis here is easy because of the characteristic location, the shape of PMF shadows, the background nodulation of the lungs, and the generalized emphysema.

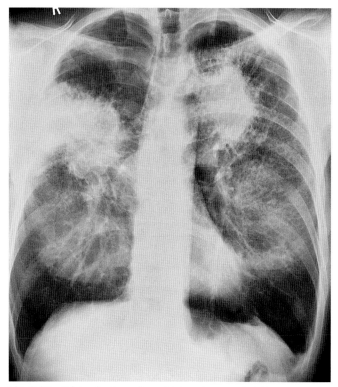

Fig. 3.96 Bilateral primary bronchial carcinoma mimicking progressive massive fibrosis.

10. Multiple nodules are a feature of coal worker's pneumoconiosis and chronic silicosis. When greater than 1 cm in diameter, they are known as progressive massive fibrosis. The presence of widespread nodulation in the rest of the lung and the characteristic shape and location of progressive massive fibrosis lead to a specific diagnosis in virtually every case (Fig. 3.95). (The nodules of Caplan syndrome may be more difficult to distinguish from metastases, because the other signs of coal worker's pneumoconiosis are often absent.) The patient's occupational history is important in diagnosing progressive massive fibrosis because, on rare occasions, neoplasms (Fig. 3.96) or inflammatory conditions such as Wegener granulomatosis can cause a similar appearance.

RING SHADOWS AND CYSTS

The causes of ring shadows and cysts are listed in Box 3.8. There is no clear distinction between cavitating consolidation, cavitary

---

Box 3.8 Pulmonary ring shadows and cysts of more than 1 cm on chest radiography

Congenital
Sequestered segment
Bronchogenic cyst
Cystic adenomatoid malformation

Infection
Bacterial abscess, notably anaerobic bacteria, *Staphylococcus*, tuberculosis
Pneumocystis jiroveci pneumonia
Fungal abscess, notably coccidioidomycosis
Echinococcus cyst

Connective tissue disease
Rheumatoid necrobiotic nodule
Wegener granulomatosis

Neoplasm
Bronchial carcinoma, notably squamous cell
Metastases, notably squamous cell
Laryngeal papillomatosis with pulmonary spread
Malignant lymphoma

Thromboembolism
Infarct, notably septic infarcts

Airway disease
Blebs and bullae
Bronchiectasis (individual ring shadows caused by dilated bronchi)

Pneumatoceles
Pulmonary laceration
Pulmonary infection, notably staphylococcal and *Pneumocystis jiroveci*
Hydrocarbon ingestion

Mimics
Bowel herniation
Empyema
Lucite plombage

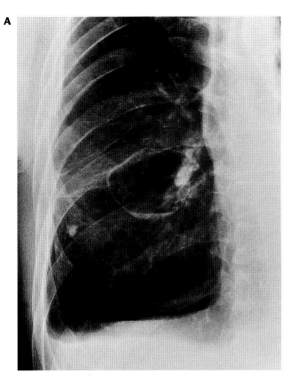
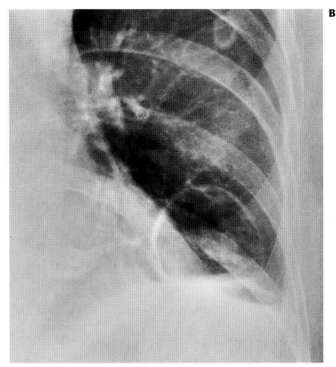

Fig. 3.97   **A**, A pneumatocele due to previous trauma. A small amount of fluid is present in the pneumatocele. **B**, A pneumatocele due to staphylococcal pneumonia. A second, smaller pneumatocele is seen in the left mid zone.

masses, and ring shadows, but the term "ring shadow" is usually restricted to discrete round or oval spaces within the lung surrounded by a thin wall less than 2 mm thick.[220] Ring shadows can be of any size and may be single or multiple, unilocular or multilocular. They may contain fluid, which is manifest as an air–fluid level. The term "cyst" is often reserved for cavitary lesions that are more than 1 cm in diameter with a thin wall (less than 4 mm) of uniform thickness. By common use the word "pneumatocele" is confined to air cysts that develop after infection (typically *Pneumocystis jiroveci* or staphylococcal pneumonia), lung trauma, and hydrocarbon ingestion (Fig. 3.97). Superimposed normal blood vessels may occasionally mimic a pneumatocele.

CT may be useful in selected cases to define more accurately the shape, position, and contents of a ring shadow. CT is particularly helpful in distinguishing between loculated pneumothorax and an intrapulmonary cyst or bleb and in demonstrating any related pulmonary disease.[221]

LINE SHADOWS AND BAND SHADOWS

The term "band shadow" is usually reserved for linear opacities more than 5 mm in diameter, whereas linear densities with a diameter less than 5 mm are simply referred to as line shadows. The causes of abnormal line and band shadows are given in Box 3.9.

Of the items listed in Box 3.9, only focal scars, mucoid impaction, septal lines, and bronchial wall thickening are discussed further in this section. The other entities are described elsewhere in this book.

Box 3.9   **Causes of line shadows and band shadows on chest radiography**

Skinfold
Clothing, tubes, etc.
Wall of a bleb or pneumatocele
Bronchial or peribronchial thickening, the causes of which are:
- Pulmonary edema
- Neoplastic infiltration
- Lymphangitis carcinomatosa
- Recurrent asthma, notably allergic bronchopulmonary aspergillosis
- Bronchiolitis
- Cystic fibrosis
- Bronchiectasis

Bronchocele (mucoid impaction)
Parenchymal or pleuro-parenchymal scar
Discoid atelectasis
Anomalous blood vessels or feeding and draining vessels to arteriovenous malformations
Thickening of pleural fissures
Pleural tail associated with pleural nodule
Septal lines (Kerley lines), the causes of which are given in Box 3.10

Focal parenchymal and pleuro-parenchymal scars

Parenchymal and pleuro-parenchymal scars are the commonest cause of line or narrow band shadows on plain chest radiographs. They are the end result of previous linear atelectasis, pulmonary infarction, or infection. Since scarring so often involves focal loss of volume and, therefore, indrawing of the pleura, the peripheral portion of the resulting line/band shadow is sometimes composed of pleura. Focal scars are of no clinical consequence.

Mucoid impaction

Mucoid impaction (bronchocele, mucocele) causes one or more branching bandlike opacities pointing to the hilum. The lesion is often 1 cm or more in diameter and is sharply marginated with branches that have been likened to fingers, the so-called "gloved finger" shadow. The presence of such shadows always implies bronchial obstruction.[222] Mucoid impactions are found typically in allergic bronchopulmonary aspergillosis (Fig. 3.98), but may be seen with a variety of obstructing lesions, provided collateral air drift maintains aeration to the affected segment. The causes are bronchial carcinoid (Fig. 3.99), carcinoma of the lung, metastases, tuberculous bronchostenosis, broncholithiasis, bronchial atresia (Fig. 3.100), sequestration, pulmonary bronchogenic cyst, foreign body aspiration, and benign stricture (Fig. 3.101).[222,223] If the surrounding lung collapses or consoli-

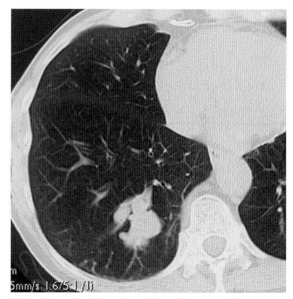

Fig. 3.99 Mucocele of bronchus in the right lower lobe due to an obstructing well-differentiated carcinoma of the bronchus. Note the branching bandlike densities.

dates, the shadow of the mucoid impaction becomes invisible because of the silhouette effect.

Septal lines

The interstitial septa of normal lungs are not visible on plain chest radiographs except in a very small minority of thin patients and then only on very high quality films. For practical purposes it is only when the septa are thickened that they become visible (Fig. 3.102).[224,225] Septal thickening on HRCT is a separate topic discussed in Chapter 4.

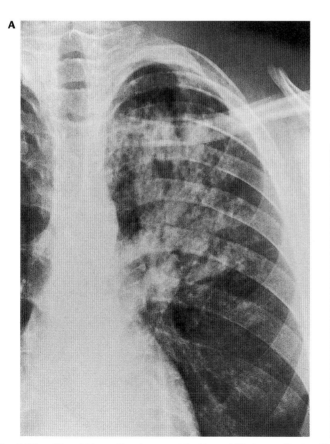

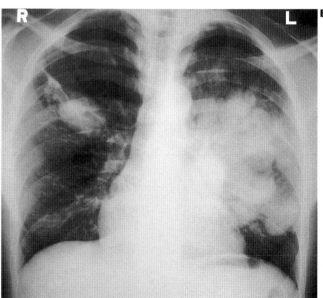

Fig. 3.98 Mucoid impaction (mucocele) of bronchi in two patients with allergic bronchopulmonary aspergillosis. **A,** The branching tubular shadows have been likened to "gloved fingers". **B,** Dilated bronchi mimicking pulmonary masses.

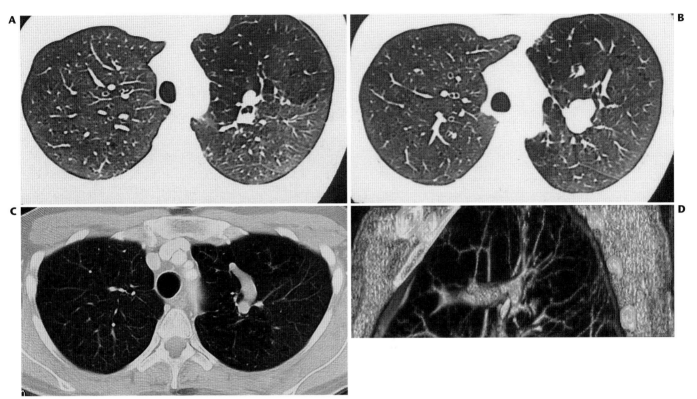

Fig. 3.100   Two young adults with a bronchocele in the left upper lobe presumed to be secondary to congenital bronchial atresia. **A** and **B,** Adjacent CT sections showing the branching pattern typical of bronchocele and emphysema distal to bronchocele. **C** and **D,** An axial section and a lateral view 3D reconstruction of a similar case.

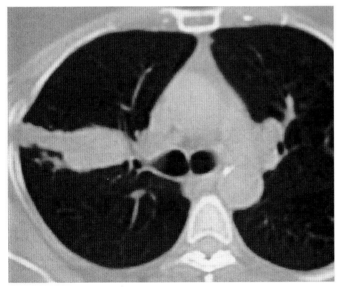

Fig. 3.101   Bronchocele (mucocele) with no visible cause at surgery other than a benign stricture. Note the branching tubular structures arising from the central ovoid mass.

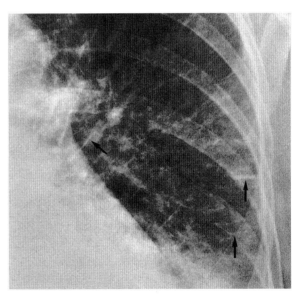

Fig. 3.102   Septal lines caused by pulmonary edema. B lines are short horizontal lines at the lung periphery (vertical arrows). A lines are lines radiating from the hila (oblique arrow).

Septal lines on chest radiographs were first described by Kerley in patients with pulmonary edema.[226] He named them A, B, and C lines because he was not certain of their anatomic basis. "Septal lines" is a more descriptive and therefore better term because the lines represent thickening of connective tissue septa within the lung.[224,227]

The septa are anatomically divided into deep septa and peripheral interlobular septa.[228] Deep septal lines (Kerley A lines) are up to 4 cm in length, radiate from the hila into the central portions of the lungs, do not reach the pleura, and are most obvious in the middle and upper zones. Interlobular septal lines (Kerley B lines) are usually less than 1 cm in length and parallel to one another at right angles to the pleura. They may be very thin and sharply defined or may be a few millimeters in width and fairly ill defined. They are located peripherally in contact with the pleura, but are generally absent along fissural surfaces.[228] They may be seen in any zone but are most frequently observed at the lung bases. The term "C lines" has been dropped, because the criss-crossing lines that Kerley designated as C lines are actually due to the superimposition of many B lines.[224]

Septal lines must be distinguished from blood vessels on plain chest radiographs. Blood vessels are not seen in the outer centimeter of the lung, whereas interlobular septa, though narrower in diameter, may be visible by virtue of having substantial depth along the trajectory of the x-ray beam. Similarly, the deep septa are seen as narrow dense lines because they are thin sheets of tissue seen end on. Blood vessels of such a narrow diameter would be either invisible or of extremely low density. Another helpful feature is that deep septal lines, though they may interconnect or superimpose, do not branch in as uniform a manner as blood vessels.

The identification of septal lines is an extremely useful diagnostic feature, since septal lines that are sufficiently thick to be visible on plain chest radiographs occur in relatively few conditions (Box 3.10). If transient or rapid in development, they are virtually diagnostic of interstitial pulmonary edema.

Bronchial wall (peribronchial) thickening

The walls of the bronchi beyond the hila are invisible on normal chest radiographs unless they are end-on to the x-ray beam, when they are seen as thin, well-defined, ringlike densities.

Box 3.10   Causes of septal lines (Kerley lines) on chest radiography

Pulmonary edema
Lymphangitis carcinomatosa and malignant lymphoma
Viral and mycoplasmal pneumonia
Pneumoconiosis
Sarcoidosis
Lymphocytic interstitial pneumonia
Late-stage idiopathic pulmonary hemorrhage
Congenital lymphangiectasia and
    lymphangioleiomyomatosis
Interstitial pulmonary fibrosis from any cause (rarely)

Portions of the walls of the lobar bronchi within the hila are also routinely visible in the healthy person. The posterior wall of the bronchus intermedius should measure less than 3 mm.[229] Since this portion of the bronchial tree is clearly seen in lateral chest radiographs and is even easier to identify on CT scans, it is a useful site at which to assess central bronchial wall thickening.

When edema or inflammatory or neoplastic cells infiltrate the peribronchial interstitial space, the combination of the bronchial wall and the widened interstitium produces so-called "bronchial wall thickening". Not only do the bronchial walls appear thick, they are also usually less well defined. Although bronchial wall thickening may resemble two adjacent blood vessels, the distinction can be made by identifying the parallelism of the walls and by observing Y-shaped branching parallel walls where the bronchi divide.

Intraparenchymal bronchial wall thickening on plain chest radiography (Fig. 3.103) is seen with pulmonary edema or

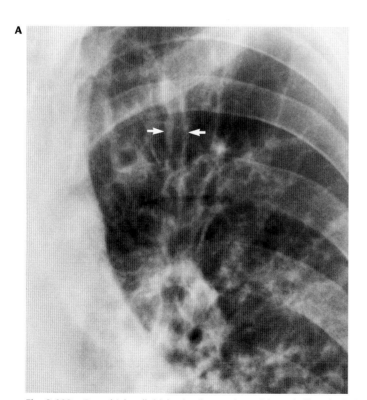
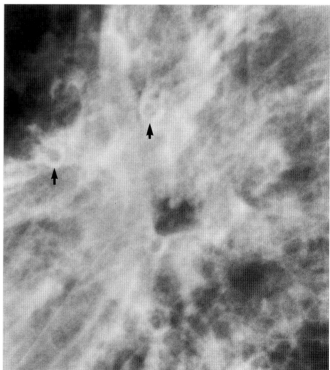

Fig. 3.103 Bronchial wall thickening in a patient with cystic fibrosis. **A,** Posteroanterior radiograph. Arrows point to parallel lines of thickened walls of a representative, moderately dilated bronchus. **B,** Lateral radiograph. Arrows point to two examples of ring shadows caused by thickened bronchial walls seen end on.

neoplastic infiltration of the peribronchial tissues (including lymphangitis carcinomatosa). It is also seen in recurrent asthma and bronchiectasis, including allergic bronchopulmonary aspergillosis and cystic fibrosis.

WIDESPREAD NODULAR, RETICULONODULAR, AND HONEYCOMB SHADOWING

Many diseases cause widespread small pulmonary opacities. Occasionally the chest radiograph provides enough information for a specific diagnosis, but usually it is just one piece of information along with clinical features and other tests. The analysis of widespread small opacities on HRCT is a separate topic discussed in Chapter 4. The following section is confined to a discussion of the appearance on plain chest radiographs.

The numerous small opacities seen on chest radiographs probably do not represent the individual lesions seen by the pathologist: the pattern appears to be produced by summation. Carstairs[230] showed that when multiple superimposed sheets of small nodules are radiographed, the resulting image is a reticulonodular pattern. This observation is important, because it suggests that the size and shape of the nodules and lines on the chest radiograph are not a precise reflection of the responsible lesion.

Many descriptive terms have been proposed for widespread small lung shadows on the plain chest radiograph; only a few are widely accepted. For diagnostic purposes, the following are recommended[231]:

1. Nodular pattern, consisting of clearly defined round or irregular opacities, ranging in diameter from 1 to 9 mm (Fig. 3.104). Such lesions may be partially or completely calcified. Above 1 cm the nodules represent individual lesions, the differential diagnosis for which is discussed on page 107.

2. Reticular or linear pattern, consisting of fine linear shadows, usually in an irregular netlike arrangement forming rings with thin walls surrounding spaces of air density (Figs 3.105 and 3.106). Septal (Kerley A and B) lines are a specific form of linear shadowing of diagnostic value because their presence is reliable evidence of interstitial thickening.

3. Reticulonodular pattern, representing a mixture of nodular and reticular patterns. The nodules are usually irregular in shape. A reticulonodular appearance is much more common than a purely reticular or purely nodular pattern.

4. Honeycomb pattern, a term used to describe a coarse reticular or reticulonodular pattern in which the criss-crossing linear elements surround small cystic airspaces. The appearance corresponds to what the pathologist calls honeycomb lung when viewing the surface of a cut section of lung (Fig. 3.106).

5. Cystic or ring pattern. Widespread ring shadows of 1 cm or more are highly suggestive of cystic bronchiectasis (Fig. 3.107).

6. Ground-glass pattern, referring to a diffuse increase in density and haziness that reduces the clarity of the pulmonary vessels but does not entirely efface their outlines. The diaphragmatic outlines may also be less distinct. The abnormality is often subtle, and the sign can be highly subjective. It is a nonspecific feature of mild airspace filling, interstitial thickening, or a combination of the two and is therefore seen in a large variety of conditions.

These six basic terms usually provide a reasonably accurate description of diffuse lung disease. They do not imply a

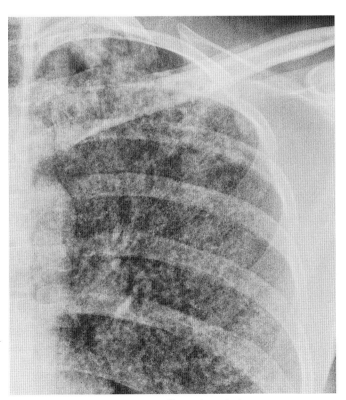

Fig. 3.104 Nodular pattern in miliary tuberculosis.

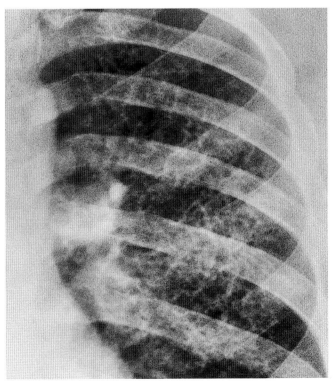

Fig. 3.105 Reticular pattern in Langerhans cell histiocytosis.

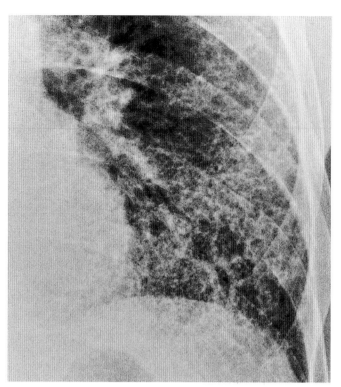

Fig. 3.106   Reticulonodular pattern interstitial pulmonary fibrosis in a patient with scleroderma.

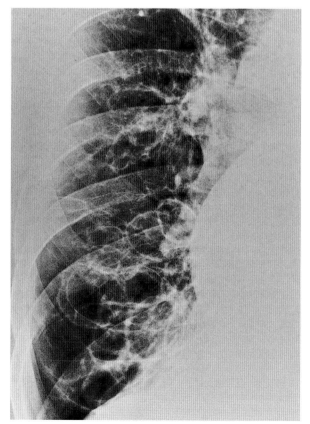

Fig. 3.107   Cystic pattern in cystic bronchiectasis.

specific disease process but are used to generate a differential diagnostic list.

Two classes of diffuse lung disease, alveolar and interstitial, based on plain radiographic findings, have been advocated. Alveolar disease is said to be manifest by opacities that are lobar, segmental, or "butterfly" in distribution.[224,232] The individual shadows have ill-defined margins (except when they contact a fissure), tend to coalesce, and may contain air bronchograms or air alveolograms. "Acinar" shadows, it is claimed, are distinctive enough to narrow the differential diagnosis of pulmonary opacities to diseases that cause filling of the alveolar airspaces. "Acinar" shadows are ill-defined coalescent nodular opacities, approximately the size of an acinus, that may initially appear as rosettes of small densities.[6] Interstitial disease, on the other hand, is manifest as a relatively well defined linear, nodular, irregular, or honeycomb pattern together with septal lines, subpleural thickening, perivascular haze, or peribronchial cuffing.

The problem with this division is that widespread small shadows are often difficult to categorize into one or the other group on plain film findings. Many diseases that are classified as alveolar by pathologists show radiographic features of interstitial disease, and conversely there is an appreciable list of so-called "interstitial diseases" that show the radiographic signs ascribed to alveolar disease. Even "acinar" shadows have been seen in interstitial processes on plain chest radiographs.[233] Nevertheless, the attempt to characterize diffuse lung disease as alveolar or interstitial has its merits. The advent of high-resolution, thin-section CT has dramatically improved the ability of radiologists to categorize diffuse lung disease into alveolar and interstitial patterns.

Nevertheless, it is equally possible,[234] and in many instances preferable, to generate a differential diagnostic list according to the combination of radiographic signs without regard to an intermediate decision as to whether the process is predominantly alveolar or interstitial (given that so many diseases have both components).

Other factors to note when deciding on differential diagnostic possibilities are zonal predominance, if any, and such signs as reduction in lung volume, bronchial wall thickening, presence of airspace shadowing, masses, lymphadenopathy, and pleural effusions. In some situations, notably industrial lung disease, the problem is not diagnosis but quantification of the severity of disease. The International Labor Office and other groups have drawn up a classification based on reference radiographs to provide standardized descriptions (see p. 441).

Boxes 3.11 to 3.13 provide a general guide to the differential diagnosis of widespread nodular, reticular, reticulonodular, and honeycomb patterns on plain chest radiography. The boxes present a simplified approach, and it is important to realize that many exceptions exist. Certain generalizations can be applied with caution:

1. Acute conditions should be considered separately. If multiple linear markings appear acutely, that is, within hours or days, the most likely diagnosis is pulmonary edema, particularly cardiogenic edema, or pneumonia. In the immunocompetent patient with fever, viral or mycoplasmal pneumonia should be the major consideration. The line shadows indicate thickening of the interstitial septa of the lung, which may produce clear-cut septal lines or if numerous may appear as a reticular pattern owing to

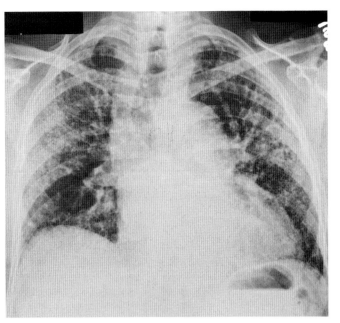

Fig. 3.108 Idiopathic pulmonary fibrosis (usual interstitial pneumonia – UIP, fibrosing alveolitis). This case demonstrates the peripheral predominance of the shadowing. Note the small-volume lungs.

Box 3.11   Diffuse bilateral small nodular opacities of the lungs (miliary pattern) on chest radiography

Miliary tuberculosis
Nontuberculous infection, notably:
- Histoplasmosis
- Blastomycosis
- Coccidioidomycosis
- Cryptococcosis
- Nocardiosis
- Viral infection
Diffuse panbronchiolitis
Pneumoconiosis, notably:
- Coal worker's pneumoconiosis
- Silicosis
- Siderosis
- Berylliosis
- Stannosis
Sarcoidosis
Metastases
Langerhans cell histiocytosis
Amyloidosis
Alveolar microlithiasis

Box 3.12   Causes of diffuse bilateral reticulonodular opacities of the lungs on chest radiography

Idiopathic pulmonary fibrosis
Rheumatoid lung disease (interstitial fibrosis)
Scleroderma, dermatomyositis, systemic lupus
   erythematosus
Drug reaction/noxious gases (acute or fibrotic stages)
Extrinsic allergic alveolitis (acute or fibrotic stages)
Pneumoconiosis, notably:
- Coal worker's pneumoconiosis
- Silicosis
- Asbestosis
- Berylliosis
Sarcoidosis
Langerhans cell histiocytosis
Interstitial pneumonia, notably:
- Fungal, particularly histoplasmosis
- *Mycoplasma pneumoniae*
- Viral
Chronic aspiration
Diffuse panbronchiolitis
Pulmonary edema
Lymphangitic spread of carcinoma or lymphoma
Lymphangioleiomyomatosis
Lymphocytic interstitial pneumonia, Waldenström
   macroglobulinemia
Amyloidosis
Hemosiderosis
- Idiopathic, Goodpasture syndrome
- Secondary to mitral valve disease
Talc granulomatosis
Alveolar proteinosis
Neurofibromatosis

---

the superimposition of many thickened septa. In the case of cardiogenic edema the other signs of circulatory overload will often be present.

2. The distribution of the shadows can be of help in differential diagnosis.

a. Reticulonodular shadows maximal at the bases and/or at the lung periphery, together with loss of lung volume but without pleural effusion or hilar adenopathy, are almost invariably due to one of the forms of interstitial pulmonary fibrosis. The major causes are usual interstitial pneumonia (such as in idiopathic pulmonary fibrosis [Fig. 3.108] or rheumatoid lung disease [Fig. 3.109]), pulmonary asbestosis, and nonspecific interstitial pneumonia, either idiopathic or associated with diseases such as scleroderma (Figs 3.106 and 3.110) and dermatomyositis. Extrinsic allergic alveolitis and drug toxicity may also show this pattern. With chronic bilateral aspiration, bronchopneumonia may convert from consolidation to interstitial fibrosis and bronchiectasis, causing reticulonodular shadowing that can closely resemble late-stage usual interstitial pneumonia.

b. Unilateral reticulonodular shadowing without zonal or lobar predominance, particularly if septal lines are obvious and pleural effusions are present, is virtually diagnostic of lymphangitis carcinomatosa (Fig. 3.111). Aspiration pneumonia may occasionally give this appearance, and usual interstitial pneumonia and sarcoidosis may very rarely cause unilateral reticulonodular shadowing.

c. Coarse reticulonodular shadowing maximal in the upper zones, particularly when associated with fibrotic contraction of the upper lobes, is seen particularly in chronic tuberculous (Fig. 3.112A) or fungal disease, notably histoplasmosis (Fig. 3.112B), the fibrotic end

Box 3.13   Signs that limit the differential diagnosis of diffuse bilateral reticulonodular opacities of the lungs on chest radiography

Acute appearance of shadows suggests:
Pulmonary edema (both cardiac and noncardiac)
Pneumonia, notably mycoplasmal, viral, or opportunistic

Lower zone predominance of the opacities together with decrease in lung volume suggests:
Idiopathic pulmonary fibrosis
Rheumatoid lung disease (interstitial fibrosis)
Scleroderma, dermatomyositis, systemic lupus erythematosus (interstitial fibrosis)
Drug reaction, noxious gases (fibrotic stage)
Hypersensitivity pneumonitis (fibrotic stage)
Asbestosis
Chronic aspiration

Mid or upper zone predominance of the opacities suggests:
Chronic tuberculous and fungal disease
Pneumoconiosis (coal worker's, silicosis, berylliosis)
Sarcoidosis
Hypersensitivity pneumonitis (fibrotic stage)
Ankylosing spondylitis (fibrosis)

Associated increase in lung volume or bullae suggests:
Underlying emphysema
Cystic fibrosis
Langerhans cell histiocytosis
Lymphangioleiomyomatosis
Neurofibromatosis

Associated septal (Kerley) lines suggest:
Pulmonary edema
Lymphangitic spread of carcinoma or lymphoma
Viral or mycoplasmal pneumonia
Sarcoidosis
Hypersensitivity pneumonitis
Interstitial pulmonary fibrosis (idiopathic, connective tissue disease, etc.)
Pneumoconiosis (notably silicosis)

Associated hilar lymphadenopathy suggests:
Sarcoidosis
Lymphangitis carcinomatosa
Lymphoma
Infections, notably:
• Tuberculosis
• Viral
Pneumoconiosis, notably:
• Silicosis
• Berylliosis

Associated hilar node calcification suggests:
Sarcoidosis
Silicosis
Chronic tuberculosis or histoplasmosis
Treated lymphoma

Associated pleural effusion suggests:
Pulmonary edema
Lymphangitic spread of carcinoma or lymphoma
Connective tissue disease
Lymphangioleiomyomatosis (particularly if effusion is chylous)
Note: Pleural effusions are notably absent in idiopathic interstitial pulmonary fibrosis

Associated pleural thickening suggests:
Asbestosis, particularly if pleural calcification is present

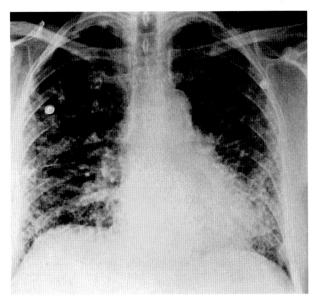

Fig. 3.109   Diffuse interstitial pulmonary fibrosis in a patient with rheumatoid arthritis. This example shows mid and lower zone predominance with only mild loss of volume.

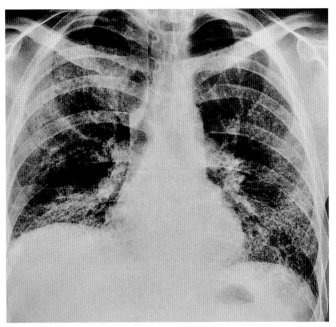

Fig. 3.110   Interstitial pulmonary fibrosis in scleroderma. The peripheral and basal predominance of shadowing, combined with small lung volumes, is typical of diffuse interstitial pulmonary fibrosis.

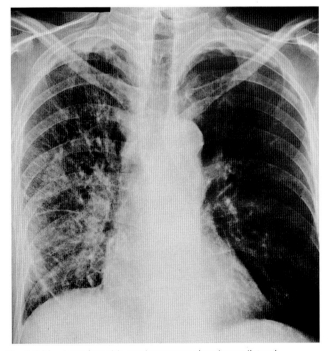

Fig. 3.111   Lymphangitis carcinomatosa showing unilateral reticulonodular shadowing. Note the fissural thickening and septal lines.

stage of extrinsic allergic alveolitis (Fig. 3.112C), sarcoidosis (Fig. 3.112D) and, occasionally, ankylosing spondylitis.

d. Clear-cut reticular shadowing with pronounced upper zone predominance strongly suggests Langerhans cell histiocytosis, particularly if airspaces greater than l cm are seen.

e. Coarse shadowing radiating from the hila into the mid and upper zones, but sparing the extreme apices, is highly suggestive of sarcoidosis (Fig. 3.113). The presence of hilar lymphadenopathy makes the diagnosis nearly certain.

f. Uniformly distributed, very small miliary nodules are virtually confined to miliary tuberculosis, sarcoidosis (Fig. 3.114), or pneumoconiosis from coal, silica, or other inorganic dusts. The presence of bilateral lymphadenopathy makes sarcoidosis much the most likely, but does not exclude the other possibilities. Signs of mitral valve disease suggest the diagnosis of secondary hemosiderosis (Fig. 3.115).

g. Small (miliary) nodules maximal in the upper zones are strongly suggestive of coal worker's pneumoconiosis, silicosis, or other mineral dust pneumoconioses. The denser the nodules, the more likely the diagnosis of pneumoconiosis.

3. The components of the pattern itself may also be of help:

a. Obvious septal lines are seen only in the conditions listed in Box 3.10. The most common cause by far is pulmonary edema; the next most frequent causes are lymphangitis carcinomatosa and viral or mycoplasmal pneumonia. Usually the other signs on the films, together with the patient's symptoms, permit one of the alternatives to be chosen, particularly if the chronicity or acuteness of the disease is known. For example, rapid appearance or disappearance of septal lines occurs only in pulmonary edema. Viral and mycoplasmal pneumonia are associated with acute febrile illness, whereas relentless progression

over a few weeks is virtually diagnostic of lymphangitis carcinomatosa.

b. True honeycomb pattern is virtually diagnostic of end-stage interstitial pulmonary fibrosis, Langerhans cell histiocytosis, and lymphangioleiomyomatosis.

c. Multiple, partially, or totally calcified small nodular shadows are seen in only a few conditions. Most of the

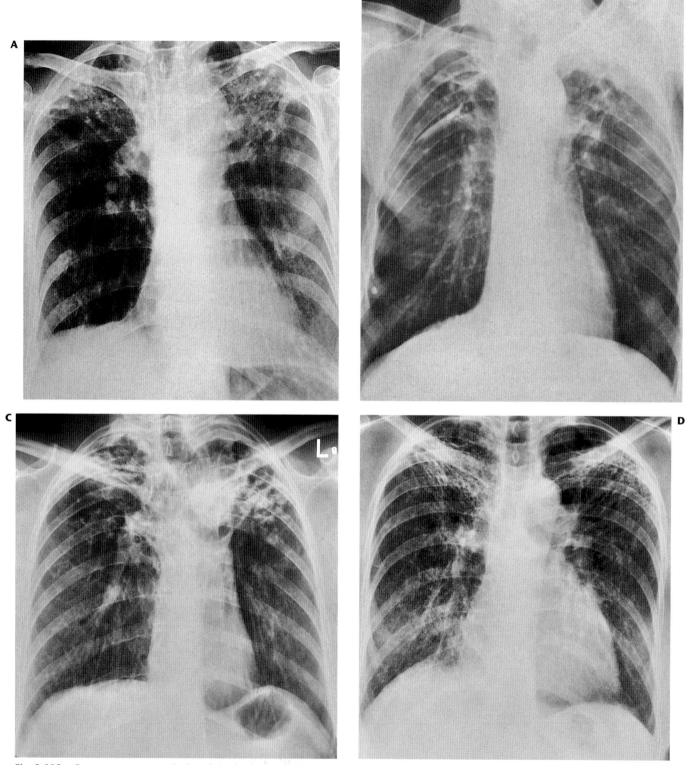

Fig. 3.112 Coarse upper zone reticulonodular shadowing with fibrotic contraction of the upper lobes. **A**, Tuberculosis. Note the patchy small calcifications within the fibrotic upper lobes. **B**, Histoplasmosis. **C**, Extrinsic allergic alveolitis: a case of bird fancier's disease. **D**, Sarcoidosis.

cases encountered will be the result of calcification of disseminated histoplasmosis, tuberculosis, or varicella infection (Fig. 3.116). Occasionally, pneumonia caused by coccidioidomycosis or blastomycosis calcifies. In each instance the responsible pneumonia will have occurred several years before. The presence of calcification indicates healing but, in the case of tuberculous and fungal infections, when there is a mixture of calcification and soft tissue densities, does not necessarily mean the disease is inactive. Radiologically visible calcification

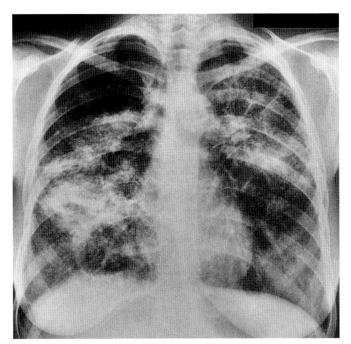

Fig. 3.113 Pulmonary fibrosis caused by sarcoidosis. The mid zone predominance radiating from the hila with relative sparing of extreme apices and bases is typical of sarcoidosis.

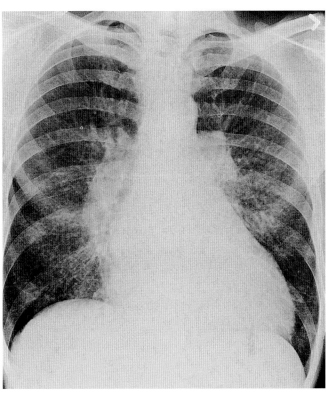

Fig. 3.115 Uniformly distributed fine nodular shadowing caused by hemosiderosis in a patient with mitral valve disease. Note the other signs of mitral valve disease.

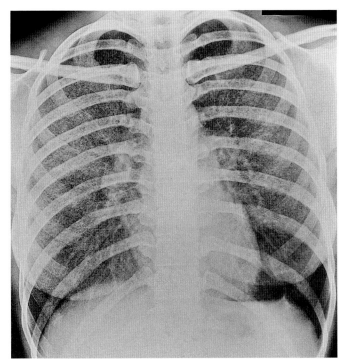

Fig. 3.114 Uniformly distributed fine nodular shadowing in sarcoidosis. Note also the bilateral hilar adenopathy.

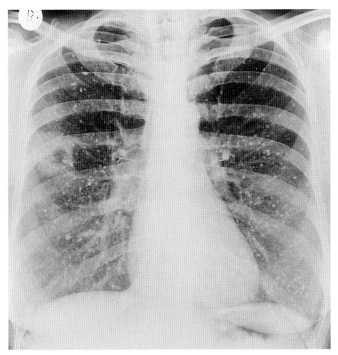

Fig. 3.116 Multiple small calcifications in the lungs caused by old healed varicella pneumonia. (The patient also has a carcinoma of the right upper lobe.)

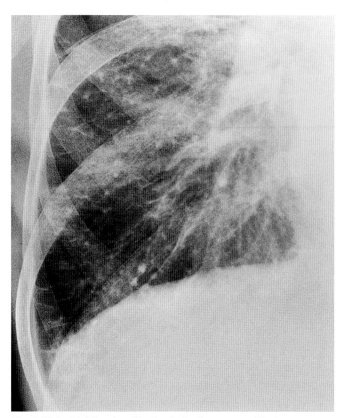

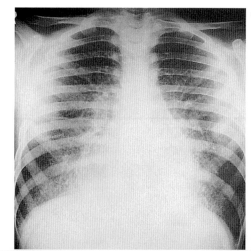

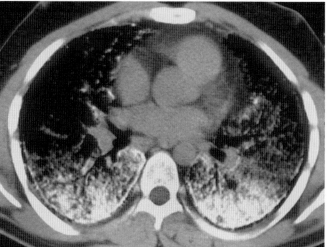

Fig. 3.117 Multifocal ossification in the lungs caused by long-standing mitral valve disease.

Fig. 3.118 Alveolar microlithiasis. **A**, The innumerable fine pulmonary calcifications are so small that they appear cloud-like on chest radiography (courtesy of Dr Michael C Pearson, London). **B**, CT in another patient shows the widespread calcification to advantage.

in miliary metastases is uncommon and for practical purposes is seen only with osteogenic sarcoma and thyroid carcinoma.

d. High-density miliary nodulation may be seen with silicosis, stannosis, baritosis, or microlithiasis. The opacity of the nodules in baritosis may be even greater than calcific density.

e. Multifocal pulmonary ossification is occasionally seen in long-standing mitral valve disease (Fig. 3.117). If the resulting small nodules clearly contain bony trabeculae, the diagnosis is easy. In most cases, however, only amorphous calcification can be recognized radiographically, and the distinction from postinfective calcification becomes impossible. Nowadays the entity is extremely rare.

f. Cloud-like punctate calcification of the lung[235,236] is seen in alveolar microlithiasis (Fig. 3.118) and in hyperparathyroidism (see, Fig. 3.38 and p. 88).

4. Certain combinations may make one diagnosis or a group of diagnoses more likely:

a. The combination of overinflation of the lung, widespread or basally predominant reticulonodular shadowing, and pleural effusion in a woman is virtually diagnostic of the rare entity lymphangioleiomyomatosis (Fig. 3.119).

b. The combination of small irregular shadows, maximal in the upper zone, with bronchial wall thickening and overinflation of the lungs in a younger patient is virtually diagnostic of cystic fibrosis (Fig. 3.120).

c. The presence of bilateral conglomerate shadows greater than l cm in diameter in the upper zones together with widespread or upper zone predominant small nodules in the lungs makes pneumoconiosis virtually certain.

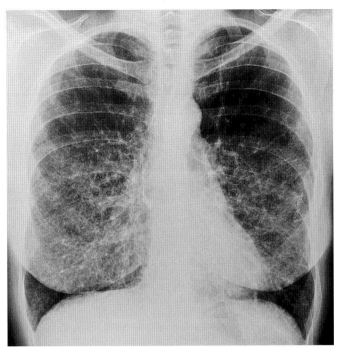

Fig. 3.119 Lymphangioleiomyomatosis of lung. A typical example in a middle-aged woman showing lower zone predominant reticulonodular shadowing and low, flat hemidiaphragms.

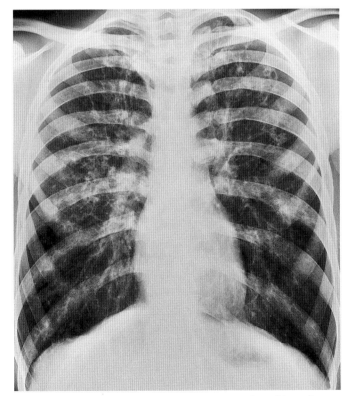

Fig. 3.120 Cystic fibrosis. Note the combination of small irregular shadows in the upper lobe, bronchial wall thickening, and overinflation of the lung in a 20-year-old man.

INCREASED TRANSRADIANCY OF THE LUNG

True increase in transradiancy of the lungs (that is, not due to technical factors) can be divided according to distribution into widespread, affecting both lungs; unilateral, affecting all or the majority of one lung; and focal, affecting a portion of one lobe only. (Increased transradiancy within a pulmonary opacity or contained with a cyst or cavity are separate topics discussed earlier in this chapter.)

Widespread increase in transradiancy of both lungs is seen in two basic conditions: airway disease, notably emphysema, bronchiolitis, and asthma; and obstruction to blood flow from the right side of the heart, usually associated with right to left cardiac shunting, such as in Fallot's tetralogy, Eisenmenger's physiology, or severe widespread peripheral pulmonary arterial stenoses. Massive pulmonary embolism is a theoretic possibility for widespread pulmonary oligemia but in practice is virtually never seen.

A focal increase in transradiancy is seen with emphysema and bullous disease in constrictive bronchiolitis and in some patients with pulmonary emboli.

Increased transradiancy of one lung (also known as unilateral hyperlucent lung) is a fairly commonly encountered radiographic finding. The causes of unilateral increased transradiancy may be broken down as follows:

1. Radiographic artifact. Output of x-rays from the x-ray tube may not be uniform across the radiographic field. This so-called "heel–toe effect" is normally adjusted vertically so that output increases from the apices to the bases. If the heel–toe effect operates across the thorax, one hemithorax may appear more penetrated (that is, more transradiant) than the other. A similar appearance may result from slight rotation of the patient; the side to which the patient is rotated is the more penetrated, regardless of whether the film has been taken PA or AP.[237] In both situations the relative exposures of the soft tissues, especially around the shoulder girdles, should be compared. A clear-cut difference in penetration of these structures indicates that the explanation for increased transradiancy is technical rather than pathological.
2. Thoracic wall and soft tissue abnormalities are the most common cause of a unilateral hyperlucent lung (notably, a mastectomy on the ipsilateral side). Other causes include a congenital defect of the pectoral muscles (Poland syndrome).
3. Diminished perfusion of the lung. A substantial reduction in perfusion of one lung may cause that lung to be abnormally lucent. The causes may be either congenital (for example, aplasia of a pulmonary artery or hypoplasia of the lung) or acquired (for example, thromboembolic disease, fibrosing mediastinitis, tumor infiltration, inhaled foreign body, or Swyer–James syndrome [Fig. 3.121]).
4. Over-expansion of the lung. The lung as a whole may be relatively hyperexpanded when compared with the opposite lung. This state may result, for example, from foreign body impaction with obstructive emphysema. On occasion, emphysema, especially with bulla formation, may be asymmetric. Lobar collapse on one side with compensatory emphysema in the rest of the lung can superficially resemble a transradiant hemithorax, particularly if the collapse is chronic and extreme, since the collapsed lobe may be a relatively inconspicuous sliver of tissue wedged

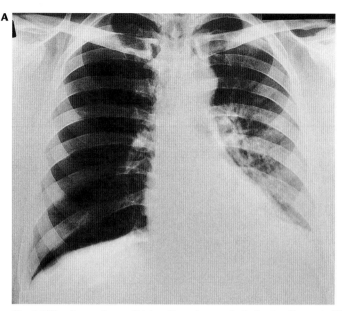
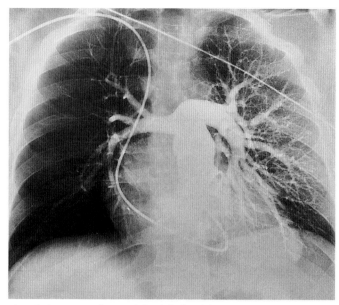

Fig. 3.121 Swyer–James (McLeod) syndrome. **A**, A chest radiograph. Note the relative transradiancy of the right hemithorax, reduction in size of the hilar vessels, and the small intrapulmonary vessels in the right lung. **B**, A pulmonary angiogram in the same patient.

against the mediastinum. Careful study of the hilar airway and vascular anatomy should resolve this confusion. On occasion, a lobar resection may have been performed, leaving remarkably little radiographic evidence of previous surgical intervention other than increased transradiancy.

5. Mild generalized increased opacity of one lung may be misinterpreted as increased transradiancy of the opposite normal lung. Examples are the filtering effect of a large pleural effusion layering out posteriorly in a supine patient and the occasional case of uniform loss of volume of a lung. The latter applies particularly to patients in intensive care who have mucus plugging. Some patchy pulmonary parenchymal density is likely to be present, indicating the true situation.

REFERENCES

1. Felson B, Felson H. Localization of intrathoracic lesions by means of the postero-anterior roentgenogram: the silhouette sign. Radiology 1950;55: 363–374.
2. Kuriyama K, Tateishi R, Doi O, et al. CT–pathologic correlation in small peripheral lung cancers. AJR Am J Roentgenol 1987;149:1139–1143.
3. Reed JC, Madewell JE. The air bronchogram in interstitial disease of the lungs. A radiological–pathological correlation. Radiology 1975;116:1–9.
4. Wilson AG. The interpretation of shadows on the adult chest radiograph. Br J Hosp Med 1987;37:526–534.
5. Tuddenham WJ. Glossary of terms for thoracic radiology: recommendations of the Nomenclature Committee of the Fleischner Society. AJR Am J Roentgenol 1984;143:509–517.
6. Ziskind MM, Weill H, Rayzant AR. The recognition and significance of acinus-filling processes of the lung. Am Rev Respir Dis 1963;87:551–559.
7. Richards PJ, Armstrong P, Parkin JM, et al. Chest imaging in AIDS. Clin Radiol 1998;53:554–566.

8. Gross BH, Glazer GM, Wimbish KJ. CT of solitary cavitary infiltrates. Semin Roentgenol 1984;19:236–242.
9. Joshi RR, Cholankeril JV. Computed tomography in lipoid pneumonia. J Comput Assist Tomogr 1985;9:211–213.
10. Lee KS, Muller NL, Hale V, et al. Lipoid pneumonia: CT findings. J Comput Assist Tomogr 1995;19:48–51.
11. Maldonado RL. The CT angiogram sign. Radiology 1999;210:323–324.
12. Im JG, Han MC, Yu EJ, et al. Lobar bronchioloalveolar carcinoma: "angiogram sign" on CT scans. Radiology 1990;176:749–753.
13. Murayama S, Onitsuka H, Murakami J, et al. "CT angiogram sign" in obstructive pneumonitis and pneumonia. J Comput Assist Tomogr 1993;17:609–612.
14. Shah RM, Friedman AC. CT angiogram sign: incidence and significance in lobar consolidations evaluated by contrast-enhanced CT. AJR Am J Roentgenol 1998;170:719–721.
15. Schuster MR, Scanlan KA. "CT angiogram sign": establishing the differential diagnosis. Radiology 1991;181:903.

16. Vincent JM, Ng YY, Norton AJ, et al. CT "angiogram sign" in primary pulmonary lymphoma. J Comput Assist Tomogr 1992;16:829–831.
17. Bressler EL, Francis IR, Glazer GM, et al. Bolus contrast medium enhancement for distinguishing pleural from parenchymal lung disease: CT features. J Comput Assist Tomogr 1987;11: 436–440.
18. Reed JC. Chest radiology: plain film patterns and differential diagnosis. Chicago: Year Book, 1987.
19. Ip M, Chen NK, So SY, et al. Unusual rib destruction in pleuropulmonary tuberculosis. Chest 1989;95:242–244.
20. Gaensler EA, Carrington CB. Peripheral opacities in chronic eosinophilic pneumonia: the photographic negative of pulmonary edema. AJR Am J Roentgenol 1977;128:1–13.
21. Mayo JR, Muller NL, Road J, et al. Chronic eosinophilic pneumonia: CT findings in six cases. AJR Am J Roentgenol 1989;153:727–730.
22. Mani TM, Lallemand D, Corone S, et al. Metastatic pulmonary calcifications after

cardiac surgery in children. Radiology 1990;174:463–467.

23. Johkoh T, Ikezoe J, Nagareda T, et al. Metastatic pulmonary calcification: early detection by high-resolution CT. J Comput Assist Tomogr 1993;17:471–473.

24. Libson E, Wechsler RJ, Steiner RM. Pulmonary calcinosis following orthotopic liver transplantation. J Thorac Imaging 1993;8:305–308.

25. Winter EM, Pollard AJ, Chapman S, et al. Case report: pulmonary calcification after liver transplantation in children. Br J Radiol 1995;68:923–925.

26. Chan ED, Morales DV, Welsh CH, et al. Calcium deposition with or without bone formation in the lung. Am J Respir Crit Care Med 2002;165:1654–1669.

27. Woodring JH, Reed JC. Types and mechanisms of pulmonary atelectasis. J Thorac Imaging 1996;11:92–108.

28. Naidich DP, McCauley DI, Khouri NF, et al. Computed tomography of lobar collapse: 2. Collapse in the absence of endobronchial obstruction. J Comput Assist Tomogr 1983;7:758–767.

29. Fleischner F. Uber das Wesen der basalen horizontalen Schattenstreifen im Lungenfeld. Wien Arch Intern Med 1936;28:461.

30. Westcott JL, Cole S. Plate atelectasis. Radiology 1985;155:1–9.

31. Nordenstrom B, Novek J. The atelectatic complex of the left lung. Acta Radiol 1960;53:177–183.

32. Price J. Linear atelectasis in the lingula as a diagnostic feature of left lower lobe collapse: Nordenstrom's sign. Australas Radiol 1991;35:56–60.

33. Molina PL, Hiken JN, Glazer HS. Imaging evaluation of obstructive atelectasis. J Thorac Imaging 1996; 11:176–186.

34. Proto AV, Tocino I. Radiographic manifestations of lobar collapse. Semin Roentgenol 1980;15:117–173.

35. Woodring JH, Reed JC. Radiographic manifestations of lobar atelectasis. J Thorac Imaging 1996;11:109–144.

36. Khoury MB, Godwin JD, Halvorsen RA Jr, et al. CT of obstructive lobar collapse. Invest Radiol 1985;20:708–716.

37. Raasch BN, Heitzman ER, Carsky EW, et al. A computed tomographic study of bronchopulmonary collapse. Radiographics 1984;4:195–232.

38. Mayr B, Ingrisch H, Haussinger K, et al. Tumors of the bronchi: role of evaluation with CT. Radiology 1989;172:647–652.

39. Naidich DP, McCauley DI, Khouri NF, et al. Computed tomography of lobar collapse: 1. Endobronchial obstruction. J Comput Assist Tomogr 1983;7:745–757.

40. Naidich DP, Lee JJ, Garay SM, et al. Comparison of CT and fiberoptic bronchoscopy in the evaluation of bronchial disease. AJR Am J Roentgenol 1987;148:1–7.

41. Woodring JH. Determining the cause of pulmonary atelectasis: a comparison of plain radiography and CT. AJR Am J Roentgenol 1988;150:757–763.

42. Golden R. The effect of bronchostenosis upon the roentgen-ray shadows in carcinoma of the bronchus. AJR Am J Roentgenol 1925;13:21–30.

43. Reinig JW, Ross P. Computed tomography appearance of Golden's "S" sign. J Comput Tomogr 1984;8: 219–223.

44. Ashizawa K, Hayashi K, Aso N, et al. Lobar atelectasis: diagnostic pitfalls on chest radiography. Br J Radiol 2001;74:89–97.

45. Glazer HS, Anderson DJ, Sagel SS. Bronchial impaction in lobar collapse: CT demonstration and pathologic correlation. AJR Am J Roentgenol 1989;153:485–488.

46. Shin MS, Ho KJ. CT fluid bronchogram: observation in postobstructive pulmonary consolidation. Clin Imaging 1992;16:109–113.

47. Herold CJ, Kuhlman JE, Zerhouni EA. Pulmonary atelectasis: signal patterns with MR imaging. Radiology 1991; 178:715–720.

48. Whalen JP, Lane EJ Jr. Bronchial rearrangements in pulmonary collapse as seen on the lateral radiograph. Radiology 1969;93:285–288.

49. Teel G, Engeler C. Computed tomography correlation in atypical (peripheral) right upper lobe collapse: the minor fissure as an explanation for the pleural-based density. J Thorac Imaging 1996;11:86–88.

50. Franken EA Jr, Klatte EC. Atypical (peripheral) upper lobe collapse. Ann Radiol (Paris) 1977;20:87–93.

51. Don C, Desmarais R. Peripheral upper lobe collapse in adults. Radiology 1989;170:657–659.

52. Gurney JW. Atypical manifestations of pulmonary atelectasis. J Thorac Imaging 1996;11:165–175.

53. Tamaki I, Pandit R, Gooding CA. Neonatal atypical peripheral atelectasis. Pediatr Radiol 1995;24:589–591.

54. Adler J, Cameron DC. CT correlation in peripheral right upper lobe collapse. J Comput Assist Tomogr 1988;12:510–511.

55. Kattan KR, Eyler WR, Felson B. The juxtaphrenic peak in upper lobe collapse. Semin Roentgenol 1980;15:187–193.

56. Cameron DC. The juxtaphrenic peak (Katten's sign) is produced by rotation of an inferior accessory fissure. Australas Radiol 1993;37:332–335.

57. Davis SD, Yankelevitz DF, Wand A, et al. Juxtaphrenic peak in upper and middle lobe volume loss: assessment with CT. Radiology 1996;198:143–149.

58. Godwin JD, Tarver RD. Accessory fissures of the lung. AJR Am J Roentgenol 1985;144:39–47.

59. Naidich DP, Ettinger N, Leitman BS, et al. CT of lobar collapse. Semin Roentgenol 1984;19:222–235.

60. Blankenbaker DG. The luftsichel sign. Radiology 1998;208:319–320.

61. Culiner MM. The right middle lobe syndrome, a non-obstructive complex. Dis Chest 1966;50:57–66.

62. Kwon KY, Myers JL, Swensen SJ, et al. Middle lobe syndrome: a clinicopathological study of 21 patients. Hum Pathol 1995;26:302–307.

63. Rosenbloom SA, Ravin CE, Putman CE, et al. Peripheral middle lobe syndrome. Radiology 1983;149:17–21.

64. Proto AV, Merhar GL. Central bronchial displacement with large posterior pleural collections. Findings on the lateral chest radiograph and CT scans. J Can Assoc Radiol 1984;35:128–132.

65. Kattan KR. Upper mediastinal changes in lower lobe collapse. Semin Roentgenol 1980;15:183–186.

66. Kattan KR, Felson B, Holder LE, et al. Superior mediastinal shift in right-lower-lobe collapse: the "upper triangle sign." Radiology 1975;116:305–309.

67. Kattan KR, Wlot JF. Cardiac rotation in left lower lobe collapse. "The flat waist sign." Radiology 1976;118:275–279.

68. Glay J, Palayew MJ. Unusual pattern of left lower lobe atelectasis. Radiology 1981;141:331–333.

69. Lee KS, Logan PM, Primack SL, et al. Combined lobar atelectasis of the right lung: imaging findings. AJR Am J Roentgenol 1994;163:43–47.

70. Saterfiel JL, Virapongse C, Clore FC. Computed tomography of combined right upper and middle lobe collapse. J Comput Assist Tomogr 1988;12:383–387.

71. Chong BW, Weisbrod GL, Herman S. Atypical collapse of the upper lobe of the right lung simulating combined right upper and middle lobe collapse: report of two cases. Can Assoc Radiol J 1990;41:358–362.

72. Blesovsky A. The folded lung. Br J Dis Chest 1966;60:19–22.

73. Cho SR, Henry DA, Beachley MC, et al. Round (helical) atelectasis. Br J Radiol 1981;54:643–650.

74. Payne CR, Jaques P, Kerr IH. Lung folding simulating peripheral pulmonary neoplasm (Blesovsky's syndrome). Thorax 1980;35:936–940.

75. Schneider HJ, Felson B, Gonzalez LL. Rounded atelectasis. AJR Am J Roentgenol 1980;134:225–232.

76. Hillerdal G. Rounded atelectasis. Clinical experience with 74 patients. Chest 1989;95:836–841.

77. Mintzer RA, Gore RM, Vogelzang RL, et al. Rounded atelectasis and its association with asbestos-induced pleural disease. Radiology 1981;139:567–570.

78. Tylen U, Nilsson U. Computed tomography in pulmonary

pseudotumors and their relation to asbestos exposure. J Comput Assist Tomogr 1982;6:229–237.

79. Stancato-Pasik A, Mendelson DS, Marom Z. Rounded atelectasis caused by histoplasmosis. AJR Am J Roentgenol 1990;155:275–276.

80. Cohen AM, Crass JR, Chung-Park M, et al. Rounded atelectasis and fibrotic pleural disease: the pathologic continuum. J Thorac Imaging 1993;8:309–312.

81. Yao L, Killam DA. Rounded atelectasis associated with end-stage renal disease. Chest 1989;96:441–443.

82. Carvalho PM, Carr DH. Computed tomography of folded lung. Clin Radiol 1990;41:86–91.

83. Munden RF, Libshitz HI. Rounded atelectasis and mesothelioma. AJR Am J Roentgenol 1998;170:1519–1522.

84. Batra P, Brown K, Hayashi K, et al. Rounded atelectasis. J Thorac Imaging 1996;11:187–197.

85. Hanke R, Kretzschmar R. Round atelectasis. Semin Roentgenol 1980;15:174–182.

86. Dernevik L, Gatzinsky P. Long term results of operation for shrinking pleuritis with atelectasis. Thorax 1985;40:448–452.

87. Menzies R, Fraser R. Round atelectasis. Pathologic and pathogenetic features. Am J Surg Pathol 1987;11:674–681.

88. Doyle TC, Lawler GA. CT features of rounded atelectasis of the lung. AJR Am J Roentgenol 1984;143:225–228.

89. Lynch DA, Gamsu G, Ray CS, et al. Asbestos-related focal lung masses: manifestations on conventional and high-resolution CT scans. Radiology 1988;169:603–607.

90. McHugh K, Blaquiere RM. CT features of rounded atelectasis. AJR Am J Roentgenol 1989;153:257–260.

91. O'Donovan PB, Schenk M, Lim K, et al. Evaluation of the reliability of computed tomographic criteria used in the diagnosis of round atelectasis. J Thorac Imaging 1997;12:54–58.

92. Stephenson N, Price J. CT appearances of rounded atelectasis. Australas Radiol 1992;36:308–312.

93. Taylor PM. Dynamic contrast enhancement of asbestos-related pulmonary pseudotumours. Br J Radiol 1988;61:1070–1072.

94. Silverman SP, Marino PL. Unusual case of enlarging pulmonary mass. Chest 1987;91:457–458.

95. Marchbank ND, Wilson AG, Joseph AE. Ultrasound features of folded lung. Clin Radiol 1996;51:433–437.

96. Verschakelen JA, Demaerel P, Coolen J, et al. Rounded atelectasis of the lung: MR appearance. AJR Am J Roentgenol 1989;152:965–966.

97. Yamaguchi T, Hayashi K, Ashizawa K, et al. Magnetic resonance imaging of rounded atelectasis. J Thorac Imaging 1997;12:188–194.

98. McAdams HP, Erasmus JJ, Patz EF, et al. Evaluation of patients with round atelectasis using 2-[18F]-fluoro-2-deoxy-D-glucose PET. J Comput Assist Tomogr 1998;22:601–604.

99. Steele JD. The solitary pulmonary nodule – report of a cooperative study of resected asymptomatic solitary pulmonary nodules in males. J Thorac Cardiovasc Surg 1963;46:21–39.

100. Good CA, Wilson TW. The solitary circumscribed pulmonary nodule: study of seven hundred and five cases encountered roentgenologically in a period of three and one half years. JAMA 1958;166:210–215.

101. Quint LE, Park CH, Iannettoni MD. Solitary pulmonary nodules in patients with extrapulmonary neoplasms. Radiology 2000;217:257–261.

102. Lillington GA, Caskey CI. Evaluation and management of solitary and multiple pulmonary nodules. Clin Chest Med 1993;14:111–119.

103. Chiles C, Sherrier RH. Analysis of the solitary pulmonary nodule by means of digital techniques. J Thorac Imaging 1990;5:55–60.

104. Higashi Y, Nakamura H, Matsumoto T, et al. Dual-energy computed tomographic diagnosis of pulmonary nodules. J Thorac Imaging 1994;9:31–34.

105. Swensen SJ, Yamashita K, McCollough CH, et al. Lung nodules: dual-kilovolt peak analysis with CT – multicenter study. Radiology 2000;214:81–85.

106. Berger WG, Erly WK, Krupinski EA, et al. The solitary pulmonary nodule on chest radiography: can we really tell if the nodule is calcified? AJR Am J Roentgenol 2001;176:201–204.

107. Swensen SJ, Morin RL, Aughenbaugh GL, et al. CT reconstruction algorithm selection in the evaluation of solitary pulmonary nodules. J Comput Assist Tomogr 1995;19:932–935.

108. Siegelman SS, Zerhouni EA, Leo FP, et al. CT of the solitary pulmonary nodule. AJR Am J Roentgenol 1980;135:1–13.

109. Proto AV, Thomas SR. Pulmonary nodules studied by computed tomography. Radiology 1985;156:149–153.

110. Siegelman SS, Khouri NF, Leo FP, et al. Solitary pulmonary nodules: CT assessment. Radiology 1986;160:307–312.

111. Zerhouni EA, Stitik FP, Siegelman SS, et al. CT of the pulmonary nodule: a cooperative study. Radiology 1986;160:319–327.

112. Goldstein MS, Rush M, Johnson P, et al. A calcified adenocarcinoma of the lung with very high CT numbers. Radiology 1984;150:785–786.

113. Jones FA, Wiedemann HP, O'Donovan PB, et al. Computerized tomographic densitometry of the solitary pulmonary nodule using a nodule phantom. Chest 1989;96:779–783.

114. Mahoney MC, Shipley RT, Corcoran HL, et al. CT demonstration of calcification in carcinoma of the lung. AJR Am J Roentgenol 1990;154:255–258.

115. Mallens WM, Nijhuis-Heddes JM, Bakker W. Calcified lymph node metastases in bronchioloalveolar carcinoma. Radiology 1986;161:103–104.

116. Stewart JG, MacMahon H, Vyborny CJ, et al. Dystrophic calcification in carcinoma of the lung: demonstration by CT. AJR Am J Roentgenol 1987;148:29–30.

117. Swensen SJ, Harms GF, Morin RL, et al. CT evaluation of solitary pulmonary nodules: value of 185-H reference phantom. AJR Am J Roentgenol 1991;156:925–929.

118. Yankelevitz DF, Henschke CI. Derivation for relating calcification and size in small pulmonary nodules. Clin Imaging 1998;22:1–6.

119. Zerhouni EA, Boukadoum M, Siddiky MA, et al. A standard phantom for quantitative CT analysis of pulmonary nodules. Radiology 1983;149:767–773.

120. Ko JP, Naidich DP. Lung nodule detection and characterization with multislice CT. Radiol Clin North Am 2003;41:575–597.

121. Nakajima R, Yokose T, Kakinuma R, et al. Localized pure ground-glass opacity on high-resolution CT: histologic characteristics. J Comput Assist Tomogr 2002;26:323–329.

122. Aoki T, Nakata H, Watanabe H, et al. Evolution of peripheral lung adenocarcinomas: CT findings correlated with histology and tumor doubling time. AJR Am J Roentgenol 2000;174:763–768.

123. Tateishi U, Nishihara H, Tsukamoto E, et al. Lung tumors evaluated with FDG-PET and dynamic CT: the relationship between vascular density and glucose metabolism. J Comput Assist Tomogr 2002;26:185–190.

124. Littleton JT, Durizch ML, Moeller G, et al. Pulmonary masses: contrast enhancement. Radiology 1990;177:861–871.

125. Swensen SJ, Brown LR, Colby TV, et al. Lung nodule enhancement at CT: prospective findings. Radiology 1996;201:447–455.

126. Swensen SJ, Viggiano RW, Midthun DE, et al. Lung nodule enhancement at CT: multicenter study. Radiology 2000;214:73–80.

127. Zhang M, Kono M. Solitary pulmonary nodules: evaluation of blood flow patterns with dynamic CT. Radiology 1997;205:471–478.

128. Potente G, Iacari V, Caimi M. The challenge of solitary pulmonary nodules:

HRCT evaluation. Comput Med Imaging Graph 1997;21:39–46.

129. Yamashita K, Matsunobe S, Tsuda T, et al. Solitary pulmonary nodule: preliminary study of evaluation with incremental dynamic CT. Radiology 1995;194:399–405.

130. Murayama S, Murakami J, Hashimoto S, et al. Noncalcified pulmonary tuberculomas: CT enhancement patterns with histological correlation. J Thorac Imaging 1995;10:91–95.

131. Guckel C, Schnabel K, Deimling M, et al. Solitary pulmonary nodules: MR evaluation of enhancement patterns with contrast-enhanced dynamic snapshot gradient-echo imaging. Radiology 1996;200:681–686.

132. Ohno Y, Hatabu H, Takenaka D, et al. Solitary pulmonary nodules: potential role of dynamic MR imaging in management initial experience. Radiology 2002;224:503–511.

133. Kono M, Adachi S, Kusumoto M, et al. Clinical utility of Gd-DTPA-enhanced magnetic resonance imaging in lung cancer. J Thorac Imaging 1993;8:18–26.

134. Sakai F, Sone S, Maruyama A, et al. Thin-rim enhancement in Gd-DTPA-enhanced magnetic resonance images of tuberculoma: a new finding of potential differential diagnostic importance. J Thorac Imaging 1992;7:64–69.

135. Chung MH, Lee HG, Kwon SS, et al. MR imaging of solitary pulmonary lesion: emphasis on tuberculomas and comparison with tumors. J Magn Reson Imaging 2000;11:629–637.

136. Menda Y, Kahn D. Somatostatin receptor imaging of non-small cell lung cancer with 99mTc depreotide. Semin Nucl Med 2002;32:92–96.

137. Blum J, Handmaker H, Lister-James J, et al. A multicenter trial with a somatostatin analog (99m)Tc depreotide in the evaluation of solitary pulmonary nodules. Chest 2000;117:1232–1238.

138. Hirano T, Otake H, Yoshida I, et al. Primary lung cancer SPECT imaging with pentavalent technetium-99m-DMSA. J Nucl Med 1995;36:202–207.

139. Minai OA, Raja S, Mehta AC, et al. Role of Tc-99m MIBI in the evaluation of single pulmonary nodules: a preliminary report. Thorax 2000;55:60-62.

140. Wang H, Maurea S, Mainolfi C, et al. Tc-99m MIBI scintigraphy in patients with lung cancer. Comparison with CT and fluorine-18 FDG PET imaging. Clin Nucl Med 1997;22:243–249.

141. Scott WJ, Schwabe JL, Gupta NC, et al. Positron emission tomography of lung tumors and mediastinal lymph nodes using [18F]fluorodeoxyglucose. The Members of the PET-Lung Tumor Study Group. Ann Thorac Surg 1994;58:698–703.

142. Patz EF Jr, Lowe VJ, Hoffman JM, et al. Focal pulmonary abnormalities: evaluation with F-18 fluorodeoxyglucose PET scanning. Radiology 1993;188:487–490.

143. Hubner KF, Buonocore E, Gould HR, et al. Differentiating benign from malignant lung lesions using "quantitative" parameters of FDG PET images. Clin Nucl Med 1996;21:941–949.

144. Gupta NC, Maloof J, Gunel E. Probability of malignancy in solitary pulmonary nodules using fluorine-18-FDG and PET. J Nucl Med 1996;37:943–948.

145. Gupta NC, Frank AR, Dewan NA, et al. Solitary pulmonary nodules: detection of malignancy with PET with 2-[F-18]-fluoro-2-deoxy-D-glucose. Radiology 1992;184:441–444.

146. Gupta N, Gill H, Graeber G, et al. Dynamic positron emission tomography with F-18 fluorodeoxyglucose imaging in differentiation of benign from malignant lung/mediastinal lesions. Chest 1998;114:1105–1111.

147. Conti PS, Lilien DL, Hawley K, et al. PET and [18F]-FDG in oncology: a clinical update. Nucl Med Biol 1996;23:717–735.

148. Lowe VJ, Hoffman JM, DeLong DM, et al. Semiquantitative and visual analysis of FDG-PET images in pulmonary abnormalities. J Nucl Med 1994;35:1771–1776.

149. Bousson V, Moretti JL, Weinmann P, et al. Assessment of malignancy in pulmonary lesions: FDG dual-head coincidence gamma camera imaging in association with serum tumor marker measurement. J Nucl Med 2000;41:1801–1807.

150. Matthies A, Hickeson M, Cuchiara A, et al. Dual time point 18F-FDG PET for the evaluation of pulmonary nodules. J Nucl Med 2002;43:871–875.

151. Lowe VJ, Fletcher JW, Gobar L, et al. Prospective investigation of positron emission tomography in lung nodules. J Clin Oncol 1998;16:1075–1084.

152. Prauer HW, Weber WA, Romer W, et al. Controlled prospective study of positron emission tomography using the glucose analogue [18f]fluorodeoxyglucose in the evaluation of pulmonary nodules. Br J Surg 1998;85:1506–1511.

153. Marom EM, Sarvis S, Herndon JE, et al. T1 lung cancers: sensitivity of diagnosis with fluorodeoxyglucose PET. Radiology 2002;223:453–459.

154. Duhaylongsod FG, Lowe VJ, Patz EF Jr, et al. Lung tumor growth correlates with glucose metabolism measured by fluoride-18 fluorodeoxyglucose positron emission tomography. Ann Thorac Surg 1995;60:1348–1352.

155. Higashi K, Ueda Y, Yagishita M, et al. FDG PET measurement of the proliferative potential of non-small cell lung cancer. J Nucl Med 2000;41:85–92.

156. Weber W, Young C, Abdel-Dayem HM, et al. Assessment of pulmonary lesions with 18F-fluorodeoxyglucose positron imaging using coincidence mode gamma cameras. J Nucl Med 1999;40:574–578.

157. Pitman AG, Hicks RJ, Binns DS, et al. Performance of sodium iodide based (18)F-fluorodeoxyglucose positron emission tomography in the characterization of indeterminate pulmonary nodules or masses. Br J Radiol 2002;75:114–121.

158. Kim S, Park CH, Han M, et al. The clinical usefulness of F-18 FDG coincidence PET without attenuation correction and without whole-body scanning mode in pulmonary lesions comparison with CT, MRI, and clinical findings. Clin Nucl Med 1999;24:945–949.

159. Coleman RE. PET in lung cancer. J Nucl Med 1999;40:814–820.

160. Goldsmith SJ, Kostakoglu L. Nuclear medicine imaging of lung cancer. Radiol Clin North Am 2000;38:511–524.

161. Shon IH, O'Doherty MJ, Maisey MN. Positron emission tomography in lung cancer. Semin Nucl Med 2002;32:240–271.

162. Gould MK, Maclean CC, Kuschner WG, et al. Accuracy of positron emission tomography for diagnosis of pulmonary nodules and mass lesions: a meta-analysis. JAMA 2001;285:914–924.

163. Higashi K, Ueda Y, Seki H, et al. Fluorine-18-FDG PET imaging is negative in bronchioloalveolar lung carcinoma. J Nucl Med 1998;39:1016–1020.

164. Lowe VJ, Naunheim KS. Current role of positron emission tomography in thoracic oncology. Thorax 1998;53:703–712.

165. Lowe VJ, Naunheim KS. Positron emission tomography in lung cancer. Ann Thorac Surg 1998;65:1821–1829.

166. Goo JM, Im JG, Do KH, et al. Pulmonary tuberculoma evaluated by means of FDG PET: findings in 10 cases. Radiology 2000;216:117–121.

167. Dewan NA, Shehan CJ, Reeb SD, et al. Likelihood of malignancy in a solitary pulmonary nodule: comparison of Bayesian analysis and results of FDG-PET scan. Chest 1997;112:416–422.

168. Gambhir SS, Shepherd JE, Shah BD, et al. Analytical decision model for the cost-effective management of solitary pulmonary nodules. J Clin Oncol 1998;16:2113–2125.

169. Goldsmith SJ, Kostakoglu L. Role of nuclear medicine in the evaluation of the solitary pulmonary nodule. Semin Ultrasound CT MR 2000;21:129–138.

170. Chahinian P. Relationship between tumor doubling time and anatomo-clinical features in 50 measurable pulmonary cancers. Chest 1992;61:340–345.

171. Garland LH, Coulson W, Wollin E. The rate of growth and apparent duration of untreated primary bronchial carcinoma. Cancer 1963;16:697–707.

172. Meyer JA. Growth rate versus prognosis in resected primary bronchogenic carcinomas. Cancer 1973;31: 1468–1472.

173. Spratt JS, Spjut HJ, Roper CI. The frequency distribution of the rates of growth and the estimated duration of primary pulmonary carcinomas. Cancer 1963;16:687–692.

174. Straus MJ. The growth characteristics of lung cancer and its application to treatment design. Semin Oncol 1974;1:167–174.

175. Usuda K, Saito Y, Sagawa M, et al. Tumor doubling time and prognostic assessment of patients with primary lung cancer. Cancer 1994;74:2239–2244.

176. Weiss W. Tumor doubling time and survival of men with bronchogenic carcinoma. Chest 1974;65:3–8.

177. Spratt JS, Meyer JS, Spratt JA. Rates of growth of human neoplasms: Part II. J Surg Oncol 1996;61:68–83.

178. Nathan MH, Collins VP, Adams RA. Differentiation of benign and malignant pulmonary nodules by growth rate. Radiology 1962;79:221–232.

179. Dunnick NR, Parker BR, Castellino RA. Rapid onset of pulmonary infiltration due to histiocytic lymphoma. Radiology 1976;118:281–285.

180. Collins VP, Loeffler RK, Tivey H. Observations on growth rates in human tumors. AJR Am J Roentgenol 1956; 76:988–1000.

181. Midthun DE, Swensen SJ, Jett JR. Approach to the solitary pulmonary nodule. Mayo Clin Proc 1993;68:378–385.

182. Huston J III, Muhm JR. Solitary pulmonary opacities: plain tomography. Radiology 1987;163:481–485.

183. Bateson EM. An analysis of 155 solitary lung lesions illustrating the differential diagnosis of mixed tumors of the lung. Clin Radiol 1965;16:51–65.

184. Toomes H, Delphendahl A, Manke HG, et al. The coin lesion of the lung. A review of 955 resected coin lesions. Cancer 1983;51:534–537.

185. Good CA. The solitary pulmonary nodule: a problem of management. Radiol Clin North Am 1963;1:429–438.

186. Zwirewich CV, Vedal S, Miller RR, et al. Solitary pulmonary nodule: high-resolution CT and radiologic–pathologic correlation. Radiology 1991;179:469–476.

187. Volterrani L, Vegni V, Pieraccini MGG, et al. Small solitary pulmonary nodule and high-resolution CT: a preliminary report. Eur Radiol 1995;5:443–447.

188. Chen SW, Price J. Focal organizing pneumonia mimicking small peripheral lung adenocarcinoma on CT scans. Australas Radiol 1998;42:360–363.

189. Bryk D. The participating tail. A roentgenographic sign of pulmonary granuloma. Am Rev Respir Dis 1969;100:406–408.

190. Hill CA. "Tail" signs associated with pulmonary lesions: critical reappraisal. AJR Am J Roentgenol 1982;139: 311–316.

191. Shapiro R, Wilson GL, Yesner R, et al. A useful roentgen sign in the diagnosis of localized bronchioloalveolar carcinoma. Am J Roentgenol Radium Ther Nucl Med 1972;114:516–524.

192. Milne EN, Zerhouni EA. Blood supply of pulmonary metastases. J Thorac Imaging 1987;2:15–23.

193. Mori K, Saitou Y, Tominaga K, et al. Small nodular lesions in the lung periphery: new approach to diagnosis with CT. Radiology 1990;177:843–849.

194. Lee KS, Kim Y, Han J, et al. Bronchioloalveolar carcinoma: clinical, histopathologic, and radiologic findings. Radiographics 1997;17:1345–1357.

195. Kuriyama K, Tateishi R, Doi O, et al. Prevalence of air bronchograms in small peripheral carcinomas of the lung on thin-section CT: comparison with benign tumors. AJR Am J Roentgenol 1991;156: 921–924.

196. Singh SP. The positive bronchus sign. Radiology 1998;209:251–252.

197. Gaeta M, Pandolfo I, Volta S, et al. Bronchus sign on CT in peripheral carcinoma of the lung: value in predicting results of transbronchial biopsy. AJR Am J Roentgenol 1991; 157:1181–1185.

198. Woodring JH, Fried AM. Significance of wall thickness in solitary cavities of the lung: a follow-up study. AJR Am J Roentgenol 1983;140:473–474.

199. Baber CE, Hedlund LW, Oddson TA, et al. Differentiating empyemas and peripheral pulmonary abscesses: the value of computed tomography. Radiology 1980;135:755–758.

200. Stark DD, Federle MP, Goodman PC, et al. Differentiating lung abscess and empyema: radiography and computed tomography. AJR Am J Roentgenol 1983;141:163–167.

201. Gaeta M, Blandino A, Scribano E, et al. Computed tomography halo sign in pulmonary nodules: frequency and diagnostic value. J Thorac Imaging 1999;14:109–113.

202. Root JD, Molina PL, Anderson DJ, et al. Pulmonary nodular opacities after transbronchial biopsy in patients with lung transplants. Radiology 1992;184: 435–436.

203. Kuhlman JE, Fishman EK, Siegelman SS. Invasive pulmonary aspergillosis in acute leukemia: characteristic findings on CT, the CT halo sign, and the role of CT in early diagnosis. Radiology 1985;157:611–614.

204. Primack SL, Hartman TE, Lee KS, et al. Pulmonary nodules and the CT halo sign. Radiology 1994;190:513–515.

205. Gaeta M, Volta S, Stroscio S, et al. CT "halo sign" in pulmonary tuberculoma. J Comput Assist Tomogr 1992;16: 827–828.

206. Caskey CI, Templeton PA, Zerhouni EA. Current evaluation of the solitary pulmonary nodule. Radiol Clin North Am 1990;28:511–520.

207. Caskey CI, Zerhouni EA. The solitary pulmonary nodule. Semin Roentgenol 1990;25:85–95.

208. Gurney JW. Determining the likelihood of malignancy in solitary pulmonary nodules with Bayesian analysis. Part I. Theory. Radiology 1993;186:405–413.

209. Webb WR. Radiologic evaluation of the solitary pulmonary nodule. AJR Am J Roentgenol 1990;154:701–708.

210. Leef JL III, Klein JS. The solitary pulmonary nodule. Radiol Clin North Am 2002;40:123–143.

211. Shaham D, Guralnik L. The solitary pulmonary nodule: radiologic considerations. Semin Ultrasound CT MR 2000;21:97–115.

212. Erasmus JJ, Connolly JE, McAdams HP, et al. Solitary pulmonary nodules: Part I. Morphologic evaluation for differentiation of benign and malignant lesions. Radiographics 2000; 20:43–58.

213. Erasmus JJ, McAdams HP, Connolly JE. Solitary pulmonary nodules: Part II. Evaluation of the indeterminate nodule. Radiographics 2000;20:59–66.

214. Gurney JW, Lyddon DM, McKay JA. Determining the likelihood of malignancy in solitary pulmonary nodules with Bayesian analysis. Part II. Application. Radiology 1993; 186:415–422.

215. Erasmus JJ, McAdams HP, Patz EF Jr. Non-small cell lung cancer: FDG-PET imaging. J Thorac Imaging 1999;14: 247–256.

216. Vourtsi A, Gouliamos A, Moulopoulos L, et al. CT appearance of solitary and multiple cystic and cavitary lung lesions. Eur Radiol 2001;11:612–622.

217. Carucci LR, Maki DD, Miller WT. Clustered pulmonary nodules: highly suggestive of benign disease. J Thorac Imaging 2001;16:103–105.

218. Ishihara T, Kikuchi K, Ikeda T, et al. Metastatic pulmonary diseases: biologic factors and modes of treatment. Chest 1973;63:227–232.

219. McGee AR, Warren R. Carcinoma metastatic from the thyroid to the lungs; a twenty-four-year radiographic follow-up. Radiology 1966;87:516–517.

220. Godwin JD, Webb WR, Savoca CJ, et al. Multiple, thin-walled cystic lesions of the lung. AJR Am J Roentgenol 1980;135:593–604.

221. Putman CE, Godwin JD, Silverman PM, et al. CT of localized lucent lung lesions. Semin Roentgenol 1984;19:173–188.

222. Felson B. Mucoid impaction (inspissated secretions) in segmental bronchial obstruction. Radiology 1979;133:9–16.

223. Woodring JH. Unusual radiographic manifestations of lung cancer. Radiol Clin North Am 1990;28:599–618.

224. Heitzman ER. The lung – radiologic–pathologic correlations. St Louis: Mosby, 1993.

225. Trapnell DH. The peripheral lymphatics of the lung. Br J Radiol 1963;36:660–672.

226. Kerley P. Radiology in heart disease. Br Med J 1933;2:594–597.

227. Trapnell DH. The differential diagnosis of linear shadows in chest radiographs. Radiol Clin North Am 1973;11:77–92.

228. Reid L. The connective tissue septa in the adult human lung. Thorax 1959; 14:138–145.

229. Proto AV, Speckman JM. The left lateral radiograph of the chest. Part 1. Med Radiogr Photogr 1979;55:29–74.

230. Carstairs LS. The interpretation of shadows in a restricted area of the lung field on a chest radiograph. Proc Roy Soc Med 1961;54:978–980.

231. Kerr IH. Interstitial lung disease: the role of the radiologist. Clin Radiol 1984; 35:1–7.

232. Felson B. The roentgen diagnosis of disseminated pulmonary alveolar diseases. Semin Roentgenol 1967; 2:3–21.

233. Itoh H, Tokunaga S, Asamoto H, et al. Radiologic–pathologic correlations of small lung nodules with special reference to peribronchiolar nodules. AJR Am J Roentgenol 1978;130: 223–231.

234. Felson B. A new look at pattern recognition of diffuse pulmonary disease. AJR Am J Roentgenol 1979;133:183–189.

235. Brown K, Mund DF, Aberle DR, et al. Intrathoracic calcifications: radiographic features and differential diagnoses. Radiographics 1994;14:1247–1261.

236. Chai JL, Patz EF Jr. CT of the lung: patterns of calcification and other high-attenuation abnormalities. AJR Am J Roentgenol 1994;162:1063–1066.

237. Joseph AE, de Lacey GJ, Bryant TH, et al. The hypertransradiant hemithorax: the importance of lateral decentring, and the explanation for its appearance due to rotation. Clin Radiol 1978;29:125–131.

Basic HRCT patterns of lung disease

The radiographic pattern of diffuse lung disease is often non-specific[1,2] and is subject to considerable observer variation.[3] Furthermore, the inability of a chest radiograph to resolve small differences in lung density makes it insensitive for the detection of early parenchymal disease.[4,5] Numerous studies have shown the fundamental superiority of high-resolution computed tomography (HRCT) over chest radiography in terms of improved detection of diffuse lung disease, provision of a histo-specific diagnosis, and the assessment of disease reversibility. The development of HRCT has resulted in a renaissance in the imaging of interstitial lung disease,[6–11] bronchiectasis,[12,13] and small airways[14,15] and other obstructive lung diseases.[16,17]

NORMAL LUNG ANATOMY ON HRCT

Before considering the individual HRCT patterns that reflect parenchymal and airways disease, an understanding of normal lung anatomy, with particular reference to the secondary pulmonary lobule, is needed. The smallest objects that can be resolved on HRCT range from 100 to 400 μm and depend on the density, geometry, and orientation of the object in relation to the voxel. The limits of spatial resolution determine the anatomy that can be identified on HRCT. Accurate interpretation of HRCT of the diseased lung requires an appreciation of the appearances of normal structures, namely the bronchi, blood vessels, and the secondary pulmonary lobule (Table 4.1).

Throughout the lung the bronchi and pulmonary arteries run and branch together. Both the bronchi and pulmonary arteries taper slightly as they travel radially; this is most obvious in bronchi running parallel and within the plane of section. At any given level, the external diameter of the bronchus is almost exactly the same diameter as its accompanying pulmonary

Table 4.1 Visibility of normal structures on HRCT

Normal lung structures visible on HRCT	Normal lung structures not visible on HRCT
Bronchi (down to eighth generation)	Lymphatic vessels
Pulmonary arteries	Alveoli and acini
Pulmonary veins	Capillary vessels
Interlobular septa (peripheral and occasional only)	Visceral pleura (nonfissural surface)
Visceral pleura (double layer as lobar fissures)	
Intrapulmonary lymph node (infrequent small nodule)	

artery: the mean ratio of external diameter of pulmonary artery to bronchus on HRCT has been reported to be 0.98, standard deviation (SD) 0.14, but the range is wide (0.53–1.39).[18] The ratio of the *internal* luminal diameter of a bronchus to the diameter of its adjacent pulmonary artery for healthy individuals has been estimated to be 0.62 ± 0.13 (mean ± SD).[19] The bronchovascular bundle is surrounded by a connective tissue sheath from its origin at the hilum to the respiratory bronchioles in the lung periphery. The concept of separate, but connected, components making up the lung interstitium, propounded by Weibel,[20] is important to the understanding of HRCT findings in interstitial lung disease (the equivalent terms applicable to HRCT are given in parenthesis): the *peripheral* interstitium (subpleural interstitium) surrounds the surface of the lung beneath the visceral pleura and penetrates the lung to surround the secondary pulmonary lobules (paraseptal interstitium). Within the lobules, a finer network of *septal* connective tissue fibers

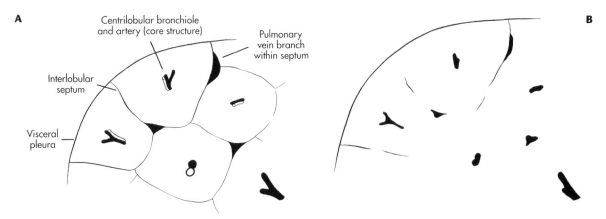

Fig. 4.1   **A**, Anatomy of a group of secondary pulmonary lobules. **B**, Features of secondary pulmonary lobules identifiable on HRCT. The centrilobular bronchioles are not resolved on HRCT and normal interlobular septa are rarely demonstrated in their entirety.

(intralobular interstitium) support the alveoli. The *axial* fibers form a sheath around the bronchovascular bundles (peribronchovascular interstitium) extending from the pulmonary hila to the lung periphery, as far out as the alveolar ducts and sacs. The connective tissue stroma of these separate components is in continuity and thus forms a fibrous skeleton for the lungs and a potential scaffold for infiltrative disease.

The interface between the bronchovascular bundle and surrounding lung is normally sharp. Any thickening of the connective tissue interstitium will result in apparent bronchial wall thickening and blurring of this interface. The size of the smallest subsegmental bronchi visible on HRCT is determined by the thickness of the bronchial wall rather than their diameter. In general, bronchi with a diameter of less than 3 mm with walls less than 300 μm thick are not identifiable on HRCT.[21,22] Airways reach this critical size approximately 3 cm from the pleural surface.

The secondary pulmonary lobule is the smallest anatomic unit of the lung surrounded by a connective tissue septum (Fig. 4.1). Within the interlobular septa are lymphatic channels and venules. Abnormal thickening of the septa between the lobules is responsible for the basal short subpleural horizontal (Kerley B) lines seen on a chest radiograph. The lobule contains approximately 12 acini, each of which measures approximately 6–10 mm in diameter. Each lobule is approximately 2 cm in diameter and is polyhedral, often resembling a truncated cone.[23–25] A defining feature of the secondary pulmonary lobule is the "core structure", comprising the supplying bronchiole and homologous pulmonary artery, which enters through the apex of the lobule.

The connective tissue interlobular septa are well developed in the subpleural regions, particularly on the diaphragmatic surfaces and anterolateral regions of the lungs, where the bases of the cone-shaped lobules lie on the visceral pleural surface. In normal individuals, these interlobular septa measure approximately 100 μm in thickness. They are not usually seen on HRCT because the lower limit of effective resolution of HRCT in vivo is approximately 200 μm. The few interlobular septa that are visible in normal individuals are inconspicuous and are seen as straight lines 1–2 cm in length terminating at a visceral pleural surface (Fig. 4.2). Sometimes several septa joining end to end are seen as a nonbranching linear structure measuring up to 4 cm[21]; these are most frequent at the lung bases overlying the

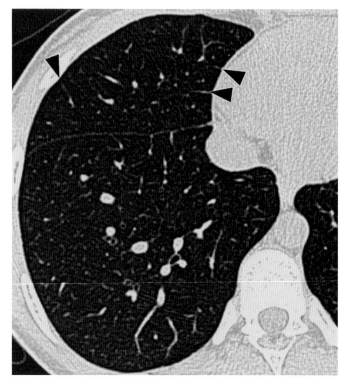

Fig. 4.2   A few peripheral interlobular septa (arrowheads) are visible in the right middle lobes and in the right lower lobe along the major fissure, in an individual with no known lung disease.

diaphragmatic surface. Deep within the lung, where the septa are less well developed, the interlobular septa are only visible when pathologically thickened.

The secondary pulmonary lobule is supplied by a centrilobular artery and bronchiole which are approximately 1 mm in diameter as they enter the lobule.[21,22,26] In the normal state the core structures, effectively the 500–1000 μm diameter centrilobular artery alone, are visible as dots 1 cm from the pleural surface. It is only when the bronchioles are considerably thickened and surrounded by exudate that they become visible as V- or Y-shaped opacities (Fig. 4.3). The lung parenchyma between the core structures and interlobular septa is usually of homogeneous low density, marginally greater than air.

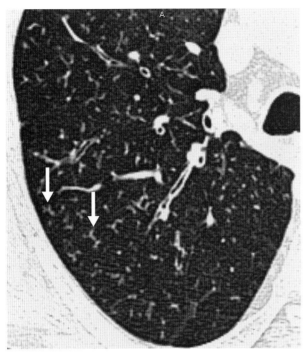

Fig. 4.3 The minute branching structures in the lung periphery (arrows) represent small airways filled and surrounded by exudate (tree-in-bud pattern) in a patient with mild cylindrical bronchiectasis.

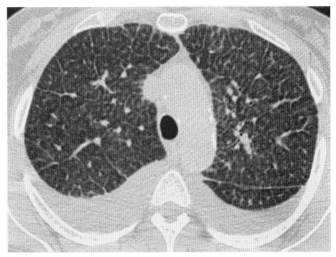

Fig. 4.4 Widespread thickening of the interlobular septa in a patient with left ventricular failure and pulmonary edema. There are also poorly defined centrilobular nodules and bilateral pleural effusions.

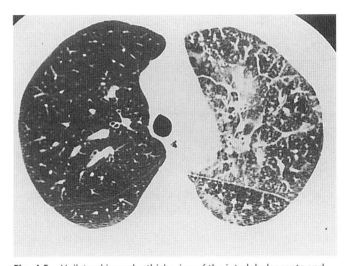

Fig. 4.5 Unilateral irregular thickening of the interlobular septa and bronchovascular bundles in a patient with lymphangitis carcinomatosa.

HRCT PATTERNS OF DIFFUSE LUNG DISEASE

The close correlation between HRCT appearances and macroscopic pulmonary abnormalities[7,27] often allows accurate anatomic terms to be used in describing patterns of diffuse lung disease. Inexact terms, often used for the description of radiographs, have largely been replaced by precise morphologic terms derived from an understanding of normal HRCT anatomy. Abnormal patterns on HRCT which denote pulmonary disease were initially given many names[28,29] but there has been convergence on the majority of terms used in HRCT terminology,[30–32] and some of the most frequently encountered terms in the HRCT lexicon, as defined by the nomenclature committee of the Fleischner Society,[32] are summarized in Table 4.2.

Diffuse abnormalities of the lung parenchyma on HRCT can be broadly categorized into one of the following four patterns: (1) reticular and short linear opacities, (2) nodular opacities, (3) increased lung opacity (ground-glass opacity or consolidation), and (4) cystic airspaces and areas of decreased lung density. While these HRCT patterns correspond to recognizable patterns on chest radiography, they are seen with much greater clarity on the cross-sectional images of HRCT, and the precise distribution of disease can be more readily appreciated.

Reticular pattern

A reticular pattern on HRCT almost always indicates significant interstitial disease. The term is purely descriptive (*reticulum* = network) and there are several morphologic variations on this basic pattern, ranging from generalized thickening of the interlobular septa to honeycomb lung destruction (Box 4.1).

A reticular pattern caused by thickening of interlobular septa is a frequent finding in many interstitial lung diseases.[33] Numerous thickened interlobular septa (which form polygonal outlines) indicate an extensive interstitial abnormality. Causes of septal thickening include infiltration with fibrosis, abnormal cells, or fluid (for example, interstitial fibrosis, lymphangitis carcinomatosa, and pulmonary edema [Fig. 4.4] respectively).

Thickened interlobular septa may appear smooth or irregular on HRCT[33,34] but this distinction is not always obvious: irregular septal thickening is a feature of lymphangitic spread of tumor (Fig. 4.5)[23,35–37] whereas pulmonary edema[38] and alveolar proteinosis cause smooth septal thickening[39–41] (Fig. 4.6). Sarcoidosis causes nodular septal thickening (Fig. 4.7) although thickened septa are not usually the dominant feature of this disease.[42] Of the common conditions that cause generalized thickening of the interlobular septa, lymphangitis carcinomatosa is characterized by the most profuse and obvious septal thick-

Table 4.2 Frequently encountered terms in HRCT of diffuse lung disease

Term	Definition
Air-trapping	Decreased attenuation of pulmonary parenchyma, especially manifest as less than normal increase in attenuation during expiration. To be differentiated from the decreased attenuation of hypoperfusion secondary to locally increased pulmonary arterial resistance. *Pathophysiology*: The retention of excess gas in all or part of the lung, especially during expiration, either as a result of complete or partial airway obstruction or as a result of local abnormalities in pulmonary compliance.
Centrilobular emphysema (centriacinar emphysema)	Centrilobular areas of decreased attenuation, usually without visible walls; of nonuniform distribution, and predominantly located in upper lung zones. *Pathology*: Emphysema that is characterized by destroyed centrilobular alveolar septa and enlargement of respiratory bronchioles.
Centrilobular structures	The pulmonary artery and its immediate branches in a secondary lobule; these arteries measure approximately 1 mm and 0.5–0.7 mm in diameter, respectively. HRCT depicts these vessels. However, a normal bronchiole supplying a secondary lobule has a wall thickness of approximately 0.15 mm, which is beyond the resolution of HRCT. Therefore, normal airways in secondary pulmonary lobules are not detected at CT examination. *Anatomy*: The central tubular structures in a secondary pulmonary lobule (i.e. the centrilobular artery and bronchiole).
Consolidation	Homogeneous increase in pulmonary parenchymal attenuation that obscures the margins of vessels and airway walls. An air bronchogram may be present.
Cyst	A round parenchymal space with a well-defined wall; usually air-containing when in the lung but without associated pulmonary emphysema; commonly used to describe enlarged airspaces in end-stage pulmonary fibrosis, Langerhans cell histiocytosis, and lymphangioleiomyomatosis.
Cystic airspace	Enlarged unit of peripheral air-containing lung, surrounded by a wall of variable thickness, which may be thin as in lymphangioleiomyomatosis, or may be thick as in idiopathic pulmonary fibrosis.
Dependent opacity	Subpleural increased attenuation in dependent lung. The increased attenuation disappears when the region of lung is nondependent. May also appear as a subpleural line.
Emphysema	Focal region or regions of low attenuation, usually without visible walls, resulting from actual or perceived enlarged airspaces and destroyed alveolar walls. May be associated with air-trapping. *Pathology*: Permanently enlarged airspaces distal to the terminal bronchiole, accompanied by destroyed alveolar walls.
Ground-glass opacity	Hazy increased attenuation of lung parenchyma, but with preservation of bronchial and vascular margins; caused by partial filling of airspaces, interstitial thickening, partial collapse of alveoli, normal expiration, or increased capillary blood volume. Bronchial tree may be conspicuous ("black bronchus"). Not to be confused with consolidation, in which bronchovascular margins are obscured.
Honeycombing	Clustered cystic airspaces, usually of comparable diameters of the order of 0.3–1.0 cm, but up to 2.5 cm diameter, often subpleural and characterized by well-defined walls, which are often thick. A CT feature of diffuse pulmonary fibrosis.
Intralobular lines	Fine linear opacities present in a lobule when the intralobular interstitium is thickened. When numerous, they may appear as a fine reticular pattern.
Irregular linear opacity	Any linear opacity of irregular thickness of 1–3 mm, distinct from interlobular septa, bronchovascular bundles, and nodular opacities. May be intralobular or extend through several adjacent secondary lobules.
Micronodule	Discrete, small, round, focal opacity of at least soft tissue attenuation and with a diameter no greater than 7 mm. Some authors have limited use of this term to a diameter of less than 3 mm. Other authors simply use the term "small nodule".
Mosaic pattern	A patchwork of regions of varied attenuation, interpreted as secondary to regional differences in perfusion. A more inclusive term than the originally described "mosaic oligemia". Air-trapping secondary to bronchial or bronchiolar obstruction may also produce focal zones of decreased attenuation, an appearance that can be enhanced by using expiratory CT.
Nodule	Round opacity, at least moderately well marginated and no greater than 3 cm in maximum diameter. Some authors use the modifier "small" if the maximum diameter of the opacity is less than 1 cm.
Panacinar emphysema (panlobular emphysema)	Emphysema that tends to show uniformly decreased parenchymal attenuation and a paucity of vessels. Severe panacinar emphysema may be indistinguishable from severe centrilobular emphysema, except on the basis of zonal distribution. *Pathology*: Emphysema that involves, more or less uniformly, all portions of the secondary lobules. It tends to predominate in the lower lobes and is the form of emphysema associated with hereditary α_1-antitrypsin deficiency.
Paraseptal emphysema	Emphysema characterized by subpleural regions of low attenuation or bullae separated by intact interlobular septa.

Table 4.2 (*cont'd*)

Term	Definition
	Pathology: Emphysema characterized by predominant involvement of alveolar ducts and sacs, characteristically in subpleural lung and adjacent to interlobular septa and vessels.
Parenchymal band	Elongated opacity, usually several millimeters wide and up to about 5 cm long, often extending to the pleura, which may be thickened and retracted at the site of contact. Originally described in asbestosis but also a sign of focal fibrosis of nonspecific cause.
Parenchymal opacification	Increase in pulmonary attenuation that may or may not obscure the margins of vessels and airway walls. "Consolidation" indicates that definition of these margins (excepting air bronchograms) is lost, whereas "ground-glass opacification" indicates a lesser increase in attenuation, in which definition of the margins is preserved. Whenever possible, use of the terms "consolidation" or "ground-glass opacity" is preferred.
Pseudoplaque	An irregular band of peripheral pulmonary opacity adjacent to visceral pleura that simulates the appearance of a pleural plaque and is formed by the coalescence of small nodules (e.g. in coal worker's pneumoconiosis).
Reticulation (reticular pattern)	Innumerable, interlacing small linear opacities that suggest a mesh. A descriptive term usually associated with interstitial lung diseases. May be fine, intermediate, or coarse.
Septal line	Thin linear opacity that corresponds to an interlobular septum; to be distinguished from centrilobular structures.
Septal thickening	Abnormal widening of an interlobular septum or septa, usually caused by edema, cellular infiltration, or fibrosis. May be smooth, irregular, or nodular.
Subpleural line	A thin curvilinear opacity, a few millimeters or less in thickness, usually less than 1 cm from the pleural surface and paralleling the pleura. A nonspecific indicator of atelectasis, edema, fibrosis, or inflammation.
Traction bronchiectasis or bronchiolectasis	Bronchial dilatation, which is commonly irregular, in association with juxtabronchial opacification that is interpreted as representing retractile pulmonary fibrosis or bronchiolar dilatation in association with peribronchiolar opacification that is interpreted as representing retractile pulmonary fibrosis.
Tree-in-bud sign	Nodular dilatation of centrilobular branching structures that resembles a budding tree and represents exudative bronchiolar dilatation (e.g. in panbronchiolitis or endobronchial spread of active pulmonary tuberculosis).

Box 4.1 Morphologic subtypes of reticular pattern

Thickened interlobular or intralobular septa
Honeycomb (fibrotic) destruction
Perilobular thickening
Conspicuous "remnant" septa (as in paraseptal or
  centrilobular emphysema)
Miscellaneous causes of intersecting linear opacities

Box 4.2 Diseases in which thickened interlobular septa are identifiable on HRCT

Dominant feature
Lymphangitis carcinomatosa[36,37]
Pulmonary edema[38]
Venoocclusive disease[43]
Pulmonary vein atresia[44]
Alveolar proteinosis[39-41]
Lipoid pneumonia[45]
Lymphocytic interstitial pneumonia[46]
Leukemic infiltration[47]
Alveolar microlithiasis[48]
Septal amyloidosis[49]
Diffuse pulmonary lymphangiomatosis[50]
Congenital lymphangiectasia[51]
Rare storage diseases including Erdheim–Chester disease[52]
  and Niemann–Pick disease[53]

Occasional feature
Sarcoidosis[42,54]
Asbestosis[55]
Pneumoconiosis and silicosis[56]
Idiopathic pulmonary hemorrhage[57]
Chronic hypersensitivity pneumonitis (fibrotic)[58]

Sometimes present
Bronchioloalveolar carcinoma[59]
Usual interstitial pneumonia[60]
Nonspecific interstitial pneumonia (crazy-paving pattern
  [case report][61])

---

ening. Conditions characterized by thickened interlobular septa are shown in Box 4.2.

As a consequence of the continuity of the various parts of the lung interstitium,[20] widespread interstitial disease which causes thickening of the interlobular septa also results in bronchovascular interstitial thickening (typified by lymphangitis carcinomatosa [Figs 4.5 and 4.8]). The bronchovascular thickening depicted on HRCT is equivalent to the peribronchial cuffing seen around end-on bronchi on chest radiography. This HRCT finding may be obvious, particularly in regional or unilateral interstitial lung disease but is sometimes quite subtle when it is minimal and diffuse. The HRCT finding of peribronchovascular thickening in isolation should be interpreted with caution since it may be a manifestation of reversible inflammatory airways disease, for example asthma. Thickening of the subsegmental and segmental bronchovascular bundles, such as that caused by lymphangitis carcinomatosa, sometimes gives the interface between the bronchial wall and surrounding lung an irregular and "feathery" appearance.

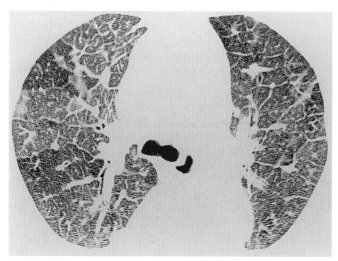

Fig. 4.6 Generalized thickening of the interlobular septa on a background of ground-glass opacification in a patient with cardiogenic pulmonary edema. There are bilateral paravertebral pleural effusions.

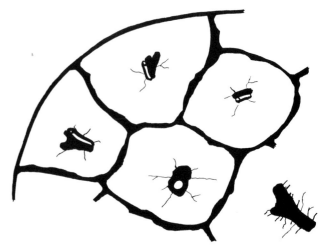

Fig. 4.8 Diagram of HRCT appearances of interstitial infiltration in lymphangitis carcinomatosa. In addition to prominent irregular thickening of the interlobular septa, there is sometimes a "feathery" appearance to the infiltrated and thickened bronchovascular bundles.

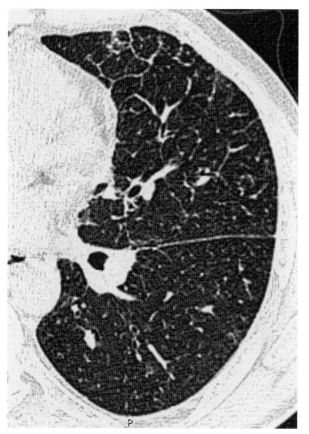

Fig. 4.7 Nodular thickening of the interlobular septa, particularly pronounced anteriorly in the lingula, in a patient with sarcoidosis.

At the level of the secondary pulmonary lobule, axial interstitial thickening of the centrilobular artery and bronchiole is seen as a prominent dot or Y-shaped opacity; there is often associated thickening of the interlobular septa. Such thickening is seen in a variety of interstitial lung diseases and is recognized as one of the earliest manifestations of asbestosis.[55,62] Diseases

involving the smallest airways can produce apparent thickening of the core structures on HRCT; in these instances, the abnormal core structure visible on HRCT is due to thickening and dilatation of the central bronchiole which is filled with and surrounded by exudate.[63,64] Distinguishing between axial interstitial disease and exudative small airways disease, both of which give rise to prominent core structures, is rarely a problem: in the latter situation the larger subsegmental and segmental bronchi are usually abnormal.

The size of network making up the reticular pattern on HRCT is determined by the level at which the interstitial thickening is most pronounced. Thickening of the intralobular septa will result in a fine reticular pattern on HRCT; such a pattern may occur in any interstitial disease but is typified by idiopathic pulmonary fibrosis.[60] Some of the very finest linear structures that make up this netlike pattern within the secondary pulmonary lobule will be so small as to be below the resolution limits of HRCT with the narrowest collimation. The result is an amorphous increase in lung density (ground-glass opacity) due to volume averaging within the section.[65] Interestingly, obvious thickening of the interlobular septa is not, contrary to expectation, a prominent feature in idiopathic pulmonary fibrosis (usual interstitial pneumonia), possibly because of the severe distortion of the lung architecture (Figs 4.9 and 4.10).

Extensive and severe pulmonary fibrosis that causes complete destruction of the architecture of the secondary pulmonary lobules results in a characteristic coarse reticular pattern made up of irregular linear opacities. The reticular pattern of end-stage fibrotic (honeycomb) lung mirrors the appearances on chest radiography and is characterized by cystic spaces, measuring a few millimeters to several centimeters across, surrounded by thick irregular walls[21,60,66,67] (Fig. 4.10). The distortion of normal lung morphology by extensive fibrosis may result in irregular dilatation of the segmental and subsegmental bronchi; in the lung periphery the dilated bronchioles may be difficult to distinguish from the surrounding parenchymal cystic airspaces[68] (Fig. 4.11). The term "traction bronchiectasis"[69] has been given to airways that are clearly dilated because of surrounding retractile pulmonary fibrosis. This phenomenon is not confined to the situation in which

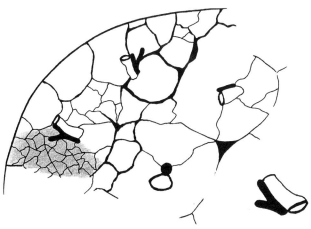

Fig. 4.9 Schematic representation of HRCT appearances in idiopathic pulmonary fibrosis. There is a coarse reticular pattern causing distortion and dilatation of the bronchi. The finer intralobular fibrosis is seen as ground-glass opacification (bottom left). Note that the coarser reticular component represents completely destroyed (honeycomb) lung and that interlobular septa are not easily identifiable.

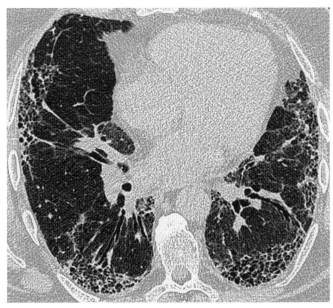

Fig. 4.10 Typical HRCT appearances of idiopathic pulmonary fibrosis. The subpleural reticular pattern consists of some destroyed lung (honeycomb). There are some small areas of ground-glass opacification. Note the lack of readily identifiable interlobular septa.

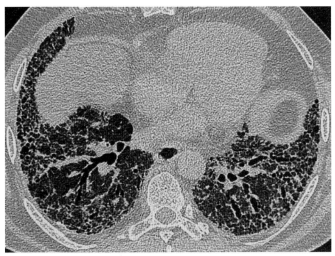

Fig. 4.11 A patient with advanced pulmonary fibrosis (histologic subtype unknown). Within the reticular pattern there are small cystic airspaces representing traction bronchiolectasis or honeycomb destruction, or both. There is obvious traction bronchiectasis affecting the more central airways.

fibrosis is seen as a reticular or honeycomb pattern on HRCT; dilatation and distortion of airways within ground-glass opacification (sometimes with a faint granular texture) is an important sign of fine intralobular fibrosis.

The positive and definite identification of honeycombing, as opposed to other forms of reticulation, is of particular relevance in patients with idiopathic pulmonary fibrosis. The positive predictive value of a subpleural basal *honeycomb* pattern on HRCT for the diagnosis of idiopathic pulmonary fibrosis (usual interstitial pneumonia at a histopathologic level) is high,[70] whereas a subpleural non-honeycomb reticular pattern may be encountered in other diseases, for example nonspecific interstitial pneumonia,[71] sarcoidosis,[54] or Wegener granuloma-

tosis.[72] Because, by definition, a honeycomb pattern is made up of cystic airspaces, an attempt should be made to confirm air density within the cysts (by comparison with air within the large bronchi), before assigning the term honeycomb (Fig. 4.10).

In some diseases a perilobular distribution[73] may give the spurious impression of thickening of the interlobular septa. The disposition of the pathologic process, such that it is "smeared" around the internal lobular surface, creates a thickened lobular margin (Fig. 4.12); this appearance may be encountered in cases of organizing pneumonia (Fig. 4.13). The crazy-paving pattern (a reticular pattern superimposed on a background of ground-glass opacity) may occasionally represent a similar perilobular distribution (e.g. idiopathic pulmonary hemorrhage),[74] rather than actually thickened interlobular septa. Another situation in which there may be apparent, rather than real, interlobular septal thickening occurs in patients with centrilobular emphysema; the residual peripheral alveoli collapse against the lobule margins and in so doing spuriously thicken the interlobular septa. Nevertheless, in cigarette smokers there may also be accompanying interstitial fibrosis, which is partly responsible for conspicuous thickening of the "remnant" interlobular septa[75] (Fig. 4.14).

In a minority of patients with interstitial fibrosis, an additional HRCT finding is a fine peripheral curvilinear line lying 1 cm from the visceral pleural surface. This dense line is extremely well defined and parallels the chest wall (Fig. 4.15). The subpleural curvilinear line caused confusion when it was first described in patients with asbestosis[76] because it was suggested that such a line was virtually pathognomonic of asbestos-induced interstitial fibrosis. However, it is now recognized that this HRCT sign is seen in patients with interstitial disease of various causes[62] and some normal individuals,[77] and it should not be regarded as specific for asbestosis.

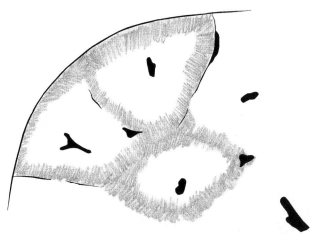

Fig. 4.12 Perilobular distribution of disease. Some pathologic processes, such as organizing pneumonia, are distributed around the internal surface of the secondary pulmonary lobule, giving the impression of thickened interlobular septa (see Fig. 4.13).

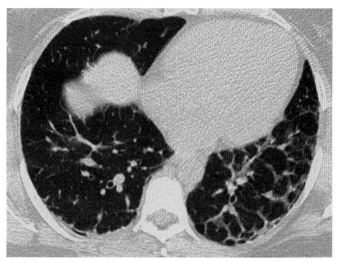

Fig. 4.13 The linear and reticular pattern in the left lower lobe represents a perilobular distribution of organizing pneumonia (this pattern regressed on follow-up HRCT, following steroid treatment).

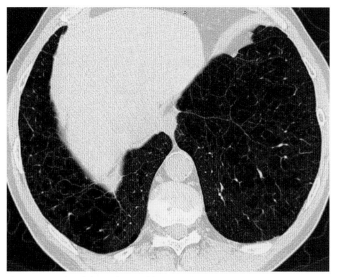

Fig. 4.14 The delicate lattice-like reticular pattern represents, in part, remnant interlobular septa in a patient with advanced centrilobular and panlobular emphysema.

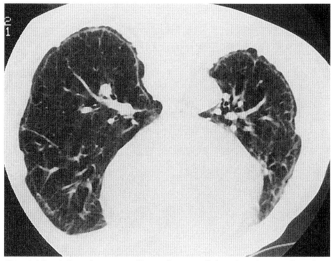

Fig. 4.15 A fine dense curvilinear line parallel to the chest wall and pleural plaques in a patient (prone position) with a history of asbestos exposure.

Nodular pattern

A nodular pattern is a feature of both interstitial and airspace disease. The localization of nodules as well as other characteristics such as their density, clarity of outline, and uniformity of size, may indicate whether the nodules are lying predominantly within the interstitium or airspaces.[78] Since many lung diseases have both interstitial and airspace components, this distinction is not always helpful in refining the differential diagnosis. Whether pulmonary nodules can be detected on CT depends upon their size, profusion, density, and the scanning technique. Narrow collimation HRCT is superior to standard CT for the detection of small nodules because there is less partial volume effect, which can average out the attenuation of such tiny nodules.[79] A further refinement is the use of maximum intensity projection (Max IP) reconstructions of contiguous thin

sections acquired by spiral CT; these images improve the depiction of minute nodules but are not routinely performed[80,81] (Fig. 4.16).

Nodules within the lung interstitium, especially those related to the lymphatic vessels, are seen in the interlobular septa, subpleural regions, and in a peribronchovascular distribution. Nodular thickening of the bronchovascular interstitium results in an irregular interface between the margins of the bronchovascular bundles and the surrounding lung parenchyma. This irregularity, which has been named the "interface sign",[82] may be seen in lymphangitis carcinomatosa,[23,36] but is most obvious in cases of sarcoidosis when a coalescence of perilymphatic granulomas results in a beaded appearance of the thickened bronchovascular bundles[42,83] (Fig. 4.17). The bronchovascular distribution of nodules, in conjunction with subpleural nodules (most obvious along the oblique fissures) and a perihilar concentration of disease is characteristic of sarcoidosis. In a few

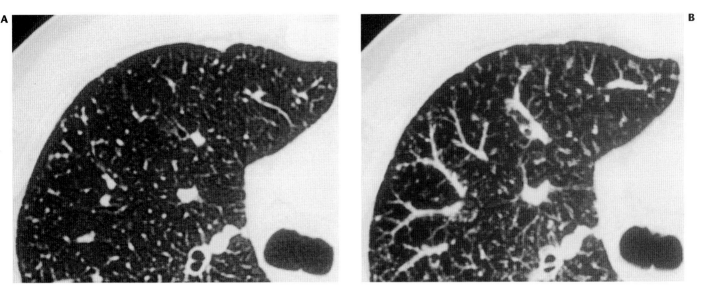

Fig. 4.16 **A**, A 1.5 mm collimation HRCT section showing a widespread micronodular pattern in a patient with sarcoidosis. **B**, A maximum intensity projection (Max IP) image comprising five contiguous thin sections showing the bronchovascular distribution of the nodules to advantage. (Courtesy of Dr M Remy-Jardin, Lille)

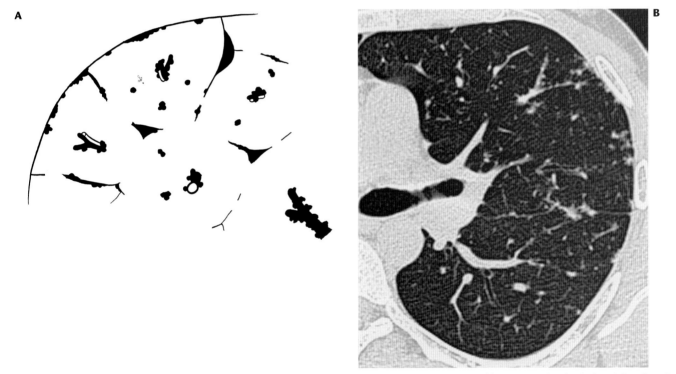

Fig. 4.17 **A**, A diagrammatic representation of the distribution of pulmonary nodules in sarcoidosis: in addition to randomly sited nodules, there is a tendency toward subpleural, septal, and bronchovascular locations. **B**, Pulmonary sarcoidosis with beading of the bronchovascular bundle and scattered small nodules. There is also nodularity along the major fissure and irregular nodularity of the pleural surface representing conglomerates of subpleural granulomas.

patients with Langerhans cell histiocytosis a centrilobular distribution of nodules has also been reported.[84] In practice, other CT features such as the size and character of the nodules aid the differentiation between these two diagnoses. The nodular pattern seen in coal worker's pneumoconiosis and silicosis is generally more uniform in distribution; the nodules may be more upper zone and subpleural in distribution, but overall tend to be more randomly spread throughout the lung parenchyma than those seen in sarcoidosis. In addition, thicken-

ing of the interlobular septa may be quite pronounced in silicosis[56,85] (Fig. 4.18).

A random distribution of small, well-defined (miliary) nodules is seen in patients with hematogenous spread of tuberculosis,[86,87] some forms of pulmonary metastases, pneumoconiosis, and rarely in pulmonary sarcoidosis (in which case there is usually some thickening of the septa and fissures). Subtle features of thickening of the interlobular and intralobular interstitium may be associated with a miliary or micronodular

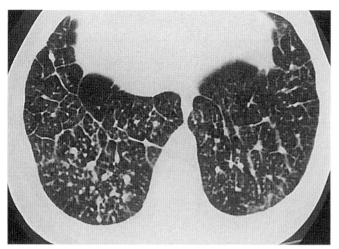

Fig. 4.18 Marked thickening of the interlobular septa with randomly distributed small nodules in an individual with silicosis.

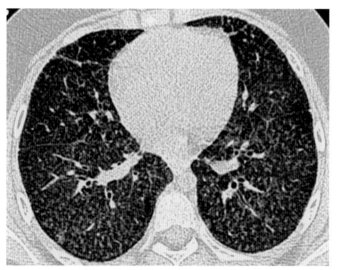

Fig. 4.19 Miliary nodules with no distribution in a patient with alveolar microlithiasis. There are a few thickened interlobular septa and there is a "black stripe" of spared subpleural lung posteriorly (an occasional feature of alveolar microlithiasis). In this case the nodules were not of calcific density on mediastinal window settings.

pattern.[88] The size and cephalocaudal distribution of miliary nodules are not generally useful characteristics for refining the differential diagnosis[89] (Fig. 4.19).

When the airspaces are filled, or partially filled, with the products of disease, individual acini may become visible on HRCT as poorly defined nodules approximately 8 mm in diameter (Fig. 4.20). Acinar nodules may merge with areas of ground-glass opacification and are often seen around the periphery of areas of dense parenchymal consolidation. Smaller, poorly defined, often centrilobular nodules are encountered in many conditions[90,91]; their centrilobular location may not be obvious when the nodules are profuse. Conditions in which centrilobular nodules of varying quality and size are found (ranging from the indistinct low-density nodules seen in subacute hypersensitivity pneumonitis [Fig. 4.21] through to the well-defined Y-shaped opacities of diffuse panbronchiolitis [Fig. 4.3]) are listed in Table 4.3.

Parenchymal opacification

Ground-glass opacity

A hazy increase in the density of the lung parenchyma on HRCT is often described as a "ground-glass" appearance. Unlike the analogous abnormality on chest radiography, in which the pulmonary vessels are often indistinct, ground-glass opacity on HRCT does not obscure the pulmonary vasculature[118,119] (Fig. 4.22). In cases in which the presence of ground-glass opacity is equivocal, it may be helpful to compare the attenuation of the lung parenchyma with air in the bronchi: in normal individuals the difference in density is marginal, whereas ground-glass opacity makes the airways more obvious (the "black bronchus" sign, Fig. 4.22). Although this HRCT abnormality is usually easily recognizable, particularly when it is interspersed with areas of normal lung parenchyma (mosaic attenuation pattern – see later section), subtle degrees of increased parenchymal opacification may not be obvious[120] (Fig. 4.23) and the conspicuity of ground-glass opacity is susceptible to alterations in window settings. Furthermore, a normal increase in lung density, indistinguishable from "pathologic" ground-glass opacification, is seen in individuals breath-holding at residual volume[120] (Fig. 4.24). There are several artifactual causes of apparent ground-glass opacification on HRCT including inappropriate (wide) window settings, contrast and brightness setting, drift on laser printers or workstation monitors, and the appearance of the lung parenchyma on images obtained on an unfamiliar CT scanner.

At a microscopic level, the changes responsible for ground-glass opacity are complex and include partial filling of the airspaces, considerable thickening of the interstitium, or a combination of the two[65,118] (Fig. 4.25). Nevertheless, the basic mechanism behind the generation of the HRCT pattern of ground-glass opacification of the lungs is nothing more or less than the displacement of air. Thickening of the intralobular interstitium by fluid or a cellular infiltrate is below the limits of resolution of HRCT and volume averaging results in an amorphous increase in lung density. Many conditions characterized by these pathologic changes result in the nonspecific pattern of ground-glass opacity.[121] Conditions that are characterized by ground-glass opacity as the dominant abnormality on HRCT are listed in Box 4.3.

Given the numerous conditions listed below, it is clearly a misconception to consider ground-glass opacity as simply representing "active alveolitis". As a generalization, the pattern of ground-glass opacity usually represents potentially reversible lung disease,[65] but there are important exceptions to this rule: widespread fine intralobular fibrosis may produce a ground-glass pattern (frequently the nonspecific interstitial pneumonia subtype of the interstitial pneumonias), but in this situation there is distortion and dilatation of the bronchi[150,151] (Fig. 4.26). The certain identification of dilatation of airways within areas of ground-glass opacification may not be easy: the increased conspicuity of such bronchi (the "black bronchus" sign) may give the spurious impression that the bronchi are dilated. There are many signs that may coexist in a patient in whom the dominant abnormality is ground-glass opacification. For example, the "texture" of ground-glass opacity, which is strictly considered to be an entirely amorphous pattern, is somewhat variable and may occasionally point towards a particular diagnosis. Ancillary features that may help to refine the diagnosis of ground-glass opacity are listed in Box 4.4.

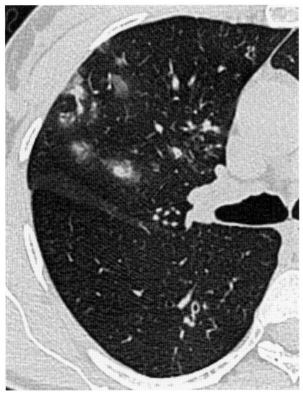

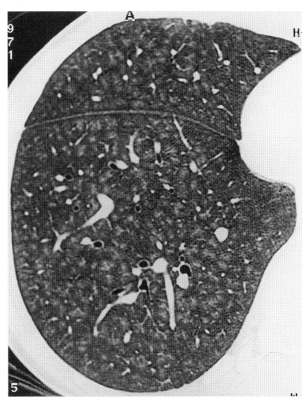

Fig. 4.20 Multiple nodules ranging from a few millimeters to "acinar" size (approximately 8 mm in diameter) in a patient with an active atypical mycobacterial infection. There were also features of cylindrical bronchiectasis on adjacent sections.

Fig. 4.21 Poorly defined, relatively low attenuation nodules of uniform size (approximately 7 mm) in a patient with subacute hypersensitivity pneumonitis.

Table 4.3 Conditions characterized by profuse centrilobular nodules on HRCT (the type of nodules vary between diseases but usually show consistent characteristics in a given condition)

Diffuse panbronchiolitis[63,64]	Peripheral Y-shaped opacities, accompanied by features of widespread cylindrical bronchiectasis.
Subacute hypersensitivity pneumonitis[92,93]	Low-density poorly defined nodules, usually superimposed on a background of ground-glass opacity.
Endobronchial spread of TB[94,95] or bacterial pneumonia[96]	Some nodules from confluent consolidation. In the case of TB, larger cavitating nodules are usually present.
Atypical mycobacterial infection[97–99]	Associated with bronchial abnormalities, 1 cm diameter nodules, and architectural distortion.
Acute *Mycoplasma pneumoniae* infection[100]	Poorly defined centrilobular nodules and tree-in-bud pattern.
Cryptogenic organizing pneumonia[101]	An unusual pattern (similar to the nodules seen in subacute hypersensitivity pneumonitis).
Respiratory bronchiolitis–interstitial lung disease (RBILD)[102–104]	Poorly defined low-density nodules associated with bronchial wall thickening, thickened interlobular septa, and mosaic pattern.
Tracheobronchial papillomatosis[105]	Indistinct nodules with or without cavitation. Involvement of larger bronchi.
Bronchioloalveolar cell carcinoma[106,107]	Rare, usually in association with areas of ground-glass opacity or consolidation.
Lymphocytic interstitial pneumonia [including follicular bronchiolitis[108]] in adults[46] or in children with AIDS[109]	Profuse micronodules with perilymphatic and subpleural distribution.
Acute silicoproteinosis[110]	Poorly defined centrilobular nodules with accompanying ground-glass and consolidation.
Various small vessel diseases[111–113]	Intravascular filling, e.g. with foreign material or tumor emboli, may result in a tree-in-bud pattern.
Aspiration[114] (specifically, lentils[115])	Tree-in-bud pattern and poorly defined nodules representing bronchiolar filling.
Primary pulmonary lymphoma[116]	Tree-in-bud pattern simulating diffuse panbronchiolitis (but without cylindrical bronchiectasis).
Fat embolism[117]	Small nodules, some related to vessels, admixed with ground-glass opacity and consolidation.

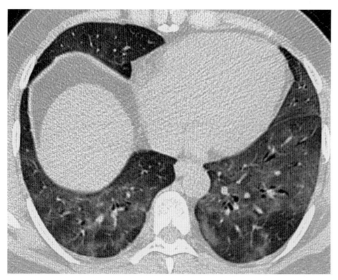

Fig. 4.22   Widespread ground-glass opacification in a patient with desquamative interstitial pneumonia. The pulmonary vasculature is not obscured by this degree of opacification and the air-filled bronchi are more conspicuous than usual (black bronchus sign) but not unduly dilated.

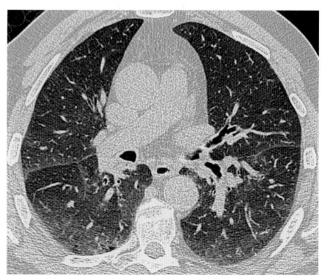

Fig. 4.24   Increase in density of the lung parenchyma on a CT section obtained at near residual volume (end-expiration) in an individual with no known lung disease.

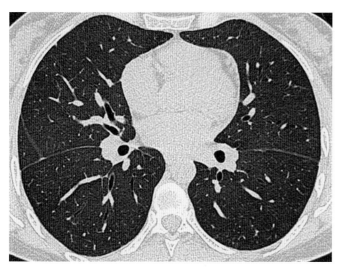

Fig. 4.23   Very subtle ground-glass opacity. This uniform increase in the attenuation of the lung parenchyma was due to cellular (non-fibrotic) nonspecific interstitial pneumonia.

Without additional signs or a distinctive distribution, and in the absence of any clinical information, widespread ground-glass opacity is truly nonspecific. In reality, a search for ancillary signs will often yield enough information to usefully limit the differential diagnosis, particularly if the clinical context is taken into account.

Mosaic attenuation pattern

The correct interpretation of an HRCT of the lungs showing patchy attenuation differences (mosaic pattern, Fig. 4.27) can be a considerable challenge.[120,152] The pattern was originally termed mosaic oligemia[153] but, less mechanistically and more descriptively, *mosaic attenuation pattern* is now the preferred term.

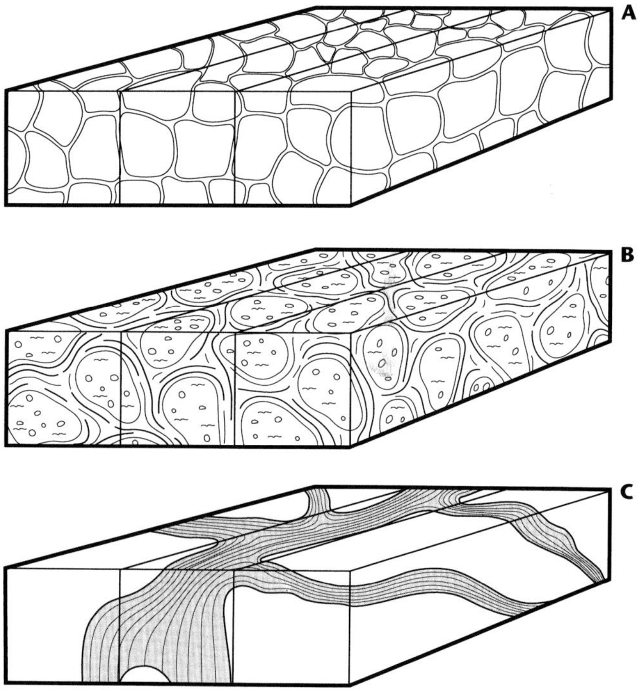

Fig. 4.25   Schematic diagram of three adjacent voxels from a HRCT section. **A**, In the normal state, most of the volume of the voxels is taken up by air. **B**, In situations in which there is gross thickening of the interstitium and/or partial filling of the airspaces with cells or fluid (causing displacement of air) there is an increase in density, seen as ground-glass opacification on HRCT. **C**, A representation of established pulmonary fibrosis: fibrotic strands occupy much of the volume of the central voxel and the pulmonary fibrosis will thus be resolved on HRCT as a reticular pattern.

Box 4.3   Conditions characterized by ground-glass opacity as the dominant HRCT abnormality

Subacute hypersensitivity pneumonitis[92,93,122,123]
Adult respiratory distress syndrome[124] and acute interstitial pneumonia[125,126]
Desquamative interstitial pneumonia[127,128]
Pneumocystis carinii, cytomegalovirus pneumonia, SARS[129–132]
Sarcoidosis[83,133]
Nonspecific interstitial pneumonia[71,134]
Pulmonary edema[38]
Idiopathic pulmonary hemorrhage[57,135]
Bronchioloalveolar cell carcinoma[106,136–138]
Eosinophilic pneumonia[139–141]
Respiratory bronchiolitis–interstitial lung disease[102,103]
Lymphocytic interstitial pneumonia[46]
Radiation pneumonitis[142,143]
Drug toxicity[144–146]
Alveolar proteinosis[39,41,147]
Sickle cell disease[148]
[Normal lung at near residual volume, particularly in children[149]]

Box 4.4   Additional useful features in conditions characterized by ground-glass opacity

Distribution (e.g. subpleural location in nonspecific interstitial pneumonia)
Texture (e.g. fine granularity may reflect intralobular fibrosis)
Superimposed nodularity (e.g. poorly defined centrilobular nodules in RB-ILD)
Background mosaic attenuation pattern (e.g. subacute hypersensitivity pneumonitis)
Interlobular septal thickening overlay (e.g. in alveolar proteinosis – "crazy-paving" sign)
Thin-walled cysts (e.g. in lymphocytic interstitial pneumonia)
Dilatation and distortion of bronchi (implies retractile fibrosis in chronic disease)
Mediastinal lymphadenopathy (e.g. sarcoidosis)

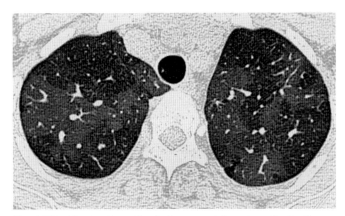

Fig. 4.27   Mosaic attenuation in the upper lobes of a patient with sickle cell disease and pulmonary hypertension. Note the increased caliber of the vessels within the increased attenuation (gray) lung compared to the decreased attenuation (black) parts of the lung, consistent with vascular cause of the mosaic attenuation pattern in this case.

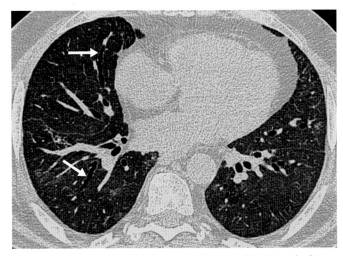

Fig. 4.26   There is generalized ground-glass opacification and a few thickened interlobular septa. Marked dilatation of the bronchi (arrows) reflects the presence of fine interstitial fibrosis. Biopsy proven nonspecific interstitial pneumonia.

Abnormal inhomogeneity of the lung parenchyma may be so slight as to be barely visible, particularly if suboptimal window settings are used. Once recognized, a mosaic pattern should be assigned to one of three basic causes (infiltrative lung disease, occlusive vascular disease, or small airways disease) before an attempt is made to refine the differential diagnosis. Understanding the pathophysiology behind the generation of a mosaic pattern will help interpretation: in patchy diffuse infiltrative disease the abnormal lung is of higher attenuation because of expansion of the interstitium and/or partial filling of the airspaces; this contrasts with the spared (blacker) areas of lung. In this situation there should be no difference in size of the pulmonary vessels within the gray versus the black lung. The major discriminating features that suggest an occlusive vascular

disease as the cause of mosaic attenuation pattern are the paucity and reduction in caliber of vessels within the areas of reduced attenuation[154] (Fig. 4.27), increased caliber segmental and central pulmonary arteries, and the lack of air-trapping on CT sections obtained at end-expiration.[152] By contrast, in small airways disease there is almost invariably at least some dilatation of the macroscopic bronchi in addition to the reduction in caliber of the vessels within the abnormal black lung. Furthermore, expiratory CTs accentuate the mosaicism because of air-trapping within the abnormal (black) lung. (See the later section on Small airways disease, p. 166.)

Nevertheless, the differentiation between the various causes of a mosaic attenuation pattern on CT is not always straightforward: in one study, subjects with a vascular cause for the mosaic attenuation pattern were the least readily identified as such by two observers.[155] Occasionally coexisting small airways and small vessels disease may both contribute to a mosaic attenuation pattern.[156] Indeed, airways abnormalities have been demonstrated in patients with thromboembolic disease, specifically dilatation of the segmental and subsegmental bronchi[157]

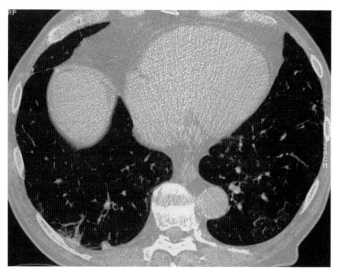

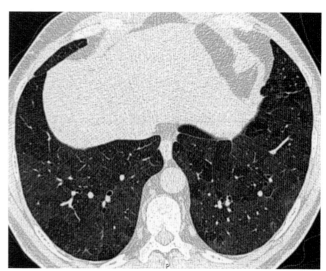

Fig. 4.28 Faint mosaic attenuation pattern (on adjacent sections) in a patient with chronic thromboembolic disease. Within the decreased attenuation of the lung there is mild dilatation of some of the bronchi – an occasional feature in thromboembolic disease. The peripheral opacities in the right lower lobe were taken to represent old infarcts.

Fig. 4.29 Mosaic attenuation pattern with the "gray" of varying intensity in this case of subacute hypersensitivity pneumonitis. At a pathologic level there is a complex combination of small airways involvement, interstitial infiltrate, and regions of relatively spared lung.

and air-trapping.[158] It is as well to be aware of this phenomenon, which may lead to the erroneous conclusion that a case showing the HRCT features of mosaic attenuation pattern and dilatation of the segmental and subsegmental bronchi is invariably the result of small airways disease (rather than an occlusive vasculopathy) (Fig. 4.28). Thus, while expiratory CT may help to clarify whether the pattern is the result of airways disease or occlusive vascular disease,[152,159] this is not always the case. Despite this caveat, if due attention is given to additional signs on inspiratory HRCT images, for example the presence of bronchial abnormalities,[160,161] the size of the proximal pulmonary arteries,[162] and changes in cross-sectional area and density of hypodense regions of lung on expiratory sections,[159] the correct category of disease can usually be selected.[155,163] The very different clinical presentations and pulmonary function test abnormalities of these three categories are a further aid in the differential diagnosis. The important discriminatory features between the three basic causes of a mosaic pattern are summarized in Table 4.4.

In a few conditions, notably subacute hypersensitivity pneumonitis and sarcoidosis, there may be a complex combination of areas of normal, increased and decreased attenuation lung (the latter two reflecting interstitial and small airways disease

components respectively, Fig. 4.29); Webb has coined, without conspicuous success, the whimsical but faintly revolting term "head cheese sign" for this pattern of mixed attenuations.[164]

Consolidation

The identification of consolidation (abnormal dense opacification of the lung parenchyma[165]) on HRCT is not a perceptual challenge. By definition, vessels are obscured by consolidated (white) lung and an air bronchogram may, or may not, be present (Fig. 4.30). Apart from an air bronchogram, consolidation is a featureless pattern and the most useful pointers to the cause of consolidation are its chronicity and distribution. For example, the rapid radiographic resolution, in less than 48 hours, of extensive consolidation is highly suggestive of pulmonary edema or hemorrhage. A subpleural and/or bronchocentric distribution of consolidation is typical of cryptogenic organizing pneumonia.[101] The distribution characteristics of consolidated lung are clearly depicted on HRCT,[166] but important information about the rate of change of this non-specific pattern should always be sought from serial chest radiographs. A bronchocentric distribution is one of the many patterns of organizing pneumonia,[167] and this distribution is

Table 4.4 Discriminatory features between the three basic causes of a mosaic pattern

	Vessels in black lung	Bronchi in black lung	Segmental arteries	Other features
Infiltrative lung disease	Equivalent to those in gray lung	Normal	Normal (unless secondary pulmonary hypertension)	Traction bronchiectasis in gray lung (if interstitial fibrosis)
Obliterative small airways disease	Reduced	Dilated and thickened	Normal	Obvious air-trapping on expiratory CT
Occlusive vascular disease	Reduced	Normal (usually)	Dilated	Peripheral scarring from previous infarcts

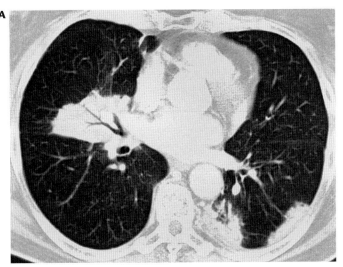 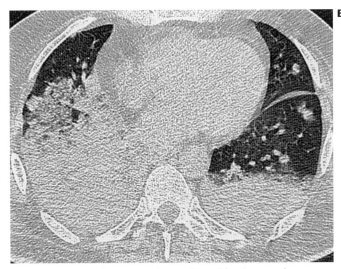

Fig. 4.30   Examples of pulmonary consolidation. **A**, Bilateral patchy consolidation on a standard CT section in a patient with primary pulmonary lymphoma. Consolidation in the right middle lobe contains an air bronchogram. **B**, Extensive bilateral consolidation, with no air bronchogram, in a patient with bronchioloalveolar carcinoma. Note the discrete nodules of consolidation in the lingula and left lower lobe.

seldom seen in, for example, chronic eosinophilic pneumonia[168]; nevertheless, discrimination on the basis of the distribution of the consolidation alone is unreliable.

The high attenuation that characterizes consolidation on HRCT results from the complete displacement of air from lung tissue; it is therefore not surprising that accompanying areas of ground-glass opacity reflect the partial filling of alveoli with the products of disease (i.e. incomplete displacement of air, Fig. 4.31). A few pathologic processes, for example lymphoma (Fig. 4.30A), are confined to the interstitium and in this situation interstitial expansion is such that the alveolar airspaces are compressed and obliterated[169] (hence, the term "airspace" consolidation is, in this situation, pedantically incorrect) (Box 4.5).

Unlike ground-glass opacity, the scope for variation in texture of completely consolidated lung is limited. Associated features such as adjacent "acinar nodules" (focal consolidation within single, or clusters of, acini [Figs 4.20 and 4.30B]) or a tree-in-bud pattern may refine the differential diagnosis in some cases,[107] but important distinctions between, for example, bronchioloalveolar carcinoma and cryptogenic organizing pneumonia or other benign causes of consolidation can rarely be made with certainty on the basis of the HRCT appearances[170,171] and a tissue diagnosis is usually necessary. Very rarely the attenuation characteristics of consolidated lung may indicate the cause: consolidation of less than usual density may be encountered in lipoid pneumonia[172,173]; conversely, high-attenuation consolidation (as seen on soft tissue window settings) is an occasional feature in patients treated with relatively high doses of amiodarone.[174] In a few patients with consolidation caused by allergic bronchopulmonary aspergillosis, mucus plugs of high attenuation may be visible on branching structures within the consolidation.[175]

Occasionally it may be difficult to determine whether small cystic airspaces within consolidation reflect dilated bronchi or true cysts. The sparing of one or more secondary pulmonary lobules within consolidated lung can give the spurious appearance of a cavity (Fig. 4.32) and, in so doing, modify the differential diagnosis; if there is any doubt, judicious manipulation of the window settings will demonstrate whether or not the "cavity" contains normal parenchymal or air density. In keeping

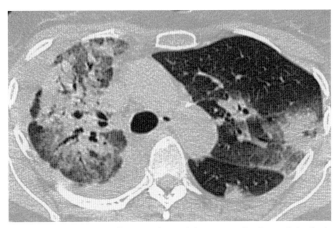

Fig. 4.31   A patient with severe bacterial pneumonia. Around the foci of consolidation there is a margin of ground-glass opacity reflecting partial filling of the airspaces.

Box 4.5   Conditions in which consolidation is the sole or dominant feature

Infective pneumonia (community acquired bacterial; tuberculosis; opportunistic)
Cryptogenic organizing pneumonia
Bronchioloalveolar cell carcinoma
Eosinophilic pneumonia (acute or chronic)
Pulmonary edema (rarely encountered on HRCT!)
Aspiration pneumonia (including lipoid pneumonia)
Acute interstitial pneumonitis and ARDS
Radiation pneumonitis
Fat embolism
Pulmonary hemorrhage (primary or aspiration)
Allergic bronchopulmonary aspergillosis
Sarcoidosis
Lymphoma

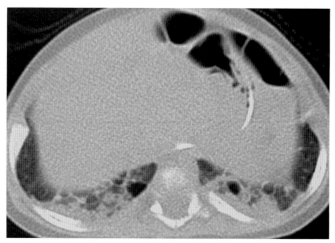

Fig. 4.32 A 9-month-old child with presumed aspiration pneumonia. Within the patchy consolidation at the lung bases, the lucent areas might be taken to represent cavitation. However, manipulation of the window settings showed that these "cavities" were of normal lung parenchymal attenuation, and therefore represented spared secondary pulmonary nodules.

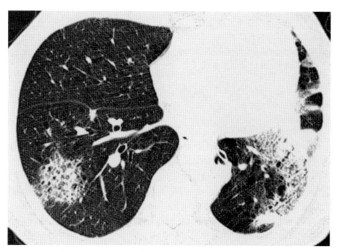

Fig. 4.33 Patchy consolidation, of unknown cause, in a cigarette smoker. The consolidation has a sponge-like texture because of the background centrilobular emphysema.

> **Box 4.6 Conditions in which cysts are a feature**
>
> *Dominant feature*
> Lymphangioleiomyomatosis
> Langerhans cell histiocytosis
> Infective pneumatoceles
> Bullous emphysema
> Usual interstitial pneumonia
>
> *Often present*
> Lymphocytic interstitial pneumonia
> Lymphoproliferative (BALT) disease
> Tracheobronchial papillomatosis
> Bronchioloalveolar cell carcinoma (cavitating form)
>
> *Rarely present*
> Sarcoidosis
> Hypersensitivity pneumonitis
> Desquamative interstitial pneumonia
> Active tuberculosis

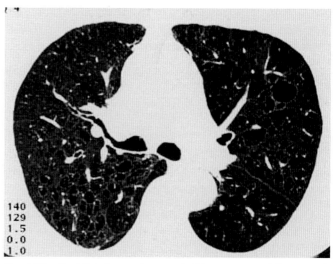

Fig. 4.34 Centrilobular emphysema. In this case some of the areas of emphysematous destruction have a definable wall – clearly seen in a large marginated cystlike lesion in the anterior segment of the left upper lobe.

with traditional teaching from the era of bronchography, dilatation of airways within acute (infective) consolidation is an expected pathophysiological response and should not be interpreted as necessarily representing underlying irreversible bronchiectasis. The morphology of consolidated lung may be modified if there is a background of honeycomb destruction or emphysema (Fig. 4.33); the presence of such coexisting patterns will usually be obvious on scrutiny of unconsolidated lung.

Cystic airspaces

The term "cystic airspace" or "lung cyst" is used to describe a clearly defined air-containing space with a definable wall. Innumerable cystic spaces may not be individually identifiable on chest radiography because of the superimposition of the thin walls that results in a delicate reticular pattern. Several conditions

are characterized by a profusion of cystic airspaces and the size, wall characteristics, and distribution of these cysts on HRCT are often helpful in suggesting a diagnosis[176–179] (Box 4.6).

Emphysematous destruction of alveolar walls produces areas of low attenuation on HRCT that often merge imperceptibly and usually have no discernible interface with normal lung.[27,180] In patients with predominantly centrilobular emphysema, there may be circular areas of lung destruction that resemble cysts, and some do indeed have an identifiable wall (Fig. 4.34); however, the centrilobular bronchovascular bundle is often visible as a dotlike structure in the center of the apparent cyst. Thin-walled bullae of varying sizes are clearly seen on HRCT in patients with emphysema, and there is usually a background of destructive emphysema, which prevents confusion with other conditions in which cystic airspaces are a prominent feature.

Cystic airspaces as the dominant abnormality are seen in relatively few conditions, most notably lymphangioleiomyo-

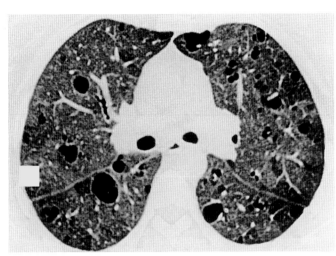

Fig. 4.35 Lymphocytic interstitial pneumonia in a patient with Sjögren syndrome. Superimposed on a background of ground-glass opacity there are several thin-walled cystic airspaces; the pathogenesis of these cysts is uncertain.

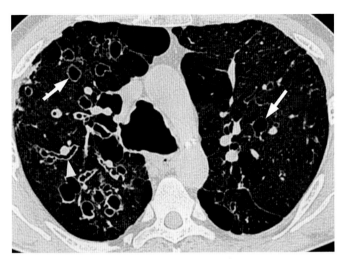

Fig. 4.37 Cystic bronchiectasis in a patient with tracheobronchomegaly (Mounier–Kuhn syndrome). Note the tracheomegaly. While some airways are clearly bronchiectatic (arrowhead), other freestanding cystic lesions are not so obviously bronchiectatic airways (arrows).

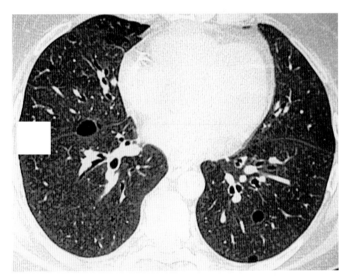

Fig. 4.36 Subacute hypersensitivity pneumonitis. In addition to the expected poorly defined low attenuation nodules and ground-glass opacification, there are a few thin-walled cystic airspaces – an occasional feature of hypersensitivity pneumonitis.

matosis,[181–183] Langerhans cell histiocytosis,[84,184] end-stage idiopathic pulmonary fibrosis,[60] and transient postinfective pneumatoceles. In the case of *Pneumocystis carinii* pneumonia, a coalescence of bizarre-shaped, sometimes thick-walled, cystic airspaces is often superimposed on a background of ground-glass opacification or frank pulmonary consolidation.[185–188] Numerous cystic airspaces may be the key HRCT finding in some rarer conditions such as lymphocytic interstitial pneumonia (LIP) associated with Sjögren syndrome (Fig. 4.35) or advanced tracheobronchial papillomatosis.[105] An occasional small cyst may be present in patients with subacute hypersensitivity pneumonitis,[189] possibly reflecting the basic similarity of the underlying pathologic process in LIP and hypersensitivity pneumonitis (i.e. a diffuse lymphocytic infiltrate) (Fig. 4.36). Unlike solid parenchymal organs, notably the kidneys,

"simple" unexplained benign cysts are distinctly uncommon in the lungs. A curious variant of cystic lung disease is the pattern of "soap-bubble" destruction in which a cluster of adjoining thin-walled cysts resembles a collection of soap bubbles; this pattern is seen in lymphoproliferative diseases, notably bronchus-associated lymphoid tissue (BALT) lymphoma.[190]

The distinction between cystic bronchiectasis and other causes of cystic parenchymal disease may occasionally be difficult, for example in cases of tracheobronchomegaly (Mounier–Kuhn syndrome, Fig. 4.37). However, bronchiectatic airways can usually be recognized as such. Expiratory CT sections have been advocated as a means of distinguishing cystic bronchiectasis from other cystic diseases[191] although collapse of cystic airspaces, whether bronchiectatic or otherwise, seems to be an almost universal finding,[192] making this observation of little discriminatory value.

In lymphangioleiomyomatosis the cysts are usually uniformly scattered throughout the lungs with normal intervening lung parenchyma[181,193] (Fig. 4.38). Even when the lung cysts are quite profuse, the pulmonary vasculature remains relatively normal without any distortion or attenuation, in contrast to emphysematous lung. Paradoxically, as lymphangioleiomyomatosis progresses, with the coalescence of larger cystic airspaces, the circumferential well-defined walls of the cysts become disrupted and the HRCT pattern of advanced lymphangioleiomyomatosis and end-stage Langerhans cell histiocytosis may be difficult to distinguish from severe centrilobular emphysema (Fig. 4.39). Nevertheless, the differentiation between these conditions using HRCT is surprisingly consistent,[194] even in advanced disease.[195] The distinction of this delicate "lacelike" pattern on HRCT from end-stage fibrosing alveolitis is usually straightforward because the cystic airspaces in honeycomb lung are smaller and have thicker walls. Furthermore, the tendency for idiopathic pulmonary fibrosis to have a peripheral distribution, even in its end stage, is often still obvious in the upper zones.

Confluent cystic airspaces giving a delicate pattern on HRCT are seen in patients with late Langerhans cell histiocytosis. However, in the earlier stages of the disease, there is often a nodular component and some of the nodules cavitate.[84,184,194]

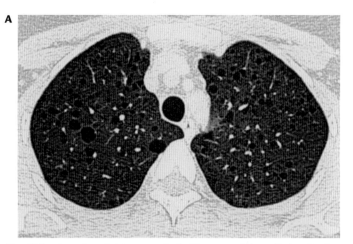

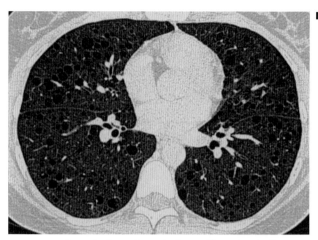

Fig. 4.38 Lymphangioleiomyomatosis. Numerous thin-walled cystic airspaces are scattered evenly throughout the lungs. There is a similar profusion of cysts in **A**, the upper, and **B**, the lower zones. The lung parenchyma and vasculature between the cysts is normal.

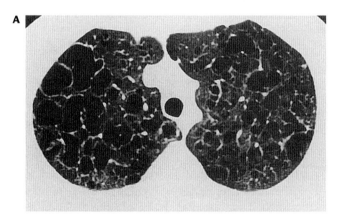

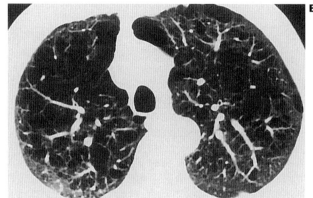

Fig. 4.39 **A**, Advanced Langerhans cell histiocytosis. Many of the cystic airspaces have merged causing widespread lung destruction. **B**, Severe centrilobular emphysema. The appearances of these two conditions may be similar in advanced cases such as these.

The constellation of HRCT findings of cavitating nodules or cysts, some of which have odd shapes, with a predominantly upper zone distribution is virtually pathognomonic for the diagnosis of Langerhans cell histiocytosis (Fig. 4.40). Serial HRCT scans show the natural history of nodules which cavitate, become cystic airspaces, and finally coalesce[196]; a notable feature of the disease is that some of the cavitating nodules and cystic airspaces may resolve with the lung parenchyma reverting to a normal appearance.[184] The strange shapes of some of the cavitating nodules in Langerhans cell histiocytosis may sometimes resemble bronchiectatic airways. Distinguishing this pattern from bronchiectasis on HRCT is usually simple because there is a lack of continuity of these lesions on adjacent sections and the segmental bronchi do not show any of the HRCT signs of bronchiectasis.

Decreased attenuation lung

Considerations of the pathologic correlate of areas of lung less than normal attenuation (black lung) are less problematic than

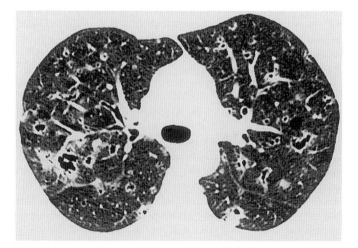

Fig. 4.40 Langerhans cell histiocytosis at a relatively early stage with numerous bizarre-shaped nodules, several of which are cavitating; the disease was concentrated in the upper lobes with sparing of the lung bases.

those that apply to ground-glass opacification. Nevertheless, areas of decreased attenuation are commonly, and over-simplistically, regarded as invariably representing air-trapping or emphysematous destruction. For example, one study of patients with bronchiectasis reported that the widespread areas of decreased attenuation identified on HRCT were caused by emphysema, which in turn accounted for the air-trapping on pulmonary function tests.[197] However, the "emphysema" seen in that study was not associated with decreased gas-diffusing capacity, the functional hallmark of emphysema. In the majority of patients with obvious bronchiectasis, it seems that areas of decreased attenuation reflect coexisting constrictive obliterative bronchiolitis,[198] which is a usual accompaniment to bronchiectasis and is readily identifiable on pathologic study of resected specimens.[199] Similarly, in non-smoking asthmatic individuals, areas of decreased attenuation, scored visually on HRCT, have been ascribed to emphysema.[200,201] However, it is more likely that the areas of decreased attenuation identified on HRCT in asthmatic individuals,[202,203] particularly on expiratory images, reflect air-trapping due to small airway obstruction, rather than emphysematous lung destruction.[204,205] Conditions which are characterized by a more or less generalized decreased in attenuation of the lungs on HRCT include:

- Emphysema (notably panacinar emphysema)
- Obliterative small airways disease
- Occlusive vascular disease (e.g. chronic thromboembolic disease)
- Bronchopulmonary dysplasia
- Congenital causes of reduced vascularization (e.g. hypoplastic lung syndromes).

In patients with severe obstructive airways disease, for example that caused by constrictive bronchiolitis, the pulmonary vessels are attenuated within areas of decreased attenuation, but are not distorted, as is the case in centrilobular emphysema. Nevertheless, the differentiation between "black lung" caused by constrictive bronchiolitis, and panacinar emphysema (in association with α_1-antitrypsin deficiency) on the basis of CT appearances alone may be especially difficult[206] (see p. 740). In one study of the discrimination between obstructive lung diseases on the basis of HRCT appearances, the most frequently miscalled distinctions were between centrilobular and panacinar emphysema, and between asthma and either normal individuals or constrictive bronchiolitis[17]; however, the consistent identification of patients with constrictive bronchiolitis was notable.[17] A useful and discriminatory functional characteristic of constrictive bronchiolitis, and indeed asthmatic individuals, is preservation of adjusted gas transfer (Kco) in most patients,[160,207] in contrast to the depression of Kco that characterizes emphysema.

Conditions characterized by areas of decreased attenuation in which expiratory CT can be used to advantage[164,208–211] to show that the phenomenon is caused by air-trapping include:

- Constrictive obliterative bronchiolitis
- Subacute hypersensitivity pneumonitis
- Acute bronchospasm, or severe irreversible changes in asthma
- Sarcoidosis
- Bronchopulmonary dysplasia

- Respiratory bronchiolitis–interstitial lung disease
- Micro-carcinoid tumorlets
- Chronic thromboembolic disease.

Distribution of infiltrative disease on HRCT

The distribution of a diffuse lung disease is often valuable in refining the differential diagnosis. The chest radiograph readily provides information about the zonal intensity of disease. Nevertheless, the radiographic pattern of distribution of diffuse lung disease may be more apparent than real. Some diseases which macroscopically have a truly uniform distribution throughout the lung parenchyma appear to have a mid and lower zone predominance on a frontal chest radiograph. As an example, in subacute hypersensitivity pneumonitis, on a chest radiograph the poorly defined nodular or ground-glass pattern appears to be most pronounced in the mid and lower zones,[212] whereas on CT it is usually uniform with no zonal predominance.[213] This misleading impression of a concentration of disease in the lower zones on chest radiography can be explained by the greater width of lung traversed by the x-ray beam in the lower zones resulting in summation of innumerable foci of disease and thus greater x-ray attenuation.[214] The cross-sectional nature of HRCT gives an accurate estimation of the uniformity or inhomogeneity of diffuse disease, in both transverse and cephalocaudal axes. Coronal reformations from volumetrically acquired data show zonal axial distribution of disease even more starkly[215,216] (Fig. 4.41). The range of distribution that a single pathologic process can have may be surprising: organizing pneumonia, which is typically basal and subpleural,[101] may also be bronchocentric, nodular, focal or perilobular in distribution.[167] As a further example, the distribution of parenchymal changes in acute respiratory distress syndrome (ARDS) is not as stereotyped as early reports suggested,[217,218] and there appear to be distribution differences depending on whether the cause of the ARDS is direct pulmonary injury or an extrapulmonary event.[219,220]

In the context of the idiopathic interstitial pneumonias, a lower zone and subpleural concentration of disease is typical of usual interstitial pneumonia and it is this distribution that is virtually pathognomonic of the disease.[60,66,70,221] By contrast, only half of patients with desquamative interstitial pneumonia show a lower zone and peripheral predominance.[127] In patients with Langerhans cell histiocytosis, the lower zone of the lungs is relatively unaffected. While this predominantly upper lobe distribution may be evident on a chest radiograph, in more advanced disease the sparing of the costophrenic recesses or the anteromedial tips of the right middle lobe and lingula may only be appreciated on CT (Fig. 4.42). Occasionally, the distribution of disease may reflect its pathogenesis, for example the basal, dependent, and sometimes bronchocentric location of aspiration pneumonia.[114] A specific example is the striking anterior distribution of a reticular pattern and associated lung distortion in patients surviving acute respiratory distress syndrome (Fig. 4.43); the anterior predilection for these changes has been ascribed to damage by mechanical ventilation to the aerated nondependent lung.[124,222]

Not only does CT confirm the general zonal distribution of disease that may be evident on chest radiography, it also gives important information about the distribution of disease in

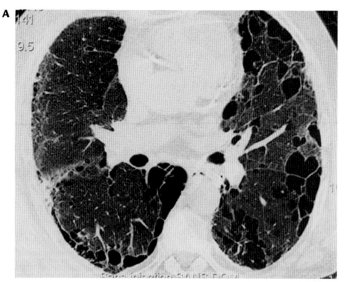
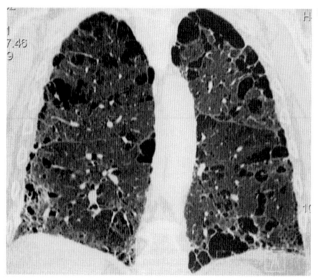

Fig. 4.41 A multidetector CT examination of a 68-year-old man with idiopathic pulmonary fibrosis and emphysema. **A**, A standard thin-section CT image through the mid zones showing a combination of emphysema and honeycomb destruction. **B**, On coronal reformation of the data the peripheral distribution of the lung destruction is easily appreciated as is the location of emphysema, which is predominantly upper zone, and fibrosis, which is predominantly basal. (With permission from Remy–Jardin M, Campistron P, Amara A, et al. Usefulness of coronal reformations in the diagnostic evaluation of infiltrative lung disease. J Comput Assist Tomogr 2003;27:266–273.)

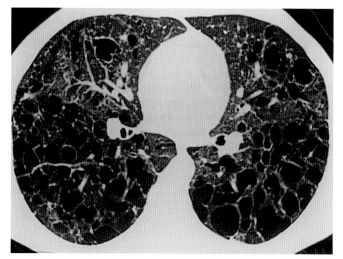

Fig. 4.42 End-stage lung in a patient with advanced Langerhans cell histiocytosis. Although there is extensive lung destruction, there is relative sparing of the anterior and medial parts of the right middle lobe and lingula. Sections through the lower zones also showed sparing of lung in the costophrenic recesses.

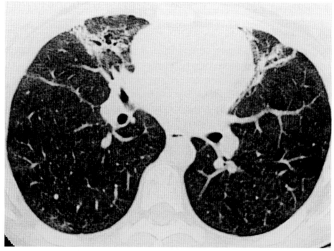

Fig. 4.43 Parenchymal opacification with a reticular element and traction bronchiectasis in an anterior distribution in a survivor of acute respiratory distress syndrome.

relation to the bronchovascular bundles, secondary pulmonary lobule and visceral pleura. For example, a nodular pattern can often be confidently categorized as perilymphatic, random, centrilobular, or associated with small airways disease.[223] The demonstration of a perilymphatic (or bronchocentric) distribution is of practical clinical use since it predicts that a transbronchial biopsy is likely to obtain diagnostic material.[224] Conditions that show a distinctly "bronchocentric" distribution

are typified by sarcoidosis, lymphangitis carcinomatosa and some cases of cryptogenic organizing pneumonia. Even in the advanced fibrotic stage of pulmonary sarcoidosis, the peribronchial distribution remains evident (Fig. 4.44). Such a striking predilection for the peribronchial regions is not usually seen in other causes of upper zone fibrosis, for example chronic hypersensitivity pneumonitis. Diseases with a more or less distinctive distribution are shown in Box 4.7.

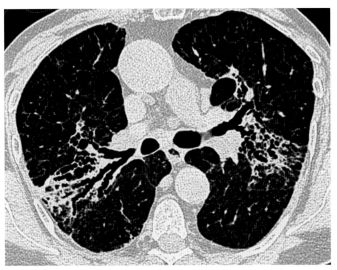

Fig. 4.44 Severe peribronchial fibrosis in the upper zones of a patient with long-standing sarcoidosis. Anteriorly there is a mild nodular thickening of some of the interlobular septa.

Box 4.7 Diseases with a tendency to a particular distribution

Upper lobe
Sarcoidosis
Pneumoconioses
Langerhans cell histiocytosis
Eosinophilic pneumonia
Tuberculosis
Respiratory bronchiolitis
Centrilobular emphysema
Cystic fibrosis
Allergic bronchopulmonary aspergillosis

Lower lobe
Usual interstitial pneumonia
Asbestosis
Cryptogenic organizing pneumonia
Nonspecific interstitial pneumonia
Aspiration pneumonia
Idiopathic bronchiectasis

Peripheral
Usual interstitial pneumonia
Asbestosis
Cryptogenic organizing pneumonia
Chronic eosinophilic pneumonia
Nonspecific interstitial pneumonia

Central
Sarcoidosis
Pulmonary edema

Bronchocentric
Sarcoidosis
Lymphangitis carcinomatosa
Leukemia/lymphoma
Cryptogenic organizing pneumonia
Follicular bronchiolitis
Tracheobronchial amyloidosis

HRCT SIGNS OF AIRWAYS DISEASE

Diseases of the large airways (most commonly bronchiectasis) and the small airways (for example, constrictive bronchiolitis) have traditionally been regarded as separate entities. However, recent HRCT observations have shown that this distinction is largely arbitrary, as these conditions often coexist. There are many causes of bronchiectasis and the entity reflects the final outcome of a number of mechanisms.[225] Bronchiectasis is the archetypal large airways disease and the term implies chronic irreversible dilatation of the bronchi. Because the definition of bronchiectasis is a morphologic one, HRCT has a key role in its identification. The ability of HRCT to demonstrate various small airways diseases is now well established[14,15,226] and the various HRCT signs of small airways dysfunction have helped to make sense of the sometimes arcane pathologic classifications. Specific forms of airways diseases are covered in Chapter 12.

Large airways diseases

In most cases of suspected bronchiectasis, HRCT technique is identical to that used in the evaluation of chronic diffuse interstitial lung disease, namely 1 or 1.5 mm sections at 10 mm intervals from apex to base.[12,13] In addition to thin sections and a high spatial resolution reconstruction algorithm, a fast acquisition time (1 second or less) is desirable to reduce artifacts caused by involuntary patient movement. Even with CT scanners capable of acquiring images in milliseconds, some artifact due to cardiac pulsation is inevitable in the right middle lobe and lingula, unless ECG gating is used. Patients are routinely scanned in the supine position, although it has been suggested that the prone position reduces motion artifact at the lung bases adjacent to the diaphragm.[227] In certain circumstances, it may be appropriate to cover the central airways with contiguous thin sections (for example, a patient who has not undergone bronchoscopy in whom an endobronchial lesion is suspected as the cause for bronchiectasis).[228]

The cardinal sign of bronchiectasis is bronchial dilatation with or without bronchial wall thickening. The major and supplementary HRCT signs of bronchiectasis are listed in Box 4.8 and shown in Figure 4.45.

HRCT criteria for the identification of abnormally dilated bronchi depend on the orientation of the bronchi in relation to

---

Box 4.8 Major and supplementary HRCT features of bronchiectasis

Major signs
Bronchial dilatation
• Signet ring sign (vertical bronchi)
• Non-tapering or flaring bronchi (horizontal bronchi)
Identification of bronchi within 1 cm of pleura (not adjacent to mediastinum)
Mucoid impaction in cystic bronchi

Supplementary signs
Bronchial wall thickening
Plugging of centrilobular bronchioles
Volume loss of affected lobe
Area of decreased attenuation (mosaic pattern)

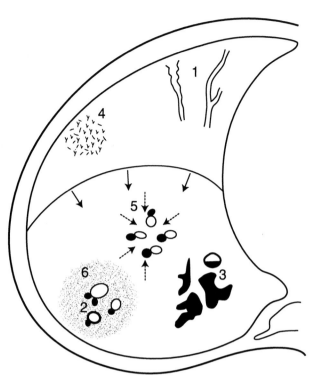

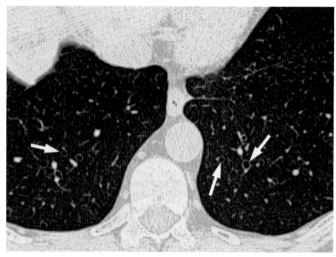

Fig. 4.46 Mild cylindrical bronchiectasis in the lower lobes. Several bronchi exhibit the "signet ring" sign (arrows).

Fig. 4.45 Major and ancillary HRCT signs of bronchiectasis: (1) non-tapering or flaring of bronchi; (2) signet ring sign; (3) mucus-filled dilated bronchi ("flame and blob" sign); (4) plugged and thickened centrilobular bronchioles ("tree-in-bud" sign); (5) crowding of bronchi with associated volume loss; (6) areas of decreased attenuation reflecting small airways obliteration.

the plane of CT section. Vertically orientated bronchi (in the lower lobes and apical segments of the upper lobes) will be seen in transverse section and reference can then be made to the accompanying pulmonary artery, which in normal individuals is of approximately the same caliber; any dilatation of the bronchus will result in the so-called "signet ring" sign (Fig. 4.46).

Although this is generally a reliable sign of abnormal bronchial dilatation, account must be taken of those conditions in which the pulmonary arteries are themselves of abnormal diameter. Furthermore, assessment of the diameter of an airway in the vicinity of a bronchial bifurcation may be misleading, particularly in the lower lobes, because the fusion of two bronchi may give the spurious impression of bronchial dilatation if the two corresponding pulmonary arteries have not fused at the same level (Fig. 4.47).

Bronchi that have a more horizontal course on CT, particularly the anterior segmental bronchi of the upper lobes and the segmental bronchi of the lingula and right middle lobe, are demonstrated along most of their length, and abnormal dilatation is seen as non-tapering parallel walls or sometimes distinct flaring of the bronchi as they course distally (Fig. 4.48). In more severe cases of bronchiectasis, the bronchi will be obviously dilated and have a varicose or cystic appearance (Fig. 4.49). Normal airways in the lung periphery are not usually visible

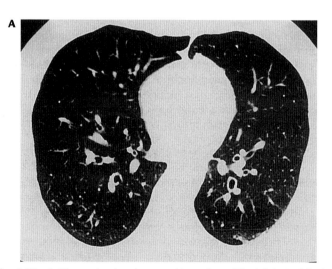

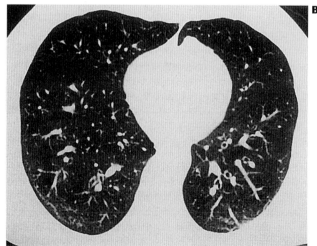

Fig. 4.47 **A,** The posterobasal segment bronchus of the left lower lobe has a larger diameter than its immediately adjacent pulmonary artery, suggesting that it is bronchiectatic. **B,** A section 10 mm below this level shows that this is a spurious appearance caused by the confluence of two subsegmental bronchi.

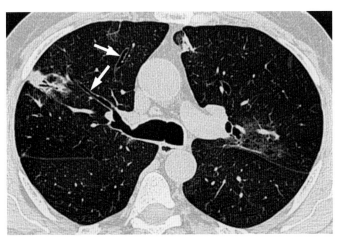

Fig. 4.48 Mild cylindrical bronchiectasis in the upper lobes of a patient with cystic fibrosis, seen as non-tapering bronchi (arrows).

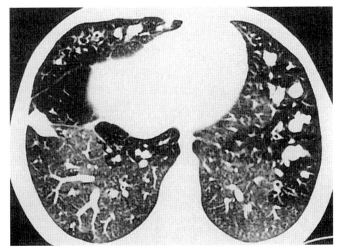

Fig. 4.50 Mucous plugging of the airways in severe bronchiectasis in a patient with cystic fibrosis. The lung surrounding the bronchiectatic airways is of decreased attenuation reflecting reduced ventilation and perfusion.

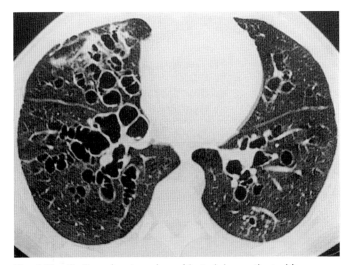

Fig. 4.49 Cystic and varicose bronchiectasis in a patient with idiopathic bronchiectasis.

Box 4.9 **Causes of misdiagnosis of bronchiectasis on HRCT**

Causes of false negative HRCT
Technical factors:
- Respiratory or cardiac motion artifact
- Inappropriate thick collimation
Inconspicuous thin-walled bronchiectasis
Obscuration of signs by adjacent fibrosis/consolidation[199]

Causes of false positive HRCT
Technical factors:
- Motion artifact (twinkling star[231] or double vessel[232] artifact)
- Confluence of subsegmental bronchi in the lower lobes
Conditions mimicking bronchiectasis:
- Langerhans cell histiocytosis[233]
- Cavitating bronchioloalveolar carcinoma[234]
- *Pneumocystis carinii* pneumonia[187]
Asthma
Acute bronchial dilatation in infective consolidation
Traction bronchiectasis

---

because their walls are below the spatial resolution of HRCT.[21] It is the presence of bronchial wall thickening and/or plugging of the lumen that renders peripheral airways visible; although a normal bronchus may occasionally be identified within 1 cm of the mediastinal pleura, airways identified within 1 cm of the costal pleura or paravertebral pleura should be regarded as bronchiectatic.[229] Bronchial wall thickening, in the absence of dilatation of the affected airways, is not a sign of bronchiectasis, which is fortunate given the wide variation between observers for this feature.[230]

Supplementary HRCT signs of bronchiectasis are crowding of the affected bronchi with obvious volume loss of the lobe as indicated by position of the fissures. Patients with bronchiectasis may show regional differences in density of the lung parenchyma due to impaired ventilation probably because of coexisting constrictive obliterative bronchiolitis.[198,199] The appearance of elliptical and circular opacities representing mucus or pus-filled dilated bronchi is a sign of gross bronchiectasis (Fig. 4.50) and is almost invariably seen in the

presence of other obviously dilated bronchi some of which may contain air–fluid levels. The most common causes of false negative and positive diagnoses of bronchiectasis on HRCT are given in Box 4.9.

False negatives are usually due to a technically imperfect examination, although subtle thin-walled bronchiectasis may be easily overlooked. A false positive diagnosis of bronchiectasis on HRCT is most frequently the result of scanning artifacts or another disease that superficially mimics bronchiectasis such as Langerhans cell histiocytosis or cavitating bronchioloalveolar carcinoma (Fig. 4.51). Despite the similarity of some cystic lung diseases to cystic bronchiectasis, the lack of continuity of these lesions between sections will usually allow their distinction

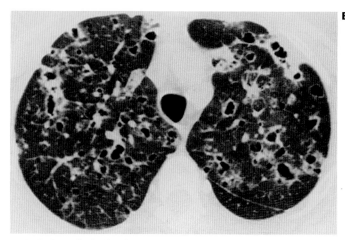

Fig. 4.51 Conditions resembling bronchiectasis. **A**, Langerhans cell histiocytosis. **B**, Bronchioloalveolar carcinoma – a relatively unusual form in which the cavitating nodules superficially resemble bronchiectatic airways.

from bronchiectatic airways to be made. In addition, normal bronchi can often be identified interspersed between non-bronchiectatic cystic lesions.

Small airways diseases

Many diffuse lung diseases are characterized by a degree of inflammation and scarring of the small airways. The pathologic type of inflammation, extent of involvement, and underlying cause all contribute to the final clinical presentation. The "bronchiolitides" are a truly heterogeneous group of disorders, such that few pathologically defined types of bronchiolitis are reflected by a distinctive clinical syndrome. This has led to much confusion because of the mismatch between pathologic, imaging, and clinical classifications of diseases of the small airways. For the purposes of HRCT imaging, the classification of small airways diseases can be greatly simplified.

Scarring and constriction of the bronchioles (constrictive bronchiolitis) may be detected indirectly on CT because regional under-ventilation results in reduced perfusion, which in turn is seen as areas of decreased attenuation of the lung parenchyma. Conversely, when there is inflammation of the bronchioles with accompanying exudate, the airways may become visible on CT, for example in cases of diffuse panbronchiolitis. In the normal state, the small airways (generally considered to be those with an internal diameter of 2 mm or less) are invisible on high-resolution CT. Because of the wide diversity of conditions which are characterized by an element of bronchiolar damage, the term "small airways disease" has much to recommend it; from the radiologist's viewpoint, there is no attempt to define the exact size of the airways included in this generic term, but it can be taken to include all airways below the resolution of HRCT in the normal state.

To reiterate, features of small airways disease on HRCT can be broadly categorized into direct and indirect patterns of disease: considerable thickening of the bronchiolar walls by inflammatory infiltrate and/or luminal and surrounding exudate render affected airways directly visible (*tree-in-bud pattern*). By contrast, cicatricial scarring of many bronchioles results in the indirect sign of patchy density differences of the lung

parenchyma, reflecting areas of under-ventilated, and consequently under-perfused lung (*mosaic attenuation pattern*). These two patterns of small airways disease account for the majority of cases encountered in clinical practice. Thus, a simple approach relies on the fundamental difference between the HRCT signs of **constrictive** (obliterative) bronchiolitis and the **exudative** form of bronchiolitis (typified by diffuse panbronchiolitis). While the two types of bronchiolitis may coexist in the same individual (for example, in a patient with cystic fibrosis), one or other pattern usually predominates in a given condition.

Standard high-resolution CT technique is satisfactory for demonstrating the signs of constrictive bronchiolitis and, at the other end of the pathologic/imaging spectrum, diffuse panbronchiolitis: the former requiring appropriate contrast resolution to demonstrate regional density differences (mosaic attenuation pattern), the latter requiring adequate spatial resolution to depict the small branching structures that characterize panbronchiolitis (tree-in-bud pattern).

A suggested protocol is thin (1–2 mm) collimation sections at 10 mm intervals from apices to costophrenic angles in the supine position. Whether expiratory CT sections (usually limited to approximately six sections taken between the aortic arch and right hemidiaphragm) need to be obtained in every case is controversial. In some centers, additional expiratory sections are obtained irrespective of the findings on the standard inspiratory HRCT sections.[163,211] If there is the opportunity to review the inspiratory HRCT of a patient with suspected small airways disease, the number of cases requiring additional expiratory sections will be small: in most patients with clinically significant constrictive bronchiolitis the HRCT features will be readily apparent on the inspiratory HRCT sections. Furthermore, in patients with diffuse panbronchiolitis the presence (or absence) of obvious air-trapping on expiratory CT sections does not alter the diagnosis, which is made on the basis of the tree-in-bud pattern on inspiratory HRCT sections. Nevertheless, it is often reassuring, particularly for clinicians, to have the sometimes subtle mosaic pattern emphasized on additional expiratory sections (Fig. 4.52).

There are other maneuvers that may enhance the appearance of air-trapping.[209] Sections obtained in quick succession at a

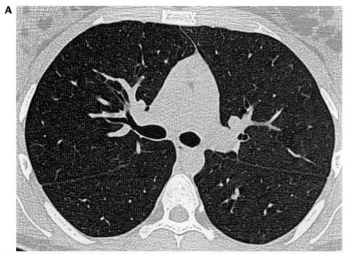

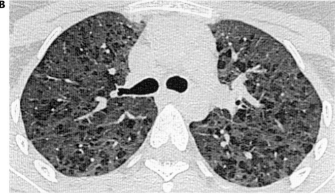

Fig. 4.52 A, There is inconspicuous regional variation in the density of lung parenchyma on HRCT section obtained with the patient breath holding at full inspiration. **B**, End-expiratory image showing obvious air-trapping at a lobular level in a patient with small airways disease as part of hypersensitivity pneumonitis.

single level during forced expiration, for example at a rate of two per second, may show areas of air-trapping that are inconspicuous or absent on sections obtained more conventionally at "end" expiration[235,236]; the physiologic reasons for the increased conspicuity of air-trapping on dynamic CT examinations are not fully understood.[237] For patients who are unable to reliably suspend respiration, specifically at end-expiration, scanning in a decubitus position has been suggested[238,239]; in this position the dependent lung is relatively restricted and so potentially mimics the state at end-expiration. The density differences that characterize the mosaic attenuation pattern on HRCT may be extremely subtle and simple image processing of adjacent thin sections may improve detection. Spiral CT can be used to acquire a "slab" of anatomically contiguous thin sections (for example, a 5 mm slab consisting of five adjacent 1 mm sections); a simple image processing algorithm is applied whereby only the lowest attenuation value of the five adjacent pixels is projected on the final image, producing a so-called "minimum intensity projection (Min IP) image". This technique improves the detection of subtle areas of low attenuation encountered in small airways disease and emphysema.[80,240] There is no doubt that Min IP and similar postprocessing of HRCT images[241] improve the conspicuity of the regional inhomogeneity of the lung parenchyma caused by small airways diseases, but they are not routinely used in clinical practice.

Constrictive bronchiolitis

Subsequent descriptions have confirmed and refined the high-resolution CT features of constrictive bronchiolitis.[14,160,226,238,242,243] The HRCT signs comprise patchy areas of reduced parenchymal density (the "mosaic attenuation pattern"), attenuation of the pulmonary vessels within areas of decreased lung density, bronchial abnormalities, and lack of change of cross-sectional area of affected parts of the lung on scans obtained at end-expiration.[159,244]

The individual CT signs of constrictive bronchiolitis are summarized in Box 4.10.

Box 4.10 HRCT features of constrictive bronchiolitis

Areas of decreased attenuation
Regions of decreased attenuation usually have poorly defined margins (Fig. 4.53), but sometimes have a sharp geographic outline (representing a collection of affected secondary pulmonary lobules, Fig. 4.54). The relatively higher attenuation regions of lung represent shunting of blood to the normally ventilated lung.
When constrictive bronchiolitis is severe, the lung may be of homogeneously decreased attenuation (so that the patchy density difference, or mosaic pattern, is lost).

Reduction in caliber of the macroscopic pulmonary vessels
In the areas of decreased attenuation, pulmonary perfusion is reduced. In *acute* bronchiolar obstruction this represents the physiologic reflex of hypoxic vasoconstriction.[245]
Over time there is vascular remodeling and the reduced perfusion becomes irreversible. In some instances the inflammatory process that causes bronchiolar scarring may synchronously affect the adjacent pulmonary artery, thus leading to vascular obliteration.
Although the vessels within areas of decreased attenuation on HRCT may be of markedly reduced caliber they are not distorted.

Bronchial abnormalities
The severity of bronchial dilatation and wall thickening is highly variable from one case to another: in immunologically mediated constrictive bronchiolitis (e.g. post transplant or associated with rheumatoid arthritis), marked dilatation of the bronchi is a frequent finding[246] (Fig. 4.55).
Some degree of bronchial thickening abnormality is the rule in most patients with constrictive bronchiolitis,[160] and seems to be pronounced in patients with postinfectious obliterative bronchiolitis.[247]

Air-trapping at expiratory CT
The regional inhomogeneity of the lung density is accentuated on sections obtained at end, or during,[236] expiration. Areas of decreased attenuation, not visible on inspiratory CT sections, may be detectable on end-expiratory CT sections[209,211,248] (Fig. 4.52, see also p. 161), and may be a normal feature, particularly in older individuals.[249]

Box 4.10 cont'd

The cross-sectional area of the affected parts of the lung does not decrease on expiratory CT.[159]

Expiratory CT may also be helpful in differentiating between the three main causes of a mosaic pattern (infiltrative lung disease, small airways disease, and occlusive pulmonary vascular disease) which may be problematic on inspiratory CT.[152,163]

An important caveat is that in patients with widespread small airways disease, end-expiratory CT sections may appear virtually identical to the standard inspiratory CT sections, simply because of the severity of the air-trapping (i.e. there is no mosaic pattern or change in cross-sectional area of the lungs).

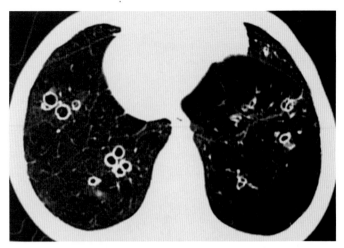

Fig. 4.55 A patient with rheumatoid arthritis and severe constrictive bronchiolitis (note the paucity of normal pulmonary vasculature); in this case there are particularly severe bronchiectatic changes.

Exudative bronchiolitis

Diffuse (Japanese) panbronchiolitis is the archetypal exudative small airways disease and the definitive pathologic and imaging studies originate from Japan.[64,250,251] The typical histopathologic features of diffuse panbronchiolitis are chronic inflammatory cell infiltration resulting in bronchiolectasis and striking hyperplasia of lymphoid follicles in the walls of the respiratory bronchioles; profuse foamy macrophages fill the bronchiolar lumens and the immediately adjacent alveoli.

The HRCT appearances reflect the pathologic distribution of disease[238]: there is a nodular pattern and small branching opacities (tree-in-bud pattern[252]) can be identified in a predominantly centrilobular distribution, corresponding to the plugged and thickened small airways (Figs 4.3 and 4.56). Accompanying cylindrical bronchiectasis, usually mild, is an almost invariable feature. Interestingly, although a mosaic attenuation pattern may be present in some cases, it is not usually a major feature; furthermore, air-trapping on expiratory CT is often surprisingly unimpressive. Nevertheless, functional studies have shown that the peripheral zone of lung is less dense than normal because of air-trapping.[253]

The HRCT features of diffuse panbronchiolitis, in the appropriate clinical setting, are virtually pathognomonic. Other conditions that may cause a similar (primarily tree-in-bud) pattern on HRCT as a result of exudates in and around the small airways include:

- Mycoplasma pneumonia (acute)[100]
- Bronchiectasis
- Allergic bronchopulmonary aspergillosis[254]
- Cystic fibrosis[255]
- Airway invasive aspergillosis[256]
- Active tuberculosis[94,257]
- Atypical mycobacterial infection (in particular *M. avium–intracellulare*)[98,258]
- Aspiration pneumonia.[114]

Although a tree-in-bud sign is relatively specific for conditions characterized by exudative small airways disease, a similar pattern is rarely encountered in small vessel or infiltrative diseases, including neoplastic emboli[112] or lymphomatous infiltrate.[116]

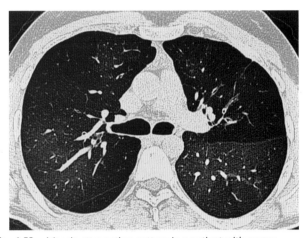

Fig. 4.53 Mosaic attenuation pattern in a patient with severe postviral constrictive bronchiolitis. The interface between the relatively normal, but over-perfused, lung and the abnormal (black) lung is indistinct.

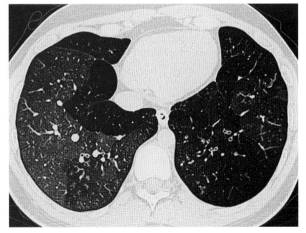

Fig. 4.54 Constrictive bronchiolitis. There are clearly defined geographic margins between the normal and affected lung. There is mild cylindrical bronchiectasis in the left lower lobe and a limited tree-in-bud pattern in both lower lobes.

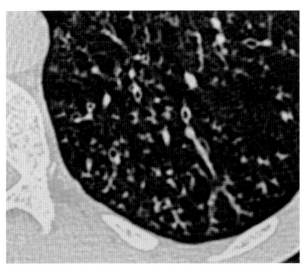

Fig. 4.56   A magnified view showing the typical tree-in-bud pattern of exudative diffuse panbronchiolitis.

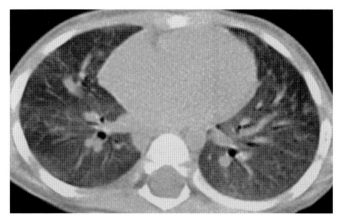

Fig. 4.57   The attenuation of normal lung parenchyma in neonates and infants is greater than that of adults, even at near total lung capacity. The appearances of the lungs in this healthy 18-month-old child give the misleading impression of pathologic ground-glass opacification.

CLINICAL ASPECTS OF HRCT

The suggested indications for HRCT that have been developed over the last fifteen years are summarized in Box 4.11.

Clinical experience and much literature confirm that HRCT has become an invaluable step in the investigation and assessment of patients with suspected or clinically obvious diffuse lung disease. The greater chance of achieving a histospecific diagnosis with HRCT means that it can be used to secure a definite diagnosis in some, but certainly not all, patients with obvious but nonspecific radiographic abnormalities. Attention has been drawn to the sometimes uncritical use of HRCT for patients in whom the certainty of diagnosis from clinical and radiographic findings does not justify the extra cost and radiation burden of HRCT.[259–261] Although the radiation received by patients from a standard HRCT examination is considerably less than that from multislice CT volumetric acquisition,[262] the radiation dose is not negligible and HRCT should therefore not be performed indiscriminately. Diagnostically satisfactory HRCT examinations can be obtained when the milliamperage is reduced between two and tenfold,[263,264] so reducing the radiation

to the patient, but this modification is seldom adopted in practice. It is likely that, with increasing awareness of the radiation burden inherent in any form of CT scanning, more stringent efforts to reduce radiation will be made in the future. This is of relevance in pediatric practice, particularly given the increasing reports of the utility of HRCT in the diagnosis of interstitial lung disease in children.[247,265–268]

Sensitivity of HRCT for the presence of diffuse lung disease

The overall frequency with which HRCT reveals pulmonary abnormalities when chest radiography (and/or pulmonary function testing) is normal is difficult to gauge. Several studies showed that HRCT scans were abnormal despite normal chest radiographs in 10% of cases of sarcoidosis,[42] 21% of cases of lymphangioleiomyomatosis,[182] 29% of cases of systemic sclerosis,[269] and approximately 30% of cases of asbestosis.[270] Subacute hypersensitivity pneumonitis is a good example of a disease which may be radiographically cryptic: in one series widespread ground-glass opacity was identified on 11 of 17 HRCT scans compared with 5 of 17 chest radiographs.[213] Taking these and other studies into account, the prevalence of normal chest radiographs in patients with abnormalities on HRCT and confirmed diffuse lung disease is in the region of 20%. A survey of many studies suggests that the sensitivity of HRCT for the detection of diffuse lung disease is approximately 94%, compared to 80% for chest radiography.[271] It is impossible to predict how often HRCT will reveal parenchymal abnormalities in the face of a normal chest radiograph, but HRCT has an important role in patients with a questionably abnormal chest radiograph, particularly if clinical findings and pulmonary function tests suggest disease. False positive diagnoses of diffuse lung disease using HRCT are relatively uncommon.[272] The situation in pediatric practice may be different; it can be difficult or impossible to differentiate, particularly in neonates, between the normal increase in lung attenuation resulting from a submaximal lung inflation and ground-glass opacification representing interstitial disease (Fig. 4.57). The position of the

---

Box 4.11   Clinical indications for HRCT of the lungs

To detect diffuse lung disease in patients with normal or equivocal radiographic abnormalities

To narrow the differential diagnosis or make a histospecific diagnosis, in patients with obvious but nonspecific radiographic abnormalities

To guide the type and site of lung biopsy

To investigate patients presenting with hemoptysis

To investigate patients with unexplained severe obstructive airways disease

To assess the distribution of emphysema in patients considered for lung volume reduction surgery

To evaluate disease reversibility, particularly in patients with fibrosing lung disease

posterior tracheal membrane may be helpful in distinguishing between the two (in the upper lobes, at least): the posterior tracheal membrane is convex outwards in inspiration, and appears horizontal or slightly concave on expiration.

Between 10% and 15% of patients with histologically proven interstitial lung disease have a normal chest radiograph.[4,273] In many studies describing the HRCT appearances of individual chronic diffuse lung diseases, a substantial proportion of patients are reported to have had normal chest radiographs. The characteristics of HRCT abnormalities likely to be encountered in patients with diffuse lung disease and a normal chest radiograph can be summarized as:

1. Subtle differences in density of the lung parenchyma (for example, subacute hypersensitivity pneumonitis[213] and the mosaic pattern seen in constrictive bronchiolitis[274]).
2. Parenchymal abnormalities involving a small volume of the lung often obscured by superimposed structures (for example, the basal subpleural distribution of fibrosing alveolitis[269]). This is of particular relevance in asbestos-exposed individuals in whom there may be considerable pleural thickening obscuring the underlying lung parenchyma on chest radiography.[77,270,275,276]
3. Structural changes requiring high spatial resolution for their demonstration (for example, the thin-walled cystic airspaces of lymphangioleiomyomatosis[277] and the sometimes fine interstitial thickening in early lymphangitis carcinomatosa[23]).

Patients with suspected diffuse lung disease on clinical grounds, but normal chest radiographs, are likely to have relatively limited changes on HRCT, and the reduced specificity of such minimal changes on HRCT should be recognized. Some normal individuals may have thickening of a few interlobular septa or parenchymal opacification mimicking early interstitial fibrosis.[77,278] Diffuse lung disease that is characterized by well-defined nodules or areas of dense pulmonary consolidation is not likely to result in the HRCT abnormalities which are invisible on chest radiography. Despite the clear improvement in sensitivity of HRCT over chest radiography, the inability of HRCT to consistently demonstrate disease that is obvious at a microscopic level, for example in some cases of hypersensitivity pneumonitis,[123,279] idiopathic pulmonary fibrosis,[280] and acute rejection following lung transplantation,[281] should be remembered. Nevertheless, clinical experience, and the paucity of reports to the contrary, suggest that patients with clinically significant diffuse lung disease very seldom have a normal HRCT examination.

Chest radiography is relatively insensitive for the detection of airways disease. In one study of adults with cystic fibrosis, only 11% of patients had evidence of bronchiectasis on chest radiography, compared with 77% on HRCT.[282] Similarly, the subtle abnormalities of some small airways diseases, notably constrictive obliterative bronchiolitis,[274] may be identifiable only on HRCT. In particular, expiratory CT may be used to identify the development of constrictive bronchiolitis in heart–lung transplant recipients,[283,284] although there is contradictory evidence about the sensitivity of HRCT for this task.[285] Although the clinical utility of detecting evidence of very early emphysema is questionable, there is no doubt that HRCT is more sensitive than chest radiography.[286–289]

Pathologic specificity of HRCT in diffuse lung disease

Given the many diseases characterized by diffuse lung shadowing on a chest radiograph, the frequency with which the correct diagnosis can be made on the basis of the radiographic appearances alone may seem surprising. This apparent success is largely a reflection of the pre-test probability of a particular diagnosis which will be heavily influenced by the known local prevalence of individual diffuse lung diseases: sarcoidosis, idiopathic pulmonary fibrosis, lymphangitis carcinomatosa and hypersensitivity pneumonitis account for the majority of non-infectious cases of diffuse lung disease encountered in most clinical practices. Nevertheless, the ability to narrow the differential diagnosis from the chest radiograph appearances in patients with diffuse lung disease is relatively limited: in one study the correct histological diagnosis was included in the first two radiological diagnoses offered by an experienced chest radiologist in only 50% of cases. Furthermore, agreement between observers about the pattern of radiographic abnormality and the severity of disease occurred in less than three quarters of cases.[1]

HRCT allows a considerable improvement in the frequency with which a correct histospecific diagnosis can be made. In the first study of its kind, Mathieson et al showed that CT enabled observers to give a correct diagnosis of a wide variety of diffuse lung diseases more often, and with more confidence, than with chest radiography alone.[224] Several studies have subsequently confirmed the superior performance of HRCT in a mixture of diffuse lung diseases[272,290,291] and in selected disease groups such as patients with AIDS[292] or diffuse cystic lung disease.[194] In the original study by Mathieson et al, a confident diagnosis was reached more than twice as often with CT compared with chest radiography (49% versus 23% respectively) and of these "confident" observations, a correct diagnosis was made in 93% of the first choice CT diagnoses as opposed to 77% of the first choice radiographic diagnoses.[224] The diagnostic benefit of HRCT is incremental: in a study by Grenier et al using Bayesian analysis which assessed the cumulative values of clinical information, chest radiography, and HRCT in patients with diffuse lung disease, an accurate diagnosis was made on the basis of clinical data alone in 27% of cases and this increased to 53% with the addition of radiographic findings and further increased to 61% with the addition of HRCT scans.[293] The majority of studies claiming to show the superior performance of HRCT over chest radiography have been retrospective with cases selected from tertiary referral patient populations. The diagnostic effectiveness of HRCT in centers with a low throughput of patients with diffuse lung disease is likely to be less striking.

The value of any diagnostic test has been defined as its ability to diminish uncertainty and, by its ability to provide a confident and correct histospecific diagnosis, HRCT can be regarded as valuable. A crucial benefit of HRCT is the added confidence it brings to the diagnosis of diffuse lung disease; nevertheless, this factor has not been evaluated in detail, partly because the statistical tools available for evaluating the subtle shades of an observer's level of confidence are relatively crude. In the few series in which observer confidence has been assessed,[224,272,293] a confident diagnosis was made more often on CT than on chest radiography and, even more importantly, a confident CT diagnosis was almost always correct. The landmark study of Mathieson et al[224] showed that a confident diagnosis of various diffuse lung diseases was made by three observers at least twice as often on CT as on chest radiography. Furthermore, the accuracy of a confident first choice diagnosis on CT was 95%, compared to 77% for chest radiography. However, when the first choice diagnosis was not made with high confidence the advantage of CT (60% accuracy in 51% of cases) over chest radiography (51% accuracy in 77% of cases) was greatly diminished. Given that the study by Mathieson et al was performed several years ago, it seems probable that the results of this widely cited study understate the diagnostic accuracy of HRCT today.

When interpreting the results of studies designed to evaluate the diagnostic accuracy of HRCT, several factors need to be borne in mind: (a) there is inevitably a selection bias with a relatively high proportion of conditions which have distinctive HRCT appearances. In this respect, the study populations are usually retrospective and drawn from tertiary referral centers and so do not reflect the case mix encountered in "normal" clinical practice, in which there will be a higher frequency of smoking-related diffuse lung disease, interstitial pulmonary edema, as well as normal individuals; an example is a study in which observers were asked to discriminate between roughly equal numbers of the individual idiopathic interstitial pneumonias[294] – an artificial proposition, in several respects, in clinical practice,[295] (b) nonrepresentative expertise, that is, observers in such studies are usually highly experienced, (c) new or "difficult" conditions are generally under-represented (for example, the idiopathic interstitial pneumonia subtype nonspecific interstitial pneumonia), (d) under-recognition of the ability of CT to exclude, rather than confirm, specific diagnoses (for example, the chest radiography shows cardiomegaly and diffuse pulmonary shadowing which on HRCT has the characteristic features of usual interstitial pneumonia, thus effectively excluding pulmonary edema), (e) the effect of pre-test clinical probability, and (f) the reported accuracy of HRCT, when given as a single result, cannot reflect the highly disease-dependent accuracy of HRCT. The last is an important point, for there are several diffuse lung diseases which, in the hands of experienced observers, are regarded as having a "diagnostic" appearance on HRCT. These include usual interstitial pneumonia (UIP), lymphangitis carcinomatosa, subacute hypersensitivity pneumonitis, sarcoidosis, Langerhans cell histiocytosis, and lymphangioleiomyomatosis.[10] Another fundamental issue is the nature of the long accepted gold standard of a histopathological diagnosis, against which the veracity of a HRCT diagnosis is usually judged. In a study of multiple biopsies taken in patients with idiopathic interstitial pneumonia, a different diagnosis (usually UIP versus NSIP) was found in different lobes in 26%.[296] Furthermore, very similar pathologic processes (i.e. histopathologic diagnoses), for example chronic eosinophilic pneumonia and organizing pneumonia, may coexist.[297] This phenomenon is particularly true of connective tissue disease-related lung disease. A further consideration is the plethora of different pathologic lesions that may coexist, in varying proportions, in a given patient with for example connective tissue disease[298,299] or smoking-related disease.[300]

> **Box 4.12** Diffuse lung diseases that often have a diagnostic appearance on HRCT
>
> Idiopathic pulmonary fibrosis (usual interstitial pneumonitis subtype)
> Centrilobular emphysema
> Sarcoidosis
> Lymphangitis carcinomatosa
> Langerhans cell histiocytosis
> Lymphangioleiomyomatosis
> Alveolar proteinosis
> Bronchiectasis
> Diffuse panbronchiolitis
> Constrictive obliterative bronchiolitis

Even without clinical information, there are a number of diffuse lung diseases that, with increasing experience, can have a "diagnostic" appearance on HRCT. In many cases the need for lung biopsy confirmation of the diagnosis can be avoided when the clinical and HRCT appearances are typical in these particular conditions, shown in Box 4.12.

The ability of HRCT to allow observers to provide correct histospecific diagnoses appears to be maintained in advanced "end-stage" disease.[195] Conversely, as a generalization HRCT is less helpful in refining the differential diagnosis of acute parenchymal disorders, for example acute infective and other pneumonic conditions.[297,301] The decision of whether or not to confirm the diagnosis of a chronic diffuse lung disease by lung biopsy is influenced by many factors, but HRCT has an increasingly influential role in this decision making.[302,303] Diffuse infiltrative lung disease in children is relatively rare and experience with HRCT in pediatric practice correspondingly slight, and the diagnostic value of HRCT in this situation is less than in adult patients.[265–268]

The greater chance of achieving a histospecific diagnosis with HRCT means that for some patients with obvious radiographic abnormalities, HRCT can be used to secure a definite diagnosis. The word "some" deserves special emphasis because not all such patients require an HRCT scan: attention has been drawn to the sometimes indiscriminate use of HRCT for patients in whom the certainty of diagnosis provided by the clinical and radiographic findings does not justify the extra cost and radiation burden of HRCT.[259–261] There is no evidence that an HRCT examination (or indeed a lung biopsy) is of diagnostic value in a patient with progressive shortness of breath, finger clubbing, crackles at the lung bases, and the typical radiographic pattern and lung function profile of idiopathic pulmonary fibrosis.

In the same way that the pattern recognition used by pathologists at a microscopic level is fallible (for example the histopathologic distinction between hypersensitivity pneumonitis and lymphocytic interstitial pneumonia may be a matter of fine judgment), so macroscopic pattern recognition in HRCT is not always reliable. Even when the HRCT abnormalities fulfill the usual criteria for, say, usual interstitial pneumonia, a very small proportion of cases may be shown to have a different diagnosis on histopathologic examination, such as chronic hypersensitivity pneumonitis.[54,221] However, the converse is occasionally true: the histopathologic diagnosis of UIP may, on occasion, be in conflict with the clinical and HRCT features, which point toward chronic hypersensitivity pneumonitis.

Some of the more distinctive HRCT patterns that were initially thought to be virtually pathognomonic of specific conditions have now been reported in other conditions. For example the "crazy-paving" pattern, first reported in cases of alveolar proteinosis, may also be encountered in other diseases[74,304] including lipoid pneumonia,[45] bronchioloalveolar carcinoma,[59] and nonspecific interstitial pneumonia.[61]

Assessment of disease reversibility with HRCT

There has been much interest in identifying patients with diffuse lung disease, particularly the fibrotic idiopathic interstitial pneumonias, who will and will not, benefit from treatment. Extensive ground-glass opacity on HRCT in patients with chronic diffuse lung disease usually represents a reversible pathologic process[65,118,305,306] (Figs 4.22 and 4.23), whereas a reticular pattern, honeycombing, and architectural distortion represent irreversible fibrosis. In patients with the diagnostic label of idiopathic pulmonary fibrosis, the concept of "disease activity" is complex and is used differently by pathologists and clinicians. The former usually consider the degree of cellularity of a lung biopsy[307,308] and the identification of histologic subsets[309] as indicators of prognosis and disease activity. More recently, attention has been paid to the prognostic significance of the profusion of fibroblastic foci in patients with an idiopathic interstitial pneumonia.[310] In contrast, clinicians tend to use more pragmatic markers, such as a patient's clinical response to treatment.[303,311] Chest radiography, lung function tests, bronchoalveolar lavage, and radionuclide techniques all have limitations in the consistent identification of patients with reversible disease.[312–315] Furthermore, only a minority of patients with fibrosing lung disease undergo lung biopsy for confirmation of the diagnosis or evaluation of disease activity.[316] As a result, there has been interest in defining the role of HRCT in identifying disease reversibility.[317]

A predominant pattern of ground-glass opacity on HRCT predicts a good response to treatment[318,319] and increased survival[320] over patients who have a reticular pattern as the dominant abnormality. Conversely, the extent of a reticular pattern on HRCT (by comparison with clinical, radiographic, and functional characteristics) is as reliable a predictor of patient survival as the severity of fibrosis on pathologic examination of a lung biopsy.[321]

The retractile property of interstitial fibrosis is reflected on HRCT images as architectural distortion, with dilatation of bronchi in areas of ground-glass opacification, well before there are macroscopic signs of honeycomb lung destruction. Nevertheless, it must be appreciated that the indirect HRCT signs of pathologic processes are not wholly reliable. Dilatation of the airways within areas of ground-glass opacification usually reflects fine intralobular fibrosis (Figs 4.26 and 4.58),[150] but the clinical context is crucial: bronchial dilatation is also seen within areas of ground-glass opacification in patients with acute respiratory distress syndrome (see p. 410), but whether these dilated airways within the milieu of acute lung inflammation and exudate truly reflect "traction bronchiectasis" due to surrounding established fibrosis has not been clarified.[151] The

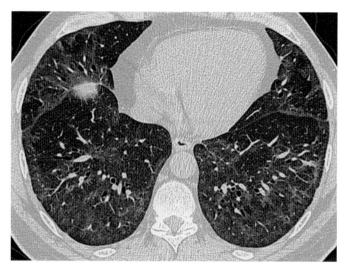

Fig. 4.58 A patient with stable nonspecific interstitial pneumonia. These HRCT appearances were unchanged over a 30-month period. Within the areas of ground-glass opacification there is slight dilatation and distortion of the airways indicating irreversible retractile fibrosis.

poor outcome seen in most patients with approximately equal proportions of ground-glass opacity and a reticular pattern on HRCT likely reflects the fact that these individuals have predominantly fibrotic disease, consisting of both fine intralobular fibrosis and coarse fibrosis (the former producing ground-glass opacification and the latter a macroscopic reticular pattern). Another assumption relates to cases in which a reticular pattern is the dominant finding on HRCT. In this context, it may be assumed when a reticular pattern (excluding a reticular pattern comprising thickened interlobular septa alone) predominates, particularly when there is associated distortion of the lung architecture, that this pattern represents "irreversible fibrosis". However, there are a few situations in which this is not the case, for example nitrofurantoin-induced lung disease[322] (Fig. 4.59). Another area of difficulty is the rapid appearance of ground-glass opacification in patients with or without known preexisting idiopathic interstitial pneumonia; opportunistic infection or pulmonary edema are differential diagnoses but in a substantial proportion of patients this development reflects a fulminant phase of the disease[323,324]; in this situation the extensive HRCT appearances of widespread ground-glass opacity and consolidation denote diffuse alveolar damage with a poor prognosis.

Similar predictions about the potential reversibility of disease on HRCT can be made in other chronic diffuse lung diseases (Box 4.13).

In patients with pulmonary sarcoidosis, nodular, ground-glass,[325–327] or airspace[328] patterns are reversible. In other conditions the identification of ground-glass opacity on HRCT, although nonspecific, usually indicates a potentially reversible disease,[65] for example hypersensitivity pneumonitis,[213] diffuse pulmonary hemorrhage,[135] and *Pneumocystis carinii* pneumonia.[129] An important exception is bronchioloalveolar carcinoma, in which there may be areas of ground-glass opacity which merge into areas of frank consolidation or a more nodular pattern[138] (Table 4.5).

Since the HRCT pattern of some diffuse lung diseases indicates disease activity and so predicts the subsequent behavior of the disease, HRCT has been used to document the evolution

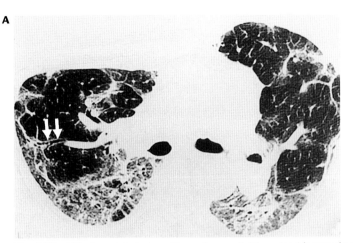
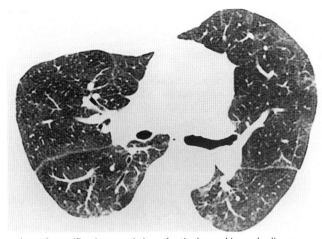

Fig. 4.59 Nitrofurantoin-induced lung disease. **A,** There is widespread parenchymal opacification consisting of reticular and irregular linear elements with associated distortion of the lung architecture, and apparent traction bronchiectasis (arrows). **B,** Several months later following cessation of nitrofurantoin and steroid treatment there has been considerable resolution of the lung abnormalities with a limited reticular pattern only remaining. The presumed pathology at presentation was organizing pneumonia with a minor component of irreversible fibrosis. (With permission from Sheehan RE, Wells AU, Milne DG, et al. Nitrofurantoin-induced lung disease: two cases demonstrating resolution of apparently irreversible CT abnormalities. J Thorac Imaging 2000;24:259–261.)

Box 4.13 Conditions in which HRCT may be used to evaluate disease reversibility

Idiopathic interstitial pneumonias (including usual, nonspecific, desquamative, and lymphoid histopathologic subtypes)
Hypersensitivity pneumonitis
Sarcoidosis
Pneumocystis carinii pneumonia
Langerhans cell histiocytosis
Eosinophilic pneumonia
Alveolar proteinosis
Wegener granulomatosis
Amiodarone-induced lung disease

Table 4.5 Summary of reversible patterns on HRCT (+ = more likelihood of reversibility, – = less likelihood of reversibility)

Ground-glass opacification	++++/–
Airspace consolidation	+++/–
Nodular pattern	++/–
Interlobular septal thickening	+/––
Reticular pattern with distortion	+/––––
Honeycomb lung destruction	––––––

of many conditions.[68,184,329–333] The limitations of predicting disease activity at a histopathologic level from HRCT appearances should always be borne in mind, for example the apparently "burnt-out" cystic appearances of late stage Langerhans cell histiocytosis may harbor active granulomatous lesions at a microscopic level.[196]

Because of the patchy nature of most diffuse lung diseases, anatomically comparable HRCT sections need to be obtained at follow-up studies for a meaningful assessment of change to be made. In practice, this may be difficult to achieve and so any judgment about change in extent or pattern of diffuse lung disease needs to take account of the comparability of sections on follow-up studies. For this reason, and because of considerations of radiation dose to patients, HRCT is not widely used for repeated clinical assessment of patients with diffuse lung disease.

REFERENCES

1. McLoud TC, Carrington CB, Gaensler EA. Diffuse infiltrative lung disease: A new scheme for description. Radiology 1983;149:353–363.
2. Felson B. A new look at pattern recognition of diffuse pulmonary disease. AJR Am J Roentgenol 1979;133:183–189.
3. Genereux GP. Pattern recognition in diffuse lung disease. A review of theory and practice. Med Radiogr Photogr 1985;61:2–31.
4. Epler GR, McLoud TC, Gaensler EA, et al. Normal chest roentgenograms in chronic diffuse infiltrative lung disease. N Engl J Med 1978;298:935–939.
5. Gaensler EA, Moister VB, Hamm J. Open lung biopsy in diffuse pulmonary disease. N Engl J Med 1964;270:1319–1331.
6. Müller NL. Clinical value of High Resolution CT in chronic diffuse lung disease. AJR Am J Roentgenol 1991;157:1163–1170.
7. Colby TV, Swensen SJ. Anatomic distribution and histopathologic patterns in diffuse lung disease: correlation with HRCT. J Thorac Imaging 1996;11:1–26.
8. Hansell DM. Computed tomography of diffuse infiltrative lung disease: value and limitations. Semin Respir Crit Care Med 1998;19:431–446.
9. Schaefer-Prokop C, Prokop M, Fleischmann D, et al. High-resolution CT of diffuse interstitial lung disease: key

findings in common disorders. Eur Radiol 2001;11:373–392.

10. Lynch DA. Imaging of diffuse infiltrative lung disease. Eur Respir Mon 2000;14: 29–54.

11. Kazerooni EA. High-resolution CT of the lungs. AJR Am J Roentgenol 2001;177: 501–519.

12. Grenier P, Cordeau MP, Beigelman C. High-resolution computed tomography of the airways. J Thorac Imaging 1993;8:213–229.

13. Hansell DM. Bronchiectasis. Radiol Clin North Am 1998;36:107–128.

14. Müller NL, Miller RR. Diseases of the bronchioles: CT and histopathologic findings. Radiology 1995;196:3–12.

15. Hansell DM. Small airways diseases: detection and insights with computed tomography. Eur Respir J 2001;17: 1294–1313.

16. Cleverley JR, Müller NL. Advances in radiologic assessment of chronic obstructive pulmonary disease. Clin Chest Med 2000;21:653–663.

17. Copley SJ, Wells AU, Müller NL, et al. Thin-section CT in obstructive pulmonary disease: discriminatory value. Radiology 2002;223:812–819.

18. Kim SJ, Im JG, Kim IO, et al. Normal bronchial and pulmonary arterial diameters measured by thin section CT. J Comput Assist Tomogr 1995;19:365–369.

19. Kim JS, Müller NL, Park CS, et al. Bronchoarterial ratio on thin section CT: comparison between high altitude and sea level. J Comput Assist Tomogr 1997;21:306–311.

20. Weibel ER. Looking into the lung: what can it tell us? AJR Am J Roentgenol 1979;133:1021–1031.

21. Webb WR, Stein MG, Finkbeiner WE, et al. Normal and diseased isolated lungs: High-resolution CT. Radiology 1988;166:81–87.

22. Murata K, Itoh H, Todo G, et al. Centrilobular lesions of the lung: demonstration by high-resolution CT and pathologic correlation. Radiology 1986;161:641–645.

23. Stein MG, Mayo J, Müller N, et al. Pulmonary lymphatic spread of carcinoma: Appearance on CT scans. Radiology 1987;162:371–375.

24. Bergin CJ, Roggli V, Coblentz C, et al. The secondary pulmonary lobule: normal and abnormal CT appearances. AJR Am J Roentgenol 1988;151:21–25.

25. Giovagnorio F, Cavallo V. HRCT evaluation of secondary lobules and acini of the lung. J Thorac Imaging 1995;10:129–133.

26. Kuhn C. Normal anatomy and histology. In: Thurlbeck WM, Churg AM, eds. Pathology of the lung. New York: Thieme Medical Publishers, 1995:1–36.

27. Hruban RH, Meziane MA, Zerhouni EA, et al. High resolution computed tomography of inflation-fixed lungs. Am Rev Respir Dis 1987;136:935–940.

28. Naidich DP. Pulmonary parenchymal high-resolution CT: To be or not to be. Radiology 1989;171:22–24.

29. Zerhouni EA, Naidich DP, Stitik FP, et al. Computed tomography of the pulmonary parenchyma. Part 2: Interstitial disease. J Thorac Imaging 1985;1:54–64.

30. Webb WR, Müller NL, Naidich DP. Standardized terms for high resolution lung CT: a proposed glossary. J Thorac Imaging 1993;8:167–175.

31. Webb WR, Müller NL, Naidich DP. An illustrated glossary of HRCT terms. High-resolution CT of the lung. Philadelphia: Lippincott Williams & Wilkins, 2001:599–618.

32. Austin JHM, Müller NL, Friedman PJ, et al. Glossary of terms for CT of the lungs: recommendations of the nomenclature committee of the Fleischner Society. Radiology 1996;200:327–331.

33. Kang EY, Grenier P, Laurent F, et al. Interlobular septal thickening: patterns at high-resolution computed tomography. J Thorac Imaging 1996;11:260–264.

34. Webb WR, Müller NL, Naidich DP. HRCT findings of lung disease. High-resolution CT of the lung. Philadelphia: Lippincott-Raven, 1996:41–108.

35. Munk PL, Müller NL, Miller RR, et al. Pulmonary lymphangitic carcinomatosis: CT and pathologic findings. Radiology 1988;166:705–709.

36. Ren H, Hruban RH, Kuhlman JE, et al. Computed tomography of inflation-fixed lungs: the beaded septum sign of pulmonary metastases. J Comput Assist Tomogr 1989;13:411–416.

37. Johkoh T, Ikezoe J, Tomiyama N, et al. CT findings in lymphangitic carcinomatosis of the lung: correlation with histologic findings and pulmonary function tests. AJR Am J Roentgenol 1992;158:1217–1222.

38. Storto ML, Kee ST, Golden JA, et al. Hydrostatic pulmonary edema: high-resolution CT findings. AJR Am J Roentgenol 1995;165:817–820.

39. Murch CR, Carr DH. Computed tomography appearances of pulmonary alveolar proteinosis. Clin Radiol 1989;40:240–243.

40. Newell JD, Underwood GHJ, Russo DJ, et al. Computed tomographic appearance of pulmonary alveolar proteinosis in adults. J Comput Tomogr 1984;8:21–29.

41. Godwin JD, Müller NL, Takasugi JE. Pulmonary alveolar proteinosis: CT findings. Radiology 1988;169:609–613.

42. Müller NL, Kullnig P, Miller RR. The CT findings of pulmonary sarcoidosis: analysis of 25 patients. AJR Am J Roentgenol 1989;152:1179–1182.

43. Swensen SJ, Tashjian JH, Myers JL, et al. Pulmonary venoocclusive disease: CT findings in eight patients. AJR Am J Roentgenol 1996;167:937–940.

44. Heyneman LE, Nolan RL, Harrison JK, et al. Congenital unilateral pulmonary vein atresia: radiologic findings in three adult patients. AJR Am J Roentgenol 2001;177:681–685.

45. Franquet T, Gimenez A, Bordes R, et al. The crazy-paving pattern in exogenous lipoid pneumonia: CT–pathologic correlation. AJR Am J Roentgenol 1998;170:315–317.

46. Johkoh T, Müller NL, Pickford HA, et al. Lymphocytic interstitial pneumonia: thin-section CT findings in 22 patients. Radiology 1999;212:567–572.

47. Heyneman LE, Johkoh T, Ward S, et al. Pulmonary leukemic infiltrates: high-resolution CT findings in 10 patients. AJR Am J Roentgenol 2000;174:517–521.

48. Melamed JW, Sostman HD, Ravin CE. Interstitial thickening in pulmonary alveolar microlithiasis: an underappreciated finding. J Thorac Imaging 1994;9:126–128.

49. Graham CM, Stern EJ, Finkbeiner WE, et al. High-resolution CT appearances of diffuse alveolar septal amyloidosis. AJR Am J Roentgenol 1992;158:265–267.

50. Swensen SJ, Hartman TE, Mayo JR, et al. Diffuse pulmonary lymphangiomatosis: CT findings. J Comput Assist Tomogr 1995;19:348–352.

51. Copley SJ, Coren M, Nicholson AG, et al. Diagnostic accuracy of thin-section CT and chest radiography of pediatric interstitial lung disease. AJR Am J Roentgenol 2000;174:549–554.

52. Wittenberg KH, Swensen SJ, Myers JL. Pulmonary involvement with Erdheim–Chester disease: radiographic and CT findings. AJR Am J Roentgenol 2000;174:1327–1331.

53. Duchateau F, Dechambre S, Coche E. Imaging of pulmonary manifestations in subtype B of Niemann–Pick disease. Br J Radiol 2001;74:1059–1061.

54. Padley SPG, Padhani AR, Nicholson A, et al. Pulmonary sarcoidosis mimicking cryptogenic fibrosing alveolitis on CT. Clin Radiol 1996;51:807–810.

55. Akira M, Yokoyama K, Yamamoto S, et al. Early asbestosis: evaluation with high-resolution CT. Radiology 1991; 178:409–416.

56. Remy-Jardin M, Degreef JM, Beuscart R, et al. Coal worker's pneumoconiosis: CT assessment in exposed workers and correlation with radiographic findings. Radiology 1990;177:363–371.

57. Primack SL, Miller RR, Müller NL. Diffuse pulmonary hemorrhage: clinical, pathologic, and imaging features. AJR Am J Roentgenol 1995;2:295–300.

58. Adler BD, Padley SP, Müller NL, et al. Chronic hypersensitivity pneumonitis:

high-resolution CT and radiographic features in 16 patients. Radiology 1992;185:91–95.

59. Tan RT, Kuzo RS. High-resolution CT findings of mucinous bronchioloalveolar carcinoma: a case of pseudopulmonary alveolar proteinosis. AJR Am J Roentgenol 1997;168:99–100.

60. Müller NL, Miller RR, Webb WR, et al. Fibrosing alveolitis: CT pathologic correlation. Radiology 1986;160:585–588.

61. Coche E, Weynand B, Noirhomme P, et al. Non-specific interstitial pneumonia showing a "crazy paving" pattern on high resolution CT. Br J Radiol 2001;74:189–191.

62. Akira M, Yamamoto S, Yokoyama K, et al. Asbestosis: High-resolution CT – pathologic correlation. Radiology 1990;176:389–394.

63. Akira M, Kitatani F, Yong-Sik L, et al. Diffuse panbronchiolitis: evaluation with high-resolution CT. Radiology 1988;168:433–438.

64. Nishimura K, Kitaichi M, Izumi T, et al. Diffuse panbronchiolitis: correlation of high-resolution CT and pathologic findings. Radiology 1992;184:779–785.

65. Leung AN, Miller RR, Müller NL. Parenchymal opacification in chronic infiltrative lung diseases: CT–pathologic correlation. Radiology 1993;188:209–214.

66. Strickland B, Strickland NH. The value of high definition, narrow section computed tomography in fibrosing alveolitis. Clin Radiol 1988;39:589–594.

67. Nishimura K, Kitaichi M, Izumi T, et al. Usual interstitial pneumonia: histologic correlation with high-resolution CT. Radiology 1992;182:337–342.

68. Akira M, Yamamoto S, Hara H, et al. Serial computed tomographic evaluation in desquamative interstitial pneumonia. Thorax 1997;52:333–337.

69. Westcott JL, Cole SR. Traction bronchiectasis in end-stage pulmonary fibrosis. Radiology 1986;161:665–669.

70. Hunninghake GW, Zimmerman MB, Schwartz DA, et al. Utility of a lung biopsy for the diagnosis of idiopathic pulmonary fibrosis. Am J Respir Crit Care Med 2001;164:193–196.

71. MacDonald SL, Rubens MB, Hansell DM, et al. Nonspecific interstitial pneumonia and usual interstitial pneumonia: comparative appearances at and diagnostic accuracy of thin-section CT. Radiology 2001;221:600–605.

72. Bicknell SG, Mason AC. Wegener's granulomatosis presenting as cryptogenic fibrosing alveolitis on CT. Clin Radiol 2000;55:890–891.

73. Johkoh T, Müller NL, Ichikado K, et al. Perilobular pulmonary opacities: high-resolution CT findings and pathologic correlation. [Review] J Thorac Imaging 1999;14:172–177.

74. Johkoh T, Itoh H, Müller NL, et al. Crazy-paving appearance at thin-section CT: spectrum of disease and pathologic findings. Radiology 1999;211:155–160.

75. Tonelli M, Stern EJ, Glenny RW. HRCT evident fibrosis in isolated pulmonary emphysema. J Comput Assist Tomogr 1997;21:322–323.

76. Yoshimura H, Hatakeyama M, Otsuji H, et al. Pulmonary asbestosis: CT study of subpleural curvilinear shadow. Radiology 1986;158:653–658.

77. Aberle DR, Gamsu G, Ray CS, et al. Asbestos-related pleural and parenchymal fibrosis: Detection with high resolution CT. Radiology 1988;166:729–734.

78. Lee KS, Kim TS, Han J, et al. Diffuse micronodular lung disease: HRCT and pathologic findings. J Comput Assist Tomogr 1999;23:99–106.

79. Remy-Jardin M, Remy J, Deffontaines C, et al. Assessment of diffuse infiltrative lung disease: comparison of conventional CT and high-resolution CT. Radiology 1991;181:157–162.

80. Bhalla M, Naidich DP, McGuinness G, et al. Diffuse lung disease: assessment with helical CT – preliminary observations of the role of maximum and minimum intensity projection images. Radiology 1996;200:341–347.

81. Remy-Jardin M, Remy J, Artaud D, et al. Diffuse infiltrative lung disease: clinical value of sliding-thin-slab maximum intensity projection CT scans in the detection of mild micronodular patterns. Radiology 1996;200:333–339.

82. Zerhouni EA. Computed tomography of the pulmonary parenchyma. An overview. Chest 1989;95:901–907.

83. Lynch DA, Webb WR, Gamsu G, et al. Computed tomography in pulmonary sarcoidosis. J Comput Assist Tomogr 1989;13:405–410.

84. Brauner MW, Grenier P, Mouelhi MM, et al. Pulmonary histiocytosis X: evaluation with high-resolution CT. Radiology 1989;172:255–258.

85. Remy-Jardin M, Beuscart R, Sault MC, et al. Subpleural micronodules in diffuse infiltrative lung diseases: evaluation with thin-section CT scans. Radiology 1990;177:133–139.

86. Hong SH, Im JG, Lee JS, et al. High resolution CT findings of miliary tuberculosis. J Comput Assist Tomogr 1998;22:220–224.

87. Andreu J, Mauleon S, Pallisa E, et al. Miliary lung disease revisited. Curr Probl Diagn Radiol 2002;31:189–197.

88. McGuinness G, Naidich DP, Jagirdar J, et al. High resolution CT findings in miliary lung disease. J Comput Assist Tomogr 1992;16:384–390.

89. Voloudaki AE, Tritou IN, Magkanas EG, et al. HRCT in miliary lung disease. Acta Radiol 1999;40:451–456.

90. Gruden JF, Webb WR, Warnock M. Centrilobular opacities in the lung on high-resolution CT: diagnostic considerations and pathologic correlation. AJR Am J Roentgenol 1994;162:569–574.

91. Gruden JF, Webb WR. Identification and evaluation of centrilobular opacities on high-resolution CT. Semin Ultrasound CT MR 1995;16:435–449.

92. Remy-Jardin M, Remy J, Wallaert B, et al. Subacute and chronic bird breeder hypersensitivity pneumonitis: sequential evaluation with CT and correlation with lung function tests and bronchoalveolar lavage. Radiology 1993;189:111–118.

93. Hansell DM, Wells AU, Padley SPG, et al. Hypersensitivity pneumonitis: correlation of individual CT patterns with functional abnormalities. Radiology 1996;199:123–128.

94. Im JG, Itoh H, Shim YS, et al. Pulmonary tuberculosis: CT findings – early active disease and sequential change with antituberculous therapy. Radiology 1993;186:653–660.

95. Hatipoglu ON, Osma E, Manisali M, et al. High resolution computed tomographic findings in pulmonary tuberculosis. Thorax 1996;51:397–402.

96. Tanaka N, Matsumoto T, Kuramitsu T, et al. High resolution CT findings in community-acquired pneumonia. J Comput Assist Tomogr 1996;20:600–608.

97. Hartman TE, Swensen SJ, Williams DE. Mycobacterium avium-intracellulare complex: evaluation with CT. Radiology 1993;187:23–26.

98. Lynch DA, Simone PM, Fox MA, et al. CT features of pulmonary Mycobacterium avium complex infection. J Comput Assist Tomogr 1995;19:353–360.

99. Tanaka D, Niwatsukino H, Oyama T, et al. Progressing features of atypical mycobacterial infection in the lung on conventional and high resolution CT (HRCT) images. Radiat Med 2001; 19:237–245.

100. Reittner P, Müller NL, Heyneman L, et al. Mycoplasma pneumoniae pneumonia: radiographic and high-resolution CT features in 28 patients. AJR Am J Roentgenol 2000;174:37–41.

101. Lee KS, Kullnig P, Hartman TE, et al. Cryptogenic organizing pneumonia: CT findings in 43 patients. AJR Am J Roentgenol 1994;162:543–546.

102. Gruden JF, Webb WR. CT findings in a proved case of respiratory bronchiolitis. AJR Am J Roentgenol 1993;161:44–46.

103. Holt RM, Schmidt RA, Godwin JD, et al. High resolution CT in respiratory bronchiolitis-associated interstitial lung disease. J Comput Assist Tomogr 1993;17:46–50.

104. Park JS, Brown KK, Tuder RM, et al. Respiratory bronchiolitis-associated

interstitial lung disease: radiologic features with clinical and pathologic correlation. J Comput Assist Tomogr 2002;26:13–20.

105. Gruden JF, Webb WR, Sides DM. Adult-onset disseminated tracheobronchial papillomatosis: CT features. J Comput Assist Tomogr 1994;18:640–642.

106. Lee KS, Kim Y, Han J, et al. Bronchioloalveolar carcinoma: clinical, histopathologic, and radiologic findings. RadioGraphics 1997;17:1345–1357.

107. Aquino SL, Chiles C, Halford P. Distinction of consolidative bronchioloalveolar carcinoma from pneumonia: do CT criteria work? AJR Am J Roentgenol 1998;171:359–363.

108. Howling SJ, Hansell DM, Wells AU, et al. Follicular bronchiolitis: thin-section CT and histologic findings. Radiology 1999;212:637–642.

109. Becciolini V, Gudinchet F, Cheseaux JJ, et al. Lymphocytic interstitial pneumonia in children with AIDS: high-resolution CT findings. Eur Radiol 2001;11:1015–1020.

110. Marchiori E, Ferreira A, Müller NL. Silicoproteinosis: high-resolution CT and histologic findings. J Thorac Imaging 2001;16:127–129.

111. Bendeck SE, Leung AN, Berry GJ, et al. Cellulose granulomatosis presenting as centrilobular nodules: CT and histologic findings. AJR Am J Roentgenol 2001;177:1151–1153.

112. Tack D, Nollevaux MC, Gevenois PA. Tree-in-bud pattern in neoplastic pulmonary emboli. AJR Am J Roentgenol 2001;176:1421–1422.

113. Nolan RL, McAdams HP, Sporn TA, et al. Pulmonary cholesterol granulomas in patients with pulmonary artery hypertension: chest radiographic and CT findings. AJR Am J Roentgenol 1999;172:1317–1319.

114. Franquet T, Gimenez A, Roson N, et al. Aspiration diseases: findings, pitfalls, and differential diagnosis. RadioGraphics 2000;20:673–685.

115. Marom EM, McAdams HP, Sporn TA, et al. Lentil aspiration pneumonia: radiographic and CT findings. J Comput Assist Tomogr 1998;22:598–600.

116. Hwang JH, Kim TS, Han J, et al. Primary lymphoma of the lung simulating bronchiolitis: radiologic findings [letter]. AJR Am J Roentgenol 1998;170:220–221.

117. Heyneman LE, Müller NL. Pulmonary nodules in early fat embolism syndrome: a case report. J Thorac Imaging 2000;15:71–74.

118. Remy-Jardin M, Remy J, Giraud F, et al. Computed tomography (CT) assessment of ground-glass opacity: semiology and significance. J Thorac Imaging 1993; 8:249–264.

119. Engeler CE, Tashjian JH, Trenkner SW, et al. Ground-glass opacity of the lung parenchyma: a guide to analysis with high-resolution CT. AJR Am J Roentgenol 1993;160:249–251.

120. Primack SL, Remy-Jardin M, Remy J, et al. High-resolution CT of the lung: pitfalls in the diagnosis of infiltrative lung disease. AJR Am J Roentgenol 1996;167:413–418.

121. Collins J, Stern EJ. Ground-glass opacity at CT: the ABCs. AJR Am J Roentgenol 1997;169:355–367.

122. Silver SF, Müller NL, Miller RR, et al. Hypersensitivity pneumonitis: Evaluation with CT. Radiology 1989;173:441–445.

123. Lynch DA, Rose CS, Way D, et al. Hypersensitivity pneumonitis: sensitivity of high-resolution CT in a population-based study. AJR Am J Roentgenol 1992;159:469–472.

124. Desai SR, Wells AU, Rubens MB, et al. Acute respiratory distress syndrome: CT abnormalities at long-term follow-up. Radiology 1999;210:29–35.

125. Primack SL, Hartman TE, Ikezoe J, et al. Acute interstitial pneumonia: radiographic and CT findings in nine patients. Radiology 1993;188:817–820.

126. Johkoh T, Müller NL, Taniguchi H, et al. Acute interstitial pneumonia: thin-section CT findings in 36 patients. Radiology 1999;211:859–863.

127. Hartman TE, Primack SL, Swensen SJ, et al. Desquamative interstitial pneumonia: thin-section CT findings in 22 patients. Radiology 1993;187:787–790.

128. Müller NL, Colby TV. Idiopathic interstitial pneumonias: high-resolution CT and histologic findings. RadioGraphics 1997;17:1016–1022.

129. Bergin CJ, Wirth RL, Berry GJ, et al. Pneumocystis carinii pneumonia: CT and HRCT observations. J Comput Assist Tomogr 1990;14:756–759.

130. Gruden JF, Huang L, Turner J, et al. High-resolution CT in the evaluation of clinically suspected Pneumocystis carinii pneumonia in AIDS patients with normal, equivocal, or nonspecific radiographic findings. AJR Am J Roentgenol 1997;169:967–975.

131. McGuinness G, Scholes JV, Garay SM, et al. Cytomegalovirus pneumonitis: spectrum of parenchymal CT findings with pathologic correlation in 21 AIDS patients. Radiology 1994;192:451–459.

132. Nicolaou S, Al Nakshabandi NA, Müller NL. SARS: Imaging of Severe Acute Respiratory Syndrome. AJR Am J Roentgenol 2003;180:1247–1249.

133. Gilman MJ, Laurens RG Jr, Somogyi JW, et al. CT attenuation values of lung density in sarcoidosis. J Comput Assist Tomogr 1983;7:407–410.

134. Kim TS, Lee KS, Chung MP, et al. Nonspecific interstitial pneumonia with fibrosis: high-resolution CT and pathologic findings. AJR Am J Roentgenol 1998;171:1645–1650.

135. Cheah FK, Sheppard MN, Hansell DM. Computed tomography of diffuse pulmonary haemorrhage with pathological correlation. Clin Radiol 1993;48:89–93.

136. Adler B, Padley S, Miller RR, et al. High-resolution CT of bronchioloalveolar carcinoma. AJR Am J Roentgenol 1992;159:275–277.

137. Jang HJ, Lee KS, Kwon OJ, et al. Bronchioloalveolar carcinoma: focal area of ground-glass attenuation at thin-section CT as an early sign. Radiology 1996;199:485–488.

138. Gaeta M, Caruso R, Barone M, et al. Ground-glass attenuation in bronchioloalveolar carcinoma: CT patterns and prognostic value. J Comput Assist Tomogr 1998;22:215–219.

139. Kim Y, Lee KS, Choi DC, et al. The spectrum of eosinophilic lung disease: radiologic findings. J Comput Assist Tomogr 1997;21:920–930.

140. King MA, Pope-Harman AL, Allen JN, et al. Acute eosinophilic pneumonia: radiologic and clinical features. Radiology 1997;203:715–719.

141. Worthy SA, Müller NL, Hansell DM, et al. Churg–Strauss syndrome: the spectrum of pulmonary CT findings in 17 patients. AJR Am J Roentgenol 1998;170:297–300.

142. Ikezoe J, Takashima S, Morimoto S, et al. CT appearance of acute radiation-induced injury in the lung. AJR Am J Roentgenol 1988;150:765–770.

143. Libshitz HI, Shuman LS. Radiation-induced pulmonary change: CT findings. J Comput Assist Tomogr 1984;8:15–19.

144. Padley SPG, Adler BD, Hansell DM, et al. High resolution computed tomography of drug-induced lung disease. Clin Radiol 1992;46:232–236.

145. Ellis SJ, Cleverley JR, Müller NL. Drug-induced lung disease: high-resolution CT findings. AJR Am J Roentgenol 2000;175:1019–1024.

146. Akira M, Ishikawa H, Yamamoto S. Drug-induced pneumonitis: thin-section CT findings in 60 patients. Radiology 2002;224:852–860.

147. Lee KN, Levin DL, Webb WR, et al. Pulmonary alveolar proteinosis: high-resolution CT, chest radiographic, and functional correlations. Chest 1997;111:989–995.

148. Bhalla M, Abboud MR, McLoud TC, et al. Acute chest syndrome in sickle cell disease: CT evidence of microvascular occlusion. Radiology 1993;187:45–49.

149. Long FR. High-resolution CT of the lungs in infants and young children. J Thorac Imaging 2001;16:251–258.

150. Remy-Jardin M, Giraud F, Remy J, et al. Importance of ground-glass attenuation in chronic diffuse infiltrative lung disease: pathologic–CT correlation. Radiology 1993;189:693–698.

151. Howling SJ, Evans TW, Hansell DM. The significance of bronchial dilatation on CT in patients with adult respiratory distress syndrome. Clin Radiol 1998; 53:105–109.

152. Stern EJ, Swensen SJ, Hartman TE, et al. CT mosaic pattern of lung attenuation: distinguishing different causes. AJR Am J Roentgenol 1995;165:813–816.

153. Martin KW, Sagel SS, Siegel BA. Mosaic oligemia simulating pulmonary infiltrates on CT. AJR Am J Roentgenol 1986;147:670–673.

154. Primack SL, Müller NL, Mayo JR, et al. Pulmonary parenchymal abnormalities of vascular origin: high-resolution CT findings. RadioGraphics 1994; 14:739–746.

155. Worthy SA, Müller NL, Hartman TE, et al. Mosaic attenuation pattern on thin-section CT scans of the lung: differentiation among infiltrative lung, airway, and vascular diseases as a cause. Radiology 1997;205:465–470.

156. Schwarz MI, Mortenson RL, Colby TV, et al. Pulmonary capillaritis. The association with progressive irreversible airflow limitation and hyperinflation. Am Rev Respir Dis 1993;148:507–511.

157. Remy-Jardin M, Remy J, Louvegny S, et al. Airway changes in chronic pulmonary embolism: CT findings in 33 patients. Radiology 1997;203:355–360.

158. Arakawa H, Kurihara Y, Sasaka K, et al. Air trapping on CT of patients with pulmonary embolism. AJR Am J Roentgenol 2002;178:1201–1207.

159. Stern EJ, Frank MS. Small-airways disease of the lungs: findings at expiratory CT. AJR Am J Roentgenol 1994;163:37–41.

160. Hansell DM, Rubens MB, Padley SPG, et al. Obliterative bronchiolitis: individual CT signs of small airways disease and functional correlation. Radiology 1997;203:721–726.

161. Im JG, Kim SH, Chung MJ, et al. Lobular low attenuation of the lung parenchyma on CT: evaluation of forty-eight patients. J Comput Assist Tomogr 1996;20:756–762.

162. Bergin CJ, Rios G, King MA, et al. Accuracy of high-resolution CT in identifying chronic pulmonary thromboembolic disease. AJR Am J Roentgenol 1996;166:1371–1377.

163. Arakawa H, Webb WR, McCowin M, et al. Inhomogeneous lung attenuation at thin-section CT: diagnostic value of expiratory scans. Radiology 1998; 206:89–94.

164. Chung MH, Edinburgh KJ, Webb EM, et al. Mixed infiltrative and obstructive disease on high-resolution CT: differential diagnosis and functional correlates in a consecutive series. J Thorac Imaging 2001;16:69–75.

165. Lee KS, Kim EA. High-resolution CT of alveolar filling disorders. Radiol Clin North Am 2001;39:1211–1230.

166. Johkoh T, Ikezoe J, Kohno N, et al. Usefulness of high-resolution CT for differential diagnosis of multi-focal pulmonary consolidation. Radiat Med 1996;14:139–146.

167. Oikonomou A, Hansell DM. Organizing pneumonia: the many morphological faces. Eur Radiol 2002; 12:1486–1496.

168. Arakawa H, Kurihara Y, Niimi H, et al. Bronchiolitis obliterans with organizing pneumonia versus chronic eosinophilic pneumonia: high-resolution CT findings in 81 patients. AJR Am J Roentgenol 2001;176:1053–1058.

169. Kinsely BL, Mastey LA, Mergo PJ, et al. Pulmonary mucosa-associated lymphoid tissue lymphoma: CT and pathologic findings. AJR Am J Roentgenol 1999;172:1321–1326.

170. Akira M, Atagi S, Kawahara M, et al. High-resolution CT findings of diffuse bronchioloalveolar carcinoma in 38 patients. AJR Am J Roentgenol 1999;173:1623–1629.

171. Jung JI, Kim H, Park SH, et al. CT differentiation of pneumonic-type bronchioloalveolar cell carcinoma and infectious pneumonia. Br J Radiol 2001;74:490–494.

172. Lee KS, Müller NL, Hale V, et al. Lipoid pneumonia: CT findings. J Comput Assist Tomogr 1995;19:48–51.

173. Laurent F, Philippe JC, Vergier B, et al. Exogenous lipoid pneumonia: HRCT, MR, and pathologic findings. Eur Radiol 1999;9:1190–1196.

174. Vernhet H, Bousquet C, Durand G, et al. Reversible amiodarone-induced lung disease: HRCT findings. Eur Radiol 2001;11:1697–1703.

175. Goyal R, White CS, Templeton PA, et al. High attenuation mucous plugs in allergic bronchopulmonary aspergillosis: CT appearance. J Comput Assist Tomogr 1992;16:649–650.

176. Kuhlman JE, Reyes BL, Hruban RH, et al. Abnormal air-filled spaces in the lung. RadioGraphics 1993;13:47–75.

177. Hartman TE. CT of cystic diseases of the lung. Radiol Clin North Am 2001;39: 1231–1244.

178. Lee KH, Lee JS, Lynch DA, et al. The radiologic differential diagnosis of diffuse lung diseases characterized by multiple cysts or cavities. J Comput Assist Tomogr 2002;26:5–12.

179. Koyama M, Johkoh T, Honda O, et al. Chronic cystic lung disease: diagnostic accuracy of high-resolution CT in 92 patients. AJR Am J Roentgenol 2003;180:827–835.

180. Webb WR. Radiology of obstructive pulmonary disease. AJR Am J Roentgenol 1997;169:637–647.

181. Templeton PA, McLoud TC, Müller NL, et al. Pulmonary lymphangioleiomyomatosis: CT and pathologic findings. J Comput Assist Tomogr 1989;13:54–57.

182. Müller NL, Chiles C, Kullnig P. Pulmonary lymphangiomyomatosis: Correlation of CT with radiographic and functional findings. Radiology 1990;175: 335–339.

183. Aberle DR, Hansell DM, Brown K, et al. Lymphangiomyomatosis: CT, chest radiographic and functional correlations. Radiology 1990;176:381–387.

184. Brauner MW, Grenier P, Tijani K, et al. Pulmonary Langerhans cell histiocytosis: evolution of lesions on CT scans. Radiology 1997;204:497–502.

185. Gurney JW, Bates FT. Pulmonary cystic disease: comparison of Pneumocystis carinii pneumatoceles and bullous emphysema due to intravenous drug abuse. Radiology 1989;173:27–31.

186. Kuhlman JE, Knowles MC, Fishman EK, et al. Premature bullous pulmonary damage in AIDS: CT diagnosis. Radiology 1989;173:23–26.

187. Feuerstein IM, Archer A, Pluda JM, et al. Thin-walled cavities cysts and pneumothorax in Pneumocystis carinii pneumonia: Further observations with histopathologic correlation. Radiology 1990;174:697–702.

188. Chow C, Templeton PA, White CS. Lung cysts associated with Pneumocystis carinii pneumonia: radiographic characteristics, natural history, and complications. AJR Am J Roentgenol 1993;161:527–531.

189. Fowler RA, Lapinsky SE, Hallett D, et al. Critically ill patients with severe acute respiratory syndrome. JAMA 2003; 290:367–373.

190. Lee DK, Im JG, Lee KS, et al. B-cell lymphoma of bronchus-associated lymphoid tissue (BALT): CT features in 10 patients. J Comput Assist Tomogr 2000;24:30–34.

191. Marti-Bonmati L, Catala FJ, Perales FR. Computed tomography differentiation between cystic bronchiectasis and bullae. J Thorac Imaging 1991;7:83–85.

192. Worthy SA, Brown MJ, Müller NL. Cystic air spaces in the lung: change in size on expiratory high-resolution CT in 23 patients. Clin Radiol 1998;53:515–519.

193. Sherrier RH, Chiles C, Roggli V. Pulmonary lymphangioleiomyomatosis: CT findings. AJR Am J Roentgenol 1989;153:937–940.

194. Bonelli FS, Hartman TE, Swensen SJ, et al. Accuracy of high-resolution CT in diagnosing lung diseases. AJR Am J Roentgenol 1997;170:1507–1512.

195. Primack SL, Hartman TE, Hansell DM, et al. End-stage lung disease: CT findings in 61 patients. Radiology 1993;189:681–686.

196. Soler P, Bergeron A, Kambouchner M, et al. Is high-resolution computed

tomography a reliable tool to predict the histopathological activity of pulmonary Langerhans cell histiocytosis? Am J Respir Crit Care Med 2000;162:264–270.

197. Loubeyre P, Paret M, Revel D, et al. Thin-section CT detection of emphysema associated with bronchiectasis and correlation with pulmonary function tests. Chest 1996;109:360–365.

198. Hansell DM, Wells AU, Rubens MB, et al. Bronchiectasis: functional significance of areas of decreased attenuation at expiratory CT. Radiology 1994;193:369–374.

199. Kang EY, Miller RR, Müller NL. Bronchiectasis: comparison of preoperative thin-section CT and pathologic findings in resected specimens. Radiology 1995;195: 649–654.

200. Paganin F, Trussard V, Seneterre E, et al. Chest radiography and high resolution computed tomography of the lungs in asthma. Am Rev Respir Dis 1992;146: 1084–1087.

201. Paganin F, Seneterre E, Chanez P, et al. Computed tomography of the lungs in asthma: influence of disease severity and etiology. Am J Respir Crit Care Med 1996;153:110–114.

202. Grenier P, Mourey-Gerosa I, Benali K, et al. Abnormalities of the airways and lung parenchyma in asthmatics: CT observations in 50 patients and inter- and intra-observer variability. Eur Radiol 1996;6:199–206.

203. Laurent F, Latrabe V, Raherison C, et al. Functional significance of air trapping detected in moderate asthma. Eur Radiol 2000;10:1404–1410.

204. King GG, Müller NL, Pare PD. Evaluation of airways in obstructive pulmonary disease using high-resolution computed tomography. Am J Respir Crit Care Med 1999;159:992–1004.

205. Gevenois PA, Scillia P, de Maertelaer V, et al. The effects of age, sex, lung size, and hyperinflation on CT lung densitometry. AJR Am J Roentgenol 1996;167:1169–1173.

206. Lynch DA. Imaging of small airways diseases. Clin Chest Med 1993;14:623–634.

207. Gelb AF, Zamel N, Hogg JC, et al. Pseudophysiologic emphysema resulting from severe small-airways disease. Am J Respir Crit Care Med 1998;158:815–819.

208. Chen D, Webb WR, Storto ML, et al. Assessment of air trapping using postexpiratory high-resolution computed tomography. J Thorac Imaging 1998;13:135–143.

209. Desai SR, Hansell DM. Small airways disease: expiratory computed tomography comes of age. Clin Radiol 1997;52:332–337.

210. Arakawa H, Niimi H, Kurihara Y, et al. Expiratory high-resolution CT:

diagnostic value in diffuse lung diseases. AJR Am J Roentgenol 2000;175: 1537–1543.

211. Arakawa H, Webb WR. Air trapping on expiratory high-resolution CT scans in the absence of inspiratory scan abnormalities: correlation with pulmonary function tests and differential diagnosis. AJR Am J Roentgenol 1998;170:1349–1353.

212. Cook PG, Wells IP, McGavin CR. The distribution of pulmonary shadowing in Farmer's Lung. Clin Radiol 1988;39: 21–27.

213. Hansell DM, Moskovic E. High-resolution computed tomography in extrinsic allergic alveolitis. Clin Radiol 1991;43:8–12.

214. Mindell HJ. Roentgen findings in Farmer's Lung. Radiology 1970;97:341–346.

215. Johkoh T, Müller NL, Nakamura H. Multidetector spiral high-resolution computed tomography of the lungs: distribution of findings on coronal image reconstructions. J Thorac Imaging 2002;17:291–305.

216. Remy-Jardin M, Campistron P, Amara A, et al. Usefulness of coronal reformations in the diagnostic evaluation of infiltrative lung disease. J Comput Assist Tomogr 2003;27:266–273.

217. Stark P, Greene R, Kott MM, et al. CT findings in ARDS. Radiologe 1987; 27:367–369.

218. Owens CM, Evans TW, Keogh BF, et al. Computed tomography in established adult respiratory distress syndrome. Chest 1994;106:1815–1821.

219. Goodman LR, Fumagalli R, Tagliabue P, et al. Adult respiratory distress syndrome due to pulmonary and extrapulmonary causes: CT, clinical, and functional correlations. Radiology 1999;213:545–552.

220. Desai SR, Wells AU, Suntharalingam G, et al. Acute respiratory distress syndrome caused by pulmonary and extrapulmonary injury: a comparative CT study. Radiology 2001;218:689–693.

221. Tung KT, Wells AU, Rubens MB, et al. Accuracy of the typical computed tomographic appearances of fibrosing alveolitis. Thorax 1993;48:334–338.

222. Nobauer-Huhmann IM, Eibenberger K, Schaefer-Prokop C, et al. Changes in lung parenchyma after acute respiratory distress syndrome (ARDS): assessment with high-resolution computed tomography. Eur Radiol 2001;11: 2436–2443.

223. Gruden JF, Webb WR, Naidich DP, et al. Multinodular disease: anatomic localization at thin-section CT – multireader evaluation of a simple algorithm. Radiology 1999;210:711–720.

224. Mathieson JR, Mayo JR, Staples CA, et al. Chronic diffuse infiltrative lung disease:

comparison of diagnostic accuracy of CT and chest radiography. Radiology 1989;171:111–116.

225. Cole P. Bronchiectasis. In: Brewis RAL, Corrin B, Geddes DM, Gibson GJ, eds. Respiratory medicine. Philadelphia: W B Saunders, 1995:1286–1316.

226. Hwang JH, Kim TS, Lee KS, et al. Bronchiolitis in adults: pathology and imaging. J Comput Assist Tomogr 1997;21:913–919.

227. Smith IE, Flower CDR. Imaging in bronchiectasis. Br J Radiol 1996; 69:589–593.

228. Naidich DP, Funt S, Ettenger NA, et al. Hemoptysis: CT–bronchoscopic correlations in 58 cases. Radiology 1990;177:357–362.

229. Kim JS, Müller NL, Park CS, et al. Cylindrical bronchiectasis: diagnostic findings on thin-section CT. AJR Am J Roentgenol 1996;168:751–754.

230. Bankier AA, Fleischmann D, de Maertelaer V, et al. Subjective differentiation of normal and pathological bronchi on thin-section CT: impact of observer training. Eur Respir J 1999;13:781–786.

231. Kuhns LR, Borlaza G. The "twinkling star" sign: an aid in differentiating pulmonary vessels from pulmonary nodules on computed tomograms. Radiology 1980;135:763–764.

232. Tarver RD, Conces DJ, Godwin JD. Motion artifacts on CT simulate bronchiectasis. AJR Am J Roentgenol 1988;151:1117–1119.

233. Moore AD, Godwin JD, Müller NL, et al. Pulmonary histiocytosis X: comparison of radiographic and CT findings. Radiology 1989;172:249–254.

234. Weisbrod GL, Chamberlain D, Herman SJ. Cystic change (pseudocavitation) associated with bronchioloalveolar carcinoma: a report of four patients. J Thorac Imaging 1995;10:106–111.

235. Stern EJ, Webb WR, Gamsu G. Dynamic quantitative computed tomography. A predictor of pulmonary function in obstructive lung diseases. Invest Radiol 1994;29:564–569.

236. Lucidarme O, Grenier PA, Cadi M, et al. Evaluation of air trapping at CT: comparison of continuous- versus suspended-expiration CT techniques. Radiology 2000;216:768–772.

237. Arakawa H, Webb WR. Expiratory high-resolution CT scan. Radiol Clin North Am 1998;36:189–209.

238. Franquet T, Stern EJ. Bronchiolar inflammatory diseases: high-resolution CT findings with histologic correlation. Eur Radiol 1999;9:1290–1303.

239. Choi SJ, Choi BK, Kim HJ, et al. Lateral decubitus HRCT: a simple technique to replace expiratory CT in children with air trapping. Pediatr Radiol 2002;32: 179–182.

240. Remy-Jardin M, Remy J, Gosselin B, et al. Sliding thin slab, minimum intensity projection technique in the diagnosis of emphysema: histopathologic–CT correlation. Radiology 1996;200:665–671.

241. Fotheringham T, Chabat F, Hansell DM, et al. A comparison of methods for enhancing the detection of areas of decreased attenuation on CT caused by airways disease. J Comput Assist Tomogr 1999;23:385–389.

242. Hartman TE, Swensen SJ, Müller NL. Bronchiolar diseases: computed tomography. In: Epler GR, ed. Diseases of the bronchioles. New York: Raven Press, 1994:43–58.

243. Padley SP, Adler BD, Hansell DM, et al. Bronchiolitis obliterans: high resolution CT findings and correlation with pulmonary function tests. Clin Radiol 1993;47:236–240.

244. Marti-Bonmati L, Ruiz Perales F, Catala F, et al. CT findings in Swyer–James syndrome. Radiology 1989;172:477–480.

245. Guckel C, Wells AU, Taylor DA, et al. Mechanism of mosaic attenuation of the lungs on computed tomography in induced bronchospasm. J Appl Physiol 1999;86:701–708.

246. Loubeyre P, Revel D, Delignette A, et al. Bronchiectasis detected with thin-section CT as a predictor of chronic lung allograft rejection. Radiology 1995;194:213–216.

247. Zhang L, Irion K, da Silva PN, et al. High-resolution computed tomography in pediatric patients with postinfectious bronchiolitis obliterans. J Thorac Imaging 1999;14:85–89.

248. Lucidarme O, Coche E, Cluzel P, et al. Expiratory CT scans for chronic airway disease: correlation with pulmonary function test results. AJR Am J Roentgenol 1998;170:301–307.

249. Lee KW, Chung SY, Yang I, et al. Correlation of aging and smoking with air trapping at thin-section CT of the lung in asymptomatic subjects. Radiology 2000;214:831–836.

250. Homma H, Yamanaka A, Shinichi T, et al. Diffuse panbronchiolitis: a disease of the transitional zone of the lung. Chest 1983;83:63–69.

251. Akira M, Higashihara S, Sakatani M, et al. Diffuse panbronchiolitis: follow-up CT examination. Radiology 1993;189:559–562.

252. Collins J, Blankenbaker D, Stern EJ. CT patterns of bronchiolar disease: what is "tree-in-bud"? AJR Am J Roentgenol 1998;171:365–370.

253. Murata K, Itoh H, Senda M, et al. Stratified impairment of pulmonary ventilation in "diffuse panbronchiolitis": PET and CT studies. J Comput Assist Tomogr 1989;13:48–53.

254. Ward S, Heyneman L, Lee MJ, et al. Accuracy of CT in the diagnosis of allergic bronchopulmonary aspergillosis in asthmatic patients. AJR Am J Roentgenol 1999;173:937–942.

255. Helbich TH, Heinz-Peer G, Eichler I, et al. Cystic fibrosis: CT assessment of lung involvement in children and adults. Radiology 1999;213:537–544.

256. Logan PM, Primack SL, Miller RR, et al. Invasive aspergillosis of the airways: radiographic, CT, and pathologic findings. Radiology 1994;193:383–388.

257. Aquino SL, Gamsu G, Webb WR, et al. Tree-in-bud pattern: frequency and significance on thin section CT. J Comput Assist Tomogr 1996;20:594–599.

258. Erasmus JJ, McAdams HP, Farrell MA, et al. Pulmonary nontuberculous mycobacterial infection: radiologic manifestations. RadioGraphics 1999;19:1487–1505.

259. Raghu G. Interstitial lung disease: a diagnostic approach. Are CT and lung biopsy indicated in every patient? Am J Respir Crit Care Med 1995;151:909–914.

260. Di Marco AF, Briones B. Is chest CT performed too often? Chest 1993;103:985–986.

261. Mana J, Teirstein AS, Mendelson DS, et al. Excessive thoracic computed tomographic scanning in sarcoidosis. Thorax 1995;50:1264–1266.

262. Schoepf UJ, Bruening RD, Hong C, et al. Multislice helical CT of focal and diffuse lung disease: comprehensive diagnosis with reconstruction of contiguous and high-resolution CT sections from a single thin-collimation scan. AJR Am J Roentgenol 2001;177:179–184.

263. Zwirewich CV, Mayo JR, Müller NL. Low dose High Resolution CT of lung parenchyma. Radiology 1991;180:413–417.

264. Mayo JR, Hartman TE, Lee KS, et al. CT of the chest: minimal tube current required for good image quality with the least radiation dose. AJR Am J Roentgenol 1995;3:603–607.

265. Copley SJ, Coren M, Nicholson AG, et al. Diagnostic accuracy of thin-section CT and chest radiography of pediatric interstitial lung disease. AJR Am J Roentgenol 2000;174:549–554.

266. Lynch DA, Hay T, Newell JD Jr, et al. Pediatric diffuse lung disease: diagnosis and classification using high-resolution CT. AJR Am J Roentgenol 1999;173:713–718.

267. Koh DM, Hansell DM. Computed tomography of diffuse interstitial lung disease in children. Clin Radiol 2000;55:659–667.

268. Copley SJ, Padley SP. High-resolution CT of paediatric lung disease. Eur Radiol 2001;11:2564–2575.

269. Schurawitzki H, Stiglbauer R, Graninger W, et al. Interstitial lung disease in progressive systemic sclerosis: High resolution CT versus radiography. Radiology 1990;176:755–759.

270. Staples CA, Gamsu G, Ray CS, et al. High resolution computed tomography and lung function in asbestos-exposed workers with normal chest radiographs. Am Rev Respir Dis 1989;139:1502–1508.

271. Padley SPG, Adler B, Müller NL. High-resolution computed tomography of the chest: current indications. J Thorac Imaging 1993;8:189–199.

272. Padley SPG, Hansell DM, Flower CDR, et al. Comparative accuracy of high resolution computed tomography and chest radiography in the diagnosis of chronic diffuse infiltrative lung disease. Clin Radiol 1991;44:227–231.

273. Gaensler EA, Carrington CB. Open lung biopsy for chronic diffuse infiltrative lung disease: clinical, roentgenographic and physiological correlations in 502 patients. Ann Thorac Surg 1980;30:411–426.

274. Sweatman MC, Millar AB, Strickland B, et al. Computed tomography in adult obliterative bronchiolitis. Clin Radiol 1990;41:116–119.

275. Friedman AC, Fiel SB, Fisher MS, et al. Asbestos-related pleural disease and asbestosis: A comparison of CT and chest radiography. AJR Am J Roentgenol 1988;150:269–275.

276. Falaschi F, Boraschi P, Neri S, et al. High-resolution computed tomography (HRCT) in the detection of "early asbestosis." Eur Radiol 1995;5:291–296.

277. Lenoir S, Grenier P, Brauner MW, et al. Pulmonary lymphangiomyomatosis and tuberous sclerosis: Comparison of radiographic and thin-section CT findings. Radiology 1990;175:329–334.

278. Bergin CJ, Castellino RA, Blank N, et al. Specificity of high-resolution CT findings in pulmonary asbestosis: do patients scanned for other indications have similar findings? AJR Am J Roentgenol 1994;163:551–555.

279. Nasser-Sharif FJ, Balter MS. Hypersensitivity pneumonitis with normal high resolution computed tomography scans. Can Respir J 2001;8:98–101.

280. Orens JB, Kazerooni EA, Fernando JM, et al. The sensitivity of high-resolution CT in detecting idiopathic pulmonary fibrosis proved by open lung biopsy: a prospective study. Chest 1995;108:109–115.

281. Gotway MB, Dawn SK, Sellami D, et al. Acute rejection following lung transplantation: limitations in accuracy of thin-section CT for diagnosis. Radiology 2001;221:207–212.

282. Santis G, Hodson ME, Strickland B. High resolution computed tomography in adult cystic fibrosis patients with mild lung disease. Clin Radiol 1991;44:20–22.

283. Bankier AA, Van Muylem A, Knoop C, et al. Bronchiolitis obliterans syndrome

in heart-lung transplant recipients: diagnosis with expiratory CT. Radiology 2001;218:533–539.

284. Leung AN, Fisher K, Valentine V, et al. Bronchiolitis obliterans after lung transplantation: detection using expiratory HRCT. Chest 1998;113: 365–370.

285. Miller WT Jr, Kotloff RM, Blumenthal NP, et al. Utility of high resolution computed tomography in predicting bronchiolitis obliterans syndrome following lung transplantation: preliminary findings. J Thorac Imaging 2001;16:76–80.

286. Bergin C, Müller N, Nichols DM, et al. The diagnosis of emphysema. A computed tomographic–pathologic correlation. Am Rev Respir Dis 1986;133:541–546.

287. Knudson RJ, Standen JR, Kaltenborn WT, et al. Expiratory computed tomography for assessment of suspected pulmonary emphysema. Chest 1991;99:1357–1366.

288. Klein JS, Gamsu G, Webb WR, et al. High-resolution CT diagnosis of emphysema in symptomatic patients with normal chest radiographs and isolated low diffusing capacity. Radiology 1992;182:817–821.

289. Gurney JW, Jones KK, Robbins RA, et al. Regional distribution of emphysema: correlation of high-resolution CT with pulmonary function tests in unselected smokers. Radiology 1992;183:457–463.

290. Grenier P, Valeyre D, Cluzel P, et al. Chronic diffuse interstitial lung disease: diagnostic value of chest radiography and high-resolution CT. Radiology 1991;179:123–132.

291. Nishimura K, Izumi T, Kitaichi M, et al. The diagnostic accuracy of high-resolution computed tomography in diffuse infiltrative lung diseases. Chest 1993;104:1149–1155.

292. Kuperman AS, Riker JB. The predicted normal maximal mid-expiratory flow. Am Rev Respir Dis 1973;107:231–238.

293. Grenier P, Chevret S, Beigelman C, et al. Chronic diffuse infiltrative lung disease: determination of the diagnostic value of clinical data, chest radiography, and CT and Bayesian analysis. Radiology 1994;191:383–390.

294. Johkoh T, Müller NL, Cartier Y, et al. Idiopathic interstitial pneumonias: diagnostic accuracy of thin-section CT in 129 patients. Radiology 1999;211:555–560.

295. Lee KS, Chung MP. Diagnostic accuracy of thin-section CT in idiopathic interstitial pneumonia. Radiology 2000;215:918–919.

296. Flaherty KR, Travis WD, Colby TV, et al. Histopathologic variability in usual and nonspecific interstitial pneumonias. Am J Respir Crit Care Med 2001;164: 1722–1727.

297. Johkoh T, Müller NL, Akira M, et al. Eosinophilic lung diseases: diagnostic accuracy of thin-section CT in 111 patients. Radiology 2000;216:773–780.

298. Saito Y, Terada M, Takada T, et al. Pulmonary involvement in mixed connective tissue disease: comparison with other collagen vascular diseases using high resolution CT. J Comput Assist Tomogr 2002;26:349–357.

299. Taouli B, Brauner MW, Mourey I, et al. Thin-section chest CT findings of primary Sjogren's syndrome: correlation with pulmonary function. Eur Radiol 2002;12:1504–1511.

300. Ryu JH, Colby TV, Hartman TE, et al. Smoking-related interstitial lung diseases: a concise review. Eur Respir J 2001;17:122–132.

301. Tomiyama N, Müller NL, Johkoh T, et al. Acute parenchymal lung disease in immunocompetent patients: diagnostic accuracy of high-resolution CT. AJR Am J Roentgenol 2000;174:1745–1750.

302. Swensen SJ, Aughenbaugh GL, Myers JL. Diffuse lung disease: diagnostic accuracy of CT in patients undergoing surgical biopsy of the lung. Radiology 1997;205:229–234.

303. Reynolds HY. Diagnostic and management strategies for diffuse interstitial lung disease. Chest 1998;113:192–202.

304. Murayama S, Murakami J, Yabuuchi H, et al. "Crazy paving appearance" on high resolution CT in various diseases. J Comput Assist Tomogr 1999;23: 749–752.

305. Müller NL, Staples CA, Miller RR, et al. Disease activity in idiopathic pulmonary fibrosis: CT and pathologic correlation. Radiology 1987;165:731–734.

306. Wells AU, Hansell DM, Corrin B, et al. High resolution computed tomography assessment of disease activity in the fibrosing alveolitis of systemic sclerosis: a histopathological correlation. Thorax 1992;47:738–742.

307. Turner-Warwick M, Burrows B, Johnson A. Cryptogenic fibrosing alveolitis: Clinical features and their influence on survival. Thorax 1980;35:171–180.

308. Cherniack RM, Colby TV, Flint A, et al. Quantitative assessment of lung pathology in idiopathic pulmonary fibrosis. Am Rev Respir Dis 1991;144: 892–900.

309. Bjoraker JA, Ryu JH, Edwin MK, et al. Prognostic significance of histopathologic subsets in idiopathic pulmonary fibrosis. Am J Respir Crit Care Med 1998;157:199–203.

310. Nicholson AG, Fulford LG, Colby TV, et al. The relationship between individual histologic features and disease progression in idiopathic pulmonary fibrosis. Am J Respir Crit Care Med 2002;166:173–177.

311. American Thoracic Society. Idiopathic pulmonary fibrosis: diagnosis and treatment. International consensus statement. American Thoracic Society (ATS), and the European Respiratory Society (ERS). Am J Respir Crit Care Med 2000;161:646–664.

312. Nugent KM, Peterson MW, Jolles H, et al. Correlation of chest roentgenograms with pulmonary function and bronchoalveolar lavage in interstitial lung disease. Chest 1989;96:1224–1228.

313. Harrison NK, Glanville AR, Strickland B, et al. Pulmonary involvement in systemic sclerosis: the detection of early changes by thin section CT scan bronchoalveolar lavage and 99mTc-DTPA clearance. Respir Med 1989; 83:1–12.

314. Pantin CF, Valind SO, Sweatman M, et al. Measures of the inflammatory response in cryptogenic fibrosing alveolitis. Am Rev Respir Dis 1990;138:1234–1241.

315. Panos RJ, Moretensen RL, Niccoli SA, et al. Clinical deterioration in patients with idiopathic pulmonary fibrosis: causes and assessment. Am J Med 1990;88:396–404.

316. Johnston ID, Prescott RJ, Chalmers JC, et al. British Thoracic Society study of cryptogenic fibrosing alveolitis: current presentation and initial management. Fibrosing Alveolitis Subcommittee of the Research Committee of the British Thoracic Society. Thorax 1997;52:38–44.

317. Hansell DM, Wells AU. State of the Art: CT evaluation of fibrosing alveolitis – applications and insights. J Thorac Imaging 1996;11:231–249.

318. Vedal S, Welsh EV, Miller RR, et al. Desquamative interstitial pneumonia: computed tomographic findings before and after treatment with corticosteroids. Chest 1988;93:215–217.

319. Lee JS, Im JG, Ahn JM, et al. Fibrosing alveolitis: prognostic implication of ground-glass attenuation at high-resolution CT. Radiology 1992;184: 451–454.

320. Wells AU, Hansell DM, Rubens MB, et al. The predictive value of thin-section computed tomography in fibrosing alveolitis. Am Rev Respir Dis 1993;148: 1076–1082.

321. Gay SE, Kazerooni EA, Toews GB, et al. Idiopathic pulmonary fibrosis: predicting response to therapy and survival. Am J Respir Crit Care Med 1998;157:1063–1072.

322. Sheehan RE, Wells AU, Milne DG, et al. Nitrofurantoin-induced lung disease: two cases demonstrating resolution of apparently irreversible CT abnormalities. J Thorac Imaging 2000;24:259–261.

323. Akira M, Hamada H, Sakatani M, et al. CT findings during phase of accelerated deterioration in patients with idiopathic

pulmonary fibrosis. AJR Am J Roentgenol 1997;168:79–83.

324. Akira M. Computed tomography and pathologic findings in fulminant forms of idiopathic interstitial pneumonia. J Thorac Imaging 1999;14:76–84.

325. Brauner MW, Lenoir S, Grenier P, et al. Pulmonary sarcoidosis: CT assessment of lesion reversibility. Radiology 1992;182:349–354.

326. Murdoch J, Müller NL. Pulmonary sarcoidosis: changes on follow-up CT examination. AJR Am J Roentgenol 1992;159:473–477.

327. Leung AN, Brauner MW, Caillat-Vigneron N, et al. Sarcoidosis activity: correlation of HRCT findings with those of ^{67}Gallium scanning, bronchoalveolar lavage, and serum angiotensin-converting enzyme assay. J Comput Assist Tomogr 1998;22:229–234.

328. Johkoh T, Ikezoe J, Takeuchi N, et al. CT findings in "pseudoalveolar" sarcoidosis. J Comput Assist Tomogr 1992;16:904–907.

329. Remy-Jardin M, Remy J, Wallaert B, et al. Pulmonary involvement in progressive systemic sclerosis: sequential evaluation with CT, pulmonary function tests, and bronchoalveolar lavage. Radiology 1993;188:499–506.

330. Wells AU, Rubens MB, Du Bois RM, et al. Serial CT in fibrosing alveolitis: prognostic significance of the initial pattern. AJR Am J Roentgenol 1993;161:1159–1165.

331. Mino M, Noma S, Taguchi Y, et al. Pulmonary involvement in polymyositis and dermatomyositis: sequential evaluation with CT. AJR Am J Roentgenol 1997;169:83–87.

332. Salaffi F, Manganelli P, Carotti M, et al. A longitudinal study of pulmonary involvement in primary Sjogren's syndrome: relationship between alveolitis and subsequent lung changes on high-resolution computed tomography. Br J Rheumatol 1998;37:263–269.

333. Hartman TE, Primack SL, Kang EY, et al. Disease progression in usual interstitial pneumonia compared with desquamative interstitial pneumonia: assessment with serial CT. Chest 1996;110:378–382.

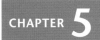

CHAPTER 5

Infections of the lungs and pleura

Pneumonias are usually classified according to the infecting organism because the cause dictates the treatment. However, imaging is usually poor at predicting even the broad category of infectious agent, let alone the specific organism.[1] Furthermore, preexisting lung disease, particularly emphysema, can modify the appearance of pulmonary consolidation. Nevertheless, imaging has many important roles in patients with suspected pulmonary infection. The plain chest radiograph is the primary method of establishing the presence of pneumonia and of determining its location and extent. Predisposing conditions, for example, bronchial carcinoma, may be visible, and complications, such as pleural effusion, empyema, and abscess formation, are readily demonstrated. Once pneumonia and its complications have been diagnosed, chest radiographs are an excellent method of following the response to treatment. In complicated cases, or in patients in whom response to treatment is unexpectedly slow, computed tomography (CT) has a role.[2]

The essential radiographic feature of pneumonia is pulmonary consolidation, which may show cavitation and may be accompanied by pleural effusion. The appearance varies almost infinitely from one or more small, ill-defined shadows to large airspace shadows involving the whole of one or more lobes. The pattern depends to some extent on the infecting organism, and on the integrity of the host defenses (see below).

Pneumonias are sometimes divided according to their chest radiographic appearances into bronchopneumonia, lobar pneumonia, spherical (round or nodular) pneumonia, and interstitial pneumonia (Table 5.1). Although widely used, these terms have limited value because the same organism may produce several patterns and because patterns often overlap in an individual patient.

In bronchopneumonia the inflammatory exudate is multifocal and centered on large inflamed airways, involving some acini and sparing others. On the chest radiograph, bronchopneumonia is characterized by patchy consolidation, loss of volume, and absence of air bronchograms (Fig. 5.1). When affected areas coalesce, the shadowing may become more uniform and resemble lobar pneumonia. Although the term "segmental consolidation" is in common use, consolidation conforming precisely to segmental anatomy is, in fact, extremely rare.

In lobar pneumonia (Fig. 5.2) the inflammatory exudate begins in the distal airspaces and spreads via the pores of Kohn across segmental boundaries, giving rise to homogeneous nonsegmental consolidation. Eventually the pneumonia may involve a whole lobe, but usually symptoms develop before the entire lobe is consolidated and then antibiotic therapy halts the process. The consolidation is usually confined to one lobe, although multilobar involvement is not uncommon. Because the airways are not primarily affected, there is little or no volume loss and visible air bronchograms are common.

Some pneumonias present as spherical or nodular consolidations (Fig. 5.3). The nodules are usually ill defined and may contain air bronchograms.

Interstitial pneumonia refers to a radiographic pattern comprising extensive peribronchial thickening and ill-defined reticulonodular shadowing of the lungs, which may be relatively localized or may be widespread (Fig. 5.4). Associated

Table 5.1 Basic radiographic patterns of infective pneumonia

Bronchopneumonia	Airways involved with filling of adjacent acini giving a nodular pattern and patchy consolidation; associated volume loss. May reflect overspill of infected secretions from tuberculous or bacterial abscess cavity
Lobar pneumonia	Homogeneous consolidation bounded by fissures, with or without air bronchogram. No volume loss. Most common manifestation of community-acquired pneumonia
Spherical (round) pneumonia	Ill-defined round area of consolidation, with or without air bronchogram. Most frequent in childhood. May progress to lobar pneumonia
Interstitial pneumonia	Widespread peribronchial thickening and interstitial shadowing. Often associated with areas of subsegmental collapse. *M. pneumoniae* or viral infections are most common causes

patchy subsegmental or discoid atelectasis is common. This pattern, although it may show a lobar or segmental distribution, is frequently independent of the lobar architecture of the lung. The usual causes are viral and *Mycoplasma pneumoniae* infections.

The chest radiograph is the most commonly ordered imaging investigation in patients with suspected pneumonia; even so, the majority of individuals with a community-acquired pneumonia are diagnosed on clinical grounds alone, without recourse to chest radiography. CT is reserved for patients with a suspected complication (for example, emphysema) or underlying cause (for example, bronchial obstruction). CT may occasionally help to refine the differential diagnosis of the causative organism,[2–4] although in general there are few CT features that discriminate between bacterial pneumonias.[2]

In children with complicated pneumonia CT may be valuable in showing significant abnormalities such as a decrease in parenchymal contrast enhancement which denotes impending cavitary necrosis.[5,6]

DIAGNOSING THE CAUSE OF PNEUMONIA

Pneumonias caused by many viruses or *M. pneumoniae* are usually self-limiting and resolve without treatment, whereas bacterial pneumonias require accurate diagnosis and therapy if serious complications, and even death, are to be avoided. It is bacterial pneumonias therefore that are most frequently encountered in hospital practice. The choice of which antibiotic to use may have to rest on a combination of clinical findings, radiographic features, and an initial gram stain of the sputum[7] because the results of bacteriologic tests may be delayed and are sometimes uninformative.[8] Many empirical factors aid the decision making in managing patients with pneumonia:

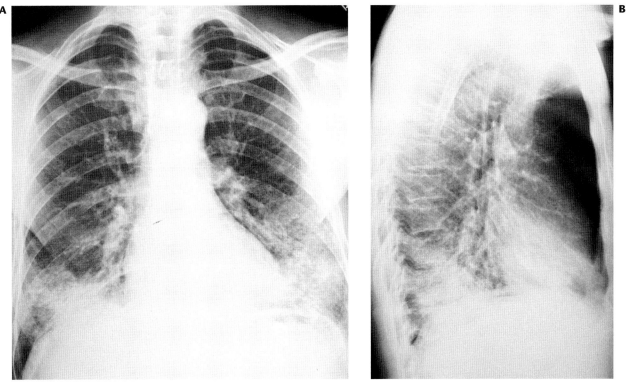

Fig. 5.1   Bronchopneumonia. Bilateral lower zone aspiration pneumonia in an alcoholic patient. **A**, Posteroanterior view. **B**, Lateral view.

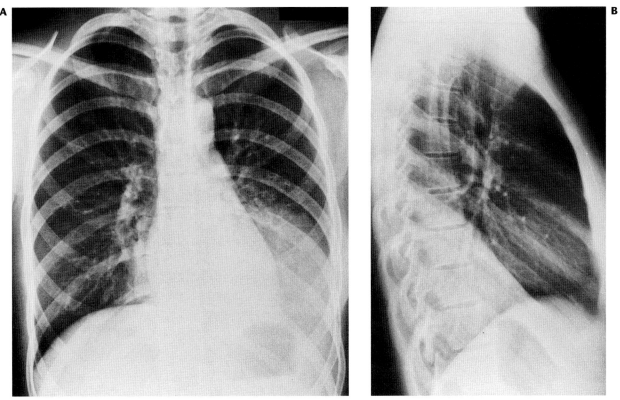

Fig. 5.2   Lobar pneumonia. Pneumococcal pneumonia involving the entire left lower lobe. **A**, Posteroanterior view. **B**, Lateral view.

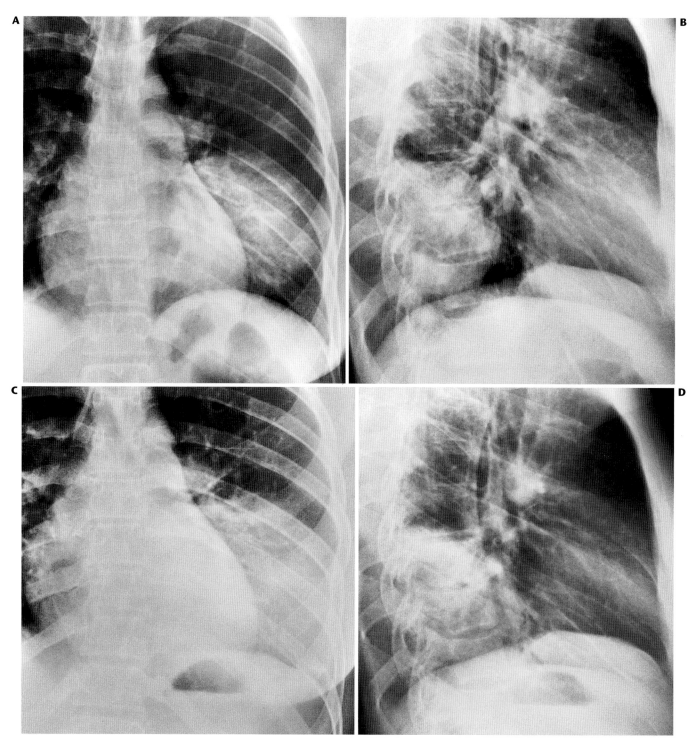

Fig. 5.3 Round pneumonia (pneumococcal) in the left lower lobe in an adult: **A**, posteroanterior and, **B**, lateral radiographs on admission to hospital; **C** and **D**, 12 hours later, the round pneumonia has progressed to become lobar in shape.

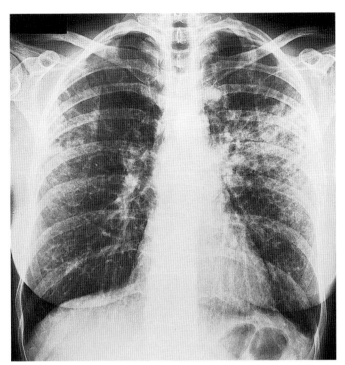

Fig. 5.4 Interstitial viral pneumonia showing bilateral poorly defined linear and nodular shadowing radiating from the hila.

1. **The age of the patient and any history of exposure to a specific organism**. In infants viral infections are the dominant cause of pneumonia, and *Mycoplasma* infection is an important cause in young children.[9] Bacterial pneumonia is relatively rare at an early age. In adults with radiographically evident pulmonary consolidation the commonest cause is bacterial infection.[7]

2. **The source of the infection, particularly whether it was acquired in the hospital or in the community**. Pneumococcal, chlamydial, mycoplasmal, and viral pneumonias are the commonest community-acquired pneumonias in adults.[10,11] *Staphylococcus aureus, Streptococcus pyogenes, Klebsiella, Rickettsia*, and *Legionella pneumophila* are less frequent agents. By contrast, gram-negative bacilli, *S. aureus*, anaerobic organisms, and pneumococci are particularly prevalent causes in hospital-acquired infections.[12,13] Nearly half the cases of hospital-acquired pneumonia have more than one pathogen.[12]

3. **The character of the illness**. Bacterial pneumonia typically presents as an acute illness with chest pain, chills, high fever, and cough productive of purulent sputum. Neutrophilia is common. *Mycoplasma* and viral pneumonias, on the other hand, usually have prodromal symptoms, mild pyrexia, and less sputum; neutrophilia is absent and the white blood cell count is usually only slightly elevated.

4. **Predisposing conditions**. The list of predisposing conditions is long and complex. For example, aspiration pneumonia, which is most often due to anaerobic organisms, gram-negative bacteria, or *S. aureus*, is particularly prevalent in patients who are alcoholics, have had recent general anesthesia or a bout of unconsciousness,

or have disturbances of swallowing.[14] Pneumococcal pneumonia is particularly likely in sickle cell disease and following splenectomy. *Pseudomonas aeruginosa* or *S. aureus* is the likely pathogen responsible for pneumonia in patients with cystic fibrosis.[15,16] Patients with chronic obstructive pulmonary disease are more prone to exacerbations caused by *Haemophilus influenzae* and *Branhamella catarrhalis*.[17] Patients who are immunocompromised present a special category and are discussed in Chapter 6.

Before considering individual pneumonias, it may be helpful to point out a few generalizations regarding pulmonary infection of the immunocompetent host:

1. Consolidation of all or most of a lobe is usually bacterial in origin (Fig. 5.2), and postobstructive pneumonia should be strongly considered, particularly in patients who may have carcinoma of the bronchus. When lobar consolidation is due to a primary bacterial infection, the usual organism is *Streptococcus pneumoniae* (pneumococcus). Occasionally the infection is due to *Klebsiella, S. aureus, Mycobacterium tuberculosis*, or *L. pneumophila* or to aspiration of anaerobic or gram-negative bacteria from the upper respiratory tract or pharynx. Expansion of the lobe is a sign that is said to suggest pneumococcal or *Klebsiella* pneumonia.

2. Aspiration pneumonia frequently causes patchy consolidation in the dependent portions of the lungs (Fig. 5.1). Consolidation is usually multilobar and bilateral in distribution.

3. Consolidation with cavitation (Fig. 5.5) suggests bacterial or fungal disease rather than viral or *Mycoplasma* infection. The bacteria that commonly cause cavitation are *S. aureus*, gram-negative bacteria (especially *Klebsiella, Proteus*, and *Pseudomonas*), anaerobic bacteria (particularly in patients with poor oral hygiene), and *M. tuberculosis*. A large solitary abscess in a patient without underlying lung disease is usually due to anaerobic bacteria. Such abscesses are usually due to aspiration of oropharyngeal secretions, alone or in combination with impairment of local or systemic host defense mechanisms.[18]
Pneumatocele formation (see p. 122) can be difficult to distinguish from cavitation (Fig. 5.6). When pneumatoceles are due to pneumonia, the responsible organism is likely to be *S. aureus*, although pneumatoceles have also been described in infants with pneumonia caused by *S. pneumoniae*.[19]
Care needs to be taken to avoid misdiagnosing cavitation or pneumatocele formation when there are focal transradiancies within consolidation due to underlying emphysema. Emphysematous bullae within the consolidated lung readily resemble cavitation.[20]
Pulmonary gangrene is a rare but interesting form of cavitation that produces sloughed lung within a large cavity secondary to thrombosis or involvement of the pulmonary vessels as they pass through the pneumonia (Fig. 5.7).[21] *S. pneumoniae* and *Klebsiella*[22,23] are the most common bacterial causes. Pulmonary gangrene has also been described with *M. tuberculosis*,[22] possibly with anaerobic bacteria,[23] with invasive *Aspergillus* infection, and with mucormycosis, particularly in the immunocompromised host.[24]

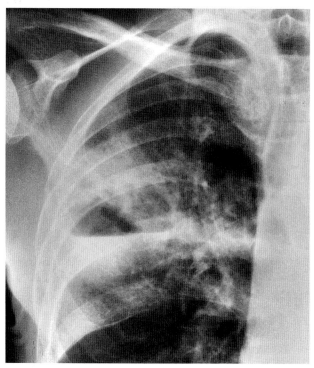

Fig. 5.5 Consolidation with extensive cavitation caused by gram-negative, presumed anaerobic, bacterial pneumonia.

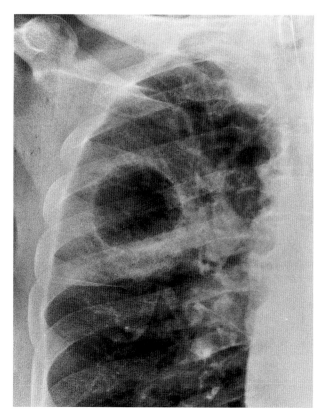

Fig. 5.6 Pneumatocele formation in staphylococcal pneumonia.

4. Nodular (spherical) pneumonia (Fig. 5.3) is usually due to pneumococcal infection[25] or *L. pneumophila, Legionella micdadei*,[26,27] Q fever,[28] or fungal disease. It may also be due to hematogenous spread of bacteria, most commonly *S. aureus*. Although spherical pneumonia can be confused with lung carcinoma, the distinction is relatively straightforward when the pneumonia is bacterial in origin, since at least part of the border of a spherical pneumonia is ill defined in almost all instances. Spherical pneumonias expand to involve the adjacent lung over the next few hours or days, may contain air bronchograms, and are associated with obvious clinical features of acute bacterial infection. They are common in childhood, an age at which lung carcinoma is nonexistent. Spherical pneumonias caused by fungal infections, however, are often chronic and may closely resemble carcinoma of the lung both clinically and radiographically.

5. Pneumonia that presents with focal or widespread, small, ill-defined reticulonodular shadows (Fig. 5.8), whether or not lobar or segmental consolidation is also present, is likely to be due to viral or mycoplasmal infection.[29,30] In exceptional cases fungal and streptococcal infections give rise to this pattern.

6. A miliary nodular pattern in the lungs has many causes. When it is due to infection, the likely organisms are *M. tuberculosis* (Fig. 5.9) and various fungi. The nodules are even in size, usually 2–4 mm in diameter, well defined, and uniformly distributed.

7. Patchy upper lobe consolidations (Fig. 5.10) are very suggestive of tuberculous or fungal infection, notably

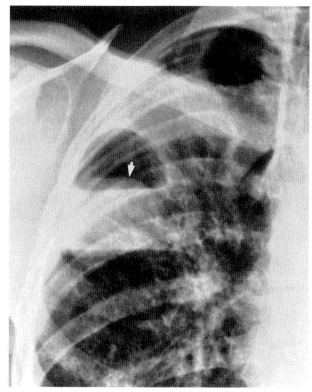

Fig. 5.7 Pulmonary gangrene. Sloughed lung (arrow) can be seen projecting above an air–fluid level in a cavity. The organism in this case was *Pseudomonas*.

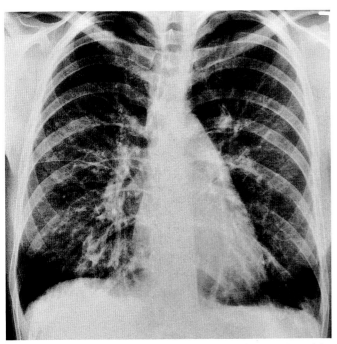

Fig. 5.8 *Mycoplasma* pneumonia showing widespread reticulonodular shadowing throughout the lungs.

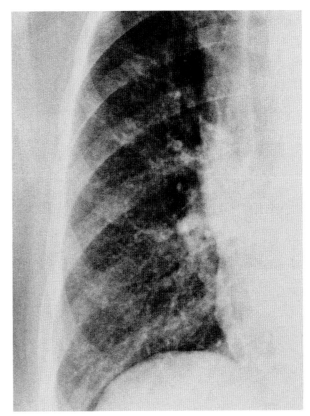

Fig. 5.9 Miliary tuberculosis.

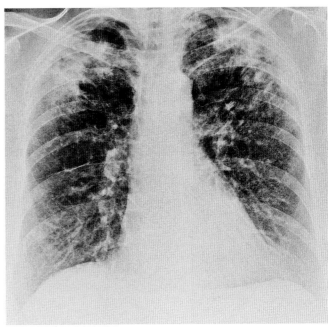

Fig. 5.10 Patchy upper lobe consolidation caused by histoplasmosis.

histoplasmosis but occasionally North American blastomycosis, cryptococcosis, and coccidioidomycosis. Patchy lower lobe consolidation together with volume loss suggests aspiration pneumonia.

8. Large pleural effusions are most commonly associated with pneumonia caused by anaerobic bacteria, gram-negative bacteria, *S. aureus*, or *S. pyogenes*. Empyemas are radiographically indistinguishable from uninfected pleural effusions, but empyema should be considered if the effusion is large, delayed in appearance, or loculated, particularly if it loculates rapidly.

9. Most pneumonias resolve radiographically within a month, often within 10–21 days, and most of the remainder by 2 months. The most indolent shadowing is seen with infection caused by tuberculosis, anaerobes, *Coxiella burnetii*, *L. pneumophila*, or *Chlamydia psittaci* and with some cases of *M. pneumoniae* pneumonia. Consolidation persisting beyond 2 months represents delayed resolution, and an explanation should be sought. The most likely reasons are that the patient is old or is not fully immunocompetent. Alternatively, the pneumonia may have been extensive or have been complicated by atelectasis, cavitation, or empyema. If none of these explanations appears satisfactory, a predisposing local cause such as obstructing neoplasm should be excluded.[31]

10. Diagnosing pneumonia in ventilated or postoperative patients can be difficult. Portable chest radiography may not disclose basal consolidation in approximately one-quarter of patients following abdominal surgery.[32] Pneumonia, edema, acute respiratory distress syndrome (ARDS), infarction, and hemorrhage have overlapping signs, so that a confident diagnosis based on radiographic features alone is often impossible.[33–35] In patients with ARDS, CT may reveal areas of cavitation or empyema, not shown on chest radiography, which are suggestive of coexisting infection.[36] CT appearances are reasonably good at distinguishing between ARDS patients with and

without ventilator-associated pneumonia, although no single CT feature is discriminatory.[37]

11. The distinction between normality and early community-acquired pneumonia is often difficult, with relatively poor interobserver agreement.[38]

BACTERIAL PNEUMONIA

Streptococcus pneumoniae pneumonia

S. pneumoniae (pneumococcal) pneumonia occurs at any age, is the most common community-acquired bacterial pneumonia,[11,39] and is the most frequent type of pneumonia that results in hospitalization.[40] Dementia, seizure disorders, institutionalization, smoking, previous splenectomy, congestive heart failure, and various chronic illnesses including HIV infection, are all predisposing factors.[41] Given a mortality rate of up to 25% of susceptible individuals, polyvalent polysaccharide pneumococcal vaccination is recommended for at-risk elderly and very young individuals.[42] The initial symptoms of pneumococcal pneumonia typically include sudden onset of high fever, pleuritic pain, and cough productive of sputum that is sometimes streaked with blood.

A variety of radiographic patterns are described. Pneumococcal pneumonia is the prototype pathologic condition for lobar consolidation (Figs 5.2 and 5.11). Bacteria are inhaled into the periphery of a lobe where they incite an intense inflammatory reaction, which is seen radiographically as an area of homogeneous nonsegmental shadowing (Fig. 5.12). Air bronchograms may be evident. The exudate spreads rapidly across interalveolar connections rather than via the bronchial tree. It crosses segmental boundaries through the pores of Kohn and therefore does not show a segmental pattern. If untreated the pneumonia may involve the whole of the lobe, which may be expanded by the intense exudate. Frequently the gravitationally dependent portions of the lobes are the most densely opacified. Sometimes more than one lobe is involved. Early in its course, before any pleural boundaries have been reached, the pneumonia

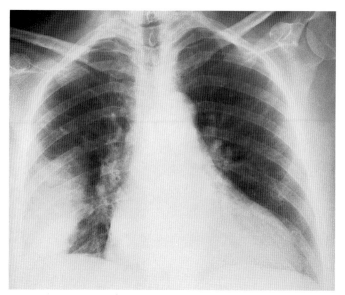

Fig. 5.12 Pneumococcal pneumonia presenting as a large area of peripheral consolidation in the right lower lobe.

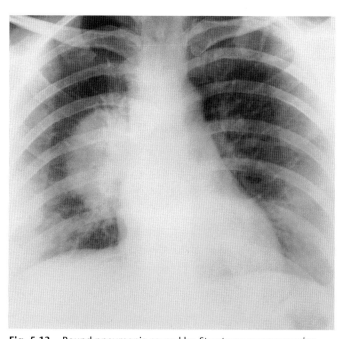

Fig. 5.13 Round pneumonia caused by *Streptococcus pneumoniae* resembling a mediastinal mass.

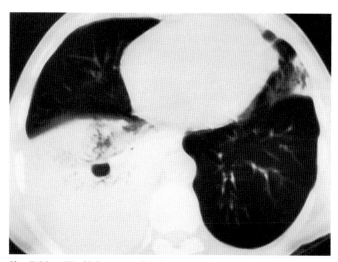

Fig. 5.11 CT of lobar consolidation caused by pneumococcal pneumonia. Note the cavity and forward bowing of the major fissure, indicating expansile consolidation.

may be spherical (Figs 5.3 and 5.13), a phenomenon seen most frequently in children.

Some reports have emphasized that the more usual pattern is patchy or peribronchial consolidation (Fig. 5.14), patterns that occurred in 57 (61%) of Ort et al's 94 patients[43] and in 28 (70%) of 40 patients in Kantor's series.[44] A widespread, small nodular and linear pattern resembling interstitial disease was seen in 22% of Kantor's patients; others do not emphasize this pattern, presumably regarding it as one of the bronchopneumonic varieties. A more recent series has emphasized that lobar consolidation remains the most frequent radiographic pattern and, interestingly, this was unaffected by HIV seropositivity.[45]

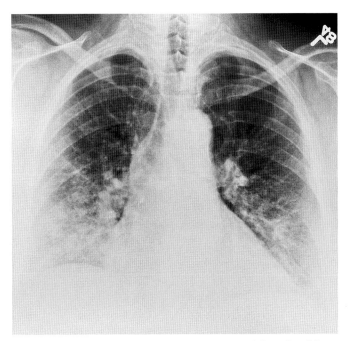

Fig. 5.14 Pneumococcal pneumonia presenting as bilateral middle and lower zone patchy consolidation.

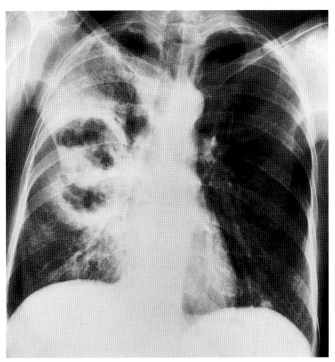

Fig. 5.15 Pneumococcal pneumonia showing extensive cavitation in lobar consolidation in the right upper and middle lobes.

With appropriate treatment the pneumonia usually clears within 14 days.

Pleural effusion is seen in up to half of patients[46] and occasionally, particularly if treatment has been delayed, the effusion turns into an empyema. The presence of parapneumonic effusions correlates with the duration of symptoms before admission, with bacteremia, and with prolonged fever after commencement of therapy.[47] Cavitation is distinctly unusual (Fig. 5.15).[41] A very rare complication is pulmonary gangrene.[23]

Streptococcus pyogenes pneumonia

S. pyogenes and other types of streptococcus cause pneumonia much less frequently than *S. pneumoniae*. In the early part of the twentieth century *S. pyogenes* was a major cause of pneumonia in both adults and children. Although comparatively rare it remains an important and potentially fatal pneumonia.[48,49] It may complicate viral infections or may follow streptococcal upper respiratory tract infections. On chest radiographs, *S. pyogenes* pneumonia appears as lower lobe predominant, confluent or patchy consolidation. Large pleural effusions and empyema are common.[50]

Staphylococcal pneumonia

Pneumonia caused by *S. aureus* usually follows aspiration of organisms from the upper respiratory tract, occurring particularly in hospitalized patients. In many hospitals *S. aureus* is becoming a problem, particularly for patients in intensive care units, because of the development of methicillin-resistant strains.[51] In a study of ventilated patients, there was a 20-fold increased mortality risk for those patients with pneumonia caused by methicillin-resistant *S. aureus* (MRSA), compared to those with nonresistant *S. aureus* pneumonia.[52] Staphylococcal

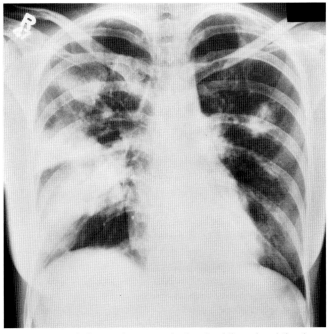

Fig. 5.16 Staphylococcal pneumonia showing bilateral multifocal consolidation.

pneumonia may also be community acquired, particularly in infants and elderly individuals, often complicating influenza. Pneumonia caused by hematogenous spread may result from endocarditis, thrombophlebitis, or staphylococcal infection of indwelling catheters. Septicemic infection is also seen in drug addicts and immunocompromised patients.

The plain chest radiograph (Fig. 5.16) typically shows patchy segmental consolidation, often with loss of volume. Air

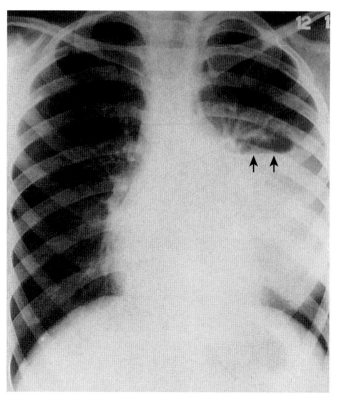

Fig. 5.17 Staphylococcal pneumonia showing confluent lobar-type consolidations with cavitation (arrows point to an air–fluid level in the superior segment of the left lower lobe).

bronchograms are rare. The consolidation may spread rapidly and become confluent, resembling lobar pneumonia (Fig. 5.17). Several lobes are usually involved,[53] and the disease may be bilateral. There do not appear to be any differences between the radiographic pattern of MRSA and that of non-MRSA infection.[54]

Abscess cavities may form within the pneumonia and are common at any age (Fig. 5.17). Pneumatoceles (Fig. 5.18) are more common in childhood than adult infection[53] and may lead to pneumothorax. Pleural effusions, which may develop rapidly, are common. Empyema formation is a frequent and serious complication, particularly in children. Septicemic staphylococcal infection, in contrast to infection following aspiration, causes multiple spherical (round) consolidations, which may cavitate.[55]

Anthrax

Anthrax is caused by *Bacillus anthracis*, a gram-positive aerobic bacillus. It is usually acquired from contact with infected goats or their products, particularly unfinished hides and wools imported from endemic areas in Asia, the Middle East, or Africa (Fig. 5.19). Indigenous anthrax is extremely rare in the United States and Europe but awareness of the disease increased sharply after its use by terrorists in 2001.[56–59] The spores may be inhaled directly into the lungs, but cutaneous anthrax is the most common clinical presentation. The spores are carried to regional lymph nodes, from which they may disseminate to the lungs and cause hemorrhagic pneumonia. Striking mediastinal widening caused by lymphadenopathy is a particularly common radiographic feature[60,61] (Fig. 5.20). Chest radiography may also show patchy consolidation, particularly at the bases, and pleural effusions. The imaging of two survivors of anthrax inhalation is described in detail by Earls et al[61]; in neither case was the diagnosis of anthrax suggested on the basis of plain radiography, nevertheless the authors emphasize the pathognomonic combination of a widened mediastinum in a previously fit individual with "flu-like" symptoms and known anthrax exposure. CT shows more extensive parenchymal and nodal involvement than plain radiography. The consolidation is often bronchocentric and perihilar (Fig. 5.21) and the enlarged

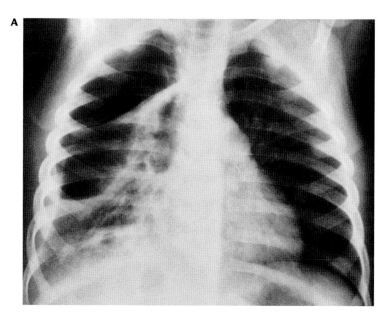
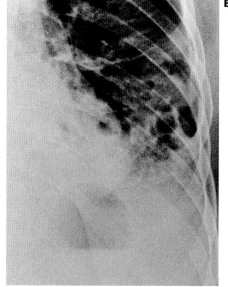

Fig. 5.18 Pneumatocele formation in staphylococcal pneumonia. **A,** A young child with a large pneumatocele in the right lung. **B,** A young adult with multiple small pneumatoceles and left lower lobe pneumonia.

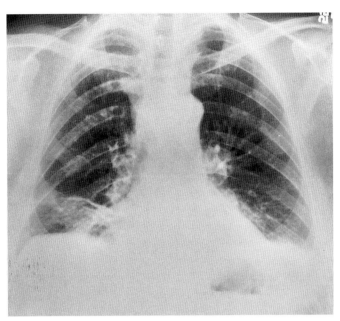

Fig. 5.19 Anthrax pneumonia in a carpet cleaner who developed pneumonia with severe fever, shaking chills, and hypotension. Bilateral basal consolidations and mediastinal lymphadenopathy are present.

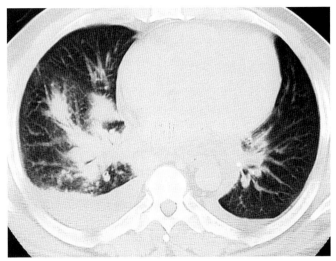

Fig. 5.21 Anthrax pneumonia. In this case the consolidation is distinctly bronchocentric. Pleural effusions are a frequent accompaniment to anthrax pneumonia. (With permission from Earls JP, Cerva D Jr, Berman E, et al. Inhalational anthrax after bioterrorism exposure: spectrum of imaging findings in two surviving patients. Radiology 2002;222:305–312.)

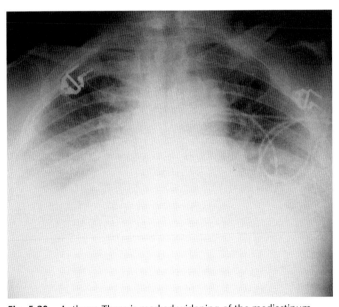

Fig. 5.20 Anthrax. There is marked widening of the mediastinum, bilateral pleural effusions, and widespread airspace consolidation. (With permission from Earls JP, Cerva D Jr, Berman E, et al. Inhalational anthrax after bioterrorism exposure: spectrum of imaging findings in two surviving patients. Radiology 2002;222:305–312.)

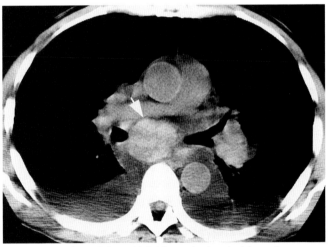

Fig. 5.22 Anthrax. Enlarged left hilar and subcarinal (arrow) hyperattenuating lymph nodes and bilateral pleural effusions. (With permission from Earls JP, Cerva D Jr, Berman E, et al. Inhalational anthrax after bioterrorism exposure: spectrum of imaging findings in two surviving patients. Radiology 2002;222:305–312.)

large airways, pericardial effusion, and opacification of the mediastinal fat by hemorrhage and edema.[62]

Gram-negative bacterial pneumonia

Many aerobic gram-negative bacteria cause pneumonia.[63] The incidence of gram-negative bacterial pneumonia has risen from less than 10% in the 1960s to approximately 20%, and these bacteria are responsible for the majority of nosocomial pneumonias.[13] The most important are Enterobacteriaceae (notably *Klebsiella, Enterobacter, Serratia marcescens, Escherichia coli,* and *Proteus mirabilis*), *P. aeruginosa, Acinetobacter, Haemophilus influenzae,* and *L. pneumophila.* Together with *S. aureus* these

lymph nodes may be of increased attenuation (on an unenhanced CT examination), presumably reflecting intranodal hemorrhage (Fig. 5.22). Similarly, hyperattenuating recent blood clot may be identifiable within pleural effusions (Fig. 5.23). Following intravenous contrast the enhancing rims of hemorrhagic lymph nodes may become visible, particularly on delayed scans.[62] Ancillary features on CT include mucosal thickening within the

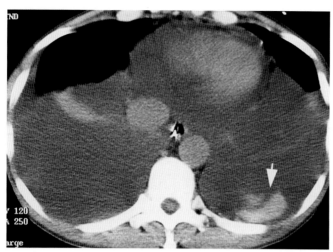

Fig. 5.23 Large pleural effusions in a patient with acute anthrax pneumonia. The increased attenuation material (arrow) within the pleural fluid represents blood clot. (With permission from Earls JP, Cerva D Jr, Berman E, et al. Inhalational anthrax after bioterrorism exposure: spectrum of imaging findings in two surviving patients. Radiology 2002;222:305–312.)

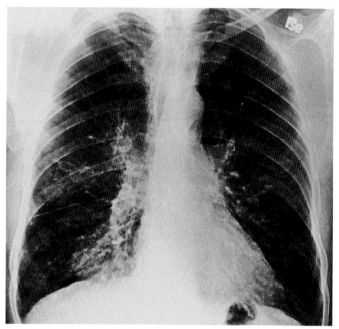

Fig. 5.24 *Haemophilus influenzae* pneumonia causing bilateral basal patchy consolidation, predominantly in the right lower lobe.

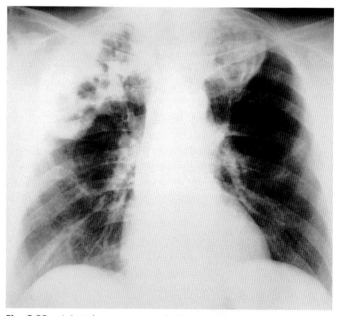

Fig. 5.25 *Acinetobacter* pneumonia showing bilateral upper lobe consolidation and abscess formation.

organisms are a major cause of morbidity and mortality to hospital patients.[13,64] These bacteria contaminate hospital equipment such as ventilators and the soaps, liquids, or jellies used to care for wounds and catheters. *Pseudomonas aeruginosa* is an opportunistic pathogen and has a propensity for colonizing bronchiectatic airways, particularly in patients with cystic fibrosis[65] but it only occasionally causes community-acquired pneumonia in otherwise healthy individuals.[66] Patients colonized with *P. aeruginosa* tend to have more severe bronchiectasis, in terms of functional deficit[67] and morphologic abnormalities on CT,[68] compared with non-colonized individuals; whether this reflects the deleterious effects of *P. aeruginosa* infections or merely the predilection of the organism for more severely damaged airways is uncertain. *Klebsiella* and *Legionella* pneumonias have features that differentiate them from other gram-negative bacterial pneumonias and are discussed separately in the next section. Affected patients usually have a known predisposing factor such as chronic obstructive pulmonary disease, a major medical condition, or recent surgery. Aspiration is believed to be the method by which the organisms most commonly enter the lungs, but pneumonia following inhalation of bacteria or spread by the bloodstream is also occasionally seen.

The radiographic pattern of the gram-negative bacterial pneumonias is entirely nonspecific and ranges from small ill-defined nodules to patchy consolidation (Fig. 5.24), which may sometimes be confluent and resemble lobar pneumonia or even pulmonary edema.[69] Usually the consolidations are multifocal, with the lower lobes nearly always affected, usually bilaterally. In approximately 50% of cases the upper and middle lobes are also involved.[70] In the specific cause of *P. aeruginosa* there may be an upper zone predominance.[71] Furthermore, on CT, a tree-in-bud pattern or centrilobular nodulation is present in half of patients with nosocomial *P. aeruginosa* infection.[71] Cavitation in gram-negative pneumonia is common (Fig. 5.25),[72] but radiographic lucencies in areas of consolidation, although often caused by abscess formation, are sometimes due to spared normal acini and lobules surrounded by pneumonia.[73] Parapneumonic pleural effusions are common in most gram-negative pneumonias, with empyema an important and fairly frequent complication.

Klebsiella pneumonia

Pneumonia caused by *Klebsiella pneumoniae* (Friedländer's pneumonia), like the other gram-negative pneumonias, usually affects people with chronic debilitating illnesses or alcoholism. The symptoms include high fever and toxemia and clinically resemble those of severe pneumococcal pneumonia. On chest radiography the consolidations are also similar to those seen with *S. pneumoniae* pneumonia: the disease is often confined to one lobe, with homogeneous nonsegmental consolidation that spreads rapidly to become a lobar pneumonia. Multilobar and bilateral consolidations may occur. Much was made of lobar expansion in early series,[74,75] but this feature is probably unusual in the modern antibiotic era. However, expansion of consolidated lobes on CT was reported in 6 of 11 patients.[76] In addition, the consolidation was described as consisting of two intermingled parts: enhancing areas and poorly marginated low-attenuation areas, the latter containing small air cavities suggesting necrosis.

Cavitation, which may occur early and progress quickly, is seen in 30–50% of cases on chest radiography (Fig. 5.26). This feature distinguishes *Klebsiella* pneumonia from pneumococcal pneumonia, in which cavitation is rare. The cavities are frequently multiple (Fig. 5.26) and may attain great size. Solitary large chronic abscesses are occasionally encountered.[77] Massive necrosis, so-called "pulmonary gangrene", is a rare but recognized phenomenon. Pleural effusion and empyema were reportedly uncommon in an early series,[63] but in another study effusions were identified in 8 of 11 patients.[76]

Legionella pneumophila pneumonia

Legionnaires' disease, which results in severe pneumonia with a high mortality (although this has markedly decreased in recent years),[78] is caused by *L. pneumophila*, an aerobic gram-negative bacillus found in aquatic environments such as reservoirs, cooling towers, water distribution systems, and humidifiers.[79] Other *Legionella* species lurk in man-made aqueous environments and can also cause pneumonia.[80] Infection comes from these sources rather than from person-to-person contact. The disease may be sporadic or occur in localized epidemics centered on an infected water source[81,82]; the most notable example was the 1976 outbreak at an American Legion convention, in which 29 of 182 affected delegates died[83] and from which the name "Legionnaires' disease" is derived. The infection is characterized by malaise, myalgia, headache, abdominal and chest pain, nausea, vomiting, diarrhea, high fever, rigors, dyspnea, and cough; the cough is usually productive and associated with hemoptysis. Bacteremic dissemination causes a variety of extrapulmonary manifestations, including endocarditis, sinusitis, brain abscess, and pancreatitis. Predisposing chronic diseases are common and may be either pulmonary, such as chronic bronchitis and emphysema, or systemic, such as malignant disease or renal failure. Coinfection with another bacterium, such as *S. pneumoniae*, is not uncommon.[84] Corticosteroid therapy is a recognized risk factor, but surprisingly patients with neutropenia or AIDS do not appear to have an undue predilection for Legionnaires' disease.[79] The organism is difficult to culture from sputum and blood, and selective culture media are required. Current diagnostic tests for *Legionella* infection are either insensitive or unable to provide a result within a clinically useful time frame.[85,86] Hyponatremia is common[87] and occurs more frequently in *L. pneumophila* pneumonia than in other pneumonias.[88]

The radiographic appearances have been reviewed in detail by Fairbank and associates.[89] The initial finding is peripherally situated patchy consolidation (Fig. 5.27), which spreads rapidly, often involving more than one lobe and becoming bilateral in

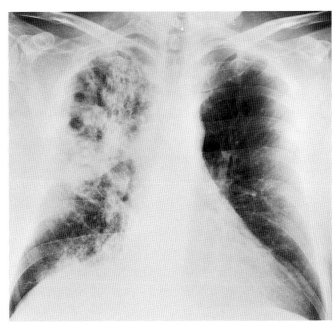

Fig. 5.26   *Klebsiella* pneumonia in the right upper lobe showing numerous cavities.

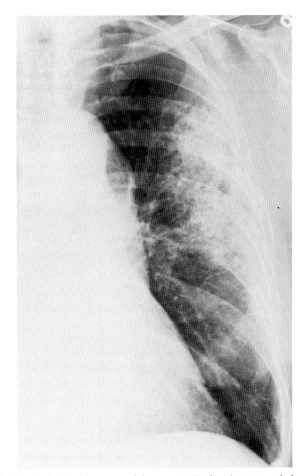

Fig. 5.27   *Legionella pneumophila* pneumonia showing a rounded peripheral area of consolidation in the left upper lobe.

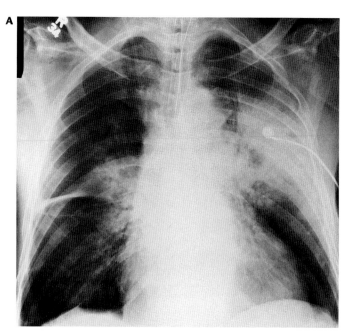

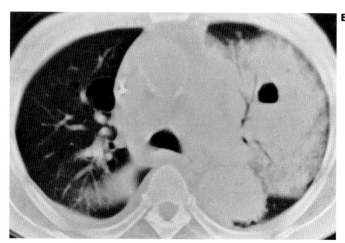

Fig. 5.28 *Legionella pneumophila* pneumonia showing multilobar confluent consolidation. Cavitation, which is visible on **A**, plain radiograph, is better demonstrated on **B**, CT.

half the cases (Fig. 5.28). There may be a slight predilection for the lower lobes, but this is not seen in all series.[90] The consolidations may assume a spherical configuration or may coalesce to resemble lobar pneumonia.[26,91] Cavitation, although reported, is unusual (Fig. 5.28)[92]; it appears to be most common in immunocompromised patients.[90,93] Pleural effusions, which are usually small but occasionally massive, are documented with variable frequency (10–66%)[82,90,92] and frank empyema formation may rarely occur.[94] Unusual radiographic features include hilar adenopathy and spontaneous pneumothorax.[89] An unusual pattern of multiple 0.5–2 cm pulmonary nodules has been reported in an infant.[95] The radiographic resolution is slow, particularly in immunocompromised patients, and lags behind the clinical improvement. The changes usually persist for at least a month after the acute illness.

L. micdadei pneumonia is considered separately in the section on immunocompromised patients on page 304.

Pertussis (whooping cough)

Whooping cough is caused by the aerobic gram-negative coccobacillus *Bordetella (Haemophilus) pertussis*. Pneumonia caused by this organism is uncommon in communities with a high uptake of immunization. Pneumonia occurs approximately four times more frequently in adults over the age of 30 years than in younger individuals.[96] In previously immunized individuals the clinical course is usually milder, with persistent cough being a prominent and distressing symptom.[97]

On chest radiographs[98–100] the striking feature is extensive peribronchial consolidation in one or more lobes. A large series, comprising 238 patients ill enough to require admission to the hospital, provides a good indication of the chest radiographic findings.[99] Sixty-three patients (26%) had abnormal findings on chest radiography. Pulmonary consolidation, which was predominantly peribronchial in distribution, was present in 50 patients, pulmonary collapse in 9, and visible lymphadenopathy in 22. The pulmonary changes showed a tendency to involve the

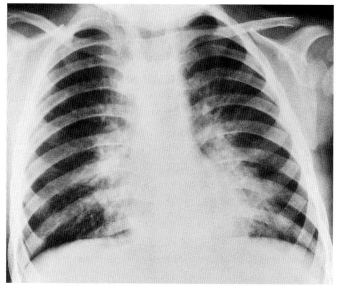

Fig. 5.29 Pertussis pneumonia showing peribronchial consolidation adjacent to the heart, giving rise to the so-called "shaggy heart sign".

right lung, particularly the lower and middle lobes. The peribronchial consolidation tends to be maximal close to the mediastinum, giving rise to an appearance that has been dubbed the shaggy heart sign (Fig. 5.29).[98] This distribution seems to be mirrored by the location of postpertussis bronchiectasis, which is said to have a predilection for the right middle lobe and lingula and occurs in a few patients.

Brucellosis

Brucellosis, an infection transmitted by inhaling infected material from domestic animals, particularly cows, pigs, and goats, or by ingesting infected animal products, such as milk,

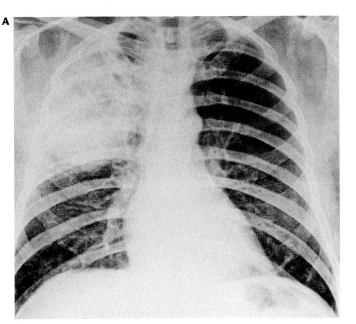
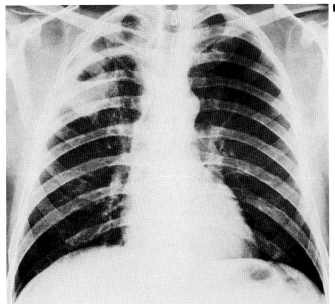

Fig. 5.30 Melioidosis pneumonia. **A,** A large area of consolidation in the right upper lobe. **B,** Six weeks later, pneumonia has partially resolved, leaving a thin walled abscess.

only occasionally causes pneumonia. The responsible organism is a gram-negative coccobacillus. The symptoms include those of systemic infection: fever, malaise, and headache. Multisystem involvement with protean symptoms is common, so that diagnosis may be elusive.[101] Symptoms of pneumonia are seen in less than half of those with abnormalities on the chest radiograph. Pneumonia as the sole manifestation of brucellosis is extremely uncommon.[102] The findings are of focal areas of consolidation, hilar adenopathy, nodular shadows, or miliary nodulation.[103] Spherical calcifications surrounded by thin lamellar calcifications may be seen in the spleen as a late manifestation.[103,104]

Melioidosis

Melioidosis[105] is caused by the aerobic gram-negative bacillus *Burkholderia pseudomallei*, an organism that resides in dust and soil. Pneumonia is rare except in the flooded fields and marshes of Southeast Asia,[106] but cases occur in Australia and nontropical countries.[107,108] Multiple organ involvement is common, with the lungs the most frequently affected organ.[106,109] The pneumonia may be acute or subacute and has a reported mortality rate of over 80%.[109] The acute form, which can be rapidly fatal, is characterized by positive blood cultures, fulminating septicemia, and high fever, with or without acute respiratory failure.[110] The subacute form consists of cough, which is usually productive, occasional hemoptysis, low grade fever, weight loss, and pleuritic chest pain. In some patients few symptoms occur and melioidosis is diagnosed only because pulmonary disease is found on chest radiography. Patients with cystic fibrosis may be more than usually susceptible to chronic melioidosis.[111]

On chest radiographs the acute pneumonia shows small, round, ill-defined areas of consolidation that are often unilateral and may coalesce to form segmental or lobar opacities (Fig. 5.30) with a striking affinity for the upper lobes. Cavitation is frequent; the cavities may be thin walled. Pleural effusion, empyema,[112]

and pneumothorax are seen in a small proportion of patients,[106] and hilar adenopathy has been reported.

In the subacute form the plain chest radiograph shows a variety of patterns, including round, segmental, or lobar consolidation, which often cavitates.[106,113] In the chronic subclinical forms the chest radiograph closely resembles postprimary tuberculosis with patchy upper lobe consolidation and cavitation. Melioidosis is relatively resistant to antimicrobial therapy and the relapse rate is high.[108]

Plague

Plague is caused by *Yersinia (Pasteurella) pestis*, a gram-negative coccobacillus still found in some areas of Asia, Africa, South America, and the southwestern United States.[114–116] Pneumonia may be primary, resulting from inhalation of infected droplets, or may spread hematogenously from infected swollen axillary or femoral lymph nodes, sometimes known as buboes. The resulting pneumonia is fulminant with high fever and death is inevitable without appropriate antibiotic treatment.[117] In fatal cases numerous petechiae and ecchymoses develop, the appearance of which gave rise to the name "Black Death" in the fearful epidemic that swept Europe in the fourteenth century.

Radiographic examination[114,118] shows rapidly progressive dense patchy consolidations that may be nodular, segmental, or lobar in shape. Eventually multiple lobes are involved and mediastinal adenopathy and pleural effusions may be present. In some cases, mediastinal and hilar adenopathy is the only radiographic finding.

P. multocida is a gram-negative rod or coccobacillus that infects cats and dogs. Respiratory infection resulting in acute bronchitis, bronchopneumonia, lung abscess, or empyema may follow inhalation of organisms or a bite. The radiographic changes include lobar, multilobar, or widespread patchy consolidation, usually sparing the upper lobes.[118] Pleural effusions occur in up to 20% of patients.

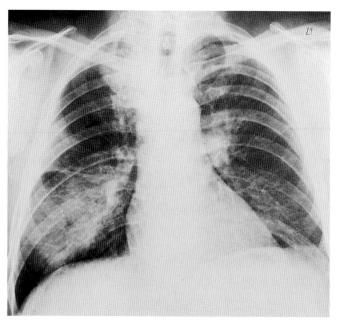

Fig. 5.31 Tularemia pneumonia showing multiple areas of consolidation in the right lung. Two weeks before this radiograph was taken, the patient had run over a rabbit while mowing his lawn.

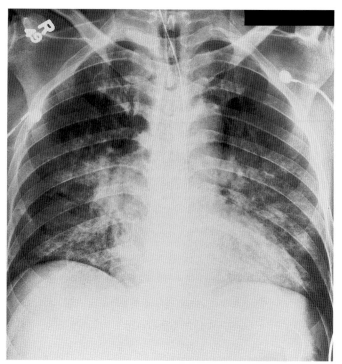

Fig. 5.32 Anaerobic aspiration pneumonia showing bilateral middle and lower zone consolidation.

Tularemia

Tularemia, named after Tulare County in California, is caused by *Francisella tularensis*, an aerobic gram-negative coccobacillus. The disease is endemic in many parts of the world, including Europe, Asia, and North America. Human infection is acquired in a variety of ways:

1. through the skin in individuals who handle infected animals (rabbits, squirrels, skunks, dogs, game birds, and many others) or their skins
2. by bites from the infected animals themselves
3. by bites from infected insect vectors, notably ticks, or mosquitoes or fleas (the latter were thought to be largely responsible for a recent outbreak in Sweden[119])
4. by inhalation of organisms from infected carcasses or even the inhalation of particles produced by lawn mowing,[120] from dust, or following laboratory accidents.

Pneumonia is a common finding in patients with tularemia.

The radiographic signs of tularemia pneumonia are lobar, segmental, rounded, oval, or patchy pulmonary consolidations, which may be unilateral or bilateral in distribution (Fig. 5.31).[121,122] The most common pattern is unilateral patchy consolidation, but widespread bronchopneumonia, lobar consolidation, a pattern resembling pulmonary edema, lung abscess, and apical opacities resembling tuberculosis are all encountered.[118] Cavitation may occur but is unusual. Miliary nodulation was reported in one case in a large series.[122] The pulmonary changes may be accompanied by cardiomegaly caused by pericarditis with pericardial effusion. Hilar adenopathy is common as are pleural effusions, both of which may be unilateral or bilateral. Empyema and bronchopleural fistula may supervene. On rare occasions the consolidation resolves with fibrosis and calcification and thus resembles tuberculosis and histoplasmosis.

Anaerobic lung infection

Most anaerobic lung infections result from aspiration of infected oral contents, and obvious periodontal disease is present in most patients.[18,123–125] Predisposing factors such as a recent episode of altered consciousness, dysphagia, or alcoholism are frequent.[18,123]

The infection is usually indolent or subacute,[126] although an acute febrile illness, closely resembling pneumococcal pneumonia but without shaking chills, may be seen.[123,127] Often the sputum is putrid, a feature not encountered in pneumonia caused by aerobic bacteria. In about half the cases anaerobic organisms alone are responsible (the common ones are *Bacteroides*, *Fusobacterium*, *Peptococcus* and *Peptostreptococcus*, microaerophilic *Streptococcus*, and *Propionibacterium*), and in the other half of cases mixed anaerobic and aerobic bacteria are found on culture. A pitfall here is that the anaerobic bacteria may not be appreciated unless especially cultured, and it may therefore be assumed that aerobic organisms alone are responsible for the pneumonia.

The radiographic appearances[123,126] can be conveniently divided into pulmonary parenchymal infection, pneumonia with cavitation, and discrete lung abscess, each of which may be associated with empyema.

Anaerobic pneumonia has a predilection for the lower lobes (Figs 5.1 and 5.32), with the right lung more commonly affected than the left. These sites are compatible with the belief that the pneumonia follows aspiration from the upper respiratory tract. There is usually one predominant focus of disease, but multilobe involvement is also common (Fig. 5.33).

Cavitation within an area of pulmonary consolidation is frequent and seen on chest radiography in up to 40% of cases. It

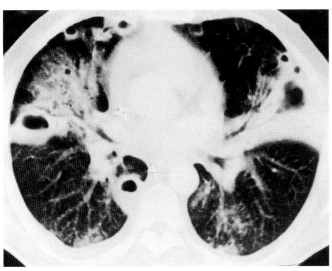

Fig. 5.33   Multiple anaerobic lung abscesses and focal areas of consolidation. The patient had swallowed a fish bone, which perforated the esophagus.

may develop while the patient is in the hospital on appropriate antibiotic therapy (Fig. 5.34). Discrete lung abscesses occur chiefly in the posterior portions of the lungs, usually in the posterior segments of the upper lobes or in the superior segments of the lower lobes. It is noted that in patients with cavitation the disease takes longer to resolve, sometimes two months or more. Hilar and mediastinal adenopathy may accompany lung abscess,[128] and such cases may therefore closely resemble carcinoma of the lung (Fig. 5.35).

One-third to one-half of patients have empyema.[123,126] Over half the patients in one series of anaerobic bacterial empyema had no apparent parenchymal disease.[126] If pleural effusion is seen in association with anaerobic lung infection, it is virtually certain to be an infected empyema.[126] The infected fluid is frequently loculated. Very large empyemas may develop and bronchopleural fistula is a recognized complication.

Syphilis

Pulmonary infection caused by *Treponema pallidum* is rare, and reports scanty.[129] Diffuse bronchopneumonia, diffuse pulmonary fibrosis, and solitary or multiple pulmonary nodules have been reported.[130]

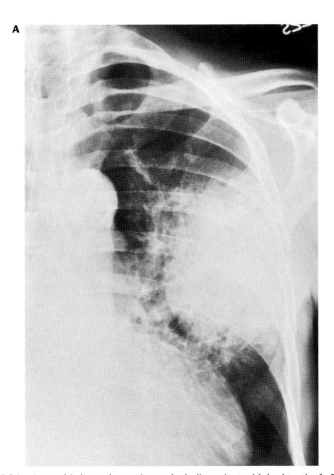
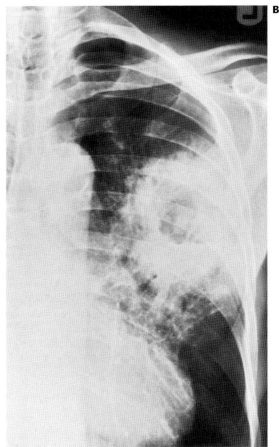

Fig. 5.34   Anaerobic lung abscess in an alcoholic patient with bad teeth. **A**, Early in the course of the disease, a rounded area of pneumonia. **B**, Two days later, a discrete lung abscess has formed.

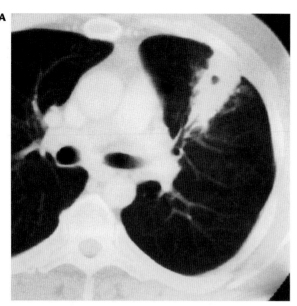

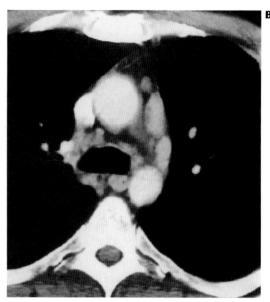

Fig. 5.35 Anaerobic lung abscess (**A**) with mediastinal adenopathy (**B**) mimicking a lung cancer.

Leptospirosis

Leptospirosis, caused by the spirochete *Leptospira*, is common in the tropics where it is the cause of Weil's disease, a syndrome comprising fever, jaundice, hemorrhage, nephritis, and meningitis. Leptospirosis follows contact with contaminated water or tissues of infected animals.

Pneumonia occurs in one-fifth to two-thirds of patients with leptospirosis.[131,132] It seems that a history of cigarette smoking may increase the risk of developing pulmonary leptospirosis.[133] The pulmonary consolidation is due to hemorrhagic pneumonitis.[134] Although one series has reported acute lung injury in 42 ventilated patients with leptospirosis, it seems probable, in the absence of other reports, that the pulmonary involvement in these cases was the expected extensive hemorrhage. Chest radiographs[131,135] show bilateral, multiple areas of pulmonary consolidation that may take the form of multiple well-defined small nodules or multifocal nonlobar consolidations with a marked tendency to peripheral predominance. These patchy areas of consolidation may be extensive and confluent in severe cases. Patchy discoid atelectasis and small pleural effusions are common. Interlobular septal thickening (Kerley lines) has been noted in a small proportion of patients.[131] Hilar and mediastinal adenopathy does not appear to be a feature. The HRCT findings are, as might be anticipated from the pathology of extensive pulmonary hemorrhage, widespread ground-glass opacification and consolidation,[136] with some poorly defined centrilobular and acinar nodules. There are no ancillary features to suggest leptospirosis as the cause of these nonspecific abnormalities.

Rickettsial infections

The most common rickettsial pneumonia is Q fever, caused by *Coxiella burnetii*. Q fever occurs worldwide and is acquired from infected dust, from cattle or sheep products, or occasionally from the bite of infected ticks or mites. The disease occurs sporadically and in epidemics.[137,138] The symptoms are sudden in onset and include a flu-like illness with fever, dry cough, myalgias, arthralgias, and headache. Pneumonia develops in less than half those infected. Many different organs may be involved, and it seems that younger patients are more prone to hepatitis whereas older, possibly less immune competent individuals,[139] or those with chronic bronchitis,[140] are more likely to develop pneumonia. The prognosis is good apart from those with myocarditis or meningoencephalitis. The usual radiographic appearance of Q fever pneumonia[28,141–143] (Fig. 5.36) is unifocal or multifocal, subsegmental, segmental, or lobar consolidation. Typically, there is a single segmental opacity in an upper lobe[143] but the radiographic findings are entirely nonspecific.[144] Spherical (round) pneumonia is also reported, particularly in epidemic cases.[145,146] Very occasionally these round pneumonias are confused with lung cancer.[145] Cavitation is rare.[147] Pleural effusions are seen in some patients, particularly in sporadic infection. CT abnormalities largely reflect radiographic findings, namely multifocal consolidation (Fig. 5.37). However, in a series of 12 patients, one patient had nodular lesions, some of which had a ground-glass halo (Fig. 5.37). The authors suggested that these might represent angioinvasion[148] (although the mechanism and evolution of septic embolism is an alternative explanation). Lymphadenopathy and small pleural effusions are more readily disclosed on CT. The disease is self-limiting, but resolution of pulmonary consolidation may take up to 6 months,[144] although the average time is 39 days.[143]

Rocky Mountain spotted fever, caused by *Rickettsia rickettsiae*, is encountered mostly in the southeastern United States, where it is transmitted through tick bites. It is an acute, often fulminant, disease in which small vessel inflammation is the basic pathologic process. The vasculitis is clinically most evident in the skin and central nervous system. In the lungs the resulting pulmonary vasculitis leads to a variety of patterns, varying from unifocal or multifocal consolidations, resembling bacterial

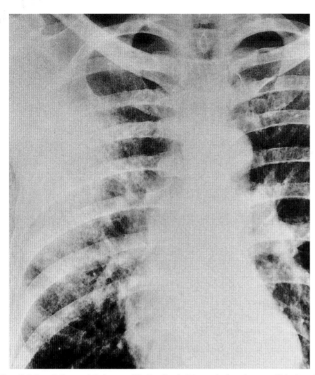

Fig. 5.36 Q fever (*C. burnetii* infection). There is focal consolidation in the right upper lobe.

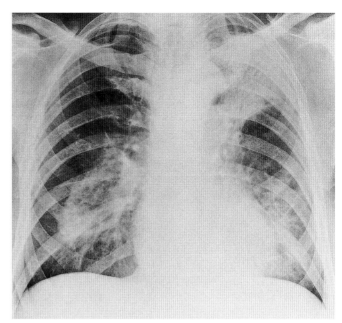

Fig. 5.38 Psittacosis pneumonia showing multifocal bilateral consolidation.

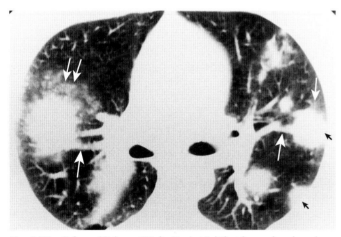

Fig. 5.37 Q fever (*C. burnetii* infection). Multifocal round and wedge-shaped areas of consolidation (arrows). Vessels enter some of these focal consolidations (large arrowheads). There is ground-glass opacity around the edges of some consolidations (small arrowheads). (With permission from Voloudaki AE, Kofteridis DP, Tritou IN, et al. Q fever pneumonia: CT findings. Radiology 2000;215:880–883.)

pneumonia, to widespread pulmonary infection, resembling pulmonary edema, combined in some cases with pleural effusions.[149,150] The pathologic result is interstitial and alveolar edema and hemorrhage, together with a mononuclear and lymphocytic interstitial infiltrate.[151] Bacterial superinfection appears to be rare.[150] The clinical diagnosis depends on recognizing a multiorgan vasculitis, notably of the skin and meninges, in an acutely febrile patient during the tick season in endemic areas. The mortality is high in patients with widespread pulmonary consolidation.

Chlamydial infections

Chlamydia psittaci infection, so-called "ornithosis" or psittacosis, is usually acquired from infected birds. Infection with the psittacosis agent may result in disease of wide clinical spectrum, ranging from completely asymptomatic infections recognized only by serologic means to respiratory failure[152] or overwhelming illness involving multiple organ systems.[153] Usually the patient complains of fever, malaise, headache, and a nonproductive cough, and the clinical picture may be indistinguishable from other acute bacterial pneumonias with pleuritic chest pain, productive cough, hemoptysis, shortness of breath, and shaking chills. In children, symptoms may closely resemble pertussis infection.[154] The chest radiograph reveals patchy pulmonary consolidation (Fig. 5.38), which can be extensive. Another described pattern is patchy reticular shadowing with lower zone predominance that appears more severe than would be expected from the clinical features. Pleural effusions have been reported in up to 50% of cases, but are usually small.[155]

Chlamydia trachomatis is a recently recognized cause of pneumonia in neonates and infants, in whom it may cause widespread streaky consolidations and air-trapping similar to that seen with acute bronchiolitis of viral origin.[156] In a few reported cases in adults the chest radiographs showed focal streaky consolidation without evidence of air-trapping. Pleural effusion, although reported, is not a striking feature.[157,158]

Chlamydia pneumoniae is now thought to be a significant but under recognized cause of community-acquired pneumonia, accounting for perhaps as many as 10% of cases of pneumonia in adults.[159,160] Antibody responses to *C. pneumoniae* are highly variable, making serologic studies of its prevalence difficult. Infection with *C. pneumoniae* may be confined to the upper respiratory tract but pneumonia of variable severity occurs in approximately half of cases. The radiographic manifestations range from focal airspace consolidation to widespread interstitial shadowing; indeed, *C. pneumoniae* has been suggested as a pathogenetic agent of nonspecific interstitial pneumonia (NSIP).[161] There appear to be differences in the radiographic appearances between first exposure infections and previously exposed individuals[162]: recurrent infections tend to be characterized by more widespread interstitial shadowing. As with other pulmonary chlamydial infections, pleural effusions occur in some patients.[163]

Septic emboli

The most common sources of septic pulmonary emboli are infected venous catheters, including pacemaker wires; tricuspid valve endocarditis (a major source in intravenous drug abusers[164]); septic thrombophlebitis (again a significant problem in drug addicts); and indwelling prosthetic devices. Immunocompromised patients are particularly vulnerable. Although rare, anaerobic infection of the lateral pharyngeal space sometimes leads to suppurative jugular vein thrombosis and septic pulmonary emboli (Lemierre syndrome).[165,166]

The diagnosis is usually established by positive blood cultures and the presence of an infected source for the emboli. It is worth noting that positive radiographic findings, particularly abnormalities seen on CT, may be present before blood cultures become positive[167] and the diagnosis may be first suggested at chest CT.[168]

The usual radiographic and CT scanning appearances[167,168] consist of multiple pulmonary opacities. As usual, CT shows more lesions and enables the radiologist to characterize these lesions with greater accuracy than is possible from plain chest radiographs. The opacities may occur in any portion of the lungs but are usually maximal in the lower zones. The lesions are usually either round (nodular) in shape or show the expected shape of a pulmonary infarct, namely a wedge-shaped density based on the pleura and pointing to the hilum. Sometimes, however, the opacities are completely nonspecific in shape. They may be any size and frequently cavitate (Fig. 5.39), a feature more easily recognized at CT. For example, in the series by Kuhlman et al,[167] 50% of the visible nodules showed cavitation. Air bronchograms are frequently seen, particularly at CT, in all types of opacity, including the nodular lesions. A relatively common CT finding of both sterile and infected infarcts, which may be helpful in differential diagnosis, is the "feeding vessel sign", a distinct vessel leading to the apex of a peripheral area of consolidation.[167–169] This sign is not specific for embolic sequelae, although it is seen more frequently with septic emboli and sterile thromboembolic infarction than in other conditions. The combination of multiple peripheral nodules or wedge-shaped consolidations, some of which have cavitated, and a distinct feeding vessel in the appropriate clinical setting is highly suggestive of the diagnosis of septic emboli.[167,168] Accompanying pleural effusion and empyema are common features.[167,168]

Identification of intraluminal filling defects in the pulmonary arteries is not an expected feature, because septic infarcts are almost invariably the consequence of very small infected emboli that lodge in the distal pulmonary vasculature.

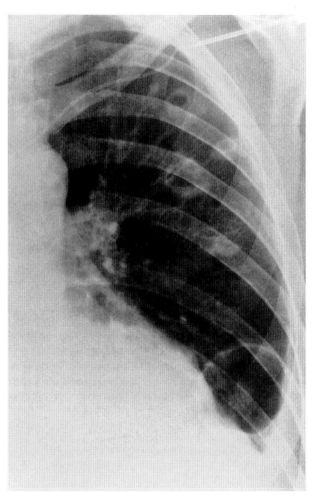

Fig. 5.39 Septic emboli caused by staphylococcal septicemia in a patient on renal dialysis with an infected dialysis shunt site. Note the multiple round pulmonary cavities with thin walls.

BACTERIAL PARAPNEUMONIC PLEURAL EFFUSIONS AND EMPYEMA

It is often impossible to distinguish between an uncomplicated parapneumonic pleural effusion and an infected collection (empyema). For conclusive proof of an empyema, positive pleural fluid cultures are needed.[170] Another definition of empyema requires that the pleural fluid must have a specific gravity greater than 1.018[171] and a white blood cell count greater than 500 cells/mm³ or a protein level greater than 2.5 g/dl. Vianna[172] defined an empyema as pleural fluid with either positive cultures for the same microorganism from at least two consecutive samples or a white blood cell count greater than 15,000 cells/mm³,[173] and a protein level above 3 g/dl. Approximately 40% of patients with pneumonia develop an effusion and, whether infected or not, consideration needs to be given as to whether the pleural effusion is likely to take a complicated or uncomplicated course[174]; the spectrum and timing of treatment options are wide, and range from the conservative to aggressive surgical intervention for multiloculated empyema.[175] The ability of imaging features alone to predict the need for surgical versus medical management is limited.[176,177]

The development of an empyema has been described in three stages, although these often merge with each other. First is the

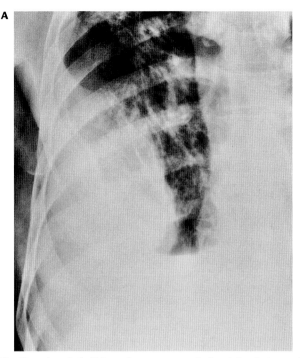
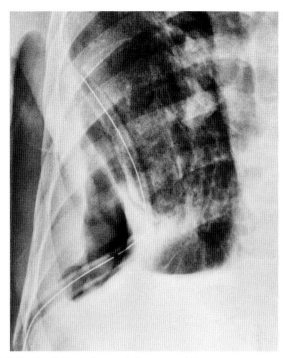

Fig. 5.40   Pleural peel. **A**, Tuberculous empyema before tube drainage. **B**, Following tube drainage, air has entered the empyema space, allowing recognition of the greatly thickened parietal and visceral pleura.

exudative stage characterized by the rapid outpouring of sterile pleural fluid into the pleural space in response to inflammation of the pleura. The associated pneumonic process is usually contiguous with the visceral pleura and results in increased permeability of the capillaries in the visceral pleura. The pleural fluid in this stage is characterized by a low white blood count, a low lactic dehydrogenase (LDH) level, a normal glucose level, and a normal pH.[178] If appropriate antibiotic therapy is instituted at this stage, the pleural effusion progresses no further, and the insertion of chest tubes is not necessary. If appropriate antibiotic therapy is not instituted, bacteria invade the pleural fluid from the contiguous pneumonic process, and the second, *fibropurulent*, stage evolves. This stage is characterized by the accumulation of large amounts of pleural fluid with many polymorphonuclear leukocytes, bacteria, and cellular debris. Fibrin is deposited in a continuous sheet covering both the visceral and parietal pleura in the involved area and the tendency is to loculation. These loculations prevent extension of the empyema but make drainage of the pleural space with chest tubes increasingly difficult. However, the demonstration of septations on ultrasonography does not inevitably predict unsuccessful chest tube drainage. As this stage progresses, the pleural fluid pH and glucose level become progressively lower and the LDH level progressively higher. Last is the *organization stage*, in which fibroblasts grow into the exudate from both the visceral and parietal pleural surfaces and produce an inelastic membrane called the pleural peel (Fig. 5.40). This pleural peel encases the lung and can render it functionless. At this stage the exudate is thick, and if the patient has remained untreated, the fluid may drain spontaneously through the chest wall or into the lung, to produce a bronchopleural fistula.

Most empyemas are associated with a recognizable pneumonia, surgery, trauma, or infradiaphragmatic infection.[179–181] The bacteria usually responsible for nontuberculous empyemas or "parapneumonic" effusions are anaerobic bacteria, *S. aureus*, *S. pneumoniae*, other streptococcal species, and various gram-negative bacteria.[182]

The clinical picture of patients with aerobic bacterial pneumonia and pleural effusion is similar to that of patients with pneumonia alone. Patients with anaerobic bacterial infections of the pleural space usually present with a subacute illness. The majority have a history of alcoholism, an episode of unconsciousness, or another reason for aspiration.

The diagnosis of parapneumonic effusion and empyema depends on recognizing the presence of fluid in the pleural cavity and aspiration of a sample for analysis. Because empyemas are rich in protein, the pleural fluid tends to loculate and therefore ultrasound or CT may be necessary to appreciate the full size of the pleural fluid collection. As a generalization, lesser quantities of fluid clear with antibiotic treatment, and therefore thoracentesis is not required.[178]

The appearance on plain chest radiographs (Figs 5.41 to 5.43)[180] varies with the evolution of the parapneumonic fluid collection. Uncomplicated, sterile effusions appear identical to pleural fluid collections that may accompany noninfectious consolidations. Previous scarring of the pleural cavity may lead to loculation, but otherwise the fluid is mobile. Fibropurulent fluid collections have a predictable tendency to loculate.

The distinction between pulmonary consolidation or abscess and infected loculated pleural fluid on conventional films can occasionally be difficult but has important therapeutic consequences. Empyema requires early drainage with obliteration

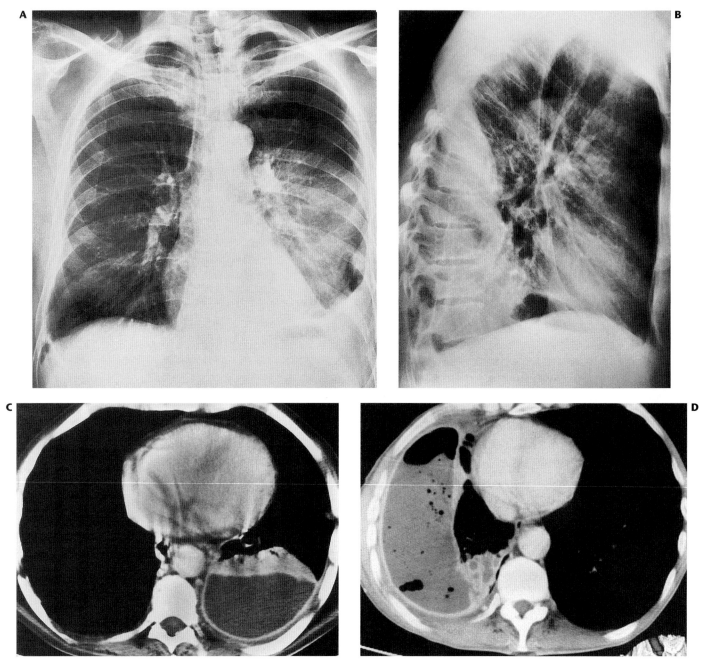

Fig. 5.41 Typical appearances of an empyema on plain radiography and CT. **A,** Frontal view. **B,** Lateral view showing lens-shaped pleural expansion. **C,** CT showing the pleural fluid collection displacing and compressing the adjacent left lower lobe. **D,** CT in another patient showing a lens-shaped fluid collection containing bubbles of air. The uniform-thickness enhancing wall is well shown. Note also edema in the adjacent extrapleural fat. (Pneumonia with abscess formation is seen in the adjacent right lower lobe.)

of the space[183] whereas adequate antibiotic therapy obviates the need for drainage in most cases of lung abscess. The radiographic features to be analyzed are shape and the appearance of any air within the opacity.[184] The shape is often the most definitive feature. Loculated collections of pleural fluid, with the exception of interlobar fluid, are based on the parietal pleura and cause an oval, lens-shaped, or rounded expansion of the pleura (Fig. 5.41). When profiled, the inner margin of the empyema is sharply defined and shows a curved, smooth interface with the adjacent lung; often, however, one or more interfaces with the lung are not tangential to the beam and the empyema therefore has an imperceptible border. Round pneumonias do not show the very smooth, well-defined interface with the adjacent lung that is seen with empyemas. Also, although they may contact the pleura, round pneumonias are rarely as broadly based on the pleura.

Interlobar loculated pleural fluid has a unique radiographic appearance. The opacity is centered on a fissure and is lens shaped with a more pronounced bulge inferiorly than superiorly, reflecting the gravitational effect of the fluid suspended within the fissure. In the lateral projection, interlobar fluid in the major fissure appears as a well-defined lens shape, whereas in frontal projection the opacity is circular and fades off in all directions. It

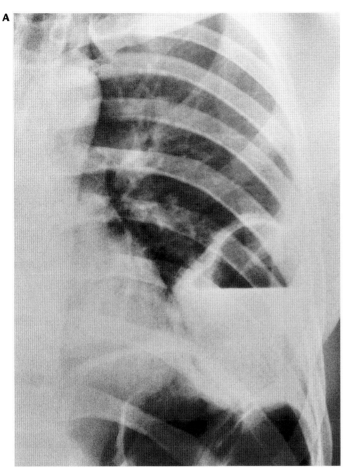

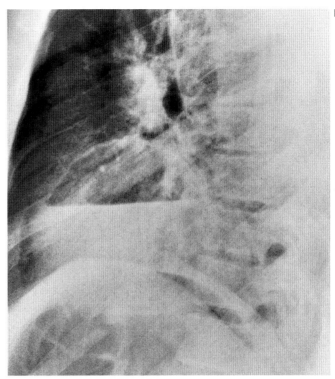

Fig. 5.42   Air–fluid level in an empyema. **A,** On the frontal view, the air–fluid level reaches the chest wall. **B,** Lateral view. Comparison of the length of the air–fluid level in the two projections shows a disparity in length, suggesting that the cavity is actually lens shaped rather than spherical.

is therefore in the frontal view that confusion with pneumonia is most likely to occur.

If an air–fluid level is present, the comparative length in frontal and lateral projections may help distinguish lung abscess and empyema (Fig. 5.42). Since empyema spaces are usually lenticular in shape, the air–fluid level is often substantially longer in one view than in the other. Intrapulmonary abscesses are usually spherical, and a spherical cavity has the same length of air–fluid level regardless of projection. Also, in empyema the air–fluid level may reach the chest wall, whereas a lung abscess is often surrounded by lung parenchyma and the air–fluid level is therefore less likely to reach the chest wall.

CT can be valuable for demonstrating empyemas and for distinguishing an empyema from a peripherally positioned lung abscess. In a large early series of 70 patients it proved possible to characterize the lesion correctly as an empyema or lung abscess in all cases.[185] The features of empyema and lung abscess at CT are described in the following paragraphs.[185–187] They are illustrated in Figures 5.41 to 5.47.

1. Shape. Empyemas, unless very large, are basically lenticular in shape. The angle formed at the interface with the chest wall is obtuse or tapering. Large collections, however, may be more spherical and may then show acute angles. Lung

abscesses, on the other hand, tend to be spherical and show acute angles at their margins with the chest wall. Also, fluid collections in the pleural space may change their shape as the patient changes position, whereas lung abscesses are fairly rigid and retain approximately the same shape in upright, supine, prone, or decubitus views.

2. Wall characteristics. The wall of an empyema is formed by thickened visceral and parietal pleura. This thickened pleura is uniform in thickness and soft tissue density, with a smooth inner and outer edge enclosing the empyema fluid; this combination of findings has been called the split pleura sign.[185] The increased thickness of the parietal pleura is particularly easy to appreciate and is not a feature of a transudate collection.[188] Normally the combined thickness of visceral and parietal pleura, together with the adjacent innermost intercostal muscle, is less than 1–2 mm. In empyemas the parietal pleura alone is 2–5 mm in some 80% of cases.[189] The thickened pleura enhances following the administration of intravenous contrast medium in almost all cases.[177,189]

The wall of a lung abscess usually has an irregular inner and outer margin. It also tends to be thicker than the wall of an empyema, may contain multiple dots of air, and may on occasion even show distorted air bronchograms.

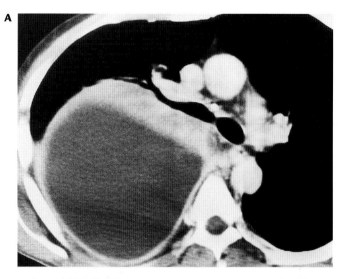

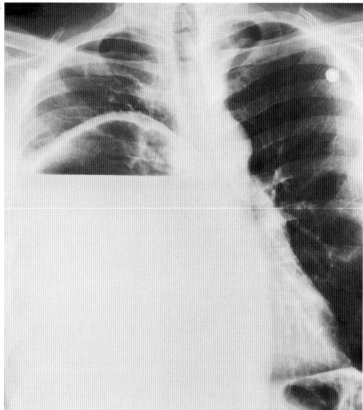

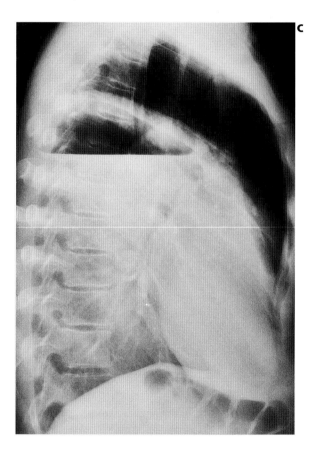

Fig. 5.43 **A**, CT of an empyema showing a homogeneous oval fluid collection based on the chest wall with a very smooth outline and no evidence of bubbles of gas in the wall of the fluid collection. Note also forward displacement of the ipsilateral central bronchi. **B**, Posteroanterior radiograph. **C**, Lateral radiograph for comparison with CT.

3. Appearance of the adjacent tissues. The lung adjacent to an empyema may be clear but is often compressed. This compression may lead to distortion of the adjacent vessels, and if the collection is very large, hilar vessels and bronchi may be displaced away from the empyema. Since lung abscesses destroy rather than displace, the adjacent vessels and bronchi tend to remain in their normal position or are pulled toward the parenchymal destruction. Consolidation adjacent to the fluid collection is of little help in differential diagnosis, since pneumonia is the primary cause of most empyemas, and lung abscesses usually form within areas of pneumonia.

The extrapleural fat adjacent to an empyema is often increased in width, and the widened fat line may show increased attenuation believed to be due to inflammatory changes in the fat,[189] especially in chronic tuberculous empyemas.[190] Similarly, the muscles of the chest wall may be swollen because of edema.[180] Moderately enlarged mediastinal lymph nodes are identifiable in approximately one-third of patients with an empyema or parapneumonic effusion,[191] but these are rarely greater than 2 cm in diameter.

Malignant neoplasms may arise in the walls of chronic, long-standing empyema cavities; this association appears to

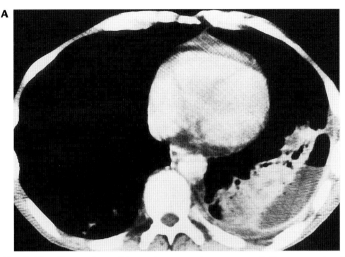
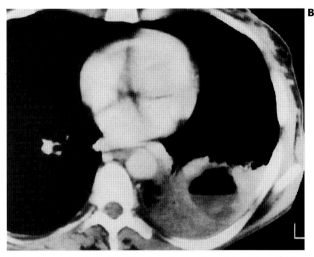

Fig. 5.44   Comparison of lung abscess and empyema. **A**, Empyema showing a lens shape, short air–fluid level, and smooth enhancing wall. There is pneumonia in the underlying lung. **B**, Lung abscess showing a spherical shape, with an irregular poorly enhancing wall imperceptibly fading into adjacent pulmonary consolidation.

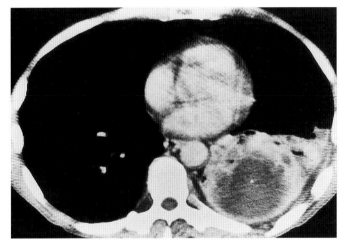
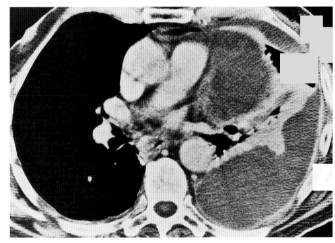

Fig. 5.45   Lung abscess that resembles empyema at CT. The wall of the abscess is relatively thick and irregular and contains bubbles of gas. The fluid collection is spherical.

Fig. 5.46   Multilocular pleural empyema. Each empyema space shows the typical CT features of pleural empyema.

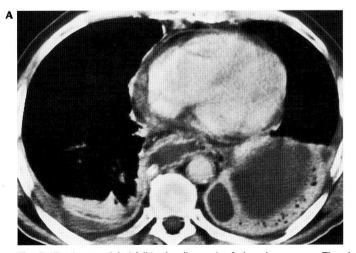
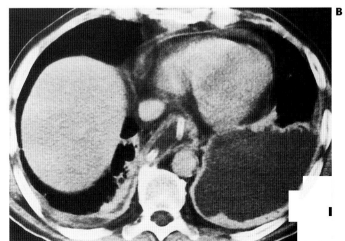

Fig. 5.47   A potential pitfall in the diagnosis of pleural empyema. The pleural empyema in this patient lies largely in a subpulmonary location. **A**, Therefore in this section, the lung is draped over the fluid collection, and air bronchograms in compressed lung are seen between the empyema and the chest wall. **B**, A lower section shows the more typical features of a pleural empyema.

Table 5.2 Comparative features of empyema and lung abscess on computed tomography

Empyema	Lung abscess
Lenticular shape	Round shape
Uniform enhancing wall (usually <5 mm thick)	Nonuniform thick wall
Compression of adjacent lung	No compression of surrounding lung
Obtuse angle with chest wall	Acute angle at interface with chest wall
Separation of pleural layers	May contain locules of gas in wall

be highest in tuberculous empyemas but is also encountered in nontuberculous infection.[192] The range of neoplasms is wide and includes non-Hodgkin lymphoma, squamous cell carcinoma, mesothelioma, and rarely sarcoma.[192] The diagnosis of neoplasm in a chronic empyema can be difficult even with CT[192] because neoplastic tissue and chronic pleural inflammatory disease both have the same density and because nodularity is seen with chronic infection as well as neoplasm. MRI may show a difference in signal intensity between mature fibrous tissues and neoplastic tissue,[192] but the diagnostic accuracy of this difference is unproven (Table 5.2).

PULMONARY TUBERCULOSIS (Box 5.1)

Recent World Health Organization estimates suggest that 1.8 billion persons worldwide are infected with tuberculosis (TB), that there are 7.9 million new cases per annum, and that 1.8 million deaths are attributable to TB each year.[193] Tuberculosis was the leading cause of death in the United States at the turn of the twentieth century. Improved public health measures and specific antituberculous chemotherapy dramatically reduced the prevalence of tuberculosis, and a near eradication of the disease seemed likely. In 1985, some 22,000 new cases were reported in the United States, representing the lowest incidence since national reporting began in 1953.[194] However, in the 1990s the incidence of tuberculosis began to increase again. The increase was widely attributed to the HIV epidemic. HIV-infected individuals, particularly intravenous drug abusers, are at considerable risk for reactivation of tuberculosis.[195] Nevertheless, the highest case rate for tuberculosis occurs in persons over 65 years of age, a group by and large not involved in the HIV epidemic. Tuberculosis in the elderly usually represents reactivation of previously acquired disease as a result of waning immunocompetence with advancing age.[196] These individuals acquired the disease at a time when it was more prevalent than it is today. Tuberculosis remains a considerable health problem in developing countries, and the United States and Europe have seen a considerable influx of immigrants and refugees from developing countries in the past two decades. Approximately a quarter of new cases of tuberculosis in the United States involve patients born outside the country,[196] and in the United Kingdom currently two-thirds of new cases occur in immigrants.[197] Tuberculosis is now more obviously an urban disease, involving

Box 5.1 Tuberculosis

Causative agent
Mycobacterium tuberculosis

Characteristics
Gram-positive pleomorphic rod $1 \times 4\ \mu m$
Acid fast (not decolored by acid)
Aerobic nonspore-bearing, nonmotile
Slow growth: 4–6 weeks

Route of infection
Via the airways causing a focal pneumonia (primary focus or Ghon focus)

Location of the primary focus
Random but with a tendency to involve the mid and lower lung zones

Pathology of the primary (Ghon) focus
Exudative reaction with infiltration of polymorphonuclear leukocytes
Extension to involve the regional lymph nodes in same reaction (Ghon or Ranke complex)
Later macrophage and lymphocyte infiltration plus fibrosis

Radiology of primary TB
Primary focus may or may not be visible
Random location – nondescript focus of airspace disease
Hilar/mediastinal adenopathy – unilateral or multiple. Occasionally very pronounced

Natural history
90% will heal, often leaving a lung calcification and/or calcified hilar nodes
10% may develop chronic progressive tuberculosis

Possible dissemination
Tuberculous meningitis
Miliary tuberculosis

Hypersensitivity to the tubercle bacillus
Develops after 6–10 weeks
Tuberculin test becomes positive
Limits the spread of disease
Associated with caseous necrosis

Secondary tuberculosis
Synonyms:
• reactivation TB
• reinfection TB
• postprimary TB

Reinfection versus reactivation
Present opinion favors reactivation

deprived population groups in particular; the incidence is high in prison populations and among the indigent and the homeless.[198] Since most of the tuberculosis sanitoria have closed, treatment of tuberculosis has devolved to the general physician. Classic pulmonary tuberculosis is readily diagnosed, but increasingly tuberculosis is encountered in the elderly, who may have other serious medical problems, making the diagnosis more challenging. Furthermore, tuberculosis in adults is increasingly a

Box 5.1 Tuberculosis—cont'd

Sites of involvement
Lung parenchyma – classically the apical and posterior
    segments of the upper lobes, superior segments of the
    lower lobes
Trachea and major bronchi – endobronchial TB
Pleura – tuberculous pleuritis

Radiology of reactivation TB
Calcified primary complex may be identified
Unilateral or bilateral disease
Apical/posterior segments of the upper lobes/superior
    segments of the lower lobes most often involved
Anterior and basal lung involvement occurs (10%)
Patchy foci of airspace disease ("cotton wool shadows")
Single or multiple cavities sometimes with air–fluid levels
With more chronic disease, scattered calcifications, fibrous
    contraction leading to hilar retraction and lobar volume
    reduction
Dissemination via the airways: overspill tuberculous
    bronchopneumonia
Hematogenous dissemination causing miliary infiltrates
Endobronchial tuberculosis – ulcers and strictures, bronchial
    obstruction leading to collapse or hyperinflation,
    bronchiectasis
Involvement of the pleura – diffuse pleural thickening,
    effusions, pneumothorax, bronchopleural fistula,
    eventually calcified pleural thickening

primary infection and by no means classic "adult" tuberculosis. A key factor in diagnosis of tuberculosis is simply awareness that this disease still lurks. Almost all cases are caused by infection with the human strain of *M. tuberculosis*, and the remainder by atypical mycobacteria, notably *M. kansasii* and *M. avium–intracellulare*.

The inflammatory response to tuberculous infection differs from the usual inflammatory response to infecting microorganisms in that it is modified substantially by a hypersensitivity reaction to components of the tubercle bacillus. The extent to which the hypersensitivity reaction is advantageous or deleterious in resisting and controlling infection is uncertain. Cellular immunity involving activated macrophages plays an important role in containing and combating tuberculosis. On the other hand, humoral immunity is minimal. When cellular immunity is impaired by disease or treatment-related immunodeficiency or when pulmonary macrophages are damaged by silica exposure, resistance to *M. tuberculosis* is reduced.

The initial response to primary tuberculosis infection is similar to the usual inflammatory reaction to bacterial infection. The response, however, relies to a greater extent on macrophages and lymphocytes, resulting in a more indolent inflammatory reaction. The macrophages become compacted and modified to form epithelioid cells and multinucleated giant cells and lymphocytes infiltrate the periphery of the tubercles. Delayed hypersensitivity develops some 4–10 weeks after the initial infection and is evidenced by a positive tuberculin reaction. The hallmark of hypersensitivity is the development of caseous necrosis in the pulmonary focus or in the involved lymph nodes. The periphery of the tubercle shows fibrocyte proliferation with the laying down

of a capsule of collagen. Inflammatory involvement of the regional lymph nodes in the hilum and mediastinum is a dominant feature of primary tuberculosis, particularly in younger individuals. In primary tuberculous infections the pulmonary focus and the adenopathy may resolve without a trace or may leave a focus of caseous necrosis, scarring, or calcification. Most primary infections are asymptomatic, and are merely characterized by conversion to a positive tuberculosis test.

Various terms are applied to the form of tuberculosis that develops and progresses under the influence of established hypersensitivity. These terms include postprimary, secondary, and reactivation tuberculosis. The term "reactivation tuberculosis", although not ideal because the disease sometimes evolves from primary tuberculosis without a latent interval, does serve to emphasize that most cases represent reactivation of endogenous infection rather than reinfection with *M. tuberculosis*.[198] Reactivation tuberculosis develops under the immediate influence of hypersensitivity, which accelerates the changes described previously. In particular, caseous necrosis occurs at an early stage in the process. Involvement of the regional lymph nodes is not a feature of reactivation tuberculosis; whether this is by virtue of the hypersensitivity reaction or acquired immunity is uncertain. Factors that predispose to reactivation of tuberculosis include aging, malnutrition, uremia, diabetes mellitus, alcoholism, silicosis, cancer, familial and acquired immune deficiency diseases, and drug-induced immunosuppression.[195]

The gross morphologic features of reactivation tuberculosis[199] can be subdivided into the following:

1. The foci of acute tuberculous infiltration in the pulmonary parenchyma.
2. Cavity formation. Airspaces in a tuberculous process may represent excavated foci of caseous necrosis or, alternatively, pneumatoceles or bullae that follow fibrous contraction or endobronchial disease.
3. Fibrosis and distortion of lung architecture. The extent of the fibrosis and damage to the lung depends on such factors as the amount of caseous necrosis and the severity of associated endobronchial and pleural disease. Fibrous tissue contracts as it matures, and even quiescent lesions may show increased contraction and distortion over an extended period of observation.
4. Calcification. Dystrophic calcification often occurs in foci of caseous necrosis. Such calcification takes a considerable time to become radiographically visible and is therefore often associated with pulmonary fibrosis (fibrocalcific disease) or tuberculoma formation.
5. Tuberculoma formation, namely a focus of tuberculosis in which the processes of activity and containment are finely balanced. The result is a fairly discrete nodule or mass in which repeated extensions of infection have created a core of caseous necrosis surrounded by a mantle of epithelioid cells and collagen with peripheral round cell infiltration.

Both primary and reactivation tuberculosis may extend to extrathoracic sites such as the gastrointestinal tract, larynx, kidneys, bones, joints, and central nervous system. In these cases it is generally thought that the primary portal of entry is the lungs, even though in many instances there is no radiographic evidence of pulmonary tuberculosis. Tuberculosis of the larynx and tuberculosis of the gastrointestinal tract have a high association with visible active pulmonary tuberculosis.[200]

Radiographic appearances of pulmonary and pleural tuberculosis

Tuberculosis may involve the lungs in disease patterns that reflect a number of factors: the host's immune status, the existence of hypersensitivity from previous infection, the method of spread of disease, and an incompletely understood tendency of the disease to affect certain portions of the lungs. The radiographic appearances can be considered under the following broad headings:

1. Primary tuberculosis
2. Reactivation tuberculosis:
   - Focal pulmonary tuberculosis
   - Tuberculous lobar pneumonia and bronchopneumonia
   - Endobronchial tuberculosis
   - Tuberculoma formation
   - Miliary tuberculosis
3. Tuberculous pleuritis.

These very broad patterns of disease may overlap or there may be transformation from one pattern to another.

Primary tuberculosis

Formerly, the initial infection with *M. tuberculosis* usually occurred in childhood, but primary tuberculosis has been increasingly encountered in an adult population. In one series[201] over half the cases of primary tuberculosis occurred in individuals 18 years of age or older, and one-quarter of adult cases were deemed to represent the primary form of the disease. The division between primary tuberculosis and postprimary or reactivation tuberculosis is by no means clear-cut; a minority of cases of primary tuberculosis may evolve without any interval into a chronic progressive form of the disease indistinguishable from reactivation tuberculosis. Classically the tubercle bacillus causes a nonspecific focal pneumonitis (Fig. 5.48). In approximately half of cases the primary pulmonary foci are never identified or documented.[202] Indeed the chest radiograph may remain entirely normal despite definite conversion of tuberculin sensitivity or the presence of positive sputum cultures.[203] The predominant radiographic feature of primary tuberculosis is the presence of adenopathy in the appropriate lymph drainage pathways (Figs 5.48 and 5.49). Radiographic evidence of lymphadenopathy was found in 92% of 191 children with primary tuberculosis in one series.[202] Foci of tuberculous pneumonitis when detected radiographically are almost invariably associated with lymphadenopathy. The resultant hilar adenopathy is usually unilateral, and any mediastinal adenopathy is contiguous to the affected hilum. In some patients hilar adenopathy is bilateral or mediastinal adenopathy occurs alone.[204] The adenopathy may be strikingly severe and extensive, particularly in individuals of African or Asian origin (Fig. 5.50), and may closely resemble lymphoma, metastatic disease, or sarcoidosis. In middle-aged and elderly patients lymph node enlargement is less common and usually less apparent than it is in children. Even in children lymphadenopathy is most striking in the very young.

The pulmonary foci of primary tuberculosis are randomly distributed and range from small ill-defined parenchymal shadows to segmental or lobar consolidation. Curiously there appears to be a predilection for involvement of the right lung.[202]

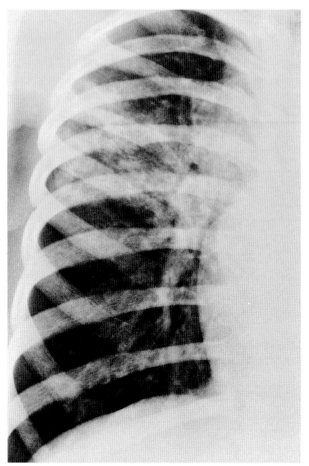

Fig. 5.48 A 10-year-old child with a primary tuberculous focus in the right upper lobe and right paratracheal adenopathy.

Slight expansion of consolidated lobes may be noted. In the absence of cavitation, consolidation of segments or lobes produces a radiographic picture indistinguishable from that of the bacterial pneumonias. The time course is, however, different; tuberculous pneumonia is much more indolent, often taking weeks or months to clear. Primary tuberculosis may be mass like and in an adult may be confused with such conditions as Wegener granulomatosis or pulmonary neoplasia (Fig. 5.51). A single pulmonary focus occurs in most instances, but multiple foci may be encountered. The reported incidence of cavitation varies, but it is unusual and probably occurs in less than 15% of cases (Fig. 5.52). The pulmonary focus frequently resolves without trace; alternatively it may evolve into a small nodule or scar that may then calcify. Such calcifications may be observed following primary tuberculosis in up to 20% of patients (Fig. 5.53). Hilar or mediastinal lymph node calcification is observed in up to one-third of cases. Single or multiple tuberculomas may develop in primary tuberculosis, but they are seen much less frequently than in reactivation tuberculosis.

Pleural effusions occur in primary tuberculosis. In cases studied in major hospitals, pleural effusions have been observed in approximately one-quarter. On the other hand, Leung and associates,[202] studying an unselected series ranging from completely asymptomatic patients to one with a tuberculous empyema, found pleural effusions in only 6%. The effusions are

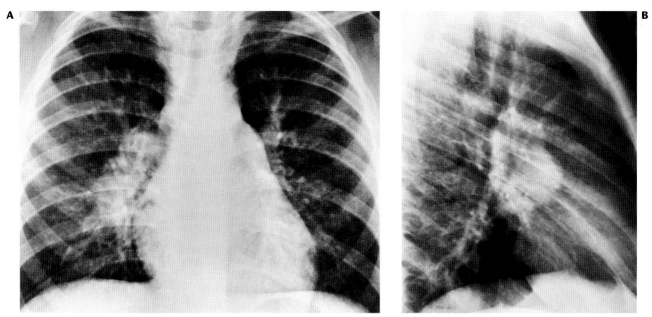

Fig. 5.49 Primary tuberculosis in a 5-year-old child with right hilar adenopathy but no pulmonary consolidation. **A**, Posteroanterior view. **B**, Lateral view.

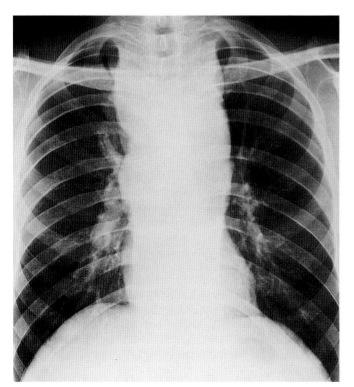

Fig. 5.50 Massive mediastinal adenopathy and slight right hilar adenopathy in a young black man with primary tuberculosis.

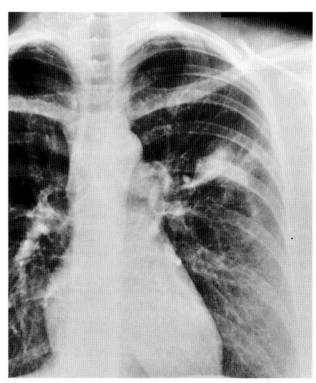

Fig. 5.51 Primary tuberculosis resembling a neoplasm in an adult. There is an area of rounded consolidation in the left upper zone together with left hilar adenopathy.

generally unilateral and are usually associated with some identifiable pulmonary parenchymal abnormality.

Segmental or lobar airway narrowing is frequent and may be caused by endobronchial tuberculosis or by extrinsic pressure from enlarged lymph nodes.[205] The result is usually segmental or lobar atelectasis, but air-trapping occurs occasionally (Fig. 5.54).[206]

CT is capable of considerable precision in the investigation of primary tuberculosis, although in most cases it is unnecessary. CT may identify foci of disease in the lung undetected on plain radiography and thereby assist the bronchoscopist in questionable cases.[207] Occult cavitation may be detected, particularly when obscured by a pleural effusion. Bronchial stenoses,

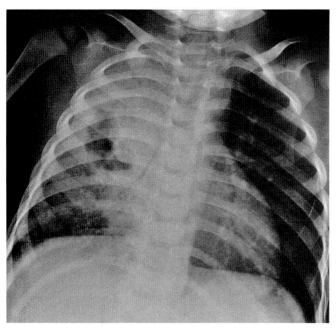

Fig. 5.52 A 15-month-old child with progressive cavitary primary tuberculosis.

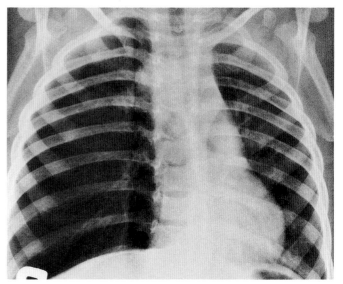

Fig. 5.54 Radiograph of a child with bronchoscopically confirmed primary endobronchial tuberculosis. There is right paratracheal adenopathy and marked hyperexpansion of the entire right lung.

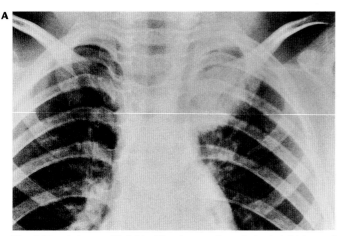
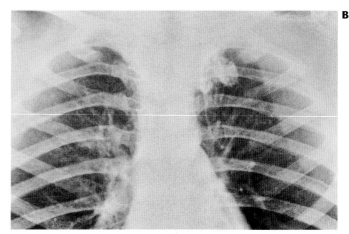

Fig. 5.53 A 6-year-old child with primary tuberculosis. **A,** Initial examination showing left apical consolidation. **B,** One year later showing apical calcification.

bronchial occlusions, and polypoid endobronchial tuberculous lesions, which may be responsible for atelectasis, can all be identified with CT.[208–211] The presence of hilar or mediastinal lymphadenopathy is readily confirmed or detected.[205] The lymph nodes in tuberculous lymphadenitis, particularly when over 2 cm in diameter, show a low density center with rim enhancement of the periphery.[205,210] Focal adenopathy of this type in a child or young adult is highly suggestive of tuberculosis. Primary tuberculosis may be complicated by tuberculous meningitis or miliary tuberculosis (Fig. 5.55), both conditions of the utmost seriousness. Miliary tuberculosis may be detected by CT, particularly high-resolution CT, at a stage when the chest radiograph may be normal.[205,212]

Pulmonary tuberculosis associated with AIDS and other immunosuppressed states such as the myelodysplastic syndromes[213] has many of the clinical and radiographic features of primary tuberculosis even when there is strong evidence that

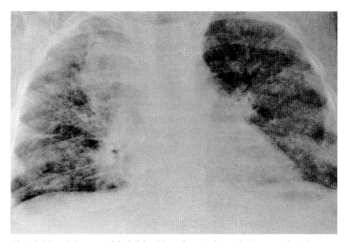

Fig. 5.55 A 3-year-old child with miliary tuberculosis complicating primary tuberculosis of the right upper lobe.

the disease represents reactivation of previously acquired infection. The hypersensitivity reaction appears to be in abeyance and caseous necrosis is much less frequent. It appears that the clinical and imaging features are related to the patient's CD4 lymphocyte count.[214] Generally speaking, with CD4 lymphocyte counts above 200/mm³ the radiographic features are those of usual reactivation tuberculosis. With CD4 lymphocyte counts falling below 200/mm³ the findings increasingly resemble primary tuberculosis, albeit often more severe than usual. Thus hilar and mediastinal adenopathy is very frequent while cavitation is much less common.[215–219] Consolidations may be noted in any part of the lung and dissemination in the form of miliary tuberculosis, tuberculous bronchopneumonia, and tuberculous pleurisy has a higher frequency with low CD4 lymphocyte counts. On the other hand Greenberg et al[220] found normal chest radiographs in 21% of AIDS patients with proven tuberculosis and CD4 lymphocyte counts of less than 200/mm³. Furthermore, in the entire series of 133 patients in this series, one-third had no chest radiographic findings suggestive of primary, reactivation, or miliary tuberculosis. Patients with AIDS are more likely to be sputum-positive for *M. tuberculosis* and have a greater tendency to extrathoracic dissemination.[221] The subject is discussed at greater length in Chapter 6.

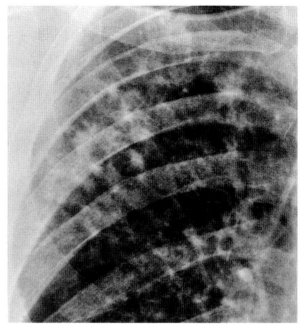

Fig. 5.56 Early reactivation tuberculosis showing patchy small shadows with ill-defined margin in the right upper lobe.

Reactivation tuberculosis

Focal pulmonary tuberculosis

In the earlier phases reactivation tuberculosis gives rise to patchy subsegmental consolidations with ill-defined margins (Fig. 5.56) and a tendency to coalesce so that there may be small satellite foci in the adjacent lung. There is a predilection for the posterior aspects of the upper lobes and the superior segments of the lower lobes (Fig. 5.57), although no portion of the lungs is immune.[222] For example, predominant or exclusive involvement of the anterior segments of the upper lobes has been described in a small percentage of patients (Fig. 5.58).[223] Bilateral and multilobar involvement is fairly frequent.

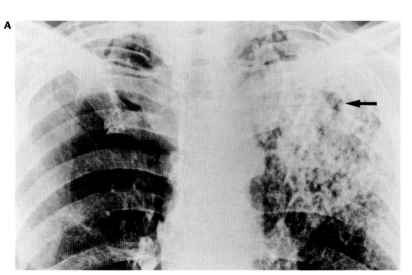

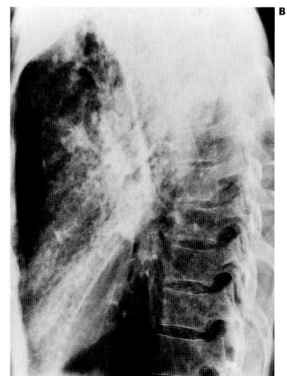

Fig. 5.57 Reactivation tuberculosis involving the left upper lobe with at least one area of cavitation (arrow). **A**, Frontal view. **B**, The lateral radiograph indicates prominent involvement of the apical and posterior segments of the left upper lobe.

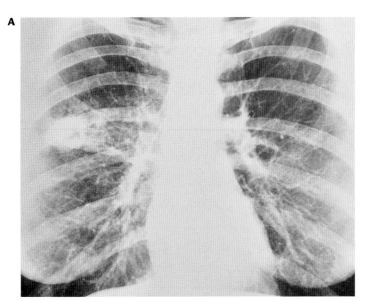
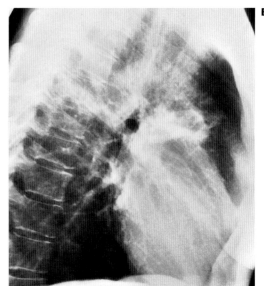

Fig. 5.58 Reactivation tuberculosis unusually confined to the anterior segment of the right upper lobe. **A**, Frontal radiograph. **B**, Lateral radiograph.

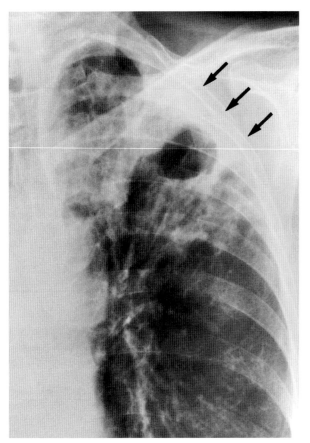

Fig. 5.59 Cavitary reactivation tuberculosis showing localized pleural thickening (arrows).

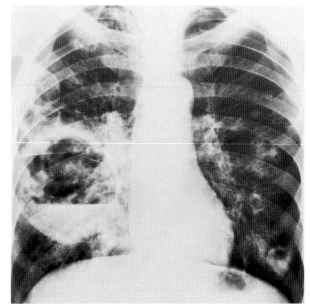

Fig. 5.60 Reactivation tuberculosis with a large right lower lobe cavitary lesion containing an air–fluid level. Other, smaller cavitary lesions are present in other lobes.

The consolidations are usually peripheral in location, and therefore air bronchograms are not present. Some focal pleural thickening may be present in the early stages even in the absence of pleural effusions (Fig. 5.59).

Cavitation is a distinct feature of reactivation tuberculosis and is a finding of considerable diagnostic significance, since it indicates a high likelihood of activity (Fig. 5.60). Even quite small pulmonary foci may cavitate, and multiple cavities of varying size may be present. Fluid levels may be seen (Fig. 5.60) and may aid in the recognition of cavities, the walls of which may be indistinct or obscured by overlying densities. Frequently, however, fluid levels are not present. Apical bullae if present may be misinterpreted as cavitation, a mistake that can often be avoided if it is borne in mind that cavities are centered within areas of consolidation and do not merely overlap them. Patients with cavitary disease represent a potential threat to those who come into contact with them, and therefore immediate infective precautions may be appropriate on the basis of the radiographic findings alone.

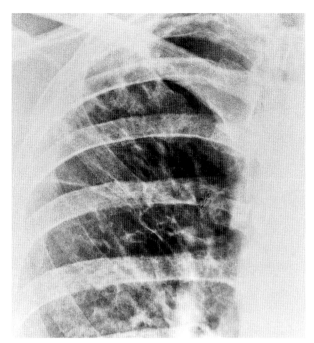

Fig. 5.61 Fibrous contraction of the right upper lobe with elevation of the minor fissure. Bronchography revealed severe bronchiectasis in this lobe.

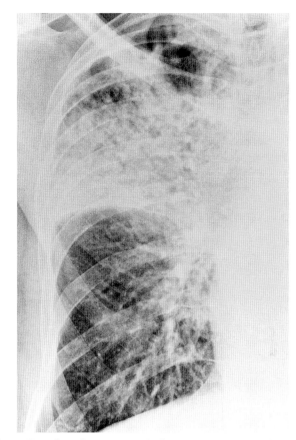

Fig. 5.62 Tuberculous pneumonia showing extensive consolidation in the right upper lobe.

Even in the absence of specific therapy, lesions often become contained by the granulomatous and fibrous response of the adjacent lung. In the pre-antibiotic era the response was prolonged and often measured in years. Specific antituberculous therapy has radically shortened the time required for healing, and the healing process is usually more complete. On radiographic examination, containment is suggested by increasing definition of the tuberculous infiltrates and the development of fibrosis in the surrounding lung. Gradual fibrous contraction of the affected segment or lobe is shown by fissural displacement or distortion of the vascular structures in the hilum (Fig. 5.61). Bronchiectasis develops in the affected lung and is often much more severe than can be appreciated from plain radiography. Calcification is often seen in areas of caseous necrosis coincident with the increasing fibrosis. Fluid levels in cavities, when present, disappear. The cavities themselves either disappear or become chronic, often with a relatively smooth inner wall.

Tuberculous lobar pneumonia and bronchopneumonia

An entire lobe can become consolidated (Fig. 5.62), and cavitation often occurs within the affected lobe. Heavy seeding of the bronchial tree is likely, particularly in the presence of cavitation, and smaller foci of disease may be found in other parts of the lungs. Although overshadowed by the lobar pneumonia, these foci may be extremely important in indicating the true nature of the process. Sequential films show that tuberculous lobar pneumonia is more chronic and indolent than the usual cavitary pneumonias.

Widespread bronchopneumonia presumably results from a breakdown in host defenses with spread of disease via the airways. It is usually patchy and bilateral (Fig. 5.63) and may involve portions of lung less commonly affected by tuberculosis,

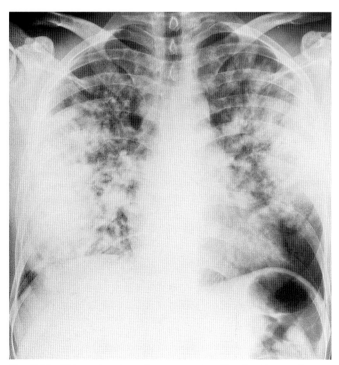

Fig. 5.63 Tuberculous bronchopneumonia without evidence of cavitation or any identifiable originating focus.

such as the middle lobe or the anterior segments of the upper lobes. Fibrocalcific changes may be seen elsewhere in the lungs if the bronchopneumonia stems from breakdown of preexisting chronic fibrocaseous tuberculosis.

In immunocompromised hosts tuberculous bronchopneumonia may become extensive and may be fatal. Cavitation may not be present in the early phases even when the patient has extensive patchy confluent perihilar consolidation.

Endobronchial tuberculosis

On occasion a tuberculous focus arises in or extends into a major bronchus. Tuberculous granulomatous cicatrization may then cause a bronchial stricture, which in turn may cause obstructive atelectasis.[224] The associated pulmonary parenchymal lesions may be obscured by the atelectasis, and the underlying cause of the atelectasis may be difficult or impossible to ascertain from the chest radiographs (Fig. 5.64).

Broncholiths represent an interesting late complication of pulmonary tuberculosis and histoplasmosis (Fig. 5.65).[225,226] A calcified lymph node may erode into an adjacent airway and be associated with hemoptysis or pneumonia. The peripheral lung may show evidence of atelectasis resulting from bronchial obstruction or areas of consolidation related to aspiration of blood or postobstructive pneumonia. On occasion, air-trapping occurs if the broncholith causes ball valve obstruction. A broncholith in one of the segmental bronchi is easy to overlook because calcifications at hilar level are assumed to be in lymph nodes outside the bronchial lumen. Broncholiths in the lobar or main bronchi may be more clearly centered within the airway, a finding that is readily confirmed by using computed tomography.[227] The node may be only partially within the lumen, but nevertheless it may be possible to forewarn the bronchoscopist even if a definite diagnosis cannot be established. Bronchoscopic removal of broncholiths may be attended by severe hemoptysis

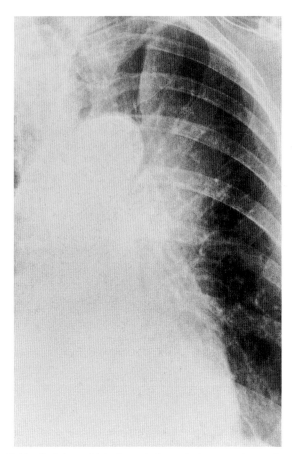

Fig. 5.64 Endobronchial tuberculosis producing complete collapse of the left upper lobe.

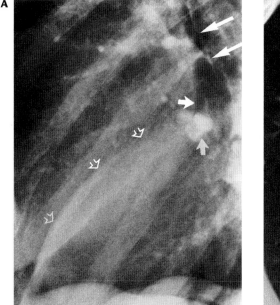

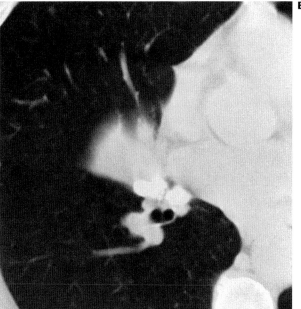

Fig. 5.65 Middle-aged female with hemoptysis caused by a broncholith. **A**, Detail of a lateral radiograph showing middle lobe collapse (open arrows) caused by calcified nodes at the orifice of the middle lobe bronchus (broad arrows). The back wall of the bronchus intermedius is indicated by long arrows. **B**, CT at the level of the right middle lobe bronchus.

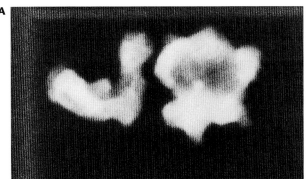

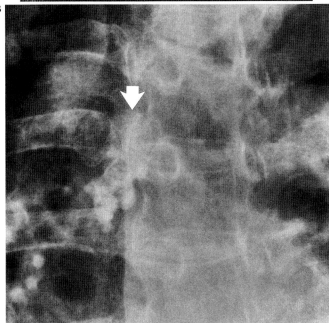

Fig. 5.66   An elderly female coughed up gritty material. **A**, Specimen radiograph of the material. **B**, A previous oblique radiograph showing calcified subcarinal nodes which were later shown to have disappeared. The carina is indicated by the arrow.

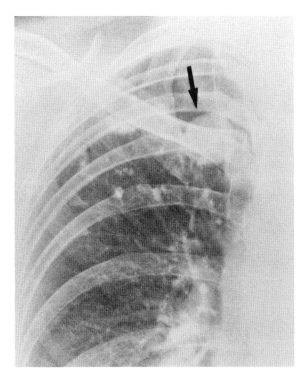

Fig. 5.67   Tuberculoma. Note the well-defined pulmonary nodule (arrow) as well as associated fibrocalcific scarring in the adjacent lung.

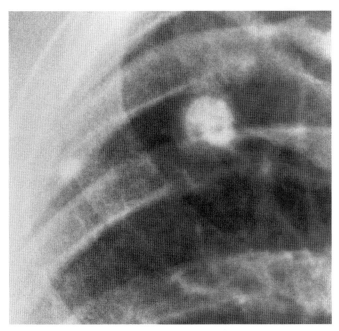

Fig. 5.68   Two apical tuberculomas. The larger tuberculoma has a low-density mantle around a large calcified core.

caused by coincident erosion of the broncholith into the accompanying branch of the pulmonary artery. Hence establishing the diagnosis noninvasively has practical significance. Broncholithiasis may also be diagnosed retrospectively if a previously documented calcification disappears. On rare occasion a patient reports recurrent lithoptysis and serial radiographs show a large central calcified node disappearing as material is discharged into the bronchus and expectorated (Fig. 5.66).

Tuberculoma formation

Tuberculomas are discrete tumorlike foci of tuberculosis in which there is a fine balance between activity and repair. The margins of tuberculomas are usually well circumscribed (Fig. 5.67), although some irregularity or focal loss of definition may occur because of adjacent fibrous changes. Tuberculomas may be multiple and on occasion become large, up to 5 cm in diameter. Some growth may be perceptible over an extended period of observation. Calcification develops in the central caseous core with time and it is often detectable radiographically. It may be amorphous, and if the core is large in relation to the cellular mantle, a nodule of uniform increased density will

result, whereas with a more confined central core of calcification a line of demarcation may be apparent (Fig. 5.68). Calcifications that are more laminar, fleck-like, or punctate also occur and are easier to appreciate because variable density is noted within the nodule. Tuberculomas show little tendency to break down, and

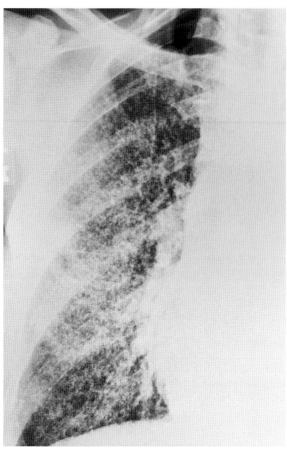

Fig. 5.69 Miliary tuberculosis showing widespread uniformly distributed fine nodulation of the lung.

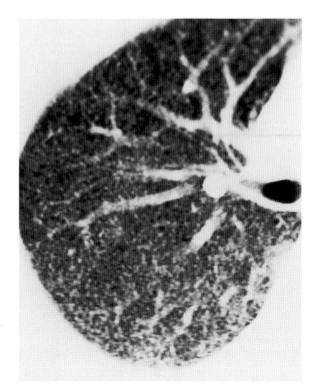

Fig. 5.70 Miliary tuberculosis. CT showing profuse fine nodulation of the lung.

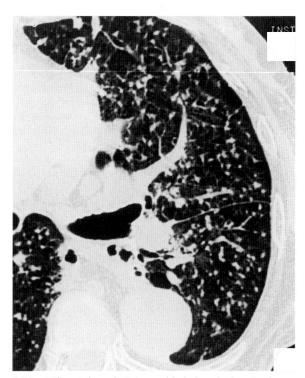

Fig. 5.71 Miliary tuberculosis in an elderly female showing less profuse and larger nodules than in Figure 5.70.

cavitation is rare. Cavitation strongly suggests reactivation. On PET scanning the majority of tuberculomas show increased FDG uptake and so may be confused with a pulmonary neoplasm.[228]

Miliary tuberculosis

Miliary tuberculosis, which results from hematogenous dissemination of the disease, is an infrequent but feared complication of both primary and reactivation tuberculosis. The lungs show a myriad of 2–3 mm granulomatous foci whimsically likened to millet seeds in size and appearance. The radiographic result is widespread fine nodules, which are uniformly distributed and equal in size (Fig. 5.69). Because there is a threshold below which the nodules are invisible, miliary tuberculosis can be present in patients with a normal chest radiograph. Kwong et al,[229] in a retrospective review of 71 patients with miliary tuberculosis, found that approximately one-third of chest radiographs at the time of diagnosis were considered normal. When the nodules reach a critical threshold in size or profusion, they become visible. On or near the threshold of visibility the nodules may appear and disappear on serial radiographs. Miliary nodules are more readily detected with HRCT (in 24 of 25 cases in one series[230]) and have a random distribution in relation to the secondary pulmonary lobule[212,231] (Figs 5.70 and 5.71); there are often patches of ground-glass opacification superimposed on the miliary pattern and when these areas are extensive they may herald the development

of ARDS.[230] Miliary tuberculosis does not leave residual calcifications. Miliary nodulation of the lung has numerous causes other than tuberculosis (see p. 129), but tuberculosis is the preeminent consideration because prompt diagnosis and treatment are vital.

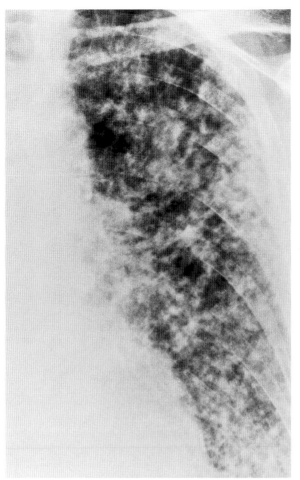

Fig. 5.72 Silicosis in an 85-year-old man. The plain chest radiograph showed widespread nodules. Autopsy showed miliary tuberculosis admixed with the silicotic nodules.

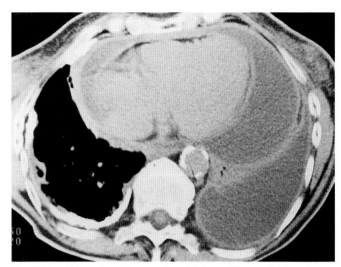

Fig. 5.73 Tuberculous pleuropericarditis in an 81-year-old female. The CT scan shows dense calcification of the right pleura indicating an old tuberculous pleurisy.

Miliary tuberculosis is a rare cause of ARDS, and in such cases the diagnosis can be extraordinarily difficult because the miliary nodules are superimposed on a more diffuse, less structured background of pulmonary density.[232,233] Equally problematic are the rare cases in which miliary tuberculosis complicates preexisting interstitial lung disease. In a case of miliary tuberculosis complicating silicosis shown in Figure 5.72, the diagnosis was not established until autopsy. Even with successful therapy the miliary nodulation may take weeks or months to clear.

Tuberculous pleuritis

Any tuberculous focus may involve the adjacent pleura, and some degree of focal pleural reaction and thickening is relatively common. Im and associates[234] studied apical tuberculosis with HRCT and made the interesting observation that the apical pleural thickening commonly seen with fibrocaseous tuberculosis is composed largely of extrapleural fat. The fat can be considered a packing material that fills space as the underlying lung undergoes fibrous contraction. Pleural effusions are not uncommon in patients with widespread tuberculosis. Tuberculous pleuritis, which may occur in the absence of a visible pulmonary focus, must be considered in the differential diagnosis of any large unilateral pleural effusion for which no adequate cause can be established radiographically, clinically, or by pleural fluid analysis (Fig. 5.73). Less commonly the pleural reaction is more cellular, resulting in diffuse irregular pleural thickening resembling pleural metastatic disease or mesothelioma.[235] CT may demonstrate a pulmonary focus that is not visible on the plain chest radiograph. Frequently, the diagnosis of tuberculous pleuritis can only be established by pleural biopsy.

The response of tuberculous pleuritis to appropriate treatment is varied. All traces of pleural reaction may clear, but it is common to see residual pleural scarring with obliteration of the costophrenic sulcus and distortion of the diaphragm. Residual thickening may be severe, and particularly in these cases the lung can become restricted by the encompassing fibrous tissue and calcification.

Tuberculous pleuritis may become localized and form a tuberculous empyema (Fig. 5.74). The empyema may break through the parietal pleura to form a subcutaneous abscess, the so-called "empyema necessitans". The empyema cavity may also be connected to the bronchial tree by a fistulous track (Fig. 5.75). Drainage of such lesions may result in a chronic bronchopleural fistula that can be extremely resistant to treatment. CT is useful in delineating foci of activity in pleural tuberculosis evidenced by fluid collections within the rind of pleural thickening. Tuberculosis was at one time a common cause of spontaneous pneumothorax, but today this complication is rare.

Assessment of activity on chest radiographs

Chest radiography plays a vital role in the detection and control of pulmonary tuberculosis. Serial radiography is important in gauging the activity of lesions and their response to treatment. It is hazardous to estimate activity on the basis of a single radiographic examination; even though fibrous infiltration and calcification may be prominent features, active foci may be present. Tuberculous foci that appear inactive over an extended period of observation may contain viable organisms with the

A

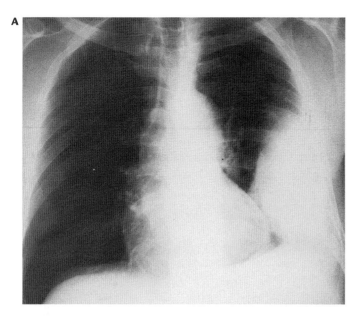

B

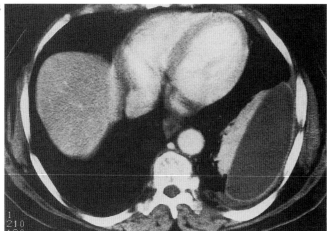

Fig. 5.74 A young Saudi Arabian male with a tuberculous empyema: **A**, chest radiograph; **B**, CT scan.

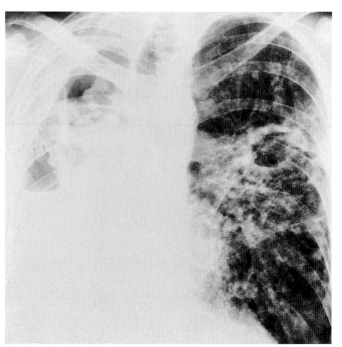

Fig. 5.75 A middle-aged alcoholic patient with widespread reactivation tuberculosis. The right lung is almost destroyed and a bronchopleural fistula has resulted in a hydropneumothorax.

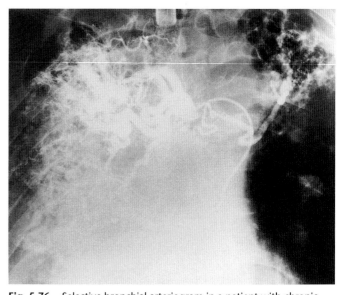

Fig. 5.76 Selective bronchial arteriogram in a patient with chronic fibrocavitary tuberculosis and hemoptysis. The proximal bronchial artery has dimensions comparable with a normal femoral artery.

potential to break down under adverse circumstances. Miliary nodulation definitely indicates activity, and cavitation is a strong indication of active disease. In practice, the physician is often obliged to base certain judgments on the findings in a single radiographic examination. For example, isolation and aggressive investigation may be urged for one patient, whereas another may be allowed to proceed to routine surgery when seemingly "inactive" fibrocalcific apical scarring is present. Nevertheless, the physician cannot afford to be too cavalier about the latter type of case, and some additional study such as comparison with any previous films or a follow-up examination is usually advisable.

Hemoptysis in pulmonary tuberculosis

Hemoptysis is an important feature of active pulmonary tuberculosis. It may also be seen in patients in whom a complication has developed: for example, a mycetoma may have developed in a tuberculous cavity, or the bleeding may be

from bronchiectasis that resulted from the tuberculous infection. The bronchial arteries supplying the bronchiectatic lung can be enormous (Fig. 5.76). Treatment of massive hemoptysis due to pulmonary tuberculosis is ideally by surgical resection but if this is precluded bronchial artery embolization is an option.[236,237] Finally, and very rarely, a mycotic aneurysm, the so-called "Rasmussen aneurysm", may have developed. Such cases can be treated by pulmonary artery embolization.[238,239]

Effects of pulmonary collapse therapy

Some of the most remarkable radiographs result from various forms of collapse therapy dating from the pre-antibiotic era. The thoracoplasty involved resecting a varied number of ribs to collapse the chest wall onto the underlying lung (Fig. 5.77). In many instances only a small portion of the lung at the base remains aerated and the majority of the lung is obliterated. There is of course at least some residual fibrocalcific thickening underlying the thoracoplasty. Various other materials or objects were inserted extrapleurally to compress the underlying lung. These included paraffin, mineral oil, and Lucite balls (Fig. 5.78).[240] Collapse therapy with pneumothoraces invariably produced some pleural thickening.

CT findings in pulmonary tuberculosis

There is little need for CT in the investigation of straightforward cases of tuberculosis when the radiographic findings are consistent with the diagnosis and tubercle bacilli have been identified in the sputum. The CT findings in the various forms of tuberculosis have been established in a series of papers on the subject.[205,208–212,234,241–253] Some of the indications for CT and the possible findings are reviewed in the following paragraphs.

The presence of cavities strongly suggests that the disease process is active, particularly if the outer margins of the cavitary process are ill defined and there are satellite centrilobular "rosettes" of infiltrates in adjacent lung (Figs 5.79 to 5.81). The inner wall of a tuberculous cavity is smooth or irregular, and the cavities usually contain only a small amount of (if any) fluid. In one series of patients with early tuberculosis, cavities were detected in 58% of the initial CT studies, whereas the corresponding figure for the radiographs was only 22%.[241] The CT detection of a cavitary process underlying and obscured by a large pleural effusion may be an important pointer to the

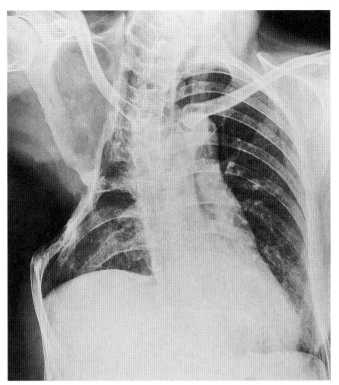

Fig. 5.77 Right thoracoplasty involving the upper eight ribs with partial collapse of the underlying lung. There was no evidence of active disease for many years.

diagnosis of tuberculous pleurisy. There may be an increased frequency of cavitation (and also unusual localization of disease) in diabetic and immunocompromised patients[254] (Fig. 5.82).

CT detects infiltrates not seen on radiographs and can help to explain the presence of hilar or mediastinal adenopathy, particularly in adult patients. The quality and pattern of

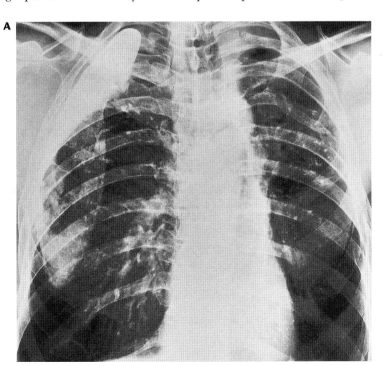

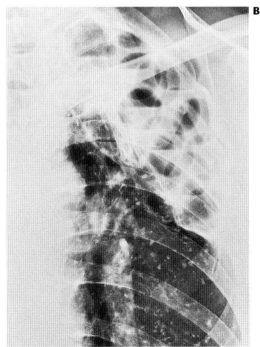

Fig. 5.78 **A**, Collapse therapy by mineral oil injection (oleothorax). **B**, Collapse therapy using Lucite balls.

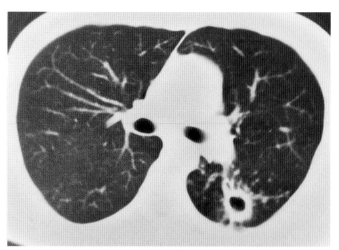

Fig. 5.79 A 33-year-old male with cavitary tuberculosis involving the superior segment of the left lower lobe.

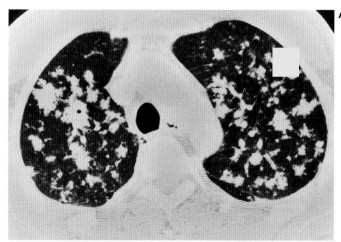

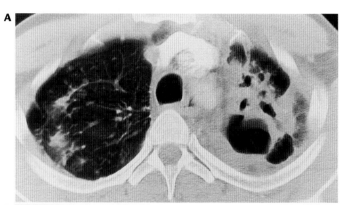

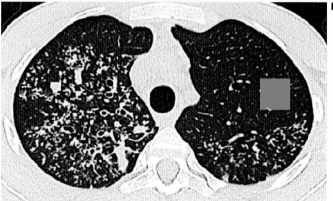

Fig. 5.81 **A**, Tuberculous bronchopneumonia in a 42-year-old male showing centrilobular rosettes likely representing coalescent "acinar" nodules. **B**, Active tuberculosis in a 23-year-old male with smaller nodules of exudate, some of which resemble a tree-in-bud pattern.

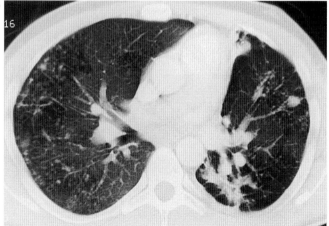

Fig. 5.80 A 24-year-old immigrant male with active tuberculosis. **A**, CT showing extensive left apical cavitary disease. **B**, CT at hilar level showing numerous centrilobular nodules of varying sizes.

pulmonary nodules is quite variable (Figs 5.80 and 5.81). The nodes themselves may show the characteristic features of central low density and rim enhancement.[245,247] At a later stage, calcification may be detected. In a series of over 40 children with tuberculosis, Kim et al[205] found that in 20% of cases the diagnosis was suggested only on the CT scans. The findings included nodules of bronchogenic spread and miliary infiltration not detected on plain radiographs. CT is more sensitive than plain radiographs in the detection of miliary TB (see p. 218).

Although hemoptysis is a classic symptom of tuberculosis, more profuse hemoptysis or recurrent hemoptysis may require additional imaging studies such as angiography or CT. Generally, tuberculosis patients with hemoptysis have disease of some chronicity with major structural changes. Fungus balls within a chronic tuberculous cavity may be associated with semiinvasive aspergillosis – such fungus balls may not always be detectable on chest radiography.[255] Reference has already been made to the use of CT in the detection of broncholithiasis. Bronchiectasis in association with tuberculosis is readily detected by CT.[256]

Complications include empyema,[257] extension of infection through the chest wall (empyema necessitans), bronchopleural fistula formation, fibrosing mediastinitis,[252] endobronchial tuberculosis leading to strictures, occlusions and fistulas,[258] pericarditis and constrictive pericarditis, and esophago-mediastinal fistulas resulting from nodal erosion into the esophagus.[224,259] The various intrathoracic complications are summarized in Box 5.2.

In terms of assessing the activity of TB a word of caution is necessary: seemingly inactive thin walled cavities with associated fibrous infiltrates and calcification may be associated with the presence of tubercle bacilli in the sputum. Nevertheless, certain CT features are highly suggestive of activity; these features are summarized in Table 5.3. Cavitation, particularly if extensive and irregular with a thick wall or in an area of consolidation, is highly

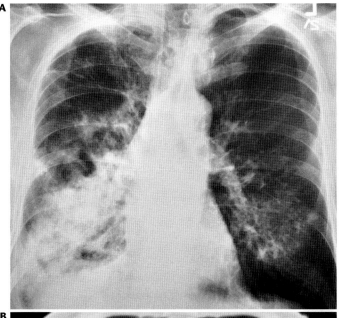

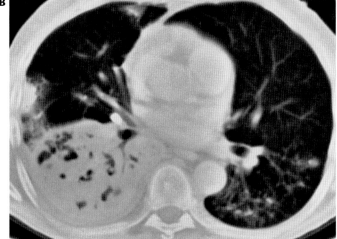

Fig. 5.82 Tuberculosis in a 63-year-old diabetic patient previously treated for cancer of the larynx showing cavitary lower lobe tuberculosis. **A**, Posteroanterior radiograph. **B**, CT scan.

suspicious. However, adjacent areas of lung should be studied with care as there may be important associated findings. These include interlobular septal thickening, ground-glass opacity and bronchovascular thickening and nodulation resulting in branching opacities, "tree-in-bud" appearance, and centrilobular rosettes of infiltration. Miliary infiltration of the lungs is an absolute indicator of activity. The association of pleural and pericardial effusions with parenchymal changes of tuberculosis is a strong indicator. In the hilum and mediastinum, activity is indicated by lymph nodes showing central low density with rim enhancement. Tracheobronchial changes indicative of activity include irregular wall thickening with narrowing or obstruction, contrast enhancement of the thickened wall, and peripheral peribronchial cuffing indicative of peripheral spread of disease. Features that indicate previous tuberculosis but do not in themselves indicate activity are also listed in Table 5.3. One should note that certain features – such as

Table 5.3 CT in the evaluation of activity in pulmonary and mediastinal tuberculosis

	Indicates or suggests activity	*Indeterminate/inactive*
Pulmonary parenchyma	Centrilobular nodule or branching structure	Calcification
	"Tree-in-bud" appearance	Bronchiectasis
	Macronodule	Bronchovascular distortion
	Ground-glass opacity	Pleural thickening or retraction
	Consolidation	Fibrosis
	Cavitation	Cavitation
	Interlobular septal thickening	
	Miliary nodules	
	Pleural/pericardial effusions	
	Pleural thickening	
Hilar and mediastinal lymph nodes	Central low attenuation	Homogeneous density
	Peripheral rim enhancement	Calcification 80%
	Calcification 20%	
Trachea and bronchi	Irregular narrowing	Generally smooth narrowing
	Wall thickening with contrast enhancement	Minimal or no wall thickening
	Obstruction with peripheral peribronchial cuffing	Obstruction without peripheral peribronchial cuffing

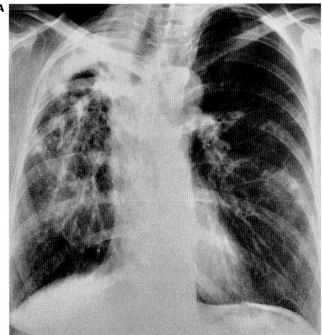

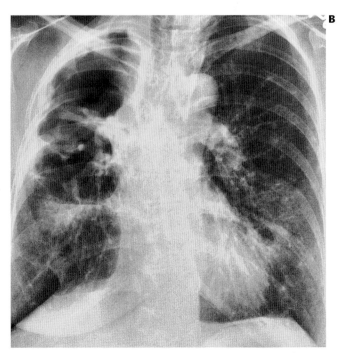

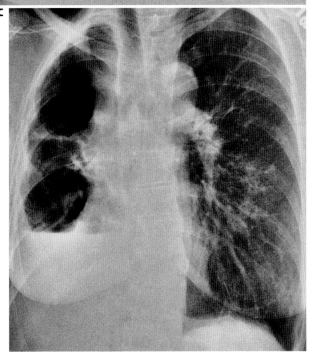

Fig. 5.83 Female with *Mycobacterium avium–intracellulare* infection. Severe progressive destruction has occurred in spite of intensive treatment. **A**, **B**, and **C** are serial radiographs (4 years between **A** and **B**; 3 years between **B** and **C**).

disease: *M. avium–intracellulare, M. kansasii, M. abscessus, M. xenopi, M. fortuitum–chelonae, M. malmoense, M. gordonae, M. szulgai, M. simiae, M. scrofulaceum,* and *M. genavense.*[261–263] The incidence of nontuberculous mycobacterial disease in the immunocompetent population is approximately 2 cases per 100,000 population, an incidence approximately one-fifth that of tuberculosis, although the proportion of nontuberculous mycobacterial infections is probably rising.[263] Nevertheless the incidence has remained fairly stable, possibly because infection occurs from the natural environment and not by person-to-person transmission. The mechanisms by which these seemingly common organisms cause progressive and potentially fatal disease in isolated individuals are ill understood. One of the problems in the study of the clinical and imaging manifestations of atypical mycobacterial infections has been that these organisms may occur as incidental contaminants.

Immunocompetent patients infected by nontuberculous mycobacteria (NTM) can be broadly divided into two groups. One comprises patients, usually older males, with preexisting lung disease such as chronic airways disease, fibrosis as a consequence of healed tuberculosis or fungal infections, bronchiectasis, and cystic fibrosis.[264] A more recently recognized group comprises predominantly elderly females, with no obvious preexisting pulmonary or systemic disease.[265,266] Immuno-compromised patients, particularly those with acquired immune deficiency syndrome[263,267,268] or following lung transplantation,[269] have an increased susceptibility to NTM infection. Compared to TB, NTM pulmonary disease is relatively indolent and runs a chronic course, sometimes remaining static for months, or indeed years: radiographic abnormalities attributable to NTM have been reported to remain stable for up to 12 years.[270] Without treatment, however, NTM pulmonary infections tend to progress and may ultimately be fatal[270] (Fig. 5.83).

calcification, cavity formation and pleural thickening – appear in both columns.

NONTUBERCULOUS MYCOBACTERIAL INFECTIONS

Many mycobacteria other than *M. tuberculosis* have been identified as causes of pulmonary infection. Mycobacteria are common in the natural environment, and numerous species exist.[260] Some of these mycobacteria have been identified as causes of pulmonary infection. These include, in approximate order of the frequency with which they cause pulmonary

Radiographic manifestations

A broad spectrum of radiographic appearances has been attributed to NTM infections; a common theme in many studies to date is the lack of imaging differences between NTM and conventional tuberculosis (Table 5.4).

However, there are radiographic features that, though not diagnostic, raise the possibility of an NTM infection, and very occasionally provide clues as to the specific species of NTM organism responsible. The radiographic features are in some respects modulated by the type of patient infected. Those with preexisting pulmonary disease, typically elderly males, tend to have upper lobe cavitary disease (Fig. 5.84) and associated reticulonodular changes with evidence of endobronchial spread as described by Christensen and colleagues in their review of *M. kansasii* infections.[271] This has been termed the "classical" appearance[272] and is very similar to conventional pulmonary TB[273] (Fig. 5.85). Clinically these patients have constitutional symptoms including weight loss, fever, malaise, cough, and hemoptysis.[262,274,275] A bias toward the reporting of cavitary disease, hence this "classical" appearance, results from the use of sputum culture to confirm diagnosis.[274,276] With the advent of more invasive diagnostic techniques such as bronchoscopic washings[277] and lung biopsy, which yield positive results despite a lower burden of mycobacterial organisms, a picture less reminiscent of typical TB has emerged.[272] This pattern is typically found in elderly females with no underlying pulmonary disease[278]; the picture is characterized by multiple nodular opacities, bronchiectasis, and focal consolidation.[279] Constitutional symptoms are absent or mild in these patients.[274]

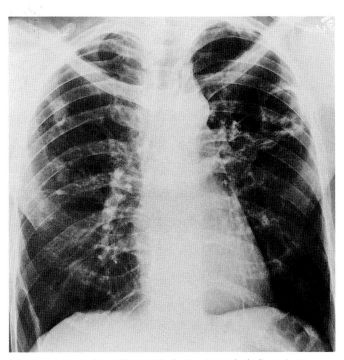

Fig. 5.84 Atypical mycobacterial infection in an alcoholic patient showing thin walled cavities bilaterally, particularly in the left upper lobe.

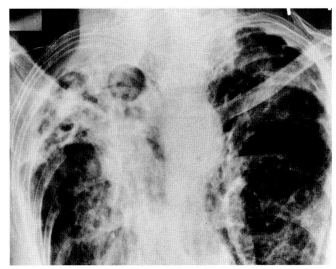

Fig. 5.85 A 79-year-old man with obstructive lung disease and fibrocavitary disease caused by *Mycobacterium avium–intracellulare*, resembling conventional reactivation TB.

Table 5.4 Comparison of radiographic features of nontuberculous (atypical) mycobacterial infections and tuberculosis

	TB	NTM	MAC	*M. kansasii*	*M. xenopi*	*M. gordonae*	*M. malmoense*	*M. chelonae*
Upper zone	+++	++	+	+++	+++	++	+++	+
Lower zone	+	++	++	+	–	+	–	++
Cavitation	++	++	+	+++	++	+	++	++
Bronchiectasis	+	+++	+++			+		+++
Micronodules (<10 mm)	+	++	++					+++
Macronodules (>10 mm)	+++	+	+					–
Airspace disease	++	+	++	+	++	++	++	+++
Adenopathy	+	+	+	–				++
Pleural effusion/thickening	+	+		+	+		+++	+
Fibrosis	++	++		++	++	++	+++	

Data accumulated from multiple papers (courtesy of Dr SM Ellis, London). The number of cases pooled as follows: TB (*n* = 148); NTM (*n* = 513); *M.avium–intracellulare* complex (MAC) (*n* = 228); *M. kansasii* (*n* = 215); *M. xenopi* (*n* = 23); *M. gordonae* (*n* = 17); *M. malmoense* (*n* = 16); *M. chelonae* (*n* = 14).
(+++ = >70%, ++ = 40–70%, + = 10–40%, – = <10%)

The radiographic appearances of the majority of NTM pulmonary infections in immunocompetent patients will reside within the spectrum of a predominantly cavitary through to a predominantly bronchiectatic/nodular pattern. It does not seem that the latter (less destructive) pattern necessarily progresses to the cavitary pattern. However, variations occur and some patients, including patients with cystic fibrosis and patients subject to repeated aspiration, such as those with esophageal achalasia or gastric outlet obstruction, have a predisposition for *M. fortuitum–chelonae* infections[280,281]; in these patients the radiographic appearances are those of large areas of confluent consolidation (Fig. 5.86). Very rarely, NTM infection may present as a focal pulmonary mass with CT features suspicious of malignancy.[270] Nevertheless, these can be regarded as very unusual presentations of NTM infection. Localized pleural reactions occur, but pleural effusions are uncommon. Adenopathy and miliary spread of disease are unusual.

Bronchiectasis is a very frequent accompaniment to NTM infection, particularly with *Mycobacterium avium–intracellulare* complex (MAC).[282] Longitudinal CT studies of patients infected with MAC have shown progression of bronchiectasis in some, suggesting MAC infection as a primary cause of bronchiectasis rather than merely an opportunistic infection of deranged airways.[283,284] MAC has also been implicated as a cause of severe small airways disease, as shown on expiratory CT, but the pathogenesis of such selective damage is unclear.[285]

Cavitation is seen in both conventional TB and NTM infections and various studies have compared the characteristics of cavitation on chest radiography in an attempt, perhaps over-optimistically, to differentiate between the two. There are conflicting reports about the size and wall thickness of cavities in NTM versus TB.[271,273,274,276,283] The reported discrepancies likely reflect the varying stages of disease, and the bottom line is that the characteristics of cavities, and particularly cavity wall thickness, do not allow discrimination between MAC infection and conventional TB in individual cases.

An increasing number of reports describe the imaging of individual NTM species and these are summarized below.

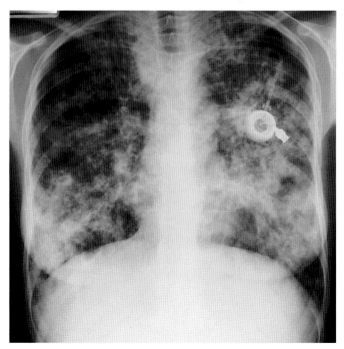

Fig. 5.86 A patient with cystic fibrosis who developed widespread consolidation over a few weeks. Sputum culture revealed heavy growth of *M. fortuitum*.

Mycobacterium avium–intracellulare complex (MAC)

The typical constellation of imaging features, shown to advantage on HRCT, of MAC infection consists of bronchiectasis (often concentrated in the right middle lobe and lingula), centrilobular nodules (usually a tree-in-bud pattern), a few scattered larger nodules approximately 1 cm diameter (one or two of which may show cavitation), and a few small foci of consolidation (Fig. 5.87).[266,276,277,279,286,287] Although these

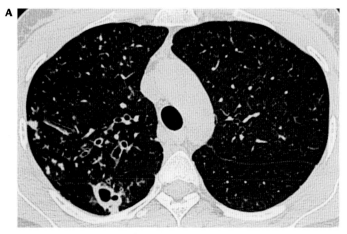
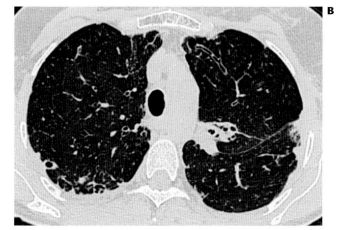

Fig. 5.87 *Mycobacterium avium–intracellulare* infection. **A**, The typical combination in the right upper lobe of mild bronchiectatic changes, tree-in-bud pattern, and a cavitating nodule. **B**, Another patient with a similar constellation of abnormalities.

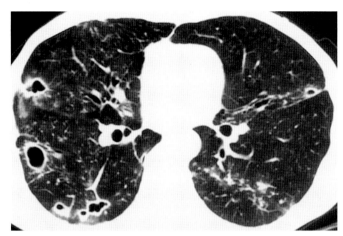

Fig. 5.88 Numerous cavitating nodules in *Mycobacterium avium–intracellulare* infection. (Courtesy of Dr M Ujita)

individual abnormalities are nonspecific, the combination, particularly in an elderly female, is very suggestive of MAC, and the radiologist is in a position to be the first to raise the possibility of MAC infection. Marked cavitation is a less frequent manifestation of MAC infection (Fig. 5.88) when compared to conventional TB.[286] When present, cavitation is associated with an increased incidence of positive sputum smears and culture.[276,288] Compared to other NTM species, bronchiectasis in patients with MAC tends to be more extensive and severe.[282]

Other *Mycobacterium* species

The radiographic appearances of *M. kansasii* infection tend to resemble those of conventional TB.[273] Infections are almost always cavitary, involving the upper lobes with coexisting fibrotic destruction and opacities. Cavities found in *M. kansasii* infection varied widely in size and wall characteristics (Fig. 5.89), offering no distinguishing features when compared to those of TB.[271,289] *M. xenopi* infections have very similar radiographic appearances to *M. kansasii*. The upper lobes are usually involved with cavitation and fibrosis and no characteristic appearances have been reported.[290] Bronchiectasis was present in all cases in one series[282] but totally absent in another.[290] The recent imaging description of *M. abscessus*[291] adds yet another mycobacterial species that has relatively nonspecific features, in this case small nodular opacities, bronchiectasis, and cavity formation.

A comparative study suggested that cavities larger than 6 cm and air–fluid levels within cavities favor *M. malmoense* infection,[292] but the previously mentioned reservation about applying this observed trend to an individual case applies. There is an important report of coexisting chronic necrotizing aspergillosis in some patients with *M. malmoense* infection[293]; the possibility of dual low grade infections in elderly or debilitated patients is always worth considering. A study of 14 patients with *Mycobacterium chelonae* described a pattern of disease similar to that of MAC with frequent bronchiectasis and nodules, although cavity formation was more common than in MAC.[294] In one series, *Mycobacterium chelonae* and *M. fortuitum* were more frequent in younger patients than the age range usually associated with MAC[282]; and these two species seem to be relatively frequent pathogens in cystic fibrosis patients.[295] In a study of 19 patients with *Mycobacterium gordonae* infection the authors concluded that there were no characteristic radiographic findings associated with *M. gordonae* infections and that in each case studied there was an alternative differential diagnosis for the radiographic findings such as community-acquired pneumonia, TB, or carcinoma.[296] *M. gordonae* is usually a nonpathogenic colonizing organism.

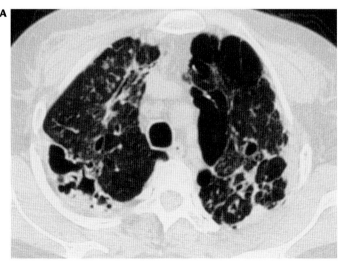

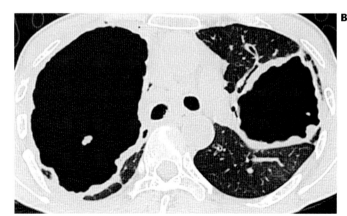

Fig. 5.89 *M. kansasii* infection. **A**, A patient with a background of severe emphysema. The cavitation and tree-in-bud pattern in the right upper lobe are nonspecific and resemble conventional reactivation TB. **B**, A different patient with unusually large cystic cavitation as a manifestation of *M. kansasii* infection.

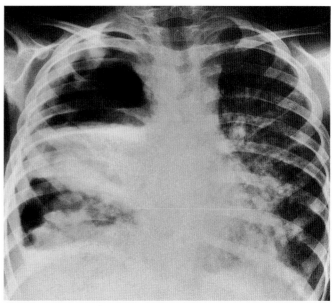

Fig. 5.90 *Nocardia asteroides* pneumonia in a child. These multifocal consolidations and the large right lung abscess developed within 1 week.

NOCARDIOSIS (Box 5.3)

Most cases of pulmonary nocardiosis are caused by *Nocardia asteroides*, although other *Nocardia* species, notably *N. brasiliensis*, are occasionally implicated. *Nocardia* is a filamentous, gram-positive, weakly acid-fast bacillus that grows very slowly on aerobic cultures. It has similarities to *Actinomyces*[297] and though infections by the *Nocardia* occur worldwide, they are rare in immunocompetent individuals. The organism grows slowly and is difficult to culture, and there is no effective serologic test. Nocardiosis is seen particularly in patients on immuno-suppressive therapy,[298] in those who have received organ transplants,[299–301] and in individuals with chronic illness, especially AIDS,[302,303] other underlying immunologic deficiency, or alveolar proteinosis.[304] Obstructive lung disease, including cystic fibrosis, seems to predispose to *Nocardia* infection.[305,306] In several series reviews a variable proportion of patients have no recognizable underlying condition.[307,308] The incidence of nocardiosis appears to be increasing, probably because of the increasing prevalence of immunocompromised patients. Dissemination from the lungs to other organs, notably the brain, may occur (in a quarter of patients in one series[309]).

In the lung, *Nocardia* typically causes single or multiple chronic cavitating lesions similar to the lesions caused by pyogenic bacteria or indeed TB.[310] Fibrosis is a late development, and pleural involvement, usually either fibrous thickening or empyema, is frequent.

The chest radiographic findings are variable.[311,312] Pulmonary consolidation is the most common feature. The consolidations are usually large and frequently cavitate (Fig. 5.90). They may be unifocal or multifocal and may be patchy, segmental, or occasionally lobar. Some patients have single or multiple round pneumonias (Fig. 5.91), which can be irregular and may cavitate, giving rise to a thick walled abscess. In such cases the distinction from bronchial carcinoma may be difficult.[313] Similarly the rare endobronchial mass caused by nocardiosis may exactly mimic a tumor radiographically and at bronchoscopy.[314] Occasionally, diffuse consolidations or widespread reticulo-nodular shadows are encountered. Pleural effusions, which may lead to empyema, and hilar and mediastinal adenopathy are reported features of the disease. Rarely, *Nocardia* forms a fungus ball similar to an aspergilloma,[315] and a nocardial mass in the anterior mediastinum of a patient with sarcoidosis has been reported.[316]

The dominant CT findings are focal nodules or masses or focal areas of consolidation showing central low attenuation, with or without cavitation[317,318] (Fig. 5.92). Extension to the pleura or even the chest wall occurs, resulting in pleural fluid, pleural thickening, or empyema. Unsurprisingly, CT detects more nodules and more cavities, and better delineates pleural and chest wall involvement. Equally unsurprising is the observation that the more immunocompromised the individual the greater the severity of the disease. This applies particularly to HIV patients.[318]

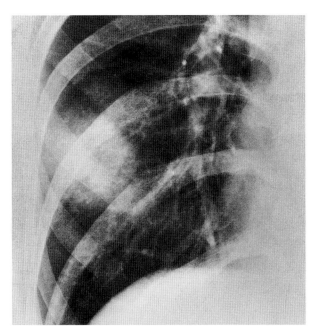

Fig. 5.91 Round pneumonia caused by *Nocardia asteroides*. Note the resemblance to bronchial carcinoma.

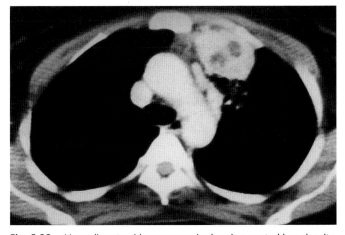

Fig. 5.92 *Nocardia asteroides* pneumonia showing central low density areas and adenopathy adjacent to the aortic arch.

ACTINOMYCOSIS (Box 5.4)

Actinomycosis is caused by *Actinomyces israelii*, an anaerobic gram-positive filamentous bacterium that was at one time erroneously classified as a fungus. Unlike the related nocardiosis, actinomycosis is not an opportunistic infection.[319] The disease occurs when local conditions favor growth, namely when organisms that reside as commensals in the mouth and oropharynx gain access to devitalized or infected tissues. Patients

---

Box 5.4 Actinomycosis

Infective agent
Actinomyces israelii – a filamentous, anaerobic, gram-positive bacillus

Route of infection
Infection of devitalized or infected tissues mainly of the jaw, gastrointestinal tract, or lung. Patients are often alcoholics with poor dental hygiene but otherwise not immunocompromised

Radiology
A suppurative pneumonia causing consolidation or a mass
Cavitation common
Spread to the pleura (empyema) or the chest wall (rib destruction or periostitis, soft tissue mass, fistula) is very characteristic
Lymphadenopathy is common
Mediastinal/spinal invasion can occur

---

are often alcoholics with poor dental hygiene, but are otherwise not immunocompromised. Once *A. israelii* is able to proliferate within the tissues, it causes a chronic inflammatory reaction characterized by abscesses that typically contain tiny sulfur granules in thick pus. The disease most commonly affects the cervicofacial region and abdomen. The lungs are infected either because of aspiration of oral debris containing the organism or because of direct spread from abdominal or cervicofacial disease. The organism produces proteolytic enzymes that allow the infection to cross fascial planes. Therefore, the pneumonia readily spreads to the pleura, producing empyema,[320] and may spread extrapleurally to give rise to abscesses and sinus tracks in the chest wall, bones of the thorax, pericardium, and mediastinum.[321] Hematogenous dissemination is rare.

The chest radiograph[322–324] and CT[325–327] usually reveal an area of persistent consolidation (Fig. 5.93) or a mass (Fig. 5.94), either of which may cavitate. The similarity to bronchogenic carcinoma[328] or tuberculosis[329,330] frequently leads to diagnostic confusion. Indeed the diagnosis may only be made following surgical resection of a presumed neoplasm (Fig. 5.95).[331,332] As with nocardiosis, actinomycosis may cause an endobronchial mass that may be confused with bronchial carcinoma at bronchoscopy.[297,333] Focal fibrosis and contraction may be striking. Widespread small nodular shadowing has been reported.[333] The infection readily transgresses the pleura and therefore crosses fissures and extends into the chest wall. Chest wall invasion is now less common, possibly because effective antibiotic therapy is available.[297,322]

Pleural involvement is manifest as pleural effusion, pleural thickening, or empyema formation but is seldom associated with large accumulations of fluid. Pleural thickening was found at CT in all 8 cases reported by Kwong and co-workers[326]; the pleural thickening was smooth and localized to the pleura

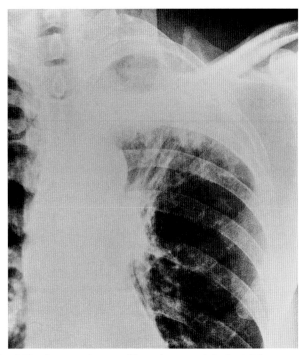

Fig. 5.93 Pneumonia caused by actinomycosis in the left lung apex. The patient complained of shoulder pain, suggesting chest wall invasion. Later a cutaneous fistula developed and discharged sulfur granules.

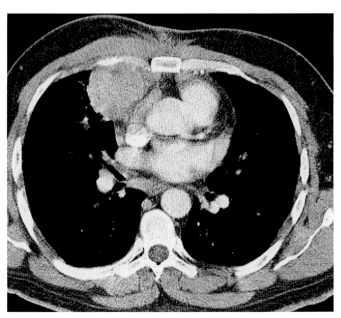

Fig. 5.95 A mass-like lesion in the right middle lobe, presumed to be lung cancer, with thickening of anterior chest wall soft tissues thought to represent tumor invasion. This was subsequently resected and confirmed to be actinomycosis pneumonia.

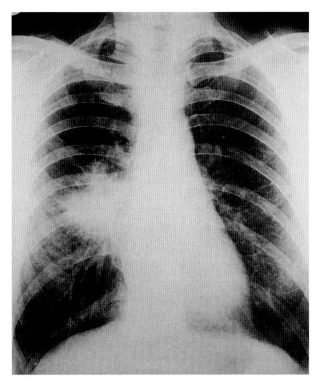

Fig. 5.94 Round pneumonia caused by actinomycosis, resembling a lung cancer.

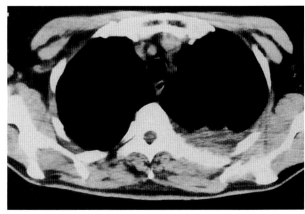

Fig. 5.96 Actinomycosis invading the chest wall. CT demonstrates periostitis of ribs and soft tissue thickening in the left posterior chest wall.

abutting the diseased lung. Rib involvement leads to lysis and visible periostitis, which may be demonstrated to advantage by CT (Fig. 5.96). Similarly, if the spine is involved, there may be a lytic lesion in the spine adjacent to the pulmonary or pleural shadowing.[326,334] Mediastinal invasion with pericardial and cardiac involvement has been reported,[321,335] but this is rare. CT can demonstrate chest wall (Fig. 5.97),[336] pleural,[326,327] mediastinal, and spinal invasion to advantage.[321] It also demonstrates intrathoracic lymphadenopathy up to 2.5 cm in diameter in a high proportion of patients.[326,336]

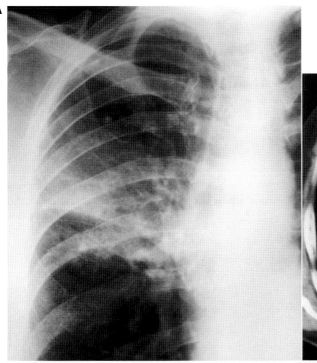

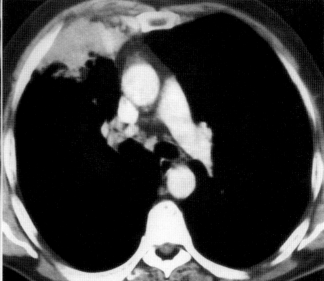

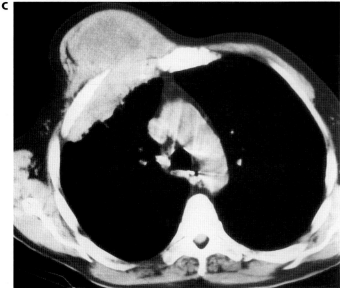

Fig. 5.97 Actinomycosis pneumonia invading the anterior chest wall. **A**, Chest radiograph showing pneumonia in the right upper lobe. **B**, CT showing consolidation and probable chest wall invasion. **C**, CT 2 months later showing obvious chest wall invasion with a large chest wall mass with a low density center.

BOTRYOMYCOSIS

Botryomycosis is a very rare chronic infectious disease that resembles actinomycosis both clinically and pathologically, in that gray-yellow granules similar to the sulfur granules of actinomycosis are a feature of the infection.[297] Reports are scant but, as with actinomycosis, some cases present as mass-like or endobronchial lesions that resemble a bronchogenic carcinoma.[337,338]

FUNGAL DISEASE

Fungi include mushrooms, molds, and yeasts but few of these organisms consistently cause pneumonia in humans.[339,340] A mold is a microscopic, multibranched tubular structure that grows at its expanding margin by the elongation of hyphal tips and by producing new branches, known as hyphae. The yeast shape is another morphologic form taken by some fungi. Yeasts are single, ovoid to spherical cells with rigid walls, in which multiplication occurs by the development of buds, with the cytoplasm and at least one nucleus moving into the bud. The distinction between certain bacteria and fungi is not clear, and some pathogenic organisms such as *Nocardia* and *Actinomyces*, originally thought of as fungi, are considered to be bacteria. Pneumonias caused by *Candida*, *Aspergillus*, and *Mucor* are predominantly seen in immunocompromised patients and are discussed on pages 289, 293 and 310. The following section discusses the agents responsible for most fungal pulmonary diseases that usually occur in endemic areas,[341] namely histoplasmosis, cryptococcosis, coccidioidomycosis, North American blastomycosis, and aspergillosis, and then briefly describes sporotrichosis and geotrichosis. It is a popular myth that fungal disease of the lung shows the same radiographic features as tuberculosis. Although this is largely true of histoplasmosis, it is a serious misstatement for cryptococcosis, coccidioidomycosis, and blastomycosis. Although these fungal diseases may resemble tuberculosis in some of their manifestations, they show a wide variety of radiographic patterns and may closely resemble bronchial carcinoma.

PULMONARY HISTOPLASMOSIS (Box 5.5)

Histoplasmosis is caused by the dimorphic fungus *Histoplasma capsulatum,* which grows as a septate mycelium in the soil in many temperate zones of the world. Birds such as chickens, starlings, and pigeons may contain the fungus in their excreta and feathers. The mixture of droppings and soil produces an enriched growth medium for the fungus. Bats are a particularly potent source of infection, but unlike birds, bats are infected and pass the yeast form in their excreta. Many reported cases occur after cleaning chicken houses or exploring bat-infested caves. Infection with the organism is particularly prevalent in the central and eastern United States, especially in the Mississippi, Ohio, and St Lawrence river valleys, Texas, Virginia, Delaware, and Maryland. Pulmonary histoplasmosis also occurs in Central and South America[342]; a variant form (*Histoplasma gondii*) is recognized in West Africa. In Europe, the disease is virtually unknown.

Box 5.5 Histoplasmosis

1. *Acute inhalational form* – massive airway inoculation leading to diffuse bronchopulmonary disease
2. *Acute disseminated form* – hematogenous dissemination to liver, CNS, lungs, bone marrow, adrenals, etc. Rare, more common in immunocompromised patients
3. *Pulmonary histoplasmosis*
   a. Fleeting focal pneumonitis with hilar and mediastinal adenopathy. Few if any symptoms. Self-limiting. Very common in endemic areas
   b. Histoplasmoma formation – single or multiple nodules with or without calcification
   c. Chronic cavitary histoplasmosis. Uncommon. Middle-aged to elderly males living in a rural environment in an endemic area. COPD is a predisposing factor
4. *Mediastinal histoplasmosis*
   a. Mediastinal adenopathy common
   b. May involve the mid esophagus – dysphagia, diverticulum formation
   c. Can extend to involve the pericardium – pericarditis, constrictive pericarditis
   d. Fibrosing mediastinitis – commonest cause in the US. Causes obstruction of the superior vena cava, major bronchi, or major central pulmonary vessels
5. *Liver and spleen granulomas* – common. A mild innocuous form of dissemination
6. *Bone involvement* – rare with *Histoplasma capsulatum* but common with *Histoplasma gondii* in Africa.

Human infection results from inhalation of airborne spores that germinate and convert to the yeast form. Other routes of infection are possible but seem infrequent. Dissemination occurs via the blood and lymphatics, and organisms are removed from the blood by the cells of the reticuloendothelial system in the liver, spleen, and bone marrow. In immunocompetent individuals the fungus multiplies intracellularly until cell-mediated immunity has developed. Macrophages can kill the fungus and this produces intense inflammation. Caseous necrosis occurs, followed by calcification. In infants, as well as in patients with reduced T-cell-mediated immunity (such as those who are taking steroids or immunosuppressive drugs or who have HIV infection), cellular immunity is overwhelmed or fails to develop and progressive dissemination occurs.[343] Acute infection in the normal host, although common, is usually asymptomatic. It has been suggested that most cases of symptomatic histoplasmosis occur in patients with either a structural defect in the lungs, such as emphysema, or some immunologic defect, which may or may not be definable.[344]

The definitive diagnosis of histoplasmosis depends on growing the organism from infected sites or demonstrating it histologically in biopsy material. Culturing *H. capsulatum* is difficult but, more important, it takes time. Therefore in acutely ill patients the diagnosis has to be made histologically. In disseminated disease the bone marrow is the best source: in one series the bone marrow examination yielded the organism in 15 of 19 cases.[345]

Several tests for histoplasmosis depend on the immune response.[346] All have the disadvantage of sometimes being negative in disseminated disease, and all may be positive in the absence of active disease, presumably because of previous exposure. Skin testing is now recommended only for epidemiologic studies, not for diagnosing active disease.[343] The complement fixation test, immunodiffusion test, radioimmunoassay, and enzyme immunoassay give more quantitative results. The first two are insensitive but specific, whereas the latter two are very sensitive but nonspecific.[343] Radioimmunoassay of antigen (rather than antibody) in urine and serum is another method. All of these tests are reasonably specific but each has recognized limitations.[346,347]

Asymptomatic infection

The widespread development of skin hypersensitivity to histoplasmin is taken as evidence that millions of people in endemic areas become infected with the fungus. More than 80% of individuals from highly endemic areas demonstrate skin test reactivity by their early twenties.[348] There is usually no definable clinical illness, but many adults in endemic areas show some radiographic evidence of infection, usually calcified foci of healed disease.

The chest radiograph findings (Fig. 5.98) of asymptomatic infection include the following[349,350]:

1. One or more patches of pneumonia that often cluster together, may be in any lobe, and may or may not be associated with symptoms. The consolidations, particularly the larger ones, often leave a calcified remnant, although they may disappear totally. In young children the calcification takes just months to occur, but in adults it occurs more slowly.[351]

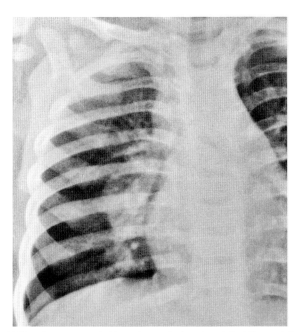

Fig. 5.98 Asymptomatic histoplasmosis showing right hilar and right paratracheal adenopathy.

2. Regional lymph node enlargement and/or calcification, both of which can be striking. The calcifications are in areas of necrosis, and since the necrosis is focal and scattered, the result is tiny nodular calcifications, sometimes called "mulberry calcification".
3. One or more histoplasmomas.

These phenomena may occur singly or in combination. Although cavitation in asymptomatic patients is unusual, it does occur.[349]

Symptomatic infection in the normal host

The major factors that determine whether symptomatic infection will occur are the burden of the airborne inoculum and, to a lesser extent, whether the host is hypersensitive before exposure. Thus individuals from endemic areas are likely to have either a mild illness or no illness at all. Symptomatic histoplasmosis usually resolves without therapy. The chest radiograph is often normal in such patients. When abnormalities are seen, they usually consist of one or more small patchy consolidations, with or without hilar adenopathy (Fig. 5.99).[343] The symptoms range from brief mild malaise to severe protracted illness. The illness resembles influenza, and the chief features are fever, headache, and muscle pains. There may also be substernal discomfort, loss of appetite, and nonproductive cough. Mediastinal adenopathy may be a cause of acute symptoms by causing pressure on and inflammation of the tracheobronchial tree (Fig. 5.100) or the esophagus. The liver and spleen may be enlarged, and other manifestations include erythema nodosum, pericarditis, and erythema multiforme.

Exceptionally heavy exposure can occur in epidemics, often from a single source. The clinical manifestations are then more severe with higher fever. Respiratory failure and death occur on rare occasions.[343] The radiographs may show multiple small nodules or irregular shadows (Fig. 5.101) less than 1 cm in diameter, which may disappear or may leave small calcifications (Fig. 5.102), or widespread fine nodular shadows 2–3 mm in size (miliary nodulation).[344,350,352–355]

Disseminated histoplasmosis

Disseminated histoplasmosis is rare. Approximately one-third of cases develop during the first year of life[356] and the rest occur in adults, especially in the sixth and seventh decades. The male predominance is approximately 4 to 1.[357]

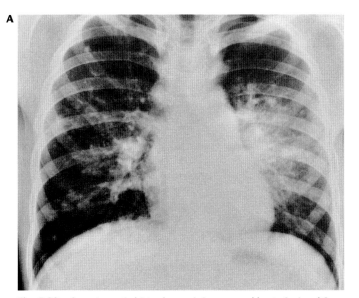
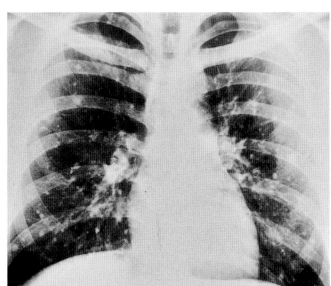

Fig. 5.99 Symptomatic histoplasmosis in a normal host. **A**, Aged 9 years. Major left lower lobe consolidation with disseminated infiltrates and adenopathy. **B**, The same patient 8 years later showing widespread calcific densities.

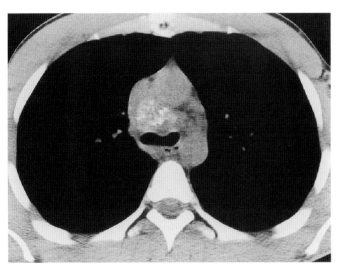

Fig. 5.100 A young male with stridor. CT shows a mass of partly calcified pretracheal lymph nodes distorting the carina; there was more compression of the distal trachea. Biopsy showed *Histoplasma capsulatum*.

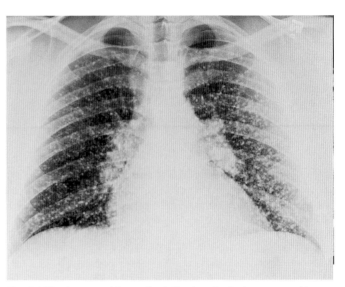

Fig. 5.102 Innumerable small calcifications in the lungs caused by previous acute inhalational histoplasmosis. There is also residual calcified adenopathy.

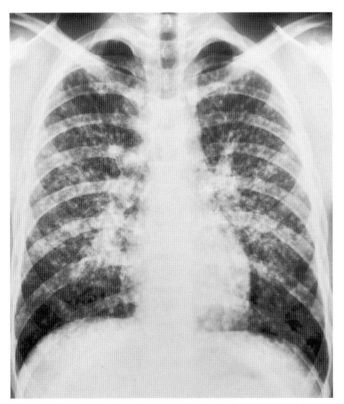

Fig. 5.101 Acute inhalational histoplasmosis in a young man who developed fever and cough after tearing down an old barn. Note the widespread perihilar ill-defined nodular densities and bilateral hilar adenopathy.

Dissemination usually indicates a failure of immune response, either because of known processes that interfere with T-cell function, such as Hodgkin disease, AIDS, or immunosuppressive therapy, or, as conjectured by Goodwin,[357,358] as "a consequence of transient defects in the immunological apparatus such as are known to complicate certain viral infections". Dissemination may

involve all organs, but it has a predilection for the reticuloendothelial system.

The chest radiograph may be normal but usually shows widespread pulmonary shadowing. The pattern varies.

Widespread miliary nodules identical to miliary tuberculosis (Fig. 5.103), interstitial shadowing, nodular shadowing, and patchy consolidations with or without cavities are all manifestations.[349] In babies the chest radiograph may remain normal despite overwhelming disease.

Chronic pulmonary histoplasmosis

Chronic pulmonary histoplasmosis can be regarded as an opportunistic infection complicating damaged (usually emphysematous) lung. It is believed that persistent infection occurs only in abnormal pulmonary airspaces. Such infection may then spread via the bronchi to produce chronic patchy pneumonitis. The colonization of large bullous spaces may produce infected cavities that are thin walled at first, but later develop thick fibrous walls. The cavities may enlarge slowly and destroy lung, exacerbating the symptoms of underlying chronic obstructive lung disease. The majority eventually heal without treatment. In the few cases that become progressive the course is relentlessly downhill. In one large study of 50 patients with relapse following treatment, 15 died.[359] The subject of mediastinal fibrosis[360] caused by histoplasmosis is discussed in Chapter 14.

The symptoms of chronic pulmonary histoplasmosis are similar to those of pulmonary tuberculosis, with mild to moderate malaise, fever, weight loss, and productive cough. Hemoptysis is common in patients with cavitary disease, and chest pain can be a distinct feature.

The radiographic appearances closely resemble postprimary tuberculosis. The multiple, small, patchy consolidations show a striking predilection for the upper lobes (Figs 5.104 and 5.105). Although the lower lobes may show evidence of infection in severe cases, they are rarely if ever involved in isolation. The consolidations may be unilateral but are frequently bilateral.

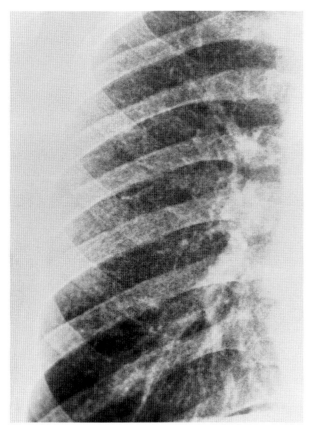

Fig. 5.103 Disseminated miliary histoplasmosis. Note the similarity to miliary tuberculosis.

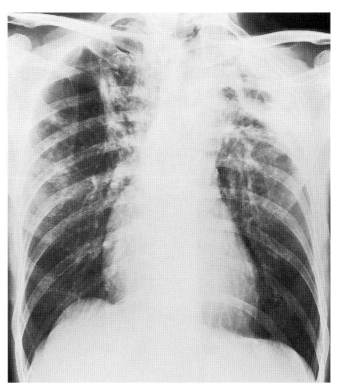

Fig. 5.104 Chronic histoplasmosis showing upper lobe consolidation, contraction, and cavitation. Note the similarity to reactivation tuberculosis.

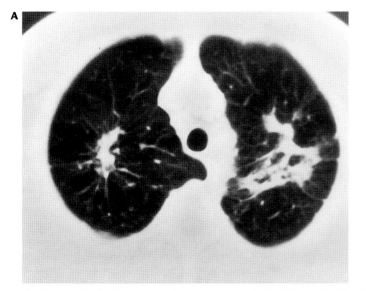

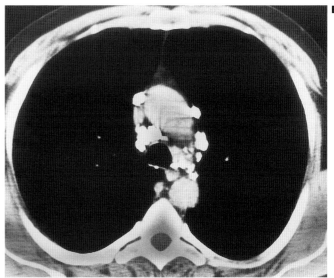

Fig. 5.105 A middle-aged man from the Shenandoah Valley of Virginia with **A**, bilateral apical fibrocavitary histoplasmosis and **B**, extensive calcification of mediastinal lymph nodes.

Cavitation, previously thought to be a common feature,[361] occurs in the minority (Fig. 5.106). The infected cavities involve the upper lobes particularly and are frequently bilateral; the cavities may resolve, but often they persist or progress. As with tuberculosis, the upper lobes contract because of scarring and destruction by the infection. Pleural effusion may occur but is rare, and lymphadenopathy is unusual.[349,350]

Histoplasmoma

On histologic examination the histoplasmoma is a small necrotic focus of infection surrounded by a massive fibrous capsule.[362] On radiologic examination the typical histoplasmoma is a well-defined spherical nodule (Fig. 5.107). It may be of soft tissue density or contain discrete calcifications. Calcification in the

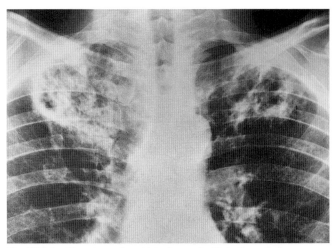

Fig. 5.106 Chronic cavitary histoplasmosis. Note the apical predominance and the large cavities.

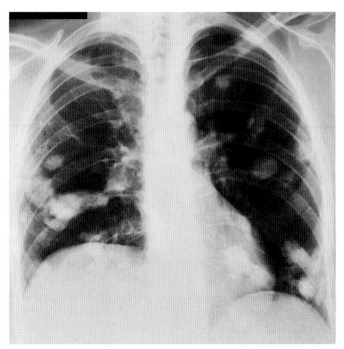

Fig. 5.108 Multiple calcified histoplasmomas. The denser nodules are heavily calcified.

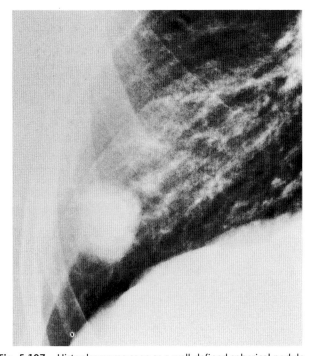

Fig. 5.107 Histoplasmoma seen as a well-defined spherical nodule containing central calcification.

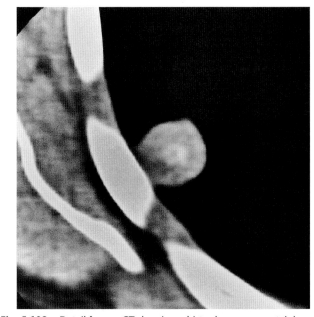

Fig. 5.109 Detail from a CT showing a histoplasmoma containing central calcification.

necrotic center is an early feature and may be seen 3 months after the lesion is first identified. As the fibrous capsule grows, calcification is laid down in laminae that may cause a general increase in density or may on occasion appear as concentric rings on radiologic examination. Histoplasmomas may be single or multiple (Fig. 5.108). The detection of increased density caused by the presence of calcification (Fig. 5.109) is the basis of the CT diagnosis of benignity in the assessment of pulmonary nodules (see p. 107).

The edge of the histoplasmoma is usually smooth or slightly lobular. There are, however, many cases on record in which the edge is irregular, sometimes markedly so. Indeed, the edge may be so shaggy that on rare occasions it is indistinguishable from the corona radiata seen with bronchial carcinoma. Occasionally

histoplasmomas, both single and multiple,[363] enlarge over the years.

The enlarging histoplasmoma, even if it is cavitary or multiple, does not appear to pose a problem of dissemination of disease. In one series[362] the increase in diameter averaged approximately 2 mm a year. This increase in size has at times led to confusion with carcinoma of the lung, particularly when the characteristic calcifications were not present. In general, however, the growth is far slower than that observed with malignant lesions.

CRYPTOCOCCOSIS (Box 5.6)

Cryptococcosis, also known as torulosis (*Torula histolytica*) or European blastomycosis, is an infection caused by inhaling spores that contain *Cryptococcus neoformans*. The organism is a non-mycelial budding yeast found in the soil and in bird droppings, particularly from pigeons. The lung, the portal of entry, is a common site of disease. From here the disease may spread to many organs, meningoencephalitis being the most serious consequence (Fig. 5.110). The disease may occur at any age but is most common in adults. The prevalence is difficult to determine because there is no wholly reliable assay for cryptococcosis, and the question of saprophytic colonization as opposed to invasive disease cannot be reliably assessed from either culture of sputum or the currently available serologic tests.[364] Nevertheless, it is suggested that patients with symptomatic disease or a positive serum cryptococcal antigen, or those who are immunocompromised should be treated.[364]

Many patients with cryptococcal pneumonia have no symptoms, and the pulmonary lesions seen radiographically heal spontaneously. Approximately one-half to two-thirds of the cases of symptomatic infection are associated with immunodeficiency from conditions such as AIDS,[365] lymphoma, leukemia, diabetes mellitus, and drug immunosuppression.

Fever, chest pain, cough, and mucoid sputum production are the usual symptoms.[366] Cryptococcal meningitis develops with a greater frequency in immunocompromised patients than those without a predisposing condition.[367] Meningeal spread is extremely common in immunocompromised individuals[365]; it was seen in 18 of 27 subjects in one series of AIDS patients.[365] In another series, most of those with meningeal involvement had no clinical features that specifically indicated pulmonary infection.[368] In some immunocompromised patients acute respiratory failure may supervene, usually in association with dissemination to extrapulmonary sites; the mortality is high.[369]

A large variety of appearances may be seen on chest radiographs. The descriptions and classifications vary considerably, as does the incidence of the various

Box 5.6 Cryptococcosis (torulosis)

*A. Immunocompetent individuals**
 (i) Single or multiple pulmonary nodules. Well-defined nodules 1–10 cm in diameter consisting of a fungal mass without reaction or an encapsulated mass with possible central necrosis. No calcification. Cavitations rare
 (ii) Single or multiple areas of segmental or lobar consolidation. Air bronchograms sometimes seen. Pleural effusions rare. Cavitation rare
 (iii) Hilar and mediastinal adenopathy may be seen
 (iv) Rarely a disseminated pattern of bronchopneumonia with nodular or irregular densities

B. Immunocompromised individuals
Immunocompromise may be mild – diabetes mellitus, alcoholism, or more severe – HIV, hematologic malignancies, organ transplantation, or chemotherapy
Findings as for A, with the following features:
 (i) Cavitation is commonly seen in both nodules and areas of consolidation (in up to 40% of cases)
 (ii) Pleural effusions frequent
 (iii) Hilar and mediastinal adenopathy is a more prominent feature
 (iv) Diffuse dissemination in the lungs is common
 (v) Systemic dissemination of infection is very common, especially to the meninges

* Symptoms may be absent or few, even with impressive radiographic findings. *C. neoformans* has a predilection for CSF – meningitis in a patient with the above findings but few chest symptoms is suggestive of cryptococcosis.

findings.[366,368,370–372] This may be due to the relative frequency and severity of immunodeficiency in the patient populations being described. There does not appear to be any difference in the range of radiographic abnormalities between HIV-infected patients, or non-HIV non-transplanted patients.[371] In general, three patterns are encountered:

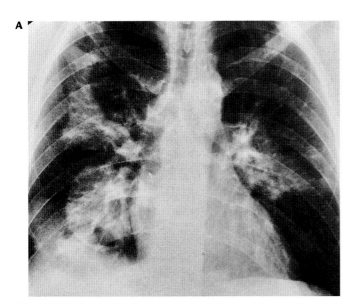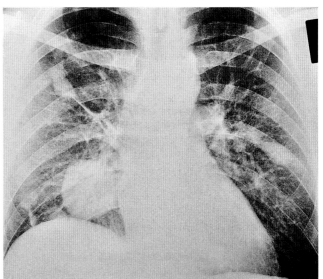

Fig. 5.110 Cryptococcal meningitis in a 27-year-old man without known immunocompromise or pulmonary symptoms. **A**, At presentation. **B**, Eight months later.

1. One or more spherical nodules or masses
2. One or more areas of patchy consolidation
3. Multiple small nodules or irregular shadows.

Hilar and mediastinal adenopathy may accompany any of these patterns, as may pleural effusions.

Nodules and masses

The size of these mass lesions varies from barely visible to huge.[373] They are usually single (Figs 5.111 and 5.112) but may be multiple, and they vary in location with no predilection for any one lobe or zone. Some are composed largely of fungus with little associated inflammatory response,[370] a form of disease that produces a well-defined mass and in the few cases reported is not associated with lymphadenopathy, cavitation, or pleural effusion. The remainder are predominantly due to fibrous tissue with central caseation and abundant organisms. These lesions are usually poorly defined and may show cavitation and associated lymphadenopathy, with both phenomena said to be more frequent in immunocompromised patients.[374]

From the preceding description it is clear that the distinction from bronchial carcinoma is often difficult (Figs 5.111 and 5.112), usually requiring biopsy. Multiple nodules can resemble metastatic disease.[375] Sputum cultures and bronchial washings that grow *C. neoformans* do not exclude the diagnosis of carcinoma. *Cryptococcus* colonizes the respiratory tract in many chronic disorders and, therefore, is often found in patients with bronchial carcinoma. CT confirms that nodules (between 5 and 20 mm) are the most common manifestation of pulmonary cryptococcosis.[376] In approximately half of the nodules there

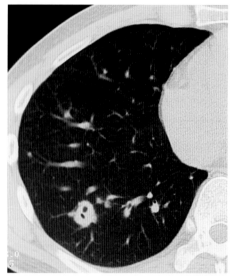

Fig. 5.112 Nonspecific cavitating nodule in the right lower lobe caused by *Cryptococcus*. (Courtesy of Dr M Ujita)

was adjacent, or surrounding, a ground-glass opacification (halo sign), thought to represent granulomatous inflammation (rather than hemorrhage).[376]

Patchy consolidation

As with the masses, the size, location, and multiplicity of consolidation vary greatly; some series have shown a predilection for the lower zones (Fig. 5.113), and some a predominance of upper lobe presentations.[377] Air bronchograms may be present. Cavitation (Fig. 5.114) and associated lymphadenopathy occur but are relatively unusual. Unlike the consolidative lesions of histoplasmosis and tuberculosis, subsequent loss of volume and calcification do not appear to be prominent features, though a single case report suggests that residual fibrosis can occur.[378] A crazy-paving pattern on CT has been reported in one case[376] and, interestingly, cryptococcosis has been reported in a patient with alveolar proteinosis (a frequent cause of crazy-paving).[379]

Widespread small nodular or irregular shadows

The pattern of widespread small shadows is the least common and is indistinguishable from a host of other interstitial diseases. When nodular it resembles miliary tuberculosis and other fungal infections.

Pleural effusions

Pleural effusions are relatively rare in pulmonary cryptococcosis either radiographically[370] or at CT.[379] When seen, they typically occur in the immunocompromised host[380] and are almost equally distributed between localized and disseminated disease.[381]

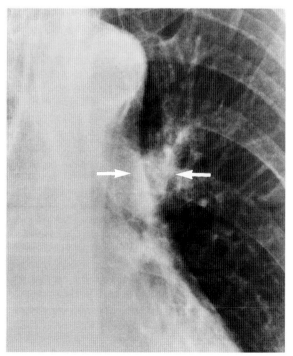

Fig. 5.111 Cryptococcal nodule. An indistinct nodule (arrows) projected over the left hilum, thought to be a lung cancer.

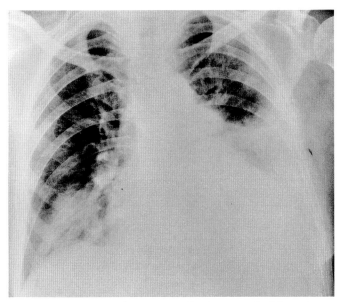

Fig. 5.113 Cryptococcal pneumonia showing extensive bilateral middle and lower zone consolidation.

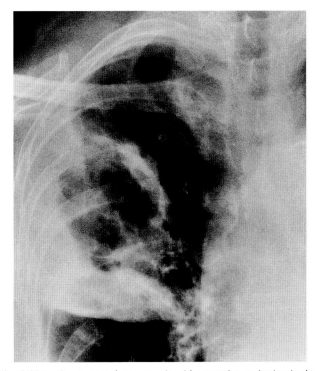

Fig. 5.114 Cryptococcal pneumonia with extensive cavitation in the right upper lobe.

Box 5.7 Coccidioidomycosis

Characteristics of *Coccidioides immitis*
A dimorphic fungus
Mycelial spore-bearing form in desert soil – the infective
　agent
Spherules – inhaled spores develop into large spherules up
　to 80 µm in diameter – the disease agent
Spherules may contain hundreds of endospores that may
　develop into further spherules when liberated by
　spherule rupture

Distribution
The arid regions of the southwestern United States and
　northern Mexico, especially the San Joaquin Valley of
　California. Highly infective in endemic areas

Portal of entry
The lungs

Clinical features
Asymptomatic infection – possibly 60% of all cases
Symptomatic infection
　(i)　Acute disease (up to 6 weeks' duration). Commonly an
　　　"influenza like" syndrome but more prolonged. If
　　　combined with erythema nodosum or erythema
　　　multiforme termed "Valley fever"
　(ii)　Chronic/chronic progressive disease (5%)
　(iii)　Disseminated disease (less than 1%). Rare in
　　　immunocompetent hosts. Multisystem involvement.
　　　High mortality

Radiographic findings
Acute disease
Normal chest radiograph or one or more of the following:
Single or multiple segmental consolidations, or perihilar
　infiltration
Single or multiple nodular foci
Pleural effusions (in less than 25% – usually small)
Hilar or mediastinal adenopathy (in less than 25%)
"Cavities" – thin walled and transient
Chronic disease
Pulmonary nodules – often single, round, well-defined,
　peripherally located, may cavitate, rarely calcify
Cavities – may be a true cavity in a nodule or consolidation
　or a very thin walled pneumatocele-like "cavity"
Stable or progressive consolidation
Apical fibrocavitary disease with lobar contraction,
　bronchiectasis, and rarely calcification – resembles
　reactivation tuberculosis
Disseminated disease
Diffuse miliary or reticulonodular pulmonary infiltration.
　Hilar and mediastinal adenopathy common. Pericardial
　effusions may occur

COCCIDIOIDOMYCOSIS (Box 5.7)

Coccidioidomycosis is caused by the fungus *Coccidioides immitis,* which is found in the soil. The disease occurs mainly in semiarid regions in the southwestern United States and Northern Mexico, where it is endemic. Pulmonary infection is acquired by inhalation of the fungus, which occurs only in the endemic areas; transmission by person-to-person contact is extremely rare. Diagnosis of cases in nonendemic areas is, understandably, often delayed.[382,383] As with histoplasmosis, the incidence of infection, as shown by coccidioidin skin test conversion, exceeds that of clinical symptoms,[384] but the incidence of symptoms is higher than in histoplasmosis. The infection usually occurs in adults and is mild and self-limiting, although occasionally it is severe and prolonged. Dissemination is rare but can occur in immunocompetent individuals. The usual combination of adverse socioeconomic factors and preexisting disease including diabetes mellitus and advanced age predispose to the development of more severe pulmonary coccidioidomycosis[385,386] with serious consequences.

The most definitive diagnosis is made by identifying or culturing the organism in body fluids (including bronchial washing[387]) or tissues, but the success rate varies greatly and recent advances in laboratory diagnosis may help to secure the diagnosis.[388] Organisms are almost always found in purulent drainage from skin and soft tissues, sometimes in sputum and lung or bronchial aspirates, and rarely in pleural fluid, although granulomas and organisms can usually be demonstrated by biopsy of the pleura.[389]

Primary coccidioidomycosis

Less than half of patients with pulmonary coccidioidomycosis become symptomatic.[384] Usually the illness is nonspecific and resembles a mild virus infection; sometimes a severe pneumonia is seen, and very occasionally the disease becomes disseminated. The usual symptoms are fatigue, nonproductive cough, and pleuritic chest pain, accompanied not infrequently by dyspnea, arthralgia, headache, and sore throat. A maculopapular rash and erythema nodosum are common skin manifestations. "Valley fever" is a relatively specific complex consisting of erythema nodosum, or erythema multiforme, and arthritis.

Radiographic examination of asymptomatic patients may show fibrous scars, small, often calcified pulmonary nodules, or calcified nodal granulomas.[390] Alternatively, the chest film may be normal.

Symptomatic patients show unifocal or multifocal segmental consolidation, or sometimes perihilar infiltration, which may take a month or two to resolve. Thin walled cavities, possibly pneumatoceles, are a rare feature. Hilar and mediastinal adenopathy and pleural effusion are each seen in very few patients, usually ipsilaterally in combination with a pulmonary shadow (Fig. 5.115). Such adenopathy may be pronounced and, if isolated, should be distinguished from sarcoidosis or lymphoma.[391] Paratracheal adenopathy may rarely be associated with granulomatous masses in the trachea or major bronchi.[392,393]

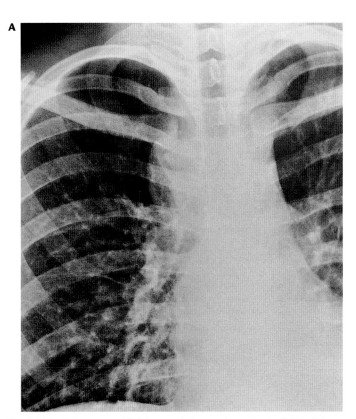

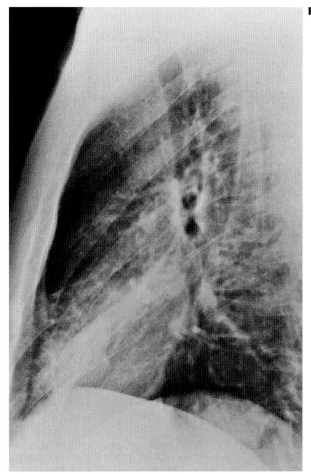

Fig. 5.115 Primary coccidioidomycosis in a patient who had visited the southwestern United States. There is consolidation in the right middle lobe and substantial right paratracheal adenopathy. **A**, Frontal radiograph. **B**, Lateral radiograph.

Persistent pulmonary coccidioidomycosis

Most patients with primary coccidioidomycosis recover within 3 weeks. Those whose symptoms or radiographic abnormalities remain after 6–8 weeks are considered to have persistent coccidioidomycosis. The most common complaint is hemoptysis. Patients with persistent and extensive pneumonia are often very sick. Fatal cases occur usually, but not always, in immunocompromised patients.

Systemic dissemination is rare except in immunocompromised patients, occurring in less than 1% of cases, but is much more common in nonwhites than in whites.[394] Dissemination occurs most frequently to skin, followed by soft tissue, synovium, bone, lymph nodes, meninges, and urinary tract.[389] In general, dissemination is accompanied by anergy to coccidioidin and by high complement fixation titers.

The radiographic findings of persistent pulmonary coccidioidomycosis are coccidioidal nodules (coccidioidoma), persistent coccidioidal pneumonia, and miliary coccidioidomycosis. Coccidioidal nodules are areas of round pneumonia. On plain chest radiographs they are usually subpleural and in an upper lobe. Cavitation is a major characteristic (Fig. 5.116). The wall may be thick but is often thin, in some cases strikingly so. On the whole the cavities are small, averaging 1.5 cm in diameter,[390] but they may reach 6 cm. Rapid change in size is a characteristic feature of the cavities and pneumothorax or pyopneumothorax may be a complication. Calcification is unusual.[394]

Patients with chronic progressive coccidioidal pneumonia have prolonged symptoms and show upper lobe fibrocavitary disease with loss of volume similar to that seen with tuberculosis or histoplasmosis (Fig. 5.117).[395] Miliary spread, a frequently fatal complication, may be an early manifestation of the disease or may complicate chronic pulmonary or extrapulmonary disease. Miliary nodulation has an appearance similar to that seen with miliary tuberculosis. Associated mediastinal lymph node enlargement is common.[394]

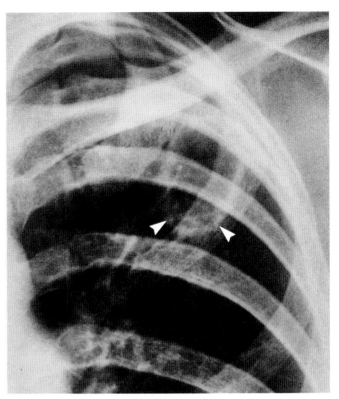

Fig. 5.116 A thin walled cavity (arrowheads) resulting from coccidioidal pneumonia.

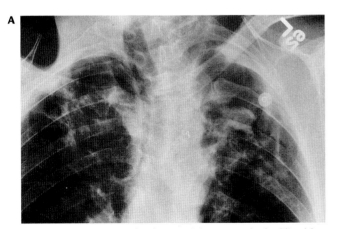

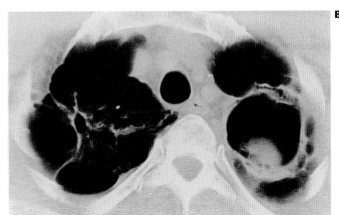

Fig. 5.117 Cavitary coccidioidomycosis in a man who had lived for years in the deserts of Arizona. The diagnosis was confirmed by pathologic examination following left upper lobectomy for severe recurrent hemoptysis. **A**, Frontal radiograph. **B**, CT showing a large left upper lobe cavity containing a fungus ball.

BLASTOMYCOSIS (Box 5.8)

Most cases of *Blastomyces dermatitidis* infection occur in the central and southeastern United States, but documented examples have been reported from Africa, the Middle East, Canada, and Central and South America.[396]

Even in endemic areas the diagnosis of blastomycosis is often overlooked. In one series of 123 cases from Mississippi, the diagnosis was suspected at initial evaluation in only 18% of patients[397]; the incorrect diagnoses entertained included other pneumonias (40%), malignancy (16%), and tuberculosis (14%), hence the reputation of blastomycosis as a great mimic.[398]

Box 5.8 Blastomycosis

Characteristics of Blastomyces dermatitidis
A dimorphic fungus
Mycelial spore-bearing form (25°C) – the infective agent
Yeast form (37°C) – the disease form. Thick walled budding yeast readily identified on histologic examination of infected tissues

Distribution of B. dermatitidis
Virtually confined to North America, particularly around the Great Lakes and in the Ohio, Mississippi, and St Lawrence River valleys. Associated with woods and rivers

Portal of entry
The lungs

Clinical features of blastomycosis
Affects: (i) Skin – raised, well-defined, and isolated maculopapular lesions often with pustulation
        (ii) Bone – a chronic destructive osteomyelitis involving one or more sites. Ribs may be involved by direct spread across the pleura
       (iii) Male genital tract – prostatitis, prostatic abscess
       (iv) Lungs:
              a. Acute form – symptoms of pneumonia
              b. Chronic form – cough, fever, weight loss, hemoptysis, chest pain

Radiographic features of pulmonary blastomycosis
 (i) Focal or multifocal consolidation. Often well-defined margins. More indolent than community-acquired pneumonias. Occasionally cavitation. Adenopathy, pleural effusions, and calcification are not features
 (ii) Focal masslike consolidation. Often mistaken for lung cancer. Up to 10 cm in diameter. Often perihilar or paramediastinal in location
(iii) Disseminated form. Diffuse reticulonodular or miliary infiltration. The originating focus of airspace consolidation may be identified

Diagnosis
Culture of the organism from sputum or biopsies
   (*B. dermatitidis* is not a commensal). Biopsy of any skin lesion is simple and effective

---

The main source of the fungus is the soil; person-to-person infection does not seem to be a mode of transmission. Blastomycosis may occur sporadically or as outbreaks from a common source. Sporadic cases show a predilection for middle-aged men, especially those exposed by occupation to the soil (for example, farmers, construction workers, and workers in the timber industry). Single-source outbreaks often follow exposure in wooded areas, particularly along rivers, and affect both sexes and all ages equally. The common thread appears to be exposure to organically rich soil in wooded areas, whether at work or play.[399,400] The usual portal of entry is the lung. After being inhaled, the organism converts from its mycelial form to the yeast form with resulting infection of the lungs and skin and to a lesser extent of the skeletal, gastrointestinal, male genitourinary, and central nervous systems.[401] The pulmonary infection is often asymptomatic. When symptoms occur, the manifestations are variable, in some cases resembling acute pneumonia. The symptoms may be similar to influenza with fever, chills, headache, myalgia, arthralgia, and cough. In the more chronic cases the disease may clinically and radiologically resemble carcinoma of the lung. Subcutaneous abscesses that grow to become maculopapular lesions with pustulation and ulceration are the most common clinical manifestations of the disease[401,402] and these skin lesions are an important clinical clue to the diagnosis. Biopsy of the skin lesions is simple and usually very rewarding. The outcome is also variable: most patients recover and remain well, but progressive pulmonary disease and dissemination may occur. Only relatively few affected patients are immunocompromised.[397,403]

Since no general screening test is available, knowledge regarding the prevalence of disease is limited. The diagnosis is only established by identification of the organism on microscopic examination of smears from infected sites or, more definitively, by culture.[404]

Pulmonary involvement is an almost constant finding at autopsy, but only 60% of patients with systemic blastomycosis demonstrate significant abnormalities on plain chest radiograph.[405] Nevertheless, in one of the largest recent series, 107 of 123 patients treated for blastomycosis had lung involvement.[406] Several series and reviews have documented the radiographic findings.[405,407–411] A major feature of acute infection is ill-defined consolidation in the lung that is indistinguishable from acute pneumonia. Screening examinations in single-source outbreaks may reveal consolidations in asymptomatic individuals. The consolidation may be unifocal or multifocal. Single-lobe involvement is somewhat more frequent than multilobar pneumonia. The consolidations range from subsegmental to lobar, occurring more frequently in the upper than the lower lobes (Figs 5.118 and 5.119). In a minority the consolidations are widespread bilaterally, and occasionally an interstitial pattern is present. Cavitation appears to be a more common manifestation of chronic disease than acute disease: the reported incidence varies from 8%[407] to 37%[409] in two large series. A pattern closely resembling fibrocavitary tuberculosis or histoplasmosis is seen in some cases of chronic blastomycosis (Fig. 5.120). In a number of cases, multiple intermediate-sized nodules develop. Intermediate-sized nodules are 2 cm or less in diameter and presumably evolve from multifocal areas of consolidation. Pleural changes are not infrequent and usually take the form of pleural thickening adjacent to the pulmonary process, but a small ipsilateral pleural effusion is present; there is a single case report of an empyema caused by *Blastomyces*.[412] Direct invasion

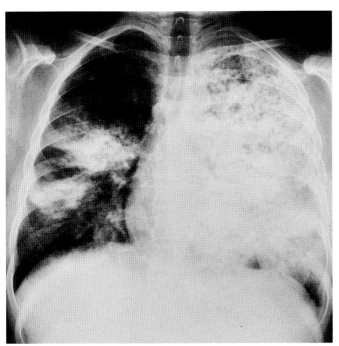

Fig. 5.118 Blastomycosis pneumonia in a 12-year-old girl, showing bilateral consolidation, predominantly in the left upper lobe.

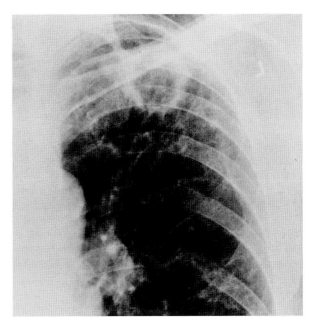

Fig. 5.120 Blastomycosis showing fibrocavitary disease in the left upper lobe.

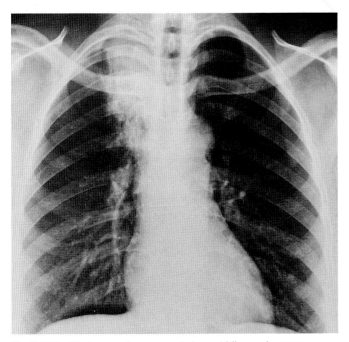

Fig. 5.119 Blastomycosis pneumonia in a middle-aged woman showing right upper lobe consolidation and loss of volume, initially thought to be postobstructive pneumonia beyond a carcinoma.

of the chest wall with the development of an extrapleural mass and rib destruction is very occasionally encountered.[413] Lytic lesions in the bones caused by hematogenous spread are more frequent than direct spread, a pattern identical to that seen with metastatic malignant neoplasm.

Some patients present with a spherical pneumonia, usually 3–8 cm in diameter. The result is a masslike lesion with ill-defined outer margins often contiguous with the hilum. The lesion is readily mistaken for a bronchial carcinoma. The presence of air bronchograms within the lesion may provide a clue that the disease is not a bronchial carcinoma, although alternative diagnoses such as bronchioloalveolar cell carcinoma and lymphoma remain. Halvorsen and co-workers[414] were unable to detect air bronchograms on the radiographs in any of the 7 masslike lesions in their series. However, Winer-Muram and associates[415] found air bronchograms by CT in 12 of 14 such lesions. Calcification is relatively infrequent in blastomycosis and is unlikely to help in excluding a malignancy. Hilar and mediastinal adenopathy, usually mild, occurs in a minority of cases. When adenopathy is associated with a mass lesion, there is a distinct risk that the findings may be attributed to a malignant process. Likewise, chest wall invasion inevitably causes confusion even in younger patients. There are no obvious differences in the acute and chronic pulmonary changes between immunocompetent and immunocompromised individuals.[411]

In a variable but small proportion of cases blastomycosis is reported as causing miliary nodulation in the lungs (Fig. 5.121), which can be indistinguishable from miliary tuberculosis. This pattern appears to be more common in immunocompromised patients.[410]

South American blastomycosis (paracoccidioidomycosis) is included here for completeness. In a large HRCT series of 41 patients with chronic pulmonary paracoccidioidomycosis, 38 had abnormalities consisting mainly of interstitial changes affecting all lung zones. The majority had interlobular septal thickening (88%), nodules ranging in size from 1 to 25 mm (83%), and features of chronic widespread fibrosis (83%). Airspace consolidation, with or without widespread cavitation, was much less frequent in this chronic condition.[416]

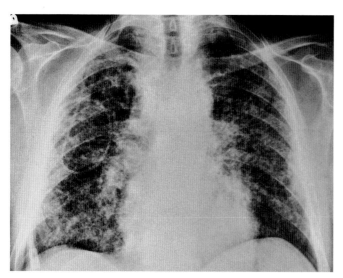

Fig. 5.121 Blastomycosis showing widespread miliary nodulation in the lungs.

PULMONARY ASPERGILLOSIS

The genus *Aspergillus* is a ubiquitous dimorphic fungus present in soil and water and abundant in decaying and moldy vegetation. There are over 300 species of *Aspergillus*, but *Aspergillus fumigatus* is by far the most common pathogen in humans.[417] It can cause a wide spectrum of pulmonary disease, ranging from simple colonization to life-threatening invasive aspergillosis, depending on the immunologic status of the host, individual susceptibility, or preexisting lung disease. It has been suggested that pulmonary aspergillosis be considered a spectrum instead of the traditional divisions of mycetoma, invasive aspergillosis, and allergic bronchopulmonary aspergillosis, particularly because these entities may overlap in an individual patient and with other *Aspergillus*-related phenomena such as mucoid impaction, eosinophilic pneumonia, bronchocentric granulomatosis, hypersensitivity pneumonitis, or asthma.[418-420] Invasion may occur with mycetoma in patients with mild immunosuppression or underlying lung disease.[421] Indeed, invasive aspergillosis can occur, albeit rarely, in apparently immunocompetent individuals with no preexisting lung damage.[422]

Saprophytic colonization is particularly seen in patients with chronic obstructive pulmonary disease who are debilitated and receiving prolonged courses of multiple antibiotics or corticosteroids. *Aspergillus* has been found in 7% of sputum cultures in patients with a wide variety of chest diseases and in 24% of sputum cultures of asthmatic patients. Some patients show evidence of an immunologic response, such as increased total immunoglobulin E, positive precipitins, and immediate or late skin reactivity to *Aspergillus* antigen.[417]

The term "aspergilloma" (mycetoma, fungus ball) is used to describe a ball of coalescent mycelial hyphae that typically colonize preexisting chronic cavities, mainly in the lung, although mycetomas may also form in chronic pleural cavities.[423,424] The fibrotic pulmonary cavities often result from sarcoidosis[425] or old healed pulmonary tuberculosis,[426] although cavities from a variety of other causes, including fungal infection, *P. jiroveci* infection, bronchiectasis, ankylosing spondylitis (Fig. 5.122), interstitial pulmonary fibrosis, postirradiation fibrosis, Wegener granulomatosis, pulmonary infarcts, lung abscesses, pulmonary neoplasms (Fig. 5.123), and cystic congenital lesions (such as pulmonary sequestration), may also be colonized by the fungus.[420,427-434]

Pathologic study of an intracavitary aspergilloma shows a compact, spherical conglomerate of hyphae that may be attached to the wall of the cavity but usually is not. On microscopic examination the fungus ball is composed of concentric or convoluted layers of radially arranged and intertwined hyphae. Although hyphae can be found along the surface and within the fibrous wall of the cavity, obvious invasion into the adjacent lung parenchyma does not occur unless host defense mechanisms are compromised, in which case the condition can take a locally destructive form known as chronic necrotizing pulmonary aspergillosis.[435] Nevertheless, thickening of the (lateral) wall of a fibrotic cavity may be seen on chest radiographs before an intracavitary mycetoma is visible[436]; whether this reflects a pleural reaction is unclear but it seems to be a reversible phenomenon with the potential for the wall thickening to regress.

Patients with mycetomas are usually over 40 years of age and are more likely to be male than female.[255] The mycetoma may be asymptomatic and first discovered incidentally on a chest radiograph, but hemoptysis is frequent and occurs in at least half of patients.[437] The mechanism of bleeding is unknown; it has been attributed to friction between the fungus ball and the hypervascular wall, to endotoxins liberated from the fungus, and to a type III reaction in the cavity wall.[417] Occasionally the hemoptysis may be massive and life-threatening. Other symptoms include productive cough, chest pain, dyspnea, weight loss, and fatigue, caused mainly by the underlying condition rather than by the mycetoma itself.[438]

The diagnosis is largely established on radiographic grounds. Skin tests and sputum cultures for *Aspergillus* may be positive, but neither is specific. Positive precipitating antibodies to *Aspergillus* antigens can be demonstrated in the serum of most patients, but again the test is not specific for mycetoma, since it is also positive in many of the forms of pulmonary aspergillosis, including temporary colonization by fungal hyphae. Also, precipitin tests are species specific; therefore the occasional negative serum precipitin test result is seen when the responsible *Aspergillus* is not *A. fumigatus*.

The essential finding on plain film is the mycetoma itself, a rounded mass of soft tissue density lying within a preexisting cavity (Fig. 5.124). Because most of the preexisting cavities are caused by sarcoidosis or previous tuberculosis, mycetomas are found most often in the upper lobes or in the superior segments of the lower lobes. Usually the mass fills only a portion of the cavity, so that air is seen between the fungus ball and the wall.

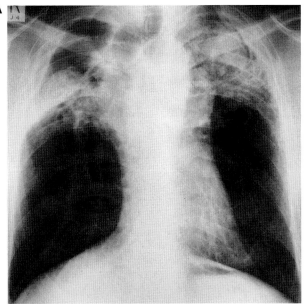

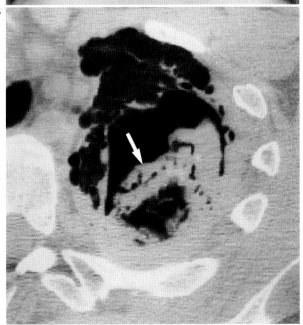

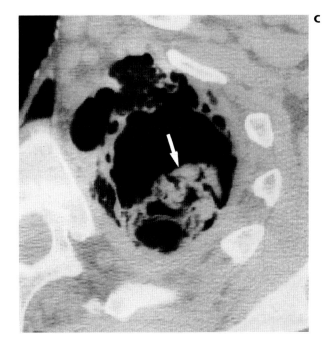

Fig. 5.122 **A**, Bilateral mycetomas within cavities secondary to upper lobe fibrosis caused by ankylosing spondylitis. **B** and **C**, HRCT through a mycetoma in the left upper lobe showing the typical folded sponge-like appearance (arrows) and adjacent pleural thickening.

The air takes the shape of a meniscus and is usually referred to as the air meniscus sign or the air crescent sign (Fig. 5.124). It should be remembered that the air crescent sign is not specific to mycetoma formation; it is also seen in patients with hematoma in a cavity,[439] sclerosing hemangioma,[440] bronchogenic carcinoma,[441] and retained surgical swabs.[442] Confusingly, the air crescent sign is also encountered in individuals with invasive (necrotizing) aspergillosis,[443,444] but in this situation there is not usually an obvious background of fibrocavitary disease. In some cases the mycetoma more or less fills the cavity and the mycetoma is no longer able to roll around.

The cavity wall is often thick (Fig. 5.125),[445] a sign that is seen most often in long-standing mycetoma with obvious intracavitary mass, but also with early colonization before the fungus ball itself is obvious.[436] An air–fluid level may be present within the cavity but is surprisingly uncommon given the inflammatory nature of the process and the theoretical possibility of superadded bacterial infection within the cavity.

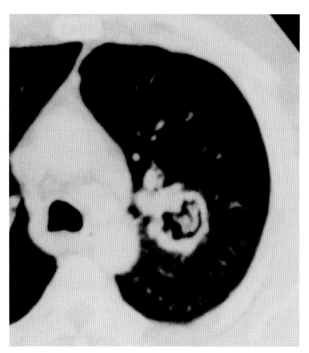

Fig. 5.123 Mycetoma in a cavitating neoplasm. The "collapsed membrane" of the mycetoma is seen within a cavitating squamous cell carcinoma.

CT shows a sponge-like mass that contains irregular airspaces (Figs 5.122 and 5.125). The air crescent sign and the wall of the preexisting cavity are well seen, and the mobility of the fungus ball can be readily demonstrated by turning the patient, although this is rarely necessary as the diagnosis is obvious in most cases. The sponge-like appearance is so characteristic that the diagnosis is secure even when the mycetoma fills the cavity and neither the air crescent sign nor evidence of mobility can be demonstrated. Flecks of calcification within the mycetoma are an occasional feature. The diagnosis of a mycetoma early in its evolution can be often made with CT by the demonstration of fungal strands either lining the cavity or within the lumen (resembling a crumpled membrane) before they have formed a ball of sufficient size to be recognized on plain chest radiograph (Fig. 5.125). Sometimes, spontaneous regression of a mycetoma occurs.[446]

In the semiinvasive form[421,447] the fungus may produce extensive local consolidation and destruction of the lung parenchyma (Fig. 5.126). There need not be a previous cavity; the appearance may simply be an area of chronic pulmonary consolidation that undergoes progressive cavitation and subsequent mycetoma formation. There is also a stable, noncavitary, nodular or masslike form of pulmonary aspergillosis in which there is no evidence of a preexisting cavity and the lesion resembles a pulmonary neoplasm on both plain film and CT examination; immunocompromise is not necessarily a prerequisite. The term *invasive aspergillosis* is most often used to describe aggressive disease in immunocompromised patients (aspergillosis in this context is dealt with in Ch. 6). However, it is important to remember that this form of aspergillus infection may be relatively indolent and can occur in apparently immunocompetent individuals, either those with preexisting mycetoma or allergic bronchopulmonary aspergillosis, or those with no obvious antecedent lung disease.[421,422,447] The sequence of invasion of structures seems to be firstly bronchial walls and subsequently the accompanying arterioles. Thus, the two main forms are somewhat arbitrarily divided into angioinvasive aspergillosis and airway invasive aspergillosis. Given the anatomic proximity of the bronchi and pulmonary arteries it is not surprising that the two forms may coexist in the same patient, and that it is not always possible to distinguish between the two types. Aspergillus may rarely invade locally mediastinal structures or the pleura.[424,448–450]

Airway invasive aspergillosis

The pathologic definition of airway invasive aspergillosis is the presence of *Aspergillus* organisms deep to the basement membrane of the bronchial tree.[451] This form of aspergillosis can be divided into acute airway invasive aspergillosis and chronic airway invasive aspergillosis (also known as semiinvasive aspergillosis or chronic necrotizing aspergillosis[447]).

Acute airway invasive aspergillosis

Acute airway invasive aspergillosis causes a spectrum of disease including acute tracheobronchitis, exudative bronchiolitis, and bronchopneumonia. It usually occurs in the same susceptible immunocompromised patients who are prone to angioinvasive aspergillosis. The HRCT findings include peribronchiolar consolidation, centrilobular micronodules (less than 5 mm; Fig. 5.127), ground-glass opacities, and lobar consolidation. It is not surprising that a positive yield of *Aspergillus* from bronchoalveolar lavage is more likely in airway than in angioinvasive aspergillosis.[452] Rarely, *Aspergillus* can invade the large airways and cause pseudomembranous necrotizing tracheal aspergillosis, which has a high mortality.[450,453,454]

Chronic airway invasive (chronic necrotizing/semiinvasive) aspergillosis

Chronic airway invasive aspergillosis is characterized by an indolent granulomatous cavitating *Aspergillus* infection and so may mimic reactivation tuberculosis radiographically.[421] This entity was first described in the early 1980s[421,447] and to this day it is probably under-diagnosed.[447,455] Patients present with a variety

A

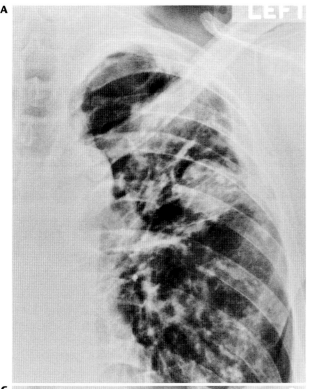

B

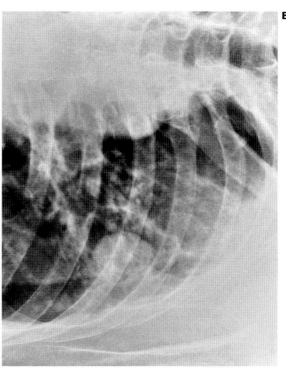

C

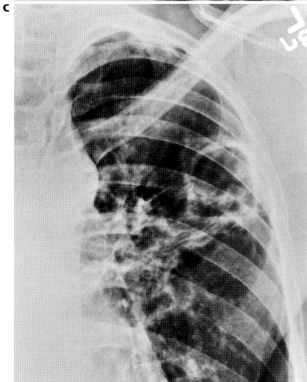

Fig. 5.124   A cavity containing an intracavitary fungus ball. Note the crescent of air above the mycetoma, adjacent pleural thickening, and movement of the fungus ball. In this case the underlying fibrocavitary disease was atypical mycobacterial infection. **A**, Frontal view. **B**, Lateral decubitus view. **C**, A frontal view 1 year earlier shows the preexisting cavity with an air–fluid level but no easily recognizable mycetoma.

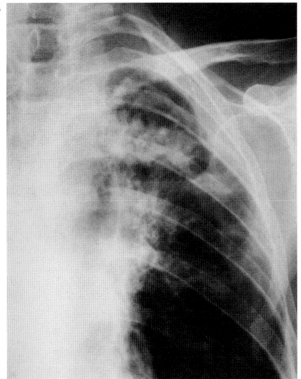

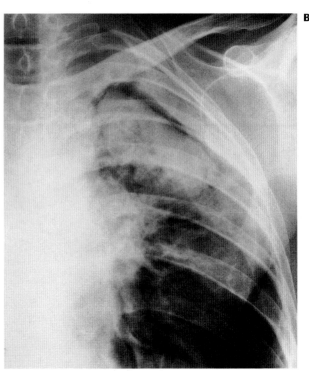

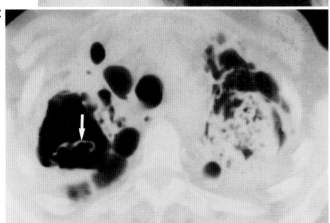

Fig. 5.125 Mycetoma growth. **A**, The initial radiograph shows an irregular mass within a cavity. **B**, One year later, the mass is larger and better defined. The air crescent sign is well demonstrated, as is thickened pleura forming the lateral wall of cavity. Bubble-like and linear lucencies within the mycetoma are visible on the chest radiograph but are better seen with CT. **C**, An early mycetoma showing the "collapsed membrane" appearance in a cavity in the right upper lobe. A small amount of fluid is present in the cavity. There is an obvious mycetoma in the left upper lobe.

of symptoms including hemoptysis, sputum production, weight loss, and fever. Many patients are debilitated and have multiple risk factors in the form of some degree of immunosuppression.[455] Chronic airway invasive aspergillosis usually starts as a focus of consolidation (Fig. 5.128) in the upper lobes and then progresses to cavitation, sometimes with subsequent aspergilloma formation and associated adjacent pleural thickening; the process develops over several months.[421,456] Mortality is between 10% and 34% (often from the underlying disease).[455] An important consideration in patients with this form of aspergillosis is the possibility of coexisting nontuberculous mycobacterial infection[293] (Fig. 5.129).

Angioinvasive aspergillosis

Angioinvasive aspergillosis is characterized by hemorrhagic bronchopneumonia, as a consequence of hyphal invasion of blood vessels with resulting infarction and necrosis. Florid angioinvasive aspergillosis is seen almost exclusively in severely immunocompromised patients (particularly those with neutropenia), most commonly following bone marrow transplant for hematologic malignancies, after solid organ transplantation, or following cytotoxic chemotherapy that induces neutropenia.

Features on chest radiography include single or multiple nodular infiltrates, segmental or subsegmental consolidation,

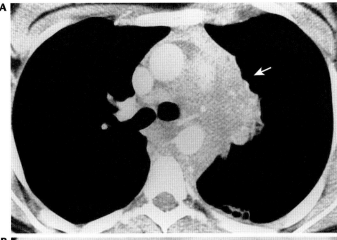

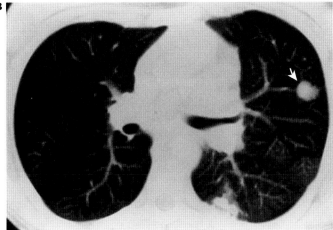

Fig. 5.126 A 19-year-old female presented with a hoarse voice and dysphagia. **A**, The mediastinal fat is completely replaced by an infiltrating soft tissue density mass (arrow) that extends out around the left hilum. **B**, Scattered pulmonary nodules (curved arrow). CT guided biopsy of the nodule showed invasive aspergillosis; mediastinal involvement was confirmed by surgical biopsy. The patient had no known immune deficiency and responded well to antifungal treatment. (With permission from Buckingham SJ, Hansell DM. Aspergillus in the lung: diverse and coincident forms. Eur Radiol 2003;13:1786–1800, ©Springer–Verlag.)

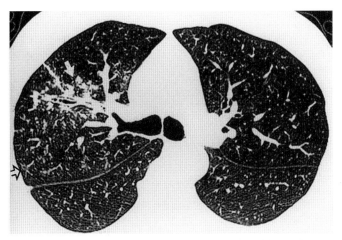

Fig. 5.127 Acute airway invasive aspergillosis with nodules and peribronchial thickening (arrow) and tree-in-bud pattern (open arrow). (With permission from Buckingham SJ, Hansell DM. Aspergillus in the lung: diverse and coincident forms. Eur Radiol 2003;13:1786–1800, ©Springer–Verlag.)

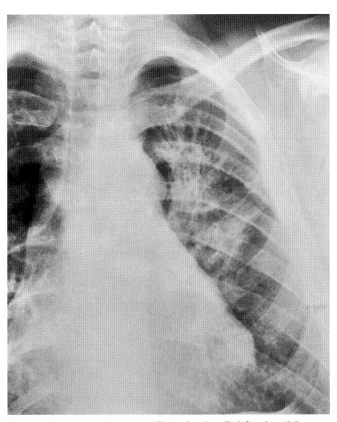

Fig. 5.128 Semiinvasive aspergillosis showing ill-defined perihilar consolidation in otherwise normal-appearing lung. The patient had no known immunocompromise.

diffuse ground-glass pattern (often progressing to consolidation), and cavitation (air crescent).[457–459] The air crescent sign in angioinvasive aspergillosis is seen in up to 48% of patients (with biopsy proven invasive aspergillosis) in the recovery phase[444] and relates to hyphal invasion of blood vessels leading to an area of infarcted lung (sequestrum), in which resorption of necrotic tissue in the periphery or retraction of the sequestrum from viable lung parenchyma leads to a crescent of air surrounding the sequestrum (Fig. 5.130). Cavitation is more likely to occur in larger areas of consolidation or nodules[444] and is associated with a higher risk of massive hemoptysis.

HRCT reveals areas of ground-glass attenuation surrounding some of the nodules (halo sign; Fig. 5.131), and areas of segmental and nonsegmental consolidation with or without a halo.[460,461] The halo sign represents hemorrhage around a nodule[462] and is seen earlier, and with greater frequency, than the air crescent sign.[462,463]

In early reports much was made of the sensitivity of the halo sign[452,460,463] in immunocompromised patients, but this sign has been reported in immunocompromised patients with mucormycosis, *Candida*, cytomegalovirus infection, herpes infection, organizing pneumonia, and pulmonary hemorrhage,[457] as well as in non-immunocompromised patients with

A

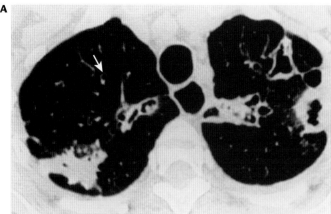

B

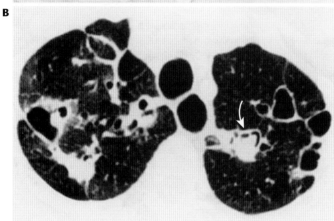

Fig. 5.129 Chronic airway invasive aspergillosis in an elderly woman with coexisting *Mycobacterium avium–intracellulare* infection. **A**, A focal area of consolidation, cavitating lesions, and bronchiectasis (arrow). **B**, Progression 4 months later with an obvious mycetoma (open arrow). Despite treatment for both aspergillosis and atypical mycobacterial infection the patient died 6 months later. (With permission from Buckingham SJ, Hansell DM. Aspergillus in the lung: diverse and coincident forms. Eur Radiol 2003;13:1786–1800, ©Springer–Verlag.)

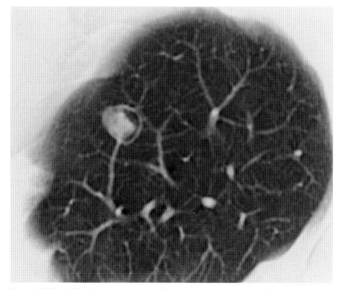

Fig. 5.130 The air crescent sign in angioinvasive aspergillosis. The infarcted lung has retracted, resulting in an air crescent. Note the normal appearance of the surrounding lung. (With permission from Buckingham SJ, Hansell DM. Aspergillus in the lung: diverse and coincident forms. Eur Radiol 2003;13:1786–1800, ©Springer–Verlag.)

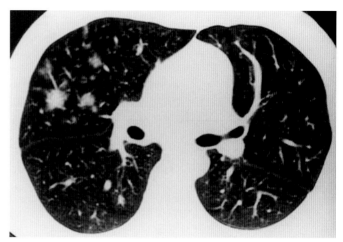

Fig. 5.131 The halo sign in invasive aspergillosis. There is a ground-glass margin to several of the nodules in the right upper lobe of this bone marrow transplant patient. (With permission from Buckingham SJ, Hansell DM. Aspergillus in the lung: diverse and coincident forms. Eur Radiol 2003;13:1786–1800, ©Springer–Verlag.)

Box 5.9 Possible transmogrifications of pulmonary aspergillosis

Mycetoma	→ Invasive aspergillosis[465]
Mycetoma	→ Allergic bronchopulmonary aspergillosis (ABPA)[466]
ABPA	→ Mycetoma[467]
ABPA	→ Chronic airway invasive aspergillosis[468]
ABPA	→ Angioinvasive aspergillosis[469]

Wegener granulomatosis, Kaposi sarcoma, and metastatic angiosarcoma.[464]

Overlap manifestations of pulmonary aspergillosis

There is considerable overlap between what are perhaps over-rigidly regarded as discrete clinicopathological entities. For example, aspergillomas can change behavior and become invasive. Other possible transmogrifications are shown in Box 5.9.

Invasive aspergillosis generally occurs in immunocompromised patients, as previously described; however, there have been several reports documenting patients with no known prior immunodeficiency, and patients with only minor immunodeficiency.[448,470,471] A case of fatal disseminated aspergillosis in an asthmatic patient in whom the only immunosuppression was a short course of corticosteroids has been reported.[472] The form taken by *Aspergillus* pulmonary infection is heavily dependent on local and systemic host immunity and the presence of underlying lung pathology, both of which can change in any given patient over time and so modify the manifestation of *Aspergillus* infection (Fig. 5.132). Some of the possible combinations of *Aspergillus* involvement in the lung are summarized schematically in Figure 5.133.

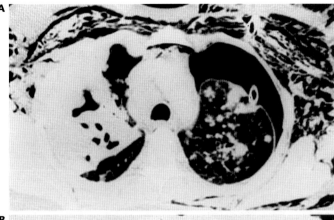

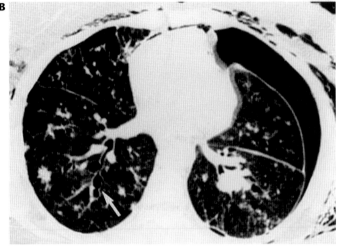

Fig. 5.132 A patient with long-standing allergic bronchopulmonary aspergillosis presented with right upper lobe consolidation which progressed on antifungal treatment and steroids. **A**, Dense consolidation in the right upper lobe with probable cavitation. Nodules and tree-in-bud pattern in the left upper lobe. Left pneumothorax and extensive surgical emphysema. **B**, Further nodules in the lower lobes and bronchiectatic proximal airways (arrow) typical of ABPA. Autopsy confirmed invasive pulmonary aspergillosis. (With permission from Buckingham SJ, Hansell DM. Aspergillus in the lung: diverse and coincident forms. Eur Radiol 2003;13:1786–1800, ©Springer–Verlag.)

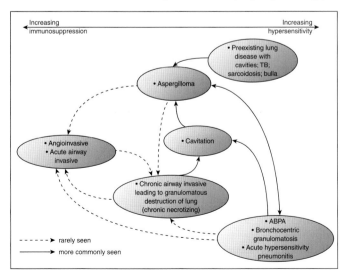

Fig. 5.133 Coincident forms and transformations of aspergillus in the lungs. (With permission of Dr SJ Buckingham, Eur Radiol 2003;13:1786, ©Springer–Verlag.)

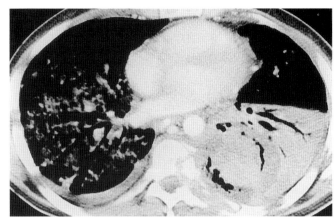

Fig. 5.134 Mucormycosis. Extensive consolidation in a diabetic patient with acute myeloid leukemia. The circle of locules of gas and adjacent low-density lung represent gangrenous infection in the left lower lobe (confirmed at autopsy). The adjacent vertebral body is involved.

MUCORMYCOSIS (ZYGOMYCOSIS)

Pulmonary mucormycosis is caused by fungi belonging to the Mucorales order. Mucormycosis occurs almost invariably in patients who are not fully immunocompetent. Patients with diabetes or a hematologic malignancy are particularly susceptible.[473,474] In diabetic patients, ketoacidosis seems to be a significant predisposing factor, possibly because in this state the functional integrity of polymorph neutrophils and bronchoalveolar macrophages is impaired.[475] Mucormycosis may present as an infection of the upper respiratory tract (particularly the sinuses) or the lungs. Individuals with pulmonary mucormycosis tend to be more severely immunosuppressed, for example recipients of bone marrow transplantation. Nevertheless, it is worth stressing that patients without apparent immunodeficiency may develop pulmonary mucormycosis,[476] albeit usually a less fulminant form of the disease.

In neutropenic patients the presentation of pulmonary mucormycosis is remarkably similar to invasive aspergillosis[477]: the typical clinical features are fever, pleuritic chest pain, and hemoptysis. Hemoptysis may be massive and fatal and is the result of pulmonary infarction caused by direct fungal angioinvasion.[478] Aggressive treatment with antifungal agents and surgical resection of necrotic pulmonary tissue may be necessary[479] but the mortality remains very high, partly because of delayed diagnosis. Bronchoalveolar lavage may be useful in securing the diagnosis.[480]

The most common radiographic abnormality is lobar consolidation.[473,481] The consolidation may be multilobar but can be focal and mass like. Less frequently, solitary or multiple pulmonary nodules may predominate. Occasionally there may be pleural effusions or hilar lymphadenopathy.[481] Bronchial occlusion and pulmonary pseudoaneurysms[482] are infrequent and are more likely to be appreciated on CT.[483] Similarly, central airway involvement can be readily demonstrated on CT.[484] Because of the angioinvasive nature of mucormycosis, the masslike lesions may show the ground-glass halo sign on CT, representing surrounding hemorrhage.[483] Once infarction has occurred, cavitation of the necrotic lung ensues, often with an air crescent within the consolidation (Fig. 5.134).[24] Over time this appearance may change to a thin walled cavity containing an intracavity body.

UNUSUAL FUNGI

Sporotrichosis is usually a lymphocutaneous infection acquired by direct implantation of the fungus *Sporothrix schenckii*. The highest incidence of the common lymphocutaneous form is in agricultural workers, nursery workers, and persons in similar occupations.[485] No skin test is available, and the serologic tests are highly specialized. The best method of diagnosis is culture of the fungus from sputum specimens, bronchial brushings or washings, or pleural biopsies. Pulmonary involvement may be secondary to skin infection, but in most cases pulmonary disease is caused by inhalation of spores and occupational exposure does not play as great a role.[485–487] Systemic dissemination may occur. The usual symptoms of pulmonary disease are productive cough and low grade fever. The chest radiographic findings (Fig. 5.135) are variable, mostly nonspecific areas of consolidation that may give rise to thin walled cavities and fibronodular densities in the upper lobes closely resembling pulmonary tuberculosis,[486,488] even to the extent that fungus balls may grow in sporotrichosis cavities.[485] The disease may respond to conventional antifungal treatment such as itraconazole.[489]

Geotrichosis is caused by *Geotrichum candidum,* a fungus that normally inhabits the pharynx and gastrointestinal tract. It may cause bronchitis, asthma, or pneumonia. In parenchymal infection the radiograph may show upper lobe consolidation and thin walled cavities.

MYCOPLASMA PNEUMONIA

Mycoplasma pneumoniae is one of the smallest of the free living microorganisms and is a common nonbacterial cause of pneumonia.[490] It usually affects previously healthy individuals between the ages of 5 and 40 years. It sometimes occurs in localized outbreaks in families, schools, or the military; the disease is spread by inhalation of droplets and has a 10–20 day incubation period. The reported prevalence of *M. pneumoniae* in adults varies from 2% to 30%.[491] The symptoms resemble a viral infection, with malaise, fever, chills, headache, sore throat, nonproductive cough, and a variety of nonrespiratory manifestations.[490,492] The physical findings on examination of the chest are often less than might be expected from the chest radiograph. Indeed, it has been estimated that *M. pneumoniae* infection is thirty times more likely to result in bronchitic symptoms than a pneumonic illness.[493] The diagnosis is usually established retrospectively on the basis of an elevated or rising cold agglutinin titer. The disease, which responds to tetracycline or erythromycin, usually runs a self-limiting course.[490] However, fatal cases have been recorded,[494] as has the development of acute lung injury,[495] interstitial fibrosis,[496,497] and constrictive obliterative bronchiolitis.[498,499]

The chest radiographic findings are variable.[490,500–505] The most common pattern is patchy consolidation that may coalesce to resemble lobar pneumonia. Usually the pneumonia is unilateral, often involving only one lobe (Fig. 5.136). Occasionally the consolidation spreads to involve other lobes.[501] There appears to be a predilection for the lower lobes[503] though solitary upper lobe involvement occurs.[501] An alternative

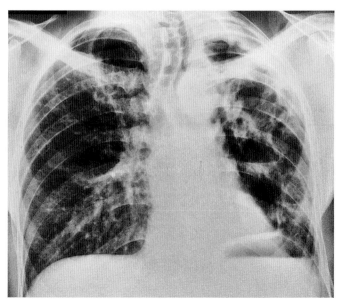

Fig. 5.135 Sporotrichosis (*Sporothrix schenckii*) showing multiple thin walled cavities containing air–fluid levels and adjacent pleural thickening. Note the close resemblance to pulmonary tuberculosis.

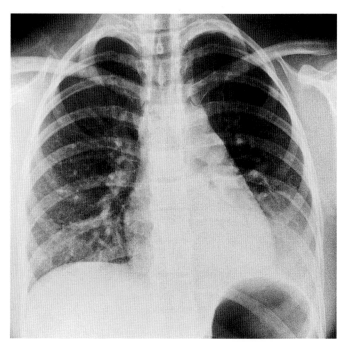

Fig. 5.136 *Mycoplasma* pneumonia. There is homogeneous nonsegmental "lobar-type" consolidation of the left lower lobe.

pattern is bilateral nodular or reticular shadowing resembling an interstitial process (Fig. 5.137). In most series this pattern has been relatively uncommon, but in one large series it was seen in the majority of patients[506] and in another it was seen in one-third of patients.[503] In the series by Putman and co-workers[502] an interstitial pattern was often associated with a longer and more indolent course, without high fever or cough.

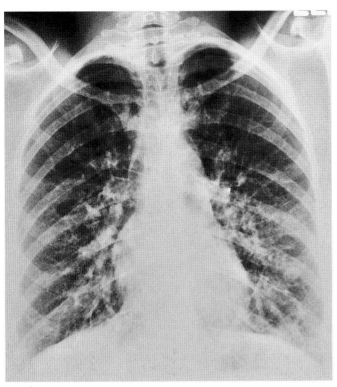

Fig. 5.137 *Mycoplasma* pneumonia showing widespread linear shadowing of interstitial type.

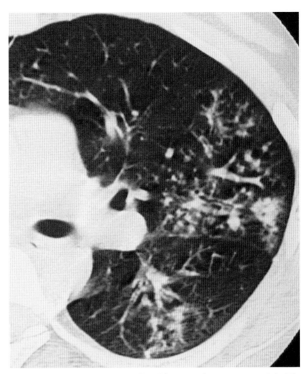

Fig. 5.139 A 29-year-old female with *Mycoplasma* pneumonia. There are small foci of consolidation and irregular nodules representing exudate, but no definite tree-in-bud pattern. (Courtesy of Dr M Ujita)

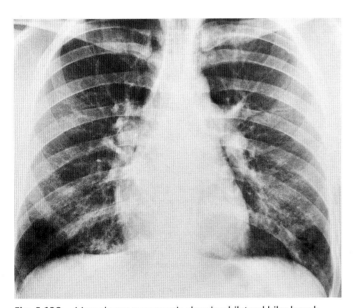

Fig. 5.138 *Mycoplasma* pneumonia showing bilateral hilar lymph node enlargement as well as pulmonary changes.

Cavitation and pneumatocele formation appear to be exceedingly rare. Pleural effusion is variously reported as rare or occurring in up to 20% of cases, but large effusions, which may be hemorrhagic, are uncommon.[502,507] Both adenopathy (Fig. 5.138) and pleural effusion are more common in children.[500,508] The chest radiograph may take several weeks to return to normal in those few patients with an interstitial pattern[496,497] and anecdotal experience suggests that some

individuals have residual fibrosis, akin to nonspecific interstitial pneumonia.

On HRCT, patchy ground-glass opacification is at least as frequently present as airspace consolidation.[504] Furthermore, centrilobular nodules and bronchial wall thickening are much more readily apparent than on chest radiography. The larger nodules may represent individual lobules filled with exudate and these are sharply outlined by surrounding aerated lung. Although some smaller nodules appear irregular, a frank tree-in-bud pattern is not, perhaps surprisingly, a usual feature (Fig. 5.139). Evidence of small airways disease, in the form of a mosaic pattern on HRCT, is particularly common in children following the acute illness.[499]

VIRAL PNEUMONIA

Viruses are the major cause of respiratory tract infection in the community, particularly in children. Droplet transmission from human to human is the usual mode of spread. The effects of infection are usually confined to the upper respiratory tract with pneumonia being relatively uncommon. In immunocompetent infants and young children the viruses that most commonly cause pneumonia are respiratory syncytial virus, parainfluenza virus, adenovirus, and influenza virus, whereas in adults influenza virus types A and B and adenovirus are the most common.[509] Viral pneumonia in immunocompromised patients is discussed in Chapter 6.

The epithelial lining of the various parts of the respiratory tract is the main target, so that tracheobronchitis, bronchiolitis, and pneumonia are the main manifestations of viral infection.

Table 5.5 Summary of CT findings in viral pneumonias

Cause of pneumonia	Centrilobular nodules	Ground-glass attenuation with or without lobular distribution	Segmental consolidation attenuation	Diffuse ground-glass
Influenza virus	+++	+++	+	+
Measles virus	++	+	+	+
Epstein–Barr virus	+	+	+	+
Adenovirus	++	+	+++	
Herpes simplex virus	+	+++	+++	
Varicella-zoster virus	+++	+		
SARS (coronavirus)	(+)	+++	++	+

Note: Plus signs indicate the relative frequency of the findings from lowest (+) to highest (+++).

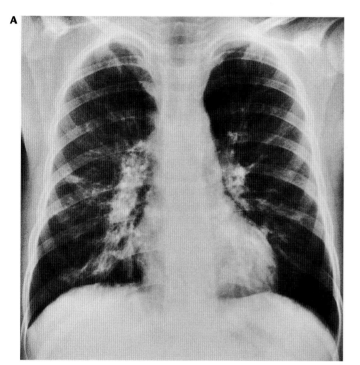

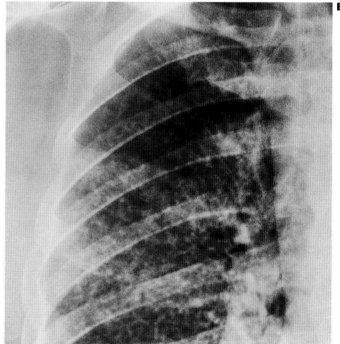

Fig. 5.140 Viral pneumonia: **A**, in a child, showing scattered small ill-defined consolidations in both middle and lower zones; **B**, in an adult, showing widespread small nodular shadows.

The pathologic course of viral pneumonia begins with destruction and sloughing of the respiratory ciliated, goblet, and mucous cells.[29] The bronchial and bronchiolar walls together with the interstitial septa of the lungs become thickened owing to edema and inflammatory cells, primarily lymphocytes. This so-called "interstitial pneumonitis" is often patchy, affecting predominantly the peribronchial portions of the lobules. With more severe inflammation the alveoli fill with inflammatory exudate, which may be hemorrhagic, and hyaline membranes may form. Resolution is the rule, but permanent mucosal damage, obliteration of small airways, and chronic interstitial fibrosis may occur.

The imaging findings of viral pneumonia[29,510–513] do not usually allow the diagnosis of a specific virus infection. Nevertheless, the combination of CT features varies somewhat between the individual viral pneumonias (Table 5.5).

The basic radiographic sign is widespread small, patchy shadows that may coalesce to a variable degree (Figs 5.140 and 5.141). Multilobar involvement is usual. Sometimes the pulmonary shadows are composed of multiple, poorly defined, 4–10 mm nodules (Figs 5.140B and 5.141B). In the specific instance of *Hantavirus* infection (described in more detail on p. 412), the appearances are indistinguishable from pulmonary edema. Bronchial wall thickening and peribronchial shadows are a striking and common feature in most viral pneumonias. Cavitation is not a feature. Air-trapping may be present in those viral infections predisposed to affect the small airways and therefore flattening of the diaphragm and increased retrosternal space are often apparent. Hilar adenopathy is variable; it is common in measles pneumonia and infectious mononucleosis but rare with other viral pneumonias. Pleural effusions are not a prominent feature, although small ones do not negate the diagnosis.

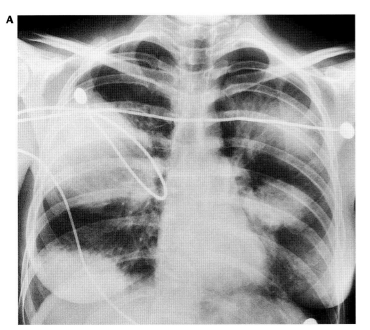
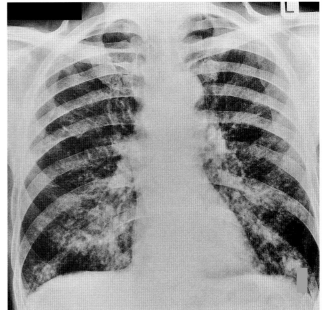

Fig. 5.141   Two examples of influenza pneumonia: **A**, multiple focal pulmonary consolidations; **B**, multiple small ill-defined nodular shadows scattered throughout the lungs, maximal at the bases.

Influenza viruses

Infections with influenza virus occur in epidemics and pandemics or sporadically. Influenza A and B are the subtypes most commonly responsible for the severe outbreaks associated with pneumonia. The symptoms include fever, dry cough, myalgias, and headaches. Rhinitis, pharyngitis, tracheo-bronchitis, and bronchiolitis may develop. When pneumonia occurs, it may be due to bacterial superinfection, most commonly by *S. aureus*, *Pneumococcus*, or *H. influenzae*. The virus itself may cause pneumonia, and when it does, the infection is often severe. Pneumonia is both more common and more serious in the very young, in those over 65 years of age, in late pregnancy, and in those with underlying disease, particularly cardiopulmonary disorders.

In one large series of more than 100 patients with influenzal pneumonia[514] the radiologic findings were multifocal, 1–2 cm, patchy consolidations that rapidly became confluent, with the majority showing bilateral consolidation and basal predominance (Fig. 5.141). Lobar and segmental consolidations were unusual, and the appearance resembled pulmonary edema in some cases. Pleural effusions, although encountered and sometimes large, were not a feature, and cavitation was notably rare. Complicating bacterial pneumonia can be difficult to distinguish from pneumonia caused by the influenza virus itself. There is no large scale CT–pathologic correlative study to date, but it seems probable that the patchy ground-glass changes and consolidation seen in severe cases reflect a combination of diffuse alveolar damage, hemorrhage, and organizing pneumonia[4,513] (Fig. 5.142).

Parainfluenza virus pneumonia occurs predominantly in winter outbreaks, mainly affecting children. Usually parain-fluenza infection causes upper respiratory symptoms, notably croup, and bronchiolitis; pneumonia is uncommon, particularly in adults. Pneumonia may be due to bacterial superinfection. The radiologic appearance is a patchy peribronchial consol-idation mainly in the lower lobes, and pleural effusions may be seen.[515]

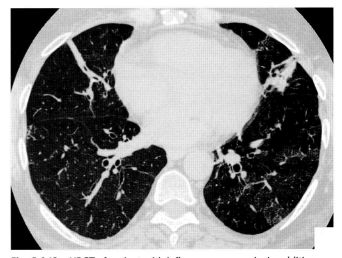

Fig. 5.142   HRCT of patient with influenza pneumonia. In addition to the foci of consolidation and peripheral tree-in-bud, there is a background mosaic attenuation pattern, perhaps reflecting acute bronchiolitis.

Respiratory syncytial virus

Respiratory syncytial virus (RSV) is a major cause of bronchiolitis and bronchopneumonia in infants and young children. It is a recognized cause of croup. It has been suggested that RSV might be associated with, if not actually responsible for, infantile lobar emphysema,[516] and more recently it has been implicated in the pathogenesis of asthma.[517,518] The virus can also cause pneumonia in adults. RSV pneumonia in adults can cause prolonged fever and require protracted stay in the hospital, but it rarely causes serious complications or death[519,520] unless the patient is immunocompromised.[521] The plain chest radiograph shows streaky peribronchial infiltrates associated with overinflation of the lungs.[522,523] Hilar adenopathy was common in some series[524,525] but rare in others.[511,522] Lobar collapse is a frequent finding and lobar consolidation is occasionally seen.[526] Reports of the CT findings are largely confined to immunocompromised adults, such as lung transplant recipients; in these individuals the acute changes are, as expected, entirely nonspecific, but chronic sequelae included a high incidence of air-trapping, bronchial dilatation, and wall thickening.[527]

Coxsackievirus, rhinovirus, and echo viruses

Coxsackievirus, rhinovirus, and echo (enteric cytopathic human orphan) viruses are all related. They usually cause a flulike illness and upper respiratory tract symptoms. Rhinovirus is thought to be a particularly common cause of (upper) respiratory tract infection.[528] Very occasionally these viruses cause pneumonia. The echo viruses usually affect infants; the other two may affect children and adults.[529] The radiologic appearance[530] is nonspecific with reticulonodular shadowing radiating from the hila predominantly into the lower zones. These shadows may become confluent. Hilar adenopathy may be present.

Severe acute respiratory syndrome (SARS)

The rapid development of an epidemic of severe pneumonia (so-called "SARS"), starting in Southern China and caused by a new pathogen – a corona virus – created considerable media attention in the first few months of 2003.[531,532] At the time of writing (June 2004) there have been no new large scale outbreaks of SARS in previous hotspots of the disease (China, Hong Kong, Singapore, Toronto) but a few isolated cases have occurred, primarily in virology laboratory environments. During the epidemic the cumulative total of cases was thought to be in the region of 8098, 774 of which were fatal (a case fatality ratio of 9.6%) [www.who.int/csr/don].

The clinical features of SARS are typically a fever (>38°C), nonproductive cough, and rapidly progressive dyspnea; lymphopenia or elevated serum liver transaminases are common. Because no single test can be used to confidently and accurately diagnose SARS, the World Health Organization provided definitions for suspected and probable cases [www.who.int/csr/sars/casedefinition/en/].

The diagnostic criteria and management guidelines for SARS were rapidly disseminated over the worldwide web, and an accessible repository of radiographic and HRCT images was established within a few weeks of the attack. The radiographic and HRCT appearances of SARS have been extensively documented.[533–538] In the prodrome the chest radiograph may be normal, but nonspecific interstitial or bilateral ground-glass opacities and patchy consolidations develop as the disease progresses (Fig. 5.143). Small nodular opacities are unusual.[533] Cavitation within the consolidation, lymphadenopathy, and pleural effusions are notably absent on chest radiography. From the various descriptions there does not appear to be a particular distribution to the radiographic abnormalities. In the majority of cases there is gradual radiographic resolution once the diffuse shadowing has reached a "peak" in deterioration. In a small proportion, perhaps less than 10%, there is progressive

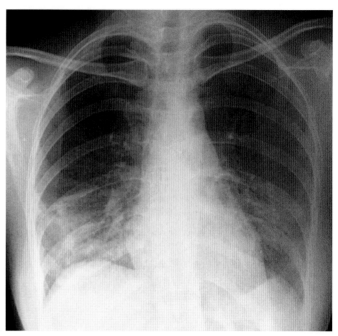

Fig. 5.143 Chest radiograph of a 26-year-old female with SARS, showing ill-defined consolidation and shadowing in the lower zones. (With permission from Antonio GE, Wong KT, Chu WCW et al. Imaging in severe acute respiratory Syndrome (SARS). Clin Rad 2003;58:825–832.)

and more confluent parenchymal opacification, analogous to diffuse alveolar damage (Fig. 5.144); such patients have a worse prognosis. Patients with suspected SARS and an abnormal chest radiograph at presentation can be monitored radiographically.

In those with a normal chest radiograph at the outset, HRCT may show early parenchymal abnormalities, typically focal areas of ground-glass opacification (Fig. 5.145). In the early phase of SARS the abnormalities on HRCT tend to be seen on the periphery of the lower zones.[536] Ancillary HRCT features include mild dilatation of the bronchi within areas of ground-glass opacity, and thickening of the inter- and intralobular septa superimposed on the ground-glass opacities (crazy-paving pattern; Fig. 5.145). HRCT features of severe SARS are less extensively documented but are likely, given the autopsy findings of diffuse alveolar damage in such cases, to resemble the appearance of ARDS with mixed ground-glass and denser opacification of the lung parenchyma. In common with other viral pneumonias there is complete radiographic resolution in the majority of patients.

Rubeola (measles) virus

Rubeola (measles) virus may cause pneumonia in addition to its other systemic and skin manifestations, particularly in children, but also occasionally in adults.[539] The pneumonia frequently contains multinucleated epithelial giant cells with inclusion bodies, a feature originally thought to be specific to measles and given the name "giant cell pneumonia". The pneumonia usually develops before or coincident with the measles skin rash. Chest radiographs of patients with pneumonia[100] show a widespread reticular pattern in the lungs, often accompanied by hilar adenopathy. Lobar atelectasis of varying degree is

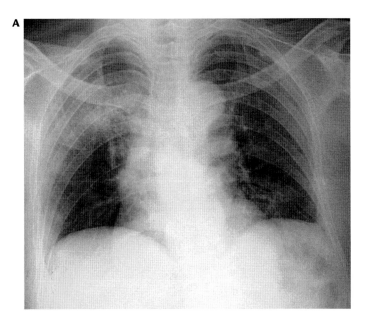

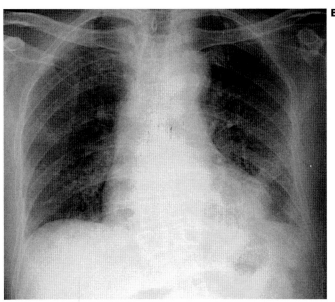

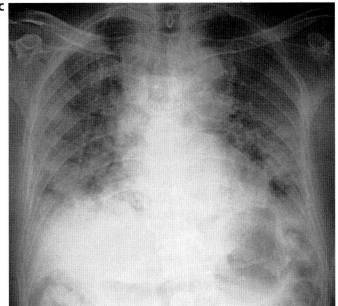

Fig. 5.144 Serial radiographs of a 75-year-old male with SARS. **A**, At presentation there is multifocal consolidation, most conspicuous in the right upper zone. **B**, 6 days later there is more diffuse shadowing. **C**, A further 4 days later there is extensive bilateral airspace consolidation similar to that seen in ARDS. (With permission from Antonio GE, Wong KT, Chu WCW et al. Imaging in severe acute respiratory Syndrome (SARS). Clin Rad 2003;58:825–832.)

common. Usually the viral pneumonia clears with the resolution of the disease, but the radiographic changes may persist for many months. The CT findings of acute measles pneumonia are patchy consolidation, ground-glass opacification, and small centrilobular nodules.[540] Early childhood measles is, along with pertussis, a potent factor in the development of bronchiectasis in adulthood.[541]

Superinfection with *S. aureus, Pneumococcus, H. influenzae*, and *S. pyogenes* may occur, in which case the pneumonia resembles bacterial pneumonia, with more focal confluent areas and sometimes cavitation.

When children who have been immunized with inactivated measles virus are exposed to the measles virus, atypical measles may develop. The radiographic appearance of pneumonia in atypical measles[542–544] differs from that seen in the usual form by showing more nodular (spherical) and segmental consolidations. The nodular consolidations may persist and be confused with pulmonary masses such as metastatic neoplasm or sequestration. Hilar adenopathy and pleural effusion frequently accompany the pneumonia in atypical measles.

Infectious mononucleosis

Infectious mononucleosis, caused by the Epstein–Barr virus, is a common infection in the community but a rare cause of pneumonia. The great majority of patients with infectious mononucleosis show no abnormalities on plain chest radiographs. The most frequent intrathoracic manifestation is mediastinal or hilar adenopathy, a phenomenon best seen with CT.[545] Pulmonary shadows are rare. When present they are usually streaky or interstitial in appearance.[546,547] Nevertheless, consolidation has been reported[548] and mononuclear cells can be identified in the interstitium and alveolar exudate.

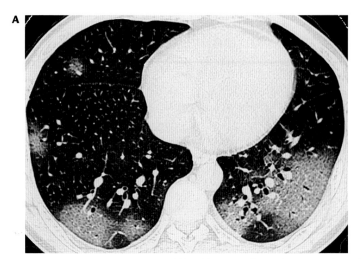

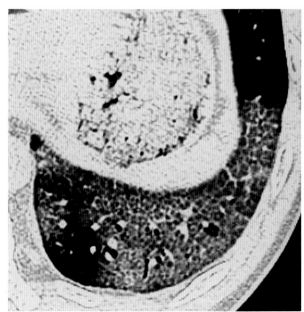

Fig. 5.145 **A**, HRCT of a 29-year-old healthcare worker with SARS, 3 days after the onset of symptoms. There are several areas of peripheral ground-glass opacification in the lower lobes and right middle lobe. **B**, In a different patient with SARS, thickened inter- and intralobular septa are superimposed on ground-glass opacity (crazy paving pattern). (With permission from Antonio GE, Wong KT, Chu WCW et al. Imaging in severe acute respiratory Syndrome (SARS). Clin Rad 2003;58:825–832.)

Adenoviruses

The adenoviruses are a relatively frequent cause of mild infection of the respiratory tract. Pneumonia is uncommon and confined largely to infants, young children, and military recruits.[549] Adenovirus pneumonia in adults can be more severe than in younger patients, particularly in immunocompromised hosts or those with COPD.[549,550] It has been proposed that latent adenoviral infection may play a part in the development of bronchiectasis in some individuals.[551] The chest radiograph shows patchy bronchopneumonic, or confluent widespread consolidation, although consolidations confined to one lobe are also encountered.[513,552,553] The presence of consolidation correlates poorly with the clinical severity of the pneumonia. Bronchial wall thickening and peribronchial shadowing are striking findings. Air-trapping is particularly common in young children, and lobar collapse is frequent. Small pleural effusions are seen in up to two-thirds of patients.[553] The infection can be highly damaging, particularly if acute infection occurs before 2 years of age, leaving bronchiectasis or obliterative bronchiolitis, and the Swyer–James/McLeod syndrome may result.[552,554]

Herpes simplex viruses

Herpes simplex viruses are divided into two basic types, one that causes mucocutaneous vesicles and another that causes genital tract infection and is spread via sexual intercourse or acquired during birth.

Pneumonia is uncommon except in immunocompromised patients and neonates.[555] However, damage to the airways, either by traumatic intubation or cigarette smoking, also seems to predispose.[556] Herpes simplex pneumonia is a particular problem for patients with AIDS (see p. 294). Herpes simplex virus 1 infection is sometimes part of polymicrobial pneumonia.

The virus causes diffuse ulceration of the tracheobronchial epithelium and sometimes necrotizing bronchopneumonia. The radiographic features include extensive bilateral lobar or generalized consolidation (resembling ARDS), lobar or segmental collapse, and small pleural effusions.[557] Occasionally there will be no radiographic abnormality despite the identification of the virus from bronchoalveolar lavage.[557] A CT study of patients with herpes simplex virus 1 pneumonia has shown that multifocal segmental and subsegmental areas of ground-glass opacification with additional patches of consolidation are the most common features.[558] In the study of Aquino et al there were no obvious radiographic or CT differences between patients with exclusive herpes simplex virus 1 pneumonia and patients with superimposed fungal or bacterial pneumonia.[558] Although herpes simplex virus 1 is frequently isolated in the respiratory secretions of severely ill patients, for example those with ARDS, it is not always clear whether the extensive pulmonary consolidation reflects a herpes simplex pneumonitis. Pleural effusions are common.

Varicella-zoster virus

Chickenpox and herpes zoster (shingles) are both caused by the varicella-zoster virus. Pneumonia caused by the virus is rare in children; pneumonia in a child with chickenpox probably results from bacterial superinfection. More than 90% of cases of varicella-zoster pneumonia occur in adults, in patients with lymphoma, and in those who are immunocompromised for a variety of reasons. Symptoms of pneumonia develop 1–6 days after the onset of the skin rash.[559] The plain chest radiograph[559,560] differs slightly from that seen with other viral infections: the pneumonia causes multiple 5–10 mm ill-defined nodules (Fig. 5.146) that may be confluent and may come and go in different areas of the lungs. Hilar adenopathy and small

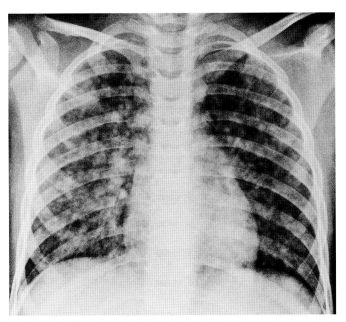

Fig. 5.146 Chickenpox pneumonia showing widespread ill-defined 5–10 mm nodular shadows.

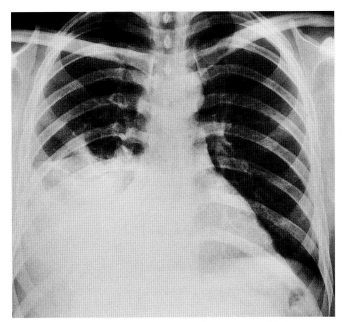

Fig. 5.147 Intrathoracic changes secondary to an amebic lung abscess. There is a large right pleural effusion with collapse and consolidation of the right lower lobe.

pleural effusions occur during the acute phase of the disease but are unusual. The small round opacities usually resolve within a week after the disappearance of the skin lesions, but they can persist for months. HRCT findings mirror the radiographic abnormalities, but smaller nodules (1–10 mm) can be identified and some have a halo of ground-glass opacification, probably representing surrounding hemorrhage.[561] In a few patients the lesions calcify and remain indefinitely as numerous, well-defined, randomly scattered, 2–3 mm, dense calcifications in otherwise normal lungs (Fig. 3.116). The appearance resembles the calcifications seen following disseminated histoplasmosis.

PROTOZOAL INFECTIONS

Amebiasis is caused by *Entamoeba histolytica*, a protozoan found worldwide. In most cases the condition is asymptomatic. Symptomatic infections are usually confined to the gastrointestinal tract and liver. Pleural effusion and lower lobe consolidation may be present contiguous to an amebic abscess in the liver or subphrenic space, just as they may accompany any other suppurative process in these sites. An amebic liver abscess may extend through the diaphragm into the pleura, giving rise to an empyema, and may even extend into the lung, causing pneumonia and lung abscess.[562,563] The most common symptoms are fever and cough, which may be productive of chocolate-colored pus. Hemoptysis and chest or abdominal pain are also frequent.[564] Fistulas may form, connecting the liver abscess to the airways, the pericardium, and very rarely the skin. The radiographic findings are empyema and adjacent consolidation or lung abscess, which may be combined with signs of an elevated hemidiaphragm (Fig. 5.147).[562,563,565] Hematogenous spread of amebic liver abscess to the lungs is rare. When it occurs, it causes transient areas of pneumonia or lung abscess.

HELMINTHIC INFECTIONS

Roundworm, hookworm, and *Strongyloides* infections

Ascaris lumbricoides (roundworm), *Ancylostoma duodenale*, *Necator americanus* (hookworm), and *Strongyloides stercoralis* are all round worms that, as part of their life cycle, pass through the lungs.[566] *Ascaris* eggs are ingested in food contaminated by infected feces and hatched in the small intestine to penetrate the bowel wall and enter the lymphatics and bloodstream. *Ancylostoma* and *Strongyloides* eggs hatch in human feces deposited in soil and penetrate the skin of the hands or feet. In some cases *Strongyloides* eggs reenter the same host via the intestinal mucosa or perianal skin. Regardless of the route by which these organisms enter the bloodstream, they are carried to the lung where they burrow through the alveolar walls to enter the airways and ascend in the tracheobronchial tree. Eventually they are swallowed into the intestine, where they grow to their adult form. *Strongyloides* may also grow to adult form within the lung itself. The clinical features are related largely to the skin and gastrointestinal tract. Pulmonary symptoms are uncommon with all three organisms and include an unproductive cough, substernal chest pain, and occasionally hemoptysis and dyspnea. The clinical manifestations of pulmonary *Strongyloides* depend largely on whether there is antecedent lung disease (which may delay the passage of the larvae through the lungs and exacerbate the infection) or impaired cellular immunity (in which case a devastating hyperinfection syndrome may occur).[567–569] Corticosteroid treatment and reduced gastric acidity because of treatment with H_2 blockers are two of the most important predisposing factors for the development of *Strongyloides* infection. The adult form of *Strongyloides* in the lung may give rise to a syndrome resembling asthma.

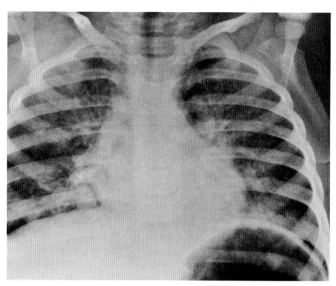

Fig. 5.148 *Toxocara canis* infection with widespread pulmonary consolidation.

In most instances no pulmonary complications occur with any of these worms, but in a few patients an allergic reaction takes place in the lung parenchyma, which manifests itself radiographically as dense transient migratory pulmonary consolidations without recognizable segmental distribution.[570] Blood and sputum eosinophilia are often present, and the entity is therefore included as one of the causes of acute pulmonary infiltrates with eosinophilia (Löffler syndrome).[571] An eosinophilic pleural effusion in association with *Strongyloides* has been reported.[572] Miliary nodulation, similar to miliary tuberculosis, may be seen.[573] Cavitation and hilar and mediastinal lymphadenopathy do not occur unless there is superadded bacterial infection, which is not uncommon (bacteria, and indeed fungi, are known to "piggy-back" on the filariform larvae).[567]

Other round worms that may cause a localized granulomatous reaction in the lung are the dog and cat worms, *Toxocara canis* and *Toxocara cati* (visceral larva migrans).[118] Symptoms include cough, wheezing, dyspnea, and a number of extrapulmonary manifestations. Infection, which is rarely diagnosed in humans, is caused by ingesting ova from contaminated hands, soil, or fomites. Young children are at greatest risk. Infection is often asymptomatic, but in approximately 50% of patients with pulmonary symptoms, chest radiographs show transient local or widespread patchy areas of consolidation, which are associated with peripheral blood eosinophilia (Fig. 5.148).

Filariasis

The most common filarial worm to cause pulmonary manifestations is *Wuchereria bancrofti*.[574] The major disease caused by this organism is the disfiguring condition of elephantiasis resulting from filarial obstruction of cutaneous lymphatics. *W. bancrofti* is also believed to be the cause of tropical eosinophilia, a syndrome consisting of cough, wheezing, and severe blood eosinophilia.[575] The chest radiograph[576,577] may be normal but usually shows widespread fine nodular or reticulonodular

shadowing. The appearance may closely resemble miliary tuberculosis. Localized consolidation is occasionally seen. The pulmonary shadowing, which corresponds to the eosinophilic infiltration,[577] is believed to be due to an immunologic response to microfilariae rather than to direct infection. Although pleural thickening may be demonstrated, pleural effusion does not appear to be a feature.[577] Generalized lymphadenopathy may occur, but radiographically visible mediastinal or hilar adenopathy is uncommon.[575] The radiographic changes usually resolve with treatment, but sometimes resolution takes months and interstitial fibrosis may supervene.[577] Although *W. bancrofti* is believed to be the major inciting organism in tropical eosinophilia, other filariae such as *Brugia malayi* are thought to be responsible for a small proportion of cases.

Very rarely the filarial worm *Dirofilaria immitis* (dog heartworm) causes pulmonary infection in humans.[578,579] It usually infects dogs and can be transferred to humans by mosquito bites. In the United States the condition is largely confined to the eastern and southern states.[580,581] The larvae travel to the walls of the right-sided cardiac chambers and may dislodge and embolize into the pulmonary vascular bed, where they cause a granulomatous reaction plus infarct that manifests itself as asymptomatic solitary or multiple 1–2 cm subpleural pulmonary nodules on chest radiograph.[581–583] The patients may have cough and hemoptysis.[581] Mostly the nodules occur in adults and are single, but in approximately 10% of patients multiple pulmonary nodules are present.[581] The nodules tend to occur in the lower lobes and are more often (76%) on the right.[584] The early lesion may be wedge shaped. Visible calcification on plain chest radiography is not recorded. Experience with CT is limited,[582] but eccentric calcification within the nodule has been demonstrated.[118] Blood eosinophilia is present in between 10% and 20% of patients, but since the blood eosinophil count is usually normal and there are no reliable skin or serologic tests, the granulomas are usually excised in the belief that they may be bronchial carcinoma.[580,581,585]

Schistosomiasis

Pulmonary disease caused by schistosomiasis is rare. Of the flukes responsible for schistosomiasis (*Schistosoma mansoni, S. japonicum,* and *S. haematobium*), *S. mansoni* and *S. haematobium* are the most likely to cause pulmonary disease. The intermediate hosts are various species of freshwater snails, which are infected by larvae hatched from eggs that reach the water in feces or urine. Cercariae, the infective larvae, leave the snails and penetrate the skin or mucous membranes of humans as they swim or paddle in the water. The cercariae migrate to the mesenteric veins or, in the case of *S. haematobium*, to the venous plexuses of the bladder, prostate, or uterus. The adult flukes mate and deposit eggs in the veins, and the eggs are carried to various sites where they induce inflammation, ulceration, and fibrosis. Deposition of eggs in the small vessels of the lungs is rare, but when it occurs the resulting granulomatous inflammation causes luminal obliteration[586] and ultimately results in increased pulmonary vascular resistance.[587] In the migratory phase from skin entrance to final habitat there may be considerable systemic upset with a marked eosinophilia (Katayama fever) and at this stage there may be nodular shadowing on a chest radiograph. This relatively early stage is more likely to be encountered by clinicians consulted by tourists

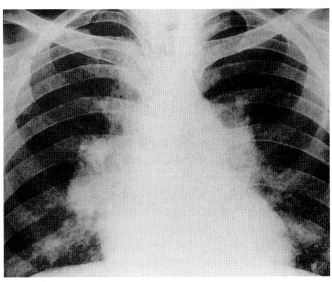

Fig. 5.149 Schistosomiasis with widespread, basally predominant, reticulonodular shadows in both lungs. Cardiac enlargement and large central pulmonary arteries are due to associated pulmonary arterial hypertension. (Courtesy Dr. Micheal C. Pearson).

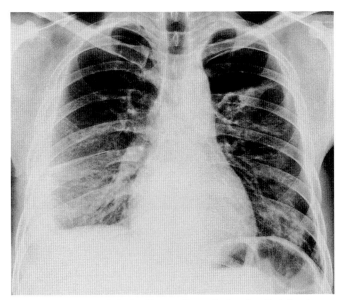

Fig. 5.150 Paragonimiasis. Chest radiograph showing ill-defined consolidation containing complex cavities.

returning from endemic areas.[588–590] In more chronic cases the major radiographic features are those of pulmonary arterial hypertension, but on occasion a widespread fine reticular nodular shadowing representing ova with surrounding inflammatory changes or fibrosis can also be seen (Fig. 5.149).[586,591] Very rarely a solitary nodule is identified.[592] There is a single report of the HRCT appearance of nodules (1–2 cm) with a ground-glass surround in a student with a relatively acute presentation[593]; the halo probably represented surrounding hemorrhage.

Paragonimiasis

Paragonimiasis is usually caused by infection with the lung fluke *Paragonimus westermani*. The disease, which is endemic in Southeast Asia, Indonesia, West Africa, and South America, is acquired by eating crustaceans and water snails that act as the intermediate host. The immature flukes penetrate the bowel wall, travel through the peritoneal cavity, and migrate through the diaphragm and pleura to enter the lung parenchyma. Infection, as documented by positive serologic tests, may be asymptomatic and show no radiographic abnormalities. Symptoms include hemoptysis, chest pain, and chronic cough, which may produce sputum containing the ova of the infecting organism; pleural involvement and empyema can occur.[594,595]

The pulmonary changes result from chronic inflammation in areas surrounding the worm. On radiographic study (Fig. 5.150)[596–598] these areas are seen as multiple round, poorly defined areas of consolidation in any lung zone but most often in the mid zones. These focal and nonspecific abnormalities are often solitary and so resemble lung cancer or tuberculosis.[595,599] The consolidations may be fleeting and associated with blood eosinophilia.[600] Linear shadows 2–4 mm thick and 3–7 cm long may be seen extending inward from the pleura on both plain films and CT scans.[601] These are believed to be worm tracks. Indeed, one case of an air-filled linear track has been reported.[602] The more chronic lesions become better defined, often appear nodular, and sometimes excavate, leaving complex cystic airspaces that may contain solid material. Im and associates[601] have postulated that the intracavitary material may represent the intracavitary worm.

Because the flukes penetrate the diaphragm and pleura, pleural effusions, pneumothorax, and hydropneumothorax are common and frequently bilateral.[596,601] The disease may also spread to distant sites such as the brain.[603]

Echinococcus infections

Hydatid disease is caused by the tapeworms *Echinococcus granulosus* and *E. multilocularis (alveolaris)*.[604] The life cycle involves primary and intermediate mammalian hosts. Dogs are the usual primary host, and the intermediate host is usually a sheep or a cow but is sometimes a human. The disease is endemic in sheep-raising areas of Australia, South America, and the Mediterranean basin, particularly North Africa and Greece. Cases are, however, occasionally encountered from infections acquired in other parts of the world, including North America and Wales. The so-called "sylvatic form"[605] has deer and moose as intermediate hosts and is endemic in the frozen north.

The adult worm lives in the small intestine of the primary host. Ova are passed in feces and ingested by the intermediate host. Larvae develop in the duodenum of the new host, where they enter the bloodstream and travel to the liver and lungs and occasionally even the systemic circulation. Pleural or pulmonary involvement may also be due to direct extension through the diaphragm from hydatid disease in the liver. The life cycle is completed when another primary host eats the remains of an infected intermediate host.

Disease in humans results from the cysts that form around the parasite. The structure of these cysts is important in understanding the radiographic findings. As hydatid cysts grow, they compress the adjacent lung into a fibrotic capsule known as the pericyst. The cyst itself has a thin smooth wall composed of two adherent layers, the laminated ectocyst and the delicate lining endocyst, from which hang the daughter cysts. The pulmonary cysts may grow rapidly, and approximately two-

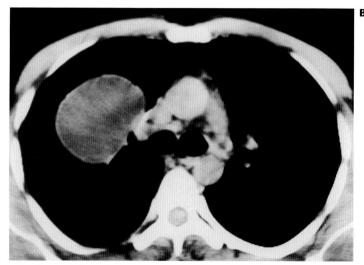

Fig. 5.151 Hydatid cyst of lung. **A**, Chest radiograph shows a well-defined, slightly lobulated mass in the right upper lobe. **B**, CT shows a homogeneous fluid density cyst.

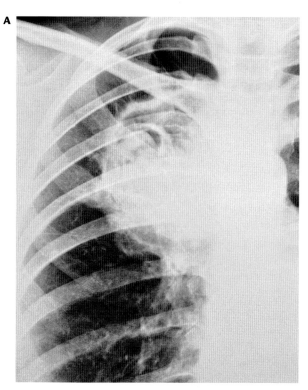

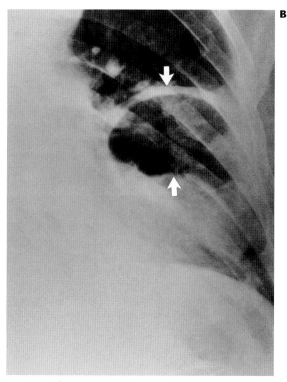

Fig. 5.152 Ruptured hydatid cyst. **A**, A complicated mass containing, from above, pericyst, ectocyst, and daughter cyst. There are air crescents between the ectocyst and pericyst and also between the daughter cyst and ectocyst. **B**, Another patient, showing pericyst (downward-pointing arrow) and ectocyst (upward-pointing arrow) with air between them.

thirds rupture. Most rupture into the surrounding lung and bronchial tree, causing secondary infection. Occasionally a cyst ruptures into the pleural cavity. Surgical resection is frequently necessary in complicated cases.[606,607] Rupture may result in an acute allergic reaction, sometimes accompanied by life-threatening hypotension. Cysts that have not ruptured usually do not give rise to symptoms, and the diagnosis is then based on a routine chest film.

A variety of serologic tests for the diagnosis of hydatid disease have been developed over the years: of these the ELISA

AgB (antigen B-rich fraction) seems to be the most sensitive and specific.[608]

The cardinal imaging features[609–611] are one or more spherical or oval well-defined smooth masses of homogeneous density in otherwise normal lung, usually in the middle or lower zone (Fig. 5.151). Multiple cysts are seen in approximately one-third of patients and are bilateral in 20%[612]; sometimes more than 10 cysts are seen. There is a predilection for the lower lobes, the posterior segments, and the right lung.[609,612] CT scanning[611,613] reveals fluid contents within the cyst, with a density close to that of water; the daughter cysts when present appear as curved septations. At CT the cyst walls range in thickness from 2 mm to 1 cm, with the wall representing the combined pericyst, ectocyst, and endocyst. The cysts may be very large: cysts of 10 cm and even 20 cm have been reported. The rate of growth may be fairly rapid, with doubling times of less than 6 months. A striking feature is that the cyst is relatively pliant and molds to adjacent structures, resulting in indentation, lobulation, or flattening. Surrounding inflammation may cause the edge of the lesion to be ill defined. Calcification, which is a common feature of hydatid cysts in the liver, is very rare in cysts arising in the lungs. Few reports of MRI in intrathoracic hydatid disease have been published.[614,615] The complex cyst contents are well displayed, and the cyst membrane, whether collapsed or not, is clearly seen as a low-intensity curvilinear structure on both short and long TR spin-echo images. MRI may be particularly helpful in revealing the exact location of a hydatid cyst in relation to the diaphragm.[616]

If the pericyst ruptures (Fig. 5.152), air dissecting between the fibrotic lung forming the pericyst and the ectocyst of the parasite leads to a visible crescent of air between the two, known as a meniscus or crescent sign. If the cyst itself ruptures, an air–fluid level results and daughter cysts may even be seen floating in the residual fluid. On rare occasions air is seen on both sides of the true cyst wall; a crescent is seen surrounding the cyst, and air–fluid levels are also present. Sometimes the cyst wall is seen to be crumpled up and floating in fluid, which lies within the non-collapsed pericyst. This pathognomonic appearance is imaginatively described as the water lily sign or the camalote sign. All these signs are particularly well demonstrated by CT (Fig. 5.152),[611,613] and CT has increased the repertoire of variant appearances of hydatid, including a sliver of air in the inferior portion of the cyst (inverse crescent sign) and blebs of air within the wall of the unruptured cyst.[617] However, a study that specifically investigated the frequency with which air bubbles and blebs are seen in the walls of perforated hydatid cysts on CT has suggested that this "air-bubble" sign is highly specific (95%) and sensitive (83%) for the detection of rupture.[618] With secondary infection the membranes may disintegrate and the walls thicken, so that the picture is indistinguishable from bacterial lung abscess on plain films. In this situation the cystic nature of the lesions may be lost and the diagnosis, on the basis of imaging characteristics, of solid complicated hydatid lesions is likely to be overlooked.[619]

Hydatid cysts may also be present in the pleura, in which case there may be secondary seeding around the pleura following rupture. In some cases the pleura is the primary site of disease. Mediastinal cysts are relatively rare. They form smooth round or oval masses in the mediastinum that may compress adjacent mediastinal structures, such as the major airways or vascular structures, or may erode the bone of the thoracic cage.[620–622] Hydatid cysts may also arise in unexpected sites such as the pericardium or wall of the thoracic aorta.[620,623] On CT these mediastinal cysts, like all hydatid cysts, have a well-defined wall and fluid contents. Rupture of cysts into the pulmonary arterial circulation can result in symptoms of pulmonary hypertension.[624–626]

REFERENCES

1. Tew J, Calenoff L, Berlin BS. Bacterial or nonbacterial pneumonia: accuracy of radiographic diagnosis. Radiology 1977;124:607–612.
2. Franquet T. Imaging of pneumonia: trends and algorithms. Eur Respir J 2001;18:196–208.
3. Katz DS, Leung AN. Radiology of pneumonia. Clin Chest Med 1999;20:549–562.
4. Tanaka N, Matsumoto T, Kuramitsu T, et al. High resolution CT findings in community-acquired pneumonia. J Comput Assist Tomogr 1996;20:600–608.
5. Donnelly LF, Klosterman LA. Pneumonia in children: decreased parenchymal contrast enhancement – CT sign of intense illness and impending cavitary necrosis. Radiology 1997;205:817–820.
6. Donnelly LF, Klosterman LA. The yield of CT of children who have complicated pneumonia and noncontributory chest radiography. AJR Am J Roentgenol 1998;170:1627–1631.
7. Levy M, Dromer F, Brion N, et al. Community-acquired pneumonia. Importance of initial noninvasive bacteriologic and radiographic investigations. Chest 1988;93:43–48.
8. Bowton DL, Bass DA. Community-acquired pneumonia: the clinical dilemma. J Thorac Imaging 1991;6:1–5.
9. Condon VR. Pneumonia in children. J Thorac Imaging 1991;6:31–44.
10. Harrison BDW. Community-acquired pneumonia in adults in British hospitals in 1982–1983: a survey of aetiology, mortality, prognostic factors and outcome. The British Thoracic Society and the Public Health Laboratory Service. Q J Med 1987;62:195–220.
11. Almirall J, Bolibar I, Vidal J, et al. Epidemiology of community-acquired pneumonia in adults: a population-based study. Eur Respir J 2000;15:757–763.
12. Bartlett JG, O'Keefe P, Tally FP, et al. Bacteriology of hospital-acquired pneumonia. Arch Intern Med 1986;146:868–871.
13. Lipchik RJ, Kuzo RS. Nosocomial pneumonia. Radiol Clin North Am 1996;34:47–58.
14. Cesar L, Gonzalez C, Calia FM. Bacteriologic flora of aspiration-induced pulmonary infections. Arch Intern Med 1975;135:711–714.
15. di Sant'agnese PA, Davis PB. Cystic fibrosis in adults. 75 cases and a review of 232 cases in the literature. Am J Med 1979;66:121–132.
16. Kulczycki LL, Murphy TM, Bellanti JA. Pseudomonas colonization in cystic fibrosis. A study of 160 patients. JAMA 1978;240:30–34.
17. Murphy TF. Lung infections. 2. Branhamella catarrhalis: epidemiological and clinical aspects of a human respiratory tract pathogen. Thorax 1998;53:124–128.
18. Groskin SA, Panicek DM, Ewing DK, et al. Bacterial lung abscess: a review of the radiographic and clinical features of 50 cases. J Thorac Imaging 1991;6:62–67.
19. Asmar BI, Thirumoorthi MC, Dajani AS. Pneumococcal pneumonia with pneumatocele formation. Am J Dis Child 1978;132:1091–1093.
20. Ziskind MM, Schwarz MI, George RB, et al. Incomplete consolidation in pneumococcal lobar pneumonia complicating pulmonary emphysema. Ann Intern Med 1970;72:835–839.
21. Reich JM. Pulmonary gangrene and the air crescent sign. Thorax 1993;48:70–74.
22. Khan FA, Rehman M, Marcus P, et al. Pulmonary gangrene occurring as a complication of pulmonary tuberculosis. Chest 1980;77:76–80.
23. O'Reilly GV, Dee PM, Otteni GV. Gangrene of the lung: successful medical

management of three patients. Radiology 1978;126:575–579.

24. Zagoria RJ, Choplin RH, Karstaedt N. Pulmonary gangrene as a complication of mucormycosis. AJR Am J Roentgenol 1985;144:1195–1196.

25. Rose RW, Ward BH. Spherical pneumonias in children simulating pulmonary and mediastinal masses. Radiology 1973;106:179–182.

26. Dietrich PA, Johnson RD, Fairbank JT, et al. The chest radiograph in legionnaires' disease. Radiology 1978;127:577–582.

27. Pope TL Jr, Armstrong P, Thompson R, et al. Pittsburgh pneumonia agent: chest film manifestations. AJR Am J Roentgenol 1982;138:237–241.

28. Millar JK. The chest film findings in 'Q' fever – a series of 35 cases. Clin Radiol 1978;29:371–375.

29. Conte P, Heitzman ER, Markarian B. Viral pneumonia. Roentgen pathological correlations. Radiology 1970;95:267–272.

30. Swischuk LE, Hayden CK Jr. Viral vs. bacterial pulmonary infections in children (is roentgenographic differentiation possible?). Pediatr Radiol 1986;16:278–284.

31. Kuru T, Lynch JP III. Nonresolving or slowly resolving pneumonia. Clin Chest Med 1999;20:623–651.

32. Beydon L, Saada M, Liu N, et al. Can portable chest x-ray examination accurately diagnose lung consolidation after major abdominal surgery? A comparison with computed tomography scan. Chest 1992;102:1697–1703.

33. Meduri GU, Mauldin GL, Wunderink RG, et al. Causes of fever and pulmonary densities in patients with clinical manifestations of ventilator-associated pneumonia. Chest 1994;106:221–235.

34. Rubin SA, Winer-Muram HT, Ellis JV. Diagnostic imaging of pneumonia and its complications in the critically ill patient. Clin Chest Med 1995;16:45–59.

35. Winer-Muram HT, Rubin SA, Ellis JV, et al. Pneumonia and ARDS in patients receiving mechanical ventilation: diagnostic accuracy of chest radiography. Radiology 1993;188:479–485.

36. Winer-Muram HT, Jennings SG, Wunderink RG, et al. Ventilator-associated Pseudomonas aeruginosa pneumonia: radiographic findings. Radiology 1995;195:247–252.

37. Winer-Muram HT, Steiner RM, Gurney JW, et al. Ventilator-associated pneumonia in patients with adult respiratory distress syndrome: CT evaluation. Radiology 1998;208:193–199.

38. Melbye H, Dale K. Interobserver variability in the radiographic diagnosis of adult outpatient pneumonia. Acta Radiol 1992;33:79–81.

39. Smith CB, Overall JC. Clinical and epidemiologic clues to the diagnosis of respiratory infections. Radiol Clin North Am 1973;11:261–278.

40. Moine P, Vercken JB, Chevret S, et al. Severe community-acquired pneumococcal pneumonia. Scand J Infect Dis 1995;27:201–206.

41. Marrie TJ. Pneumococcal pneumonia: epidemiology and clinical features. Semin Respir Infect 1999;14:227–236.

42. Mufson MA. Pneumococcal pneumonia. Curr Infect Dis Rep 1999;1:57–64.

43. Ort S, Ryan JL, Barden G, et al. Pneumococcal pneumonia in hospitalized patients. Clinical and radiological presentations. JAMA 1983;249:214–218.

44. Kantor HG. The many radiologic facies of pneumococcal pneumonia. AJR Am J Roentgenol 1981;137:1213–1220.

45. Shah RM, Gupta S, Angeid-Backman E, et al. Pneumococcal pneumonia in patients requiring hospitalization: effects of bacteremia and HIV seropositivity on radiographic appearance. AJR Am J Roentgenol 2000;175:1533–1536.

46. Light RW, Girard WM, Jenkinson SG, et al. Parapneumonic effusions. Am J Med 1980;69:507–512.

47. Taryle DA, Potts DE, Sahn SA. The incidence and clinical correlates of parapneumonic effusions in pneumococcal pneumonia. Chest 1978;74:170–173.

48. Barnham M, Weightman N, Anderson A, et al. Review of 17 cases of pneumonia caused by Streptococcus pyogenes. Eur J Clin Microbiol Infect Dis 1999;18:506–509.

49. Birch C, Gowardman J. Streptococcus pyogenes: a forgotten cause of severe community-acquired pneumonia. Anaesth Intensive Care 2000;28:87–90.

50. Basiliere JL, Bistrong HW, Spence WF. Streptococcal pneumonia. Recent outbreaks in military recruit populations. Am J Med 1968;44:580–589.

51. Haddadin AS, Fappiano SA, Lipsett PA. Methicillin resistant Staphylococcus aureus (MRSA) in the intensive care unit. Postgrad Med J 2002;78:385–392.

52. Rello J, Torres A, Ricart M, et al. Ventilator-associated pneumonia by Staphylococcus aureus. Comparison of methicillin-resistant and methicillin-sensitive episodes. Am J Respir Crit Care Med 1994;150:1545–1549.

53. Macfarlane J, Rose D. Radiographic features of staphylococcal pneumonia in adults and children. Thorax 1996;51:539–540.

54. Gonzalez C, Rubio M, Romero-Vivas J, et al. Bacteremic pneumonia due to Staphylococcus aureus: A comparison of disease caused by methicillin-resistant and methicillin-susceptible organisms. Clin Infect Dis 1999;29:1171–1177.

55. Naraqi S, McDonnell G. Hematogenous staphylococcal pneumonia secondary to soft tissue infection. Chest 1981;79: 173–175.

56. Traeger MS, Wiersma ST, Rosenstein NE, et al. First case of bioterrorism-related inhalational anthrax in the United States, Palm Beach County, Florida, 2001. Emerg Infect Dis 2002;8:1029–1034.

57. Borio L, Frank D, Mani V, et al. Death due to bioterrorism-related inhalational anthrax: report of 2 patients. JAMA 2001;286:2554–2559.

58. Mayer TA, Bersoff-Matcha S, Murphy C, et al. Clinical presentation of inhalational anthrax following bioterrorism exposure: report of 2 surviving patients. JAMA 2001;286:2549–2553.

59. Ketai L, Alrahji AA, Hart B, et al. Radiologic manifestations of potential bioterrorist agents of infection. AJR Am J Roentgenol 2003;180: 565–575.

60. Vessal K, Yeganehdoust J, Dutz W, et al. Radiological changes in inhalation anthrax. A report of radiological and pathological correlation in two cases. Clin Radiol 1975;26:471–474.

61. Earls JP, Cerva D Jr, Berman E, et al. Inhalational anthrax after bioterrorism exposure: spectrum of imaging findings in two surviving patients. Radiology 2002;222:305–312.

62. Krol CM, Uszynski M, Dillon EH, et al. Dynamic CT features of inhalational anthrax infection. AJR Am J Roentgenol 2002;178:1063–1066.

63. Pierce AK, Sanford JP. Aerobic gram-negative bacillary pneumonias. Am Rev Respir Dis 1974;110:647–658.

64. Costa SF, Newbaer M, Santos CR, et al. Nosocomial pneumonia: importance of recognition of aetiological agents to define an appropriate initial empirical therapy. Int J Antimicrob Agents 2001;17:147–150.

65. Wilson R, Dowling RB. Lung infections. 3. Pseudomonas aeruginosa and other related species. Thorax 1998;53:213–219.

66. Vikram HR, Shore ET, Venkatesh PR. Community acquired Pseudomonas aeruginosa pneumonia. Conn Med 1999;63:271–273.

67. Evans SA, Turner SM, Bosch BJ, et al. Lung function in bronchiectasis: the influence of Pseudomonas aeruginosa. Eur Respir J 1996;9:1601–1604.

68. Miszkiel KA, Wells AU, Rubens MB, et al. Effects of airway infection by Pseudomonas aeruginosa: a computed tomographic study. Thorax 1997;52: 260–264.

69. Iannini PB, Claffey T, Quintiliani R. Bacteremic Pseudomonas pneumonia. JAMA 1974;230:558–561.

70. Unger JD, Rose HD, Unger GF. Gram-negative pneumonia. Radiology 1973;107:283–291.

71. Shah RM, Wechsler R, Salazar AM, et al. Spectrum of CT findings in nosocomial

Pseudomonas aeruginosa pneumonia. J Thorac Imaging 2002;17:53–57.

72. Mays B, Thomas G, Leonard J, et al. Gram-negative bacillary necrotizing pneumonia: a bacteriologic and histopathologic correlation. J Infect Dis 1969;120:687–697.

73. Renner RR, Coccaro AP, Heitzman ER, et al. Pseudomonas pneumonia: a prototype of hospital-based infection. Radiology 1972;105:555–562.

74. Felson L, Rosenberg L, Hamburger M. Roentgen findings in acute Friedlander's pneumonia. Radiology 1949;53:559–565.

75. Holmes R. Friedlander's pneumonia. AJR Am J Roentgenol 1956;75:728–747.

76. Moon WK, Im JG, Yeon KM, et al. Complications of Klebsiella pneumonia: CT evaluation. J Comput Assist Tomogr 1995;19:176–181.

77. Reed WP. Indolent pulmonary abscess associated with Klebsiella and Enterobacter. Am Rev Respir Dis 1973;107:1055–1059.

78. Benin AL, Benson RF, Besser RE. Trends in legionnaires disease, 1980–1998: declining mortality and new patterns of diagnosis. Clin Infect Dis 2002;35:1039–1046.

79. Nguyen ML, Yu VL. Legionella infection. Clin Chest Med 1991;12:257–268.

80. Muder RR, Yu VL. Infection due to Legionella species other than L. pneumophila. Clin Infect Dis 2002;35:990–998.

81. Ruggles L. Legionella pneumonia. Can Fam Physician 2001;47:1737–1739.

82. Fernandez JA, Lopez P, Orozco D, et al. Clinical study of an outbreak of Legionnaire's disease in Alcoy, Southeastern Spain. Eur J Clin Microbiol Infect Dis 2002;21:729–735.

83. Fraser DW, Tsai TR, Orenstein W, et al. Legionnaires' disease: description of an epidemic of pneumonia. N Engl J Med 1977;297:1189–1197.

84. Tan MJ, Tan JS, File TM Jr. Legionnaires disease with bacteremic coinfection. Clin Infect Dis 2002;35:533–539.

85. Murdoch DR. Diagnosis of Legionella infection. Clin Infect Dis 2003;36:64–69.

86. Waterer GW, Baselski VS, Wunderink RG. Legionella and community-acquired pneumonia: a review of current diagnostic tests from a clinician's viewpoint. Am J Med 2001;110:41–48.

87. Kirby BD, Snyder KM, Meyer RD, et al. Legionnaires' disease: report of sixty-five nosocomially acquired cases of review of the literature. Medicine Balt 1980;59:188–205.

88. Yu VL, Kroboth FJ, Shonnard J, et al. Legionnaires' disease: new clinical perspective from a prospective pneumonia study. Am J Med 1982;73:357–361.

89. Fairbank JT, Patel MM, Dietrich PA. Legionnaires' disease. J Thorac Imaging 1991;6:6–13.

90. Meenhorst PL, Mulder JD. The chest X-ray in Legionella Pneumonia (Legionnaires' disease). Eur J Radiol 1983;3:180–186.

91. Evans AF, Oakley RH, Whitehouse GH. Analysis of the chest radiograph in Legionnaires' disease. Clin Radiol 1981;32:361–365.

92. Kroboth FJ, Yu VL, Reddy SC, et al. Clinicoradiographic correlation with the extent of Legionnaire disease. AJR Am J Roentgenol 1983;141:263–268.

93. Moore EH, Webb WR, Gamsu G, et al. Legionnaires' disease in the renal transplant patient: clinical presentation and radiographic progression. Radiology 1984;153:589–593.

94. Randolph KA, Beekman JF. Legionnaires' disease presenting with empyema. Chest 1979;75:404–406.

95. Quagliano PV, Das Narla L. Legionella pneumonia causing multiple cavitating pulmonary nodules in a 7-month-old infant. AJR Am J Roentgenol 1993;161:367–368.

96. De Serres G, Shadmani R, Duval B, et al. Morbidity of pertussis in adolescents and adults. J Infect Dis 2000;182:174–179.

97. Yaari E, Yafe-Zimerman Y, Schwartz SB, et al. Clinical manifestations of Bordetella pertussis infection in immunized children and young adults. Chest 1999;115:1254–1258.

98. Barnhard H, Kniker W. Roentgenologic findings in pertussis with particular emphasis on the "shaggy heart" sign. AJR Am J Roentgenol 1960;84:445–450.

99. Bellamy EA, Johnston ID, Wilson AG. The chest radiograph in whooping cough. Clin Radiol 1987;38:39–43.

100. Fawcitt J, Parry H. Lung changes in pertussis and measles in childhood: a review of 1894 cases with a follow up study of the pulmonary complications. Br J Radiol 1957;30:76–82.

101. Piampiano P, McLeary M, Young LW, et al. Brucellosis: unusual presentations in two adolescent boys. Pediatr Radiol 2000;30:355–357.

102. Abu-Ekteish F, Kakish K. Pneumonia as the sole presentation of brucellosis. Respir Med 2001;95:766–767.

103. Gurney JW, Unger JM, Dorby CA, et al. Agricultural disorders of the lung. RadioGraphics 1991;11:625–634.

104. Arcomano JP, Pizzolato NF, Singer R, et al. A unique type of calcification in chronic brucellosis. AJR Am J Roentgenol 1977;128:135–137.

105. Dance DA. Melioidosis. Curr Opin Infect Dis 2002;15:127–132.

106. Dhiensiri T, Puapairoj S, Susaengrat W. Pulmonary melioidosis: clinical–radiologic correlation in 183 cases in northeastern Thailand. Radiology 1988;166:711–715.

107. Inglis TJ, Garrow SC, Adams C, et al. Acute melioidosis outbreak in Western Australia. Epidemiol Infect 1999;123:437–443.

108. Ip M, Osterberg LG, Chau PY, et al. Pulmonary melioidosis. Chest 1995;108:1420–1424.

109. Tan AP, Pui MH, Tan LK. Imaging patterns in melioidosis. Australas Radiol 1995;39:260–264.

110. Puthucheary SD, Vadivelu J, Wong KT, et al. Acute respiratory failure in melioidosis. Singapore Med J 2001;42:117–121.

111. Schulin T, Steinmetz I. Chronic melioidosis in a patient with cystic fibrosis. J Clin Microbiol 2001;39:1676–1677.

112. Tsang TY, Lai ST. A case of thoracic empyema due to suppurative melioidosis. Hong Kong Med J 2001;7:201–204.

113. Sweet R, Wilson E, Chandler B. Melioidosis manifested by cavitary lung disease. AJR Am J Roentgenol 1968;103:543–547.

114. Alsofrom DJ, Mettler FA Jr, Mann JM. Radiographic manifestations of plague in New Mexico, 1975–1980. A review of 42 proved cases. Radiology 1981;139:561–565.

115. Crook LD, Tempest B. Plague. A clinical review of 27 cases. Arch Intern Med 1992;152:1253–1256.

116. Boisier P, Rahalison L, Rasolomaharo M, et al. Epidemiologic features of four successive annual outbreaks of bubonic plague in Mahajanga, Madagascar. Emerg Infect Dis 2002;8:311–316.

117. Gradon JD. Plague pneumonia. Curr Infect Dis Rep 2002;4:244–248.

118. Winer-Muram HT, Rubin SA. Pet-associated lung diseases. J Thorac Imaging 1991;6:14–30.

119. Eliasson H, Lindback J, Nuorti JP, et al. The 2000 tularemia outbreak: a case-control study of risk factors in disease-endemic and emergent areas, Sweden. Emerg Infect Dis 2002;8:956–960.

120. Feldman KA, Enscore RE, Lathrop SL, et al. An outbreak of primary pneumonic tularemia on Martha's Vineyard. N Engl J Med 2001;345:1601–1606.

121. Overholt E, Tiggert W. Roentgenographic manifestations of pulmonary tularemia. Radiology 1960;74:758–765.

122. Rubin SA. Radiographic spectrum of pleuropulmonary tularemia. AJR Am J Roentgenol 1978;131:277–281.

123. Bartlett JG, Finegold SM. Anaerobic infections of the lung and pleural space. Am Rev Respir Dis 1974;110:56–77.

124. Mojon P. Oral health and respiratory infection. J Can Dent Assoc 2002;68:340–345.

125. Levison ME. Anaerobic pleuropulmonary infection. Curr Opin Infect Dis 2001;14:187–191.

126. Landay MJ, Christensen EE, Bynum LJ, et al. Anaerobic pleural and pulmonary infections. AJR Am J Roentgenol 1980;134:233–240.

127. Bartlett JG. Anaerobic bacterial pneumonitis. Am Rev Respir Dis 1979;119:19–23.

128. Rohlfing BM, White EA, Webb WR, et al. Hilar and mediastinal adenopathy caused by bacterial abscess of the lung. Radiology 1978;128:289–293.

129. Guseinov GK, Guseinov AG. [A case of tertiary syphilis of the lungs and spine masking as tuberculosis]. Probl Tuberk 2001;52–53.

130. Cholankeril JV, Greenberg AL, Matari HM, et al. Solitary pulmonary nodule in secondary syphilis. Clin Imaging 1992;16:125–128.

131. Im JG, Yeon KM, Han MC, et al. Leptospirosis of the lung: radiographic findings in 58 patients. AJR Am J Roentgenol 1989;152:955–959.

132. Carvalho CR, Bethlem EP. Pulmonary complications of leptospirosis. Clin Chest Med 2002;23:469–478.

133. Martinez Garcia MA, de Diego DA, Menendez VR, et al. Pulmonary involvement in leptospirosis. Eur J Clin Microbiol Infect Dis 2000;19:471–474.

134. Bethlem EP, Carvalho CR. Pulmonary leptospirosis. Curr Opin Pulm Med 2000;6:436–441.

135. Lee RE, Terry SI, Walker TM, et al. The chest radiograph in leptospirosis in Jamaica. Br J Radiol 1981;54:939–943.

136. Marchiori E, Müller NL. Leptospirosis of the lung: high-resolution computed tomography findings in five patients. J Thorac Imaging 2002;17:151–153.

137. Sampere M, Font B, Font J, et al. Q Fever in adults: review of 66 clinical cases. Eur J Clin Microbiol Infect Dis 2003;22:108–110.

138. Stein A, Raoult D. Pigeon pneumonia in Provence: a bird-borne Q fever outbreak. Clin Infect Dis 1999;29:617–620.

139. Raoult D, Tissot-Dupont H, Foucault C, et al. Q fever 1985–1998. Clinical and epidemiologic features of 1,383 infections. Medicine Balt 2000;79:109–123.

140. Domingo P, Munoz C, Franquet T, et al. Acute Q fever in adult patients: report on 63 sporadic cases in an urban area. Clin Infect Dis 1999;29:874–879.

141. Gordon J, McKeen A, Maric T, et al. The radiographic features of epidemic and sporadic Q fever pneumonia. J Can Assoc Rad 1984;35:293–296.

142. Pickworth FE, el Soussi M, Wells IP, et al. The radiological appearances of 'Q' fever pneumonia. Clin Radiol 1991;44:150–153.

143. Gikas A, Kofteridis D, Bouros D, et al. Q fever pneumonia: appearance on chest radiographs. Radiology 1999;210:339–343.

144. Smith DL, Wellings R, Walker C, et al. The chest X ray in Q-fever: a report on 69 cases from the 1989 West Midlands outbreak. Br J Radiol 1991;64:1101–1108.

145. Janigan DT, Marrie TJ. An inflammatory pseudotumor of the lung in Q fever pneumonia. N Engl J Med 1983;308:86–88.

146. Lipton JH, Fong TC, Gill MJ, et al. Q fever inflammatory pseudotumor of the lung. Chest 1987;92:756–757.

147. Seggev JS, Levin S, Schey G. Unusual radiological manifestations of Q fever. Eur J Respir Dis 1986;69:120–122.

148. Voloudaki AE, Kofteridis DP, Tritou IN, et al. Q fever pneumonia: CT findings. Radiology 2000;215:880–883.

149. Lees RF, Harrison RB, Willamson BR, et al. Radiographic findings in Rocky Mountain spotted fever. Radiology 1978;129:17–20.

150. Donohue JF. Lower respiratory tract involvement in Rocky Mountain spotted fever. Arch Intern Med 1980;140:223–227.

151. Martin W III, Choplin RH, Shertzer ME. The chest radiograph in Rocky Mountain spotted fever. AJR Am J Roentgenol 1982;139:889–893.

152. Soni R, Seale JP, Young IH. Fulminant psittacosis requiring mechanical ventilation and demonstrating serological cross-reactivity between Legionella longbeachae and Chlamydia psittaci. Respirology 1999;4:203–205.

153. Schaffner W, Drutz DJ, Duncan GW, et al. The clinical spectrum of endemic psittacosis. Arch Intern Med 1967;119:433–443.

154. Hagiwara K, Ouchi K, Tashiro N, et al. An epidemic of a pertussis-like illness caused by Chlamydia pneumoniae. Pediatr Infect Dis J 1999;18:271–275.

155. Sahn SA. Pleural effusions in the atypical pneumonias. Semin Respir Infect 1988;3:322–334.

156. Radkowski MA, Kranzler JK, Beem MO, et al. Chlamydia pneumonia in infants: radiography in 125 cases. AJR Am J Roentgenol 1981;137:703–706.

157. Edelman RR, Hann LE, Simon M. Chlamydia trachomatis pneumonia in adults: radiographic appearance. Radiology 1984;152:279–282.

158. Stutman HR, Rettig PJ, Reyes S. Chlamydia trachomatis as a cause of pneumonitis and pleural effusion. J Pediatr 1984;104:588–591.

159. Thom DH, Grayston JT. Infections with Chlamydia pneumoniae strain TWAR. Clin Chest Med 1991;12:245–256.

160. Blasi F, Cosentini R, Tarsia P. Chlamydia pneumoniae respiratory infections. Curr Opin Infect Dis 2000;13:161–164.

161. Fujita J, Bandoh S, Tokuda M, et al. Non-specific interstitial pneumonia and Chlamydia pneumoniae infection. Jpn J Infect Dis 2001;54:225–228.

162. McConnell CTJ, Plouffe JF, File TM, et al. Radiographic appearance of Chlamydia pneumoniae (TWAR strain) respiratory infections. CBPIS Study Group. Community-based Pneumonia Incidence Study. Radiology 1994;192:819–824.

163. Toorians AW, Pneumatikos JA, Zaaijer HL, et al. Bilateral pleural effusion and a subsegmental infiltrate due to Chlamydia pneumoniae in a mechanically ventilated patient. Neth J Med 2001;59:62–65.

164. Julander I. Staphylococcal septicaemia and endocarditis in 80 drug addicts. Aspects on epidemiology, clinical and laboratory findings and prognosis. Scand J Infect Dis Suppl 1983;41:49–55.

165. Hughes CE, Spear RK, Shinabarger CE, et al. Septic pulmonary emboli complicating mastoiditis: Lemierre's syndrome revisited. Clin Infect Dis 1994;18:633–635.

166. Screaton NJ, Ravenel JG, Lehner PJ, et al. Lemierre syndrome: forgotten but not extinct – report of four cases. Radiology 1999;213:369–374.

167. Kuhlman JE, Fishman EK, Teigen C. Pulmonary septic emboli: diagnosis with CT. Radiology 1990;174:211–213.

168. Huang RM, Naidich DP, Lubat E, et al. Septic pulmonary emboli: CT–radiographic correlation. AJR Am J Roentgenol 1989;153:41–45.

169. Ren H, Kuhlman JE, Hruban RH, et al. CT of inflation-fixed lungs: wedge-shaped density and vascular sign in the diagnosis of infarction. J Comput Assist Tomogr 1990;14:82–86.

170. Light RW. Pleural diseases, 3rd edn. Philadelphia: Lea & Febiger, 1990.

171. Weese WC, Shindler ER, Smith IM, et al. Empyema of the thorax then and now. A study of 122 cases over four decades. Arch Intern Med 1973;131:516–520.

172. Vianna NJ. Nontuberculous bacterial empyema in patients with and without underlying diseases. JAMA 1971;215:69–75.

173. Light RW. Parapneumonic effusions and empyema. Clin Chest Med 1985;6:55–62.

174. Hamm H, Light RW. Parapneumonic effusion and empyema. Eur Respir J 1997;10:1150–1156.

175. Colice GL, Curtis A, Deslauriers J, et al. Medical and surgical treatment of parapneumonic effusions: an evidence-based guideline. Chest 2000;118:1158–1171.

176. de Souza A, Offner PJ, Moore EE, et al. Optimal management of complicated empyema. Am J Surg 2000;180:507–511.

177. Kearney SE, Davies CW, Davies RJ, et al. Computed tomography and ultrasound in parapneumonic effusions and empyema. Clin Radiol 2000;55:542–547.

178. Light RW. Management of parapneumonic effusions. Arch Intern Med 1981;141:1339–1341.

179. Alfageme I, Munoz F, Pena N, et al. Empyema of the thorax in adults.

Etiology, microbiologic findings, and management. Chest 1993;103:839–843.

180. Hanna JW, Reed JC, Choplin RH. Pleural infections: a clinical–radiologic review. J Thorac Imaging 1991;6:68–79.

181. Choe DH, Lee JH, Lee BH, et al. Postpneumonectomy empyema. CT findings in six patients. Clin Imaging 2001;25:28–31.

182. Brook I, Frazier EH. Aerobic and anaerobic microbiology of empyema. A retrospective review in two military hospitals. Chest 1993;103:1502–1507.

183. Wallenhaupt SL. Surgical management of thoracic empyema. J Thorac Imaging 1991;6:80–88.

184. Friedman PJ, Hellekant CA. Radiologic recognition of bronchopleural fistula. Radiology 1977;124:289–295.

185. Stark DD, Federle MP, Goodman PC, et al. Differentiating lung abscess and empyema: radiography and computed tomography. AJR Am J Roentgenol 1983;141:163–167.

186. Leung AN, Müller NL, Miller RR. CT in differential diagnosis of diffuse pleural disease. AJR Am J Roentgenol 1990;154:487–492.

187. Shin MS, Ho KJ. Computed tomographic characteristics of pleural empyema. J Comput Tomogr 1983;7:179–182.

188. Aquino SL, Webb WR, Gushiken BJ. Pleural exudates and transudates: diagnosis with contrast-enhanced CT. Radiology 1994;192:803–808.

189. Waite RJ, Carbonneau RJ, Balikian JP, et al. Parietal pleural changes in empyema: appearances at CT. Radiology 1990;175:145–150.

190. Kim HY, Song KS, Lee HJ, et al. Parietal pleura and extrapleural space in chronic tuberculous empyema: CT–pathologic correlation. J Comput Assist Tomogr 2001;25:9–15.

191. Kearney SE, Davies CW, Tattersall DJ, et al. The characteristics and significance of thoracic lymphadenopathy in parapneumonic effusion and empyema. Br J Radiol 2000;73:583–587.

192. Minami M, Kawauchi N, Yoshikawa K, et al. Malignancy associated with chronic empyema: radiologic assessment. Radiology 1991;178:417–423.

193. Dye C, Scheele S, Dolin P, et al. Consensus statement. Global burden of tuberculosis: estimated incidence, prevalence, and mortality by country. WHO Global Surveillance and Monitoring Project. JAMA 1999; 282:677–686.

194. CDC tuberculosis – United States 1985. MMWR 1986;35:669–703.

195. Pitchenik AE, Rubinson HA. The radiographic appearance of tuberculosis in patients with the acquired immune deficiency syndrome (AIDS) and pre-AIDS. Am Rev Respir Dis 1985;131: 393–396.

196. Buckner CB, Leithiser RE, Walker CW, et al. The changing epidemiology of tuberculosis and other mycobacterial infections in the United States: implications for the radiologist. AJR Am J Roentgenol 1991;156:255–264.

197. Rose AM, Watson JM, Graham C, et al. Tuberculosis at the end of the 20th century in England and Wales: results of a national survey in 1998. Thorax 2001;56:173–179.

198. Stead WW. Special problems in tuberculosis. Tuberculosis in the elderly and in residents of nursing homes, correctional facilities, long-term care hospitals, mental hospitals, shelters for the homeless, and jails. Clin Chest Med 1989;10:397–405.

199. Pratt PC. Pathology of tuberculosis. Semin Roentgenol 1979;14:196–203.

200. Bailey CM, Windle-Taylor PC. Tuberculous laryngitis: a series of 37 patients. Laryngoscope 1981;91:93–100.

201. Woodring JH, Vandiviere HM, Fried AM, et al. Update: the radiographic features of pulmonary tuberculosis. AJR Am J Roentgenol 1986;146:497–506.

202. Leung AN, Müller NL, Pineda PR, et al. Primary tuberculosis in childhood: radiographic manifestations. Radiology 1992;182:87–91.

203. Delacourt C, Mani TM, Bonnerot V, et al. Computed tomography with normal chest radiograph in tuberculous infection. Arch Dis Child 1993;69:430–432.

204. Baran R, Tor M, Tahaoglu K, et al. Intrathoracic tuberculous adenopathy: clinical and bronchoscopic features in 17 adults without parenchymal lesions. Chest 1996;51:87–89.

205. Kim WS, Moon WK, Kim IO, et al. Pulmonary tuberculosis in children: evaluation with CT. AJR Am J Roentgenol 1997;168:1005–1009.

206. Niggemann B, Klettke U, Magdorf K, et al. Two cases of pulmonary tuberculosis presenting with unilateral pulmonary hyperinflation in infancy. Eur J Pediatr 1995;154:413–415.

207. Kuhlman JE, Deutsch JH, Fishman EK, et al. CT features of thoracic mycobacterial disease. RadioGraphics 1990;10:413–431.

208. Lee KS, Im JG. CT in adults with tuberculosis of the chest: characteristic findings and role in management. AJR Am J Roentgenol 1995;164:1361–1367.

209. Lee KS, Hwang JW, Chung MP, et al. Utility of CT in the evaluation of pulmonary tuberculosis in patients without AIDS. Chest 1996;110:977–984.

210. Kim Y, Lee KS, Yoon JH, et al. Tuberculosis of the trachea and main bronchi: CT findings in 17 patients. AJR Am J Roentgenol 1997;168:1051–1056.

211. Beigelman C, Sellami D, Brauner M. CT of parenchymal and bronchial tuberculosis. Eur Radiol 2000;10:699–709.

212. Oh YW, Kim YH, Lee NJ, et al. High-resolution CT appearance of miliary tuberculosis. J Comput Assist Tomogr 1994;18:862–866.

213. Kim HC, Goo JM, Kim HB, et al. Tuberculosis in patients with myelodysplastic syndromes. Clin Radiol 2002;57:408–414.

214. Yabuuchi H, Murayama S, Murakami J, et al. Correlation of immunologic status with high-resolution CT and distributions of pulmonary tuberculosis. Acta Radiol 2002;43:44–47.

215. Haramati LB, Jenny-Avital ER, Alterman DD. Effect of HIV status on chest radiographic and CT findings in patients with tuberculosis. Clin Radiol 1997;52: 31–35.

216. Leung AN, Brauner MW, Gamsu G, et al. Pulmonary tuberculosis: comparison of CT findings in HIV-seropositive and HIV-seronegative patients. Radiology 1996;198:687–691.

217. Post F, Wood R, Pillay G. Pulmonary tuberculosis in HIV infection: radiographic appearance is related to CD4+ T-lymphocyte count. Tubercle Lung Dis 1995;76:518–521.

218. Perlman DC, el Sadr WM, Nelson ET, et al. Variation of chest radiographic patterns in pulmonary tuberculosis by degree of human immunodeficiency virus-related immunosuppression. The Terry Beirn Community Programs for Clinical Research on AIDS (CPCRA). The AIDS Clinical Trials Group (ACTG). Clin Infect Dis 1997;25:242–246.

219. Saurborn DP, Fishman JE, Boiselle PM. The imaging spectrum of pulmonary tuberculosis in AIDS. J Thorac Imaging 2002;17:28–33.

220. Greenberg SD, Frager D, Suster B, et al. Active pulmonary tuberculosis in patients with AIDS: spectrum of radiographic findings (including a normal appearance). Radiology 1994;193:115–119.

221. Alpert PL, Munsiff SS, Gourevitch MN, et al. A prospective study of tuberculosis and human immunodeficiency virus infection: clinical manifestations and factors associated with survival. Clin Infect Dis 1997;24:661–668.

222. Berger HW, Granada MG. Lower lung field tuberculosis. Chest 1974;65:522–526.

223. Spencer D, Yagan R, Blinkhorn R, et al. Anterior segment upper lobe tuberculosis in the adult. Occurrence in primary and reactivation disease. Chest 1990;97:384–388.

224. Kim HY, Song KS, Goo JM, et al. Thoracic sequelae and complications of tuberculosis. RadioGraphics 2001;21: 839–858.

225. Vix VA. Radiographic manifestations of broncholithiasis. Radiology 1978;128: 295–299.

226. Seo JB, Song KS, Lee JS, et al. Broncholithiasis: review of the causes with radiologic–pathologic correlation. RadioGraphics 2002;22:S199–S213.

227. Kowal LE, Goodman LR, Zarro VJ, et al. CT diagnosis of broncholithiasis. J Comput Assist Tomogr 1983;7:321–323.

228. Goo JM, Im JG, Do KH, et al. Pulmonary tuberculoma evaluated by means of FDG PET: findings in 10 cases. Radiology 2000;216:117–121.

229. Kwong JS, Carignan S, Kang EY, et al. Miliary tuberculosis. Diagnostic accuracy of chest radiography. Chest 1996;110:339–342.

230. Hong SH, Im JG, Lee JS, et al. High resolution CT findings of miliary tuberculosis. J Comput Assist Tomogr 1998;22:220–224.

231. Lee KS, Kim TS, Han J, et al. Diffuse micronodular lung disease: HRCT and pathologic findings. J Comput Assist Tomogr 1999;23:99–106.

232. Dee P, Teja K, Korzeniowski O, et al. Miliary tuberculosis resulting in adult respiratory distress syndrome: a surviving case. AJR Am J Roentgenol 1980;134:569–572.

233. Penner C, Roberts D, Kunimoto D, et al. Tuberculosis as a primary cause of respiratory failure requiring mechanical ventilation. Am J Respir Crit Care Med 1995;151:867–872.

234. Im JG, Webb WR, Han MC, et al. Apical opacity associated with pulmonary tuberculosis: high resolution CT findings. Radiology 1991;178:727–731.

235. Nyman RS, Brismar J, Hugosson C, et al. Imaging of tuberculosis – experience from 503 patients. I. Tuberculosis of the chest. Acta Radiol 1996;37:482–488.

236. Lampmann LE. Control of massive hemoptysis due to pulmonary tuberculosis with bronchial arterial embolization. Radiology 1997;204: 875–876.

237. Ramakantan R, Bandekar VG, Gandhi MS, et al. Massive hemoptysis due to pulmonary tuberculosis: control with bronchial artery embolization. Radiology 1996;200:691–694.

238. Remy J, Smith M, Lemaitre L, et al. Treatment of massive hemoptysis by occlusion of a Rasmussen aneurysm. AJR Am J Roentgenol 1980;135: 605–606.

239. Santelli ED, Katz DS, Goldschmidt AM, et al. Embolization of multiple Rasmussen aneurysms as a treatment of hemoptysis. Radiology 1994;193: 396–398.

240. Moore NR, Phillips MS, Shneerson JM, et al. Appearances on computed tomography following thoracoplasty for pulmonary tuberculosis. Br J Radiol 1988;61:573–578.

241. Im JG, Itoh H, Shim YS, et al. Pulmonary tuberculosis: CT findings – early active

disease and sequential change with antituberculous therapy. Radiology 1993;186:653–660.

242. Lee KS, Song KS, Lim TH, et al. Adult-onset pulmonary tuberculosis: findings on chest radiographs and CT scans. AJR Am J Roentgenol 1993;160:753–758.

243. Im JG, Itoh H, Han MC. CT of pulmonary tuberculosis. Semin Ultrasound CT MR 1995;16:420–434.

244. Hatipoglu ON, Osma E, Manisali M, et al. High resolution computed tomographic findings in pulmonary tuberculosis. Thorax 1996;51:397–402.

245. Moon WK, Im JG, Yeon KM, et al. Tuberculosis of the central airways: CT findings of active and fibrotic disease. AJR Am J Roentgenol 1997;169:649–653.

246. Poey C, Verhaegen F, Giron J, et al. High resolution chest CT in tuberculosis: evolutive patterns and signs of activity. J Comput Assist Tomogr 1997;21:601–607.

247. Moon WK, Im JG, Yeon KM, et al. Mediastinal tuberculous lymphadenitis: CT findings of active and inactive disease. AJR Am J Roentgenol 1998;170:715–718.

248. Akira M, Sakatani M. Clinical and high-resolution computed tomographic findings in five patients with pulmonary tuberculosis who developed respiratory failure following chemotherapy. Clin Radiol 2001;56:550–555.

249. Park S, Hong YK, Joo SH, et al. CT findings of pulmonary tuberculosis presenting as segmental consolidation. J Comput Assist Tomogr 1999;23: 736–742.

250. Tateishi U, Kusumoto M, Akiyama Y, et al. Role of contrast-enhanced dynamic CT in the diagnosis of active tuberculoma. Chest 2002;122:1280–1284.

251. Goo JM, Im JG. CT of tuberculosis and nontuberculous mycobacterial infections. Radiol Clin North Am 2002;40:73–87, viii.

252. Atasoy C, Fitoz S, Erguvan B, et al. Tuberculous fibrosing mediastinitis: CT and MRI findings. J Thorac Imaging 2001;16:191–193.

253. Lee JY, Lee KS, Jung KJ, et al. Pulmonary tuberculosis: CT and pathologic correlation. J Comput Assist Tomogr 2000;24:691–698.

254. Ikezoe J, Takeuchi N, Johkoh T, et al. CT appearance of pulmonary tuberculosis in diabetic and immunocompromised patients: comparison with patients who had no underlying disease. AJR Am J Roentgenol 1992;159:1175–1179.

255. Roberts CM, Citron KM, Strickland B. Intrathoracic aspergilloma: Role of CT in diagnosis and treatment. Radiology 1987;165:123–128.

256. Shin MS, Ho KJ. Computed tomography of bronchiectasis in association with tuberculosis. Clin Imaging 1989;13: 36–43.

257. Sahn SA, Iseman MD. Tuberculous empyema. Semin Respir Infect 1999;14:82–87.

258. Yilmaz E, Akkoclu A, Sevinc C. CT and MRI appearance of a fistula between the right and left main bronchus caused by tracheobronchial tuberculosis. Br J Radiol 2001;74:1056–1058.

259. Im JG, Kim JH, Han MC, et al. Computed tomography of esophagomediastinal fistula in tuberculous mediastinal lymphadenitis. J Comput Assist Tomogr 1990;14:89–92.

260. Falkinham JO III. Nontuberculous mycobacteria in the environment. Clin Chest Med 2002;23:529–551.

261. Ellis SM, Hansell DM. Imaging of non-tuberculous (atypical) mycobacterial pulmonary infection. Clin Radiol 2002;57:661–669.

262. Contreras MA, Cheung OT, Sanders DE, et al. Pulmonary infection with nontuberculous mycobacteria. Am Rev Respir Dis 1988;137:149–152.

263. O'Brien RJ. The epidemiology of nontuberculous mycobacterial disease. Clin Chest Med 1989;10:407–418.

264. Ebert DL, Olivier KN. Nontuberculous mycobacteria in the setting of cystic fibrosis. Clin Chest Med 2002;23:655–663.

265. Chalermskulrat W, Gilbey JG, Donohue JF. Nontuberculous mycobacteria in women, young and old. Clin Chest Med 2002;23:675–686.

266. Swensen SJ, Hartman TE, Williams DE. Computed tomographic diagnosis of Mycobacterium avium-intracellulare complex in patients with bronchiectasis. Chest 1994;105:49–52.

267. Gold JA, Rom WN, Harkin TJ. Significance of abnormal chest radiograph findings in patients with HIV-1 infection without respiratory symptoms. Chest 2002;121:1472–1477.

268. El-Solh AA, Nopper J, Abul-Khoudoud MR, et al. Clinical and radiographic manifestations of uncommon pulmonary nontuberculous mycobacterial disease in AIDS patients. Chest 1998;114:138–145.

269. Malouf MA, Glanville AR. The spectrum of mycobacterial infection after lung transplantation. Am J Respir Crit Care Med 1999;160:1611–1616.

270. Woodring JH, Vandiviere HM. Pulmonary disease caused by nontuberculous mycobacteria. J Thorac Imaging 1990;5:64–76.

271. Christensen EE, Dietz GW, Ahn CH, et al. Radiographic manifestations of pulmonary Mycobacterium kansasii infections. AJR Am J Roentgenol 1978;131:985–993.

272. Miller WTJ, Miller WTS. Pulmonary infections with atypical mycobacteria in the normal host. Semin Roentgenol 1993;28:139–149.

273. Evans AJ, Crisp AJ, Hubbard RB, et al. Pulmonary Mycobacterium kansasii

infection: comparison of radiological appearances with pulmonary tuberculosis. Thorax 1996;51:1243–1247.

274. Albelda SM, Kern JA, Marinelli DL, et al. Expanding spectrum of pulmonary disease caused by nontuberculous mycobacteria. Radiology 1985;157: 289–296.

275. Obayashi Y, Fujita J, Suemitsu I, et al. Successive follow-up of computed tomography in patients with *Mycobacterium avium-intracellulare* complex. Respir Med 1999;93:11–15.

276. Lynch DA, Simone PM, Fox MA, et al. CT features of pulmonary Mycobacterium avium complex infection. J Comput Assist Tomogr 1995;19:353–360.

277. Tanaka E, Amitani R, Niimi A, et al. Yield of computed tomography and bronchoscopy for the diagnosis of Mycobacterium avium complex pulmonary disease. Am J Respir Crit Care Med 1997;155:2041–2046.

278. Bailey WC. Treatment of atypical mycobacterial disease. Chest 1983;84:625–628.

279. Hartman TE, Swensen SJ, Williams DE. Mycobacterium avium-intracellulare complex: evaluation with CT. Radiology 1993;187:23–26.

280. Varghese G, Shepherd R, Watt P. Fatal infection with *Mycobacterium fortuitum* associated with oesophageal achalasia. Thorax 1988;43:151–152.

281. Aronchick JM, Miller WT, Epstein DM, et al. Association of achalasia and pulmonary Mycobacterium fortuitum infection. Radiology 1986;160:85–86.

282. Hollings NP, Wells AU, Wilson R, et al. Comparative appearances of non-tuberculous mycobacteria species: a CT study. Eur Radiol 2002;12:2211–2217.

283. Moore EH. Atypical mycobacterial infection in the lung: CT appearance. Radiology 1993;187:777–782.

284. Obayashi Y, Fujita J, Suemitsu I, et al. Successive follow-up of chest computed tomography in patients with Mycobacterium avium-intracellulare complex. Respir Med 1999;93:11–15.

285. Kubo K, Yamazaki Y, Masubuchi T, et al. Pulmonary infection with Mycobacterium avium-intracellulare leads to air trapping distal to the small airways. Am J Respir Crit Care Med 1998;158:979–984.

286. Primack SL, Logan PM, Hartman TE, et al. Pulmonary tuberculosis and Mycobacterium avium-intracellulare: a comparison of CT findings. Radiology 1995;194:413–417.

287. Wittram C, Weisbrod GL. Mycobacterium avium complex lung disease in immunocompetent patients: radiography–CT correlation. Br J Radiol 2002;75:340–344.

288. Obayashi Y, Fujita J, Suemitsu I, et al. Clinical features of non-tuberculous mycobacterial disease: comparisons between smear-positive and smear-negative cases, and between Mycobacterium avium and Mycobacterium intracellulare. Int J Tuberc Lung Dis 1998;2:597–602.

289. Anderson DH, Grech P, Townshend RH, et al. Pulmonary lesions due to opportunistic mycobacteria (review includes 30 cases of M.kansasii infections). Clin Radiol 1975;26: 461–469.

290. Wittram C, Weisbrod GL. *Mycobacterium xenopi* pulmonary infection: Evaluation with CT. J Comput Assist Tomogr 1998;22:225–228.

291. Han D, Lee KS, Koh WJ, et al. Radiographic and CT findings of nontuberculous mycobacterial pulmonary infection caused by Mycobacterium abscessus. AJR Am J Roentgenol 2003;181:513–517.

292. Evans AJ, Crisp AJ, Colville A, et al. Pulmonary infections caused by *Mycobacterium malmoense* and *Mycobacterium tuberculosis*: Comparison of radiographic features. AJR Am J Roentgenol 1993;161:733–737.

293. Hafeez I, Muers MF, Murphy SA, et al. Non-tuberculous mycobacterial lung infection complicated by chronic necrotising pulmonary aspergillosis. Thorax 2000;55:717–719.

294. Hazelton TR, Newell JD Jr, Cook JL, et al. CT findings in 14 patients with Mycobacterium chelonae pulmonary infection. AJR Am J Roentgenol 2000;175:413–416.

295. Oliver A, Maiz L, Canton R, et al. Nontuberculous mycobacteria in patients with cystic fibrosis. Clin Infect Dis 2001;32:1298–1303.

296. Eckburg PB, Buadu EO, Stark P, et al. Clinical and chest radiographic findings among persons with sputum culture positive for Mycobacterium gordonae: a review of 19 cases. Chest 2000;117: 96–102.

297. de Montpreville VT, Nashashibi N, Dulmet EM. Actinomycosis and other bronchopulmonary infections with bacterial granules. Ann Diagn Pathol 1999;3:67–74.

298. Baracco GJ, Dickinson GM. Pulmonary nocardiosis. Curr Infect Dis Rep 2001;3:286–292.

299. Krick JA, Stinson EB, Remington JS. Nocardia infection in heart transplant patients. Ann Intern Med 1975;82:18–26.

300. Munoz P, Palomo J, Guembe P, et al. Lung nodular lesions in heart transplant recipients. J Heart Lung Transplant 2000;19:660–667.

301. Raby N, Forbes G, Williams R. Nocardia infection in patients with liver transplants or chronic liver disease: radiologic findings. Radiology 1990;174:713–716.

302. Lee CC, Loo LW, Lam MS. Case reports of nocardiosis in patients with human immunodeficiency virus (HIV) infection. Ann Acad Med Singapore 2000;29: 119–126.

303. Aviram G, Fishman JE, Sagar M. Cavitary lung disease in AIDS: etiologies and correlation with immune status. AIDS Patient Care STDS 2001;15: 353–361.

304. Rubin E, Weisbrod GL, Sanders DE. Pulmonary alveolar proteinosis: relationship to silicosis and pulmonary infection. Radiology 1980;135:35–41.

305. Mari B, Monton C, Mariscal D, et al. Pulmonary nocardiosis: clinical experience in ten cases. Respiration 2001;68:382–388.

306. Lumb R, Greville H, Martin J, et al. Nocardia asteroides isolated from three patients with cystic fibrosis. Eur J Clin Microbiol Infect Dis 2002;21:230–233.

307. Curry WA. Human nocardiosis. A clinical review with selected case reports. Arch Intern Med 1980;140:818–826.

308. Pintado V, Gomez-Mampaso E, Fortun J, et al. Infection with Nocardia species: clinical spectrum of disease and species distribution in Madrid, Spain, 1978–2001. Infection 2002;30:338–340.

309. Dorman SE, Guide SV, Conville PS, et al. Nocardia infection in chronic granulomatous disease. Clin Infect Dis 2002;35:390–394.

310. Subhash HS, Christopher DJ, Roy A, et al. Pulmonary nocardiosis in human immunodeficiency virus infection: a tuberculosis mimic. J Postgrad Med 2001;47:30–32.

311. Feigin DS. Nocardiosis of the lung: chest radiographic findings in 21 cases. Radiology 1986;159:9–14.

312. Grossman CB, Bragg DG, Armstrong D. Roentgen manifestations of pulmonary nocardiosis. Radiology 1970;96:325–330.

313. Brown A, Geyer S, Arbitman M, et al. Pulmonary nocardiosis presenting as a bronchogenic tumor. South Med J 1980;73:660–663.

314. Henkle JQ, Nair SV. Endobronchial pulmonary nocardiosis. JAMA 1986;256:1331–1332.

315. Murray JF, Finegold SM, Froman S. The changing spectrum of nocardiosis. Am Rev Respir Dis 1961;83:315–330.

316. Jastrzembski SA, Teirstein AS, Herman SD, et al. Nocardiosis presenting as an anterior mediastinal mass in a patient with sarcoidosis. Mt Sinai J Med 2002;69:350–353.

317. Yoon HK, Im JG, Ahn JM, et al. Pulmonary nocardiosis: CT findings. J Comput Assist Tomogr 1995;19:52–55.

318. Buckley JA, Padhani AR, Kuhlman JE. CT features of pulmonary nocardiosis. J Comput Assist Tomogr 1995;19:726–732.

319. von Lichtenberg F. Infectious diseases. In: Cotran R, Kumar V, Collins T, eds. Robbins' Pathologic basis of disease, 4th edn. Philadelphia: W B Saunders, 1998:349–350.

320. Mabeza GF, Macfarlane J. Pulmonary actinomycosis. Eur Respir J 2003;21: 545–551.

321. Morgan DE, Nath H, Sanders C, et al. Mediastinal actinomycosis. AJR Am J Roentgenol 1990;155:735–737.

322. Frank P, Strickland B. Pulmonary actinomycosis. Br J Radiol 1974;47:373–378.

323. Flynn M, Felson B. The roentgen manifestations of thoracic actinomycosis. AJR Am J Roentgenol 1970;110:707–716.

324. Slade PR, Slesser BV, Southgate J. Thoracic actinomycosis. Thorax 1973;28:73–85.

325. Allen HA III, Scatarige JC, Kim MH. Actinomycosis: CT findings in six patients. AJR Am J Roentgenol 1987;149:1255–1258.

326. Kwong JS, Müller NL, Godwin JD, et al. Thoracic actinomycosis: CT findings in eight patients. Radiology 1992;183: 189–192.

327. Cheon JE, Im JG, Kim MY, et al. Thoracic actinomycosis: CT findings. Radiology 1998;209:229–233.

328. Moore WR, Scannell JG. Pulmonary actinomycosis simulating cancer of the lung. J Thorac Cardiovasc Surg 1968;55:193–195.

329. Goussard P, Gie R, Kling S, et al. Thoracic actinomycosis mimicking primary tuberculosis. Pediatr Infect Dis J 1999;18:473–475.

330. Lee SH, Shim JJ, Kang EY, et al. Endobronchial actinomycosis simulating endobronchial tuberculosis: a case report. J Korean Med Sci 1999;14: 315–318.

331. Tastepe AI, Ulasan NG, Liman ST, et al. Thoracic actinomycosis. Eur J Cardiothorac Surg 1998;14:578–583.

332. Endo S, Murayama F, Yamaguchi T, et al. Surgical considerations for pulmonary actinomycosis. Ann Thorac Surg 2002;74:185–190.

333. Ariel I, Breuer R, Kamal NS, et al. Endobronchial actinomycosis simulating bronchogenic carcinoma. Diagnosis by bronchial biopsy. Chest 1991;99:493–495.

334. Young W. Actinomycosis with involvement of the vertebral column: case report and review of the literature. Clin Radiol 1960;11:175–182.

335. Shinagawa N, Yamaguchi E, Takahashi T, et al. Pulmonary actinomycosis followed by pericarditis and intractable pleuritis. Intern Med 2002;41:319–322.

336. Poey C, Giron J, Verhaegen F, et al. [X-ray computed tomographic and radiographic aspects of thoracic actinomycosis]. J Radiol 1996;77: 177–183.

337. Kathir K, Dennis C. Primary pulmonary botryomycosis: an important differential diagnosis for lung cancer. Respirology 2001;6:347–350.

338. Tuggey JM, Hosker HS, DaCosta P. Primary pulmonary botryomycosis: a late complication of foreign body aspiration. Thorax 2000;55:1068–1069.

339. Saubolle MA. Fungal pneumonias. Semin Respir Infect 2000;15:162–177.

340. Wheat LJ, Goldman M, Sarosi G. State-of-the-art review of pulmonary fungal infections. Semin Respir Infect 2002; 17:158–181.

341. Goldman M, Johnson PC, Sarosi GA. Fungal pneumonias. The endemic mycoses. Clin Chest Med 1999;20: 507–519.

342. Severo LC, Oliveira FM, Irion K, et al. Histoplasmosis in Rio Grande do Sul, Brazil: a 21-year experience. Rev Inst Med Trop Sao Paulo 2001;43:183–187.

343. Johnson P, Sarosi G. Histoplasmosis. Semin Respir Med 1987;9:145–151.

344. Goodwin RA, Loyd JE, Des Prez RM. Histoplasmosis in normal hosts. Medicine Balt 1981;60:231–266.

345. Davies SF, McKenna RW, Sarosi GA. Trephine biopsy of the bone marrow in disseminated histoplasmosis. Am J Med 1979;67:617–622.

346. Wheat LJ. Laboratory diagnosis of histoplasmosis: update 2000. Semin Respir Infect 2001;16:131–140.

347. Wheat LJ, Kohler RB, Tewari RP. Diagnosis of disseminated histoplasmosis by detection of Histoplasma capsulatum antigen in serum and urine specimens. N Engl J Med 1986;314:83–88.

348. Edwards LB, Acquaviva FA, Livesay VT, et al. An atlas of sensitivity to tuberculin, PPD-B, and histoplasmin in the United States. Am Rev Respir Dis 1969;99 (suppl 4):1–32.

349. Connell JV, Muhm JR. Radiographic manifestations of pulmonary histoplasmosis: a 10-year review. Radiology 1976;121:281–285.

350. Schwarz J, Baum G. Pulmonary histoplasmosis. Semin Roentgenol 1970;5:13–28.

351. Palayew MJ, Frank H, Sedlezky I. Our experience with histoplasmosis: an analysis of seventy cases with follow-up study. J Can Assoc Radiol 1966;17:142–150.

352. Chick EW, Bauman DS. Editorial: Acute cavitary histoplasmosis – fact or fiction? Chest 1974;65:497–480.

353. Babbit D, Waisbren B. Epidemic pulmonary histoplasmosis. AJR Am J Roentgenol 1960;83:236–250.

354. Murray JF, Lurie H, Kaye J. Benign pulmonary histoplasmosis (cave disease) in South Africa. S Afr Med J 1957;31: 245–253.

355. Ward JI, Weeks M, Allen D, et al. Acute histoplasmosis: clinical, epidemiologic and serologic findings of an outbreak associated with exposure to a fallen tree. Am J Med 1979;66:587–595.

356. Riggs W, Nelson P. The roentgenographic findings in infantile and childhood histoplasmosis. AJR Am J Roentgenol 1966;181–185.

357. Goodwin RA Jr, Shapiro JL, Thurman GH, et al. Disseminated histoplasmosis: clinical and pathologic correlations. Medicine Balt 1980;59:1–33.

358. Goodwin RA Jr, Des Prez RM. State of the art: histoplasmosis. Am Rev Respir Dis 1978;117:929–956.

359. Parker JD, Sarosi GA, Doto IL, et al. Treatment of chronic pulmonary histoplasmosis. N Engl J Med 1970;283:225–229.

360. Rossi SE, McAdams HP, Rosado-de-Christenson ML, et al. Fibrosing mediastinitis. RadioGraphics 2001;21:737–757.

361. Baum G, Schwarz J. Chronic pulmonary histoplasmosis. Am J Med 1962;33: 873–879.

362. Goodwin RA Jr, Snell JD Jr. The enlarging histoplasmoma. Concept of a tumor-like phenomenon encompassing the tuberculoma and coccidioidoma. Am Rev Respir Dis 1969;100:1–12.

363. Palayew MJ, Frank H. Benign progressive multinodular pulmonary histoplasmosis. A radiological and clinical entity. Radiology 1974;111: 311–314.

364. Aberg JA, Mundy LM, Powderly WG. Pulmonary cryptococcosis in patients without HIV infection. Chest 1999; 115:734–740.

365. Kovacs JA, Kovacs AA, Polis M, et al. Cryptococcosis in the acquired immunodeficiency syndrome. Ann Intern Med 1985;103:533–538.

366. Kerkering TM, Duma RJ, Shadomy S. The evolution of pulmonary cryptococcosis: clinical implications from a study of 41 patients with and without compromising host factors. Ann Intern Med 1981;94:611–616.

367. Balmes JR, Hawkins J. Pulmonary cryptococcosis. Semin Respir Med 1987;9:180–186.

368. Miller WT Jr, Edelman JM, Miller WT. Cryptococcal pulmonary infection in patients with AIDS: radiographic appearance. Radiology 1990;175: 725–728.

369. Vilchez RA, Linden P, Lacomis J, et al. Acute respiratory failure associated with pulmonary cryptococcosis in non-aids patients. Chest 2001;119:1865–1869.

370. Feigin DS. Pulmonary cryptococcosis: radiologic–pathologic correlates of its three forms. AJR Am J Roentgenol 1983;141:1262–1272.

371. Lacomis JM, Costello P, Vilchez R, et al. The radiology of pulmonary cryptococcosis in a tertiary medical

center. J Thorac Imaging 2001;16: 139–148.

372. Woodring JH, Ciporkin G, Lee C, et al. Pulmonary cryptococcosis. Semin Roentgenol 1996;31:67–75.

373. Pantongrag-Brown L. Pulmonary cryptococcoma. Semin Roentgenol 1991;26:101–103.

374. Khoury MB, Godwin JD, Ravin CE, et al. Thoracic cryptococcosis: immunologic competence and radiologic appearance. AJR Am J Roentgenol 1984;142:893–896.

375. Sun LM, Chen TY, Chen WJ, et al. Cryptococcus infection in a patient with nasopharyngeal carcinoma: imaging findings mimicking pulmonary metastases. Br J Radiol 2002;75:275–278.

376. Zinck SE, Leung AN, Frost M, et al. Pulmonary cryptococcosis: CT and pathologic findings. J Comput Assist Tomogr 2002;26:330–334.

377. Gordonson J, Birnbaum W, Jacobson G, et al. Pulmonary cryptococcosis. Radiology 1974;112:557–561.

378. Lam CL, Lam WK, Wong Y, et al. Pulmonary cryptococcosis: a case report and review of the Asian-Pacific experience. Respirology 2001;6:351–355.

379. Lee YC, Chew GT, Robinson BW. Pulmonary and meningeal cryptococcosis in pulmonary alveolar proteinosis. Aust N Z J Med 1999;29:843–844.

380. Conces DJ Jr, Vix VA, Tarver RD. Pleural cryptococcosis. J Thoracic Imaging 1990;5:84–86.

381. Young EJ, Hirsh DD, Fainstein V, et al. Pleural effusions due to Cryptococcus neoformans: a review of the literature and report of two cases with cryptococcal antigen determinations. Am Rev Respir Dis 1980;121:743–747.

382. Desai SA, Minai OA, Gordon SM, et al. Coccidioidomycosis in non-endemic areas: a case series. Respir Med 2001;95:305–309.

383. Feldman BS, Snyder LS. Primary pulmonary coccidioidomycosis. Semin Respir Infect 2001;16:231–237.

384. Bayer AS. Fungal pneumonias; pulmonary coccidioidal syndromes (Part I). Primary and progressive primary coccidioidal pneumonias – diagnostic, therapeutic, and prognostic considerations. Chest 1981;79:575–583.

385. Rosenstein NE, Emery KW, Werner SB, et al. Risk factors for severe pulmonary and disseminated coccidioidomycosis: Kern County, California, 1995–1996. Clin Infect Dis 2001;32:708–715.

386. Arsura EL, Kilgore WB. Miliary coccidioidomycosis in the immunocompetent. Chest 2000;117:404–409.

387. Sarosi GA, Lawrence JP, Smith DK, et al. Rapid diagnostic evaluation of bronchial washings in patients with suspected coccidioidomycosis. Semin Respir Infect 2001;16:238–241.

388. Lin J, Hamill RJ. Coccidioidomycosis pulmonary infection. Curr Infect Dis Rep 2001;3:274–278.

389. Levine B. Coccidioidomycosis. Semin Respir Med 1987;9:152–158.

390. McGahan JP, Graves DS, Palmer PE, et al. Classic and contemporary imaging of coccidioidomycosis. AJR Am J Roentgenol 1981;136:393–404.

391. Greendyke W, Resnick D, Harvey W. Roentgen manifestations of coccidioidomycosis. AJR Am J Roentgenol 1970;109:491–499.

392. Moskowitz PS, Sue JY, Gooding CA. Tracheal coccidioidomycosis causing upper airway obstruction in children. AJR Am J Roentgenol 1982;139: 596–600.

393. Polesky A, Kirsch CM, Snyder LS, et al. Airway coccidioidomycosis – report of cases and review. Clin Infect Dis 1999;28:1273–1280.

394. Schwarz J, Baum GL. Coccidioidomycosis. Semin Roentgenol 1970;5:29–39.

395. Sarosi GA, Parker JD, Doto IL, et al. Chronic pulmonary coccidioidomycosis. N Engl J Med 1970;283:325–329.

396. Chick EW. Epidemiologic aspects of the pulmonary mycoses. Semin Respir Med 1987;9:123–129.

397. Lemos LB, Baliga M, Guo M. Blastomycosis: The great pretender can also be an opportunist. Initial clinical diagnosis and underlying diseases in 123 patients. Ann Diagn Pathol 2002;6:194–203.

398. Wallace J. Pulmonary blastomycosis: a great masquerader. Chest 2002; 121:677–679.

399. Klein BS, Vergeront JM, DiSalvo AF, et al. Two outbreaks of blastomycosis along rivers in Wisconsin. Isolation of Blastomyces dermatitidis from riverbank soil and evidence of its transmission along waterways. Am Rev Respir Dis 1987;136:1333–1338.

400. Proctor ME, Klein BS, Jones JM, et al. Cluster of pulmonary blastomycosis in a rural community: evidence for multiple high-risk environmental foci following a sustained period of diminished precipitation. Mycopathologia 2002; 153:113–120.

401. Sarosi GA, Davies SF. Blastomycosis. Am Rev Respir Dis 1979;120:911–938.

402. Assaly RA, Hammersley JR, Olson DE, et al. Disseminated blastomycosis. J Am Acad Dermatol 2003;48:123–127.

403. Recht LD, Davies SF, Eckman MR, et al. Blastomycosis in immunosuppressed patients. Am Rev Respir Dis 1982;125: 359–362.

404. Lemos LB, Guo M, Baliga M. Blastomycosis: organ involvement and etiologic diagnosis. A review of 123 patients from Mississippi. Ann Diagn Pathol 2000;4:391–406.

405. Alkrinawi S, Reed MH, Pasterkamp H. Pulmonary blastomycosis in children: findings on chest radiographs. AJR Am J Roentgenol 1995;165:651–654.

406. Lemos LB, Baliga M, Guo M. Acute respiratory distress syndrome and blastomycosis: presentation of nine cases and review of the literature. Ann Diagn Pathol 2001;5:1–9.

407. Brown LR, Swensen SJ, Van Scoy RE, et al. Roentgenologic features of pulmonary blastomycosis. Mayo Clin Proc 1991;66:29–38.

408. Laskey W, Sarosi GA. The radiological appearance of pulmonary blastomycosis. Radiology 1978;126:351–357.

409. Sheflin JR, Campbell JA, Thompson GP. Pulmonary blastomycosis: findings on chest radiographs in 63 patients. AJR Am J Roentgenol 1990;154:1177–1180.

410. Stelling CB, Woodring JH, Rehm SR, et al. Miliary pulmonary blastomycosis. Radiology 1984;150:7–13.

411. Patel RG, Patel B, Petrini MF, et al. Clinical presentation, radiographic findings, and diagnostic methods of pulmonary blastomycosis: a review of 100 consecutive cases. South Med J 1999;92:289–295.

412. Wiesman IM, Podbielski FJ, Hernan MJ, et al. Thoracic blastomycosis and empyema. JSLS 1999;3:75–78.

413. Hawley C, Felson B. Roentgenographic aspects of intrathoracic blastomycosis. AJR Am J Roentgenol 1956;75:751–757.

414. Halvorsen RA, Duncan JD, Merten DF, et al. Pulmonary blastomycosis: radiologic manifestations. Radiology 1984;150:1–5.

415. Winer-Muram HT, Beals DH, Cole FH Jr. Blastomycosis of the lung: CT features. Radiology 1992;182:829–832.

416. Funari M, Kavakama J, Shikanai-Yasuda MA, et al. Chronic pulmonary paracoccidioidomycosis (South American blastomycosis): high-resolution CT findings in 41 patients. AJR Am J Roentgenol 1999;173:59–64.

417. Johnson J. Pulmonary aspergillosis. Semin Respir Med 1987;9:187–199.

418. Greene R. The pulmonary aspergilloses: three distinct entities or a spectrum of disease. Radiology 1981;140:527–530.

419. Buckingham SJ, Hansell DM. Aspergillus in the lung: diverse and coincident forms. Eur Radiol 2003;13:1786–1800.

420. Gotway MB, Dawn SK, Caoili EM, et al. The radiologic spectrum of pulmonary Aspergillus infections. J Comput Assist Tomogr 2002;26:159–173.

421. Gefter WB, Weingrad TR, Epstein DM, et al. "Semi-invasive" pulmonary aspergillosis: a new look at the spectrum of aspergillus infections of the lung. Radiology 1981;140:313–321.

422. Kang EY, Kim DH, Woo OH, et al. Pulmonary aspergillosis in immunocompetent hosts without

underlying lesions of the lung: radiologic and pathologic findings. AJR Am J Roentgenol 2002;178:1395–1399.

423. Costello P, Rose RM. CT findings in pleural aspergillosis. J Comput Assist Tomogr 1985;9:760–762.

424. Meredith HC, Cogan BM, McLaulin B. Pleural aspergillosis. AJR Am J Roentgenol 1978;130:164–166.

425. Wollschlager C, Khan F. Aspergillomas complicating sarcoidosis. A prospective study in 100 patients. Chest 1984;86: 585–588.

426. Aspergilloma and residual tuberculous cavities – the results of a resurvey. Tubercle 1970;51:227–245.

427. Franquet T, Müller NL, Gimenez A, et al. Spectrum of pulmonary aspergillosis: histologic, clinical, and radiologic findings. RadioGraphics 2001;21: 825–837.

428. Schwarz J, Baum GL, Straub M. Cavitary histoplasmosis complicated by fungus ball. Am J Med 1961;31:692–700.

429. Torrents C, Alvarez-Castells A, de Vera PV, et al. Postpneumocystis aspergilloma in AIDS: CT features. J Comput Assist Tomogr 1991;15:304–307.

430. Fujimoto K, Meno S, Nishimura H, et al. Aspergilloma within cavitary lung cancer: MR imaging findings. AJR Am J Roentgenol 1994;163:565–567.

431. Uppal MS, Kohman LJ, Katzenstein AL. Mycetoma within an intralobar sequestration. Evidence supporting acquired origin for this pulmonary anomaly. Chest 1993;103:1627–1628.

432. Regnard JF, Icard P, Nicolosi M, et al. Aspergilloma: a series of 89 surgical cases. Ann Thorac Surg 2000;69:898–903.

433. Schouwink JH, Weigel HM, Blaauwgeers JL, et al. Aspergilloma formation in a pneumatocele associated with Pneumocystis carinii pneumonia. AIDS 1997;11:135–137.

434. Le Thi HD, Wechsler B, Chamuzeau JP, et al. Pulmonary aspergilloma complicating Wegener's granulomatosis. Scand J Rheumatol 1995;24:260.

435. Yousem SA. The histological spectrum of chronic necrotizing forms of pulmonary aspergillosis. Hum Pathol 1997;28: 650–656.

436. Sansom HE, Baque-Juston M, Wells AU, et al. Lateral cavity wall thickening as an early radiographic sign of mycetoma formation. Eur Radiol 2000;10:387–390.

437. Jewkes J, Kay PH, Paneth M, et al. Pulmonary aspergilloma: analysis of prognosis in relation to haemoptysis and survey of treatment. Thorax 1983;38:572–578.

438. Rafferty P, Biggs BA, Crompton GK, et al. What happens to patients with pulmonary aspergilloma? Analysis of 23 cases. Thorax 1983;38:579–583.

439. Knower MT, Kavanagh P, Chin JR. Intracavitary hematoma simulating mycetoma formation. J Thorac Imaging 2002;17:84–88.

440. Nam JE, Ryu YH, Cho SH, et al. Air-trapping zone surrounding sclerosing hemangioma of the lung. J Comput Assist Tomogr 2002;26:358–361.

441. Cubillo-Herguera E, McAlister WH. The pulmonary meniscus sign in a case of bronchogenic carcinoma. Radiology 1969;92:1299–1300.

442. Sheehan RE, Sheppard MN, Hansell DM. Retained intrathoracic surgical swab: CT appearances. J Thorac Imaging 2000;15:61–64.

443. Vincent L, Biron F, Jardin P, et al. Pulmonary mucormycosis in a diabetic patient. Ann Med Interne (Paris) 2000;151:669–672.

444. Kim MJ, Lee KS, Kim J, et al. Crescent sign in invasive pulmonary aspergillosis: frequency and related CT and clinical factors. J Comput Assist Tomogr 2001;25:305–310.

445. Lipinski JK, Weisbrod GL, Sanders DE. Unusual manifestations of pulmonary aspergillosis. J Can Assoc Radiol 1978;29:216–220.

446. Hammerman KJ, Christianson CS, Huntington I, et al. Spontaneous lysis of aspergillomata. Chest 1973;64:679.

447. Binder RE, Faling LJ, Pugatch RD, et al. Chronic necrotizing pulmonary aspergillosis: a discrete clinical entity. Medicine Balt 1982;61:109–124.

448. Ahmad M, Weinstein AJ, Hughes JA, et al. Granulomatous mediastinitis due to Aspergillus flavus in a nonimmunosuppressed patient. Am J Med 1981;70:887–890.

449. Koral K, Hall TR. Mycotic pseudoaneurysm of the aortic arch: an unusual complication of invasive pulmonary aspergillosis. Clin Imaging 2000;24:279–282.

450. Franquet T, Serrano F, Gimenez A, et al. Necrotizing Aspergillosis of large airways: CT findings in eight patients. J Comput Assist Tomogr 2002;26: 342–345.

451. Logan PM, Primack SL, Miller RR, et al. Invasive aspergillosis of the airways: radiographic, CT, and pathologic findings. Radiology 1994;193:383–388.

452. Brown MJ, Worthy SA, Flint JD, et al. Invasive aspergillosis in the immunocompromised host: utility of computed tomography and bronchoalveolar lavage. Clin Radiol 1998;53:255–257.

453. Ducreux D, Chevallier P, Perrin C, et al. Pseudomembranous aspergillus bronchitis in a double-lung transplanted patient: unusual radiographic and CT features. Eur Radiol 2000;10:1547–1549.

454. Hines DW, Haber MH, Yaremko L, et al. Pseudomembranous tracheobronchitis caused by Aspergillus. Am Rev Respir Dis 1991;143:1408–1411.

455. Saraceno JL, Phelps DT, Ferro TJ, et al. Chronic necrotizing pulmonary aspergillosis: approach to management. Chest 1997;112:541–548.

456. Franquet T, Müller NL, Gimenez A, et al. Semiinvasive pulmonary aspergillosis in chronic obstructive pulmonary disease: radiologic and pathologic findings in nine patients. AJR Am J Roentgenol 2000;174:51–56.

457. Won HJ, Lee KS, Cheon JE, et al. Invasive pulmonary aspergillosis: prediction at thin-section CT in patients with neutropenia – a prospective study. Radiology 1998;208:777–782.

458. Curtis AM, Smith GJ, Ravin CE. Air crescent sign of invasive aspergillosis. Radiology 1979;133:17–21.

459. Herbert DH. The roentgen features of Eaton agent pneumonia. Am J Roentgenol Radium Ther Nucl Med 1966;98:300–304.

460. Kuhlman JE, Fishman EK, Siegelman SS. Invasive pulmonary aspergillosis in acute leukemia: characteristic findings on CT, the CT halo sign, and the role of CT in early diagnosis. Radiology 1985;157:611–614.

461. Kuhlman JE, Fishman EK, Burch PA, et al. CT of invasive pulmonary aspergillosis. AJR Am J Roentgenol 1988;150:1015–1020.

462. Hruban RH, Meziane MA, Zerhouni EA, et al. Radiologic–pathologic correlation of the CT halo sign in invasive pulmonary aspergillosis. J Comput Assist Tomogr 1987;11:534–536.

463. Kuhlman JE, Fishman EK, Burch PA, et al. Invasive pulmonary aspergillosis in acute leukemia. The contribution of CT to early diagnosis and aggressive management. Chest 1987;92:95–99.

464. Primack SL, Hartman TE, Lee KS, et al. Pulmonary nodules and the CT halo sign. Radiology 1994;190:513–515.

465. Leggat PO, De Kretser DM. Aspergillus pneumonia in association with an aspergilloma. Br J Dis Chest 1968;62: 147–150.

466. Ein ME, Wallace RJ Jr, Williams TW Jr. Allergic bronchopulmonary aspergillosis-like syndrome consequent to aspergilloma. Am Rev Respir Dis 1979;119:811–820.

467. McCarthy DS, Simon G, Hargreave FE. The radiological appearances in allergic bronchopulmonary aspergillosis. Clin Radiol 1970;21:366–375.

468. Riley DJ, Mackenzie JW, Uhlman WE, et al. Allergic bronchopulmonary aspergillosis: evidence of limited tissue invasion. Am Rev Respir Dis 1975;111: 232–236.

469. Anderson CJ, Craig S, Bardana EJ Jr. Allergic bronchopulmonary aspergillosis and bilateral fungal balls terminating in disseminated aspergillosis. J Allergy Clin Immunol 1980;65:140–144.

470. Cook DJ, Achong MR, King DE. Disseminated aspergillosis in an apparently healthy patient. Am J Med 1990;88:74–76.

471. Cooper JA, Weinbaum DL, Aldrich TK, et al. Invasive aspergillosis of the lung and pericardium in a nonimmunocompromised 33 year old man. Am J Med 1981;71:903–907.

472. Lake KB, Browne PM, Van Dyke JJ, et al. Fatal disseminated aspergillosis in an asthmatic patient treated with corticosteroids. Chest 1983;83:138–139.

473. Rubin SA, Chaljub G, Winer-Muram HT, et al. Pulmonary zygomycosis: a radiographic and clinical spectrum. J Thorac Imaging 1992;7:85–90.

474. Lee FY, Mossad SB, Adal KA. Pulmonary mucormycosis: the last 30 years. Arch Intern Med 1999;159:1301–1309.

475. Chinn R, Diamind R. Generation of chemotactic factors by *Rhyzopus oryzae* in the presence and absence of serum; relationship to hypal damage mediated by human neutrophils and effects of hyperglycemia and ketoacidosis. Infect Immun 1982;38:1123–1129.

476. Majid AA, Yii NW. Granulomatous pulmonary zygomycosis in a patient without underlying illness. Computed tomographic appearances and treatment by pneumonectomy. Chest 1991;100:560–561.

477. Libshitz HI, Pagani JJ. Aspergillosis and mucormycosis: two types of opportunistic fungal pneumonia. Radiology 1981;140:301–306.

478. Loevner LA, Andrews JC, Francis IR. Multiple mycotic pulmonary artery aneurysms: a complication of invasive mucormycosis. AJR Am J Roentgenol 1992;158:761–762.

479. Donado-Una JR, Diaz-Hellin V, Lopez-Encuentra A, et al. Persistent cavitations in pulmonary mucormycosis after apparently successful amphotericin B. Eur J Cardiothorac Surg 2002;21:940–942.

480. Glazer M, Nusair S, Breuer R, et al. The role of BAL in the diagnosis of pulmonary mucormycosis. Chest 2000;117:279–282.

481. McAdams HP, Rosado de Christenson M, Strollo DC, et al. Pulmonary mucormycosis: radiologic findings in 32 cases. AJR Am J Roentgenol 1997;168:1541–1548.

482. Merlino J, Temes RT, Joste NE, et al. Invasive pulmonary mucormycosis with ruptured pseudoaneurysm. Ann Thorac Surg 2003;75:1332.

483. Jamadar DA, Kazerooni EA, Daly BD, et al. Pulmonary zygomycosis: CT appearance. J Comput Assist Tomogr 1995;19:733–738.

484. Kim KH, Choi YW, Jeon SC, et al. Mucormycosis of the central airways: CT findings in three patients. J Thorac Imaging 1999;14:210–214.

485. Rohwedder J. Pulmonary sporotrichosis. Semin Respir Med 1987;9:176–179.

486. Bennett J. Sporothrix schenckii. In: Mandell G, Douglas R, Bennett J, eds. Principles and practice of infectious diseases, 2nd edn. New York: John Wiley & Sons, 1995.

487. Mohr JA, Patterson CD, Eaton BG, et al. Primary pulmonary sporotrichosis. Am Rev Respir Dis 1972;106:260–264.

488. Comstock C, Wolson A. Roentgenology of sporotrichosis. AJR Am J Roentgenol 1975;125:651–655.

489. Ramirez J, Byrd RP Jr, Roy TM. Chronic cavitary pulmonary sporotrichosis: efficacy of oral itraconazole. J Ky Med Assoc 1998;96:103–105.

490. Mansel JK, Rosenow EC III, Smith TF, et al. Mycoplasma pneumoniae pneumonia. Chest 1989;95:639–646.

491. Hammerschlag MR. Mycoplasma pneumoniae infections. Curr Opin Infect Dis 2001;14:181–186.

492. Murray HW, Masur H, Senterfit LB, et al. The protean manifestations of Mycoplasma pneumoniae infection in adults. Am J Med 1975;58:229–242.

493. Leigh MW, Clyde WA Jr. Chlamydial and mycoplasmal pneumonias. Semin Respir Infect 1987;2:152–158.

494. Koletsky RJ, Weinstein AJ. Fulminant Mycoplasma pneumoniae infection. Report of a fatal case, and a review of the literature. Am Rev Respir Dis 1980;122:491–496.

495. Radisic M, Torn A, Gutierrez P, et al. Severe acute lung injury caused by Mycoplasma pneumoniae: potential role for steroid pulses in treatment. Clin Infect Dis 2000;31:1507–1511.

496. Kaufman JM, Cuvelier CA, Van der SM. Mycoplasma pneumonia with fulminant evolution into diffuse interstitial fibrosis. Thorax 1980;35:140–144.

497. Tablan OC, Reyes MP. Chronic interstitial pulmonary fibrosis following Mycoplasma pneumoniae pneumonia. Am J Med 1985;79:268–270.

498. Coultas DB, Samet JM, Butler C. Bronchiolitis obliterans due to Mycoplasma pneumoniae. West J Med 1986;144:471–474.

499. Kim CK, Chung CY, Kim JS, et al. Late abnormal findings on high-resolution computed tomography after Mycoplasma pneumonia. Pediatrics 2000;105:372–378.

500. Cameron DC, Borthwick RN, Philp T. The radiographic patterns of acute mycoplasma pneumonitis. Clin Radiol 1977;28:173–180.

501. Finnegan OC, Fowles SJ, White RJ. Radiographic appearances of mycoplasma pneumonia. Thorax 1981;36:469–472.

502. Putman CE, Curtis AM, Simeone JF, et al. Mycoplasma pneumonia. Clinical and roentgenographic patterns. Am J Roentgenol Radium Ther Nucl Med 1975;124:417–422.

503. Guckel C, Benz-Bohm G, Widemann B. Mycoplasmal pneumonias in childhood. Roentgen features, differential diagnosis and review of literature. Pediatr Radiol 1989;19:499–503.

504. Reittner P, Müller NL, Heyneman L, et al. Mycoplasma pneumoniae pneumonia: radiographic and high-resolution CT features in 28 patients. AJR Am J Roentgenol 2000;174:37–41.

505. John SD, Ramanathan J, Swischuk LE. Spectrum of clinical and radiographic findings in pediatric mycoplasma pneumonia. RadioGraphics 2001;21:121–131.

506. Stenstrom R, Jansson E, Von Essen R. Mycoplasma pneumonias. Acta Radiol Diagn (Stockh) 1972;12:833–841.

507. Fine NL, Smith LR, Sheedy PF. Frequency of pleural effusions in mycoplasma and viral pneumonias. N Engl J Med 1970;283:790–793.

508. Grix A, Giammona ST. Pneumonitis with pleural effusion in children due to Mycoplasma pneumoniae. Am Rev Respir Dis 1974;109:665–671.

509. Greenberg SB. Viral pneumonia. Infect Dis Clin North Am 1991;5:603–621.

510. Janower ML, Weiss EB. Mycoplasmal, viral, and rickettsial pneumonias. Semin Roentgenol 1980;15:25–34.

511. Osborne D. Radiologic appearance of viral disease of the lower respiratory tract in infants and children. AJR Am J Roentgenol 1978;130:29–33.

512. Ruben FL, Nguyen ML. Viral pneumonitis. Clin Chest Med 1991;12:223–235.

513. Kim EA, Lee KS, Primack SL, et al. Viral pneumonias in adults: radiologic and pathologic findings. RadioGraphics 2002;22 Spec No:S137–S149.

514. Galloway R, Miller R. Lung changes in the recent influenza epidemic. Br J Radiol 1959;32:28–31.

515. Wenzel RP, McCormick DP, Beam WE Jr. Parainfluenza pneumonia in adults. JAMA 1972;221:294–295.

516. Newman B, Yunis E. Lobar emphysema associated with respiratory syncytial virus pneumonia. Pediatr Radiol 1995;25:646–648.

517. Cohen L, Castro M. The role of viral respiratory infections in the pathogenesis and exacerbation of asthma. Semin Respir Infect 2003;18:3–8.

518. Wennergren G, Kristjansson S. Relationship between respiratory syncytial virus bronchiolitis and future obstructive airway diseases. Eur Respir J 2001;18:1044–1058.

519. Vikerfors T, Grandien M, Olcen P. Respiratory syncytial virus infections in adults. Am Rev Respir Dis 1987;136:561–564.

520. Walsh EE, Falsey AR, Hennessey PA. Respiratory syncytial and other virus infections in persons with chronic cardiopulmonary disease. Am J Respir Crit Care Med 1999;160:791–795.

521. Englund JA, Sullivan CJ, Jordan MC, et al. Respiratory syncytial virus infection in immunocompromised adults. Ann Intern Med 1988;109:203–208.

522. Rice RP, Loda F. A roentgenographic analysis of respiratory syncytial virus pneumonia in infants. Radiology 1966;87:1021–1027.

523. Simpson W, Hacking PM, Court SD, et al. The radiological findings in respiratory syncytial virus infection in children. II. The correlation of radiological categories with clinical and virological findings. Pediatr Radiol 1974;2:155–160.

524. Eriksson J, Nordshus T, Carlsen KH, et al. Radiological findings in children with respiratory syncytial virus infection: relationship to clinical and bacteriological findings. Pediatr Radiol 1986;16:120–122.

525. Odita JC, Nwankwo M, Aghahowa JE. Hilar enlargement in respiratory syncytial virus pneumonia. Eur J Radiol 1989;9:155–157.

526. Quinn SF, Erickson S, Oshman D, et al. Lobar collapse with respiratory syncytial virus pneumonitis. Pediatr Radiol 1985;15:229–230.

527. Ko JP, Shepard JA, Sproule MW, et al. CT manifestations of respiratory syncytial virus infection in lung transplant recipients. J Comput Assist Tomogr 2000;24:235–241.

528. Greenberg SB. Respiratory consequences of rhinovirus infection. Arch Intern Med 2003;163:278–284.

529. George RB, Mogabgab WJ. Atypical pneumonia in young men with rhinovirus infections. Ann Intern Med 1969;71:1073–1078.

530. George RB, Weill H, Rasch JR, et al. Roentgenographic appearance of viral and mycoplasmal pneumonias. Am Rev Respir Dis 1967;96:1144–1150.

531. Ksiazek TG, Erdman D, Goldsmith CS, et al. A novel coronavirus associated with severe acute respiratory syndrome. N Engl J Med 2003;348:1953–1966.

532. Kuiken T, Fouchier RA, Schutten M, et al. Newly discovered coronavirus as the primary cause of severe acute respiratory syndrome. Lancet 2003;362:263–270.

533. Nicolaou S, Al Nakshabandi NA, Müller NL. SARS: Imaging of severe acute respiratory syndrome. AJR Am J Roentgenol 2003;180:1247–1249.

534. Antonio GE, Wong KT, Hui DS, et al. Thin-section CT in patients with severe acute respiratory syndrome following hospital discharge: preliminary experience. Radiology 2003;228:810–815.

535. Wong KT, Antonio GE, Hui DS, et al. Severe acute respiratory syndrome: radiographic appearances and pattern of progression in 138 patients. Radiology 2003;228:401–406.

536. Wong KT, Antonio GE, Hui DS, et al. Thin-section CT of severe acute respiratory syndrome: evaluation of 73 patients exposed to or with the disease. Radiology 2003;228:395–400.

537. Antonio GE, Wong KT, Hui DS, et al. Imaging of severe acute respiratory syndrome in Hong Kong. AJR Am J Roentgenol 2003;181:11–17.

538. Grinblat L, Shulman H, Glickman A, et al. Severe acute respiratory syndrome: radiographic review of 40 probable cases in Toronto, Canada. Radiology 2003; 228:802–809.

539. Gremillion DH, Crawford GE. Measles pneumonia in young adults. An analysis of 106 cases. Am J Med 1981;71:539–542.

540. Tanaka H, Honma S, Yamagishi M, et al. Clinical features of measles pneumonia in adults: usefulness of computed tomography. Nihon Kyobu Shikkan Gakkai Zasshi 1993;31:1129–1133.

541. Pasteur MC, Helliwell SM, Houghton SJ, et al. An investigation into causative factors in patients with bronchiectasis. Am J Respir Crit Care Med 2000;162: 1277–1284.

542. Margolin FR, Gandy TK. Pneumonia of atypical measles. Radiology 1979;131: 653–655.

543. Martin DB, Weiner LB, Nieburg PI, et al. Atypical measles in adolescents and young adults. Ann Intern Med 1979;90:877–881.

544. Young LW, Smith D, Glasgow L. Pneumonia of atypical measles: residual nodular lesions. AJR Am J Roentgenol 1970;110:439–448.

545. Garten AJ, Mendelson DS, Halton KP. CT manifestations of infectious mononucleosis. Clin Imaging 1992;16:114–116.

546. Andiman WA, McCarthy P, Markowitz RI, et al. Clinical, virologic, and serologic evidence of Epstein-Barr virus infection in association with childhood pneumonia. J Pediatr 1981;99:880–886.

547. Lander P, Palayew MJ. Infectious mononucleosis – a review of chest roentgenographic manifestations. J Can Assoc Radiol 1974;25:303–306.

548. Miyake H, Matsumoto A, Komatsu E, et al. Infectious mononucleosis with pulmonary consolidation. J Thorac Imaging 1996;11:158–160.

549. Zahradnik JM. Adenovirus pneumonia. Semin Respir Infect 1987;2:104–111.

550. Retalis P, Strange C, Harley R. The spectrum of adult adenovirus pneumonia. Chest 1996;109: 1656–1657.

551. Bateman ED, Hayashi S, Kuwano K, et al. Latent adenoviral infection in follicular bronchiectasis. Am J Respir Crit Care Med 1995;151:170–176.

552. Osborne D, White P. Radiology of epidemic adenovirus 21 infection of the lower respiratory tract in infants and young children. AJR Am J Roentgenol 1979;133:397–400.

553. Han BK, Son JA, Yoon HK, et al. Epidemic adenoviral lower respiratory tract infection in pediatric patients: radiographic and clinical characteristics. AJR Am J Roentgenol 1998;170:1077–1080.

554. Teper AM, Kofman CD, Maffey AF, et al. Lung function in infants with chronic pulmonary disease after severe adenoviral illness. J Pediatr 1999; 134:730–733.

555. Hubbell C, Dominguez R, Kohl S. Neonatal herpes simplex pneumonitis. Rev Infect Dis 1988;10:431–438.

556. Graham BS, Snell JD Jr. Herpes simplex virus infection of the adult lower respiratory tract. Medicine Balt 1983;62:384–393.

557. Umans U, Golding RP, Duraku S, et al. Herpes simplex virus 1 pneumonia: conventional chest radiograph pattern. Eur Radiol 2001;11:990–994.

558. Aquino SL, Dunagan DP, Chiles C, et al. Herpes simplex virus 1 pneumonia: patterns on CT scans and conventional chest radiographs. J Comput Assist Tomogr 1998;22:795–800.

559. Triebwasser JH, Harris RE, Bryant RE, et al. Varicella pneumonia in adults. Report of seven cases and a review of literature. Medicine Balt 1967;46:409–423.

560. Sargent EN, Carson M, Reilly E. Roentgenographic manifestations of varicella pneumonia with postmortem correlation. AJR Am J Roentgenol 1966;98:305–317.

561. Kim JS, Ryu CW, Lee SI, et al. High-resolution CT findings of varicella-zoster pneumonia. AJR Am J Roentgenol 1999;172:113–116.

562. Ibarra-Perez C. Thoracic complications of amebic abscess of the liver: report of 501 cases. Chest 1981;79:672–677.

563. Shamsuzzaman SM, Hashiguchi Y. Thoracic amebiasis. Clin Chest Med 2002;23:479–492.

564. Stephen SJ, Uragoda CG. Pleuro-pulmonary amoebiasis. A review of 40 cases. Br J Dis Chest 1970;64:96–106.

565. Wilson E. Pleuropulmonary amebiasis. AJR Am J Roentgenol 1971;111:518–524.

566. Barrett-Connor E. Parasitic pulmonary disease. Am Rev Respir Dis 1982;126: 558–563.

567. Woodring JH, Halfhill H, Reed JC. Pulmonary strongyloidiasis: clinical and imaging features. AJR Am J Roentgenol 1994;162:537–542.

568. Purtilo DT, Meyers WM, Connor DH. Fatal strongyloidiasis in immunosuppressed patients. Am J Med 1974;56:488–493.

569. Scowden EB, Schaffner W, Stone WJ. Overwhelming strongyloidiasis: an unappreciated opportunistic infection. Medicine Balt 1978;57:527–544.

570. Bean W. Recognition of ascariasis by routine chest or abdomen roentgenograms. AJR Am J Roentgenol 1965;94:379–384.

571. Gelpi AP, Mustafa A. Ascaris pneumonia. Am J Med 1968;44:377–389.

572. Emad A. Exudative eosinophilic pleural effusion due to Strongyloides stercoralis in a diabetic man. South Med J 1999; 92:58–60.

573. Krysl J, Müller NL, Miller RR, et al. Patient with miliary nodules and diarrhea. Can Assoc Radiol J 1991;42:363–366.

574. Dunn IJ. Filarial diseases. Semin Roentgenol 1998;33:47–56.

575. Neva FA, Ottesen EA. Tropical (filarial) eosinophilia. N Engl J Med 1978;298:1129–1131.

576. Herlinger H. Pulmonary changes in tropical eosinophilia. Br J Radiol 1963;36:889–901.

577. Udwadia F. Tropical eosinophilia. Prog Respir Res 1975;7:35–155.

578. Echeverri A, Long RF, Check W, et al. Pulmonary dirofilariasis. Ann Thorac Surg 1999;67:201–202.

579. Shah MK. Human pulmonary dirofilariasis: review of the literature. South Med J 1999;92:276–279.

580. Risher WH, Crocker EF Jr, Beckman EN, et al. Pulmonary dirofilariasis. The largest single-institution experience. J Thorac Cardiovasc Surg 1989;97:303–308.

581. Ro JY, Tsakalakis PJ, White VA, et al. Pulmonary dirofilariasis: the great imitator of primary or metastatic lung tumor. A clinicopathologic analysis of seven cases and a review of the literature. Hum Pathol 1989;20:69–76.

582. Cholankeril J, Napolitano J, Ketyer S. Computed tomography in the evaluation of *Dirofiliaria immitus* granuloma of the lung. J Comput Tomogr 1983;7:305–309.

583. Levinson ED, Ziter FM Jr, Westcott JL. Pulmonary lesions due to Dirofilaria immitis (dog heartworm). Report of four cases with radiologic findings. Radiology 1979;131:305–307.

584. Flieder DB, Moran CA. Pulmonary dirofilariasis: a clinicopathologic study of 41 lesions in 39 patients. Hum Pathol 1999;30:251–256.

585. Gomez-Merino E, Chiner E, Signes-Costa J, et al. Pulmonary dirofilariasis mimicking lung cancer. Monaldi Arch Chest Dis 2002;57:33–34.

586. Jawahiry K, Karpas L. Pulmonary schistosomiasis: a detailed clinicopathologic study. Am Rev Respir Dis 1963;88:517–527.

587. Garcia-Palmieri M, Marcial-Rojas R. The protean manifestations of Schistosomiasis mansoni: a clinicopathologic correlation. Ann Intern Med 1962;57:763–775.

588. Schwartz E. Pulmonary schistosomiasis. Clin Chest Med 2002;23:433–443.

589. Cooke GS, Lalvani A, Gleeson FV, et al. Acute pulmonary schistosomiasis in travelers returning from Lake Malawi, sub-Saharan Africa. Clin Infect Dis 1999;29:836–839.

590. Salanitri J, Stanley P, Hennessy O. Acute pulmonary schistosomiasis. Australas Radiol 2002;46:435–437.

591. De Leon EP, Pardo de Tavera M. Pulmonary schistosomiasis in the Philippines. Dis Chest 1968;53:154–161.

592. Paul R. Pulmonary "coin" lesion of unusual pathology. Radiology 1960;75:118–120.

593. Waldman AD, Day JH, Shaw P, et al. Subacute pulmonary granulomatous schistosomiasis: high resolution CT appearances – another cause of the halo sign. Br J Radiol 2001;74:1052–1055.

594. DeFrain M, Hooker R. North American paragonimiasis: case report of a severe clinical infection. Chest 2002;121:1368–1372.

595. Mukae H, Taniguchi H, Matsumoto N, et al. Clinicoradiologic features of pleuropulmonary Paragonimus westermani on Kyusyu Island, Japan. Chest 2001;120:514–520.

596. Johnson RJ, Johnson JR. Paragonimiasis in Indochinese refugees. Roentgenographic findings with clinical correlations. Am Rev Respir Dis 1983;128:534–538.

597. Ogakwu M, Nwokolo C. Radiological findings in pulmonary paragonimiasis as seen in Nigeria: a review based on one hundred cases. Br J Radiol 1973;46:699–705.

598. Taylor CR, Swett HA. Pulmonary paragonimiasis in Laotian refugees. Radiology 1982;143:411–412.

599. Tomita M, Matsuzaki Y, Nawa Y, et al. Pulmonary paragonimiasis referred to the department of surgery. Ann Thorac Cardiovasc Surg 2000;6:295–298.

600. Bahk Y. Pulmonary paragonimiasis as a cause for Loeffler's syndrome. Radiology 1962;78:598–601.

601. Im JG, Whang HY, Kim WS, et al. Pleuropulmonary paragonimiasis: radiologic findings in 71 patients. AJR Am J Roentgenol 1992;159:39–43.

602. Singcharoen T, Silprasert W. CT findings in pulmonary paragonimiasis. J Comput Assist Tomogr 1987;11:1101–1102.

603. Singcharoen T, Rawd-Aree P, Baddeley H. Computed tomography findings in disseminated paragonimiasis. Br J Radiol 1988;61:83–86.

604. Gottstein B, Reichen J. Hydatid lung disease (echinococcosis/hydatidosis). Clin Chest Med 2002;23:397–408, ix.

605. Cuthbert R. Sylvatic pulmonary hydatid disease a radiologic survey. J Can Assoc Radiol 1975;26:132–138.

606. Dakak M, Genc O, Gurkok S, et al. Surgical treatment for pulmonary hydatidosis (a review of 422 cases). J R Coll Surg Edinb 2002;47:689–692.

607. Kilani T, El Hammami S. Pulmonary hydatid and other lung parasitic infections. Curr Opin Pulm Med 2002;8:218–223.

608. Sbihi Y, Rmiqui A, Rodriguez-Cabezas MN, et al. Comparative sensitivity of six serological tests and diagnostic value of ELISA using purified antigen in hydatidosis. J Clin Lab Anal 2001;15:14–18.

609. Balikian JP, Mudarris F. Hydatid disease of the lungs: a roentgenologic study of 50 cases. AJR Am J Roentgenol 1974; 122:692–707.

610. McPhail JL, Arora TS. Intrathoracic hydatid disease. Dis Chest 1967; 52:772–781.

611. Kervancioglu R, Bayram M, Elbeyli L. CT findings in pulmonary hydatid disease. Acta Radiol 1999;40:510–514.

612. Beggs I. The radiology of hydatid disease. AJR Am J Roentgenol 1985;145:639–648.

613. Saksouk FA, Fahl MH, Rizk GK. Computed tomography of pulmonary hydatid disease. J Comput Assist Tomogr 1986;10:226–232.

614. von Sinner WN. New diagnostic signs in hydatid disease; radiography, ultrasound, CT and MRI correlated to pathology. Eur J Radiol 1991;12:150–159.

615. von Sinner WN, Rifai A, te Strake L, et al. Magnetic resonance imaging of thoracic hydatid disease. Correlation with clinical findings, radiography, ultrasonography, CT and pathology. Acta Radiol 1990;31:59–62.

616. Prieto A, Diaz A, Calvo J, et al. MR imaging of pulmonary hydatid disease. Eur J Radiol 1996;23:85–87.

617. Koul PA, Koul AN, Wahid A, et al. CT in pulmonary hydatid disease: unusual appearances. Chest 2000;118:1645–1647.

618. Kokturk O, Ozturk C, Diren B, et al. "Air bubble": a new diagnostic CT sign of perforated pulmonary hydatid cyst. Eur Radiol 1999;9:1321–1323.

619. Tor M, Ozvaran K, Ersoy Y, et al. Pitfalls in the diagnosis of complicated pulmonary hydatid disease. Respir Med 2001;95:237–239.

620. von Sinner WN, Linjawi T, al watban JA. Mediastinal hydatid disease: report of three cases. Can Assoc Radiol J 1990;41:79–82.

621. Solli P, Carbognani P, Cattelani L, et al. Unusually located hydatid cysts miming a pulmonary tumor invaliding the spine. J Cardiovasc Surg (Torino) 2001;42:147–149.

622. Kakrani AL, Chowdhary VR, Bapat VM. Disseminated pulmonary hydatid

disease presenting as multiple cannon ball shadows in human immunodeficiency virus infection. J Assoc Physicians India 2000;48: 1208–1209.

623. Hendaoui L, Siala M, Fourati A, et al. Case report: hydatid cyst of the aorta. Clin Radiol 1991;43:423–425.

624. Lahdhili H, Hachicha S, Ziadi M, et al. Acute pulmonary embolism due to the rupture of a right ventricle hydatic cyst. Eur J Cardiothorac Surg 2002;22:462.

625. Lioulias A, Kotoulas C, Kokotsakis J, et al. Acute pulmonary embolism due to multiple hydatid cysts. Eur J Cardiothorac Surg 2001;20:197–199.

626. Smith GJ, Irons S, Schelleman A. Hydatid pulmonary emboli. Australas Radiol 2001;45:508–511.

The immunocompromised patient

AIDS

The human immunodeficiency virus (HIV) responsible for AIDS is a retrovirus that attaches to the CD4 surface glycoprotein of helper T lymphocytes, monocytes, macrophages, and other antigen presenting cells. It fuses with the cell, injects its RNA (ribonucleic acid), makes a DNA (deoxyribonucleic acid) copy, and integrates into the host DNA. The virus replicates within the helper T lymphocytes and eventually destroys the infected cells. It also causes "bystander" killing of uninfected cells by autoimmune destruction and apoptosis, resulting in the characteristic CD4 lymphocyte depletion. Cell-mediated immunity becomes progressively impaired as the CD4 lymphocyte count falls. The types of infection to which HIV-positive patients become susceptible vary as cell-mediated immunity becomes less effective at eradicating viruses, fungi, protozoa, and facultative intracellular bacteria such as *Mycobacterium tuberculosis*. Knowledge of the CD4 lymphocyte count can thus be helpful for interpretation of radiological images in AIDS patients.[1-3] The normal CD4 lymphocyte count is greater than 450 cells/mm³. As the CD4 lymphocyte count falls, tuberculous infection, bacterial pneumonia, and oral *Candida albicans* become increasingly common, as do virus-associated tumors such as Kaposi sarcoma. *Pneumocystis jiroveci* (previously known as Pneumocystis carinii) is the most common cause of pneumonia in the West when the CD4 lymphocyte count is 200/mm^3 or less (assuming no antibiotic prophylaxis). With counts below this level, HIV infection becomes frank AIDS and the CD8-cytotoxic lymphocyte count also falls. When the CD4 count falls below 100 cells/mm^3, toxoplasmosis, disseminated herpes zoster, crypto-coccosis, esophageal candidiasis, cytomegalovirus (CMV), atypical mycobacterial infections, and Epstein–Barr virus-related non-Hodgkin disease become common.

The morbidity and mortality of AIDS continue to fall in the western world. Reasons for this improvement are multifactorial and include the aggressive use of prophylactic antimicrobial therapies and so-called "highly active antiretroviral therapy" (HAART).[4–10] The pattern of disease in patients with AIDS is changing with the introduction of more effective therapies[11] and, therefore, the radiologic manifestations are also changing.[12] For example, an entirely new manifestation of disease, the immune restoration syndrome, has been recently described in AIDS patients receiving HAART.[5–10] Despite these recent advances, however, pulmonary disease remains one of the prime modes of presentation and a major cause of life-threatening illness in patients with AIDS.

Bacterial infection

Pyogenic pneumonia

Although T-cell defects are the major cause of immune deficiency in patients with HIV infection, B-cell function and antibody production are also affected, particularly in children. This deficiency in humoral immunity, in addition to the reduction in CD4 lymphocyte counts, increases susceptibility to pyogenic bacterial infection. Other factors that may predispose AIDS patients to pyogenic infection include: (i) poor drainage of lung due to endobronchial obstruction by Kaposi sarcoma; and (ii) bone marrow suppression from drugs used to treat cytomegalovirus infection and various tumors. In particular, neutropenia due to bone marrow suppression may predispose AIDS patients to gram-negative bacterial pneumonia.

In one large prospective North American series, pyogenic bacterial pneumonia was six times more common in HIV-positive than HIV-negative patients.[13] Pyogenic organisms are responsible for up to 45% of pulmonary infections in AIDS patients at some stage of their illness with an even higher incidence when AIDS is contracted through intravenous drug abuse.[14,15] However, the overall incidence of pyogenic bacterial pneumonia in AIDS patients appears to be declining.

Many types of community-acquired pyogenic infection are encountered in patients with AIDS. Most infections are caused by encapsulated bacteria such as *Streptococcus pneumoniae*,[16] *Haemophilus influenzae*, *Moraxella* species,[15,17] and *Pseudomonas aeruginosa*.[18] Infection with *Rhodococcus equi* is being increasingly reported.[19–21]

The radiologic findings of pyogenic pneumonia in AIDS patients are similar to those seen in immunocompetent patients. Focal homogeneous segmental or lobar consolidation is probably the most common pattern (Fig. 6.1).[14,22] However, either localized

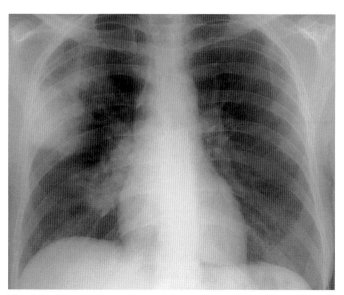

Fig. 6.1 *Streptococcus* pneumonia in an AIDS patient with cough and fever. A frontal chest radiograph shows focal homogeneous opacities in the right lung.

or diffuse heterogeneous opacities, sometimes indistinguishable from the findings of Pneumocystis pneumonia, are seen in up to half of patients, especially those infected with *Haemophilus influenzae* and *Pseudomonas aeruginosa*.[15,18] Other radiologic findings of pyogenic bacterial infection include pleural effusion, lung nodules or masses, and pulmonary cavitation (Fig. 6.2).[14,15,18,23]

Hematogenous spread of pyogenic bacterial pneumonia can cause septicemia, multifocal pulmonary infection, and systemic septic emboli to skin and solid organs. These complications are more common in patients with AIDS than in immunocompetent individuals. Sepsis may result in diffuse homogeneous pulmonary opacities on chest radiographs and lead to adult respiratory distress syndrome (ARDS). Septic pulmonary emboli are a particularly common complication in intravenous drug abusers with AIDS. Septic pulmonary emboli manifest on chest radiographs and CT as peripheral wedge-shaped opacities and cavitary lung nodules (Fig. 6.3). The cavities can be quite thin-walled.

Nocardia asteroides only causes clinically significant infection in AIDS patients with a very low CD4 count (mean of 80 cells/mm^3). The organisms can be identified on biopsy samples, sputum cultures, and bronchoalveolar lavage aspirates. *Nocardia* infection manifests radiologically (Fig. 6.4) as consolidation, large masses, or multiple nodules, all of which may cavitate.[24,25] The upper lobes are more commonly affected than the lower lobes. Rapid enlargement and progression of pulmonary abnormalities is typical, as are associated pleural effusions.

Bacillary angiomatosis is a vasoproliferative infection in patients with AIDS. It is caused by *Bartonella* (previously *Rochalimaea*) species. The main risk factor is exposure to cats, cat fleas, and lice. The skin is the most common site of involvement. Bacillary angiomatosis in the thorax can manifest as mediastinal lymph node enlargement, lung nodules or masses, endobronchial lesions, chest wall masses, or pleural effusions.[26,27] Because of their vascularity, the mass lesions may enhance intensely on CT after administration of intravenous contrast material.

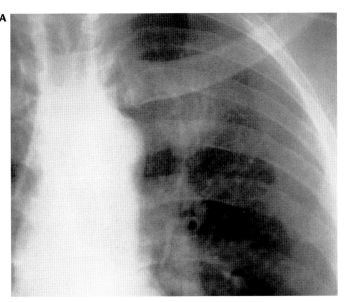
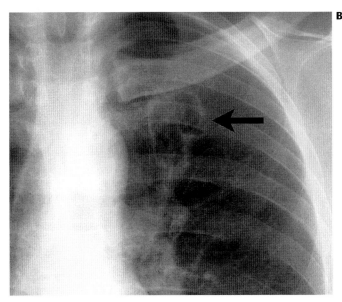

Fig. 6.2   *Rhodococcus equi* pneumonia in an AIDS patient. **A**, A coned-down view from a frontal chest radiograph shows a poorly marginated rounded opacity in the left upper lobe. **B**, A radiograph obtained 2 weeks later shows cavitation (black arrow). Sputum cultures showed *R. equi*.

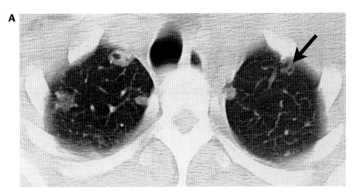

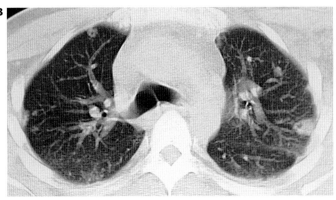

Fig. 6.3   *Staphylococcus aureus* emboli in an intravenous drug abuser with AIDS. **A** and **B**, Adjacent CT sections show multiple peripheral cavitary lung nodules. Some cavities (black arrow on **A**) have very thin walls.

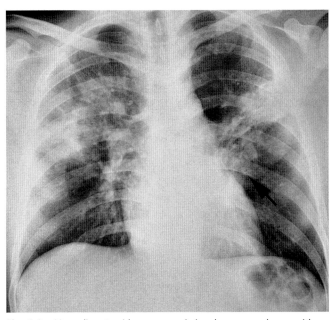

Fig. 6.4   *Nocardia asteroides* pneumonia in a homosexual man with AIDS. A frontal chest radiograph shows scattered ill-defined opacities in the right lung, a more masslike opacity in the left lung, and hilar lymphadenopathy (black arrow).

Mycobacterial infection

Tuberculosis

In most developed countries, the incidence of tuberculosis steadily declined until 1985. After 1985, the incidence began to rise again, at least partly due to the advent of widespread HIV infection. In developed countries, the incidence again leveled off in the mid 1990s and began to decline slowly thereafter. Nevertheless, *Mycobacterium tuberculosis* remains an important pathogen in the AIDS population in developed countries, and is still the most common pulmonary pathogen in AIDS patients in

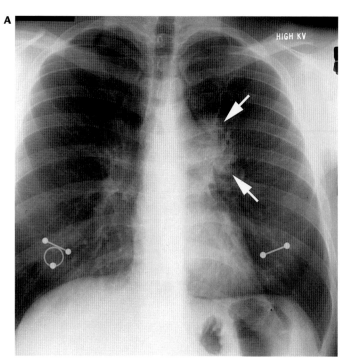

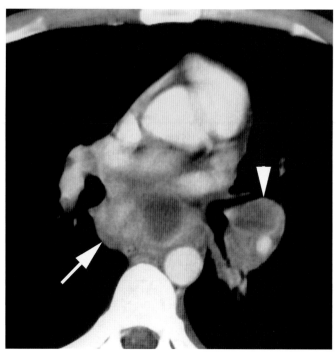

Fig. 6.5 Tuberculosis in a man with AIDS. **A**, A frontal chest radiograph shows a left hilar mass (white arrows). **B**, Contrast-enhanced CT shows enlarged subcarinal (white arrow) and left hilar lymph nodes (white arrowhead). Note the low-attenuation centers and subtle rim enhancement.

Africa. The risk of tuberculous infection depends on the concentration of tubercle bacilli in the environment, which is heavily dependent on social conditions. The high rate of multi-drug resistant tuberculosis in HIV-positive patients in cities such as New York is of increasing significance both to those with HIV infection and to the immunocompetent population.[28] Patients with AIDS-related tuberculosis[29] are more likely to be nonwhite and also more likely to be heterosexual drug users than AIDS patients without tuberculosis.[30] In AIDS, tuberculosis is more often disseminated and up to 60% of patients have at least one extrapulmonary site of disease, a much higher incidence than in patients who do not have AIDS.[30]

The diagnosis of tuberculosis in AIDS patients can be difficult. The various tuberculin tests, which rely on an intact cell-mediated response, are falsely negative in 50–70% of patients with advanced AIDS. Up to half of AIDS patients with culture-proven tuberculosis have false negative sputum and bronchoalveolar lavage samples for acid-fast bacilli. Prompt diagnosis therefore requires a high index of clinical suspicion.

The radiographic features of tuberculosis in AIDS patients are more commonly those of primary rather than postprimary disease. As such, the disease typically manifests with focal homogeneous lobar or segmental opacities and enlarged hilar or mediastinal lymph nodes (Fig. 6.5).[31–36] In some patients, lymphadenopathy may be the dominant radiologic feature; tuberculous and nontuberculous mycobacterial infection is a common cause of isolated lymphadenopathy on chest radiographs in HIV-infected patients (Fig. 6.5).[37]

Numerous comparisons of chest radiographic findings in tuberculosis in HIV-positive and HIV-negative patients have been published.[31,32,34–40] Hilar and mediastinal lymphadenopathy (Fig. 6.5) is more common in HIV-positive patients (17–60%) than in HIV-negative patients (3–23%) with tuberculosis. Other features seen more frequently in HIV-positive patients include

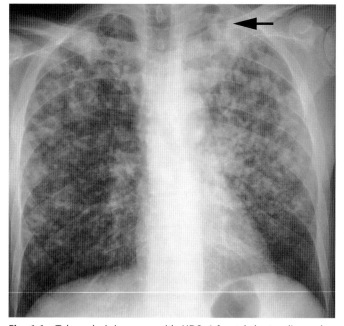

Fig. 6.6 Tuberculosis in a man with AIDS. A frontal chest radiograph shows a cavity in the left upper lobe (arrow) and diffuse poorly defined 5–8 mm nodules, consistent with endobronchial spread of infection.

consolidation in the lower and middle lobes, disseminated tuberculosis (Figs 6.6 and 6.7), and pleural effusions. A comparative study of 42 HIV-positive and 42 HIV-negative patients with tuberculosis showed a lower incidence of localized parenchymal disease and a higher incidence of disseminated disease in HIV-positive patients.[41]

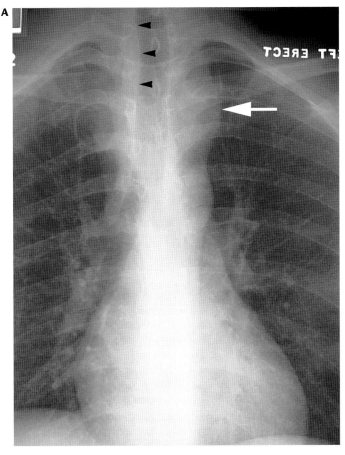

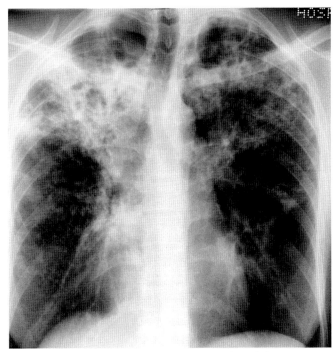

Fig. 6.8 Tuberculosis in a woman with AIDS. A frontal chest radiograph shows consolidation and cavitation in the right upper lobe and heterogeneous opacities in the left upper lobe, a pattern typical of postprimary tuberculosis.

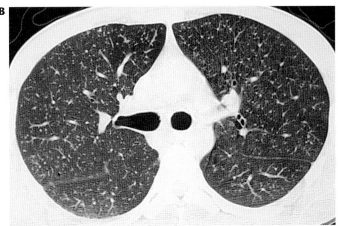

Fig. 6.7 Tuberculosis in a man with AIDS. **A**, The frontal chest radiograph shows bilateral mediastinal (arrow) and right supraclavicular lymphadenopathy. Note the mass effect on the trachea (arrowheads). **B**, CT (lung window) shows diffuse tiny nodules consistent with miliary tuberculosis.

The level of depression of cellular immunity, as reflected by the CD4 lymphocyte count, may influence the radiographic appearance of tuberculosis in AIDS patients. Keiper et al[39] evaluated 35 patients with AIDS and tuberculosis and correlated radiographic findings with CD4 lymphocyte count. In their series, 8 of 9 (89%) patients with CD4 lymphocyte counts of greater than 200 cells/mm³ had chest radiographic

findings characteristic of postprimary tuberculosis (Fig. 6.8). Furthermore, 24 of 26 (92%) patients with CD4 counts of less than 200 cells/mm³ had "atypical findings" on chest radiographs. These "atypical findings" included diffuse and lower lobar opacities (Fig. 6.6), pleural effusion, mediastinal adenopathy (Fig. 6.7A), a miliary pattern (Fig. 6.7B), and a normal chest radiograph. Greenberg et al,[38] in a study of 133 patients, reached similar conclusions to Keiper et al[39] but also found that AIDS patients with a CD4 count less than 200 cells/mm³ were more likely to have a normal chest radiograph despite culture-proven tuberculosis than were patients with a CD4 count greater than 200 cells/mm³. In that series, 32% of AIDS patients with culture-proven tuberculosis had a normal chest radiograph.

CT has a limited role in the evaluation of AIDS patients with tuberculosis. CT can be used: (1) to confirm the presence of parenchymal abnormalities suspected on chest radiographs; (2) to further characterize abnormalities such as miliary or endobronchial spread of disease (Fig. 6.7); (3) to identify cavitation or other complications of infection; and (4) to evaluate suspected hilar or mediastinal lymphadenopathy (Fig. 6.5). Laissy et al[42] compared CT findings in 29 patients with and 47 patients without HIV infection, all of who had culture-proven active pulmonary tuberculosis. Patients with HIV infection had significantly less cavitation and bronchial wall thickening than non-HIV-infected patients. Centrilobular nodules, presumably due to endobronchial spread, were also less common in non-HIV patients. HIV-positive patients with CD4 counts less than 200 cells/mm³ had less cavitation and more lymphadenopathy than patients with CD4 counts greater than 200 cells/mm³. Tuberculous lymph nodes often contain low-attenuation centers

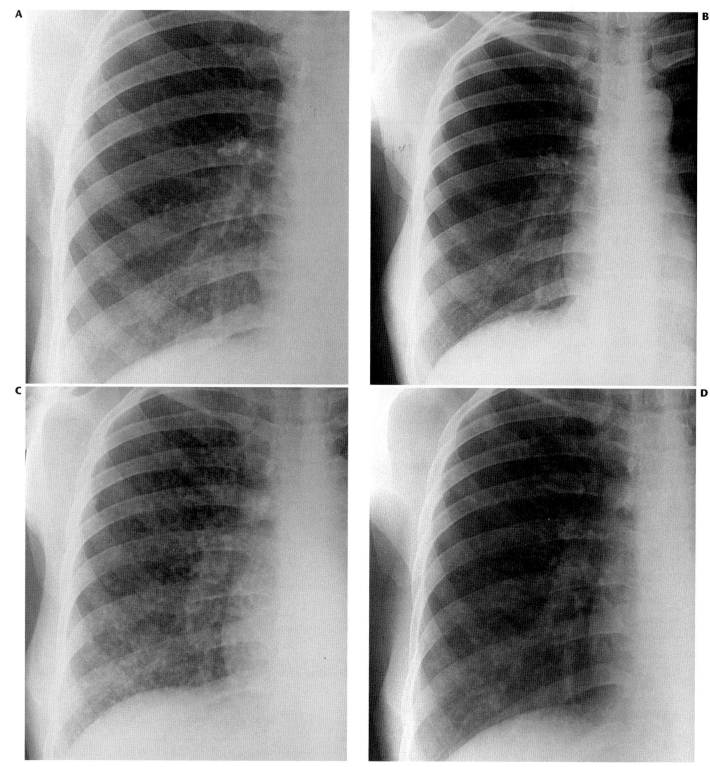

Fig. 6.9 Tuberculosis in a woman with AIDS on highly active antiretroviral therapy (HAART). **A,** A coned-down view of a frontal chest radiograph obtained at admission shows diffuse fine nodular opacities and calcified hilar lymph nodes. **B,** A radiograph obtained after 1 month of antituberculous treatment shows resolution of opacities. **C,** A radiograph obtained after 1 month of HAART shows increased opacities. The patient now had fever and progressive cervical lymphadenopathy. **D,** A radiograph obtained 2 months after cessation of antituberculous therapy and HAART shows radiographic and clinical improvement. (With permission from Fishman JE, Saraf-Lavi E, Narita M, et al. Pulmonary tuberculosis in AIDS patients: transient chest radiographic worsening after initiation of antiretroviral therapy. AJR Am J Roentgenol 2000;174:43–49.)

(Fig. 6.5).[43–46] In one study of 25 patients with tuberculous adenopathy, over 80% of affected lymph nodes had low-attenuation centers and a quarter showed marked peripheral rim enhancement.[46] However, Laissy et al[42] found that low-attenuation adenopathy was significantly less common in HIV-infected patients with tuberculosis than in non-HIV-infected patients.

After diagnosis and the institution of appropriate anti-tuberculous therapy, serial radiographs usually demonstrate rapid clearing within months, with no evidence of residual disease.[47] Transient worsening of radiologic findings may occur after institution of antiretroviral therapy (Fig. 6.9)[48]; improvement usually occurs within several weeks, however. If there is no clinical and radiographic improvement on appropriate treatment, concurrent opportunistic infection, tumor, or multidrug resistant tuberculosis should be considered. Noncompliance with anti-tuberculous medications is also a problem in this population and is a further cause of treatment failure. Directly observed therapy may be required in this setting.[49–51]

Nontuberculous (atypical) mycobacterial infection

Nontuberculous mycobacteria, also known as atypical mycobacteria, include *Mycobacterium avium–intracellulare* (MAI), also known as *M. avium* complex (MAC), and *M. kansasii*. These organisms are present worldwide, being found particularly in water and soil. When nontuberculous mycobacterial infection occurs in an immunocompetent patient, the disease is usually confined to the chest. When it occurs in patients with AIDS, disease is usually extrathoracic and commonly involves the gut, liver, lymph nodes, and bone marrow. Infection confined to the thorax is rare in AIDS patients, but has been reported.[52]

Infection due to *M. avium–intracellulare* is thought to enter via the gastrointestinal tract causing systemic upset and chronic diarrhea; clinically significant pneumonia is uncommon in the AIDS population.[53,54] Organisms may be found in bronchoalveolar lavage fluid or sputum, blood, bone marrow, stool, and urine cultures; however, culture of the organism does not always correlate with clinical disease.

The chest radiograph is normal in most AIDS patients with disseminated *M. avium–intracellulare* disease, even when the organism is cultured from respiratory secretions.[55] When radiographic findings are present (Fig. 6.10), the predominant features are hilar and mediastinal lymphadenopathy and diffuse pulmonary opacities that often have upper lung predominance.[53,56,57] Less frequent manifestations include intrapulmonary nodules and pleural effusions,[56] endobronchial masses, possibly from erosion by hilar lymph nodes, and rarely, cavitary upper lobe disease.[53] CT, particularly high-resolution CT, may demonstrate ground-glass opacities and bronchial wall and interlobular septal thickening.[57,58]

The second most common atypical mycobacterium, *M. kansasii*, has a greater predilection for the lungs and causes disease that is clinically similar to infection with *M. tuberculosis* (Fig. 6.11). A variety of radiographic appearances are found in AIDS patients with *M. kansasii* infection, including focal homogeneous segmental or lobar opacities which may cavitate, focal or diffuse reticulonodular opacities, and thin-

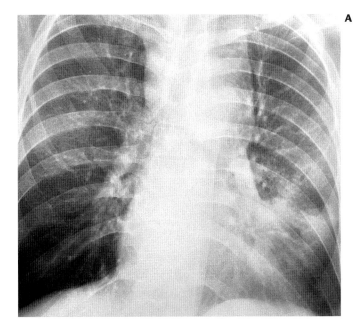

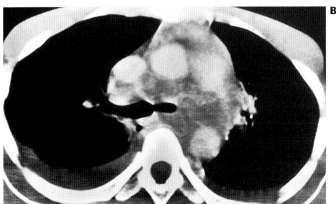

Fig. 6.10 Nontuberculous mycobacterial infection in a man with AIDS. **A**, A frontal chest radiograph shows bilateral mediastinal adenopathy and an ill-defined lingular opacity. **B**, CT shows extensive low-attenuation mediastinal adenopathy and bilateral pleural effusions.

walled cavities.[59,60] Pleural effusions are uncommon.[59] Intrathoracic lymphadenopathy is seen in 25% of patients and lymphadenopathy is the only radiographic finding of infection in 12%.[59]

The less common atypical mycobacteria, including *M. gordonae, M. xenopi, M. fortuitum, M. chelonae,* and *M. malmoense* (Fig. 6.12), may also cause symptomatic pulmonary disease in HIV-infected patients.[61,62] A variety of radiographic patterns have been described with these infections, including interstitial opacities, scattered peribronchial opacities, miliary nodules, and parenchymal consolidation.[63,64]

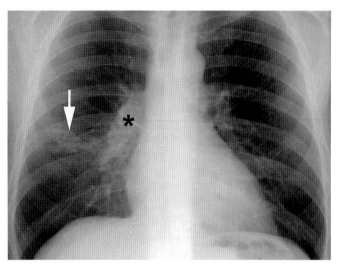

Fig. 6.11 *Mycobacterium kansasii* infection in an AIDS patient. A frontal chest radiograph shows an ill-defined right lung opacity (arrow) and right hilar enlargement (*).

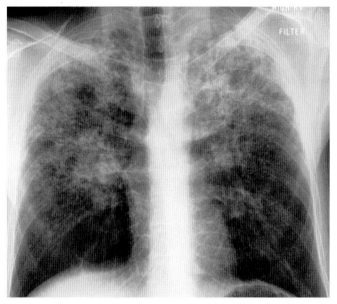

Fig. 6.12 *Mycobacterium malmoense* infection in an AIDS patient. A frontal chest radiograph shows bilateral linear and coarse nodular opacities in a mid and upper lobe distribution, a pattern indistinguishable from postprimary tuberculosis.

Fungal infection

Fungi are ubiquitous and commonly cause recurrent symptoms during the course of AIDS-related illnesses because efficient eradication of fungi requires a competent cell-mediated immune response.

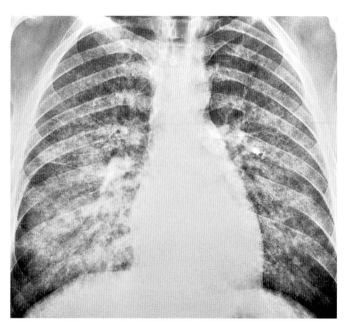

Fig. 6.13 *Pneumocystis jiroveci* pneumonia in a man with AIDS. A frontal chest radiograph shows typical perihilar heterogeneous opacities.

Pneumocystis jiroveci pneumonia

The organism that causes Pneumocystis pneumonia in humans, formerly known as P. carinii, was renamed *P. jiroveci* in order to better reflect its distinctiveness from the organism that infects animals[65]. Further, although previously thought to be a protozoan, the organism is now widely believed to be a fungus[65]. Because of the confusion attendant to this change in nomenclature, the abbreviation PCP is still commonly accepted for the pneumonia caused by *P. jiroveci*. Prior to the widespread use of antibiotic prophylaxis, *Pneumocystis jiroveci* caused pneumonia in over half of all patients with AIDS at some point in the course of their disease. Many AIDS-related deaths were due to respiratory failure directly attributable to PCP. The overall incidence of symptomatic infection has declined due to effective prophylaxis, earlier recognition, and more effective therapy.[66] The mortality from PCP is now approximately 5%.

P. jiroveci pneumonia usually occurs in HIV-infected patients who are not on prophylaxis and who have CD4 lymphocyte counts less than 200/mm³. The clinical prodrome, which may last from a few days to a few weeks, consists of fever, malaise, and weight loss. Patients then develop either a nonproductive cough or a cough productive of frothy white phlegm associated with increased respiratory rate and arterial desaturation on exertion.

On chest radiographs, *P. jiroveci* pneumonia typically manifests with diffuse or perihilar fine reticular and ill-defined ground-glass opacities (Figs 6.13 and 6.14). Untreated, these opacities may progress to diffuse homogeneous opacification in 3–4 days (Figs 6.15 and 6.16). Coarse reticular opacities may

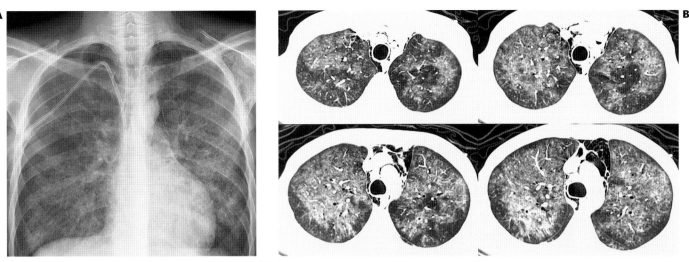

Fig. 6.14 *Pneumocystis jiroveci* pneumonia in a man with AIDS. **A**, A frontal chest radiograph shows bilateral perihilar ground-glass opacities. Note the extensive pneumomediastinum and subcutaneous air. **B**, CT shows diffuse ground-glass opacities and pneumomediastinum. Note the peripheral sparing, a typical CT feature of severe PCP.

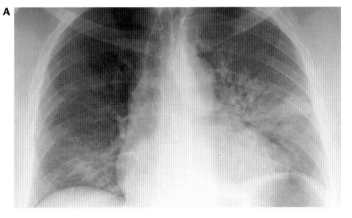

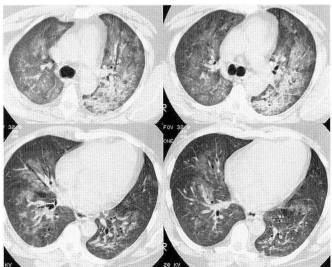

Fig. 6.15 *Pneumocystis jiroveci* pneumonia in a man with AIDS. **A**, A frontal chest radiograph shows left perihilar consolidation and more heterogeneous opacities in the right lung. **B**, CT images show diffuse perihilar ground-glass opacity. Note the peripheral sparing, a typical CT feature of severe PCP.

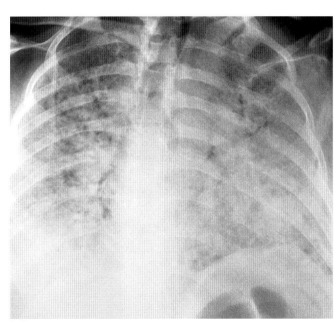

Fig. 6.16 Severe *Pneumocystis jiroveci* pneumonia in a hemophilia patient with AIDS. A frontal chest radiograph shows diffuse pulmonary opacification.

develop if infection persists[14,15,67,68] (Figs 6.17 and 6.18). The chest radiograph is normal at presentation in up to 6% of symptomatic patients.[69] Hilar or mediastinal lymphadenopathy is rare, as is pleural fluid in the absence of extrapulmonary pneumocystosis.

Atypical radiographic features are seen in 5–18% of cases of *P. jiroveci* pneumonia.[67,70–73] Isolated segmental or lobar consolidation (Fig. 6.19) that can be mistaken for pyogenic pneumonia is occasionally seen. Focal nodular opacities with or

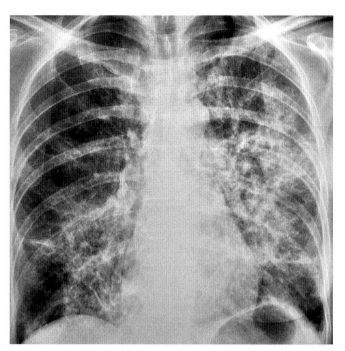

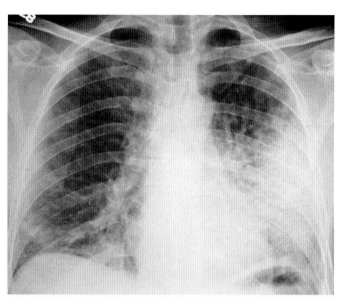

Fig. 6.19 *Pneumocystis jiroveci* pneumonia in a young man with AIDS. A frontal chest radiograph shows focal homogeneous opacity in the left lung, mimicking community-acquired pneumonia.

Fig. 6.17 *Pneumocystis jiroveci* pneumonia in a middle-aged woman with AIDS. A frontal chest radiograph shows scattered coarse linear and more confluent pulmonary opacities.

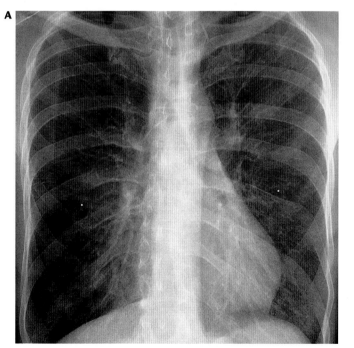

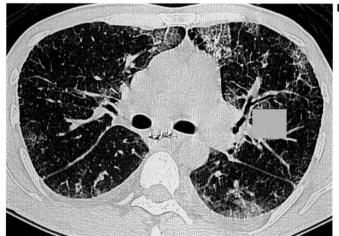

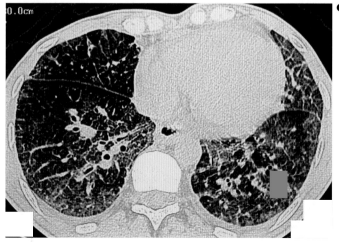

Fig. 6.18 Recurrent *Pneumocystis jiroveci* pneumonia. **A**, A frontal chest radiograph shows bilateral reticular opacities. **B** and **C**, CT shows scattered ground-glass opacities, coarse linear opacities, and septal thickening.

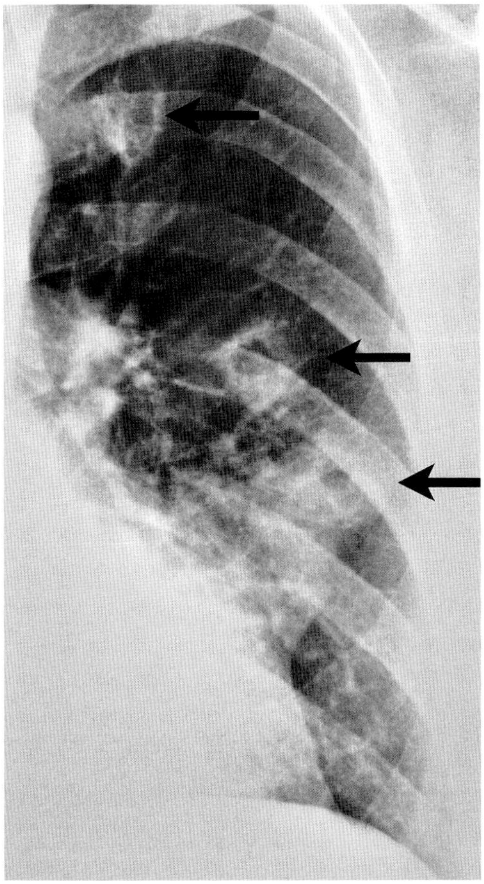

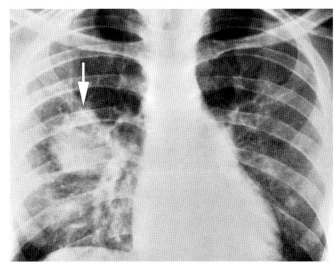

Fig. 6.20 *Pneumocystis jiroveci* pneumonia in a 47-year-old man with AIDS. Coned-down view of a frontal chest radiograph shows multiple cavitary lung nodules (arrows). (Courtesy of Drs P Needelman and B Suster, New York)

Fig. 6.21 *Pneumocystis jiroveci* pneumonia in an intravenous drug abuser with AIDS. A frontal chest radiograph shows a large right mid-lung mass (arrow) with ill-defined margins, mimicking neoplasm. Transbronchial lung biopsy yielded only *Pneumocystis jiroveci* organisms and the lesion resolved with treatment. (Case courtesy of Drs P Needelman and B Suster, New York)

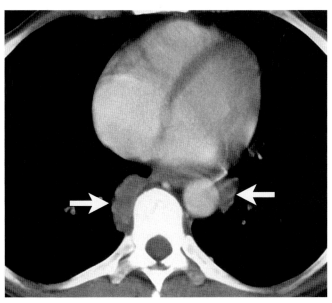

Fig. 6.22 *Pneumocystis jiroveci* pneumonia in a patient with AIDS. Contrast-enhanced CT shows bilateral smoothly marginated soft tissue masses (arrows), mimicking lymphoma. Transthoracic needle aspiration biopsy showed only *Pneumocystis jiroveci* organisms.

without cavitation can occur (Fig. 6.20) and be confused with lung cancer (Fig. 6.21), lymphoma (Fig. 6.22), or metastases.[72,74] *P. jiroveci* pneumonia may rarely manifest as miliary nodules (Fig. 6.23), pleural effusion,[70,71,75] endobronchial mass, or hilar and mediastinal lymphadenopathy,[67,70,71,73,76] which may be calcified.[77,79] Upper lobe disease mimicking tuberculosis (Fig. 6.24) can be seen[71,80] in patients using aerosolized pentamidine because of relative undertreatment of the lung apices.[79,80] Extrapulmonary disease involving the abdominal viscera is occasionally encountered.[77]

The CT, and in particular, the HRCT findings of *P. jiroveci* pneumonia include scattered or diffuse ground-glass opacities, consolidation, and thickening of interlobular septa.[82,83] The CT findings may reflect disease chronicity with ground-glass opacities predominating in the early stages of the disease and with linear opacities predominating in cases of more chronic, repetitive, or under-treated infection (Fig. 6.14).[70] In practice, however, the disease affects both interstitium and airspaces in an unpredictable way[84,85]; thickening of interlobular septa can be the sole CT manifestation of PCP.[86]

CT is usually not necessary in symptomatic patients with classic findings on chest radiographs. However, CT, particularly HRCT, can be quite useful for evaluating patients with suspected

P. jiroveci pneumonia and a normal chest radiograph, or patients who have atypical radiographic findings for PCP. In this setting, CT may show typical ground-glass opacities and can be used to direct invasive diagnostic procedures (Figs 6.25 and 6.26).[82,86–89] Conversely, a normal HRCT is good evidence that *P. jiroveci* pneumonia is not the cause of symptoms.[86,88] Gallium-67 and DTPA radionuclide scans are sensitive but non-

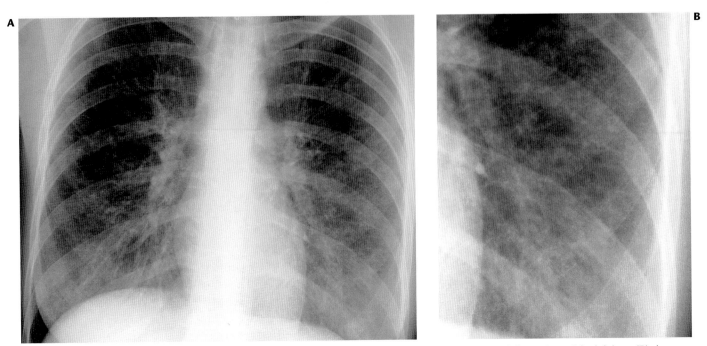

Fig. 6.23 *Pneumocystis jiroveci* pneumonia in a man with AIDS. A frontal chest radiograph (**A**) and a coned-down view of the left lung (**B**) show bilateral fine nodular opacities (miliary pattern).

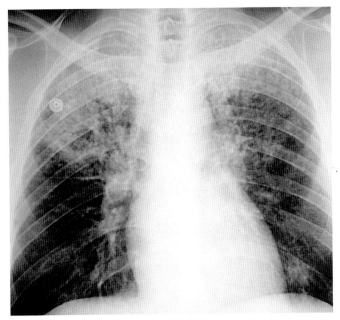

Fig. 6.24 *Pneumocystis jiroveci* pneumonia in a patient with AIDS receiving aerosolized pentamidine. A frontal chest radiograph shows bilateral homogeneous opacities in the upper lobes, mimicking tuberculosis.

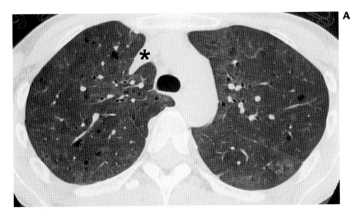

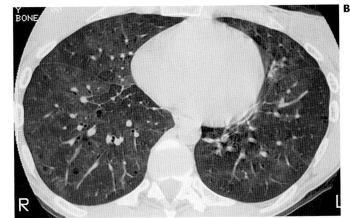

Fig. 6.25 *Pneumocystis jiroveci* pneumonia in a patient with AIDS and a normal chest radiograph. **A** and **B**, CT shows scattered ground-glass opacities in a geographic distribution and thin walled air-filled cysts. Note the azygos fissure (* on **A**).

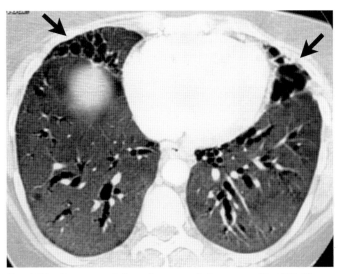

Fig. 6.26 *Pneumocystis jiroveci* pneumonia in a man with AIDS. The chest radiograph was normal. CT shows diffuse ground-glass opacities, clustered air-filled cysts in the middle lobe and lingula (arrows), and strikingly dilated bronchi in the lower lobes.

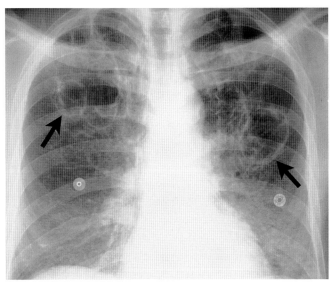

Fig. 6.27 *Pneumocystis jiroveci* pneumonia in a patient receiving aerosolized pentamidine. A frontal chest radiograph shows scattered thin walled pneumatoceles (arrows) of various sizes. Note the upper lung distribution.

specific for diagnosing *P. jiroveci* pneumonia.[90–92] Both are time-consuming and expensive, may be poorly tolerated by debilitated patients, and are thus rarely used for this purpose.

Up to one-third of patients with *P. jiroveci* pneumonia develop thin walled air-containing cysts (pneumatoceles), either in the acute or postinfective period (Figs 6.27 to 6.29).[67,71,75,93,94] The incidence in one series of patients examined by CT was 38%.[70] The cysts are round, oval, or crescent-shaped, and range in size from 1 to 8.5 cm; they are usually multiple but may be solitary.[93–97] They may occur at any location, although there was a predilection for the upper lobes in several series,[70,93,95,98] especially in patients on prophylactic aerosolized pentamidine (Fig. 6.27).[71,81] The etiology of *Pneumocystis*-related pneumatoceles is unclear, although a number of possible mechanisms have been suggested[95,96,99,100]: (1) *Pneumocystis jiroveci* infection may stimulate macrophages to release elastase, tissue necrosis factor, and other toxins that cause cystic destruction of lung parenchyma; (2) vascular invasion by *Pneumocystis jiroveci* may cause tissue necrosis and cavitation; and (3) obstruction of small airways may lead to a ball valve effect on distal lung. A history of intravenous drug abuse[101] and repeated prior infections are also likely to be associated with cystic change. The cysts usually resolve within 7 months of treatment, usually without sequela.[94] However, cysts that persist up to 3 years have been reported.[102,103] Spontaneous pneumothorax due to cyst (Fig. 6.30) or subpleural bleb rupture may complicate the course of infected patients.[67,70,71,93,95,99,104–106]

Candida albicans

The yeast *Candida albicans* is a normal commensal organism of the skin and mouth. In advanced cases of AIDS, it initially causes oral, then esophageal, candidiasis. Patients with esophageal candidiasis may present with severe, painful dysphagia. Barium swallow examination may show focal or diffuse irregular narrowing of the esophagus and diffuse ulceration. Although candida is isolated from the airways or lungs of 2% of all patients

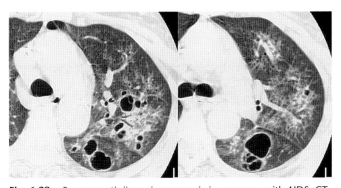

Fig. 6.28 *Pneumocystis jiroveci* pneumonia in a woman with AIDS. CT (lung window) shows both thin and thick walled air-filled cysts in the left lung and ground-glass and denser opacities.

with AIDS,[107] pulmonary candidiasis is a late, often preterminal, manifestation of HIV infection. It usually occurs in the setting of widely disseminated disease[108] and nearly always occurs in AIDS patients who also have profound neutropenia. Histopathological evidence of tissue invasion is required for definitive diagnosis of *Candida* pneumonia. In less severely immunocompromised patients, the organism may occasionally colonize preexisting tuberculous cavities or cystic spaces due to *P. jiroveci* infection. The radiologic manifestations of pulmonary candidiasis are nonspecific and include diffuse heterogeneous or homogeneous pulmonary opacities. Nodules and thick walled cavities are less common.[109]

Cryptococcus neoformans

Cryptococcus neoformans is a ubiquitous fungus that infects up to 2% of patients with AIDS. Cryptococcal infection in this

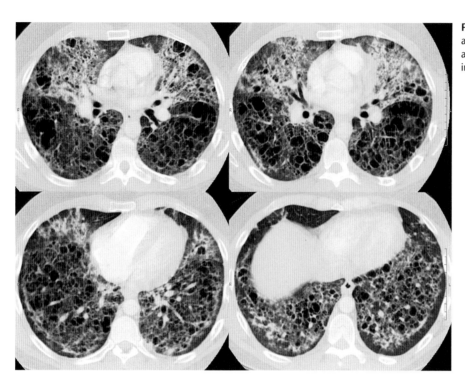

Fig. 6.29 *Pneumocystis jiroveci* pneumonia in an AIDS patient. CT shows diffuse thin walled air-filled cysts (pneumatoceles), thickened interlobular septa, and ground-glass opacity.

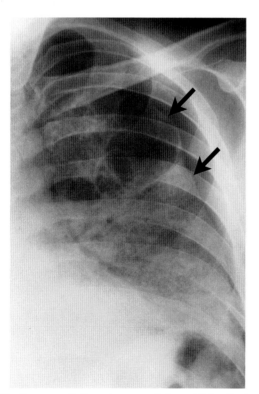

Fig. 6.30 *Pneumocystis jiroveci* pneumonia in an AIDS patient. Coned-down view of a frontal chest radiograph shows diffuse pulmonary opacities, multiple thin walled cysts, and a moderate left pneumothorax (arrows).

population usually manifests with meningitis. Most cases occur in conjunction with other opportunistic infections; cryptococcosis is the sole manifestation of AIDS in less than 4% of patients.[107] The clinical presentation of cryptococcal meningitis is often nonspecific. Patients may complain of vague symptoms and have a prolonged prodrome lasting from 1 to 4 months. Typical features of bacterial meningitis are usually absent. Less than half of patients complain of nausea and vomiting and only a quarter complain of neck stiffness or photophobia at diagnosis. The organism must be isolated from body fluids or tissues for definitive diagnosis.[107] The serologic test for cryptococcal capsular polysaccharide antigen is both sensitive and specific for invasive infection.

Cryptococcus accounts for 2–15% of all respiratory tract infections in patients with AIDS. A variety of radiologic patterns are described for pulmonary cryptococcal infection (Figs 6.31 to 6.33).[110–114] Diffuse heterogeneous or reticulonodular opacities are common.[115] Infection can also manifest as solitary or multiple nodules varying from several millimeters to centimeters in diameter, with or without cavitation. Miliary disease, indistinguishable from tuberculosis, has been reported.[116] Intrathoracic lymphadenopathy is a common feature and may be the sole radiographic manifestation of disease. Pleural effusions are rare, occurring in less than 10% of cases in most series. Normal chest radiographs do not exclude the diagnosis.[114]

Coccidioides immitis

Coccidioides immitis is endemic in the semiarid regions of North America. It is widely distributed by the wind and then inhaled.[107] Symptoms are nonspecific and include night sweats, fatigue, and weight loss. Cough and dyspnea are reported in up to 50% of patients. Neurologic complications, typically menin-

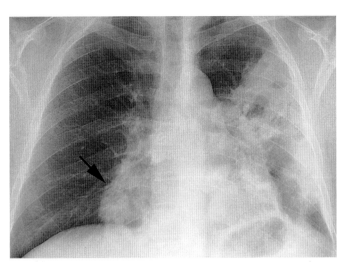

Fig. 6.31 Cryptococcal pneumonia in a patient with AIDS. A frontal chest radiograph shows cavitary consolidation in the left lung and masslike consolidation in the right middle lobe (arrow).

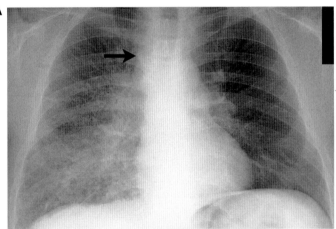

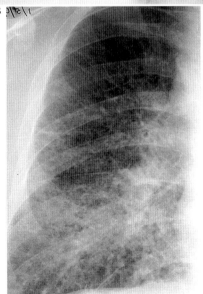

Fig. 6.32 Cryptococcal pneumonia in a patient with AIDS. Frontal (**A**) and coned-down (**B**) chest radiographs show heterogeneous opacities and septal thickening in the right lung. Note the evidence of right hilar and mediastinal (arrow) lymphadenopathy. (With permission from Connolly JE Jr, McAdams HP, Erasmus JJ, et al. Opportunistic fungal pneumonia. J Thorac Imaging 1999;14:51–62.)

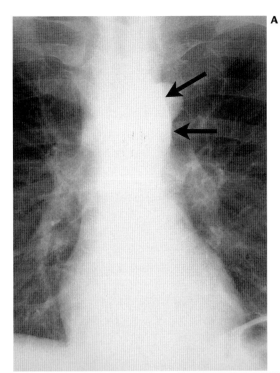

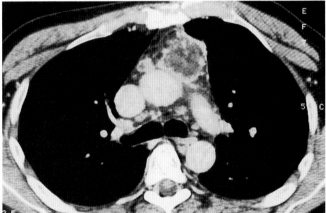

Fig. 6.33 *Cryptococcus neoformans* infection in a patient with AIDS who presented with headache. **A**, The frontal chest radiograph suggests an anterior mediastinal mass (arrows). **B**, CT shows an anterior mediastinal abscess. Aspiration confirmed *C. neoformans* infection. (With permission from Connolly JE Jr, McAdams HP, Erasmus JJ, et al. Opportunistic fungal pneumonia. J Thorac Imaging 1999;14:51–62.)

goencephalitis or brain abscess, occur less commonly than in cases of cryptococcosis. When such complications occur, however, they are quite difficult to treat and have a very poor prognosis. Disseminated coccidioidomycosis usually occurs in the setting of low CD4 lymphocyte counts (less than 200 cells/mm^3) and has very high mortality (up to 70%).[107] Radiographs of affected patients show focal or diffuse homogeneous or heterogeneous pulmonary opacities.[117] Less common findings include discrete nodules, hilar or mediastinal lymphadenopathy, cavitation, and bilateral pleural effusions (1%).

A

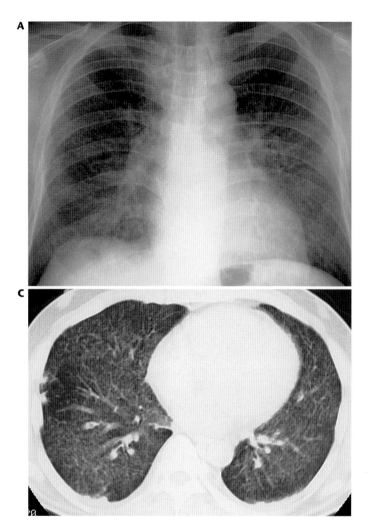

C

B

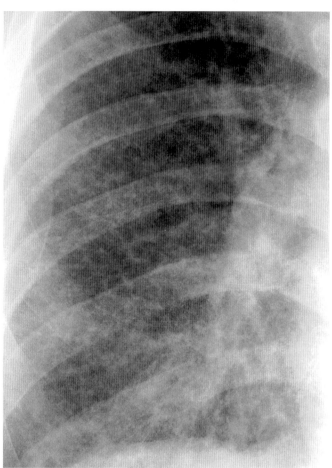

Fig. 6.34 Disseminated histoplasmosis in an AIDS patient. Frontal (**A**) and coned-down (**B**) chest radiographs show diffuse small nodular opacities (miliary pattern), confirmed on **C**, CT.

Histoplasma capsulatum

Histoplasma capsulatum is found throughout the world, but histoplasmosis is rare except in North America and the Caribbean. In immunocompetent individuals, it may cause a flu-like illness that resolves spontaneously in almost all cases. In patients with impaired T-cell function, progressive extra-pulmonary infection leads to a systemic, debilitating febrile illness known as progressive disseminated histoplasmosis. Infection occurs in 2–5% of AIDS patients in endemic areas.[118] Affected patients complain of cough, dyspnea, and weight loss, and 10% are frankly septic with lymphadenopathy and hepatosplenomegaly.[107] It is not clear whether pulmonary disease in AIDS patients results from reactivation of latent infection or from new exposure. As in tuberculosis, the intradermal skin test is negative in advanced disease and a positive antibody or prick test does not establish active current infection.[107] The highest diagnostic yields are from bronchoalveolar lavage samples or bone marrow aspiration and biopsy.[119] Identification of *Histoplasma* capsular polysaccharide antigen in blood and urine specimens is a rapid and relatively sensitive and specific means for diagnosing disseminated infection and for following patients during treatment.[118–121]

Up to half of AIDS patients with disseminated histoplasmosis have normal chest radiographs.[122,123] Radiographs in the remainder may show diffuse small nodules (miliary pattern; Fig. 6.34), linear opacities, and focal or diffuse homogeneous opacities.[122] Small pleural effusions and septal thickening may also be seen. On HRCT, the disease usually manifests with perivascular, paraseptal, and subpleural nodules as well as intra- and interlobular septal thickening – findings that are indistinguishable from those of miliary tuberculosis.[124] Medi-astinal lymphadenopathy, which may be calcified, is noted in up to 13% of cases.[122–123] After treatment, parenchymal findings usually resolve completely.[122]

Blastomyces dermatitidis

Blastomyces dermatitidis is endemic in North America. Disseminated infection in patients with AIDS produces clinical features indistinguishable from other fungal infections or tuberculosis: notably fever, weight loss, cough, and dyspnea.[125] Typically, other concurrent AIDS-defining illnesses are present at the time of diagnosis and the CD4 lymphocyte count is below 200 cells/mm³. Disseminated blastomycosis is characterized by multiorgan involvement, including the central nervous system, and has high mortality (over 30%). Pulmonary involvement can lead to acute respiratory distress syndrome. There are very few reports regarding the radiologic manifestations of *Blastomyces* infection in AIDS patients. Pappas et al reported the chest radiographic manifestations of blastomycosis in 15 AIDS patients.[125] In that series, a diffuse reticulonodular or fine nodular (miliary) pattern was most common. However, chest radiographs were normal in 27% of AIDS patients with disseminated blastomycosis.

Aspergillus

The incidence of *Aspergillus* infection in HIV-positive patients is less than 1%.[126,127] This is in contrast to the very high incidence (up to 41%) reported in patients with acute leukemia.[128] This difference is because the neutrophil is the primary effector cell against *Aspergillus* species. Thus, patients with AIDS are not particularly susceptible to *Aspergillus* infection until they become very severely immunocompromised. *Aspergillus* infection usually occurs only when the CD4 count falls below 50 cells/mm^3,[126,127,129,130] or when the patient becomes secondarily neutropenic due to use of bone marrow suppressive drugs. Use of aerosolized pentamidine may be an independent risk factor.[130] Hemoptysis is a common and often fatal complication.[127]

The radiographic manifestations of pulmonary aspergillosis in AIDS patients are quite varied, with several types of infection often present in the same patient. The most common pattern seen in the AIDS population resembles the type of infection described as chronic necrotizing aspergillosis. In this form, *Aspergillus* infection manifests with progressive cavitary pneumonia, usually in the upper lobes (Fig. 6.35). Cavitary lesions are reported in 20–80% of patients with AIDS and aspergillosis.[126,127,130,133] Intracavitary masses, due either to true mycetomas or infarcted lung, may develop. Noncavitating nodules, secondary to tissue invasion with or without infarction, have been reported in up to one-third of cases (Fig. 6.36).[127,130,131,133] Invasive aspergillosis may also cause pulmonary consolidation and vascular invasion with infarction in AIDS patients.[126,127,130,132,133] Colonization of preexisting cavities or pneumatoceles may result in intracavitary aspergillomas.[131,134] Other reported features of aspergillosis in AIDS patients include pleural effusion,[130,131] pneumothorax,[126,127] lymphadenopathy,[130] cardiomegaly,[133] pericardial effusion,[133] and pericardial thickening.[131]

There are several reports of a distinctive form of airway infection in AIDS patients known as obstructing bronchopulmonary aspergillosis.[127,132,135] In this unusual form of the disease, invasive airway infection leads to pseudomembranes and obstructing mucus plugs in the large airways. Chest radiographs of affected patients may be normal or show mucoid impaction, atelectasis, or obstructive pneumonia.[136,141] CT may show circumferential airway wall thickening, intramural sinus tracts, and large mucus plugs (Fig. 6.37).[135]

Protozoal infection

Toxoplasma

The protozoan *Toxoplasma gondii* is the most frequent cause of focal neurological abnormalities in patients with AIDS, but is an extremely rare cause of pulmonary infection. Nonspecific fever

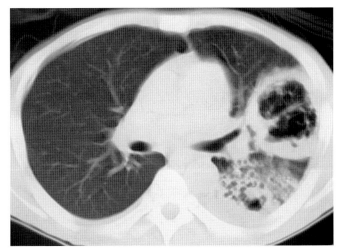

Fig. 6.35 Aspergillosis in an AIDS patient. CT shows a cavitary mass in the left upper lobe and ground-glass opacities in the left lower lobe.

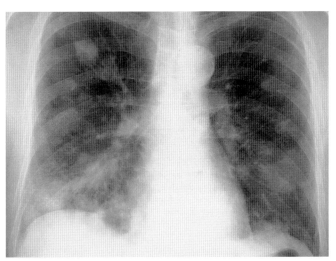

Fig. 6.36 Disseminated aspergillosis in an AIDS patient. A frontal chest radiograph shows bilateral pulmonary nodules with ill-defined margins.

is the typical presenting manifestation when the thorax is affected. Occasionally, an acute disseminated form occurs that manifests with septic shock.[136] Affected patients are typically severely immunosuppressed with a mean CD4 lymphocyte count of 32 cells/mm^3.[137] Diagnosis may be difficult because, in this setting, there may be no specific IgM *Toxoplasma* antibody response. The diagnosis is made by identifying the organism in bronchoalveolar lavage fluid or lung biopsy specimens.[137]

The radiographic findings of pulmonary toxoplasmosis[136,138] can be very similar to severe *P. jiroveci* pneumonia but usually show a more coarse nodular pattern. Small pleural effusions are occasionally encountered, but mediastinal or hilar adenopathy is not a feature.

Cryptosporidium

The protozoan *Cryptosporidium* is an unusual pathogen in the immunocompetent patient, being limited to farm workers or to

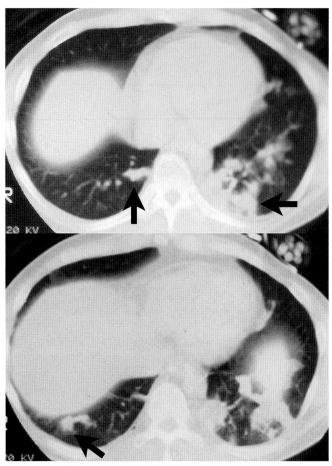

Fig. 6.37 Obstructing bronchopulmonary aspergillosis in an AIDS patient. CT shows tubular opacities (arrows) in both lower lobes consistent with mucus plugs. (With permission from Connolly JE Jr, McAdams HP, Erasmus JJ, et al. Opportunistic fungal pneumonia. J Thorac Imaging 1999;14:51–62.)

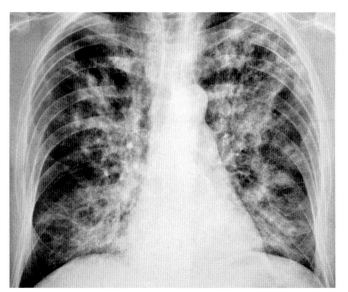

Fig. 6.38 Cytomegalovirus and *Pneumocystis jiroveci* pneumonia in a homosexual man with AIDS. A frontal chest radiograph shows bilateral, diffuse coarse heterogeneous opacities and scattered pneumatoceles.

individuals drinking contaminated water. In patients with AIDS, *Cryptosporidium* infection causes severe protracted diarrhea that is resistant to therapy. The organism passes from the gut into the biliary system and causes a form of sclerosing cholangitis. Pulmonary infection is quite uncommon, and, when it occurs, is thought to be due to aspiration of trophozoites during episodes of vomiting. The radiographic manifestations of *Cryptosporidium* pneumonia are quite nonspecific and include focal or diffuse airspace opacities that cannot be differentiated from other causes of pneumonia.

Human Herpes virus infections

The Herpes virus family of DNA viruses includes three viruses that cause pneumonia: cytomegalovirus, herpes simplex, and varicella-zoster. The Epstein–Barr virus, also in the Herpes virus family, does not cause pneumonia but is associated with a number of lymphoproliferative diseases in immunocompromised patients, including AIDS-related lymphoma and posttransplant lymphoproliferative disorder.[139]

Cytomegalovirus (CMV) infection in immunocompetent adults typically results in either subclinical infection or in mild symptoms that resemble those of infectious mononucleosis. CMV infection in AIDS patients is usually more severe and manifests with retinitis, colitis, encephalitis, or radiculopathy. Over 90% of HIV-positive patients have latent infection, but clinically apparent disease only emerges when the CD4 count is less than 60 cells/mm³. The clinical significance of CMV as a pulmonary pathogen in AIDS patients is controversial[140] as there are frequently many other concurrent pathogens, especially *P. jiroveci* (Fig. 6.38).[141] Most clinicians require evidence of CMV-related lung damage, such as cytomegalic inclusions in biopsy specimens, for definitive diagnosis.[142] Viral culture from respiratory secretions is considered less reliable evidence of infection.[143] The use of the newer antiretroviral drugs, in particular the protease inhibitors, is associated with a marked reduction in the development of CMV disease and an increase in survival for those with infection.[144]

Very few reports have described the imaging manifestations of symptomatic CMV pneumonia in AIDS patients. The largest published series studied 21 patients in whom CMV was the sole pathogen.[140] Solitary or multiple nodules or masses, seen in 57% of cases, were the most common radiographic findings. The nodules varied in size from 2 mm to 3 cm in diameter. Pathologically, the lesions were due to focal areas of dense consolidation, alveolar injury, hemorrhage and fibrin collections, atypical necrotic lymphoid cells, or clusters of cytomegalic cells with focal necrosis. Ground-glass opacities were seen on CT in 43% of patients. Less common features included irregular linear opacities, bronchial wall thickening, bronchiectasis, and pleural effusion. Although the chest radiograph was normal in three patients, CT showed consolidation in two and ground-glass opacity in one. Endobronchial CMV causing circumferential narrowing and ulceration of the trachea has also been reported.[145]

Failure of cell-mediated immunity in patients with AIDS allows reactivation of latent herpes simplex and varicella-zoster infections and usually manifests with cutaneous eruptions. Pneumonitis is less common. The radiographic manifestations of pulmonary infection with these organisms are similar to those of

CMV pneumonia: focal or diffuse homogeneous consolidation, diffuse heterogeneous opacities, or multiple lung nodules.

AIDS-associated airway disease

Bronchiectasis has been reported in both HIV-positive and AIDS patients[146–150] and is attributed to inflammation of the airways caused by *P. jiroveci* infection or recurrent pyogenic pneumonia (Fig. 6.39).[82] As discussed below, bronchiectasis is also seen in children with AIDS and lymphocytic interstitial pneumonia (LIP). Organizing pneumonia has also been reported in association with HIV infection and may represent a response to undiagnosed infection.[149,151]

Immune restoration syndrome

In recent years, the morbidity and mortality of HIV infection has dramatically declined, due in no small part to the introduction of highly active antiretroviral therapy (HAART).[8,152–154] Patients receiving HAART have both a qualitative and quantitative improvement in T-cell function, as reflected by the CD4 lymphocyte count.[8,153] However, as the immune system reconstitutes, clinical and radiographic manifestations of previously latent opportunistic infections may become apparent, a phenomenon known as the immune restoration syndrome.[5–7,9,10,152,154–157] The reported incidence of immune restoration syndrome varies from 3.6%[154] to 25%[5] of AIDS patients treated with HAART. The clinical and radiologic features of immune restoration syndrome are thought to be the result of renewed potency of the immune response to latent subclinical infection, particularly to atypical mycobacteria, fungi, and viruses.[9] Although the disease is frequently self-limited, antimicrobial therapy may be required. Fatal cases, though rare, are reported, particularly with central nervous system disease.[155] Affected patients usually begin to exhibit signs and symptoms of infection within 3 months of institution of HAART,[154] as the CD4 lymphocyte count rises. Radiographic findings of disease are similar to those reported for these infections in the non-AIDS population, including mediastinal lymphadenopathy (Fig. 6.40), lytic bone lesions, localized abscesses, and parenchymal lung disease.[5,7,9,10,152,154,156,157]

Typical clinical, radiologic, and histopathologic features of sarcoidosis have also been reported in AIDS patients after beginning HAART.[158–160] It is thus possible that sarcoidosis represents a distinct manifestation of the immune restoration syndrome. Furthermore, transient worsening of existing clinical infection, particularly tuberculosis and *P. jiroveci* pneumonia, has also been reported following initiation of HAART.[7,161]

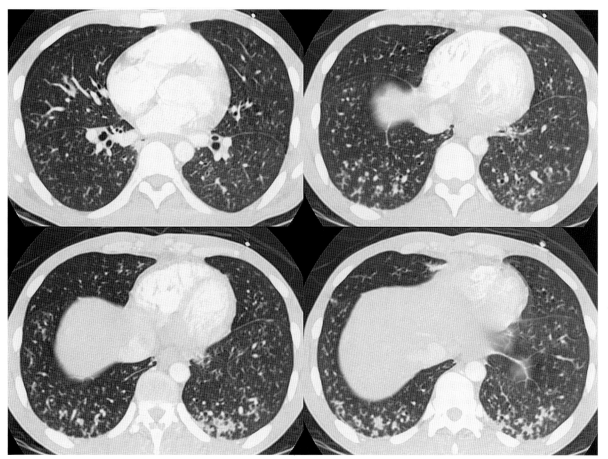

Fig. 6.39 AIDS-related airway disease. CT shows basal bronchiectasis, centrilobular nodules, and tree-in-bud opacities. Sputum cultures grew *S. pneumoniae*.

Thoracic neoplasms and noninfectious complications

Kaposi sarcoma and non-Hodgkin disease are the major neoplasms encountered in patients with AIDS and are likely mediated by viral infection. They may therefore be considered a complication of opportunistic infection. It is also possible that decreased cytotoxic T-cell and natural killer cell function may contribute to development of neoplasms in patients with AIDS.

AIDS-related lymphoma

Non-Hodgkin rather than Hodgkin disease predominates in patients with AIDS, being invariably of high grade and usually of B-cell or non-B, non-T-cell origin.[162] The disease is typically extranodal and is in most cases associated with Epstein–Barr virus (EBV).[139] EBV-driven polyclonal B-cell proliferations, similar to those seen in organ transplant patients, and body cavity lymphomas associated with the herpes virus HHV-8 have also been reported in patients with HIV infection.[162]

Thoracic involvement is reported in up to 40% of patients with AIDS-related lymphoma.[164,165] Extranodal pulmonary involvement in the setting of disseminated disease is the usual pattern, but primary pulmonary lymphoma has been reported.[166,167] The presence of extranodal disease predicts a poor outcome, with most affected patients surviving less than one year.[168] Parenchymal lymphoma usually manifests with solitary or multiple lung nodules or masses of varying size (Fig. 6.41).[164–166,169,170] Cavitation is rare; one case of cavitation with an intracavitary mass resembling mycetoma has been reported.[164]

Pleural fluid is also common in patients with thoracic AIDS-related lymphoma. Effusions may be unilateral or bilateral and are usually moderate to large in size.[164–166] The pleura are sometimes the only site of disease (Fig. 6.42).[165] Mediastinal and hilar lymphadenopathy is not necessarily a predominant radiologic feature. Although reported in up to 45% of cases, adenopathy is not usually bulky or always multi-compartmental. The nodes are often less than 1 cm in diameter and may therefore only be seen on CT.[164–166,171]

Kaposi sarcoma

Prior to the advent of the AIDS epidemic, Kaposi sarcoma was a rare neoplasm seen primarily in endemic form in sub-Saharan Africa, in elderly people in the Eastern Mediterranean, and

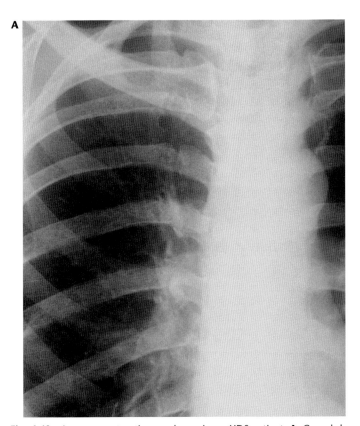
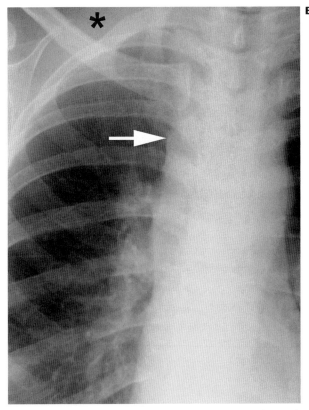

Fig. 6.40 Immune restoration syndrome in an AIDS patient. **A,** Coned-down view of a frontal chest radiograph is normal. **B,** Chest radiograph obtained 1 week after institution of HAART shows lymphadenopathy in the right paratracheal region (white arrow) and supraclavicular fossa (*). Biopsy showed granulomas and cultures showed *M. tuberculosis*. (With permission from Fishman JE, Saraf-Lavi E, Narita M, et al. Pulmonary tuberculosis in AIDS patients: transient chest radiographic worsening after initiation of antiretroviral therapy. AJR Am J Roentgenol 2000;174:43–49.)

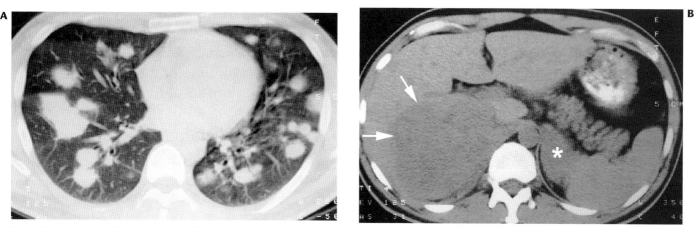

Fig. 6.41   Non-Hodgkin disease in an AIDS patient. **A**, CT shows bilateral lung masses and nodules. **B**, CT through the upper abdomen shows right renal (arrows) and left adrenal (*) masses.

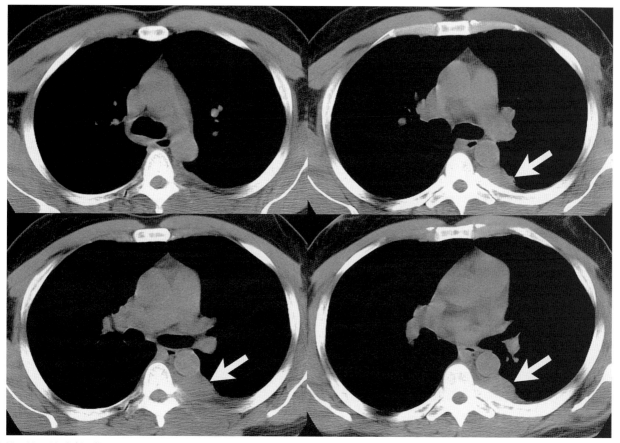

Fig. 6.42   Non-Hodgkin disease in an AIDS patient with chest pain. CT shows extranodal lymphoma (arrows) involving the posterior left pleural space and paraspinal muscles.

A

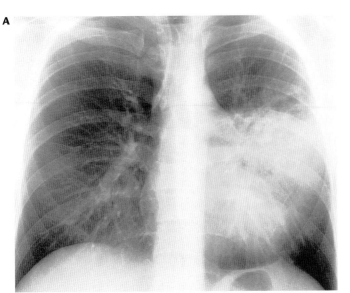

B

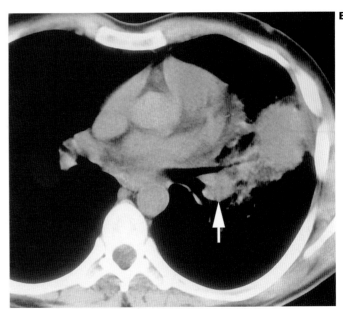

Fig. 6.43 Kaposi sarcoma in a patient with AIDS. **A**, A frontal chest radiograph shows a masslike lingular consolidation, mimicking pneumonia. **B**, CT shows a homogeneous lingular mass, adjacent consolidation and left hilar lymph node enlargement (arrow).

in heavily immunosuppressed patients. It had a relatively benign course and caused purple nodular lesions on the skin of the lower limbs; other forms of the disease were quite rare.[172] In patients with AIDS, Kaposi sarcoma is a multifocal polyclonal neoplasm with distinct histopathologic features. It is composed of a proliferation of vascular or lymphatic endothelial cells with associated spindle cells and atypical mitotic nuclear figures. The tumor forms multiple slitlike spaces that trap erythrocytes, a feature that accounts for the purple coloration of the lesion.

Kaposi sarcoma in AIDS patients particularly affects homosexual or bisexual men and individuals from Africa. It is uncommon in patients who acquire HIV infection transplacentally, through needle sharing, or from blood products. The incidence has decreased since the disease was first described in AIDS; this reduction occurred at the same time as the increased practice of safe sex and is presumed to be due to a decrease in the sexually transmitted form of the disease. A close association has been documented between human herpes virus type 8 (HHV-8) infection and Kaposi sarcoma.[173] The great majority of affected AIDS patients have cutaneous disease and over half also have oropharyngeal lesions[174]; a much smaller proportion have bronchopulmonary Kaposi sarcoma.[175] The clinical manifestations of pulmonary involvement are often nonspecific. Affected patients usually have advanced AIDS with a median CD4 count of 34 cells/mm³,[174] and present with fever and recurrent pneumonia. In most cases, cutaneous findings of Kaposi sarcoma precede visceral involvement.

On chest radiographs and CT, focal Kaposi sarcoma may cause segmental, lobar-shaped, or masslike opacities due to the tumor itself (Fig. 6.43). Endobronchial disease may cause atelectasis or postobstructive pneumonia.[176] Disseminated pulmonary disease is seen more frequently. This form of the disease is distinctly bronchocentric in distribution as the lesions spread via the bronchial mucosa. Chest radiographs typically show nodular or coalescent masslike opacities in a perihilar and distinctively peribronchovascular distribution (Figs 6.44 and 6.45).[175,177,178] On CT,[174,176,179–181] lesions are usually nodular in

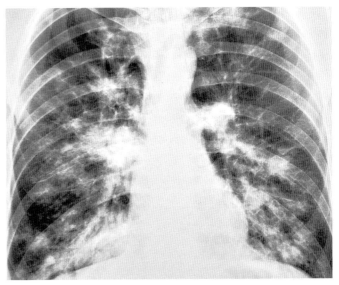

Fig. 6.44 Kaposi sarcoma in a young homosexual man with AIDS. A frontal chest radiograph shows ill-defined peribronchovascular nodules in a basal distribution.

shape with either well- or ill-defined borders (Figs 6.45 and 6.46). Such lesions are sometimes described as "flame-shaped" (Fig. 6.47). The lesions vary in size from 1 cm to well over 2 cm in diameter. The larger masses may contain air bronchograms (Fig. 6.46) and may have a surrounding rim of ground-glass opacity. Smooth or nodular thickening of bronchovascular bundles is seen in two-thirds of cases. Thickened interlobular septa and nodularity along the fissures are also common.[180] Up to half of affected patients have either unilateral or bilateral pleural effusions, which may be quite large. Hilar and mediastinal lymph node enlargement is seen in a substantial proportion of patients. While any of these findings may be seen in

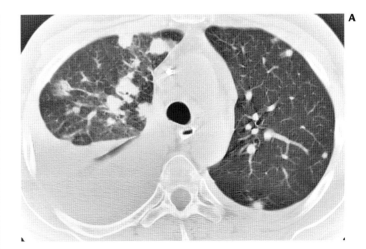

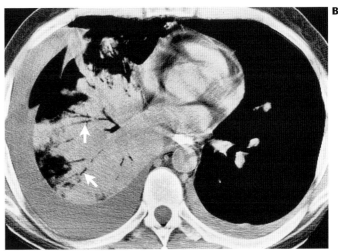

Fig. 6.46 Kaposi sarcoma in a young homosexual man with AIDS. **A**, CT shows bilateral pleural effusions and spiculated nodules. **B**, CT at a lower level shows masslike consolidation in the right lower lung. Note the air bronchogram signs (arrows). (Courtesy of Drs P Needelman and B Suster, New York)

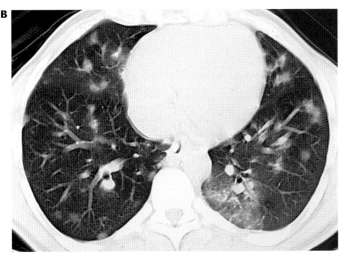

Fig. 6.45 Kaposi sarcoma in a patient with AIDS. **A**, A frontal chest radiograph shows ill-defined peribronchovascular nodules in a basal distribution. **B**, CT shows ill-defined nodules in a peribronchovascular distribution and scattered ground-glass opacities.

isolation, multiple findings are present in the great majority of patients.[179]

MR findings of Kaposi sarcoma were reported in a series of 10 cases.[182] In that series, the lesions were of high signal intensity on T1-weighted images and of low signal intensity on T2-weighted images. These findings were suggestive of hemorrhage within the lesions (Fig. 6.48). The masses also enhanced following intravenous administration of a gadolinium-based contrast agent.

Strictly speaking, either transbronchial or thoracoscopic lung biopsy is required for definitive diagnosis of pulmonary Kaposi sarcoma. Neither pleural fluid analysis nor pleural biopsy is diagnostic. In practice, however, the presence of typical radiologic features (poorly defined nodules in a peribronchovascular distribution) and findings of endobronchial Kaposi sarcoma at bronchoscopy are regarded as evidence of pulmonary involvement.

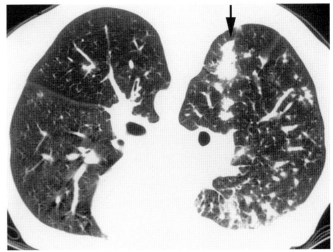

Fig. 6.47 Kaposi sarcoma in a patient with AIDS. Prone HRCT shows spiculated nodules in a peribronchovascular distribution. Note the flame-shaped nodule (arrow) in the right lower lobe.

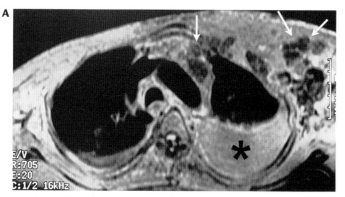

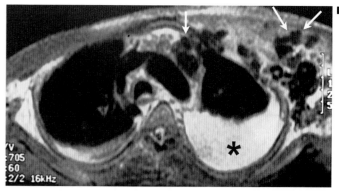

Fig. 6.48 Kaposi sarcoma in a patient with AIDS. Axial T1- (**A**) and T2-weighted (**B**) MR images show an infiltrating mass in the left anterior chest wall and lymphadenopathy (arrows) in the left anterior mediastinum and axilla. Note the loss of signal in the nodes on both pulse sequences due to hemosiderin deposition and large left pleural effusion (*).

Lymphocytic interstitial pneumonia and other pulmonary lymphoproliferative disorders

Lymphocytic bronchiolitis,[183] lymphocytic alveolitis,[184] and lymphocytic interstitial pneumonia (LIP) form a spectrum of atypical lymphoproliferative disorders encountered in patients with AIDS. Along with nonspecific interstitial pneumonia (see below), these pulmonary complications of HIV infection may occur in the absence of a detectable opportunistic infection or neoplasm.[185]

LIP is an AIDS-defining illness in children less than 13 years of age.[186] LIP frequently occurs as part of a widespread syndrome of lymphocytic infiltration of parotid glands, stomach, thymus, liver, kidneys, and spleen. This syndrome is thought, in many cases, to be a reactive immune response to the Epstein–Barr virus.[139] It responds well to antiretroviral therapy and has a relatively good prognosis. Although the radiographic features of LIP may persist unchanged for a long while, they may also resolve as the level of immunosuppression worsens.[187] Affected patients may be asymptomatic or present with subacute dyspnea and cough. Diagnosis in children rarely requires biopsy and is often based on the clinical and radiographic features alone.

LIP in adults with AIDS is very uncommon and is thought to represent a specific pulmonary response to HIV infection.[188] Symptoms are nonspecific and include cough, dyspnea, and fever.[189] Histopathologic specimens show polyclonal proliferations of lymphocytes and micronodular lymphoid aggregates that diffusely infiltrate alveolar septa and bronchovascular bundles.[188,189]

The radiologic features of LIP are similar to, and often indistinguishable from, those of other infectious and noninfectious conditions that occur in patients with AIDS. Reticulonodular opacities are the most common finding on chest radiographs; the nodules vary from 1 to 5 mm in size (Figs 6.49 and 6.50).[188–191] Lobar or segmental homogeneous opacities have also been described.[188] CT, especially HRCT, typically confirms the presence of small nodules in a diffuse distribution. Ground-glass opacities, bronchial wall thickening, and findings of bronchiolitis may also be seen.[190] Bronchiectasis, observed in children with LIP,[150] probably results from lymphocytic infiltration of the bronchioles leading to wall thickening, destruction, fibrosis, and dilatation.[192] CT may also demonstrate small, thin walled, air-filled cysts in cases of LIP.[193] The cysts may be related to partial obstruction of bronchioles from lymphocytic infiltration.

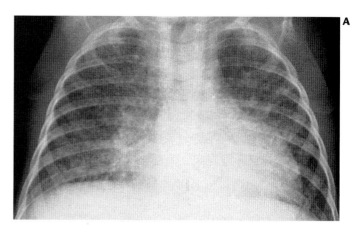

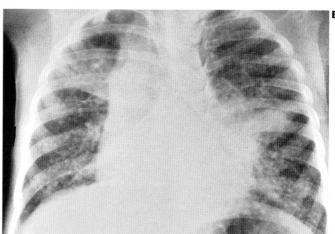

Fig. 6.49 Lymphocytic interstitial pneumonia in two different children with AIDS. **A**, A frontal chest radiograph shows diffuse small nodules. Note the absence of lymphadenopathy. **B**, A frontal chest radiograph in a second child shows more coarse nodules, confluent opacities in the right upper lobe and lingula, and possible lymphadenopathy.

Lymphadenopathy is seen in 25% of cases.[188] Gallium scanning may be positive but is rarely performed.[194]

Pulmonary nodules measuring approximately 5–6 mm in diameter are also seen in cases of bronchus-associated lymphoid tissue hyperplasia.[190,195] Ground-glass opacities and bronchiectasis may also be seen in this condition.[190]

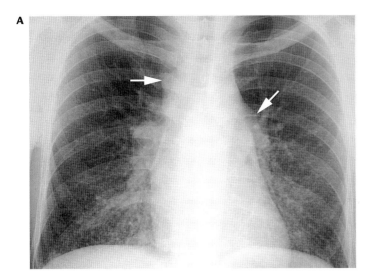

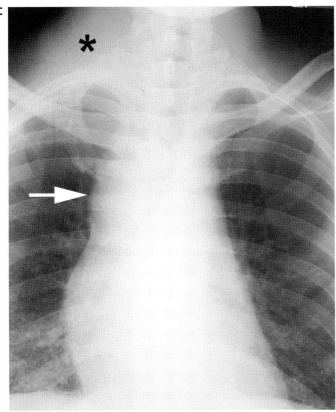

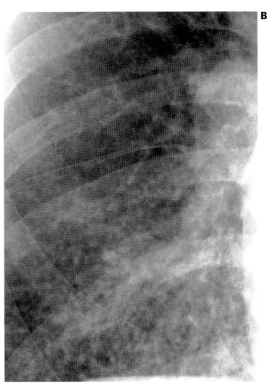

Fig. 6.50 Lymphocytic interstitial pneumonia in an AIDS patient. Frontal (**A**) and coned-down (**B**) chest radiographs show bilateral small nodular opacities in a lower lobe distribution. Note the evidence of mediastinal (arrows) and possibly hilar lymphadenopathy. Lung biopsy showed lymphocytic interstitial pneumonia. **C**, A radiograph obtained 1 year later shows progressive mediastinal (arrow) and supraclavicular (*) adenopathy. Lymph node biopsy now showed non-Hodgkin disease.

Nonspecific interstitial pneumonia

Nonspecific interstitial pneumonia (NSIP), a noninfectious pneumonia that may be clinically indistinguishable from *P. jiroveci* pneumonia, has been described in patients with AIDS.[185,196–199] Affected patients present with cough, dyspnea, and pyrexia. Histopathologic specimens show diffuse alveolar damage, an increased number of alveolar macrophages, alveolar hemorrhage, interstitial inflammation, and fibrin deposition. No causative agent can be identified, though patients may have a recent history of *P. jiroveci* pneumonia, Kaposi sarcoma, drug therapy, or drug abuse.

The reported incidence of NSIP in patients with AIDS varies. Sattler et al[198] evaluated lung biopsy specimens from 351 HIV-positive patients with presumed *P. jiroveci* pneumonia. Of the 67 patients who did not have PCP, 16 (24%) had findings of NSIP. Clinical symptoms, physical examination findings, and blood gas values were similar in patients with NSIP and patients with *P. jiroveci*. Patients with NSIP tended to present earlier in the course of their disease and had higher CD4+ lymphocyte counts (492 cells/mm^3 versus 57 cells/mm^3) than patients with *P. jiroveci* pneumonia. These authors concluded that NSIP may be the most common entity that mimics *P. jiroveci* pneumonia in AIDS patients. They also found that NSIP tended to improve during empiric therapy for PCP. Ognibene et al[199] evaluated 23 consecutive HIV-positive patients with no pulmonary symptoms, normal chest radiographs, no history of *P. jiroveci* pneumonia, and no prior treatment with anti-*Pneumocystis* prophylaxis. None of the patients had evidence of *P. jiroveci* or other infectious pathogens by stains of bronchoalveolar lavage fluid and histopathological examination of lung biopsy specimens. However, transbronchial lung biopsy specimens showed findings of NSIP in 11 of 23 (48%) patients. It would thus appear that NSIP can exactly mimic the clinical features of *P. jiroveci* pneumonia or be found by transbronchial lung biopsy in asymptomatic AIDS patients with normal chest radiographs.

Over half of symptomatic AIDS patients with biopsy-proven NSIP have a normal chest radiograph. Diffuse reticular opacities are noted in the remainder.[196] Radiographic findings vary in severity from minimal perihilar opacities to severe bilateral pulmonary consolidation, frequently associated with pleural effusion. Although the disease usually resolves without sequela, repeated episodes may cause permanent lung injury and may contribute to longterm pulmonary dysfunction in patients with AIDS.

Persistent generalized lymphadenopathy

Persistent generalized lymphadenopathy is a feature of early but otherwise asymptomatic HIV infection. It characteristically affects the peripheral lymph nodes and, though documented in the nasopharyngeal lymphoid tissue, rarely causes significant hilar or mediastinal lymph node enlargement.

Bronchogenic carcinoma

Bronchogenic carcinoma is increasingly reported in HIV-positive patients.[200–205] Many,[202,204,205] but not all[203] investigators have reported an increased incidence of lung cancer in AIDS patients, especially among women. However, whether the incidence of bronchogenic carcinoma in patients with HIV infection is truly increased or not continues to be debated.[205–207]

Patients with AIDS and lung cancer are typically smokers, with an average age at diagnosis of approximately 40 years. Lung carcinoma frequently occurs early in the course of disease, sometimes before seropositivity for HIV infection is known. Rapid progression of carcinoma is the rule and the prognosis is extremely poor, with an increased proportion of poorly differentiated carcinomas.[208] The lung cancers are predominantly found in the upper lobes[201,209] and have frequently spread to lymph nodes in the adjacent mediastinum or hilum.[208] Extensive pleural disease from adenocarcinoma was present in 35% of HIV-positive patients with lung carcinoma in one study.[201]

Imaging diagnosis of pulmonary complications of AIDS

There is considerable overlap in the radiologic manifestations of the various pulmonary complications of AIDS. Furthermore, the chest radiograph may be normal even when a pulmonary complication has developed. However, by carefully correlating clinical, laboratory, and radiographic findings with results of sputum analysis, bronchoalveolar lavage, or transbronchial biopsy results, a diagnosis can be made with confidence in most cases.[2,109] CT can be useful for either diagnosing or excluding pulmonary complications in symptomatic patients with normal or equivocal chest radiographs.[86,124,140] CT may also help to limit the differential diagnosis when the chest radiograph is abnormal.[2,109,210–213]

Tuberculosis, bacterial pneumonia, *P. jiroveci* pneumonia, Kaposi sarcoma, AIDS-related lymphoma, and septic emboli are the disorders most likely to be confidently diagnosed by chest radiography (Table 6.1) or CT (Box 6.1). The radiographic findings of other infectious or noninfectious complications are less specific and have extensive differential diagnoses. Several studies have

Table 6.1 Radiographic patterns in patients with AIDS

Cause	Focal consolidation	Interstitial/ nodules <5 mm	Nodules ≥5 mm	Cavity/cysts	Airways (CT)	Lymphadenopathy	Pleural effusions
Bacterial							
Bacterial pneumonia	++++	–	+	++	–	+	++
Bronchitis, bronchiolitis	–	++	+	–	+++	–	–
Mycobacterial							
Tuberculosis	++++	++	+++	++	++	+++	+++
MAC	+	++	++	++	+	++++	–
Fungal							
Histoplasmosis	++	++++	++	++	–	++	++
Cryptococcosis	+	+++	+++	++	–	+++	++
Aspergillosis	+++	+	++++	++++	++	+	–
Pneumocystis jiroveci	++	++++	+	+++	–	–	–
Viral	+	+++	++	+	++	+	+
Malignancies							
Kaposi sarcoma	++	+++	++++	–	+++	++	+++
Lymphoma	+++	+	+++	+	+	+++	+++
Lung cancer	++++	+	+++	+++	+++	+++	+++

+, uncommon; ++, moderately common; +++, common; ++++, typical
Adapted from Haramati LB, Jenny-Avital ER. Approach to the diagnosis of pulmonary disease in patients infected with the human immunodeficiency virus. J Thorac Imaging 1998;13:247–260.

investigated the diagnostic accuracy of chest radiography for specific AIDS-related pulmonary infections.[14,69,210] These studies show that findings of diffuse bilateral ground-glass, fine reticular, or airspace opacities are most likely due to *P. jiroveci* pneumonia; however, other infections including bacterial pneumonia can rarely cause this pattern. Conversely, segmental or lobar consolidation suggests bacterial pneumonia; however, a small percentage of cases of PCP can manifest in this way. Scattered, dependent acinar nodules, particularly when seen in association with pulmonary cavities and enlarged hilar or mediastinal lymph nodes, strongly suggest tuberculosis. It should be noted that the diagnostic accuracy of chest radiography is significantly diminished when more than one complication is present.[210]

Because these studies were limited to patients with single pulmonary complications and the observers were blinded to clinical and laboratory data, their results may not be directly applicable to everyday practice. This is certainly true for patients with more than one complication. Bearing these caveats in mind, Boiselle et al[69] showed in a series of 163 patients with a variety of pulmonary complications that the accuracy of a confident radiologic diagnosis was 84% for tuberculosis, 75% for *P. jiroveci* pneumonia, and 64% for bacterial pneumonia.

OTHER FORMS OF IMMUNOCOMPROMISE

Pulmonary infection in immunocompromised patients

The ability of an individual to combat infections can be impaired in a variety of ways (Table 6.2 on page 316) that include:

- **Neutropenia.** Neutrophils are an essential line of defense against many microorganisms. Deficiencies in neutrophil numbers weaken host defenses. Neutropenia may be a feature of the disease itself or, more commonly, a consequence of drug or radiation therapy. The incidence of pulmonary infection rises steeply as the absolute neutrophil count falls below 1000 cells/mm^3.
- **Reduced cell-mediated immunity.** T-lymphocyte-dependent immune responses are an important line of defense, particularly against obligate intracellular parasites and ordinarily nonpathogenic commensal organisms in the respiratory tract.
- **Reduced humoral immunity.** Impairment of B-lymphocyte function reduces the antibody response to infective agents, diminishing host resistance. A reduction in circulating antibodies is a feature of the various hypoglobulinemic states. Similarly, thymic aplasia, asplenia, or splenectomy can result in humoral immunodeficiency, leading to marked susceptibility to infection with encapsulated organisms such as *Streptococcus pneumoniae*.
- **Incompetence of cellular elements.** An enzymatic defect in the neutrophils of patients with chronic granulomatous disease renders them incapable of combating certain microorganisms. Because silica particles can impair pulmonary macrophage function, patients with silicosis may not mount an adequate response to microorganisms such as *M. tuberculosis* or fungi.[214,215]
- **Nonspecific reduction in host resistance.** Advanced age, alcoholism, diabetes mellitus, starvation or malnutrition, cancer, or other debilitating diseases can reduce an individual's ability to combat infection.

The immunocompromised patient with fever and new pulmonary opacities is a very common clinical problem. Before the differential diagnosis is discussed in more detail, a few generalizations are applicable[216–219]:

- Seventy-five percent of pulmonary complications in immunocompromised patients are due to infection. When the patient has severe neutropenia or when there are focal pulmonary lesions, the proportion increases to 90%. In the remaining few, complications are due to pulmonary drug reactions, pulmonary manifestations of the underlying disease, or unrelated processes such as edema or pulmonary emboli. In up to 30% of cases, more than one pulmonary complication is present.
- New diffuse pulmonary opacities on chest radiographs in this population are associated with an overall mortality approaching 50%. Establishing the exact nature of the complication improves the outcome by no more than 10–20%. Even at autopsy, the exact diagnosis is not established in 15–20% of cases.

The chest radiograph yields a specific diagnosis in a minority of cases. In most instances, all that can be expected is a reasonable differential diagnosis that must be correlated with clinical and laboratory findings. Boxes 6.2 to 6.4 outline conditions that should be considered when chest radiographs show segmental or lobar disease, nodular or masslike opacities, and diffuse lung disease, respectively.

Bacterial pneumonia

Bacteria are the most frequent cause of pneumonia in immunocompromised patients. In general terms, the clinical and radio-

---

Box 6.2 Lobar or segmental opacities* on chest radiographs

Infectious causes
Gram-negative bacilli
- *Klebsiella pneumoniae*
- *Serratia marcescens*
- *Escherichia coli*
- *Pseudomonas aeruginosa*
- *Legionella pneumophila*

Gram-positive bacilli
- *Streptococcus pneumoniae*
- *Staphylococcus aureus*
- *Proteus mirabilis*
- *Haemophilus influenzae*

Noninfectious causes
Pulmonary infarction
Lymphoproliferative disorders

*Solitary or multiple foci, with or without cavitation, with or without pleural fluid.

Box 6.3 Diffuse pulmonary opacities on chest radiographs

Infectious causes
Protozoal
- *Strongyloides stercoralis*

Mycobacteria
- *Mycobacterium tuberculosis*
- Atypical mycobacteria

Viruses
- Cytomegalovirus
- Varicella-zoster virus
- Herpes simplex virus
- Respiratory viruses*

Fungi
- *Aspergillus* species
- *Candida* species
- *Histoplasma capsulatum*
- *P. jiroveci*

Noninfectious causes
Nonspecific interstitial pneumonia
Drug reactions
Pulmonary hemorrhage
Radiation pneumonitis
Pulmonary edema
Lymphangitic spread of tumor
Leukemic infiltration

*Respiratory syncytial virus, adenovirus, influenza, and parainfluenza viruses.

Box 6.4 Nodular opacities with or without cavitation on chest radiographs

Infectious causes
Nocardia asteroides
Legionella micdadei
Aspergillus species
Cryptococcus neoformans
Mucor species

Noninfectious causes
Pulmonary infarction
Lymphoproliferative disorders

---

graphic features of pneumonia caused by organisms such as *Streptococcus pneumoniae*, *Staphylococcus aureus*, and *Pseudomonas aeruginosa* do not differ from those seen in the general population.[220] Patients with neutropenia may show a slight lag in the appearance of pulmonary consolidation, and in the group as a whole, pleural effusions and empyema are uncommon. On occasion, bacterial pneumonias become widely disseminated in the lungs of immunocompromised patients, something that is unusual in otherwise healthy individuals. Immunocompromised patients may be infected with bacteria almost never encountered in the general population such as *Rhodococcus equi*.

Patients receiving corticosteroid therapy and renal transplant recipients are particularly susceptible to *Legionella* organisms, including *L. pneumophila* and *L. micdadei* (Pittsburgh agent). *L. pneumophila* pneumonia is a rapidly progressive disease that begins with focal consolidation and may spread to involve both lungs diffusely (Fig. 6.51). Cavitation and pleural effusion are uncommon in the immunocompetent population, but are more common in immunocompromised patients.[23] *L. micdadei* pneumonia is particularly associated with renal dialysis patients. It has a fairly characteristic radiographic pattern[221] consisting of fairly well circumscribed nodular densities with a distinct tendency to cavitate (Fig. 6.52). The number of opacities is variable and the distribution may be widespread and random.

Tuberculosis and atypical mycobacterial infections, important pulmonary complications in AIDS patients, are uncommon in other immunocompromised patients. This presumably reflects the decline of tuberculosis in the general population. Reported cases likely represent reactivation of quiescent lesions; consequently, there is often a history of prior tuberculosis or a positive tuberculin skin test. Tuberculosis in non-AIDS immunocompromised patients is usually clinically and radiographically indistinguishable from postprimary tuberculosis.[222] On rare occasions, tuberculosis disseminates in a fulminant fashion, resulting in diffuse pulmonary disease (Fig. 6.53). The radiographic features of tuberculosis are more thoroughly discussed in Chapter 5.

Nocardia asteroides infection is fairly common in immunocompromised hosts, particularly in patients receiving corticosteroids and immunosuppressive agents (Fig. 6.54). The clinical presentation is subacute, and the radiographic abnormalities progress slowly. The radiographic features of *Nocardia asteroides* infection are discussed on page 228.

Fungal infection

Aspergillus fumigatus is a rare cause of pneumonia in the general population but is an important pathogen in immunocompromised patients, particularly those with lymphoma or leukemia.[223,224] *Aspergillus* infections are particularly problematic in patients with neutropenia or defects in neutrophil function such as chronic granulomatous disease. The pulmonary manifestations of aspergillosis form a broad spectrum of disease that ranges from allergic bronchopulmonary aspergillosis in hyperimmune hosts to mycetoma formation in preexisting lung cavities of otherwise normal patients (see p. 244) to invasive

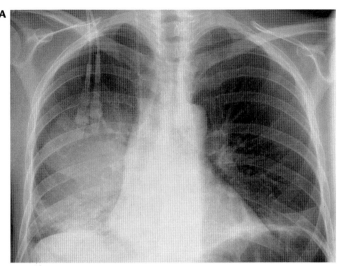

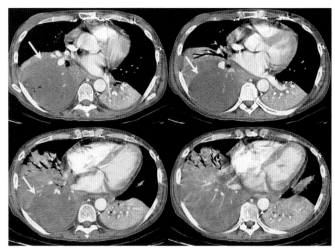

Fig. 6.51 *Legionella pneumophila* pneumonia in an immunocompromised patient. **A,** A frontal chest radiograph shows homogeneous right lower lobe consolidation. **B,** Contrast-enhanced CT shows a large round area (arrows) of non-enhancement in the right lower lobe consistent with necrosis.

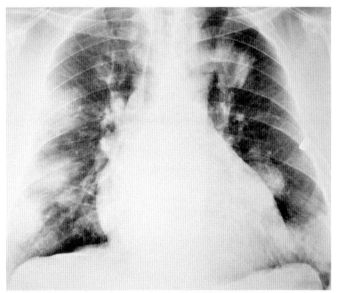

Fig. 6.52 *Legionella micdadei* pneumonia in a renal transplant recipient. A frontal chest radiograph shows multifocal rounded areas of consolidation.

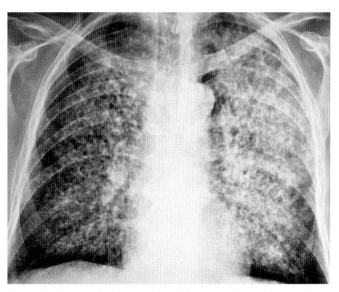

Fig. 6.53 Tuberculosis in a patient with acute leukemia. A frontal chest radiograph shows bilateral, confluent, coarse nodular opacities. A chest radiograph obtained 1 month earlier was normal.

aspergillosis in immunocompromised hosts.[225] Overlap between these entities occurs: "semiinvasive" or chronic necrotizing aspergillosis has been described in patients with mild degrees of immune dysfunction and underlying lung disease.[226] The following discussion is confined to the acute invasive forms of pulmonary aspergillosis that occur in severely immuno-compromised patients: airway-invasive and angioinvasive aspergillosis (Boxes 6.5 and 6.6).

Airway infection by *Aspergillus* in neutropenic patients causes a necrotizing tracheobronchitis that can result in either focal or diffuse bronchopneumonia or, on occasion, even lobar pneumonia.[227,228] The disease is centered on the airways with direct invasion of the airway wall and adjacent lung. The findings on chest radiography and CT vary depending on the stage, severity, and extent of disease. In early stages, these

examinations may be normal.[228,229] As disease progresses, either localized or diffuse heterogeneous or nodular opacities are seen on chest radiographs (Figs 6.55 and 6.56). CT usually shows airway-centered abnormalities consisting of bronchial wall thickening, peribronchial consolidation or ground-glass opacity, centrilobular nodules, and occasionally bronchiectasis (Fig. 6.56).[228] Sinus tracts in the airway walls have also been described in patients with airway-invasive aspergillosis. Progressive infection may result in homogeneous segmental or lobar consolidation. Focal nodular opacities representing circumscribed areas of consolidation or abscess formation can also occur.[228,230]

Angioinvasive aspergillosis, the most feared form of pul-monary aspergillosis, occurs in only the most severely immuno-compromised patients. Disease does not typically occur until the

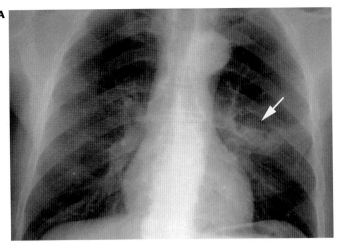

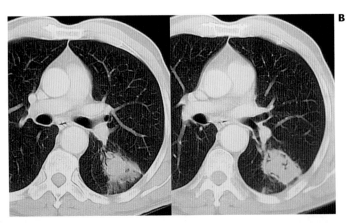

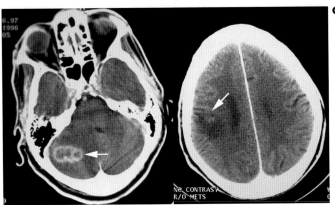

Fig. 6.54 *Nocardia asteroides* infection in a renal transplant recipient with headache and ataxia. **A,** A frontal chest radiograph shows a focal cavitary lesion (arrow) in the left lung, confirmed on CT (**B**). **C,** Contrast-enhanced cranial CT shows multiple ring-enhancing lesions (arrows) consistent with cerebral abscesses. Aspiration showed *N. asteroides* infection.

Box 6.5 Aspergillosis in immunocompromised patients

Infective agents
A. fumigatus (most common)
A. niger

Predisposing conditions
Severe, prolonged neutropenia
Hematologic malignancies
Bone marrow transplant recipients

Clinical types
Airway-invasive aspergillosis
Angioinvasive aspergillosis

Clinical manifestations
Cough, fever, chest pain, hemoptysis
Progressive respiratory failure
Mortality up to 70%

Box 6.6 Aspergillosis in immunocompromised patients – CT and radiographic findings

Airway-invasive aspergillosis: CT findings
Mucosal sinus tracts or fistulas in central airways
Diffuse bronchial wall thickening
Centrilobular nodules ("tree-in-bud")
Peribronchial ground-glass opacity or consolidation

Angioinvasive aspergillosis: radiographic findings
Initial: scattered poorly defined nodules or masses
Late: more confluent opacities, cavitation (air crescent sign)
Air crescent sign: late finding seen during neutrophil recovery, associated with good prognosis

Angioinvasive aspergillosis: CT findings
Scattered nodules or masses with rims of ground-glass opacity (CT halo sign)
Scattered or diffuse ground-glass opacities or consolidation

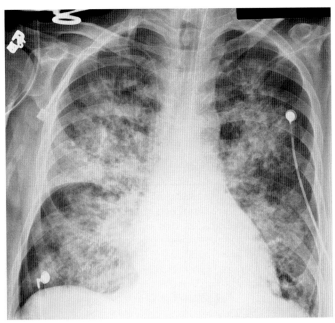

Fig. 6.55 Aspergillosis in a patient with chronic leukemia. A frontal chest radiograph shows bilateral, perihilar heterogeneous and nodular opacities. Note the focal peripheral right upper lobe opacity.

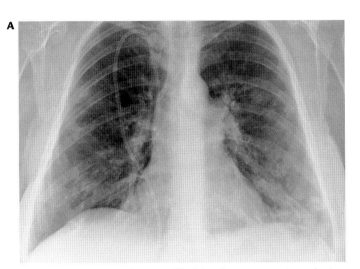

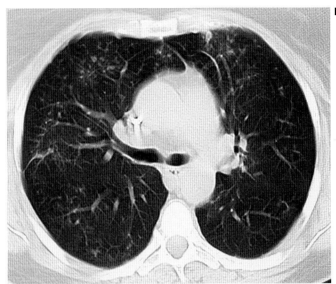

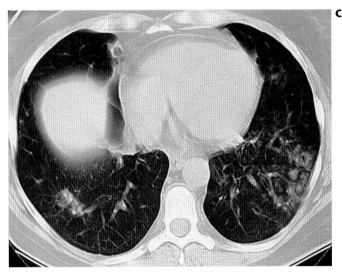

Fig. 6.56 Airway-invasive aspergillosis in a bone marrow transplant patient. **A**, A frontal chest radiograph shows heterogeneous lower lobe opacities. **B** and **C**, CT shows scattered centrilobular nodules, ground-glass opacities, and mild cylindrical bronchiectasis in the left lower lobe.

absolute neutrophil count is below 500 cells/mm³ for several weeks. This form of the disease is characterized by invasion of small and medium-sized blood vessel walls leading to *in situ* pulmonary infarction, hemorrhage, and systemic dissemination. The typical clinical history is that of a severely neutropenic patient with new onset fever, chest pain, and dyspnea. Initial chest radiographs are normal in up to one-third of cases.[229] CT can be very useful in this setting by demonstrating subtle opacities indicative of early infection – opacities not evident on the chest radiograph.[231–235] Eventually, however, chest radiographs will show one or more rounded areas of homogeneous opacification. The opacities are typically several centimeters in diameter, random in distribution, peripheral in location, and have poorly-defined margins (Figs 6.57 and 6.58).[236] These opacities are due to a peculiar form of pulmonary infarction that occurs in cases of angioinvasive fungal infection – the so-called "round" or "target" infarction.[237,238] This type of infarction is characterized by a round central region of coagulative necrosis, a rim of pulmonary hemorrhage, and a peripheral thrombosed pulmonary artery. Later, with neutrophil recovery, an inflammatory reaction is found in the rim as well. CT demonstrates well the rounded nature of the opacities and the rim of ground-glass opacity around the

lesions, resulting in the so-called "CT halo sign" (Figs 6.57 and 6.58). The "halo" is due to hemorrhage around the central lesion, is best seen with HRCT, and though a very consistent finding, is not specific for invasive aspergillosis.[239,240] In the clinical setting of severe neutropenia and fever, however, the CT halo sign is very suggestive of early angioinvasive aspergillosis.[233,241] On isolated occasions, an air bronchogram sign is seen within the opacity as well.

Over the course of several weeks, the rounded opacities tend to enlarge slowly and coalesce into larger homogeneous, sometimes wedge-shaped, opacities. Associated pulmonary hemorrhage can result in diffuse pulmonary opacification. Hilar or mediastinal lymphadenopathy is not a feature of the disease and pleural effusions are generally seen only if hemorrhagic infarction results in bleeding into the pleural space. Invasion of chest wall or mediastinal structures is described but is quite rare.[242,243] After several weeks, the lesions may begin to cavitate. The earliest finding of cavitation is the so-called "air crescent sign" in which a crescent of air develops along one margin of the lesion (Fig. 6.59).[244] The lucency then enlarges to form a true cavity with an intracavitary mass (Figs 6.59 to 6.61).[245] The mass is due to necrotic lung and is usually adherent to the wall of the

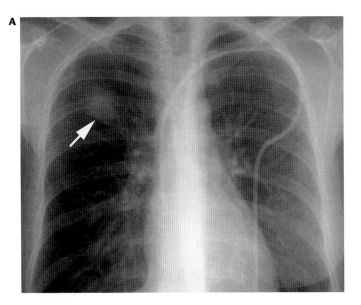

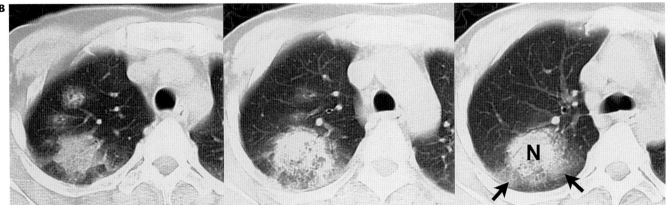

Fig. 6.57 Invasive aspergillosis in a febrile neutropenic patient. **A,** A frontal chest radiograph shows an ill-defined nodule (white arrow) in the right upper lobe. **B,** CT shows multiple right upper lobe nodules (N) with surrounding rims (black arrows) of ground-glass opacity (the CT halo sign).

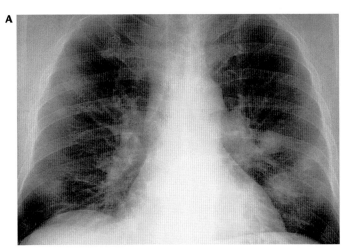

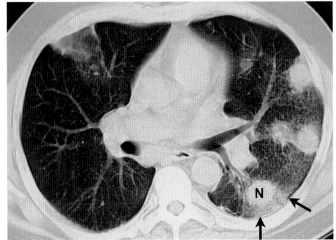

Fig. 6.58 Invasive aspergillosis in a febrile neutropenic patient. **A,** A frontal chest radiograph shows multiple, bilateral ill-defined nodules. **B,** CT shows multiple nodules (N) with rims (black arrows) of ground-glass opacity (the CT halo sign). (With permission from Connolly JE Jr, McAdams HP, Erasmus JJ, et al. Opportunistic fungal pneumonia. J Thorac Imaging 1999;14:51–62.)

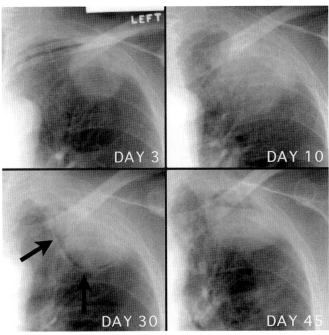

Fig. 6.59 Invasive aspergillosis in a febrile neutropenic patient. Sequential coned-down views of the left upper lobe show progression from rounded consolidation to cavitation. Note the air crescent sign (black arrows) medially.

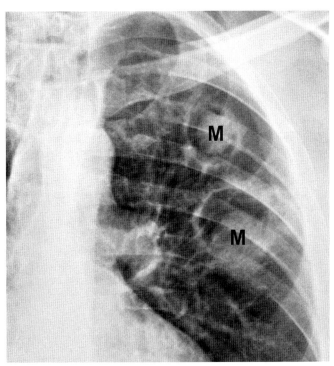

Fig. 6.61 Angioinvasive aspergillosis in a patient with leukemia. Coned-down view of a frontal chest radiograph shows two cavitary lesions in the left upper lobe with intracavitary masses (M) due to lung necrosis. Note the crescents of air around masses resulting in the characteristic "air crescent" sign. Note also that the masses are not always dependent in position.

cavity – it is not typically gravity-dependent like a mycetoma. Cavitation is usually a late, not an early, finding of infection and occurs as neutrophil counts recover and the host begins to mount an immune response against the fungus. Gefter et al[246] evaluated 25 patients with acute leukemia and invasive aspergillosis. Cavitation occurred in half the patients. Two-thirds of the patients who had cavitation survived their infection, as opposed to only 8% of the patients who did not have cavitation. Thus, cavitation is

a favorable prognostic sign in patients with invasive aspergillosis as it is indicative of a vigorous host response.

Magnetic resonance imaging has been used to investigate patients with angioinvasive aspergillosis.[247,248] The MRI characteristics depend on the age of the lesion. Early lesions, defined

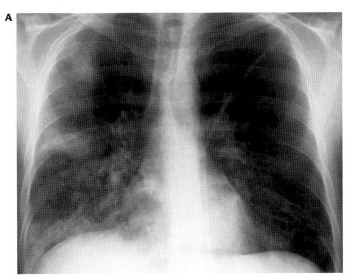

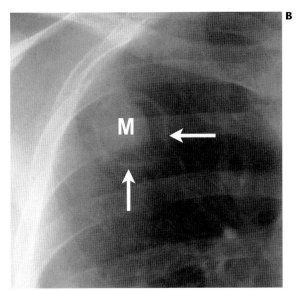

Fig. 6.60 Invasive aspergillosis in a febrile neutropenic patient. **A**, A frontal chest radiograph shows an ill-defined nodule in the right upper lobe and scattered lower lobe opacities. **B**, The coned-down view of a frontal radiograph obtained 2 weeks later shows cavitation in the right upper lobe nodule (arrows) with an intracavitary mass (M) resulting in the characteristic "air crescent" sign. (With permission from Connolly JE Jr, McAdams HP, Erasmus JJ, et al. Opportunistic fungal pneumonia. J Thorac Imaging 1999;14:51–62.)

by Blum et al[247] as being of less than 10 days duration, showed uniform low or intermediate signal intensity on T1-weighted images and high signal intensity on T2-weighted images. Early lesions uniformly enhanced with gadolinium-DTPA. There was no MRI correlate to the CT halo sign at this stage. With later evolution of the lesions, a targetlike appearance was seen on MRI consisting of a low signal intensity center and an isointense or hyperintense rim on T1- and T2-weighted images. Areas of aging hemorrhage resulted in foci of hyperintensity within the low signal intensity center.[248] Gadolinium enhancement of the rim became manifest at this stage, presumably indicating an inflammatory reaction at the margin. While these reports are interesting, the utility of MRI for diagnosis of angioinvasive aspergillosis in these critically ill patients is doubtful.

Disseminated aspergillosis may arise de novo or complicate the course of either pulmonary form. Pulmonary opacities in these patients range from a miliary to a more coarsely nodular pattern.[236,247] Hematogenous dissemination from a distant focus, as might be expected, results in diffusely distributed opacities in the lungs, whereas a heavy airway inoculum may give a more central, unevenly distributed pattern of bronchopneumonia.

Candida albicans species may cause pneumonia alone, but more commonly do so in association with other fungal pathogens, particularly *Aspergillus*.[224] A significant proportion of patients with *C. albicans* pneumonia have leukemia or lymphoma, often in the later stages of treatment.[249] The majority of patients have widespread systemic dissemination of the organism.[250] *Candida* pneumonia without systemic involvement is rare.[251] Diagnosis of *C. albicans* pneumonia is difficult, partly because pneumonia caused by other opportunistic organisms may also be present and partly because the presence of superficial colonization by *Candida* species may be discounted clinically. Typically the patient with disseminated candidiasis has severe and prolonged neutropenia, persistent fever despite antibacterial therapy, hepatomegaly, obvious colonies of *C. albicans* on the mucous membranes, and diffuse pulmonary opacities on chest radiographs. Buff et al[249] analyzed chest radiographic findings of 20 histopathologically proven cases of "pure" pulmonary candidiasis. Most cases were identified at autopsy, and the chest radiographs, obtained within 48 hours of death, presumably reflected advanced disease. Chest radiographs in nearly half the patients showed diffuse, bilateral, nonsegmental scattered heterogeneous opacities. The remainder showed unilateral or bilateral lobar or segmental consolidation. Cavitation, adenopathy, masslike opacities, or diffuse miliary nodules were not observed. In contrast, Pagani and Libshitz[252] described a pattern of diffuse miliary nodules in cases of pulmonary candidiasis (Fig. 6.62). It is possible that this pattern represents an earlier manifestation of pulmonary candidiasis. All the patients in the series of Buff et al[249] died of disseminated candidiasis. Dubois et al[253] failed to find any specific radiographic pattern in patients with pulmonary candidiasis, partly because of the high frequency of other pulmonary infections, edema, and hemorrhage. These authors stressed the need for early institution of antifungal therapy based primarily on clinical grounds.

Mucormycosis (also known as zygomycosis) is the third most common opportunistic fungal infection of the lungs (Boxes 6.7 and 6.8). The infective agents belong to the class Zygomycetes, order Mucorales, and include fungi of the genera *Rhizopus, Mucor, Absidia,* and *Cunninghamella*.[224] The most striking histopathologic feature of mucormycosis is vascular invasion resulting in infarction.[254,255] The diagnosis depends on identifying the organism by culture or by more directly showing histologic

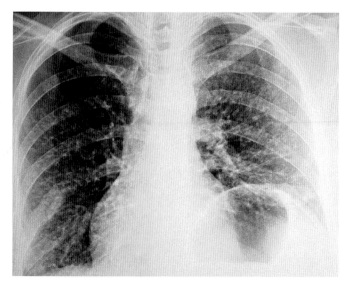

Fig. 6.62 Disseminated pulmonary candidiasis in a man with immunoblastic lymphoma. A frontal chest radiograph shows bilateral small to medium-sized nodules and an elevated left hemidiaphragm.

Box 6.7 Mucormycosis (zygomycosis) in immunocompromised patients

Infective agents
Fungi of class Zygomycetes, order Mucorales
Genera *Rhizopus, Mucor, Mortierella, Absidia, Basidiobolus, Cunninghamella*

Predisposing conditions
Diabetes mellitus, especially with ketoacidosis
Hematologic malignancies
Solid organ transplant recipients
Severe burns
Deferoxamine therapy

Clinical types
Rhinocerebral (most common)
Pulmonary
Abdominopelvic
Cutaneous (burn patients)
Disseminated

Clinical manifestations
Occasionally asymptomatic in diabetic patients
Cough, fever, chest pain, hemoptysis
Progressive respiratory failure
Mortality without aggressive early treatment approaches 80%

---

evidence of fungal invasion on biopsy. The fungal hyphae are broad, nonseptate, and branch at right angles. Furthermore, they can be readily seen on sections stained with hematoxylin and eosin. Diagnosis is critical because of the very high mortality in the absence of specific treatment with amphotericin B. Three particular groups of patients are particularly susceptible to mucormycosis: diabetics, patients undergoing treatment for hematologic malignancies, and recipients of solid organ trans-

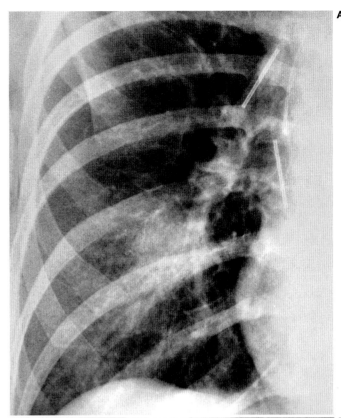

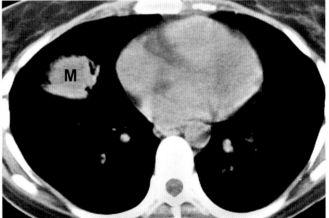

Box 6.8 Mucormycosis (zygomycosis) in immunocompromised patients – CT and radiographic findings

Radiographic findings
Lobar or segmental consolidation, either unifocal or multifocal
Solitary or multiple nodules
Cavitation is frequent
Air crescent sign occurs
Pleural effusions
Rapid progression

CT findings
As above with additional features in some cases:
Air bronchograms
Central low attenuation indicating necrosis
Early detection of air crescent sign and cavitation
Halo sign around nodules
Endobronchial masses
Hilar and mediastinal adenopathy
Extrapulmonary invasion
Pulmonary artery pseudoaneurysms

plants. Ketoacidosis is the critical predisposing factor in diabetic patients. Deferoxamine therapy may also be associated with mucormycosis (see p. 509).

There are five clinical types of mucormycosis: rhinocerebral, pulmonary, abdominopelvic, cutaneous (seen primarily in burn patients), and disseminated. The pulmonary form is the second most common form after rhinocerebral mucormycosis. The imaging findings of pulmonary mucormycosis (Figs 6.63 to 6.65) are diverse. The disease most commonly manifests with either focal or multifocal pulmonary opacities that vary in shape from round to segmental or lobar.[256,257] Pulmonary mucormycosis tends to be localized in diabetic patients and has a relatively good prognosis. Conversely, mucormycosis in patients with hematologic malignancies tends to be multifocal or diffuse in distribution and carries a very poor prognosis.[258] The pulmonary opacities frequently cavitate. CT can show central low attenuation foreshadowing the development of cavitation.[258,259] Nodular opacities may show a halo sign on CT akin to that seen with invasive aspergillosis.[259] An air crescent sign may be seen in the initial stages of cavitation.[258] Intracavitary masses are common and are due to sloughed necrotic lung (Fig. 6.65). On occasion, the infection is so overwhelming as to cause pulmonary gangrene in which a large portion of lung sloughs into a thin walled cavity.[260] Other CT features include endobronchial masses, hilar or mediastinal adenopathy, and pleural effusions. An unusual complication of mucormycosis is the development of multiple pulmonary artery pseudoaneurysms.[258,259,261] Extrapulmonary spread of disease to the spine and mediastinum is described but appears to be uncommon. Prompt diagnosis, usually with biopsy proof of disease, is essential because aggressive treatment with amphotericin B and surgical excision of necrotic lung can reduce the mortality rate from around 80% to as low as 25%.[258]

Cryptococcus neoformans pneumonia occurs in immunocompromised patients (Fig. 6.66), although the pneumonia is

Fig. 6.63 Mucormycosis in a patient with lymphoma. **A,** A coned-down view from a frontal chest radiograph shows an ill-defined mass in the right middle lobe. **B,** CT shows that the mass (M) is of homogeneous attenuation.

often overshadowed by cryptococcal meningitis. Cryptococcal pulmonary infection is discussed in detail on pages 237 and 289.

Widespread dissemination of blastomycosis, coccidioidomycosis, and histoplasmosis occurs in immunocompromised patients and has serious consequences (Fig. 6.67). However, given the frequency of these diseases in certain geographic areas it is surprising that these fungi are so rarely implicated as opportunistic infective agents. Specific diagnostic features are lacking, and the clinical thrust is likely to be toward excluding infection with the more common opportunistic fungi.

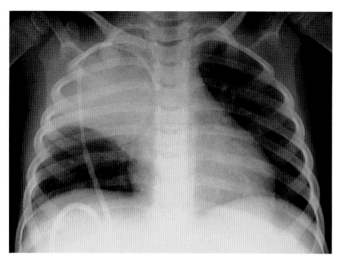

Fig. 6.64 Mucormycosis in a child with leukemia. A frontal chest radiograph shows homogeneous consolidation in the right upper lobe. (With permission from McAdams HP, Rosado de Christenson M, Strollo DC, et al. Pulmonary mucormycosis: radiologic findings in 32 cases. AJR Am J Roentgenol 1997;168:1541–1548.)

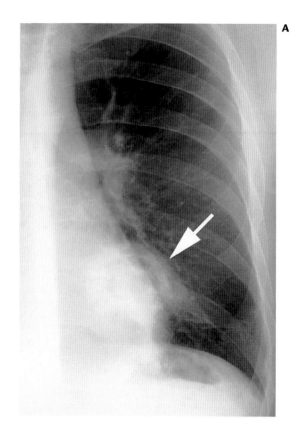

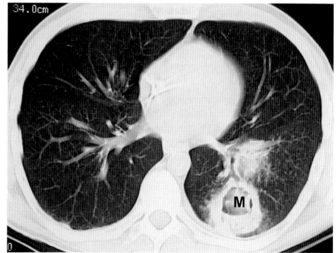

Fig. 6.65 Mucormycosis in a renal transplant recipient. **A**, The coned-down view from a frontal chest radiograph shows a masslike opacity (arrow) in the left lower lobe. **B**, CT shows cavitation and an intracavitary mass (M).

Viral infection

Cytomegalovirus (CMV) is the most common viral pathogen in immunocompromised patients. Infection results from defects in cell-mediated immunity and most frequently occurs in patients with AIDS or hematologic malignancies or in organ transplant recipients.[262] Diagnosis is complicated by the fact that CMV infection is very common in the general population and many immunosuppressed patients are latent carriers of the virus.[143] Distinction of the carrier state from active infection is difficult. This diagnostic difficulty is further compounded by the fact that the clinical manifestations of infection are quite variable, ranging from completely asymptomatic to catastrophic infection. Furthermore, clinical symptoms and radiologic features of infection are nonspecific and are often indistinguishable from other complications. Cytomegalovirus pneumonia may also coexist with or even predispose to other pneumonias, especially *P. jiroveci* pneumonia.[263] Rapid culture (shell-vial technique) of virus from respiratory secretions or biopsy material is considered suggestive of infection, as are positive CMV serologies.[143] However, demonstration of characteristic CMV cellular inclusion bodies is considered more definitive for diagnosis of active infection.[262] Even then a response to antiviral therapy is often required for full confirmation. Quantification of viral load by pp65 antigenemia and quantitative polymerase chain reaction (PCR) techniques is also helpful for deciding when to treat and to identify high risk patients for prophylactic therapy.[143]

The radiographic findings of CMV pneumonia are varied and overlap those of other opportunistic infections.[264] On chest radiographs, CMV pneumonia most commonly manifests with bibasilar heterogeneous opacities, often with a slightly nodular character (Fig. 6.68). Although the opacities are usually bilateral, focal opacities mimicking bacterial pneumonia are occasionally seen,[265] as are pleural effusions. Less common manifestations include diffuse fine (miliary) nodular opacities. Spontaneous pneumothorax and pneumomediastinum can occur in cases of advanced CMV pneumonia.[264] The chest radiograph may also be normal despite biopsy-proven infection. The CT manifestations of CMV pneumonia are equally varied and include scattered or diffuse ground-glass opacities, nodules up to 5 mm in size, masses, consolidation, and reticular opacities.[140,266,267] Multiple small nodules and ground-glass opacities are the most suggestive findings on CT (Fig. 6.68).[266] Pleural fluid is common on CT.[267] CT in affected patients usually shows more extensive abnormalities than are seen radiographically. CT may also be normal in patients with biopsy-proven disease.[266]

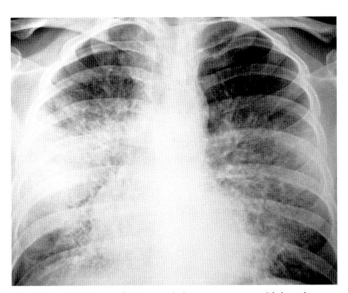

Fig. 6.66 Cryptococcal pneumonia in a young man with lymphoma. A frontal chest radiograph shows homogeneous right lung consolidation and heterogeneous perihilar opacities in the left lung.

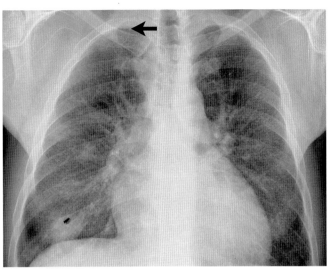

Fig. 6.67 Disseminated histoplasmosis in a renal transplant recipient. A frontal chest radiograph shows diffuse small nodular opacities (miliary pattern). Note the malpositioned right central catheter (arrow).

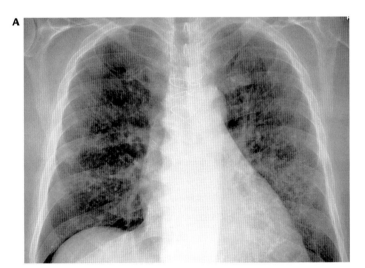

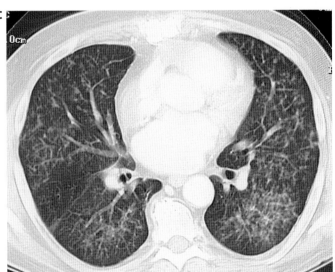

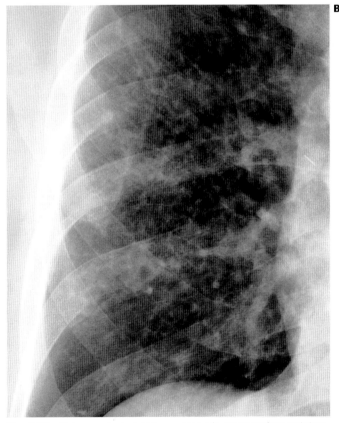

Fig. 6.68 Cytomegalovirus pneumonia in a heart transplant recipient. Frontal (**A**) and coned-down (**B**) chest radiographs show diffuse small nodular and ground-glass opacities. **C**, CT (lung window) shows peribronchovascular nodules and ground-glass opacities.

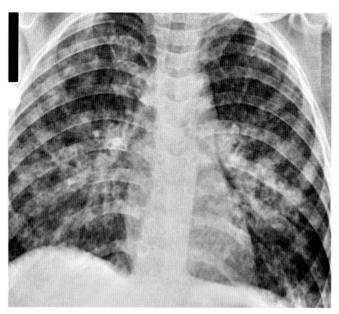

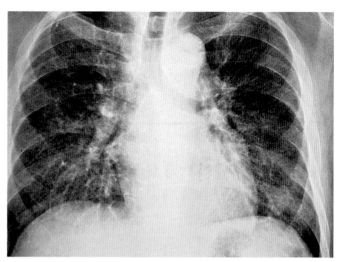

Fig. 6.70 *Pneumocystis jiroveci* pneumonia in a patient with leukemia. A frontal chest radiograph shows bilateral fine reticular opacities.

Fig. 6.69 Varicella pneumonia in a man with acute myelocytic leukemia. A frontal chest radiograph shows bilateral coarse nodular opacities that are confluent in the perihilar regions.

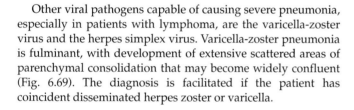

Other viral pathogens capable of causing severe pneumonia, especially in patients with lymphoma, are the varicella-zoster virus and the herpes simplex virus. Varicella-zoster pneumonia is fulminant, with development of extensive scattered areas of parenchymal consolidation that may become widely confluent (Fig. 6.69). The diagnosis is facilitated if the patient has coincident disseminated herpes zoster or varicella.

Pneumocystis jiroveci infection

As mentioned earlier, *P. Jiroveci* is the new name for the organism previously known as *P. carinii*. It has also been variably classified as a parasite and as a fungus, although recent evidence argues for a fungal origin. And, as previously discussed *P. jiroveci* is an important opportunistic agent in AIDS patients. However, *P. jiroveci* is also an important pathogen in other groups of immunocompromised patients, including malnourished infants, children with primary immune deficiencies, organ transplant recipients, and patients being treated for inflammatory or collagen–vascular disorders, hematologic malignancies, or brain neoplasms.[268–273] An important risk factor in many of these patients is prolonged, high dose corticosteroid therapy. Yale et al,[274] in a study of 116 cases of PCP, found 37 patients whose only cause of immune compromise was corticosteroid therapy for a variety of inflammatory conditions, including sarcoidosis and Wegener granulomatosis. The median dose of steroids in these patients was 40 mg per day. Nevertheless, 25% of the patients were on half these doses for 8 weeks or less before diagnosis. Brain tumor patients receiving high dose dexamethasone and concomitant chemotherapy are at particular risk for developing *P. jiroveci* pneumonia.[269,271,273] Risk factors include duration of therapy greater than 5 weeks and lymphopenia.[269,271,273] Some authors have reported a particular propensity for pneumonia

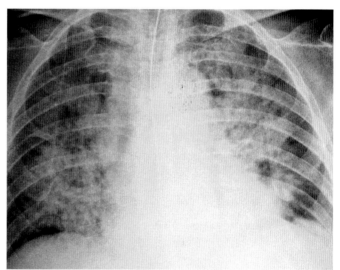

Fig. 6.71 *Pneumocystis jiroveci* pneumonia in a patient with lymphoma. A frontal chest radiograph shows diffuse consolidation.

to occur during steroid taper. Patients with endogenous corticosteroid production (Cushing syndrome) are also at risk for PCP.[272]

Diagnosis of *P. jiroveci* pneumonia can be difficult because the entity may not be considered in non-AIDS patients. Also, many affected patients have conditions such as sarcoidosis or Wegener granulomatosis, diseases whose radiographic manifestations could mask the appearance of PCP. The radiologic findings of *P. jiroveci* pneumonia in the non-AIDS patient are similar to those seen in AIDS patients (Figs 6.70 and 6.71), as discussed on page 284. However, PCP in this population can be more fulminant than is typically seen in AIDS patients, perhaps because the diagnosis is not suspected until later in the course

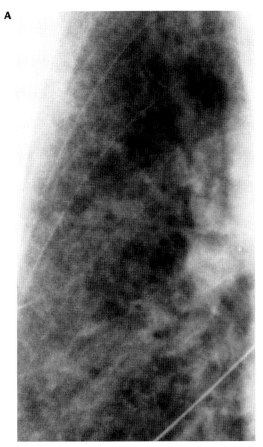

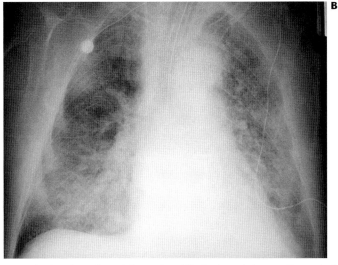

Fig. 6.72 *Strongyloides stercoralis* superinfection in an immunocompromised patient. Coned-down view (**A**) of a frontal chest radiograph of the shows diffuse small nodules. **B**, A radiograph obtained 1 week later shows progression to bilateral diffuse opacification.

of the disease. Mortality up to 50% has been reported for PCP in the non-AIDS population.[268] Prompt diagnosis therefore requires knowledge of the important risk factors for PCP in the non-AIDS patient and a high index of suspicion. The diagnosis should be strongly suspected in patients treated with high dose corticosteroids who develop dry cough, dyspnea, and hypoxemia as well as new bilateral opacities on chest radiographs.

Protozoal infection

Strongyloides stercoralis is a common intestinal parasite in many parts of the world. Infection confined to the intestinal tract may be asymptomatic or cause nonspecific complaints such as diarrhea, weight loss, or abdominal pain. Severe compromise of the immune system may lead to massive proliferation of the organism in the gastrointestinal tract. The filariform larva then penetrate the colonic wall or the perianal skin and migrate into the lungs. An overwhelming burden of larvae may result in systemic dissemination, for example, to the central nervous system. The chest radiograph in patients with disseminated strongyloidiasis may be normal or show widespread pulmonary opacities (Fig. 6.72).[275–278] Eosinophilia, a feature of helminthic infections, is often present. The organisms may be detected in sputum, small bowel aspirates, or stool.[279] There may be an accompanying gram-negative bacteremia, and this, together with the patient's intestinal symptoms, may provide a clue to the diagnosis.

Radiologic evaluation and differential diagnosis of pulmonary opacities in immunocompromised patients

Fever and new pulmonary opacities are commonly encountered problems in immunocompromised patients. Elucidation of their cause requires consideration of the following: (1) cause of immune impairment (see Table 6.2); (2) results of previous tuberculin testing; (3) whether the infection was acquired in or out of hospital; (4) whether there is any known potential source of infection; and (5) results of blood or sputum cultures and serologic testing. In an autopsy study of patients with leukemia, Winer-Muram et al[219] found that chest radiography was valuable for detecting pulmonary abnormalities but that its ability to discriminate between causes of those abnormalities was poor, with the exception of adult respiratory distress syndrome (ARDS). However, most of their 45 patients were critically ill with more than one infectious or noninfectious complication; only 7 patients had a single complication (either ARDS or pulmonary hemorrhage). In a less critically ill group of non-AIDS patients with a wide range of causes of immune compromise, Logan et al[217] found that a correct diagnosis was made on the basis of the chest radiograph in 34% of cases. Winer-Muram et al,[218] in a later paper involving less critically ill patients with hematologic malignancies, had better results with chest radiography, particularly with fungal pneumonia and cryptogenic organizing pneumonia.

Table 6.2 Impairment of human immunity to infection

Impaired cell	Nature of immunocompromise	Causes of immunocompromise	Common infecting organisms
Granulocyte	Altered inflammatory response	Acute and chronic myelocytic leukemia Steroids Chemotherapeutic agents Irradiation Chronic granulomatous disease	**Bacteria** *Escherichia coli* *Staphylococcus aureus* *Serratia marcescens* *Pseudomonas aeruginosa* *Klebsiella pneumoniae* *Enterobacter* species *Proteus* species *Legionella pneumophila* *Nocardia asteroides* **Fungi** *Aspergillus* species *Mucor* species
T lymphocyte	Reduced cell-mediated immunity	Lymphoma Acquired immune deficiency syndrome Steroids Chemotherapeutic agents Irradiation Renal insufficiency Solid organ transplant	**Bacteria** *Legionella micdadei* *Salmonella* species *N. asteroides* *Mycobacterium tuberculosis* **Viruses** Cytomegalovirus Varicella-zoster virus Herpes simplex virus Respiratory syncytial virus **Fungi** *Aspergillus* species *Cryptococcus neoformans* *Histoplasma capsulatum* *Coccidioides immitis* *Pneumocystis jiroveci* **Parasites** *Toxoplasma gondii* Helminths *Strongyloides stercoralis*
B lymphocyte	Reduced antibody formation	Lymphoma Acute and chronic lymphocytic leukemia Multiple myeloma Hypogammaglobulinemia Steroids Chemotherapeutic agents	**Bacteria** *E. coli* *P. aeruginosa* *K. pneumonia* *Streptococcus pneumoniae* *Haemophilus influenzae* **Viruses** Cytomegalovirus Respiratory syncytial virus **Fungi** *P. jiroveci*
Macrophage	Impaired granulomatous response	Silica	**Bacteria** *M. tuberculosis* **Fungi** *Blastomyces dermatitidis* *H. capsulatum*

CT may play an important role in the evaluation of persistently febrile immunosuppressed patients. The two best-studied populations in this regard are patients with AIDS and severely neutropenic patients. As previously noted, CT, particularly HRCT, can be useful in AIDS patients with symptoms of pneumonia and a normal or equivocal chest radiograph. In this setting, CT can be useful for either diagnosing or excluding pulmonary complications such as *P. jiroveci* pneumonia.[82,86,89,124,140]

In the febrile patient with neutropenia, CT may be useful to show findings of pneumonia when the chest radiograph is normal or equivocal[280] and to better characterize the nature of radiographically evident abnormalities.[281] Heussel et al[282] prospectively studied 87 patients with febrile neutropenia for

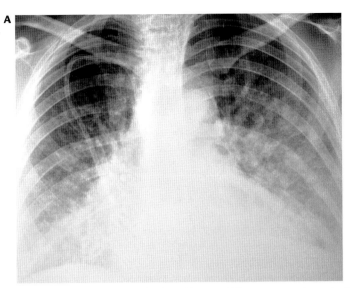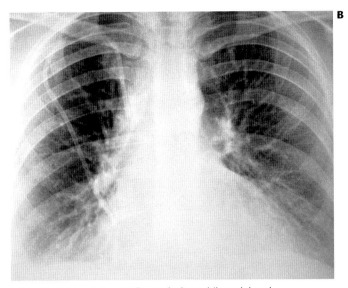

Fig. 6.73 Transfusion reaction in a 40-year-old bone marrow transplant recipient. **A**, A frontal chest radiograph shows bilateral, basal heterogeneous opacities consistent with edema. **B**, A radiograph obtained 12 hours later after treatment with corticosteroids shows near complete resolution of edema.

more than 2 days despite empiric antibiotics. Of the patients with a normal chest radiograph, almost half had findings suggestive of pneumonia on HRCT. In a separate study, the same authors reported that CT showed findings of pneumonia in 60% of 112 persistently febrile neutropenic patients with normal chest radiographs.[283] In both studies, CT showed findings of pneumonia approximately 5 days earlier than did chest radiographs, leading the authors to conclude that all febrile neutropenic patients with normal chest radiographs should undergo CT. Barloon et al[284] evaluated 33 febrile neutropenic patients with HRCT. Chest radiographs in one-third were normal and in the remainder were interpreted as "nonspecific". In this study, CT findings resulted in a change in clinical management in one-third of patients, whereas no additional information was provided in 45%. Gulati et al[285] assessed the utility of HRCT in 21 consecutive renal transplant recipients with suspected pulmonary infection. Compared to chest radiography, HRCT revealed additional findings suggestive of the correct diagnosis in 11 (50%) patients. Mori et al[286] found that CT was helpful for predicting the nature of pulmonary complications in febrile bone marrow transplant (BMT) recipients. When CT showed nodular opacities, pulmonary fungal infection (usually aspergillosis) was the cause. When the CT was negative, bacteremia or nonpulmonary fungal infection was usually the cause. Janzen and co-workers,[287] however, found that CT was no more sensitive than chest radiography in non-AIDS immunocompromised patients with acute pulmonary complications. They did find, however, that CT was distinctly better for predicting the cause of those abnormalities.

The morbidity and mortality of *Aspergillus* infection in neutropenic patients has led several authors to advocate the use of CT for early diagnosis. Kami et al[288] showed that CT was better than either the latex agglutination (LA) test or plasma (1,3)-β-D-glucan (BDG) levels for early diagnosis of aspergillosis in BMT recipients. In that series, CT showed abnormalities at least a week before these tests became positive. In two separate studies, Caillot et al[231,289] reported that the systemic use of CT allowed very early recognition of *Aspergillus* infection in at-risk

patients. In one of the studies, mean time to diagnosis was reduced from 7 to 2 days.[289] They also reported that earlier diagnosis and aggressive management could improve outcome.[231,289]

Thus, it would seem that CT can be useful in patients with febrile neutropenia and normal chest radiographs. In this setting, a normal CT suggests a nonpulmonary complication. An abnormal CT suggests a pulmonary complication, may suggest the nature of that complication, and may direct further invasive testing such as bronchoalveolar lavage or transbronchial biopsy. The role of CT in patients with definitely abnormal radiographs is less clear. Whether or not this approach improves patient outcome, however, is not yet known.

It should also be remembered that a host of noninfectious complications can cause pulmonary problems in immuno-compromised patients. These include, but are not limited to, neoplastic involvement of the lung (see Ch. 13), drug or radiation-induced toxicity (see Ch. 9), transfusion reactions, pulmonary edema, and pulmonary hemorrhage. Transfusion reactions are usually acute and the temporal relationship to the transfusion of blood or blood products is clear. The reaction may simply be one of volume overload and pulmonary edema. More capricious are the agglutinin reactions resulting from an excess of antibodies in the donor serum directed against the recipient's cells, particularly granulocytes. The result is the abrupt onset of fever, chills, tachypnea, and tachycardia coincident with the development of varying patterns of pulmonary edema (Fig. 6.73). The edema pattern may persist for 24–48 hours, and a response to corticosteroid therapy may occur. Leukemia may be associated with pulmonary hemorrhage. The clinical features may clearly indicate the bleeding tendency, and the abrupt appearance of scattered homogeneous opacities with hemoptysis and a fall in the hematocrit may allow confident diagnosis. The incidence of pulmonary hemorrhage in leukemia is difficult to ascertain, particularly because the coagulopathy may preclude biopsy. Pulmonary hemorrhage varying from microscopic to massive is seen in some three-quarters of leukemic patients at autopsy.[290] Pulmonary hemorrhage may be associated not only with a bleeding tendency, but also with infection or diffuse alveolar damage.[290,291] Tenholder and Hooper[292] suggest that the incidence of pulmonary hemorrhage as a sole cause of pulmonary opacities in leukemic patients may be as high as 40%. This seems a high figure, but it does serve to emphasize that pulmonary hemorrhage is probably under-diagnosed.

Nonspecific interstitial pneumonia and organizing pneumonia

Exhaustive clinical investigation may fail to establish the etiology of pulmonary opacities in immunocompromised patients. Lung biopsy, either by video-assisted thoracoscopy or by fiberoptic bronchoscopy, may be required in the most problematic cases. In a significant number of patients, however, histopathological examination of affected lung only shows findings of diffuse alveolar damage, nonspecific interstitial pneumonia (NSIP), or organizing pneumonia (OP); etiological agents cannot be identified. Nonspecific interstitial pneumonia (NSIP) is found in some 30–45% of biopsies in this clinical setting.[293–295] It is likely that lung injury in these patients is multifactorial and may be a manifestation of undiagnosed infection, pulmonary drug toxicity, radiation therapy, sepsis, etc. Organizing pneumonia (OP) is probably less commonly encountered in this setting than NSIP but responds well to corticosteroids and has a more favorable prognosis. The radiographic and CT findings of organizing pneumonia are discussed in detail on page 552. Because the imaging findings of OP are quite similar to those of other pulmonary complications in immunocompromised patients, the diagnosis is typically made at biopsy.[296–299] Organizing pneumonia should be distinguished from obliterative bronchiolitis, a distinct condition that results in irreversible airway occlusion in bone marrow and lung transplant recipients. Transplant-related obliterative bronchiolitis has a very poor prognosis (see below).[300]

Bone marrow transplantation

Many thousands of bone marrow transplants (BMT) are performed annually for a diverse range of conditions (Box 6.9).[301] Bone marrow transplant recipients are in a much more precarious position than are recipients of solid organ transplants. Pulmonary complications are seen in 40–60% of BMT recipients

---

Box 6.10 Bone marrow transplantation: pulmonary complications

Noninfectious complications
Acute graft versus host disease
Chronic graft versus host disease
Interstitial pneumonia
Pulmonary edema
Pulmonary hemorrhage
Acute tracheobronchitis
Pulmonary venoocclusive disease

Infectious complications
Viral, especially cytomegalovirus
Bacterial
Fungal, especially *Aspergillus* species
Pneumocystis jiroveci

---

and many of the complications (Box 6.10) have significant mortality.[302,303]

Bone marrow transplantation involves intravenous infusion of hematopoietic elements into a patient whose bone marrow has been ablated by high dose chemotherapy and total body irradiation (the conditioning regimen). The patient may receive radiation to the entire lungs and the chemotherapeutic doses used are formidable, sometimes 10 times greater than used for other malignancies. The conditioning regimen employed is therefore a major factor contributing to pulmonary complications. Pneumonitis in the first 100 days following bone marrow transplantation may be induced by drugs or radiation, as may be oropharyngeal ulceration and tracheobronchitis.

The transplanted marrow used may be the patient's own marrow harvested before conditioning (autologous transplant), marrow harvested from an HLA-matched donor (allogeneic transplant), or stem cells harvested from peripheral blood (stem cell transplant). Autologous transplant recipients have a much lower incidence of cytomegalovirus and fungal infections and idiopathic pneumonia syndrome. Furthermore, they are not subject to graft versus host disease and obliterative bronchiolitis is rare.[304] More recently, techniques of stem cell transfusion (cord blood, peripheral stem cells) have been developed whose complications are less severe than those of traditional allogeneic transplants. Furthermore, "mini" transplant techniques that use more moderate conditioning regimens combined with post-transplant immunosuppression have been developed. Complications of these transplants are expected to be less severe than those of traditional allogeneic transplants.

A 2–3 week period of profound bone marrow dysfunction before the graft "takes" (engraftment) is common to most marrow transplant procedures. Red blood cells and platelets can be supplied by transfusion, but the consequent neutropenia renders the patient susceptible to bacterial and fungal infection during this period. Neutrophil production usually begins to accelerate after approximately 2 weeks and the period of severe neutropenia usually lasts only approximately 4 weeks. Neutropenia is less severe and less prolonged in patients receiving autologous transplants. Hence, their risk for opportunistic infection in the first month is reduced compared to patients receiving stem cell or conventional allogeneic transplants. However, neutropenia is only a part of the immune deficit in these patients. Lymphocytes, for example, are the most radiosensitive cellular element in the

---

Box 6.9 Bone marrow transplantation: indications

Acute leukemia
Chronic myelogenous leukemia
Chronic lymphatic leukemia in younger patients
Disease – Hodgkin and non-Hodgkin
Multiple myeloma
Aplastic anemia
Hemoglobinopathies – sickle cell disease, thalassemia
Myelodysplastic syndrome
Immunodeficiency disorders
Solid tumors, e.g. breast, testicular cancers, neuroblastoma
Miscellaneous genetic disorders, e.g. Gaucher disease,
    osteopetrosis

body and may also be depleted. After the first month, there is a continuous recovery of immune function that is usually complete at about 1 year.

Complications are customarily divided into those occurring in the first month (neutropenic phase), those occurring between the first 30–100 days after the transplant (early phase) and those occurring thereafter (later phase). The advantage of this temporal division is that certain complications, although their clinical and radiologic manifestations may be similar, tend to occur during specific time periods after transplantation. The temporal relationships between bone marrow transplantation and pulmonary complications are illustrated in Table 6.3.

Complications in the first month

Patients are usually profoundly neutropenic and immuno-suppressed in the first month after stem cell or conventional allogeneic BMT. The complications that occur in this period may be either infectious or noninfectious in origin. The most common infections are caused by bacterial, *Aspergillus*, or *Candida* species. Common noninfectious complications include pulmonary edema, hemorrhage, and drug toxicity.[305] As noted above, patients treated with autologous transplants are not as profoundly neutropenic, nor as heavily immunosuppressed, and are therefore less

susceptible to opportunistic infection during this period. They are, however, at risk for many of the same noninfectious complications as allogeneic transplant recipients. In fact, complications in autologous recipients during this period are often noninfectious in nature.[306]

Bacterial sepsis occurs in up to 50% of BMT recipients, particularly in the first 2 weeks before marrow engraftment takes place. Gram-negative organisms predominate, presumably due to seeding from the gastrointestinal tract. Gram-positive bacteremia is becoming more common, likely due to the use of central venous catheters. The common presence of oral and tracheobronchial ulceration is an additional predisposing factor to bacterial infection in this population. Presumably because of the routine use of prophylactic antibiotics, radiographically evident bacterial pneumonia is uncommon in this period. When it occurs, however, radiographic manifestations are nonspecific and similar to those seen in other groups of immunocompromised patients. Pneumonia initially manifests as focal or multifocal consolidation; rapid progression to more diffuse opacification may occur.

Candida and *Aspergillus* infections are the most common fungal infections in this period.[307,308] *Candida* uncommonly causes isolated pneumonia. More commonly, it causes gastrointestinal or genitourinary infection or results in systemic

Table 6.3 Timing of complications following BMT

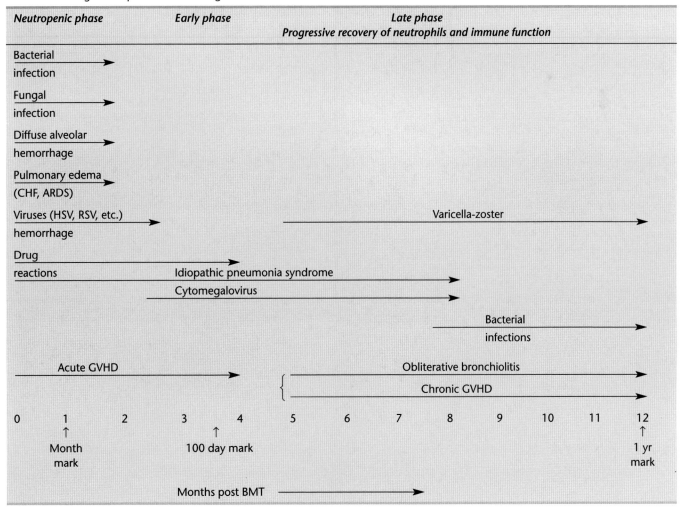

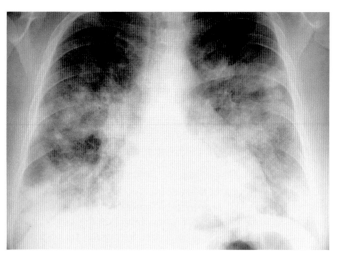

Fig. 6.74 Herpes pneumonia in a bone marrow transplant recipient with rash and severe oropharyngeal ulceration. A frontal chest radiograph shows scattered bilateral homogeneous opacities.

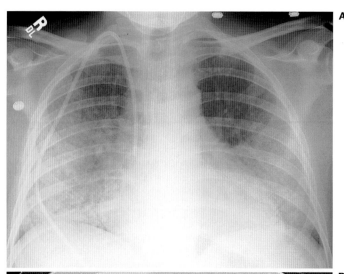

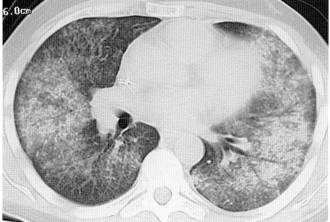

Fig. 6.75 Diffuse pulmonary hemorrhage in a bone marrow transplant recipient. **A**, A frontal chest radiograph shows diffuse bilateral homogeneous opacities. **B**, CT shows diffuse reticular and ground-glass opacities. Bronchoalveolar lavage revealed hemorrhage.

dissemination. Conversely, *Aspergillus* has a predilection for the respiratory tract, including the paranasal sinuses. The imaging features of invasive aspergillosis have been previously discussed. Both airway-invasive and angioinvasive forms of the disease are encountered during this period (see Figs 6.56 to 6.61).

Viral infections are uncommon causes of pulmonary disease in the neutropenic phase. Some viruses, however, may cause pneumonia either as a direct pathogen or by indirectly potentiating bacterial infection in the first few weeks after bone marrow transplantation. Herpes simplex virus primarily causes oropharyngeal ulceration in this setting. Such infection is a risk factor for both bacterial sepsis and for herpes simplex pneumonia, which may result from contiguous spread from the airways. Pneumonia acquired in this fashion manifests with focal or multifocal bronchocentric opacities. Conversely, pneumonia acquired by viremia manifests with more diffuse pulmonary opacities. Herpes simplex pneumonia should always be considered in BMT recipients with evidence of extrapulmonary herpetic infection (Fig. 6.74). Respiratory viruses such as respiratory syncytial virus, adenovirus, influenza, and parainfluenza have also been implicated in cases of early posttransplant pneumonias.[309–312]

Pulmonary edema, either due to cardiac failure, fluid overload, or capillary leak, is a frequent cause of symptoms and radiographic abnormalities in the immediate posttransplant period.[305] The so-called "engraftment syndrome" occurs in this early period and is characterized by fever, skin rash, and capillary leak.[313,314] It occurs in one-third[313] to one-half[314] of patients; autologous and allogeneic recipients are affected equally. Alterations in renal and hepatic function are common. Pulmonary edema occurs in about half of affected patients.[313,314] Radiographic findings are nonspecific and include bilateral homogeneous opacities, septal thickening, and pleural fluid. The syndrome is usually self-limited and does not progress to ARDS.[313] Sepsis and/or preexisting capillary injury from conditioning regimens may potentiate edema, as may profound hypoalbuminemia. Pulmonary venoocclusive disease leading to edema has also been reported in BMT recipients.[315]

Diffuse alveolar hemorrhage occurs in up to 21% of transplant patients[305] and has a high mortality, between 50%

and 80%.[316,317] It occurs after either autologous or allogeneic transplants, usually within the first month. There does not appear to be any association between alveolar hemorrhage in this setting and disorders of coagulation. Hemorrhage occurs at the time of engraftment and may represent a complication of leukostasis caused by the sudden influx of neutrophils into the lungs. There is evidence that early treatment with corticosteroids may reduce mortality.[318] Affected patients present with dyspnea, cough, and sometimes fever. Hemoptysis is quite rare. Diagnosis is established by bronchoalveolar lavage that yields progressively more bloody aliquots. Chest radiographs usually show diffuse consolidation (Fig. 6.75), but approximately one-third show diffuse reticular opacities (Fig. 6.76).[319] CT can show scattered or diffuse ground-glass opacities that may progress to consolidation (Fig. 6.75).[320–322] These findings are frequently indistinguishable from other complications, particularly drug toxicity and opportunistic pneumonia. Furthermore, diffuse pulmonary hemorrhage tends to occur at about the same time as pulmonary edema; the two conditions can usually be distinguished on clinical grounds.

Conditioning regimens prior to bone marrow transplantation typically involve some degree of total body irradiation and

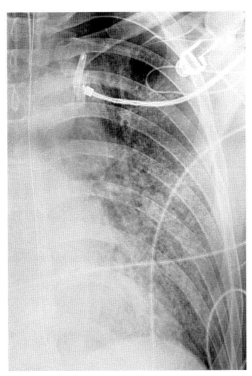

Fig. 6.76 Pulmonary hemorrhage in a bone marrow transplant recipient. The coned-down view of a frontal chest radiograph shows diffuse reticular opacities. Bronchoalveolar lavage revealed hemorrhage.

intensive cytotoxic chemotherapy. These regimens may result in pulmonary toxicity, often in the form of diffuse alveolar damage. These effects may be latent and not manifest for some time after transplantation and may potentiate the effects of previously described complications. Drug toxicity should always be considered in the differential diagnosis of pulmonary complications in the first few months after BMT and may be a dominant cause of complications in autologous transplant recipients.[306] The histopathologic, clinical, and radiologic manifestations of drug- and radiation-induced lung disease are discussed in Chapter 9.

Early phase complications

Early phase complications (30–100 days after transplantation) occur during a period of depressed cellular and humoral immunity. The two most important pulmonary complications in this phase are cytomegalovirus (CMV) pneumonia and the idiopathic pneumonia syndrome. Acute graft versus host disease (GVHD) also occurs in this period. GVHD results from transplantation of immunocompetent donor lymphocytes that attack the recipient's tissues. Acute graft versus host disease occurs 20–100 days after transplantation in 25–75% of patients.[323,324] The effects are predominantly extrapulmonary and include exfoliative dermatitis, diarrhea, and liver dysfunction. Pulmonary manifestations are usually minimal. However, acute GVHD may potentiate the effects of more common pulmonary complications such as infection. Of course, GVHD does not occur in autologous bone marrow transplant recipients.

CMV pneumonia is, overall, the most significant pathogen in BMT recipients, in terms of both morbidity and mortality.[325] At least 70% of recipients develop clinical or subclinical infection with CMV. The clinical manifestations of CMV infection are extremely varied and include retinitis, encephalitis, esophagitis and enterocolitis, hepatitis, and nephritis. Pneumonia is the most serious manifestation of CMV infection with an incidence of 10–40% following allogeneic transplantation; mortality rates up to 85% in this setting have been reported.[301] Early diagnosis and treatment with acyclovir or ganciclovir and immunoglobulin can halve the mortality. Diagnosis of CMV infection is discussed on page 294, as are the radiologic manifestations of CMV pneumonia.

Other viral pathogens can cause pneumonia during this period, including herpes simplex virus (Fig. 6.74) and the respiratory viruses (Fig. 6.77).[309–312] Respiratory virus infection is more common in allogeneic than autologous transplant recipients and is an uncommon cause of death in these patients. Mortality in affected patients can be substantial, however. In one series,[311] direct RSV and influenza A associated mortality was 17% and 15%, respectively. Others have reported lower mortality rates, however.[310] Adenovirus is apparently an increasingly important viral pathogen in bone marrow transplant recipients, particularly in the pediatric population.[326] Adenovirus can cause

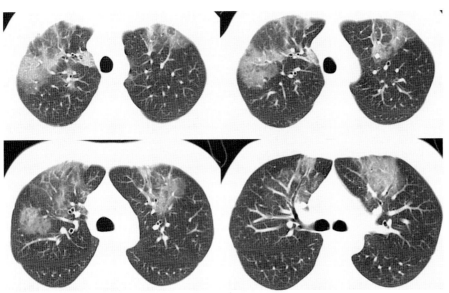

Fig. 6.77 Respiratory syncytial virus pneumonia in a bone marrow transplant recipient with cough, fever, and a normal chest radiograph. CT shows geographic ground-glass opacities in the upper lobes.

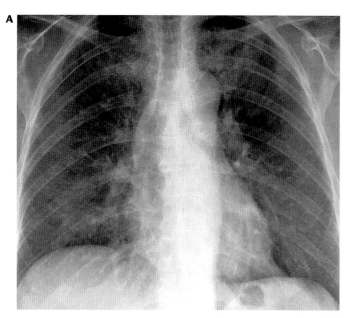

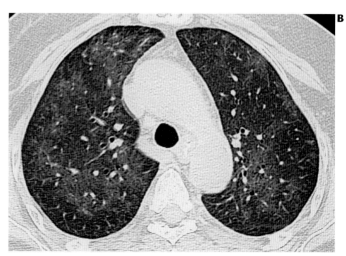

Fig. 6.78 Idiopathic pneumonia syndrome after bone marrow transplant for multiple myeloma. **A,** A frontal chest radiograph shows bilateral heterogeneous opacities. **B,** HRCT confirms diffuse ground-glass opacities. Transbronchial lung biopsies and bronchoalveolar lavage showed no evidence of infection or hemorrhage.

hepatitis, hemorrhagic cystitis, and pneumonia in affected individuals.[326–331] Reported mortality rates vary from 1% in patients with localized disease[331] to 73% in patients with pneumonia.[329] Pediatric patients and patients with GVHD are at greater risk for severe adenoviral infection after BMT.

Pneumonia accounts for over 40% of transplant-related deaths. Of these, approximately one-half are noninfectious (or at least no infectious agent can be identified). This condition in bone marrow transplant recipients is known as the idiopathic pneumonia syndrome (IPS). IPS is slightly more common in allogeneic than autologous transplant recipients. Mortality is high (>70%). IPS manifests histopathologically with progressive diffuse alveolar damage. The precise pathogenesis is unknown, but IPS likely results from multiple types and episodes of lung injury, including drug toxicity, radiation-induced injury, undiagnosed infection (viral or fungal), and GVHD. Affected patients present with worsening dyspnea and fever. Chest radiographs show scattered or diffuse opacities that may progress to diffuse consolidation (Fig. 6.78). CT shows ground-glass opacities in the early stages; later stages may show more linear opacities with evidence of architectural distortion. The diagnosis is typically one of exclusion; infection must, as far as possible, be excluded. Clark et al[332] defined the following criteria for clinical diagnosis of IPS: (1) signs and symptoms of pneumonia; (2) chest radiograph shows multilobar opacities; (3) abnormal pulmonary physiology manifested by an increased alveolar to arterial oxygen gradient and restrictive pulmonary function test abnormalities; (4) rigorous exclusion of infectious pathogens by bronchoalveolar lavage or lung biopsy.

Late phase complications

Occurring more than 100 days after transplantation, the major late phase complication is chronic GVHD in allogeneic bone marrow transplants.[333] The risk for idiopathic pneumonia syndrome, respiratory viral and CMV pneumonia also persists

for several more months into this phase in both autologous and allogeneic transplant recipients.

Chronic GVHD occurs in one-third to one-half of patients surviving the first 100 days after allogeneic bone marrow transplantation.[323,334] The clinical manifestations are similar to those of the autoimmune diseases; scleroderma, primary biliary cirrhosis, and the sicca syndrome may result. The precise incidence of pulmonary disease resulting from chronic GVHD is not well known. Ten percent of patients in the series of Palmas et al[335] developed late noninfectious pulmonary complications that were thought to be related to chronic GVHD. In that series,[334] 50% of the patients with late complications had NSIP or diffuse alveolar damage (DAD) on biopsy, 28% had obliterative bronchiolitis (OB), and 17% had organizing pneumonia (OP). Trisolini et al[336] reported progression from NSIP to OP and OB in a single patient with chronic GVHD. In the study of Palmas et al,[334] enhanced immunosuppression resulted in long term clinical improvement in all patients with OP and half of patients with DAD or NSIP on biopsy. Improvement was seen in only one patient with OB. Others have reported similar encouraging results in patients with OP in this setting.[337,338] However, progressive fibrosis leading to death from respiratory failure is reported in patients with chronic GVHD as well.[339]

Chest radiographs in patients with chronic GVHD are often normal despite clinical evidence of pulmonary dysfunction (Fig. 6.79).[340] When disease progresses, heterogeneous or consolidative opacities may be seen (Fig. 6.80).[341] The clinical and radiologic manifestations of OB in allogeneic bone marrow transplant recipients are similar to those of OB in lung transplant recipients and are discussed below on page 338. The clinical and radiologic manifestations of OP in bone marrow transplant recipients are also similar to those of cryptogenic OP and are discussed in Chapter 10. In short, chest radiographs show scattered, almost nodular areas of pulmonary consolidation. CT may show, in addition, centrilobular nodules and tree-in-bud opacities. It should be remembered that although OP in this

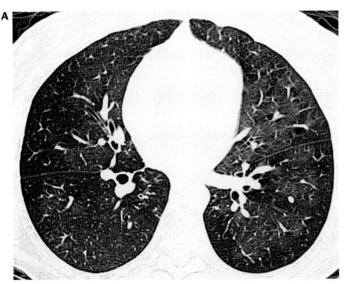

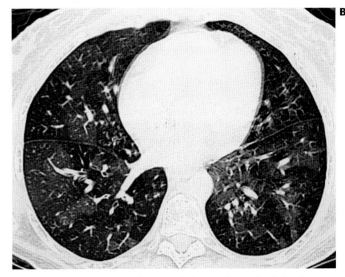

Fig. 6.79 Graft versus host disease in a bone marrow transplant recipient with progressive dyspnea and a normal chest radiograph. **A**, Inspiratory HRCT (lung window) shows subtle mosaic attenuation. **B**, Expiratory HRCT (lung window) shows air-trapping consistent with obliterative bronchiolitis.

setting may be part of a response to chronic GVHD, it may also be a manifestation of pulmonary drug toxicity or undiagnosed infection.

There is an association between the development of chronic GVHD and bacterial pneumonia, probably because of associated lung and airway injury. Thus, there is an increased incidence of bacterial infections in the late phase after bone marrow transplantation. On the other hand, fungal infections are rarely encountered during this period. Varicella-zoster infection also occurs in this time frame and most cases appear to represent reactivation of previous infection. Varicella only accounts for approximately 15% of all infections in bone marrow transplant recipients and the majority of the manifestations are cutaneous.[301] Nevertheless, varicella infection may be associated with systemic dissemination and varicella pneumonia (see Fig. 6.69).

Heart transplantation

According to the most recent registry data from the International Society of Heart and Lung Transplantation (www.ishlt.org/registries), over 3000 heart transplants were performed worldwide in 2003, down from almost 4500 in 1994. The 5-year actuarial survival rate for all heart transplants was slightly less than 70%, and approximately half of patients were alive at 9 years. The most common indications for transplantation in adult heart recipients were cardiomyopathy (45%) and coronary artery disease (45%). Combined heart–lung transplants are performed mainly for pulmonary hypertension and complex congenital heart disease. Fewer than 100 such transplants were performed worldwide in 2003, down from a peak of almost 250 in 1989. The 5-year actuarial survival rate for heart–lung recipients was 40%; only half of patients survived 3 years. For more recent data, the interested reader is referred to the ISHLT website (www.ishlt.org/registries).

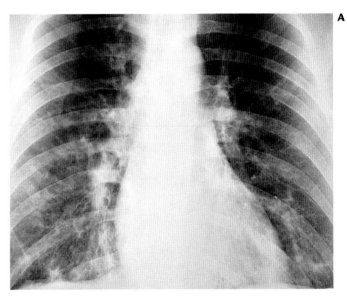

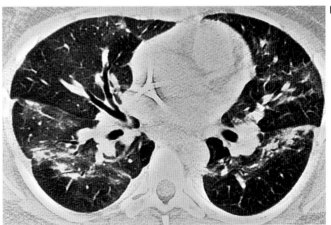

Fig. 6.80 Graft versus host disease in a bone marrow transplant recipient. **A**, A frontal chest radiograph shows predominantly basal peribronchovascular opacities. **B**, CT more clearly demonstrates the peribronchial distribution of disease. Note also mild bronchiectasis and mosaic attenuation consistent with obliterative bronchiolitis.

The majority of heart and heart–lung transplant patients encounter problems common to all patients undergoing open heart surgery. A description of all of the possible radiographic findings following thoracic surgery is beyond the scope of this text, but a brief summary is given here as a prelude to a discussion of the pulmonary problems encountered with heart and heart–lung transplantation. Pleural effusions and basal atelectasis are almost inevitable, particularly at the left lung base.[342,343] Pleural effusions may be a response to manipulation of the pleura during surgery. Atelectasis may be related to the local compressive effect of the effusions, although postoperative chest pain may play a part. The left lower lobe is particularly prone to atelectasis, possibly because of the compressive effect of the heart, the decreased effectiveness of endotracheal suction in this region, and the comparative frequency of a transient postoperative paresis of the left hemidiaphragm following cardioplegia.[344,345] In the immediate postoperative period the mediastinum should be observed for undue widening, which may indicate postoperative mediastinal hemorrhage.[342] Air in pleural and mediastinal spaces is routinely observed but is rarely significant unless a large pneumothorax develops. Evidence of persisting anterior mediastinal gas collections or a pericardial effusion may be seen in association with anterior mediastinitis.

The transplanted heart, particularly the right-sided chambers, may not function fully in the immediate postoperative period. This may be related to transient ischemic damage. Inotropic support usually tides the patient over this period. Nevertheless, pulmonary edema frequently occurs in the immediate postoperative period. The edema may have other or additional causes, including renal insufficiency, excessive fluid administration, or the acute respiratory distress syndrome. However, on occasion, acute right-sided failure with decline in the cardiac output ensues because of preexisting pulmonary hypertension. This acute right-sided failure cannot be detected radiographically.

Inevitably, immunosuppressed patients are at risk of infective complications, either locally in the mediastinum and pleura as a direct result of the surgery or in the lungs. The prophylactic use of antimicrobial agents substantially reduces these complications.[346] Just as important is the fine tuning of immunosuppressive regimens allowed by the more liberal use of endomyocardial biopsy to detect early rejection. The infective complications following heart transplantation have no particular features to distinguish them from infections in the other states of immune compromise (Figs 6.81 and 6.82). The use of cyclosporine and prophylactic antimicrobial agents has elevated the importance of viruses, especially CMV (Fig. 6.82) and herpes simplex virus, as a cause of infection.[265]

Acute and chronic rejection is indicated by clinical, hemodynamic, and radiographic evidence of biventricular dysfunction. Radiographic changes include an increase in the transverse cardiac diameter with signs of pulmonary vascular congestion, interstitial and alveolar edema, and pericardial and pleural effusions. Hyperacute rejection may occur in the immediate perioperative period but is uncommon. Acute rejection commonly occurs 2 weeks to 3 months following transplantation. Chronic rejection may occur at any time in the following months or years. Other remote complications include accelerated atherosclerosis in the graft,[347,348] postpericardiectomy syndrome (Dressler syndrome), lymphoproliferative disorders, and malignancies (Fig. 6.83).[349,352] Posttransplant lymphoproliferative disease is discussed on page 345.

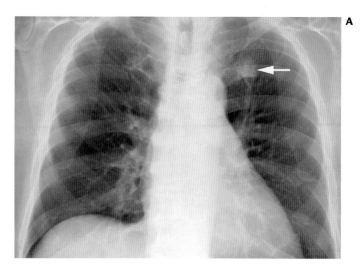

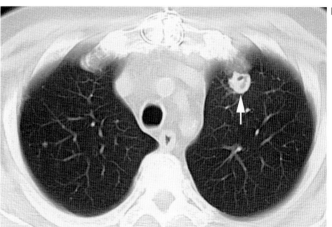

Fig. 6.81 Pulmonary cryptococcosis in an asymptomatic heart transplant recipient. **A**, A surveillance chest radiograph shows a left upper lobe nodule (arrow). **B**, CT shows a well-circumscribed nodule (arrow) in the left upper lobe. Biopsy confirmed *C. neoformans* infection.

Lung transplantation

Dr Hardy performed the first "successful" human lung transplant at the University of Mississippi in 1963.[353] Unfortunately, the patient survived only a few weeks and died of postoperative sepsis; at autopsy, however, the graft was found to be functioning. The next two decades of research on human lung transplantation were fraught with difficulty. Two main problems quickly became apparent.[354] First, it was difficult to maintain adequate immunosuppression and yet avoid infection. The lung, after all, is the only organ transplant exposed directly to the environment. Second, interruption of the bronchial circulation made a satisfactory and durable airway anastomosis difficult to achieve. High dose corticosteroids used for immunosuppression further aggravated this problem. The introduction of cyclosporine proved to be a major advance in this regard. Not only was the degree of immunosuppression more satisfactory, but the doses of corticosteroids could be radically reduced, improving tissue healing. The second decisive step was the introduction of new techniques for performing the bronchial anastomosis. Early approaches involved wrapping the anastomosis with intercostal

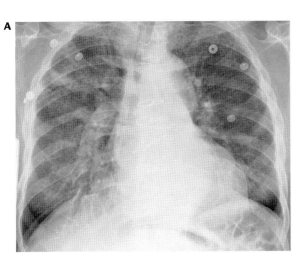

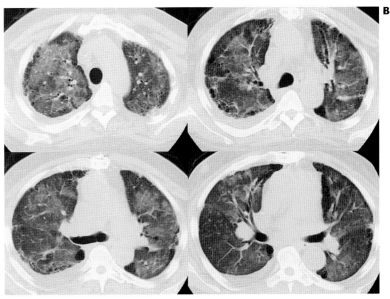

Fig. 6.82 Cytomegalovirus pneumonia in a heart transplant recipient with dyspnea and fever. **A**, A frontal chest radiograph shows bilateral heterogeneous opacities. **B**, CT shows diffuse ground-glass opacities superimposed upon preexisting pulmonary fibrosis. Lung biopsy showed CMV infection.

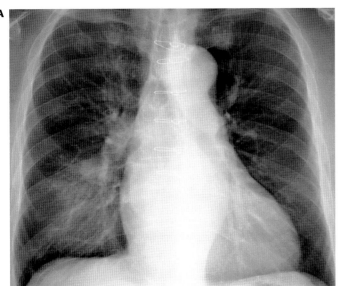

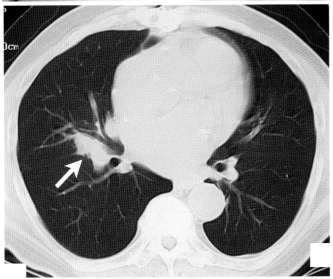

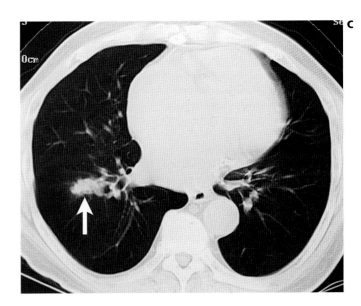

Fig. 6.83 Kaposi sarcoma in an asymptomatic heart transplant recipient. **A**, A surveillance chest radiograph shows a poorly defined opacity in the right lower lobe. **B** and **C**, CT scans show peribronchovascular nodules (arrows) in the right lower lobe. Biopsy showed Kaposi sarcoma.

muscle or with omentum brought up into the chest through an anterior diaphragmatic tunnel.[355,356] These procedures increased vascularity in the region of anastomosis, greatly enhanced bronchial healing. These two major advances ushered in the modern era of lung transplantation. The first clinically successful single lung transplants with reasonable postoperative survival were reported from the University of Toronto in the early 1980s.[357]

According to the most recent registry data from the International Society of Heart and Lung Transplantation (www.ishlt.org/registries), over 1600 lung transplants were performed worldwide in 2003, the most ever reported. The 5-year actuarial survival rate for all lung transplants was slightly less than 50% and approximately half of patients were alive at 4 years. The most common indications for transplantation in adult lung recipients were emphysema/COPD (39%), idiopathic pulmonary fibrosis (17%), cystic fibrosis (16%), α_1-antiprotease deficiency (9%), and primary pulmonary hypertension (5%) (Box 6.11).

Types of lung transplants

There are two major types of lung transplantation: single (SLT) and bilateral (BLT). Decisions regarding the use of single versus double lung transplants involve three major considerations: availability of donor lungs, the underlying disease, and longterm function. The only absolute contraindications to single lung transplantation are suppurative lung disease (bronchiectasis, cystic fibrosis) and uncorrectable heart disease.[358,359] Because the major factor limiting lung transplantation is the limited availability of donor lungs,[360–364] SLT gained popularity for treating patients with fibrosis and emphysema/COPD because this procedure maximized the number of treated patients (one donor, two treated patients). An additional advantage favoring SLT over BLT was a slightly lower initial morbidity and mortality (www.ishlt.org/registries).[365] In the early to mid 1990s, SLT was performed much more often than BLT for these indications. This trend may be changing, however. Actuarial survival data accumulated over the last ten years suggest a small but distinct longterm survival advantage for patients with emphysema/COPD and α_1-antiprotease deficiency treated with BLT. Potential reasons for this survival difference include: (1) BLT recipients tolerate obliterative bronchiolitis better than do SLT recipients[366,367]; (2) BLT recipients have greater pulmonary reserve than SLT recipients[366,367]; and (3) patients with giant bullous emphysema may have fewer difficulties with native lung herniation and mediastinal shift following BLT.[367–369] Perhaps for these reasons, the number of BLTs performed for COPD/emphysema has steadily increased over the last few years.[361] Furthermore, although good results have been achieved using SLT to treat pulmonary hypertension, many centers preferentially now use BLT in this setting to minimize hemodynamic instability.[358,359,366,370] Large patients may also require BLT because of the shortage of suitably sized donors for SLT.[367] In 2003, the number of BLTs surpassed the number of SLTs performed worldwide (www.ishlt.org/registries).

Others have argued, however, that the survival advantage for BLT over SLT is small and may be accounted for by bias in selection of younger and less severely ill patients for BLT.[361] Weill and Keshavjee[361] suggest that, given the persistent shortage of donor lungs and absence of more compelling data favoring BLT in patients with emphysema/COPD, SLT should still be the preferred transplant option. At the present time, these decisions remain very much dependent on the institution.

Surgical technique

Surgical techniques have evolved significantly over the last two decades. Morbidity and mortality have been greatly reduced and cardiopulmonary bypass is rarely required except in patients with pulmonary hypertension. Single lung transplants are performed through a standard posterolateral thoracotomy. Bilateral lung transplants are performed either by transverse thoracosternotomy ("clam-shell" incision) or by bilateral thoracotomy.[359,366,367] Either lung may be used for SLT, although there is a slight technical bias for the left lung, since the left bronchus is longer and easier to anastomose and a greater cuff of the left atrium is left, facilitating the separate use of the heart for transplantation. Implantation of the allograft begins with the bronchial anastomosis. Two types of bronchial anastomosis are currently performed: telescoping and end-to-end.[359,367,371–373] As noted above, the telescoping bronchial anastomosis was developed to eliminate the need for an omental wrap procedure – obviating laparotomy and eliminating the risk for late diaphragmatic herniation.[372,373] Omental wrapping is thus no longer routinely performed. When a telescoping anastomosis is performed, the donor bronchus is divided two rings proximal to the upper lobe orifice and the membranous bronchus is approximated using a continuous suture. The smaller cartilaginous bronchus is intussuscepted one or two rings into the larger bronchus and sutured into position. More recently, improvements in surgical technique and donor lung preservation have allowed end-to-end anastomosis to be performed without an omental wrap with good clinical success.[374] Following bronchial anastomosis, the pulmonary arterial and venous anastomoses are performed.

Donor selection

Proper donor selection is an important process.[375,376] The ideal donor is less than 55 years of age, has no significant smoking history, and has normal cardiac function and a normal chest radiograph.[359,365,368,377,378] Bronchoscopy should be performed

---

Box 6.11 Indications for lung transplantation

Single or bilateral lung transplantation
Chronic obstructive pulmonary disease/emphysema
α_1-Antiprotease deficiency
Idiopathic pulmonary fibrosis
Pulmonary artery hypertension
Sarcoidosis
Langerhans cell histiocytosis
Lymphangioleiomyomatosis
Hypersensitivity pneumonitis

Bilateral lung transplantation (only)
Cystic fibrosis
Bronchiectasis

Heart–lung transplantation
Coexisting severe left ventricular dysfunction
Uncorrectable congenital heart disease

with negative results. The donor is screened serologically for HIV, hepatitis B, and cytomegalovirus, and must be ABO compatible with the recipient. There should be reasonable size matching between donor lung and recipient thorax. Size matching is done using either height and age normograms or anteroposterior chest radiographs.[378] Lung sizes are approximated by comparing the height (from lung apex to diaphragm in the midclavicular line) and width (at the level of the diaphragm) of the donor and recipient lungs.[378] Significantly undersized donor lungs can result in excessive mediastinal shift compromising graft function. Oversized donor lungs can be intraoperatively reduced to match the recipient. Unfortunately, only 5–25% of donors of other solid organs are found suitable for lung donation.[367,377,378] Increased experience and the shortage of suitable donor lungs has resulted in a relaxation of some of these requirements, particularly the requirement for a normal donor chest radiograph.[367] Donor lungs with marginal oxygenation and/or pulmonary opacities due to contusion or edema have been successfully transplanted.[367,379,380] The use of BLT provides a greater degree of safety if donor lung function is suboptimal.[367,379]

The vast majority of lung transplants are performed using cadaveric organs. Over the last few years, the technique of living related donor (LRD) transplantation has evolved.[363] This type of transplantation is reserved for patients with a rapidly deteriorating clinical course who cannot wait for cadaveric organs. Most such patients have cystic fibrosis. Because this procedure is usually performed as a BLT, two donors are required – a right lower lobe from one and a left lower lobe from the other (Fig. 6.84). Most donors are thus family members. Very few outcome data for this procedure have been reported. Barr et al[363] reported their results in 97 patients

undergoing living related donor transplantation. Preliminary data indicate acceptable morbidity and no mortality on the part of the donors, and actuarial survival in the recipient as good or better than that reported for cadaveric transplantation. Interestingly, the incidence of obliterative bronchiolitis at 5 years (14%) was significantly less than that reported for recipients of cadaveric lungs. Donors typically undergo thorough medical screening, complete serotyping, appropriate cardiac evaluation, quantitative ventilation–perfusion scintigraphy, and chest CT to exclude underlying lung disease.

Recipient evaluation

Proper recipient selection and preparation is also critical. Potential recipients should have end-stage pulmonary disease with a very limited life expectancy. Criteria have been developed to facilitate the selection of appropriate candidates for lung transplantation and to ensure the best possible allocation of organs.[358,368] Patients less than 65 and 55 years of age are considered for SLT and BLT, respectively. Patients must have a realistic understanding of the posttransplant medical regimen and the intensity and necessity of rehabilitation.[358,368] Patients who have demonstrated a pattern of noncompliance or who have a psychiatric illness or drug or ethanol dependence are not considered candidates for transplantation.[358,365,368,377] Potential transplant recipients should be ambulatory and able to undergo comprehensive pre- and postoperative rehabilitation.[368] Because of the vigor of rehabilitation, severe malnourishment or obesity can preclude transplantation if not corrected.[358,365] Patients with multisystem disease that limits the expected benefits or increases the risks of transplantation are considered poor candidates for

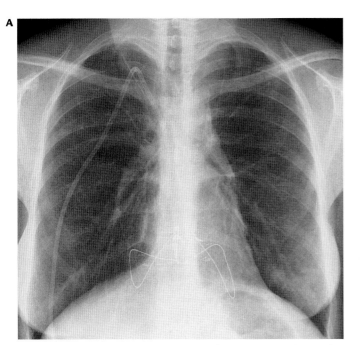
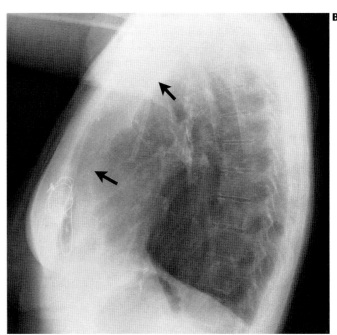

Fig. 6.84 Living related donor lung transplantation in a patient with cystic fibrosis. Cadaveric transplant was precluded by the presence of anti-HLA antibodies. Lower lobes from two closely matched relatives were used. Frontal (**A**) and lateral (**B**) chest radiographs show typical findings after LRD transplantation. Note the characteristic sternal wiring after transverse thoracosternotomy ("clam-shell" incision). The anterior soft tissue opacity on the lateral radiograph (arrows on **B**) is due to a size mismatch between the donor lungs and the recipient thorax.

lung transplantation.[367,368] Patients with preoperative pulmonary infection by pan-antibiotic resistant *Pseudomonas*, *Burkholderia* or mycobacterial species have high rates of reinfection after transplantation and increased mortality. Some transplantation programs consider these infections to be contraindications to transplantation.[358,367,381] Active extrapulmonary infection is also a relative contraindication to transplantation.[368,377]

Preoperative radiologic evaluation of the transplant candidate typically includes posteroanterior and lateral chest radiographs, chest CT, quantitative ventilation–perfusion scintigraphy, and a thorough assessment of cardiac function, as clinically indicated. Because active malignancy is considered an absolute contraindication to lung transplantation, many candidates undergo screening chest CT (Fig. 6.85).[382] Kazerooni et al[382] evaluated 190 potential lung transplant candidates with CT and found 3 small lung malignancies, 2 of which were seen only by CT. Because candidates with COPD/emphysema are at increased risk for lung cancer, any noncalcified nodule detected on CT in this population must be further evaluated. Depending upon the size of the lesion and the overall clinical scenario, transthoracic needle aspiration biopsy, FDG-PET imaging or shortterm interval radiologic follow up may be recommended. Because of the shortage of lung donors, transplantation may not occur for up to two years following the initial assessment. Kazerooni et al[382] recommend that chest radiographs be performed routinely at 3-month intervals during this period. Furthermore, they recommend repeat CT prior to transplantation to detect small interval malignancies if the period to transplantation is extended.

Selection of the proper lung for replacement is important for success of SLT procedures. The choice depends upon the severity of the underlying lung disease and the presence of pleural disease from previous infection, thoracotomy, or pleurodesis.[359] It is theoretically preferable to replace the more diseased lung. However, unilateral pleural disease can preclude SLT on that side.[359] CT can be useful for determining the most appropriate side for SLT. Kazerooni et al[382] found that CT changed the lung selected for SLT in 16% of candidates. Radionuclide imaging is also important in selection of the lung for SLT. In the absence of extensive pleural disease, the lung with less function, based on quantitative perfusion scintigraphy, is usually replaced.[359,381] It should be noted, however, that CT is not useful for pretransplant evaluation of patients with cystic fibrosis.[383] These patients are typically young, not at risk for lung malignancy, and must undergo BLT. CT rarely if ever shows findings that have significant impact on decisions regarding transplantation.[383]

Complications of lung transplantation

Early complications

Complications after lung transplantation may be divided into those occurring in the first month after the transplant and those occurring after this time. The most common causes of death in the first month after transplantation include graft failure (31%), infection (25%), cardiac disease (9%), technical problems (8%), and acute rejection (6%) (www.ishlt.org/registries). From a radiologic perspective, the most important early complications are ischemia/reperfusion edema, acute rejection, bronchial anastomotic complications, and infection (Box 6.12).

Early graft failure is the most common cause of death in the early postoperative period (www.ishlt.org/registries). Causes of graft failure include hyperacute rejection, severe ischemia/

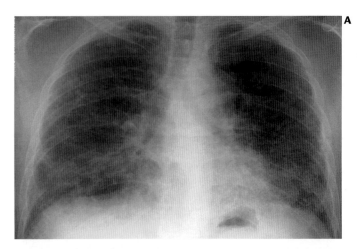

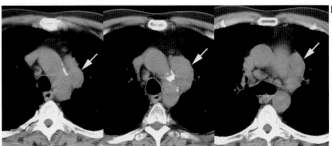

Fig. 6.85 Lung cancer discovered during pretransplant screening. **A**, A frontal chest radiograph shows findings of end-stage pulmonary fibrosis. **B**, CT shows extensive anterior mediastinal lymphadenopathy (arrows). Biopsy revealed metastatic cancer. (With permission from Erasmus JJ, McAdams HP, Tapson VF, et al. Radiologic issues in lung transplantation for end-stage pulmonary disease. AJR Am J Roentgenol 1997;169:69–78.)

Box 6.12 Important early complications after lung transplantation

First week
Ischemia/reperfusion injury
Hyperacute rejection
Bronchial anastomotic dehiscence
Vascular anastomotic stenoses or occlusion
Acute native lung overinflation (after SLT)

First month
Acute rejection
Infection (particularly bacterial pneumonia)

---

reperfusion injury, and problems with the vascular anastomoses. Hyperacute rejection is fortunately quite rare but occurs in patients with preformed circulating antibodies that attack the graft.[384–386] Edema and graft failure develop within hours of implantation. Initial radiographs usually show diffuse opacification of the allograft (Fig. 6.86). Unfortunately, most affected patients die or require immediate retransplant; rare cases of successful treatment by plasmapheresis have been reported.[384]

Ischemia/reperfusion edema, also known as the reimplantation response, is caused by allograft ischemia and subsequent

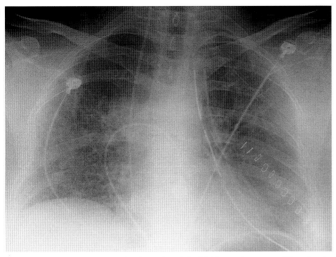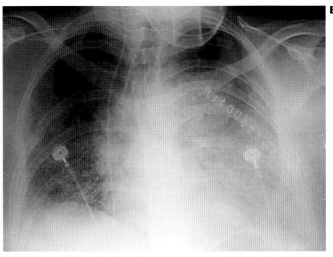

Fig. 6.86   Hyperacute rejection after left SLT for pulmonary fibrosis. **A**, The initial chest radiograph shows heterogeneous opacities in the left lung allograft. Note fibrosis in the native right lung. **B**, A repeat radiograph obtained 12 hours later shows diffuse homogeneous opacification of the graft. The patient underwent immediate retransplantation but subsequently died.

reperfusion, which results in increased microvascular permeability in the first 24–48 hours after the transplantation. It may be exacerbated by decreased lymphatic clearance due to severance of the central lymphatic pathways and the effects of lung denervation.[367,369] Ischemia/reperfusion edema occurs to a variable degree in virtually all transplants.[387–389] Anderson et al[389] reported that 97% of over 100 lung transplant recipients in their series developed radiologic evidence of reperfusion edema. In up to 15% of cases, ischemia/reperfusion injury is severe enough to cause graft failure, resulting in death or immediate retransplantation (Fig. 6.87). In such cases, findings of diffuse alveolar damage (DAD) are seen at histopathologic examination of explanted tissue.[390]

The clinical manifestations of ischemia/reperfusion edema depend upon the severity of lung injury. Most patients are only minimally symptomatic; a minority are severely dyspneic and hypoxemic. Ischemia/reperfusion edema manifests on chest radiographs with heterogeneous opacities, usually in a basal distribution. Edema is typically most severe in the first lung implanted during a BLT procedure and in allografts of patients treated with SLT for pulmonary hypertension.[367,369] The opacities typically appear within 24–48 hours after transplantation and may worsen for several days but usually begin to clear between 5 and 10 days post transplantation[389,391] (Figs 6.88 and 6.89). Persistent or worsening opacities after 5 days suggest a new complication such as acute rejection or infection. Strategies to

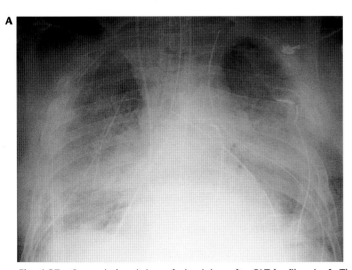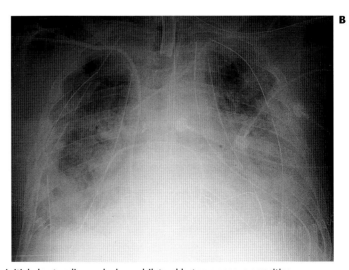

Fig. 6.87   Severe ischemia/reperfusion injury after BLT for fibrosis. **A**, The initial chest radiograph shows bilateral heterogeneous opacities. **B**, A repeat radiograph obtained 2 weeks later shows persistent and progressive opacities. A lung biopsy showed findings of DAD. The patient became ventilator-dependent and died of sepsis.

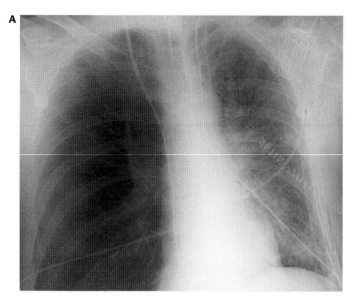

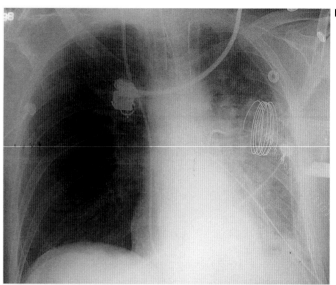

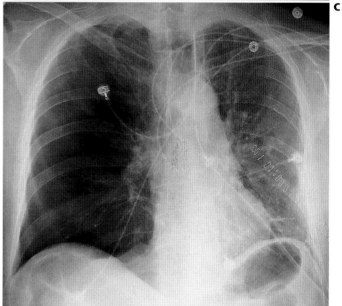

Fig. 6.88 Ischemia/reperfusion edema after left SLT for emphysema. **A**, The initial chest radiograph shows minimal heterogeneous opacities in the left lung allograft. Note findings of emphysema in the native right lung. **B**, A repeat radiograph obtained 24 hours later shows progressive perihilar consolidation in the allograft. **C**, A radiograph obtained 4 days later shows near-complete resolution of edema.

minimize the severity of edema include better donor preservation techniques, limiting the ischemic time, and reducing the volume of fluids administered to the patient in the first 48–72 hours after surgery.

Technical problems with the **vascular anastomoses** can cause early graft failure but fortunately occur in less than 5% of lung transplant recipients.[392] Significant stenosis or frank occlusion occurs more frequently at the arterial than the venous anastomosis, can be diagnosed by early postoperative perfusion scintigraphy, and can be treated by balloon dilation and stenting (Fig. 6.90).[393,394]

Acute rejection (AR) is very common in the first month after transplantation and may be difficult to distinguish clinically from reperfusion/ischemia edema, infection, or pulmonary edema resulting from fluid overload.[395] The first episode of AR usually occurs between 5 and 10 days after transplantation.[396] Affected patients are frequently febrile, hypoxemic, and have a greater than 10% decrease in forced expiratory volume in 1 second (FEV_1) from baseline.[396,397] Histopathologically, AR is diagnosed on the basis of perivascular and interstitial mononuclear infiltrates and is graded from 0 to 4 depending upon the severity of the reaction.[398,399] The reported sensitivity

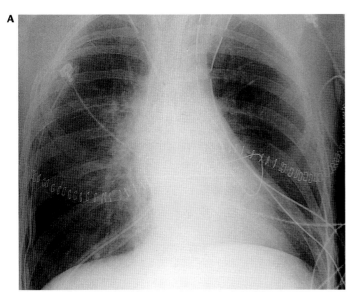

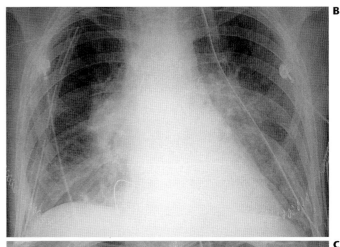

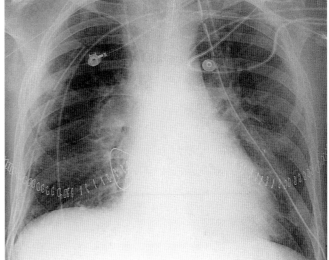

Fig. 6.89 Ischemia/reperfusion edema after BLT for cystic fibrosis. **A**, The initial chest radiograph shows minimal bilateral heterogeneous opacities. **B**, A repeat radiograph obtained 24 hours later shows progressive perihilar consolidation. **C**, A radiograph obtained 5 days later shows near-complete resolution of edema.

of transbronchial biopsy for diagnosis of AR ranges from 72% to 94%, but can be limited by the focal nature of the process.[397] Typical radiographic findings of AR include heterogeneous basal lung opacities, septal lines, and new or increasing pleural effusions (Figs 6.91 and 6.92). Bergin et al[400] suggest that these findings, together with absence of an increase in heart size or redistribution of pulmonary blood flow, usually indicate AR. However, Millet et al[401] and Anderson et al[389] showed that up to 25% of affected patients had normal chest radiographs despite lung biopsy proof of AR. Acute rejection may occur beyond the first month after transplantation; at that time, there is an increasing tendency for the chest radiograph to remain normal or unchanged despite biopsy proof of AR.[401]

The radiographic findings of acute rejection are similar to those of ischemia/reperfusion edema and infection. Ischemia/reperfusion edema is distinguished from AR by time course; the former occurs within the first 5 days after surgery whereas the latter typically occurs beyond this time period. Infection is distinguished from AR by transbronchial biopsy.[390,402,403] Transbronchial biopsy is performed freely in the early postoperative period because both acute rejection and infection are common complications at this time. Rapid clinical and radiographic response to bolus injection of high dose methylprednisolone is additional evidence for acute rejection[365,397] (Fig. 6.91).

CT has been investigated as a means for detecting and grading acute rejection in lung transplant recipients. Loubeyre et al[404] found that scattered or diffuse ground-glass opacities were the most frequent CT findings in patients with AR (Fig. 6.92). These findings were only 65% sensitive for mild to moderate acute rejection, however. Ikonen et al[405] evaluated CT in an experimental animal model of acute rejection. They reported four CT stages that correlated with histopathologic severity of rejection: (1) ill-defined centrilobular nodules or minimal

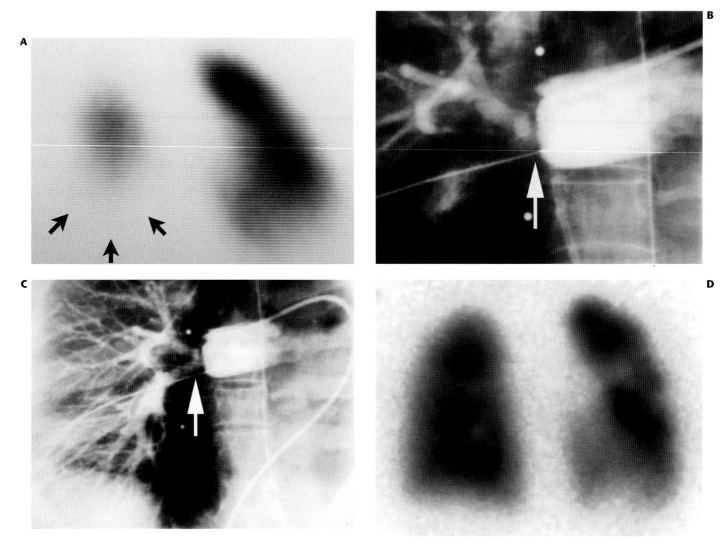

Fig. 6.90 Pulmonary arterial anastomotic stenosis after right SLT for sarcoidosis. **A,** The anterior view from an initial perfusion scintigram shows no perfusion to the right lower lung (arrows). **B,** Arteriogram shows focal stenosis at the vascular anastomosis with occlusion of the interlobar artery (arrow). **C,** A repeat arteriogram after balloon dilation and stent placement shows improved flow (arrow) to the right middle and lower lobes. **D,** A repeat scintigram confirms normal right lung perfusion. (With permission from Murray JG, McAdams HP, Erasmus JJ, et al. Complications of lung transplantation: radiologic findings. AJR Am J Roentgenol 1996;166:1405–1411.)

scattered ground-glass opacities; (2) diffuse small nodules or extensive ground-glass opacities and bronchial wall thickening; (3) lung volume loss and diffuse ground-glass opacities; and (4) consolidation of the lung. In their series, CT was 86.7% sensitive and 85.6% specific for the diagnosis of AR. Gotway et al[406] evaluated 34 patients with histopathologically proved acute rejection. In their series, CT was only 35% sensitive and 73% specific for the diagnosis of AR. No individual CT finding was significantly associated with acute rejection. They concluded that HRCT had limited accuracy for the diagnosis of acute rejection following lung transplantation. From a clinical standpoint, CT is rarely performed to either diagnose or grade the severity of acute rejection.

Infection is the second most common cause of early mortality in lung transplant recipients and is, overall, the most

common complication encountered in these patients. Most infections involve the allograft(s). Native lung infection in SLT recipients is uncommon in the early postoperative period.[407] The patient's overall susceptibility to infection is increased because of potent immune suppression in the early postoperative period. The allograft is uniquely susceptible to infection because it is exposed to the environment, mucociliary clearance is impaired after bronchial transection, and the cough reflex is absent due to denervation.[369,408,409] Diaphragmatic paralysis, fortunately a very uncommon complication, may also increase risk of infection.[410]

Bacteria account for over 60% of posttransplantation pneumonia and for most pneumonia in the first month after transplantation. Although the incidence of bacterial pneumonia is highest in the first month, it continues to be a major cause of

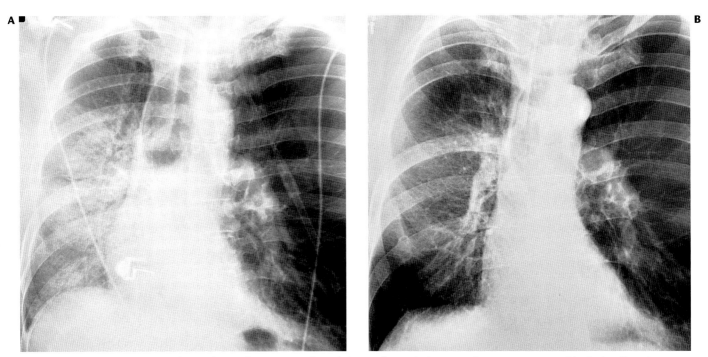

Fig. 6.91 Acute rejection after right SLT for emphysema. **A,** A frontal chest radiograph shows new heterogeneous opacities in the allograft. Biopsies showed acute rejection. **B,** A repeat radiograph obtained 72 hours after bolus corticosteroid therapy shows complete resolution of opacities.

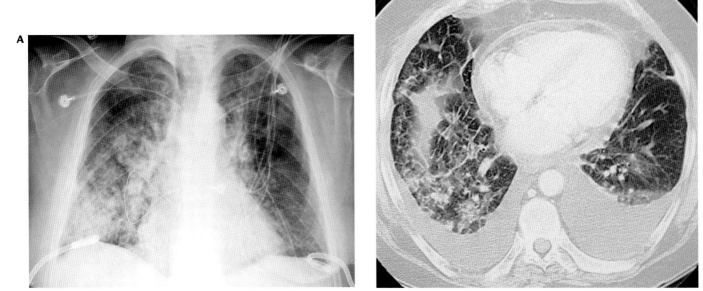

Fig. 6.92 Acute rejection 2 weeks after BLT for emphysema. **A,** A frontal chest radiograph shows bilateral heterogeneous opacities in a perihilar distribution. Note the bilateral pigtail catheters placed to drain the associated pleural effusions. **B,** CT shows ground-glass opacities and interlobular septal thickening, particularly in the right lung. Note the bilateral effusions. Biopsy showed grade 3 acute rejection.

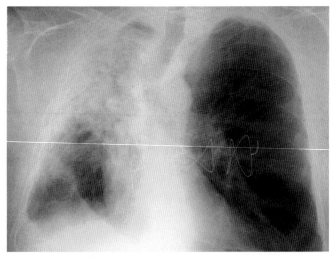

Fig. 6.93 *Staphylococcus aureus* pneumonia one month after right SLT for emphysema. A frontal chest radiograph shows homogeneous right upper lobe consolidation. (With permission from Murray JG, McAdams HP, Erasmus JJ, et al. Complications of lung transplantation: radiologic findings. AJR Am J Roentgenol 1996;166:1405–1411.)

morbidity and mortality throughout the recipient's life (www.ishlt.org/registries).[409] Opportunistic infections are less common during this period, with the possible exception of bronchial anastomotic infection by *Aspergillus* or *Candida* species. *Pneumocystis jiroveci* pneumonia has been virtually eliminated by routine prophylaxis.[409] Most early bacterial pneumonias are caused by *S. aureus* (frequently methicillin-resistant), *Enterobacter*, *P. aeruginosa*, or other gram-negative organisms. The incidence of serious bacterial pneumonia in the early period has been decreased by the routine use of broad-spectrum antibiotic prophylaxis.[409,411] The radiographic manifestations of bacterial pneumonia are similar to those in other hospitalized patients and include lobar or diffuse consolidation, cavitation, and lung nodules (Figs 6.93 and 6.94).[390,409,412–414]

Airway complications after lung transplantation are relatively common. As noted previously, bronchial anastomotic healing is inhibited by airway ischemia, low cardiac output, acute allograft rejection, and prolonged postoperative ventilation. Complications include dehiscence of the bronchial anastomosis, bronchomalacia, and bronchial stenosis.[381,415,416] The overall incidence of airway complications has steadily declined and is now approximately 12–17% per anastomosis, with an overall mortality of 2–3%.[415–417]

Complete dehiscence of the bronchial anastomosis is a catastrophic and frequently lethal event that is now quite rare. Complete dehiscence is usually an early posttransplant complication. Presumably, this is because bronchial arteries regenerate with time and the anastomosis becomes revascularized.[418] Affected patients may become acutely dyspneic and develop hemoptysis. Chest radiographs are limited in their ability to show dehiscence; persistent air leaks, mediastinal emphysema, or pneumothorax are important ancillary findings. CT can be useful for showing the site of dehiscence (Fig. 6.95).[419,420] Complete dehiscence requires surgical repair by wrapping the anastomosis with omentum or intercostal muscle to promote healing. Omental wraps are readily identified by fatty CT attenuation measurements and should not be confused with fluid collections or inflammatory masses.[421]

More commonly, small areas of limited airway wall necrosis occur in the immediate postoperative period. Such patients may be completely asymptomatic, with the defects discovered either at routine fiberoptic bronchoscopy or by CT. CT can diagnose limited bronchial dehiscence by demonstrating extrabronchial air collections in the vicinity of the anastomosis.[388,395,419] CT may also show the actual defect in the bronchial wall.[388,389] Many of these small foci of airway necrosis will resolve with time and can be treated conservatively, though the risk of late stenosis is increased.[416,420]

The telescoping bronchial anastomosis has a distinctive appearance on HRCT. The site of anastomosis is identified on CT as a bandlike focal constriction of the bronchial lumen.[422] Because the donor bronchus is invaginated into the recipient bronchus, a

A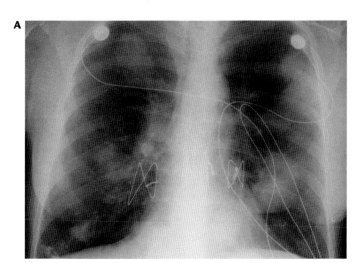

B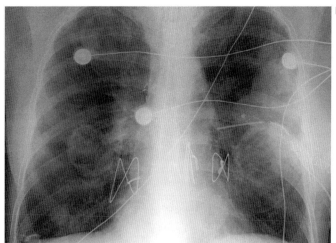

Fig. 6.94 *Pseudomonas aeruginosa* infection after BLT for cystic fibrosis. **A**, A frontal chest radiograph shows bilateral masses and nodules. **B**, A repeat radiograph one week later shows cavitation. (With permission from Murray JG, McAdams HP, Erasmus JJ, et al. Complications of lung transplantation: radiologic findings. AJR Am J Roentgenol 1996;166:1405–1411.)

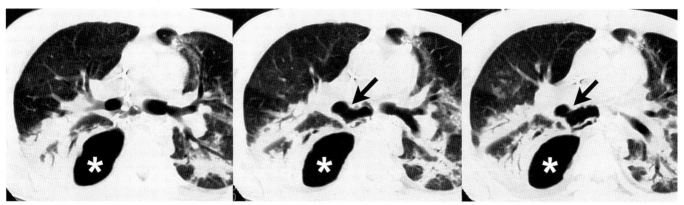

Fig. 6.95 Bronchial anastomotic dehiscence after BLT for cystic fibrosis. CT shows features suggestive of necrosis of the bronchus intermedius (arrows) at the anastomosis with a bronchopleural fistula. Note the loculated pneumothorax (*). The airway was successfully repaired with an intercostal muscle flap. (With permission from McAdams HP, Murray JG, Erasmus JJ, et al. Telescoping bronchial anastomoses for unilateral or bilateral sequential lung transplantation: CT appearance. Radiology 1997;203:202–206.)

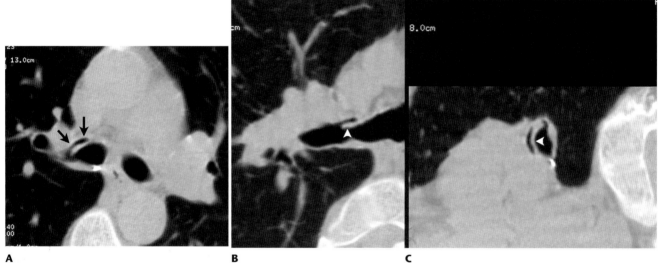

Fig. 6.96 Telescoping bronchial anastomosis after right SLT for emphysema. **A**, Axial CT shows an anterior perianastomotic air collection (arrows). Reformatted images in oblique axial (**B**) and coronal (**C**) planes show that the anterior air collection is due to the invaginated recipient bronchus (arrowheads). (With permission from McAdams HP, Murray JG, Erasmus JJ, et al. Telescoping bronchial anastomoses for unilateral or bilateral sequential lung transplantation: CT appearance. Radiology 1997;203:202–206.)

small curvilinear pocket of air may develop along the superior, anterior, and inferior aspect of the anastomosis (Fig. 6.96).[423] This finding should not be misinterpreted as that of dehiscence.

Late stenosis occurs at approximately 10% of bronchial anastomoses and may be increased at telescoping anastomoses.[417] Although bronchial anastomotic stenoses can be inferred by clinical symptoms or pulmonary function testing, they are usually diagnosed by bronchoscopy.[367,424] CT can also be useful for diagnosing and sizing airway stenoses and for monitoring stent placement.[419,420,422] Two- and three-dimensional reconstructions from helical CT data sets well demonstrate the location and length of stenoses (Figs 6.97 and 6.98).[422,425] Bronchomalacia or stenosis may require dilation with or without stent placement. Both silastic and expandable metallic mesh stents are used to treat anastomotic stenoses.[416] Silastic stents have the advantage of being removable. However, they have a small, fixed lumen and secretions tend to accumulate distal to the stent.[416] Expandable metallic mesh stents are larger and

interfere less with clearance of secretions. They are, however, more difficult to remove or reposition.[426] There is an increasing trend toward the use of expandable metallic mesh stents in the posttransplant population.[426]

Late complications

Complications of lung transplantation that occur after the first month include opportunistic infection, acute rejection, obliterative bronchiolitis, stenoses of bronchial or vascular anastomoses, recurrence of primary disease, and malignancy including posttransplant lymphoproliferative disorder (Box 6.13). The most common causes of death in the first year after transplant include infection (42%), graft failure (17%), and lymphoproliferative disorders (3%) (www.ishlt.org/registries). After the first year, mortality due to obliterative bronchiolitis and non-lymphoproliferative malignancy steadily increases. Infection remains an important cause of morbidity and mortality throughout the posttransplant period. Acute rejection

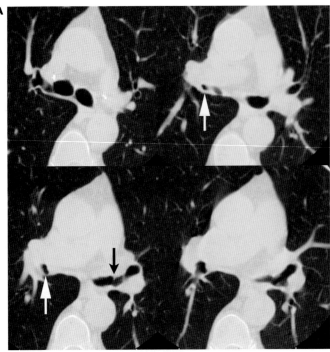

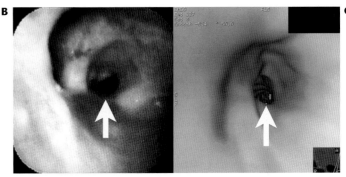

Fig. 6.97 Bronchial anastomotic stenosis after BLT for cystic fibrosis. **A**, CT shows severe stenosis of the bronchus intermedius (white arrows) at the anastomosis. Note the web (black arrow) at the left anastomosis due to the telescoping procedure. **B**, Fiberoptic and **C**, simulated ("virtual") bronchoscopic views show the right-sided stenosis (arrows). (With permission from McAdams HP, Palmer SM, Erasmus JJ, et al. Bronchial anastomotic complications in lung transplant recipients: virtual bronchoscopy for noninvasive assessment. Radiology 1998;209:689–695.)

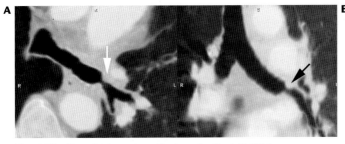

Fig. 6.98 Bronchial anastomotic stenosis after left SLT for emphysema. Reformatted CT images in oblique axial (**A**) and coronal (**B**) planes show a focal high grade stenosis (arrows) of the left bronchial anastomosis.

Box 6.13 Important late complications after lung transplantation

First year
Opportunistic infection
- CMV
- Fungi
Acute rejection
Posttransplant lymphoproliferative disorder
Bronchial anastomotic stenosis

Beyond the first year
Bronchiolitis obliterans syndrome (BOS)
Posttransplant lymphoproliferative disorder
Other malignancies
Infection
Recurrent disease

---

and airway/vascular anastomotic stenoses are discussed above. Opportunistic infection, obliterative bronchiolitis, recurrence of primary disease, and posttransplant malignancy are discussed below.

Opportunistic infection. As previously noted, lung allografts are uniquely susceptible to infection, which is the most common cause of morbidity and mortality in lung transplant recipients. Bacterial infections predominate in the early period after transplantation; opportunistic fungal and viral infections become more common thereafter.

Opportunistic infection occurs in 34–59% of lung transplant recipients.[409] Cytomegalovirus (CMV) is the most common opportunistic pathogen.[427] Most CMV infections occur between 1 and 12 months after transplantation with a peak incidence between 1 and 3 months.[369,409,427] CMV infection is rare after the first year. CMV infection accounts for 4% of deaths in the first year after transplant; its influence as a cause of mortality declines thereafter (www.ishlt.org/registries). CMV infection may be acquired de novo, by transmission of virus from an infected graft, or by reactivation of latent virus in the recipient. Primary CMV infection in a seronegative host, either by de novo infection, or more commonly, by transmission of virus from an infected, seropositive allograft, is much more clinically significant than reactivation of latent infection in the recipient.[428] Infection develops in over 90% of these patients and is serious in 50–60%[367,369]; such primary infection can be fatal. For these reasons, care is taken to match CMV status between donor and recipient. The worst possible combination is a seronegative host and a seropositive donor.[429–433] If such a transplant must be performed, the patient is treated prophylactically with an antiviral agent such as ganciclovir and anti-CMV immune globulin. Secondary infection from reactivation of latent virus in

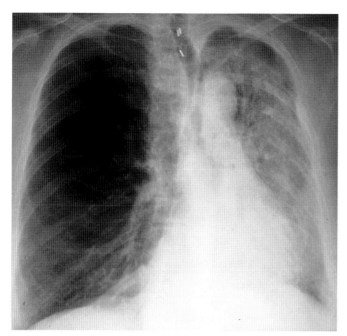

Fig. 6.99 Cytomegalovirus pneumonia after left SLT for emphysema. A frontal chest radiograph shows diffuse heterogeneous opacities in the left lung. Biopsy showed CMV infection. (With permission from Erasmus JJ, McAdams HP, Tapson VF, et al. Radiologic issues in lung transplantation for end-stage pulmonary disease. AJR Am J Roentgenol 1997;169:69–78.)

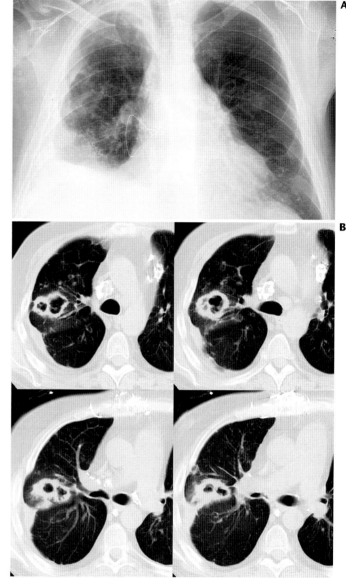

Fig. 6.100 Mucormycosis after BLT for emphysema. **A**, A frontal chest radiograph shows new heterogeneous opacities in the right lung and a right pleural effusion. **B**, CT shows cavitary masses in the right lung. Resection showed *Rhizopus* infection.

the recipient is usually less serious than primary infection.[369,428]

The clinical and radiographic manifestations of CMV pneumonia in lung transplant recipients are highly variable. Affected patients may be asymptomatic or minimally symptomatic and have normal chest radiographs, only to have CMV infection shown on biopsy.[369,428] Others have fulminant pneumonia, presenting with dyspnea, fever, malaise, and leukopenia (Fig. 6.99), progressing to respiratory failure and death.[263,434] Ganciclovir or anti-CMV immune globulin prophylaxis can delay the onset of pneumonia and attenuate the clinical course.[367,427]

There are few reports concerning specific radiologic manifestations of CMV pneumonia in the lung transplant population (Fig. 6.99). It is likely that the radiographic and CT features do not differ significantly from those seen in other immunocompromised patients, as discussed above on pages 294 and 312. These manifestations include diffuse reticular or reticulonodular opacities, ground-glass opacities, nodules, consolidation, and small effusions.[140,266,427] In the series of Shreeniwas et al,[427] CMV pneumonia manifested on chest radiographs as either diffuse (60%) or focal (33%) ground-glass opacities or focal consolidation (7%). Others have described nodules of varying size.[435] Chest radiographs can be normal with active infection.[428] Diagnosis of active infection can be difficult to establish for reasons previously discussed (p. 312), but usually requires bronchoscopy with bronchoalveolar lavage (BAL) and transbronchial biopsy.

Other viral pathogens can cause significant respiratory infection in the lung transplant population, including herpes simplex virus, adenovirus, influenza, parainfluenza, and respiratory syncytial virus.[369,409,436–438] The clinical and radiologic manifestations of respiratory viral infection in lung transplant recipients are similar to those reported in other immunocompromised patients.

Opportunistic fungal pneumonia, caused by *Aspergillus* species, *C. albicans*, *C. neoformans*, or the agents of mucormycosis, is less common than CMV pneumonia but has higher mortality.[409,439,440] These infections usually occur between 10 and 60 days following transplantation.[367,409] *Aspergillus* infection can present as an indolent pneumonia or as fulminant invasive infection with systemic dissemination.[369,439,440] *Aspergillus* species can also cause ulcerative tracheobronchitis that is usually radiographically occult but can lead to anastomotic dehiscence.[365,367,439] *Candida* species frequently colonize the airways but invasive pulmonary infection is uncommon.[367] The clinical and radiologic manifestations of opportunistic fungal infection in lung transplant recipients (Fig. 6.100) are similar to those reported in other immunocompromised patients and are

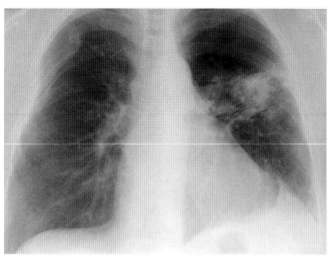

Fig. 6.101 *Cladosporium* infection after right SLT for emphysema. Frontal chest radiograph shows a masslike opacity in the native left lung.

discussed above (pp. 304–312). Fungi should be remembered as an important cause of lung nodules or masses in lung transplant recipients (Fig. 6.101).[441] Fungal anastomotic infection or pneumonia is suspected on the basis of positive sputum or bronchoalveolar lavage smears and cultures. However, because these organisms may colonize the donor lung, definitive diagnosis of invasive fungal infection may require biopsy.[440]

Mycobacterial infection is considered uncommon in lung transplant recipients.[442–446] Malouf and Glanville[443] reviewed their experience with 261 lung or heart–lung transplant recipients and found that 9% had evidence of mycobacterial infection. Most infections were diagnosed more than a year after transplantation and most were caused by atypical mycobacteria, usually *M. avium–intracellulare* complex. Kesten and Chaparro[444] reviewed their experience with 219 patients and reported a much lower incidence of mycobacterial infection. *M. tuberculosis* caused the only symptomatic mycobacterial infection in their series. Tuberculosis may be acquired by transmission of latent infection in the allograft.[427,447–449] Although experience is limited, findings of mycobacterial disease in the lung transplant recipient do not seem to differ significantly from those in nontransplant patients. Mycobacteria should be remembered as a potential cause of lung nodules or masses in lung transplant recipients (Fig. 6.102).[441,443–445,449,450]

Box 6.14 Bronchiolitis obliterans syndrome (BOS)

Etiology
Chronic immunologic rejection

Risk factors
Multiple episodes of acute rejection
Severe episodes of acute rejection
CMV infection

Histopathology
Obliterative bronchiolitis
Lymphocytic bronchiolitis/bronchitis

Prevalence
15–50% of all lung transplant recipients
50% of 5-year survivors have BOS

Diagnosis
>20% decrement in postoperative FEV_1 or characteristic findings on lung biopsy

CT findings
Mosaic attenuation
Bronchial wall thickening
Bronchiectasis
Air-trapping*

*Most sensitive finding for early BOS.

Obliterative bronchiolitis is the most important cause of morbidity and mortality in heart–lung and lung transplant recipients who survive more than one year (Box 6.14). It is now the major factor limiting longterm survival after transplantation.[451,453] Obliterative bronchiolitis accounts for 30% of deaths between 1 and 3 years post transplant and 33% of deaths thereafter (www.ishlt.org/registries). The prevalence of BOS in long term survivors is between 15% and 50% and the mortality rate is 29–50%.[365,397,452] It usually develops within 6–18 months after transplantation, but may occur as early as the second month.[397,454] At 5 years, approximately 50% of transplant recipients will have developed obliterative bronchiolitis. The disease is about equally prevalent in recipients of heart–lung, single, and bilateral lung transplants.[453]

Obliterative bronchiolitis is thought to result from chronic immunologic rejection.[453,455] However, other factors including viral infection, acute rejection, environmental exposures, and

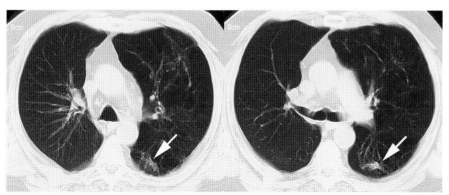

Fig. 6.102 *Mycobacterium avium–intracellulare* complex infection after right SLT for emphysema. CT shows spiculated nodules (arrows) in the native left lung. Cultures from lung biopsy specimens showed MAC.

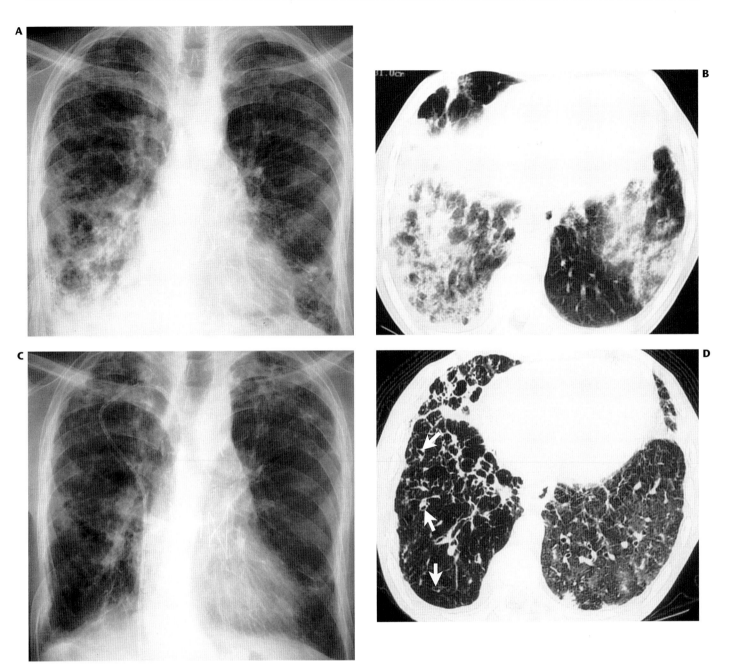

Fig. 6.103 Acute rejection and subsequent bronchiolitis obliterans syndrome after BLT for cystic fibrosis. **A,** A frontal chest radiograph obtained after the patient discontinued cyclosporine (against medical advice) and presented with fever and dyspnea shows bilateral, right greater than left, heterogeneous opacities and a right pleural effusion. **B,** CT shows diffuse ground-glass opacities and consolidation. Lung biopsy showed grade 4 acute rejection. The patient was treated for acute rejection with symptomatic improvement. **C,** A chest radiograph obtained 1 year later when the patient presented with worsening dyspnea and declining FEV_1 shows resolution of consolidation but increased diffuse coarse reticular opacities. **D,** HRCT shows decreased lung attenuation and bronchial dilatation (white arrows) in the right lower lobe consistent with obliterative bronchiolitis. The patient clinically had BOS-2.

graft aging may play a role.[453] Estenne et al[453] reviewed the literature regarding risk factors for developing obliterative bronchiolitis. They concluded that acute rejection, lymphocytic bronchitis or bronchiolitis, CMV pneumonia, and medication noncompliance were the most important risk factors for subsequent development of obliterative bronchiolitis. There is a significant correlation between frequency and severity of episodes of acute rejection and development of obliterative bronchiolitis (Fig. 6.103).[456] Estenne et al[453] also noted that the

risk inferred by CMV pneumonia was more significant in the early transplant era, perhaps because of less effective therapies or prophylaxis. Potential risk factors for which they[453] found less substantial evidence include CMV infection without pneumonia, organizing pneumonia, bacterial, fungal, and non-CMV viral pneumonia, and longer graft ischemic times. Other putative risk factors for which there is little solid evidence include underlying disease, HLA mismatching, genetic susceptibility, and gastroesophageal reflux with aspiration.[453]

Obliterative bronchiolitis, as the name implies, primarily affects the small airways of the lung. Early histopathologic manifestations include lymphocytic infiltration of the airway wall, a nonspecific inflammatory reaction with neutrophils, and intraluminal polyps composed of granulation tissue.[453] Later on, complete obliteration of the airway lumen by fibrous scar is seen. Because the process is heterogeneous, random lung biopsies may show a more active, but less specific, bronchocentric inflammatory process rather than the more specific fibrous lesions. For this reason, transbronchial lung biopsy may not be diagnostic of obliterative bronchiolitis, particularly in the early stages.[452,455,457,458]

Obliterative bronchiolitis clinically manifests with worsening dyspnea and progressive loss of lung function. Affected patients experience a significant reduction in quality of life and increased risk for death.[454,456] The disease pursues a variable course, however. Some patients experience a rapid inexorable decline to death. Others experience periods of decline followed by periods of stability or even improvement.[453] Obliterative bronchiolitis in patients who have been retransplanted for OB can pursue an accelerated course.[459] Early diagnosis of obliterative bronchiolitis is important because some reports suggest that initiation of augmented immunosuppressive therapy can stabilize or improve lung function.[460,461]

Because transbronchial lung biopsies are frequently nondiagnostic, obliterative bronchiolitis is typically diagnosed clinically. The term "bronchiolitis obliterans syndrome" (BOS) is now used for lung transplant recipients who experience an otherwise unexplained loss of lung function that is presumed to be due to obliterative bronchiolitis.[453,455] Although the exact criteria used to diagnose BOS are in flux, the current standard for diagnosis is a 20% or greater decrease in FEV_1 in the posttransplant period.[455] BOS is graded from BOS-0 to BOS-3 depending upon the severity of lung dysfunction by using the ratio of current FEV_1 to best posttransplant FEV_1.[455] Recent data, however, suggest that the 20% cut-off point used to differentiate BOS-0 (no disease) from BOS-1 may not be sensitive enough to detect early BOS. Furthermore, these data suggest that a decline in FEF_{25-75}, a marker for small airway dysfunction, may be a more sensitive indicator of early BOS. Thus, Estenne et al[453]

suggest a category of BOS-0p to denote patients with potential BOS who have a 10–19% decline in FEV_1 or who have a greater than 25% decline in FEF_{25-75} without a change in FEV_1. Diagnosis of BOS requires exclusion of other causes of graft dysfunction such as central airway stenosis, acute rejection, infection, progressive underlying lung disease, and heart failure.[453]

Chest radiographic findings of BOS are usually subtle or nonspecific, and frequently nonexistent. The chest radiograph is likely to be normal in the early stages and may remain normal throughout the course of the disease. Skeens et al[462] reported chest radiographic findings in 11 patients with histopathologically proven obliterative bronchiolitis after heart–lung transplantation. Presumably, all patients had very advanced disease. The most distinctive finding in this group was central bronchiectasis, seen in 9 patients. Findings of reticular or reticulonodular opacities in a peripheral or basal distribution, seen in all patients, were less specific (Fig. 6.103C). Pulmonary hyperinflation, reflecting air-trapping, is occasionally noted.

There has been intense interest in the use of CT to diagnose obliterative bronchiolitis/BOS. Typical CT findings include bronchial wall thickening, bronchial dilatation, mosaic attenuation, and air-trapping on expiratory images (Figs 6.103 to 6.105).[463–471] Numerous investigators have shown that air-trapping on expiratory CT is the most sensitive predictor of BOS[465,467] in lung transplant recipients (Fig. 6.104). Bankier et al,[467] for example, prospectively studied 38 transplant recipients and found that air-trapping was 83% sensitive and 89% specific for the diagnosis of BOS in patients with clinically evident disease. Siegel et al,[465] studying a smaller group of pediatric transplant recipients with BOS, reported a sensitivity of 100% and a specificity of 71% for air-trapping. Both groups also reported an extremely high negative predictive value for air-trapping on expiratory CT. Several studies have further suggested that CT may be useful for early diagnosis of BOS, prior to onset of clinical symptoms and decline in respiratory function.[463,465,467,471] Bankier et al[467] found that patients without clinical BOS who had air-trapping involving greater than 32% of the lung were at significantly increased risk for developing BOS. Knollmann et al[463] used spirometrically gated CT to investigate 49 lung transplant recipients without clinical BOS.

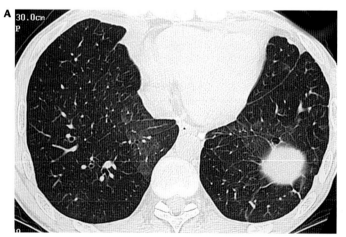
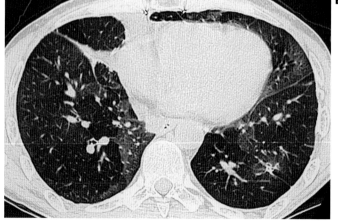

Fig. 6.104 Mild bronchiolitis obliterans syndrome (BOS-1) after BLT for pneumoconiosis. **A,** Inspiratory HRCT shows subtle mosaic attenuation. The airways appear normal. **B,** Expiratory HRCT shows marked air-trapping consistent with BOS. The patient eventually required retransplantation for progressive BOS.

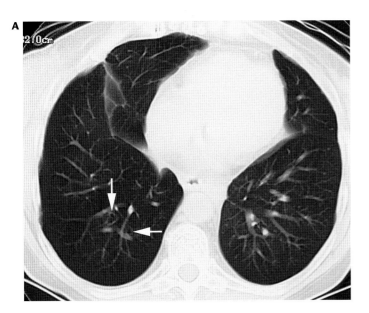

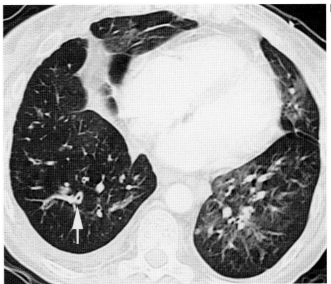

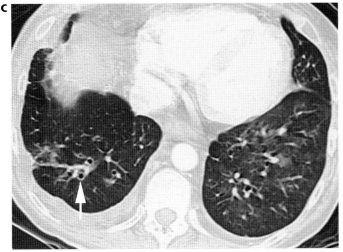

Fig. 6.105 Severe bronchiolitis obliterans syndrome (BOS-3) after BLT for lymphangioleiomyomatosis. **A**, Conventional CT shows decreased attenuation in the right lower lung and mild bronchiectasis (arrows). **B** and **C**, HRCT obtained 3 months after **A** shows increased bronchial wall thickening and bronchiectasis (arrows) in the right lower lobe.

They found that mean lung attenuation was significantly lower in the patients who subsequently developed BOS than in the patients who maintained normal lung function.

Other investigators have questioned the ability of CT to diagnose BOS. Lee et al[472] reported limited accuracy in diagnosing early obliterative bronchiolitis using CT in a small series of lung transplant recipients. Loubeyre et al[473] studied 40 lung transplant recipients (14 with BOS) and concluded that although CT findings were supportive of the diagnosis when pulmonary function impairment was limited, the diagnosis of BOS should be primarily based on pulmonary function testing. Miller et al[466] found that none of the typical CT findings associated with established BOS (bronchial dilatation, bronchial wall thickening, mosaic attenuation, and air-trapping) was sensitive or specific for prediction of subsequent BOS. Furthermore, Choi et al,[464] in a large series of transplant recipients with BOS, found only limited correlation between CT findings and severity of BOS. Possible reasons for these disparate results include the small sample size used in many studies (rarely more than 20 patients with BOS), markedly different patient selection criteria used for inclusion in the studies, differences in CT technique, and variability in diagnosis of BOS. Some studies included only patients with histopathologically proved

BO[468,470,472] whereas others included patients with clinical BOS without histopathologic proof.[465–467] These conflicting results mean that the precise role of CT for diagnosis of BOS (particularly early disease) remains uncertain.[464]

Hyperpolarized gas enhanced MR imaging has been investigated for diagnosis of BOS in lung transplant recipients[474–478]: helium-3 is the gas most commonly used. Following inhalation of gas, a significant increase in MR signal is seen in normal lung. Preliminary data suggest that this technique can identify ventilation defects in patients with BOS,[474] that the number of the defects correlates with severity of BOS (Fig. 6.106),[474] and that more defects are seen by MR than expiratory CT.[476] Furthermore, defects can be seen in patients without BOS, suggesting that the technique could prove useful for early diagnosis of BOS.[478] However, the utility of this technique for diagnosis of BOS is unknown at this time.

Complications after single lung transplantation

Most complications that occur after single lung transplantation, such as acute graft dysfunction, reperfusion edema, and acute or chronic rejection, occur exclusively in the allograft.[407] Others, such as posttransplant lymphoproliferative disorder (see

A

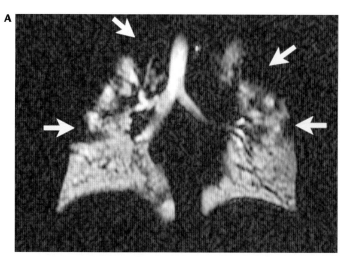

B

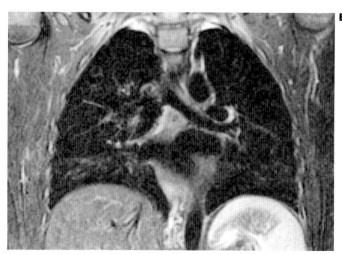

Fig. 6.106 Mild bronchiolitis obliterans syndrome (BOS-1) after BLT for cystic fibrosis. Chest CT was normal. **A**, A helium-3 enhanced coronal MR image shows multiple, peripheral, and predominantly upper lobe ventilation defects (arrows). **B**, A coronal FSE proton MR image is shown for anatomic correlation. (Reprinted from ref 478a by courtesy of Marcel Dekker Inc.)

below) and infection, occur more frequently in the allograft than in the native lung.[479,480] However, complications that primarily involve the native lung occur in up to 25% of single lung transplant recipients.[407,481] These complications include both acute and chronic hyperinflation of the native lung in patients with emphysema,[482,483] infection,[407,479,481] lung cancer,[407,481,484] and pulmonary embolism.[407] These complications are associated with high morbidity and mortality. Twenty-five percent of patients in one series[481] experienced significant morbidity and mortality from native lung complications; 29% of patients in a second series[407] died from complications originating in the native lung.

In the immediate postoperative period, the native lung of patients transplanted for emphysema may acutely over-inflate, resulting in problems with ventilation and gas exchange. Hemodynamic collapse due to tamponade of the heart and allograft can also occur.[361,434] Fortunately, this severe outcome is quite uncommon. Weill et al[482] reviewed their experience with 51 consecutive SLT procedures for emphysema: 16 patients (31%) had radiographic evidence of acute native lung hyperinflation but only 8 (16%) were symptomatic. All patients responded well to conservative medical and ventilator management; none had adverse late effects on graft function. Some patients with emphysema treated by SLT experience gradual native lung hyperinflation and apparent graft shrinkage.[485] Malchow et al[483] evaluated 32 SLT recipients treated for emphysema and found that half had evidence of progressive native lung hyperinflation (and graft shrinkage) on postoperative radiographs (Fig. 6.107).[483] Some patients with native lung hyperinflation experience a significant decline in postoperative lung function.[361,486] For instance, Malchow et al[483] found that the hyperinflated group in their series fared poorly compared to the non-hyperinflated group based on serial FEV_1 measurements. Whether this decline or decrement in lung function is the result of chronic native lung hyperinflation and graft compression or the result of chronic graft infection or rejection is often difficult to determine *a priori*.[482,485] Some patients with native lung hyperinflation and declining lung function show clinical improvement following contralateral lung volume reduction surgery,[487–489] whereas

others do not. Identifying which patients with native lung hyperexpansion will benefit from lung volume reduction surgery and which will not has proved a difficult task.

While native lung infection is clearly not as common as allograft infection, it can be associated with high morbidity and mortality. Infection accounts for most serious native lung complications and deaths.[407,481,490] Bacteria and opportunistic fungi are the most frequent pathogens (Figs 6.101 and 6.102). Interestingly, opportunistic viral pneumonia, particularly CMV, is quite uncommon in the native lung.[407,481] Bacterial pneumonia in the native lung manifests in typical fashion, with acute onset of cough, fever, and dyspnea. Chest radiographs usually show focal opacities in a segmental or lobar distribution.[407]

Non-small cell cancer is an important, but uncommon, complication that has been reported almost exclusively in the native lung of SLT recipients (Fig. 6.108).[481,484,491,492] Collins et al[484] reviewed 2168 consecutive transplant recipients at seven transplant centers who survived one month or more. Twenty-four (1%) SLT recipients developed cancers that always arose in the native lung. Cancer developed twice as frequently in native fibrotic lungs than emphysematous lungs. As expected, cancer in the native lung most commonly manifested as a pulmonary nodule or mass (Fig. 6.108). Less common manifestations included mediastinal mass or lobar atelectasis.

Recurrent disease

Many diseases, including sarcoidosis,[493] lymphangioleiomyomatosis,[494] diffuse panbronchiolitis,[495] giant cell interstitial pneumonia,[496] Langerhans cell histiocytosis,[497,498] and alveolar proteinosis[499] can recur in the transplanted lung. The radiologic manifestations of recurrent disease in the allograft are generally similar to those of the original disease and can mimic other posttransplant complications, including infection, rejection, and posttransplant lymphoproliferative disorder (PTLD). The risk, however, seems to be quite small. Collins et al[500] reviewed 1394 transplant recipients and found 15 (1%) with biopsy-proven recurrent disease in the allograft. Sarcoidosis was the most common disease to recur (35% of 26 patients transplanted for

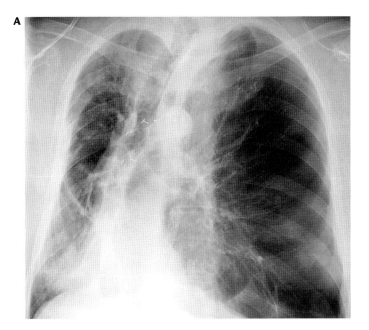

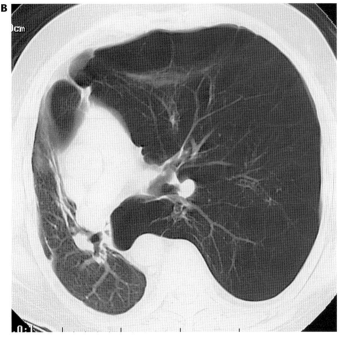

Fig. 6.107 Hyperinflation of the native lung after left SLT for emphysema. **A**, A frontal chest radiograph shows marked hyperinflation of the native right lung. **B**, CT demonstrates the severity of the allograft (right lung) compression. The patient had declining respiratory function but refused left lung volume reduction surgery.

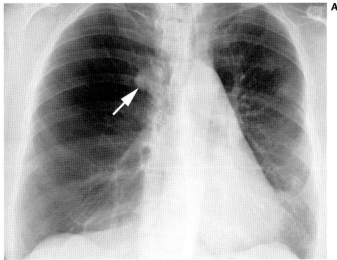

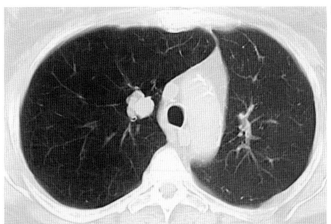

Fig. 6.108 Lung cancer arising in the native lung after left SLT for emphysema. Frontal chest radiograph (**A**) and CT (**B**) show a nodule (arrow on **A**) in the right upper lobe. Note the native lung emphysema. Resection confirmed stage 1 non-small cell lung cancer.

sarcoidosis). Interestingly, most (66%) of the cases of recurrent sarcoid were clinically and radiologically occult; disease was found on routine surveillance lung biopsies (Fig. 6.109).

Pleural complications

Significant pleural complications after lung transplantation are seen in up to 22% of patients and include empyema, parapneumonic effusion, hemothorax, and chylothorax.[369,501] Because BLT or heart–lung transplantation frequently results in a single communicating pleural space (so-called "buffalo chest"[502]), these air and fluid collections are often bilateral (Fig. 6.110).[369,503,504] Such pneumothoraces may preferentially accumulate in the retrosternal region, and a lateral radiograph may be needed to accurately assess their size.[369]

Pleural effusion occurs in virtually all lung transplant recipients in the early postoperative period.[387] Most early effusions are self-limited and resolve within two weeks of transplantation.[387,505] Causes of early effusions include increased capillary permeability due to ischemia/reperfusion injury,[506] disruption of lymphatic flow in the allograft,[507] hemorrhage, and acute lung rejection.[400,406] If pleural fluid decreases and the patient shows clinical improvement in the first two weeks after transplantation, examination or drainage of small-to-moderate pleural fluid collections is usually not necessary.[505]

New pleural effusions or those persisting beyond the first two weeks are more concerning. Potential etiologies for such late effusions include empyema or parapneumonic effusion, acute rejection (see Fig. 6.92), organizing pleural hematoma, lymphoproliferative disorder, and cardiac or renal failure. Marom et al[508] studied 31 transplant recipients referred for radiology-guided drainage of pleural fluid. In their series, half

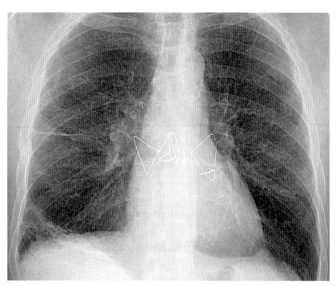

Fig. 6.109 Recurrent sarcoidosis after BLT. Surveillance lung biopsies showed findings of recurrent sarcoidosis 9 months after transplantation. A frontal chest radiograph (not shown) obtained at that time was normal. The chest radiograph (shown) obtained 18 months after surgery shows diffuse small nodular opacities (miliary pattern). Biopsy reconfirmed sarcoidosis and excluded infection.

of the effusions were due to infection; the remainder were related to acute lung rejection or cardiac or renal failure. Empyema is a potentially disastrous complication in lung transplant recipients, especially in BLT recipients in whom both pleural spaces may directly communicate.[509] Empyema in one thorax must be rapidly diagnosed and adequately drained so that infected pleural contents do not contaminate the contralateral pleural space (Fig. 6.111). Mortality from empyema is high in lung transplant recipients, ranging from 28% to 44%.[501,508,510]

Late effusions are often managed aggressively for several reasons. First, it is clearly important to diagnose and treat pleural space infection as rapidly as possible. Second, an uninfected effusion may be drained in order to prevent secondary infection, a phenomenon that has been reported in immunocompetent hosts.[511,512] Third, an effusion may be drained to improve pulmonary function. Data in non-transplant patients suggests that even small effusions can cause significant respiratory compromise and hypoxemia[513] and that their evacuation may relieve dyspnea and improve lung function.[514] Thus, if the transplant recipient is symptomatic, the fluid is usually drained. Finally, effusions may be drained to prevent the potential late complication of fibrothorax. Fibrothorax, it is assumed, could result from persistent undrained pleural fluid and could cause shortness of breath, chest pain, and a late decline in FEV_1, mimicking rejection. Although there is evidence to this effect in non-transplant patients,[515–517] this rationale for drainage in lung transplant recipients is unproven.

Marom et al[508] reported success with radiology-guided small-bore catheter drainage of pleural fluid in lung transplant recipients. In that series, partial or complete resolution of fluid occurred in over 90% of treated patients. Because the effusions were frequently loculated, the authors found that effective drainage often required multiple tubes and fibrolytic therapy with streptokinase. Drainage was also typically prolonged.

Miscellaneous complications

Phrenic nerve paralysis is an uncommon complication (less than 4%) of lung transplantation.[410] Recent transbronchial lung biopsy can result in focal lung nodules or cavities that must be distinguished from infection or malignancy (Fig. 6.112).[518,519] Up

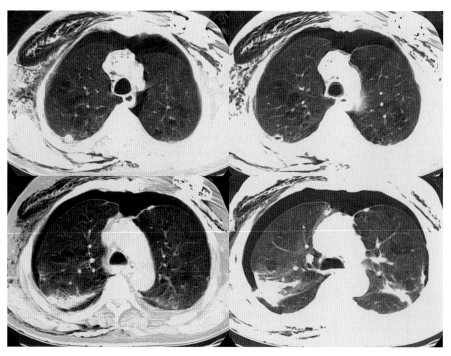

Fig. 6.110 Communicating pleural spaces ("buffalo chest") after BLT for emphysema. CT shows that pleural spaces communicate anteriorly. Note the extensive subcutaneous emphysema.

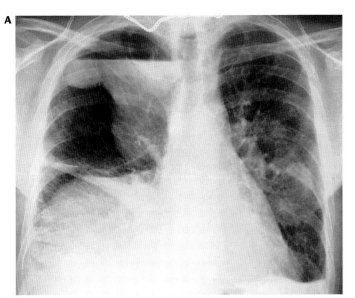

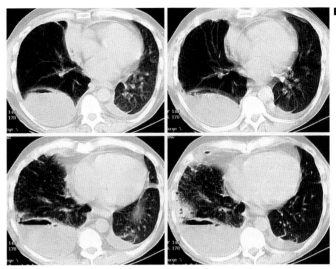

Fig. 6.111 Empyema after left SLT for emphysema. Frontal chest radiograph (**A**) and CT (**B**) show loculated right pleural fluid collections. Aspiration confirmed bacterial empyema.

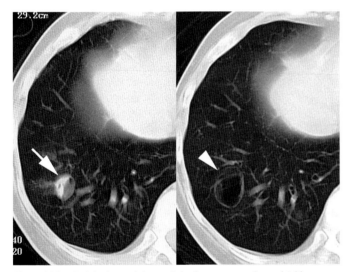

Fig. 6.112 A right lower lobe nodule due to a transbronchial lung biopsy after right SLT for pulmonary fibrosis. Sequential CT images obtained 2 months apart show a right lower lobe nodule (arrow) after lung biopsy. Repeat CT shows an enlarging pneumatocele at the site of previous biopsy (arrowhead).

to 5% of patients with an omental wrap procedure to either prevent or repair bronchial anastomotic dehiscence may require an emergency laparotomy to correct intrathoracic herniation of abdominal contents.[520] The omental wrap can also simulate a hilar or mediastinal mass on chest radiographs; CT is useful for showing the fatty nature of this abnormality.[413] Living related donor transplants present particular problems in postoperative management. Because of frequent size mismatch between donor lobe and recipient hemithorax, postoperative air leaks and pleural fluid drainage may be prolonged. Reperfusion edema may also be more severe in these patients.[363]

Differential diagnosis of new pulmonary opacities in lung transplant recipients

The differential diagnosis of new pulmonary opacities in lung transplant recipients is extensive. The differential can be appropriately tailored, however, by consideration of the nature of the opacities and the time course of presentation after transplantation. The following "rules of thumb" may be helpful[375]:

- Pulmonary opacities in the first week after transplantation are usually the result of ischemia/reperfusion edema. Persistent, new, or worsening opacities after that time suggest infection or acute rejection.
- Pleural fluid is common in the first two weeks after transplantation. Persistent, new, or worsening effusions after that time suggest acute rejection, infection, or malignancy. The diagnosis must be aggressively pursued.
- Bacterial pneumonia is most common in the first month after transplantation; opportunistic infection with CMV or fungus becomes more common thereafter.
- Nodular opacities or masses suggest infection (bacterial, fungal, mycobacterial) or malignancy (PTLD or cancer). The diagnosis must be aggressively pursued. Occasionally, hematoma from recent transbronchial biopsy can result in a focal lung nodule.
- Bronchiolitis obliterans syndrome manifests on HRCT with mosaic attenuation, air-trapping, and progressive bronchial dilatation. Air-trapping is the most sensitive CT finding for early BOS.

Lymphoproliferative disease in organ transplant recipients

Posttransplant lymphoproliferative disorder (PTLD) is an important cause of morbidity and mortality in transplant recipients (Box 6.15).[521] Overall, between 1% and 10% of

Box 6.15 Posttransplant lymphoproliferative disorder

Incidence
1–10%, highest in lung transplant recipients

Histopathology
Variable
Most of B-cell origin

Etiology
EBV-infected B cells

Risk factors
EBV infection
Severity and type of immune suppression

Mortality
40–70%

Prognosis
Depends on number of sites involved

Time to onset
Median 6 months in solid organ transplant recipients
Median 60–90 days in bone marrow recipients

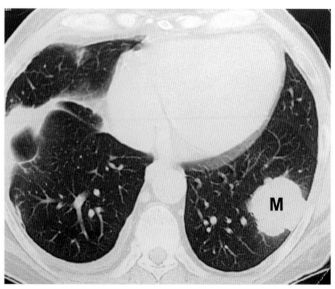

Fig. 6.113 Posttransplant lymphoproliferative disorder after BLT for emphysema. CT shows a lobulated mass (M) in the left lower lobe. No other sites of disease were found.

transplant recipients develop PTLD.[352,522,523] It occurs in all transplant populations, both solid organ and hematopoietic, but the highest incidence is in the lung transplant population.[521,524] The overall mortality of PTLD is difficult to assess due to the heterogeneity of the disease (see below) and the variety of associated co-morbidities. Mortality rates of 40–70% have been reported in recipients of solid organ transplants.[524] PTLD accounts for about 3% of deaths in lung transplant recipients in the first year after surgery; its importance as a cause of death declines thereafter (www.ishlt.org/registries). Although time of onset varies, most cases occur within two years of transplantation.[525,526] The median time to onset is 6 months in the solid organ transplant population and 60–90 days in the allogeneic bone marrow transplant population.[524] Late-onset cases, which may not be EBV-related (see below), are increasingly reported.[525]

PTLD is a heterogeneous disease that varies from a mononucleosis-type illness with nonspecific polyclonal lymphoid proliferation to a monoclonal, cytologically atypical proliferation that resembles immunoblastic lymphoma.[522,525,527–529] The histopathologic classification of PTLD is currently in flux.[524] PTLD is strongly associated with both the type and degree of immune suppression as well as infection with Epstein–Barr virus (EBV).[530–532] EBV-negative serology prior to transplantation and EBV seroconversion after transplantation is a major risk factor for development of PTLD.[533,534] Further risk factors in solid organ transplant recipients include lung or heart–lung transplantation, specific antilymphocyte therapy (tacrolimus, antithymocyte globulin) and high levels of immune suppression.[523,524] Current theories of pathogenesis suggest that PTLD results from proliferation of EBV-infected B cells in the setting of defective T-cell function.[524] Most cases (90%) are thus of donor B-cell lymphocyte origin. Evidence suggests that at least some cases respond favorably to reduction of immune suppression and administration of antiviral agents.[349,524,535] Nevertheless, as noted above, PTLD can be lethal and early diagnosis is considered vital.

The histopathologic pattern of disease is not as reliable a predictor of clinical behavior and prognosis as is the anatomic extent of disease.[525,529,536] The number of disease sites correlates better with overall tumor burden than does the Ann Arbor stage.[521,525,537] Patients with multifocal disease have a worse prognosis than do patients with anatomically limited disease.[529] PTLD is frequently extranodal in location: the central nervous system, tonsils, gastrointestinal tract, and lungs are the common sites of disease.[350] The allograft is frequently affected as well.[524] The number of disease sites influences treatment. Local therapy, such as resection or limited field irradiation, can result in longterm remission in patients with anatomically limited PTLD. Patients with more widespread disease usually require more aggressive systemic therapy.[536] Thus, accurate depiction of disease extent, or staging, is of critical importance.[525]

The clinical manifestations of PTLD are heterogeneous. Some patients present with a mononucleosis-type illness and complain of fever, night sweats, and weight loss. Others present with complaints related to mass effect or organ system dysfunction due to PTLD. Still others are asymptomatic at presentation, with disease detected on routine surveillance studies such as chest radiographs. The exact incidence of thoracic involvement is uncertain and probably varies by transplant population. In one small series encompassing a variety of transplant and other immunosuppressed populations, approximately half of cases involved the thorax.[139] The incidence of thoracic disease may be higher in lung transplant recipients than in recipients of other solid organs.[538] At least 70% of lung transplant recipients with PTLD have thoracic disease.[480,521,538]

Thoracic PTLD most commonly manifests as solitary or multiple well-circumscribed pulmonary nodules or masses (Figs 6.113 and 6.114; Box 6.16).[350,351,527,529,539] The nodules typically range in size from 0.3 to 5 cm in diameter, predominantly occur in the middle and lower lobes, are peribronchovascular in distribution, and grow slowly.[139,480,527,528] On CT, a subtle halo of ground-glass attenuation is sometimes seen around the nodule.[167,527] Dodd et al[349] reported that the nodules were

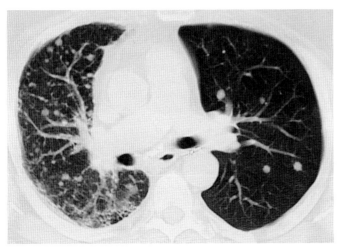

Fig. 6.114 Posttransplant lymphoproliferative disorder after left SLT for pulmonary fibrosis. CT shows multiple nodules in both lungs.

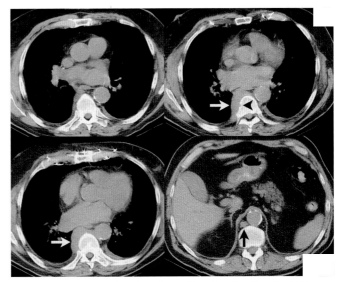

Fig. 6.115 Posttransplant lymphoproliferative disorder after BLT for COPD. CT shows an infiltrative right paravertebral mass (white arrows). Note the subtle vertebral body invasion (arrowhead) and retrocrural lymphadenopathy (black arrow).

Box 6.16 Thoracic posttransplant lymphoproliferative disorder

Incidence
Variable
70% in lung transplant recipients

Common radiologic manifestations
Nodules or masses (most common)
Lymphadenopathy

Uncommon radiologic manifestations
Focal or diffuse consolidation
Septal thickening
Endobronchial lesion
Thymic enlargement
Pericardial or pleural thickening or effusion

---

typically solid on CT; evidence of central necrosis was exceptional and suggested an inflammatory etiology. The reported incidence of thoracic hilar and mediastinal lymphadenopathy varies: Dodd et al[349] reported a very high incidence, Collins et al[139] reported an incidence of 38%, and Rappaport et al[527] reported a very low incidence in lung transplant recipients with PTLD. Less common manifestations of PTLD in the thorax include focal or diffuse consolidation, ground-glass opacity, septal thickening, endobronchial lesions, thymic enlargement, pericardial or pleural thickening, or effusion (Fig. 6.115).[139,349,480,527,538] Pickhardt et al[480] noted a marked survival difference based upon the radiographic appearance of disease. Patients in whom PTLD manifested as a solitary nodule had much better survival at 1 year (89%) than those who presented with multifocal disease (35%). Abdominal disease is also common at presentation.[538] Typical abdominal manifestations include bowel wall thickening, lymphadenopathy, and focal masses involving multiple organs.[538,540]

REFERENCES

1. Shah RM, Kaji AV, Ostrum BJ, et al. Interpretation of chest radiographs in AIDS patients: usefulness of CD4 lymphocyte counts. RadioGraphics 1997;17:47–58, discussion 59–61.
2. Haramati LB, Jenny-Avital ER. Approach to the diagnosis of pulmonary disease in patients infected with the human immunodeficiency virus. J Thorac Imaging 1998;13:247–260.
3. Reiter GS. Clinical correlates of human immunodeficiency virus (HIV)-related immunosuppression. Semin Ultrasound CT MR 1998;19:128–132.
4. Palella FJ Jr, Delaney KM, Moorman AC, et al. Declining morbidity and

mortality among patients with advanced human immunodeficiency virus infection. HIV Outpatient Study Investigators. N Engl J Med 1998;338:853–860.
5. French MA, Lenzo N, John M, et al. Immune restoration disease after the treatment of immunodeficient HIV-infected patients with highly active antiretroviral therapy. HIV Med 2000;1:107–115.
6. Jenny-Avital ER, Abadi M. Immune reconstitution cryptococcosis after initiation of successful highly active antiretroviral therapy. Clin Infect Dis 2002;35:e128–133.

7. Kunimoto DY, Chui L, Nobert E, et al. Immune mediated 'HAART' attack during treatment for tuberculosis. Highly active antiretroviral therapy. Int J Tuberc Lung Dis 1999;3:944–947.
8. Lederman MM, Valdez H. Immune restoration with antiretroviral therapies: implications for clinical management. JAMA 2000;284:223–228.
9. Price P, Mathiot N, Krueger R, et al. Immune dysfunction and immune restoration disease in HIV patients given highly active antiretroviral therapy. J Clin Virol 2001;22:279–287.
10. Trevenzoli M, Cattelan AM, Rea F, et al. Mediastinitis due to cryptococcal

infection: a new clinical entity in the HAART era. J Infect 2002;45:173–179.

11. Reiter GS. Human immunodeficiency virus (HIV) in America, 1981 to 1997: epidemiologic and therapeutic considerations. Semin Ultrasound CT MR 1998;19:122–127.

12. McGuinness G. Changing trends in the pulmonary manifestations of AIDS. Radiol Clin North Am 1997;35: 1029–1082.

13. Hirschtick RE, Glassroth J, Jordan MC, et al. Bacterial pneumonia in persons infected with the human immunodeficiency virus. Pulmonary Complications of HIV Infection Study Group. N Engl J Med 1995;333:845–851.

14. Amorosa JK, Nahass RG, Nosher JL, et al. Radiologic distinction of pyogenic pulmonary infection from Pneumocystis carinii pneumonia in AIDS patients. Radiology 1990;175:721–724.

15. Magnenat JL, Nicod LP, Auckenthaler R, et al. Mode of presentation and diagnosis of bacterial pneumonia in human immunodeficiency virus-infected patients. Am Rev Respir Dis 1991;144: 917–922.

16. Janoff EN, Breiman RF, Daley CL, et al. Pneumococcal disease during HIV infection. Epidemiologic, clinical, and immunologic perspectives. Ann Intern Med 1992;117:314–324.

17. Daley CL. Pyogenic bacterial pneumonia in the acquired immunodeficiency syndrome. J Thorac Imaging 1991;6: 36–42.

18. Traill ZC, Miller RF, Ali N, et al. Pseudomonas aeruginosa bronchopulmonary infection in patients with advanced human immunodeficiency virus disease. Br J Radiol 1996;69:1099–1103.

19. Linares MJ, Lopez-Encuentra A, Perea S. Chronic pneumonia caused by Rhodococcus equi in a patient without impaired immunity. Eur Respir J 1997;10:248–250.

20. Johnson DH, Cunha BA. Rhodococcus equi pneumonia. Semin Respir Infect 1997;12:57–60.

21. Mayor B, Jolidon RM, Wicky S, et al. Radiologic findings in two AIDS patients with Rhodococcus equi pneumonia. J Thorac Imaging 1995;10:121–125.

22. Amin Z, Miller RF, Shaw PJ. Lobar or segmental consolidation on chest radiographs of patients with HIV infection. Clin Radiol 1997;52:541–545.

23. Mirich D, Gray R, Hyland R. Legionella lung cavitation. Can Assoc Radiol J 1990;41:100–102.

24. Kramer MR, Uttamchandani RB. The radiographic appearance of pulmonary nocardiosis associated with AIDS. Chest 1990;98:382–385.

25. Uttamchandani RB, Daikos GL, Reyes RR, et al. Nocardiosis in 30 patients with advanced human immunodeficiency virus infection: clinical features and outcome. Clin Infect Dis 1994;18: 348–353.

26. Coche E, Beigelman C, Lucidarme O, et al. Thoracic bacillary angiomatosis in a patient with AIDS. AJR Am J Roentgenol 1995;165:56–58.

27. Moore EH, Russell LA, Klein JS, et al. Bacillary angiomatosis in patients with AIDS: multiorgan imaging findings. Radiology 1995;197:67–72.

28. Neville K, Bromberg A, Bromberg R. The third epidemic – multidrug-resistant tuberculosis. Chest 1994;105:45–48.

29. Goodman PC. Tuberculosis and AIDS. Radiol Clin North Am 1995;33:707–717.

30. Chaisson RE, Schecter GF, Theuer CP, et al. Tuberculosis in patients with the acquired immunodeficiency syndrome. Clinical features, response to therapy, and survival. Am Rev Respir Dis 1987;136:570–574.

31. Colebunders RL, Ryder RW, Nzilambi N, et al. HIV infection in patients with tuberculosis in Kinshasa, Zaire. Am Rev Respir Dis 1989;139:1082–1085.

32. Gutierrez J, Miralles R, Coll J, et al. Radiographic findings in pulmonary tuberculosis: the influence of human immunodeficiency virus infection. Eur J Radiol 1991;12:234–237.

33. Hill AR, Premkumar S, Brustein S, et al. Disseminated tuberculosis in the acquired immunodeficiency syndrome era. Am Rev Respir Dis 1991;144: 1164–1170.

34. Long R, Maycher B, Scalcini M, et al. The chest roentgenogram in pulmonary tuberculosis patients seropositive for human immunodeficiency virus type 1. Chest 1991;99:123–127.

35. Saks AM, Posner R. Tuberculosis in HIV positive patients in South Africa: a comparative radiological study with HIV negative patients. Clin Radiol 1992;46:387–390.

36. Asimos AW, Ehrhardt J. Radiographic presentation of pulmonary tuberculosis in severely immunosuppressed HIV-seropositive patients. Am J Emerg Med 1996;14:359–363.

37. Haramati LB, Jenny-Avital ER, Alterman DD. Effect of HIV status on chest radiographic and CT findings in patients with tuberculosis. Clin Radiol 1997;52: 31–35.

38. Greenberg SD, Frager D, Suster B, et al. Active pulmonary tuberculosis in patients with AIDS: spectrum of radiographic findings (including a normal appearance). Radiology 1994;193:115–119.

39. Keiper MD, Beumont M, Elshami A, et al. CD4 T lymphocyte count and the radiographic presentation of pulmonary tuberculosis. A study of the relationship between these factors in patients with human immunodeficiency virus infection. Chest 1995;107:74–80.

40. Tshibwabwa-Tumba E, Mwinga A, Pobee JO, et al. Radiological features of pulmonary tuberculosis in 963 HIV-infected adults at three Central African Hospitals. Clin Radiol 1997;52:837–841.

41. Leung AN, Brauner MW, Gamsu G, et al. Pulmonary tuberculosis: comparison of CT findings in HIV-seropositive and HIV-seronegative patients. Radiology 1996;198:687–691.

42. Laissy JP, Cadi M, Boudiaf ZE, et al. Pulmonary tuberculosis: computed tomography and high-resolution computed tomography patterns in patients who are either HIV-negative or HIV-seropositive. J Thorac Imaging 1998;13:58–64.

43. Haramati LB, Choi Y, Widrow CA, et al. Isolated lymphadenopathy on chest radiographs of HIV-infected patients. Clin Radiol 1996;51:345–349.

44. Hartman TE, Primack SL, Müller NL, et al. Diagnosis of thoracic complications in AIDS: accuracy of CT. AJR Am J Roentgenol 1994;162:547–553.

45. Perich J, Ayuso MC, Vilana R, et al. Disseminated lymphatic tuberculosis in acquired immunodeficiency syndrome: computed tomography findings. Can Assoc Radiol J 1990;41:353–357.

46. Pastores SM, Naidich DP, Aranda CP, et al. Intrathoracic adenopathy associated with pulmonary tuberculosis in patients with human immunodeficiency virus infection. Chest 1993;103:1433–1437.

47. Small PM, Hopewell PC, Schecter GF, et al. Evolution of chest radiographs in treated patients with pulmonary tuberculosis and HIV infection. J Thorac Imaging 1994;9:74–77.

48. Fishman JE, Saraf-Lavi E, Narita M, et al. Pulmonary tuberculosis in AIDS patients: transient chest radiographic worsening after initiation of antiretroviral therapy. AJR Am J Roentgenol 2000;174:43–49.

49. Schluger NW, Burzynski J. Tuberculosis and HIV infection: epidemiology, immunology, and treatment. HIV Clin Trials 2001;2:356–365.

50. Sterling TR, Lehmann HP, Frieden TR. Impact of DOTS compared with DOTS-plus on multidrug resistant tuberculosis and tuberculosis deaths: decision analysis. BMJ 2003;326:574.

51. Volmink J, Garner P. Directly observed therapy for treating tuberculosis. Cochrane Database Syst Rev 2003:CD003343.

52. Hocqueloux L, Lesprit P, Herrmann JL, et al. Pulmonary Mycobacterium avium complex disease without dissemination in HIV-infected patients. Chest 1998;113:542–548.

53. Kalayjian RC, Toossi Z, Tomashefski JF Jr, et al. Pulmonary disease due to

infection by Mycobacterium avium complex in patients with AIDS. Clin Infect Dis 1995;20:1186–1194.

54. Kotloff RM. Infection caused by nontuberculous mycobacteria: clinical aspects. Semin Roentgenol 1993;28:131–138.

55. MacDonell KB, Glassroth J. Mycobacterium avium complex and other nontuberculous mycobacteria in patients with HIV infection. Semin Respir Infect 1989;4:123–132.

56. Marinelli DL, Albelda SM, Williams TM, et al. Nontuberculous mycobacterial infection in AIDS: clinical, pathologic, and radiographic features. Radiology 1986;160:77–82.

57. Sider L, Gabriel H, Curry DR, et al. Pattern recognition of the pulmonary manifestations of AIDS on CT scans. RadioGraphics 1993;13:771–784; discussion 785–786.

58. Laissy JP, Cadi M, Cinqualbre A, et al. Mycobacterium tuberculosis versus nontuberculous mycobacterial infection of the lung in AIDS patients: CT and HRCT patterns. J Comput Assist Tomogr 1997;21:312–317.

59. Fishman JE, Schwartz DS, Sais GJ. Mycobacterium kansasii pulmonary infection in patients with AIDS: spectrum of chest radiographic findings. Radiology 1997;204:171–175.

60. Levine B, Chaisson RE. Mycobacterium kansasii: a cause of treatable pulmonary disease associated with advanced human immunodeficiency virus (HIV) infection. Ann Intern Med 1991;114:861–868.

61. Claydon EJ, Coker RJ, Harris JR. Mycobacterium malmoense infection in HIV positive patients. J Infect 1991;23:191–194.

62. Shafer RW, Sierra MF. Mycobacterium xenopi, Mycobacterium fortuitum, Mycobacterium kansasii, and other nontuberculous mycobacteria in an area of endemicity for AIDS. Clin Infect Dis 1992;15:161–162.

63. El-Solh AA, Nopper J, Abdul-Khoudoud MR, et al. Clinical and radiographic manifestations of uncommon pulmonary nontuberculous mycobacterial disease in AIDS patients. Chest 1998;114:138–145.

64. Bankier AA, Stauffer F, Fleischmann D, et al. Radiographic findings in patients with acquired immunodeficiency syndrome, pulmonary infection, and microbiologic evidence of Mycobacterium xenopi. J Thorac Imaging 1998;13:282–288.

65. Stringer JR, Beard CB, Miller RF, et al. A new name (Pneumocystis jiroveci) for Pneumocystis from humans. Emerg Infect Dis 2002;8:891–6.

66. Peters BS, Coleman D, Beck EJ, et al. Changing disease patterns in AIDS. BMJ 1991;302:726.

67. DeLorenzo LJ, Huang CT, Maguire GP, et al. Roentgenographic patterns of Pneumocystis carinii pneumonia in 104 patients with AIDS. Chest 1987;91:323–327.

68. Naidich DP, Garay SM, Leitman BS, et al. Radiographic manifestations of pulmonary disease in the acquired immunodeficiency syndrome (AIDS). Semin Roentgenol 1987;22:14–30.

69. Boiselle PM, Tocino I, Hooley RJ, et al. Chest radiograph interpretation of Pneumocystis carinii pneumonia, bacterial pneumonia, and pulmonary tuberculosis in HIV-positive patients: accuracy, distinguishing features, and mimics. J Thorac Imaging 1997;12:47–53.

70. Kuhlman JE, Kavuru M, Fishman EK, et al. Pneumocystis carinii pneumonia: spectrum of parenchymal CT findings. Radiology 1990;175:711–714.

71. Chaffey MH, Klein JS, Gamsu G, et al. Radiographic distribution of Pneumocystis carinii pneumonia in patients with AIDS treated with prophylactic inhaled pentamidine. Radiology 1990;175:715–719.

72. Kuhlman JE. Pneumocystic infections: the radiologist's perspective. Radiology 1996;198:623–635.

73. Goodman PC, Gamsu G. Radiographic findings in AIDS. Postgrad Radiol 1987;7:3–15.

74. Eagar GM, Friedland JA, Sagel SS. Tumefactive Pneumocystis carinii infection in AIDS: report of three cases. AJR Am J Roentgenol 1993;160:1197–1198.

75. Sivit CJ, Miller CR, Rakusan TA, et al. Spectrum of chest radiographic abnormalities in children with AIDS and Pneumocystis carinii pneumonia. Pediatr Radiol 1995;25:389–392.

76. Mayor B, Schnyder P, Giron J, et al. Mediastinal and hilar lymphadenopathy due to Pneumocystis carinii infection in AIDS patients: CT features. J Comput Assist Tomogr 1994;18:408–411.

77. Radin DR, Baker EL, Klatt EC, et al. Visceral and nodal calcification in patients with AIDS-related Pneumocystis carinii infection. AJR Am J Roentgenol 1990;154:27–31.

78. Groskin SA, Massi AF, Randall PA. Calcified hilar and mediastinal lymph nodes in an AIDS patient with Pneumocystis carinii infection. Radiology 1990;175:345–346.

79. Feuerstein IM, Francis P, Raffeld M, et al. Widespread visceral calcifications in disseminated Pneumocystis carinii infection: CT characteristics. J Comput Assist Tomogr 1990;14:149–151.

80. Abd AG, Nierman DM, Ilowite JS, et al. Bilateral upper lobe Pneumocystis carinii pneumonia in a patient receiving inhaled pentamidine prophylaxis. Chest 1988;94:329–331.

81. Edelstein H, McCabe RE. Atypical presentations of Pneumocystis carinii pneumonia in patients receiving inhaled pentamidine prophylaxis. Chest 1990;98:1366–1369.

82. Moskovic E, Miller R, Pearson M. High resolution computed tomography of Pneumocystis carinii pneumonia in AIDS. Clin Radiol 1990;42:239–243.

83. Naidich DP, McGuinness G. Pulmonary manifestations of AIDs. CT and radiographic correlations. Radiol Clin North Am 1991;29:999–1017.

84. Leung AN, Miller RR, Müller NL. Parenchymal opacification in chronic infiltrative lung diseases: CT–pathologic correlation. Radiology 1993;188:209–214.

85. Remy-Jardin M, Remy J, Giraud F, et al. Computed tomography assessment of ground-glass opacity: semiology and significance. J Thorac Imaging 1993;8:249–264.

86. Richards PJ, Riddell L, Reznek RH, et al. High resolution computed tomography in HIV patients with suspected Pneumocystis carinii pneumonia and a normal chest radiograph. Clin Radiol 1996;51:689–693.

87. Bergin CJ, Wirth RL, Berry GJ, et al. Pneumocystis carinii pneumonia: CT and HRCT observations. J Comput Assist Tomogr 1990;14:756–759.

88. Gruden JF, Huang L, Turner J, et al. High-resolution CT in the evaluation of clinically suspected Pneumocystis carinii pneumonia in AIDS patients with normal, equivocal, or nonspecific radiographic findings. AJR Am J Roentgenol 1997;169:967–975.

89. Hartelius H, Gaub J, Ingemann Jensen L, et al. Computed tomography of the lungs in acquired immunodeficiency syndrome. An early indicator of interstitial pneumonia. Acta Radiol 1988;29:641–644.

90. Kramer EL, Sanger JJ, Garay SM, et al. Gallium-67 scans of the chest in patients with acquired immunodeficiency syndrome. J Nucl Med 1987;28:1107–1114.

91. O'Doherty MJ, Page CJ, Bradbeer CS, et al. The place of lung 99mTc DTPA aerosol transfer in the investigation of lung infections in HIV positive patients. Respir Med 1989;83:395–401.

92. Barron TF, Birnbaum NS, Shane LB, et al. Pneumocystis carinii pneumonia studied by gallium-67 scanning. Radiology 1985;154:791–793.

93. Chow C, Templeton PA, White CS. Lung cysts associated with Pneumocystis carinii pneumonia: radiographic characteristics, natural history, and complications. AJR Am J Roentgenol 1993;161:527–531.

94. Sandhu JS, Goodman PC. Pulmonary cysts associated with Pneumocystis carinii pneumonia in patients with AIDS. Radiology 1989;173:33–35.

95. Feurestein IM, Archer A, Pluda JM, et al. Thin-walled cavities, cysts, and pneumothorax in Pneumocystis carinii pneumonia: further observations with histopathologic correlation. Radiology 1990;174:697–702.

96. Travis WD, Pittaluga S, Lipschik GY, et al. Atypical pathologic manifestations of Pneumocystis carinii pneumonia in the acquired immune deficiency syndrome. Review of 123 lung biopsies from 76 patients with emphasis on cysts, vascular invasion, vasculitis, and granulomas. Am J Surg Pathol 1990;14:615–625.

97. Tung KT. Cystic pulmonary lesions in AIDS. Clin Radiol 1992;45:149–152.

98. Gurney JW, Bates FT. Pulmonary cystic disease: comparison of Pneumocystis carinii pneumatoceles and bullous emphysema due to intravenous drug abuse. Radiology 1989;173:27–31.

99. Coker RJ, Moss F, Peters B, et al. Pneumothorax in patients with AIDS. Respir Med 1993;87:43–47.

100. Murry CE, Schmidt RA. Tissue invasion by Pneumocystis carinii: a possible cause of cavitary pneumonia and pneumothorax. Hum Pathol 1992; 23:1380–1387.

101. Kuhlman JE, Knowles MC, Fishman EK, et al. Premature bullous pulmonary damage in AIDS: CT diagnosis. Radiology 1989;173:23–26.

102. Evlogias NE, Leonidas JC, Rooney J, et al. Severe cystic pulmonary disease associated with chronic Pneumocystis carinii infection in a child with AIDS. Pediatr Radiol 1994;24:606–608.

103. Wassermann K, Pothoff G, Kirn E, et al. Chronic Pneumocystis carinii pneumonia in AIDS. Chest 1993; 104:667–672.

104. Tumbarello M, Tacconelli E, Pirronti T, et al. Pneumothorax in HIV-infected patients: role of Pneumocystis carinii pneumonia and pulmonary tuberculosis. Eur Respir J 1997;10:1332–1335.

105. Newsome GS, Ward DJ, Pierce PF. Spontaneous pneumothorax in patients with acquired immunodeficiency syndrome treated with prophylactic aerosolized pentamidine. Arch Intern Med 1990;150:2167–2168.

106. Slabbynck H, Kovitz KL, Vialette JP, et al. Thoracoscopic findings in spontaneous pneumothorax in AIDS. Chest 1994;106: 1582–1586.

107. Stansell JD. Fungal disease in HIV-infected persons: cryptococcosis, histoplasmosis, and coccidioidomycosis. J Thorac Imaging 1991;6:28–35.

108. Murray JF, Mills J. Pulmonary infectious complications of human immunodeficiency virus infection. Part I. Am Rev Respir Dis 1990;141:1356–1372.

109. Kuhlman JE. Pulmonary manifestations of acquired immunodeficiency syndrome. Semin Roentgenol 1994;29:242–274.

110. Cameron ML, Bartlett JA, Gallis HA, et al. Manifestations of pulmonary cryptococcosis in patients with acquired immunodeficiency syndrome. Rev Infect Dis 1991;13:64–67.

111. Chechani V, Kamholz SL. Pulmonary manifestations of disseminated cryptococcosis in patients with AIDS. Chest 1990;98:1060–1066.

112. Miller WT Jr, Edelman JM, Miller WT. Cryptococcal pulmonary infection in patients with AIDS: radiographic appearance. Radiology 1990;175:725–728.

113. Sider L, Westcott MA. Pulmonary manifestations of cryptococcosis in patients with AIDS: CT features. J Thorac Imaging 1994;9:78–84.

114. Suster B, Akerman M, Orenstein M, et al. Pulmonary manifestations of AIDS: review of 106 episodes. Radiology 1986;161:87–93.

115. Friedman EP, Miller RF, Severn A, et al. Cryptococcal pneumonia in patients with the acquired immunodeficiency syndrome. Clin Radiol 1995;50:756–760.

116. Douketis JD, Kesten S. Miliary pulmonary cryptococcosis in a patient with the acquired immunodeficiency syndrome. Thorax 1993;48:402–403.

117. Fish DG, Ampel NM, Galgiani JN, et al. Coccidioidomycosis during human immunodeficiency virus infection. A review of 77 patients. Medicine (Baltimore) 1990;69:384–391.

118. Wheat J. Histoplasmosis in the acquired immunodeficiency syndrome. Curr Top Med Mycol 1996;7:7–18.

119. Corti ME, Cendoya CA, Soto I, et al. Disseminated histoplasmosis and AIDS: clinical aspects and diagnostic methods for early detection. AIDS Patient Care STDS 2000;14:149–154.

120. Wheat LJ. Laboratory diagnosis of histoplasmosis: update 2000. Semin Respir Infect 2001;16:131–140.

121. Sarosi GA, Johnson PC. Disseminated histoplasmosis in patients infected with human immunodeficiency virus. Clin Infect Dis 1992;14 Suppl 1:S60–67.

122. Conces DJ Jr, Stockberger SM, Tarver RD, et al. Disseminated histoplasmosis in AIDS: findings on chest radiographs. AJR Am J Roentgenol 1993;160:15–19.

123. Wheat LJ, Connolly-Stringfield PA, Baker RL, et al. Disseminated histoplasmosis in the acquired immune deficiency syndrome: clinical findings, diagnosis and treatment, and review of the literature. Medicine (Baltimore) 1990;69:361–374.

124. McGuinness G, Naidich DP, Jagirdar J, et al. High resolution CT findings in miliary lung disease. J Comput Assist Tomogr 1992;16:384–390.

125. Pappas PG, Pottage JC, Powderly WG, et al. Blastomycosis in patients with the acquired immunodeficiency syndrome. Ann Intern Med 1992;116:847–853.

126. Klapholz A, Salomon N, Perlman DC, et al. Aspergillosis in the acquired immunodeficiency syndrome. Chest 1991;100:1614–1618.

127. Miller WT Jr, Sais GJ, Frank I, et al. Pulmonary aspergillosis in patients with AIDS. Clinical and radiographic correlations. Chest 1994;105:37–44.

128. Meyer RD, Young LS, Armstrong D, et al. Aspergillosis complicating neoplastic disease. Am J Med 1973;54:6–15.

129. Keating JJ, Rogers T, Petrou M, et al. Management of pulmonary aspergillosis in AIDS: an emerging clinical problem. J Clin Pathol 1994;47:805–809.

130. Lortholary O, Meyohas MC, Dupont B, et al. Invasive aspergillosis in patients with acquired immunodeficiency syndrome: report of 33 cases. French Cooperative Study Group on Aspergillosis in AIDS. Am J Med 1993;95:177–187.

131. Staples CA, Kang EY, Wright JL, et al. Invasive pulmonary aspergillosis in AIDS: radiographic, CT, and pathologic findings. Radiology 1995;196:409–414.

132. Denning DW, Follansbee SE, Scolaro M, et al. Pulmonary aspergillosis in the acquired immunodeficiency syndrome. N Engl J Med 1991;324:654–662.

133. Mylonakis E, Barlam TF, Flanigan T, et al. Pulmonary aspergillosis and invasive disease in AIDS: review of 342 cases. Chest 1998;114:251–262.

134. Torrents C, Alvarez-Castells A, de Vera PV, et al. Postpneumocystis aspergilloma in AIDS: CT features. J Comput Assist Tomogr 1991;15:304–307.

135. Flores KM, White CS, Wisniewski P, et al. Invasive pulmonary aspergillosis: CT diagnosis of a peribronchial sinus track in an AIDS patient. J Comput Assist Tomogr 1994;18:495–496.

136. Rottenberg GT, Miszkiel K, Shaw P, et al. Case report: fulminant Toxoplasma gondii pneumonia in a patient with AIDS. Clin Radiol 1997;52:472–474.

137. Oksenhendler E, Cadranel J, Sarfati C, et al. Toxoplasma gondii pneumonia in patients with the acquired immunodeficiency syndrome. Am J Med 1990;88:18N–21N.

138. Goodman PC, Schnapp LM. Pulmonary toxoplasmosis in AIDS. Radiology 1992;184:791–793.

139. Collins J, Müller NL, Leung AN, et al. Epstein-Barr-virus-associated lymphoproliferative disease of the lung: CT and histologic findings. Radiology 1998;208:749–759.

140. McGuinness G, Scholes JV, Garay SM, et al. Cytomegalovirus pneumonitis: spectrum of parenchymal CT findings with pathologic correlation in 21 AIDS patients. Radiology 1994;192:451–459.

141. Stover DE, White DA, Romano PA, et al. Spectrum of pulmonary diseases associated with the acquired immunodeficiency syndrome. Am J Med 1985;78:429–437.

142. Waxman AB, Goldie SJ, Brett-Smith H, et al. Cytomegalovirus as a primary pulmonary pathogen in AIDS. Chest 1997;111:128–134.

143. Tendero DT. Laboratory diagnosis of cytomegalovirus (CMV) infections in immunodepressed patients, mainly in patients with AIDS. Clin Lab 2001;47:169–183.

144. Deayton JR. Changing trends in cytomegalovirus disease in HIV-infected patients. Herpes 2001;8:37–40.

145. Imoto EM, Stein RM, Shellito JE, et al. Central airway obstruction due to cytomegalovirus-induced necrotizing tracheitis in a patient with AIDS. Am Rev Respir Dis 1990;142:884–886.

146. Holmes AH, Trotman-Dickenson B, Edwards A, et al. Bronchiectasis in HIV disease. Q J Med 1992;85:875–882.

147. McGuinness G, Naidich DP, Garay S, et al. AIDS associated bronchiectasis: CT features. J Comput Assist Tomogr 1993;17:260–266.

148. King MA, Neal DE, St John R, et al. Bronchial dilatation in patients with HIV infection: CT assessment and correlation with pulmonary function tests and findings at bronchoalveolar lavage. AJR Am J Roentgenol 1997;168:1535–1540.

149. McGuinness G, Gruden JF, Bhalla M, et al. AIDS-related airway disease. AJR Am J Roentgenol 1997;168:67–77.

150. Sheikh S, Madiraju K, Steiner P, et al. Bronchiectasis in pediatric AIDS. Chest 1997;112:1202–1207.

151. Allen JN, Wewers MD. HIV-associated bronchiolitis obliterans organizing pneumonia. Chest 1989;96:197–198.

152. Bachmeyer C, Blum L, Stelianides S, et al. Mycobacterium xenopi pulmonary infection in an HIV infected patient under highly active antiretroviral treatment. Sex Transm Infect 2002;78:60–61.

153. Lederman MM. Immune restoration and CD4+ T-cell function with antiretroviral therapies. AIDS 2001;15 Suppl 2:S11–15.

154. Rodriguez-Rosado R, Soriano V, Dona C, et al. Opportunistic infections shortly after beginning highly active antiretroviral therapy. Antivir Ther 1998;3:229–231.

155. Safdar A, Rubocki RJ, Horvath JA, et al. Fatal immune restoration disease in human immunodeficiency virus type 1-infected patients with progressive multifocal leukoencephalopathy: impact of antiretroviral therapy-associated immune reconstitution. Clin Infect Dis 2002;35:1250–1257.

156. Bartley PB, Allworth AM, Eisen DP. Mycobacterium avium complex causing endobronchial disease in AIDS patients after partial immune restoration. Int J Tuberc Lung Dis 1999;3:1132–1136.

157. French M, Price P. Immune restoration disease in HIV patients: aberrant immune responses after antiretroviral therapy. J HIV Ther 2002;7:46–51.

158. Haramati LB, Lee G, Singh A, et al. Newly diagnosed pulmonary sarcoidosis in HIV-infected patients. Radiology 2001;218:242–246.

159. Gomez V, Smith PR, Burack J, et al. Sarcoidosis after antiretroviral therapy in a patient with acquired immunodeficiency syndrome. Clin Infect Dis 2000;31:1278–1280.

160. Mirmirani P, Maurer TA, Herndier B, et al. Sarcoidosis in a patient with AIDS: a manifestation of immune restoration syndrome. J Am Acad Dermatol 1999;41:285–286.

161. Dean GL, Williams DI, Churchill DR, et al. Transient clinical deterioration in HIV patients with Pneumocystis carinii pneumonia after starting highly active antiretroviral therapy: another case of immune restoration inflammatory syndrome. Am J Respir Crit Care Med 2002;165:1670.

162. Ioachim HL, Cooper MC, Hellman GC. Lymphomas in men at high risk for acquired immune deficiency syndrome (AIDS). A study of 21 cases. Cancer 1985;56:2831–2842.

163. Morassut S, Vaccher E, Balestreri L, et al. HIV-associated human herpesvirus 8-positive primary lymphomatous effusions: radiologic findings in six patients. Radiology 1997;205:459–463.

164. Blunt DM, Padley SP. Radiographic manifestations of AIDS related lymphoma in the thorax. Clin Radiol 1995;50:607–612.

165. Sider L, Weiss AJ, Smith MD, et al. Varied appearance of AIDS-related lymphoma in the chest. Radiology 1989;171:629–632.

166. Shin MS, McElvein RB, Listinsky CM, et al. CT manifestation of non-Hodgkin's lymphoma as a solitary pulmonary nodule in a patient with acquired immunodeficiency syndrome. Clin Imaging 1993;17:279–281.

167. Carignan S, Staples CA, Müller NL. Intrathoracic lymphoproliferative disorders in the immunocompromised patient: CT findings. Radiology 1995;197:53–58.

168. Kaplan LD, Abrams DI, Feigal E, et al. AIDS-associated non-Hodgkin's lymphoma in San Francisco. JAMA 1989;261:719–724.

169. Polish LB, Cohn DL, Ryder JW, et al. Pulmonary non-Hodgkin's lymphoma in AIDS. Chest 1989;96:1321–1326.

170. Eisner MD, Kaplan LD, Herndier B, et al. The pulmonary manifestations of AIDS-related non-Hodgkin's lymphoma. Chest 1996;110:729–736.

171. Dodd GD III, Greenler DP, Confer SR. Thoracic and abdominal manifestations of lymphoma occurring in the immunocompromised patient. Radiol Clin North Am 1992;30:597–610.

172. Nyberg DA, Federle MP. AIDS-related Kaposi sarcoma and lymphomas. Semin Roentgenol 1987;22:54–65.

173. Martin JN, Ganem DE, Osmond DH, et al. Sexual transmission and the natural history of human herpesvirus 8 infection. N Engl J Med 1998;338:948–954.

174. Gruden JF, Huang L, Webb WR, et al. AIDS-related Kaposi sarcoma of the lung: radiographic findings and staging system with bronchoscopic correlation. Radiology 1995;195:545–552.

175. Miller RF, Tomlinson MC, Cottrill CP, et al. Bronchopulmonary Kaposi's sarcoma in patients with AIDS. Thorax 1992;47:721–725.

176. Naidich DP, Tarras M, Garay SM, et al. Kaposi's sarcoma. CT–radiographic correlation. Chest 1989;96:723–728.

177. Davis SD, Henschke CI, Chamides BK, et al. Intrathoracic Kaposi sarcoma in AIDS patients: radiographic–pathologic correlation. Radiology 1987;163:495–500.

178. Sivit CJ, Schwartz AM, Rockoff SD. Kaposi's sarcoma of the lung in AIDS: radiologic–pathologic analysis. AJR Am J Roentgenol 1987;148:25–28.

179. Khalil AM, Carette MF, Cadranel JL, et al. Intrathoracic Kaposi's sarcoma. CT findings. Chest 1995;108:1622–1626.

180. Traill ZC, Miller RF, Shaw PJ. CT appearances of intrathoracic Kaposi's sarcoma in patients with AIDS. Br J Radiol 1996;69:1104–1107.

181. Wolff SD, Kuhlman JE, Fishman EK. Thoracic Kaposi sarcoma in AIDS: CT findings. J Comput Assist Tomogr 1993;17:60–62.

182. Khalil AM, Carette MF, Cadranel JL, et al. Magnetic resonance imaging findings in pulmonary Kaposi's sarcoma: a series of 10 cases. Eur Respir J 1994;7:1285–1289.

183. Ettensohn DB, Mayer KH, Kessimian N, et al. Lymphocytic bronchiolitis associated with HIV infection. Chest 1988;93:201–202.

184. Guillon JM, Autran B, Denis M, et al. Human immunodeficiency virus-related lymphocytic alveolitis. Chest 1988;94:1264–1270.

185. Travis WD, Fox CH, Devaney KO, et al. Lymphoid pneumonitis in 50 adult patients infected with the human immunodeficiency virus: lymphocytic interstitial pneumonitis versus nonspecific interstitial pneumonitis. Hum Pathol 1992;23:529–541.

186. Revision of the CDC surveillance case definition for acquired immunodeficiency syndrome. Council of State and Territorial Epidemiologists; AIDS Program, Center for Infectious

Diseases. MMWR Morb Mortal Wkly Rep 1987;36 Suppl 1:1S–15S.

187. Prosper M, Omene JA, Ledlie, et al. Clinical significance of resolution of chest X-ray findings in HIV-infected children with lymphocytic interstitial pneumonitis (LIP). Pediatr Radiol 1995;25 Suppl 1:S243–S246.

188. Oldham SA, Castillo M, Jacobson FL, et al. HIV-associated lymphocytic interstitial pneumonia: radiologic manifestations and pathologic correlation. Radiology 1989;170:83–87.

189. Conces DJ Jr, Tarver RD. Noninfectious and nonmalignant pulmonary disease in AIDS. J Thorac Imaging 1991;6:53–59.

190. McGuinness G, Scholes JV, Jagirdar JS, et al. Unusual lymphoproliferative disorders in nine adults with HIV or AIDS: CT and pathologic findings. Radiology 1995;197:59–65.

191. Griffiths MH, Miller RF, Semple SJ. Interstitial pneumonitis in patients infected with the human immunodeficiency virus. Thorax 1995;50:1141–1146.

192. Amorosa JK, Miller RW, Laraya-Cuasay L, et al. Bronchiectasis in children with lymphocytic interstitial pneumonia and acquired immune deficiency syndrome. Plain film and CT observations. Pediatr Radiol 1992;22:603–606.

193. Ichikawa Y, Kinoshita M, Koga T, et al. Lung cyst formation in lymphocytic interstitial pneumonia: CT features. J Comput Assist Tomogr 1994;18:745–748.

194. Schiff RG, Kabat L, Kamani N. Gallium scanning in lymphoid interstitial pneumonitis of children with AIDS. J Nucl Med 1987;28:1915–1919.

195. Heitzman ER. Pulmonary neoplastic and lymphoproliferative disease in AIDS: a review. Radiology 1990;177:347–351.

196. Simmons JT, Suffredini AF, Lack EE, et al. Nonspecific interstitial pneumonitis in patients with AIDS: radiologic features. AJR Am J Roentgenol 1987;149:265–268.

197. Suffredini AF, Ognibene FP, Lack EE, et al. Nonspecific interstitial pneumonitis: a common cause of pulmonary disease in the acquired immunodeficiency syndrome. Ann Intern Med 1987;107:7–13.

198. Sattler F, Nichols L, Hirano L, et al. Nonspecific interstitial pneumonitis mimicking Pneumocystis carinii pneumonia. Am J Respir Crit Care Med 1997;156:912–917.

199. Ognibene FP, Masur H, Rogers P, et al. Nonspecific interstitial pneumonitis without evidence of Pneumocystis carinii in asymptomatic patients infected with human immunodeficiency virus (HIV). Ann Intern Med 1988;109:874–879.

200. Braun MA, Killam DA, Remick SC, et al. Lung cancer in patients seropositive for

human immunodeficiency virus. Radiology 1990;175:341–343.

201. White CS, Haramati LB, Elder KH, et al. Carcinoma of the lung in HIV-positive patients: findings on chest radiographs and CT scans. AJR Am J Roentgenol 1995;164:593–597.

202. Alshafie MT, Donaldson B, Oluwole SF. Human immunodeficiency virus and lung cancer. Br J Surg 1997;84:1068–1071.

203. Serraino D, Boschini A, Carrieri P, et al. Cancer risk among men with, or at risk of, HIV infection in southern Europe. AIDS 2000;14:553–559.

204. Phelps RM, Smith DK, Heilig CM, et al. Cancer incidence in women with or at risk for HIV. Int J Cancer 2001;94:753–757.

205. Parker MS, Leveno DM, Campbell TJ, et al. AIDS-related bronchogenic carcinoma: fact or fiction? Chest 1998;113:154–161.

206. Chan TK, Aranda CP, Rom WN. Bronchogenic carcinoma in young patients at risk for acquired immunodeficiency syndrome. Chest 1993;103:862–864.

207. Demopoulos BP, Vamvakas E, Ehrlich JE, et al. Non-acquired immunodeficiency syndrome-defining malignancies in patients infected with human immunodeficiency virus. Arch Pathol Lab Med 2003;127:589–592.

208. Gruden JF, Webb WR, Yao DC, et al. Bronchogenic carcinoma in 13 patients infected with the human immunodeficiency virus (HIV): clinical and radiographic findings. J Thorac Imaging 1995;10:99–105.

209. Fishman JE, Schwartz DS, Sais GJ, et al. Bronchogenic carcinoma in HIV-positive patients: findings on chest radiographs and CT scans. AJR Am J Roentgenol 1995;164:57–61.

210. Kang EY, Staples CA, McGuinness G, et al. Detection and differential diagnosis of pulmonary infections and tumors in patients with AIDS: value of chest radiography versus CT. AJR Am J Roentgenol 1996;166:15–19.

211. Logan PM, Finnegan MM. Pulmonary complications in AIDS: CT appearances. Clin Radiol 1998;53:567–573.

212. Mason AC, Müller NL. The role of computed tomography in the diagnosis and management of human immunodeficiency virus (HIV)-related pulmonary diseases. Semin Ultrasound CT MR 1998;19:154–166.

213. Shah RM, Salazar AM. CT manifestations of human immunodeficiency virus (HIV)-related pulmonary infections. Semin Ultrasound CT MR 1998;19:167–174.

214. Allison AC, Hart PD. Potentiation by silica of the growth of Mycobacterium tuberculosis in macrophage cultures. Br J Exp Pathol 1968;49:465–476.

215. Heppleston AG. The fibrogenic action of silica. Br Med Bull 1969;25:282–287.

216. Rosenow EC III, Wilson WR, Cockerill FR III. Pulmonary disease in the immunocompromised host. 1. Mayo Clin Proc 1985;60:473–487.

217. Logan PM, Primack SL, Staples C, et al. Acute lung disease in the immunocompromised host. Diagnostic accuracy of the chest radiograph. Chest 1995;108:1283–1287.

218. Winer-Muram HT, Arheart KL, Jennings SG, et al. Pulmonary complications in children with hematologic malignancies: accuracy of diagnosis with chest radiography and CT. Radiology 1997;204:643–649.

219. Winer-Muram HT, Rubin SA, Fletcher BD, et al. Childhood leukemia: diagnostic accuracy of bedside chest radiography for severe pulmonary complications. Radiology 1994;193:127–133.

220. Conces DJ Jr. Bacterial pneumonia in immunocompromised patients. J Thorac Imaging 1998;13:261–270.

221. Pope TL Jr, Armstrong P, Thompson R, et al. Pittsburgh pneumonia agent: chest film manifestations. AJR Am J Roentgenol 1982;138:237–241.

222. Washington L, Miller WT Jr. Mycobacterial infection in immunocompromised patients. J Thorac Imaging 1998;13:271–281.

223. Herbert PA, Bayer AS. Fungal pneumonia (Part 4): invasive pulmonary aspergillosis. Chest 1981;80:220–225.

224. Connolly JE Jr, McAdams HP, Erasmus JJ, et al. Opportunistic fungal pneumonia. J Thorac Imaging 1999;14:51–62.

225. Greene R. The pulmonary aspergilloses: three distinct entities or a spectrum of disease. Radiology 1981;140:527–530.

226. Gefter WB, Weingrad TR, Epstein DM, et al. "Semi-invasive" pulmonary aspergillosis: a new look at the spectrum of aspergillus infections of the lung. Radiology 1981;140:313–321.

227. Logan PM, Müller NL. High-resolution computed tomography and pathologic findings in pulmonary aspergillosis: a pictorial essay. Can Assoc Radiol J 1996;47:444–452.

228. Logan PM, Primack SL, Miller RR, et al. Invasive aspergillosis of the airways: radiographic, CT, and pathologic findings. Radiology 1994;193:383–388.

229. Young RC, Bennett JE, Vogel CL, et al. Aspergillosis. The spectrum of the disease in 98 patients. Medicine (Baltimore) 1970;49:147–173.

230. Brown MJ, Miller RR, Müller NL. Acute lung disease in the immunocompromised host: CT and pathologic examination findings. Radiology 1994;190:247–254.

231. Caillot D, Mannone L, Cuisenier B, et al. Role of early diagnosis and aggressive surgery in the management of invasive

pulmonary aspergillosis in neutropenic patients. Clin Microbiol Infect 2001;7 Suppl 2:54–61.

232. Hauggaard A, Ellis M, Ekelund L. Early chest radiography and CT in the diagnosis, management and outcome of invasive pulmonary aspergillosis. Acta Radiol 2002;43:292–298.

233. Kami M, Kishi Y, Hamaki T, et al. The value of the chest computed tomography halo sign in the diagnosis of invasive pulmonary aspergillosis. An autopsy-based retrospective study of 48 patients. Mycoses 2002;45:287–294.

234. Brown MJ, Worthy SA, Flint JD, et al. Invasive aspergillosis in the immunocompromised host: utility of computed tomography and bronchoalveolar lavage. Clin Radiol 1998;53:255–257.

235. Won HJ, Lee KS, Cheon JE, et al. Invasive pulmonary aspergillosis: prediction at thin-section CT in patients with neutropenia – a prospective study. Radiology 1998;208:777–782.

236. Libshitz HI, Pagani JJ. Aspergillosis and mucormycosis: two types of opportunistic fungal pneumonia. Radiology 1981;140:301–306.

237. Orr DP, Myerowitz RL, Dubois PJ. Patho-radiologic correlation of invasive pulmonary aspergillosis in the compromised host. Cancer 1978;41:2028–2039.

238. Hruban RH, Meziane MA, Zerhouni EA, et al. Radiologic–pathologic correlation of the CT halo sign in invasive pulmonary aspergillosis. J Comput Assist Tomogr 1987;11:534–536.

239. Primack SL, Hartman TE, Lee KS, et al. Pulmonary nodules and the CT halo sign. Radiology 1994;190: 513–515.

240. Kim Y, Lee KS, Jung KJ, et al. Halo sign on high resolution CT: findings in spectrum of pulmonary diseases with pathologic correlation. J Comput Assist Tomogr 1999;23:622–626.

241. Kuhlman JE, Fishman EK, Siegelman SS. Invasive pulmonary aspergillosis in acute leukemia: characteristic findings on CT, the CT halo sign, and the role of CT in early diagnosis. Radiology 1985;157:611–614.

242. Altman AR. Thoracic wall invasion secondary to pulmonary aspergillosis: a complication of chronic granulomatous disease of childhood. AJR Am J Roentgenol 1977;129:140–142.

243. Luce JM, Ostenson RC, Springmeyer SC, et al. Invasive aspergillosis presenting as pericarditis and cardiac tamponade. Chest 1979;76:703–705.

244. Curtis AM, Smith GJ, Ravin CE. Air crescent sign of invasive aspergillosis. Radiology 1979;133:17–21.

245. Gross BH, Spitz HB, Felson B. The mural nodule in cavitary opportunistic pulmonary aspergillosis. Radiology 1982;143:619–622.

246. Gefter WB, Albelda SM, Talbot GH, et al. Invasive pulmonary aspergillosis and acute leukemia. Limitations in the diagnostic utility of the air crescent sign. Radiology 1985;157:605–610.

247. Blum U, Windfuhr M, Buitrago-Tellez C, et al. Invasive pulmonary aspergillosis. MRI, CT, and plain radiographic findings and their contribution for early diagnosis. Chest 1994;106:1156–1161.

248. Herold CJ, Kramer J, Sertl K, et al. Invasive pulmonary aspergillosis: evaluation with MR imaging. Radiology 1989;173:717–721.

249. Buff SJ, McLelland R, Gallis HA, et al. Candida albicans pneumonia: radiographic appearance. AJR Am J Roentgenol 1982;138:645–648.

250. DeGregorio MW, Lee WM, Linker CA, et al. Fungal infections in patients with acute leukemia. Am J Med 1982;73: 543–548.

251. Rose HD, Sheth NK. Pulmonary candidiasis. A clinical and pathological correlation. Arch Intern Med 1978;138: 964–965.

252. Pagani JJ, Libshitz HI. Opportunistic fungal pneumonias in cancer patients. AJR Am J Roentgenol 1981;137:1033–1039.

253. Dubois PJ, Myerowitz RL, Allen CM. Pathoradiologic correlation of pulmonary candidiasis in immunosuppressed patients. Cancer 1977;40:1026–1036.

254. Meyer RD, Rosen P, Armstrong D. Phycomycosis complicating leukemia and lymphoma. Ann Intern Med 1972;77:871–879.

255. Reich J, Renzetti AD Jr. Pulmonary phycomycosis. Report of a case of bronchocutaneous fistula formation and pulmonary arterial mycothrombosis. Am Rev Respir Dis 1970;102:959–964.

256. Gale AM, Kleitsch WP. Solitary pulmonary nodule due to phycomycosis (mucormycosis). Chest 1972;62:752–755.

257. Record NB Jr, Ginder DR. Pulmonary phycomycosis without obvious predisposing factors. JAMA 1976;235:1256–1257.

258. McAdams HP, Rosado de Christenson M, Strollo DC, et al. Pulmonary mucormycosis: radiologic findings in 32 cases. AJR Am J Roentgenol 1997;168:1541–1548.

259. Jamadar DA, Kazerooni EA, Daly BD, et al. Pulmonary zygomycosis: CT appearance. J Comput Assist Tomogr 1995;19:733–738.

260. Zagoria RJ, Choplin RH, Karstaedt N. Pulmonary gangrene as a complication of mucormycosis. AJR Am J Roentgenol 1985;144:1195–1196.

261. Loevner LA, Andrews JC, Francis IR. Multiple mycotic pulmonary artery aneurysms: a complication of invasive mucormycosis. AJR Am J Roentgenol 1992;158:761–762.

262. de la Hoz RE, Stephens G, Sherlock C. Diagnosis and treatment approaches of CMV infections in adult patients. J Clin Virol 2002;25 Suppl 2:S1–S12.

263. Wilczek B, Wilczek HE, Heurlin N, et al. Prognostic significance of pathological chest radiography in transplant patients affected by cytomegalovirus and/or pneumocystis carinii. Acta Radiol 1996;37:727–731.

264. Olliff JF, Williams MP. Radiological appearances of cytomegalovirus infections. Clin Radiol 1989;40: 463–467.

265. Austin JH, Schulman LL, Mastrobattista JD. Pulmonary infection after cardiac transplantation: clinical and radiologic correlations. Radiology 1989;172:259–265.

266. Kang EY, Patz EF Jr, Müller NL. Cytomegalovirus pneumonia in transplant patients: CT findings. J Comput Assist Tomogr 1996;20: 295–299.

267. Moon JH, Kim EA, Lee KS, et al. Cytomegalovirus pneumonia: high-resolution CT findings in ten non-AIDS immunocompromised patients. Korean J Radiol 2000;1:73–78.

268. Mathew BS, Grossman SA. Pneumocystis carinii pneumonia prophylaxis in HIV negative patients with primary CNS lymphoma. Cancer Treat Rev 2003;29:105–119.

269. Wen PY, Marks PW. Medical management of patients with brain tumors. Curr Opin Oncol 2002;14:299–307.

270. Russian DA, Levine SJ. Pneumocystis carinii pneumonia in patients without HIV infection. Am J Med Sci 2001; 321:56–65.

271. Schiff D. Pneumocystis pneumonia in brain tumor patients: risk factors and clinical features. J Neurooncol 1996;27:235–240.

272. McQuillen DP, Sugar AM. Pneumocystis carinii pneumonia associated with solid ectopic corticotropin-producing tumors. Arch Neurol 1992;49:1012.

273. Henson JW, Jalaj JK, Walker RW, et al. Pneumocystis carinii pneumonia in patients with primary brain tumors. Arch Neurol 1991;48:406–409.

274. Yale SH, Limper AH. Pneumocystis carinii pneumonia in patients without acquired immunodeficiency syndrome: associated illness and prior corticosteroid therapy. Mayo Clin Proc 1996;71:5–13.

275. Purtilo DT, Meyers WM, Connor DH. Fatal strongyloidiasis in immunosuppressed patients. Am J Med 1974;56:488–493.

276. Scowden EB, Schaffner W, Stone WJ. Overwhelming strongyloidiasis: an unappreciated opportunistic infection. Medicine (Baltimore) 1978;57:527–544.

277. Wehner JH, Kirsch CM. Pulmonary manifestations of strongyloidiasis. Semin Respir Infect 1997;12:122–129.

278. Lemos LB, Qu Z, Laucirica R, et al. Hyperinfection syndrome in strongyloidiasis: Report of two cases. Ann Diagn Pathol 2003;7:87–94.

279. Kramer MR, Gregg PA, Goldstein M, et al. Disseminated strongyloidiasis in AIDS and non-AIDS immunocompromised hosts: diagnosis by sputum and bronchoalveolar lavage. South Med J 1990;83:1226–1229.

280. Ninane V. Radiological and invasive diagnosis in the detection of pneumonia in febrile neutropenia. Int J Antimicrob Agents 2000;16:91–92.

281. Maschmeyer G. Pneumonia in febrile neutropenic patients: radiologic diagnosis. Curr Opin Oncol 2001;13:229–235.

282. Heussel CP, Kauczor HU, Heussel G, et al. Early detection of pneumonia in febrile neutropenic patients: use of thin-section CT. AJR Am J Roentgenol 1997;169:1347–1353.

283. Heussel CP, Kauczor HU, Heussel GE, et al. Pneumonia in febrile neutropenic patients and in bone marrow and blood stem-cell transplant recipients: use of high-resolution computed tomography. J Clin Oncol 1999;17:796–805.

284. Barloon TJ, Galvin JR, Mori M, et al. High-resolution ultrafast chest CT in the clinical management of febrile bone marrow transplant patients with normal or nonspecific chest roentgenograms. Chest 1991;99:928–933.

285. Gulati M, Kaur R, Jha V, et al. High-resolution CT in renal transplant patients with suspected pulmonary infections. Acta Radiol 2000;41:237–241.

286. Mori M, Galvin JR, Barloon TJ, et al. Fungal pulmonary infections after bone marrow transplantation: evaluation with radiography and CT. Radiology 1991; 178:721–726.

287. Janzen DL, Padley SP, Adler BD, et al. Acute pulmonary complications in immunocompromised non-AIDS patients: comparison of diagnostic accuracy of CT and chest radiography. Clin Radiol 1993;47:159–165.

288. Kami M, Tanaka Y, Kanda Y, et al. Computed tomographic scan of the chest, latex agglutination test and plasma (1AE3)-beta-D-glucan assay in early diagnosis of invasive pulmonary aspergillosis: a prospective study of 215 patients. Haematologica 2000;85:745–752.

289. Caillot D, Casasnovas O, Bernard A, et al. Improved management of invasive pulmonary aspergillosis in neutropenic patients using early thoracic computed tomographic scan and surgery. J Clin Oncol 1997;15:139–147.

290. Maile CW, Moore AV, Ulreich S, et al. Chest radiographic–pathologic correlation in adult leukemia patients. Invest Radiol 1983;18:495–499.

291. Smith LJ, Katzenstein AL. Pathogenesis of massive pulmonary hemorrhage in acute leukemia. Arch Intern Med 1982;142:2149–2152.

292. Tenholder MF, Hooper RG. Pulmonary infiltrates in leukemia. Chest 1980;78:468–473.

293. Katzenstein AL, Askin FB. Interpretation and significance of pathologic findings in transbronchial lung biopsy. Am J Surg Pathol 1980;4:223–234.

294. Leight GS Jr, Michaelis LL. Open lung biopsy for the diagnosis of acute, diffuse pulmonary infiltrates in the immunosuppressed patient. Chest 1978;73:477–482.

295. Rossiter SJ, Miller C, Churg AM, et al. Open lung biopsy in the immunosuppressed patient. Is it really beneficial? J Thorac Cardiovasc Surg 1979;77:338–345.

296. d'Alessandro MP, Kozakewich HP, Cooke KR, et al. Radiologic–pathologic conference of Children's Hospital Boston: new pulmonary nodules in a child undergoing treatment for a solid malignancy. Pediatr Radiol 1996;26:19–21.

297. Helton KJ, Kuhn JP, Fletcher BD, et al. Bronchiolitis obliterans–organizing pneumonia (BOOP) in children with malignant disease. Pediatr Radiol 1992;22:270–274.

298. Lee KS, Kullnig P, Hartman TE, et al. Cryptogenic organizing pneumonia: CT findings in 43 patients. AJR Am J Roentgenol 1994;162:543–546.

299. Logan PM, Miller RR, Müller NL. Cryptogenic organizing pneumonia in the immunocompromised patient: radiologic findings and follow-up in 12 patients. Can Assoc Radiol J 1995;46:272–279.

300. Hansell DM. What are bronchiolitis obliterans organizing pneumonia (BOOP) and cryptogenic organizing pneumonia (COP)? Clin Radiol 1992;45:369–370.

301. Sable CA, Donowitz GR. Infections in bone marrow transplant recipients. Clin Infect Dis 1994;18:273–281.

302. Chan CK, Hyland RH, Hutcheon MA, et al. Small-airways disease in recipients of allogeneic bone marrow transplants. An analysis of 11 cases and a review of the literature. Medicine (Baltimore) 1987;66:327–340.

303. Krowka MJ, Rosenow EC III, Hoagland HC. Pulmonary complications of bone marrow transplantation. Chest 1985; 87:237–246.

304. Paz HL, Crilley P, Patchefsky A, et al. Bronchiolitis obliterans after autologous bone marrow transplantation. Chest 1992;101:775–778.

305. Gosselin MV, Adams RH. Pulmonary complications in bone marrow transplantation. J Thorac Imaging 2002;17:132–144.

306. Patz EF Jr, Peters WP, Goodman PC. Pulmonary drug toxicity following high-dose chemotherapy with autologous bone marrow transplantation: CT findings in 20 cases. J Thorac Imaging 1994;9:129–134.

307. Pirsch JD, Maki DG. Infectious complications in adults with bone marrow transplantation and T-cell depletion of donor marrow. Increased susceptibility to fungal infections. Ann Intern Med 1986;104:619–631.

308. Meunier F. Fungal infections in the immunocompromised host. In: Rubin R, Young L, eds. Clinical approach to infection in the compromised host. New York: Plenum, 1981:193–220.

309. Champlin RE, Whimbey E. Community respiratory virus infections in bone marrow transplant recipients: the M.D. Anderson Cancer Center experience. Biol Blood Marrow Transplant 2001;7 Suppl:8S–10S.

310. Machado CM, Boas LS, Mendes AV, et al. Low mortality rates related to respiratory virus infections after bone marrow transplantation. Bone Marrow Transplant 2003;31:695–700.

311. Ljungman P, Ward KN, Crooks BN, et al. Respiratory virus infections after stem cell transplantation: a prospective study from the Infectious Diseases Working Party of the European Group for Blood and Marrow Transplantation. Bone Marrow Transplant 2001;28:479–484.

312. Ghosh S, Champlin RE, Ueno NT, et al. Respiratory syncytial virus infections in autologous blood and marrow transplant recipients with breast cancer: combination therapy with aerosolized ribavirin and parenteral immunoglobulins. Bone Marrow Transplant 2001;28:271–275.

313. Ravenel JG, Scalzetti EM, Zamkoff KW. Chest radiographic features of engraftment syndrome. J Thorac Imaging 2000;15:56–60.

314. Cahill RA, Spitzer TR, Mazumder A. Marrow engraftment and clinical manifestations of capillary leak syndrome. Bone Marrow Transplant 1996;18:177–184.

315. Hackman RC, Madtes DK, Petersen FB, et al. Pulmonary venoocclusive disease following bone marrow transplantation. Transplantation 1989;47:989–992.

316. Ettinger NA, Trulock EP. Pulmonary considerations of organ transplantation. Part 2. Am Rev Respir Dis 1991;144: 213–223.

317. Robbins RA, Linder J, Stahl MG, et al. Diffuse alveolar hemorrhage in autologous bone marrow transplant recipients. Am J Med 1989;87:511–518.

318. Chao NJ, Duncan SR, Long GD, et al. Corticosteroid therapy for diffuse

alveolar hemorrhage in autologous bone marrow transplant recipients. Ann Intern Med 1991;114:145–146.

319. Witte RJ, Gurney JW, Robbins RA, et al. Diffuse pulmonary alveolar hemorrhage after bone marrow transplantation: radiographic findings in 39 patients. AJR Am J Roentgenol 1991;157:461–464.

320. Marasco WJ, Fishman EK, Kuhlman JE, et al. Acute pulmonary hemorrhage. CT evaluation. Clin Imaging 1993;17:77–80.

321. Primack SL, Miller RR, Müller NL. Diffuse pulmonary hemorrhage: clinical, pathologic, and imaging features. AJR Am J Roentgenol 1995;164:295–300.

322. Worthy S, Kang EY, Müller NL. Acute lung disease in the immunocompromised host: differential diagnosis at high-resolution CT. Semin Ultrasound CT MR 1995;16:353–360.

323. Ferrara JL, Deeg HJ. Graft-versus-host disease. N Engl J Med 1991;324:667–674.

324. Soubani AO, Miller KB, Hassoun PM. Pulmonary complications of bone marrow transplantation. Chest 1996;109:1066–1077.

325. Meyers JD, Thomas ED. Infection complicating bone marrow transplantation. In: Rubin R, Young L, eds. Clinical approach to infection in the compromised host. New York: Plenum, 1988:525–555.

326. Walls T, Shankar AG, Shingadia D. Adenovirus: an increasingly important pathogen in paediatric bone marrow transplant patients. Lancet Infect Dis 2003;3:79–86.

327. Wang WH, Wang HL. Fulminant adenovirus hepatitis following bone marrow transplantation. A case report and brief review of the literature. Arch Pathol Lab Med 2003;127:e246–248.

328. Fassas AB, Buddharaju LN, Rapoport A, et al. Fatal disseminated adenoviral infection associated with thrombotic thrombocytopenic purpura after allogeneic bone marrow transplantation. Leuk Lymphoma 2001;42:801–804.

329. Akiyama H, Kurosu T, Sakashita C, et al. Adenovirus is a key pathogen in hemorrhagic cystitis associated with bone marrow transplantation. Clin Infect Dis 2001;32:1325–1330.

330. La Rosa AM, Champlin RE, Mirza N, et al. Adenovirus infections in adult recipients of blood and marrow transplants. Clin Infect Dis 2001; 32:871–876.

331. Baldwin A, Kingman H, Darville M, et al. Outcome and clinical course of 100 patients with adenovirus infection following bone marrow transplantation. Bone Marrow Transplant 2000;26: 1333–1338.

332. Clark JG, Hansen JA, Hertz MI, et al. NHLBI workshop summary. Idiopathic pneumonia syndrome after bone marrow transplantation. Am Rev Respir Dis 1993;147:1601–1606.

333. Sanders JE. Chronic graft-versus-host disease and late effects after hematopoietic stem cell transplantation. Int J Hematol 2002;76 Suppl 2:15–28.

334. Lum LG, Storb R. Bone marrow transplantation. In: Flye Mea, ed. Principles of organ transplantation. Philadelphia: WB Saunders, 1989:478–499.

335. Palmas A, Tefferi A, Myers JL, et al. Late-onset noninfectious pulmonary complications after allogeneic bone marrow transplantation. Br J Haematol 1998;100:680–687.

336. Trisolini R, Bandini G, Stanzani M, et al. Morphologic changes leading to bronchiolitis obliterans in a patient with delayed non-infectious lung disease after allogeneic bone marrow transplantation. Bone Marrow Transplant 2001;28: 1167–1170.

337. Kanamori H, Mishima A, Tanaka M, et al. Bronchiolitis obliterans organizing pneumonia (BOOP) with suspected liver graft-versus-host disease after allogeneic bone marrow transplantation. Transpl Int 2001;14:266–269.

338. Ishii T, Manabe A, Ebihara Y, et al. Improvement in bronchiolitis obliterans organizing pneumonia in a child after allogeneic bone marrow transplantation by a combination of oral prednisolone and low dose erythromycin. Bone Marrow Transplant 2000;26:907–910.

339. Wolff D, Reichenberger F, Steiner B, et al. Progressive interstitial fibrosis of the lung in sclerodermoid chronic graft-versus-host disease. Bone Marrow Transplant 2002;29:357–360.

340. Pagani JJ, Kangarloo H, Gyepes MT, et al. Radiographic manifestations of bone marrow transplantation in children. AJR Am J Roentgenol 1979;132:883–890.

341. Graham NJ, Müller NL, Miller RR, et al. Intrathoracic complications following allogeneic bone marrow transplantation: CT findings. Radiology 1991;181:153–156.

342. Carter AR, Sostman HD, Curtis AM, et al. Thoracic alterations after cardiac surgery. AJR Am J Roentgenol 1983;140:475–481.

343. Thorsen MK, Goodman LR. Extracardiac complications of cardiac surgery. Semin Roentgenol 1988;23:32–48.

344. Benjamin JJ, Cascade PN, Rubenfire M, et al. Left lower lobe atelectasis and consolidation following cardiac surgery: the effect of topical cooling on the phrenic nerve. Radiology 1982;142:11–14.

345. Wheeler WE, Rubis LJ, Jones CW, et al. Etiology and prevention of topical cardiac hypothermia-induced phrenic nerve injury and left lower lobe atelectasis during cardiac surgery. Chest 1985;88:680–683.

346. Andreone PA, Olivari MT, Elick B, et al. Reduction of infectious complications following heart transplantation with triple-drug immunotherapy. J Heart Transplant 1986;5:13–19.

347. Gao SZ, Schroeder JS, Hunt S, et al. Retransplantation for severe accelerated coronary artery disease in heart transplant recipients. Am J Cardiol 1988;62:876–881.

348. Uys CJ, Rose AG. Pathologic findings in long-term cardiac transplants. Arch Pathol Lab Med 1984;108:112–116.

349. Dodd GD III, Ledesma-Medina J, Baron RL, et al. Posttransplant lymphoproliferative disorder: intrathoracic manifestations. Radiology 1992;184:65–69.

350. Harris KM, Schwartz ML, Slasky BS, et al. Posttransplantation cyclosporine-induced lymphoproliferative disorders: clinical and radiologic manifestations. Radiology 1987;162:697–700.

351. Honda H, Barloon TJ, Franken EA Jr, et al. Clinical and radiologic features of malignant neoplasms in organ transplant recipients: cyclosporine-treated vs untreated patients. AJR Am J Roentgenol 1990;154:271–274.

352. Penn I. Malignancies associated with immunosuppressive or cytotoxic therapy. Surgery 1978;83:492–502.

353. Hardy JD, Webb WR, Dalton ML. Lung homotransplantation in man: report of an initial case. JAMA 1963;186:1065–1074.

354. Cooper JD. The evolution of techniques and indications for lung transplantation. Ann Surg 1990;212:249–255; discussion 255–256.

355. Cooper JD, Pearson FG, Patterson GA, et al. Technique of successful lung transplantation in humans. J Thorac Cardiovasc Surg 1987;93:173–181.

356. Schafers HJ, Haydock DA, Cooper JD. The prevalence and management of bronchial anastomotic complications in lung transplantation. J Thorac Cardiovasc Surg 1991;101:1044–1052.

357. Unilateral lung transplantation for pulmonary fibrosis. Toronto Lung Transplant Group. N Engl J Med 1986;314:1140–1145.

358. Waters PF. Lung transplantation: recipient selection. Semin Thorac Cardiovasc Surg 1992;4:73–78.

359. Waters PF. Single lung transplant: indications and technique. Semin Thorac Cardiovasc Surg 1992;4:90–94.

360. Meyers BF, Patterson GA. Lung transplantation versus lung volume reduction as surgical therapy for emphysema. World J Surg 2001; 25:238–243.

361. Weill D, Keshavjee S. Lung transplantation for emphysema: two lungs or one. J Heart Lung Transplant 2001;20:739–742.

362. Schmidt F, McGiffin DC, Zorn G, et al. Management of congenital abnormalities of the donor lung. Ann Thorac Surg 2001;72:935–937.

363. Barr ML, Baker CJ, Schenkel FA, et al. Living donor lung transplantation: selection, technique, and outcome. Transplant Proc 2001;33:3527–3532.

364. Harringer W, Haverich A. Heart and heart-lung transplantation: standards and improvements. World J Surg 2002;26:218–225.

365. Jenkinson SG, Levine SM. Lung transplantation. Dis Mon 1994;40:1–38.

366. Patterson GA. Bilateral lung transplant: indications and technique. Semin Thorac Cardiovasc Surg 1992;4:95–100.

367. Davis RD Jr, Pasque MK. Pulmonary transplantation. Ann Surg 1995;221:14–28.

368. Lung transplantation. Report of the ATS workshop on lung transplantation. American Thoracic Society, Medical Section of the American Lung Association. Am Rev Respir Dis 1993;147:772–776.

369. De Hoyos A, Maurer JR. Complications following lung transplantation. Semin Thorac Cardiovasc Surg 1992;4:132–146.

370. Pasque MK, Kaiser LR, Dresler CM, et al. Single lung transplantation for pulmonary hypertension. Technical aspects and immediate hemodynamic results. J Thorac Cardiovasc Surg 1992;103:475–481; discussion 481–482.

371. Pasque MK, Cooper JD, Kaiser LR, et al. Improved technique for bilateral lung transplantation: rationale and initial clinical experience. Ann Thorac Surg 1990;49:785–791.

372. Bolman RM III, Shumway SJ, Estrin JA, et al. Lung and heart-lung transplantation. Evolution and new applications. Ann Surg 1991;214:456–468; discussion 469–470.

373. Calhoon JH, Grover FL, Gibbons WJ, et al. Single lung transplantation. Alternative indications and technique. J Thorac Cardiovasc Surg 1991;101:816–824; discussion 824–825.

374. Khaghani A, Tadjkarimi S, al-Kattan K, et al. Wrapping the anastomosis with omentum or an internal mammary artery pedicle does not improve bronchial healing after single lung transplantation: results of a randomized clinical trial. J Heart Lung Transplant 1994;13:767–773.

375. Erasmus JJ, McAdams HP, Tapson VF, et al. Radiologic issues in lung transplantation for end-stage pulmonary disease. AJR Am J Roentgenol 1997;169:69–78.

376. Garg K, Zamora MR, Tuder R, et al. Lung transplantation: indications, donor and recipient selection, and imaging of complications. RadioGraphics 1996;16:355–367.

377. Dark JH. Lung transplantation. Transplant Proc 1994;26:1708–1709.

378. Winton TL. Lung transplantation: donor selection. Semin Thorac Cardiovasc Surg 1992;4:79–82.

379. Puskas JD, Winton TL, Miller JD, et al. Unilateral donor lung dysfunction does not preclude successful contralateral single lung transplantation. J Thorac Cardiovasc Surg 1992;103:1015–1017; discussion 1017–1018.

380. Sundaresan S, Semenkovich J, Ochoa L, et al. Successful outcome of lung transplantation is not compromised by the use of marginal donor lungs. J Thorac Cardiovasc Surg 1995;109:1075–1079; discussion 1079–1080.

381. de Hoyos AL, Patterson GA, Maurer JR, et al. Pulmonary transplantation. Early and late results. The Toronto Lung Transplant Group. J Thorac Cardiovasc Surg 1992;103:295–306.

382. Kazerooni EA, Chow LC, Whyte RI, et al. Preoperative examination of lung transplant candidates: value of chest CT compared with chest radiography. AJR Am J Roentgenol 1995;165:1343–1348.

383. Marom EM, McAdams HP, Palmer SM, et al. Cystic fibrosis: usefulness of thoracic CT in the examination of patients before lung transplantation. Radiology 1999;213:283–288.

384. Bittner HB, Dunitz J, Hertz M. Hyperacute rejection in single lung transplantation – case report of successful management by means of plasmapheresis and antithymocyte globulin treatment. Transplantation 2001;71:649–651.

385. Choi JK, Kearns J, Palevsky HI, et al. Hyperacute rejection of a pulmonary allograft. Immediate clinical and pathologic findings. Am J Respir Crit Care Med 1999;160:1015–1018.

386. Frost AE, Jammal CT, Cagle PT. Hyperacute rejection following lung transplantation. Chest 1996;110:559–562.

387. Chiles C, Guthaner DF, Jamieson SW, et al. Heart-lung transplantation: the postoperative chest radiograph. Radiology 1985;154:299–304.

388. Herman SJ, Rappaport DC, Weisbrod GL, et al. Single-lung transplantation: imaging features. Radiology 1989;170:89–93.

389. Anderson DC, Glazer HS, Semenkovich JW, et al. Lung transplant edema: chest radiography after lung transplantation – the first 10 days. Radiology 1995;195:275–281.

390. Paradis IL, Duncan SR, Dauber JH, et al. Distinguishing between infection, rejection, and the adult respiratory distress syndrome after human lung transplantation. J Heart Lung Transplant 1992;11:S232–S236.

391. Marom EM, Choi YW, Palmer SM, et al. Reperfusion edema after lung transplantation: effect of daclizumab. Radiology 2001;221:508–514.

392. Clark SC, Levine AJ, Hasan A, et al. Vascular complications of lung transplantation. Ann Thorac Surg 1996;61:1079–1082.

393. Gaubert JY, Moulin G, Thomas P, et al. Anastomotic stenosis of the left pulmonary artery after lung transplantation: treatment by percutaneous placement of an endoprosthesis. AJR Am J Roentgenol 1993;161:947–949.

394. Murray JG, McAdams HP, Erasmus JJ, et al. Complications of lung transplantation: radiologic findings. AJR Am J Roentgenol 1996;166:1405–1411.

395. Herman SJ, Weisbrod GL, Weisbrod L, et al. Chest radiographic findings after bilateral lung transplantation. AJR Am J Roentgenol 1989;153:1181–1185.

396. Kirby TJ, Mehta A, Rice TW, Gephardt GN. Diagnosis and management of acute and chronic lung rejection. Semin Thorac Cardiovasc Surg 1992;4:126–131.

397. Trulock EP. Management of lung transplant rejection. Chest 1993;103:1566–1576.

398. Yousem SA, Berry GJ, Cagle PT, et al. Revision of the 1990 working formulation for the classification of pulmonary allograft rejection: Lung Rejection Study Group. J Heart Lung Transplant 1996;15:1–15.

399. Yousem S. A perspective on the Revised Working Formulation for the grading of lung allograft rejection. Transplant Proc 1996;28:477–479.

400. Bergin CJ, Castellino RA, Blank N, et al. Acute lung rejection after heart-lung transplantation: correlation of findings on chest radiographs with lung biopsy results. AJR Am J Roentgenol 1990;155:23–27.

401. Millet B, Higenbottam TW, et al. The radiographic appearances of infection and acute rejection of the lung after heart-lung transplantation. Am Rev Respir Dis 1989;140:62–67.

402. Scott JP, Fradet G, Smyth RL, et al. Prospective study of transbronchial biopsies in the management of heart-lung and single lung transplant patients. J Heart Lung Transplant 1991;10:626–636.

403. Tazelaar HD, Nilsson FN, Rinaldi M, et al. The sensitivity of transbronchial biopsy for the diagnosis of acute lung rejection. J Thorac Cardiovasc Surg 1993;105:674–678.

404. Loubeyre P, Revel D, Delignette A, et al. High-resolution computed tomographic findings associated with histologically diagnosed acute lung rejection in heart-lung transplant recipients. Chest 1995;107:132–138.

405. Ikonen T, Kivisaari L, Taskinen E, et al. Acute rejection diagnosed with computed tomography in a porcine experimental lung transplantation model. Scand Cardiovasc J 1997;31:25–32.

406. Gotway MB, Dawn SK, Sellami D, et al. Acute rejection following lung transplantation: limitations in accuracy of thin-section CT for diagnosis. Radiology 2001;221:207–212.

407. McAdams HP, Erasmus JJ, Palmer SM. Complications (excluding hyperinflation) involving the native lung after single-lung transplantation: incidence, radiologic features, and clinical importance. Radiology 2001;218:233–241.

408. Herve P, Silbert D, Cerrina J, et al. Impairment of bronchial mucociliary clearance in long-term survivors of heart/lung and double-lung transplantation. The Paris-Sud Lung Transplant Group. Chest 1993;103:59–63.

409. Dauber JH, Paradis IL, Dummer JS. Infectious complications in pulmonary allograft recipients. Clin Chest Med 1990;11:291–308.

410. Maziak DE, Maurer JR, Kesten S. Diaphragmatic paralysis: a complication of lung transplantation. Ann Thorac Surg 1996;61:170–173.

411. Low DE, Kaiser LR, Haydock DA, et al. The donor lung: infectious and pathologic factors affecting outcome in lung transplantation. J Thorac Cardiovasc Surg 1993;106:614–621.

412. End A, Helbich T, Wisser W, et al. The pulmonary nodule after lung transplantation. Cause and outcome. Chest 1995;107:1317–1322.

413. O'Donovan PB. Imaging of complications of lung transplantation. RadioGraphics 1993;13:787–796.

414. Flume PA, Egan TM, Paradowski LJ, et al. Infectious complications of lung transplantation. Impact of cystic fibrosis. Am J Respir Crit Care Med 1994;149:1601–1607.

415. Date H, Trulock EP, Arcidi JM, et al. Improved airway healing after lung transplantation. An analysis of 348 bronchial anastomoses. J Thorac Cardiovasc Surg 1995;110:1424–1432; discussion 1432–1433.

416. Ramirez J, Patterson GA. Airway complications after lung transplantation. Semin Thorac Cardiovasc Surg 1992;4:147–153.

417. Shennib H, Massard G. Airway complications in lung transplantation. Ann Thorac Surg 1994;57:506–511.

418. Schoenberger JA, Darcy MD. Bronchial artery embolization for hemoptysis in a lung transplant recipient. J Vasc Interv Radiol 1995;6:354–356.

419. Semenkovich JW, Glazer HS, Anderson DC, et al. Bronchial dehiscence in lung transplantation: CT evaluation. Radiology 1995;194:205–208.

420. Schlueter FJ, Semenkovich JW, Glazer HS, et al. Bronchial dehiscence after lung transplantation: correlation of CT findings with clinical outcome. Radiology 1996;199:849–854.

421. Glazer HS, Anderson DJ, Cooper JD, et al. Omental flap in lung transplantation. Radiology 1992;185:395–400.

422. Quint LE, Whyte RI, Kazerooni EA, et al. Stenosis of the central airways: evaluation by using helical CT with multiplanar reconstructions. Radiology 1995;194:871–877.

423. McAdams HP, Murray JG, Erasmus JJ, et al. Telescoping bronchial anastomoses for unilateral or bilateral sequential lung transplantation: CT appearance. Radiology 1997;203:202–206.

424. Anzueto A, Levine SM, Tillis WP, et al. Use of the flow-volume loop in the diagnosis of bronchial stenosis after single lung transplantation. Chest 1994;105:934–936.

425. McAdams HP, Palmer SM, Erasmus JJ, et al. Bronchial anastomotic complications in lung transplant recipients: virtual bronchoscopy for noninvasive assessment. Radiology 1998;209:689–695.

426. Higgins R, McNeil K, Dennis C, et al. Airway stenoses after lung transplantation: management with expanding metal stents. J Heart Lung Transplant 1994;13:774–778.

427. Shreeniwas R, Schulman LL, Berkmen YM, et al. Opportunistic bronchopulmonary infections after lung transplantation: clinical and radiographic findings. Radiology 1996;200:349–356.

428. Anderson DC. Role of the imaging specialist in the detection of opportunistic infection after lung transplantation: are we out of the loop? Radiology 1996;200:325–326.

429. Zamora MR. Use of cytomegalovirus immune globulin and ganciclovir for the prevention of cytomegalovirus disease in lung transplantation. Transpl Infect Dis 2001;3 Suppl 2:49–56.

430. Valantine HA, Luikart H, Doyle R, et al. Impact of cytomegalovirus hyperimmune globulin on outcome after cardiothoracic transplantation: a comparative study of combined prophylaxis with CMV hyperimmune globulin plus ganciclovir versus ganciclovir alone. Transplantation 2001;72:1647–1652.

431. Avery RK. Special considerations regarding CMV in lung transplantation. Transpl Infect Dis 1999;1 Suppl 1:13–18.

432. Salomon N, Perlman DC. Cytomegalovirus pneumonia. Semin Respir Infect 1999;14:353–358.

433. Metras D, Viard L, Kreitmann B, et al. Lung infections in pediatric lung transplantation: experience in 49 cases. Eur J Cardiothorac Surg 1999;15:490–494; discussion 495.

434. Collins J, Kuhlman JE, Love RB. Acute, life-threatening complications of lung transplantation. RadioGraphics 1998;18:21–43; discussion 43–47.

435. Munoz P, Palomo J, Guembe P, et al. Lung nodular lesions in heart transplant recipients. J Heart Lung Transplant 2000;19:660–667.

436. Matar LD, McAdams HP, Palmer SM, et al. Respiratory viral infections in lung transplant recipients: radiologic findings with clinical correlation. Radiology 1999;213:735–742.

437. Garantziotis S, Howell DN, McAdams HP, et al. Influenza pneumonia in lung transplant recipients: clinical features and association with bronchiolitis obliterans syndrome. Chest 2001;119:1277–1280.

438. Ko JP, Shepard JA, Sproule MW, et al. CT manifestations of respiratory syncytial virus infection in lung transplant recipients. J Comput Assist Tomogr 2000;24:235–241.

439. Guillemain R, Lavarde V, Amrein C, et al. Invasive aspergillosis after transplantation. Transplant Proc 1995;27:1307–1309.

440. Kanj SS, Welty-Wolf K, Madden J, et al. Fungal infections in lung and heart-lung transplant recipients. Report of 9 cases and review of the literature. Medicine (Baltimore) 1996;75:142–156.

441. Schulman LL, Htun T, Staniloae C, et al. Pulmonary nodules and masses after lung and heart-lung transplantation. J Thorac Imaging 2000;15:173–179.

442. Paciocco G, Martinez FJ, Kazerooni EA, et al. Tuberculous pneumonia complicating lung transplantation: case report and review of the literature. Monaldi Arch Chest Dis 2000;55:117–121.

443. Malouf MA, Glanville AR. The spectrum of mycobacterial infection after lung transplantation. Am J Respir Crit Care Med 1999;160:1611–1616.

444. Kesten S, Chaparro C. Mycobacterial infections in lung transplant recipients. Chest 1999;115:741–745.

445. Baldi S, Rapellino M, Ruffini E, et al. Atypical mycobacteriosis in a lung transplant recipient. Eur Respir J 1997;10:952–954.

446. Trulock EP, Bolman RM, Genton R. Pulmonary disease caused by Mycobacterium chelonae in a heart-lung transplant recipient with obliterative bronchiolitis. Am Rev Respir Dis 1989;140:802–805.

447. Carlsen SE, Bergin CJ. Reactivation of tuberculosis in a donor lung after transplantation. AJR Am J Roentgenol 1990;154:495–497.

448. Miller RA, Lanza LA, Kline JN, et al. Mycobacterium tuberculosis in lung transplant recipients. Am J Respir Crit Care Med 1995;152:374–376.

449. Schulman LL, Scully B, McGregor CC, et al. Pulmonary tuberculosis after lung transplantation. Chest 1997;111:1459–1462.

450. Collins J, Müller NL, Kazerooni EA, et al. CT findings of pneumonia after lung transplantation. AJR Am J Roentgenol 2000;175:811–818.

451. Keenan RJ, Zeevi A. Immunologic consequences of transplantation. Chest Surg Clin N Am 1995;5:107–120.

452. Nathan SD, Ross DJ, Belman MJ, et al. Bronchiolitis obliterans in single-lung transplant recipients. Chest 1995; 107:967–972.

453. Estenne M, Maurer JR, Boehler A, et al. Bronchiolitis obliterans syndrome 2001: an update of the diagnostic criteria. J Heart Lung Transplant 2002;21: 297–310.

454. Keller CA, Cagle PT, Brown RW, et al. Bronchiolitis obliterans in recipients of single, double, and heart-lung transplantation. Chest 1995;107:973–980.

455. Cooper JD, Billingham M, Egan T, et al. A working formulation for the standardization of nomenclature and for clinical staging of chronic dysfunction in lung allografts. International Society for Heart and Lung Transplantation. J Heart Lung Transplant 1993;12:713–716.

456. Girgis RE, Tu I, Berry GJ, et al. Risk factors for the development of obliterative bronchiolitis after lung transplantation. J Heart Lung Transplant 1996;15:1200–1208.

457. Kramer MR, Stoehr C, Whang JL, et al. The diagnosis of obliterative bronchiolitis after heart-lung and lung transplantation: low yield of transbronchial lung biopsy. J Heart Lung Transplant 1993;12:675–681.

458. Cagle PT, Brown RW, Frost A, et al. Diagnosis of chronic lung transplant rejection by transbronchial biopsy. Mod Pathol 1995;8:137–142.

459. Novick RJ, Schafers HJ, Stitt L, et al. Seventy-two pulmonary retransplantations for obliterative bronchiolitis: predictors of survival. Ann Thorac Surg 1995;60:111–116.

460. Burke CM, Theodore J, Dawkins KD, et al. Post-transplant obliterative bronchiolitis and other late lung sequelae in human heart-lung transplantation. Chest 1984;86:824–829.

461. Verleden GM. Bronchiolitis obliterans syndrome after lung transplantation: medical treatment. Monaldi Arch Chest Dis 2000;55:140–145.

462. Skeens JL, Fuhrman CR, Yousem SA. Bronchiolitis obliterans in heart-lung transplantation patients: radiologic findings in 11 patients. AJR Am J Roentgenol 1989;153:253–256.

463. Knollmann FD, Ewert R, Wundrich T, Bronchiolitis obliterans syndrome in lung transplant recipients: use of spirometrically gated CT. Radiology 2002;225:655–662.

464. Choi YW, Rossi SE, Palmer SM, et al. Bronchiolitis obliterans syndrome in lung transplant recipients: Correlation of computed tomography findings with bronchiolitis obliterans syndrome stage. J Thorac Imaging 2003;18:72–79.

465. Siegel MJ, Bhalla S, Gutierrez FR, et al. Post-lung transplantation bronchiolitis obliterans syndrome: usefulness of expiratory thin-section CT for diagnosis. Radiology 2001;220:455–462.

466. Miller WT Jr, Kotloff RM, Blumenthal NP, et al. Utility of high resolution computed tomography in predicting bronchiolitis obliterans syndrome following lung transplantation: preliminary findings. J Thorac Imaging 2001;16:76–80.

467. Bankier AA, Van Muylem A, Knoop C, et al. Bronchiolitis obliterans syndrome in heart-lung transplant recipients: diagnosis with expiratory CT. Radiology 2001;218:533–539.

468. Leung AN, Fisher K, Valentine V, et al. Bronchiolitis obliterans after lung transplantation: detection using expiratory HRCT. Chest 1998;113:365–370.

469. Lau DM, Siegel MJ, Hildebolt CF, et al. Bronchiolitis obliterans syndrome: thin-section CT diagnosis of obstructive changes in infants and young children after lung transplantation. Radiology 1998;208:783–788.

470. Worthy SA, Park CS, Kim JS, et al. Bronchiolitis obliterans after lung transplantation: high-resolution CT findings in 15 patients. AJR Am J Roentgenol 1997;169:673–677.

471. Ikonen T, Kivisaari L, Taskinen E, et al. High-resolution CT in long-term follow-up after lung transplantation. Chest 1997;111:370–376.

472. Lee ES, Gotway MB, Reddy GP, et al. Early bronchiolitis obliterans following lung transplantation: accuracy of expiratory thin-section CT for diagnosis. Radiology 2000;216:472–477.

473. Loubeyre P, Revel D, Delignette A, et al. Bronchiectasis detected with thin-section CT as a predictor of chronic lung allograft rejection. Radiology 1995;194:213–216.

474. McAdams HP, Palmer SM, Donnelly LF, et al. Hyperpolarized 3He-enhanced MR imaging of lung transplant recipients: preliminary results. AJR Am J Roentgenol 1999;173:955–959.

475. Markstaller K, Kauczor HU, Puderbach M, et al. 3He-MRI-based vs. conventional determination of lung volumes in patients after unilateral lung transplantation: a new approach to regional spirometry. Acta Anaesthesiol Scand 2002;46:845–852.

476. Gast KK, Viallon M, Eberle B, et al. MRI in lung transplant recipients using hyperpolarized 3He: comparison with CT. J Magn Reson Imaging 2002;15: 268–274.

477. Salerno M, Altes TA, Mugler JP III, et al. Hyperpolarized noble gas MR imaging of the lung: potential clinical applications. Eur J Radiol 2001;40:33–44.

478. McAdams HP, Hatabu H, Donnelly LF, et al. Novel techniques for MR imaging of pulmonary airspaces. Magn Reson Imaging Clin N Am 2000;8:205–219.

478a. McAdams HP, Donnelly LF, MacFall JR. Hyperpolarized gas-enhanced MR imaging of the lungs. In: Boiselle PM, White CS, eds. New techniques in thoracic imaging: 265–288. Marcel Dekker, Inc. NY; 2002.

479. Horvath J, Dummer S, Loyd J, et al. Infection in the transplanted and native lung after single lung transplantation. Chest 1993;104:681–685.

480. Pickhardt PJ, Siegel MJ, Anderson DC, et al. Chest radiography as a predictor of outcome in posttransplantation lymphoproliferative disorder in lung allograft recipients. AJR Am J Roentgenol 1998;171:375–382.

481. Speziali G, McDougall JC, Midthun DE, et al. Native lung complications after single lung transplantation for emphysema. Transpl Int 1997;10: 113–115.

482. Weill D, Torres F, Hodges TN, et al. Acute native lung hyperinflation is not associated with poor outcomes after single lung transplant for emphysema. J Heart Lung Transplant 1999;18:1080–1087.

483. Malchow SC, McAdams HP, Palmer SM, et al. Does hyperexpansion of the native lung adversely affect outcome after single lung transplantation for emphysema? Preliminary findings. Acad Radiol 1998;5:688–693.

484. Collins J, Kazerooni EA, Lacomis J, et al. Bronchogenic carcinoma after lung transplantation: frequency, clinical characteristics, and imaging findings. Radiology 2002;224:131–138.

485. Moy ML, Loring SH, Ingenito EP, et al. Causes of allograft dysfunction after single lung transplantation for emphysema: extrinsic restriction versus intrinsic obstruction. Brigham and Women's Hospital Lung Transplantation Group. J Heart Lung Transplant 1999;18:986–993.

486. Yonan NA, el-Gamel A, Egan J, et al. Single lung transplantation for emphysema: predictors for native lung hyperinflation. J Heart Lung Transplant 1998;17:192–201.

487. Anderson MB, Kriett JM, Kapelanski DP, et al. Volume reduction surgery in the native lung after single lung transplantation for emphysema. J Heart Lung Transplant 1997;16:752–757.

488. Kapelanski DP, Anderson MB, Kriett JM, et al. Volume reduction of the native lung after single-lung transplantation for emphysema. J Thorac Cardiovasc Surg 1996;111:898–899.

489. Kuno R, Kanter KR, Torres WE, et al. Single lung transplantation followed by contralateral bullectomy for bullous emphysema. J Heart Lung Transplant 1996;15:389–394.

490. Venuta F, Boehler A, Rendina EA, et al. Complications in the native lung after single lung transplantation. Eur J Cardiothorac Surg 1999;16:54–58.

491. Spiekerkoetter E, Krug N, Hoeper M, et al. Prevalence of malignancies after lung transplantation. Transplant Proc 1998;30:1523–1524.

492. Svendsen CA, Bengtson RB, Park SJ, et al. Stage I adenocarcinoma presenting in the pneumonectomy specimen at the time of single lung transplantation. Transplantation 1998;66:1108–1109.

493. Kazerooni EA, Jackson C, Cascade PN. Sarcoidosis: recurrence of primary disease in transplanted lungs. Radiology 1994;192:461–464.

494. Nine JS, Yousem SA, Paradis IL, et al. Lymphangioleiomyomatosis: recurrence after lung transplantation. J Heart Lung Transplant 1994;13:714–719.

495. Baz MA, Kussin PS, Van Trigt P, et al. Recurrence of diffuse panbronchiolitis after lung transplantation. Am J Respir Crit Care Med 1995;151:895–898.

496. Frost AE, Keller CA, Brown RW, et al. Giant cell interstitial pneumonitis. Disease recurrence in the transplanted lung. Am Rev Respir Dis 1993;148:1401–1404.

497. Gabbay E, Dark JH, Ashcroft T, et al. Recurrence of Langerhans cell granulomatosis following lung transplantation. Thorax 1998;53:326–327.

498. Habib SB, Congleton J, Carr D, et al. Recurrence of recipient Langerhans cell histiocytosis following bilateral lung transplantation. Thorax 1998;53:323–325.

499. Parker LA, Novotny DB. Recurrent alveolar proteinosis following double lung transplantation. Chest 1997;111:1457–1458.

500. Collins J, Hartman MJ, Warner TF, et al. Frequency and CT findings of recurrent disease after lung transplantation. Radiology 2001;219:503–509.

501. Herridge MS, de Hoyos AL, Chaparro C, et al. Pleural complications in lung transplant recipients. J Thorac Cardiovasc Surg 1995;110:22–26.

502. Schorlemmer GR, Khouri RK, Murray GF, et al. Bilateral pneumothoraces secondary to iatrogenic buffalo chest. An unusual complication of median sternotomy and subclavian vein catheterization. Ann Surg 1984;199:372–374.

503. Paranjpe DV, Wittich GR, Hamid LW, et al. Frequency and management of pneumothoraces in heart-lung transplant recipients. Radiology 1994;190:255–256.

504. Lee YC, McGrath GB, Chin WS, et al. Contralateral tension pneumothorax following unilateral chest tube drainage of bilateral pneumothoraces in a heart-lung transplant patient. Chest 1999;116:1131–1133.

505. Judson MA, Handy JR, Sahn SA. Pleural effusions following lung transplantation. Time course, characteristics, and clinical implications. Chest 1996;109:1190–1194.

506. Siegleman SS, Sinha SB, Veith FJ. Pulmonary reimplantation response. Ann Surg 1973;177:30–36.

507. Ruggiero R, Fietsam R Jr, Thomas GA, et al. Detection of canine allograft lung rejection by pulmonary lymphoscintigraphy. J Thorac Cardiovasc Surg 1994;108:253–258.

508. Marom EM, Palmer SM, Erasmus JJ, et al. Pleural effusions in lung transplant recipients: image-guided small-bore catheter drainage. Radiology 2003;228:241–245.

509. Spaggiari L, Rusca M, Carbognani P, et al. Contralateral spontaneous pneumothorax after single lung transplantation for fibrosis. Acta Biomed Ateneo Parmense 1993;64:29–31.

510. Nunley DR, Grgurich WF, Keenan RJ, et al. Empyema complicating successful lung transplantation. Chest 1999;115:1312–1315.

511. Personne C, Hertzog P, Toty L. Les poches pleurales calcifees. Risques evolutifs et possibilites therapeutiques. Rev Tuberc Pneumol 1959;23:394–406.

512. Personne C. Suppuration des poches pleurales calcifees. Rev Tuberc Pneumol 1963;27:604–609.

513. Nishida O, Arellano R, Cheng DC, et al. Gas exchange and hemodynamics in experimental pleural effusion. Crit Care Med 1999;27:583–587.

514. Zerahn B, Jensen BV, Olsen F, et al. The effect of thoracentesis on lung function and transthoracic electrical bioimpedance. Respir Med 1999;93:196–201.

515. Bourbeau J, Ernst P, Chrome J, et al. The relationship between respiratory impairment and asbestos-related pleural abnormality in an active work force. Am Rev Respir Dis 1990;142:837–842.

516. McGavin CR, Sheers G. Diffuse pleural thickening in asbestos workers: disability and lung function abnormalities. Thorax 1984;39:604–607.

517. Yates DH, Browne K, Stidolph PN, et al. Asbestos-related bilateral diffuse pleural thickening: natural history of radiographic and lung function abnormalities. Am J Respir Crit Care Med 1996;153:301–306.

518. Kazerooni EA, Cascade PN, Gross BH. Transplanted lungs: nodules following transbronchial biopsy. Radiology 1995;194:209–212.

519. Root JD, Molina PL, Anderson DJ, et al. Pulmonary nodular opacities following transbronchial biopsy in patients with lung transplants. Radiology 1992;184:435–436.

520. Smith PC, Slaughter MS, Petty MG, Abdominal complications after lung transplantation. J Heart Lung Transplant 1995;14:44–51.

521. Paranjothi S, Yusen RD, Kraus MD, et al. Lymphoproliferative disease after lung transplantation: comparison of presentation and outcome of early and late cases. J Heart Lung Transplant 2001;20:1054–1063.

522. Armitage JM, Kormos RL, Stuart RS, et al. Posttransplant lymphoproliferative disease in thoracic organ transplant patients: ten years of cyclosporine-based immunosuppression. J Heart Lung Transplant 1991;10:877–886; discussion 886–887.

523. Herzig KA, Juffs HG, Norris D, et al. A single-centre experience of post-renal transplant lymphoproliferative disorder. Transpl Int 2003;16:529–536.

524. Loren AW, Porter DL, Stadtmauer EA, et al. Post-transplant lymphoproliferative disorder: a review. Bone Marrow Transplant 2003;31:145–155.

525. Nalesnik MA. Clinicopathologic characteristics of post-transplant lymphoproliferative disorders. Recent Results Cancer Res 2002;159:9–18.

526. Opelz G, Henderson R. Incidence of non-Hodgkin lymphoma in kidney and heart transplant recipients. Lancet 1993;342:1514–1516.

527. Rappaport DC, Chamberlain DW, Shepherd FA, et al. Lymphoproliferative disorders after lung transplantation: imaging features. Radiology 1998;206:519–524.

528. Rappaport DC, Weisbrod GL, Herman SJ. Cyclosporine-induced lymphoma following a unilateral lung transplant. The Toronto Lung Transplant Group. Can Assoc Radiol J 1989;40:110–111.

529. Fraser RS, Müller NL, Colman N, et al. Post-transplantation lymphoproliferative disorder. In: Fraser RS, Müller NL, Colman N, et al, eds. Fraser and Pare's Diagnosis of diseases of the chest, 4th edn. Philadelphia: W B Saunders, 1999:1711–1713.

530. List AF, Greco FA, Vogler LB. Lymphoproliferative diseases in immunocompromised hosts: the role of Epstein-Barr virus. J Clin Oncol 1987;5:1673–1689.

531. Montone KT, Litzky LA, Wurster A, et al. Analysis of Epstein-Barr virus-associated posttransplantation lymphoproliferative disorder after lung transplantation. Surgery 1996;119:544–551.

532. Nalesnik MA, Makowka L, Starzl TE. The diagnosis and treatment of posttransplant lymphoproliferative

disorders. Curr Probl Surg 1988;25:367–472.

533. Ho M, Miller G, Atchison RW, et al. Epstein-Barr virus infections and DNA hybridization studies in posttransplantation lymphoma and lymphoproliferative lesions: the role of primary infection. J Infect Dis 1985;152:876–886.

534. Walker RC, Paya CV, Marshall WF, et al. Pretransplantation seronegative Epstein-Barr virus status is the primary risk factor for posttransplantation lymphoproliferative disorder in adult heart, lung, and other solid organ transplantations. J Heart Lung Transplant 1995;14:214–221.

535. Starzl TE, Nalesnik MA, Porter KA, et al. Reversibility of lymphomas and lymphoproliferative lesions developing under cyclosporin-steroid therapy. Lancet 1984;1:583–587.

536. Swinnen LJ. Diagnosis and treatment of transplant-related lymphoma. Ann Oncol 2000;11:45–48.

537. Leblond V, Dhedin N, Mamzer Bruneel MF, et al. Identification of prognostic factors in 61 patients with posttransplantation lymphoproliferative disorders. J Clin Oncol 2001;19:772–778.

538. Lim GY, Newman B, Kurland G, et al. Posttransplantation lymphoproliferative disorder: manifestations in pediatric thoracic organ recipients. Radiology 2002;222:699–708.

539. Tubman DE, Frick MP, Hanto DW. Lymphoma after organ transplantation: radiologic manifestations in the central nervous system, thorax, and abdomen. Radiology 1983;149:625–631.

540. Pickhardt PJ, Siegel MJ. Abdominal manifestations of posttransplantation lymphoproliferative disorder. AJR Am J Roentgenol 1998;171:1007–1013.

541. McAdams HP, Donnelly LF, MacFall JR. Hyperpolarized gas-enhanced MR imaging of the lungs. In: Boiselle PM, White CS, eds. New Techniques in thoracic imaging. New York: Marcel Dekker Inc; 2002:265–288.

CHAPTER 7

Pulmonary vascular diseases and pulmonary edema

PULMONARY THROMBOEMBOLISM

Just how frequently pulmonary embolism occurs is difficult to establish, but pulmonary thromboembolism appears to be the sole or major cause of death in 10–15% of adults dying in the acute care wards of general hospitals.[1] However, there is some evidence to suggest that the incidence of pulmonary embolism is declining.[2] Community-based studies suggest that the overall annual incidence of pulmonary embolism is 65 cases per 100,000.[3,4]

Essentially, there appears to be a clear correlation between increasing age and the incidence of pulmonary embolism, but little difference between gender or race.[5] Well-known predisposing factors for pulmonary embolism are a hypercoagulable state,[6,7] orthopedic surgery, malignancy, medical illness,[8] and pregnancy. However, the exact incidence is difficult to gauge even in these recognized higher risk groups; for example, in pregnancy the risk of thromboembolism is probably rather higher ante partum – the incidence during pregnancy may have been overstated in the past.[9] The majority of emboli arise from the deep veins of the legs but other sites, such as the upper limbs, may be a source of emboli, particularly in patients with indwelling venous catheters.[10]

Almost all pulmonary emboli lodge within the branches of the pulmonary arteries, but a few straddle the bifurcation of the main pulmonary artery (saddle emboli), and occasionally one lodges in the right side of the heart. The effects of emboli are primarily due to vascular obstruction.[11,12] The bronchial circulation alone can sustain the lung parenchyma, so preventing embolic infarction.[13,14] Animal studies have shown that bronchial arteries start to dilate within days after pulmonary arterial occlusion,[15,16] and are hypertrophic with collateral vessels developing over the succeeding months.[17,18] Why some emboli cause pulmonary infarction whereas others do not is uncertain, but it would appear that infarction occurs only when the combined bronchial and pulmonary arterial circulation is inadequate, a situation that applies particularly when emboli lodge peripherally in the pulmonary arterial tree and also when emboli occur in patients with heart failure or circulatory shock.[13,19]

No more than 15% of emboli cause true infarction.[11] On pathologic study pulmonary infarction is characterized by ischemic necrosis of alveolar walls, bronchioles, and blood vessels within an area of hemorrhage. Most infarcts occur in the lower lobes, and the majority are multiple. Usually they are cone-shaped areas of hemorrhage and edema that point toward the hilum and are based on the pleura, which is often covered by a fibrinous exudate. Following infarction, fibrous replacement converts the infarct into a contracted scar, with indrawing of the pleura. The resultant parenchymal scarring is only rarely extensive enough to cause lung restriction.[20] In some cases hemorrhage is the dominant finding and there is no evidence of tissue necrosis; these lesions resolve without residual scar formation.

In very few individuals, pulmonary embolism causes pulmonary edema. Such patients usually have heart disease, and it seems probable that in these patients the pulmonary emboli precipitate left ventricular failure.[21] In massive pulmonary embolism the edema may be due to over-perfusion of nonoccluded portions of the pulmonary circulation.[22,23]

Emboli usually resolve, and the vessel lumen is restored.[11,24–26] The main mechanism is presumed to be intravascular lysis and fragmentation. In a few patients emboli do not lyse[27,28] and the presence of repeated, unresolved emboli may lead to chronic pulmonary hypertension,[24] although the inevitability of this cause and effect has recently been questioned.[29] The effects of pulmonary embolism are summarized in Box 7.1.

> ### Box 7.1 Possible pathophysiologic consequences of pulmonary embolism
>
> Pulmonary infarction
> - Subsequent parenchymal scarring
>
> Local pulmonary hemorrhage
>
> Exudative pleural effusion
> - Subsequent pleural thickening
>
> Pulmonary edema
> - Either precipitated LVF or over-perfusion of nonembolized lung
>
> Pulmonary hypertension following repeated unresolved emboli

Since the clinical manifestations of pulmonary embolism are protean and largely nonspecific[5,30] it is unsurprising that the diagnosis is often missed. They range from no symptoms to silent emboli[31] to sudden death. The symptoms and signs include dyspnea, chest pain that is often pleuritic but is sometimes anginal, cough, hemoptysis, tachypnea, hypotension, tachycardia, fever, and a pleural friction rub.[12,32] Because so many of the clinical features of pulmonary embolism are nonspecific, the diagnosis is often overlooked.[33]

Primarily serologic tests such as D-dimer levels may be useful for excluding venous thrombosis.[34,35] In some centers, the relatively high sensitivity of the ELISA D-dimer test[36] has led to its adoption, in conjunction with a careful assessment of clinical probability, as a means of ruling out the need for further investigations in patients with a negative D-dimer result.[37–40] Nevertheless, false negative results do occur in patients with pulmonary embolism, particularly those with subsegmental emboli.[41] A meta-analysis of the second generation of rapid D-dimer tests indicates sensitivity within the range of 87–98%.[42] The poor specificity of D-dimer, resulting in raised levels in many disparate conditions (including pregnancy, cancer, inflammatory disorders, and increasing age), is now well recognized and means that its usefulness lies in ruling out, not in, venous thromboembolism. Various forms of D-dimer assay are under development that will doubtless improve the accuracy and, most importantly, the negative predictive value of the test.[43,44]

Every potential diagnosis of pulmonary thromboembolism must be carefully considered because anticoagulant[45,46] and thrombolytic[47] therapy carries significant risks that would not be justified in the absence of pulmonary embolism; conversely, the consequences of undiagnosed pulmonary embolism may be dire.

Imaging of pulmonary emboli

Imaging tests that have been brought to bear on the diagnosis of pulmonary embolism include plain chest radiography, radionuclide lung scanning, pulmonary angiography, computed tomography, and magnetic resonance imaging. Over the last ten years the emphasis placed on the efficacy of individual tests has shifted considerably; no single technique is flawless and, for the foreseeable future, it seems probable that more than one diagnostic test, combined with clinical judgment, will be used to make the diagnosis of pulmonary embolism.

Chest radiography

Radiographic signs of pulmonary embolism and infarction have been extensively described.[48–55] Before discussion of these signs it is important to state clearly that none is specific and that the sensitivity of the signs is poor.[53,56–58] Even in patients with life-threatening pulmonary embolism, the chest radiograph can appear normal.[59] In one large series of 152 patients suspected of having pulmonary emboli, the overall sensitivity of the chest radiograph was 33% and the overall specificity was 59%.[57] Therefore the major role of the chest film is to exclude other diagnoses that might mimic pulmonary embolism, such as pneumothorax, pneumonia, or rib fractures, and to provide information that helps in interpreting the radionuclide scans.[60,61] There will, however, be some cases in which the chest radiograph will suggest the diagnosis, and it is therefore important to

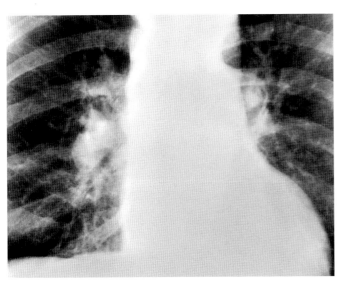

Fig. 7.1 Westermark's sign of pulmonary embolism. The right hilum is large, and vessels beyond the hilum in the right lower lobe are small.

appreciate the radiographic signs, despite their low sensitivity and specificity. A useful framework for discussing the radiographic abnormalities in acute pulmonary embolism is to divide them into (1) pulmonary embolism without infarction, and (2) pulmonary embolism with infarction.

Acute pulmonary embolism without infarction

Since most emboli do not cause infarction, as discussed earlier, the plain film signs of acute pulmonary embolism without infarction or hemorrhage are confined to oligemia of the lung beyond the occluded vessel (Westermark's sign; Fig. 7.1), an increase in the size of the main pulmonary artery or of one of the descending pulmonary trunks, and elevation of a hemidi-

aphragm.[49,50,52,54,62,63] The lack of specificity of these signs is self-evident; chronic obstructive pulmonary disease may cause similar pulmonary vascular changes, and the position of the diaphragm is influenced by numerous factors, of which pulmonary embolism is just one.

In some patients linear densities[64] may be a manifestation of pulmonary embolism (Fig. 7.2). These shadows represent atelectatic lung, not pulmonary infarcts,[65,66] and are secondary to elevation of the diaphragm, inhibition of ventilation, and possibly depletion of surfactant.[1]

Acute pulmonary embolism with infarction

Typically, pulmonary infarction gives rise to radiographically detectable consolidation, which is usually multifocal and is predominant in the lower lung zones.[13] Such shadows usually occur 12–24 hours after the embolic episode, although their appearance may be delayed for several days.[67] The resulting opacity (Fig. 7.3) may assume a variety of shapes depending on the location and underlying lobular architecture of the lung.[68,69] Consolidation of an entire lobe is, however, unusual.[70]

Hampton and Castleman[68] described their famous "hump" in an early paper that correlated the pathologic findings with the postmortem chest radiograph. They emphasized that "infarcts are always in contact with pleural surfaces and that the shadows are rarely, if ever, triangular in shape" (a point worth knowing in the context of CT interpretation). They noticed that the central margin of the infarct shadow might be rounded, hence the term "hump" (Fig. 7.3). In fact, a Hampton's hump is relatively unusual[71] and is, in any event, a nonspecific finding. An air bronchogram within the hump is rarely seen on plain radiography.[72] Frequently, the clinical features point to one or another diagnosis; if they do not, the radiographic appearance of the opacity cannot be relied on to offer a distinction between the various causes of consolidation.

A theoretical, rather than practical, distinction between non-infarctive and infarctive consolidation can be made from the

A
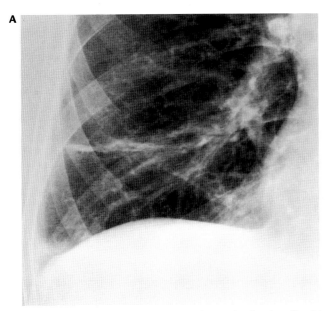

B
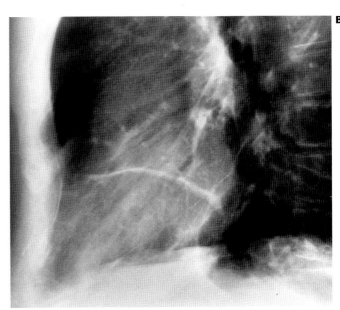

Fig. 7.2 **A**, Posteroanterior and **B**, lateral radiographs showing discoid atelectasis in a patient with pulmonary embolism.

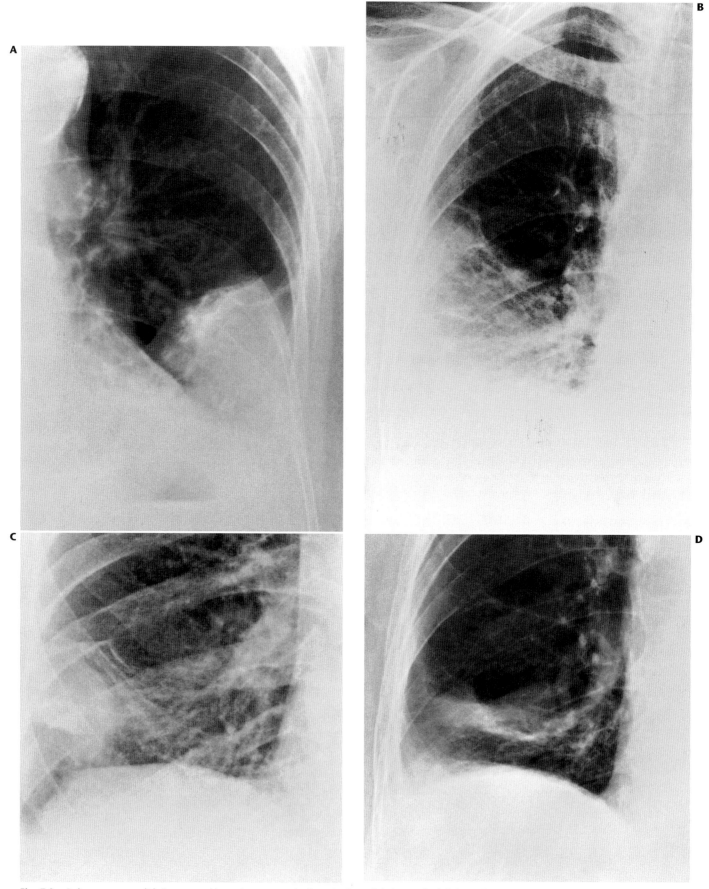

Fig. 7.3 Pulmonary consolidation caused by pulmonary embolism. **A**, Consolidation at the left base shows a rounded, truncated, cone shape (Hampton's hump). **B**, Consolidation in the right lung in the same patient, showing segmental configuration. Appearance of right-sided consolidation **C**, 2½ weeks later and **D**, 5½ weeks later showing gradual resolution "from the periphery".

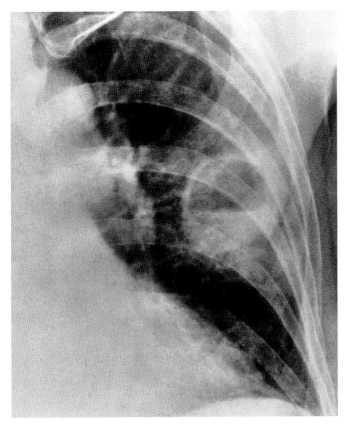

Fig. 7.4 A cavitating pulmonary infarct.

Knowledge about the frequency with which pleural effusions accompany pulmonary embolism comes from a carefully conducted prospective study that showed that approximately half of patients with pulmonary embolism also had a pleural effusion, and these were often bloody.[80] In one-third of the cases the effusion was an isolated finding, and in the remaining two-thirds it was accompanied by radiographic evidence of pulmonary infarction or hemorrhage. Typically, the effusions are small and unilateral and appear soon after the onset of symptoms, but occasionally effusions are bilateral and large.[53] It is interesting to note that almost all patients who had a pleural effusion had chest pain on the same side.[80] It appears probable that pleural effusions following pulmonary embolism are caused by infarction of the lung and that, in those cases in which no infarct shadow is visible on plain chest radiograph, the infarct is present but is hidden from view by the effusion[80] (Box 7.3).

Box 7.3 Pleural effusions in pulmonary embolism

Small unilateral pleural effusion is a common accompaniment to pulmonary embolism
Pleural effusion reflects underlying infarction and is usually hemorrhagic
Pleural effusion may be the only manifestation of pulmonary embolism on plain chest radiography (~30% of cases)
CT shows subpleural pulmonary infarct in most cases in which an effusion is present

---

observation that when the consolidation is the result of pulmonary hemorrhage without true infarction, radiographic clearing occurs quickly, often within a week, whereas infarction takes several months to resolve[73] and frequently leaves permanent linear scars.[74] By 3 months, infarct shadows either have totally resolved or show no more than linear scarring or pleural thickening.[75] As infarcts resolve, they tend to "melt away like an ice cube" (Fig. 7.3), whereas acute pneumonia disappears in a patchy fashion.[76] It may therefore be possible to suggest the diagnosis retrospectively, but this sign has no value at the time when it is most needed.

Notably, cavitation within an infarct is rare (Fig. 7.4). It may be seen in the absence of infection[77,78] but usually cavitary infarcts are either secondarily infected or result from septic emboli in the first place. Aseptic cavitation is more likely to occur in an area of infarction greater than 4 cm in diameter and usually occurs 2 weeks after the appearance of the focal consolidation.[79] The plain radiographic signs of pulmonary embolism are summarized in Box 7.2.

Box 7.2 Plain radiographic signs of acute pulmonary embolism

Normal radiographic appearances (!)
Regional oligemia
Increase in size of a proximal pulmonary artery
Elevated hemidiaphragm
• Associated linear atelectasis
Focal consolidation (infarcts)
• Usually basal, rarely cavitate
Pleural effusion

Radionuclide imaging

Years have passed since diagnostic scintigraphy was first used in cases of suspected pulmonary embolism. This venerable test involves the simultaneous imaging of the distributions of pulmonary blood flow and alveolar ventilation. The combined study is called a ventilation–perfusion ($\dot{V}/Q$) scan and remains a widely available[81] and cost-effective[82] test. The principle underlying the diagnosis of pulmonary embolism is that whereas pulmonary perfusion is abnormal, the pulmonary parenchyma usually remains intact and ventilation remains normal. This gives rise to the so-called "mismatched perfusion defect", the hallmark of pulmonary embolic disease. If embolism results in pulmonary infarction, a defect of ventilation also appears, corresponding to the perfusion defect.

Perfusion scanning

One part of the $\dot{V}/Q$ scan is perfusion imaging which consists of the intravenous injection of microparticles labeled with technetium-99m (^{99m}Tc). These microembolize in the lung vascular bed and are trapped on first pass (Fig. 7.5). Particles of macroaggregated human serum albumin (MAA), which have a size range of 10–100 µm, are most commonly used. In patients with pulmonary hypertension there is a risk of further occlusion of an already depleted vascular bed. However, the number of capillaries (of the order of 300 million) far outnumbers the number of particles administered (200,000 to 500,000), even in pulmonary vascular disease, so there is a wide safety margin. The particles are biodegradable and have a biological half life in the lung of less than 8 hours. The ^{99m}Tc elutes from the particles faster than this, and by 24 hours most of the remaining activity is visible

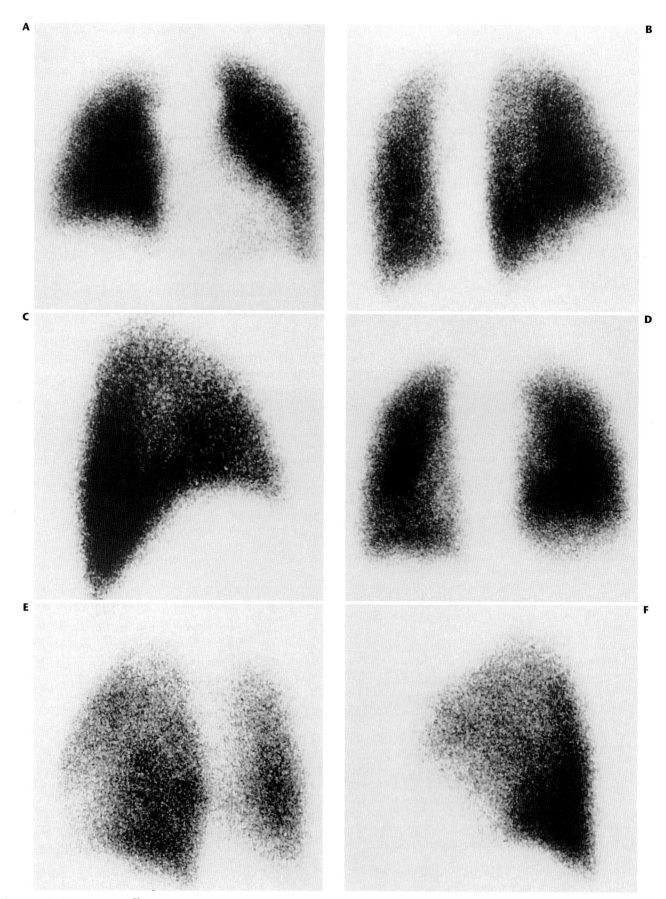

Fig. 7.5 (*Left page*) Normal ^{99m}Tc perfusion scans of the lungs: **A**, anterior; **B**, right posterior oblique; **C**, right lateral; **D**, posterior; **E**, left posterior oblique; **F**, left lateral view.

in the gut and kidneys. Provided the particles mix completely in the blood prior to microembolization, the distribution of radioactivity is proportional to the distribution of pulmonary blood flow (Fig. 7.5). Not only is photon emission itself a random event, so also is the distribution of the particles. A distribution of radioactivity which is proportional to the distribution of pulmonary blood flow is, therefore, also dependent on the injection of a sufficiently large number of particles as well as the amount of injected radioactivity.[83]

Usually the supine (rather than prone) position is used to promote even delivery of particles to the apices, which, in the erect position, are poorly visualized because of the normal gravity-dependent distribution of pulmonary blood flow.[84] Of the administered [99mTc], 95–99% is trapped in the lungs[85]; the majority of the non-trapped radioactivity is probably unbound [99mTc]. A [99mTc] lung perfusion scan gives an effective radiation dose equivalent of 1 mSv/100 MBq. The usual imaging dose is 75 MBq (approximately 2 mCi). Since the material is "sticky", injection through long lines should be avoided because a considerable fraction is likely to be retained in the line.

Ventilation scanning

Despite their very different properties (and availability), two classes of agents are used for ventilation imaging: the radioactive inert gases xenon-133 and krypton-81m (^{133}Xe, [81m]Kr) and the radiolabeled aerosols. Worldwide, aerosols are now the most frequently used agent. The ultrashort-lived inert gas [81m]Kr is probably the optimal agent for ventilation imaging, but it is expensive and has limited availability. Because of the very short half life of [81m]Kr, the technique of [81m]Kr imaging is fundamentally different from that of xenon imaging. Xenon-133 has a half life of 5.3 days and, although cheap and easily available, gives images of poor resolution because of its low photon energy of 80 KeV. Following a short period of inhalation, the so-called "wash-in phase", it gives an image of the regional distribution of ventilation. With continuing inhalation the distribution of radio-activity increasingly reflects regional lung volume. Eventually the wash-in rate becomes equal to the wash-out rate, and during this equilibrium phase the image portrays regional lung volume. Because of its very short half life of 13 seconds, [81m]Kr (190 KeV) effectively gives information only for wash-in studies since it has decayed by the time it is exhaled. Krypton-81m is the metastable daughter of rubidium-81 ([81]Rb), which is delivered in a canister from a cyclotron unit. The canister is connected to an air cylinder and has an outlet port through which cylinder air is delivered to the patient for continuous inhalation. Rubidium-81 has a half life of 4.7 hours, giving a [81m]Kr generator a useful life span of 1 working day. The attraction of [81m]Kr is that it can be continuously administered and images acquired in any projection with minimal patient cooperation. Perfusion and ventilation images can be obtained without moving the patient, either in sequence by alternating the photopeak settings on the gamma camera between [81m]Kr and [99mTc], or simultaneously by dual photon acquisition. For the sequential approach, switching off the [81m]Kr supply prevents "down-scatter" of the higher energy photons of [81m]Kr into the [99mTc] window. Residual gas clears rapidly, mainly by radioactive decay, and does not therefore interfere with the [99mTc] images.

Aerosol ventilation imaging has become popular largely because of technical improvements in the delivery systems and reduction in aerosol particle size. Aerosols are generally made from [99mTc]-diethylenetriaminepentaacetic acid (DTPA). Their administration requires the patient to breathe through a mouthpiece, with a nose clip in place, for several minutes. Most users give the aerosol before the administration of [99mTc]-MAA, although some give it after, only to patients with abnormal perfusion scans. If they are given in close succession, some form of image subtraction may be necessary. As with [81m]Kr, images can be acquired in multiple projections, facilitating comparison with the subsequent perfusion images. The regional distribution of radioactivity depicts regional ventilation at the instant of inhalation. In this respect, aerosol imaging is similar to [99mTc]-MAA perfusion imaging in that the distribution of agent is "frozen" at the time of administration, unlike [81m]Kr, which continuously and dynamically depicts the distribution of ventilation as the patient breathes the gas.

Versions of available aerosols include an agent called "Technegas".[86] This is an ultrafine dispersion of [99mTc]-labeled carbon particles generated by combustion of pertechnetate at 2500°C in a graphite crucible in an atmosphere of 100% argon within the Technegas "generator". This agent gives ventilation images with a quality approaching that of [81m]Kr,[87] but is otherwise similar to the conventional DTPA aerosols in terms of convenience and availability. Once the generator has been purchased, ventilation imaging can be performed immediately on request. Deposition of particles in the central airways, which is a problem with conventional DTPA aerosols, particularly in patients with chronic lung disease, appears to be less with Technegas because of the smaller particle size. As with [99mTc]-DTPA aerosols, subtraction of the Technegas signal from the subsequent perfusion signal (or vice versa) may be necessary.

In healthy, nonsmoking subjects, [99mTc]-DTPA clears from the lungs with a half life of about 80 minutes. In smokers it is up to three times faster. By the time the perfusion scans are performed, activity is often already visible in the renal collecting systems, especially in smokers (because of increased epithelial permeability of their lungs). It is also usually visible, as swallowed activity, in the upper gastrointestinal tract as a result of particle deposition in the mouth, and in the proximal airways of patients with chronic lung disease as a result of particle deposition caused by turbulent airflow.

Dedicated anterior, posterior, and both posterior oblique views, as a minimum, are recommended for $\dot{V}/Q$ scanning. Occasionally, laterals and anterior obliques may also be useful. Single photon emission computed tomography (SPECT) may have a role in $\dot{V}/Q$ lung scanning,[88] particularly when ventilation imaging is performed with [81m]Kr[89] or Technegas.[90] It has been suggested that chest radiography may substitute for the ventilation scan in $\dot{V}/Q$ imaging, but that further evidence is needed before this recommendation is generally adopted.[91] If clinically relevant, $\dot{V}/Q$ lung imaging should be performed with little hesitation in pregnant women because of the obvious undesirability of anticoagulation in such circumstances. The radiation dose to the fetus is small and perfusion-only lung imaging may be adequate, provided the patient is a non-smoker, has a normal chest radiograph, and has no history of chronic lung disease.

Interpretation of the $\dot{V}/Q$ scan

Having an appreciation of how "defects" on perfusion and ventilation scintigraphy are generated greatly helps in the correct interpretation of the $\dot{V}/Q$ scan. The diagnostic feature of pulmonary embolism in a $\dot{V}/Q$ lung scan is a perfusion defect in a region of normally ventilated lung – the so-called "mismatched perfusion defect" (Figs 7.6 and 7.7). The size of the defect may range from appreciably smaller than a segment (subsegmental), to about the size of a segment (segmental), or even a lobe or whole lung. A nonsegmental defect is one that does not correspond to segmental anatomy. The pathologic basis of the mismatched perfusion defect is that in uncomplicated pulmonary embolism the pulmonary architecture remains intact and ventilation therefore continues as normal. However, when embolism is followed by lung infarction, a ventilation defect appears, although it is usually smaller than the perfusion defect because the lung around the periphery of the perfusion defect continues to ventilate. The diagnostic feature of a pulmonary infarct, therefore, is an incompletely matched perfusion defect (Fig. 7.7) in association with an appropriate radiographic abnormality. The positive identification of a pulmonary infarct on a $\dot{V}/Q$ lung scan depends on high quality, multiprojection imaging, and can be improved with SPECT imaging.[88]

A perfusion scan showing two or more defects of segmental size or larger in the presence of a normal ventilation scan (Fig. 7.8) and the appropriate clinical setting signifies a high probability (greater than 90%) of recent pulmonary embolism, whereas a normal perfusion scan effectively excludes embolism (likelihood <<5%), whatever the ventilation scan shows.[92–94] Very often, however, patients with suspected pulmonary embolism have coincidental cardiopulmonary disease and it becomes more difficult to rule in or rule out the diagnosis.

Not only single, but several, matched defects may be seen on the ventilation and perfusion scans (Fig. 7.9). Complete matching is seen in obstructive airways disease, either acute as in bronchial

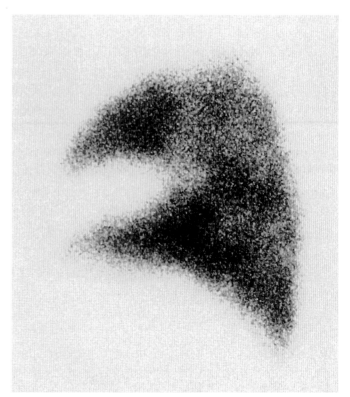

Fig. 7.6 Perfusion defect. Technetium-99m scan; right lateral view. The typical segmental-shaped perfusion defect is pointing to the hilum and is based on the pleura. The defect in this case corresponds to the entire middle lobe and is due to a pulmonary embolus. The ventilation scan was normal.

A

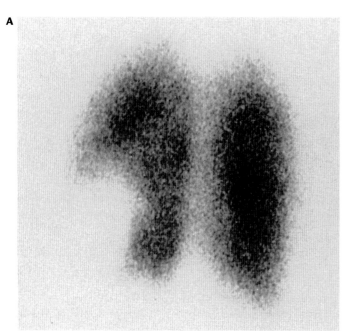

B

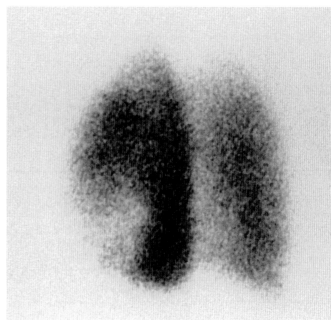

Fig. 7.7 Pulmonary infarct. **A,** A perfusion defect is visible in the lingular region of the left lung (left posterior oblique view). **B,** A ^{81m}Kr ventilation scan shows a defect at the same site, but it is clearly smaller than the corresponding perfusion defect, typical of pulmonary infarction.

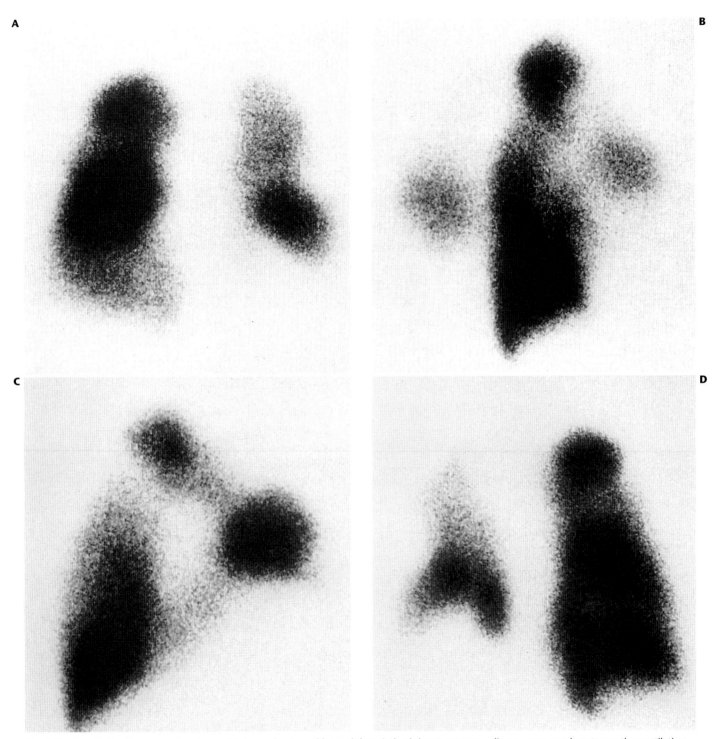

Fig. 7.8 A perfusion lung scan showing multiple moderate and large defects in both lungs corresponding to segmental anatomy; the ventilation images were normal, thereby indicating a high probability of pulmonary embolism. Four projections are shown: **A**, anterior; **B**, right posterior oblique; **C**, posterior; **D**, left posterior oblique.

asthma, or chronic as in chronic obstructive airways disease. It is complete because of efficient hypoxic vasoconstriction, a defense mechanism that prevents pulmonary arterial blood from circulating through nonventilated lung. Hypoxic vasoconstriction may nevertheless be incomplete, in which case a region of lung may be better perfused than ventilated – a so-called *"reversed mismatch"* (Box 7.4).

Several chest diseases are characterized by reversed mismatching, including pleural effusions and fluid in the fissures, lobar pneumonia, collapsed and consolidated lung, and gross

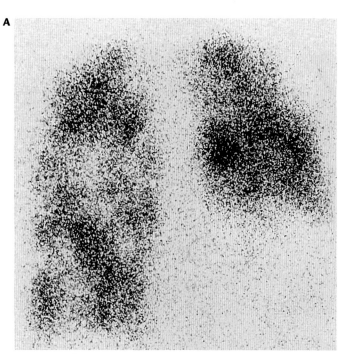
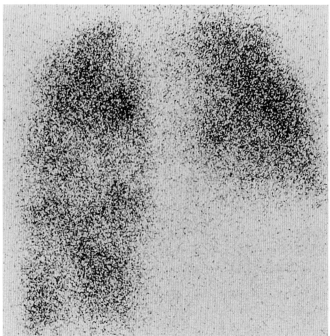

Fig. 7.9 A V̇/Q scan indicating low probability of pulmonary embolism. The perfusion scan is on the left (**A**) and ^{81m}Kr ventilation scan on the right (**B**). There are multiple perfusion defects which are matched on the corresponding ventilation images.

Box 7.4 **Causes of a reversed V̇/Q mismatch**

Basal pleural effusion
Lobar pneumonia
Lobar collapse
Acute partial bronchial obstruction
Chronic obstructive airways disease

---

cardiomegaly (which compresses the adjacent lung).[95–97] The phenomenon is also seen in acute partial bronchial obstruction, in which the chest radiograph may appear normal, and in chronic obstructive airways disease, especially in acute exacerbations.[98] In these conditions, hypoxic vasoconstriction fails or is incomplete. Completely matched defects are seen in destructive parenchymal disease, such as bullous or fibrosing lung disease and pulmonary abscess.

Exact language to convey the likelihood of pulmonary embolism, on the basis of the V̇/Q appearances, has proved elusive and several diagnostic algorithms have been proposed for the interpretation and reporting of V̇/Q lung scans.[92,93,99–102] These algorithms express the likelihood of embolism on a verbal probability scale as low, intermediate, and high. The probability or likelihood that an abnormal scan is due to pulmonary embolism is the positive predictive value of the test, defined as the ratio of true positives:all positives. It is highly dependent on the prevalence of the disease in the patient population studied. Before discussing these algorithms, it should be emphasized that they have been based largely on ventilation imaging using ^{133}Xe and generally ignore the pretest clinical likelihood of pulmonary embolism. Summarizing the

literature, an abnormal V̇/Q scan indicating a low probability for pulmonary embolism is one in which the individual perfusion defects are: (1) smaller than 25% of a segment (that is, subsegmental), regardless of the chest radiographic and ventilation scan appearances; or (2) are matched on the ventilation scan or are accompanied by larger chest radiographic abnormalities. Prominent, nonpulmonary intrathoracic structures, such as an enlarged hilum, cardiac chamber, or aorta, are described as giving matched defects, but they are readily identifiable from the chest radiograph and should not be described as "defects".

Least problematic is a V̇/Q scan indicating a high probability of recent pulmonary embolism, in which there are two or more perfusion defects, not matched by corresponding ventilation defects or chest radiographic abnormalities, including at least one of segmental or larger size (Fig. 7.8). In the appropriate clinical setting, a high-probability V̇/Q scan indicates a probability of pulmonary embolism exceeding 90%.

Less satisfactory is an intermediate-probability V̇/Q scan, also described in the literature as an indeterminate scan, which does not fit into the low- or high-probability categories. In essence, the probability of pulmonary embolism in patients with intermediate-probability scans is likely to be similar to what it was before the scan, and the patient will need further investigation. In general, V̇/Q scans indicating an intermediate probability for recent pulmonary embolism have been classified in the literature as those (1) with perfusion defects that, although matched, correspond in size and shape to an area of consolidation on the chest radiograph (and may therefore represent infarction – so-called "triple match"), or (2) with perfusion defects in areas of severe obstructive lung disease, pulmonary edema, or pleural effusion. Good quality ventilation imaging has the potential to reduce the number of scans placed in the intermediate category. For example, in the second of the above criteria for intermediate probability, the perfusion abnormalities should be seen on multiple projection ventilation imaging to be matched by, or be smaller than, the corresponding ventilation defects and so be categorized as "low probability".

A follow-up study is often helpful, even when the $\dot{V}/Q$ scan indicates a high probability of embolism, for two reasons: first, because unresolved pulmonary embolism is probably not uncommon, and second, to establish a new baseline in the event of incomplete resolution. It seems probable that some long-standing perfusion defects will, on the basis of a single $\dot{V}/Q$ scan, be interpreted as representing acute pulmonary embolism and thus result in unnecessary anticoagulation.[103]

Within nuclear medicine reporting practice, the probability stratification approach, with its specified criteria, is exclusive to the $\dot{V}/Q$ scan performed for suspected pulmonary embolism. It is not unreasonable to suggest that this has grown out of the philosophy that the only reason for performing a $\dot{V}/Q$ lung scan is to diagnose pulmonary embolism. Several early reports comparing scintigraphy with pulmonary angiography have failed to take into account the clinical and imaging evidence of deep venous thrombosis, early follow-up of abnormal scans, and the pretest likelihood of the disease. This last consideration was brought out by the PIOPED study,[92] in which it was shown that the incidence of abnormal pulmonary angiography was greater, in all probability categories, when the prescan clinical likelihood of pulmonary embolism was high compared with when it was it low. This means that the $\dot{V}/Q$ scan can be regarded as a *screening* test which increases the pretest likelihood of embolism, decreases it, or leaves it unchanged. Thus a patient without risk factors for pulmonary embolism, who presents with sudden onset of pleuritic chest pain and is deemed to have a low clinical likelihood of embolism, and who then has a $\dot{V}/Q$ scan indicating a low probability of embolism on scintigraphic criteria, can be deemed to have a post-$\dot{V}/Q$ scan likelihood which is even lower and which for clinical purposes rules out the need for anticoagulation. Conversely, a patient with a risk factor for pulmonary embolism, such as recent surgery or a history of previous deep vein thrombosis, who then has a low-probability $\dot{V}/Q$ scan retains an overall likelihood of embolism in the region of 10–20%, or even higher.[104]

In the context of the patient with suspected pulmonary embolism, an important function of the chest radiograph, apart from providing anatomic landmarks, is to avoid missing pulmonary infarction. A matched defect without a corresponding radiographic abnormality has a low probability for pulmonary embolism: the appearance of a corresponding radiographic abnormality moves the $\dot{V}/Q$ scan into the intermediate category because it increases the likelihood of infarction. Partial mismatching typical of infarction with an appropriate radiographic abnormality further increases the likelihood. An important question that remains unanswered is how often an infarct can give a completely matched defect. Nevertheless, a matched defect can be relegated to low probability, irrespective of the chest radiograph.

Rather than listing the criteria for categorizing a lung scan on a verbal probability scale, it may be more useful to identify those features on the $\dot{V}/Q$ lung scan that have been most contentious and cause difficulty in diagnosing pulmonary embolism. These are (1) the solitary unmatched perfusion defect, (2) symmetric segmental unmatched perfusion defects, (3) the matched perfusion defect with a similar-sized corresponding

radiographic opacity, (4) multiple unmatched but subsegmental perfusion defects, and (5) unmatched segmental perfusion defects not clearly seen on any projection to extend to the periphery of the lung (the so-called "stripe sign"). In this setting it is important to appreciate that the unmatched perfusion defect points to pulmonary vascular disease and not specifically to embolic disease. There are several diseases other than pulmonary embolism in which the $\dot{V}/Q$ scan may show mismatched perfusion abnormalities. A mismatched defect indicates pulmonary vascular disease, which usually, although not always, is due to pulmonary embolism. The causes of mismatched perfusion defects are listed in Box 7.5.

> **Box 7.5 Causes of $\dot{V}/Q$ mismatching**
>
> Pulmonary embolism
> - Acute
> - Chronic
>
> Pulmonary thrombosis
> Primary pulmonary hypertension
> Pulmonary venoocclusive disease
> Vasculitis of medium-sized arteries
> Ventilated bullous disease
> External compression of pulmonary artery
> - Carcinoma of the bronchus
> - Lymphoma
>
> Focal obliteration of pulmonary capillaries
> - Fibrosing lung disease
> - Emphysema
> - Irradiation
>
> Congenital pulmonary artery hypoplasia
> Sequestrated segment
> Artifactual (may be posture-dependent)
> - Unstable ventilation
> - Related to pleural fluid
>
> Upper lobe diversion (in heart disease)
> Previous vascular surgery with creation of intravascular shunts
> Intraluminal obstruction (e.g. catheters, *Dirofilaria immitis*)
> Pulmonary arteriovenous malformations (especially following therapeutic embolization)

Important causes include: carcinoma of the bronchus, which often gives rise to the characteristic finding of a completely nonperfused lung or lobe with a normally perfused opposite lung and normal ventilation (Fig. 7.10); bullae, which occasionally ventilate[105] but are usually evident on the chest radiograph; pulmonary vasculitis involving medium-sized arteries, which may be indistinguishable from embolism; and idiopathic pulmonary fibrosis, which usually involves the lower zones symmetrically[106] (Fig. 7.11). In children, in whom pulmonary embolism is rarely diagnosed, unmatched perfusion defects are more likely to be due to sequestered segments, congenital anomalies of the pulmonary artery, and previous surgery for congenital cardiovascular anomalies. Caution is occasionally required in this last setting with regard to the venous site used for injecting the microparticles.

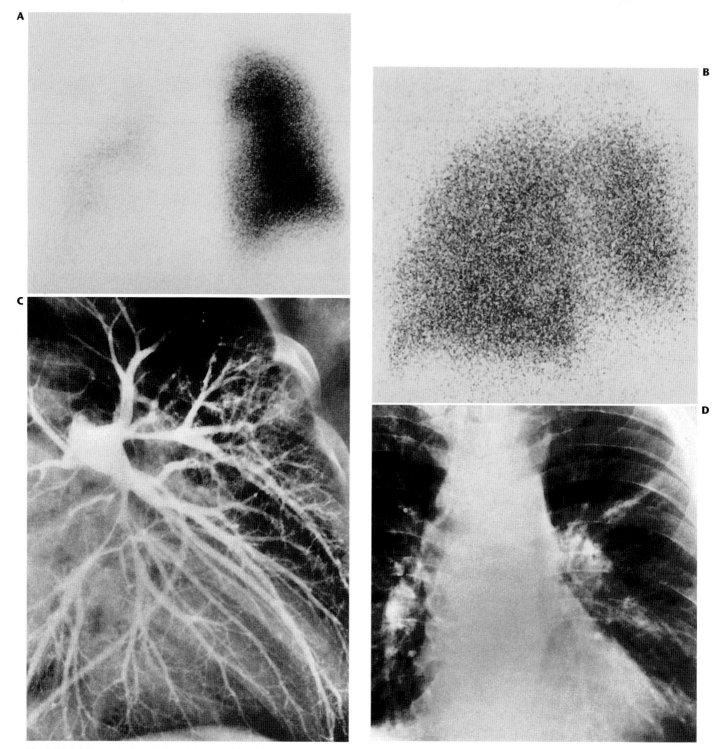

Fig. 7.10 Mismatched perfusion defect resulting from a carcinoma of the bronchus involving the major divisions of the left pulmonary artery. **A,** A ^{99m}Tc scan, posterior view. **B,** A ^{133}Xe ventilation scan, left posterior oblique. **C,** Pulmonary arteriogram illustrates involvement of the central pulmonary arteries by the tumor. **D,** Posteroanterior radiograph.

Pulmonary angiography

The morbidity and mortality of pulmonary angiography have probably been exaggerated over the years. In the PIOPED study there were only 5 deaths (0.5%) out of the 1111 patients who underwent pulmonary angiography.[107] In some large series no deaths are reported,[108,109] and in others the rate is less than 1% and usually under 0.5%.[51,110–112] More recent studies have confirmed the low morbidity and negligible mortality of pulmonary angiography, particularly when it is used in carefully selected patients.[113,114] Pulmonary hypertension is the major predisposing factor for increased mortality: 9 of the 10 patients reported by

A 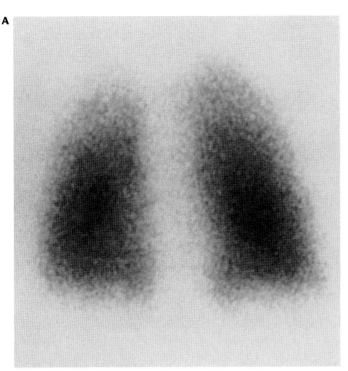 B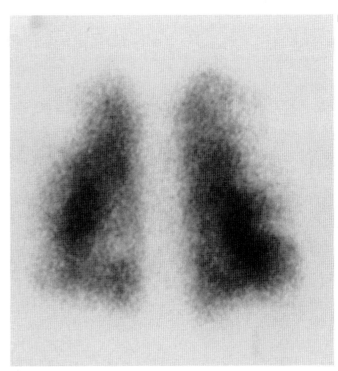

Fig. 7.11 Idiopathic pulmonary fibrosis. This disease is one of several, other than pulmonary embolic disease, that may give rise to unmatched perfusion defects. This V̇/Q scan (posterior view) shows extensive, fairly symmetrical, perfusion abnormalities (**B**) but a normal ⁸¹ᵐKr ventilation image (**A**).

Goodman[115] had proved or presumed pulmonary hypertension. Of the nonfatal complications, arrhythmias are the most common, followed by cardiac perforation. Cardiac perforation, although it may lead to pericardial tamponade, frequently resolves without incident, particularly if there is no associated myocardial intravasation. Such nonfatal complications occur in 1–5% of patients.[107,114] Elderly patients are more at risk of renal failure but otherwise have the same low complication rate as younger patients.[116] When a perfusion lung scan has been performed, the angiographic examination can be tailored to search for emboli in the areas of perfusion defect. Thus the perfusion scan helps in performing the study and may also reduce complications by justifying a more limited examination than would otherwise be necessary.[113,117,118] The advantages of digital subtraction angiography are increased contrast resolution and greater safety, but these advantages may be offset by poor spatial resolution and motion artifact.[119–121] Image quality has improved to the extent that interobserver agreement and confidence for digital subtraction pulmonary angiography has been reported to be superior to that for conventional selective angiography.[122,123]

The two major angiographic signs of acute pulmonary embolism are (Figs 7.12 and 7.13)[55,124–126]:

1. Intraluminal filling defects within the opacified arterial tree. These filling defects are caused by opacified blood flowing around the thrombus. Sometimes, the contrast medium flows past the thrombus to opacify the distal vessels. At other times only the trailing edge of a thrombus impacted in a downstream arterial branch is seen.
2. Complete occlusion of a pulmonary artery branch. Occlusion is a nonspecific sign and may be seen in a variety of conditions, including congenital malformations, organized thrombus from a previous embolus, in situ

thrombosis, mediastinal fibrosis, occlusion from direct involvement by a neoplasm or a variety of inflammatory diseases.

The other arteriographic sign of pulmonary embolism is focal reduction or delay in the opacification of the pulmonary arterial branches,[124] equivalent to the perfusion defect seen at radionuclide imaging. Clearly, reduced perfusion, regardless of how it is demonstrated, is a less specific sign than an intraluminal filling defect or an abrupt occlusion of a vessel.[127,128] It will be seen in any condition that destroys lung parenchyma, notably emphysema, bronchiectasis, or pulmonary scarring, and in any condition that leads to focal hypoxic vasoconstriction.

Pulmonary thromboemboli usually lyse following the embolic episode. In dogs, experimentally produced emboli can disappear within days,[129,130] and rapid resolution has also been recorded in humans.[131] In general, however, it appears that thromboemboli are detectable angiographically for weeks or months following the acute event.[115] Some emboli do not lyse completely. They may leave residual webs, which can be seen angiographically,[132,133] or they may form permanent occlusions. Filling defects representing recent emboli are often more difficult to find and may not be detectable.

Historically, opinions about the place of pulmonary angiography in the diagnosis of pulmonary embolism have always varied.[33,108,134–138] Despite its accuracy and apparent safety, pulmonary angiography is too expensive to be considered a cost-effective first-line investigation in all cases of suspected pulmonary embolism.[139] It has recently been pointed out that the radiation dose of pulmonary angiography is higher than that delivered by computed tomography pulmonary angiography (CTPA).[140] In the absence of CTPA or magnetic resonance angiography, pulmonary angiography may be indicated when:

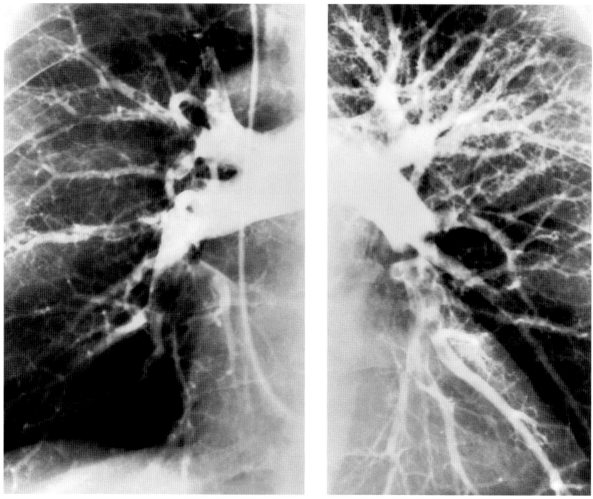

Fig. 7.12 Pulmonary emboli. There are multiple filling defects and occlusions of branches of the pulmonary arteries on pulmonary angiography. **A**, Right and **B**, left pulmonary arteriograms.

1. the $\dot{V}/Q$ scan is abnormal but cannot be placed into either high- or low-probability categories, for example, in patients with underlying chronic obstructive lung disease[141]
2. the identification of subsegmental emboli is regarded as vital, usually in patients with severely limited cardiopulmonary reserve
3. in situ thrombolysis of central pulmonary emboli is contemplated.

Pulmonary angiography is regarded as "gold standard" for the diagnosis of pulmonary embolism during life,[110,124,136] and has been used as a reference standard when evaluating newer techniques such as CTPA.[142] It is self-evident, however, that there are both false positive and false negative interpretations of pulmonary angiograms. Nevertheless, it appears that life-threatening emboli are very infrequently missed.[143] Furthermore, small subsegmental emboli can be detected, albeit with less reliability.[122,144,145] Novelline and associates,[109] Cheely and co-workers,[108] and the PIOPED study[146] all followed large groups of patients clinically suspected of having pulmonary embolism who had normal pulmonary angiograms. Had significant pulmonary emboli been overlooked, it seems likely that some of these patients would have had further embolic episodes in the ensuing years. In fact, none of Novelline's 167 patients did (and

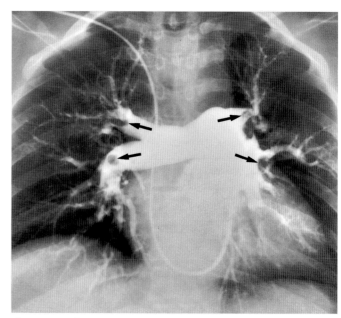

Fig. 7.13 Pulmonary emboli. The pulmonary angiogram shows multiple filling defects. The trailing ends of the occluding thromboemboli are particularly well shown (arrows).

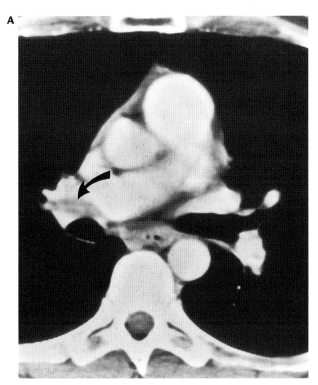

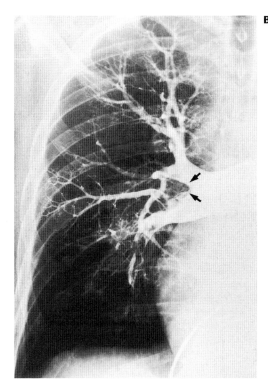

Fig. 7.14 Pulmonary emboli. **A**, The arrow points to an intraluminal defect in the right pulmonary artery on a conventional contrast-enhanced CT scan. **B**, A corresponding pulmonary angiogram shows a large embolus straddling the bifurcation of the right pulmonary artery (arrows) and multiple emboli occluding the right lower lobe artery and its branches.

they were not receiving anticoagulant therapy); in 3 cases small incidental emboli were found in patients dying from other causes.[109] In Cheely's series, 4 of 144 patients with negative angiograms subsequently developed emboli, but in none were they the cause of death.[108] In the PIOPED study, surveillance of 675 patients with negative angiograms revealed 4 (0.06%) patients with pulmonary embolism.[146] The problem of false positive diagnoses is more difficult to evaluate.[126] Despite the evidence that pulmonary angiography is relatively safe and highly sensitive, the provision of pulmonary angiography is often lacking.[134] However, pulmonary angiography may be more accessible than CTPA in some countries.[81,147,148]

Computed tomography pulmonary angiography (CTPA)

Large emboli in the main pulmonary arteries and their major branches may, by chance, be visible on contrast-enhanced CT (Fig. 7.14),[149–154] but their serendipitous detection depends on catching the intravascular bolus of contrast at the right time.[155] Very rarely a large acute embolus may be seen as an area of relatively high attenuation within a central pulmonary artery on an unenhanced CT,[156] but this is exceptional (Fig. 7.15). The advent of continuous volumetric (spiral or helical) scanning[157] paved the way for the improved demonstration of pulmonary

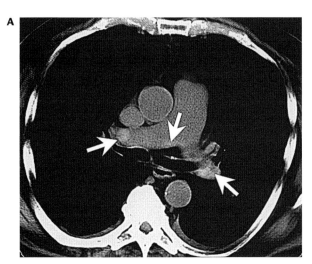

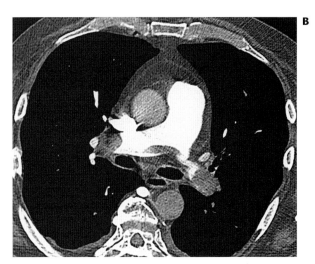

Fig. 7.15 **A**, Unenhanced CT of a patient with a history of a syncopal episode 1 month after surgery for cancer of the colon. There are bilateral high-attenuation central emboli (arrows) **B**, confirmed on the contrast-enhanced CT. (With permission from Kanne JP, Gotway MB, Thoongsuwan N, et al: six cases of acute central pulmonary embolism revealed on unenhanced multidetector CT of the chest. AJR Am J Roentgenol 2003;180:1661–1664. Reprinted with permission.)

embolism on contrast-enhanced CT. Imaging the entire thorax in a single breath hold is now routine and volumetric scanning allows contrast to be administered more economically and timed more precisely, thus giving more consistent vascular opacification. There have now been numerous studies to evaluate the ability of contrast-enhanced CTPA to identify pulmonary embolism.[158–175] This surge of interest should not by itself be regarded as an index of the diagnostic efficacy of CTPA, and the debate about its place in the diagnostic hierarchy has not been finally settled.[139,176–181] Nevertheless, the rapid emergence of CTPA and the enthusiasm with which it has been adopted – before complete evidence of its superiority over existing tests has been gathered – is a dramatic example of "technology creep"; even when the shortcomings of CTPA are, in due course, fully appreciated it seems unlikely that the popularity of this test will diminish. The availability of this noninvasive test is a major factor in ensuring that it will remain in demand.

Technical considerations

Many factors contribute to a technically satisfactory CTPA examination for the diagnosis of pulmonary embolism.[182–186] The steady refinement of scanning protocols, in particular ever-narrower collimation and faster data acquisition, possible with multidetector CT, has improved the detection of segmental and subsegmental emboli.[187] Early studies using 5 mm collimation[161,162,188,189] showed that CTPA was unable to demonstrate reliably emboli in pulmonary arteries below the fourth (segmental) generation. Subsequent investigations have focused on two related questions: how far can the detection of small subsegmental emboli be improved by narrowing collimation? What are the management implications of a negative (optimal) CTPA? (The second question is dealt with on p. 382). With respect to the first question, multidetector CT has undoubtedly improved the ability to detect peripheral emboli by virtue of the increased acquisition speed, which allows thin (~1 mm) sections to be obtained in a single breath hold.[190–194] In a study by Schoepf et al the 1 mm collimation image set increased the detection of subsegmental emboli by 40% compared to 3 mm collimation images.[191]

The iodine concentration, injection rate, and timing of the bolus of contrast have an important bearing on the degree of opacification of the pulmonary arteries. There are, broadly, two options: low-concentration contrast injected at a high flow rate, or a high concentration at a low flow rate.[184] The problem associated with a high-concentration contrast medium (350 mg/ml iodine, or greater) is streak artifact from the superior vena cava which may obscure the immediately adjacent right pulmonary artery (Fig. 7.16). The most obvious solution to this problem (the severity of which is to some extent determined by the characteristics of the CT scanner) is to reduce the flow rate and/or the concentration. However, low flow rates may not produce sufficient contrast enhancement of the segmental arteries (Fig. 7.17). Various iodine concentration protocols have been evaluated ranging from 120 to 140 ml of 15–30% iodine concentration contrast medium injected at a flow rate of 3–5 ml/s.[171,185,192,195] The novel use of gadolinium for CTPA, in a patient in whom iodinated contrast medium was contraindicated, has been reported.[196]

The appropriate delay between the injection of contrast and the start of scanning is largely governed by the patient's circulation time. For most patients, an 8–20 second delay is usually adequate. Contrary to what might be expected, patients with pulmonary

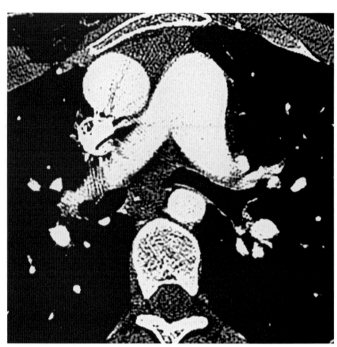

Fig. 7.16 Streak artifact from the column of contrast medium within the superior vena cava. This artifact has the potential to obscure filling defects within the right pulmonary artery.

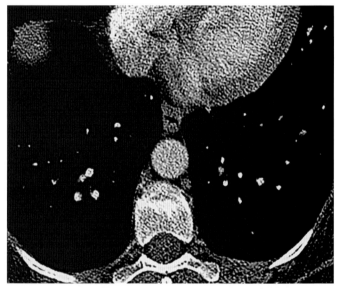

Fig. 7.17 Suboptimal contrast opacification of the segmental and subsegmental pulmonary arteries in the lower lobes. Contributing factors include a low flow rate of contrast medium (2.5 ml/s) and substantial quantum noise.

hypertension do not have a significantly reduced transit time through their lungs, unless there are overt clinical signs of right-sided heart failure.[197] Nevertheless, the time at which the central and segmental and pulmonary arteries are optimally opacified is not always predictable and there are no readily available clinical parameters that predict transit time.[198] To overcome this, a "scout" time–density curve can be performed after the injection of a small bolus of contrast to determine the time at which maximal

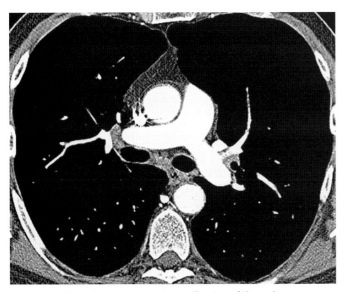

Fig. 7.18 CTPA showing optimal opacification of the pulmonary arteries. In this case the scan acquisition was triggered automatically by detection of a pre-set rise in attenuation in a region of interest placed over the main pulmonary artery. Note the typical appearances of the normal lymph node straddling the right pulmonary artery. This CTPA was negative.

opacification of the pulmonary arteries occurs.[185] Modern CT scanners have a facility that triggers scanning once predetermined levels of enhancement (e.g. a rise in attenuation of 100 HU) have been reached within a region of interest (i.e. the central pulmonary arteries) and this considerably improves the chances of optimal vascular opacification (Fig. 7.18). Nevertheless, in one study a fixed scan delay of 20 seconds provided equally satisfactory vascular opacification compared to individualized contrast timing.[198]

Pulmonary arteries that run obliquely to the plane of section (notably the lingular and right middle lobe arteries and their branches) may be difficult to visualize on transverse CT images.

Reformatted images that depict such vessels in longitudinal axis can be useful.[199] Such reformation of the volumetric data is best performed by localizing the artery in question from a three-dimensional shaded surface display which allows precise delineation of the long axis of the artery. Remy-Jardin et al found that such reconstructions were most helpful in confirming the absence of pulmonary emboli in oblique vessels, that is, they reduced the number of inconclusive CT scans (Fig. 7.19). Such postprocessing did not add anything to the routine transverse CT scans that were classified confidently as either negative or positive for pulmonary emboli.[199]

Window settings have a significant effect on the ease with which pulmonary emboli are detected. It has been suggested that conventional mediastinal window settings may result in some filling defects being overlooked.[182] By modifying the window settings to encompass the whole gray scale of thrombus through to the opacified vessel in question, the conspicuity of filling defects may be increased. A disadvantage of this maneuver is that it may make the detection of an embolus that completely occludes a pulmonary artery more difficult.[182] Image reconstruction with a very high spatial frequency algorithm should be avoided because of the possibility of producing an artifactual high-attenuation rim, simulating contrast, around the margin of vertically running vessels.[200]

There are very few patient-related factors that will prevent the acquisition of a diagnostic study. The most obvious anatomic causes for suboptimal opacification of the pulmonary arteries include obstruction of the superior vena cava, a substantial left-to-right shunt, or a patent foramen ovale – all of which will reduce opacification (the abnormality responsible will be readily identifiable on CT). The examination of patients who are unable to breath hold will result in suboptimal CT scans for two reasons. First, pulmonary arterial flow rate changes with the phase of respiration: pulmonary arterial pressure is raised at both end-expiration and end-inspiration[84] so that arterial opacification is variable. Second, marked motion artifact from breathing causes image degradation.

The range of nondiagnostic CTPA for pulmonary embolism is reported to be between 2% and 9%.[166,171] This is in contrast to the rate of nondiagnostic V̇/Q scans, which varies considerably

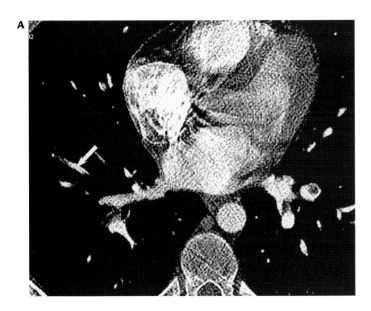

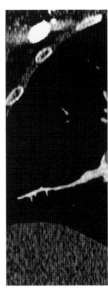

Fig. 7.19 Positive CTPA with **A**, filling defects within pulmonary arteries of the left lower lobe. There was a questionable linear filling defect within a subsegmental pulmonary artery in the right lower lobe (arrow). **B**, A freehand multiplanar reconstruction through the long axis of this artery excluded an embolus within this vessel.

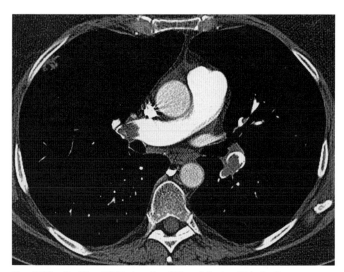

Fig. 7.20 Positive CTPA showing filling defects within both pulmonary arteries and a segmental lingular artery. The peripheral opacity in the right lung anteriorly had the appearances of a pulmonary infarct on lung window settings.

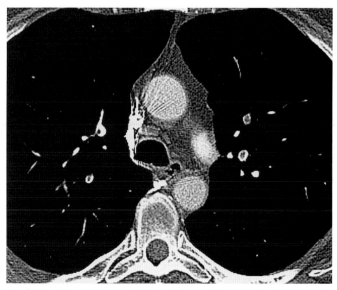

Fig. 7.21 There are several filling defects within opacified segmental and subsegmental pulmonary arteries in the upper lobes, representing pulmonary emboli.

between studies (range 28%[166] to 87%[164]). The rate of non-diagnostic pulmonary arteriograms is comparable to that of CTPA: approximately 3% according to the PIOPED study.[146]

CTPA signs of acute pulmonary embolism

The cardinal sign of acute pulmonary embolism, that is, a filling defect within an opacified pulmonary artery, is straightforward and analogous to the arteriographic sign of pulmonary embolism (Fig. 7.20).[185,186,201] When contrast can flow around an embolus, the appearance is of a central or eccentrically placed filling defect within the artery lumen on perpendicular sections (Fig. 7.21) or a "tram-track" if the artery lies parallel and within the plane of section (Fig. 7.22). If there is complete occlusion of a small pulmonary artery by clot, such that there is no surrounding contrast medium, a pulmonary embolus may be less conspicuous (Fig. 7.23). A semiquantitative score of the extent of pulmonary artery obstruction by emboli correlates well with echocardiographic estimation of disease severity.[202] Ancillary signs of thromboembolic disease such as a small dependent pleural effusion or focal consolidation in the costophrenic recess, although nonspecific, provide important additional evidence of pulmonary embolism.[203] A mosaic attenuation pattern in the lung parenchyma, analogous to the regional inhomogeneity seen on a radionuclide perfusion scan, is sometimes present but is often subtle: in one study this feature was identified in only 1 out of 13 patients who had pulmonary embolism and an accompanying HRCT.[204] However, CT densitometry and postprocessing of contrast-enhanced CT images can show measurable differences between perfused and under-perfused lung.[205,206] Variation in the caliber of segmental and subsegmental pulmonary arteries can be striking, even in the absence of identifiable embolism on CTPA at that level (Fig. 7.24). The presence or absence of parenchymal and pleural abnormalities on CT in patients with suspected pulmonary embolism is largely nondiscriminatory in determining the diagnosis of pulmonary embolism.[207] Nevertheless, scrutiny of the lung window settings of the entire volume included is important because ancillary signs of pulmonary embolism, such as small peripheral infarcts, pleural effusions, or a

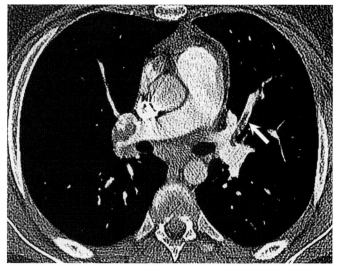

Fig. 7.22 CTPA showing bilateral filling defects. Within the left upper lobe anterior segmental pulmonary artery, the linear embolus is outlined by contrast giving the appearance of a "tram-track" (arrow).

mosaic perfusion pattern,[203] may be revealed (Fig. 7.25). Furthermore, CT may show other abnormalities that provide an alternative explanation for the patient's symptoms.[159,166,174,208]

Infarcts in the lung on CT may show a pleura-based truncated cone or triangular configuration – a shape that corresponds to the Hampton's hump described in the section on plain chest radiography. While CT cross-sectional images show the wedge shape of pulmonary infarction to advantage[209] (Figs 7.25 and 7.26), a postmortem HRCT study of 83 fixed lungs with subpleural densities (12 containing pulmonary infarcts and 71 a variety of pathologic conditions including pneumonia, hemorrhage, and tumor) showed that there was no significant difference in the frequency of wedge shaped opacities on CT between the lungs with infarcts and those with other disorders. A "vascular sign" (a vessel running into the apex of the wedge) was slightly more

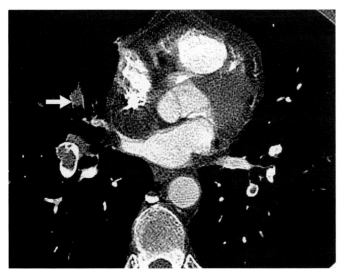

Fig. 7.23 There are several obvious filling defects within opacified vessels bilaterally. An embolus completely occupies the lumen of the right middle lobe pulmonary artery (arrow) so that there is no surrounding contrast medium, making it less conspicuous than the other emboli.

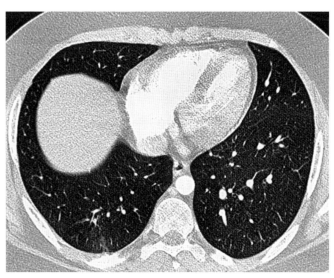

Fig. 7.24 Lung window setting image from a CTPA examination that showed emboli in the central pulmonary arteries. There is a marked discrepancy in the size of the segmental and subsegmental pulmonary arteries between the two sides. No filling defects were identified within the lower lobe pulmonary arteries; there were appearances consistent with a pulmonary infarct at the right lung base posteriorly.

A

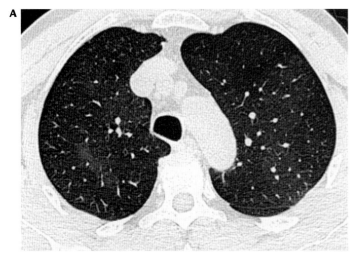

B

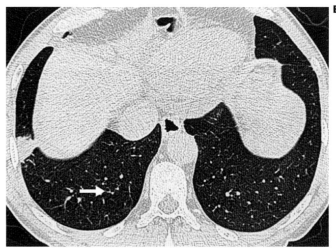

Fig. 7.25 A patient with recurrent pulmonary embolism. **A**, There is mosaic attenuation pattern in the upper lobes and a striking reduction in the caliber of the pulmonary vessels within the under-perfused lung (e.g. anterior left lung). **B**, A section through the lower lobes shows a pulmonary infarct in the periphery of the right lung. Note the dilated subsegmental bronchus (arrow), an occasional feature in pulmonary embolism, particularly in chronic thromboembolic disease.

A

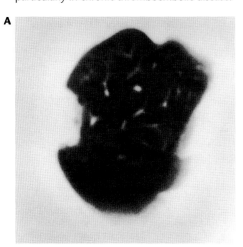

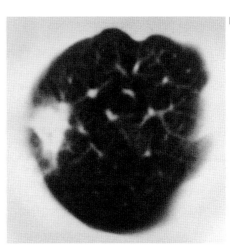

B Fig. 7.26 CT of a pulmonary infarct in the right upper lobe. **A** and **B**, Adjacent sections illustrate a truncated cone shape based on the pleura.

common in the infarct group.[210] However, some infarcts do not have the truncated wedge configuration but have a more rounded form without a broad base in contact with the pleura.[149,151]

The distinction between acute versus chronic pulmonary embolism on CTPA is, as with other tests, not always possible. The hemodynamic consequences of recurrent pulmonary emboli may be seen as dilatation of the proximal pulmonary arteries, tortuosity of the segmental arteries, and narrowing of the peripheral pulmonary vessels with a mosaic attenuation pattern.[211] Chronic pulmonary embolism usually appears as crescentic thrombus adhering to the arterial wall (Fig. 7.27); the thrombus may contain calcifications and may show signs of recanalization.[211–213] In more severe cases there may be hypertrophy of the systemic supply to the lungs, particularly the bronchial arteries[214] (Fig. 7.28). Although it is hard to establish the exact prevalence, changes in the lung periphery, reflecting previous pulmonary infarcts, are present in most patients with chronic thromboembolism.

The causes of false negative results in the segmental and central pulmonary arteries are almost invariably due to technique.[215] Conversely, mimics of pulmonary embolism causing false positive results are less frequent and more often due to anatomical variants or unrelated pathology (Box 7.6).

Small or moderately enlarged lymph nodes immediately adjacent to the central and segmental pulmonary arteries are a potent cause of false positive diagnoses of pulmonary embolism, particularly if beam collimation greater than 3 mm is used. An intimate knowledge of the precise location of these

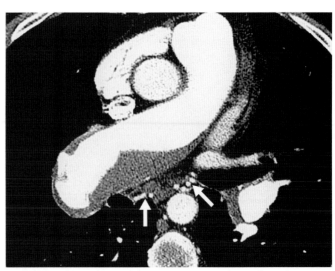

Fig. 7.28 Dilated bronchial arteries (arrows) in a patient with long-standing and severe thromboembolic disease.

Box 7.6 Causes of false negative and positive diagnoses of pulmonary embolism on CTPA

False negatives

Inadequate opacification of pulmonary arteries (factors: flow rate, concentration of contrast, and scan delay; Fig. 7.17)

Emboli confined to peripheral subsegmental pulmonary arteries

Unfavorable patient hemodynamics (e.g. cardiomyopathy, patent foramen ovale, left-to-right shunt, SVC obstruction)

Motion artifact degrading image (severe respiratory movement or cardiac pulsation artifact)

Partial volume effect (inappropriate thick collimation)

Low signal-to-noise ratio (insufficient milliamperage for large patient; Fig. 7.17)

False positives

Hilar and bronchopulmonary lymph nodes (Fig. 7.29), (especially N1b, N2a and 2b lymph nodes adjacent to the right main pulmonary artery; Fig. 7.29)

Partial opacification of pulmonary arteries or veins (e.g. insufficient scan delay resulting in pseudofilling defects in pulmonary arteries, partial opacification of pulmonary veins; Fig. 7.30)

Partial volume effect (e.g. adjacent mediastinal fat, obliquely running pulmonary vessels; Fig. 7.31)

Artifactual high-attenuation collar around vertically orientated arteries (caused by inappropriate use of high spatial frequency reconstruction algorithm)

Bronchiectatic airways (when viewed on mediastinal window settings; Fig. 7. 32)

Any cause of focal reduced pulmonary perfusion (i.e. reduced blood flow, and thus vascular opacification, in consolidated lung)

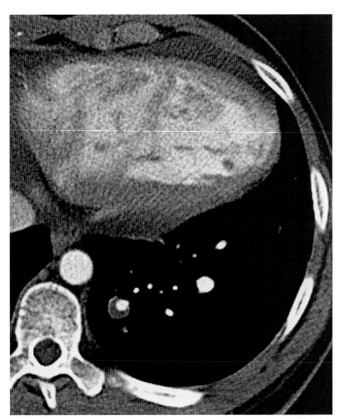

Fig. 7.27 A patient with chronic thromboembolic disease. There is a crescentic filling defect within a dilated lower lobe pulmonary artery.

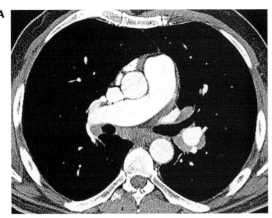 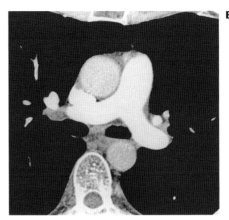

Fig. 7.29 Hilar lymph nodes mimicking pulmonary emboli. **A**, A collar of lymph nodes surrounding the posterior aspect of the left pulmonary artery might be misinterpreted as crescentic thrombus within the artery (note the subcarinal and contralateral hilar lymph nodes). **B**, A prominent fibrofatty lymph node (N1b) lying on the superolateral aspect of the right main pulmonary artery mimicked a filling defect (immediately contiguous sections did not show an intravascular filling defect).

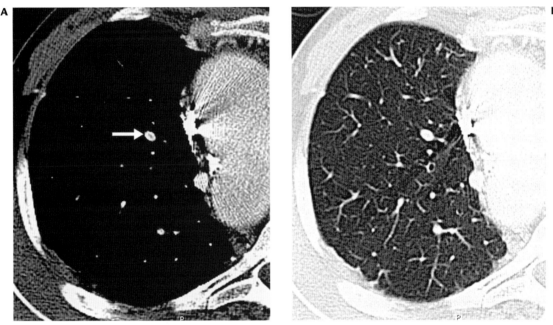

Fig. 7.30 **A**, An apparent filling defect in a right upper lobe vessel (arrow) suggestive of a pulmonary embolus in a patient with pulmonary atresia and a ventricular septal defect. **B**, When this vessel was followed on contiguous images on window settings it became apparent that it was a pulmonary vein (note the lack of an accompanying bronchus).

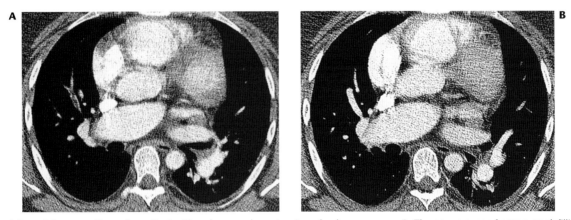

Fig. 7.31 Adjacent 3 mm sections of a patient with pulmonary hypertension of unknown cause. **A**, The appearance of a tram-track filling defect within a vessel in the right mid zone. **B**, An immediately adjacent section shows that the spurious appearance in **A** is due to partial volume effect (the vessel is a normal pulmonary vein).

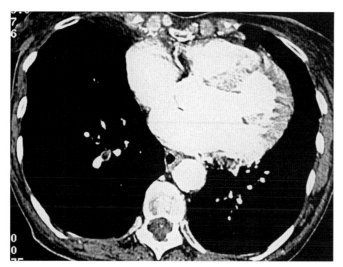

Fig. 7.32 A patient with known bronchiectasis and suspected pulmonary embolism. The apparently opacified vessel in the right lower lobe was confirmed on lung window settings to be a mucus-filled bronchiectatic airway.

lymph nodes is desirable[216]; of all these lymph nodes, the most frequently identified (and also the most convincing mimic of an intravascular filling defect) lies on the superolateral aspect of the right main pulmonary artery. This fibrofatty lymph node, classified as N1b, may be identified in up to 80% of patients[216] (Fig. 7.29B). Other bronchopulmonary lymph nodes lying around the more vertically orientated lower lobe and segmental pulmonary arteries are more readily identified as such because of their eccentric disposition around the circumference of the arteries. Pulmonary veins, if they are partially opacified, may also cause interpretative problems. However, the identification of pulmonary veins as such can usually be made by studying contiguous sections on lung window settings.

Accuracy of computed tomography pulmonary angiography

It is difficult to reach final conclusions about the accuracy of CTPA because of differences in patient populations studied, technical factors (notably collimation), location of emboli, and chosen "gold standard". In a systematic review of published studies up to November 1999, the culled sensitivity of CTPA ranged from 53% to 100% (specificity 81% to 100%).[217] Although some of the pre-2000 studies of CTPA have been criticized on methodologic grounds, it is worth noting that they are more numerous and robust than those that led, in an earlier era, to the adoption of scintigraphy for the diagnosis of pulmonary embolism. In the landmark study of Remy-Jardin et al in 1992, the sensitivity and specificity of CTPA for the detection of acute *central* pulmonary embolism was 100% and 96%, respectively.[161] The same group later reported a sensitivity and specificity of 91% and 76% in a larger group of patients.[171] The discrepancy between the two studies occurred because of the exclusion of technically unsatisfactory CTPAs in the first study. Later studies (of comparable methodology) mirrored these figures: the range of sensitivity for CTPA is 75%[164] to 100%[161] and the range of specificity is 78%[171] to 100%.[164] These early studies were constrained by relatively small patient numbers but the results of

a large European multicenter study broadly confirmed earlier results (sensitivity 88%, specificity 94%).[175] Furthermore, inter-observer agreement appears to be good for CTPA, compared with ventilation–perfusion scanning.[170] In the European study, observer agreement for CTPA (kappa 0.72) was superior to pulmonary angiography (kappa 0.46) which was in turn superior to ventilation–perfusion scanning (kappa 0.39).[175] Similar results of good observer agreement for CTPA continue to be reported.[218–220]

The emergence of CTPA for the detection of pulmonary embolism has highlighted the problems of comparing a new diagnostic technique with an established, but fallible, test. Although pulmonary angiography has been regarded as the standard to which CTPA should aspire (pulmonary angiography has an estimated sensitivity of 98% and specificity of 97%),[173] CTPA can occasionally detect pulmonary embolism in the face of a technically adequate negative pulmonary angiogram.[221]

The early studies of the accuracy of CTPA for the diagnosis of pulmonary embolism highlighted the inability of CTPA to detect small emboli. In 20 patients with indeterminate $\dot{V}/Q$ scans, pulmonary arteriography showed emboli in 11 patients, 4 of whom had emboli limited to the subsegmental vessels,[162] and CTPA was positive in only one of these 4 patients. Although it is now technically feasible to increase the diagnostic yield of subsegmental emboli,[190–192,222] many centers do not routinely employ this technique. The anatomic level down to which emboli can be "chased", in small subsegmental vessels, has not yet been established. Although pulmonary arteriography allows detection of subsegmental clot, observer disagreement at this anatomic level may be unacceptably high. Agreement on the presence or absence of subsegmental embolism on pulmonary arteriography is between 45% and 66% of cases.[107,223] In other words, sub-segmental emboli can be overlooked on pulmonary arteriography. The important questions about the prevalence of emboli confined to the subsegmental pulmonary arteries (anywhere between 2% and 36%[183,224]) cannot easily be answered. The hemodynamic effects of a small subsegmental embolus will be negligible in normal individuals but may be more severe in patients with preexisting severe cardiopulmonary disease. Moreover, whether such small emboli should be regarded as heralding a larger, possibly fatal, embolus is far from certain. Nevertheless, much effort has gone into the investigation of the implications of a negative CTPA in patients suspected of having pulmonary embolism.[225–232] In the absence of a reliable gold standard diagnostic test, there is much merit in what are, in effect, patient outcome studies. Not only does the negative predictive value of CTPA appear to be good,[225,226,233] even in the presence of an underlying lung disease,[231] the CT examination may provide alternative diagnoses in up to half of patients with a negative CTPA.[225,232,234] Inevitably, a negative CTPA cannot absolutely exclude the possibility of a future embolic episode; in one study, venous thromboembolism subsequently occurred in 3 of 215 (1.4%) of patients with a negative CTPA, one of whom died from pulmonary embolism.[227] In another study, pulmonary embolism occurred in 4 of 441 (1%) patients with a negative CTPA during a 3-month follow-up period: in 2 of the 4 patients, the embolism contributed to the patient's death.[228] In the largest study of this type, Swensen et al[230] reported that 8 of 993 (0.08%) patients with a negative CTPA developed venous thrombosis or pulmonary embolism (3 died from embolism). Thus the inference has been made that anticoagulation can be safely withheld in most patients with a negative CTPA; the caveat that patients with poor cardiopulmonary reserve should also undergo leg Doppler ultrasonography or CT venography has been adopted in some centers.[235]

With increasing experience of CTPA, the question now arises as to where CTPA should be placed in the various diagnostic pathways that have already been developed.[100,236,237] The debate began with a controversial editorial by Goodman and Lipchik in 1996,[238] which suggested that in many situations CTPA should be the first investigation in patients with suspected pulmonary embolism. More recent studies have largely supported this recommendation,[218] but there are contradictory views.[239] The undesirability of simply adding a new test to what is already a long list of more or less inadequate tests is clear.[240,241] Many of the diagnostic algorithms proposed in the past have built-in assumptions and biases,[242] such as the equivalent availability and cost of various tests, the same pre-test probability of pulmonary embolism,[243] and the same significance of identifying large versus small emboli in all patients. Nevertheless, local differences in the availability of scintigraphy and CTPA are likely the single most important determinant of which tests are used, and this is recognized in some published recommendations[244] (Fig. 7.33).

An in-depth debate about the emerging role of CTPA in the detection of acute pulmonary embolism can be found in a series of responses from experts[245–248] to a commentary by Goodman.[249] The approach favored by Goodman relies on the high specificity of a normal perfusion scintigram and the stratification of patients into outpatients (typically patients with a low pre-test probability of pulmonary embolism and no pulmonary disease apparent on chest radiography) and inpatients (patients with a higher probability of pulmonary embolism and often with preexisting cardiopulmonary disease). For patients with symptoms of deep venous thrombosis and pulmonary embolism, ultrasound of the lower limbs is the first test. Goodman emphasized at the time that his approach should not be regarded as a rigid algorithm.[249] Although the potential place of CTPA has already been widely debated in the radiologic journals, continuous refinement of the

technique[142] and the interpolation of other techniques, such as D-dimer testing[39,250,251] and CT phlebography,[252] mean that there can be no definitive recommendation, however desirable that may be for practising clinicians.[253]

There are currently few studies that attempt to address the cost-effectiveness of diagnostic algorithms.[82,254,255] However, in an analysis of 15 combinations of the diagnostic tests (CTPA, lower limb ultrasonography, $\dot{V}$/Q scanning, pulmonary arteriography and D-dimer plasma levels), the authors found that the five strategies that were most effective (least mortality at 3 months and lowest associated costs per life saved) all included CTPA, usually in combination with lower limb ultrasonography.[173] Using CTPA as the initial test, with or without subsequent leg ultrasonography is undoubtedly an expensive option, but is associated with improved survival[256]; Perrier et al[255] have convincingly argued that CTPA used alone is not cost-effective, but becomes so when it is used in combination with D-dimer testing and lower limb ultrasonography.

Many centers have investigated the feasibility of combining CT venography of the deep veins of the legs with CTPA,[252,257–262] the rationale being that pulmonary embolism and deep venous thrombosis (DVT) are part of the same process, and that the detection of either is important. Furthermore, demonstration of DVT on CT may, on occasion, "salvage" a suboptimal CTPA. The CT signs of DVT are, as might be expected, low-attenuation clot within a distended vein[263,264] (Fig. 7.34). In acute DVT there may be enhancement of the vein wall, reflecting the arterial vasa vasorum. Occasionally there are features suggesting perivenous soft tissue edema.[265] The first comprehensive study of the combined technique of CTPA followed by CT venography by Loud et al in 1998[169] indicated that no extra contrast material was needed, and that a delay of up to 3.5 minutes was necessary to allow opacification of the veins of the legs and pelvis. More recent studies have suggested that peak venous opacification occurs earlier, at about 2 minutes,[266] although the timing for optimal opacification does not appear to be critical, and a 3 minute

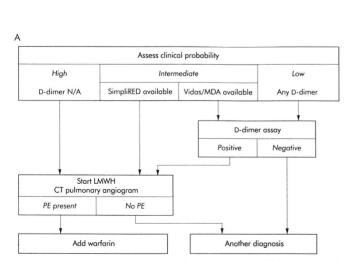

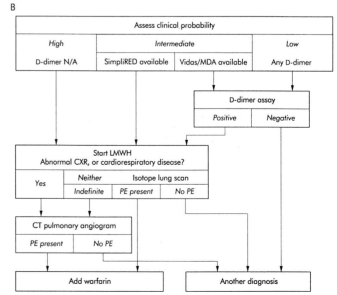

Fig. 7.33 Suggested flowcharts for the management of the suspected pulmonary embolism (non-massive): **A**, in the situation where scintigraphy is not available on site and **B**, where scintigraphy is available on site. (With permission from British Thoracic Society guidelines for the management of suspected acute pulmonary embolism. Thorax 2003;58:470–483.)

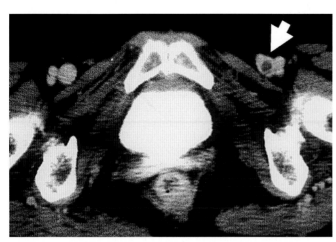

Fig. 7.34 Indirect CT venography showing thrombus in the left common femoral vein (arrow). (With permission from Cham MD, Yankelevitz DF, Shaham D, et al. Deep venous thrombosis: detection by using indirect CT venography. The Pulmonary Angiography–Indirect CT Venography Cooperative Group. Radiology 2000;216:744–751.)

delay seems satisfactory.[267] Widely interspaced (4–5 cm) 10 mm collimation sections from the diaphragm to the ankles are recommended.[268] Studies using contiguous sections[252] through the pelvis are clearly associated with a considerably higher radiation burden than interspaced sections. Windows narrower than usual width (100 as opposed to 400 HU for abdominal examinations) improve the often low contrast encountered in CT venography.

The sensitivity, specificity, and observer agreement for CT venography so far reported appear to be good and the attraction of a "one-stop shop" examination for the diagnosis of venous thromboembolism is obvious, but concerns have been voiced, particularly about the added radiation of CT venography.[269,270] The increased diagnostic yield from CT venography, that is the proportion of patients with positive CT venography but negative CTPA, is reported to be between 3% and 5%.[252,259,262] Whether such individuals represent the very small proportion of patients with a negative CTPA who subsequently have pulmonary embolism is a matter of speculation. Now it is known that CT venography is a comparatively accurate test, outcome studies are awaited to establish whether it should be routinely performed in conjunction with CTPA.

Magnetic resonance imaging

Magnetic resonance (MR) imaging is an alternative to CTPA for the noninvasive diagnosis of pulmonary embolism and has the advantage that it does not use ionizing radiation or necessarily require iodinated contrast medium. However, the rapid development of MR angiography techniques has meant that few large scale studies have been performed, using a single standardized MR imaging protocol, to compare its diagnostic efficacy with other currently available tests. The data available from clinical studies published in the early 1990s suggested that the sensitivity of MR for the detection of acute pulmonary embolism in large pulmonary arteries ranged from 85% to 90%, with a specificity of 62% to 77%.[271–273] More recent studies, including investigations using animal models, indicate that, in ideal circumstances, the accuracy of MR angiography is nearly equivalent to CTPA[274–278] (Fig. 7.35). Nevertheless, earlier expectations that CTPA would be replaced by MR angiography have, for a variety of reasons (not least the great progress CTPA has made in detecting small emboli), receded.[279]

There are several fundamentally different MR techniques that can be used for the detection of pulmonary embolism.[280] In this context, the three most commonly described "traditional" approaches to MRI demonstration of pulmonary embolism are:

1. Spin-echo technique in which thrombotic emboli are seen as white objects, whereas fast flowing blood is black.
2. Gradient recalled echo (GRE) technique with flow compensation in which emboli are dark and flowing blood is white.
3. Phase-contrast technique which can be used to clarify that an intraluminal signal (gray) is due to a thrombotic embolus rather than slow flowing blood.[281]

Although these relatively simple techniques can be performed on most MR scanners, motion artifact, together with pulsatile and turbulent flow patterns, conspire to reduce the effectiveness of these techniques for imaging subsegmental emboli.

There has been much interest in developing MR angiography to a state equivalent to a noninvasive conventional pulmonary angiogram. In essence, MR pulse sequences that emphasize the signal of flowing blood, and at the same time suppress signal from static structures, are used and the resulting blood signal is postprocessed to produce a 2D or 3D angiogram.[271,282–285] Intravenous gadolinium contrast media may be used to enhance further the blood signal[277,286–289] (Fig. 7.36). In addition, defects in

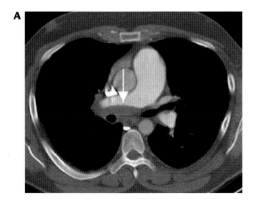

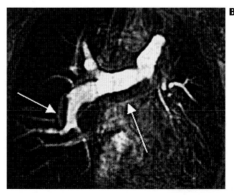

Fig. 7.35 Comparison of **A**, contrast-enhanced MR angiography and **B**, CTPA in a patient with chronic thromboembolic disease. The organized thrombus (arrows) is shown clearly by both techniques. (With permission from Ley S, Kauczor HU, Heussel CP, et al. Value of contrast-enhanced MR angiography and helical CT angiography in chronic thromboembolic pulmonary hypertension. Eur Radiol 2003;13:2365–2371.)

A 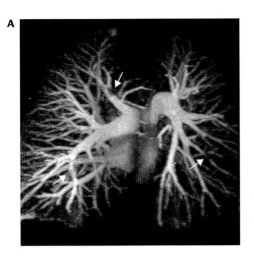 **B**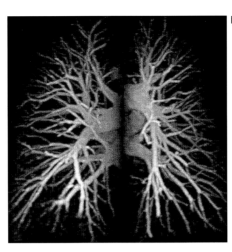

Fig. 7.36 High-resolution 3D gadolinium-enhanced magnetic resonance angiography acquired in deep inspiration during two separate breath holds for each lung. **A**, A maximum-intensity projection rendering, showing multiple pulmonary emboli (arrows) and **B**, subsequent resolution of the emboli following anticoagulation. (Reprinted with permission from Elsevier. Lancet 2002;359:1643–1647.)

pulmonary perfusion, analogous to the cardinal sign of pulmonary embolism on radionuclide perfusion scanning, may also be demonstrated on noncontrast[290] gadolinium-enhanced MR angiography.[291,292] Various forms of ventilation scanning are now possible with MR imaging[293–295] so that a combination of these techniques could theoretically replace conventional radionuclide V̇/Q scanning.[290,296] In the same way that the role of CT venography in patients with suspected pulmonary embolism is being explored, the utility of detecting pelvic and leg thrombosis with MR angiography has now been described.[297]

TUMOR EMBOLISM

Hemodynamically significant tumor emboli are rare[298,299] but can occasionally be the presenting feature of neoplastic disease.[300,301] They occlude small pulmonary vessels and can give rise to severe dyspnea, which usually develops over a matter of days[302] but sometimes increases over several weeks.[303] Pleuritic chest pain is relatively common, and fatigue, weight loss, cough, hemoptysis, and syncope are seen in a few patients. The mortality of the condition is very high.

On physical examination most patients show signs of right ventricular overload, but just as with pulmonary thromboembolism there may be relatively few respiratory findings. The condition differs from widespread bloodborne metastases in that a "regular" metastasis represents tumor that has invaded the vessel wall and acquired its own blood supply, whereas tumor emboli are clumps of cells that are lodged within the lumen of small pulmonary arteries and have not yet invaded the vessel wall but are acting as obstructing emboli similar to thromboemboli. The patients are hypoxemic, have increased alveolar–arterial oxygen gradients, and have pulmonary arterial hypertension, sometimes severe.[304,305] Tumor emboli are a fairly frequent finding at autopsy, but the condition is rarely diagnosed ante mortem. Chan et al,[298] in their extensive review of the literature on the subject, found a wide distribution of types of malignancy. The primary tumors associated with tumor embolism are hepatoma, bronchioloalveolar cell carcinoma,[305] breast[304] and renal carcinoma,[301] gastric and prostate cancers, and choriocarcinoma.[306,307] The diagnosis of pulmonary endovascular choriocarcinoma in young female patients is particularly important because it is potentially curable with chemotherapy.[308]

The chest radiograph is usually normal and signs of pulmonary arterial hypertension are rarely recognizable. A few patients show nonspecific pulmonary shadows, possibly infarcts. Radionuclide lung scans show multiple, small, peripheral, subsegmental perfusion defects with a normal ventilation scan. Dilated and beaded pulmonary arteries have been described in one CT report of 4 cases[309]; this appearance reflects distension by intravascular tumor. Occasionally pulmonary infarcts may be the most conspicuous abnormality on CT.[310] An unusual pathologic response to microscopic tumor emboli is thrombotic microangiopathy[311] in which minute tumor emboli cause dramatic fibrocellular proliferation of the intima with resulting thrombosis and luminal obliteration. The HRCT correlate is prominence of otherwise inconspicuous small peripheral pulmonary arteries, resembling a tree-in-bud pattern[312] (Fig. 7.37).

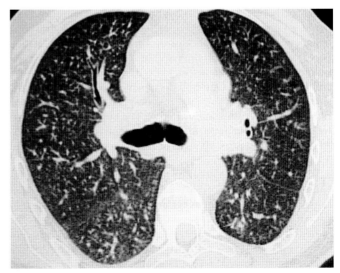

Fig. 7.37 Neoplastic thrombotic microangiography. HRCT shows profuse small nodules, some of which are coalescent and resemble a tree-in-bud pattern (most obvious in the superior segment of the right lower lobe). (Courtesy of Dr T Franquet, Barcelona)

PULMONARY ARTERIAL HYPERTENSION

Pulmonary artery pressure is a function of blood flow and the resistance across the pulmonary vascular system, the resistance to flow depending predominantly on the cross-sectional area of the perfused vascular bed. The pulmonary vascular bed has a much lower resistance than the systemic circuit and can respond to increasing flow by opening up additional vascular channels. Pulmonary arterial hypertension occurs when the flow increases to such an extent that the available extra channels are saturated, or because of vasoconstriction or structural change in the small pulmonary vessels. It is defined as pulmonary artery pressures above a mean of 25 mmHg at rest or above the mean value of 30 mmHg on exercise.

The imaging features of pulmonary arterial hypertension are discussed before the various causes are described because the same signs are seen regardless of the cause of the hypertension. Over the years the classification of the various causes and associations of pulmonary arterial hypertension has been refined; below is a synthesis loosely based on one proposed at a WHO symposium in 1998[313] (Box 7.7).

Although the clinical presentation and treatment for advanced pulmonary hypertension are largely the same, whatever the cause, there are clear risk factors, of differing certainty, that can be screened for in any individual found to have pulmonary hypertension (Box 7.8):

The well-known basic signs of pulmonary hypertension are cardiac enlargement (caused by right ventricular enlargement), enlargement of the central pulmonary arteries, and rapid tapering of the vessels as they proceed distally (Fig. 7.38). The distal vessels may be large, normal, or reduced in caliber. The important point is the disparity in the relative size of the central and distal vessels. The terms "central" and "distal" are inevitably vague because there is no precise anatomic definition of central and distal (peripheral) vessels, but the term "central arteries" refers to the main pulmonary artery and its branches approximately down to segmental level. The term "distal vessels" refers to vessels beyond the segmental level. The criteria of central vessel dilatation on plain chest radiographs are, with one exception, also poorly defined. On a PA chest radiograph the main pulmonary artery forms the border for less than half of its circumference, and this border represents a portion of the vessel that is traveling obliquely upward and backward. Thus, diagnosing dilatation based on increased prominence or convexity of the main pulmonary artery segment of the cardiac contour is at best a crude measurement. One well-documented measurement of the size of the pulmonary arterial tree on plain films is that of the right descending pulmonary artery.[314] The upper limit of normal for transverse diameter at the mid point of this vessel is 16–17 mm. Thus measurements of 17 mm or greater are taken to indicate dilatation (Fig. 7.39).

The degree of dilatation of the central pulmonary arteries varies considerably, not only among the various entities that cause pulmonary arterial hypertension, but also from patient to patient with the same condition. Therefore, although the radiographic changes are reasonably specific, they are not sensitive nor do they correlate well with the severity of the hypertension. Indeed, severe pulmonary arterial hypertension can be present in patients with a normal-appearing chest radiograph. Probably because more precise measurement of the main pulmonary artery is possible with CT, Kuriyama and associates[315] found good correlation between the calculated cross-sectional area of the main pulmonary artery, adjusted for body surface area, and mean pulmonary artery pressure. Nevertheless, the caveat that rarely some individuals may have idiopathic dilatation of the pulmonary artery needs to be remembered.[316] Another study has confirmed that there is a reasonable correlation between pulmonary artery pressure and CT measurements of various parts of the proximal pulmonary arterial tree.[317] A mean pulmonary artery diameter (measured at its widest point within 3 cm of its bifurcation) of greater than or equal to 29 mm has been shown to have a positive predictive value of 0.97 (positive likelihood ratio of 7.91) for predicting

---

Box 7.7 Classification of pulmonary hypertension

Increased resistance to pulmonary venous drainage
Congenital narrowing of pulmonary veins
Mediastinal fibrosis involving the pulmonary veins
Pulmonary venoocclusive disease
Left atrial obstruction – mitral valve disease, cor triatriatum, left atrial myxoma
Left ventricular dysfunction
Constrictive pericarditis (rarely)

Increased resistance due to disease in the arterial-arteriolar wall or lumen
Primary pulmonary hypertension (sporadic or familial)
Emboli: thrombotic and others (including e.g. sickle cell disease)
Eisenmenger syndrome
Persistent pulmonary hypertension of the newborn
Drug or chemically induced vasculopathy (particularly anorexigens)
Pulmonary vasculitides (especially related to collagen vascular disease, e.g. systemic sclerosis)
HIV infection
Schistosomiasis
Portal hypertension
Congenital stenosis
Pulmonary capillary hemangiomatosis
Hypogenesis or aplasia
Surgical resection of lung

Increased pulmonary vascular resistance secondary to pleuropulmonary disease
Chronic obstructive pulmonary disease
Interstitial fibrosis of the lungs
Sarcoidosis
Pneumoconioses
Granulomatous infections
Alveolar capillary dysplasia
Pleural fibrothorax

Increased pulmonary blood flow
Left-to-right shunts (atrial septal defect, ventricular septal defect, patent ductus arteriosus)

Hypoventilation
Obesity/hypoventilation syndromes
Pharyngeal or tracheal obstructions
High altitude
Neuromuscular disorders affecting ventilation
Chest wall deformity including severe kyphoscoliosis

Box 7.8 Classification of risk for pulmonary hypertension

Drugs and toxins
Definite
e.g. Toxic rapeseed oil, aminorex, fenfluramine
Very likely
e.g. Amphetamines
Possible
e.g. Cocaine, some chemotherapies
Unlikely
e.g. Antidepressants, cigarette smoking, oral contraceptives

Demographic and medical conditions
Definite
Female gender
Possible
Pregnancy, systemic hypertension
Unlikely
Obesity

Diseases
Definite
HIV infection
Very likely
Portal hypertension/liver disease
Collagen vascular diseases
Systemic–pulmonary cardiac shunts
Possible
Thyroid disease

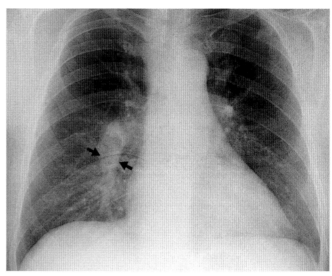

Fig. 7.39 Pulmonary arterial hypertension (primary) in a 43-year-old man showing increased transverse diameter of the right lower lobe pulmonary artery (arrows), which measures 23 mm.

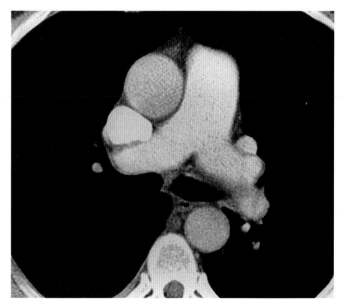

Fig. 7.40 Dilated main pulmonary artery (36 mm at maximum diameter) in a patient with known pulmonary arterial hypertension caused by chronic thromboembolic disease.

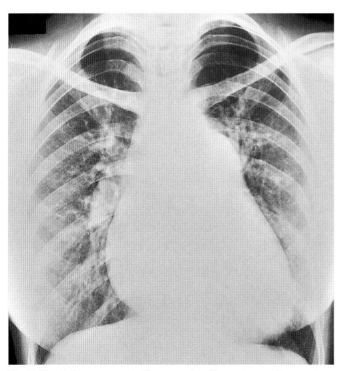

Fig. 7.38 Pulmonary arterial hypertension illustrating cardiomegaly and enlargement of the main pulmonary artery and hilar arteries. Vessels beyond the hilum are normal or small, notably in the lower zones. The patient, a 19-year-old woman, had severe primary pulmonary hypertension.

pulmonary arterial hypertension (Fig. 7.40).[318] In another CT study in which the main pulmonary artery was measured close to its bifurcation, the mean diameter in 100 normal individuals was found to be 2.72 cm (standard deviation 3 mm) compared with 3.47 cm (standard deviation 3.3 mm) in 12 patients with pulmonary arterial hypertension of greater than 20 mmHg (mean pulmonary artery pressure).[319] The authors proposed that a main pulmonary artery diameter greater than 3.32 cm is highly suggestive of pulmonary arterial hypertension (specificity 95%). However, this value is associated with a relatively low sensitivity (58%).[319] The relationship between main pulmonary artery diameter and pressure is not entirely predictable: in the latter study there was no linear correlation between the degree of pulmonary arterial hypertension and main pulmonary artery diameter.[318] Despite the obvious complexity underlying this relationship, a useful empiric rule reported by Ng et al[320] is that pulmonary arterial hypertension is likely when the diameter of the main pulmonary artery on CT exceeds that of the adjacent ascending aorta (positive predictive value 93%) (Fig. 7.41). However, the negative predictive value of this observation is relatively low (44%) and a nondilated main pulmonary artery, by reference to the aorta, does not necessarily exclude pulmonary arterial hypertension. Just over half (53%) of patients with a mean pulmonary artery pressure of more than 35 mm, that is severe pulmonary arterial hypertension, have evidence of pericardial thickening or effusion on CT[321] (Figs 7.41 and 7.42), whatever the cause of pulmonary hypertension. The pathophysiologic mechanism is unclear.

MRI measures of pulmonary artery diameter, flow characteristics, and other variables have been reported in patients with pulmonary artery hypertension.[322–325] In a study that examined the ratio of the diameter of the main pulmonary artery to the diameter of the mid descending thoracic aorta, Murray et al[325] showed a significantly higher ratio in patients with pulmonary arterial hypertension. Pulmonary artery distensibility, as judged by changes in pulmonary artery caliber on MRI, is significantly diminished in patients with pulmonary arterial hypertension.[322] Velocity mapping with cine MRI shows inhomogeneity of flow in the main pulmonary arteries in pulmonary hypertension.[323]

Prolonged severe pulmonary arterial hypertension may lead to atheroma formation in the central pulmonary arteries or their branches (Fig. 7.43) (atheroma is not seen in the pulmonary circuit with normal pulmonary artery pressures). The atheroma may be seen as curvilinear calcification identical to that seen with

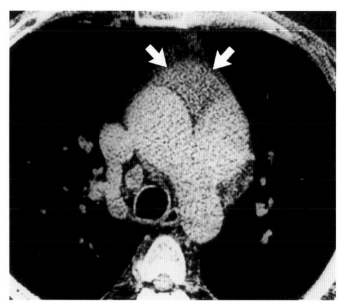

Fig. 7.42 Pericardial effusion accumulating in the anterior superior pericardial recess (arrows) in a patient with severe primary pulmonary arterial hypertension (mean pulmonary artery pressure 60 mmHg).

atheromatous change in the aorta and its branches. In practice, atheromatous calcification of the pulmonary artery is very rare indeed and is seen only in Eisenmenger syndrome and in a few patients with very prolonged pulmonary hypertension. Dissection of the pulmonary artery occurs even more rarely and may be recognized on echocardiography, contrast-enhanced CT or, as described in a single case report, on MRI.[326]

Pulmonary hypertension secondary to increased resistance to pulmonary venous drainage

Restriction of flow through the pulmonary venous system or through the left atrium and mitral valve raises pulmonary venous pressure, which in turn leads to elevation of pulmonary arterial pressure. With a healthy right ventricle, increases in mean left atrial pressure up to 25 mmHg are accompanied by a proportional increase in pulmonary artery pressure to maintain a constant mean gradient of approximately 10 mmHg.

When the mean venous pressure is chronically greater than 25 mmHg, a disproportionate elevation of pulmonary arterial pressure is observed, indicating an increase in pulmonary arteriolar resistance (mitral stenosis is a good example: just under one-third of patients with stenosis sufficiently severe to chronically elevate pulmonary venous pressure above 25 mmHg develop systolic pressures of 80 mmHg or greater). The mechanism for the elevation of pulmonary arterial pressure is unclear. Both vasoconstriction and structural changes play a part. Microscopic examination shows distension of the pulmonary capillaries, thickening and rupture of the basement membranes of the endothelial cells, and minor degrees of hemorrhage into the alveoli.

The changes of pulmonary arterial hypertension secondary to chronic impedance of pulmonary venous drainage are visible radiographically only when the pulmonary arterial pressures are very high. Such high pressures are almost never encountered in left ventricular failure, reduced left ventricular compliance, or

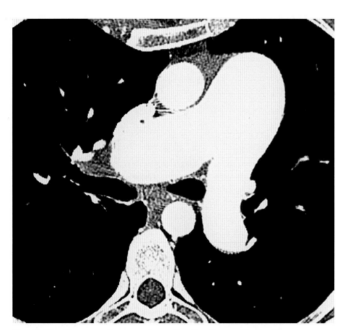

Fig. 7.41 Severe pulmonary hypertension in a patient with Eisenmenger syndrome: The main pulmonary artery is approximately twice the diameter of the ascending aorta. Note the conspicuous bronchial arteries around the left main bronchus and the fluid in the anterior pericardial recess, between the ascending aorta and main pulmonary artery; a pericardial effusion frequently accompanies severe pulmonary hypertension.

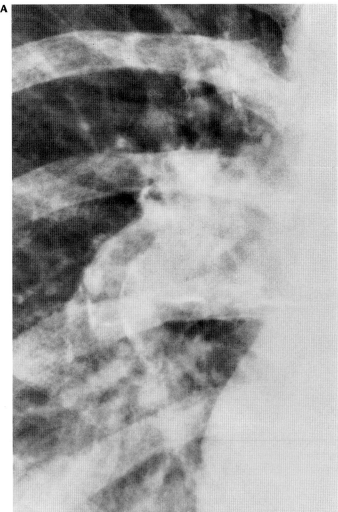

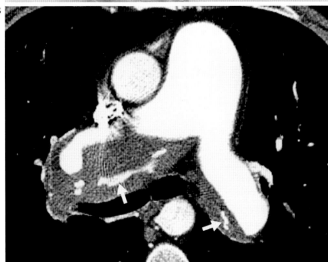

Fig. 7.43 Atheromatous calcification in the pulmonary arteries. **A**, A chest radiograph in a patient with prolonged severe pulmonary hypertension caused by a patent ductus arteriosus with Eisenmenger syndrome. **B**, In another patient with Eisenmenger syndrome the calcifications (arrows) can be seen within extensive mural thrombus. This appearance resembles recanalization, but appropriate window settings confirmed the calcific density.

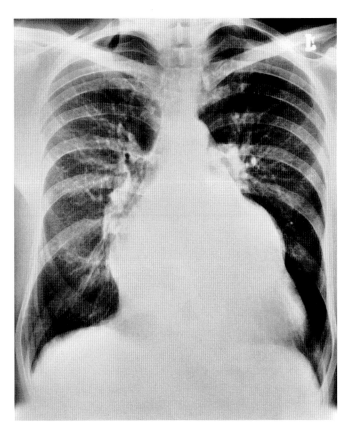

Fig. 7.44 Pulmonary arterial hypertension secondary to mitral stenosis. Note the large hilar arteries and small arteries beyond the hila. The upper zone vessels are large because of elevation of the pulmonary venous pressure, and the left atrium is massively dilated.

constrictive pericarditis. Thus, when radiographic features of pulmonary arterial hypertension are evident in an adult, the conditions to be considered in the category of increased impedance to pulmonary venous drainage are mitral valve disease, left atrial myxoma, cor triatriatum (which may develop in adulthood), and pulmonary venoocclusive disease.

The radiographic changes reflect a combination of pulmonary arterial and pulmonary venous hypertension together with the features of the primary condition (Figs 7.44 and 7.45). The central pulmonary arteries are dilated, tapering to normal caliber at or beyond segmental level. The upper zone vessels are enlarged because of upper zone blood diversion. In mitral stenosis the left atrium is enlarged and may show calcification either in its wall or in left atrial thrombus. Although the left atrium is almost invariably enlarged in cases of mitral valve disease with pulmonary arterial hypertension, it may not be strikingly big, and enlargement should therefore be looked for carefully on the plain chest radiograph. The chest radiograph in left atrial myxoma is identical to that of mitral stenosis except that occasionally it is possible to recognize focal calcifications within the tumor mass.

Pulmonary hypertension secondary to thromboembolism

Pulmonary hypertension may follow acute pulmonary embolism when the emboli occlude enough of the pulmonary arterial bed. The mechanisms are complex, consisting of a mixture of

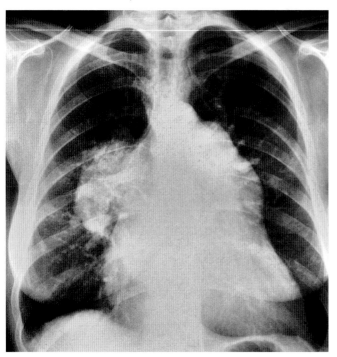

Fig. 7.45 Pulmonary arterial hypertension caused by mitral stenosis. Dilatation of the central pulmonary arteries is particularly striking in this 59-year-old woman with systemic pressures in her pulmonary circuit. Note the enlarged left atrium.

mechanical obstruction and vasoconstriction. These acute changes in pulmonary artery pressure do not produce radiographically visible pulmonary arterial hypertension, in part because a previously normal right ventricle can only produce right ventricular systolic pressures up to 45–55 mmHg. Higher pressures indicate preexisting right ventricular hypertrophy.

Repetitive thromboembolism without intervening lysis of thrombi may lead to chronic elevation of pulmonary artery pressure. The condition is rare, being seen in less than 1% of patients following acute embolism. Sometimes there is an obvious source for recurrent pulmonary emboli, such as a ventriculoatrial shunt catheter.[327]

There is, however, the debate about whether pulmonary hypertension caused by chronic obstruction of the pulmonary arterial blood flow is actually the result of recurrent pulmonary emboli rather than thrombotic occlusion of the pulmonary microvasculature.[29,328] Infarction is not usually a feature, and the condition frequently is not diagnosed until widespread and progressive occlusion of the pulmonary vascular bed has led to symptomatic pulmonary arterial hypertension. It is these patients who may show the radiographic changes of pulmonary arterial hypertension. Surgical thromboendarterectomy may be undertaken in carefully selected patients with substantial success.[211,329,330]

At pathologic study, organized thrombi are seen in both elastic and muscular arteries. The thrombi in the smaller vessels show recanalization, forming a lattice of fibrous trabeculae lined by endothelium. New blood vessels may form within the thrombi, and medial hypertrophy occurs secondarily. Plexiform lesions (see the description in the following section) are absent, although organizing thrombi may on occasion be difficult to distinguish from plexiform lesions.

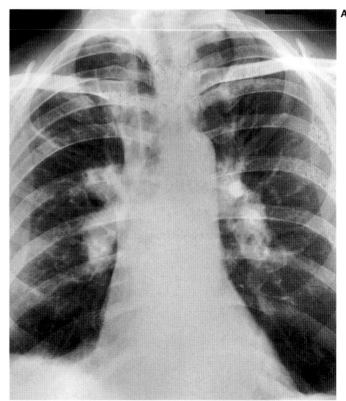

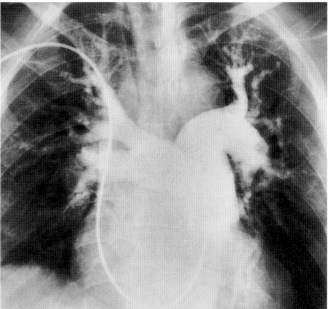

Fig. 7.46 Pulmonary arterial hypertension caused by chronic thromboembolism. **A,** A chest radiograph showing enlargement of the hilar arteries with peripheral oligemia. **B,** A pulmonary angiogram showing central vessel dilatation with occlusion of multiple branch vessels and an increase in size of the unobstructed pulmonary arterial branches.

The plain chest radiograph shows cardiomegaly and central vessel dilatation, with regional peripheral oligemia in the majority of patients[331,332] (Fig. 7.46). A few patients have normal or near-normal radiographs. Others show only changes such as atelectasis, pleural thickening, or pleural effusion, with no radiographic signs of pulmonary hypertension.

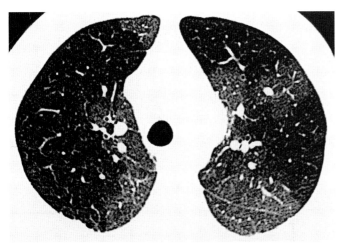

Fig. 7.47 Mosaic attenuation pattern (mosaic oligemia) in a patient with chronic thromboembolic disease. Note the more prominent vessels in the denser (relatively over-perfused) regions of the lung. The subpleural irregularity posteriorly in the right upper lobe likely reflects a previous pulmonary infarct.

Box 7.9 Features of pulmonary hypertension secondary to thromboembolism

Cardiac
Features of right heart strain (dilated right ventricle and bulging of interventricular septum)

Vascular
Dilated proximal pulmonary arteries (intraluminal thrombus, rarely calcification in artery walls)
Hypertrophied bronchial arteries
Filling defects in pulmonary arteries representing emboli/thrombus
Weblike filling defects in pulmonary arteries
Outpouching/aneurysmal pulmonary arteries (rare)

Parenchymal
Mosaic attenuation pattern
Regional variation in caliber of subsegmental pulmonary arteries
Basal subpleural linear and irregular opacities reflecting previous infarcts
Dilatation of bronchi and air-trapping (occasional feature)

The features shown on CT can be broadly divided into cardiac, vascular, and parenchymal abnormalities.[333,334] Dilatation of the right ventricular cavity and deviation of the interventricular septum may be clearly evident on contrast-enhanced CT. Marked dilatation of the proximal pulmonary arteries, which may have calcified walls, and intraluminal thrombus are clearly demonstrated on CT,[211] and contrast-enhanced CT or MRI is probably superior to pulmonary arteriography for the detection of central thrombus, particularly when it is lamellar, in patients being considered for thromboendarterectomy[212,278] (Figs 7.29 and 7.35). Bronchial artery hypertrophy usually accompanies chronic thromboembolic disease and the enlarged vessels may be readily identified on contrast-enhanced CT[214,333,335] (Fig. 7.28).

Areas of low attenuation of the lung parenchyma caused by hypoperfusion secondary to the pulmonary vascular occlusion, the mosaic oligemia or mosaic attenuation pattern,[334,336,337] may be a striking feature (Fig. 7.47). The intervening normal lung may appear abnormally dense, because of relatively increased perfusion, and these areas may be misinterpreted as having an abnormal ground-glass pattern due to another cause.[338,339] A mosaic attenuation pattern appears to be an almost invariable finding in patients with chronic thromboembolic disease and this, coupled with disparities in the size of segmental pulmonary arteries, may differentiate such patients from those with other causes of pulmonary arterial hypertension.[340] Dilatation of bronchi in areas of reduced perfusion (hypoxic bronchodilatation) is an interesting ancillary CT sign that has been reported in some patients with chronic thromboembolic disease[341] (Fig. 7.25B). Furthermore, expiratory CT has been reported to show patchy air-trapping (not necessarily in segments with occluded supplying vessels) in over half of patients with acute pulmonary embolism[342]; the degree to which this phenomenon is responsible for the mosaic pattern seen in patients with chronic thromboembolic disease is uncertain (Box 7.9).

Ventilation–perfusion lung scans in pulmonary hypertension secondary to chronic thromboembolic disease show multiple segmental mismatched perfusion defects indistinguishable from high-probability scans in acute pulmonary embolism.[343] The appearances remain unchanged on sequential imaging. It is not uncommon to find patients referred for V̇/Q scintigraphy for the first time with suspected acute pulmonary embolism who show mismatched perfusion defects that do not resolve on repeat scans performed several weeks later.

Pulmonary angiography[331] reveals filling defects caused by thrombi in the lobar or segmental arteries, with occlusions of large and medium-sized vessels. If the thrombus in the main pulmonary arteries is laminated, the typical angiographic signs of filling defects may be absent.[344] The central vessels are usually dilated, with rapid distal tapering. Web-shaped filling defects are occasionally seen. "Pouching" of partially or completely occluded pulmonary arteries is also reported in chronic thromboembolic disease.[345]

Primary pulmonary hypertension

The term "primary pulmonary hypertension" refers to a group of patients who have pulmonary arterial hypertension with no clinically discernible cause, a normal pulmonary arterial wedge pressure, and no evidence of left-to-right shunt on cardiac catheterization. Pulmonary hypertension at rest reflects extensive obliteration (>70%) of the pulmonary vascular bed. Primary pulmonary hypertension has traditionally been classified into three subtypes based on the histologic appearances of the vascular bed[346,347]: (1) plexogenic arteriopathy, (2) recurrent pulmonary thromboembolism, and (3) pulmonary venoocclusive disease. The latter is seen in less than 10% of patients and, because the lesion of intimal proliferation is confined to the pulmonary veins, it is usually considered a separate entity.

Prolonged vasoconstriction is believed to be the first stage of plexogenic pulmonary arteriopathy (classic primary pulmonary hypertension); the next stage is structural change in the arterial wall. On pathologic study,[348,349] the initial structural manifestations are medial hypertrophy of the muscular pulmonary arteries and muscularization of the arterioles. This is followed by concentric laminar fibrosis in a so-called "onionskin" configuration. The walls of the muscular pulmonary arteries may show necrotizing arteritis with fibrinoid necrosis. Plexiform lesions are a striking and diagnostically important finding, consisting of a network of capillary-like channels within a dilated segment of a muscular pulmonary artery. The lesions are seen only in patients with severe pulmonary arterial hypertension. They are not a feature of pulmonary venoocclusive disease or of recurrent pulmonary thromboembolism.

Aminorex fumarate, an appetite suppressant, produced an identical picture to primary pulmonary hypertension in those few subjects who used the drug, as does the "bush tea" of native West Indians, in which *Crotalaria fulva* is believed to be responsible. Identical clinical and pathologic features to those encountered in primary pulmonary hypertension have been reported in patients with the toxic oil syndrome.[350] The striking female-to-male ratio of patients with primary pulmonary hypertension and the fact that the disease is often encountered shortly after puberty suggest that female sex hormones may be important in the etiology of the condition. Familial cases of primary pulmonary hypertension have also been reported,[351] and it has been postulated that the disease may be related to an inherited tendency to increased pulmonary vascular reactivity.

The age range is wide; most patients are adults or older children, but cases have been described in young children and infants. In a large series of 156 patients the average age was 33 (range 16–69) and the female-to-male ratio was 4:1.[352] The patients complain of weakness, dyspnea, and chest pain. Arrhythmias are common in the later stages. Physical examination reveals all the expected signs of right ventricular pressure overload and elevated systemic venous pressure. The murmur of pulmonary regurgitation may be heard on auscultation.

The radiographic features of primary pulmonary hypertension (Figs 7.38 and 7.48) are dilatation of the main pulmonary artery and the other central arteries with rapid tapering to oligemic peripheral lung. The peripheral lung vessels are narrow and inconspicuous. The average width of the right descending pulmonary artery was twice the diameter of that in normal control subjects in one review of 54 patients with primary pulmonary hypertension,[353] but as with all types of pulmonary hypertension, the plain chest radiographs may show relatively little dilatation of central vessels (Fig. 7.49).

V̇/Q scintigraphy in primary pulmonary hypertension may be normal or show multiple small unmatched perfusion defects throughout both lungs.[343,354,355] The appearances are, in other words, quite different from those in chronic, unresolved, pulmonary embolism. Wilson and co-workers[356] noted that patients with normal scans were predominantly young women, whereas there was an equal sex distribution in those with multiple perfusion defects. This observation is consistent with a later one by Rich and co-workers[355] who correlated the perfusion scan with the histology of the lung. Their category of plexogenic hypertension was seen in women and associated with a normal scan, while their histologic category, microthrombotic, was seen in both sexes, was associated with multiple small defects, and seems to correspond to Wilson's group with a similar perfusion pattern. The concept that this latter form of primary pulmonary hypertension arises from previously unrecognized microthrombosis is an attractive one but remains unproven.

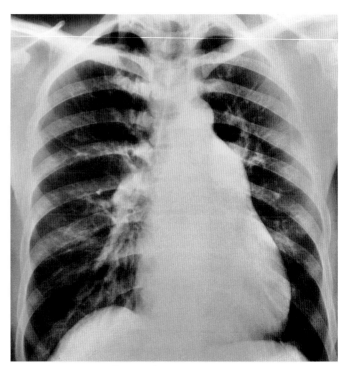

Fig. 7.48 Primary pulmonary hypertension in a 37-year-old man. There is cardiomegaly, an enlarged main pulmonary artery, and enlarged hilar arteries. In this instance, the arteries beyond hilar are normal in size.

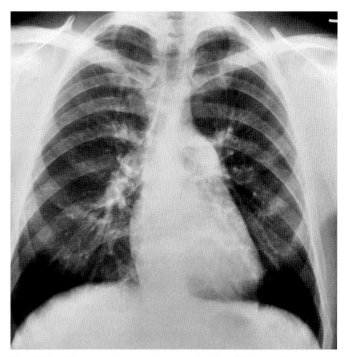

Fig. 7.49 Primary pulmonary hypertension in a 25-year-old man. The chest is almost normal despite a pulmonary artery pressure of 93 mmHg systolic and a mean pressure of 62 mmHg. The heart is normal in size and shape. The only abnormal finding is enlargement of the main pulmonary artery.

Pressure measurements at cardiac catheterization confirm the diagnosis. The pulmonary vascular resistance is extremely high. The pulmonary capillary wedge pressure, if it can be measured, is normal, and the left-sided pressures are also normal. Right-to-left shunting through a patent foramen ovale may be present. Pulmonary arteriography is used to exclude intraluminal filling defects caused by thromboembolism rather than to make the diagnosis. The pulmonary arterial tree shows dilatation of the central vessels. The peripheral vessels taper to an abnormal degree[357] and are reduced in number. Delayed clearance of contrast material from the arterial tree was seen in 22 of 25 patients in one series.[358]

There is relatively little in the HRCT literature on the effects of primary pulmonary hypertension on the appearances of the lung parenchyma. This reflects both the rarity of the condition and the nonspecific and subtle changes that occur. While the mosaic attenuation pattern on HRCT is an expected feature of chronic thromboembolic disease,[333] anecdotal experience suggests that it is less prevalent or conspicuous in primary pulmonary hypertension. In a study of 64 patients with pulmonary artery hypertension of various causes, only 4 had primary pulmonary hypertension but all of these had some regional inhomogeneity of the attenuation of lung parenchyma (13 of 15 patients with thromboembolic disease had a mosaic attenuation pattern).[336] Whether the distribution of the pathologic process in primary pulmonary hypertension (relatively uniform involvement of the small muscular pulmonary arteries, in comparison to patchy thrombotic occlusion of larger generations of pulmonary arteries in thromboembolic disease) is responsible for different HRCT manifestations, for example, loss of the normal gravity-dependent density gradient in non-thromboembolic pulmonary hypertension[359] rather than the obvious mosaic attenuation pattern seen in chronic thromboembolic pulmonary hypertension,[340] is uncertain. In some patients with advanced primary pulmonary hypertension there is scintigraphic evidence of reversed mismatching, that is pulmonary perfusion of areas of lung showing little or no ventilation. A CT study has shown that such areas show normal or engorged pulmonary vasculature with areas of increased parenchymal attenuation which are shown to have ventilatory defects on scintigraphy.[360]

Inconspicuous small, poorly defined, low-attenuation, centrilobular nodules (similar to those seen in subacute hypersensitivity pneumonitis) are sometimes seen on HRCT (Fig. 7.50) in patients with pulmonary arterial hypertension of various causes.[361] On histologic examination these nodules may contain cholesterol granulomas, thought to be the consequence of macrophage ingestion of red blood cells following repeated pulmonary hemorrhage. Two of the 5 patients included in this report had primary pulmonary hypertension; the presence of a widespread nodular pattern on HRCT clearly raises the possibility of a secondary (diffuse parenchymal) cause for pulmonary hypertension, for example conditions characterized by a nodular pattern with a propensity to cause pulmonary hypertension, such as Langerhans cell histiocytosis[362] (Fig. 7.51) or pulmonary capillary hemangiomatosis[363]; the latter deserves special mention as this rare condition may be overlooked in patients thought to have primary pulmonary hypertension (Box 7.10).

Pulmonary capillary hemangiomatosis is characterized by widespread abnormal proliferation of thin walled capillary channels in the pulmonary interstitium. There is associated obstruction of small venules (so that the histologic picture in

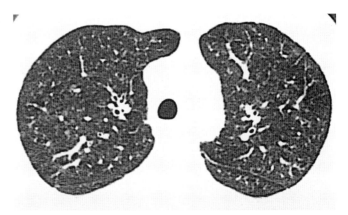

Fig. 7.50 CT showing poorly defined, relatively low-attenuation nodules in a patient with severe pulmonary hypertension of unknown cause.

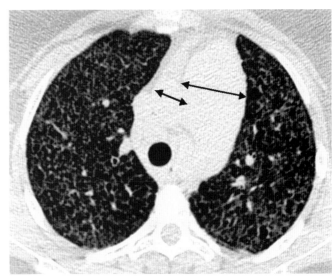

Fig. 7.51 Severe pulmonary hypertension in a patient with Langerhans cell histiocytosis. There are micronodular and reticular patterns, concentrated in the upper lobes. The main pulmonary artery is markedly dilated (longer double-headed arrow) by comparison with the ascending aorta (shorter double-headed arrow), reflecting severe pulmonary hypertension.

Box 7.10 Features of primary pulmonary hypertension on CT

Dilatation of proximal and segmental pulmonary arteries
Small pericardial effusion (with severe pulmonary hypertension, mean pressure >35 mmHg)
Subtle mosaic attenuation pattern
Small, poorly defined centrilobular nodules (rare)
May be signs of coexisting left ventricular failure

---

some ways resembles pulmonary venoocclusive disease), resulting in pulmonary hypertension.[364,365] This proliferation of fragile capillary-sized vessels, prone to bleed, is responsible for the CT picture of poorly defined small nodular opacities, thickened interlobular septa, and areas of ground-glass opacification[363,366] (Fig. 7.52). The authors of one study[366] state

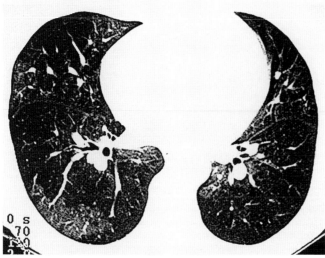

Fig. 7.52 Capillary hemangiomatosis. The patient had severe pulmonary hypertension and was on the waiting list for transplantation. The well-defined areas of ground-glass opacification reflect, at a microscopic level, the abnormal capillary proliferation. (Courtesy of Dr L Mitchell, Newcastle upon Tyne)

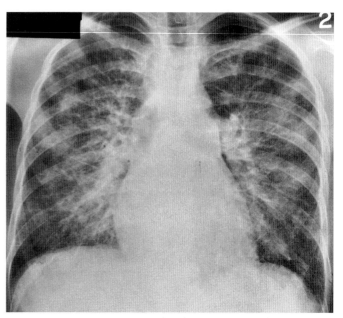

Fig. 7.53 Pulmonary venoocclusive disease. A chest radiograph of a 16-year-old boy with a 4-month history of increasing dyspnea. The patient died 3 days later. There is alveolar and interstitial edema and signs of pulmonary arterial hypertension.

that nodules were not seen in patients with primary pulmonary hypertension, although only 5 were evaluated; nevertheless similar nodules (representing cholesterol granulomas, as described above) are said to be an occasional feature in "pure" primary pulmonary hypertension.[361] The distinction between capillary hemangiomatosis and primary pulmonary hypertension is important because the treatment of primary pulmonary hypertension with epoprostenol can precipitate fatal pulmonary edema in patients with capillary hemangiomatosis.[367–369]

There is some overlap between the HRCT–pathologic features of pulmonary capillary hemangiomatosis and those of pulmonary venoocclusive disease,[366,370] simply because of the size and site of the pulmonary vessels involved (capillaries and adjoining venules respectively).

Pulmonary venoocclusive disease

Pulmonary venoocclusive disease is a very rare disorder, and its cause is unknown.[371,372] Occasionally the disease may be inherited and a single study has suggested a pathogenetic link with primary pulmonary hypertension.[373] The pulmonary veins thrombose and develop intimal fibrosis. Occlusion of the pulmonary veins leads to pulmonary venous and capillary congestion, pulmonary edema, rarely acute pulmonary hemorrhage,[374] alveolar hemosiderin deposits, and pulmonary arterial hypertension that may be very severe.[375] The muscular pulmonary arteries develop medial hypertrophy, and there is muscularization of the small pulmonary veins and arterioles.[376] Thrombi, which may be recent, organized, or recanalized, may be seen in these vessels, but plexiform lesions are absent. The pulmonary arteriolar wedge pressure is usually normal, and if abnormal is only mildly elevated[377–379]: one reason why pulmonary venoocclusive disease has historically been included in the category of primary pulmonary hypertension. The outcome is almost invariably fatal, and in most cases the only curative treatment is lung transplantation.[380] Apart from a

report of 2 patients who developed venoocclusive disease following bone marrow transplantation and who responded to high-dose methylprednisolone,[381] steroid therapy seems to be ineffective. There are a few reports of individual patients showing sustained response to vasodilators[382] and specifically nifedipine.[383] However, prostacyclin therapy has been associated with acute and fatal pulmonary edema in one patient with venoocclusive disease,[384] similar to the more recent reports of adverse response to prostaglandin treatment in patients with capillary hemangiomatosis.[367,368]

The chest radiographic appearances are those of pulmonary arterial hypertension, usually with signs of pulmonary edema. Both alveolar edema and interstitial edema are commonly seen in this condition (Fig. 7.53). In one review of the radiographic features of 26 cases, 20 patients showed pulmonary edema.[377] The left atrium is not enlarged, an important point of difference from mitral valve disease, left atrial myxoma, and cor triatriatum. Surprisingly, there is usually no evidence of upper zone blood diversion.

The CT features of venoocclusive disease mirror the radiographic abnormalities: ground-glass opacity, reflecting interstitial and early airspace edema, is the most frequent finding and smooth thickening of the interlobular septa is almost invariably present[385,386] (Fig. 7.54). Mediastinal adenopathy is an inconstant feature.[387] Of the 8 patients described by Swensen et al,[386] 5 had bilateral pleural effusions and 4 showed a mosaic attenuation pattern; the central pulmonary arteries were judged to be dilated in 7 patients (whereas the pulmonary veins were not). Although this constellation of HRCT features is suggestive of pulmonary venoocclusive disease, the authors concluded that a lung biopsy is required to confirm the diagnosis[386]; others have suggested that the clinical findings may be sufficiently characteristic to avoid the need for biopsy confirmation.[372]

Radionuclide perfusion scans are diagnostically nonspecific and are either normal or show small bilateral wedge-shaped

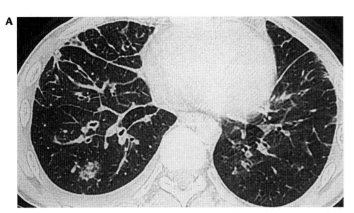
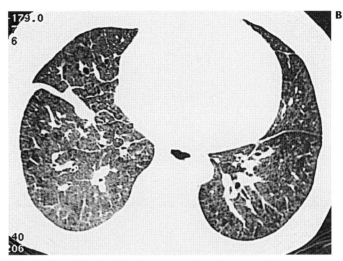

Fig. 7.54 HRCT of pulmonary venoocclusive disease. **A**, There is widespread thickening of the interlobular septa and patchy ground-glass opacification (courtesy of Dr S Swensen, Mayo Clinic, Rochester). **B**, In another case the ground-glass opacification is more intense and there is a small pleural effusion tracking into the right major fissure.

perfusion defects.[388] Pulmonary angiography shows dilatation of the proximal pulmonary arteries and slow circulation through the pulmonary vascular bed.[388] The venous phase does not help in making the diagnosis but does help to exclude other causes of pulmonary arterial hypertension, such as congenital stenosis of the pulmonary veins, left atrial myxoma, and cor triatriatum[379] (Box 7.11).

> **Box 7.11** **Imaging features of pulmonary venoocclusive disease**
>
> Signs of pulmonary arterial hypertension
> Radiographic signs of (interstitial) pulmonary edema
> – no upper lobe blood diversion
> Pleural effusions
> Mediastinal lymphadenopathy (an occasional CT finding)
> Ground-glass opacity and thickened interlobular septa
> (conspicuous) on HRCT

Pulmonary hypertension secondary to pulmonary vasculitis

Pulmonary arterial hypertension may be caused by a large variety of extremely rare pulmonary vasculitides.

Mostly these conditions affect the small vessels and they are discussed in Chapter 10. Large vessel vasculitis is recognized but is much less common.[389] Takayasu disease is the best-known example of a large vessel vasculitis causing pulmonary hypertension.

Takayasu arteritis (Takayasu disease, pulseless disease) is an arteritis of medium and large arteries that most commonly affects segments of the aorta and its main branches. The vessel wall becomes fibrosed and thickened, usually causing luminal stenosis rather than aneurysm. Takayasu arteritis occurs chiefly in women, and is manifested between 10 and 20 years of age in 75% of patients.[390,391] The presenting features are constitutional

symptoms, fever, arthralgia, and symptoms of local ischemia with absent pulses or bruits. Moderate systemic hypertension is common and is usually due to renal ischemia.[390] The course is variable, with episodic remissions or progression; death occurs in about 25% of cases.

Involvement of pulmonary arteries occurs in approximately half the patients[392,393] and there appears to be a correlation between the frequency of pulmonary and systemic artery lesions.[394] The pulmonary hypertension is usually mild, and pulmonary symptoms are unusual.[393] The plain chest radiograph, in addition to showing the features of pulmonary arterial hypertension, may reveal oligemic areas beyond the obstructed arteries.[395] The plain chest radiograph may also show the features of aortic arteritis, namely irregular outline to the aorta, aortic ectasia, calcification of the aortic wall, or even rib notching.[395,396] Angiography reveals obstructions or stenoses of the lobar and segmental branches of the pulmonary arteries, and there may also be focal areas of dilatation.[393,395] Endovascular stenting, sometimes with numerous stents, may alleviate symptoms.[397,398] Both MRI and CTPA can show vessel wall abnormalities to advantage[399,400] (Fig. 7.55). Precontrast CT scans may reveal the aortic wall to be of higher than normal attenuation, with or without obvious calcification. The thickened walls of involved vessels sometimes show early or delayed enhancement following the injection of contrast medium.[400]

Pulmonary hypertension secondary to pleuropulmonary disease

Pulmonary hypertension is a common phenomenon in chronic pulmonary diseases, notably in chronic obstructive pulmonary disease (COPD), and interstitial fibrotic lung disease (Figs 7.56 and 7.57). The acquired immunodeficiency syndrome is a recognized cause of pulmonary hypertension,[401–403] but the mechanism by which HIV infection causes pulmonary hypertension remains unclear.[404,405] Fibrothorax and lung destruction resulting from infection are less frequent causes of pulmonary hypertension.

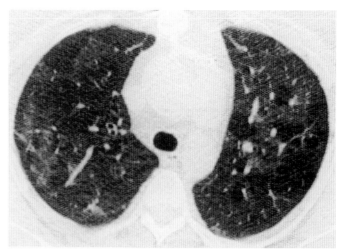

Fig. 7.55 Takayasu arteritis in a 43-year-old female. **A,** The main pulmonary artery and ascending aorta are dilated and their walls are abnormally thickened. Adjacent sections showed an aneurysmal pouch arising from the anterior aspect of the main pulmonary artery. **B,** Mosaic perfusion pattern in the upper lobes, presumed to reflect arteritic involvement and/or thrombosis of the medium-sized and smaller pulmonary vessels.

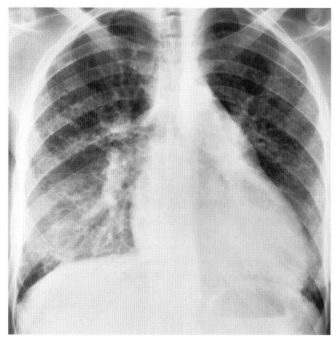

Fig. 7.56 Pulmonary arterial hypertension secondary to interstitial fibrosis, in this case associated with dermatomyositis.

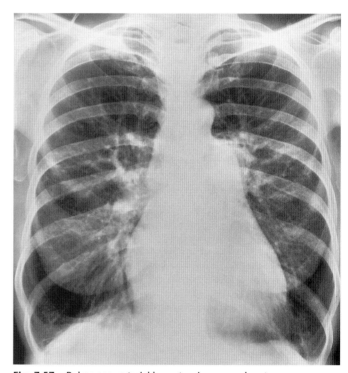

Fig. 7.57 Pulmonary arterial hypertension secondary to severe chronic obstructive pulmonary disease: pulmonary hypertension (cardiomegaly, central arterial dilatation, and upper zone vessel enlargement) and signs of COPD (over-inflated lungs and patchy vessel deficiency).

The common factor responsible for the elevated pulmonary vascular resistance in all these conditions is probably hypoxia, the most efficient known vasoconstrictor. Hypercapnia, acidemia, erythrocythemia, and increased blood volume may all contribute to the pulmonary hypertension. In disorders such as emphysema and interstitial fibrosis there is the added possibility that destruction of the lung vasculature may play a role.[406] The relationship between lung destruction and raised pulmonary vascular resistance is not simple. No direct correlation between the severity of the emphysema and the degree of right ventricular hypertrophy (the pathologist's criterion of long-standing pulmonary arterial hypertension) at autopsy has been

shown.[407,408] However, in vivo studies using MRI have demonstrated right ventricular hypertrophy in patients considered to have mild and even trivial chronic obstructive pulmonary disease.[409,410] Conversely, COPD as a cause of severe pulmonary hypertension, as judged by its low prevalence in a population of 600 patients with documented pulmonary hypertension, is noteworthy.[411] Doppler echocardiography provides indirect evidence of pulmonary arterial hypertension in patients with a variety of disorders such as chronic obstructive pulmonary disease,[412,413] and the pulmonary vasculopathy associated with systemic sclerosis,[414] but there may be problems in consistently obtaining pressure gradient readings with continuous wave Doppler.[415]

The radiographic features consist of a combination of the signs of the responsible pleuropulmonary disease and the signs of pulmonary arterial hypertension, often with evidence of associated biventricular cardiac failure.

Pulmonary hypertension secondary to increased pulmonary blood flow

Pulmonary artery pressure can be elevated even without a rise in pulmonary vascular resistance if the pulmonary arterial blood flow is large enough. Sustained very high flows of this order are seen only with left-to-right shunts. The increased vessel size resulting from the massive blood flow dominates the radiographic picture. The elevations of pulmonary artery pressure are mild and do not contribute in a recognizable fashion to the radiographic appearances.

The term "Eisenmenger reaction" refers to raised pulmonary vascular resistance secondary to left-to-right shunting of blood, the usual causes of which are atrial septal defect (ASD),

ventricular septal defect (VSD), and patent ductus arteriosus (PDA). The arterial changes on histologic examination consist of varying degrees of hypertrophy of the media of the small muscular arteries and arterioles, together with intimal proliferation; plexiform lesions and necrotizing arteritis may also be seen in the advanced cases.

The radiographic features of left-to-right shunt are cardiac enlargement and enlargement of all the pulmonary vessels, both central and peripheral, in all lung zones. With normal pulmonary vascular resistance the distension of the pulmonary vascular tree is approximately proportional to the increased flow. With a fully established Eisenmenger syndrome (reversal of shunt owing to elevation of pulmonary vascular resistance) the central vessels show disproportionate enlargement with rapid tapering at segmental level and beyond. It can be difficult to recognize mild or moderate elevation of pulmonary vascular resistance because the diagnosis depends on evaluating the relative size of the vessels and there are no acceptable measurements or ratios on which to base this judgment. The pattern varies according to the defect. Rees and Jefferson[416] noted that in Eisenmenger ASD the chest radiograph shows massive enlargement of the central vessels with rapid tapering beyond hilar level (Fig. 7.58), whereas with Eisenmenger VSD the degree of dilatation of the central vessels is usually mild and sometimes even unrecognizable (Fig. 7.59). Thus, with ventricular septal

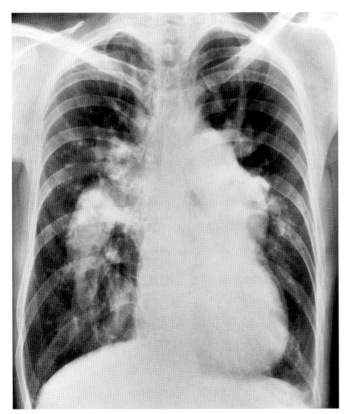

Fig. 7.58 Pulmonary arterial hypertension in a middle-aged man caused by an atrial septal defect with Eisenmenger syndrome, showing truly massive enlargement of the central pulmonary arteries.

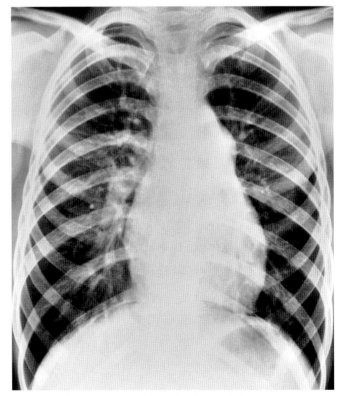

Fig. 7.59 Pulmonary arterial hypertension in a 14-year-old boy caused by ventricular septal defect with Eisenmenger syndrome, illustrating the relatively mild dilatation of the main pulmonary artery and hilar arteries seen with this condition even when, as in this case, the pulmonary arterial pressure is at systemic levels.

defect, even in cases with systemic pressures in the pulmonary circuit, the rapid tapering of vessel size is often not present. In fact, the appearances are often similar to a mild or moderate left-to-right shunt with no recognizable evidence of pulmonary arterial hypertension. It is even possible to see a normal or near-normal radiograph in Eisenmenger VSD. Eisenmenger PDA shows moderate dilatation of the aortic arch and the main pulmonary artery, and mild dilatation of the right and left hilar arteries. (The ductus itself may calcify.) The explanation for the different appearances of Eisenmenger ASD, VSD, and PDA is conjectural.

Pulmonary hypertension caused by alveolar hypoventilation without underlying lung disease

Alveolar hypoventilation can lead to hypoxia, and hypoxia is the most potent known stimulus for pulmonary vasoconstriction.[417] Hypoxic pulmonary vasoconstriction normally helps match blood flow and ventilation, diverting blood flow away from poorly ventilated areas.[418] When only a small portion of the lung is hypoxic, this response improves arterial oxygen saturation by reducing blood flow to the poorly ventilated segments without increasing pulmonary artery pressure. However, with widespread alveolar hypoxia, this normally protective response causes a large fraction of the pulmonary vasculature to constrict, increasing pulmonary artery pressure.[418]

Alveolar hypoventilation without underlying disease is seen in morbid obesity.[402] The effects of morbid obesity on lung ventilation are complex, consisting of (1) obstructive sleep apnea (almost invariably), and (2) hypoventilation (hypoxemia and hypercapnia) even while awake and breathing room air. The mechanisms of hypoventilation include a marked increase in abdominal contents that push the diaphragm up, increased chest wall compliance, weakness of inspiratory muscles, and altered hypoxic and hypercapnic responsiveness.[419,420] Most patients with the sleep apnea and alveolar hypoventilation syndromes are markedly obese, but there are exceptions. Conversely, many very obese patients do not suffer from either syndrome. On radiographic study the appearances are those of pulmonary arterial hypertension with cardiomegaly and dilatation of the central pulmonary arteries in an obese subject. Biventricular cardiac failure is a frequent cause of death in these patients.[421]

A consequence of chronic hypoxia has been elegantly demonstrated in a radiographic study of individuals living at sea level, at 1400 m, and at 2600 m above sea level. The width of the right descending pulmonary artery, presumed to reflect pulmonary artery pressure, was independently related to residence at elevated altitude.[422]

PULMONARY ARTERY ANEURYSM

Pulmonary artery aneurysms are very rare. They may be congenital in origin or acquired. Reports of idiopathic pulmonary artery aneurysms are limited to single case reports. Mycotic aneurysms are the most frequently encountered.[423] Those that develop in the walls of tuberculous cavities are known as Rasmussen aneurysms.[424] Mycotic aneurysms may also occur in association with lung abscess or septicemia, particularly in drug addicts. Behçet disease, described on page 601, is a potent cause of lobar and segmental artery aneurysms,[425] and segmental pulmonary artery aneurysms are a feature of the rare Hughes–Stovin syndrome (see p. 601). Posttraumatic false aneurysm[426] (more recently reported as a complication of Swan–Ganz catheter placement[427,428]), dissecting aneurysm of a pulmonary artery,[429] postembolic aneurysm,[430] bronchial carcinoma,[431] and myxomatous emboli from a right atrial myxoma[432] are all very rare causes of pulmonary artery aneurysm. Very rarely the main pulmonary artery, but not the right or left, may appear aneurysmally dilated in otherwise normal individuals[316]; only with prolonged follow-up care can such cases be regarded as idiopathic and of no clinical consequence.

Hemoptysis is the principal complication and is frequently fatal. The largest series were reported before the advent of antituberculous therapy. In one autopsy series,[424] rupture of the aneurysm was the immediate cause of death in 38 of the 45 tuberculosis patients examined. In only 2 cases were the aneurysms believed to be incidental.

It is rare to see the aneurysm as a discrete mass in an otherwise normal lung. Usually the aneurysm is adjacent to, or surrounded by, the infection that caused it, and it may therefore be very difficult to appreciate. On chest radiography, Rasmussen aneurysms may occasionally resemble mycetomas. Because both cause hemoptysis, the true diagnosis is easily overlooked. The clue may be the rapid change in size of a mass resulting from an aneurysm. CT scanning with contrast clearly shows the vascular nature of pulmonary artery aneurysms.[423,433,434]

HEPATOPULMONARY SYNDROME

It has been known for a long time that patients with severe chronic liver disease of any cause may develop a form of angiodysplasia of the lungs.[435,436] The hepatopulmonary syndrome comprises chronic hepatic dysfunction, intrapulmonary vascular dilatation, and arterial hypoxemia.[437] The abnormal intrapulmonary vessels, which have been likened to spider nevi, are randomly distributed through the lungs with a predilection for the subpleural regions.

The pathophysiology behind the hypoxemia is complex and cannot entirely be ascribed to right-to-left shunting through the abnormal vessels.[437,438] Despite the increased blood flow through the pulmonary vasculature, pulmonary artery pressure is not usually greatly raised. Krowka and Cortese have classified the vascular lesions of the hepatopulmonary syndrome as either type 1 (minimal) – the more common type with a spidery appearance of the peripheral vessels on angiography and some response (decreased shunting) to 100% oxygen, or type 2 (accounting for approximately 15% of cases), which are essentially small, but macroscopic, arteriovenous fistulas which do not respond to inspired oxygen.[439]

The chest radiograph may be normal or may show increased vascular markings or small nodular shadows in the lower zones (the latter may resemble interstitial disease; Fig. 7.60). Radionuclide perfusion lung scanning shows extensive extrapulmonary uptake caused by the bypassing of the pulmonary arteriolar bed,[440] and radionuclide shunt calculations have shown that more than half of the pulmonary blood flow may bypass the alveoli.[441] Pulmonary angiography shows dilatation of the large and medium-sized arteries, with a myriad of abnormal spidery branches in the lung periphery and rapid filling of enlarged pulmonary veins. On HRCT the nature of the minute nodular opacities seen on chest radiography is clearly displayed: the terminal pulmonary arterial branches are abnormally profuse and dilated[442,443] (Fig. 7.61). Some of these abnormally dilated peripheral vessels can be seen to abut the pleural surface. These vessels are not found in normoxic cirrhotic patients.[443]

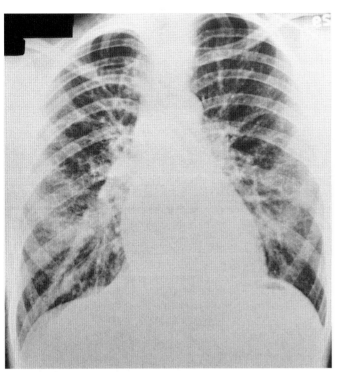

Fig. 7.60 Hepatopulmonary syndrome in a 20-year-old man with cirrhosis from childhood who was severely hypoxic. The lungs show a widespread increase in vessel size and background nodularity.

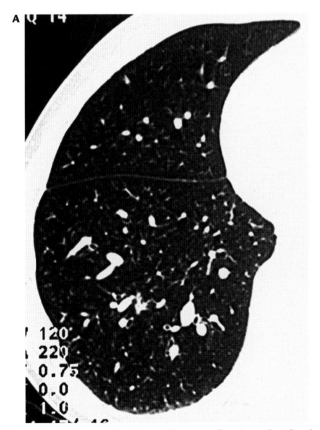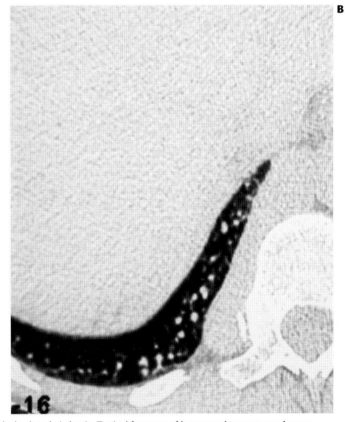

Fig. 7.61 A 43-year-old patient with a recent liver transplant for alcohol-related cirrhosis. Typical features of hepatopulmonary syndrome: **A**, marked dilatation of the segmental pulmonary arteries in the lower lobes and slightly increased nodularity in the subpleural lung posteriorly; **B**, obvious enlargement of the extremely peripheral pulmonary vessels nestling in the costophrenic recess. (Courtesy of Dr S R Desai, London)

SICKLE CELL DISEASE

Patients with sickle cell anemia are at increased risk for pneumonia and pulmonary infarction.[444] Distinguishing between these two entities both clinically and radiologically can be difficult.[445,446] Because of this difficulty the more general term "acute chest syndrome" is often applied to describe fever, clinical findings of a pulmonary process, and radiological evidence of new pulmonary consolidation in a patient with sickle cell hemoglobinopathy.[447] The acute chest syndrome is one of the most common reasons for hospitalization and is a significant cause of mortality in these patients.[447–450]

A large survey of children who required hospital admission during a 10 year period[448] showed that bacterial pneumonia, particularly pneumococcal pneumonia, was responsible for the acute event in some 40% of patients, and the authors speculated that the true incidence of bacterial pneumonia was much higher. Another survey revealed a similar incidence of pulmonary infections but a much lower proportion of bacterial pneumonia and relatively few cases of pneumococcal pneumonia.[447] Viral pneumonia and mycoplasmal pneumonia were approximately as frequent as bacterial pneumonia. The lower incidence of bacterial pneumonia in the more recent study may have reflected the use of penicillin prophylaxis and pneumococcal immunization.[447] In both of these series the precise cause of more than half the episodes could not be determined, and they were presumed to result from pulmonary infarction, atelectasis, or missed infection.

In a more recent study, no identifiable cause for the acute chest syndrome was discovered in 87% of patients (median age 14 years)[451] and fat embolism has been suggested as a noninfective cause for the acute chest syndrome.[449,452]

Pulmonary infarction, which is much more frequent in adults than in children,[453,454] is often associated with other evidence of sickle cell crisis such as abdominal or musculoskeletal pain.[448] Pulmonary infarction is rare in children under 12 years of age. Autopsy series, which clearly represent the severe end of the spectrum of pulmonary disease, show a high prevalence of pulmonary infarcts, even in infants and young children.[455] The autopsy findings consist of (1) pneumonia, (2) pulmonary infarction with necrosis of alveolar walls, (3) pulmonary vascular thrombosis with pulmonary hypertension, and (4) bone marrow embolization from areas of ischemic bone necrosis.[444]

On radiographic examination[456] there are confluent lobar or segmental consolidations that may be accompanied by pleural effusion. The consolidations resolve more slowly than in the general population, and recurrence is common. Distinguishing consolidation resulting from infection from that caused by infarction is often impossible. One clue to the diagnosis of infarction may be the late development of a pulmonary shadow; consolidation resulting from pneumonia is likely to be present on the initial film. If the shadowing is clearly interstitial in character and the patient has fever, viral or mycoplasmal pneumonia is the likely diagnosis. Pulmonary edema, either interstitial or alveolar, may be present and can be confused with pneumonia and infarction. The edema may be the result of treatment with analgesics such as morphine or may be the consequence of heart failure. Bone infarcts in ribs may sometimes be identified on chest radiographs, but radionuclide bone scans are far more sensitive.[457,458]

In addition to the pulmonary features of the acute chest syndrome, the heart may show nonspecific enlargement and the pulmonary blood vessels are frequently enlarged. Several hemodynamic factors are at work, and the relative role of each may be difficult to unravel in an individual case. Chronic anemia of any cause gives rise to a sustained increase in cardiac output even when the patient is at rest.[459] Chronic high cardiac output can be recognized on plain chest radiographs as nonspecific cardiomegaly and increase in the size of the pulmonary blood vessels. Increased left ventricular mass has been well documented by echocardiography.[460] Myocardial damage or ischemia from sickle cell disease may also contribute to the cardiac enlargement and to cardiac dysfunction.[461] Pulmonary hypertension similar to that seen in primary pulmonary hypertension may develop secondary to obstruction of the pulmonary vascular bed.[462,463]

As might be anticipated, the most frequent finding on CT in patients with acute chest syndrome is areas of "hypoperfusion",[464] that is, areas of decreased attenuation within which there are fewer pulmonary vessels than expected (Fig. 7.62). In addition, there may be areas of ground-glass opacification[446]; in the study by Bhalla et al, these areas of ground-glass opacity were identified only in segments which showed features of "hypoperfusion", and possibly represented areas of hemorrhagic oedema caused by reversible ischemia.[464] By contrast, denser areas of consolidation reflect either true tissue infarction or, less likely, infective consolidation responsible for precipitation of the acute chest syndrome. Chronic changes are seen in individuals with repeated acute episodes, with approximately half showing evidence of interstitial disease, most probably reflecting scarring from small pulmonary infarcts[465] (Fig. 7.63). The nature of the chronic changes seen on HRCT, such as diffuse uniform ground-glass opacification, has not been characterized at a histologic level. Ultimately, if there is sufficient and permanent occlusion of the microvascular bed, cor pulmonale develops with dilatation of the central pulmonary arteries and evidence of right ventricular hypertrophy. In this situation, an obvious mosaic attenuation pattern, similar to that seen in chronic thromboembolic disease, may develop (Fig. 7.64; Box 7.12).

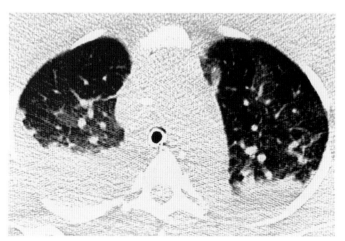

Fig. 7.62 Acute chest syndrome in a patient with sickle cell disease; the patient required ventilation. There are bilateral pleural effusions with adjacent atelectasis. Within the aerated lung there is a mosaic attenuation pattern.

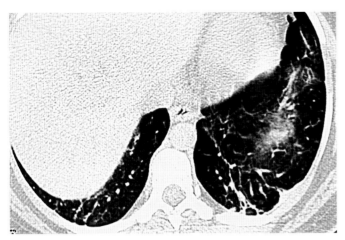

Fig. 7.63 Patient with repeated sickle cell crises. The parenchymal distortion suggests some interstitial fibrosis and the linear pleural-based opacities would be consistent with pulmonary infarcts.

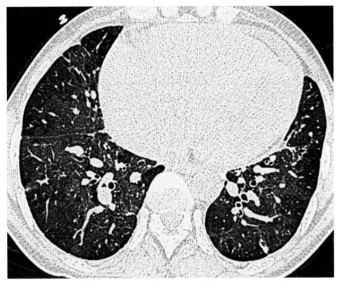

Fig. 7.64 Chronic sickle cell disease. In addition to a mosaic attenuation pattern there are signs of pulmonary hypertension, including dilatation of the proximal pulmonary arteries, an enlarged heart, and a pericardial effusion, reflecting the severe pulmonary hypertension.

Box 7.12 Features of chronic sickle cell disease on HRCT

Mosaic attenuation pattern
- Decreased attenuation areas reflecting hypoperfusion
- Ground-glass opacity, ?hemorrhagic edema

Reticular pattern, subpleural opacities
- Residual scarring from infection or infarction

Signs of pulmonary hypertension

PULMONARY EDEMA

Pulmonary edema is most often caused by one of two mechanisms[466–469]: elevated pulmonary venous pressure or increased permeability of the alveolar-capillary membrane. In some instances a combination of factors contributes to the development of pulmonary edema; for example, patients receiving immunomodulatory therapy for advanced malignancy often have renal insufficiency, fluid overload, and increased alveolar–capillary permeability.[470] Occasionally the edema is related to decreased plasma oncotic pressure or lymphatic insufficiency. Finally there are those disorders in which the mechanism is unknown or incompletely understood; even here, increased vascular permeability is probably a major factor.

This division of pulmonary edema into "cardiogenic" and "noncardiogenic", although convenient, is not always clear-cut,[467] and, it has been suggested that at least four categories are needed to encompass most types of pulmonary edema: (1) hydrostatic edema, (2) acute respiratory distress syndrome (permeability edema), (3) permeability edema without alveolar damage, and (4) mixed hydrostatic and permeability edema.[469,471] Despite the inevitable imprecision, the concept of dividing pulmonary edema into conditions in which the cause is primarily hydrostatic and those in which the cause is primarily increased permeability caused by capillary damage (such as acute respiratory distress syndrome; see discussion in a later section) has some considerable merit, since treatment is fundamentally different.

Raised pulmonary venous pressure

The signs of raised pulmonary venous pressure frequently precede or accompany cardiogenic pulmonary edema and are therefore described first.

Normally, in the upright subject, particularly on a film taken with deep inspiration, the vessels in the lower zones are larger than the equivalent vessels in the upper zones. With elevation of the pulmonary venous pressure the upper zone vessels enlarge. If, when the patient is erect, the upper zone vessels have a diameter equal to or larger than the equivalent lower zone vessels, elevation of the pulmonary venous pressure should be strongly considered[472] (Fig. 7.65).

It has been suggested that, as an absolute measurement, vessels in the first intercostal space on standard upright films should not exceed 3 mm in diameter.[473] In some patients one can measure the diameter of the vessels that accompany a bronchus. For example, the anterior segmental bronchus of one or the other upper lobe can often be identified end on as a ring shadow. The accompanying segmental artery is normally much the same diameter as the bronchus. Woodring has established that the pulmonary artery:bronchus (seen end on) ratio on the erect chest radiograph in normal individuals is 0.85 (standard deviation 0.15) in the upper zones and 1.34 (standard deviation 0.25) in the lower zones.[474] In patients with left ventricular failure the ratios reverse and become 1.5 in the upper zones and 0.87 in the lower zones; this relationship is maintained on supine radiographs of patients with left ventricular failure. However, reliable identification of an end-on pulmonary artery and its accompanying bronchus in both the upper and lower zones on a portable radiograph is often impossible.

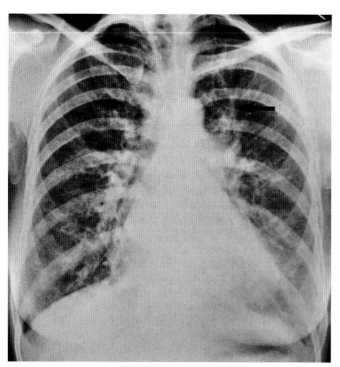

Fig. 7.65 Raised pulmonary venous pressure in a patient with mitral stenosis. Note that the vessels in the upper zones (arrow) are large compared with equivalent vessels in the lower zones.

The sign of upper zone vessel dilatation is believed to reflect increased blood flow to the upper zones.[475] The most widely accepted explanation for redistribution of pulmonary blood flow in subjects with elevated pulmonary venous pressure is that of West and associates,[475] who suggested that in the upright subject there is preferential development of pulmonary edema in the lower lobes. This basal interstitial edema, although not visible radiographically, is believed to form a perivascular cuff, which acts as a buffer between the vessels and the distending forces being transmitted through the lungs, with resultant redistribution of blood flow to the upper zones.[472]

The assessment of the signs of redistribution of blood flow requires technically good radiographs and is therefore easier when films obtained with fixed equipment are used, although acceptable interpretations can often be made from images taken with portable equipment. It is not surprising that there is considerable interobserver variation for the signs of mild raised pulmonary venous pressure.[476] It is essential that the patient be upright and that the film be exposed on inspiration. In normal supine subjects blood flow is fairly equal in the upper and lower zones, and redistribution of blood flow is therefore much more difficult to recognize on examinations with the patient supine. Furthermore, a similar pattern of redistribution occurs in several other conditions, particularly lower zone predominant emphysema.

The radiographic sign of upper zone redistribution of blood flow is reasonably accurate in predicting the pulmonary venous pressure in chronic valvular heart disease and chronic heart disease[477]; however, it should be appreciated that there is a significant proportion of patients with chronic ischemic heart disease causing left ventricular end-diastolic pressures higher than 24 mmHg who do not show visible upper zone vessel dilatation or, for that matter, any of the other radiographic signs of congestive heart failure.[477] The presence of upper lobe redistribution of flow is of limited value in the differential diagnosis of pulmonary shadows, when pulmonary edema is just one of several diagnoses being considered. In one large series only 50% of the patients with pulmonary edema resulting from heart disease showed redistribution of flow.[478] We also have seen many examples of cardiogenic pulmonary edema in which the vascular redistribution could not be recognized. Frequently the vessels cannot be adequately seen because of surrounding edema; sometimes they can be readily identified, but no redistribution is present.

Cardiogenic pulmonary edema

Under normal circumstances the pulmonary interstitium and alveoli are kept relatively dry. Increased quantities of tissue fluid resulting from elevated pulmonary venous pressure lead at first to increased lymphatic drainage. Once the capacity of the pulmonary lymphatics is exceeded, pulmonary edema results. Fluid collects first in the interstitium and then leaks into the airspaces.

The major causes of hydrostatic pulmonary edema are cardiac disease, overhydration, and fluid retention as a result of renal failure. Clinically the major effects are dyspnea and tachypnea. With the development of alveolar flooding, severe hypoxemia and hypocapnia or hypercapnia occur. In extreme cases blood-tinged foam is expectorated. Wheezing, the demand for an upright posture, and sweating are all prominent symptoms.

The radiographic signs of cardiogenic pulmonary edema are usually divided into interstitial and alveolar patterns, even though these phenomena are in reality a continuum. Interstitial edema may be seen without alveolar fluid, but if alveolar edema is present, the interstitium must also be edematous, whether or not it can be seen on the radiograph.

Plain chest radiography is sensitive for the diagnosis of pulmonary edema and can even demonstrate edema in patients who have not developed symptoms.[479] Conversely, it should be realized that pulmonary edema may be visible radiographically long after the hemodynamic factors have returned to normal.[480]

Interstitial pulmonary edema

Interstitial pulmonary edema causes a variety of radiographic signs,[469,481] the most readily recognized of which are septal lines, bronchial wall thickening, and subpleural pulmonary edema (Fig. 7.66). All of these features are even more clearly depicted on HRCT images[469,482–484] (Fig. 7.67).

Septal lines

The appearance of septal lines is discussed in detail in Chapter 3. The identification of septal lines is an extremely useful indicator of pulmonary edema. If transient or rapid in development, they are virtually diagnostic of interstitial pulmonary edema. Septal lines may not be particularly prominent even in florid pulmonary edema. Occasionally septal lines persist after pulmonary edema has resolved.

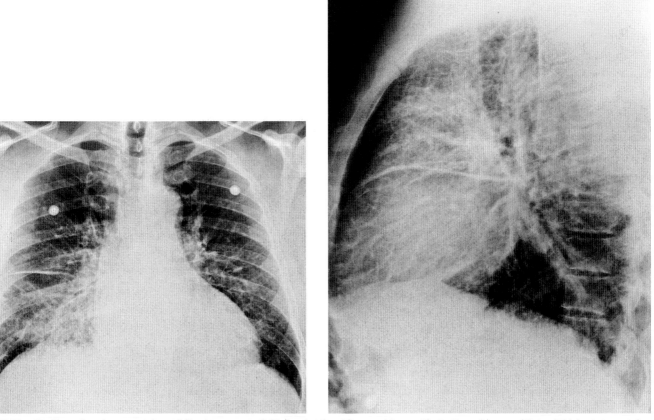

Fig. 7.66   Cardiogenic pulmonary edema following myocardial infarction in a 52-year-old man, illustrating widespread fissural thickening, septal lines, and lack of clarity of the intrapulmonary vessels. There is frank alveolar edema in the right lower zone. The fissural thickening caused by subpleural edema is particularly striking. **A**, Frontal view. **B**, Lateral view.

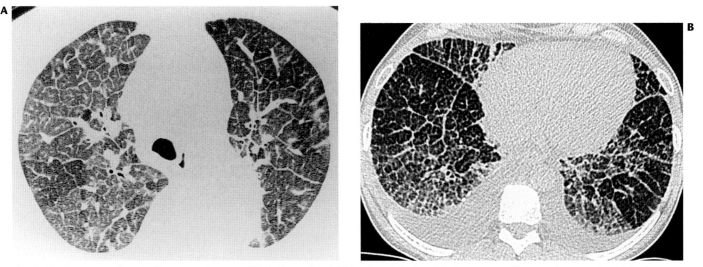

Fig. 7.67   Two examples of pulmonary edema on CT. **A**, Generalized thickening of the interlobular septa and increased attenuation of the lung parenchyma on HRCT in a patient with left ventricular failure. There are bilateral paravertebral pleural effusions. **B**, Standard CT of a different patient with cardiogenic pulmonary edema showing similar features.

Bronchial wall thickening

In normal chest radiographs the walls of the bronchi within the lung substance are invisible unless end on to the x-ray beam, when they are seen to have a very thin and well-defined ringlike wall. If edema collects in the peribronchial interstitial space, the combined shadow of the edematous bronchial wall and the thickened interstitium results in visible bronchial wall thickening.[485] Not only do the end-on bronchial walls become much thicker, the walls of those that are not end on may become visible. The posterior wall of the bronchus intermedius, as seen in the lateral chest radiograph, is another site at which wall thickening caused by edema can be assessed (it should normally measure less than 3 mm[486]).

Subpleural pulmonary edema

Fluid can accumulate in the loose connective tissue beneath the visceral pleura. The pulmonary septa communicate freely with this space, and edema can therefore flow peripherally to dissect beneath the pleura. Subpleural edema is seen radiographically as a sharply defined band of increased density that, when adjacent to a fissure, makes the fissure appear thick[71] (Fig. 7.66) and when in the costophrenic angles produces a lamella-shaped fluid collection resembling pleural effusion. It is the lamellar shape with the shadow conforming to the pleural boundary that suggests pulmonary rather than pleural fluid (Fig. 7.68). A well-defined curvilinear opacity in a subpleural distribution on CT has been described in some patients with left ventricular failure. The bandlike opacity, possibly representing engorged lymphatics, is separated from the visceral pleural surface by a few millimeters and disappears after diuretic therapy.[487]

Lack of clarity of the intrapulmonary and hilar vessels (hilar haze)

The hilar and pulmonary blood vessels may appear indistinct because of surrounding edema. This sign, which is often subtle, is one of the most consistent findings with interstitial pulmonary edema.[481] Comparison with previous radiographs to establish the normal appearance for a particular patient is frequently needed. Often the sign can only be appreciated retrospectively on follow-up films once the edema has resolved.

Generalized increase in density of the lung parenchyma

Generalized increase in density of the lung parenchyma is another subtle feature of pulmonary edema. The density of the lung on a plain chest radiograph is dependent on so many anatomic and technical factors that the sign is of little use in clinical assessment. Density measurement by CT and signal characteristics at MRI are more objective methods of quantitating the amount of fluid present in the lungs,[482,488,489] although they are of little practical use for making the diagnosis of early pulmonary edema.

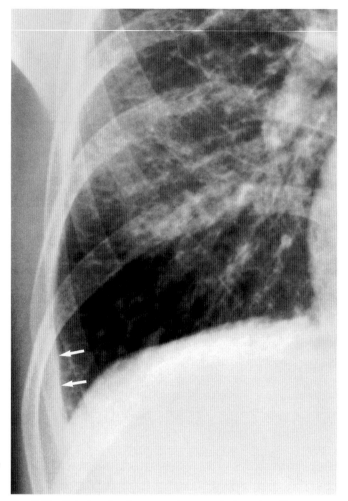

Fig. 7.68 Subpleural pulmonary edema producing a lamellar homogeneous density parallel to the chest wall (arrows).

Enlarged mediastinal lymph nodes and mediastinal fat opacification

An interesting CT observation in patients with clinical signs of heart failure is the increased prevalence of enlarged mediastinal lymph nodes (55%) (Fig. 7.69) and hazy opacification of the mediastinal fat (33%).[490] In patients with raised pulmonary capillary wedge pressure (mean 23 mmHg), enlargement of mediastinal lymph nodes on CT occurred in 82% of patients and fat opacification was identified in 59%. These phenomena are reversible on treatment of the heart failure.

Alveolar edema

Alveolar edema represents spill of fluid from the interstitium into the alveolar airspaces. The cardinal radiographic sign is therefore shadowing with the characteristics of airspace filling

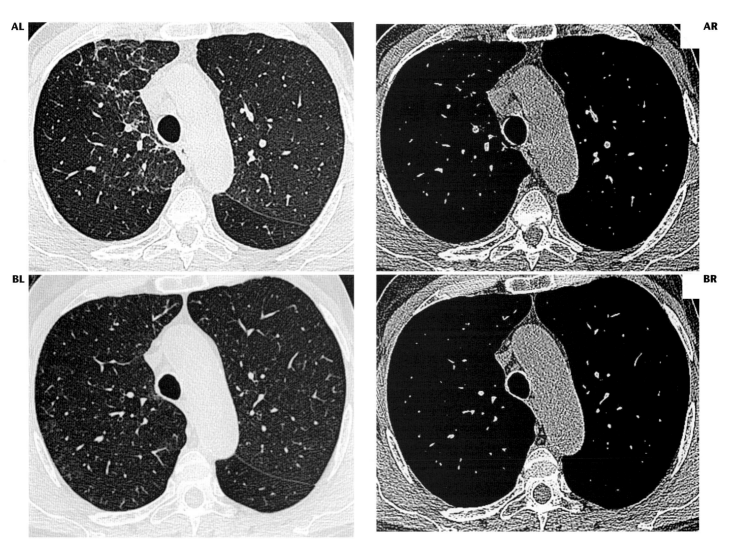

Fig. 7.69 A patient with chronic left ventricular failure. **A**, Left, the lung window settings show changes compatible with mild interstitial pulmonary edema. Right, on mediastinal settings there is a moderately enlarged pretracheal lymph node. **B**, 5 months later following treatment for heart failure the pulmonary changes have receded and the mediastinal lymph node has decreased in size (there were several other central mediastinal lymph nodes which showed a similar decrease in size).

(Fig. 7.70). The margins are poorly defined, although larger collections may show a well-defined boundary. The distribution is patchy and widespread, and the shadows tend to coalesce. Usually the shadowing is bilateral, occasionally unilateral, and rarely lobar. When unilateral, there is a striking and unexplained predisposition for the right lung[491] (Fig. 7.71). In patients with pulmonary edema associated with mitral regurgitation, there is a higher than expected occurrence (9%) of pulmonary edema localized to the right upper lobe.[492] Many more or less predictable factors such as the presence of accessory lobes,[493] pulmonary fibrosis,[494] Swyer–James syndrome[495] or the effects of mechanical ventilation[496] modify the usual distribution of pulmonary edema. Air bronchograms or air alveolograms may be evident, particularly when the edema is confluent. The acinar shadow of pulmonary edema has been emphasized; the appearance is due

to the contrast between fluid-filled acini surrounded by aerated acini. The resulting shadow is a 5–10 mm moderately ill-defined nodule. Sometimes the nodules are smaller and resemble a miliary pattern.

The terms "bat's wing" and "butterfly" shadowing have been coined to describe the appearance of perihilar shadowing that is predominantly in the central portions of the lobes and fades out peripherally, leaving an aerated outer "cortex" (Fig. 7.70). This pattern is best seen on frontal views; the distribution is less easy to define on the lateral views. The mechanism responsible for this characteristic distribution is uncertain. One suggestion is that lymphatic drainage is better in the outer portions of the lungs. Another is that the greater change in volume of the outer lung during each respiratory cycle in some way helps prevent edema. Despite the emphasis given to the bat's wing pattern, it

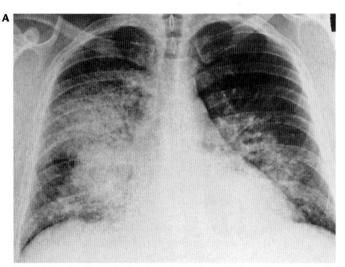

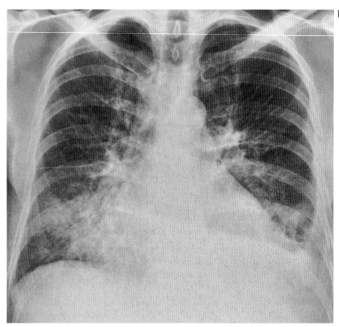

Fig. 7.70 Cardiogenic alveolar edema. **A**, Butterfly pattern. **B**, Bibasilar edema in a different patient showing septal lines and a left pleural effusion. Note also the bronchial wall thickening and thickening of the minor fissure.

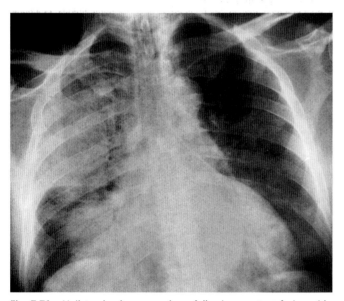

Fig. 7.71 Unilateral pulmonary edema following overtransfusion with intravenous fluids, showing an alveolar filling process almost entirely confined to the right lung. Note the air bronchograms.

should be realized that most patients show a more diffuse and random distribution, with some lobes more severely affected than others. Although it is true that the shadowing of pulmonary edema often spares the extreme upper and lower zones, the classic bat's wing pattern is seen in only a minority of patients.

Whatever the pattern, a striking feature of cardiogenic pulmonary edema is rapid change on radiographs taken over short intervals; rapid clearing is particularly suggestive of the diagnosis. An extension of this phenomenon is the change in distribution of pulmonary edema when patients alter their position for a few hours, for example, by lying on one side.[497]

ACUTE RESPIRATORY DISTRESS SYNDROME (ARDS)

Acute respiratory distress syndrome (the preferred term, supplanting "adult" respiratory distress syndrome[498]) is a common disorder with a high mortality.[499] It is due to increased pulmonary vascular permeability and develops in response to lung injury. A large variety of insults may precipitate the disorder, particularly bacterial sepsis, pneumonia, aspiration of gastric contents, circulatory shock, trauma, burns, and drug overdose. A list of causes, not exhaustive, is given in Box 7.13.

The clinical syndrome is characterized by acute, severe, progressive respiratory distress, widespread pulmonary opacification on chest radiography, significant hypoxemia despite a high inspired oxygen concentration, and decreased compliance of the lungs. In most cases these features are present within 24 hours of the inciting events, and in 90% of patients the syndrome is evident within 72 hours.[498] There is a trend towards distinguishing between inciting injuries that are direct (pulmonary ARDS) and those that are indirect (extrapulmonary ARDS).[500] While this has attractions in terms of understanding the pathogenesis of the disease and possibly for predicting the outcome, there is clearly an overlap in many situations (for example, a patient with an aspiration-related lung abscess and consequent septicemia). Patients with less severe disease – as judged by the arterial oxygenation to fraction of inspired oxygen – may be considered to have acute lung injury (ALI) rather than full-blown ARDS.[498]

The mechanism of damage to the pulmonary vascular endothelium that characterizes ARDS remains under intensive investigation, and although the neutrophil appears to be a crucial effector cell,[501] numerous other mediators are involved and no pathogenetic sequence completely accounts for the acute alveolar damage that characterizes ARDS.[502,503]

Whatever the mechanism, the end result is damage to the alveolar capillary membrane leading to increased permeability to protein and interstitial edema. As the process continues, proteinaceous fluid spills into the alveoli. Eventually alveolar disruption and hemorrhage occur; surfactant is reduced and the alveoli tend to collapse. Unlike cardiogenic pulmonary edema, the edema is prolonged because the oncotic forces for resorption of fluid are not present. On pathologic study[504] the alveoli and the perivascular and peribronchial spaces are congested and edematous.[503] Widespread pulmonary microthrombosis is a feature in approximately 75% of patients with posttraumatic ARDS.[505] The alveoli are inhomogeneously filled with proteinaceous hemorrhagic fluid, neutrophils, and debris. The morphologic features can be divided conveniently, but arbitrarily, into the following stages:

1. In stage 1 (first 24 hours) there is capillary congestion, endothelial cell swelling, and extensive microatelectasis. During this stage fluid leakage is minimal and limited to the interstitium. The respiratory distress is largely due to decreased pulmonary compliance.
2. In stage 2 (1–5 days) there is fluid leakage and fibrin deposition, and hyaline membranes develop. Alveolar consolidation by hemorrhagic fluid becomes extensive, and severe hypoxemia develops.
3. In stage 3 (after 5 days) there is alveolar cell and fibroblastic proliferation, collagen deposition, and microvascular destruction. The type II pneumonocytes become hyperplastic in an attempt to cover the denuded alveolar surfaces. In the later recovery phase the normal parenchymal architecture may be restored but in some individuals extensive interstitial fibrosis, in part induced by mechanical ventilation, develops.[506,507]

The radiographic changes may be delayed by 12 hours or more following the onset of clinical symptoms – an important difference from cardiogenic pulmonary edema where the chest radiograph is frequently abnormal before or coincident with the onset of symptoms. Some patients do not develop significant pulmonary shadowing even though they become profoundly hypoxemic.[508]

The major features of established ARDS on plain chest radiography (Figs 7.72 and 7.73) have been widely

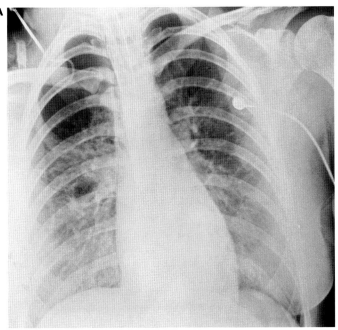
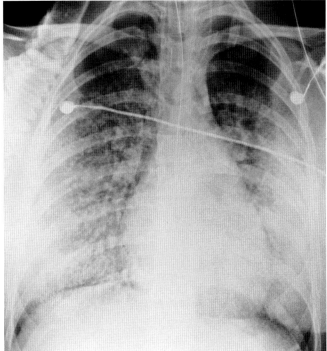

Fig. 7.72 Acute respiratory distress syndrome in a 19-year-old woman: **A**, early phase showing perihilar shadowing; **B**, 24 hours later there is widespread, fairly uniformly distributed airspace shadowing.

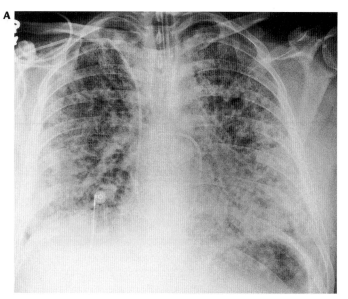

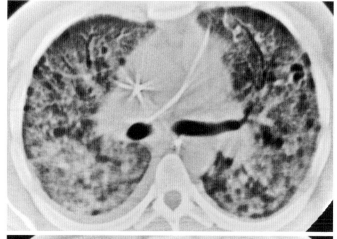

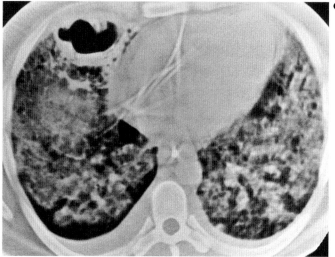

Fig. 7.73 Lung abscess complicating acute respiratory distress syndrome (ARDS). **A**, A plain chest radiograph shows features of ARDS, but a complicating pneumonia with abscess formation is difficult to recognize. **B**, CT shows widespread but patchy distribution of the airspace shadows. **C**, CT section at a lower level shows a large abscess in the middle lobe. Sputum cultures revealed mixed gram-positive and gram-negative bacteria.

reviewed[480,509–511] and comprise bilateral, widespread, patchy, ill-defined lung opacification, usually without cardiomegaly, upper zone blood diversion, or pleural effusion. The densities progress in severity to produce confluent airspace opacification, the distribution of which is variable, but usually all lung zones are involved both centrally and peripherally. Air bronchograms may be a prominent feature. Signs of interstitial edema, namely hilar haze and lack of clarity of lung vessels, are usually present, particularly early on in the evolution of the disease. Occasionally the shadowing appears exclusively interstitial, but septal lines are very rare.[480] Pistolesi and co-workers[480] have pointed out that right ventricular dilatation and enlargement of the main pulmonary artery are common. The basic radiographic abnormality of diffuse pulmonary opacification usually stabilizes after a few days and the development of any further, more focal, parenchymal density raises the possibility of, for example, pulmonary infarction or nosocomial infection.[512] An unusual asymmetric distribution of ARDS has recently been reported in some patients undergoing lobectomy[513]: the remaining lung on the operated side seems to be protected and does not develop ARDS of the severity seen in the contralateral lung (Fig. 7.74).

Patients with abnormal radiographs are severely hypoxic and require assisted ventilation. There is usually reasonable correlation between the radiographic severity of the pulmonary edema and the arterial Po_2. Furthermore, the extent of lung involvement as judged by standardized reading of chest radiographs has been shown to correlate well with densitometric measurements on CT.[514] Nevertheless there is, not surprisingly, some observer variation inherent in applying radiographic criteria suggested by the American-European Consensus Conference (AECC).[498,515] The clinical uses of chest radiography in patients with ARDS include:

- Corroboration of the diagnosis of ARDS (part of the AECC criteria)
- Monitoring the progress of pulmonary opacification
- Confirmation of clinically suspected pulmonary complication (e.g. pneumothorax)
- Demonstration of complication (e.g. misplaced device).

Despite the widespread practice of obtaining daily chest radiographs on patients with established ARDS,[516,517] no compelling evidence about the cost-effectiveness of this habit exists.

CT studies of the lungs of patients with ARDS, notably by Gattinoni and co-workers, have resulted in several important new insights into the evolution, distribution, and pathophysiology of the disease.[518,519] The cross-sectional images of computed tomography have shown that the distribution of disease in ARDS is not as homogeneous as chest radiography suggests, particularly in patients scanned in the early phases of the disease.[520–523] The distribution of densely opacified lung tends to be gravity dependent and is thought to be due to compression by the generalized increase in weight of the overlying lung; this

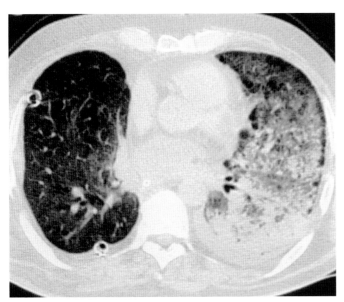

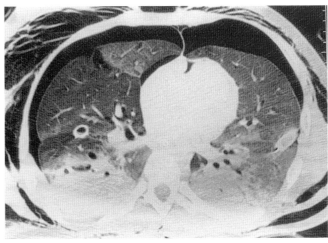

Fig. 7.75 Typical distribution of parenchymal changes in ARDS. There is dense opacification in the dependent parts of the lungs with more generalized ground-glass opacification of the nondependent lung, and subcutaneous emphysema and bilateral pneumothoraces secondary to mechanical ventilation. There are bilateral chest tubes within the oblique fissures.

Fig. 7.74 Asymmetric distribution of ARDS in a patient who had undergone a right lobectomy (hence the chest drainage tubes). The appearances of the left lung are typical of ARDS with an exaggerated nondependent to dependent density gradient and dense opacification posteriorly. The mechanism by which the lung of the operated side is protected is unknown. (With permission from Padley SP, Jordan SJ, Goldstraw P, et al. Asymmetric ARDS following pulmonary resection: CT findings initial observations. Radiology 2002;223:468–473.)

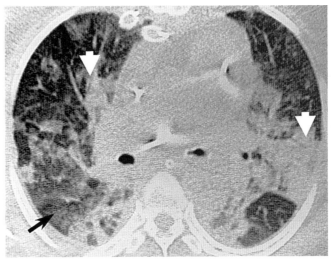

Fig. 7.76 A patient fulfilling the clinical criteria for ARDS, the consequence of a bacterial pneumonia. The pattern of disease is not the relatively uniform distribution seen in "extrapulmonary" ARDS. In this case, there are patchy areas of dense opacification in the nondependent lung (arrowheads) as well as the expected areas of ground-glass opacification (arrow). (With permission from Desai SR, Wells AU, Suntharalingam G, et al. Acute respiratory distress syndrome caused by pulmonary and extrapulmonary injury: a comparative CT study. Radiology 2001;218:689–693.)

phenomenon is exaggerated in ARDS.[524] Thus, in the supine patient, the greatest volume of dense parenchymal opacification is usually seen in the posterobasal segments of the lower lobes (Fig. 7.75). There is also a craniocaudal gradient with increasing density from lung apices to bases.[525] The rapid redistribution of apparently densely consolidated lung on repositioning supine patients with ARDS to a prone position has been well documented[524,526,527–530] and favors the hypothesis that atelectasis is the dominant process. More recently, it has been suggested that the lung mechanics and distribution of consolidation may be different depending on whether the ARDS is caused by pulmonary or extrapulmonary disease.[500] On CT, patients with an extrapulmonary, or indirect, cause for their ARDS (for example, acute pancreatitis) tend to have more diffuse parenchymal abnormalities, that is the "classic" ARDS appearance of an enhanced gravity dependent density gradient with symmetrical dense opacification in the posterobasal segments. By contrast, with a direct pulmonary insult (for example, a severe bacterial pneumonia) multifocal areas of consolidation, not confined to the dependent lung, are an expected feature[500,531,532] (Fig. 7.76). Nevertheless, given the regional and temporal inhomogeneity of the disease (and the possibility of coexisting processes, for example aspiration pneumonia on a background of extrapulmonary ARDS), it is not surprising that CT appearances alone cannot reliably distinguish between pulmonary and extrapulmonary causes of ARDS.[531] However, there appear to be trends that suggest differences in the outcome of patients with these different CT patterns of ARDS.[532]

Away from areas of dense opacification, most of the remaining lung is of increased attenuation producing ground-glass opacification (Figs 7.75 to 7.77). The ground-glass opacification of the lung parenchyma reflects a decrease in the overall air content: this may be the result of an outpouring of cells or exudate into the airspaces (short of causing frank pulmonary consolidation), interstitial thickening, or merely underinflation of the lung. Rarely, thickened interlobular septa may be conspicuous and produce a crazy-paving pattern.[533] Little, if any, of the lung parenchyma is of entirely normal lung density; paradoxically, some of the nondependent lung may be of abnormally low attenuation if mechanical ventilation has

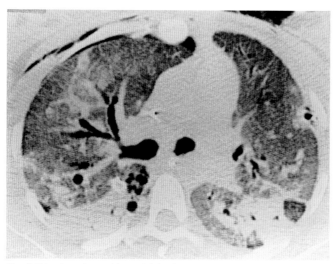

Fig. 7.77 A patient with established ARDS at 5 weeks following intubation. Note the abnormal dilatation of the bronchi within the right upper lobe. Some of the small cystic airspaces represent cavitating bacterial abscesses.

caused alveolar distension and disruption. The segmental and subsegmental bronchi may be dilated within areas of ground-glass opacification[534] and this appears to be a fixed phenomenon (Fig. 7.77). Whether this airway dilatation represents traction bronchiectasis, and thus a surrogate marker for the development of interstitial fibrosis, is uncertain. The CT features of established ARDS are listed in Box 7.14.

Box 7.14 CT findings in ARDS

Early established phase
Generalized increased opacification (ground-glass opacification and consolidation)
Exaggerated gravity dependent density gradient
• Dense opacification (atelectasis) in the posterobasal segments
Prominent air bronchogram in consolidated lung
• Interlobular septal thickening (sparse)
• Cysts and subpleural blebs

Chronic/recovery phase
Reticular pattern with parenchymal distortion
• Anterior distribution in all zones
• Residual ground-glass opacification (?fine fibrosis)

Deciding which of the many pathologic processes is responsible for the pattern of ground-glass opacification is not easy and, in the case of acute lung injury, there are many variables at play (for example, the method of ventilation, fluid-balance status, and phase of the disease). For this reason, although the overall lung weight can be precisely measured from analysis of CT density of the lung parenchyma (with an error of about 1%),[535] interpretation of regional density measurements in isolation must be guarded. Nevertheless, using estimates of the lung weight and frequency distribution of CT measures of lung density, fractions of normally aerated, poorly aerated, and unaerated lung can be calculated.[519,535,536] Comparing these data with functional measurements of static lung compliance, shunt fraction, and arterial oxygen tension can produce informative correlations between structure and function of the injured lung. Such data from CT indicate that static lung compliance correlates well with the amount of normally aerated lung, but not with the proportion of poorly or unaerated lung and is thus a useful indicator of the fraction of residual healthy lung in ARDS. Both arterial oxygen tension and shunt fraction are inversely correlated to the fraction of unaerated lung tissue quantified by CT. Increasing the level of positive end expiratory pressure (PEEP) from 5 to 15 cm of water increases the fraction of normally aerated lung "as quantified by CT" showing that recruitment of previously collapsed alveoli occurs with this maneuver. Accompanying this phenomenon is a decrease in shunt fraction indicating that improved arterial oxygenation is due to recruitment of otherwise nonventilated, but still perfused, alveolar units. In the analyses of morphologic changes in relation to different methods of ventilation, Gattinoni et al have shown with CT densitometry that the increased hydrostatic pressure superimposed on an area of lung is responsible for its atelectasis and this may be prevented when the PEEP is equal to or greater than this pressure.[537,538] Predictably, if PEEP is able to inflate the most dependent atelectatic parts of the lung, the nondependent, relatively normal lung becomes markedly overdistended. Puybasset et al have shown that patients with more diffuse parenchymal opacification show greater alveolar recruitment with PEEP, compared to those with patchy "lobar" opacification (and in these latter patients there was associated overdistension of previously normally aerated lung).[539] A potential role for CT densitometry is the precise titration of pressure and volume variables to achieve optimal non-injurious ventilation.[540] After the first week or two, blebs and bullae, mostly subpleural, develop usually, but not exclusively, in the nondependent lung[541]; these are presumed to be the result of prolonged ventilation.[519]

The distinction between cardiogenic and noncardiogenic pulmonary edema on radiographic grounds alone, can, particularly in the context of the critically ill patient, be difficult, but certain features may point in one direction or another.[480,542] In cardiogenic edema the radiographic shadowing caused by pulmonary edema is present coincident with the onset of symptoms, shows a central predominance, and may be associated with peribronchial cuffing and septal lines. Air bronchograms are relatively rare in cardiogenic edema, occurring one-third as frequently as in ARDS. The extent and density of the radiographic shadowing changes rapidly on serial films by contrast to the "stuck" generalized opacification of ARDS. Pleural effusions are common. It has been suggested that even in ventilated supine patients the ancillary signs of increased cardiothoracic ratio (>0.52) and widened vascular pedicle (>63 mm) are more indicative of hydrostatic cardiogenic edema than increased permeability edema.[542] ARDS is rarely associated with septal lines, and peribronchial cuffing is less common than with cardiogenic pulmonary edema. The central and peripheral pulmonary vascular pattern is normal in ARDS, though the main pulmonary artery may appear large. Pleural effusions are small and are only occasionally seen on plain chest radiography.[478]

Complications of acute respiratory distress syndrome

ARDS results in high mortality, but survival rates have improved over the years.[543,544] As might be expected, patients with ARDS are subject to many complications. Septicemia is common and in many instances results from a pneumonia that complicates the ARDS. Multiple organ failure is a major cause of death. It is not clear whether organs such as the kidney, liver, and central nervous system are damaged by the same process that initiates the ARDS or whether multiple organ failure results from complications that follow the pulmonary injury, but it would appear that, with modern critical care facilities, death from respiratory failure is less common than death from multiple organ failure.

Diagnosing infective pneumonia from the chest radiograph in the presence of extensive pulmonary shadowing is clearly a difficult task[512,545,546] (Fig. 7.73). Increasing consolidation in one area of the lung in a patient with clinical features that suggest pneumonia is an important, but not wholly reliable, radiographic finding. The distinction from edema and atelectasis is often impossible. Cavitation is fairly specific to pneumonia, but even here there is still the difficulty of distinguishing abscess formation from a pneumatocele or a cavitating sterile infarct. CT can be helpful in this regard[547] (Fig. 7.73). However, in one study no single CT feature was significantly more frequent in ARDS patients who had developed pneumonia. Nevertheless, observers were reasonably successful at identifying patients without pneumonia.[548] The main indications for CT, which should be reserved as a problem-solving tool in patients with ARDS, are shown in Box 7.15.

Box 7.15 Indications for CT in patients with ARDS

To detect complications (e.g. radiographically cryptic pneumothorax or abscess) in patients who are deteriorating

For the quantification of the extent of lung involvement in patients with equivocal radiographic and/or physiologic signs

As an aid to determining the cause (i.e. pulmonary or extrapulmonary) of ARDS

For the demonstration of significant areas of dependent atelectasis – patients in whom PEEP and/or prone nursing may be beneficial

For the follow-up of survivors to identify the morphologic consequences of ARDS (e.g. barotrauma)

During the acute phase many patients suffer barotrauma caused by positive-pressure ventilation with relatively non-compliant lungs.[506] Pneumothorax and pneumomediastinum are common, and in severe cases air dissects from the mediastinum into the neck and chest wall and even into the retroperitoneum or peritoneal cavity (Fig. 7.78). Interstitial emphysema is common, and pneumatoceles may develop within the lungs (Fig. 7.79).

The long-term outlook for survivors of ARDS is poorly documented. Alberts, Priest, and Moser,[549] in their review of the literature, found descriptions of follow-up chest radiographs in only 81 patients. In the great majority the chest radiograph returned to normal, a few showed some degree of hyperinflation, and 11% showed residual interstitial shadowing. The true rate of conversion of ARDS to established interstitial fibrosis is unknown. Functional impairment is frequent in ARDS survivors but is mild in most.[550] Follow-up study with HRCT has provided some insights into the nature of the residual morphologic damage in

survivors of ARDS.[507,534,551,552] In long-term ARDS survivors, the most frequent abnormality is a reticular pattern which, although limited in extent, has a strikingly anterior distribution (Fig. 7.80). It seems likely that this distribution reflects the fact that the nondependent part of the lung bears the brunt of barotrauma caused by mechanical ventilation, whereas the nonaerated dependent lung is protected.[507,552]

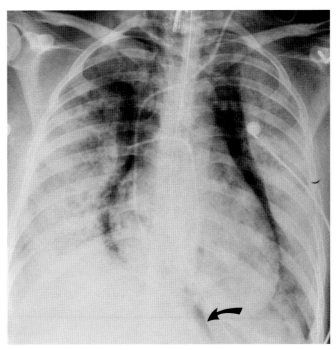

Fig. 7.78   Pneumomediastinum in a patient with ARDS receiving positive-pressure ventilation. Air has tracked into the neck and retroperitoneum (arrow).

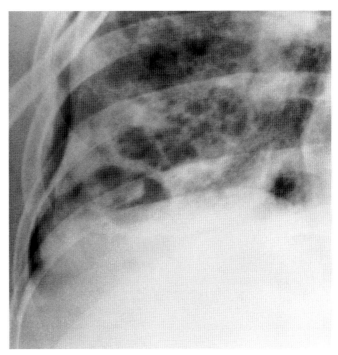

Fig. 7.79   Pneumatoceles that have developed in a patient with ARDS. (There is also a right pneumothorax and a chest drainage tube.)

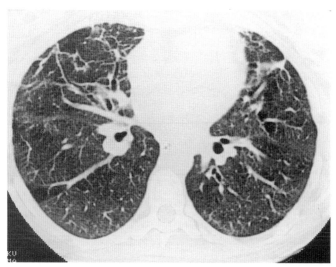

Fig. 7.80 A long-term survivor of ARDS. Note the striking anterior (nondependent) distribution of the coarse reticular pattern. These changes are thought to represent damage caused by ventilatory barotrauma to the aerated lung.

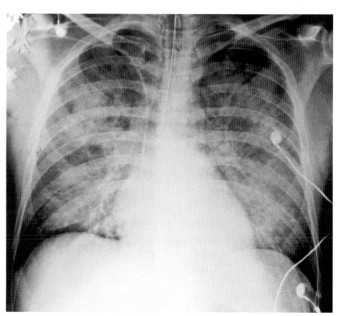

Fig. 7.81 Pulmonary edema caused by increased intracranial pressure following a subarachnoid hemorrhage caused by a ruptured aneurysm.

PULMONARY EDEMA FROM NEUROGENIC CAUSES, HIGH ALTITUDE, HANTAVIRUS INFECTION, AND ACUTE AIRWAY OBSTRUCTION

These four forms of pulmonary edema are considered separately because the edema in these conditions shows certain differences from the other varieties of noncardiogenic pulmonary edema.

Neurogenic pulmonary edema

A number of intracranial conditions, including head trauma, seizures, intracranial hemorrhage, tumors,[553] and less obvious conditions such as enterovirus encephalitis,[554] can be associated with acute pulmonary edema, even in patients who have no detectable heart or lung disease. The mechanism of the edema is debated.[555,556] Because the edema can occur within a minute, it has been suggested that a sudden burst of neural activity stimulates the sympathetic nervous system, increasing the pulmonary blood volume and raising the pulmonary venous pressure.[556] The edema becomes proteinaceous, suggesting that endothelial damage also plays a part, but the cause of this damage is obscure.

The radiographic picture[557] is indistinguishable from that of cardiogenic pulmonary edema except that the heart is not enlarged (Fig. 7.81). Although the edema may appear quickly, it may take up to 24 hours to be radiologically apparent. Unlike the usual forms of noncardiogenic pulmonary edema, the lungs usually clear within 24–48 hours.[555]

High-altitude pulmonary edema

High-altitude pulmonary edema (mountain sickness) is seen predominantly in children or young adults who ascend rapidly to heights of 2700–3500 m or greater. The entity is seen more frequently in individuals who undertake heavy physical exercise shortly after arrival at altitude, and there seems to be an individual susceptibility,[558] young persons being at greater risk.[559] Pulmonary edema may occur at altitudes as low as 1400 m, well within the range of many ski slopes – a salutary thought for cautious radiologists on vacation.[560] Symptoms of pulmonary edema develop 3–48 hours after achieving high altitude, and the majority of patients experience symptoms within 24 hours.[561] The most frequent early symptoms are shortness of breath, dry cough, and restlessness. The edema is extremely responsive to treatment with oxygen and a return to lower altitudes.[561]

The mechanism remains unclear. Lockhart and Saiag[558] divided the potential causes into the consequences of high pulmonary arterial pressure secondary to hypoxia and the effect of increased capillary permeability. Pulmonary capillary wedge pressures are near normal,[562] although transient elevations at the time of edema cannot be excluded. The presence of hyaline membranes and fibrin-like material in the alveoli at autopsy suggests a protein-rich edema fluid.[561,563] However, another study did not confirm increased capillary permeability in subjects exposed to high altitudes.[564]

The chest radiographic appearances are those of acute alveolar edema.[565] High-altitude pulmonary edema tends to be more severe in the lung bases, particularly on the right, but the pattern of distribution is usually unpredictable; recurrent episodes generally show a different distribution.[566] The heart remains normal in size, but the main pulmonary artery becomes prominent, decreasing in size with recovery.[561]

Hantavirus cardiopulmonary syndrome

An unusual cause of increased permeability pulmonary edema is Hantavirus, a zoonotic infection that occurs in rural North and South America. The recently described Hantavirus cardiopulmonary syndrome is characterized by cardiogenic shock with severe damage to the pulmonary capillary endothelium and is fatal in more than 40% of cases.[567] Because of systemic capillary leakage, possibly mediated by gamma interferon and tumor necrosis factor,[568] patients with Hantavirus cardio-pulmonary syndrome are volume depleted and so have a low capillary wedge pressure, even when cardiac dysfunction develops. Diffuse alveolar damage and hyaline membrane formation, the defining pathologic features of the archetypal increased permeability condition, ARDS, are absent in Hantavirus pulmonary syndrome. Not all patients progress to such fulminant pulmonary disease: in one series (from Canada) 7 of 20 patients experienced a mild form of the disease with little radiographic abnormality.[569] Radiographic appearances mirror this difference: features of interstitial, rather than airspace, pulmonary edema predominate because of the endothelium-centered damage[570] (Fig. 7.82). In a study that sought to identify radiographic differences between Hantavirus cardio-pulmonary syndrome and ARDS, experienced observers were moderately successful in distinguishing between the two conditions.[571] The radiographic sequence of interstitial pulmonary edema that rapidly progresses to predominantly perihilar or basal airspace pulmonary edema is typical of Hantavirus cardio-pulmonary syndrome.[570,571] The diagnosis is difficult to secure even with a high level of suspicion, but a distinctive combination of hematologic features on peripheral blood smear may help to make the diagnosis.[572]

Pulmonary edema associated with upper airway obstruction

Pulmonary edema can on rare occasion be associated with acute upper airway obstruction caused by such conditions as

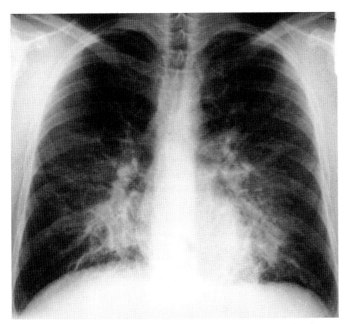

Fig. 7.82 A 21-year-old male oil-field worker who presented with a 5 day history of dyspnea and flulike symptoms. Hantavirus infection was confirmed serologically. The chest radiograph at presentation shows the features of interstitial pulmonary edema and some perihilar consolidation. (With permission from Boroja M, Barrie JR, Raymond GS. Radiographic findings in 20 patients with Hantavirus pulmonary syndrome correlated with clinical outcome. AJR Am J Roentgenol 2002;178:159–163. Reprinted with permission.)

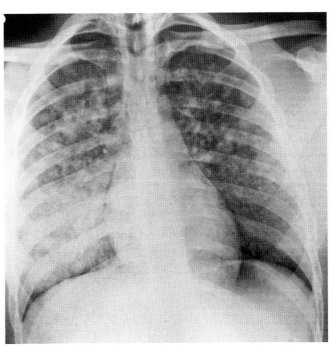

Fig. 7.83 Pulmonary edema caused by acute severe laryngospasm following general anesthesia.

laryngospasm[573] (Fig. 7.83), croup,[574] epiglottitis,[574] sleep apnea,[575] adenotonsillectomy,[576] or strangulation.[575] The mechanism is not clear. The possibilities include hypoxia or sympathomimetic overactivity, and these processes may act in concert.[574] The extremely negative intrathoracic pressures in a patient struggling to overcome upper airway obstruction may lead to transudation of fluid on a mechanical basis, whereas severe hypoxemia may damage the small intrapulmonary vessels directly or may act by means of extreme vasoconstriction, elevation of pulmonary pressure, and excess sympathomimetic activity.

Pulmonary edema may, conversely, occur after the relief of upper airway obstruction[577]; this has been reported in the context of general anesthesia when patients with laryngospasm-induced negative-pressure pulmonary edema are extubated[578,579] and in patients with obstructive sleep apnea treated by tracheotomy.[580]

REEXPANSION PULMONARY EDEMA

Following drainage of a pneumothorax or large pleural effusion the reexpanded lung may become acutely edematous.[581,582] The phenomenon may also occur as a complication of thoracoscopic surgery.[583,584] The mechanism is obscure, some authors suggesting that it is related to surfactant depletion[585] and others that it results from hypoxic capillary damage, leading to increased capillary permeability or, more recently, a marked increase in cardiac output immediately prior to the development of pulmonary edema.[586] The fact that reexpansion pulmonary edema is concentrated mainly in the reinflated lower lobes, following pleural effusion aspiration, has led to the suggestion that hypoxic damage, rather than mechanical stress, is the dominant mechanism.[587] Against this is the fact that "contralateral reexpansion edema" has been reported.[588] The edema usually develops within 2 hours of reexpansion and can progress for 1

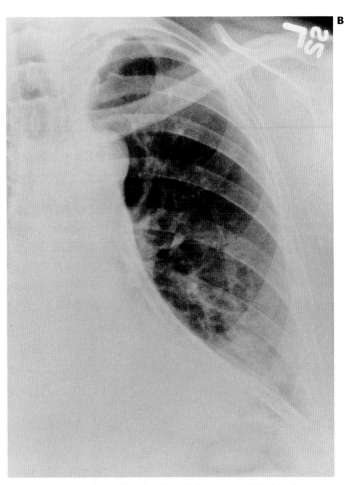

Fig. 7.84 Reexpansion pulmonary edema: **A**, a chest radiograph showing acute pulmonary edema that developed after a large left pleural effusion was drained; **B**, 25 hours later, the pulmonary edema has cleared.

or 2 days, resolving within 5–7 days. Reexpansion edema generally causes little morbidity, but patients can become hypotensive and hypoxic,[589,590] and at least one death has been recorded.[591] It is generally held that complete pneumothoraces with gross lung collapse, chronicity of the pneumothorax, and high negative aspiration pressures are predisposing factors. Most pneumothoraces have been complete and present for at least 3 days but exceptions of shorter duration have been reported.[592] In many patients expansion has been rapid because negative aspiration was used[593] but this has by no means been universal.[594,595] The chest radiograph shows ipsilateral airspace shadowing (Fig. 7.84). Rarely, recurrent edema may accompany recurrent pneumothoraces.[596]

It is worth noting that rapid reperfusion of a lung, for example after thrombolysis of a massive pulmonary embolus[23] or following thromboendarterectomy,[597] may also cause acute pulmonary edema.[23] The occurrence of pulmonary edema following talc pleurodesis has been reported, and it seems unlikely that the cause is invariably pulmonary reexpansion in these cases.[598,599]

AMNIOTIC FLUID EMBOLISM

Under normal circumstances no amniotic fluid enters the maternal circulation during pregnancy or labor. Amniotic fluid contains fetal cellular debris and mucin, and it is the squames from the fetal skin and the mucin from fetal meconium that appear to be responsible for the syndrome of amniotic fluid embolism[600] although the pathogenesis is not fully understood and its management difficult.[601] On reaching the lungs these materials incite hemodynamic shock with dyspnea, frothy blood-tinged sputum, and cyanosis.[602] Right-sided heart catheterization characteristically shows elevated central venous pressure, elevated pulmonary arterial pressure, and elevated capillary wedge pressure, and it may be possible to identify amniotic fluid debris in blood samples taken through the right heart catheter.[563]

The condition is rare but frequently fatal (in one review of the literature the fatality rate was found to be 86%[563] but in a more recent report it was 26%[603]). There is a high correlation with intrauterine death and fetal distress, suggesting that it is the amniotic fluid contents – particularly mucin – that incite the harm. At autopsy the lungs are edematous with widespread atelectasis. It is not possible on gross examination to recognize that amniotic fluid embolism has occurred, but histologic examination with special stains reveals fetal squames or mucin.[600]

The radiographic appearances are those of pulmonary edema, which is indistinguishable from the two other conditions that need to be considered in women during labor, acute cardiogenic edema and massive gastric aspiration.

REFERENCES

1. Moser KM. Venous thromboembolism: state of the art. Am Rev Respir Dis 1990;141:235–249.

2. Bergqvist D. Incidence of pulmonary embolism: is it declining? Semin Vasc Surg 2000;13:167–170.

3. Oger E. Incidence of venous thromboembolism: a community-based study in Western France. EPI-GETBP Study Group. Groupe d'Etude de la Thrombose de Bretagne Occidentale. Thromb Haemost 2000;83:657–660.

4. Heit JA, Melton LJ III, Lohse CM, et al. Incidence of venous thromboembolism in hospitalized patients vs community residents. Mayo Clin Proc 2001;76: 1102–1110.

5. Stein PD, Huang H, Afzal A, et al. Incidence of acute pulmonary embolism in a general hospital: relation to age, sex, and race. Chest 1999;116:909–913.

6. Provenzale JM, Ortel TL. Anatomic distribution of venous thrombosis in patients with antiphospholipid antibody: imaging findings. AJR Am J Roentgenol 1995;165:365–368.

7. Gilkeson RC, Patz EFJ, Culhane D, et al. Thoracic imaging features of patients with antiphospholipid antibodies. J Comput Assist Tomogr 1998;22:241–244.

8. Liu HS, Kho BC, Chan JC, et al. Venous thromboembolism in the Chinese population – experience in a regional hospital in Hong Kong. Hong Kong Med J 2002;8:400–405.

9. Gherman RB, Goodwin TM, Leung B, et al. Incidence, clinical characteristics, and timing of objectively diagnosed venous thromboembolism during pregnancy. Obstet Gynecol 1999;94:730–734.

10. Black MD, French GJ, Rasuli P, et al. Upper extremity deep venous thrombosis. Underdiagnosed and potentially lethal. Chest 1993;103:1887–1890.

11. Moser KM. Pulmonary embolism: state of the art. Am Rev Respir Dis 1977;115: 829–852.

12. Wolfe WG, Sabiston DC. Pulmonary embolism. Philadelphia: WB Saunders, 1980.

13. Dalen JE, Haffajee CI, Alpert JS III, et al. Pulmonary embolism, pulmonary hemorrhage and pulmonary infarction. N Engl J Med 1977;296:1431–1435.

14. Im JG, Choi YW, Kim HD, et al. Thin-section CT findings of the lungs: experimentally induced bronchial and pulmonary artery obstruction in pigs. AJR Am J Roentgenol 1996;167:631–636.

15. Malik AB, Tracy SE. Bronchovascular adjustments after pulmonary embolism. J Appl Physiol 1980;49:476–481.

16. Weibel ER. Early stages in the development of collateral circulation to the lung in the rat. Circ Res 1960;8: 353–376.

17. Sherrier RH, Chiles C, Newman GE. Chronic multiple pulmonary emboli: regional response of the bronchial circulation. Invest Radiol 1989;24:437–441.

18. Remy J, Deschildre F, Artaud D, et al. Bronchial arteries in the pig before and after permanent pulmonary artery occlusion. Invest Radiol 1997; 32:218–224.

19. Tsao MS, Schraufnagel D, Wang NS. Pathogenesis of pulmonary infarction. Am J Med 1982;72:599–606.

20. Morris TA, Auger WR, Ysrael MZ, et al. Parenchymal scarring is associated with restrictive spirometric defects in patients with chronic thromboembolic pulmonary hypertension. Chest 1996;110:399–403.

21. Yuceoglu YZ, Rubler S, Eshwar KP, et al. Pulmonary edema associated with pulmonary embolism: a clinicopathological study. Angiology 1971;22:501–510.

22. Hyers TM, Fowler AA, Wicks AB. Focal pulmonary edema after massive pulmonary embolism. Am Rev Respir Dis 1981;123:232–233.

23. Ward BJ, Pearse DB. Reperfusion pulmonary edema after thrombolytic therapy of massive pulmonary embolism [published erratum appears in Am Rev Respir Dis 1989;139:572]. Am Rev Respir Dis 1988;138:1308–1311.

24. Dalen JE, Alpert JS. Natural history of pulmonary embolism. Prog Cardiovasc Dis 1975;17:257–270.

25. Fred HL, Axelrad MA, Lewis JM, et al. Rapid resolution of pulmonary thromboemboli in man. An angiographic study. JAMA 1966;196:1137–1139.

26. Mathur VS, Dalen JE, Evans H, et al. Pulmonary angiography one to seven days after experimental pulmonary embolism. Invest Radiol 1967;2:304–312.

27. Chait A, Summers D, Krasnow N, et al. Observation on the fate of large pulmonary emboli. AJR Am J Roentgenol 1967;100:364–373.

28. Tilkian AG, Schroeder JS, Robin ED. Chronic thromboembolic occlusion of main pulmonary artery or primary branches. Case report and review of the literature. Am J Med 1976;60:563–570.

29. Egermayer P, Peacock AJ. Is pulmonary embolism a common cause of chronic pulmonary hypertension? Limitations of the embolic hypothesis. Eur Respir J 2000;15:440–448.

30. Hampson NB, Culver BH. Clinical aspects of pulmonary embolism. Semin Ultrasound CT MR 1997;18:314–322.

31. Meignan M, Rosso J, Gauthier H, et al. Systematic lung scans reveal a high frequency of silent pulmonary embolism in patients with proximal deep venous thrombosis. Arch Intern Med 2000;160: 159–164.

32. Bell WR, Simon TL, DeMets DL. The clinical features of submassive and massive pulmonary emboli. Am J Med 1977;62:355–360.

33. Rosenow EC III, Osmundson PJ, Brown ML. Pulmonary embolism. Mayo Clin Proc 1981;56:161–178.

34. Bounameaux H, de Moerloose P, Perrier A, et al. D-dimer testing in suspected venous thromboembolism: an update. Q J Med 1997;90:437–442.

35. Egermayer P, Town GI, Turner JG, et al. Usefulness of D-dimer, blood gas, and respiratory rate measurements for excluding pulmonary embolism. Thorax 1998;53:830–834.

36. Brown MD, Rowe BH, Reeves MJ, et al. The accuracy of the enzyme-linked immunosorbent assay D-dimer test in the diagnosis of pulmonary embolism: a meta-analysis. Ann Emerg Med 2002;40:133–144.

37. Wells PS, Anderson DR, Rodger M, et al. Excluding pulmonary embolism at the bedside without diagnostic imaging: management of patients with suspected pulmonary embolism presenting to the emergency department by using a simple clinical model and d-dimer. Ann Intern Med 2001;135:98–107.

38. Kruip MJ, Slob MJ, Schijen JH, et al. Use of a clinical decision rule in combination with D-dimer concentration in diagnostic workup of patients with suspected pulmonary embolism: a prospective management study. Arch Intern Med 2002;162:1631–1635.

39. Burkill GJ, Bell JR, Chinn RJ, et al. The use of a D-dimer assay in patients undergoing CT pulmonary angiography for suspected pulmonary embolus. Clin Radiol 2002;57:41–46.

40. Mac Gillavry MR, Lijmer JG, Sanson BJ, et al. Diagnostic accuracy of triage tests to exclude pulmonary embolism. Thromb Haemost 2001;85:995–998.

41. De Monye W, Sanson BJ, Mac Gillavry MR, et al. Embolus location affects the sensitivity of a rapid quantitative D-dimer assay in the diagnosis of pulmonary embolism. Am J Respir Crit Care Med 2002;165:345–348.

42. Kline JA, Johns KL, Colucciello SA, et al. New diagnostic tests for pulmonary embolism. Ann Emerg Med 2000;35:168–180.

43. Kovacs MJ, MacKinnon KM, Anderson D, et al. A comparison of three rapid D-dimer methods for the diagnosis of venous thromboembolism. Br J Haematol 2001;115:140–144.

44. Reber G, Bounameaux H, Perrier A, et al. Performances of a new, automated latex assay for the exclusion of venous thromboembolism. Blood Coagul Fibrinolysis 2001;12:217–220.

45. Mant MJ, O'Brien BD, Thong KL, et al. Haemorrhagic complications of heparin therapy. Lancet 1977;1:1133–1135.

46. Porter J, Jick H. Drug-related deaths among medical inpatients. JAMA 1977;237:879–881.

47. Goldhaber SZ. Recent advances in the diagnosis and lytic therapy of pulmonary embolism. Chest 1991;99:173S–179S.

48. Chang CH. Radiological considerations in pulmonary embolism. Clin Radiol 1967;18:301–309.

49. Fleischner FG. Pulmonary embolism. Clin Radiol 1962;13:169–182.

50. Kerr IH, Simon G, Sutton GC. The value of the plain radiograph in acute massive pulmonary embolism. Br J Radiol 1971;44:751–757.

51. Moses DC, Silver TM, Bookstein JJ. The complementary roles of chest radiography, lung scanning, and selective pulmonary angiography in the diagnosis of pulmonary embolism. Circulation 1974;49:179–188.

52. Palla A, Donnamaria V, Petruzzelli S, et al. Enlargement of the right descending pulmonary artery in pulmonary embolism. AJR Am J Roentgenol 1983;141:513–517.

53. Talbot S, Worthington BS, Roebuck EJ. Radiographic signs of pulmonary embolism and pulmonary infarction. Thorax 1973;28:198–203.

54. Westermark N. On the roentgen diagnosis of lung embolism. Acta Radiol 1938;19:357–372.

55. Wiener SN, Edelstein J, Charms B. Observations on pulmonary embolism and the pulmonary angiogram. AJR Am J Roentgenol 1966;98:859–873.

56. Buckner CB, Walker CW, Purnell GL. Pulmonary embolism: chest radiographic abnormalities. J Thorac Imaging 1989;4:23–27.

57. Greenspan RH, Ravin CE, Polansky SM, et al. Accuracy of the chest radiograph in diagnosis of pulmonary embolism. Invest Radiol 1982;17:539–543.

58. Szucs MM Jr, Brooks HL, Grossman W, et al. Diagnostic sensitivity of laboratory findings in acute pulmonary embolism. Ann Intern Med 1971;74:161–166.

59. Wenger NK, Stein PD, Willis PW III. Massive acute pulmonary embolism. The deceivingly nonspecific manifestations. JAMA 1972;220:843–844.

60. Tourassi GD, Floyd CE, Coleman RE. Improved noninvasive diagnosis of acute pulmonary embolism with optimally selected clinical and chest radiographic findings. Acad Radiol 1996;3:1012–1018.

61. Forbes KP, Reid JH, Murchison JT. Do preliminary chest X-ray findings define the optimum role of pulmonary scintigraphy in suspected pulmonary embolism? Clin Radiol 2001;56:397–400.

62. Teplick JG, Haskin ME, Steinberg SB. Changes in the main pulmonary artery segment following pulmonary embolism. AJR Am J Roentgenol 1964;92:557–560.

63. Chang CH, Davis WC. A roentgen sign of pulmonary infarction. Clin Radiol 1965;16:141–147.

64. Fleischner FG, Hampton AO, Castleman B. Linear shadows in the lung. AJR Am J Roentgenol 1941;46:610–618.

65. Tudor J, Maurer BJ, Wray R, et al. Lung shadows after acute myocardial infarction. Clin Radiol 1973;24:365–369.

66. Westcott JL, Cole S. Plate atelectasis. Radiology 1985;155:1–9.

67. Vix VA. The usefulness of chest radiographs obtained after a demonstrated perfusion scan defect in the diagnosis of pulmonary emboli. Clin Nucl Med 1983;8:497–500.

68. Hampton AO, Castleman B. Correlations of post mortem chest teleroentgenograms with autopsy findings with special reference to pulmonary embolism and infarction. AJR Am J Roentgenol 1940;43:305–326.

69. Heitzman ER, Markarian B, Dailey ET. Pulmonary thromboembolic disease. A lobular concept. Radiology 1972; 103:529–537.

70. Jacoby CG, Mindell HJ. Lobar consolidation in pulmonary embolism. Radiology 1976;118:287–290.

71. Groskin SA. Heitzman's The lung: radiologic–pathologic correlations, 3rd edn. St Louis: Mosby, 1993.

72. Bachynski JE. Absence of the air bronchogram sign. A reliable finding in pulmonary embolism with infarction or hemorrhage. Radiology 1971;100: 547–552.

73. Figley MM, Gerdes AJ, Ricketts HJ. Radiographic aspects of pulmonary embolism. Semin Roentgenol 1967;2:389–405.

74. Simon G. Further observations on the long line shadow across a lower zone of the lung. Br J Radiol 1970;43:327–332.

75. McGoldrick PJ, Rudd TG, Figley MM, et al. What becomes of pulmonary infarcts? AJR Am J Roentgenol 1979;133: 1039–1045.

76. Woesner ME, Sanders I, White GW. The melting sign in resolving transient pulmonary infarction. AJR Am J Roentgenol 1971;111:782–790.

77. Grieco MH, Ryan SF. Aseptic cavitary pulmonary infarction. Am J Med 1968;45:811–816.

78. Scharf J, Nahir AM, Munk J, et al. Aseptic cavitation in pulmonary infarction. Chest 1971;59:456–458.

79. Wilson AG, Joseph AEA, Butland RJA. The radiology of aseptic cavitation in pulmonary infarction. Clin Radiol 1986;37:327–333.

80. Bynum LJ, Wilson JE. Radiographic features of pleural effusions in pulmonary embolism. Am Rev Respir Dis 1978;117:829–834.

81. Burkill GJ, Bell JR, Padley SP. Survey on the use of pulmonary scintigraphy, spiral CT and conventional pulmonary angiography for suspected pulmonary embolism in the British Isles. Clin Radiol 1999;54:807–810.

82. Hull RD, Pineo GF, Stein PD, et al. Cost-effectiveness of currently accepted strategies for pulmonary embolism diagnosis. Semin Thromb Hemost 2001;27:15–23.

83. Heck LL, Duley JW Jr. Statistical considerations in lung imaging with 99mTc albumin particles. Radiology 1974;113:675–679.

84. Hughes JMB, Glazier JB, Maloney JE, et al. Effects of lung volume on the distribution of pulmonary blood flow in man. Respir Physiol 1968;4:58–72.

85. Whyte MK, Peters AM, Hughes JM, et al. Quantification of right to left shunt at rest and during exercise in patients with pulmonary arteriovenous malformations. Thorax 1992;47:790–796.

86. Burch WM, Sullivan PJ, McLaren CJ. Technegas – a new ventilation agent for lung scanning. Nucl Med Commun 1986;7:865–871.

87. James JM, Lloyd JJ, Leahy BC, et al. 99Tcm-Technegas and krypton-81m ventilation scintigraphy: a comparison in known respiratory disease. Br J Radiol 1992;65:1075–1082.

88. Collart JP, Roelants V, Vanpee D, et al. Is a lung perfusion scan obtained by using single photon emission computed tomography able to improve the radionuclide diagnosis of pulmonary embolism? Nucl Med Commun 2002;23:1107–1113.

89. Wiener CM, McKenna WJ, Myers MJ, et al. Left lower lobe ventilation is reduced in patients with cardiomegaly in the supine but not the prone position. Am Rev Respir Dis 1990;141:150–155.

90. Lemb M, Oei TH, Sander U. Ventilation-perfusion lung SPECT in the diagnosis of pulmonary thromboembolism. Eur J Nucl Med 1989;14:422.

91. de Groot MR, Turkstra F, van Marwijk KM, et al. Value of chest X-ray combined with perfusion scan versus ventilation/perfusion scan in acute pulmonary embolism. Thromb Haemost 2000;83:412–415.

92. Value of the ventilation/perfusion scan in acute pulmonary embolism. Results of the prospective investigation of pulmonary embolism diagnosis (PIOPED). The PIOPED Investigators. JAMA 1990;263:2753–2759.

93. Sostman HD, Coleman RE, Delong DM, et al. Evaluation of revised criteria for ventilation-perfusion scintigraphy in patients with suspected pulmonary embolism. Radiology 1994;193:103–107.

94. Bajc M, Albrechtsson U, Olsson CG, et al. Comparison of ventilation/perfusion scintigraphy and helical CT for diagnosis of pulmonary embolism; strategy using clinical data and ancillary findings. Clin Physiol Funct Imaging 2002;22:392–397.

95. Cunningham DA, Lavender JP. Krypton 81m ventilation scanning in chronic obstructive airways disease. Br J Radiol 1981;54:110–116.

96. Carvalho P, Lavender JP. The incidence and etiology of the ventilation/perfusion reverse mismatch defect. Clin Nucl Med 1989;14:571–576.

97. Alexander MS, Peters AM, Cleland JP, et al. Impaired left lower lobe ventilation in patients with cardiomegaly. An isotope study of mechanisms. Chest 1992;101:1189–1193.

98. Lavender JP, Irving H, Armstrong JD. Krypton-81m ventilation scanning: acute respiratory disease. AJR Am J Roentgenol 1981;136:309–316.

99. Spies WG, Burstein SP, Dillehay GL, et al. Ventilation-perfusion scintigraphy in suspected pulmonary embolism: correlation with pulmonary angiography and refinement of criteria for interpretation. Radiology 1986;159:383–390.

100. Hull RD, Raskob GE, Coates G, et al. A new non-invasive management strategy for patients with suspected pulmonary embolism. Arch Intern Med 1989;149:2549–2555.

101. Braun SD, Newman GE, Ford K, et al. Ventilation-perfusion scanning and pulmonary angiography: correlation in clinical high-probability pulmonary embolism. AJR Am J Roentgenol 1984;143:977–980.

102. Robinson PJ. Lung scintigraphy – doubt and certainty in the diagnosis of pulmonary embolism. Clin Radiol 1989;40:557–560.

103. Gotthardt M, Schipper M, Franzius C, et al. Follow-up of perfusion defects in pulmonary perfusion scanning after pulmonary embolism: are we too careless? Nucl Med Commun 2002;23:447–452.

104. Bone RC. The low-probability lung scan. A potentially lethal reading. Arch Intern Med 1993;153:2621–2622.

105. Cunningham DA, Mitchell DM. Well ventilated bullae: a potential confusion on ventilation/perfusion scanning. Br J Radiol 1991;64:56–60.

106. Strickland NH, Hughes JM, Hart DA, et al. Cause of regional ventilation-perfusion mismatching in patients with idiopathic pulmonary fibrosis: a combined CT and scintigraphic study. AJR Am J Roentgenol 1993;161:719–725.

107. Stein PD, Athanasoulis C, Alavi A, et al. Complications and validity of pulmonary angiography in acute pulmonary embolism. Circulation 1992;85:462–468.

108. Cheely R, McCartney WH, Perry JR, et al. The role of non-invasive tests versus pulmonary angiography in the diagnosis of pulmonary embolism. Am J Med 1981;70:17–22.

109. Novelline RA, Baltarowich OH, Athanasoulis CA, et al. The clinical course of patients with suspected pulmonary embolism and a negative pulmonary arteriogram. Radiology 1978;126:561–567.

110. Bell WR, Simon TL. Current status of pulmonary thromboembolic disease: pathophysiology, diagnosis, prevention, and treatment. Am Heart J 1982;103:239–262.

111. Marsh JD, Glynn M, Torman HA. Pulmonary angiography. Application in a new spectrum of patients. Am J Med 1983;75:763–770.

112. Mills SR, Jackson DC, Older RA, et al. The incidence, etiologies and avoidance of complications of pulmonary angiography in a large series. Radiology 1980;136:295–299.

113. van Beek EJ, Reekers JA, Batchelor DA, et al. Feasibility, safety and clinical utility of angiography in patients with suspected pulmonary embolism. Eur Radiol 1996;6:415–419.

114. Zuckerman DA, Sterling KM, Oser RF. Safety of pulmonary angiography in the 1990s. J Vasc Interv Radiol 1996;7:199–205.

115. Goodman PC. Pulmonary angiography. Clin Chest Med 1984;5:465–477.

116. Stein PD, Gottschalk A, Saltzman HA, et al. Diagnosis of acute pulmonary embolism in the elderly. J Am Coll Cardiol 1991;18:1452–1457.

117. Dunnick NR, Newman GE, Perlmutt LM, et al. Pulmonary embolism. Curr Probl Diagn Radiol 1988;17:197–237.

118. Davey NC, Smith TP, Hanson MW, et al. Ventilation-perfusion lung scintigraphy as a guide for pulmonary angiography in the localization of pulmonary emboli. Radiology 1999;213:51–57.

119. Blinder RA, Coleman RE. Evaluation of pulmonary embolism. Radiol Clin North Am 1985;23:391–405.

120. Ferris EJ, Holder JC, Lim WN, et al. Angiography of pulmonary emboli: digital studies and balloon-occlusion cineangiography. AJR Am J Roentgenol 1984;142:369–373.

121. Hirji M, Gamsu G, Webb WR, et al. EKG-gated digital subtraction angiography in the detection of pulmonary emboli. Radiology 1984;152:19–22.

122. van Beek EJ, Bakker AJ, Reekers JA. Pulmonary embolism: interobserver agreement in the interpretation of conventional angiographic and DSA images in patients with nondiagnostic lung scan results. Radiology 1996;198:721–724.

123. Johnson MS, Stine SB, Shah H, et al. Possible pulmonary embolus: evaluation with digital subtraction versus cut-film angiography – prospective study in 80 patients. Radiology 1998;207:131–138.

124. Dalen JE, Brooks HL, Johnson LW, et al. Pulmonary angiography in acute pulmonary embolism: indications, techniques, and results in 367 patients. Am Heart J 1971;81:175–185.

125. Ferris EJ, Steinzler RM, Rowke JA, et al. Pulmonary angiography in pulmonary embolic disease. AJR Am J Roentgenol 1967;100:355–363.

126. Stein PD, O'Connor JF, Dalen JE, et al. The angiographic diagnosis of acute pulmonary embolism: evaluation of criteria. Am Heart J 1967;73:730–741.

127. Bookstein JJ, Silver TM. The angiographic differential diagnosis of acute pulmonary embolism. Radiology 1974;110:25–33.

128. Sagel SS, Greenspan RH. Nonuniform pulmonary arterial perfusion. Pulmonary embolism? Radiology 1971;99:541–548.

129. Dalen JE, Mathur VS, Evans H, et al. Pulmonary angiography in experimental pulmonary embolism. Am Heart J 1966;72:509–520.

130. Moser KM, Guisan M, Bartimmo EE, et al. In vivo and post mortem dissolution rates of pulmonary emboli and venous thrombi in the dog. Circulation 1973;48:170–178.

131. Sautter RD, Fletcher FW, Ousley JL, et al. Extremely rapid resolution of a pulmonary embolus. Report of a case. Dis Chest 1967;52:825–827.

132. Korn D, Core I, Blenke A, et al. Pulmonary arterial bands and webs: an unrecognized manifestation of organized pulmonary emboli. Am J Pathol 1962;40:129–151.

133. Peterson KL, Fred HL, Alexander JK. Pulmonary arterial webs. A new angiographic sign of previous thromboembolism. N Engl J Med 1967;277:33–35.

134. Cooper TJ, Hayward MW, Hartog M. Survey on the use of pulmonary scintigraphy and angiography for suspected pulmonary thromboembolism in the UK. Clin Radiol 1991;43:243–245.

135. Newman GE. Pulmonary angiography in pulmonary embolic disease. J Thorac Imag 1989;4:28–39.

136. Robin ED. Overdiagnosis and overtreatment of pulmonary embolism: the emperor may have no clothes. Ann Intern Med 1977;87:775–781.

137. Sostman HD, Ravin CE, Sullivan DC, et al. Use of pulmonary angiography for suspected pulmonary embolism: influence of scintigraphic diagnosis. AJR Am J Roentgenol 1982;139:673–677.

138. Schluger N, Henschke C, King T, et al. Diagnosis of pulmonary embolism at a large teaching hospital. J Thorac Imag 1994;9:180–184.

139. Henschke CI, Yankelevitz DF, Sicherman N. Evaluation of algorithms for the diagnosis of pulmonary embolism. Semin Ultrasound CT MR 1997;18: 376–382.

140. Diederich S. Radiation dose in helical CT for detection of pulmonary embolism. Eur Radiol 2003;13:1491–1493.

141. Lippmann M, Fein A. Pulmonary embolism in the patient with chronic obstructive pulmonary disease: a diagnostic dilemma. Chest 1981; 79:39–42.

142. Harvey RT, Gefter WB, Hrung JM, et al. Accuracy of CT angiography versus pulmonary angiography in the diagnosis of acute pulmonary embolism: evaluation of the literature with summary ROC curve analysis. Acad Radiol 2000;7:786–797.

143. van Beek EJ, Brouwerst EM, Song B, et al. Clinical validity of a normal pulmonary angiogram in patients with suspected pulmonary embolism – a critical review. Clin Radiol 2001;56: 838–842.

144. Stein PD. Opinion response to acute pulmonary embolism: the role of computed tomographic imaging. J Thorac Imaging 1997;12:86–89.

145. Stein PD, Henry JW, Gottschalk A. Reassessment of pulmonary angiography for the diagnosis of pulmonary embolism: relation of interpreter agreement to the order of the involved pulmonary arterial branch. Radiology 1999;210:689–691.

146. The PIOPED investigators. Value of ventilation/perfusion scan in acute pulmonary embolism. JAMA 1990;263:2753–2759.

147. Hagen PJ, van Strijen MJ, Kieft GJ, et al. Availability of diagnostic facilities in the Netherlands for patients with suspected pulmonary embolism. ANTELOPE Study Group. Advances in New Technologies Evaluating the Localisation of Pulmonary Embolism. Neth J Med 2000;57:142–149.

148. Schibany N, Fleischmann D, Thallinger C, et al. Equipment availability and diagnostic strategies for suspected pulmonary embolism in Austria. Eur Radiol 2001;11:2287–2294.

149. Balakrishnan J, Meziane MA, Siegelman SS, et al. Pulmonary infarction: CT appearance with pathologic correlation. J Comput Assist Tomogr 1989;13:941–945.

150. Breatnach E, Stanley RJ. CT diagnosis of segmental pulmonary artery embolism. J Comput Assist Tomogr 1984;8:762–764.

151. Chintapalli K, Thorsen MK, Olson DL, et al. Computed tomography of pulmonary thromboembolism and infarction. J Comput Assist Tomogr 1988;12:553–559.

152. Godwin JD, Webb WR, Gamsu G, et al. Computed tomography of pulmonary embolism. AJR Am J Roentgenol 1980;135:691–695.

153. Kalebo P, Wallin J. Computed tomography in massive pulmonary embolism. Acta Radiol 1989;30:105–107.

154. Kereiakes DJ, Herfkens RJ, Brundage BH, et al. Computerized tomography in chronic thromboembolic pulmonary hypertension. Am Heart J 1983;106: 1432–1436.

155. Verschakelen JA, Vanwijck E, Bogaert J, et al. Detection of unsuspected central pulmonary embolism with conventional contrast-enhanced CT. Radiology 1993;188:847–850.

156. Kanne JP, Gotway MB, Thoongsuwan N, et al. Six cases of acute central pulmonary embolism revealed on unenhanced multidetector CT of the chest. AJR Am J Roentgenol 2003;180:1661–1664.

157. Kalender WA, Seissler W, Klotz E, et al. Spiral volumetric CT with single-breath-hold technique, continuous transport, and continuous scanner rotation. Radiology 1990;176:181–183.

158. van Rossum AB, Pattynama PM, Ton ER, et al. Pulmonary embolism: validation of spiral CT angiography in 149 patients. Radiology 1996;201:467–470.

159. Cross JJ, Kemp PM, Walsh CG, et al. A randomized trial of spiral CT and ventilation perfusion scintigraphy for the diagnosis of pulmonary embolism. Clin Radiol 1998;53:177–182.

160. Ferretti GR, Bosson JL, Buffaz PD, et al. Acute pulmonary embolism: role of helical CT in 164 patients with intermediate probability at ventilation-perfusion scintigraphy and normal results at duplex US of the legs. Radiology 1997;205:453–458.

161. Remy-Jardin M, Remy J, Wattinne L, et al. Central pulmonary thromboembolism: diagnosis with spiral volumetric CT with the single-breath-hold technique – comparison with pulmonary angiography. Radiology 1992;185:381–387.

162. Goodman LR, Curtin JJ, Mewissen MW, et al. Detection of pulmonary embolism in patients with unresolved clinical and scintigraphic diagnosis: helical CT versus angiography. AJR Am J Roentgenol 1995;164:1369–1374.

163. Teigen CL, Maus TP, Sheedy PF, et al. Pulmonary embolism: diagnosis with electron-beam CT. Radiology 1993; 188:839–845.

164. Teigen CL, Maus TP, Sheedy PF, et al. Pulmonary embolism: diagnosis with contrast-enhanced electron-beam CT and comparison with pulmonary angiography. Radiology 1995;194:313–319.

165. Blum AG, Delfan F, Grignon B, et al. Spiral-computed tomography versus pulmonary angiography in the diagnosis of acute massive pulmonary embolism. Am J Cardiol 1994;74:96–98.

166. van Rossum AB, Treurniet FE, Kieft GJ, et al. Role of spiral volumetric computed tomographic scanning in the assessment of patients with clinical suspicion of pulmonary embolism and an abnormal ventilation/perfusion lung scan. Thorax 1996;51:23–28.

167. Garg K, Welsh CH, Feyerabend AJ, et al. Pulmonary embolism: diagnosis with spiral CT and ventilation-perfusion scanning – correlation with pulmonary angiographic results or clinical outcome. Radiology 1998;208:201–208.

168. Gosselin MV, Rubin GD, Leung AN, et al. Unsuspected pulmonary embolism: prospective detection on routine helical CT scans. Radiology 1998;208:209–215.

169. Loud PA, Grossman ZD, Klippenstein DL, et al. Combined CT venography and pulmonary angiography: a new diagnostic technique for suspected thromboembolic disease. AJR Am J Roentgenol 1998;170:951–954.

170. Mayo JR, Remy-Jardin M, Müller NL, et al. Pulmonary embolism: prospective comparison of spiral CT with ventilation-perfusion scintigraphy. Radiology 1997;205:447–452.

171. Remy-Jardin M, Remy J. Spiral CT of pulmonary embolism. In: Remy-Jardin M, Remy M, eds. Spiral CT of the chest. Berlin: Springer, 1996:201–230.

172. Sostman HD, Layish DT, Tapson VF, et al. Prospective comparison of helical CT and MR imaging in clinically suspected acute pulmonary embolism. J Magn Reson Imaging 1996;6:275–281.

173. van Erkel AR, van Rossum AB, Bloem JL, et al. Spiral CT angiography for suspected pulmonary embolism: a cost-effectiveness analysis. Radiology 1996;201:29–36.

174. van Rossum AB, Pattynama PM, Mallens WM, et al. Can helical CT replace scintigraphy in the diagnostic process in suspected pulmonary embolism? A retrolective-prolective cohort study focusing on total diagnostic yield. Eur Radiol 1998;8:90–96.

175. Herold CJ, Remy-Jardin M, Grenier PA, et al. Prospective evaluation of pulmonary embolism: initial results of the European multicenter trial (ESTIPEP). Radiology 1998;123(S):334.

176. ACCP Consensus Committee on Pulmonary Embolism. Opinions regarding the diagnosis and management of venous thromboembolic disease. ACCP Consensus Committee on Pulmonary Embolism. American College of Chest Physicians. Chest 1998;113: 499–504.

177. Goodman LR, Lipchik RJ, Kuzo RS. Acute pulmonary embolism: the role of computed tomographic imaging. J Thorac Imaging 1997;12:83–86.

178. Hansell DM, Padley SPG, Padley SP. Continuous volume computed

tomography in pulmonary embolism: the answer, or just another test? Thorax 1996;51:1–2.

179. Robinson PJ. Ventilation-perfusion lung scanning and spiral computed tomography of the lungs: competing or complementary modalities? Eur J Nucl Med 1996;23:1547–1553.

180. Rubin GD. Helical CT for the detection of acute pulmonary embolism: experts debate. J Thorac Imaging 1997;12:81–82.

181. Tapson VF. Pulmonary embolism: the diagnostic repertoire. Chest 1997;112:578–580.

182. Brink JA, Woodard PK, Horesh L, et al. Depiction of pulmonary emboli with spiral CT: optimization of display window settings in a porcine model. Radiology 1997;204:703–708.

183. Remy-Jardin M, Remy J, Artaud D, et al. Spiral CT of pulmonary embolism: technical considerations and interpretive pitfalls. J Thorac Imaging 1997;12:103–117.

184. Remy-Jardin M, Remy J, Artaud D, et al. Peripheral pulmonary arteries: optimization of the spiral CT acquisition protocol. Radiology 1997;204:157–163.

185. Kuzo RS, Goodman LR. CT evaluation of pulmonary embolism: technique and interpretation. AJR Am J Roentgenol 1997;169:959–965.

186. Remy-Jardin M, Remy J, Artaud D, et al. Spiral CT of pulmonary embolism: diagnostic approach, interpretive pitfalls and current indications. Eur Radiol 1998;8:1376–1390.

187. Raptopoulos V, Boiselle PM. Multi-detector row spiral CT pulmonary angiography: comparison with single-detector row spiral CT. Radiology 2001;221:606–613.

188. Remy-Jardin M, Remy J, Deschildre F, et al. Diagnosis of pulmonary embolism with spiral CT: comparison with pulmonary angiography and scintigraphy. Radiology 1996;200:699–706.

189. Drucker EA, Rivitz SM, Shepard JA, et al. Acute pulmonary embolism: assessment of helical CT for diagnosis. Radiology 1998;209:235–241.

190. Ghaye B, Szapiro D, Mastora I, et al. Peripheral pulmonary arteries: how far in the lung does multi-detector row spiral CT allow analysis? Radiology 2001;219:629–636.

191. Schoepf UJ, Holzknecht N, Helmberger TK, et al. Subsegmental pulmonary emboli: improved detection with thin-collimation multi-detector row spiral CT. Radiology 2002;222:483–490.

192. Remy-Jardin M, Tillie-Leblond I, Szapiro D, et al. CT angiography of pulmonary embolism in patients with underlying respiratory disease: impact of multislice CT on image quality and negative predictive value. Eur Radiol 2002;12:1971–1978.

193. Coche E, Pawlak S, Dechambre S, et al. Peripheral pulmonary arteries: identification at multi-slice spiral CT with 3D reconstruction. Eur Radiol 2003;13:815–822.

194. Patel S, Kazerooni EA, Cascade PN. Pulmonary embolism: optimization of small pulmonary artery visualization at multi-detector row CT. Radiology 2003;227:455–460.

195. Schnyder P, Meuli P, Wicky S, et al. Injection techniques in helical CT of the chest. Eur Radiol (Suppl) 1995;5:26.

196. Coche EE, Hammer FD, Goffette PP. Demonstration of pulmonary embolism with gadolinium-enhanced spiral CT. Eur Radiol 2001;11:2306–2309.

197. Sostman HD, MacFall JR, Foo TKF et al. Pulmonary arteries and veins. In: Potchen EJ, Haacke EM, Siebert JE, Gottschalk A, eds. Magnetic resonance angiography: concepts and applications. St Louis: Mosby, 1993:546–572.

198. Hartmann IJ, Lo RT, Bakker J, et al. Optimal scan delay in spiral CT for the diagnosis of acute pulmonary embolism. J Comput Assist Tomogr 2002;26:21–25.

199. Remy-Jardin M, Remy J, Cauvain O, et al. Diagnosis of central pulmonary embolism with helical CT: role of two-dimensional multiplanar reformations. AJR Am J Roentgenol 1995;5:1131–1138.

200. Swensen SJ, Morin RL, Aughenbaugh GL, et al. CT reconstruction algorithm selection in the evaluation of solitary pulmonary nodules. J Comput Assist Tomogr 1995;19:932–935.

201. Greaves SM, Hart EM, Brown K, et al. Pulmonary thromboembolism: spectrum of findings on CT. AJR Am J Roentgenol 1995;165:1359–1363.

202. Mastora I, Remy-Jardin M, Masson P, et al. Severity of acute pulmonary embolism: evaluation of a new spiral CT angiographic score in correlation with echocardiographic data. Eur Radiol 2003;13:29–35.

203. Coche EE, Müller NL, Kim KI, et al. Acute pulmonary embolism: ancillary findings at spiral CT. Radiology 1998;207:753–758.

204. Johnson PT, Wechsler RJ, Salazar AM, et al. Spiral CT of acute pulmonary thromboembolism: evaluation of pleuroparenchymal abnormalities. J Comput Assist Tomogr 1999;23:369–373.

205. Groell R, Peichel KH, Uggowitzer MM, et al. Computed tomography densitometry of the lung: a method to assess perfusion defects in acute pulmonary embolism. Eur J Radiol 1999;32:192–196.

206. Schoepf UJ, Bruening R, Konschitzky H, et al. Pulmonary embolism: comprehensive diagnosis by using electron-beam CT for detection of emboli and assessment of pulmonary blood flow. Radiology 2000;217:693–700.

207. Shah AA, Davis SD, Gamsu G, et al. Parenchymal and pleural findings in patients with and patients without acute pulmonary embolism detected at spiral CT. Radiology 1999;211:147–153.

208. Gotway MB, Nagai BK, Reddy GP, et al. Incidentally detected cardiovascular abnormalities on helical CT pulmonary angiography: spectrum of findings. AJR Am J Roentgenol 2001;176:421–427.

209. Sinner WN. Computed tomographic patterns of pulmonary thromboembolism and infarction. J Comput Assist Tomogr 1978;2:395–399.

210. Ren H, Kuhlman JE, Hruban RH, et al. CT of inflation-fixed lungs: wedge-shaped density and vascular sign in the diagnosis of infarction. J Comput Assist Tomogr 1990;14:82–86.

211. Schwickert HC, Schweden F, Schild HH, et al. Pulmonary arteries and lung parenchyma in chronic pulmonary embolism: preoperative and postoperative CT findings. Radiology 1994;191:351–357.

212. Bergin CJ, Sirlin CB, Hauschildt JP, et al. Chronic thromboembolism: diagnosis with helical CT and MR imaging with angiographic and surgical correlation. Radiology 1997;204:695–702.

213. Roberts HC, Kauczor HU, Schweden F, et al. Spiral CT of pulmonary hypertension and chronic thromboembolism. J Thorac Imaging 1997;12:118–127.

214. Kauczor HU, Schwickert HC, Mayer E, et al. Spiral CT of bronchial arteries in chronic thromboembolism. J Comput Assist Tomogr 1994;18:855–861.

215. Gotway MB, Patel RA, Webb WR. Helical CT for the evaluation of suspected acute pulmonary embolism: diagnostic pitfalls. J Comput Assist Tomogr 2000;24:267–273.

216. Remy-Jardin M, Duyck P, Remy J, et al. Hilar lymph nodes: identification with spiral CT and histologic correlation. Radiology 1995;196:387–394.

217. Rathbun SW, Raskob GE, Whitsett TL. Sensitivity and specificity of helical computed tomography in the diagnosis of pulmonary embolism: a systematic review. Ann Intern Med 2000;132:227–232.

218. Blachere H, Latrabe V, Montaudon M, et al. Pulmonary embolism revealed on helical CT angiography: comparison with ventilation-perfusion radionuclide lung scanning. AJR Am J Roentgenol 2000;174:1041–1047.

219. Chartrand-Lefebvre C, Howarth N, Lucidarme O, et al. Contrast-enhanced helical CT for pulmonary embolism detection: inter- and intraobserver agreement among radiologists with variable experience. AJR Am J Roentgenol 1999;172:107–112.

220. Domingo ML, Marti-Bonmati L, Dosda R, et al. Interobserver agreement in the

diagnosis of pulmonary embolism with helical CT. Eur J Radiol 2000;34:136–140.

221. Winston CB, Wechsler RJ, Salazar AM, et al. Incidental pulmonary emboli detected at helical CT: effect on patient care. Radiology 1996;201:23–27.

222. Remy-Jardin M, Remy J, Baghaie F, et al. Clinical value of thin collimation in the diagnostic workup of pulmonary embolism. AJR Am J Roentgenol 2000;175:407–411.

223. Diffin DC, Leyendecker JR, Johnson SP, et al. Effect of anatomic distribution of pulmonary emboli on interobserver agreement in the interpretation of pulmonary angiography. AJR Am J Roentgenol 1998;171:1085–1089.

224. Stein PD, Henry JW. Prevalence of acute pulmonary embolism in central and subsegmental pulmonary arteries and relation to probability interpretation of ventilation/perfusion lung scans. Chest 1997;111:1246–1248.

225. Garg K, Sieler H, Welsh CH, et al. Clinical validity of helical CT being interpreted as negative for pulmonary embolism: implications for patient treatment. AJR Am J Roentgenol 1999;172:1627–1631.

226. Goodman LR, Lipchik RJ, Kuzo RS, et al. Subsequent pulmonary embolism: risk after a negative helical CT pulmonary angiogram – prospective comparison with scintigraphy. Radiology 2000; 215:535–542.

227. Gottsater A, Berg A, Centergard J, et al. Clinically suspected pulmonary embolism: is it safe to withhold anticoagulation after a negative spiral CT? Eur Radiol 2001;11:65–72.

228. Nilsson T, Olausson A, Johnsson H, et al. Negative spiral CT in acute pulmonary embolism. Acta Radiol 2002;43:486–491.

229. Ost D, Rozenshtein A, Saffran L, et al. The negative predictive value of spiral computed tomography for the diagnosis of pulmonary embolism in patients with nondiagnostic ventilation-perfusion scans. Am J Med 2001;110:16–21.

230. Swensen SJ, Sheedy PF, Ryu JH, et al. Outcomes after withholding anticoagulation from patients with suspected acute pulmonary embolism and negative computed tomographic findings: a cohort study. Mayo Clin Proc 2002;77:130–138.

231. Tillie-Leblond I, Mastora I, Radenne F, et al. Risk of pulmonary embolism after a negative spiral CT angiogram in patients with pulmonary disease: 1-year clinical follow-up study. Radiology 2002;223:461–467.

232. van Strijen MJ, De Monye W, Schiereck J, et al. Single-detector helical computed tomography as the primary diagnostic test in suspected pulmonary embolism: a multicenter clinical management study

of 510 patients. Ann Intern Med 2003; 138:307–314.

233. Lomis NN, Yoon HC, Moran AG, et al. Clinical outcomes of patients after a negative spiral CT pulmonary arteriogram in the evaluation of acute pulmonary embolism. J Vasc Interv Radiol 1999;10:707–712.

234. Kim KI, Müller NL, Mayo JR. Clinically suspected pulmonary embolism: utility of spiral CT. Radiology 1999;210: 693–697.

235. Woodard PK. CT scan negative for pulmonary embolism: where do we go from here? Radiology 2000;215:325–326.

236. Kelley MA, Carson JL, Palevsky HI, et al. Diagnosing pulmonary embolism: new facts and strategies. Ann Intern Med 1991;114:300–306.

237. Hyers TM. Diagnosis of pulmonary embolism. Thorax 1995;50:930–932.

238. Goodman LR, Lipchik RJ. Diagnosis of acute pulmonary embolism: time for a new approach. Radiology 1996;199:25–27.

239. Perrier A, Howarth N, Didier D, et al. Performance of helical computed tomography in unselected outpatients with suspected pulmonary embolism. Ann Intern Med 2001;135:88–97.

240. Lorut C, Ghossains M, Horellou MH, et al. A noninvasive diagnostic strategy including spiral computed tomography in patients with suspected pulmonary embolism. Am J Respir Crit Care Med 2000;162:1413–1418.

241. Perrier A, Bounameaux H. Diagnosis of pulmonary embolism in outpatients by sequential noninvasive tools. Semin Thromb Hemost 2001;27:25–32.

242. Hartmann IJ, Prins MH, Buller HR, et al. Acute pulmonary embolism: impact of selection bias in prospective diagnostic studies. ANTELOPE Study Group. Advances in New Technologies Evaluating the Localization of Pulmonary Embolism. Thromb Haemost 2001;85:604–608.

243. Ghali WA, Cornuz J, Perrier A. New methods for estimating pretest probability in the diagnosis of pulmonary embolism. Curr Opin Pulm Med 2001;7:349–353.

244. British Thoracic Society guidelines for the management of suspected acute pulmonary embolism. Thorax 2003;58:470–483.

245. Gefter WB, Palevsky HI. Opinion response to acute pulmonary embolism: the role of computed tomographic imaging. J Thorac Imaging 1997; 12:97–100.

246. Mayo JR. Opinion response to acute pulmonary embolism: the role of computed tomographic imaging. J Thorac Imaging 1997;12:95–97.

247. Sostman HD. Opinion response to acute pulmonary embolism: the role of computed tomographic imaging.

J Thorac Imaging 1997;12:89–92.

248. Remy-Jardin M, Remy J, Artaud D, et al. Opinion response to acute pulmonary embolism: the role of computed tomographic imaging. J Thorac Imaging 1997;12:92–95.

249. Goodman LR. CT of acute pulmonary emboli: where does it fit? RadioGraphics 1997;17:1037–1042.

250. Carman TL, Deitcher SR. Advances in diagnosing and excluding pulmonary embolism: spiral CT and D-dimer measurement. Cleve Clin J Med 2002;69:721–729.

251. Irwin GA, Luchs JS, Donovan V, et al. Can a state-of-the-art D-dimer test be used to determine the need for CT imaging in patients suspected of having pulmonary embolism? Acad Radiol 2002;9:1013–1017.

252. Cham MD, Yankelevitz DF, Shaham D, et al. Deep venous thrombosis: detection by using indirect CT venography. The Pulmonary Angiography-Indirect CT Venography Cooperative Group. Radiology 2000;216:744–751.

253. Donkers-van Rossum AB. Diagnostic strategies for suspected pulmonary embolism. Eur Respir J 2001;18:589–597.

254. Larcos G, Chi KK, Shiell A, et al. Suspected acute pulmonary emboli: cost-effectiveness of chest helical computed tomography versus a standard diagnostic algorithm incorporating ventilation-perfusion scintigraphy. Aust N Z J Med 2000;30:195–201.

255. Perrier A, Nendaz MR, Sarasin FP, et al. Cost-effectiveness analysis of diagnostic strategies for suspected pulmonary embolism including helical computed tomography. Am J Respir Crit Care Med 2003;167:39–44.

256. Paterson DI, Schwartzman K. Strategies incorporating spiral CT for the diagnosis of acute pulmonary embolism: a cost-effectiveness analysis. Chest 2001;119: 1791–1800.

257. Peterson DA, Kazerooni EA, Wakefield TW, et al. Computed tomographic venography is specific but not sensitive for diagnosis of acute lower-extremity deep venous thrombosis in patients with suspected pulmonary embolus. J Vasc Surg 2001;34:798–804.

258. Walsh G, Redmond S. Does addition of CT pelvic venography to CT pulmonary angiography protocols contribute to the diagnosis of thromboembolic disease? Clin Radiol 2002;57:462–465.

259. Coche EE, Hamoir XL, Hammer FD, et al. Using dual-detector helical CT angiography to detect deep venous thrombosis in patients with suspicion of pulmonary embolism: diagnostic value and additional findings. AJR Am J Roentgenol 2001;176:1035–1039.

260. Duwe KM, Shiau M, Budorick NE, et al. Evaluation of the lower extremity veins

in patients with suspected pulmonary embolism: a retrospective comparison of helical CT venography and sonography. 2000 ARRS Executive Council Award I. American Roentgen Ray Society. AJR Am J Roentgenol 2000;175:1525–1531.

261. Garg K, Kemp JL, Wojcik D, et al. Thromboembolic disease: comparison of combined CT pulmonary angiography and venography with bilateral leg sonography in 70 patients. AJR Am J Roentgenol 2000;175:997–1001.

262. Loud PA, Katz DS, Bruce DA, et al. Deep venous thrombosis with suspected pulmonary embolism: detection with combined CT venography and pulmonary angiography. Radiology 2001;219:498–502.

263. Baldt MM, Zontsich T, Stumpflen A, et al. Deep venous thrombosis of the lower extremity: efficacy of spiral CT venography compared with conventional venography in diagnosis. Radiology 1996;200:423–428.

264. Ciccotosto C, Goodman LR, Washington L, et al. Indirect CT venography following CT pulmonary angiography: spectrum of CT findings. J Thorac Imaging 2002;17:18–27.

265. Lomas DJ, Britton PD. CT demonstration of acute and chronic iliofemoral thrombosis. J Comput Assist Tomogr 1991;15:861–862.

266. Yankelevitz DF, Gamsu G, Shah A, et al. Optimization of combined CT pulmonary angiography with lower extremity CT venography. AJR Am J Roentgenol 2000;174:67–69.

267. Bruce D, Loud PA, Klippenstein DL, et al. Combined CT venography and pulmonary angiography: how much venous enhancement is routinely obtained? AJR Am J Roentgenol 2001;176:1281–1285.

268. Katz DS, Loud PA, Bruce D, et al. Combined CT venography and pulmonary angiography: a comprehensive review. RadioGraphics 2002;22 Spec No:S3–19.

269. Rademaker J, Griesshaber V, Hidajat N, et al. Combined CT pulmonary angiography and venography for diagnosis of pulmonary embolism and deep vein thrombosis: radiation dose. J Thorac Imaging 2001;16:297–299.

270. Mayo JR, Ketai LH. Invited commentary. RadioGraphics 2002;22:20S–24S.

271. Schiebler ML, Holland GA, Hatabu H, et al. Suspected pulmonary embolism: prospective evaluation with pulmonary MR angiography. Radiology 1993;189:125–131.

272. Erdman WA, Peshock RM, Redman HC, et al. Pulmonary embolism: comparison of MR images with radionuclide and angiographic studies. Radiology 1994;190:499–508.

273. Grist TM, Sostman HD, MacFall JR, et al. Pulmonary angiography with MR imaging: preliminary clinical experience. Radiology 1993;189:523–530.

274. Reittner P, Coxson HO, Nakano Y, et al. Pulmonary embolism: comparison of gadolinium-enhanced MR angiography with contrast-enhanced spiral CT in a porcine model. Acad Radiol 2001;8:343–350.

275. Hurst DR, Kazerooni EA, Stafford-Johnson D, et al. Diagnosis of pulmonary embolism: comparison of CT angiography and MR angiography in canines. J Vasc Interv Radiol 1999;10:309–318.

276. Haage P, Piroth W, Krombach G, et al. Pulmonary embolism: comparison of angiography with spiral CT, MRA and real-time MR imaging. Am J Respir Crit Care Med 2003;167:729–734.

277. Oudkerk M, van Beek EJ, Wielopolski P, et al. Comparison of contrast-enhanced magnetic resonance angiography and conventional pulmonary angiography for the diagnosis of pulmonary embolism: a prospective study. Lancet 2002;359:1643–1647.

278. Ley S, Kauczor HU, Heussel CP, et al. Value of contrast-enhanced MR angiography and helical CT angiography in chronic thromboembolic pulmonary hypertension. Eur Radiol 2003;13:2365–2371.

279. Hatabu H, Uematsu H, Nguyen B, et al. CT and MR in pulmonary embolism: A changing role for nuclear medicine in diagnostic strategy. Semin Nucl Med 2002;32:183–192.

280. Erdman WA, Clarke GD. Magnetic resonance imaging of pulmonary embolism. Semin Ultrasound CT MR 1997;18:338–348.

281. Erdman WA. Magnetic resonance imaging. In: Talbot S, Oliver MA, eds. Techniques of venous imaging. Pasadena, CA: Appleton-Davies, 1992:175–185.

282. Gefter WB, Hatabu H. Evaluation of pulmonary vascular imaging and blood flow by magnetic resonance. J Thorac Imaging 1993;8:122–136.

283. Foo TK, MacFall JR, Sostman HD, et al. Single-breath-hold venous or arterial flow-suppressed pulmonary vascular MR imaging with phased-array coils. J Magn Reson Imag 1993;3:611–616.

284. Gefter WB, Hatabu H, Holland GA, et al. Pulmonary thromboembolism: recent developments in diagnosis with CT and MR imaging. Radiology 1995;197:561–574.

285. Hatabu H, Gaa J, Kim D, et al. Pulmonary perfusion and angiography: evaluation with breath-hold enhanced three-dimensional fast imaging steady-state precession MR imaging with short TR and TE. AJR Am J Roentgenol 1996;167:653–655.

286. Loubeyre P, Revel D, Douek P, et al. Dynamic contrast-enhanced MR angiography of pulmonary embolism: comparison with pulmonary angiography. AJR Am J Roentgenol 1994;162:1035–1039.

287. Meaney JFM, Weg JG, Chenevert TL, et al. Diagnosis of pulmonary embolism with magnetic resonance angiography. N Engl J Med 1997;336:1422–1427.

288. Li KC, Pelc LR, Napel SA, et al. MRI of pulmonary embolism using Gd-DTPA-polyethylene glycol polymer enhanced 3D fast gradient echo technique in a canine model. Magn Reson Imaging 1997;15:543–550.

289. Vrachliotis TG, Bis KG, Shetty AN, et al. Contrast-enhanced three-dimensional MR angiography of the pulmonary vascular tree. Int J Cardiovasc Imaging 2002;18:283–293.

290. Suga K, Ogasawara N, Okada M, et al. Lung perfusion impairments in pulmonary embolic and airway obstruction with noncontrast MR imaging. J Appl Physiol 2002;92:2439–2451.

291. Hatabu H, Gaa J, Kim D, et al. Pulmonary perfusion: qualitative assessment with dynamic contrast-enhanced MRI using ultra-short TE and inversion recovery turbo FLASH. Magn Reson Med 1996;36:503–508.

292. Amundsen T, Kvaerness J, Jones RA, et al. Pulmonary embolism: detection with MR perfusion imaging of lung – a feasibility study. Radiology 1997;203:181–185.

293. Kauczor HU, Hofmann D, Kreitner KF, et al. Normal and abnormal pulmonary ventilation: visualization at hyperpolarized He-3 MR imaging. Radiology 1996;201:564–568.

294. Edelman RR, Hatabu H, Tadamura E, et al. Noninvasive assessment of regional ventilation in the human lung using oxygen-enhanced magnetic resonance imaging. Nat Med 1996;2:1236–1239.

295. Suga K, Ogasawara N, Tsukuda T, et al. Assessment of regional lung ventilation in dog lungs with Gd-DTPA aerosol ventilation MR imaging. Acta Radiol 2002;43:282–291.

296. Lipson DA, Roberts DA, Hansen-Flaschen J, et al. Pulmonary ventilation and perfusion scanning using hyperpolarized helium-3 MRI and arterial spin tagging in healthy normal subjects and in pulmonary embolism and orthotopic lung transplant patients. Magn Reson Med 2002;47:1073–1076.

297. Stern JB, Abehsera M, Grenet D, et al. Detection of pelvic vein thrombosis by magnetic resonance angiography in patients with acute pulmonary embolism and normal lower limb compression ultrasonography. Chest 2002;122:115–121.

298. Chan CK, Hutcheon MA, Hyland RH, et al. Pulmonary tumor embolism: a

critical review of clinical, imaging, and hemodynamic features. J Thorac Imaging 1987;2:4–14.

299. Hadfield JW, Sterling JC, Wraight EP. Multiple tumour emboli simulating a massive pulmonary embolus. Postgrad Med J 1982;58:792–793.

300. Burchard KW, Carney WI Jr. Tumor embolism as the first manifestation of cancer. J Surg Oncol 1984;27:26–30.

301. Daughtry JD, Stewart BH, Golding LA, et al. Pulmonary embolus presenting as the initial manifestation of renal cell carcinoma. Ann Thorac Surg 1977;24:178–181.

302. Soares FA, Landell GA, de Oliveira JA. Pulmonary tumor embolism to alveolar septal capillaries. An unusual cause of sudden cor pulmonale. Arch Pathol Lab Med 1992;116:187–188.

303. He XW, Tang YH, Luo ZQ, et al. Subacute cor pulmonale due to tumor embolization to the lungs. Angiology 1989;40:11–17.

304. Hibbert M, Braude S. Tumour microembolism presenting as "primary pulmonary hypertension." Thorax 1997;552:1016–1017.

305. Singh SP, Nath H, Pinkard NB, et al. Bronchioloalveolar carcinoma causing pulmonary hypertension: a unique manifestation. AJR Am J Roentgenol 1994;162:30–32.

306. Evans KT, Cockshott WP, Hendrickse PdV, et al. Pulmonary changes in malignant trophoblastic disease. Br J Radiol 1965;38:161–171.

307. Graham JP, Rotman HH, Weg JG. Tumor emboli presenting as pulmonary hypertension. A diagnostic dilemma. Chest 1976;69:229–230.

308. Seckl MJ, Rustin GJ, Newlands ES, et al. Pulmonary embolism, pulmonary hypertension, and choriocarcinoma. Lancet 1991;338:1313–1315.

309. Shepard JA, Moore EH, Templeton PA, et al. Pulmonary intravascular tumor emboli: dilated and beaded peripheral pulmonary arteries at CT. Radiology 1993;187:797–801.

310. Kim AE, Haramati LB, Janus D, et al. Pulmonary tumor embolism presenting as infarcts on computed tomography. J Thorac Imaging 1999;14:135–137.

311. Yao DX, Flieder DB, Hoda SA. Pulmonary tumor thrombotic microangiopathy: an often missed antemortem diagnosis. Arch Pathol Lab Med 2001;125:304–305.

312. Franquet T, Gimenez A, Prats R, et al. Thrombotic microangiopathy of pulmonary tumors: a vascular cause of tree-in-bud pattern on CT. AJR Am J Roentgenol 2002;179:897–899.

313. Peacock AJ. Primary pulmonary hypertension. Thorax 1999;54:1107–1118.

314. Chang CH. The normal roentgenographic measurement of the right descending pulmonary artery in 1085 cases. AJR Am J Roentgenol 1962;87:929–935.

315. Kuriyama K, Gamsu G, Stern RG, et al. CT determined pulmonary artery diameters in predicting pulmonary hypertension. Invest Radiol 1984;19:16–22.

316. Ring NJ, Marshall AJ. Idiopathic dilatation of the pulmonary artery. Br J Radiol 2002;75:532–535.

317. Haimovici JB, Trotman-Dickenson B, Halpern EF, et al. Relationship between pulmonary artery diameter at computed tomography and pulmonary artery pressures at right-sided heart catheterization. Massachusetts General Hospital Lung Transplantation Program. Acad Radiol 1997;4:327–334.

318. Tan RT, Kuzo R, Goodman LR, et al. Utility of CT scan evaluation for predicting pulmonary hypertension in patients with parenchymal lung disease. Medical College of Wisconsin Lung Transplant Group. Chest 1998;113:1250–1256.

319. Edwards PD, Bull RK, Coulden R. CT measurement of main pulmonary artery diameter. Br J Radiol 1998;71:1018–1020.

320. Ng CS, Wells AU, Padley SP. A CT sign of chronic pulmonary arterial hypertension: the ratio of main pulmonary artery to aortic diameter. J Thorac Imaging 1999;14:270–278.

321. Baque-Juston MC, Wells AU, Hansell DM. Pericardial thickening or effusion in patients with pulmonary artery hypertension: a CT study. AJR Am J Roentgenol 1999;172:361–364.

322. Bogren HG, Klipstein RH, Mohiaddin RH, et al. Pulmonary artery distensibility and blood flow patterns: a magnetic resonance study of normal subjects and of patients with pulmonary arterial hypertension. Am Heart J 1989;118:990–999.

323. Kondo C, Caputo GR, Masui T, et al. Pulmonary hypertension: pulmonary flow quantification and flow profile analysis with velocity-encoded cine MR imaging. Radiology 1992;183:751–758.

324. Frank H, Globits S, Glogar D, et al. Detection and quantification of pulmonary artery hypertension with MR imaging: results in 23 patients. AJR Am J Roentgenol 1993;161:27–31.

325. Murray TI, Boxt LM, Katz J, et al. Estimation of pulmonary artery pressure in patients with primary pulmonary hypertension by quantitative analysis of magnetic resonance images. J Thorac Imaging 1994;9:198–204.

326. Stern EJ, Graham C, Gamsu G, et al. Pulmonary artery dissection: MR findings. J Comput Assist Tomogr 1992;16:481–483.

327. Piatt JH Jr, Hoffman HJ. Cor pulmonale: a lethal complication of ventriculoatrial CSF diversion. Childs Nerv Syst 1989;5:29–31.

328. Rich S, Levitsky S, Brundage BH. Pulmonary hypertension from chronic pulmonary thromboembolism. Ann Intern Med 1988;108:425–434.

329. Moser KM, Auger WR, Fedullo PF, et al. Chronic thromboembolic hypertension: clinical picture and surgical treatment. Eur Respir J 1992;5:334–342.

330. Bergin CJ. Chronic thromboembolic pulmonary hypertension: the disease, the diagnosis, and the treatment. Semin Ultrasound CT MR 1997;18:383–391.

331. Woodruff WW III, Hoeck BE, Chitwood WR Jr, et al. Radiographic findings in pulmonary hypertension from unresolved embolism. AJR Am J Roentgenol 1985;144:681–686.

332. Schmidt HC, Kauczor HU, Schild HH, et al. Pulmonary hypertension in patients with chronic pulmonary thromboembolism: chest radiograph and CT evaluation before and after surgery. Eur Radiol 1996;6:817–825.

333. King MA, Ysrael M, Bergin CJ. Chronic thromboembolic pulmonary hypertension: CT findings. AJR Am J Roentgenol 1998;170:955–960.

334. King MA, Bergin CJ, Yeung DW, et al. Chronic pulmonary thromboembolism: detection of regional hypoperfusion with CT. Radiology 1994;191:359–363.

335. Ley S, Kreitner KF, Morgenstern I, et al. Bronchopulmonary shunts in patients with chronic thromboembolic pulmonary hypertension: evaluation with helical CT and MR imaging. AJR Am J Roentgenol 2002;179:1209–1215.

336. Sherrick AD, Swensen SJ, Hartman TE. Mosaic pattern of lung attenuation on CT scans: frequency among patients with pulmonary artery hypertension of different causes. AJR Am J Roentgenol 1997;169:79–82.

337. Falaschi F, Palla A, Formichi B, et al. CT evaluation of chronic thromboembolic pulmonary hypertension. J Comput Assist Tomogr 1992;16:897–903.

338. Martin KW, Sagel SS, Siegel BA. Mosaic oligemia simulating pulmonary infiltrates on CT. AJR Am J Roentgenol 1986;147:670–673.

339. Worthy SA, Müller NL, Hartman TE, et al. Mosaic attenuation pattern on thin-section CT scans of the lung: differentiation among infiltrative lung, airway, and vascular diseases as a cause. Radiology 1997;205:465–470.

340. Bergin CJ, Rios G, King MA, et al. Accuracy of high-resolution CT in identifying chronic pulmonary thromboembolic disease. AJR Am J Roentgenol 1996;166:1371–1377.

341. Remy-Jardin M, Remy J, Louvegny S, et al. Airway changes in chronic pulmonary embolism: CT findings in 33 patients. Radiology 1997;203:355–360.

342. Arakawa H, Kurihara Y, Sasaka K, et al. Air trapping on CT of patients with

pulmonary embolism. AJR Am J Roentgenol 2002;178:1201–1207.

343. Lisbona R, Kreisman H, Novales-Diaz J, et al. Perfusion lung scanning: differentiation of primary from thromboembolic pulmonary hypertension. AJR Am J Roentgenol 1985;144:27–30.

344. Brown KT, Bach AM. Paucity of angiographic findings despite extensive organized thrombus in chronic thromboembolic pulmonary hypertension. J Vasc Interv Radiol 1992;3:99–102.

345. Auger WR, Fedullo PF, Moser KM, et al. Chronic major-vessel thromboembolic pulmonary artery obstruction: appearance at angiography. Radiology 1992;182:393–398.

346. Primary pulmonary hypertension: WHO committee report. Geneva: World Health Organization, 1975.

347. Edwards WD, Edwards JE. Clinical primary pulmonary hypertension: three pathologic types. Circulation 1977;56:884–888.

348. Bjornsson J, Edwards WD. Primary pulmonary hypertension: a histopathologic study of 80 cases. Mayo Clin Proc 1985;60:16–25.

349. Wagenvoort CA. Primary pulmonary hypertension: pathology. In: Peacock AJ, ed. Pulmonary circulation. London: Chapman and Hall, 1996:325–328.

350. Gomez-Sanchez MA, Mestre de Juan MJ, Gomez-Pajuelo C, et al. Pulmonary hypertension due to toxic oil syndrome. A clinicopathologic study. Chest 1989;95:325–331.

351. Scherpereel A, Steenhouwer F, Quandalle P, et al. Primary familial pulmonary arterial hypertension. Rev Mal Respir 1997;14:409–412.

352. Wagenvoort CA, Wagenvoort N. Primary pulmonary hypertension: a pathologic study of the lung vessels in 156 clinically diagnosed cases. Circulation 1970;42:1163–1184.

353. Kanemoto N, Furuya H, Etoh T, et al. Chest roentgenograms in primary pulmonary hypertension. Chest 1979;76:45–49.

354. Powe JE, Palevsky HI, McCarthy KE, et al. Pulmonary arterial hypertension: value of perfusion scintigraphy. Radiology 1987;164:727–730.

355. Rich S, Pietra GG, Kieras K, et al. Primary pulmonary hypertension: radiographic and scintigraphic patterns of histologic subtypes. Ann Intern Med 1986;105:499–502.

356. Wilson AG, Harris CN, Lavender JP, et al. Perfusion lung scanning in obliterative pulmonary hypertension. Br Heart J 1973;35:917–930.

357. Boxt LM, Rich S, Fried R, et al. Automated morphologic evaluation of pulmonary arteries in primary pulmonary hypertension. Invest Radiol 1986;21:906–909.

358. Gupta BD, Moodie DS, Hodgman JR. Primary pulmonary hypertension in adults; clinical features, catheterization findings and long-term follow up. Cleve Clin Q 1980;47:275–284.

359. Cailes JB, Du Bois RM, Hansell DM. Density gradient of the lung parenchyma on CT in patients with lone pulmonary hypertension and systemic sclerosis. Acad Radiol 1996;3:724–730.

360. Engeler CE, Kuni CC, Tashjian JH, et al. Regional alterations in lung ventilation in end-stage primary pulmonary hypertension: correlation between CT and scintigraphy. AJR Am J Roentgenol 1995;164:831–835.

361. Nolan RL, McAdams HP, Sporn TA, et al. Pulmonary cholesterol granulomas in patients with pulmonary artery hypertension: chest radiographic and CT findings. AJR Am J Roentgenol 1999;172:1317–1319.

362. Fartoukh M, Humbert M, Capron F, et al. Severe pulmonary hypertension in histiocytosis X. Am J Respir Crit Care Med 2000;161:216–223.

363. Lippert JL, White CS, Cameron EW, et al. Pulmonary capillary hemangiomatosis: radiographic appearance. J Thorac Imaging 1998;13:49–51.

364. Eltorky MA, Headley AS, Winer-Muram H, et al. Pulmonary capillary hemangiomatosis: a clinicopathologic review. Ann Thorac Surg 1994;57:772–776.

365. Pycock CJ, Thomas AJ, Marshall AJ, et al. Capillary haemangiomatosis: a rare cause of pulmonary hypertension. Respir Med 1994;88:153–155.

366. Dufour B, Maitre S, Humbert M, et al. High-resolution CT of the chest in four patients with pulmonary capillary hemangiomatosis or pulmonary venoocclusive disease. AJR Am J Roentgenol 1998;171:1321–1324.

367. Humbert M, Maitre S, Capron F, et al. Pulmonary edema complicating continuous intravenous prostacyclin in pulmonary capillary hemangiomatosis. Am J Respir Crit Care Med 1998;157:1681–1685.

368. Resten A, Maitre S, Humbert M, et al. Pulmonary arterial hypertension: thin-section CT predictors of epoprostenol therapy failure. Radiology 2002;222:782–788.

369. Almagro P, Julia J, Sanjaume M, et al. Pulmonary capillary hemangiomatosis associated with primary pulmonary hypertension: report of 2 new cases and review of 35 cases from the literature. Medicine (Baltimore) 2002;81:417–424.

370. Katzenstein AL, Askin FB. Pulmonary hypertension and other vascular disorders. In: Bennington JL, ed. Surgical pathology of non-neoplastic lung disease, 2nd edn. Philadelphia: W B Saunders, 1990:432–467.

371. Mandel J, Mark EJ, Hales CA. Pulmonary veno-occlusive disease. Am J Respir Crit Care Med 2000; 162:1964–1973.

372. Holcomb BW Jr, Loyd JE, Ely EW, et al. Pulmonary veno-occlusive disease: a case series and new observations. Chest 2000;118:1671–1679.

373. Runo JR, Vnencak-Jones CL, Prince M, et al. Pulmonary veno-occlusive disease caused by an inherited mutation in bone morphogenetic protein receptor II. Am J Respir Crit Care Med 2003;167:889–894.

374. Cohn RC, Wong R, Spohn WA, et al. Death due to diffuse alveolar hemorrhage in a child with pulmonary veno-occlusive disease. Chest 1991;100:1456–1458.

375. Wagenvoort CA, Wagenvoort N. The pathology of pulmonary veno-occlusive disease. Virchows Arch A Pathol Anat Histol 1974;364:69–79.

376. Harris P, Heath D. The human pulmonary circulation, 3rd edn. Edinburgh: Churchill Livingstone, 1986.

377. Rambihar VS, Fallen EL, Cairns JA. Pulmonary veno-occlusive disease: antemortem diagnosis from roentgenographic and hemodynamic findings. Can Med Assoc J 1979; 120:1519–1522.

378. Rosenthal A, Vawter G, Wagenvoort CA. Intrapulmonary veno-occlusive disease. Am J Cardiol 1973;31:78–83.

379. Shackelford GD, Sacks EJ, Mullins JD, et al. Pulmonary venoocclusive disease: case report and review of the literature. AJR Am J Roentgenol 1977;128:643–648.

380. de Vries TW, Weening JJ, Roorda RJ. Pulmonary veno-occlusive disease: a case report and a review of therapeutic possibilities. Eur Respir J 1991;4: 1029–1032.

381. Hackman RC, Madtes DK, Petersen FB, et al. Pulmonary venoocclusive disease following bone marrow transplantation. Transplantation 1989;47:989–992.

382. Palevsky HI, Pietra GG, Fishman AP. Pulmonary veno-occlusive disease and its response to vasodilator agents. Am Rev Respir Dis 1990;142:426–429.

383. Salzman GA, Rosa UW. Prolonged survival in pulmonary veno-occlusive disease treated with nifedipine. Chest 1989;95:1154–1156.

384. Palmer SM, Robinson LJ, Wang A, et al. Massive pulmonary edema and death after prostacylin infusion in a patient with pulmonary veno-occlusive disease. Chest 1998;113:237–240.

385. Cassart M, Gevenois PA, Kramer M, et al. Pulmonary venoocclusive disease: CT findings before and after single-lung transplantation. AJR Am J Roentgenol 1993;160:759–760.

386. Swensen SJ, Tashjian JH, Myers JL, et al. Pulmonary venoocclusive disease: CT findings in eight patients. AJR Am J Roentgenol 1996;167:937–940.

387. Veeraraghavan S, Koss MN, Sharma OP. Pulmonary veno-occlusive disease. Curr Opin Pulm Med 1999;5:310–313.

388. Thadani U, Burrow C, Whitaker W, et al. Pulmonary veno-occlusive disease. Q J Med 1975;44:133–159.

389. Okubo S, Kunieda T, Ando M, et al. Idiopathic isolated pulmonary arteritis with chronic cor pulmonale. Chest 1988;94:665–666.

390. Lupi-Herrera E, Sanchez-Torres G, Marcushamer J, et al. Takayasu's arteritis. Clinical study of 107 cases. Am Heart J 1977;93:94–103.

391. Creager MA. Takayasu arteritis. Rev Cardiovasc Med 2001;2:211–214.

392. Kawai C, Ishikawa K, Kato M, et al. "Pulmonary pulseless disease": pulmonary involvement in so-called Takayasu's disease. Chest 1978;73:651–657.

393. Lupi E, Sanchez G, Horwitz S, et al. Pulmonary artery involvement in Takayasu's arteritis. Chest 1975;67:69–74.

394. Yamada I, Shibuya H, Matsubara O, et al. Pulmonary artery disease in Takayasu's arteritis: angiographic findings. AJR Am J Roentgenol 1992;159:263–269.

395. Yamato M, Lecky JW, Hiramatsu K, et al. Takayasu arteritis: radiographic and angiographic findings in 59 patients. Radiology 1986;161:329–334.

396. Berkmen YM, Lande A. Chest roentgenography as a window to the diagnosis of Takayasu's arteritis. AJR Am J Roentgenol 1975;125:842–846.

397. Gradden C, McWilliams R, Gould D, et al. Multiple stenting in Takayasu arteritis. J Endovasc Ther 2002;9:936–940.

398. Both M, Jahnke T, Reinhold-Keller E, et al. Percutaneous management of occlusive arterial disease associated with vasculitis: a single center experience. Cardiovasc Intervent Radiol 2003; 26:19–26.

399. Yamada I, Numano F, Suzuki S. Takayasu arteritis: evaluation with MR imaging. Radiology 1993;188:89–94.

400. Park JH, Chung JW, Im JG, et al. Takayasu arteritis: evaluation of mural changes in the aorta and pulmonary artery with CT angiography. Radiology 1995;196:89–93.

401. Speich R, Jenni R, Opravil M, et al. Primary pulmonary hypertension in HIV infection. Chest 1991;100:1268–1271.

402. Petrosillo N, Pellicelli AM, Boumis E, et al. Clinical manifestation of HIV-related pulmonary hypertension. Ann N Y Acad Sci 2001;946:223–235.

403. Bugnone AN, Viamonte M Jr, Garcia H. Imaging findings in human immunodeficiency virus-related pulmonary hypertension: report of five cases and review of the literature. Radiology 2002;223:820–827.

404. Mette SA, Palevsky HI, Pietra GG, et al. Primary pulmonary hypertension in association with human immunodeficiency virus infection. A possible viral etiology for some forms of hypertensive pulmonary arteriopathy. Am Rev Respir Dis 1992;145:1196–1200.

405. Pellicelli AM, Palmieri F, Cicalini S, et al. Pathogenesis of HIV-related pulmonary hypertension. Ann N Y Acad Sci 2001; 946:82–94.

406. Matthay RA, Berger HJ. Cardiovascular function in cor pulmonale. Clin Chest Med 1983;4:269–295.

407. Cromie JB. Correlation of anatomic pulmonary emphysema and right ventricular hypertrophy. Am Rev Respir Dis 1961;84:657–662.

408. Hicken P, Heath D, Brewer D. The relation between the weight of the right ventricle and the percentage of abnormal air space in the lung in emphysema. J Pathol Bacteriol 1966;92:519–528.

409. Pattynama PM, Willems LN, Smit AH, et al. Early diagnosis of cor pulmonale with MR imaging of the right ventricle. Radiology 1992;182:375–379.

410. Turnbull LW, Ridgway JP, Biernacki W, et al. Assessment of the right ventricle by magnetic resonance imaging in chronic obstructive lung disease. Thorax 1990;45:597–601.

411. Stevens D, Sharma K, Szidon P, et al. Severe pulmonary hypertension associated with COPD. Ann Transplant 2000;5:8–12.

412. Migueres M, Escamilla R, Coca F, et al. Pulsed Doppler echocardiography in the diagnosis of pulmonary hypertension in COPD. Chest 1990;98:280–285.

413. Zompatori M, Battaglia M, Rimondi MR, et al. Hemodynamic estimation of chronic cor pulmonale by Doppler echocardiography. Clinical value and comparison with other noninvasive imaging techniques. Rays 1997;22:73–93.

414. Denton CP, Cailes JB, Phillips GD, et al. Comparison of Doppler echocardiography and right heart catheterization to assess pulmonary hypertension in systemic sclerosis. Br J Rheumatol 1997;36:239–243.

415. Torbicki A, Skwarski K, Hawrylkiewicz I, et al. Attempts at measuring pulmonary arterial pressure by means of Doppler echocardiography in patients with chronic lung disease. Eur Respir J 1989;2:856–860.

416. Rees RS, Jefferson KE. The Eisenmenger syndrome. Clin Radiol 1967;18:366–371.

417. Fishman AP. State of the art: chronic cor pulmonale. Am Rev Respir Dis 1976; 114:775–794.

418. Michael JR, Summer WR. Pulmonary hypertension. Lung 1985;163:65–82.

419. Sugerman HJ. Pulmonary function in morbid obesity. Gastroenterol Clin North Am 1987;16:225–237.

420. Zwillich CW, Sutton FD, Pierson DJ, et al. Decreased hypoxic ventilatory drive in the obesity-hypoventilation syndrome. Am J Med 1975;59:343–348.

421. Ahmed Q, Chung-Park M, Tomashefski JF Jr. Cardiopulmonary pathology in patients with sleep apnea/obesity hypoventilation syndrome. Hum Pathol 1997;28:264–269.

422. Ghio AJ, Meyer GA, Crapo RO. Association of pulmonary artery size on chest radiograph with residence at elevated altitudes. J Thorac Imaging 1996;11:53–57.

423. Remy J, Lemaitre L, Lafitte JJ, et al. Massive hemoptysis of pulmonary arterial origin: diagnosis and treatment. AJR Am J Roentgenol 1984;143:963–969.

424. Auerbach O. Pathology and pathogenesis of pulmonary arterial aneurysm in tuberculous cavities. Am Rev Tuberc 1939;39:99–115.

425. Gibson RN, Morgan SH, Krauz T, et al. Pulmonary artery aneurysms in Behcet's disease. Br J Radiol 1985;58:79–82.

426. Dillon WP, Taylor AT, Mineau DE, et al. Traumatic pulmonary artery pseudoaneurysm simulating pulmonary embolism. AJR Am J Roentgenol 1982;139:818–819.

427. Ferretti GR, Thony F, Link KM, et al. False aneurysm of the pulmonary artery induced by a Swan–Ganz catheter: clinical presentation and radiologic management. AJR Am J Roentgenol 1996;167:941–945.

428. Guttentag AR, Shepard JA, McLoud TC. Catheter-induced pulmonary artery pseudoaneurysm: the halo sign on CT. AJR Am J Roentgenol 1992;158:637–639.

429. Shilkin KB, Low LP, Chen BT. Dissecting aneurysm of the pulmonary artery. J Pathol 1969;98:25–29.

430. Hartshorne MF, Eisenberg B. CT diagnosis of a giant central pulmonary artery aneurysm arising quickly after pulmonary embolic disease [letter]. AJR Am J Roentgenol 1989;153:190–191.

431. Oliver TB, Stevenson AJ, Gillespie IN. Pulmonary artery pseudoaneurysm due to bronchial carcinoma. Br J Radiol 1997;70:950–951.

432. Geddes DM, Kerr IH. Pulmonary arterial aneurysms in association with a right ventricular myxoma. Br J Radiol 1976;49:374–376.

433. Iula G, Ziviello R, Del Vecchio W. Aneurysms of proximal pulmonary arteries: CT diagnosis and preoperative assessment. Eur Radiol 1996;6:730–733.

434. Iula G, Ziviello R, Del Vecchio W. Aneurysms of proximal pulmonary arteries: CT diagnosis and preoperative assessment. Eur Radiol 1996;6:730–733.

435. Berthelot P, Walker JG, Sherlock S, et al. Arterial changes in the lungs in cirrhosis of the liver – lung spider nevi. N Engl J Med 1966;274:291–298.

436. Sano A, Kuroda Y, Moriyasu F, et al. Porto-pulmonary venous anastomosis in

portal hypertension demonstrated by percutaneous transhepatic cine-portography. Radiology 1982;144: 479–484.

437. Lange PA, Stoller JK. The hepatopulmonary syndrome. Ann Intern Med 1995;122:521–529.

438. Krowka MJ. Pathophysiology of arterial hypoxemia in advanced liver disease. Liver Transpl Surg 1996;2:308–312.

439. Krowka MJ, Cortese DA. Hepatopulmonary syndrome. Current concepts in diagnostic and therapeutic considerations. Chest 1994;105: 1528–1537.

440. Bank ER, Thrall JH, Dantzker DR. Radionuclide demonstration of intrapulmonary shunting in cirrhosis. AJR Am J Roentgenol 1983;140:967–969.

441. Wolfe JD, Tashkin DP, Holly FE, et al. Hypoxemia of cirrhosis: detection of abnormal small pulmonary vascular channels by a quantitative radionuclide method. Am J Med 1977;63:746–754.

442. McAdams HP, Erasmus J, Crockett R, et al. The hepatopulmonary syndrome: radiologic findings in 10 patients. AJR Am J Roentgenol 1996;166:1379–1385.

443. Lee KN, Lee HJ, Shin WW, et al. Hypoxemia and liver cirrhosis (hepatopulmonary syndrome) in eight patients: comparison of the central and peripheral pulmonary vasculature. Radiology 1999;211:549–553.

444. Haupt HM, Moore GW, Bauer TW, et al. The lung in sickle cell disease. Chest 1982;81:332–337.

445. Barrett-Connor E. Pneumonia and pulmonary infarction in sickle cell anemia. JAMA 1973;224:997–1000.

446. Leong CS, Stark P. Thoracic manifestations of sickle cell disease. J Thorac Imaging 1998;13:128–134.

447. Poncz M, Kane E, Gill FM. Acute chest syndrome in sickle cell disease: etiology and clinical correlates. J Pediatr 1985;107:861–866.

448. Barrett-Connor E. Acute pulmonary disease and sickle cell anemia. Am Rev Respir Dis 1971;104:159–165.

449. Maitre B, Habibi A, Roudot-Thoraval F, et al. Acute chest syndrome in adults with sickle cell disease. Chest 2000;117:1386–1392.

450. Platt OS. The acute chest syndrome of sickle cell disease. N Engl J Med 2000;342:1904–1907.

451. Martin L, Buonomo C. Acute chest syndrome of sickle cell disease: radiographic and clinical analysis of 70 cases. Pediatr Radiol 1997;27:637–641.

452. Vichinsky EP, Neumayr LD, Earles AN, et al. Causes and outcomes of the acute chest syndrome in sickle cell disease. National Acute Chest Syndrome Study Group. N Engl J Med 2000;342:1855–1865.

453. Charache S, Scott JC, Charache P. "Acute chest syndrome" in adults with sickle cell anemia. Microbiology, treatment, and prevention. Arch Intern Med 1979;139:67–69.

454. Davies SC, Luce PJ, Win AA, et al. Acute chest syndrome in sickle-cell disease. Lancet 1984;1:36–38.

455. Oppenheimer EH, Esterly JR. Pulmonary changes in sickle cell disease. Am Rev Respir Dis 1971;103:858–859.

456. Smith JA. Cardiopulmonary manifestations of sickle cell disease in childhood. Semin Roentgenol 1987;22:160–167.

457. Gelfand MJ, Daya SA, Rucknagel DL, et al. Simultaneous occurrence of rib infarction and pulmonary infiltrates in sickle cell disease patients with acute chest syndrome. J Nucl Med 1993; 34:614–618.

458. Cockshott WP. Rib infarcts in sickling disease. Eur J Radiol 1992;14:63–66.

459. Varat MA, Adolph RJ, Fowler NO. Cardiovascular effects of anemia. Am Heart J 1972;83:415–426.

460. Balfour IC, Covitz W, Davis H, et al. Cardiac size and function in children with sickle cell anemia. Am Heart J 1984;108:345–350.

461. Lindsay J Jr, Meshel JC, Patterson RH. The cardiovascular manifestations of sickle cell disease. Arch Intern Med 1974;133:643–651.

462. Castro O, Hoque M, Brown BD. Pulmonary hypertension in sickle cell disease: cardiac catheterization results and survival. Blood 2003;101:1257–1261.

463. Haque AK, Gokhale S, Rampy BA, et al. Pulmonary hypertension in sickle cell hemoglobinopathy: a clinicopathologic study of 20 cases. Hum Pathol 2002;33: 1037–1043.

464. Bhalla M, Abboud MR, McLoud TC, et al. Acute chest syndrome in sickle cell disease: CT evidence of microvascular occlusion. Radiology 1993;187:45–49.

465. Aquino SL, Gamsu G, Fahy JV, et al. Chronic pulmonary disorders in sickle cell disease: findings at thin-section CT. Radiology 1994;193:807–811.

466. Matthay MA. Pathophysiology of pulmonary edema. Clin Chest Med 1985;6:301–314.

467. Sprung CL, Rackow EC, Fein IA, et al. The spectrum of pulmonary edema: differentiation of cardiogenic, intermediate, and noncardiogenic forms of pulmonary edema. Am Rev Respir Dis 1981;124:718–722.

468. Goodman LR. Congestive heart failure and adult respiratory distress syndrome. New insights using computed tomography. Radiol Clin North Am 1996;34:33–46.

469. Gluecker T, Capasso P, Schnyder P, et al. Clinical and radiologic features of pulmonary edema. RadioGraphics 1999;19:1507–1531.

470. Saxon RR, Klein JS, Bar MH, et al. Pathogenesis of pulmonary edema during interleukin-2 therapy: correlation of chest radiographic and clinical findings in 54 patients. AJR Am J Roentgenol 1991;156:281–285.

471. Ketai LH, Godwin JD. A new view of pulmonary edema and acute respiratory distress syndrome. J Thorac Imaging 1998;13:147–171.

472. Turner AF, Lau FYK, Jacobson G. A method for the estimation of pulmonary venous and arterial pressures from the routine chest roentgenograms. AJR Am J Roentgenol 1972;116:97–106.

473. Jefferson K, Rees S, eds. Clinical cardiac radiology. London: Butterworths, 1973.

474. Woodring JH. Pulmonary artery-bronchus ratios in patients with normal lungs pulmonary vascular plethora, and congestive heart failure. Radiology 1991;179:115–122.

475. West JB, Dollery CT, Heard BE. Increased pulmonary vascular resistance in the dependent zone of isolated dog lung caused by perivascular edema. Circ Res 1965;17:191–206.

476. Norgaard H, Gjorup T, Brems-Dalgaard E, et al. Interobserver variation in the detection of pulmonary venous hypertension in chest radiographs. Eur J Radiol 1990;11:203–206.

477. Baumstark A, Swensson RG, Hessel SJ, et al. Evaluating the radiographic assessment of pulmonary venous hypertension in chronic heart disease. AJR Am J Roentgenol 1984;141:877–884.

478. Milne ENC, Pistolesi M, Miniati M, et al. The radiologic distinction of cardiogenic and noncardiogenic edema. AJR Am J Roentgenol 1985;144:879–894.

479. Harrison MO, Conte PJ, Heitzman ER. Radiological detection of clinically occult cardiac failure following myocardial infarction. Br J Radiol 1971;44: 265–272.

480. Pistolesi M, Miniati M, Milne ENC, et al. The chest roentgenogram in pulmonary edema. Clin Chest Med 1985;6:315–344.

481. Pistolesi M, Giuntini C. Assessment of extravascular lung water. Radiol Clin North Am 1978;16:551–574.

482. Storto ML, Kee ST, Golden JA, et al. Hydrostatic pulmonary edema: high-resolution CT findings. AJR Am J Roentgenol 1995;165:817–820.

483. Brasileiro FC, Vargas FS, Kavakama JI, et al. High-resolution CT scan in the evaluation of exercise-induced interstitial pulmonary edema in cardiac patients. Chest 1997;111:1577–1582.

484. Primack SL, Müller NL, Mayo JR, et al. Pulmonary parenchymal abnormalities of vascular origin: high-resolution CT findings. RadioGraphics 1994;14:739–746.

485. Don C, Johnson R. The nature and significance of peribronchial cuffing in pulmonary edema. Radiology 1977;125:577–582.

486. Schnur MJ, Winkler B, Austin JH. Thickening of the posterior wall of the bronchus intermedius. A sign on lateral radiographs of congestive heart failure, lymph node enlargement, and neoplastic infiltration. Radiology 1981;139:551–559.

487. Arai K, Takashima T, Matsui O, et al. Transient subpleural curvilinear shadow caused by pulmonary congestion. J Comput Assist Tomogr 1990;14:87–88.

488. Kato S, Nakamoto T, Iizuka M. Early diagnosis and estimation of pulmonary congestion and edema in patients with left-sided heart diseases from histogram of pulmonary CT number. Chest 1996;109:1439–1445.

489. Mayo JR, MacKay AL, Whittall KP, et al. Measurement of lung water content and pleural pressure gradient with magnetic resonance imaging. J Thorac Imaging 1995;10:73–81.

490. Slanetz PJ, Truong M, Shepard JA, et al. Mediastinal lymphadenopathy and hazy mediastinal fat: new CT findings of congestive heart failure. AJR Am J Roentgenol 1998;171:1307–1309.

491. Youngberg AS. Unilateral diffuse lung opacity; Differential diagnosis with emphasis on lymphangitic spread of cancer. Radiology 1977;123:277–281.

492. Schnyder PA, Sarraj AM, Duvoisin BE, et al. Pulmonary edema associated with mitral regurgitation: prevalence of predominant involvement of the right upper lobe. AJR Am J Roentgenol 1993;161:33–36.

493. Greatrex KV, Fisher MS. Sparing of some accessory lobes in diffuse pulmonary edema. J Thorac Imaging 1997;12:78–79.

494. Zwikler MP, Peters TM, Michel RP. Effects of pulmonary fibrosis on the distribution of edema. Computed tomographic scanning and morphology. Am J Respir Crit Care Med 1994;149:1266–1275.

495. Saleh M, Miles AI, Lasser RP. Unilateral pulmonary edema in Swyer-James syndrome. Chest 1974;66:594–597.

496. Iancu DM, Zwikler MP, Michel RP. Distribution of alveolar edema in ventilated and unventilated canine lung lobes. Invest Radiol 1996;31:423–432.

497. Zimmerman JE, Goodman LR, St Andre AC, et al. Radiographic detection of mobilizable lung water: the gravitational shift test. AJR Am J Roentgenol 1982;138:59–64.

498. Bernard GR, Artigas A, Brigham KL, et al. The American-European Consensus Conference on ARDS. Definitions, mechanisms, relevant outcomes, and clinical trial coordination. Am J Respir Crit Care Med 1994;149:818–824.

499. Divertie MB. The adult respiratory distress syndrome. Mayo Clin Proc 1982;57:371–378.

500. Goodman LR, Fumagalli R, Tagliabue P, et al. Adult respiratory distress syndrome due to pulmonary and extrapulmonary causes: CT, clinical, and functional correlations. Radiology 1999;213:545–552.

501. Aldridge AJ. Role of the neutrophil in septic shock and the adult respiratory distress syndrome. Eur J Surg 2002;168:204–214.

502. Greene R. Adult respiratory distress syndrome: acute alveolar damage. Radiology 1987;163:57–66.

503. Tomashefski JF Jr. Pulmonary pathology of the adult respiratory distress syndrome. Clin Chest Med 1990;11:593–619.

504. Bachofen M, Weibel ER. Structural alterations of lung parenchyma in the adult respiratory distress syndrome. Clin Chest Med 1982;3:35–56.

505. Vesconi S, Rossi GP, Pesenti A, et al. Pulmonary microthrombosis in severe adult respiratory distress syndrome. Crit Care Med 1988;16:111–113.

506. Pinhu L, Whitehead T, Evans T, et al. Ventilator-associated lung injury. Lancet 2003;361:332–340.

507. Desai SR, Wells AU, Rubens MB, et al. Acute respiratory distress syndrome: CT abnormalities at long-term follow-up. Radiology 1999;210:29–35.

508. Wegenius G, Erjkson U, Borg T, et al. Value of chest radiography in adult respiratory distress syndrome. Acta Radiol 1984;25:177–184.

509. Iannuzzi M, Petty TL. The diagnosis, pathogenesis, and treatment of adult respiratory distress syndrome. J Thorac Imaging 1986;1:1–10.

510. Goodman PC. Radiographic findings in patients with acute respiratory distress syndrome. Clin Chest Med 2000;21:419–33, vii.

511. Desai SR. Acute respiratory distress syndrome: imaging of the injured lung. Clin Radiol 2002;57:8–17.

512. Winer-Muram HT, Rubin SA, Ellis JV, et al. Pneumonia and ARDS in patients receiving mechanical ventilation: diagnostic accuracy of chest radiography. Radiology 1993;188:479–485.

513. Padley SP, Jordan SJ, Goldstraw P, et al. Asymmetric ARDS following pulmonary resection: CT findings initial observations. Radiology 2002;223:468–473.

514. Bombino M, Gattinoni L, Pesenti A, et al. The value of portable chest roentgenography in adult respiratory distress syndrome. Comparison with computed tomography. Chest 1991;100:762–769.

515. Rubenfeld GD, Caldwell E, Granton J, et al. Interobserver variability in applying a radiographic definition for ARDS. Chest 1999;116:1347–1353.

516. Bekemeyer WB, Calhoon S, Crapo RO, et al. Efficacy of chest radiography in a respiratory intensive care unit. Chest 1985;88:691–696.

517. Strain DS, Kinasewitz GT, Vereen LE, et al. Value of routine daily chest x-rays in the medical intensive care unit. Crit Care Med 1985;13:534–536.

518. Tagliabue M, Casella TC, Zincone GE, et al. CT and chest radiography in the evaluation of adult respiratory distress syndrome. Acta Radiol 1994;35:230–234.

519. Gattinoni L, Caironi P, Pelosi P, et al. What has computed tomography taught us about the acute respiratory distress syndrome? Am J Respir Crit Care Med 2001;164:1701–1711.

520. Maunder RJ, Shuman WP, McHugh JW, et al. Preservation of normal lung regions in the adult respiratory distress syndrome: analysis by computed tomography. JAMA 1986;255:2463–2465.

521. Marini JJ. Lung mechanics in the adult respiratory distress syndrome: recent conceptual advances and implications for management. Clin Chest Med 1990;11:673–690.

522. Marini JJ. New approaches to the ventilatory management of the adult respiratory distress syndrome. J Crit Care 1992;7:256–267.

523. Puybasset L, Cluzel P, Gusman P, et al. Regional distribution of gas and tissue in acute respiratory distress syndrome. I. Consequences for lung morphology. CT Scan ARDS Study Group. Intensive Care Med 2000;26:857–869.

524. Gattinoni L, Pelosi P, Vitale G, et al. Body position changes redistribute lung computed-tomographic density in patients with acute respiratory failure. Anesthesiology 1991;74:15–23.

525. Puybasset L, Cluzel P, Chao N, et al. A computed tomography scan assessment of regional lung volume in acute lung injury. The CT Scan ARDS Study Group. Am J Respir Crit Care Med 1998;158:1644–1655.

526. Gattinoni L, Pelosi P, Pesenti A, et al. CT scan in ARDS: clinical and physiopathological insights. Acta Anaesthesiol Scand 1991;35 (Suppl 95):87–96.

527. Langer M, Mascheroni D, Marcolin R, et al. The prone position in ARDS patients. Chest 1988;94:103–107.

528. Gattinoni L, Tognoni G, Pesenti A, et al. Effect of prone positioning on the survival of patients with acute respiratory failure. N Engl J Med 2001;345:568–573.

529. Pelosi P, Brazzi L, Gattinoni L. Prone position in acute respiratory distress syndrome. Eur Respir J 2002;20:1017–1028.

530. Gattinoni L, Pesenti A, Bombino M, et al. Relationships between lung computed tomography density, gas exchange, and PEEP in acute respiratory failure. Anesthesiology 1988;69:824–832.

531. Desai SR, Wells AU, Suntharalingam G, et al. Acute respiratory distress syndrome caused by pulmonary and extrapulmonary injury: a comparative CT study. Radiology 2001;218:689–693.

532. Rouby JJ, Puybasset L, Cluzel P, et al. Regional distribution of gas and tissue in acute respiratory distress syndrome. II. Physiological correlations and definition of an ARDS Severity Score. CT Scan ARDS Study Group. Intensive Care Med 2000;26:1046–1056.

533. Murayama S, Murakami J, Yabuuchi H, et al. "Crazy paving appearance" on high resolution CT in various diseases. J Comput Assist Tomogr 1999;23: 749–752.

534. Howling SJ, Evans TW, Hansell DM. The significance of bronchial dilatation on CT in patients with adult respiratory distress syndrome. Clin Radiol 1998; 53:105–109.

535. Gattinoni L, Presenti A, Torresin A, et al. Adult respiratory distress syndrome profiles by computed tomography. J Thorac Imaging 1986;1:25–30.

536. Gattinoni L, Pesenti A, Avalli L, et al. Pressure-volume curve of total respiratory system in acute respiratory failure. Computed tomographic scan study. Am Rev Respir Dis 1987;136:730–736.

537. Gattinoni L, D'Andrea L, Pelosi P, et al. Regional effects and mechanism of positive end-expiratory pressure in early adult respiratory distress syndrome. JAMA 1993;269:2122–2127.

538. Bone RC. The ARDS lung. New insights from computed tomography. JAMA 1993;269:2134–2135.

539. Puybasset L, Gusman P, Müller JC, et al. Regional distribution of gas and tissue in acute respiratory distress syndrome. III. Consequences for the effects of positive end-expiratory pressure. CT Scan ARDS Study Group. Adult Respiratory Distress Syndrome. Intensive Care Med 2000;26: 1215–1227.

540. Prella M, Feihl F, Domenighetti G. Effects of short-term pressure-controlled ventilation on gas exchange, airway pressures, and gas distribution in patients with acute lung injury/ARDS: comparison with volume-controlled ventilation. Chest 2002;122:1382–1388.

541. Gattinoni L, Bombino M, Pelosi P, et al. Lung structure and function in different stages of severe adult respiratory distress syndrome. JAMA 1994;271: 1772–1779.

542. Thomason JW, Ely EW, Chiles C, et al. Appraising pulmonary edema using supine chest roentgenograms in ventilated patients. Am J Respir Crit Care Med 1998;157:1600–1608.

543. Petty TL. Indicators of risk, course, and prognosis in adult respiratory distress syndrome (ARDS). Am Rev Respir Dis 1985;132:471.

544. Abel SJ, Finney SJ, Brett SJ, et al. Reduced mortality in association with the acute respiratory distress syndrome (ARDS). Thorax 1998;53:292–294.

545. Andrews CP, Coalson JJ, Smith JD, et al. Diagnosis of nosocomial bacterial pneumonia in acute, diffuse lung injury. Chest 1981;80:254–258.

546. Henschke CI, Yankelevitz DF, Wand A, et al. Accuracy and efficacy of chest radiography in the intensive care unit. Radiol Clin North Am 1996;34:21–31.

547. Winer-Muram HT, Jennings SG, Wunderink RG, et al. Ventilator-associated Pseudomonas aeruginosa pneumonia: radiographic findings. Radiology 1995;195:247–252.

548. Winer-Muram HT, Steiner RM, Gurney JW, et al. Ventilator-associated pneumonia in patients with adult respiratory distress syndrome: CT evaluation. Radiology 1998;208: 193–199.

549. Alberts WM, Priest GR, Moser KM. The outlook for survivors of ARDS. Chest 1983;84:272–274.

550. Ghio AJ, Elliott G, Crapo RO, et al. Impairment after adult respiratory distress syndrome. Am Rev Respir Dis 1989;139:1158–1162.

551. Owens CM, Evans TW, Keogh BF, et al. Computed tomography in established adult respiratory distress syndrome. Chest 1994;106:1815–1821.

552. Nobauer-Huhmann IM, Eibenberger K, Schaefer-Prokop C, et al. Changes in lung parenchyma after acute respiratory distress syndrome (ARDS): assessment with high-resolution computed tomography. Eur Radiol 2001;11: 2436–2443.

553. Simon RP, Gean-Marton AD, Sander JE. Medullary lesion inducing pulmonary edema: a magnetic resonance imaging study. Ann Neurol 1991;30:727–730.

554. Lin TY, Chang LY, Hsia SH, et al. The 1998 enterovirus 71 outbreak in Taiwan: pathogenesis and management. Clin Infect Dis 2002;34 (Suppl 2):S52–S57.

555. Colice GL, Matthay MA, Bass E, et al. Neurogenic pulmonary edema. Am Rev Respir Dis 1984;130:941–948.

556. Simon RP. Neurogenic pulmonary edema. Neurol Clin 1993;11:309–323.

557. Felman AH. Neurogenic pulmonary edema: observations in 6 patients. AJR Am J Roentgenol 1971;112:393–396.

558. Lockhart A, Saiag B. Altitude and the human pulmonary circulation. Clin Sci (Lond) 1981;60:599–605.

559. Hultgren HN. High-altitude pulmonary edema: current concepts. Ann Rev Med 1996;47:267–284.

560. Gabry AL, Ledoux X, Mozziconacci M, et al. High-altitude pulmonary edema at moderate altitude (< 2,400 m; 7,870 feet): a series of 52 patients. Chest 2003;123: 49–53.

561. Marticorena E, Tapia FA, Dyer J, et al. Pulmonary edema by ascending to high altitudes. Dis Chest 1964;45:273–283.

562. Hultgren HN, Lopez CE, Lundberg E, et al. Physiologic studies of pulmonary edema at high altitude. Circulation 1985;29:393–408.

563. Mulder JI. Amniotic fluid embolism: an overview and case report. Am J Obstet Gynecol 1985;152:430–435.

564. Kleger GR, Bartsch P, Vock P, et al. Evidence against an increase in capillary permeability in subjects exposed to high altitude. J Appl Physiol 1996;81: 1917–1923.

565. Maldonado D. High altitude pulmonary edema. Radiol Clin North Am 1978;16: 537–549.

566. Vock P, Brutsche MH, Nanzer A, et al. Variable radiomorphologic data of high altitude pulmonary edema. Features from 60 patients. Chest 1991;100:1306–1311.

567. Khan AS, Khabbaz RF, Armstrong LR, et al. Hantavirus pulmonary syndrome: the first 100 US cases. J Infect Dis 1996;173:1297–1303.

568. Peters CJ, Simpson GL, Levy H. Spectrum of hantavirus infection: hemorrhagic fever with renal syndrome and hantavirus pulmonary syndrome. Annu Rev Med 1999;50:531–545.

569. Boroja M, Barrie JR, Raymond GS. Radiographic findings in 20 patients with Hantavirus pulmonary syndrome correlated with clinical outcome. AJR Am J Roentgenol 2002;178:159–163.

570. Ketai LH, Williamson MR, Telepak RJ, et al. Hantavirus pulmonary syndrome: radiographic findings in 16 patients. Radiology 1994;191:665–668.

571. Ketai LH, Kelsey CA, Jordan K, et al. Distinguishing Hantavirus pulmonary syndrome from acute respiratory distress syndrome by chest radiography: are there different radiographic manifestations of increased permeability. J Thorac Imaging 1998;13:172–177.

572. Koster F, Foucar K, Hjelle B, et al. Rapid presumptive diagnosis of hantavirus cardiopulmonary syndrome by peripheral blood smear review. Am J Clin Pathol 2001;116:665–672.

573. Jackson FN, Rowland V, Corssen G. Laryngospasm-induced pulmonary edema. Chest 1980;78:819–821.

574. Travis KW, Todres ID, Shannon DC. Pulmonary edema associated with croup and epiglottitis. Pediatrics 1977;59: 695–698.

575. Chaudhary BA, Ferguson DS, Speir WA Jr. Pulmonary edema as a presenting feature of sleep apnea syndrome. Chest 1982;82:122–124.

576. Oudjhane K, Bowen A, Oh KS, et al. Pulmonary edema complicating upper airway obstruction in infants and children. Can Assoc Radiol J 1992;43:278–282.

577. Van Kooy MA, Gargiulo RF. Postobstructive pulmonary edema. Am Fam Physician 2000;62:401–404.

578. Cascade PN, Alexander GD, Mackie DS. Negative-pressure pulmonary edema after endotracheal intubation. Radiology 1993;186:671–675.

579. Lathan SR, Silverman ME, Thomas BL, et al. Postoperative pulmonary edema. South Med J 1999;92:313–315.

580. Burke AJ, Duke SG, Clyne S, et al. Incidence of pulmonary edema after tracheotomy for obstructive sleep apnea. Otolaryngol Head Neck Surg 2001;125:319–323.

581. Tarver RD, Broderick LS, Conces DJ Jr. Reexpansion pulmonary edema. J Thorac Imaging 1996;11:198–209.

582. Sherman SC. Reexpansion pulmonary edema: a case report and review of the current literature. J Emerg Med 2003;24:23–27.

583. Iqbal M, Multz AS, Rossoff LJ, et al. Reexpansion pulmonary edema after VATS successfully treated with continuous positive airway pressure. Ann Thorac Surg 2000;70:669–671.

584. Yanagidate F, Dohi S, Hamaya Y, et al. Reexpansion pulmonary edema after thoracoscopic mediastinal tumor resection. Anesth Analg 2001;92:1416–1417.

585. Sewell RW, Fewel JG, Grover FL, et al. Experimental evaluation of reexpansion pulmonary edema. Ann Thorac Surg 1978;26:126–132.

586. Tan HC, Mak KH, Johan A, et al. Cardiac output increases prior to development of pulmonary edema after re-expansion of spontaneous pneumothorax. Respir Med 2002;96:461–465.

587. Woodring JH. Focal reexpansion pulmonary edema after drainage of large pleural effusions: clinical evidence suggesting hypoxic injury to the lung as the cause of edema. South Med J 1997;90:1176–1182.

588. Heller BJ, Grathwohl MK. Contralateral reexpansion pulmonary edema. South Med J 2000;93:828–831.

589. Henderson AF, Banham SW, Moran F. Re-expansion pulmonary oedema: a potentially serious complication of delayed diagnosis of pneumothorax. Br Med J (Clin Res Ed) 1985;291:593–594.

590. Jenkinson SG. Pneumothorax. Clin Chest Med 1985;6:153–161.

591. Sautter RD, Dreher WH, MacIndoe JH, et al. Fatal pulmonary edema and pneumonitis after reexpansion of chronic pneumothorax. Chest 1971;60:399–401.

592. Sherman S, Ravikrishnan KP. Unilateral pulmonary edema following re-expansion of pneumothorax of brief duration. Chest 1980;77:714.

593. Ziskind MM, Weill H, George RA. Acute pulmonary edema following the treatment of spontaneous pneumothorax with excessive negative intrapleural pressure. Am Rev Respir Dis 1965;92:632–636.

594. Humphreys RL, Berne AS. Rapid re-expansion of pneumothorax. A cause of unilateral pulmonary edema. Radiology 1970;96:509–512.

595. Waqaruddin M, Bernstein A. Re-expansion pulmonary oedema. Thorax 1975;30:54–60.

596. Shaw TJ, Caterine JM. Recurrent re-expansion pulmonary edema. Chest 1984;86:784–786.

597. Miller WT, Osiason AW, Langlotz CP, et al. Reperfusion edema after thromboendarterectomy: radiographic patterns of disease. J Thorac Imaging 1998;13:178–183.

598. de Campos JR, Vargas FS, de Campos WE, et al. Thoracoscopy talc poudrage: a 15-year experience. Chest 2001;119:801–806.

599. Scalzetti EM. Unilateral pulmonary edema after talc pleurodesis. J Thorac Imaging 2001;16:99–102.

600. Peterson EP, Taylor HB. Amniotic fluid embolism. An analysis of 40 cases. Obstet Gynecol 1970;35:787–793.

601. Davies S. Amniotic fluid embolus: a review of the literature. Can J Anaesth 2001;48:88–98.

602. Green BT, Umana E. Amniotic fluid embolism. South Med J 2000;93:721–723.

603. Gilbert WM, Danielsen B. Amniotic fluid embolism: decreased mortality in a population-based study. Obstet Gynecol 1999;93:973–977.

Inhalational lung disease

Inhaled agents may cause injury to any part of the tracheo-bronchial tree or the lung parenchyma, depending on the physical characteristics of the agent (especially its physical state and particle size). Many inhaled agents will affect more than one compartment of the lung. For instance, inhaled cigarette smoke, the most common cause of inhalational lung injury, may cause tracheitis, bronchitis, bronchiolitis, and parenchymal inflammation and destruction. Other inhaled agents include mineral dusts which cause pneumoconiosis, organic agents causing hypersensitivity pneumonitis, noxious fumes, and aspirated fluids or solids.

SMOKING RELATED LUNG DISEASES

Respiratory bronchiolitis/respiratory bronchiolitis-interstitial lung disease

Respiratory bronchiolitis (RB) is a histopathologic lesion found in cigarette smokers, characterized by the presence of pigmented intraluminal macrophages within first and second order respiratory bronchioles. It is usually asymptomatic, and the histologic finding of RB is present at autopsy in virtually all cigarette smokers dying of incidental causes.[1] This histologic finding persists after stopping smoking, and was found in one-third of patients 5 years after discontinuing smoking, and in one patient who had stopped 32 years before.[2] Although usually due to cigarette smoking, RB may also be found in other inhalational lung diseases such as asbestosis.[3]

Respiratory bronchiolitis-interstitial lung disease (RB-ILD) occurs in heavy smokers when RB is extensive enough to cause symptoms and physiologic evidence of interstitial lung disease.[4–7] When a lung biopsy is performed, RB is the only histologic lesion identified. RB, RB-ILD, and desquamative interstitial pneumonia (DIP) are best regarded as a part of a continuum of smoking related lung injury (Table 8.1).[8,9] RB-ILD usually affects heavy smokers, with average exposures of over 30 pack years of cigarette smoking.

The radiographic findings of smoking related RB or RB-ILD are subtle and nonspecific. Airway wall thickening is usually present. The associated parenchymal abnormality is subtle and difficult to describe. It defies illustration. It has been variously described as reticular, reticulonodular, or ground-glass pattern.[4,7,10,11] Some have used the term "dirty lung"[12] to describe the prominence of bronchovascular structures, and slight blurring of bronchovascular outlines commonly seen in heavy smokers. This parenchymal abnormality appears to be due to a combination of thickening of the walls of bronchi and bronchioles, emphysema, and patchy ground-glass abnormality due to RB-ILD.[12]

On CT scanning, patients with asymptomatic RB generally show mild centrilobular nodularity and small patches of ground-glass attenuation (Fig. 8.1).[13] In RB-ILD, both of these findings, particularly the ground-glass attenuation, become more extensive (Fig. 8.2).[10] Emphysema and areas of decreased lung attenuation are commonly also present.[11] When patchy abnormalities of this type are present in heavy smokers with impaired pulmonary function, RB-ILD may be diagnosed with a high degree of confidence. The CT findings of RB-ILD are at least partially reversible in patients who stop smoking.[11] Remy-Jardin et al,[14] in a longitudinal study of smoking related CT changes, found that in patients with centrilobular micronodules who continued to smoke, these nodules most commonly either increased in profusion or evolved into areas of emphysema. Emphysema and ground-glass abnormality also increased in prevalence in those who continued to smoke. The presence of emphysema and/or ground-glass abnormality on a baseline scan was associated with a significantly more rapid decline in physiologic indices of airway obstruction.

The CT features of RB-ILD may be similar to those of hypersensitivity pneumonitis, DIP, and nonspecific interstitial

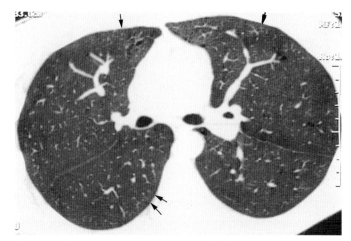

Fig. 8.1   Biopsy proven respiratory bronchiolitis in a young cigarette smoker. CT shows a few scattered, poorly defined centrilobular nodules (arrows).

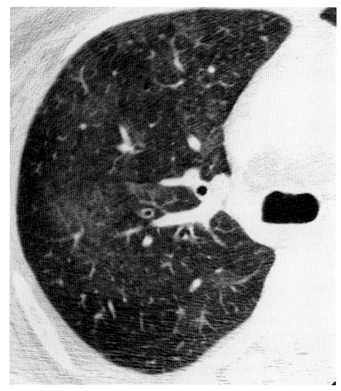

Fig. 8.2   Respiratory bronchiolitis interstitial lung disease. CT shows bronchial wall thickening, with patchy ground-glass abnormality and centrilobular nodules.

Table 8.1   Continuum of smoking related interstitial lung diseases[a]

	Symptoms	Physiologic impairment	Pathologic findings	Imaging features
RB	Minimal or absent	None	Intraluminal pigmented macrophages	Centrilobular nodules, small areas of ground-glass attenuation
RB-ILD	Significant	Significant	More extensive peribronchiolar macrophages and interstitial thickening	Widespread centrilobular nodules and ground glass
DIP	Significant	Significant	Diffuse intraalveolar macrophages and interstitial thickening	Widespread ground-glass abnormality, cysts ±

[a]Langerhans histiocytosis is not included in this table, because its imaging and pathologic findings are different from RB, RB-ILD, and DIP.
RB = respiratory bronchiolitis; RB-ILD = respiratory bronchiolitis-interstitial lung disease; DIP = desquamative interstitial pneumonia.

pneumonia (NSIP). RB-ILD differs from DIP in that the ground-glass attenuation of RB-ILD is usually less extensive, more patchy, and more poorly defined. Centrilobular nodules are uncommon in DIP. However, RB-ILD may be indistinguishable from DIP and hypersensitivity pneumonitis. Clinical differentiation of RB-ILD from hypersensitivity pneumonitis is facilitated by the fact that most patients with hypersensitivity pneumonitis are non-smokers.[15, 16]

Desquamative interstitial pneumonia

DIP was one of the first conditions to be differentiated histologically and prognostically from usual interstitial pneumonia (UIP).[17] More recent studies of the natural history of UIP and DIP have shown that UIP differs from DIP in its radiologic findings, and in its natural history.[18,19] Histologically, it is characterized by diffuse accumulation of large cells within the alveoli, previously thought to be desquamated pneumocytes, but now known to represent alveolar macrophages.[20] There is a variable amount of associated inflammatory change in the alveolar walls. Typically, the disease is relatively homogeneous at a microscopic level, with little lung fibrosis. It occurs almost entirely in cigarette smokers, and is thought to represent an idiosyncratic response to inhalation of cigarette smoke. Unlike most inhalational lung diseases, it does not have a peribronchiolar predominance, and therefore is characterized on CT by a diffuse ground-glass pattern, rather than centrilobular nodules.

The clinical presentation of DIP is similar to that of the other interstitial pneumonias, such as UIP and NSIP.[18] Symptoms of exertional breathlessness and a nonproductive cough are most common.

On the chest radiograph, the findings of DIP are relatively nonspecific, with reticulonodular abnormality or ground-glass attenuation being the salient features (Fig. 8.3).[21] The chest radiograph may be normal in up to 20% of cases.[22] The CT findings in DIP are much more specific than those on the chest radiograph. Ground-glass attenuation is seen in all patients,[23] with lower lobe predominance in about 75% (Fig. 8.4). Peripheral

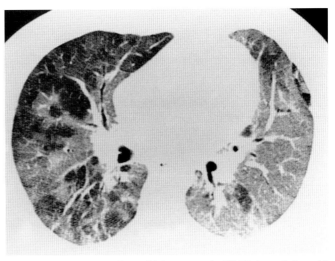

Fig. 8.4 Desquamative interstitial pneumonia. HRCT through the mid lungs shows diffuse ground-glass abnormality, diffuse on the left, but more geographic on the right.

predominance is seen in about 60%. Signs of lung fibrosis with anatomic distortion are seen in about 50% of cases, while traction bronchiectasis and honeycombing are seen in about one-third. Micronodules are seen in a small number of patients, perhaps a reflection of associated RB. An unusual feature seen in some patients with DIP is the presence of small cysts (Fig. 8.3), which differ from honeycomb cysts in that they are not clustered and do not occur in areas of underlying fibrosis.[24] Some of these cysts resolve with time. The combination of cysts and ground-glass attenuation should suggest the diagnosis of DIP or lymphoid interstitial pneumonia (LIP). The pathologic basis of these cysts is unclear.

When patients with DIP are followed over time, the ground-glass attenuation usually regresses or stays stable in response to treatment. Progression to a UIP pattern is uncommon.[19,24] However, some patients with DIP do progress despite treatment and may ultimately require lung transplantation.

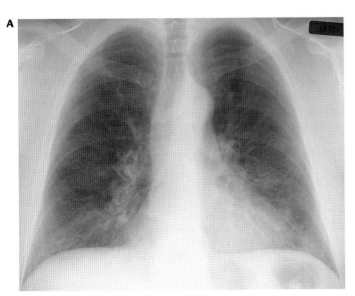

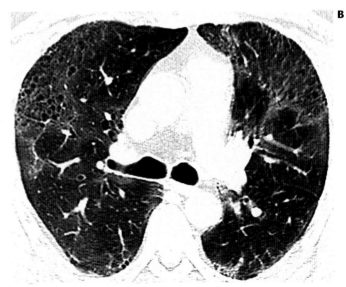

Fig. 8.3 Desquamative interstitial pneumonia. **A**, Chest radiograph shows patchy basal ground-glass abnormality. **B**, CT of the same patient shows bilateral peripheral predominant ground-glass abnormality. The areas of ground glass contain multiple small cysts.

Because of the significant overlap between the clinical, imaging, and histologic features of DIP and RB-ILD, there is increasing agreement that these entities should be grouped together as smoking related interstitial lung diseases (Table 8.1).[9] Some cases of NSIP may also be smoking related.[25] Some patients with DIP or RB-ILD also have lesions of Langerhans histiocytosis. For these reasons, the use of the term smoking related interstitial lung disease has been advocated as a global term to encompass these overlapping entities.[25]

Langerhans histiocytosis

Langerhans histiocytosis (previously called histiocytosis X or eosinophilic granuloma of the lung) is an idiopathic disorder characterized by the abnormal proliferation of the Langerhans cell, a mononuclear cell, in the lung. Histologically, the disease centers on the bronchioles, with associated involvement of the interstitium and pulmonary vasculature.[26]

Langerhans histiocytosis is a disease of smokers, with an impressive tobacco use history present in 90–100% of cases.[26,27] Most are under 40 years of age. Cough and dyspnea are the most common presenting complaints.[28] The presence of asymptomatic chest radiographic abnormalities occasionally precipitates the evaluation. Twenty-five percent of patients will develop a pneumothorax at some time during the course of their disease (Fig. 8.5), and this may be the presenting complaint. Because Langerhans histiocytosis may involve other organs, symptoms related to bony lesions or diabetes insipidus may rarely occur. There are several case reports and series suggesting a relationship between Langerhans histiocytosis and malignancy, particularly hematologic malignancies.[29] However, this association appears to be rare.

In children, Langerhans histiocytosis tends to present with multisystem involvement, particularly involving bone, lung, pituitary, and skin.[30] Because of the aggressive nature of the disease in children it is often treated with chemotherapy. Pulmonary involvement occurs in about 40% of cases.[31]

The physiologic abnormality of Langerhans histiocytosis evolves over time. At presentation the physiology may be normal, or may show a mixed restrictive–obstructive pattern. With progressive disease, there is an obstructive ventilatory defect with marked airflow limitation and increased lung volumes.[27] Because of the tendency of this disease to involve the pulmonary vasculature, the diffusing capacity for carbon monoxide (DLco) is often markedly reduced, and gas exchange is abnormal with hypoxemia. Blood chemistry evaluation is unhelpful. A firm histologic diagnosis generally requires an open or thoracoscopic lung biopsy, though identification of Birbeck granules on electron microscopic evaluation of the cell pellet from a bronchoalveolar lavage can be diagnostic. The prognosis is variable, but with smoking cessation, physiologic stabilization will occur in the majority of patients.

Imaging features

The chest radiographic appearance of Langerhans histiocytosis is often strongly suggestive of this diagnosis (Figs 8.6 and 8.7, Box 8.1).[32] The characteristic radiographic features are a combination of cysts and nodules (the nodules are usually easier to see than the cysts). There is mid and upper zone predominance, with sparing of the costophrenic sulci, and preservation of lung volumes. In the acute phase, the nodules are often poorly defined (Fig. 8.5), but later become well defined.

> ### Box 8.1 Langerhans histiocytosis: radiographic and CT features
>
> Nodules are usually poorly defined, may be cavitary
> Cysts – often irregular in shape
> Upper and mid lung predominance
> Sparing of costophrenic sulci
> Preserved or increased lung volumes
> Pulmonary arterial enlargement at later stage

HRCT contributes further to the accuracy of diagnosis of Langerhans histiocytosis. Grenier et al[33] showed that a first choice diagnosis of Langerhans histiocytosis had a 60% likelihood of being correct when made from the chest radiograph, but had a 90% likelihood of correctness on CT scanning. The combination of pulmonary nodules and cysts is virtually diagnostic of Langerhans histiocytosis (Fig. 8.8).[32,34,35] A study by Bonelli et al[36] showed that Langerhans histiocytosis can be confidently diagnosed in 84% of cases: confident diagnoses were correct in 100% of cases. Similar results were found in a more recent paper by Koyama et al.[37] Langerhans histiocytosis may be distinguished from lymphangiomyomatosis by the presence of nodules and sparing of the lung bases.

On HRCT, the nodules of Langerhans histiocytosis may be poorly or well defined and are typically most prominent in the upper lobes (Fig. 8.8). They are usually <5 mm in diameter, but may be up to 1 cm. Cavities with thin or thick walls may be seen (Figs 8.8 and 8.9).[38] These are not due to necrosis, but probably result from progressive bronchiolar dilation. The cysts in this disorder are invariably well defined (Fig. 8.10) and again are usually most profuse in the upper lobes, with relative sparing of the costophrenic sulci (Fig. 8.11).[36] The cysts are often irregular in outline (Fig. 8.9). By three-dimensional histologic reconstruction of lesions of Langerhans histiocytosis, Kambouchner et

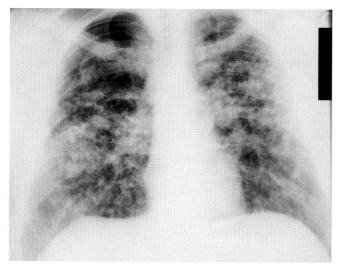

Fig. 8.5 Langerhans histiocytosis presenting with pneumothorax in a young cigarette smoker. Chest radiograph shows bilateral poorly defined nodules, sparing the lung bases, and a right pneumothorax.

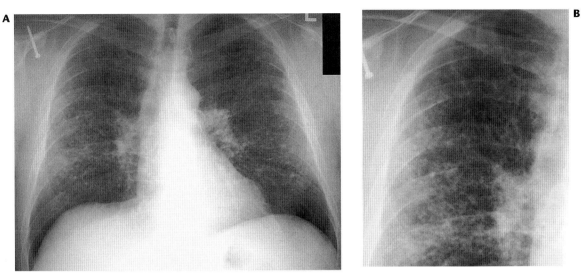

Fig. 8.6 **A**, Chest radiograph with **B**, magnified view shows characteristic features of Langerhans histiocytosis. There is a diffuse parenchymal abnormality due to cysts and nodules, with upper and mid lung predominance, and sparing of costophrenic sulci. Lung volumes are preserved. Enlargement of central pulmonary arteries suggests pulmonary arterial hypertension.

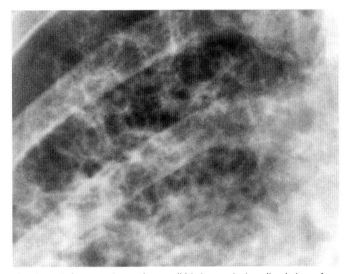

Fig. 8.7 Pulmonary Langerhans cell histiocytosis. Localized view of right mid lung shows multiple small cysts.

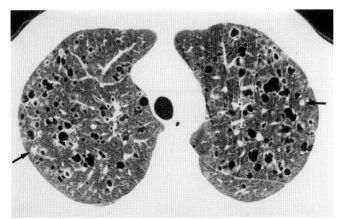

Fig. 8.8 Pulmonary Langerhans cell histiocytosis. CT through the upper lungs shows a characteristic combination of thin walled cysts and poorly defined nodules. Two of the nodules are just beginning to cavitate (arrows) – cavitation is thought to be the earliest stage of cyst formation.

al[39] demonstrated that the cavities and cysts occurring in Langerhans histiocytosis are due to destruction of the bronchiolar wall and progressive dilatation of the lumen, subsequently circumscribed by fibrous tissue, accounting for the tubular or irregular outline of these lesions.[39]

HRCT is also useful in following the progression or regression of Langerhans histiocytosis. Regression of the chest radiographic findings of Langerhans histiocytosis occurs in about one-third of cases.[40] A study of serial HRCT scans in 21 patients with this disease showed that the lung nodules and cavities tend to regress over time, while cysts and linear abnormalities remain the same or progress.[41] Nodules predominate on early CT scans, while cysts tend to predominate on follow-up scans. Parenchymal abnormality resolved completely in one of 21 patients in this study. The disease may recur in a small number of patients, usually those who continue to smoke or take up smoking

again. Tazi et al[42] described four patients who developed recurrent nodules 7 months to 7 years after initial presentation.

Patients with advanced Langerhans histiocytosis may have marked enlargement of the pulmonary arteries with severe pulmonary hypertension (Figs 8.6 and 8.12),[43] probably because Langerhans histiocytosis substantially involves the pulmonary vasculature.[44,45] In one series of 21 patients with advanced Langerhans histiocytosis, the mean pulmonary artery pressure was 59 mmHg, significantly higher than in patients with advanced chronic obstructive pulmonary disease or idiopathic pulmonary fibrosis (IPF).[46]

The CT features of pulmonary involvement in children are similar to those in adults, but mediastinal masses are more common.[47,48] When Bernstrand et al[49] used HRCT to evaluate patients a median of 16 years after the diagnosis of pediatric Langerhans histiocytosis, they found lung lesions (cysts or

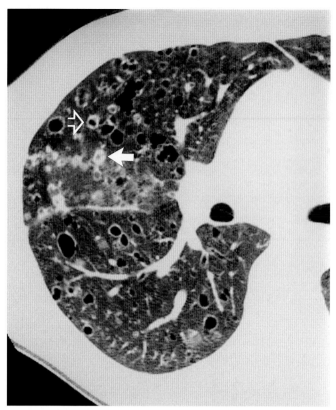

Fig. 8.9 Pulmonary Langerhans cell histiocytosis. CT through the right mid lung shows a combination of small poorly defined nodules, cavitary nodules with thin and thick walls (arrows), and thin walled cysts.

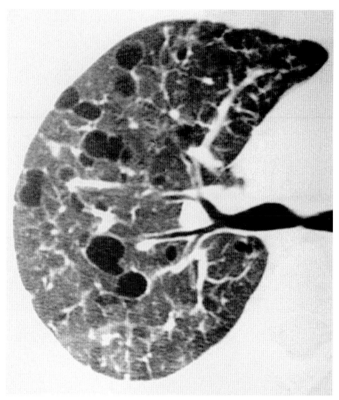

Fig. 8.10 Pulmonary Langerhans cell histiocytosis. CT shows multiple irregularly shaped cysts ranging in size from 3 to 20 mm. A few small nodules are visible.

emphysema) in 10 of 41 patients, mainly in those who had multisystem involvement at presentation, in those who had received chemotherapy, and in cigarette smokers.[49]

Other smoking affected diseases

The commonly recognized smoking related lung diseases such as lung cancer, emphysema, and chronic obstructive lung disease are discussed elsewhere. However, cigarette smoking is also a risk factor for a number of other respiratory diseases.[50] It appears to increase the risk of respiratory infections, including the common cold, influenza, bacterial pneumonia, varicella pneumonia, and tuberculosis.[50] Smoking is associated with a greatly increased risk of pulmonary hemorrhage (Goodpasture syndrome) in patients with antiglomerular basement membrane antibodies,[51] perhaps because it causes mild alveolar injury, allowing the antibodies access to the basement membrane.

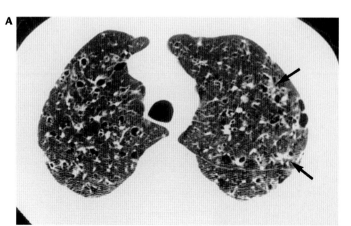

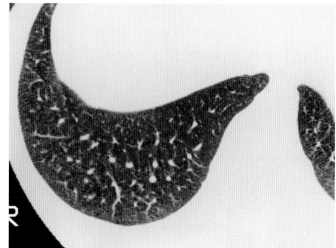

Fig. 8.11 Pulmonary Langerhans cell histiocytosis, present for 3 years. **A**, CT through the upper lungs shows irregular nodules thought to be due to scarring (arrows). **B**, CT through the lower lungs shows relative sparing of costophrenic sulci.

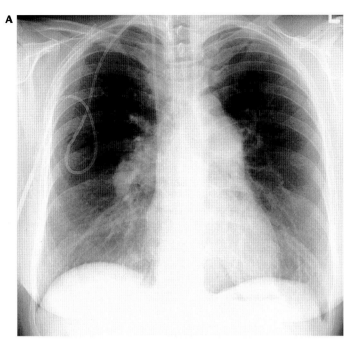 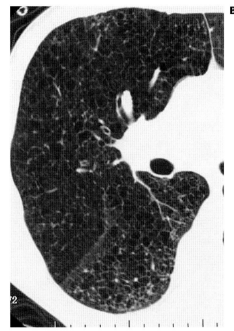

Fig. 8.12   Burnt-out Langerhans histiocytosis in a patient presenting with pulmonary hypertension. **A**, Chest radiograph shows mild hyperinflation, with a fine reticular pattern. The pulmonary arteries are markedly enlarged. **B**, CT shows an upper lung predominant pattern of fine irregular cysts and nodules.

There are numerous case reports suggesting that acute eosinophilic pneumonia often occurs within 1–2 weeks of initiation of cigarette smoking.[52,53]

Women with breast cancer who smoke have a twofold increase in risk of pulmonary metastasis.[54] However, there is no documented increase in risk of metastases from other malignancies in smokers.

Cigarette smoking is a major risk factor for spontaneous pneumothorax[55] and recurrent pneumothorax. The occurrence of pneumothorax in cigarette smokers may be related to the development of subpleural emphysematous blebs, and also to underlying RB.[56] About 70% of patients with IPF are current or former cigarette smokers, and the odds ratio for development of IPF in smokers is 1.6, with a higher risk for those with heavier exposures.[57] Smoking may also be associated with development of fibrosis in asbestos workers and patients with rheumatoid arthritis, but evaluation of this issue is confounded by the difficulty in separating the radiographic and physiologic effects of cigarette smoking from those of lung fibrosis.[50]

Smoking is consistently negatively associated with the development of hypersensitivity pneumonitis.[16,58] However, smokers who develop hypersensitivity pneumonitis may have a more insidious onset, and a worse prognosis, than non-smokers.[59] The prevalence of sarcoidosis is probably lower in cigarette smokers than in non-smokers, but its severity does not appear to differ.[60]

HYPERSENSITIVITY PNEUMONITIS

Hypersensitivity pneumonitis, also known as extrinsic allergic alveolitis, is a pulmonary syndrome caused by repeated exposure and sensitization to a variety of organic and chemical antigens. Diagnosis relies on a constellation of findings, including antigen exposure, characteristic signs and symptoms, pulmonary function abnormalities, radiologic abnormalities, and, frequently, characteristic histologic findings.[61]

Etiology

The extensive list of agents known to cause hypersensitivity pneumonitis can be organized into three main categories: microbial agents, animal proteins, and low molecular weight chemicals (Table 8.2). Regardless of the antigen, typically only a

Table 8.2 Major causes of hypersensitivity pneumonitis

Agent	Source	Disease
Aspergillus, thermophilic actinomyces	Moldy hay, compost	Farmer's lung Mushroom worker's lung
Trichosporum asahii	Tatami mats	Japanese summer-type hypersensitivity pneumonitis
Mycobacterium avium complex	Hot tubs Metal working fluids	Hot tub lung Metal worker's lung
Bird proteins	Bird feathers, excrement, especially doves, parakeets	Bird fancier's lung
Isocyanates	Paint sprays, plastics	Isocyanate hypersensitivity pneumonitis

minority of exposed and/or sensitized individuals will develop hypersensitivity pneumonitis.

As a group, various bacteria and fungi represent the most common causative agents.[61] Among bacteria, multiple species of thermophilic actinomyces are the most frequently reported. Thermophilic actinomyces contaminate decaying vegetable matter and are causally associated with farmer's lung (the prototypical example of hypersensitivity pneumonitis) and composting (including mushroom worker's lung).[62,63] They may also cause disease by contaminating ventilation systems and humidifiers.[64] More recently, nontuberculous mycobacteria contaminating hot tubs or metal-working fluids have been implicated as a likely cause of hypersensitivity pneumonitis.[65–67]

Multiple fungi have been shown to cause hypersensitivity pneumonitis, including various species of *Aspergillus*, *Mucor*, *Penicillium*, *Basidiospores*, and *Trichosporon*. Summer-type hypersensitivity pneumonitis, the most common form of hypersensitivity pneumonitis in Japan, is caused by *Trichosporon asahii* (formerly *T. cutaneum*).[68]

Antigens from avian dander and excreta are the most common animal proteins associated with hypersensitivity pneumonitis. Exposure to live birds is not required as cases have been reported related to the use of a feather duvet.[69]

Occupational exposure to isocyanate compounds is an important cause of occupational asthma and hypersensitivity pneumonitis.[70–72] The chemicals are thought to combine as haptens with human proteins to form complete antigens.[63] Other rare chemical causes include acid anhydrides, pesticide pyrethrum, Pauli's reagent (sodium diazobenzenesulfate), and copper sulfate.[61]

The immune system, host, and exposure related factors all play a role in the pathogenesis of hypersensitivity pneumonitis. Pathogenesis involves repeated antigen exposure leading to immunologic sensitization and subsequent immune mediated lung inflammation. Although previous reports implicated an immune complex mediated pathogenesis, it is now generally agreed that hypersensitivity pneumonitis is mediated primarily by cell-mediated immunity.[73,74]

The prevalence of hypersensitivity pneumonitis in exposed populations varies dramatically. For example, the reported prevalence of farmer's lung ranges from 0.02% in Scandinavia to 9% in parts of Scotland.[61] The incidence of hypersensitivity pneumonitis may be higher than this in building related outbreaks. Environmental risk factors, including antigen concentration, duration of exposure before symptom onset, frequency and intermittency of exposure, particle size, antigen solubility and potency, use of respiratory protection, and variability in work practices may influence disease prevalence, latency, and severity.[75] Since only a small percent of individuals with similar levels of exposure develop hypersensitivity pneumonitis, individual host factors must also play a role in the development of disease, but these remain poorly defined.

Clinical features

Classically, the presentation of hypersensitivity pneumonitis has been divided into acute, subacute, and chronic forms. However, significant overlap between the classic presentations exists. In acute hypersensitivity pneumonitis, systemic symptoms of fever, chills, and myalgias occur, along with respiratory symptoms of cough and dyspnea. These symptoms typically occur 4–12 h after heavy exposure to the inciting antigen. The subacute and chronic forms typically present with an insidious onset of respiratory symptoms, often with nonspecific systemic symptoms such as malaise, fatigue, or weight loss. Usually, the temporal relationship between symptoms and exposure is difficult to elicit. A high degree of clinical suspicion is required to confirm the diagnosis and initiate appropriate management. In a case series from Japan, the most frequent symptoms in chronic hypersensitivity pneumonitis were cough and dyspnea.[68] Fever (low grade) occurred in only half of the patients.

Hypersensitivity pneumonitis must be distinguished clinically from the organic toxic dust syndrome, which is characterized by flulike symptoms occurring after heavy organic dust exposures. This syndrome does not relate to a specific antigen, and the chest radiograph is usually said to be normal or near normal, though to this author's knowledge there are no specific descriptions of the CT appearances.

The finding of specific IgG precipitating antibodies in the serum of a patient with suspected hypersensitivity pneumonitis is a helpful diagnostic clue but is neither sensitive nor specific and is no longer thought of as a hallmark of hypersensitivity pneumonitis. Serum precipitins are found in 3–30% of asymptomatic farmers and in up to 50% of asymptomatic pigeon breeders.[76,77] Precipitins are thus a marker of exposure sufficient to generate a humoral immune response. However, they have no role in the pathogenesis of hypersensitivity pneumonitis.

There is no single characteristic pattern of pulmonary function abnormalities in hypersensitivity pneumonitis. Physiology may be predominantly restrictive, predominantly obstructive, or mixed. Lalancette et al[78] found obstructive abnormalities in 42% of farmers after 6 years of follow up. Others have confirmed the high prevalence of airways obstruction, even after accounting for the effects of smoking.[79]

The classic histopathology of hypersensitivity pneumonitis features the triad of cellular bronchiolitis, a lymphoplasmocytic interstitial infiltrate, and poorly formed non-necrotizing granulomas.[80] However, the complete triad is not always present. Additional features may include giant cells and organizing pneumonia. Pathologic features may vary with disease stage.[81] A fibrotic pattern very similar to UIP[81] or NSIP[82] is frequently seen in chronic, fibrotic hypersensitivity pneumonitis. In addition, the classic granulomas are only seen in 60–70% of acute cases and in <50% of chronic cases.[68,83]

Radiologic features

The radiographic findings of acute hypersensitivity pneumonitis include diffuse ground-glass opacification (Fig. 8.13) and a fine nodular or reticulonodular pattern, often with lower lung predominance. Consolidation is almost never seen,[84] and should lead to consideration of alternative diagnoses such as cryptogenic organizing pneumonia. A nodular or reticulonodular pattern becomes more prominent in the subacute phase (Fig. 8.14).[85] In chronic hypersensitivity pneumonitis, fibrosis with upper lobe retraction, reticular opacity, volume loss, and honeycombing may be seen (Figs 8.15 and 8.16).[68]

The prevalence of an abnormal chest radiograph in population based studies of patients with hypersensitivity pneumonitis is only about 10%.[86,87] This relatively low sensitivity is probably due to the lack of conspicuity of the typical features of hypersensitivity pneumonitis, and also to use of more sensitive

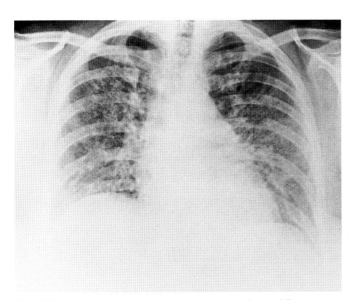

Fig. 8.13   Acute farmer's lung. Chest radiograph shows diffuse parenchymal ground-glass pattern with some areas of consolidation. The severity of parenchymal opacification in this case is unusual.

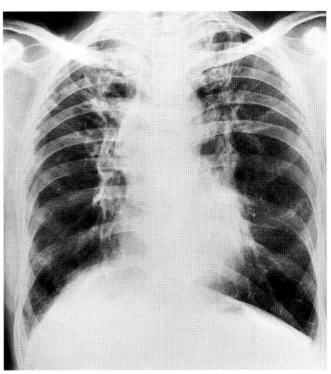

Fig. 8.15   Chronic farmer's lung. The patient had recurrent acute episodes of hypersensitivity pneumonitis over a 15 year period. He then discontinued farming and this radiograph was obtained 10 years later. It shows marked bilateral upper lobe volume loss with linear scarring.

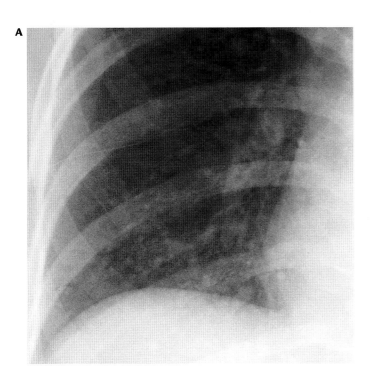

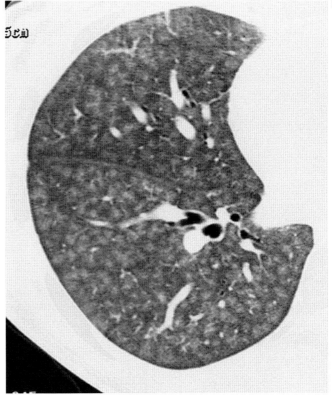

Fig. 8.14   Subacute hypersensitivity pneumonitis related to mold exposure. **A**, Detail view of chest radiograph shows poorly defined nodules. **B**, CT shows profuse poorly defined centrilobular nodules of ground-glass attenuation, typical of hypersensitivity pneumonitis.

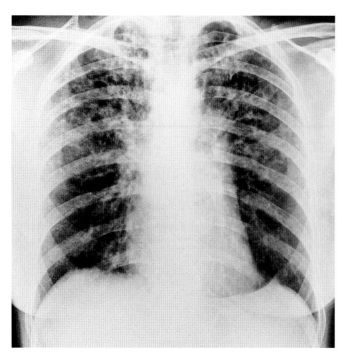

Fig. 8.16 Chronic bird fancier's lung, resulting from parakeet exposure. There is bilateral upper lung reticulonodular pattern. The hilar elevation and left diaphragmatic juxtaphrenic peak indicate upper lobe volume loss.

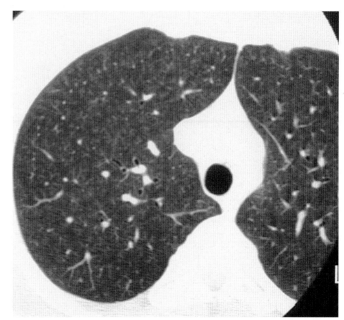

Fig. 8.17 Subacute hypersensitivity pneumonitis in a swimming pool lifeguard exposed to a bioaerosol from pool fountains. Chest radiograph was normal. CT shows profuse fine micronodules.

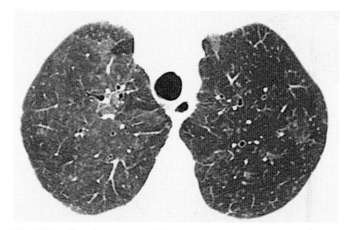

Fig. 8.18 Chronic hypersensitivity pneumonitis due to *Mycobacterium avium* complex (hot tub lung). HRCT shows extensive ground-glass abnormality in the right lung, with centrilobular nodules. The left lung shows decreased attenuation reflecting small airways disease.

diagnostic techniques, especially fiberoptic bronchoscopy. The sensitivity of high-resolution CT (HRCT) for the detection of hypersensitivity pneumonitis is significantly better than plain radiographs, but less than that of biopsy.[88–90]

Computed tomography

A variety of HRCT patterns have been described in hypersensitivity pneumonitis (Box 8.2).[91,92] Each of these is discussed in more detail below. Most of these patterns have been correlated with histologic findings and some with pulmonary function abnormalities.[85] Up to 50% of patients have mediastinal lymphadenopathy,[93] but the adenopathy typically is not diffuse and the enlarged nodes are almost always smaller than 20 mm (short axis diameter).[93] Lymph node enlargement is therefore usually not visible on the chest radiograph.

Box 8.2 Hypersensitivity pneumonitis: CT features

Poorly defined centrilobular nodules
Ground-glass abnormality
Mosaic attenuation
Reticular abnormality

The nodules seen in hypersensitivity pneumonitis are round, poorly defined, and <5 mm in diameter (Figs 8.14 and 8.17).[84] They are typically centrilobular[90] and profuse throughout the lung but a mid to lower lung zone predominance has been variably reported.[94] In contrast to the centrilobular nodules of silicosis and other inhalational diseases, they are usually of ground-glass attenuation rather than of soft tissue attenuation. Profuse nodules of this type can be diagnostic of hypersensitivity pneumonitis in the correct clinical context. Although the nodules are centrilobular in the sense that they spare the periphery of the secondary pulmonary lobule, a true tree-in-bud pattern indicative of cellular bronchiolitis is quite uncommon.[90,94,95] The nodules usually regress with removal from exposure.[89,90]

Ground-glass attenuation (Fig. 8.18) is most common in acute hypersensitivity pneumonitis but may also be seen in subacute and chronic hypersensitivity pneumonitis, especially if there is ongoing exposure.[96] The ground-glass opacification may be patchy or diffuse and some authors report a middle lung zone predominance.[94] Ground-glass opacification may resolve with removal from exposure.[90] It is usually associated with restrictive

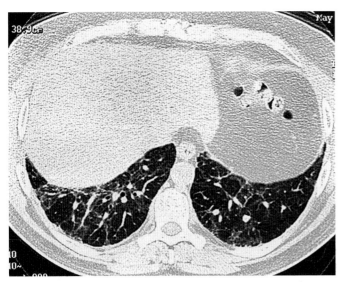

Fig. 8.19 Chronic hypersensitivity pneumonitis with nonspecific pattern. HRCT shows basal predominant ground-glass abnormality associated with reticular abnormality and traction bronchiectasis, a pattern suggestive of nonspecific interstitial pneumonia.

physiology and impaired gas exchange on pulmonary function testing.[97] Ground-glass opacification is frequently found in association with other CT abnormalities such as centrilobular nodules or air-trapping. Lung cysts, similar to those seen in lymphoid interstitial pneumonia, may be seen in about 10% of cases of subacute hypersensitivity pneumonitis.[98]

In chronic hypersensitivity pneumonitis, fibrosis is signified by irregular linear opacities, traction bronchiectasis, lobar volume loss, and honeycombing that may be seen in hypersensitivity pneumonitis (Fig. 8.19).[91] In some cases, there is a mid zone predominance with sparing of the apices and the costophrenic angles, but the fibrotic appearance may also be seen in the

upper or lower lobes.[94] In the transverse plane, the fibrotic changes are randomly distributed but a subpleural predominance has been described in some patients.[94] Honeycombing (Fig. 8.20) has been found in up to 50% of patients with chronic bird fancier's lung[90] but may be less common in chronic hypersensitivity pneumonitis of other etiologies.[68]

A mosaic attenuation pattern is common in hypersensitivity pneumonitis (Figs 8.18 and 8.21). Nineteen of 22 patients in a series reported by Hansell et al[97] displayed this finding. Likewise, 15 of 20 patients in a study by Small et al[99] had this pattern. In hypersensitivity pneumonitis, the mosaic pattern may be due to either patchy areas of ground glass or air-trapping, or often to a combination of these. Air-trapping on expiratory imaging is seen in many cases of hypersensitivity pneumonitis (Fig. 8.21),[99] and may be the predominant or only feature. HRCT evidence of air-trapping correlates with evidence of obstruction on pulmonary function testing.[97,100] The air-trapping and mosaic attenuation are presumed to be due to bronchiolitis. Thus, a mosaic pattern and air-trapping provide supportive evidence for the diagnosis of hypersensitivity pneumonitis, especially when they occur in association with the abnormalities described above.[91]

Radiographic evidence of emphysema in patients with chronic hypersensitivity pneumonitis was first noted by Barbee et al in 1968.[62] Remy-Jardin et al[90] noted emphysematous changes on HRCT in 50% of patients with chronic bird fancier's hypersensitivity pneumonitis. In addition, Lalancette et al[78] reported that emphysema occurred more commonly than fibrosis in chronic farmer's lung. A more recent study by Cormier et al[96] confirmed that emphysema is more prevalent than fibrosis in chronic farmer's lung, even after accounting for the effects of tobacco abuse. Another study showed an increased prevalence of emphysema in patients with farmer's lung compared to control farmers matched for age, sex, and smoking status.[92] In this study, 13 of 20 patients with farmer's lung and emphysema had never been smokers. The available studies do not clearly describe or illustrate the pattern of emphysema, and its significance therefore remains unclear.

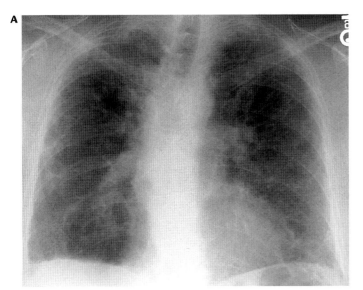

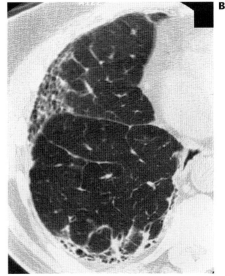

Fig. 8.20 Chronic hypersensitivity pneumonitis of unclear etiology, with a usual interstitial pneumonia pattern. **A,** Chest radiograph shows diffuse reticular abnormality, with slight basal predominance. **B,** HRCT shows peripheral reticular abnormality and honeycombing. Subtle areas of decreased attenuation are a clue to the diagnosis of hypersensitivity pneumonitis (see p. 438 for similar example).

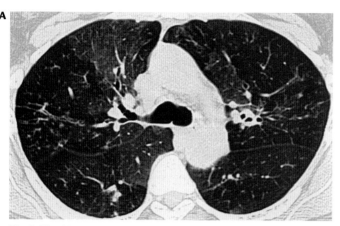 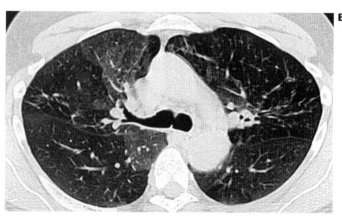

Fig. 8.21 Hypersensitivity pneumonitis with marked air-trapping. **A,** Inspiratory CT shows mosaic attenuation, with areas of ground-glass abnormality and decreased attenuation. The mild cylindric bronchiectasis in the right upper lobe is not a usual feature of hypersensitivity pneumonitis. **B,** Expiratory CT shows marked air-trapping.

Relationship between imaging findings and phase of disease

Hypersensitivity pneumonitis is often divided into acute, sub-acute, and chronic phases, based on the duration of the patient's symptoms. However, the imaging findings do not necessarily correlate with the duration of symptoms. Centrilobular nodules, ground-glass attenuation, and mosaic attenuation may all be found at any phase of the disease, and may be the sole finding even in patients with clinically chronic hypersensitivity pneumonitis. Findings of fibrosis or emphysema are usually found only in chronic hypersensitivity pneumonitis.

Radiologic differential diagnosis

The radiologic differential diagnosis of hypersensitivity depends on the imaging findings. Profuse poorly defined nodules of ground-glass attenuation are virtually pathognomonic of hypersensitivity pneumonitis (Figs 8.14 and 8.17). The differential diagnosis may include smoking related respiratory bronchio-litis, but in this condition the nodules are usually more patchy and sparse. If the nodules are of soft tissue attenuation, sarcoidosis, berylliosis, or pneumoconiosis would be more likely than hypersensitivity pneumonitis. A patchy or unilateral distribution of nodules should suggest infection.[95]

When ground-glass attenuation is present as the only sign of hypersensitivity pneumonitis, it may be indistinguishable from other conditions characterized by ground-glass attenuation such as viral infection, organizing pneumonia, DIP, or NSIP. The differential diagnosis of mixed ground-glass attenuation and air-trapping should include sarcoidosis, another disease characterized by mixed obstructive and restrictive physiology.

Patients with chronic hypersensitivity pneumonitis may exhibit a histologic and imaging pattern of NSIP (Fig. 8.19) or UIP (Fig. 8.20). Hypersensitivity pneumonitis should always be considered in the differential diagnosis of NSIP[82] and of UIP.[101] Imaging features which favor hypersensitivity pneumonitis over IPF include upper or mid zone predominance, presence of ground-glass abnormality or air-trapping, and absence of honeycombing.[101] However, hypersensitivity pneumonitis should always be considered in the differential diagnosis even when the imaging features are typical of UIP (Fig. 8.20).

Diagnosis

Because the clinical presentation of hypersensitivity pneumonitis may be nonspecific, and because the diagnosis of hypersensitivity pneumonitis may have profound implications for the lifestyle of the patient, it is important to have criteria for establishing the diagnosis. Although there are multiple published diagnostic criteria, none have been validated. A history of exposure to a known antigen, or the presence of circulating precipitins, is inadequate evidence for the diagnosis of hypersensitivity pneumonitis. The temporal relationship between exposure and symptoms is important, but does not always occur, especially in chronic hypersensitivity pneumonitis. It should always be also demonstrated either that the patient has physiologic impairment (decreased lung volumes, impaired diffusing capacity, or abnormal gas exchange at rest or exercise), or that the patient has a radiographic or CT abnormality compatible with hypersensitivity pneumonitis. If the diagnosis remains equivocal, bronchoscopy may be helpful by demonstrating lymphocytosis on bronchoalveolar lavage or granulomas on transbronchial biopsy. Surgical lung biopsy is primarily used for cases in which there is no clear history of exposure, or where there is concern for other lung diseases.

BYSSINOSIS

Byssinosis in cotton workers is characterized by respiratory symptoms which are most severe on the first day of the working week, and improve as the week progresses. Descriptions of the radiologic findings of this entity have been sparse, but a recent report showed basal predominant ground-glass abnormality on the chest radiograph, with associated centrilobular nodules on CT.[102]

PNEUMOCONIOSIS

The term "pneumoconiosis", which means "dusty lungs", is generally used to describe the non-neoplastic reactions of the lungs to inhaled dust particles. In general, the term excludes diseases due to organic dusts, such as hypersensitivity pneumonitis or organic toxic dust syndrome. It also excludes asthma, bronchitis, and emphysema,[103] which are common causes of symptoms and physiologic impairment in dust exposed workers.

The character and severity of the reaction of lung tissue to inhaled dust are determined by five basic factors:

- Properties of the inhaled dust, particularly the particle size and the degree to which the dust is fibrogenic.
- Amount of dust retained in the lungs (respirable particles measuring between 0.5 and 5 μm are usually most likely to be retained, but asbestos fibers and talc particles may be larger than this).
- Duration and intensity of exposure.
- Interval since the onset of exposure. A long latency from first exposure (20–30 years) is characteristic of pneumoconioses.
- Individual idiosyncrasy.

The pneumoconioses are best classified according to the mineral dust responsible (Box 8.3). This classification is not always easy because industrial exposure may involve more than one dust known to be fibrogenic. For example, silica is so plentiful in the rocks of the earth's crust that some exposure to silica is inevitable in many forms of mining. Also, workers may be exposed to more than one type of dust during their careers.

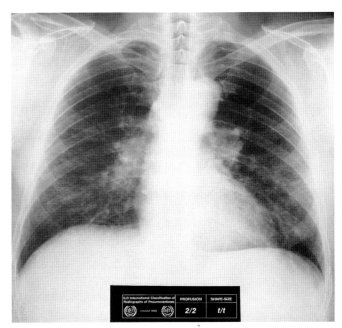

Fig. 8.22 International Labor Organization standard radiograph for t type small irregular opacities, profusion 2/2.

> **Box 8.3 The pneumoconioses**
>
> *Due to dusts which are usually inert*
> Iron – siderosis
> Tin – stannosis
> Barium – baritosis
>
> *Due to dusts which cause interstitial fibrosis*
> Beryllium – berylliosis
> Aluminum – aluminosis (Shaver's disease)
> Asbestos – asbestosis
>
> *Due to dust causing nodules. May progress to pulmonary massive fibrosis*
> Coal – anthracosis, coal worker's pneumoconiosis
> Silica – silicosis
> Talc (may be contaminated with asbestos) – talcosis
> Kaolin – kaolinosis
> Graphite – graphitosis

Radiographic classification

Occupational physicians have long recognized the need for quantitative techniques for evaluation of occupational lung diseases. This led to the development of the International Labor Organization (ILO) classification scheme for chest radiographs.[104,105] In this system, the size, shape, and profusion of opacities on radiographs of patients with pneumoconiosis are classified in a detailed fashion by trained observers using a set of standard radiographs (Fig. 8.22). Regular (round) opacities are graded as p (<1.5 mm diameter), q (1.5–3 mm), or r (3–10 mm). Irregular opacities are classified as s, t, or u, using the same size criteria. Larger opacities are classified according to their size. The system also scores the extent and thickness of pleural

plaques and pleural thickening, and provides symbols for other abnormalities such as fissural thickening and calcified nodules.

For each type of opacity, four standard radiographs are available: 0/0, 1/1, 2/2, and 3/3. Opacities with profusion matching the standard radiographs are classified as 0/0, 1/1, 2/2, or 3/3. If a radiograph shows a profusion greater than the 1/1 standard, but does not reach the level of the 2/2 standard, then it is classified as 1/2 if it is closer to the 1/1 standard, or as 2/1 if it is closer to the 2/2 standard. In this system, the digit before the slash indicates the standard to which the radiograph is closest. Creation of subcategories in this way has allowed the development of a 12 point profusion scale (0/–, 0/0, 0/1, 1/0, 1/1, 1/2, 2/1, 2/2, 2/3, 3/2, 3/3, 3/+).

Although initially introduced for epidemiologic studies and industrial surveys, the ILO classification system is now widely used in medical screening programs for occupational lung disease, and to define the extent of occupational lung disease for purposes of compensation. The ILO classification, and the accompanying standard radiographs, provides valuable epidemiologic information about the prevalence of radiographic evidence of disease in workers with a wide range of occupations, and in many countries.[106–109] It has also been used to document radiographic progression over 20–40 years.[110]

The value of the ILO classification system is that it provides a standardized, semiquantitative assessment of the extent of radiographic abnormality. It is the only large scale system for standardized radiology reporting which requires proficiency testing as a condition for being certified as a reader, and regular reassessment to ensure continued competency. The ILO system forces the reader to record the presence and extent of radiographic opacities consistent with pneumoconiosis.

The ILO classification system has been validated by correlation with autopsy specimens and with physiologic impairment. The classification of profusion of p and q type opacities in patients with coal worker's pneumoconiosis correlates quite well with the number of fibrotic lung lesions at autopsy and with the total dust content of the lung.[111] The profusion of opacities correlates with impairment of pulmonary function both for irregular[112,113] and rounded opacities.[114]

The classification of pneumoconiosis under the ILO system has substantial prognostic significance. The relative risk of developing progressive massive fibrosis in coal workers with normal radiographs is 3.7%, compared with 17% in coal workers with category 1 profusion, 20% in those with category 2 profusion, and 47% in coal workers who have category 3 profusion.[115] More recently, Bourgkard et al[116] have shown that coal miners with borderline chest radiographs (0/1 or 1/0) were more likely to develop progressive pneumoconiosis than those with normal radiographs. Similarly, in gold miners with silicosis, the rate of deterioration of lung function was much more rapid in patients with a higher profusion of opacities, and the degree of radiographic profusion was a significant determinant of the forced expiratory volume in 1 s (FEV_1) measured 5 years later.[117] In a study of 354 asbestos miners who applied for compensation for asbestosis, median survival was 17 years for workers with category 1 disease, 12 years in category 2 disease, and 3 years in category 3 disease.[118] Similarly, in a population of 2609 asbestos exposed insulators, the 10 year risk of death from asbestosis rose dramatically from 0.9% in those who had an initial chest radiographic category of 0 to 35.4% in those with a category 3 disease on their initial chest radiograph.[119]

The limitations of the ILO classification scheme as a system for determining disease extent are clearly recognized. The radiographic standards and the test cases were developed and validated between 1950 and 1980, and have not been updated. Correlation between the measures of profusion and the degree of physiologic impairment are in general weak, particularly in patients with simple coal worker's pneumoconiosis or silicosis.[120] Pleural disease is scored by an unnecessarily elaborate and arbitrary system, and it is difficult to accurately distinguish between pleural plaque and extrapleural fat. Despite the extensive quality assurance, there is substantial interobserver variation in scoring of profusion, and it is probably impossible to score profusion accurately within one subcategory. For this reason, multiple readers are usually required in epidemiologic studies.

The category of small irregular opacities poses particular problems. Indeed, the whole concept of irregular opacities is misleading, since CT and pathologic studies show that most of these opacities are part of a reticular network, rather than being discrete small opacities. It is clear from several studies[121–125] that the presence of small irregular opacities by ILO criteria on the chest radiograph is strongly related to a history of cigarette smoking. These observations serve to emphasize the fact that the diagnosis of asbestosis cannot be based on a radiographic profusion score alone. The presence of small irregular opacities on antemortem chest radiographs is a poor predictor of pathologic asbestosis.[126] Similarly in coal workers, small round opacities are not always associated with CT evidence of pneumoconiosis.[127,128]

One of the unavoidable problems with the use of the ILO system relates to the invisibility of early lung disease on the chest radiograph. In coal worker's pneumoconiosis,[129] silicosis,[130] and asbestosis,[131] the chest radiograph is insensitive for mild lesions of pneumoconiosis. This lack of sensitivity is a particular problem in asbestos workers, where patients with normal parenchyma on radiographs can have a significantly reduced forced vital capacity.[113]

Perhaps the most difficult issue in the radiographic evaluation of patients with occupational lung disease is the evaluation of the patient whose radiograph shows borderline evidence of pneumoconiosis (0/1 and 1/0 by the ILO classification system). Where should the line be drawn between normal and abnormal? In an autopsy based study of South African miners, Hnizdo et al[130] showed that silicosis was present in 78% of those with an ILO grade of 0/1 or more, 89% of those with an ILO grade of 1/0 or more, and 96% of those with an ILO grade of 1/1 or more. Conversely, the use of cut-off points of 0/1, 1/0, and 1/1 resulted in detection of 60, 50 and 37% of cases of silicosis, respectively. This study makes it clear that the choice of a cut-off point has a critical impact on sensitivity and specificity for disease, and that the chest radiograph is relatively insensitive for the diagnosis of silicosis. It is necessary to accept that the borderline between normal and abnormal is blurred. CT may help clarify the presence or absence of nodules in patients with borderline chest radiographs.[128,132,133] However, the sensitivity and specificity of CT for pneumoconiosis has not been documented by correlation with pathologic findings.

A revision of the ILO system has recently been introduced.[134] Although there are no changes in the overall scoring system, there are slight changes in the standard radiographs and in the reporting form, which incorporates some new abbreviations for entities such as round atelectasis. It is expected that this will simplify the assessment of the pleura, clarify that costophrenic angle blunting is required in order to call diffuse pleural thickening, and incorporate an abbreviation for rounded atelectasis. However, there are no plans to introduce standards based on CT scanning, or to clarify the issues surrounding borderline chest radiographs.

The most prevalent misuse of the ILO classification system occurs when this primarily descriptive, epidemiologic system is used to define the diagnosis of pneumoconiosis for medicolegal purposes, to determine whether the worker will receive compensation for occupational lung disease.[134] The ILO system cannot be used in isolation to make or refute the diagnosis of pneumoconiosis. Radiographic profusion in the absence of additional clinical data may be misleading in individual patients.[135]

Silicosis

Inhalation of free silica (silicon dioxide) can cause a variety of clinical abnormalities (Box 8.4). Free silica is present in many rocks in the earth's crust. It occurs in amorphous and crystalline forms, with quartz being the most important crystal. Exposed individuals usually work in quarries, drill or tunnel quartz containing rocks, cut or polish masonry, clean boilers or castings in iron and steel foundries (fettlers), or are exposed to sandblasting. Silica exposure may also occur in ceramics workers. Although the incidence of silicosis has fallen since its peak during World War II, it is still a major cause of pulmonary impairment in at-risk workers. The continued incidence of silicosis may be due to the inadequacy of current respirable dust limits, or to failure to use appropriate respiratory protection.

The clinical presentation of silicosis may be acute, accelerated, or chronic, depending on the amount of dust exposure. The usual chronic form of the disease requires exposure to high dust concentrations for 20 years or more before radiographic abnormality is visible.[136] With very high concentrations of dust,

Box 8.4 Effects of silica exposure

Simple silicosis
- Diffuse upper zone predominant nodules, centrilobular on CT
- Calcification in pulmonary nodules and hilar and mediastinal nodes (often eggshell)

Progressive massive fibrosis
- Conglomeration of nodules in the posterior upper lobes
- Peripheral cicatricial emphysema

Acute silicoproteinosis

Chronic bronchitis

Emphysema

Tuberculosis and atypical mycobacterial infection

Lung cancer

Scleroderma

radiographic changes may be visible in 4–10 years (accelerated silicosis).[136,137] Acute silicoproteinosis is a clinically distinct entity that occurs with severe exposure, particularly in enclosed spaces.

Patients with simple silicosis may be asymptomatic, or may have symptoms of chronic bronchitis. Symptoms are more common in those with greater profusion of disease. Most patients with complicated pneumoconiosis (progressive massive fibrosis) have shortness of breath. Patients with acute or accelerated silicosis generally have significant respiratory impairment.

Pathogenesis and pathology

Silica dust particles of appropriately small size are deposited on the alveolar walls and ingested by macrophages. They may enter the pulmonary lymphatics, or they may be transported to bronchioles by the mucociliary escalator. The silica particle is directly cytotoxic to macrophages. The dying macrophages induce fibrosis by releasing oxidants, proinflammatory cytokines, and stimulants of fibroblast proliferation.[138]

The basic histologic lesion of silicosis is the hyalinized nodule. The silica particles, nearly all of which are 1–2 mm in diameter, are found fixed within the silicotic nodules. These nodules are usually more prominent in the upper zones and lie close to the bronchioles, small vessels, and lymphatics. They consist of concentric layers of collagen-containing silica particles surrounded by a fibrous capsule. The outer zone is made up of irregularly dispersed connective tissue that also contains crystalline silica. Silica in this peripheral zone sets up a further reaction, resulting in enlargement of nodules and creation of new nodules. The fibrosis seen with silicosis is both more abundant and more collagenous than that seen with other mineral dusts, such as coal. Silica-laden macrophages that reach the hilar and mediastinal nodes form granuloma-like lesions in the nodes.

Silicosis is often complicated by massive fibrotic lesions that are the result of the conglomeration of nodules matted together by fibrosis. These masses, which contain obliterated blood vessels and bronchi, may cavitate. Mycobacterial infection coexists in some cases.[139] The pulmonary macrophage, important in the granulomatous response to the tubercle bacillus, is damaged by silica particles rendering the silicotic individual more susceptible to infection.

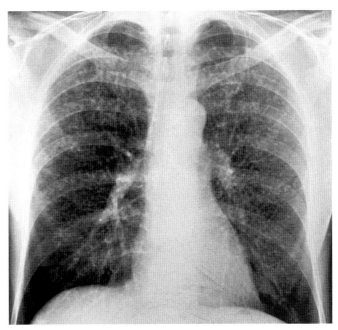

Fig. 8.23 Simple silicosis. There are widespread 2–3 mm nodules, with middle and upper zone predominance.

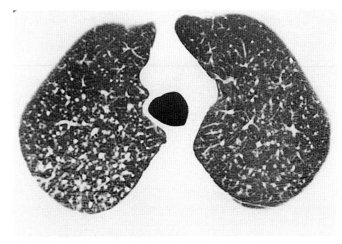

Fig. 8.24 CT in a patient with silicosis. A scan through the upper lobes shows diffuse centrilobular nodules.

Simple silicosis

The earliest changes of silicosis are 1–3 mm round, well-defined nodules, especially in the posterior portions of the upper two-thirds of the lungs (Fig. 8.23).[140,141] A reticular pattern may also be seen, either alone or in combination with the nodules. As the process advances, the nodules increase in size and number and become more widespread, involving all zones. Usually the nodulation is symmetric. Sometimes the nodules are calcified.

On CT scanning, the micronodules are usually shown to be centrilobular (Fig. 8.24).[142] As the disease evolves, there is spread anteriorly and inferiorly, though the upper zone preponderance is usually maintained. The upper lung preponderance is thought to be due to poor lymphatic clearance from the upper lobes.[143] Nodules may also be seen subpleurally, where they may cluster to form "pseudoplaques" (Fig. 8.25).[144] Larger

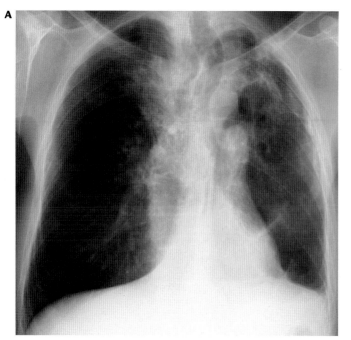

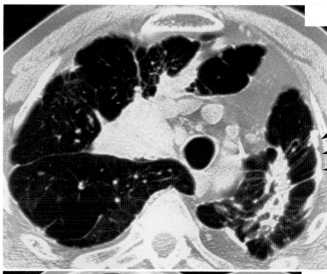

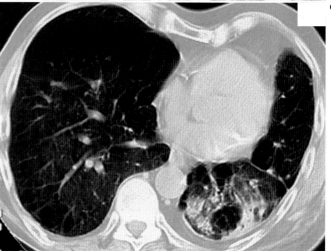

Fig. 8.25 Silicosis with progressive massive fibrosis. **A**, Chest radiograph shows bilateral upper lobe masses. The left upper lobe mass is relatively peripheral, and associated with marked volume loss with leftward herniation of the trachea and right lung. The more central right upper lobe mass is partially obscured by the overlying sternum. There is moderate background nodularity. Pleural thickening and calcification are evident on the left. **B**, CT shows a large mass in the medial right upper lobe, with a smaller mass on the left. There is centrilobular emphysema, and bilateral peripheral cicatricial emphysema. Scattered small nodules are predominantly subpleural. Subpleural clustering of nodules on the left has created a pseudoplaque (arrowheads). **C**, CT through the lower lobe shows typical appearances of rounded atelectasis, related to an area of pleural thickening.

nodules may also be seen, and these may calcify. Interlobular septal thickening may be present.

Hilar and mediastinal lymph node enlargement is not uncommon in silicosis. Calcification, sometimes of the eggshell type, may be seen in the nodes, either on the chest radiograph (Fig. 8.26) or CT.[145]

Progressive massive fibrosis

Progressive massive fibrosis (PMF), also called complicated silicosis and conglomerate silicosis, is defined as nodules >1 cm in diameter. Recognition of PMF is important because it indicates that the patient is likely to be symptomatic and physiologically impaired. Typically, PMF starts as a round or oval mass near the periphery of the lung (Fig. 8.25), often with a well-defined lateral border that parallels the lateral chest wall. A lateral view confirms the posterior location and the lens shaped appearance of the conglomerate mass (Fig. 8.27). As the nodules coalesce and the upper lobes contract, the hila retract and compensatory emphysema occurs in the lower lobes. Apical pleural thickening is frequently seen.

CT confirms the architectural distortion associated with PMF, with a peripheral zone of paracicatricial emphysema,

though there may also be fibrous bands extending to the pleural surface (Fig. 8.25). PMF may be rounded in contour, but ovoid masses are more usual. The outer margin of PMF often parallels the contour of the adjacent chest wall. Large lesions (5 cm or greater in diameter) often show irregular low-attenuation regions indicative of avascular necrosis, and cavitation may occur. Lesions may also show irregular punctate calcifications. Asymmetry between the lungs may occur in early PMF, with unilateral involvement on occasion. The larger lesions exhibit reasonable side-to-side symmetry.

PMF is discussed further in the section Coal Worker's Pneumoconiosis (p. 447).

Other complications of silica exposure

While chronic simple silicosis refers to the development of silicosis between 10 and 30 years after exposure, *accelerated silicosis* refers to the development of silicosis within 10 years of exposure (usually related to more intense exposure[146]). The radiologic appearance of this entity is similar to that of chronic simple silicosis. However, workers with accelerated silicosis are at high risk for the development of complications such as PMF.[147]

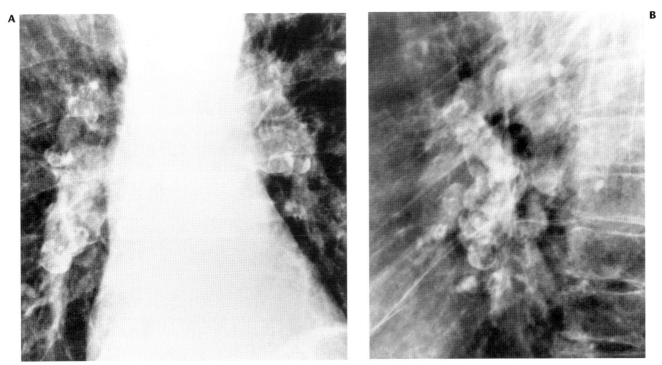

Fig. 8.26   Eggshell nodal calcification in silicosis. **A**, Anteroposterior and **B**, lateral views.

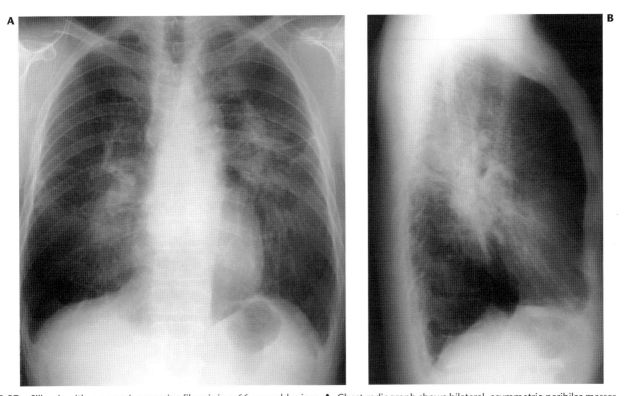

Fig. 8.27   Silicosis with progressive massive fibrosis in a 66-year-old miner. **A**, Chest radiograph shows bilateral, asymmetric perihilar masses. **B**, Lateral radiograph confirms the posterior location of the masses.

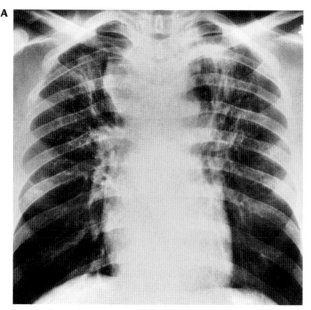
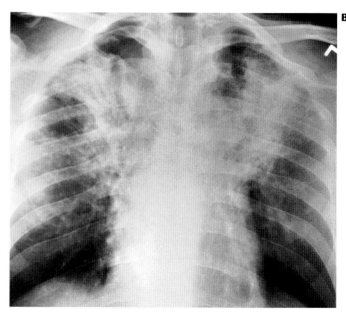

Fig. 8.28 Acute silicoproteinosis in a young man employed for 2 years as a sandblaster. **A**, Mediastinal adenopathy and upper zone opacity after 2 years of exposure. **B**, One year later there is dense consolidation of upper zones with air bronchograms. Death ensued shortly thereafter.

Intense exposure to silica dust may result in lung damage after only weeks or months, called *acute silicosis* or *silicoproteinosis*. In these cases, usually in sandblasters, there is a marked cellular and exudative alveolar reaction[148] and death may ensue within 1–3 years. The dominant feature is the presence of an alveolar proteinaceous exudate, similar to that found in pulmonary alveolar proteinosis, hence the term "acute silicoproteinosis".[149]

On radiographic examination of patients with silicoproteinosis there is widespread alveolar opacity that progresses over a period of months.[150] The opacity is quite symmetric, but central and upper zone predominance is frequent (Fig. 8.28). Air bronchograms may be noted, and contraction of the lungs may be minimal at first, suggesting consolidation of the lungs. Hilar and mediastinal adenopathy may be seen, but the hila are often obscured by the parenchymal opacities. Peripheral air-trapping, bulla formation, lung volume loss, and distortion of mediastinal structures all indicate increasing fibrosis. Pneumothorax may occur. Silicoproteinosis may present with recurrent episodes of apparent pneumonia.[151] In a report of the CT findings in two workers with silicoproteinosis,[152] hilar enlargement, centrilobular nodules, and patchy consolidation were described, but the crazy-paving pattern typically found in pulmonary alveolar proteinosis was not identified. However, a crazy-paving pattern was illustrated in another case described by Kim et al.[102]

The relative risk of *lung cancer* in silica exposed individuals ranges from 1.3 to 6.9, depending on the population,[151] but some of this excess risk is accounted for by cigarette smoking. Analysis is also complicated by the carcinogenic effect of radon gas exposure in miners. Nevertheless, both the American Thoracic Society,[151] and the International Agency for Research on Cancer,[153] have issued statements indicating that silica is a probable carcinogen and cause of lung cancer. It has not been established whether the risk is related to silica itself or to the pulmonary fibrosis induced by the silica.

Chronic bronchitis is probably the most common complication of silica exposure, often associated with airway obstruction. It has no radiographic manifestations, apart from airway wall thickening.

Silica exposure may be associated with *emphysema* (Fig. 8.25). However, as with lung cancer, the confounding effect of cigarette smoking complicates analysis. Non-smokers exposed to silica may develop emphysema,[117] particularly if they also have silicosis,[154] but the extent and physiologic significance of this emphysema are disputed.[155] It is clear, however, that in patients with simple silicosis, the degree of impairment of pulmonary function is more closely related to the presence and severity of emphysema on CT than to the profusion of nodules.[141,156] Most emphysema seen in association with silicosis is centrilobular, but cicatricial emphysema commonly occurs in association with PMF (Fig. 8.25).

Inhalation of silica predisposes to *mycobacterial infection*, both with *M. tuberculosis* and a wide range of nontuberculous mycobacteria (Fig. 8.29).[139] The relative risk of tuberculosis in workers with chronic silicosis is increased threefold compared with a control group.[151] The risk of mycobacterial infection is even greater in those with accelerated or acute silicosis, and in those with PMF. Mycobacterial infection in silicotics may be pulmonary or extrapulmonary. Pulmonary mycobacterial infection should always be suspected when cavitation or consolidation develops in a patient with silicosis (Fig. 8.29).

Silica workers have an increased risk of usual interstitial pneumonia.[157,158] They are also at increased risk of scleroderma,[159,160] and perhaps rheumatoid arthritis.[151]

Although silicosis is not usually associated with pleural abnormality, there have been several case reports of the development of *pleural thickening* and *rounded atelectasis* in patients with silicosis (Fig. 8.25).[161,162]

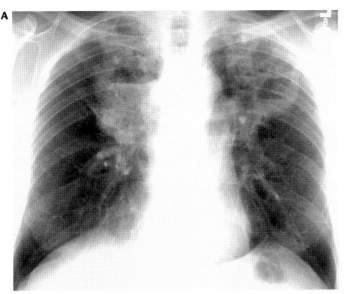

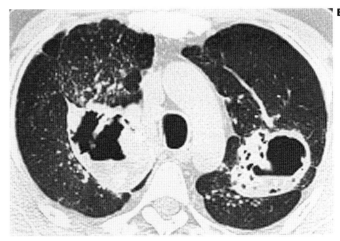

Fig. 8.29   Progressive massive fibrosis complicated by infection with *Mycobacterium terrae*. **A**, Chest radiograph shows cavitation in upper lobe masses. **B**, CT confirms cavitation, with associated nodules.

Coal worker's pneumoconiosis

The factors governing the degree of lung damage caused by inhaling coal dust are not fully understood. Probably the most important factor is the amount of dust of suitable particle size that is inhaled.[163] What is less certain is the importance of the silica content of the dust. That coal dust alone could cause classic PMF was shown many years ago in coal trimmers who, because they worked in the hulls of ships, were exposed only to coal dust containing virtually no free silica. At postmortem examination their disease was found to be due to coal dust alone.[164] Later epidemiologic studies showed that the radiographic changes in miners are closely related to coal dust exposure,[165] but poorly related to the silica content of the coal. It is generally agreed that silica plays little part in simple coal worker's pneumoconiosis,[163,166] though some dispute this.[167,168] However, there is reasonable evidence that silica plays a part in the development of PMF in some cases,[169,170] and that PMF can develop in miners exposed to coal dust with negligible quantities of silica.[171]

With excessive dust load of appropriate size, clearance by the mucociliary escalator is overwhelmed and dust-laden macrophages aggregate in the respiratory bronchioles and alveoli. After a time fibroblasts lay down reticulin. The aggregation of dust and fibroblasts leads to the basic lesion of simple pneumoconiosis – the coal macule. If silica is released, collagenous fibrosis is stimulated. The coal macule develops around bronchioles, weakening the bronchiolar wall and leading to proximal acinar or focal emphysema,[172,173] a form of centrilobular emphysema believed to be clinically unimportant.[166] The extent to which clinically important panacinar emphysema is caused by coal dust is debated.[172–176]

Despite the similarity of their radiographic appearances, coal worker's pneumoconiosis and silicosis are different pathologically. The coal macule does not have a hyaline center, nor does it show the laminated collagen typical of the silicotic nodule.

The massive nodules (defined as those with a diameter >1 cm) in coal worker's pneumoconiosis are ill-defined, amorphous, inhomogeneous collections of proteinaceous material, mineral dust, and calcium phosphates. The mass lesions may cavitate with or without infection.

Clinical features

It has been stated that simple coal worker's pneumoconiosis is symptom free.[166] However, as with silica workers, coal miners commonly have symptoms of bronchitis and emphysema, features that are excluded from the definition of pneumoconiosis, but are responsible for significant symptoms and physiologic impairment. The extent to which these two processes are due to coal dust exposure or other factors such as smoking is contentious.[103,166,177]

PMF category A (<5 cm) appears not to cause symptoms or signs. PMF categories B and C may be associated with respiratory disability and deterioration in ventilatory function tests.[166] Cough and sputum sometimes occur. Hemoptysis is rare. Jet black sputum (melanoptysis) caused by ischemic rupture of PMF into a bronchus is occasionally reported.

Radiographic appearances

The radiographic and CT signs of coal worker's pneumoconiosis are usually indistinguishable from those described above for silicosis (Figs 8.30 and 8.31). Statistically, the main differences between coal worker's pneumoconiosis and silicosis are that the nodules in coal worker's pneumoconiosis tend to be smaller, and that silicosis is more likely to progress to PMF.

PMF is uncommon in coal workers with <20 years' experience in and around the mines.[178] Its appearance in coal workers is identical to that seen in silicosis (Fig. 8.32). Masses of PMF, as the name implies, enlarge with time. The rate of growth is, however, very slow, an observable increase in diameter taking

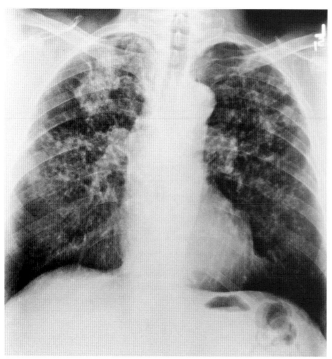

Fig. 8.30 Coal worker's pneumoconiosis. A typical example showing widespread middle and upper zone small nodules with category A progressive massive fibrosis (PMF). PMF opacities are larger on the right than on the left.

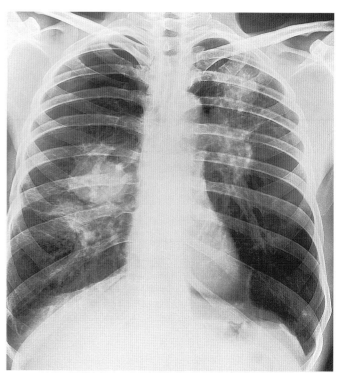

Fig. 8.32 Coal worker's pneumoconiosis with progressive massive fibrosis (PMF). There has been substantial medial migration of the right PMF opacity. Note the punctate calcification in the left-sided masses and also accompanying severe emphysema.

years, not months, as is the case with carcinoma. In some cases PMF lesions migrate medially toward the hilum, leaving a rim of peripheral cicatricial emphysema (Fig. 8.32). The migration is slow, taking 10 or more years to reach the hilum. Severe emphysema accompanies such migration. Cavitation may be visible, and the cavities may empty and fill over a period of time.[179] Cavitation may be associated with expectoration of jet black sputum (melanoptysis). When this occurs, CT or MRI may show a fluid–fluid level within the cavity, and may show rim enhancement.[180] The presence of cavitation should always raise the suspicion of mycobacterial superinfection.

A 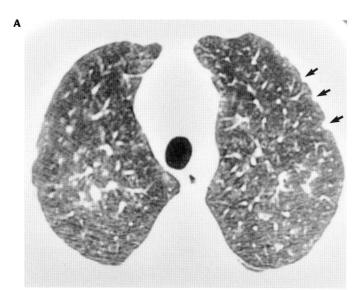 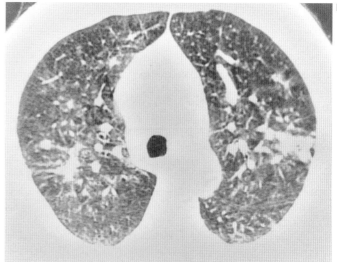 **B**

Fig. 8.31 Coal worker's pneumoconiosis. **A**, HRCT shows subpleural nodules (arrows) and micronodules. **B**, HRCT at a lower level shows developing conglomerate opacities of progressive massive fibrosis in the posterior and lateral aspects of the upper lobes. (Courtesy of Dr Martin Wastie, Nottingham, UK)

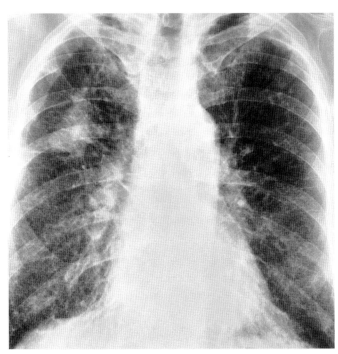

Fig. 8.33 Unilateral progressive massive fibrosis in a West Virginia coal miner.

Since PMF is frequently bilateral and accompanied by widespread nodules in the remainder of the lungs (Fig. 8.30), the diagnosis is rarely in doubt. There are cases, however, where the mass is completely or predominantly unilateral (Fig. 8.33) and background nodules may be minimal or absent. In such cases the differential diagnosis from lung carcinoma becomes particularly important. In a patient with a long history of exposure, a lens shaped density is virtually diagnostic of PMF if it is peripherally situated in an upper lobe close to and parallel to the major fissure, and has a well-defined outer margin paralleling the chest wall. Another important feature that distinguishes PMF from bronchial carcinoma is small irregular calcifications that may be seen within PMF; sometimes the mass has a calcified rim. The presence of upper lobe volume loss and peripheral emphysema may also be helpful. MRI has been used to distinguish lung cancer from PMF.[181] Lung cancer is associated with high signal intensity on both T1- and T2-weighted sequences, in contrast to the low intensity of PMF. In addition to lung cancer, sarcoidosis must be considered in the imaging differential diagnosis of PMF, as its radiographic and CT features may be very similar.

A minority (perhaps 10–20%) of coal miners develop diffuse lung fibrosis, characterized on the chest radiograph by small irregular opacities (Fig. 8.34).[182,183] These irregular opacities correlate better than rounded opacities with the extent of physiologic impairment.[184] On chest CT scans, this entity is characterized by reticular abnormality often associated with honeycombing, similar to UIP or NSIP.[185,186] This abnormality may or may not be associated with pneumoconiotic nodules. This pattern of diffuse interstitial fibrosis appears to be associated with a high prevalence of lung cancer.[186]

The chest radiograph reflects fairly well the extent and severity of the macules and masses found pathologically and is therefore a good tool for diagnosing and following the progression of coal worker's pneumoconiosis.[120,140,165,174,179,187–189] The radiographic findings correlate well with the amount of dust to which the worker was exposed[167] and the quantity of dust found in the lungs at postmortem examination.[190] However, the correlation between the chest radiograph and lung function is poor, except in patients with large conglomerate masses,[191] probably because the radiograph substantially underdiagnoses the associated emphysema.[169,173] The degree of functional disability appears to correlate far better with the severity of emphysema than it does with the presence of macules or PMF.[141,173,188,192] The etiologic role of smoking in coal worker's emphysema is debated. Some studies have shown that coal miners have a degree of emphysema that is excessive even if allowance is made for age and smoking history.[193,194] This applies particularly to patients with PMF. At lesser degrees of pulmonary involvement, smoking may play a more significant role in the causation of the emphysema and hence the patient's symptoms.[141,195]

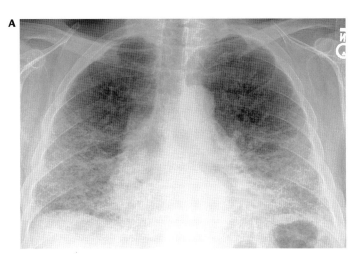
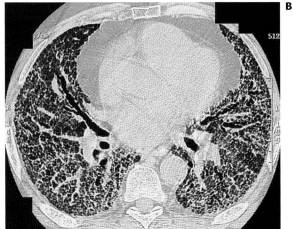

Fig. 8.34 Coal miner with diffuse lung fibrosis. **A**, Chest radiograph shows basal predominant reticular abnormality, with a substantial decrease in lung volumes. **B**, HRCT shows marked basal reticular abnormality with traction bronchiectasis and honeycombing. No nodules were seen.

Asbestos related diseases

Asbestos is composed of a group of fibrous silicates with differing chemical and physical properties but with the notable common property of heat resistance (Box 8.5). Chemical differences such as solubility and acid resistance, and physical differences such as fiber length, brittleness, and texture, are probably important determinants of the distribution and severity of deleterious effects on the lungs and pleura. Asbestos is divided into two principal subgroups based on the physical properties of the fibers: the serpentines; and the amphiboles. Serpentine asbestos has long, curly, flexible, smooth fibers composed of fibrillary subunits. The only serpentine asbestos used commercially is chrysotile, which accounts for >90% of the asbestos used in the United States today.[196] The amphiboles have straight, needlelike fibers of varying length, diameter, brittleness, and texture. The main types in use are crocidolite (blue asbestos), amosite (brown asbestos), tremolite, and anthophyllite. The longer, less soluble amphibole fibers tend to be very slow to clear from the lung, compared with chrysotile. A major reason for the decline in the use of the amphiboles was the recognition that the amphiboles, particularly crocidolite, have a much greater fibrogenic and carcinogenic potential than the serpentine form chrysotile.[197,198] It has even been suggested that chrysotile in its pure form has a minimal carcinogenic potential, and that contamination with the tremolite is the main reason for the carcinogenicity and fibrogenicity of the chrysotile forms of asbestos.[199–201] However, there is increasing evidence to support the contrary hypothesis that uncontaminated chrysotile is carcinogenic.[202–205]

Box 8.5 Asbestos

A family of naturally occurring fibrous silicates highly resistant to physical or chemical destruction

Two fiber types
Serpentine asbestos – long curly fibers composed of fibrillary subunits
- Chrysotile

Amphibole asbestos – straight shorter needlelike fibers
- Crocidolite
- Amosite
- Anthophyllite
- Tremolite

Uses
- Manufacture of cement, bricks, tiles, paints, fireproof felts and textiles
- Furnace and oven linings
- Insulation of steam pipes and electric lines
- Brake lining manufacture
- Fire proofing and insulation of buildings

World production and use of asbestos have expanded to an extraordinary degree over the past century. Production expanded from 50 tons per annum in the 1860s to a peak of >5 million tons per annum in the early 1970s.[206] Asbestos production has now declined somewhat as alternative materials have become available. Nevertheless, with the long latency which exists before the adverse effects of asbestos exposure become manifest (Box 8.6, Table 8.3), and with the vast tonnages of the material now in place or in use, asbestos is likely to remain one of the major environmental hazards well into the twenty-first century. A recent outbreak of asbestos related pleural disease and mesothelioma related to a vermiculite mine in Libby, Montana, illustrates the need for continued vigilance for asbestos related disease. The vermiculite was thought to be safe, but was contaminated with small amounts of tremolite, which was sufficient to cause a significant increase in mortality from lung cancer, mesothelioma, and asbestosis.[207,208]

Box 8.6 Adverse effects of asbestos exposure

Benign asbestos related pleural effusion(s)
Diffuse pleural thickening
Pleural plaque formation
Rounded atelectasis
Asbestosis
Malignancies
- Lung cancer and other epithelial malignancies – larynx, gastrointestinal tract
- Mesothelioma – pleural, peritoneal, pericardial

Benign asbestos related pleural effusion

Benign asbestos related pleural effusion is one of the less common manifestations of asbestos exposure, but it has the shortest latency period (Box 8.7).[209,210] The transient, often asymptomatic nature of these effusions and the lack of specific markers to indicate their cause undoubtedly accounted for the delayed recognition of this condition. Indeed the diagnosis is one of exclusion and should conform to the following criteria: (1) a history of occupational or environmental asbestos exposure; (2) no other cause for the effusion; and (3) no evidence of malignancy within 3 years of detecting the effusion.

In the noteworthy epidemiologic study by Epler et al,[209] the overall incidence of benign pleural effusion was 3.1%, with a 7% incidence among individuals having a heavy occupational exposure and a 0.2% incidence in environmentally exposed

Table 8.3 Frequency and latency of asbestos-related diseases (adapted with permission from Lynch et al. Imaging of diffuse lung disease. Hamilton: BC Decker, 2000)[a]

Finding	Latency (years)	Approximate frequency in asbestos workers (%)
Asbestos related effusion	5–20	3
Noncalcified plaques	15–30	15–80
Calcified plaques	30–40	10–50
Diffuse pleural thickening	10–40	10
Asbestosis	20–40	15–30
Lung cancer	>15	20–40[b]
Mesothelioma	15–40	10[b]

[a]The above figures are provided only as approximate guidelines. The prevalence or incidence of disease depends on the duration and intensity of exposure.
[b]Lifetime incidence.

Box 8.7 Pleural changes related to asbestos exposure

Benign asbestos related pleural effusion(s)
- May be the first manifestation of asbestos exposure
- Unilateral or bilateral
- Often asymptomatic; otherwise fever, pleuritic chest pain, or dyspnea
- Usually small but may be >500 ml
- Fluid – exudative often blood tinged
- Usually resolves completely but may leave diffuse pleural thickening

Diffuse pleural thickening
- Usually follows effusion
- Costophrenic sulcus blunted
- Usually asymptomatic but may cause pulmonary restriction

Pleural plaques
- Usually located on parietal pleura
- Most commonly seen between the fourth and eighth ribs
- No functional significance – they are a marker of asbestos exposure

Malignant mesothelioma

individuals. Effusions may be unilateral or bilateral and tend to recur. The amount of fluid is usually small; effusions >500 ml are uncommon. The fluid has the characteristics of an exudate and may be blood tinged. Symptoms include pleuritic pain, fever, and an elevated white blood cell count, but many patients have only mild symptoms or no symptoms at all. Indeed the presence of significant chest pain should lead to concern for mesothelioma.

Benign pleural effusion is the most common abnormality seen within 10 years of the onset of asbestos exposure. However, it may occur up to 58 years after initial exposure.[211] No direct causal relationship between benign effusions and the

subsequent development of malignant pleural effusion has been postulated, but in one study of 70 cases of malignant mesothelioma,[212] five cases were preceded by what were regarded as successive benign pleural effusions for up to 7 years. In asbestos workers with pleural effusions, the diagnosis of benign effusion should be a diagnosis of exclusion.

Mesothelioma should be considered in any patient with a latency longer than 10 years, or in any patient with chest wall pain. In one series of 312 cases of mesothelioma, the latency periods ranged from 14 to 72 years with a mean of 48 years.[213] There appeared to be a relationship to the intensity of exposure with, for example, a mean latency period of 30 years for insulators as opposed to 52 years for domestically exposed women.

Benign pleural effusions are associated with the subsequent development of diffuse pleural thickening (Fig. 8.35).[214,215] McLoud et al[216] found that just over 50% of their patients with benign pleural effusions subsequently developed diffuse basal pleural thickening, an association also emphasized by Cookson et al.[217] As discussed later, there is a possible association between benign pleural effusions and the subsequent development of rounded atelectasis.[218] Diffuse pleural thickening frequently results in some restrictive impairment of pulmonary function.[219, 220] This is not usually progressive over time.[219,220] On rare occasion the degree and extent of the subsequent pleural thickening may be such that the resulting impairment of lung function necessitates surgical decortication.[120,221]

Asbestos related pleural plaques

Irregular pleural thickening and calcification were first positively related to exposure to asbestos in 1955,[218] and the occurrence of noncalcified, asbestos induced plaques was first reported in 1967.[222] Considerable attention has since been paid to these changes, as they represent the most frequent radiographic manifestation of exposure to asbestos. Although the incidence of pleural plaque formation increases with dose, the elapsed time from initial exposure is a more important factor.[223] Pleural

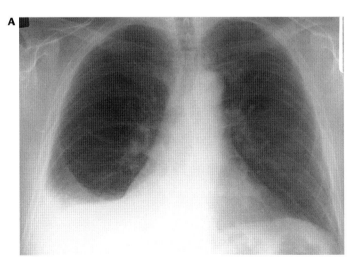
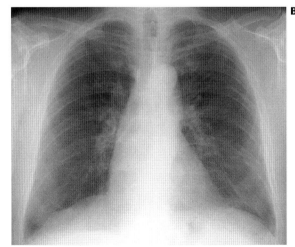

Fig. 8.35 Diffuse pleural thickening occurring as a sequel of benign asbestos related effusion. **A**, Chest radiograph shows an asymptomatic benign asbestos related effusion on the right. **B**, Chest radiograph 5 years later shows clearing of the effusion, but residual pleural thickening evident by blunting of the right costophrenic sulcus.

plaques are usually first identified >20–30 years after the initial asbestos exposure.[224] Asbestos induced pleural plaques occur on the parietal pleura, especially over the diaphragm and along the posterolateral chest wall. The apices, the costophrenic sulci, and the mediastinal surfaces tend to be spared. The plaques are composed of elevated areas of hyalinized fibrous tissue and frequently lie beneath the ribs. Although usually isolated, they may enlarge, spread, and coalesce. Dystrophic calcification within plaques is common and is more frequent as the plaques age and enlarge. Electron microscopy studies have identified asbestos fibers in the plaques on the parietal pleura, indicating that transpleural migration and assimilation of inhaled asbestos fibers must occur.[225] There is evidence that the widely used, more benign form of asbestos, chrysotile, is particularly associated with this transpleural migration, while the more fibrogenic and carcinogenic amphiboles, crocidolite and amosite, tend to be retained in the lung parenchyma.[224,226] This may account for the widespread finding of asbestos related pleural disease unassociated with parenchymal fibrosis or intrathoracic malignancy.

Population surveys in industrial regions and in asbestos mining areas have revealed a surprisingly high incidence of pleural plaques even in individuals who have only a remote connection with asbestos.[227–229] The use of asbestos is so widespread that many individuals are exposed unknowingly, and therefore accurate data are difficult to obtain. In autopsy based studies of unselected populations, pleural plaques may be found in up to 20% of patients, and a history of asbestos exposure is lacking in most of these,[230, 231] particularly where the plaques are small or unilateral.[231] Therefore, the possibility of another, as yet unidentified, environmental agent as a cause of pleural plaque formation cannot be discounted. In an exhaustive study of pleural plaque formation in a rural region of Czechoslovakia, Rous and Studeny[232] were adamant that asbestos could not be implicated in their cases. Pleural plaque formation and calcification have been noted to occur after contact with other nonasbestos fibrous minerals, such as erionite in Turkey[233] and sepiolite in Bulgaria.[234]

On radiographic examination, noncalcified pleural plaques are irregular, smooth elevations of the pleura most easily identified in profile along the chest wall or over the diaphragm (Fig. 8.36). Plaques are less easily seen en face unless they are large or calcified. Plaques seen en face are seen as amorphous areas of increased density. They are relatively flat in relation to their width, and the density of the opacity projected over the lungs is therefore less than would be expected for a parenchymal lesion of equivalent size. Furthermore, one margin of the lesion is likely to be indistinct as it smooths off into normal pleura. Plaques are usually multiple and bilateral. Although Hu et al[235] reported that pleural plaques detected on chest radiographs

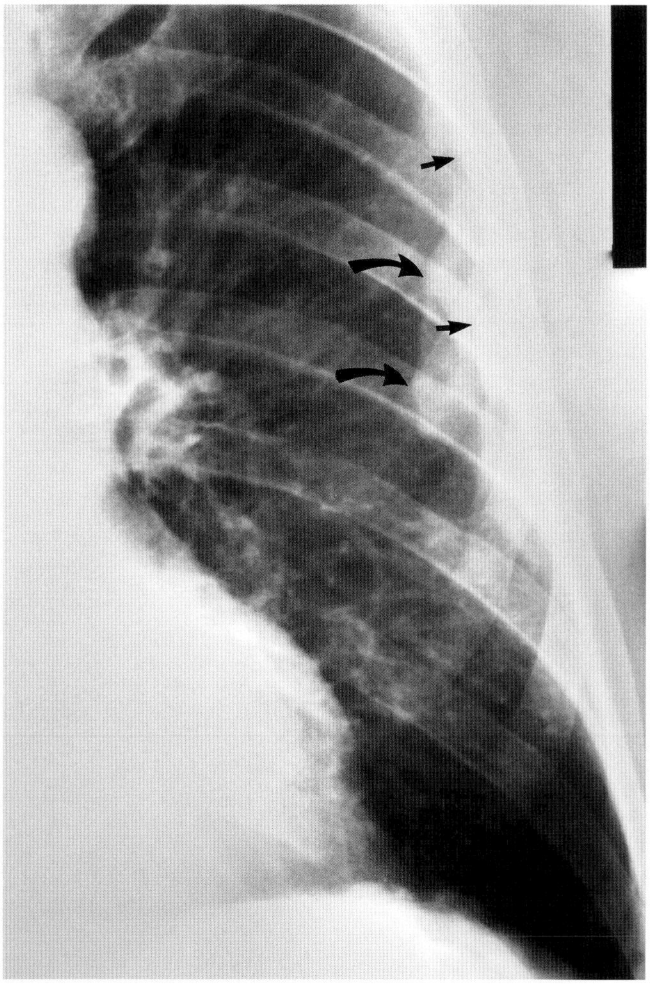

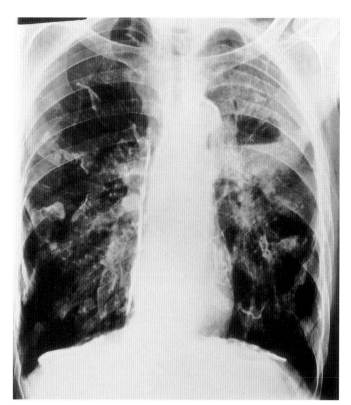

Fig. 8.36 Noncalcified pleural plaques seen in profile (straight arrows) and en face (curved arrows) in an asbestos exposed individual. Note the typical location between the fourth and eighth ribs, and the sparing of the costophrenic sulcus.

Fig. 8.37 Linear calcification in pleural plaques over the diaphragm and in the right paravertebral region. There is also calcified plaque formation seen en face, as well as a left upper lobe cavitating bronchial carcinoma.

were statistically more common on the left, a left-sided predominance was not confirmed in a CT based study.[236]

Calcification in pleural plaques is linear when seen in profile (Fig. 8.37), but when seen en face, its appearance is variable (Fig. 8.38), the most common type being "holly leaf" calcification (Fig. 8.39). Extensive pleural calcification in association with parenchymal fibrosis may be lacelike (Fig. 8.40). Enlargement and spreading of plaques result in thick irregular sheets of pleural thickening, which are often calcified. Pleural plaques may occur on the visceral pleura, but these can usually only be identified when a plaque is present in an interlobar fissure (Fig. 8.41).[237,238] Smooth visceral pleural thickening due to plaque must be distinguished from the more irregular subpleural fibrosis which occurs in patients with asbestosis.[239]

Asbestos exposure may be associated with pericardial fibrosis, with or without calcification or effusion.[240,241] Yazicioglu,[242] in a study of 511 cases of pleural disease secondary to environmental exposure to chrysolite asbestos in Turkey, found that 1.7% of cases had coincident pericardial calcification. Asbestos related pericardial fibrosis may lead to constrictive pericarditis.[240,243]

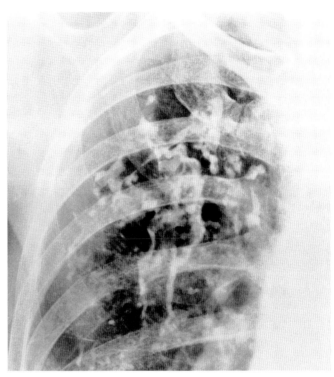

Fig. 8.39 "Holly leaf" calcification in asbestos related plaques seen en face.

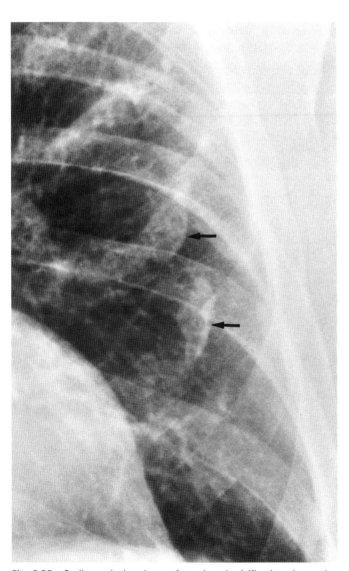

Fig. 8.38 Radiograph showing en face pleural calcifications (arrows).

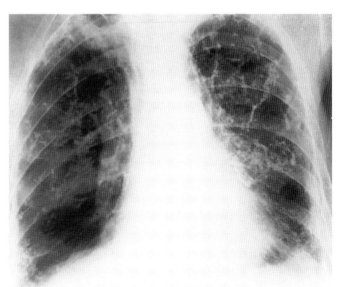

Fig. 8.40 Lacelike asbestos related pleural plaque formation seen en face.

Visualization of pleural plaques is improved by optimal radiographic technique. Oblique views can substantially increase the rate of plaque detection by throwing posterolateral plaques into profile.[244]

The differential diagnosis of pleural plaques includes extrapleural fat deposition in obesity,[245] extrapleural thickening in relation to multiple rib fractures, postinflammatory pleural thickening, and pleural metastases. In practice, the most frequent simulator of asbestos related pleural plaque formation is extra-

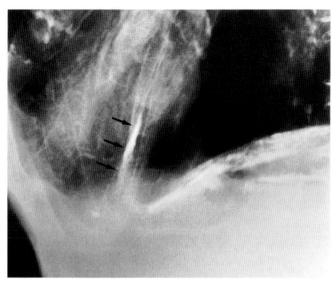

Fig. 8.41 Detail view of lateral chest radiograph shows calcified plaque formation in a major fissure (arrows). Calcification must be in the visceral pleura. There is also extensive diaphragmatic pleural calcification.

pleural fat deposition.[246] Extrapleural fat may be differentiated from pleural plaques by its lower density, its smooth, undulating outline, and by the fact that it typically extends all the way to the lung apices (Fig. 8.42). Fat is most abundant over the fourth to eighth ribs and does not involve the costophrenic sulci. Of course, CT will readily distinguish the soft tissue density of pleural plaques from extrapleural fat.

Although the presence of pleural plaques is associated with less physiologic impairment than diffuse pleural thickening, several studies have indicated that identification of plaques on chest radiographs is associated with evidence of pulmonary restriction, independent of the presence or extent of radiographic parenchymal abnormality.[220,247–250] However, it seems likely that

at least some of this association is explained by the presence of subradiographic asbestosis.[251,252]

CT is substantially more sensitive than the chest radiograph for detection of pleural plaques (Fig. 8.43).[253–256] Contiguous CT imaging maximizes sensitivity for plaques.[257] CT is also more sensitive than radiographs for detecting calcification in plaques.[258] Elevated plaques may indent the adjacent lung, and may even cause ground-glass abnormality by interfering with local pulmonary expansion. Thinner plaques may be difficult to distinguish from the intercostal musculature, but may be identified by recognizing that they overlay ribs as well as intercostal spaces (Fig. 8.44).

Diffuse pleural thickening

It is important to distinguish between asbestos related diffuse pleural thickening and pleural plaques because patients with diffuse pleural thickening commonly have significant impairment of pulmonary function. The radiographic definition of diffuse pleural thickening has varied. The ILO classification defines it as pleural thickening that involves the costophrenic sulci (Figs 8.35 and 8.45),[105] while McLoud et al[216] also included patients in whom pleural plaques occupied more than one-quarter of the chest wall. Most studies have used the more restrictive ILO definition. On CT scanning, the definition of diffuse pleural thickening has also varied. Lynch et al[239] defined it as an area of pleural thickening >3 mm thick, >5 cm in transverse dimension, and >8 cm in craniocaudal dimension.[239] However, Copley et al[259] defined diffuse pleural thickening as pleural thickening with tapered margins, in contrast to pleural plaques, which were required by this definition to have well-defined margins. Since diffuse pleural thickening, by all definitions, is associated with physiologic impairment, it seems likely that the precise definition of this entity is of little importance.

Asbestos related diffuse pleural thickening must be distinguished from the visceral pleural and subpleural fibrosis which occurs in patients with many forms of lung fibrosis (including

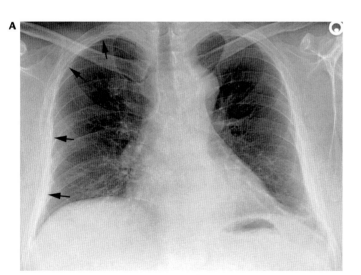
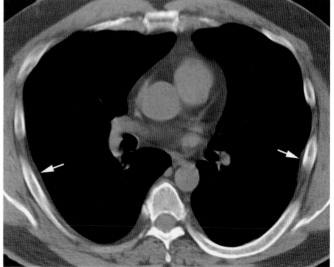

Fig. 8.42 Extrapleural fat. **A**, Chest radiograph shows soft tissue thickening extending in an undulating fashion all the way to the apices (arrows). The costophrenic sulci are not involved. **B**, CT confirms extrapleural fat (arrows).

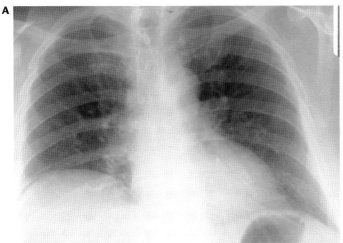

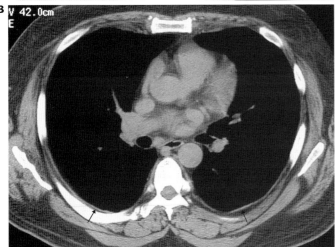

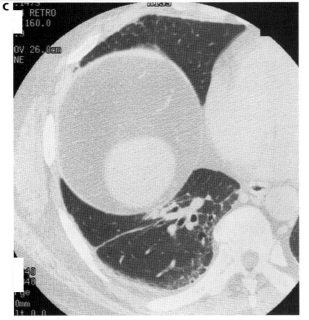

Fig. 8.43 A 60-year-old male with radiographically occult pleural plaques and asbestosis. **A**, Chest radiograph is normal apart from elevated right hemidiaphragm and mild cardiomegaly. **B**, CT shows pleural plaques (arrows) which are not visible on the chest radiograph because they are posterior. **C**, Supine HRCT shows fine parenchymal reticular abnormality with traction bronchiectasis. Septal thickening is seen in the nondependent anterior right lung.

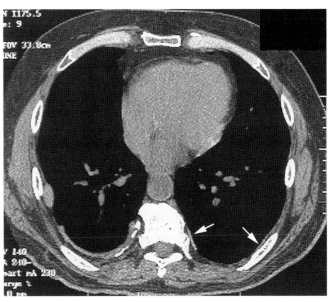

Fig. 8.44 A 68-year-old man with asbestos related pleural plaques. CT shows bilateral plaques. The plaques on the right are easy to recognize because they are elevated and the more medial plaque is partly calcified. The linear plaques on the left (arrows) are more subtle; the more medial plaque is recognizable because it is hyperdense, while the more lateral plaque is distinguishable from intercostal muscles because it overlies a rib.

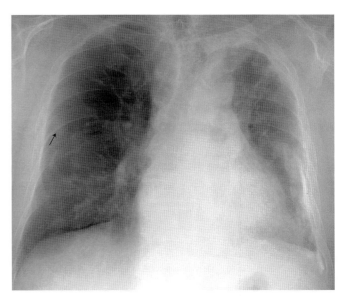

Fig. 8.45 Diffuse pleural thickening. Chest radiograph shows diffuse pleural thickening around the left hemithorax, associated with calcification, and blunting of the costophrenic sulcus. A noncalcified plaque is seen en face on the right (arrow).

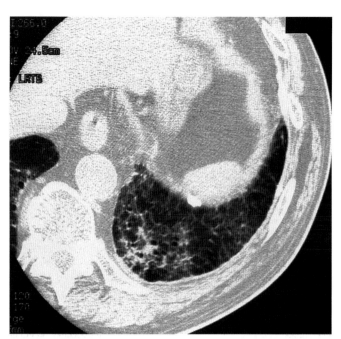

Fig. 8.46 Visceral pleural thickening in asbestosis. HRCT shows reticular abnormality with traction bronchiectasis. Note the fine irregularity of the visceral pleura, which differs from the smooth interface seen with parietal pleural plaques.

asbestosis). Pure parietal pleural thickening is usually sharply defined on CT, while visceral pleural fibrosis is associated with fine fibrous strands extending into the underlying lung, giving a "blurred" or "fluffy" demarcation to the pleural process (Fig. 8.46).[239,260] Visceral pleural fibrosis is usually, but not always, associated with other evidence of lung fibrosis. Visceral pleural/subpleural fibrosis can sometimes be identified on the chest radiograph as thickening of the interlobar fissures (scored as "pi" in the ILO classification system).[261] Asbestos related diffuse pleural thickening often cannot be differentiated from pleural thickening due to prior empyema, infection, or other cause. Interestingly, patients with asbestos related diffuse pleural thickening were found to have a more frequent history of coronary bypass surgery than other asbestos exposed individuals, suggesting that thoracic surgery may have a synergistic role in the development of this complication.[262] Diffuse pleural thickening can usually be differentiated from mesothelioma by the absence of pleural effusion or pleural masses.

The relationship between asbestos related pleural disease and physiologic impairment has been extensively evaluated. It is clear from numerous studies using both chest radiographs[220] and chest CT[259,262] that diffuse pleural thickening, however defined, is associated with substantial restriction of pulmonary function.

Rounded atelectasis

Rounded atelectasis, also called folded lung,[263] is a masslike area of lung collapse occurring in relation to an area of pleural thickening. The condition is not unique to asbestos related pleural thickening, and may also be seen with any other cause of exudative or organizing pleural disease. Although typically associated with benign pleural disease, it may sometimes be seen with mesothelioma.[264]

Hanke and Kretzschmar[265] proposed that rounded atelectasis occurs when an atelectatic area of lung becomes infolded during resorption of a pleural effusion. Other authors,[266,267] noting that rounded atelectasis is not always preceded by a pleural effusion, have suggested that it may result from centripetal contraction of a focus of visceral pleural fibrosis, causing buckling of the pleura and collapse of the underlying lung parenchyma.

The radiographic findings are characteristic (Box 8.8, Fig. 8.47). Rounded atelectasis typically presents with a masslike area adjacent to the pleura. Despite its name, rounded atelectasis is not usually round, but may be oval, lenticular, or irregular in shape. Acute angles are usually visible at the pleural margins and indicate an intraparenchymal location. The mass is usually separated from the diaphragm by interposed lung. The pleura is thickened, particularly in the vicinity of the lesion, and the costophrenic sulci are usually blunted or obliterated. The pathognomonic feature, however, is the characteristic pattern of distortion of the vessels and bronchi in the vicinity of the lesion. The vessels leading toward the mass are crowded, but as they reach the mass, they tend to arc around the undersurface of the mass before merging with it. This appearance has been described as the "comet tail" sign.[268] Rounded atelectasis may be solitary

---

Box 8.8 Rounded atelectasis

Causes
Asbestos related pleural fibrosis (70%)
Tuberculous pleuritis or any nonspecific pleuritis
Dressler syndrome or chronic heart failure

Radiographic features
Intraparenchymal mass
Single or multiple
Juxtapleural location, often posterior and basal
Subjacent pleural thickening
Convergence of bronchovascular bundles into the mass –
   "comet tail"
Stability over time

CT features
Mass directly related to pleural thickening
Curving of bronchi and vessels into medial, lateral, and
   inferior aspects of mass
Homogeneous enhancement
Lobar volume loss (fissural displacement)

---

or multiple,[268] and is most commonly found in one of the lower lobes posteriorly or posteromedially.[269] The lingula or the middle lobe may also be involved (Fig. 8.48), but upper lobe involvement is less common.[266,270]

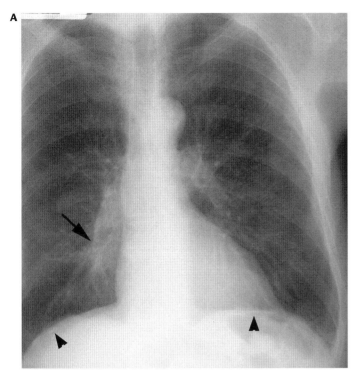

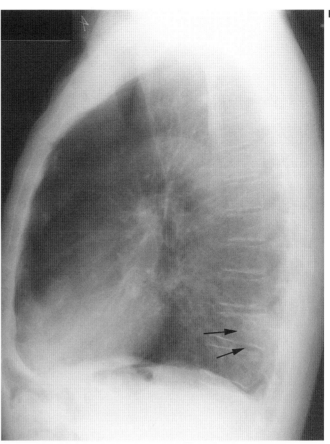

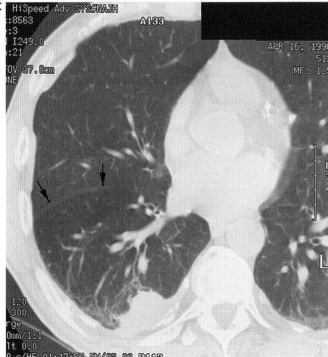

Fig. 8.47 Rounded atelectasis. **A**, Frontal chest radiograph shows a subtle increase in density on the right (arrow). Linear plaque calcification is evident along each hemidiaphragm (arrowheads). **B**, Lateral chest radiograph shows a rounded mass along the posterior pleura (arrows). **C**, CT shows a rounded mass adjacent to an area of pleural thickening, with a vessel curving into its lateral aspect. Lobar volume loss is evident from the posterior displacement of the major fissure (arrows).

CT is usually employed to confirm the diagnosis of rounded atelectasis. The characteristic CT signs of rounded atelectasis are the direct relationship of the mass to an area of pleural thickening, the presence of lobar volume loss with fissural displacement, and the curving of bronchi and vessels into the medial and lateral aspects of the mass (Fig. 8.49).[270–273] The margin directed toward the hilum is usually indistinct, though the other margins are well defined. An air bronchogram may be noted in the lesion. Like most types of atelectasis, rounded atelectasis enhances homogeneously after intravenous

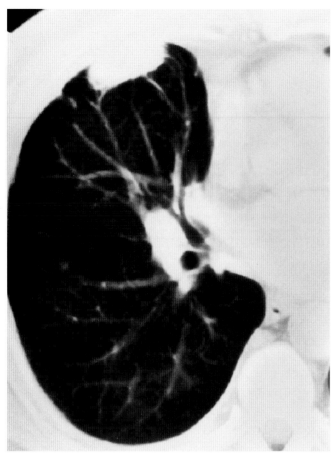

Fig. 8.48 Rounded atelectasis in the middle lobe of a middle-aged man with a previous asbestos related pleural effusion.

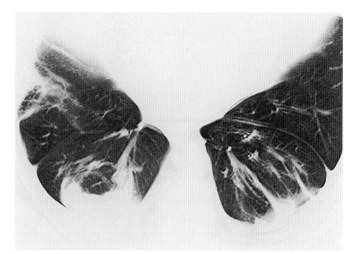

Fig. 8.49 CT in the prone position (but oriented as if supine) showing bilateral posterior basal rounded atelectasis. Note the marked bilateral posterior fissural displacement.

Asbestosis

Asbestosis is one of the main health hazards related to asbestos exposure, second only to bronchogenic carcinoma.[221] It was first identified with certainty at the turn of the century,[278] and by the mid 1980s an estimated 65,000 individuals in the United States had clinically diagnosable asbestosis.[279] The term "asbestosis" is generally reserved for asbestos induced pulmonary fibrosis (Box 8.9). Pleural abnormalities are excluded by definition, being regarded more as an indication of such exposure than as a significant disease entity. Asbestosis is related to the cumulative dust exposure whereas the parietal pleural changes are more related to the length of time since the initial exposure.[196] The time interval between the initial exposure and the development of evidence of asbestosis is extremely variable, but 20–30 years is usual. Intense exposures can cause asbestosis in as short a period as 3 years, but this is exceptional. The most fibrogenic form of asbestos is crocidolite, and in descending order of fibrogenicity are amosite, anthophyllite, and chrysotile.

administration of contrast material.[274] Multiplanar reconstruction can provide an excellent depiction of the converging bronchovascular pattern (Fig. 8.50).

The appearance of rounded atelectasis on MRI has been described.[275] The lesion had a signal intensity similar to liver on T1-weighted images, and blood vessels and bronchi were seen to curve into the mass. On ultrasound, Marchbank et al[276] were able to identify a highly echogenic line extending into the mass from the pleural surface in 12 of 14 patients. These authors postulated that this line represented the scarred invaginated pleura.

The main differential diagnosis of rounded atelectasis is peripheral bronchogenic carcinoma, and biopsy may be necessary to exclude bronchogenic carcinoma where the CT features are atypical for rounded atelectasis. The necessity for continued follow up of cases of rounded atelectasis should be emphasized. Rounded atelectasis is ordinarily a static or very slowly growing process. O'Donovan et al,[277] in an evaluation of the reliability of CT in distinguishing rounded atelectasis from other pleural based masses, found that no single CT feature allowed perfect discrimination. They found the convergence of bronchovascular markings to be the best discriminator, but one case was encountered in which lung cancer developed within an area of rounded atelectasis.

Box 8.9 Asbestosis

Pulmonary fibrosis related to asbestos exposure

Chest radiograph
Small irregular opacities with basal and subpleural predominance
Benign asbestos related pleural changes and rounded atelectasis may be present

Computed tomography
Prone imaging is essential to detect early changes
Peripheral, basal, and posterior predominance
Interlobular septal thickening
Centrilobular thickening
Reticular abnormality
Honeycombing
Subpleural curvilinear density

A

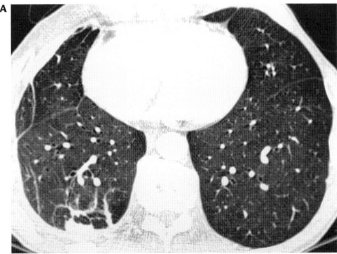

Fig. 8.50 A 76-year-old man with pleural disease and rounded atelectasis related to exposure to vermiculite contaminated with tremolite asbestos. **A**, Axial thin section shows a rounded mass adjacent to an area of pleural thickening, with bronchi and vessels curving into the medial and lateral aspects of the mass. Volume loss is confirmed by the posterior fissural displacement, and rightward mediastinal shift. **B**, Parasagittal maximum intensity projection reconstruction of contrast enhanced image shows the enhancing atelectatic lung (arrows) adjacent to the posterior pleural thickening (arrowheads). **C**, Corresponding lung windows show the "comet tail" of vessels curving into the inferior aspect of the mass.

B

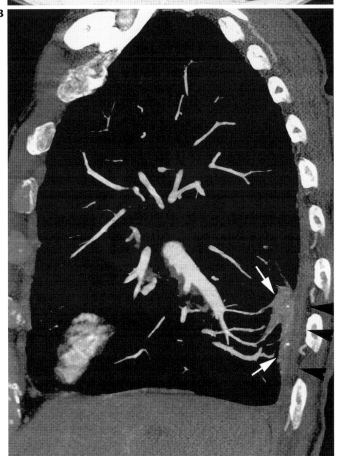

C

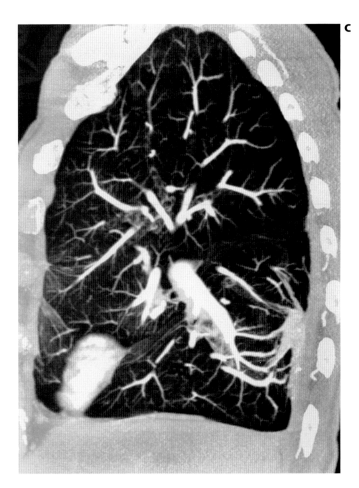

Asbestos causes interstitial pulmonary fibrosis, spreading centrifugally from the region of the terminal bronchioles and the alveolar ducts,[280] with histologic features that are indistinguishable from those of IPF. The changes predominate in the subpleural portions of the lungs and at the lung bases. Visceral pleural thickening occurs, particularly over the regions of maximum fibrosis. Established asbestos induced pulmonary fibrosis tends to progress with time even after cessation of exposure.[281-283] Symptoms of dyspnea and dry cough usually develop approximately 20 years following initial exposure. Characteristic functional abnormalities consist of progressive reduction of both vital capacity and diffusing capacity.[221]

The diagnosis of asbestosis must not be based on imaging features alone. It requires consideration of the occupational history or possible environmental exposure, the clinical features (breathlessness, clubbing, lung crackles), the results of pulmonary function tests, and the chest radiographic and CT appearances.

On the chest radiograph, asbestosis typically presents with basal predominant reticular interstitial abnormality (small irregular opacities according to the ILO classification), which may later extend up the lateral chest wall (Figs 8.51 and 8.52). Progressive disease leads to honeycombing and lower lobe volume loss. Associated pleural abnormalities facilitate the diagnosis, but may be absent on the chest radiograph in 10% of cases.[284] Coarse or fine linear bands of fibrosis are commonly seen radiating from pleural surfaces. Conglomerate opacities akin to PMF have been reported in asbestosis,[285,286] but may relate to concomitant exposure to silica or talc.[287] A limitation of chest radiographic assessment of asbestosis is the questionable physiologic and pathologic significance of the small irregular opacities which are the chest radiographic hallmark of early asbestosis. In at least some cases these small irregular opacities appear to be related to a combination of cigarette smoke and asbestos exposure.[125]

The main indications for the use of CT in asbestosis are: (1) identification of pulmonary fibrosis as distinct from emphysema or diffuse pleural disease[254]; (2) identification of asbestosis in workers with normal parenchyma on chest radiographs[256,288]; (3) identification of pulmonary fibrosis for compensation purposes when the chest radiographs and pulmonary function tests give conflicting results; and (4) investigation of suspected pleural or parenchymal masses and guidance for their biopsy.

Early asbestosis is manifested on HRCT by prominent centrilobular structures, interlobular septal thickening, intra-lobular lines, curvilinear subpleural lines, and peripheral reticular opacities (Fig. 8.53).[253,256] Because of the posterior and basal predominance of the lesions of early asbestosis, examination of the lung bases in the prone position is critical for confirming the fixed nature of septal thickening and curvilinear subpleural lines. More advanced asbestosis is characterized by parenchymal bands of fibrosis, honeycombing, and traction bronchiectasis (Figs 8.46 and 8.54). None of these features is specific for asbestosis, and similar changes may be seen in other

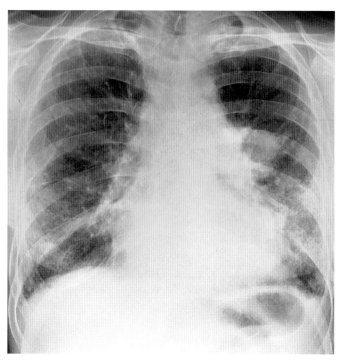

Fig. 8.52 Asbestosis with a bronchogenic carcinoma in the left lung. Note basal predominant fibrosis. There is slight blunting of the costophrenic sulci; otherwise, pleural changes are lacking in this case.

lung diseases such as IPF.[289] When CT scans of patients with asbestosis are compared with those of patients with IPF, patients with asbestosis have a higher prevalence of parenchymal bands, centrilobular nodules, and subpleural curvilinear lines, while the prevalence of traction bronchiolectasis and honeycombing is lower.[290,291] Copley et al[292] have recently

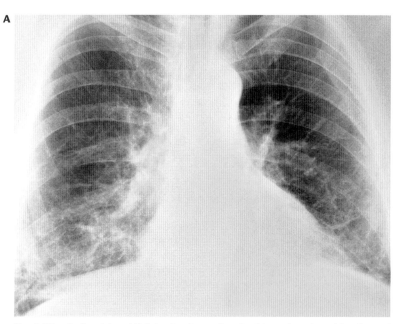
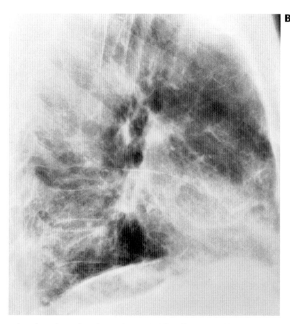

Fig. 8.51 **A**, Frontal and **B**, lateral radiographs of a shipyard worker with asbestosis showing basal predominant interstitial pulmonary fibrosis. There is widespread pleural calcification.

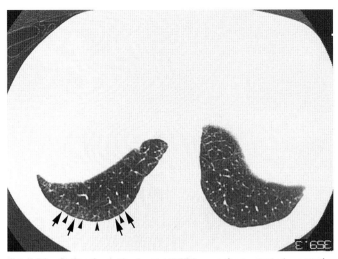

Fig. 8.53 Early asbestosis. Prone HRCT image shows posterior septal thickening (arrows) and centrilobular thickening (arrowheads). The changes were present bilaterally and at multiple levels.

shown that asbestosis shows a coarser pattern of fibrosis on CT than that found in UIP or NSIP.

The chest radiograph is relatively insensitive for detection of asbestosis[22,120,131,293] (Fig. 8.43). Staples et al[288] studied HRCT in asbestos exposed subjects with normal lung parenchyma on chest radiographs. Both vital capacity and diffusing capacity (percent predicted) were significantly lower in those who had abnormal HRCT scans. Similarly, in a study by Oksa et al,[294] an HRCT score for parenchymal abnormalities correlated significantly with diffusing capacity and total lung capacity in patients who had normal lung parenchyma on chest radiographs. Neri et al[295] showed that the presence of parenchymal abnormality on CT was associated with a significantly lower FVC in non-smoking asbestos exposed subjects. Thus, parenchymal abnormalities seen on CT in asbestos workers are clearly associated with physiologic impairment, even in those with normal chest radiographs.

The radiographic and CT changes of asbestosis usually progress over time, but the rate of progression is usually less than that seen in IPF. Akira et al[296] in a serial study of 23 asbestos exposed patients with minimal or no abnormalities on chest radiographs, demonstrated that the changes of early asbestosis progressed in two of seven patients who were reexamined between 10 and 19 months after the first CT scan, and in six of eight patients who were examined between 20 and 39 months after the first CT examination. This evidence of progression on CT was accompanied by decrease in lung diffusing capacity in three of four patients in whom serial pulmonary function tests were available. Progression of disease by HRCT criteria appeared to be more prominent in cigarette smokers. Using post mortem HRCT scans these authors also demonstrated that the centrilobular nodules and branching structures corresponded histologically to fibrosis around the bronchioles, which subsequently involved the alveolar ducts. Pleural based nodular irregularities corresponded histologically to subpleural fibrosis. Hazy patches of increased attenuation tended to correspond to fibrotic thickening of the alveolar walls and interlobular septa.

A study by Gamsu et al[297] shows that the CT findings of early asbestosis are neither sensitive nor specific. Some patients with abnormal lung parenchyma on CT have no histologic evidence of asbestosis, while some with normal CT or minor parenchymal abnormalities have histologic asbestosis. However, the study showed that asbestosis can be diagnosed with confidence when parenchymal changes are bilateral or present at multiple levels.

The relationship between asbestosis and lung cancer is controversial. Histologic asbestosis is almost invariably seen in asbestos workers who develop lung cancer.[131] Although there is a strong association between lung cancer and the presence of radiographic asbestosis[298,299] (Figs 8.55 and 8.56), asbestosis is not always visible on the chest radiograph or chest CT when lung cancer is present.[131,297,300,301]

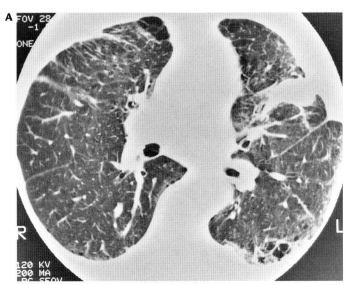

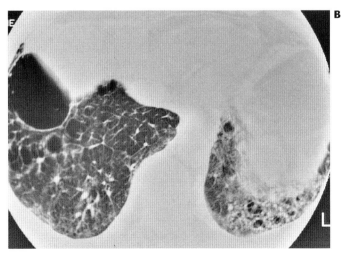

Fig. 8.54 Asbestosis. **A**, HRCT shows coarse bands of fibrous tissue extending into the lung from the pleural surface. Some of these bands emanate from a pleural plaque. **B**, HRCT at a lower level shows a right anterior bulla, with left basal reticular abnormality, traction bronchiectasis, and honeycombing. (Courtesy of Dr C Fuhrman, Pittsburgh)

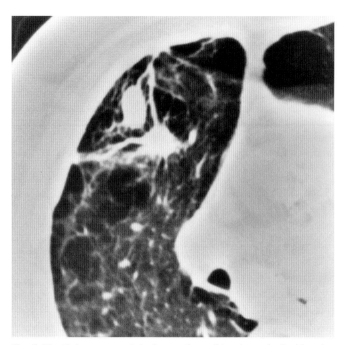

Fig. 8.55 Pulmonary nodules in a patient with asbestosis. Excisional biopsy revealed squamous cell carcinoma. Note the subpleural bleb formation and a subpleural linear density paralleling the chest wall. There are also coarse linear fibrotic bands in the vicinity of the nodules.

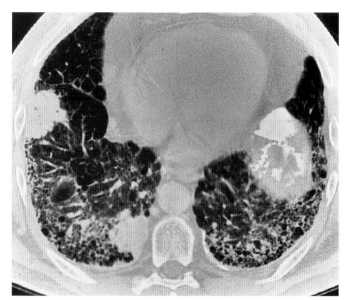

Fig. 8.56 HRCT in a pipe fitter with asbestosis. Two synchronous primary bronchial carcinomas are seen in the right lung. Note the honeycombing and a large calcified pleural plaque on the left diaphragm.

Less common pneumoconioses

Talcosis

Talc is a hydrated magnesium silicate that has widespread use as a cosmetic, industrial lubricant, and filling agent in the pharmaceutical industry. Geologically, talc is often associated with asbestos and silica, and this has resulted in problems in determining the extent to which radiographic and pathologic changes can be attributed to talc exposure.[302] Feigin[287] correlated the radiographic and pathologic findings in a series of individuals exposed to talc of varying degrees of purity. Mineralogic analysis of the talc gave an estimate of the extent of contamination by asbestos and silica. Feigin[287] described four categories of disease: talcoasbestosis, talcosilicosis, pure talcosis, and intravenous talcosis. Intravenous talcosis is considered on page 493. Talcoasbestosis and talcosilicosis show the classic features of exposure to asbestos and silica discussed above; the changes attributable to talc are completely overshadowed. On chest radiography, pure talcosis is seen as a reticulonodular infiltration of the lungs, either diffuse or lower zone predominant. Hilar adenopathy may occur. Pleural thickening and calcification are not features of pure talcosis, contrary to previous descriptions.

Kaolinosis

Kaolin, a hydrated aluminum silicate, causes a pneumoconiosis with features similar to coal worker's pneumoconiosis, including a tendency to develop PMF and even Caplan syndrome.[303] The radiographic changes of kaolinosis occur in a minority of exposed workers, and progression of the lesions is slow.[304,305] The most frequent abnormality is a fine nodulation of the lungs with some basal predominance. The nodules become larger and more numerous with prolonged exposure, and a reticular element may become apparent. Enlargement and condensation of the nodules into PMF occur in only a small minority of cases, some 1% in Oldham's estimate.[305]

Siderosis/arc welder's lung

Welding is associated with a variety of adverse health effects, including metal fume fever, asthma, asbestos related conditions, lung cancer, and siderosis. Siderosis is the accumulation of iron particles within the lung (Fig. 8.57). Usually, these particles are inert, but occasionally there is associated fibrosis. On CT scanning of patients with welder's lung, small centrilobular nodules are the most common finding, with ground-glass abnormality or reticular abnormality being less common.[306–308]

Hard metal pneumoconiosis

Hard metal pneumoconiosis is caused by exposure to cobalt in combination with tungsten carbide and diamond dust.[309] These compounds are used in engine manufacturing, drills, and polishing tools. Exposure causes an unusual histologic entity called giant cell interstitial pneumonia. Hard metal pneumoconiosis is characterized on CT by ground-glass

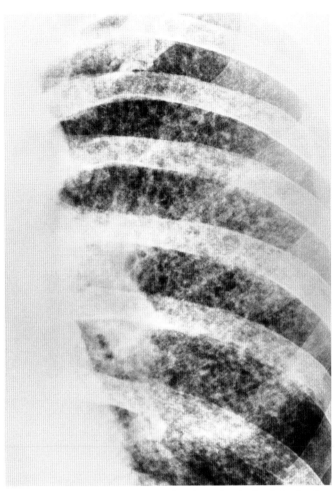

Fig. 8.57 Siderosis in a hematite miner from Cumberland, England. (Courtesy of Dr Peter Hacking, Newcastle upon Tyne, UK)

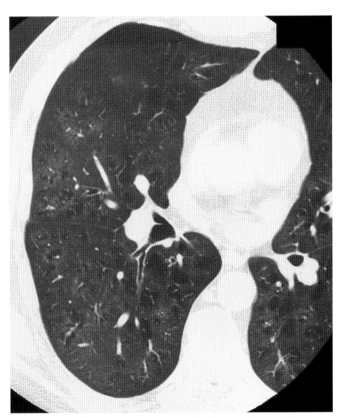

Fig. 8.58 Hard metal pneumoconiosis. A 47-year-old man with giant cell pneumonitis due to cobalt lung. HRCT shows patchy ground-glass abnormality, with background emphysema.

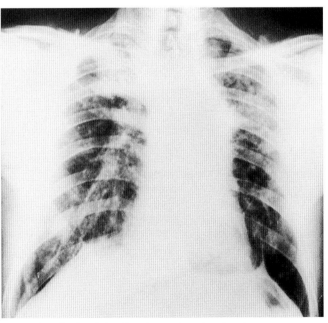

Fig. 8.59 Aluminosis in a bauxite smelter, showing dense upper zone pulmonary fibrosis.

attenuation and consolidation (Fig. 8.58). Cysts and reticular abnormality may also occur.[310]

Aluminosis

The inhalation of aluminum and its oxides has been associated with the development of pulmonary fibrosis in aluminum workers. Only a few are affected, and these are usually involved with particular processes. For example, Shaver and Riddell[311] described a form of pneumoconiosis, which is basically the prototype of the condition aluminosis, in workers involved in the smelting of aluminum ore (bauxite) to produce corundum. The condition is therefore sometimes known as Shaver's disease.

The role of aluminum and aluminum oxides in causing pulmonary disease is difficult to assess because workers are also exposed to silica and mineral oils in dusts and fumes.[312] Exposure to the fumes may be acute and intense, resulting in

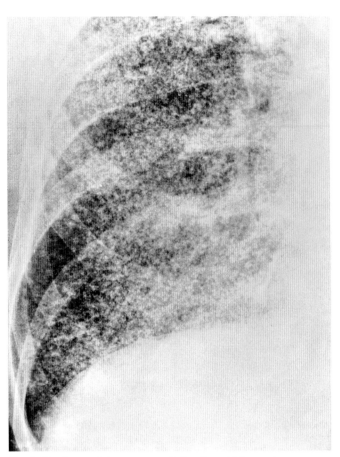

Fig. 8.60 Stannosis in an apparently healthy middle-aged man. Detail of chest radiograph shows extensive fine nodular abnormality due to metal deposition.

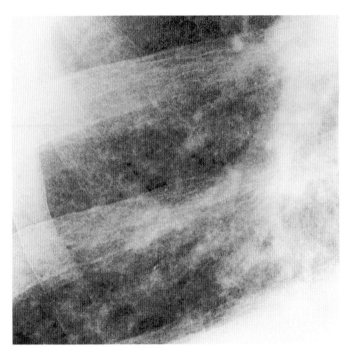

Fig. 8.61 Detailed view of right lung base in an antimony refiner. Note the fine diffuse increase in the lung markings, representing antimony dust deposition.

acute tracheobronchitis and even pulmonary edema. The pulmonary edema pattern in such individuals usually evolves over subsequent weeks or months into a diffuse reticulonodular pattern, indicating diffuse lung damage with fibrosis. Shaver and Riddell's patients[311] were subjected to chronic exposure to fumes over periods ranging from 3 to 15 years, and the result was a coarse interstitial pulmonary fibrosis with reduced lung volumes. The upper zones were more severely involved, and honeycombing and bleb formation were frequent findings (Fig. 8.59). Pneumothorax was strikingly common. Widening of the mediastinum with distortion of the tracheobronchial structures was common and was presumably related to the fibrosis. Less intense exposures may cause an asthma-like syndrome after single or repeated exposures. On CT, reticular and small nodular opacities and fibrosis predominate.[307] Vahlensieck et al[313] described the CT finding of high-attenuation mediastinal lymph nodes in an aluminum worker.

Inert dust pneumoconioses

A number of inorganic dusts are inert and fail to excite any fibrous response when taken up into the lung parenchyma. The dust accumulates in the lung parenchyma and may become radiographically visible, often dramatically so. The most frequently encountered inert dusts are the following:

- Tin (stannosis). The main occupational exposure occurs during the smelting of tin ores (Fig. 8.60).
- Barium (baritosis). This condition is encountered in miners and handlers of the ore baryta.
- Antimony. Antimony pneumoconiosis is encountered as a result of the mining, milling, and refining of antimony ores (Fig. 8.61).

Pathologic examination shows some dust at the alveolar level, but the major accumulations are seen in aggregations of dust-laden macrophages in the interstitium of the lung and along the lymphatic pathways. Radiographic visibility depends on the atomic number of the dust and the severity of dust accumulation. Relatively small dust accumulations may be visible as a very fine, low density stippling of the lung parenchyma. Dusts of high atomic number, such as iron, may result in much more remarkable radiographic changes if the dust accumulation is considerable. The pattern tends to be reticulonodular with the nodular element predominating. The changes are most pronounced in the central portion of the lungs, reflecting perhaps the greater amount of interstitial tissue in the perihilar regions. The unusually high radiographic density of the nodules may be more evident if comparison is made with the density of the ribs. In many industrial circumstances the workers receive a concomitant exposure to silica dust and therefore the changes of silicosis may also be present (Fig. 8.62).

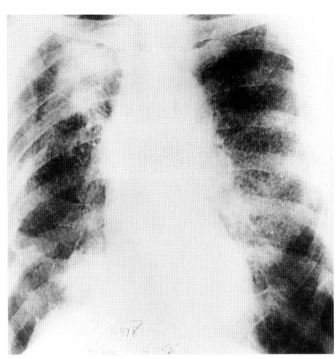

Fig. 8.62 Siderosilicosis in a hematite miner from Cumberland, England. There is diffuse fine nodular abnormality, presumed due to siderosis, with a conglomerate mass of silicosis in the right upper lobe.

BERYLLIOSIS

Although berylliosis (Box 8.10) technically meets the definition of pneumoconiosis, it differs from pneumoconiosis for the following reasons: (1) it represents a granulomatous hypersensitivity response to inhaled beryllium; and (2) its incidence and severity is not always related to the intensity and duration of exposure; in fact, it may occur with relatively trivial exposure (see Fig. 8.66).

Box 8.10 Berylliosis

Causative agent – elemental beryllium, used in lightweight alloys

Exposure – aerospace industry, ceramics, dental alloys, nuclear weapons manufacture

Bystanders with minimal exposure may develop disease

Radiologically and pathologically identical to sarcoidosis

Hilar and mediastinal adenopathy

Peribronchovascular nodules

Ground-glass abnormality

Upper lobe fibrosis

Granulomatous skin rashes

Granulomatous infiltration of the liver and spleen

Exposure to beryllium occurs in a variety of industries (including aerospace, ceramics, dentistry, and nuclear weapons and reactors) where workers may be at risk for disease from either direct or indirect exposure to the metal. The pulmonary sequelae of beryllium exposure include acute pneumonitis, tracheobronchitis, chronic beryllium disease, and increased risk of lung cancer. Acute berylliosis,[314] which usually results from a single intense exposure, is now rare with appropriate workplace protection. It manifests as an acute tracheobronchitis and pulmonary edema.

Between 1 and 15% of those exposed develop chronic beryllium disease.[315,316] The disease may develop with relatively trivial exposure. Latency from time of first exposure to clinical illness ranges from a few months to 40 years. The most common presenting symptoms include gradual onset of exertional dyspnea, cough, chest discomfort, and fatigue. Disease is usually limited to the lung and thoracic lymph nodes. Extrathoracic disease is rare. Physiologic abnormalities include exercise related gas exchange abnormalities as well as airflow obstruction, sometimes with a mixed restrictive pattern, and more severe restriction in later disease stages.

The histologic appearance of chronic beryllium disease is indistinguishable from sarcoidosis, with noncaseating granulomas accompanied by mononuclear cell infiltrates and variable interstitial fibrosis. The beryllium lymphocyte proliferation test (BeLPT) quantitates the beryllium specific cellular immune response in peripheral blood and bronchoalveolar lavage lymphocytes, and identifies >90% of individuals who have chronic beryllium disease.[315] Diagnostic criteria for chronic beryllium disease include: (1) a history of beryllium exposure; (2) demonstration of a beryllium specific cell-mediated immune response; and (3) granulomas and/or mononuclear cell infiltrates on biopsy in the absence of infection.

With early diagnosis, no treatment may be needed. With symptomatic, progressive, or impairing chronic beryllium disease, oral corticosteroids are used. Other immunosuppressive agents and lung transplantation should be considered if there is no response to corticosteroids. Removal from further beryllium exposure is essential.

The radiographic and CT appearances of chronic beryllium disease are similar to those of sarcoidosis (Fig. 8.63), though mediastinal and hilar lymphadenopathy is less common. Adenopathy is seen in about 25% of cases.[317] On the chest radiograph, the most common parenchymal abnormality is lung nodules, seen in about 40% (Fig. 8.64).[317] In advanced disease there is progressive volume loss and hilar distortion, with conglomerate masses.

On HRCT, nodules are seen in about 60% of cases, often clustered together around the bronchi, interlobular septa, or in the subpleural region (Fig. 8.63).[317] Subpleural clusters of nodules may form pseudoplaques (Fig. 8.65). Ground-glass opacity (Fig. 8.66), bronchial wall thickening, and thickening of interlobular septa are common CT features.[317, 318] Reticular opacity and architectural distortion may occur, but honeycombing is relatively uncommon. In advanced disease, subpleural cysts and conglomerate masses may be found. Bronchial stenoses may rarely occur.[319]

In a study by Newman et al,[317] the sensitivity of the chest radiograph for biopsy proven chronic beryllium disease was about 45%, compared with about 75% for HRCT. HRCT findings of chronic beryllium disease correlate significantly (though weakly) with evidence of lung restriction and impaired gas exchange.[320]

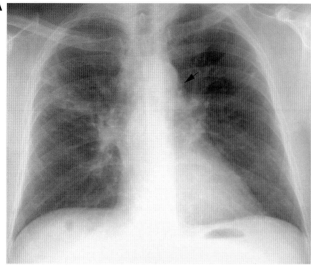

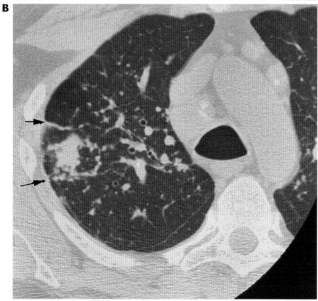

Fig. 8.63 Chronic beryllium disease. **A**, Chest radiograph shows bilateral hilar and mediastinal adenopathy, with lung nodules and a right upper lung mass. The arrow indicates aortopulmonary window adenopathy. **B** and **C**, CT images show a peribronchovascular conglomerate mass in the right upper lobe, with nodular thickening of the interlobular septa (arrows). The appearances are indistinguishable from those of sarcoidosis.

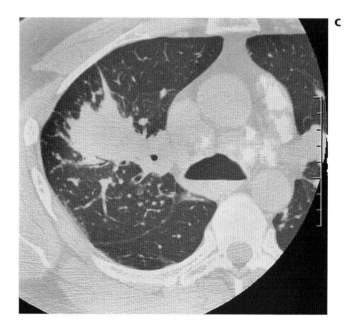

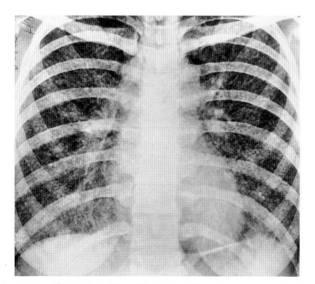

Fig. 8.64 Chronic berylliosis. There are diffuse fine nodules with hilar and mediastinal adenopathy.

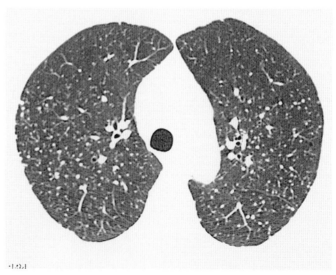

Fig. 8.65 Chronic beryllium disease. CT shows upper lobe nodules, with subpleural clustering.

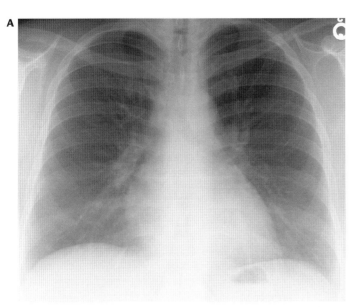

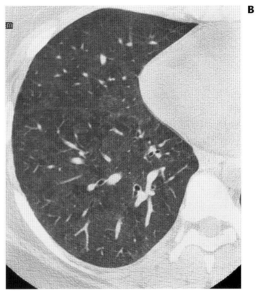

Fig. 8.66 Chronic beryllium disease due to relatively minor "bystander" exposure. Diffuse ground-glass abnormality are seen on **A**, chest radiograph and **B**, chest CT in a secretary who worked at a beryllium plant. There is hilar and mediastinal adenopathy.

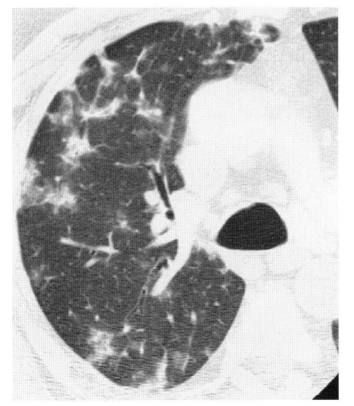

Fig. 8.67 Flock worker's lung. CT shows patchy areas of ground-glass abnormality and consolidation.

OTHER OCCUPATIONAL LUNG DISEASES

Flock worker's lung

Flock is a fine nylon fiber which is applied to backing to produce the plush material used in luxury upholstery, wallpaper, greeting cards, and many other products. The manufacture of this product may result in a dust of tiny respirable fibers that can reach the alveoli. Some flock workers develop a respiratory illness called flock worker's lung, characterized pathologically by a pattern of lymphocytic bronchiolitis and peribronchiolitis with lymphoid hyperplasia.[321] On HRCT scanning, flock worker's lung is characterized by a combination of ground-glass attenuation (Fig. 8.67) and centrilobular nodularity, sometimes appearing similar to the findings in hypersensitivity pneumonitis or respiratory bronchiolitis.[322] HRCT may identify similar findings in symptomatic patients who do not meet current criteria for flock worker's lung.

Flavor worker's lung

Clusters of severe obstructive lung disease have been reported in workers who manufacture flavoring agents, particularly the flavoring agent used in microwave popcorn.[323] On CT scanning, these patients have appearances characteristic of constrictive bronchiolitis, with cylindric bronchiectasis, decreased lung attenuation, and air trapping (Fig. 8.68).

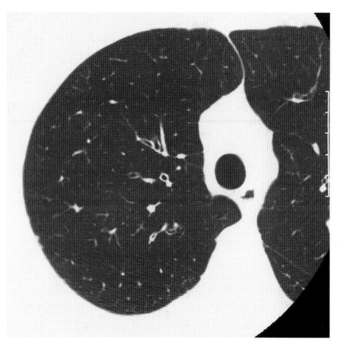

Fig. 8.68 Flavor worker's lung in a woman who worked at a microwave popcorn flavoring manufacturing plant. She presented with severe obstructive lung disease. HRCT shows marked airway wall thickening, decreased lung attenuation, and mild cylindric bronchial dilation.

ACUTE INHALATIONAL INJURY

Injury to the airways and lung parenchyma may result from the inhalation of a variety of noxious substances (Box 8.11). The result may be chemical tracheobronchitis, pulmonary edema, or pneumonia severe enough in some cases to cause death. The intensity of exposure to the inhaled agent is a key determinant of the severity of damage.[324] Other important factors which determine the site and severity of injury include the nature of the noxious agent and its water solubility.

Box 8.11 Common causes of acute inhalational injury

Smoke and fire products
Nitrogen dioxide/tetroxide (silo filler's lung)
Sulfur dioxide
Ammonia
Chlorine
Phosgene
Ozone

Smoke and fire injury

Fire accidents are the most frequent cause of severe acute inhalational injury. Approximately 6000 persons die in fires in the United States every year, and a much greater number require hospital treatment. More than 50% of the deaths occur as a result of inhalational injury.[325] Victims of fire accidents may be divided into three categories: those suffering only cutaneous injury; those with cutaneous and inhalational injury; and those

with inhalational injury alone. Extensive or severe cutaneous injury may result in sepsis and fluid balance problems with possible pulmonary edema or acute respiratory distress syndrome (ARDS). The greatest problems are, however, encountered with inhalational injury to the airways. In a study of patients with cutaneous burns complicated by inhalational injury, Darling et al[326] found that pulmonary complications accounted for nearly 80% of all deaths in the series. An abnormal chest radiograph in the first 48 h after injury was stated to be a poor prognostic indicator. Complications included ARDS, pneumonia, and problems with fluid balance.

The pathophysiology of inhalational injury is complex, but three main causes of injury can be identified[327]:

- *Thermal injury to the upper airways.* Except in the rare cases when inhalational injury is caused by steam or explosive gases, thermal damage below the subglottic region does not appear to occur.[328] Nevertheless, thermal damage to the larynx may lead to serious respiratory compromise requiring tracheotomy.
- *Carbon monoxide poisoning.* Carbon monoxide poisoning is thought to be an important direct or indirect cause of death from fire. As an indirect cause it may cause loss of consciousness or disorientation, preventing the victim from escaping the fire. There are no direct radiographic manifestations of carbon monoxide poisoning.
- *Noxious effects of the products of combustion.* The composition of smoke may be extremely complex and may include volatilized plastics and their breakdown products, as well as simpler noxious agents such as oxides of nitrogen, cyanides, and aldehydes.[329]

The noxious products of combustion induce a laryngotracheobronchitis that may be severe enough to be hemorrhagic, ulcerative, or necrotizing. Less severe degrees of damage may show edema, bronchospasm, and inhibition of ciliary action. At alveolar level, there may be damage to the alveolar macrophages, increasing the susceptibility to infection. Surfactant and the surfactant producing type II pneumocytes may be destroyed or damaged, leading to a loss of lung compliance. Finally, the vascular endothelium may be damaged, leading to an increased microvascular permeability with resultant edema.

Radiographic findings are variable in their severity and extent. Some 60[330]–75%[331] of patients in specialized burn units have some chest radiographic abnormality during the course of their hospitalization (Fig. 8.69). The radiographic findings may be divided into those occurring immediately (within the first 24 h) and those occurring in a delayed fashion. The significance of the presence or absence of radiographic findings in the immediate postinjury period is disputed. Earlier reports suggested that the chest radiograph is an insensitive indicator of the severity of inhalational injury.[332] Other authors have placed more reliance on the radiograph as a predictor of outcome and the likely need for ventilation support.[330,331,333,334]

The immediate radiographic findings include subglottic edema, tracheal narrowing (Fig. 8.69), diffuse peribronchial infiltration, frank interstitial or alveolar pulmonary edema, areas of atelectasis developing as a result of bronchial occlusions, and barotrauma resulting from intubation and positive pressure ventilation. Lee and O'Connell[331] found subglottic edema that caused a conical narrowing of the airway in nearly one-third of patients from a major fire disaster. In two-thirds of patients there was evidence of diffuse peribronchial thickening,

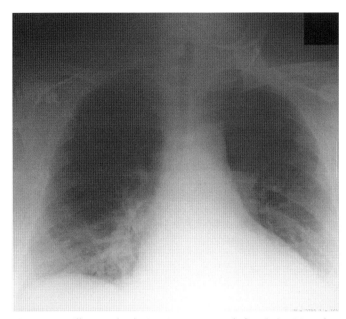

Fig. 8.69 Diffuse tracheal injury in a young male fire victim. Note the diffuse narrowing of the intrathoracic trachea, diffuse bronchial wall thickening, and bibasal opacity thought to represent lung injury edema.

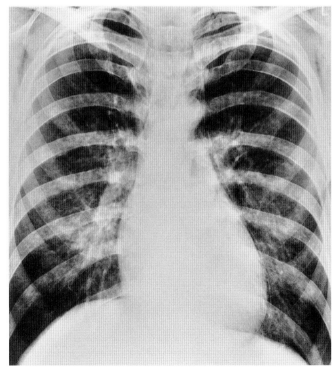

Fig. 8.71 Lung injury edema. Radiograph of an intubated patient who had sustained severe smoke inhalation injury 36 h previously shows diffuse fine nodules, most likely due to evolving lung injury edema.

which progressed to frank edema in seven of 45 cases. Teixidor et al[334] found evidence of alveolar and mixed interstitial and alveolar edema in nearly one-half of cases admitted for smoke inhalation to a burn unit over a 1 year period (Fig. 8.70). Areas of atelectasis may develop rapidly and may be present on admission. Patients with only airway damage may never develop radiographic changes. On the other hand, severe inhalational injury involving the pulmonary parenchyma produces more widespread radiographic changes that may be present on admission or wax during the first 24 h (Fig. 8.71).[330]

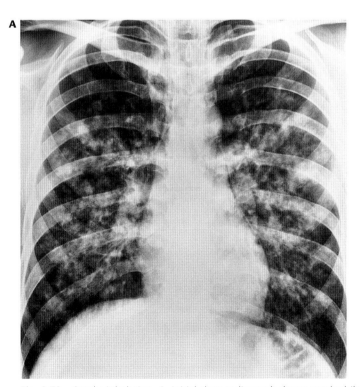

Fig. 8.70 Smoke inhalation. **A**, Initial chest radiograph shows patchy bilateral consolidation, thought to be due to lung injury edema. **B**, Prompt recovery after 72 h. Pneumomediastinum is present on both images. (Courtesy of Dr K Simpkins, Leeds, UK)

After the first 24 h, pulmonary manifestations of inhalational injury include pneumonia, ARDS, barotrauma, atelectasis, and fluid overload.[333,334] In severely burned patients in intensive care units it may be difficult to discriminate among these various components of the radiographic picture. Even with the aid of clinical data such as pulmonary wedge pressures, the nature of the tracheal aspirates, ventilatory pressures, and blood gas data, anything more than an educated guess may not be possible. In general, the more rapid the radiographic improvement, the more favorable the prognosis. Previous reports indicated that obliterative bronchiolitis may develop 2–6 weeks following inhalational injury. However, it is unclear from published reports whether this represents true obliterative bronchiolitis, bronchiolitis obliterans with organizing pneumonia, or some combination of both. The radiographic features described in such cases include fine patchy interstitial opacity – mainly peripheral in location and fairly symmetric in distribution. These changes wane over a period of days or weeks, leaving no visible sequelae, though the patient may continue to have respiratory deficits.

Airway and lung injury from toxic fume inhalation

Depending on the concentration and solubility of the fumes, toxic fume inhalation (Box 8.11) may cause injury to the upper airway, larynx, trachea, bronchi (Fig. 8.72), small airways (Fig. 8.73), or lung parenchyma. Of these, "bronchiolitis obliterans" has been most frequently emphasized in the past, though there are few descriptions in the more recent literature.

Silo filler's lung, due to inhalation of high concentrations of oxides of nitrogen which have accumulated in poorly ventilated silos, is a classic model of acute inhalational disease, and illustrates the biphasic nature of the injury.[335–337] In the acute phase, immediately after exposure, upper airway symptoms predominate, and pulmonary edema may develop. The chest radiograph at this point may be normal, or may show signs of edema (Fig. 8.74). Although sometimes fatal, the pulmonary edema usually responds to corticosteroid treatment. Those who survive the first phase, or those who have few initial symptoms, may develop a syndrome of progressive airway obstruction

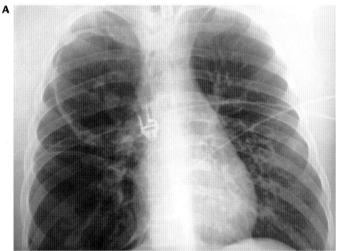

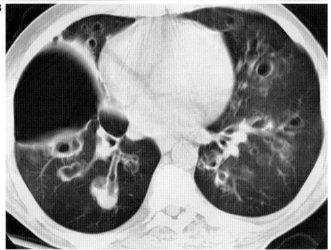

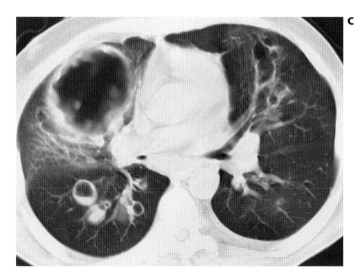

Fig. 8.72 Diffuse bronchiectasis from inhalational injury due to an explosion at a refinery. **A**, Chest radiograph shows widespread perihilar bronchiectasis, with a large pneumatocele in the right upper lung. **B** and **C**, CT confirms widespread varicose and cystic bronchiectasis.

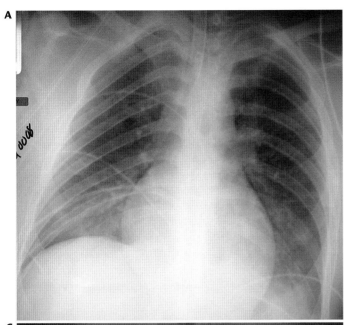

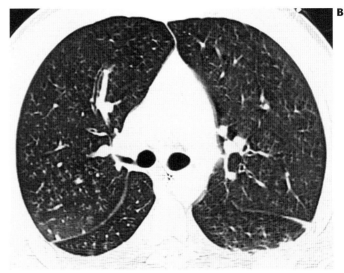

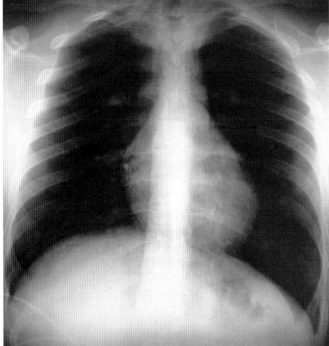

Fig. 8.73 Obliterative bronchiolitis due to inhalational injury from an unknown substance in an automobile paint workshop. **A**, Initial chest radiograph shows that the patient is intubated for respiratory failure, with bibasal consolidation. **B**, CT shows widespread centrilobular nodularity with a tree-in-bud pattern of cellular bronchiolitis. **C**, Follow-up chest radiograph 8 weeks later shows hyperinflation.

with obliterative bronchiolitis after 2–6 weeks. The chest radiograph at this point may show fine nodularity or coarser opacities, or may be normal. CT findings of this entity have not been described.

Reactive airways disease syndrome

The most common respiratory complication of occupational exposure to noxious fumes, gases, or mists is reactive airways disease, often occurring in patients who have no previous history of asthma. This entity is called reactive airway dysfunction syndrome (RADS), or work related asthma. Like other forms of reactive airways disease, the radiographic manifestations of this

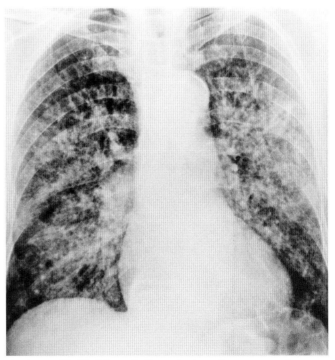

Fig. 8.74 Silo filler's lung. Radiograph of a patient overcome by fumes in a silo several hours previously shows bilateral patchy opacity compatible with lung injury edema.

entity are limited to airway wall thickening. On CT imaging, these patients may show mosaic lung attenuation with air-trapping on expiratory imaging.[338]

SPECTRUM OF PULMONARY ASPIRATION SYNDROMES

The term aspiration refers to the intake of solid or liquid materials into the airways and lungs. Although the lung is quite effective at clearing small amounts of aspirated fluid, aspiration of larger amounts of fluid, or of solid materials, commonly produces disease. A wide range of pulmonary syndromes has been associated with aspiration (Table 8.4).

Near drowning

Each year an estimated 150,000 persons worldwide die from drowning.[339] The number of episodes of near drowning cannot be estimated. Unless prevented by laryngeal spasm, the drowning fluid penetrates the lungs, where it may be radiographically demonstrable as pulmonary edema. Laryngeal spasm, which is particularly common in children, may prevent ingress of fluid but may prove fatal because of cerebral hypoxia from inadequate ventilation. In one series of 12 children requiring mechanical ventilation, four did not have radiographic evidence of pulmonary edema on admission.[340] Nevertheless, two of these four children subsequently died.

The initial radiographic appearances vary from complete normality through varying degrees of pulmonary edema (Fig. 8.75).[341] However, an initially normal chest radiograph may be associated with significant hypoxia, and furthermore radiographic deterioration may occur in the first 72 h.[342] This delayed pattern of lung edema may be due to negative pressure lung edema from laryngospasm (see p. 413).

Although the common drowning fluids, fresh and salt water, are capable of damaging the pneumocytes and dispersing or inactivating lung surfactant, no such effect is demonstrable in most cases of near drowning and the aspirated fluid may be promptly absorbed or otherwise dispersed.[343] Nevertheless, in more severe cases there may be a significant decrease in lung compliance and alterations in ventilation–perfusion matching, necessitating mechanical ventilation. Mechanical ventilation, or

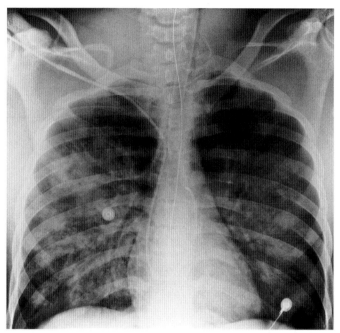

Fig. 8.75 Near drowning. Radiograph of a young man following an episode of near drowning, showing pulmonary edema pattern.

aspiration of gastric contents during resuscitation, may modify the radiographic picture during subsequent examinations. Pneumothorax and pneumomediastinum occur commonly in victims of near drowning on ventilator support. Neurogenic pulmonary edema or ARDS may supervene.[344]

Massive aspiration

Massive aspiration of gastric contents typically occurs during periods of altered consciousness. Predisposing factors may include general anesthesia, deep sedation, drug or alcohol abuse, or head injury. The clinical features are abrupt in onset and consist of cough, wheezing, cyanosis, dyspnea, and tachypnea. Massive aspiration of gastric contents around the time of childbirth is known as Mendelson syndrome.[345] A number of factors make pregnant patients more liable to aspiration.

Table 8.4 Syndromes of pulmonary aspiration

Aspirated material	Clinical consequence	Imaging appearances
Foreign bodies	Bronchial obstruction	Atelectasis, hyperinflation, abscess
Hydrocarbon	Chemical pneumonia	Consolidation, pneumatoceles
Lipid	Lipoid pneumonia	Consolidation, masses
Water	Near drowning	Airspace opacity
Gastric contents (acute)	Chemical pneumonitis	Airspace opacity, cavity
	Secondary anaerobic infection	
	Lung abscess	
Gastric contents (chronic/recurrent)	Recurrent aspiration	Migratory opacities
	Bronchiolitis	Centrilobular nodules or air trapping
	Bronchiectasis	Airways disease
Legumes	Granulomatous pneumonitis	Centrilobular nodules
Microaspiration	Asthma, lung fibrosis (possible)	

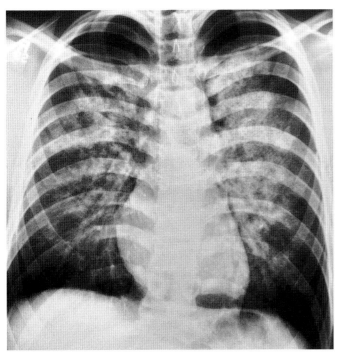

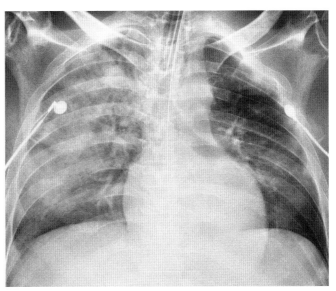

Fig. 8.77 Predominantly unilateral opacity following an episode of massive gastric aspiration in a 43-year-old man.

Fig. 8.76 Massive gastric aspiration during general anesthesia. Chest radiograph shows diffuse bilateral consolidation.

During pregnancy the volume and acidity of gastric secretions increase and relative atony of the stomach with delayed emptying occurs. The gastroesophageal sphincter is relatively lax, and the administration of some form of anesthetic, often with the patient in an "unprepared" state, is common.

If the aspirated fluid is bland and has a neutral pH, it can be reabsorbed quite rapidly, without clinical sequel. However, if the aspirated material has a pH <2.5, a chemical tracheobronchitis and pneumonitis develops, and may evolve into ARDS. After 2–3 days, secondary bacterial infection (usually anaerobic), commonly develops, sometimes with abscess formation.

The classic radiographic finding of acute massive aspiration is diffuse perihilar alveolar consolidation similar to cardiogenic pulmonary edema (Fig. 8.76). Landay et al[346] reviewed 60 patients who had suffered acute aspiration of gastric contents and found a remarkable variability in the radiographic findings. This study showed that the severity of the pulmonary changes depended on the volume of fluid aspirated, and experimental evidence indicates that the severity of the process is also related to the pH of the aspirate.[347] Almost all patients have radiographic abnormalities following an episode of massive aspiration, and some worsening is usual in the first 36 h. In uncomplicated cases the chest radiograph clears over the next 4–5 days. Secondary bacterial pneumonia with severe underlying pulmonary disease and the development of ARDS are adverse features that may lead to a fatal outcome even after an initial period of improvement. The parenchymal densities are often ill-defined acinar airspace opacities, which are frequently confluent. The distribution of the densities is generally perihilar or bibasilar, though there is considerable variation, depending in part on the patient's position during the episode of aspiration. The pulmonary opacities can be entirely unilateral (Fig. 8.77).[348] Pleural effusions are uncommon. The more severe and extensive the shadowing on the initial examination, the worse

the prognosis. However, relatively minor initial changes may progress to a fatal outcome.

Chronic or recurrent aspiration

Chronic or recurrent aspiration typically occurs in patients with an impaired swallowing mechanism or esophageal abnormalities. Because of laryngeal desensitization, the patient is often unaware of the aspiration. Aspiration commonly occurs during sleeping. Clinical presentations of chronic aspiration include recurrent pneumonia, chronic cough (often nocturnal), and episodic wheezing.

Chest radiographic manifestations of recurrent aspiration may include migratory pulmonary opacities (Fig. 8.78) and basal predominant airway wall thickening. On CT, chronic aspiration should be suggested when an at risk patient has basal predominant bronchiectasis (Figs 8.78 and 8.79). Chemical bronchiolitis due to aspiration can cause a tree-in-bud pattern on CT, suggestive of cellular bronchiolitis, or may also cause a pattern of constrictive bronchiolitis.[349]

Chronic aspiration of legumes such as lentils (often mashed and fed to nursing home residents) can lead to a granulomatous pneumonitis called lentil aspiration pneumonia, which is associated with radiographic and CT evidence of poorly defined nodules measuring up to 1 cm in diameter.[350]

Microaspiration

Normal individuals commonly aspirate small amounts of nasal contents into the lungs during sleep.[351] This has no clinical effect, being presumably eliminated by the normal clearance mechanisms. Microaspiration of gastric contents is common in patients with hiatal hernias or gastroesophageal reflux,[352] and has been implicated in the development of asthma[353] and pulmonary fibrosis,[354] though both of these hypotheses are controversial.

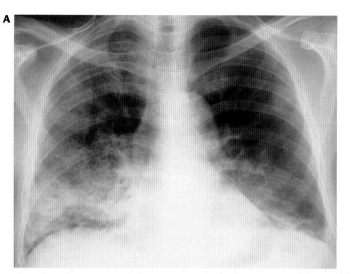

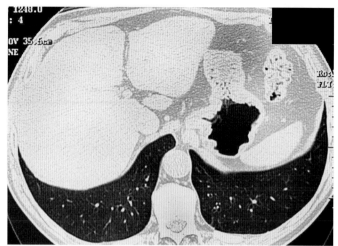

Fig. 8.78 Recurrent aspiration in a neurologically competent 66-year-old male with gastroesophageal reflux. **A,** Chest radiograph shows right lung consolidation. **B,** HRCT after recovery shows cylindrical bronchiectasis.

Hydrocarbon aspiration

Volatile hydrocarbons, when aspirated, may result in a widespread chemical pneumonia.[355] Radiographic abnormalities are commonly present on admission or develop within the first 12 h. These radiographic abnormalities correlate poorly with clinical symptoms and signs. Many patients with radiographic abnormalities have no symptoms, or their symptoms resolve before the radiographic changes clear. Chest radiographs show scattered pulmonary densities that are almost invariably bilateral with middle and lower zone predominance (Fig. 8.80). Initially the densities are often mottled, but with time they may become confluent. The pulmonary opacity commonly worsens somewhat over the first 72 h following aspiration. Usually the pulmonary densities then clear over the next few days. On occasion, however, radiographic changes take weeks or months to clear, particularly in adults. Obstructive emphysema with peripheral air-trapping may be seen, and pneumatoceles are occasionally observed. Segmental or subsegmental atelectasis is common.

Most cases of hydrocarbon pneumonia occur in children, particularly young children. The prognosis, both immediate and longterm, is good. Few children have damage to the lungs, though there may be minor residual pulmonary function abnormalities.[356] In adults, hydrocarbon aspiration can occur in those who siphon fuel, and may also occur in fire eaters, who use liquid hydrocarbons such as petroleum as part of their act.[357] Some adults suffer permanent damage, with chronic organizing pneumonia, fibrosis, and bronchiectasis.

Inhalation of foreign bodies

The usual foreign materials inhaled into the lungs are food and broken fragments of teeth; a nut is the single most common object. Inhalation of foreign bodies occurs most frequently in the first 3 years of life, with a peak incidence at 1–2 years of age. It is rare before 6 months of age. Foreign bodies usually lodge in

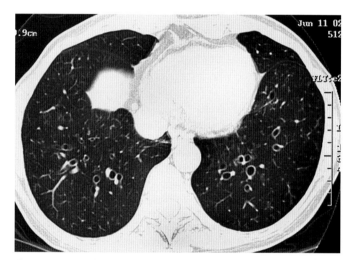

Fig. 8.79 Bronchiectasis due to chronic aspiration. CT shows marked bilateral lower lobe cylindrical bronchiectasis, with mild centrilobular thickening.

the left or right main bronchus; neither side is involved significantly more often than the other. The next most common site is the trachea, followed by a lobar bronchus.[358–360]

Although in most cases aspiration of a foreign body is diagnosed within 2–3 days of the event, the diagnosis may not be made for weeks or sometimes even months, as was the case in approximately one-third of children in two large series.[358,359] In >80% of cases,[358,360–362] a definite event of aspiration or choking is followed by cough or wheezing, which may persist, usually without respiratory distress. In time the cough may disappear. However, an interval of hours, months, or years may occur during which time the child is asymptomatic following the initial event.[363]

The most common complication of foreign body aspiration is pneumonia or atelectasis, which occurs in approximately one-quarter of cases when the foreign body lodges in a

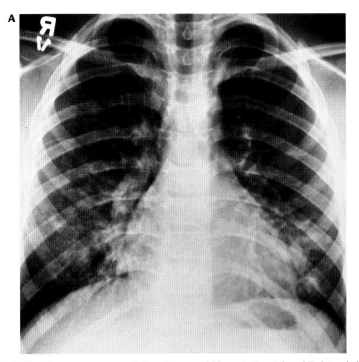

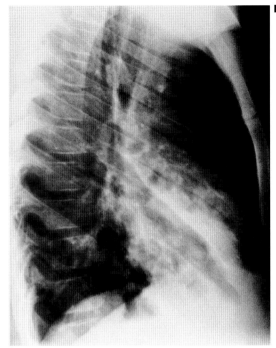

Fig. 8.80 Kerosene pneumonia in a 12-year-old boy. **A**, Frontal and **B**, lateral chest radiographs show patchy bibasilar consolidation.

bronchus; consolidation/collapse is rare when the object lodges in the trachea. Bronchiectasis may result from the prolonged retention of a bronchial foreign body. Pneumothorax and pneumomediastinum are rare.

Bronchoscopy is the usual method of final diagnosis and also permits removal of the foreign body in most cases. Thoracotomy or other surgical intervention is rarely required. Blazer et al[358] emphasized that 15% of their patients who had inhaled foreign bodies required a second or third bronchoscopy, demonstrating that foreign bodies may be missed at bronchoscopy and that the finding of one foreign body does not exclude the presence of another.

The chest radiograph shows a radiopaque foreign body in 5–15% of cases (Fig. 8.81). Occasionally the foreign body is seen as an opacity of soft tissue density in one of the larger airways. However, the cardinal sign of foreign inhaled body soon after aspiration is obstructive overinflation or air-trapping of the affected lobe or lobes (Fig. 8.82).[358,361,362] Air-trapping with or without contralateral shift of the mediastinum is best demonstrated on radiographs taken during expiration. Such radiographs can be difficult to obtain in young children, and air-trapping and mediastinal shift are often easier to demonstrate with fluoroscopy. Alternative techniques that do not require fluoroscopy include assisted expiratory radiographs[364] and lateral decubitus examinations.[365] Lateral decubitus radiographs facilitate detection of inhaled foreign bodies because the dependent lung is normally less inflated than the uppermost lung, whereas air-trapping renders the dependent lung hyperlucent.

The other major feature of foreign body aspiration into the airway is atelectasis or pneumonia distal to the obstructing

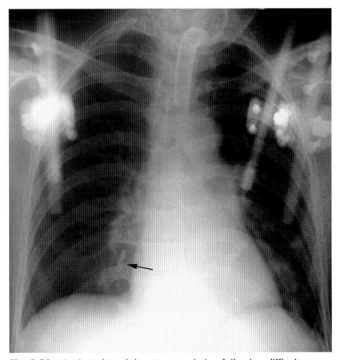

Fig. 8.81 Aspirated tooth in a trauma victim, following difficult intubation and subsequent emergency tracheostomy. The tooth is seen in the medial right lower lobe (arrow).

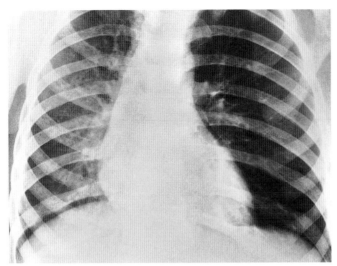

Fig. 8.82 Inhaled foreign body lodged in the left main bronchus in a young child. Chest radiograph shows hyperlucent left lung, with decreased vascularity, due to obstructive air-trapping in the left lung.

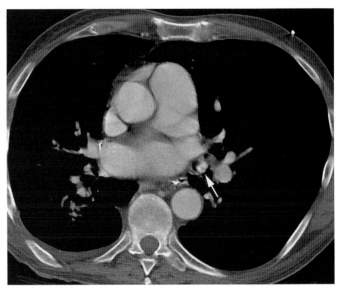

Fig. 8.84 Aspirated pill in a lung transplant patient. The radiodense pill is impacted at the bifurcation of the left main bronchus (arrow).

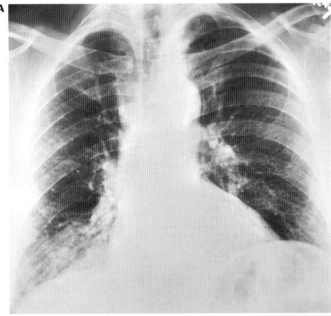

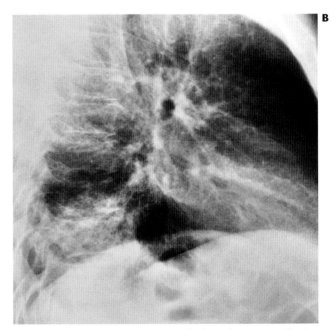

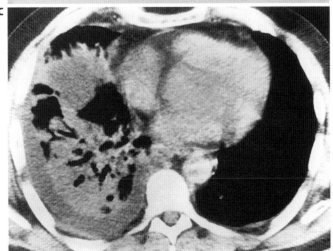

Fig. 8.83 Inhaled peanut lodged in the bronchus intermedius in an adult, causing postobstructive collapse and consolidation of the right middle and lower lobes, which had been present for 2 months. Prebronchoscopic diagnosis was carcinoma of lung. **A** and **B**, Radiographs show right middle lobe and right lower lobe consolidation. **C**, CT shows consolidation with bronchiectasis and effusion.

foreign body (Fig. 8.83). These signs were seen in 20–45% of patients in the larger series.[358,360–362] A pneumothorax or a pneumomediastinum may be present, but both are surprisingly uncommon (<2% of patients) following aspiration of a foreign body.[358,362]

Normal inspiratory and expiratory chest radiographs can be expected in about one-quarter of cases. In the series of 200 patients reported by Blazer et al,[358] 15.6% of those with bronchial foreign bodies and 60.6% of those with tracheal foreign bodies showed no abnormalities on inspiratory and expiratory films. CT can be quite helpful in identifying the presence and location of an inhaled foreign body when inspiratory and expiratory radiographs are normal or equivocal, or when the diagnosis is not anticipated (Fig. 8.84).[366]

REFERENCES

1. Niewoehner DE, Kleinerman J, Rice DB. Pathologic changes in the peripheral airways of young cigarette smokers. N Engl J Med 1974;291:755–758.
2. Fraig M, Shreesha U, Savici D, et al. Respiratory bronchiolitis: a clinicopathologic study in current smokers, ex-smokers, and never-smokers. Am J Surg Pathol 2002;26:647–653.
3. Freemer M, King T. Connective tissue diseases. In: Schwarz M, King T, eds. Interstitial lung disease, 4th edn. Toronto: Brian C Decker, 2003:535–598.
4. King TE Jr. Respiratory bronchiolitis-associated interstitial lung disease. Clin Chest Med 1993;14:693–698.
5. Myers JL, Veal CJ, Shin MS, et al. Respiratory bronchiolitis causing interstitial lung disease. A clinicopathologic study of six cases. Am Rev Respir Dis 1987;135:880–884.
6. Epler GR, Colby TV, McLoud TC, Carrington CB, Gaensler EA. Respiratory bronchiolitis-associated interstitial lung disease and its relationship to desquamative interstitial pneumonia. Mayo Clin Proc 1989;64:1373–1380.
7. Yousem SA, Colby TV, Gaensler EA. Respiratory bronchiolitis-associated interstitial lung disease and its relationship to desquamative interstitial pneumonia. Mayo Clin Proc 1989;64:1373–1380.
8. Heyneman LE, Ward S, Lynch DA, et al. Respiratory bronchiolitis, respiratory bronchiolitis-associated interstitial lung disease, and desquamative interstitial pneumonia: different entities or part of the spectrum of the same disease process? AJR Am J Roentgenol 1999;173:1617–1622.
9. Moon J, du Bois RM, Colby TV, et al. Clinical significance of respiratory bronchiolitis on open lung biopsy and its relationship to smoking related interstitial lung disease. Thorax 1999;54:1009–1014.
10. Holt R, Schmidt R, Godwin J, et al. High resolution CT in respiratory bronchiolitis-associated interstitial lung disease. J Comput Assist Tomogr 1993;1993:46–50.
11. Park JS, Brown KK, Tuder RM, et al. Respiratory bronchiolitis-associated interstitial lung disease: radiologic features with clinical and pathologic correlation. J Comput Assist Tomogr 2002;26:13–20.
12. Gückel C, Hansell DM. Imaging the 'dirty lung' has high resolution computed tomography cleared the smoke? Clin Radiol 1998;53:717–722.
13. Remy-Jardin M, Remy J, Gosselin B, et al. Lung parenchymal changes secondary to cigarette smoking: pathologic-CT correlations. Radiology 1993;186:643–651.
14. Remy-Jardin M, Edme JL, Boulenguez C, et al. Longitudinal follow-up study of smoker's lung with thin-section CT in correlation with pulmonary function tests. Radiology 2002;222:261–270.
15. Dalphin JC, Debieuvre D, Pernet D, et al. Prevalence and risk factors for chronic bronchitis and farmer's lung in French dairy farmers. Br J Ind Med 1993;50:941–944.
16. Warren C. Extrinsic allergic alveolitis: a disease commoner in nonsmokers. Thorax 1977;32:567–573.
17. Carrington CB, Gaensler EA, Coutu RE, et al. Natural history and treated course of usual and desquamative interstitial pneumonia. N Engl J Med 1978;298:801–809.
18. Bjoraker J, Ryu J, Edwin M, et al. Prognostic significance of histopathologic subsets in idiopathic pulmonary fibrosis. Am J Respir Crit Care Med 1998;157:199–203.
19. Hartman TE, Primack SL, Kang EY, et al. Disease progression in usual interstitial pneumonia compared with desquamative interstitial pneumonia. Assessment with serial CT. Chest 1996;110:378–382.
20. Valdivia E, Hensley G, Leory EP, et al. Morphology and pathogenesis of desquamative interstitial pneumonitis. Thorax 1977;32:7–18.
21. Feigin D, Friedman P. Chest radiography in desquamative interstitial pneumonitis: a review of 37 patients. AJR Am J Roentgenol 1980;134:91–99.
22. Epler GR, McLoud TC, Gaensler EA, et al. Normal chest roentgenograms in chronic diffuse infiltrative lung disease. N Engl J Med 1978;298:934–939.
23. Hartman TE, Primack SL, Swensen SJ, et al. Desquamative interstitial pneumonia: thin-section CT findings in 22 patients. Radiology 1993;187:787–790.
24. Akira M, Yamamoto S, Hara H, et al. Serial computed tomographic evaluation in desquamative interstitial pneumonia. Thorax 1997;52:333–337.
25. Hansell DM, Nicholson AG. Smoking-related interstitial lung disease: HRCT-pathologic correlation. Semin Respir Crit Care Med 2003; 24: 377–391.
26. Travis WD, Borok Z, Roum JH, et al. Pulmonary Langerhans cell granulomatosis (histiocytosis X). A clinicopathologic study of 48 cases. Am J Surg Pathol 1993;17:971–986.
27. Hance AJ, Cadranel J, Soler P, et al. Pulmonary and extra pulmonary Langerhan cell granulomatosis (Histiocytosis X). Semin Respir Med 1988;9:349–368.
28. Lewis JG. Eosinophilic granuloma and its variants with special reference to lung involvement: a report of 12 patients. Q J Med 1964;131:337–359.
29. Egeler RM, Neglia JP, Puccetti DM, et al. Association of Langerhans cell histiocytosis with malignant neoplasms. Cancer 1993;71:865–873.
30. A multicentre retrospective survey of Langerhans cell histiocytosis: 348 cases observed between 1983 and 1993. The French Langerhans Cell Histiocytosis Study Group. Arch Dis Childhood 1996;75:17–24.
31. Ha SY, Helms P, Fletcher M, et al. Lung involvement in Langerhans cell histiocytosis: prevalence, clinical features, and outcome. Pediatrics 1992;89:466–469.
32. Kulwiec E, Lynch D, Aguayo S, et al. Imaging of pulmonary histiocytosis X. RadioGraphics 1992;12:515–526.
33. Grenier P, Valeyre D, Cluzel P, et al. Chronic diffuse interstitial lung disease: diagnostic value of chest radiography and high-resolution CT. Radiology 1991;179:123–132.
34. Brauner MW, Grenier P, Mouelhi MM, et al. Pulmonary histiocytosis X: evaluation with high-resolution CT. Radiology 1989;172:255–258.
35. Moore A, Godwin J, Müller N, et al. Pulmonary histiocytosis X: Comparison of radiographic and CT findings. Radiology 1989;172:249–254.

36. Koyama M, Johkoh T, Honda O, et al. Chronic cystic lung disease: diagnostic accuracy of high-resolution CT in 92 patients. AJR Am J Roentgenol 2003;180:827–835.

37. Taylor DB, Joske D, Anderson J, et al. Cavitating pulmonary nodules in histiocytosis-X high resolution CT demonstration. Australas Radiol 1990;34:253–255.

38. Bonelli FS, Hartman TE, Swensen SJ, et al. Accuracy of high-resolution CT in diagnosing lung diseases. AJR Am J Roentgenol 1998;170:1507–1512.

39. Kambouchner M, Basset F, Marchal J, et al. Three-dimensional characterization of pathologic lesions in pulmonary Langerhans cell histiocytosis. Am J Respir Crit Care Med 2002;166:1483–1490.

40. Marcy T, Reynolds H. Pulmonary histiocytosis X. Lung 1985;163:129–150.

41. Brauner MW, Grenier P, Tijani K, et al. Pulmonary Langerhans cell histiocytosis: evolution of lesions on CT scans. Radiology 1997;204:497–502.

42. Tazi A, Montcelly L, Bergeron A, et al. Relapsing nodular lesions in the course of adult pulmonary Langerhans cell histiocytosis. Am J Respir Crit Care Med 1998;157:2007–2010.

43. Harari S, Brenot F, Barberis M, et al. Advanced pulmonary histiocytosis X is associated with severe pulmonary hypertension. Chest 1997;111:1142–1144.

44. Crausman RS, Jennings CA, Tuder RM, et al. Pulmonary histiocytosis X: pulmonary function and exercise pathophysiology. Am J Respir Crit Care Med 1996;153:426–435.

45. Crausman RS, King TE Jr. Pulmonary vascular involvement in pulmonary histiocytosis X [letter; comment]. Chest 1997;112:1714.

46. Fartoukh M, Humbert M, Capron F, et al. Severe pulmonary hypertension in histiocytosis X. Am J Respir Crit Care Med 2000;161:216–223.

47. Smets A, Mortele K, de Praeter G, et al. Pulmonary and mediastinal lesions in children with Langerhans cell histiocytosis. Pediatr Radiol 1997;27:873–876.

48. Odagiri K, Nishihira K, Hatekeyama S, et al. Anterior mediastinal masses with calcifications on CT in children with histiocytosis-X (Langerhans cell histiocytosis). Report of two cases. Pediatr Radio 1991;21:550–551.

49. Bernstrand C, Cederlund K, Sandstedt B, et al. Pulmonary abnormalities at long-term follow-up of patients with Langerhans cell histiocytosis. Med Pediatr Oncol 2001;36:459–468.

50. Murin S, Bilello KS, Matthay R. Other smoking-affected pulmonary diseases. Clin Chest Med 2000;21:121–137.

51. Herody M, Bobrie G, Gouarin C, et al. Anti-GBM disease: predictive value of clinical, histological and serological data. Clin Nephrol 1993;40:249–255.

52. Watanabe K, Fujimura M, Kasahara K, et al. Acute eosinophilic pneumonia following cigarette smoking: a case report including cigarette-smoking challenge test. Intern Med 2002;41:1016–1020.

53. Miki K, Miki M, Okano Y, et al. Cigarette smoke-induced acute eosinophilic pneumonia accompanied with neutrophilia in the blood. Intern Med 2002;41:993–996.

54. Murin S, Inciardi J. Cigarette smoking and the risk of pulmonary metastasis from breast cancer. Chest 2001;119:1635–1640.

55. Bense L, Eklund G, Wiman LG. Smoking and the increased risk of contracting spontaneous pneumothorax. Chest 1987;92:1009–1012.

56. Cottin V, Streichenberger N, Gamondes JP, et al. Respiratory bronchiolitis in smokers with spontaneous pneumothorax. Eur Respir J 1998;12:702–704.

57. Baumgartner KB, Samet JM, Stidley CA, et al. Cigarette smoking: a risk factor for idiopathic pulmonary fibrosis. Am J Respir Crit Care Med 1997;155:242–248.

58. Arima K, Ando M, Ito K, et al. Effect of cigarette smoking on prevalence of summer-type hypersensitivity pneumonitis caused by Trichosporon cutaneum. Arch Environ Health 1992;47:274–278.

59. Ohtsuka Y, Munakata M, Tanimura K, et al. Smoking promotes insidious and chronic farmer's lung disease, and deteriorates the clinical outcome. Intern Med 1995;34:966–971.

60. Valeyre D, Soler P, Clerici C, et al. Smoking and pulmonary sarcoidosis: effect of cigarette smoking on prevalence, clinical manifestations, alveolitis, and evolution of the disease. Thorax 1988;43:516–524.

61. Selman M. Hypersensitivity pneumonitis. In: Schwarz MI, King TE, eds. Interstitial lung disease, 4th edn. Hamilton: BC Decker, 2003:452–484.

62. Barbee RA, Callies Q, Dickie HA, et al. The long-term prognosis in farmer's lung. Am Rev Respir Dis 1968;97:223–231.

63. Grammer LC. Occupational allergic alveolitis. Ann Allergy Asthma Immunol 1999;83:602–606.

64. Ganier M, Lieberman P, Fink J, et al. Humidifier lung. An outbreak in office workers. Chest 1980;77:183–187.

65. Aksamit TR. Hot tub lung: infection, inflammation, or both? Semin Respir Infect 2003;18:33–39.

66. Hodgson MJ, Bracker A, Yang C, et al. Hypersensitivity pneumonitis in a metal-working environment. Am J Ind Med 2001;39:616–628.

67. Wallace Jr RJ Jr., Zhang Y, Wilson RW, et al. Presence of a single genotype of the newly described species Mycobacterium immunogenum in industrial metalworking fluids associated with hypersensitivity pneumonitis. Appl Environ Microbiol 2002;68:5580–5584.

68. Yoshizawa Y, Ohtani Y, Hayakawa H, et al. Chronic hypersensitivity pneumonitis in Japan: a nationwide epidemiologic survey. J Allergy Clin Immunol 1999;103:315–320.

69. Haitjema T, van V, Blad H, van Velzen Blad H, van den Bosch JM, et al. Extrinsic allergic alveolitis caused by goose feathers in a duvet. Thorax 1992;47:990–991.

70. Baur X. Hypersensitivity pneumonitis (extrinsic allergic alveolitis) induced by isocyanates. J Allergy Clin Immunol 1995;95:1004–1010.

71. Simpson C, Garabrant D, Torrey S, et al. Hypersensitivity pneumonitis-like reaction and occupational asthma associated with 1,3-bis(isocyanatomethyl) cyclohexane pre-polymer. Am J Ind Med 1996;30:48–55.

72. Nakashima K, Takeshita T, Morimoto K. Occupational hypersensitivity pneumonitis due to isocyanates: mechanisms of action and case reports in Japan. Ind Health 2001;39:269–279.

73. Schuyler M, Gott K, Cherne A. Mediators of hypersensitivity pneumonitis. J Lab Clin Med 2000;136:29–38.

74. Schuyler M, Gott K, Cherne A, et al. Th1 CD4+ cells adoptively transfer experimental hypersensitivity pneumonitis. Cell Immunol 1997;177:169–175.

75. Glazer CS, Rose CS, Lynch DA. Clinical and radiologic manifestations of hypersensitivity pneumonitis. J Thorac Imaging 2002;17:261–272.

76. Roberts RC, Zais DP, Emanuel DA. The frequency of precipitins to trichloroacetic acid-extractable antigens from thermophilic actinomycetes in farmer's lung patients and asymptomatic farmers. Am Rev Respir Dis 1976;114:23–28.

77. McSharry C, Banham SW, Lynch PP, et al. Antibody measurement in extrinsic allergic alveolitis. Eur J Respir Dis 1984;65:259–265.

78. Lalancette M, Carrier G, Laviolette M, et al. Farmer's lung. Long-term outcome and lack of predictive value of bronchoalveolar lavage fibrosing factors. Am Rev Respir Dis 1993;148:216–221.

79. Bourke SJ, Banham SW, Carter R, et al. Longitudinal course of extrinsic allergic alveolitis in pigeon breeders. Thorax 1989;44:415–418.

80. Coleman A, Colby TV. Histologic diagnosis of extrinsic allergic alveolitis. Am J Surg Pathol 1988;12:514–518.

81. Hayakawa H, Shirai M, Sato A, et al. Clinicopathological features of chronic hypersensitivity pneumonitis. Respirology 2002;7:359–364.

82. Katzenstein AL, Fiorelli RF. Nonspecific interstitial pneumonia/fibrosis. Histologic features and clinical significance. Am J Surg Pathol 1994;18:136–147.

83. Ando M, Arima K, Yoneda R, et al. Japanese summer-type hypersensitivity pneumonitis. Geographic distribution, home environment, and clinical characteristics of 621 cases. Am Rev Respir Dis 1991;144:765–769.

84. Silver S, Müller N, Miller R, et al. Hypersensitivity pneumonitis: evaluation with CT. Radiology 1989;173:441–445.

85. Matar LD, McAdams HP, Sporn TA. Hypersensitivity pneumonitis. AJR Am J Roentgenol 2000;174:1061–1066.

86. Lynch DA, Rose CS, Way D, et al. Hypersensitivity pneumonitis: sensitivity of high-resolution CT in a population-based study. AJR Am J Roentgenol 1992;159:469–472.

87. Frank J, Schleuter D, Sosman A, et al. Clinical survey of pigeon breeders. Chest 1972;62:277–281.

88. Buschman DL, Gamsu G, Waldron J, et al. Chronic hypersensitivity pneumonitis: use of CT in diagnosis. AJR Am J Roentgenol 1992;159:957–960.

89. Akira M, Kita N, Higashihara T, et al. Summer-type hypersensitivity pneumonitis: comparison of high-resolution CT and plain radiographic findings. AJR Am J Roentgenol 1992;158:1223–1228.

90. Remy-Jardin M, Remy J, Wallaert B, et al. Subacute and chronic bird breeder hypersensitivity pneumonitis: sequential evaluation with CT and correlation with lung function tests and bronchoalveolar lavage. Radiology 1993;189:111–118.

91. Patel RA, Sellami D, Gotway MB, et al. Hypersensitivity pneumonitis: patterns on high-resolution CT. J Comput Assist Tomogr 2000;24:965–970.

92. Erkinjuntti-Pekkanen R, Rytkonen H, Kokkarinen JI, et al. Long-term risk of emphysema in patients with farmer's lung and matched control farmers. Am J Respir Crit Care Med 1998;158:662–665.

93. Niimi H, Kang EY, Kwong JS, et al. CT of chronic infiltrative lung disease: prevalence of mediastinal lymphadenopathy. J Comput Assist Tomogr 1996;20:305–308.

94. Adler BD, Padley SP, Müller NL, et al. Chronic hypersensitivity pneumonitis: high-resolution CT and radiographic features in 16 patients. Radiology 1992;185:91–95.

95. Tomiyama N, Müller NL, Johkoh T, et al. Acute parenchymal lung disease in immunocompetent patients: diagnostic accuracy of high-resolution CT. AJR Am J Roentgenol 2000;174:1745–1750.

96. Cormier Y, Brown M, Worthy S, et al. High-resolution computed tomographic characteristics in acute farmer's lung and in its follow-up. Eur Respir J 2000;16:56–60.

97. Hansell DM, Wells AU, Padley SP, et al. Hypersensitivity pneumonitis: correlation of individual CT patterns with functional abnormalities. Radiology 1996;199:123–128.

98. Franquet T, Hansell DM, Senbanjo T, et al. Lung cysts in subacute hypersensitivity pneumonitis. J Comput Assist Tomogr 2003;27:475–478.

99. Small JH, Flower CD, Traill ZC, et al. Air-trapping in extrinsic allergic alveolitis on computed tomography. Clin Radiol 1996;51:684–688.

100. Lucidarme O, Coche E, Cluzel P, et al. Expiratory CT scans for chronic airway disease: correlation with pulmonary function test results. AJR Am J Roentgenol 1998;170:301–307.

101. Lynch D, Newell J, Logan P, et al. Can CT distinguish idiopathic pulmonary fibrosis from hypersensitivity pneumonitis? AJR Am J Roentgenol 1995;165:807–811.

102. Kim KI, Kim CW, Lee MK, et al. Imaging of occupational lung disease. RadioGraphics 2001;21:1371–1391.

103. Parkes WR. Occupational lung disorders, 2nd edn. London: Butterworths, 1982.

104. Guidelines for the use of ILO international classification of radiographs of pneumoconioses. Revised Edition 1980. Geneva: International Labour Office, 1980.

105. Classification of radiographs of the pneumoconioses. Med Radiogr Photogr 1981;57:2–17.

106. Chien VC, Chai SK, Hai DN, et al. Pneumoconiosis among workers in a Vietnamese refractory brick facility. Am J Ind Med 2002;42:397–402.

107. Finkelstein MM. Radiographic silicosis and lung cancer risk among workers in Ontario. Am J Indust Med 1998;34:244–251.

108. Parihar YS, Patnaik JP, Nema BK, et al. Coal workers' pneumoconiosis: a study of prevalence in coal mines of eastern Madhya Pradesh and Orissa states of India. Ind Health 1997;35:467–473.

109. Ogle CJ, Rundle EM, Sugar ET. China clay workers in the south west of England: analysis of chest radiograph readings, ventilatory capacity, and respiratory symptoms in relation to type and duration of occupation. Br J Ind Med 1989;46:261–270.

110. Ogawa S, Imai H, Ikeda M. A 40-year follow-up of whetstone cutters on silicosis. Ind Health 2003;41:69–76.

111. Fernie JM, Ruckley VA. Coalworkers' pneumoconiosis: correlation between opacity profusion and number and type of dust lesions with special reference to opacity type. Br J Ind Med 1987;44:273–277.

112. Rosenstock L, Barnhart S, Heyer NJ, et al. The relation among pulmonary function, chest roentgenographic abnormalities, and smoking status in an asbestos-exposed cohort. Am Rev Respir Dis 1988;138:272–277.

113. Miller A, Lilis R, Godbold J, et al. Relationship of pulmonary function to radiographic interstitial fibrosis in 2,611 long-term asbestos insulators. An assessment of the International Labour Office profusion score. Am Rev Respir Dis 1992;145:263–270.

114. Ng TP, Chan SL. Lung function in relation to silicosis and silica exposure in granite workers. Eur Respir J 1992;5:986–991.

115. Maclaren WM, Soutar CA. Progressive massive fibrosis and simple pneumoconiosis in ex-miners. Br J Ind Med 1985;42:734–740.

116. Bourgkard E, Bernadac P, Chau N, et al. Can the evolution to pneumoconiosis be suspected in coal miners? A longitudinal study. Am J Respir Crit Care Med 1998;158:504–509.

117. Cowie RL, Hay M, Thomas RG. Association of silicosis, lung dysfunction, and emphysema in gold miners. Thorax 1993;48:746–749.

118. Cookson WO, Musk AW, Glancy JJ, et al. Compensation, radiographic changes, and survival in applicants for asbestosis compensation. Br J Ind Med 1985;42:461–468.

119. Markowitz SB, Morabia A, Lilis R, et al. Clinical predictors of mortality from asbestosis in the North American Insulator Cohort, 1981 to 1991. Am J Respir Crit Care Med 1997;156:101–108.

120. Gaensler E, Carrington C, Coutu R, et al. Pathologic, physiologic, and radiologic correlations in the pneumoconioses. Ann NY Acad Sci 1972;200:574–607.

121. Blanc P, Golden J, Gamsu G. Asbestos exposure-cigarette smoking interactions among shipyard workers. JAMA 1988;259:370–373.

122. Blanc PD, Gamsu G. The effect of cigarette smoking on the detection of small radiographic opacities in inorganic dust diseases. J Thorac Imag 1988;3:51–56.

123. Hnizdo E, Sluis-Cremer GK. Effect of tobacco smoking on the presence of asbestosis at postmortem and on the reading of irregular opacities on roentgenograms in asbestos-exposed workers. Am Rev Resp Dis 1988;138:1207–1212.

124. Kilburn K, Lilis R, Anderson H, et al. Interaction of asbestos, age, and cigarette smoking in producing radiographic evidence of diffuse pulmonary fibrosis. Am J Med 1986;80:377–381.

125. Weiss W. Cigarette smoke, asbestos, and small irregular opacities. Am Rev Respir Dis 1984;130:293–301.

126. Sluis-Cremer GK, Hessel PA, Hnizdo E. Factors influencing the reading of small irregular opacities in a radiological survey of asbestos miners in South Africa. Arch Environ Health 1989;44:237–243.

127. Akira M, Higashihara T, Yokoyama K, et al. Radiographic type p pneumoconiosis: high-resolution CT. Radiology 1989;171:117–123.

128. Gevenois PA, Pichot E, Dargent F, et al. Low grade coal worker's pneumoconiosis. Comparison of CT and chest radiography. Acta Radiol 1994;35:351–356.

129. Vallyathan V, Brower PS, Green FH, et al. Radiographic and pathologic correlation of coal workers' pneumoconiosis. Am J Respir Crit Care Med 1996;154:741–748.

130. Hnizdo E, Murray J, Sluis-Cremer GK, et al. Correlation between radiological and pathological diagnosis of silicosis: an autopsy population based study. Am J Ind Med 1993;24:427–445.

131. Kipen HM, Lilis R, Suzuki Y, et al. Pulmonary fibrosis in asbestos insulation workers with lung cancer: a radiological and histopathological evaluation. Br J Ind Med 1987;44:96–100.

132. Begin R, Ostiguy G, Fillion R, et al. Computed tomography in the early detection of silicosis. Am Rev Respir Dis 1991;144:697–705.

133. Harkin TJ, McGuinness G, Goldring R, et al. Differentiation of the ILO boundary chest roentgenograph (0/1 to 1/0) in asbestosis by high-resolution computed tomography scan, alveolitis, and respiratory impairment. J Occup Environ Med 1996;38:46–52.

134. Henry D. The ILO classification system in the age of imaging: relevant or redundant? J Thorac Imag 2002;17:179–188.

135. Jacobsen M. The International Labour Office classification: use and misuse. Ann N Y Acad Sci 1991;643:100–107.

136. Ziskind M, Jones RN, Weill H. Silicosis. Am Rev Respir Dis 1976;113:643–665.

137. Seaton A, Legge JS, Henderson J, et al. Accelerated silicosis in Scottish stonemasons. Lancet 1991;337:341–344.

138. Castranova V, Vallyathan V. Silicosis and coal workers' pneumoconiosis. Environ Health Perspect 2000;108 Suppl 4:675–684.

139. Sonnenberg P, Murray J, Glynn JR, et al. Risk factors for pulmonary disease due to culture-positive *M. tuberculosis* or nontuberculous mycobacteria in South African gold miners. Eur Respir J 2000;15:291–296.

140. Prendergrass EP. Silicosis and a few of the other pneumoconioses: observations on certain aspects of the problem with emphasis in the role of the radiologist. AJR Am J Roentgenol 1958;80:1–41.

141. Bergin CJ, Müller NL, Vedal S, et al. CT in silicosis: correlation with plain films and pulmonary function tests. AJR Am J Roentgenol 1986;146:477–483.

142. Remy-Jardin M, Degreef JM, Beuscart R, et al. Coal worker's pneumoconiosis: CT assessment in exposed workers and correlation with radiographic findings. Radiology 1990;177:363–371.

143. Gurney JW, Schroeder BA. Upper lobe lung disease: physiologic correlates. Radiology 1988;167:359–366.

144. Remy-Jardin M, Beuscart R, Sault MC, et al. Subpleural micronodules in diffuse infiltrative lung diseases: evaluation with thin-section CT scans. Radiology 1990;177:133–139.

145. Jacobson GJ, Felson B, Pendergrass EP, et al. Eggshell calcifications in coal and metal miners. Semin Roentgenol 1967;2:276–282.

146. Jiang CQ, Xiao LW, Lam TH, et al. Accelerated silicosis in workers exposed to agate dust in Guangzhou, China. Am J Ind Med 2001;40:87–91.

147. Weissman D, Banks D. Silicosis. In: Schwarz MI, King TE, eds. Interstitial lung disease, 4th edn. Hamilton: BC Decker, 2003:387–401.

148. Suratt PM, Winn WC Jr, Brody AR, et al. Acute silicosis in tombstone sandblasters. Am Rev Respir Dis 1977;115:521–529.

149. Buechner HA, Ansari A. Acute silico-proteinosis. A new pathologic variant of acute silicosis in sandblasters, characterized by histologic features resembling alveolar proteinosis. Dis Chest 1969;55:274–278.

150. Dee P, Suratt P, Winn W. The radiographic findings in acute silicosis. Radiology 1978;126:359–363.

151. American Thoracic Society. Adverse effects of crystalline silica exposure. Am J Respir Crit Care Med 1997;155:761–765.

152. Marchiori E, Ferreira A, Müller NL. Silicoproteinosis: high-resolution CT and histologic findings. J Thorac Imaging 2001;16:127–129.

153. International Agency for Research on Cancer. Silica, some silicates, coal dust and para-aramid fibrils. Lyon: IARC, 1997.

154. Begin R, Filion R, Ostiguy G. Emphysema in silica- and asbestos-exposed workers seeking compensation. A CT scan study. Chest 1995;108:647–655.

155. Hnizdo E, Sluis CG, Baskind E, et al. Emphysema and airway obstruction in non-smoking South African gold miners with long exposure to silica dust. Occup Environ Med 1994;51:557–563.

156. Gevenois PA, Sergent G, De Maertelaer V, et al. Micronodules and emphysema in coal mine dust or silica exposure: relation with lung function. Eur Respir J 1998;12:1020–1024.

157. Honma K, Chiyotani K. Diffuse interstitial fibrosis in nonasbestos pneumoconiosis: a pathological study. Respiration 1993;60:120–126.

158. Baumgartner KB, Samet JM, Coultas DB, et al. Occupational and environmental risk factors for idiopathic pulmonary fibrosis: a multicenter case-control study. Collaborating Centers. Am J Epidemiol 2000;152:307–315.

159. Englert H, Small-McMahon J, Davis K, et al. Male systemic sclerosis and occupational silica exposure-a population-based study. Australas N Z J Med 2000;30:215–220.

160. Steen VD. Occupational scleroderma. Curr Opin Rheumatol 1999;11:490–494.

161. Shida H, Chiyotani K, Honma K, et al. Radiologic and pathologic characteristics of mixed dust pneumoconiosis. RadioGraphics 1996;16:483–498.

162. Honma K, Shida H, Chiyotani K. Rounded atelectasis associated with silicosis. Wien Klin Wochenschr 1995;107:585–589.

163. Hurley JF, Burns J, Copland L, et al. simple pneumoconiosis and exposure to dust at 10 British coalmines. Br J Ind Med 1982;39:120–127.

164. Gough J. Pneumoconiosis of coal trimmers. J Path Bacteriol 1940;51:277–285.

165. Rivers D, Wise ME, King ES, et al. Dust content, radiology, and pathology in simple pneumoconiosis of coal workers. Br J Ind Med 1960;17:87–108.

166. Morgan WK, Lapp NL. Respiratory disease in coal miners. Am Rev Respir Dis 1976;113:531–559.

167. Jacobsen M. New data on the relationship between simple pneumoconiosis and exposure to coal mine dust. Chest 1980;78:408–410.

168. Seaton A, Dick JA, Dodgson J, et al. Quartz and pneumoconiosis in coalminers. Lancet 1981;2:1272–1275.

169. Naeye RL, Dellinger WS. Coal workers' pneumoconiosis. Correlation of roentgenographic and postmortem findings. JAMA 1972;220:223–227.

170. Pratt PC. Role of silica in progressive massive fibrosis. In coal workers' pneumoconiosis. Arch Environ Health 1968;16:734–737.

171. Nagelschmidt G, Rivers D, King EJ, et al. Dust and collagen content of lungs of coal workers with progressive massive fibrosis. Br J Ind Med 1963;20:181–191.

172. Heppleston AG. The pathological recognition and pathogenesis of emphysema and fibrocystic disease of the lung with special reference to coal

workers. Ann N Y Acad Sci 1972;200: 347–369.

173. Ryder R, Lyons JP, Campbell H, et al. Emphysema in coal workers' pneumoconiosis. Br Med J 1970;3:481–487.

174. Caplan A. Correlation of radiological category with lung pathology in coal worker's pneumoconiosis. Br J Ind Med 1962;19:171–179.

175. Leigh J, Outhred KG, McKenzie HI, et al. Quantified pathology of emphysema, pneumoconiosis, and chronic bronchitis in coal workers. Br J Ind Med 1983;40:258–263.

176. Lyons JP, Ryder R, Campbell H, et al. Pulmonary disability in coal workers' pneumoconiosis. Br Med J 1972;1:713–716.

177. Oxman AD, Muir DC, Shannon HS, et al. Occupational dust exposure and chronic obstructive pulmonary disease. A systematic overview of the evidence. Am Rev Respir Dis 1993;148:38–48.

178. Williams JL, Moller GA. Solitary mass in the lungs of coal miners. Am J Roentgenol Radium Ther Nucl Med 1973;117:765–770.

179. Greening RR, Heslep JH. The roentgenology of silicosis. Semin Roentgenol 1967;2:265–275.

180. Kirchner J, Kirchner EM. Melanoptysis: findings on CT and MRI. Br J Radiol 2001;74:1003–1006.

181. Matsumoto S, Mori H, Miyake H, et al. MRI signal characteristics of progressive massive fibrosis in silicosis. Clinical Radiology 1998;53:510–514.

182. Cockcroft A, Lyons JP, Andersson N, et al. Prevalence and relation to underground exposure of radiological irregular opacities in South Wales coal workers with pneumoconiosis. Br J Ind Med 1983;40:169–172.

183. Trapnell DH. Septal lines in pneumoconiosis. Br J Radiol 1964;37:805–810.

184. Cockcroft A, Berry G, Cotes JE, et al. Shape of small opacities and lung function in coalworkers. Thorax 1982;37:765–769.

185. Brichet A, Wallaert B, Gosselin B, et al. "Primary" diffuse interstitial fibrosis in coal miners: a new entity? Study Group on Interstitial Pathology of the Society of Thoracic Pathology of the North. Revue des Maladies Respiratoires 1997;14: 277–285.

186. Katabami M, Dosaka-Akita H, Honma K, et al. Pneumoconiosis-related lung cancers: preferential occurrence from diffuse interstitial fibrosis-type pneumoconiosis. Am J Respir Crit Care Med 2000;162:295–300.

187. Gough J, James WRL, Wentworth JE. A comparison of the radiological and pathological changes in coal worker's pneumoconiosis. J Fac Radiol 1949; 1:28–60.

188. Heitzman ER, Naeye RL, Markarian B. Roentgen pathological correlations in coal workers' pneumoconiosis. Ann N Y Acad Sci 1972;200:510–526.

189. Ruckley VA, Fernie JM, Chapman JS, et al. Comparison of radiographic appearances with associated pathology and lung dust content in a group of coalworkers. Br J Ind Med 1984;41: 459–467.

190. Rossiter CE. Relation of lung dust content to radiological changes in coal workers. Ann N Y Acad Sci 1972;200: 465–477.

191. Newell DJ, Browne RC. Symptomatology and radiology in pneumoconiosis: a survey in the Durham coalfield. J Fac Radiol 1955;7:20–28.

192. Lyons JP, Ryder RC, Campbell H, et al. Significance of irregular opacities in the radiology of coalworkers' pneumoconiosis. Br J Ind Med 1974;31:36–44.

193. Cockcroft A, Seal RM, Wagner JC, et al. Post-mortem study of emphysema in coalworkers and non-coalworkers. Lancet 1982;2:600–603.

194. Ruckley VA, Gauld SJ, Chapman JS, et al. Emphysema and dust exposure in a group of coal workers. Am Rev Respir Dis 1984;129:528–532.

195. Kinsella M, Müller N, Vedal S, et al. Emphysema in silicosis. A comparison of smokers with nonsmokers using pulmonary function testing and computed tomography. Am Rev Respir Dis 1990;141:1497–1500.

196. Casey KR, Rom WN, Moatamed F. Asbestos-related diseases. Clin Chest Med 1981;2:179–202.

197. Talcott JA, Thurber WA, Kantor AF, et al. Asbestos-associated diseases in a cohort of cigarette-filter workers. N Engl J Med 1989;321:1220–1223.

198. Weill H, Hughes JM. Asbestos as a public health risk: disease and policy. Annu Rev Publ Health 1986;7:171–192.

199. McDonald JC, McDonald AD, Hughes JM. Chrysotile, tremolite and fibrogenicity. Ann Occup Hyg 1999;43:439–442.

200. Keller CA, Naunheim KS, Osterloh J, et al. Histopathologic diagnosis made in lung tissue resected from patients with severe emphysema undergoing lung volume reduction surgery. Chest 1997;111:941–947.

201. Cullen MR. Chrysotile asbestos: enough is enough. Lancet 1998; 351:1377–1378.

202. Frank AL, Dodson RF, Williams MG. Carcinogenic implications of the lack of tremolite in UICC reference chrysotile. Am J Ind Med 1998;34:314–317.

203. Nicholson WJ. The carcinogenicity of chrysotile asbestos: a review. Ind Health 2001;39:57–64.

204. Smith AH, Wright CC. Chrysotile asbestos is the main cause of pleural mesothelioma. Am J Ind Med 1996;30:252–266.

205. Stayner LT, Dankovic DA, Lemen RA. Occupational exposure to chrysotile asbestos and cancer risk: a review of the amphibole hypothesis. Am J Public Health 1996;86:179–186.

206. Becklake MR. Asbestos-related diseases of the lung and other organs: their epidemiology and implications for clinical practice. Am Rev Respir Dis 1976;114:187–227.

207. Amandus HE, Wheeler R. The morbidity and mortality of vermiculite miners and millers exposed to tremolite-actinolite: Part II. Mortality. Am J Ind Med 1987;11:15–26.

208. Centers for Disease Control. Mortality from asbestosis in Libby, Montana, 1979–1998. http://www.atsdr.cdc.gov/HAC/PHA/libby/lib_p1.html, 2003.

209. Epler G, McLoud T, Gaensler E. Prevalence and incidence of benign asbestos pleural effusion in a working population. JAMA 1982;247:617–622.

210. Gaensler EA, Kaplan AI. Asbestos pleural effusion. Ann Intern Med 1971;74:178–191.

211. Hillerdal G, Ozesmi M. Benign asbestos pleural effusion: 73 exudates in 60 patients. Eur J Respir Dis 1987;71:113–121.

212. Delajartre M, Delajartre A. Mesothelioma on the coast of Brittany, France. Ann N Y Acad Sci 1979;330:323–332.

213. Bianchi C, Giarelli L, Grandi G, et al. Latency periods in asbestos-related mesothelioma of the pleura. Eur J Cancer Prev 1997;6:162–166.

214. Lilis R, Lerman Y, Selikoff IJ. Symptomatic benign pleural effusions among asbestos insulation workers: residual radiographic abnormalities. Br J Ind Med 1988;45:443–449.

215. Hillerdal G. Non-malignant asbestos pleural disease. Thorax 1981;669–675.

216. McLoud TC, Woods BO, Carrington CB, et al. Diffuse pleural thickening in an asbestos-exposed population: Prevalence and causes. AJR Am J Roentgenol 1985;144:9–18.

217. Cookson WO, De Klerk NH, Musk AW, et al. Benign and malignant pleural effusions in former Wittenoom crocidolite millers and miners. Aust N Z J Med 1985;15:731–737.

218. Jacob B, Bohlig, H. Die roentgenologische Komplikationen der lungen Asbestose. Fortrschr roentgenstr 1955;83:515–525.

219. Yates DH, Browne K, Stidolph PN, et al. Asbestos-related bilateral diffuse pleural thickening: natural history of radiographic and lung function abnormalities. Am J Respir Crit Care Med 1996;153:301–306.

220. Schwartz DA, Fuortes LJ, Galvin JR, et al. Asbestos-induced pleural fibrosis and impaired lung function. Am Rev Respir Dis 1990;141:321–326.

221. Gefter WB, Conant EF. Issues and controversies in the plain-film diagnosis of asbestos-related disorders in the chest. J Thorac Imaging 1988;3:11–28.

222. Anton HC. Multiple pleural plaques. Br J Radiol 1967;40:685–690.

223. Wain S, Roggli V, Foster W. Parietal pleural plaques, asbestos bodies, and neoplasia: A clinical, pathologic, and roentgenographic correlation of 25 consecutive cases. Chest 1984; 86:707–713.

224. Rudd RM. New developments in asbestos-related pleural disease. Thorax 1996;51:210–216.

225. Kannerstein M. Recent advances and perspectives relevant to the pathology of asbestos-related diseases in man. IARC Sci Publ 1980:149–162.

226. Sebastien P, Janson X, Gaudichet A, et al. Asbestos retention in human respiratory tissues: comparative measurements in lung parenchyma and in parietal pleura. IARC Sci Publ 1980:237–246.

227. Albelda SM, Epstein DM, Gefter WB, et al. Pleural thickening: its significance and relationship to asbestos dust exposure. Am Rev Respir Dis 1982;126:621–624.

228. Hilt B, Lien JT, Lund-Larsen PG, et al. Asbestos-related findings in chest radiographs of the male population of the county of Telemark, Norway: a cross-sectional study. Scand J Work Environ Health 1986;12:567–573.

229. Sider L, Holland EA, Davis TM Jr, et al. Changes on radiographs of wives of workers exposed to asbestos. Radiology 1987;164:723–726.

230. Churg A. Asbestos fibers and pleural plaques in a general autopsy population. Am J Pathol 1982;109:88–96.

231. Mollo F, Andrion A, Bellis D, et al. Screening of autopsy populations for previous occupational exposure to asbestos. Arch Environ Health 1987;42:44–50.

232. Rous V, Studeny J. Aetiology of pleural plaques. Thorax 1970;25: 270–284.

233. Baris I, Simonato L, Artvinli M, et al. Epidemiological and environmental evidence of the health effects of exposure to erionite fibres: a four-year study in the Cappadocian region of Turkey. Int J Cancer 1987;39:10–17.

234. Stephens M, Gibbs AR, Pooley FD, et al. Asbestos induced diffuse pleural fibrosis: pathology and mineralogy. Thorax 1987;42:583–588.

235. Hu H, Beckett L, Kelsey K, et al. The left-sided predominance of asbestos-related pleural disease. Am Rev Resp Dis 1993;148:981–984.

236. Gallego JC. Absence of left-sided predominance in asbestos-related pleural plaques: a CT study. Chest 1998;113:1034–1036.

237. Rockoff S, Kagan E, Schwartz A, et al. Visceral pleural thickening in asbestos exposure: The occurrence and implications of thickened interlobar fissures. J Thorac Imag 1987;2:58–66.

238. Webb WR, Cooper C, Gamsu G. Interlobar pleural plaque mimicking a lung nodule in a patient with asbestos exposure. J Comput Assist Tomogr 1983;7:135–136.

239. Lynch D, Gamsu G, Aberle D. Conventional and high resolution CT in the diagnosis of asbestos-related diseases. RadioGraphics 1989;9:523–551.

240. Davies D, Andrews MI, Jones JS. Asbestos induced pericardial effusion and constrictive pericarditis. Thorax 1991;46:429–432.

241. Cooper M, Johnson K, Delany DJ. Case report: asbestos related pericardial disease. Clin Radiol 1996;51:656–657.

242. Yazicioglu S. Pleural calcification associated with exposure to chrysotile asbestos in southeast Turkey. Chest 1976;70:43–47.

243. Fischbein L, Namade M, Sachs RN, et al. Chronic constrictive pericarditis associated with asbestosis. Chest 1988;94:646–647.

244. Baker E, Greene R. Incremental value of oblique chest radiographs in the diagnosis of asbestos-induced pleural disease. Am J Ind Med 1982;3:17–22.

245. Sargent E, Boswell W, Ralls P, et al. Subpleural fat pads in patients exposed to asbestos: Distinction from non-calcified pleural plaques. Radiology 1984;152:273–277.

246. Vix VA. Extrapleural costal fat. Radiology 1974;112:563–565.

247. Kouris SP, Parker DL, Bender AP, et al. Effects of asbestos-related pleural disease on pulmonary function. Scand J Work Environ Health 1991;17:179–183.

248. Broderick A, Fuortes LJ, Merchant JA, et al. Pleural determinants of restrictive lung function and respiratory symptoms in an asbestos-exposed population. Chest 1992;101:684–691.

249. Kilburn KH, Warshaw R. Pulmonary functional impairment associated with pleural asbestos disease. Circumscribed and diffuse thickening. Chest 1990;98: 965–672.

250. Bourbeau J, Ernst P, Chrome J, et al. The relationship between respiratory impairment and asbestos-related pleural abnormality in an active work force. Am Rev Respir Dis 1990;142:837–842.

251. Schwartz DA, Galvin JR, Dayton CS, et al. Determinants of restrictive lung function in asbestos-induced pleural fibrosis. J Appl Physiol 1990;68:1932–1937.

252. Shih JF, Wilson JS, Broderick A, et al. Asbestos-induced pleural fibrosis and impaired exercise physiology. Chest 1994;105:1370–1376.

253. Aberle DR, Gamsu G, Ray CS, et al. Asbestos-related pleural and parenchymal fibrosis: detection with high-resolution CT. Radiology 1988;166:729–734.

254. Friedman AC, Fiel SB, Fisher MS, et al. Asbestos-related pleural disease and asbestosis: A comparison of CT and chest radiography. AJR Am J Roentgenol 1988;150:269–275.

255. Kreel L. Computer tomography in the evaluation of pulmonary asbestosis. Acta Radiol 1976;17:405–412.

256. Aberle DR, Gamsu G, Ray CS. High-resolution CT of benign asbestos-related diseases: clinical and radiographic correlation. AJR Am J Roentgenol 1988;151:883–891.

257. Gevenois PA, de Vuyst P, Dedeire S, et al. Conventional and high-resolution CT in asymptomatic asbestos-exposed workers. Acta Radiologica 1994;35: 226–229.

258. Sperber M, Mohan KK. Computed tomography: a reliable diagnostic modality in pulmonary asbestosis. Comput Radiol 1984;8:125–132.

259. Copley SJ, Wells AU, Rubens MB, et al. Functional consequences of pleural disease evaluated with chest radiography and CT. Radiology 2001;220:237–243.

260. Solomon A. Radiological features of asbestos-related visceral pleural changes. Am J Ind Med 1991; 19: 339–355.

261. Solomon A, Irwig L, Sluis-Cremer G, et al. Thickening of pulmonary interlobar fissures: exposure-response relationship in crocidolite and amosite miners. Br J Ind Med 1979;36:195–198.

262. Kee ST, Gamsu G, Blanc P. Causes of pulmonary impairment in asbestos-exposed individuals with diffuse pleural thickening. Am J Respir Crit Care Med 1996;154:789–793.

263. Blesovsky A. The folded lung. Br J Dis Chest 1966;60.

264. Munden RF, Libshitz HI. Rounded atelectasis and mesothelioma. AJR Am J Roentgenol 1998;170:1519–1522.

265. Hanke R, Kretzschmar R. Rounded atelectasis. Semin Roentgenol 1980;15:174–182.

266. Hillerdal G, Hemmingsson A. Pulmonary pseudotumours and asbestos. Acta Radiologica 1979;21:615–620.

267. Menzies R, Fraser R. Round atelectasis. Pathologic and pathogenetic features. Am J Surg Pathol 1987;11:674–681.

268. Schneider HJ, Felson B, Gonzales LL. Rounded atelectasis. AJR Am J Roentgenol 1980;134:225–232.

269. Voisin C, Fisekci F, Voisin-Saltiel S, et al. Asbestos-related rounded atelectasis. Radiologic and mineralogic data in 23 cases. Chest 1995;107:477–481.

270. Carvalho PM, Carr DH. Computed tomography of folded lung. Clin Radiol 1990;41:86–91.

271. Doyle TC, Lawler GA. CT features of rounded atelectasis of the lung. AJR Am J Roentgenol 1984;143:225–228.

272. Lynch D, Gamsu G, Ray C, et al. Asbestos-related focal lung masses: manifestations on conventional and high-resolution CT scans. Radiology 1988;169:603–607.

273. McHugh K, Blaquiere RM. CT features of rounded atelectasis. AJR Am J Roentgenol 1989;153:257–260.

274. Taylor PM. Dynamic contrast enhancement of asbestos-related pulmonary pseudotumours. Br J Radiol 1988;61:1070–1072.

275. Verschakelen JA, Demaerel P, Coolen J, et al. Rounded atelectasis of the lung: MR appearance. AJR Am J Roentgenol 1989;152:965–966.

276. Marchbank ND, Wilson AG, Joseph AE. Ultrasound features of folded lung. Clin Radiol 1996;51:433–437.

277. O'Donovan PB, Schenk M, Lim K, et al. Evaluation of the reliability of computed tomographic criteria used in the diagnosis of round atelectasis. J Thorac Imaging 1997;12:54–58.

278. Cooke WE. Pulmonary asbestosis. Br Med J 1927;2:1024–1025.

279. Walker AM, Loughlin JE, Friedlander ER, et al. Projections of asbestos-related disease 1980–2009. J Occup Med 1983; 25:409–425.

280. Craighead JE, Mossman BT. The pathogenesis of asbestos-associated diseases. N Engl J Med 1982;306: 1446–1455.

281. Gregor A, Parkes RW, du Bois R, et al. Radiographic progression of asbestosis: preliminary report. Ann N Y Acad Sci 1979;330:147–156.

282. Rubino GF, Newhouse M, Murray R, et al. Radiologic changes after cessation of exposure among chrysotile asbestos miners in Italy. Ann N Y Acad Sci 1979;330:157–161.

283. Shepherd JR, Hillerdal G, McLarty J. Progression of pleural and parenchymal disease on chest radiographs of workers exposed to amosite asbestos. Occup Environ Med 1997;54:410–415.

284. Gefter W, Epstein D, Miller W. Radiographic evaluation of asbestos-related chest disorders. CRC Crit Rev Diagn Imaging 1984;21:123–181.

285. Green RA, Dimcheff DG. Massive bilateral upper lobe fibrosis secondary to asbestos exposure. Chest 1974;65:52–55.

286. Hillerdal G. Asbestos exposure and upper lobe involvement. AJR Am J Roentgenol 1982;139:1163–1166.

287. Feigin DS. Talc: understanding its manifestations in the chest. AJR Am J Roentgenol 1986;146:295–301.

288. Staples CA, Gamsu G, Ray CS, et al. High resolution computed tomography and lung function in asbestos-exposed workers with normal chest radiographs. Am Rev Respir Dis 1989;139: 1502–1508.

289. Bergin CJ, Castellino RA, Blank N, et al. Specificity of high-resolution CT findings in pulmonary asbestosis: do patients scanned for other indications have similar findings? AJR Am J Roentgenol 1994;163:551–555.

290. al Jarad N, Strickland B, Pearson MC, et al. High resolution computed tomographic assessment of asbestosis and cryptogenic fibrosing alveolitis: a comparative study. Thorax 1992;47: 645–650.

291. Akira M, Yamamoto S, Inoue Y, et al. High-resolution CT of asbestosis and idiopathic pulmonary fibrosis. AJR Am J Roentgenol 2003;181:163–169.

292. Copley S, Wells A, Sivakumaran P, et al. Asbestosis and idiopathic pulmonary fibrosis: comparison thin-section CT features. Radiology 2003;229:731–736.

293. Rockoff SD, Schwartz A. Roentgenographic underestimation of early asbestosis by international labor organization classification. Chest 1988;93:1988–1991.

294. Oksa P, Suoranta H, Koskinen H, et al. High-resolution computed tomography in the early detection of asbestosis. Int Arch Occ Envir Health 1994;65: 299–304.

295. Neri S, Boraschi P, Antonelli A, et al. Pulmonary function, smoking habits, and high resolution computed tomography (HRCT) early abnormalities of lung and pleural fibrosis in shipyard workers exposed to asbestos. Am J Ind Med 1996;30:588–595.

296. Akira M, Yokoyama K, Yamamoto S, et al. Early asbestosis: evaluation with high-resolution CT. Radiology 1991; 178:409–416.

297. Gamsu G, Salmon CJ, Warnock ML, et al. CT quantification of interstitial fibrosis in patients with asbestosis: a comparison of two methods. AJR Am J Roentgenol 1995;164:63–68.

298. Hughes JM, Weill H. Asbestosis as a precursor of asbestos related lung cancer: results of a prospective mortality study. Br J Ind Med 1991;48:229–233.

299. Weiss W. Asbestosis: a marker for the increased risk of lung cancer among workers exposed to asbestos. Chest 1999;115:536–549.

300. Wilkinson P, Hansell DM, Janssens J, et al. Is lung cancer associated with asbestos exposure when there are no small opacities on the chest radiograph?

[see comments]. Lancet 1995;345: 1074–1078.

301. Finkelstein MM. Radiographic asbestosis is not a prerequisite for asbestos-associated lung cancer in Ontario asbestos-cement workers. Am J Ind Med 1997;32:341–348.

302. Scancarello G, Romeo R, Sartorelli E. Respiratory disease as a result of talc inhalation. J Occup Environ Med 1996;38:610–614.

303. Wells IP, Bhatt RC, Flanagan M. Kaolinosis: a radiological review. Clin Radiol 1985;36:579–582.

304. Kennedy T, Rawlings W Jr, Baser M, et al. Pneumoconiosis in Georgia kaolin workers. Am Rev Respir Dis 1983;127:215–220.

305. Oldham PD. Pneumoconiosis in Cornish china clay workers. Br J Ind Med 1983;40:131–137.

306. Han D, Goo JM, Im JG, et al. Thin-section CT findings of arc-welders' pneumoconiosis. Korean J Radiol 2000;1:79–83.

307. Akira M. Uncommon pneumoconioses: CT and pathologic findings. Radiology 1995;197:403–409.

308. Yoshii C, Matsuyama T, Takazawa A, et al. Welder's pneumoconiosis: diagnostic usefulness of high-resolution computed tomography and ferritin determinations in bronchoalveolar lavage fluid. Intern Med 2002;41:1111–1117.

309. Mapel D, Coultas DB. Disorders due to metals other than silica, coal, asbestos, to metals. In: Hendrick D, Burge P, Beckett W, Churg A, eds. Occupational disorders of the lungs: recognition, management, and prevention. London: Harcourt, 2002:163–191.

310. Kim CK, Kim SW, Kim JS, et al. Bronchiolitis obliterans in the 1990s in Korea and the United States. Chest 2001;120:1101–1106.

311. Shaver CG, Riddell AR. Lung changes associated with the manufacture of alumina abrasive. J Ind Hyg 1947;29: 145–157.

312. Brooks SM. Lung disorders resulting from the inhalation of metals. Clin Chest Med 1981;2:235–254.

313. Vahlensieck M, Overlack A, Müller KM. Computed tomographic high-attenuation mediastinal lymph nodes after aluminum exposition. Eur Radiol 2000;10:1945–1946.

314. Hooper WF. Acute beryllium lung disease. N C Med J 1981;42:551–553.

315. Kreiss K, Wasserman S, Mroz MM, et al. Beryllium disease screening in the ceramics industry. Blood lymphocyte test performance and exposure-disease relations. J Occup Med 1993;35:267–274.

316. Kreiss K, Mroz MM, Zhen B, et al. Epidemiology of beryllium sensitization and disease in nuclear workers. Am Rev Respir Dis 1993;148:985–991.

317. Newman LS, Buschman DL, Newell JD, et al. Beryllium disease: assessment with CT. Radiology 1994;190:835–840.

318. Harris KM, McConnochie K, Adams H. The computed tomographic appearances in chronic berylliosis. Clin Radiol 1993;47:26–31.

319. Iles PB. Multiple bronchial stenoses: treatment by mechanical dilatation. Thorax 1981;36:784–786.

320. Daniloff E, Lynch D, Bartelson B, et al. Observer variation and relationship of computed tomography to severity of beryllium disease. Am J Resp Crit Care Med 1997;155:2047–2056.

321. Kern DG, Crausman RS, Durand KT, et al. Flock worker's lung: chronic interstitial lung disease in the nylon flocking industry. Ann Intern Med 1998;129:261–272.

322. Weiland DA, Lynch DA, Jensen SP, et al. Thin-section CT findings in flock worker's lung, a work-related interstitial lung disease. Radiology 2003;227: 222–231.

323. Kreiss K, Gomaa A, Kullman G, et al. Clinical bronchiolitis obliterans in workers at a microwave-popcorn plant. N Engl J Med 2002;347:330–338.

324. Rabinowitz PM, Siegel MD. Acute inhalation injury. Clin Chest Med 2002;23:707–715.

325. Heimbach DM, Waeckerle JF. Inhalation injuries. Ann Emerg Med 1988;17: 1316–1320.

326. Darling GE, Keresteci MA, Ibanez D, et al. Pulmonary complications in inhalation injuries with associated cutaneous burn. J Trauma 1996;40:83–89.

327. Fein A, Leff A, Hopewell PC. Pathophysiology and management of the complications resulting from fire and the inhaled products of combustion: review of the literature. Crit Care Med 1980;8:94–98.

328. Hathaway PB, Stern EJ, Harruff RC, et al. Steam inhalation causing delayed airway occlusion. AJR Am J Roentgenol 1996;166:322.

329. Demling RH. Smoke inhalation injury. Postgrad Med 1987;82:63–68.

330. Teixidor HS, Novick G, Rubin E. Pulmonary complications in burn patients. J Can Assoc Radiol 1983;34:264–270.

331. Lee MJ, O'Connell DJ. The plain chest radiograph after acute smoke inhalation. Clin Radiol 1988;39:33–37.

332. Putman CE, Loke J, Matthay RA, et al. Radiographic manifestations of acute smoke inhalation. AJR Am J Roentgenol 1977;129:865–870.

333. Kangarloo H, Beachley MC, Ghahremani GG. The radiographic spectrum of pulmonary complications in burn victims. AJR Am J Roentgenol 1977;128:441–445.

334. Teixidor HS, Rubin E, Novick GS, et al. Smoke inhalation: radiologic manifestations. Radiology 1983;149:383–387.

335. Morrissey WL, Gould IA, Carrington CB, et al. Silo-filler's disease. Respiration 1975;32:81–92.

336. Ramirez J, Dowell AR. Silo-filler's disease: nitrogen dioxide-induced lung injury. Long-term follow-up and review of the literature. Ann Intern Med 1971;74:569–576.

337. Scott EG, Hunt WB Jr. Silo filler's disease. Chest 1973;63:701–706.

338. Bardana EJ Jr. Reactive airways dysfunction syndrome (RADS): guidelines for diagnosis and treatment and insight into likely prognosis. Ann Allergy Asthma Immunol 1999;83:583–586.

339. Wunderlich P, Rupprecht E, Trefftz F, et al. Chest radiographs of near-drowned children. Pediatr Radiol 1985;15:297–299.

340. Fandel I, Bancalari E. Near-drowning in children: clinical aspects. Pediatrics 1976;58:573–579.

341. Hunter TB, Whitehouse WM. Fresh-water near-drowning: radiological aspects. Radiology 1974;112:51–56.

342. Putman CE, Tummillo AM, Myerson DA, et al. Drowning: another plunge. Am J Roentgenol Radium Ther Nucl Med 1975;125:543–548.

343. Pearn J. Pathophysiology of drowning. Med J Aust 1985;142:586–588.

344. Effmann EL, Merten DF, Kirks DR, et al. Adult respiratory distress syndrome in children. Radiology 1985;157:69–74.

345. Mendelson CL. The aspiration of stomach contents into the lungs during obstetric anesthesia. Am J Obstet Gynecol 1946;52:191–205.

346. Landay MJ, Christensen EE, Bynum LJ. Pulmonary manifestations of acute aspiration of gastric contents. AJR Am J Roentgenol 1978;131:587–592.

347. Bynum LJ, Pierce AK. Pulmonary aspiration of gastric contents. Am Rev Respir Dis 1976;114:1129–1136.

348. Youngberg AS. Unilateral diffuse lung opacity; Differential diagnosis with emphasis on lymphangitic spread of cancer. Radiology 1977;123:277–281.

349. Franquet T, Gimenez A, Roson N, et al. Aspiration diseases: findings, pitfalls, and differential diagnosis. Radiographics 2000;20:673–685.

350. Marom EM, McAdams HP, Sporn TA, et al. Lentil aspiration pneumonia: radiographic and CT findings. J Comput Assist Tomogr 1998;22:598–600.

351. Gleeson K, Eggli DF, Maxwell SL. Quantitative aspiration during sleep in normal subjects. Chest 1997;111: 1266–1272.

352. Jack CI, Calverley PM, Donnelly RJ, et al. Simultaneous tracheal and oesophageal pH measurements in asthmatic patients with gastro-oesophageal reflux. Thorax 1995;50:201–204.

353. Harding SM. Nocturnal asthma: role of nocturnal gastroesophageal reflux. Chronobiol Int 1999;16:641–662.

354. Tobin RW, Pope CE 2nd, Pellegrini CA, et al. Increased prevalence of gastroesophageal reflux in patients with idiopathic pulmonary fibrosis. Am J Respir Crit Care Med 1998;158: 1804–1808.

355. Eade NR, Taussig LM, Marks MI. Hydrocarbon pneumonitis. Pediatrics 1974;54:351–357.

356. Gurwitz D, Kattan M, Levison H, et al. Pulmonary function abnormalities in asymptomatic children after hydrocarbon pneumonitis. Pediatrics 1978;62:789–794.

357. Brander PE, Taskinen E, Stenius-Aarniala B. Fire-eater's lung. Eur Respir J 1992;5:112–114.

358. Blazer S, Naveh Y, Friedman A. Foreign body in the airway. A review of 200 cases. Am J Dis Child 1980; 134:68–71.

359. Cohen SR, Herbert WI, Lewis GB Jr, et al. Foreign bodies in the airway. Five-year retrospective study with special reference to management. Ann Otol Rhinol Laryngol 1980;89:437–442.

360. Kim IG, Brummitt WM, Humphry A, et al. Foreign body in the airway: a review of 202 cases. Laryngoscope 1973;83:347–354.

361. Brown BST, Ma H, Dunbar JS, et al. Foreign bodies in the tracheobronchial tree in childhood. J Can Assoc Radiol 1963;14:158–171.

362. Rothmann BF, Boeckman CR. Foreign bodies in the larynx and tracheobronchial tree in children. A review of 225 cases. Ann Otol Rhinol Laryngol 1980;89:434–436.

363. Pyman C. Inhaled foreign bodies in childhood. A review of 230 cases. Med J Aust 1971;1:62–68.

364. Wesenberg RL, Blumhagen JD. Assisted expiratory chest radiography: an effective technique for the diagnosis of foreign-body aspiration. Radiology 1979;130:538–539.

365. Capitanio MA, Kirkpatrick JA. The lateral decubitus film. An aid in determining air-trapping in children. Radiology 1972;103:460–462.

366. Zissin R, Shapiro-Feinberg M, Rozenman J, et al. CT findings of the chest in adults with aspirated foreign bodies. Eur Radiol 2001;11:606–611.

CHAPTER 9

Drug and radiation induced lung disease

DRUG INDUCED LUNG DISEASE

Many commonly used drugs, including both cytotoxic and noncytotoxic agents, can adversely affect the lungs. Drug induced lung injury is a common cause of acute and chronic lung disease,[1–10] and most commonly occurs with cytotoxic agents used to treat hematologic and solid organ malignancies. This is not surprising since cancer chemotherapy is essentially a form of controlled cellular poisoning. Lung injury caused by noncytotoxic drugs occurs less frequently and is less predictable.

Diagnosis of drug induced lung disease is difficult because the clinical manifestations are often nonspecific and may be attributed to infection, radiation pneumonitis, or recurrence of the underlying disease. Reduction in diffusing capacity for carbon monoxide (DLco) is an important and early clinical finding of drug induced lung injury.[11] Early recognition is important because undiagnosed injury can be progressive and fatal, whereas cessation of therapy can result in stabilization or even reversal of disease. The radiologic and histopathologic manifestations of drug induced lung disease are, with the possible exception of amiodarone toxicity,[12] nonspecific. Prompt diagnosis of drug induced lung disease requires first and foremost a high index of clinical suspicion. Diagnosis also requires careful correlation of clinical symptoms, history of drug exposure, reduction in DLco, appropriate radiologic findings, exclusion of other causes of injury, and response to therapy (see Box 9.1). Many, if not most, cases are diagnosed clinically, without histopathologic confirmation. Lung biopsy specimens may be obtained, however, not necessarily to diagnose drug toxicity, but to exclude other causes of lung injury prior to institution of therapy. The mainstays of treatment are withdrawal of the offending agent, supportive care, and in some instances, administration of corticosteroids.

Box 9.1 Diagnosis of drug-induced lung disease

Appropriate history of drug exposure
Clinical signs and symptoms
- Dyspnea
- Cough
- Fever
- Decreased gas transfer
Compatible radiologic findings
Exclusion of alternate diagnoses
- Infection
- Malignancy
Response to therapy
- Withdrawal of offending agent
- Corticosteroids

Chest radiography is the mainstay for imaging patients with suspected drug induced lung disease. CT can also be useful in this regard.[13–18] CT, particularly high-resolution CT (HRCT), can detect findings of drug induced lung disease at an earlier stage than can chest radiography. CT may also better categorize the type of pulmonary reaction. Padley et al,[15] for example, were able to distinguish drug induced cases of diffuse alveolar damage (DAD) from hypersensitivity reactions using CT. Amiodarone toxicity, however, may be the only condition in which CT can be definitive by virtue of the high-attenuation values of amiodarone deposits in the lung.[19–21]

Although the radiologic features of drug induced lung injury are nonspecific, they may reflect the underlying histopathologic pattern of lung injury. These patterns are fairly stereotypical and are often associated with specific drugs.[22] Thus, knowledge of these patterns and of the drugs most frequently involved can facilitate diagnosis of drug induced lung disease. Table 9.1 and Box 9.2 summarize some of the more important histopathologic and clinicopathologic manifestations of drug induced lung injury. This chapter will first review the most important clinical, histopathologic, and radiologic manifestations of drug induced lung injury and then discuss selected drugs.

Mechanisms of injury

Lung injury due to direct toxic action on lung tissue

The mechanisms of direct toxic action of drugs on the lung are complex and poorly understood.[23–25] The production of excessive reactive oxygen metabolites and a disturbance of the complex oxidant/antioxidant system may result in damage to cells and cell membranes. Alveolar macrophages, polymorphonuclear leukocytes, and lymphocytes may be damaged, resulting in the release of leukokines, lymphokines, and other humoral factors with chemotactic, cytotoxic, or immune modulating effects. The balance between collagen production and collagen lysis may be altered, causing excess collagen deposition and thus leading to pulmonary fibrosis. The collagen itself may be disordered either by damage to the fibroblasts or by the action of anticollagen

Table 9.1 Common histopathologic manifestations of drug induced lung injury

Histopathology	Drugs
Diffuse alveolar damage	Bleomycin, busulfan, carmustine (BCNU), cyclophosphamide, mitomycin, melphalan, gold salts
Interstitial pneumonia	Amiodarone, methotrexate, BCNU, chlorambucil
Organizing pneumonia	Bleomycin, gold salts, methotrexate, amiodarone, nitrofurantoin, penicillamine, sulfasalazine, cyclophosphamide
Eosinophilic pneumonia	Penicillamine, sulfasalazine, nitrofurantoin, nonsteroidal antiinflammatory drugs, paraaminosalicylic acid
Pulmonary hemorrhage	Anticoagulants, amphotericin B, cytosine arabinoside (Ara-C), penicillamine, cyclophosphamide

---

Box 9.2 Important clinicopathologic manifestations of drug induced lung toxicity

Injury due to direct toxic action on lung tissue
Diffuse alveolar damage (see Table 9.1)
Interstitial pneumonia (see Table 9.1)
Organizing pneumonia (see Table 9.1)

Injury due to hypersensitivity reactions
Drug induced asthma (see Box 9.3)
Eosinophilic pneumonia (see Table 9.1)

Injury due to neural or humoral mechanisms
Drug induced pulmonary edema (see Box 9.4)
Drug induced asthma (see Box 9.3)

Injury due to autoimmune mechanisms
Drug induced lupus (see Box 9.5)
Drug induced vasculitis (see Box 9.6)

Drug induced pulmonary granulomatosis
Granulomatous vasculitis (see Box 9.7)
Exogenous lipoid pneumonia (see Box 9.7)
Drug induced sarcoidosis (see Box 9.7)

Miscellaneous
Drug induced pulmonary hemorrhage (see Table 9.1)
Drug induced vasospasm
Drug induced pulmonary thromboembolism
Drug induced pulmonary calcification
Drug related pleural effusions and fibrosis
Drug related lymphadenopathy

---

antibodies. Inflammatory cells release proteolytic enzymes, and a complex antiprotease system exists to combat the effects of these enzymes. Inhibition of the antiprotease systems can also result in toxicity.

Direct toxic action on lung tissue usually takes some time to reach a clinically appreciable threshold, and thus the effects may not be apparent for weeks or months after treatment has begun. In many cases the effect is dose related, a relationship that is most

A

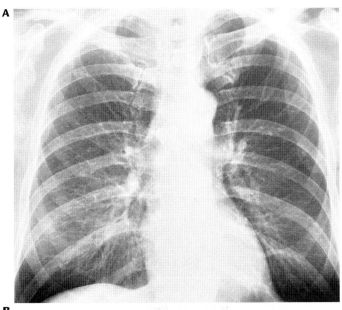

B

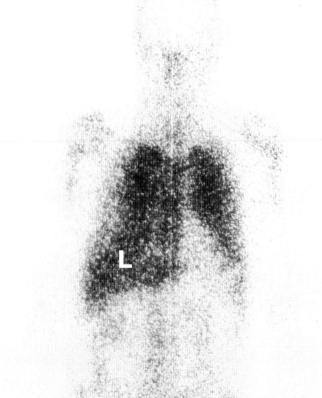

Fig. 9.1 BCNU induced diffuse alveolar damage (DAD) in a patient with a decreased diffusing capacity for carbon monoxide (DLco). **A**, The frontal chest radiograph is normal. **B**, ^{67}Ga scan shows diffuse pulmonary uptake consistent with toxicity, likely acute DAD. L = liver.

evident with the cytotoxic agents bleomycin, busulfan, and carmustine (BCNU). Lung toxicity may be accentuated by other factors such as increasing age, decreased renal function, radiation therapy, oxygen therapy, and other cytotoxic drug therapy.[23] Direct toxic action of drugs on the lung manifests histopathologically with at least three important patterns of lung injury: DAD, interstitial pneumonia (IP), and organizing pneumonia (OP).

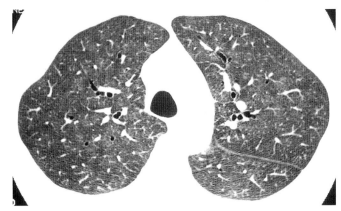

Fig. 9.2 BCNU induced diffuse alveolar damage (DAD) in a patient with a decreased diffusing capacity for carbon monoxide (DLco). The chest radiograph was normal. HRCT shows subtle, scattered ground-glass opacities. Lung biopsy showed early DAD. DLco normalized after cessation of BCNU therapy. (With permission from Rossi SE, Erasmus JJ, McAdams HP, Sporn TA, Goodman PC. Pulmonary drug toxicity: radiologic and pathologic manifestations. RadioGraphics 2000;20: 1245–1259.)

Diffuse alveolar damage

DAD is a descriptive term for the sequence of events that occurs after acute severe lung injury and results in necrosis of type I pneumocytes and alveolar endothelial cells.[22] Drugs that most frequently cause DAD include bleomycin, busulfan, BCNU, cyclophosphamide, melphalan, methotrexate, mitomycin, and gold salts (see Table 9.1).[12,26] At least two histopathologic phases of DAD are recognized: an acute exudative phase and an organizing reparative phase.[26,27] The exudative phase occurs in the first week after lung injury and is characterized by edema and intraalveolar membranes composed of necrotic epithelial cells and protein rich fluid.[22,26,27] The reparative phase typically occurs after 1 or 2 weeks and is characterized by proliferation of type II pneumocytes and fibrosis.[22,26–28] Depending on the severity of the injury, DAD can progress to end-stage fibrosis. DAD is, however, sometimes reversible and many survivors have minimal residual functional abnormalities.[22]

The chest radiograph is often normal in early drug induced DAD. In this setting, however, gallium or CT scans, pulmonary function tests, or lung biopsies can show direct or indirect evidence of lung toxicity (Figs 9.1 and 9.2). As disease progresses, however, chest radiographs show bilateral, scattered or diffuse heterogeneous or homogeneous opacities (Fig. 9.3). These may be more apparent in the lung bases. Segmental or lobar consolidation is not a typical feature and pleural effusion is rare. HRCT can be quite useful in early drug induced DAD by showing scattered or diffuse ground-glass opacities when the chest radiograph is normal (Figs 9.1, 9.2, and 9.4) or equivocal. HRCT performed in the late, reparative phase of DAD may show findings of fibrosis, such as irregular linear opacities, architectural distortion, and traction bronchiectasis (Fig. 9.5).

Because most cases of drug induced DAD occur in patients with malignancy, the differential diagnosis includes lymphangitis carcinomatosa, leukemic or lymphomatous infiltration of the lung, opportunistic infections such as *Pneumocystis* pneumonia, and pulmonary hemorrhage (see Ch. 6). The clinical circumstances and sequence of events may suggest drug induced DAD as the cause. Lung biopsy may, however, be necessary to confidently distinguish drug toxicity from other conditions.

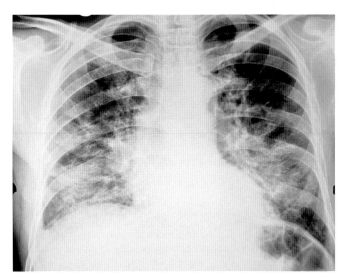

Fig. 9.3 Bleomycin induced diffuse alveolar damage. The frontal chest radiograph shows bibasilar heterogeneous pulmonary opacities.

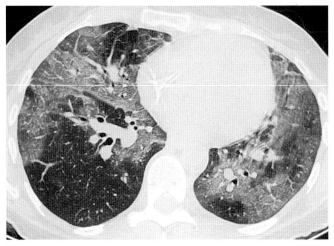

Fig. 9.4 Cyclophosphamide induced diffuse alveolar damage (DAD) in a patient with dyspnea and decreased diffusing capacity for carbon monoxide (DLco). CT shows extensive bilateral ground-glass opacities. Biopsy showed early DAD. Symptoms and functional abnormalities resolved after cessation of therapy.

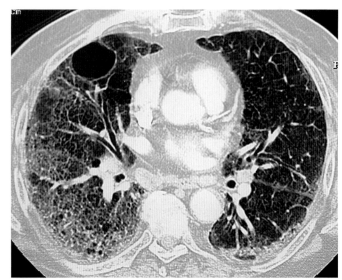

Fig. 9.5 BCNU induced diffuse alveolar damage in a patient with severe dyspnea. HRCT shows ground-glass and coarse reticular opacities, more prominent in the right lower lobe, and architectural distortion.

Interstitial pneumonia

Nonspecific interstitial pneumonia (NSIP) is a term used to describe interstitial inflammation and fibrosis that does not fulfill diagnostic criteria for usual, desquamative, or acute IP. NSIP is characterized histopathologically by scattered infiltrates of mononuclear inflammatory cells, mild interstitial fibrosis, and reactive hyperplastic type II pneumocytes.[26] Use of the term NSIP in the setting of drug induced lung disease is controversial, however. Some authors prefer to reserve the term NSIP for cases of idiopathic interstitial fibrosis and to use the term cellular IP (CIP) or just IP for cases of drug induced fibrosis. For clarity, the term IP will be used for the remainder of this chapter.

IP is probably the most common form of fibrosing pneumonia associated with drug administration. The drugs most frequently associated with IP are amiodarone, bleomycin, methotrexate,

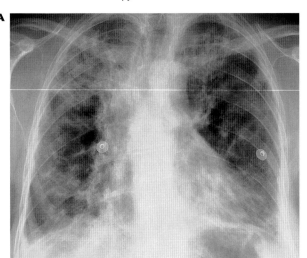

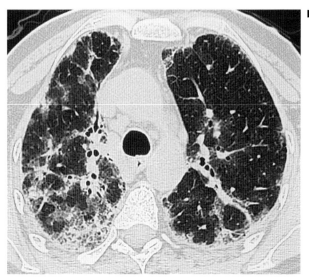

Fig. 9.6 Nitrofurantoin induced interstitial pneumonia in a patient with progressive dyspnea. **A,** The frontal chest radiograph shows bilateral scattered poorly defined opacities with preservation of lung volumes. **B,** HRCT shows scattered ground-glass and irregular linear opacities in a peribronchovascular distribution. Note also the mild architectural distortion. Biopsy showed interstitial pneumonia.

A

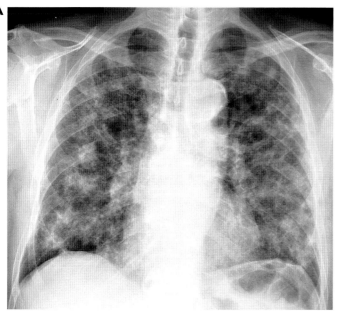

B

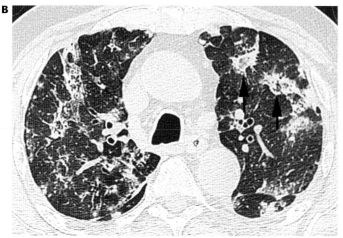

C

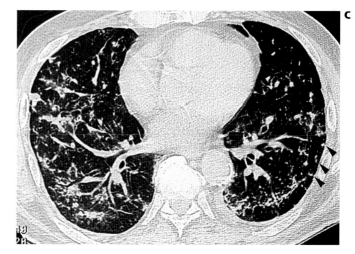

Fig. 9.7   Amiodarone induced organizing pneumonia. **A**, The frontal chest radiograph demonstrates bilateral poorly defined pulmonary opacities. Lung volumes are preserved. **B** and **C**, HRCT demonstrates scattered, almost rounded, areas of consolidation (arrows) and centrilobular nodules (arrowheads).

and BCNU (see Table 9.1).[22,23,26–30] Gold salts and chlorambucil are less common causes of drug induced IP.[22] Drug induced IP manifests on chest radiographs with heterogeneous opacities that are either diffuse or basal in distribution (Fig. 9.6).[22,23,29,31] HRCT shows scattered areas of ground-glass opacity, focal areas of consolidation, and irregular linear opacities, often in a basal and peribronchovascular distribution.[32]

Organizing pneumonia

OP is a term used to describe inflammatory infiltration and fibrosis that predominantly involves the airspaces. OP is characterized histopathologically by fibroblastic plugs (Masson bodies) within the respiratory bronchioles, alveolar ducts, and adjacent alveolar spaces, and accumulation of lipid laden macrophages in the distal airspaces.[33] The drugs most commonly implicated are bleomycin, methotrexate, cyclophosphamide, and gold salts (see Table 9.1).[1,22,26] Amiodarone, nitrofurantoin, penicillamine, and sulfasalazine are less common causes of drug induced OP.[1] OP manifests on chest radiographs with rounded, scattered, and often peripheral areas of consolidation (Fig. 9.7).[22,23,31] HRCT usually shows bilateral scattered areas of ground-glass opacification or consolidation that are often

peripheral in distribution. Centrilobular nodules, branching linear opacities, and bronchial dilation are common associated findings.[33]

Lung injury due to hypersensitivity reactions

Because the molecular size of most drugs is too small to provoke an immune response, it is likely that they act as haptenes in combination with endogenous protein.[34,35] The provoked immune responses are most commonly type I (immediate hypersensitivity) or type III (immune complex) reactions. Drugs most commonly associated with hypersensitivity reactions are shown in Box 9.3. Hypersensitivity reactions are usually immediate and may become clinically apparent within hours or days after institution of drug therapy (Fig. 9.8). Fever and peripheral eosinophilia suggest the diagnosis. Withdrawal of the offending drug and administration of corticosteroids usually results in prompt and complete resolution of symptoms. Hypersensitivity reactions to drugs may predominantly affect the airways or the lung parenchyma.

Airway hypersensitivity results in bronchial constriction, mucus hypersecretion and inspissation, and mucosal edema

Box 9.3 Drugs that can cause hypersensitivity reactions

Antiarthritics
Aurothioglucose (gold salts)

Antiasthmatics
Sodium cromoglycate

Antibacterials
Erythromycin
Nitrofurantoin
Paraaminosalicylic acid
Isoniazid
Penicillin
Sulfonamides

Antidepressants
Imipramine

Antihypertensives
Mecamylamine
Hydralazine

Central nervous system stimulants
Methylphenidate

Cytotoxic agents
Bleomycin
Methotrexate
Procarbazine
Azathioprine
Paclitaxel

Hypoglycemic agents
Chlorpropamide

Muscle relaxants
Dantrolene

Chelating agents
Penicillamine

Antiinflammatory agents
Sulfasalazine
Nonsteroidal antiinflammatory drugs

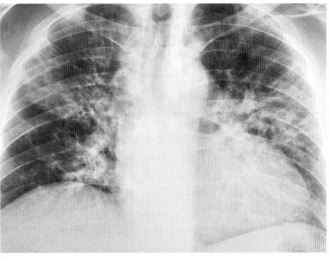

Fig. 9.8   Desipramine induced hypersensitivity reaction in a patient with acute dyspnea following drug administration. The frontal chest radiograph shows predominantly upper lobe and perihilar heterogeneous opacities that rapidly resolved following cessation of therapy and administration of corticosteroids.

with eosinophilic infiltration. This clinically manifests as drug induced asthma and lacks specific radiographic features. Pulmonary parenchymal involvement can result in either acute or chronic eosinophilic pneumonia (EP).[36] Although many drugs can cause EP, the agents most commonly implicated are penicillamine, sulfasalazine, nitrofurantoin, paraaminosalicylic acid and nonsteroidal antiinflammatory drugs (see Table 9.1).[1,22,26,27,37–43] EP is characterized histopathologically by accumulation of eosinophils and macrophages in alveolar spaces.[27] There is usually an accompanying infiltrate of eosinophils, lymphocytes, and plasma cells within alveolar septa and adjacent interstitium. Eosinophilia is often present in the peripheral blood. Drug induced EP manifests on chest radiographs with scattered areas of subsegmental consolidation, often in the periphery of the lung (Fig. 9.9). The extent of consolidation varies and distribution within the peripheral

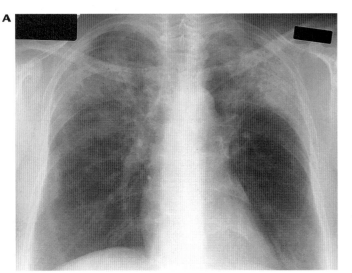
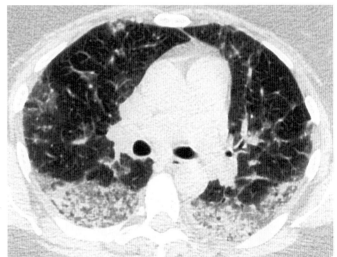

Fig. 9.9   Nonsteroidal antiinflammatory agent induced eosinophilic pneumonia. **A**, The frontal chest radiograph shows predominantly upper lobe homogeneous opacities. Note the preservation of lung volumes. **B**, CT shows subpleural ground-glass opacities and consolidation, findings typical of eosinophilic pneumonia.

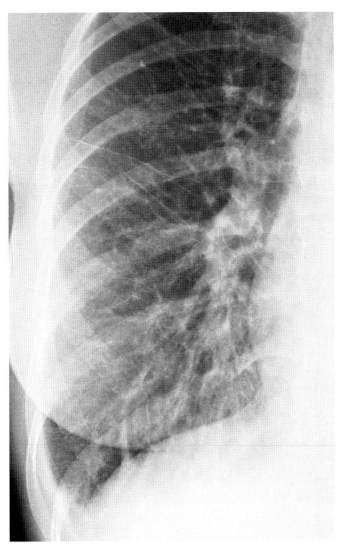

Fig. 9.10   Nitrofurantoin induced hypersensitivity reaction in a patient who developed dyspnea and tachypnea a few hours after a single dose of the drug. The coned down view of a frontal chest radiograph shows thickened interlobular septa in the right lower lobe and a small right pleural effusion. Symptoms and radiologic abnormalities resolved rapidly.

lungs is random. The opacities tend to be fleeting – resolving in one area of the lung only to reappear in another. HRCT shows ground-glass opacities and consolidation that is typically peripheral and upper lobe in distribution (Fig. 9.9).[44]

A hyperacute hypersensitivity reaction has been described in patients receiving bleomycin,[45,46] methotrexate,[47,48] and carbamazepine,[49] particularly after previous exposure to the drug. In these cases, the patient presents with acute onset of respiratory symptoms and chest radiographs show diffuse heterogeneous or homogeneous opacities (Fig. 9.10). Response to discontinuation of the offending drug is usually prompt, but a similar reaction after readministration of the drug may be expected.

Lung injury due to neural or humoral mechanisms

Drugs can cause noncardiogenic pulmonary edema in a number of ways.[50,51] Central nervous system depressants can cause neurogenic pulmonary edema. In such cases, pulmonary capillary permeability is altered, either by direct toxic action on the lung or

by impulses from the brainstem and hypothalamus,[52–54] and fluid leaks into the pulmonary interstitium and alveoli. However, not all cases of drug induced pulmonary edema operate through these mechanisms. Some drugs cause water and salt retention, leading to fluid imbalance and edema. Edema caused by drug toxicity is indistinguishable from other forms of edema both in its radiologic appearance and in the rapidity of onset and clearing (Fig. 9.11). Drugs most commonly associated with pulmonary edema are shown in Box 9.4.

Box 9.4 Drugs that can cause pulmonary edema

Analgesics
Acetylsalicylic acid
Codeine
Pentazocine

Antibacterials
Nitrofurantoin

Antidepressants
Amitryptyline
Doxepine
Desipramine
Imipramine

Antiinflammatories
Phenylbutazone

Insecticides
Oxyphenbutazone

β-Adrenergic agonists
Ritodrine
Terbutaline

Cytotoxic agents
Cyclophosphamide
Methotrexate
Cytosine arabinoside

Immune suppressants
Interleukin-2
OKT3

Phenothiazines
Chlorpromazine

Sedatives
Chlordiazepoxide
Ethchlorvynol

Opiates
Heroin
Propoxyphene
Methadone

Organophosphates
Parathion
Malathion

Diuretics
Hydrochlorothiazide

Miscellaneous
Iodinated contrast media
Dextran
Colchicine
Epinephrine

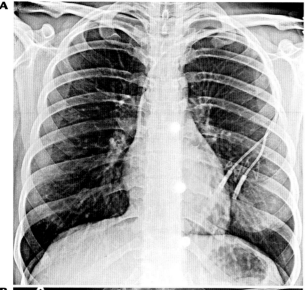

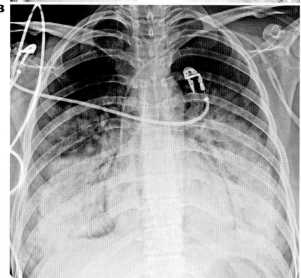

Fig. 9.11 Cytosine arabinoside (Ara-C) induced pulmonary edema. **A,** The frontal chest radiograph obtained just prior to drug administration is normal. **B,** The chest radiograph obtained several hours after drug administration shows diffuse bilateral homogeneous opacities consistent with edema.

Drug induced asthma may also result from neurohumoral mechanisms. Certain drugs, including β-adrenergic antagonists such as propranolol and parasympatheticomimetics such as neostigmine, cause asthma by directly affecting bronchial innervation. Acetylsalicylic acid may cause asthma by inhibiting prostaglandin synthesis.[55]

Lung injury due to autoimmune mechanisms

Drug induced lupus

Many drugs can trigger an autoimmune response and cause systemic lupus erythematosus.[56–58] At least 90% of cases of drug induced lupus are associated with procainamide, hydralazine, isoniazid, or phenytoin. Antinuclear antibodies are usually detectable in the serum of affected patients and are often found in patients taking these drugs in the absence of clinical or radiographic evidence of lupus. Drugs most commonly associated with systemic lupus erythematosus are shown in Box 9.5.

Box 9.5 Drugs that can cause systemic lupus erythematosis

Antibacterials
Griseofulvin
Nitrofurantoin
Paraaminosalicylic acid
Penicillin
Streptomycin
Sulfonamides

Anticonvulsants
Carbamazepine
Ethosuximide
Methsuximide
Phenytoin
Primidone
Trimethadone

Antiinflammatories
Phenylbutazone
Oxyphenbutazone

Cardiovascular agents
Clofibrate
Digitalis
Isoniazid
Hydralazine
Methyldopa
Procainamide
Propranolol
Reserpine
Quinidine

Diuretics
Chlorthalidone
Thiazides

Thyroid blockers
Thiouracil
Propylthiouracil

Miscellaneous
Phenothiazines
Penicillamine
Methysergide
Gold salts
Levodopa

Drug induced lupus does not differ in its pleural or pulmonary manifestations from the idiopathic form of the disease. Pleural effusion is by far the most common radiologic manifestation of this condition and there may be a concomitant pericardial effusion (Fig. 9.12). Lung parenchymal involvement is uncommon but, when it occurs, typically manifests with bilateral basal heterogeneous opacities. Because some of the drugs that cause this condition are used to treat cardiac disease, and because the manifestations of cardiac disease can be similar to those of drug induced lupus, diagnosis can be difficult and is often delayed.

Drug induced vasculitis

Although the list of potential causative drugs is extensive,[59,60] the association between pulmonary vasculitis and drugs is

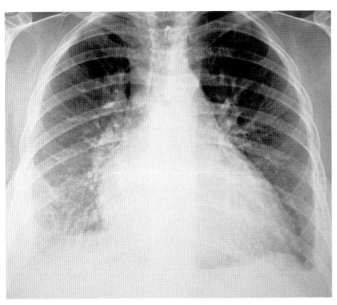

Fig. 9.12 Procainamide induced systemic lupus erythematosus. The frontal chest radiograph shows enlargement of the cardiopericardial silhouette suggestive of pericardial effusion and bilateral pleural effusions.

Box 9.6 Drugs that can cause pulmonary vasculitis

Antiasthmatics
Sodium cromoglycate

Antibacterials
Sulfonamides
Penicillin

Anticonvulsants
Phenytoin

Antiinflammatories
Phenylbutazone

Cardiovascular agents
Quinidine
Hydralazine

Cytotoxic agents
Busulfan

Thyroid blockers
Thiouracil
Propylthiouracil

Tranquillizers
Phenothiazines

---

perhaps strongest with the sulfonamides (see Box 9.6). Drug induced vasculitis may be an expression of a type III (immune complex) or a type IV (cell mediated) hypersensitivity response. Pulmonary involvement is usually associated with, and often overshadowed by, systemic vasculitis that particularly involves the skin, kidneys, and liver. Drug induced pulmonary vasculitis can result in pulmonary infarction and hemorrhage. Diagnosis of drug induced pulmonary vasculitis usually requires evidence of

---

Box 9.7 Drugs that can cause pulmonary granulomatosis

Granulomatous vasculitis ("drug abuser's lung")
Intravenous talc injection
Intravenous starch injection
Intravenous cellulose injection

Exogenous lipid pneumonia
Mineral oil
Oily nasal drops
Occupational exposure

Drug induced sarcoidosis
Interferon
Methotrexate

---

vasculitis on lung biopsy and a history of appropriate drug exposure.

Radiologic findings of drug induced pulmonary vasculitis are variable and nonspecific. Scattered areas of subsegmental consolidation in a peripheral distribution may occur in a pattern similar to that seen in cases of drug induced eosinophilic pneumonia. In other patients, more diffuse heterogeneous or homogeneous opacities are seen. Cavitation may occur in areas of infarction. Pleural effusion is rare.

Drug induced pulmonary granulomatosis

Granulomas are aggregates of pulmonary macrophages that are reacting to certain microorganisms, foreign particles, various drugs such as methotrexate and nitrofurantoin, or other unknown stimuli. There are a number of granulomatous pulmonary reactions related to drug therapy, including granulomatous vasculitis, exogenous lipoid pneumonia and drug induced sarcoidosis (see Box 9.7).

Granulomatous vasculitis

Intravenous administration of illicit drugs can cause a granulomatous vasculitis and pulmonary hypertension ("drug abuser's lung"). Vasculitis in these cases is caused by a foreign body giant cell reaction to contaminants or suspending agents, such as talc, starch, or cellulose.[61,62] Distinctive pathologic features include: (1) medial hypertrophy of muscular pulmonary arteries with thrombosis and recanalization; and (2) foreign body giant cell granulomas containing doubly refractile particles in the lumina and arterial walls, in the perivascular connective tissues, and in the alveolar septa. Patients may be asymptomatic when the condition is discovered. Many eventually progress to severe respiratory insufficiency. Typical radiologic findings include pulmonary hyperinflation, diffuse small nodular opacities, large bulla, and vascular and cardiac changes of pulmonary hypertension (Fig. 9.13). With time, the nodules may enlarge and coalesce into large, often perihilar conglomerate masses in the mid to upper lungs, similar to those seen in cases of silicosis.[63–69]

Exogenous lipoid pneumonia

Exogenous lipoid pneumonia (ELP) is a fairly common form of granulomatous pneumonitis that results from chronic aspiration of mineral oils or other lipids. Because mineral oil is inert and is

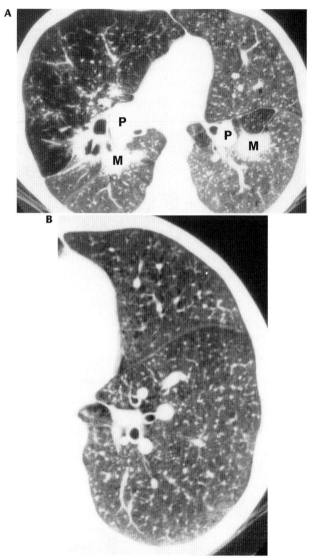

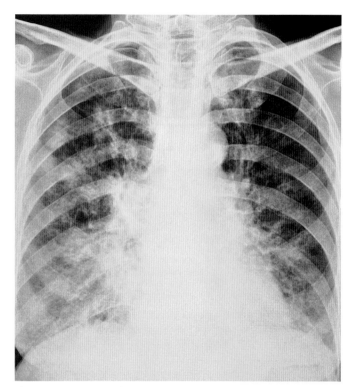

Fig. 9.14 Exogenous lipoid pneumonia in an elderly woman with a hiatal hernia and chronic constipation treated with mineral oils. The frontal chest radiograph shows bilateral, predominantly lower lobe, heterogeneous opacities and scattered poorly defined nodules in the upper right lung.

Fig. 9.13 Talc induced granulomatosis in an intravenous drug abuser. **A**, HRCT shows severe emphysema in the right upper lobe, diffuse tiny nodules and perihilar conglomerate masses (M). The central pulmonary arteries (P) are enlarged, consistent with pulmonary hypertension. **B**, The coned view of the left lung shows the diffuse nodules to better advantage. (Courtesy of Laura Heynernan, MD, Durham, NC)

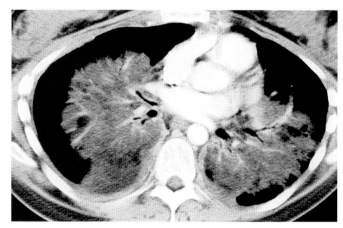

Fig. 9.15 Exogenous lipid pneumonia due to chronic mineral oil aspiration. CT shows bilateral low attenuation areas of consolidation. Region of interest measurements showed −70 to −100 HU, consistent with fat.

not hydrolyzed by lipase, it causes a foreign body giant cell reaction in the lung. ELP most frequently occurs in elderly patients with swallowing disorders or hiatal hernias and who use either mineral oil as a laxative or oily nose drops. It can also result from occupational exposure to oil mist. Because patients regard the use of mineral oils as something normal and inconsequential, they often fail to volunteer this information. Thus, the diagnosis of ELP can be difficult. Although the diagnosis can sometimes be suggested radiologically, it is more often made by pathologic examination of affected lung. Staining of bronchoalveolar lavage fluid for neutral fats can also be diagnostic.

Most patients with ELP are asymptomatic. In these cases, the condition is discovered on "routine" chest radiographs. A few patients complain of chronic cough or chest pain. Long-standing, recurrent aspiration can result in fibrosis that manifests with

severe, progressive dyspnea. Three patterns have been described on chest radiographs. First, acute aspiration of a large volume of oil can result in diffuse airspace consolidation. Affected patients are typically quite ill and have marked respiratory distress. This type of ELP is fortunately quite rare. Second, chronic low grade aspiration of oil over a long period of time can result in either focal or multifocal homogeneous opacities or consolidation (Figs 9.14 and 9.15). Affected patients can be asymptomatic

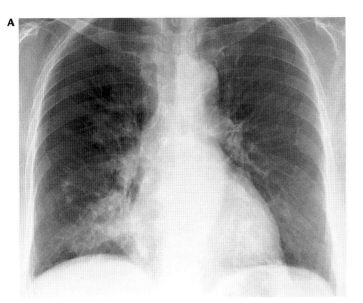

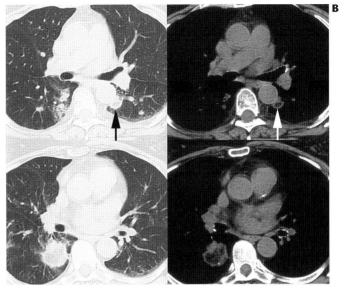

Fig. 9.16   Exogenous lipoid pneumonia due to mineral oil aspiration. **A**, The frontal chest radiograph shows a poorly defined opacity in the right mid lung and scattered small nodular opacities. **B**, CT shows multifocal pulmonary masses and nodules. Note that the large superior segment mass has an irregular rim of soft tissue and contains abundant central fat. Note also that the second small periaortic nodule on the left (arrows) has similar features.

despite impressive radiographic abnormalities and late fibrosis can result. Third, aspiration of oil can result in one or more pulmonary masses (Fig. 9.16). Affected patients are also typically asymptomatic and differentiation from bronchogenic carcinoma can be difficult (see Figs 10.10 and 10.11).[70–72] Cavitation is uncommon in cases of ELP and, when present, is usually due to superinfection by atypical mycobacteria, particularly *M. fortuitum* or *M. chelonei*.

On CT, ELP can manifest with airspace consolidation or irregular masslike opacities. Superimposed fibrosis with irregular linear opacities, traction bronchiectasis, and honeycombing can also be seen. A distinctive and frequently diagnostic finding of ELP on CT is fat within the consolidation or mass (Figs 9.15 and 9.16). The "crazy paving" appearance on HRCT has also been described in patients with ELP (Fig. 9.17).[73]

Drug induced sarcoidosis

Sarcoidosis is a granulomatous disease of unknown etiology. Its pathologic hallmark is the presence of interstitial noncaseating granulomas that typically involve the lymphatics of the bronchovascular bundles. While the exact pathogenesis of sarcoidosis remains in doubt, a number of immune modulators have been implicated, including interferons. Recent reports suggest that interferon therapy for malignant and nonmalignant conditions (such as hepatitis) may cause sarcoidosis.[74–77] In the largest series to date, 7% of patients treated with interferon-2a developed sarcoidosis that regressed with discontinuation of interferon.[74] Prognosis for interferon induced sarcoidosis seems to be good, provided that the medication can be discontinued. Sarcoidosis induced by methotrexate therapy has also been reported.[78,79]

The radiologic findings of drug induced sarcoidosis are similar to those of idiopathic sarcoid: hilar and mediastinal lymphadenopathy, fine nodular opacities (miliary pattern), reticulation, or, less commonly, airspace opacities (Fig. 9.18).[74,80] These findings typically predominate in the mid to upper

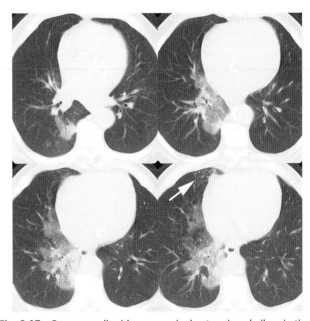

Fig. 9.17   Exogenous lipoid pneumonia due to mineral oil aspiration. CT shows focal dependent ground-glass opacity with superimposed septal thickening ("crazy paving" appearance). Note also the small centrilobular nodules in the right middle lobe (arrow).

lungs. CT frequently demonstrates a distinctly bronchovascular distribution of abnormalities.

Miscellaneous forms of drug induced lung injury

Drug induced pulmonary hemorrhage

Drug related pulmonary hemorrhage is usually the consequence of a drug induced coagulopathy. In some cases, as in oxyphenbutazone or quinidine induced thrombocytopenia, the

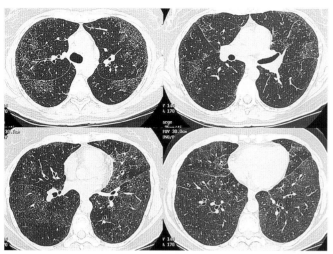

Fig. 9.18 Sarcoidosis induced by γ-interferon therapy for hepatitis. HRCT shows scattered and diffuse tiny nodules as well as ground-glass opacity in the lower lobes. Lung biopsy showed findings consistent with sarcoidosis.

coagulopathy is unexpected and idiosyncratic. More commonly, however, hemorrhage results from anticoagulant therapy and is not entirely unexpected.

Less commonly, hemorrhage occurs as a toxic reaction to drug therapy. Diffuse pulmonary hemorrhage (DPH) is an uncommon complication of drug therapy. Drugs most commonly associated with DPH are anticoagulants, amphotericin B, high dose cyclophosphamide, mitomycin, cytarabine (Ara-C), and penicillamine (see Table 9.1).[1,22,26] Penicillamine can cause a syndrome of pulmonary hemorrhage with or without renal failure.[81] Penicillamine induced pulmonary hemorrhage is thought to be an immune complex disorder. Affected patients are typically dyspneic and have a falling hematocrit. Hemoptysis may or may not occur.

Chest radiographs in patients with drug induced pulmonary hemorrhage show scattered airspace consolidation of variable severity that is generally rapid in onset and clears fairly quickly. HRCT usually shows bilateral, scattered, or diffuse, ground-glass opacities (Fig. 9.19).[82] There are no associated pleural, hilar, or mediastinal abnormalities. Drug induced pulmonary hemorrhage is usually an isolated event; fibrosis, as is seen in patients with idiopathic pulmonary hemosiderosis or Goodpasture syndrome and repeated episodes of hemorrhage, is uncommon. Fiberoptic bronchoscopy with bronchoalveolar lavage that yields increasingly bloody aliquots of fluid is characteristic.

Drug induced pulmonary vasospasm

Drug induced pulmonary vasospasm appears to be rare. The first documented case of this complication occurred in the 1960s when Aminorex, an over the counter appetite suppressant, was marketed in Europe. Pulmonary arteriolar vasospasm induced by Aminorex caused pulmonary arterial hypertension and cor pulmonale.[83] More recently, several amphetamine-like appetite suppressant drugs, particularly the fenfluramines, have been implicated in cases of pulmonary arterial hypertension.[84–86] These drugs may also cause valvular heart disease involving both right and left sided valves.[87]

Drug induced thromboembolism

Venous thromboembolism is associated with the use of oral contraceptives and hormone replacement therapy (HRT).[88–90] Randomized trials have shown a two- to threefold increased risk of venous thromboembolism in postmenopausal women treated with HRT.[88,89] Although the risk is highest in the first year of treatment, increased risk persists after the first year if treatment continues.[89] Furthermore, it is also clear that newer birth control pill formulations (so-called third generation pills) are associated with a greater risk of thromboembolism than older formulations.[88]

Oil embolism occurs to some extent in all properly conducted lymphangiography examinations. Only when patients have poor

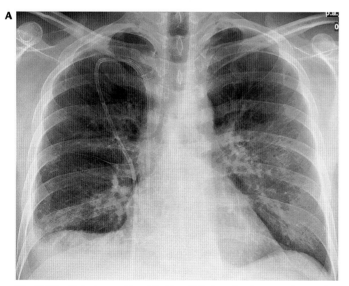

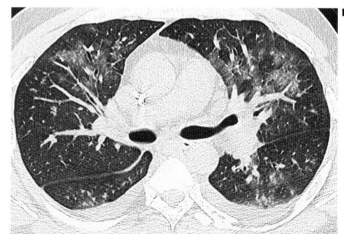

Fig. 9.19 Cytosine arabinoside (Ara-C) induced pulmonary hemorrhage. **A**, The frontal chest radiograph shows bilateral scattered heterogeneous opacities. **B**, HRCT shows scattered ground-glass opacities and small bilateral pleural effusions. Bronchoalveolar lavage was diagnostic for pulmonary hemorrhage.

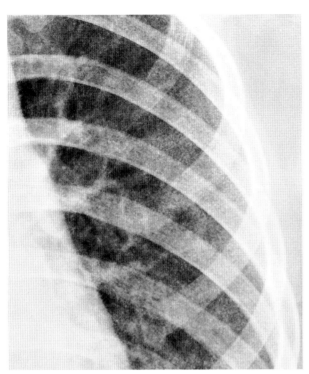

Fig. 9.20 Oil embolization after ethiodol lymphangiography. Coned down view of a chest radiograph taken 24 h after lymphography shows diffuse fine nodular opacities (miliary pattern).

pulmonary reserve or when excessive amounts of the contrast medium are administered is there any potential for harm. For this reason, patients with poor respiratory function should not undergo lymphangiography. Chest radiographs obtained 24–48 h after administration of the contrast medium may show a very fine nodular (miliary) pattern (Fig. 9.20). At the same time, the patient may experience mild fever and slight shortness of breath on exertion. These clinical and radiographic findings are usually transient.[91]

Drug induced obliterative bronchiolitis

Obliterative bronchiolitis (OB) is a process that results in permanent, fibrous occlusion of small airways. It is an important manifestation of chronic graft versus host disease in bone marrow transplant recipients and of chronic rejection in lung transplant recipients (see Ch. 6). OB can also be the result of toxic fume inhalation and is a rare manifestation of pulmonary drug toxicity. Penicillamine[92–94] and consumption of uncooked leaves of *Sauropus androgynus*[95] have been reported to cause OB. Radiologic findings of OB are more fully discussed in Chapter 12 and include pulmonary hyperinflation, mosaic attenuation on inspiratory HRCT, lobular air-trapping on expiratory CT, and bronchiectasis.[96–99]

Drug induced pulmonary calcification

Pulmonary calcification usually occurs in the setting of an abnormal calcium phosphorous product (typically >70 mg^2/dl^2). Alkaline environments favor calcium deposition; hence, the lung apices are more commonly affected than the bases. Calcium predominately deposits in alveolar and bronchial walls and in the walls of pulmonary vessels. When severe,

calcification can produce fibrosis or invoke a foreign body response. The most frequent cause of pulmonary parenchymal calcification is hyperparathyroidism. Pulmonary calcification can also occur after prolonged vitamin D and calcium therapy and in the milk alkali syndrome. Most patients with metastatic pulmonary calcification are asymptomatic, a minority has nonspecific respiratory complaints, and a few develop lethal respiratory distress. Chest radiographs are usually normal. When abnormal, bilateral confluent nodular opacities or consolidation is seen. The calcific nature of the opacities is often not evident on the chest radiograph. The radiographic pattern can be mistaken for pneumonia or pulmonary edema.

CT, especially HRCT, can detect pulmonary involvement when the chest radiograph is normal.[100] The most common findings of metastatic pulmonary calcification on HRCT are 3–10 mm diameter, poorly marginated, centrilobular nodules.[101–103] Many, though not all, nodules are of increased attenuation on CT or may be frankly calcified. Septal thickening and irregular linear opacities are uncommon. CT can also show calcification in chest wall vessels, a helpful adjunctive finding. Up to 60% of patients with chronic renal failure and a normal chest radiograph have pulmonary uptake on ^{99m}Tc bone scintigraphy,[104,105] a finding which is considered diagnostic of metastatic pulmonary calcification. Diagnosis can also be made at lung biopsy. There is a single case report of MRI of pulmonary calcification.[106] Unexpectedly, high signal intensity was noted on T1-weighted images. This was explained by more rapid relaxation of water protons on the surface of diamagnetic calcium crystals.

Drug induced pleural effusion and fibrosis

Drug induced pleural effusion usually occurs in the setting of the systemic lupus erythematosus syndrome.[107] Over 50% of patients with drug induced lupus develop pleural effusions at some stage of their illness. Effusions may also occur in the setting of hypersensitivity reactions to nitrofurantoin,[10,108,109] methotrexate,[110] and procarbazine.[111] These effusions usually resolve without sequelae. However, treatment with methysergide is associated with both pleural fluid and pleural fibrosis.[112] Irregular masses of pleural fibrosis may be interspersed with loculated pleural fluid and there may be associated mediastinal fibrosis. Ergotamine, ergonovine maleate, bromocriptine, amiodarone,[113] and pergolide can produce similar effects.[114,115]

Drug induced lymphadenopathy

A few drugs are known to cause hilar or mediastinal adenopathy, including phenytoin and methotrexate. Phenytoin can cause a pseudolymphoma syndrome with generalized adenopathy, fever, skin rashes, eosinophilia, and hepatosplenomegaly.[116] There is a slightly increased risk of lymphoma in patients taking this drug. Adenopathy in the setting of methotrexate therapy is frequently granulomatous in nature and may represent a form of drug induced sarcoidosis (see above).[78,79,117] Since methotrexate is used in the treatment of malignancy, the possibility of mistaking methotrexate induced adenopathy for metastatic disease is real.

Specific drugs and their adverse effects

Certain drugs are discussed here in further detail either because their adverse effects are relatively common or serious, or have noteworthy features.

Cytotoxic drugs

Drug induced lung injury affects up to 10% of patients receiving chemotherapy.[22,23,118,119] Cyclophosphamide, busulfan, BCNU, bleomycin, and methotrexate are the drugs that most commonly cause lung injury.

All-trans *retinoic acid*

All-*trans* retinoic acid induces maturation of leukemic cells in patients with acute promyelocytic leukemia. Between 15 and 25% of treated patients develop "retinoic acid syndrome".[120,121] This syndrome, which develops within 5–15 days of initiation of therapy, is characterized by fever, respiratory distress, anasarca, cardiac decompensation, and hypotension. The etiology is uncertain, but is probably related to lung tissue infiltration by maturing leukocytes that release vasoactive cytokines, causing increased capillary permeability. Retinoic acid syndrome is usually associated with a rise in the white blood cell count to >20,000 cells/mm^3 and its severity correlates with the peak white blood cell count.[121] It is potentially fatal, although prompt treatment with corticosteroids resolves symptoms.[121,122] Chest radiographs in affected patients usually show diffuse heterogeneous or homogeneous opacities and pleural effusions.[120,121]

Bacillus Calmette-Guerin

Intravesical bacillus Calmette-Guerin (BCG) therapy is used to treat superficial bladder cancer. Both early and late complications of BCG therapy have been reported.[123–127] Early complications generally occur within 3 months of instillation and are probably due to a hypersensitivity reaction.[128,129] Affected patients present with constitutional complaints, hepatitis,[130] diffuse pneumonitis, or pericarditis. Noncaseating granulomas are found on biopsy in most cases. Chest radiographs or CT may be normal or show either diffuse heterogeneous or fine nodular opacities (miliary pattern) (Fig. 9.21).[127,131–134] Treatment includes antituberculous drugs and, in cases where features of hypersensitivity predominate, corticosteroids.[125,135] Prognosis is generally good, although fatalities have been reported.[136–139] DAD is rarely reported as a complication of BCG therapy.[140] Late complications occur more than a year after BCG treatment. Disease usually manifests as focal mycobacterial infection of the genitourinary tract. Infection at other sites, such as the spine, kidneys, or retroperitoneal soft tissues, can also occur.[125]

Bleomycin (Box 9.8)

The cytotoxic antibiotic bleomycin is used to treat a variety of neoplasms, including squamous cell carcinoma, lymphoma, and testicular malignancies. It is concentrated in the lung, which is therefore a primary target for adverse effects. Toxicity is related to the cumulative dose. Risk of toxicity increases significantly when doses exceed a total of 400 IU.[141] The reported incidence of overt pulmonary toxicity varies from 4%[46] to 15%.[142] The risk and severity of pulmonary toxicity increases with age, prior or concomitant radiation therapy, concomitant treatment with other chemotherapeutic agents, oxygen therapy, decreased renal function, or bleomycin readministration within 6 months of discontinuation.[23,142] DAD is the most common histopathologic manifestation of bleomycin induced lung toxicity (see Fig. 9.3); IP and OP are less common manifestations.[118] An acute hypersensitivity reaction to low doses of bleomycin has also been reported.[23]

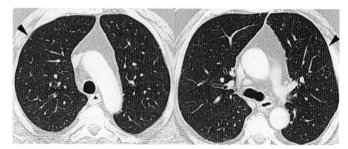

Fig. 9.21 An elderly man with fever and dyspnea after intravesical BCG therapy. The chest radiograph was normal. CT demonstrates peripheral multiple 2–3 mm nodules (arrowheads) in both lungs consistent with toxicity. (Courtesy of Jeremy Erasmus, MD, Houston, TX)

Box 9.8 Bleomycin induced lung injury

Commonly used for treatment of
Germ cell neoplasms
Kaposi sarcoma
Lymphoma
Squamous cell carcinoma

Toxicity
Risk increases with total dose >400 IU
Risk enhanced by O_2 therapy

Histopathology
Diffuse alveolar damage common
Interstitial and organizing pneumonia less common

Radiology
Early chest x-ray – basal reticulonodular opacities in costophrenic angles
Early CT – basal ground-glass opacities, subpleural linear opacities (prone imaging useful)
Late – progressive fibrosis, loss of lung volume
Uncommon – pulmonary nodules simulating metastases

Bleomycin toxicity can be quite serious, with mortality rates up to 25% reported. However, early detection may result in a substantial improvement in prognosis because mild injury may respond to discontinuation of bleomycin and corticosteroid administration.[2] The earlier the toxic effects are detected, the greater the likelihood of a favorable response to treatment. Hence, strict surveillance of patients under treatment with bleomycin, as with all patients undergoing chemotherapy, is imperative. Bleomycin toxicity ordinarily becomes apparent within 3 months of initiation of therapy and manifests clinically with progressive dyspnea and cough.[2] Reduction in DLco appears to be the most sensitive means for detecting early lung toxicity. However, reduction in DLco may occur in patients receiving bleomycin who never develop clinically apparent toxicity.[143] The chest radiograph is often normal in early toxicity despite a decreased DLco, abnormal lung accumulation of ^{67}Ga, ground-glass opacities on HRCT, or abnormal bronchoalveolar lavage fluid or lung biopsy findings.[144,145] It has thus been suggested that HRCT may be useful for evaluating patients with clinical findings of early pulmonary drug toxicity who have normal chest radiographs.[16,22,23,146] In this setting, new linear or ground-glass opacities in a basal and frequently subpleural distribution suggest the diagnosis (Fig. 9.22).

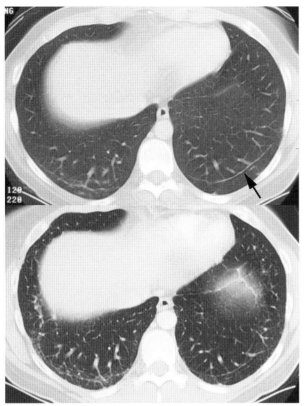

Fig. 9.22 Bleomycin toxicity in a man with a testicular malignancy who is asymptomatic but has a declining diffusing capacity for carbon monoxide (DLco). The chest radiograph is normal. CT (top frame) performed 3 months after starting bleomycin shows bilateral subpleural bandlike opacities (arrow). CT (bottom frame) performed 3 months later shows increasing subpleural opacities consistent with progressive toxicity. At this point, bleomycin therapy was stopped and the DLco normalized.

The earliest findings of bleomycin toxicity on chest radiographs are basal reticulonodular opacities (Figs 9.23 and 9.24). Balikian et al[147] noted that the earliest findings consistently appeared in the costophrenic sulci and subpleural regions of the lungs. These authors also noted a high incidence of associated pleural thickening in the costophrenic angles and in the interlobar fissures. Reduction of lung volumes, indicated by diaphragmatic elevation, is also a common manifestation of early bleomycin toxicity. Progressive toxicity may result in more homogeneous pulmonary opacities and lead to irreversible pulmonary fibrosis.

On occasion, discrete pulmonary nodules simulating metastases are seen on chest radiographs or CT.[148–150] These nodules are usually peripheral in location, 5 mm to 3.0 cm in diameter and either sharply or poorly marginated (Fig. 9.25).[23,146,148,150–154] In most cases, these lesions can be clinically differentiated from pulmonary metastases based upon appearance of the lesions (they usually have more ill defined margins than typical metastases), their relationship to bleomycin treatment, and the overall clinical scenario (lesions may appear while known tumor masses are decreasing in size). However, on occasion, confident differentiation of nodular bleomycin toxicity from metastases may require lung biopsy.

Acute hypersensitivity to bleomycin manifests with rapidly appearing scattered pulmonary opacities that mimic pulmonary

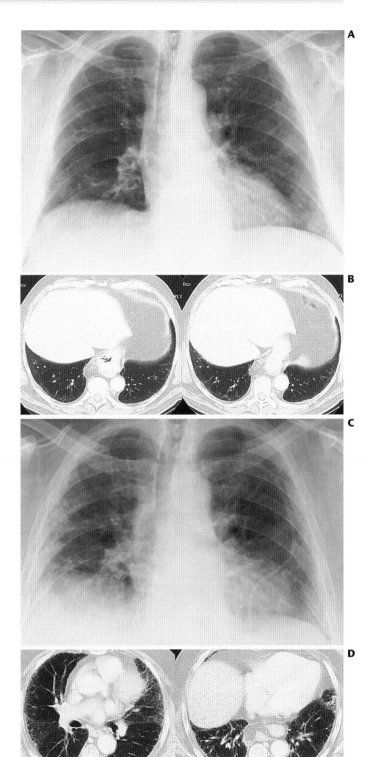

Fig. 9.23 Bleomycin toxicity in a man with a testicular germ cell malignancy. **A**, The frontal chest radiograph obtained 3 months after starting bleomycin is normal. **B**, CT performed at the same time demonstrates subtle subpleural ground-glass and reticular opacities. Although the patient was asymptomatic at this time, diffusing capacity for carbon monoxide (DLco) had diminished to 70% of predicted. Nevertheless, bleomycin therapy was continued. **C**, The radiograph obtained 9 months later shows progressive loss of lung volume and bibasilar coarse heterogeneous opacities, consistent with progressive fibrosis. **D**, CT now shows more advanced findings of bleomycin toxicity. (With permission from Rossi SE, Erasmus JJ, McAdams HP, Sporn TA, Goodman PC. Pulmonary drug toxicity: radiologic and pathologic manifestations. RadioGraphics 2000;20:1245–1259.)

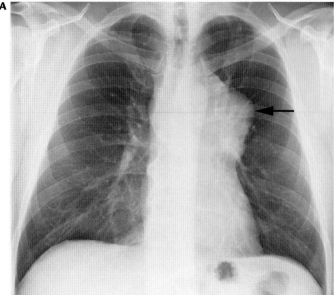

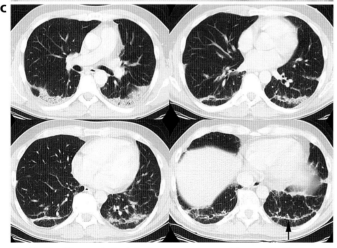

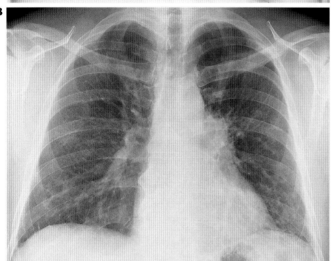

Fig. 9.24 Bleomycin toxicity in a young man with a mediastinal germ cell malignancy. **A**, The frontal chest radiograph demonstrates a large, lobulated anterior mediastinal mass (arrow). The lung parenchyma is normal. **B**, The radiograph obtained 4 months after starting bleomycin shows marked improvement in the mediastinal mass. Note, however, the new basilar heterogeneous opacities and loss of lung volume. **C**, CT shows bibasilar ground-glass opacities, thickened interlobular and intralobular septa, and subpleural bandlike opacities (arrow), consistent with bleomycin toxicity.

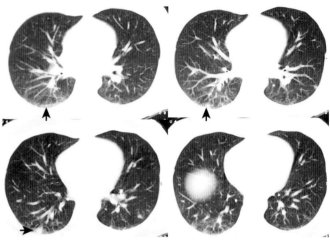

Fig. 9.25 Bleomycin toxicity in a young man with a germ cell malignancy who presented with cough, dyspnea, and decreased diffusing capacity for carbon monoxide (DLco). CT shows peripheral, poorly defined pulmonary nodules (arrowheads) that were not seen on prior CT scans. Transthoracic needle aspiration biopsy was negative for malignancy and the nodules resolved after cessation of bleomycin therapy. (With permission from Rossi SE, Erasmus JJ, McAdams HP, Sporn TA, Goodman PC. Pulmonary drug toxicity: radiologic and pathologic manifestations. RadioGraphics 2000;20:1245–1259.)

edema. These findings usually resolve quickly when therapy is discontinued.

Busulfan

Busulfan, one of the earliest chemotherapeutic agents, is still used for the treatment of chronic myelogenous leukemia.[155] The reported incidence of pulmonary toxicity ranges from 2 to 10% and typically occurs in patients who have received a total dose of >500 mg.[23,146,151] Lung injury can, however, occur at low doses if the patient has had prior cytotoxic therapy.[23,156] Evidence of pulmonary toxicity may be detected within months of starting treatment, but some patients do not show signs or symptoms of toxicity for several years. This variability makes the existence of a true dose/response relationship uncertain. DAD seems to be the most common histopathologic manifestation of busulfan induced lung disease (Fig. 9.26).[22,157,158] IP is less common and typically occurs only after prolonged administration of high doses of busulfan.[22,159]

Cyclophosphamide (Box 9.9)

Cyclophosphamide (Cytoxan) is an alkylating agent used to treat a wide range of malignancies as well as benign conditions such as glomerulonephritis and Wegener granulomatosis. DAD is the most commonly reported histopathologic manifestation of cyclophosphamide induced lung disease (Fig. 9.27, see also Fig. 9.4).[22,119,160,161] IP and OP are less common (Fig. 9.28).[22] Despite the widespread use of this drug, cyclophosphamide induced lung injury seems to be rare.[146] However, the fact that it is rarely used alone has made it difficult to gather data on its potential toxic side effects.

Careful analysis of a limited number of patients treated with cyclophosphamide alone suggests two distinct patterns of disease.[119] The first is an early onset pneumonitis that develops within 6 months of initiating therapy. Affected patients present with dyspnea, cough, and fever.[119] Chest radiographs

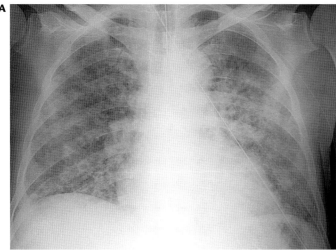

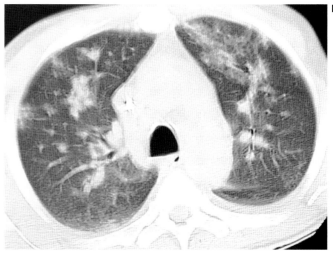

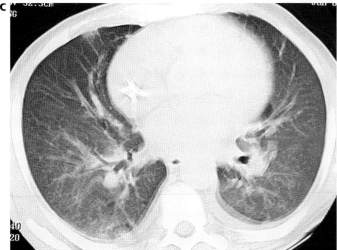

Fig. 9.26 Busulfan toxicity in a bone marrow transplant patient. **A**, The frontal chest radiograph shows bilateral heterogeneous pulmonary opacities. **B** and **C**, CT demonstrates scattered, almost nodular, areas of consolidation in the upper lobes and more diffuse ground-glass opacities in the lower lobes.

Box 9.9 Cyclophosphamide induced lung injury

Commonly used for treatment of
Nonmalignant conditions: nephrotic syndrome, interstitial pneumonia, collagen vascular diseases, Wegener granulomatosis
Malignancies: lymphoma, leukemia, breast and ovarian carcinoma

Toxicity
Occurs anytime from 2 weeks to 13 years after initiation of treatment
Not clearly related to dose or duration

Histopathology
Diffuse alveolar damage most common
Interstitial and organizing pneumonia less frequent

Radiology
Nonspecific
Basal reticulonodular opacities
Pleural thickening can be a prominent feature

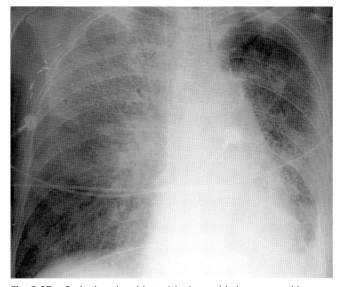

Fig. 9.27 Cyclophosphamide toxicity in an elderly woman with a breast malignancy. The frontal chest radiograph shows bilateral heterogeneous and homogeneous pulmonary opacities. Lung biopsy showed advanced diffuse alveolar damage and the patient eventually succumbed due to respiratory failure. (With permission from Rossi SE, Erasmus JJ, McAdams HP, Sporn TA, Goodman PC. Pulmonary drug toxicity: radiologic and pathologic manifestations. RadioGraphics 2000;20:1245–1259.)

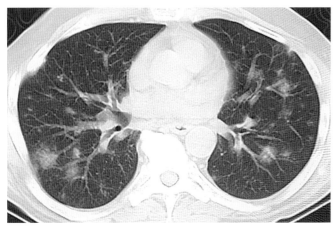

Fig. 9.28 Cyclophosphamide toxicity. CT shows scattered poorly defined nodular opacities. Lung biopsy showed organizing pneumonia that resolved following drug cessation and treatment with corticosteroids.

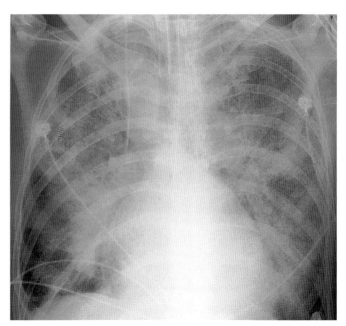

Fig. 9.29 Interleukin-2 (IL-2) toxicity in a young man with melanoma. The frontal chest radiograph obtained shortly after administration of IL-2 shows bilateral homogeneous opacities consistent with pulmonary edema. Radiographic findings rapidly resolved after cessation of drug therapy.

show nonspecific basilar reticular or reticulonodular opacities. This patient group responds well to discontinuation of cyclophosphamide therapy and corticosteroid administration. The second pattern of disease is a chronic pneumonitis that occurs several months or years after prolonged treatment with cyclophosphamide. Clinical onset is insidious with progressive dyspnea and cough.[119] This form of toxicity has a much poorer prognosis, usually does not respond to corticosteroid treatment, and can lead to end-stage fibrosis (Fig. 9.27).[119] Radiographic findings are nonspecific, but bilateral pleural thickening may be a prominent feature.[119]

Cytosine arabinoside

Cytosine arabinoside (Ara-C) is an antimetabolite that inhibits DNA synthesis. It is effective in the treatment of acute leukemia in adults but can cause serious side effects depending on the total dose used.[162] Andersson et al[162] reported a 22% incidence of subacute pulmonary toxicity occurring 2–21 days (median 6 days) after initiation of therapy. Toxicity primarily manifests as permeability pulmonary edema, although the precise mechanism of injury has not been established.[163–165] The radiographic findings are those of pulmonary edema and include diffuse bilateral heterogeneous opacities that progress to diffuse homogeneous opacification (see Fig. 9.11).[166] Small pleural effusions can be seen but are an insignificant feature. Following cessation of drug therapy and possible corticosteroid administration, chest radiographs may show clearing over a period of 1–3 weeks.

Interleukin-2

Interleukin-2 (IL-2) is used in the treatment of disseminated malignancies, notably renal cell carcinoma and malignant melanoma. IL-2 can cause a diffuse capillary leak syndrome due to toxic effects on the vascular endothelium.[167] Direct toxic effects on the myocardium[168] can also contribute to edema, but pulmonary capillary wedge pressure usually remains normal.[169] Consequent depletion of intravascular volume can result in a clinical state analogous to the toxic shock syndrome, with diminished peripheral vascular resistance, hypotension, severe tachycardia, and decreased cardiac output.

The reported incidence of IL-2 toxicity varies. Abnormalities are noted on chest radiographs in 50–80% of treated patients.[170–173] However, White et al[174] found that only 4% of almost 200 patients undergoing treatment with IL-2 had clinical or physiologic evidence of significant respiratory compromise. They also found that the pulmonary side effects, which included diffuse edema and hypoxia, reversed rapidly with cessation of therapy.

The onset of signs and symptoms of toxicity is usually closely related to the initiation of therapy. In the series of Saxon et al,[173] radiologic abnormalities developed within 4 days in 50% of patients, within 8 days in 75%, and beyond 8 days in only 25%. The radiologic findings are essentially those of diffuse pulmonary edema (Fig. 9.29). Saxon et al[173] described focal lobar or segmental consolidation in about one-quarter of their patients but attributed these findings to nosocomial infection rather than IL-2 toxicity, an association also noted by Snydman et al.[175] Pleural effusions occur in >50% of treated patients. The signs and symptoms of IL-2 toxicity usually resolve completely within 2 weeks of cessation of therapy.[176] Although the incidence of toxicity may be high, deaths attributable solely to IL-2 therapy are rare.

Methotrexate (Box 9.10)

Methotrexate, a folic acid analog, is used extensively in the treatment of hematologic and other malignancies, and also a number of benign conditions, such as rheumatoid arthritis and psoriasis. According to the most reliable estimate, pulmonary toxicity occurs in 7% of treated patients[177] and is not related to duration of therapy or total cumulative dose.[23] The incidence of toxicity depends upon the condition being treated. Patients with acute lymphocytic leukemia have a higher incidence of toxicity than patients with trophoblastic tumors or osteogenic sarcoma.[178] A 14% incidence of toxicity has been reported in

Box 9.10 Methotrexate induced lung injury

Commonly used for treatment of
Nonmalignant conditions: collagen vascular disease,
   interstitial pneumonia
Malignancies: lymphoma, leukemia, and breast carcinoma

Toxicity
Uncommon
Idiosyncratic
Not clearly related to dose or duration

Histopathology
Interstitial pneumonia most common
Organizing pneumonia, diffuse alveolar damage less
   common
Acute hypersensitivity is a rare manifestation

Radiology
Variable, nonspecific
Basal reticulonodular opacities

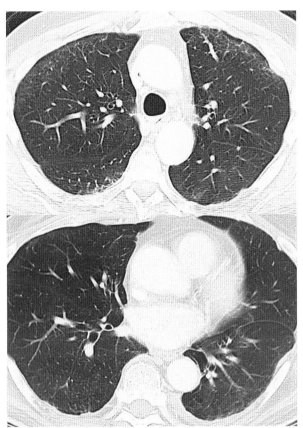

Fig. 9.30 Methotrexate toxicity in an elderly man with leukemia. CT shows subpleural ground-glass and subtle reticular opacities consistent with early methotrexate toxicity.

patients with primary biliary cirrhosis.[179] However, patients treated with low dose methotrexate for rheumatoid arthritis seem to have a much lower, if nonexistent, incidence of pulmonary toxicity.[180]

The histopathologic, clinical, and radiologic manifestations of methotrexate toxicity are variable. IP is the most common histopathologic manifestation (Figs 9.30 and 9.31); OP and DAD are less common.[181,182] Fibrosis occurs in up to 10% of patients with methotrexate induced pulmonary toxicity. A hypersensitivity response accompanied by pulmonary opacities and peripheral eosinophilia is also fairly common. Affected patients typically present with subacute symptoms of fever, malaise,

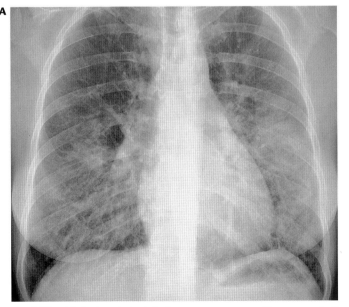

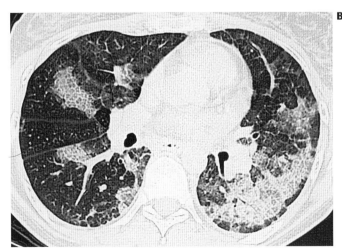

Fig. 9.31 Methotrexate toxicity in a young woman with severe arthritis who presented with dyspnea. **A**, The frontal chest radiograph shows bilateral, predominantly lower lobe, heterogeneous pulmonary opacities. Note the preservation of lung volumes. **B**, CT shows scattered ground-glass opacities with superimposed septal thickening ("crazy paving" appearance). Symptoms and radiologic findings resolved after cessation of drug therapy and treatment with corticosteroids. (With permission from Rossi SE, Erasmus JJ, McAdams HP, Sporn TA, Goodman PC. Pulmonary drug toxicity: radiologic and pathologic manifestations. RadioGraphics 2000;20:1245–1259)

cough, and dyspnea. A skin eruption is frequently seen. The hypersensitivity response occurs within weeks of starting therapy and can usually be successfully treated with high dose corticosteroid therapy.[182] The pulmonary opacities are usually bilateral and reticulonodular in character. Occasionally, more localized airspace opacities are seen, sometimes with a nodular or masslike appearance. Hilar and mediastinal adenopathy may also occur in the setting of a hypersensitivity reaction to methotrexate. Pleural effusions can occur in association with manifestations of lung injury due to development of acute pleuritis associated with high dose therapy.[143,164,183,184] Intrathecal administration of methotrexate has also been associated with pulmonary edema.[185]

The prognosis of methotrexate induced lung injury is generally favorable, with an overall mortality of approximately 10%. This represents <1% of all patients receiving methotrexate therapy. Corticosteroids may help in cases of hypersensitivity reactions. In some cases, toxicity resolves despite continued use of the drug, and in others readministration does not cause a recurrence of toxic manifestations.

Mitomycin

Mitomycin is a cytotoxic antibiotic derived from a species of *Streptomyces*. It acts by inhibiting DNA synthesis and is used in the treatment of gastrointestinal, gynecologic, and breast malignancies. Toxic side effects are dose related and generally occur at cumulative dose levels of 30 mg/m^2 or above. The overall incidence of toxicity is <10% when mitomycin is used alone.[186] The incidence increases to >35% when mitomycin is used in combination with the vinca alkaloids vinblastine and vindesine.[143,164,187] This is noteworthy because the vinca alkaloids do not cause pulmonary toxicity when used alone. Mitomycin toxicity primarily manifests as IP that can lead to fibrosis if the drug is not discontinued. However, the prognosis is relatively good with a mortality of <10%.[143]

Microangiopathic hemolytic anemia with renal failure, thrombocytopenia, and pulmonary edema is a less common, and possibly unique, form of drug toxicity associated with mitomycin therapy.[188–190] This form of hemolytic uremic syndrome occurs in <5% of treated patients, but has a very high mortality.[190] Onset of symptoms is frequently delayed, occurring many months after initiation of treatment, often when the patient is in remission.

Acute bronchospasm is a second rare and idiosyncratic effect of mitomycin therapy that only occurs when the drug is used with the vinca alkaloids. The reaction is immediate and recurs upon readministration of the drug. Affected patients usually recover with supportive therapy but there are reports of progression to severe respiratory failure.[164]

Nitrosoureas (Box 9.11)

The nitrosoureas (BCNU, CCNU) are used in the treatment of cerebral glioma, lymphoma, and melanoma. There is a direct relationship between cumulative dose and lung injury with the incidence of toxicity increasing to 50% if the cumulative dose is >1500 mg/m^2.[23,191] In the series of Weinstein et al,[192] no patient receiving a total dose of <900 mg/m^2 developed pulmonary toxicity. The risk of toxicity with total doses of 1400–1900 mg/m^2 was 3–11 times that of patients receiving 900 mg/m^2.[192] Lung injury can, however, occur at lower doses if the patient has had prior thoracic radiation. Other risk factors include preexisting pulmonary disease, smoking, or combination therapy with other cytotoxic agents. Age at the time of treatment is also a risk

---

Box 9.11 BCNU induced lung injury

Commonly used for treatment of
CNS malignancies (gliomas)
Myeloablative therapy prior to bone marrow transplantation

Toxicity
Risk increases when total dose >900 mg/m^2
Risk enhanced by prior thoracic radiation or preexisting lung disease

Histopathology
Diffuse alveolar damage most common
Interstitial pneumonia less common

Radiology
Chest radiography
- Initially normal
- Progression to basal heterogeneous opacities
Thin-section CT
- Scattered or diffuse ground-glass opacities

---

factor: children under 7 years of age are more likely to develop pulmonary toxicity than adults.[193] Pulmonary toxicity due to nitrosourea therapy is quite serious with mortality between 30 and 40%.[143] DAD is the most common histopathologic manifestation of nitrosourea induced lung disease; IP is less common.[30,194] Affected patients present with dry cough and dyspnea. DLco may decline prior to onset of symptoms and radiographic findings. Chest radiographs may be normal initially, but HRCT may show scattered or diffuse ground-glass opacities (see Fig. 9.2). With progression, chest radiographs show predominantly basal heterogeneous opacities that may progress to fibrosis (Fig. 9.32, see also Fig. 9.5). In some individuals, particularly those treated in childhood, an apical predominance has been described.[195,196] These patients also seem to have a high incidence of spontaneous pneumothorax.[197]

Because BCNU treatment can effectively cure some central nervous system tumors in children, unusually prolonged follow up after treatment with this agent is feasible. O'Driscoll et al[198] and Taylor et al[199] evaluated 30 adolescents aged 13–17 years after treatment of central nervous system tumors. They reported six delayed deaths from pulmonary fibrosis in their study group. These patients had fibrosis in a mainly upper zone and peripheral distribution.

New agents

New cytotoxic agents are brought on the market every year. Among the most promising of the last few years are the taxoid derivatives paclitaxel[11] and docetaxel,[200–202] fludarabine,[203] gemcitabine,[200,201,204,205] vinorelbine,[206] gefitinib,[207] topotecan, and etoposide.[208] These agents can effectively treat a variety of malignancies, such as breast, lung, and ovarian carcinoma. Preliminary experience indicates that many, if not all, of these agents can also cause lung injury.[209,210] The precise incidence of toxicity with these agents, and spectrum of histopathologic, clinical, and radiologic features of toxicity, are not well understood as many are given in combination with multiple other agents as well as radiation therapy.

Inoue et al[207] reported four patients with severe lung toxicity due to gefitinib, an inhibitor of the epidermal growth factor

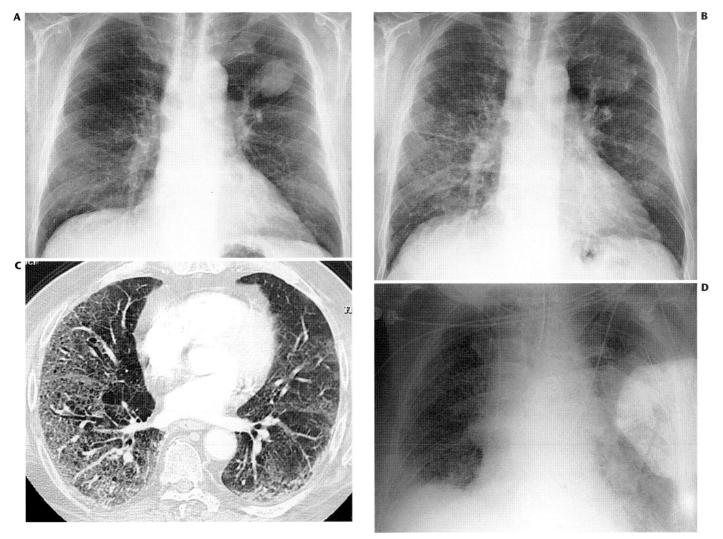

Fig. 9.32 BCNU toxicity in a patient with metastatic melanoma (same patient as in Fig. 9.5). **A**, The frontal chest radiograph obtained prior to treatment shows a large left upper lobe mass and normal lungs. **B**, The radiograph obtained 6 months after starting BCNU shows bilateral heterogeneous opacities. The mass has enlarged. **C**, CT obtained at the same time shows diffuse ground-glass and coarse reticular opacities and architectural distortion in the right lung. **D**, The radiograph obtained 3 months later shows progression to diffuse pulmonary opacification. The patient eventually succumbed due to respiratory failure.

receptor tyrosine kinase. In this small series, all affected patients developed diffuse ground-glass opacities suggestive of DAD. Half of the patients recovered following administration of corticosteroids and half died from progressive respiratory insufficiency.

Gemcitabine, a nucleoside analog used to treat solid tumors such as nonsmall cell lung and breast cancer, appears to cause lung toxicity (Fig. 9.33). Because it is usually given in combination with other agents, the precise incidence of toxicity is difficult to determine. Although dyspnea is reported in up to 8% of recipients,[204] the best estimates suggest that serious toxicity is rare, affecting perhaps no more than 0.45% of treated individuals.[205] Numerous cases of fatal pneumonitis (presumably DAD) caused by gemcitabine, either given alone[204,211] or in combination with other agents (docetaxol,[200,201] pacitaxel,[212] or vinorelbine[212]), have been reported.

The taxol derivatives, paclitaxel, docetaxol, and carbtaxol (Fig. 9.34) have also been implicated as potential causes of lung toxicity. Again, because these drugs are frequently given in combination with other agents, the precise incidence of toxicity is

difficult to determine. Dimopoulou et al[11] studied 33 patients receiving paclitaxel and carboplatin and found significant declines in DLco; none of the patients developed respiratory symptoms or radiologic evidence of toxicity. Read et al[202] reported four patients who developed severe IP due to docetaxol; half of the patients died from progressive respiratory insufficiency. Severe toxicity when used in combination with gemcitabine has also been reported.[200,201]

Noncytotoxic drugs

Amiodarone (Box 9.12)

Amiodarone, an iodinated benzofuran derivative, is used to treat a variety of cardiac rhythm disturbances. It contains 37% iodine by weight, is concentrated in the lung and liver, and has a relatively long tissue half life. This may account for the relatively delayed appearance of pulmonary toxic effects after commencement of therapy (median 6 months) and slow resolution after cessation (median 3 months).[213] Furthermore, the latent period between beginning drug therapy and onset of

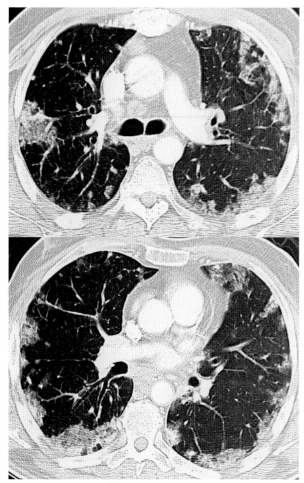

Fig. 9.33 Gemcitabine toxicity in a man with pancreatic cancer. CT shows bilateral, predominantly subpleural foci of ground-glass opacity and consolidation. The CT pattern is suggestive of organizing pneumonia. These findings resolved after cessation of drug therapy and treatment with corticosteroids.

Box 9.12 Amiodarone induced lung injury

Commonly used for treatment of
Ventricular arrhythmias
Atrial arrhythmias (increasingly used)

Toxicity
Risk increases with dose >400 mg/day
Toxicity does occur at lower doses (200 mg/day)

Histopathology
Interstitial pneumonia, diffuse alveolar damage most common
Organizing pneumonia less common
"Foamy" macrophages suggest exposure to drug, not necessarily toxicity

Radiology
Usually nonspecific, but may be consolidation resembling pulmonary edema
High-attenuation pleural or parenchymal opacities suggestive
Increased liver, spleen attenuation indicates exposure
Occasional pleural effusion or thickening

---

signs and symptoms of toxicity is variable, and may be quite prolonged. Toxicity from amiodarone appears to be dose related.[12,29,214] The incidence of amiodarone toxicity ranges from 5 to 10% in patients treated with high doses (>400 mg daily) and is approximately 2% in patients treated with low doses (400 mg or less daily). The risk of lung injury is also increased in elderly patients[12] and in patients receiving high levels of inspired oxygen during and after surgery.[20,215] For example, patients treated preoperatively with amiodarone have an increased risk of acute respiratory distress syndrome after cardiac surgery.[216]

IP is the most common histopathologic manifestation of amiodarone induced lung disease; DAD and OP are less common (see Fig. 9.7).[31,217] Amiodarone toxicity is somewhat unusual in that a specific histopathologic finding (intraalveolar accumulation of macrophages with foamy cytoplasm) is considered characteristic. However, such macrophages can be

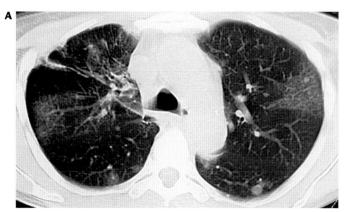

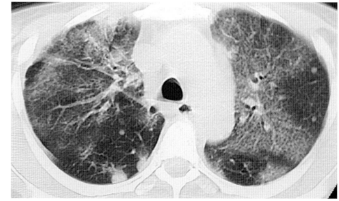

Fig. 9.34 Carbotaxol toxicity in a young woman with a breast malignancy. **A**, CT obtained several months after starting treatment shows bilateral ground-glass opacities. **B**, CT obtained several months later shows progressive ground-glass opacity, increasing reticulation and architectural distortion, particularly in the right upper lobe, suggestive of fibrosis. Note also the evidence of progressive metastatic disease.

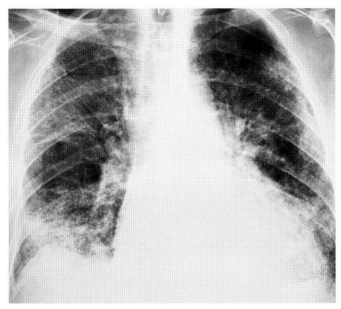

Fig. 9.35 Amiodarone toxicity. The chest radiograph shows bilateral coarse reticular opacities in a peripheral and basal distribution.

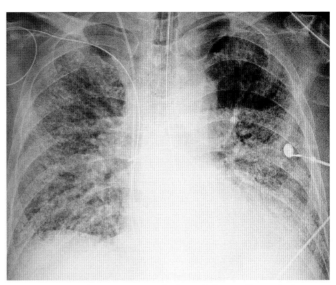

Fig. 9.37 Amiodarone toxicity. The frontal chest radiograph shows diffuse heterogeneous pulmonary opacities, likely due to advanced diffuse alveolar damage.

also found in asymptomatic patients receiving amiodarone who have no clinical or radiologic evidence of disease. Thus, this "characteristic" histopathologic finding may indicate nothing more than exposure to the drug.

The most common presenting complaint of amiodarone toxicity is dyspnea. Less common complaints include pleuritic chest pain, cough, fever, and weight loss.[218] DLco is usually reduced.[214] As is the case with many drugs, chest radiographs

may be normal in some patients with early signs or symptoms of amiodarone toxicity. In this setting, HRCT can be useful for showing findings of early lung injury.[219]

The chest radiographic findings of more advanced amiodarone toxicity are quite variable. Chest radiographs of affected patients frequently show multiple peripheral areas of consolidation – findings that resemble those seen in patients with hypersensitivity reactions (Figs 9.35 and 9.36). However, there is usually no evidence of either blood or tissue eosinophilia. Less commonly, amiodarone toxicity manifests with diffuse heterogeneous opacities (Figs 9.37 and 9.38), focal or multifocal homogeneous opacities (Fig. 9.39), or scattered nodular opacities on chest radiographs. Pleural effusions can occur in association with manifestations of lung injury due to the development of pleural inflammation (Fig. 9.40).[220]

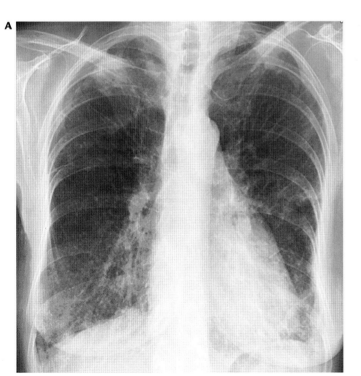

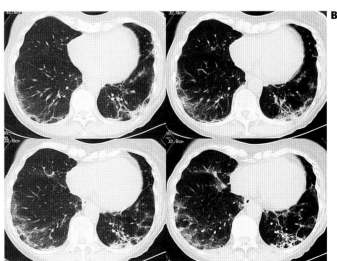

Fig. 9.36 Amiodarone toxicity in an elderly woman with a ventricular arrhythmia. **A,** The frontal chest radiograph demonstrates bilateral, predominantly peripheral and subpleural, heterogeneous opacities. Note the preservation of lung volumes. **B,** CT shows subpleural ground-glass and irregular linear opacities, and occasional subpleural bands.

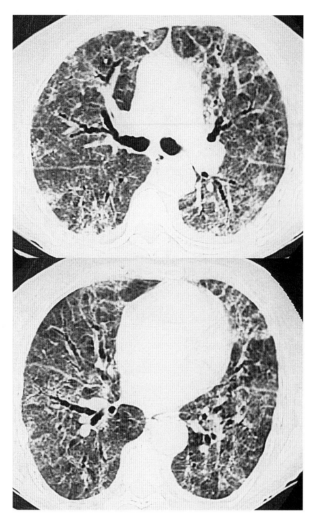

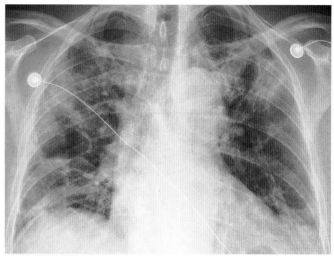

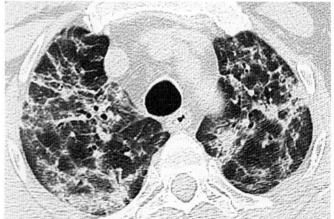

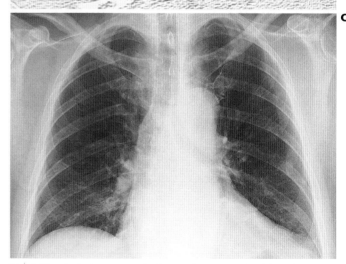

Fig. 9.38 Amiodarone toxicity. CT shows bilateral ground-glass and coarse reticular opacities and traction bronchiectasis, consistent with fibrosis. Lung biopsy showed advanced diffuse alveolar damage. (Courtesy of Santiago Rossi, MD, Buenos Aires, Argentina)

Because patients treated with amiodarone usually have significant cardiac disease, the clinical and radiographic findings of amiodarone toxicity can be difficult to distinguish from those of heart failure. Lack of response to treatment for heart failure and lack of shortterm fluctuations in pulmonary opacities suggests amiodarone toxicity. Since amiodarone contains iodine by weight and is concentrated in the liver and lung, CT attenuation of these tissues may be consequently increased in patients receiving the drug.[19,221] As is the case with finding foamy macrophages on histopathologic specimens, increased attenuation on CT is more likely a marker of drug exposure than toxicity. Nevertheless, the finding of high-attenuation pleural or parenchymal lesions and increased liver attenuation on CT suggests the diagnosis of amiodarone toxicity *in the appropriate clinical setting* (Fig. 9.40).[19,21]

Amiodarone toxicity is potentially fatal if untreated, but may be reversible if diagnosed and treated early.[222] Stringent monitoring of patients receiving amiodarone therapy is therefore essential. Sunderji et al[222] recommend that baseline chest radiographs and pulmonary function tests should be obtained prior to institution of amiodarone therapy. They further recommend that follow-up radiographs at 3–6 month intervals

Fig. 9.39 Amiodarone toxicity in a patient treated with low dose therapy for an atrial arrhythmia who presents with fever and dyspnea. **A,** The frontal chest radiograph shows bilateral heterogeneous and homogeneous pulmonary opacities and loss of lung volume. **B,** CT shows bilateral diffuse ground-glass and coarse reticular opacities and possible bronchiectasis. Lung biopsy showed both organizing and interstitial pneumonia. **C,** The radiologic abnormalities resolved after cessation of drug therapy and administration of corticosteroids.

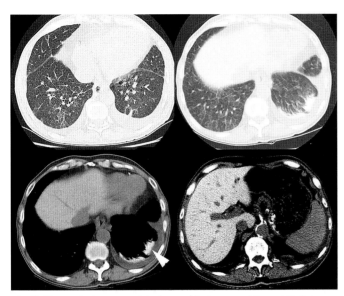

Fig. 9.40 Amiodarone toxicity in an elderly man with ventricular arrhythmia who presented with mild, progressive dyspnea. CT (top left) shows subtle ground-glass opacity, septal thickening, and small bilateral pleural effusions. CT (upper right and bottom left) shows a high-attenuation parenchymal opacity (arrowhead) in the left lower lobe adjacent to the pleural fluid. CT (bottom right) shows that the liver is of high attenuation consistent with amiodarone exposure.

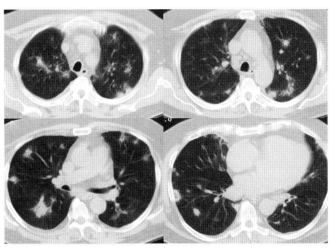

Fig. 9.41 Amiodarone toxicity in a patient treated with low dose therapy for an atrial arrhythmia who presents with fever and dyspnea. CT shows scattered, poorly defined nodules, a pattern suggestive of organizing pneumonia. Symptoms and CT findings resolved after cessation of drug therapy and administration of corticosteroids.

be obtained, but suggest that repeat lung function testing or CT should be reserved for patients who develop new symptoms or radiographic abnormalities.

Recently, low dose amiodarone (<400 mg daily) has gained popularity for treating refractory atrial arrhythmias, including atrial fibrillation.[223] Although the incidence of toxicity in these patients is significantly less than that of patients receiving higher doses, it is not insignificant (Figs 9.39 and 9.41).[217,218,222–225] Because these patients are on low dose therapy, however, the association between symptoms, radiologic abnormalities and amiodarone may be overlooked. Ott et al[224] reported eight patients on low dose therapy who developed signs and symptoms of toxicity. Seven responded to cessation of therapy and administration of corticosteroids, but one died of progressive respiratory failure.

Bromocriptine

Bromocriptine, an ergot alkaloid derivative, is an extremely effective and valuable treatment for Parkinson disease and prolactinemia. Its chemical structure is similar to that of methysergide, which may account for the fact that pleural effusions and pleural fibrosis occur in a small minority of patients receiving bromocriptine. Less than 5% of treated patients are affected and all reported patients have been men.[226,227] Adverse effects appear to be confined to the pleura and adjacent lung. Symptoms and radiographic signs of effusion and pleural fibrosis usually take months or years to evolve. Slow resolution occurs after cessation of treatment, although it appears that the situation will stabilize if continuation of treatment is necessary.

Deferoxamine

Deferoxamine is a chelating agent used to treat systemic overload of metals, such as iron and aluminum, particularly in patients

undergoing dialysis. Many microbes require free iron for growth. Normally, the amount of free iron available *in vivo* is quite low. Some organisms have mechanisms such as siderophores that enable them to compete for iron in the host. Siderophores trap iron and deliver it to the microorganism, enhancing its growth and virulence.[228] Because deferoxamine acts as a siderophore, it can enhance the growth of certain microorganisms. Thus, patients receiving deferoxamine therapy are at increased risk for infection with organisms such as *Yersinia enterocolitica* and mucormycosis. Dialysis patients who receive deferoxamine therapy seem to be at particular risk for mucormycosis.[229]

Diphenylhydantoin

The hydantoin derivatives such as diphenylhydantoin (Dilantin) are effective and widely prescribed antiseizure medications. Dilantin can cause diverse adverse reactions, including gingival hyperplasia, hyperostosis, rashes, and lymphadenopathy.[230–233] The most common site of adenopathy is in the cervical region but other nodal groups, including the hilar and mediastinal nodes, may be involved (Fig. 9.42). Clinically, Dilantin-induced lymphadenopathy has features of a hypersensitivity reaction. Affected patients typically present with maculopapular rash, hepatosplenomegaly, eosinophilia, and lymphadenopathy.[231,232] The time of onset varies from 1 week to 30 years (median 5 years) after institution of therapy.[116] Biopsy of affected lymph nodes in these patients may show a spectrum of histopathologic patterns from reactive hyperplasia to immunoblastic hyperplasia. Progression to frank lymphoma, either Hodgkin or non-Hodgkin, is rare.

Fenfluramines

A group of anorectic drugs, including fenfluramine and dexfenfluramine and possibly phentermine, have been shown to cause pulmonary arterial hypertension and valvular heart disease.[234,235] In patients taking these drugs for prolonged periods, the risk of pulmonary arterial hypertension is estimated to be 30 times that of the general population.[84] Not unexpectedly, these patients tend to be young women who are thereby

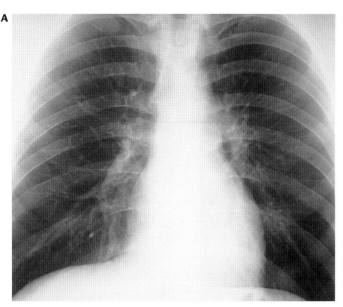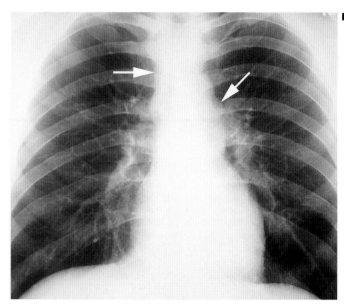

Fig. 9.42 Dilantin (diphenylhydantoin) toxicity. **A**, The frontal chest radiograph obtained prior to starting therapy is normal. **B**, The radiograph obtained after several years of treatment shows new mediastinal lymphadenopathy (arrows).

exposed to the risk of a potentially fatal disorder. Furthermore, these drugs have been shown to damage heart valves leading to valve incompetence. Valve injury is probably related to abnormal serotonin metabolism – a mechanism similar to that of the malignant carcinoid syndrome. However, unlike the malignant carcinoid syndrome, both right and left sided valves can be damaged. Some patients have required valve replacement or repair.[87]

Gold salts

Gold salts used in the treatment of rheumatoid arthritis probably cause pulmonary toxicity in about 1% of patients.[29,143,236] Pulmonary toxicity is overshadowed by the far more frequent complications of stomatitis and dermatitis. Pulmonary toxicity occurs within 3 months of beginning of therapy and usually develops subacutely. The most common reaction is a hypersensitivity response. Chest radiographs show scattered or diffuse reticulonodular or more homogeneous pulmonary opacities (Fig. 9.43).[236–238] Patients may show evidence of a hypersensitivity reaction in other organ systems, with fever, proteinuria, or a skin rash. Such manifestations of hypersensitivity may precede the pulmonary abnormalities and be associated with peripheral eosinophilia. DAD leading to fibrosis is also reported, but is much less common. Lupus caused by gold salts is quite rare. The major differential diagnostic problem is that the underlying disease, rheumatoid arthritis, can also cause lung disease. However, pulmonary opacities due to gold salts resolve in most instances after cessation of therapy, particularly if corticosteroids are administered. Pulmonary disease related to gold therapy also tends to be more acute in onset, whereas pulmonary involvement in rheumatoid arthritis is more insidious in onset and tends to be progressive.

Hydrochlorothiazide

Adverse reactions to the widely used diuretic hydrochlorothiazide are extremely rare. Nevertheless, the acute onset of a form of pulmonary edema within hours of taking the drug is well described.[239] Because hydrochlorothiazide is typically used

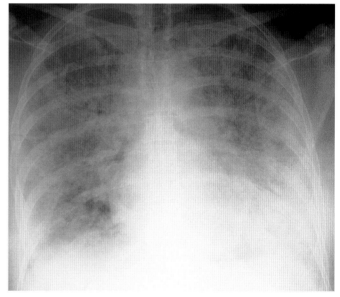

Fig. 9.43 Gold toxicity in a patient with rheumatoid arthritis. The frontal chest radiograph obtained shortly after starting therapy shows bilateral homogenous pulmonary opacities consistent with pulmonary edema. These findings resolved after cessation of drug therapy.

to treat hypertension and heart disease, which can also cause pulmonary edema, the presence of this adverse drug reaction may not be recognized until readministration elicits the same reaction.

Methysergide

Methysergide, an ergot alkaloid, can cause chronic pleuritis that results in chronic pleural effusion, irregular pleural thickening,[112] and, in some cases, rounded atelectasis. These manifestations develop between 6 months and several years after therapy begins. Affected patients typically complain of chest pain and dyspnea, depending on the extent of lung entrapment. Depending on the extent of the pleural fibrosis, a variable degree of regression occurs after cessation of therapy. Improvement, though slow, may be remarkable in many cases.[240] Endomyocardial, mediastinal, and retroperitoneal fibrosis can also occur with methysergide therapy.[241] Ergotamine tartrate, another ergot derivative, used in the treatment of migraine headaches, can also cause pleural effusion and fibrosis.[242]

Narcotics (Box 9.13)

Overdoses of heroin, methadone, and propoxyphene are well known causes of pulmonary edema. Edema develops in as many as one-third of individuals with signs of opiate overdose.[243] The

exact mechanism of pulmonary injury has not been elucidated, but possibilities include direct effects on the central nervous system leading to neurogenic edema, hypoxemic or direct drug toxic effects on the alveolar/capillary membrane, allergic responses, and immunologic activation. The radiographic findings are the same as those seen with pulmonary edema from any other cause (Fig. 9.44).

Because intravenous drug abusers are often careless about antiseptic precautions, septic cardiopulmonary complications may be encountered.[64,65,244,245] These include endocarditis, particularly involving the tricuspid valve, septic pulmonary emboli (Figs 9.45 and 9.46), and mycotic aneurysms (Fig. 9.47).

Box 9.13 Thoracic complications of intravenous drug abuse

Noninfectious pulmonary
Pulmonary edema (especially narcotics)
Hypersensitivity pneumonitis (particularly inhaled "crack")
Pulmonary hemorrhage (particularly inhaled "crack")
Pulmonary granulomatosis (see Box 9.7)

Infection
Thrombophlebitis
Septic emboli
Tricuspid valve endocarditis
Mycotic pulmonary artery aneurysms
Osteomyelitis
Septic arthritis
Aspiration pneumonia

Cardiac (particularly cocaine)
Arrhythmias
Myocarditis
Endocarditis
Cardiomyopathy

Pneumothorax
Pneumomediastinum

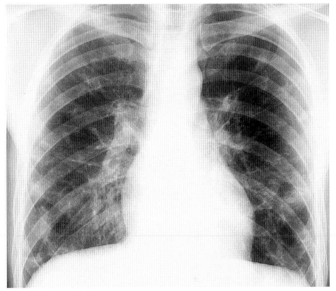

Fig. 9.45 Septic pulmonary emboli in an intravenous drug abuser. The frontal chest radiograph demonstrates bilateral, predominantly peripheral, pulmonary nodules consistent with septic emboli. Echocardiography (not shown) confirmed right sided endocarditis and blood cultures showed *Staphylococcus aureus* infection.

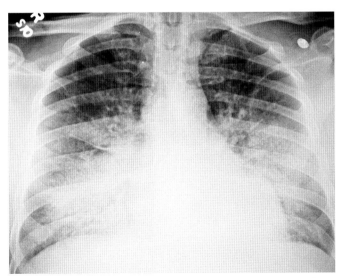

Fig. 9.44 Pulmonary edema due to intravenous administration of cocaine. The frontal chest radiograph shows bilateral homogeneous opacities consistent with edema. The patient recovered promptly with only supportive care.

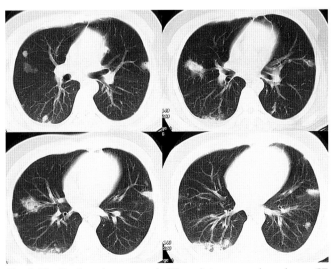

Fig. 9.46 Septic pulmonary emboli in an intravenous drug abuser. CT shows bilateral, predominantly subpleural, pulmonary nodules, some with central cavitation. Echocardiography (not shown) confirmed right sided endocarditis and blood cultures showed *Staphylococcus aureus* infection.

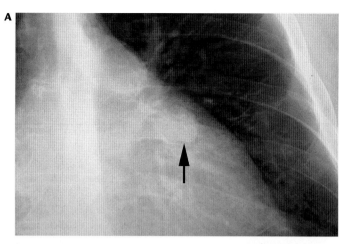

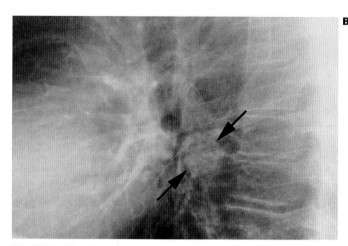

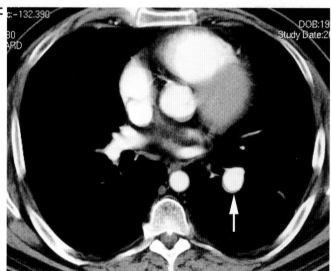

Fig. 9.47 Mycotic pulmonary artery aneurysm in an intravenous drug abuser with right sided endocarditis. **A,** The coned down views of frontal and **B,** lateral chest radiographs demonstrate a well defined mass in the left hilum (arrows). **C,** Contrast-enhanced CT confirms that the mass is due to a aneurysm (arrow) of the left lower lobe pulmonary artery.

Addicts may resort to direct injection into the subclavian or jugular veins as peripheral veins become sclerosed, which may result in mediastinal hematoma or mycotic or traumatic pseudoaneurysms. Other problems encountered include bronchopneumonia after aspiration during drug induced stupor and hematogenous spread of infection to the musculoskeletal system. Thus, septic arthritis involving sternoclavicular joints or osteomyelitis of the thoracic spine may result.

Cocaine hydrochloride, the acidic form of the drug, has been used in the Western world as a recreational drug for decades. In this form, the drug is either insufflated intranasally or injected intravenously. Cocaine is known to induce a range of cardiac problems, including arrhythmias, myocarditis, endocarditis, and cardiomyopathy.[246–254] The alkaloid form of cocaine, "crack", is highly addictive, is smoked and produces a rapid, intense, but short lived effect. Apart from the central toxic effects common to illicit drugs, there are specific toxic effects of inhaled crack cocaine. Pneumothorax and pneumomediastinum may occur, possibly as a result of explosive coughing and straining.[255–259] Focal airspace disease and atelectasis may be seen, which may be related to distal airway damage or to a hypersensitivity reaction.[260] Pulmonary hemorrhage has been described, and hemoptysis is a relatively common symptom.[251] Pulmonary edema is well described in crack addicts (Fig. 9.48), although the overall incidence is probably much lower than in intravenous cocaine abusers (see Fig. 10.19).[254,255]

Nitrofurantoin (Box 9.14)

Nitrofurantoin has been widely used in the treatment of urinary tract infections. Over 80% of cases of nitrofurantoin induced pulmonary toxicity occur in women, largely because of their higher incidence of urinary tract infection.[261] The incidence of adverse reactions is probably not high; the large number of reported cases reflects the extensive use of the drug.

Two distinct patterns of toxicity are noted: an acute and a chronic form. The acute form is likely a hypersensitivity reaction, is far more common, and accounts for about 90% of reactions to

Box 9.14 Nitrofurantoin induced lung injury
Commonly used for treatment of Chronic urinary tract infection
Toxicity Uncommon
Histopathology Interstitial pneumonia most common Diffuse alveolar damage and organizing pneumonia less common
Acute toxicity (<6 months) Fever, chest pain, dyspnea Peripheral eosinophilia common Basal opacities may progress to diffuse edema pattern Rapid improvement with drug cessation
Chronic (>6 months) Insidious onset dyspnea Basal reticulonodular opacities Can progress to fibrosis

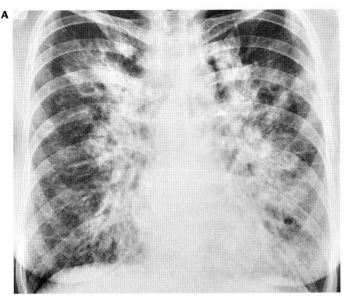

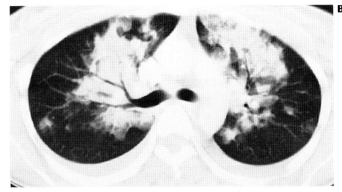

Fig. 9.48 "Crack lung" in a young female with severe dyspnea after smoking crack. **A**, The frontal chest radiograph shows perihilar heterogeneous and homogeneous opacities. **B**, CT confirms extensive perihilar consolidation with prominent air bronchogram signs.

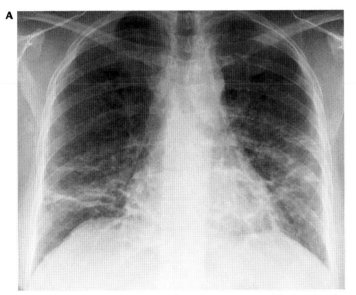

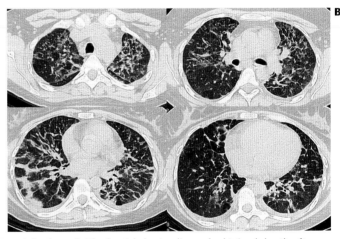

Fig. 9.49 Nitrofurantoin toxicity in a young woman with chronic urinary tract infections. **A**, The frontal chest radiograph obtained shortly after starting therapy shows bilateral, predominantly lower lobe, heterogeneous opacities. **B**, CT, however, demonstrates more diffuse reticular and ground-glass opacities. Note also the small bilateral pleural effusions. Symptoms and radiologic abnormalities resolved after cessation of drug therapy and treatment with corticosteroids.

this drug.[261] Histopathologically, findings of either DAD or OP are reported.[262] Symptoms usually develop within 1 month of beginning therapy or sooner (often within 24 h) if the patient has been previously sensitized. Symptoms include fever, chest pain, dyspnea, nonproductive cough, arthralgias, and rashes. Peripheral eosinophilia is common.[22] Chest radiographs show basally predominant heterogeneous opacities (Figs 9.49 and 9.50). Pleural effusions occur fairly frequently and are usually small. In severe acute and hyperacute cases, the radiographic pattern may resemble cardiogenic pulmonary edema. Response to withdrawal of the drug is prompt and almost invariably complete.[15]

The chronic form of toxicity usually develops after at least 6 months of nitrofurantoin therapy. In many instances, the patient has had several years of therapy before developing clinical manifestations of toxicity. This form manifests clinically with insidious onset dyspnea and cough. IP is the most common histopathologic manifestation of chronic nitrofurantoin toxicity.[182] Chest radiographs show bilateral basal reticular or reticulonodular opacities and loss of lung volume. CT may show either diffuse or subpleural reticular opacities, often with a distinct peribronchovascular distribution. More consolidative opacities, suggesting a component of OP, are sometimes seen on CT as

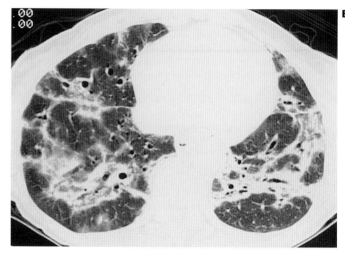

Fig. 9.50 Nitrofurantoin toxicity in an elderly woman with chronic urinary tract infections. **A,** The frontal chest radiograph demonstrates predominantly peripheral and basilar heterogeneous opacities with preservation of lung volume. **B,** CT demonstrates marked architectural distortion with ground-glass opacity, consolidation, and traction bronchiectasis in a peribronchovascular distribution. Lung biopsy showed interstitial pneumonia. (With permission from Rossi SE, Erasmus JJ, McAdams HP, Sporn TA, Goodman PC. Pulmonary drug toxicity: radiologic and pathologic manifestations. RadioGraphics 2000;20:1245–1259.)

well. Improvement usually follows discontinuation of nitrofurantoin therapy, an important diagnostic feature.[263] Depending on the duration and severity of the changes, resolution may not be complete, and approximately 10% of affected patients die of progressive respiratory insufficiency.[261]

OKT3

OKT3 is a monoclonal antibody used in the treatment of acute rejection of allografts. It interacts with the T3 antigen of human T cells, thereby blocking the rejection reaction. OKT3 toxicity is manifested as acute pulmonary edema, usually occurring within hours of the commencement of therapy.[264–266] Fluid is restricted prior to administration of OKT3 to limit this toxic side effect.

Oxygen

Oxygen has significant toxic effects on the lungs, particularly when administered in very high concentrations.[267] It has been estimated that 100% inspired oxygen causes damage within 48 h; lesser concentrations take a proportionally longer time. Patients receiving high levels of oxygen for extended periods almost invariably have significant pulmonary abnormalities from other causes and thus it may be difficult or impossible to determine how much additional change can reasonably be attributed to oxygen therapy.

The effects of oxygen toxicity differ between the mature and immature lung. In the mature lung, the most significant damage occurs at alveolar level and manifests histopathologically with findings of DAD and hyaline membrane formation. As with DAD of any cause, pulmonary fibrosis may ensue. Other effects of oxygen in the mature lung include damage to the terminal airways and inhibition of phagocytosis, resulting in a predisposition to infection.

The effects of oxygen toxicity in the immature lung are more distinctive, both clinically and radiographically, and result in bronchopulmonary dysplasia (BPD). The damage is frequently more apparent in the terminal airways with epithelial cell necrosis and squamous metaplasia. Damage to the alveoli is less obvious but may, with time, prove more significant because lung growth and pulmonary vascular development may be impaired. Premature infants, with birth weights <2000 g, are at high risk for respiratory distress syndrome and subsequent BPD. Respiratory distress syndrome is, however, not a necessary precursor to the development of BPD.[268] The major risk factors are pulmonary immaturity and assisted ventilation with supplemental oxygen. Thus, initial radiographs are normal in perhaps as many as 50% of patients.[269] The evolution of BPD may not be recognized in the early stages because of preexisting pulmonary disease. Many of the features of BPD, such as hyperexpansion of the lungs, pulmonary interstitial emphysema, atelectasis, and pneumonia, also occur in other diffuse pulmonary diseases involving premature infants. The development of progressively coarse reticular opacities, irregular cystlike spaces, coarse stranding, and pulmonary hyperexpansion suggests BPD (Figs 9.51 and 9.52). With time, these findings become increasingly "fixed", i.e. the basic radiographic pattern does not show any significant day-to-day variation other than changes related to varying radiographic technique or incidental complications such as atelectasis or barotrauma.

Severe cases of BPD are often fatal but the condition is of variable severity and there are many longterm survivors. For example, in the series of Lanning et al,[270] two patients with BPD died at the age of 3 months but there were 26 patients who survived. It has been conclusively shown that the changes of BPD improve to a greater or lesser extent during infancy with

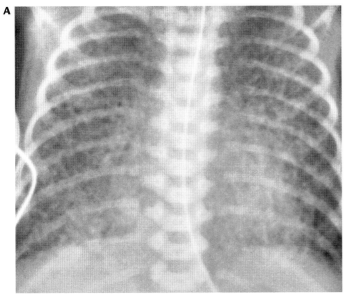

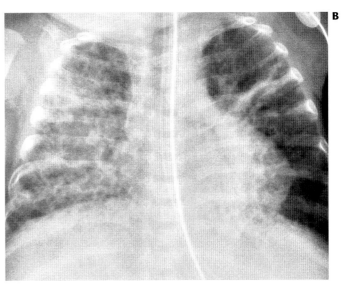

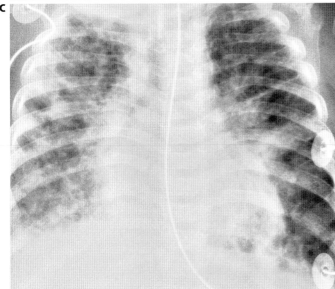

Fig. 9.51 Bronchopulmonary dysplasia in an infant treated with high levels of inspired oxygen for hyaline membrane disease. **A**, The frontal chest radiograph at 10 days of age shows bilateral coarse granular opacities and pulmonary hyperinflation. **B**, The radiograph at 3 months of age shows persistent opacities in the right lung with development of round, well circumscribed lucencies in both lungs. **C**, The radiograph at 7 months of age shows slight overall improvement with persistent hyperinflation, coarse heterogeneous opacities, and lung cysts.

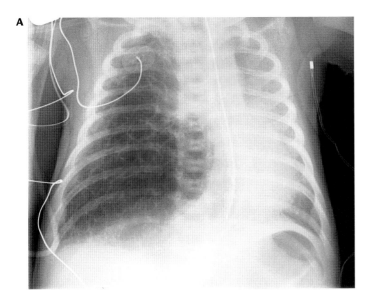

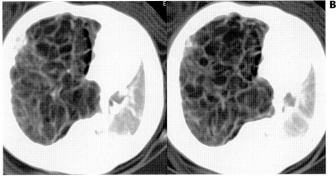

Fig. 9.52 Severe bronchopulmonary dysplasia (BPD) in an infant treated with high levels of inspired oxygen for hyaline membrane disease. **A**, The frontal chest radiograph demonstrates marked hyperexpansion of the right lung with shift of mediastinum to the left. **B**, CT shows findings of severe BPD affecting the right lung only. Note the ground-glass opacity in the left lung, presumably due to residual hyaline membrane disease.

further development of the lung. Lanning et al[270] found that normalization of the chest radiograph usually occurred between 3 and 6 months of age. Mortensson et al[271] noted an increased susceptibility to lower respiratory tract infections in infancy and observed that the changes of BPD cleared or almost cleared in the first 2 years. Nevertheless, longterm sequelae are seen, particularly in severe cases and with use of CT.[272,273] Chest radiographs may show hyperexpansion, hyperlucent areas, irregular linear densities representing fibrous stranding, and a relatively flat chest with a decreased anteroposterior diameter.[268] CT shows multifocal areas of hyperaeration with linear bands of fibrosis extending to the pleural surface and triangular pleural densities resulting from puckering of the lung surface.[273] CT in adult survivors may show multifocal areas of decreased lung attenuation and perfusion, and bronchial wall thickening.[274] Air-trapping may be a prominent feature on expiratory CT.[275]

Penicillamine

Penicillamine is used to treat lead poisoning, Wilson disease, cystinuria, and, on occasion, connective tissue disorders such as rheumatoid arthritis. It is not a commonly used drug, however, and pulmonary toxicity is rare. Recognized forms of toxicity include DAD, hypersensitivity pneumonitis[236] and obliterative bronchiolitis.[92–94] Penicillamine may also cause a relatively unique form of pulmonary toxicity, hemorrhagic pneumonitis with acute glomerulonephritis, that is clinically and radiographically indistinguishable from Goodpasture syndrome.[276] Onset is typically acute and chest radiographs show bilateral diffuse homogeneous pulmonary opacities. Renal dysfunction develops synchronously.

Salicylates

Salicylates probably exert their adverse effects on the lung by inhibiting prostaglandin synthesis. In some patients, this leads to bronchospasm. In others, capillary permeability is altered, resulting in pulmonary edema.[277,278] Salicylate induced edema generally occurs only with blood levels >30 mg/dl and may be related to acute intoxication.[55] The radiographic features of salicylate induced pulmonary edema are indistinguishable from those of cardiogenic edema. Increasing age and smoking are risk factors. Neurologic disturbances and proteinuria are common associated features and possibly indicate alterations in capillary permeability elsewhere.

While most salicylate induced pulmonary toxicity is associated with acute intoxication, Leatherman et al[279] and Chalasani et al[280] described a clinical presentation similar to toxic shock syndrome in patients with chronic salicylate intoxication. In this setting, extravascular fluid loss resulted in tachycardia, reduced systemic vascular resistance, hypotension, and multiple organ system failure, including acute respiratory distress syndrome.

Tricyclic antidepressants

Widespread use of tricyclic antidepressants in a population prone to attempted suicide probably explains why tricyclic antidepressant overdose is a common cause of admission to intensive care units. Pulmonary problems in these patients are overshadowed by problems of coma, seizure, and cardiac arrhythmia. In addition to aspiration pneumonia and atelectasis, the tricyclic antidepressants can cause interstitial pulmonary edema and acute respiratory distress syndrome.[10,281–285] Pulmonary edema develops in approximately 10% of patients and is more likely to occur with severe overdoses. The mechanism of edema production is unknown, although it does not appear to be cardiac in origin.[283,284] Most affected patients recover quickly and only transiently require intensive care.

RADIATION INDUCED LUNG INJURY

Radiation therapy is widely used in the treatment of pulmonary and mediastinal malignancies. Normal tissues are inevitably included in the radiation field and are subject to damage. Radiation effects on the lung are commonly seen on chest radiographs and CT, and abnormalities may also be noted in other structures such as the thoracic skeleton, pleura, or heart. The severity and extent of damage to normal lung tissue depend on a number of factors[286–290]:

1. The volume of normal lung irradiated is related to field size. Lung damage typically does not occur outside the field of irradiation, which is purposely kept as small as adequate therapy permits. On average only one-quarter to one-third of a lung is included in the field, but on occasion very large tumors necessitate irradiation of much larger lung volumes. The administration of 30 Gy to all of both lungs will kill most individuals, whereas the same or even higher doses administered to a portion of one lung may not even produce symptoms.

2. The total dose and the fractionation of that dose are of critical importance. The effect of a single large dose is more severe than the effect of the same dose divided into a series of fractions given over 2–3 weeks. There is, of course, no threshold at which deleterious effects become manifest, but they do become more apparent and inevitable with increasing total doses. With modern radiation therapy there are no significant differences in the effects of radiation from different sources, e.g. from cobalt sources as opposed to linear accelerators.

3. Individual susceptibility to radiation is variable and unpredictable. Clinical or radiographic evidence of radiation pneumonitis may develop in one patient but not in another receiving similar treatment. The preexisting state of the lungs may also play a role in determining the full clinical effects of radiation. For example, a patient with severe chronic obstructive pulmonary disease and poor respiratory reserve may be severely affected by even minimal radiation pneumonitis.

4. Previous or concomitant therapy may influence the timing and the severity of the radiation changes. A second course of radiation therapy produces earlier and more severe changes than the first. Certain cytotoxic agents, such as bleomycin, cyclophosphamide, mitomycin, and vincristine, heighten the effects of radiation.[291] Other agents, such as actinomycin D and adriamycin, that do not in themselves cause pulmonary toxicity, accentuate the effects of radiation.[292,293] Corticosteroids dampen the effects of irradiation as they do in other inflammatory processes.[294]

5. Furthermore, there is increasing evidence that portions of the lungs (and likely other structures) that are outside the field may be adversely affected by external beam radiation. Crestani et al[295] reported a group of 15 patients who had been treated with radiation therapy for breast cancer and who developed recurrent pulmonary opacities outside of the radiation field associated with dyspnea and fever. Histopathology in one-third showed findings of OP. All

responded well to corticosteroid therapy, but the majority suffered relapses when therapy was discontinued. Others have reported a similar association between OP and previous irradiation.[296,297] Arbetter et al[297] suggested that an immunologically mediated lymphocytic alveolitis was responsible for the recurrent migratory OP in these cases.

Histopathology

Knowledge of the underlying pathologic changes is useful for understanding the radiographic manifestations of radiation induced lung injury. A series of phases is recognized by pathologic, clinical, and radiographic criteria.[298] In the initial 24–48 h, the lymphoid follicles degenerate, the bronchial mucosa becomes hyperemic and edematous, and leukocytes infiltrate the bronchial wall. Ordinarily these changes are undetectable clinically or radiographically. In rare cases a central tumor may have narrowed the bronchial lumen so critically that the mucosal swelling and reaction produce clinically and radiographically detectable effects. This reaction subsides and a latent phase ensues.

The phase of acute radiation pneumonitis develops 1–6 months after the therapy. Histopathologic findings include thickening of the alveolar septa by edema and round cell infiltration, hyperplasia, and desquamation of the alveolar lining cells, fibrinous alveolar exudation leading to hyaline membrane formation, endothelial cell damage with engorgement and thrombus formation, and evidence of arteritis. Depending on the severity of reaction a variable degree of interstitial and alveolar fibrosis is seen. A simultaneous reaction occurs in the bronchial mucosa, with hyperemia, edema, and cessation of mucus gland and cilia function. These changes peak and merge into a regenerative phase in which the exudates and edema disperse, the alveolar lining cells regenerate, and the capillary endothelial cells become normal. Fibrosis, however, progresses, consolidates, and contracts over the following weeks and months. In addition, there may be progressive sclerosis of the pulmonary vascular bed and bronchial structural damage. The latter changes may lead to bronchiectasis and altered perfusion of the affected portions of the lung.[299]

Clinical features

If any symptoms related to pulmonary irradiation occur, they are seen during the phase of acute radiation pneumonitis or develop much later as a consequence of fibrosis and lung contraction. The severity of symptoms depends on the extent and severity of the post irradiation changes and on the presence of underlying lung disease. The usual symptoms in the acute phase are dyspnea, cough, production of tenacious sputum, and sometimes fever and night sweats. These symptoms may persist for several weeks. In the fibrotic phase, the patient is usually asymptomatic. If fibrosis is severe and extensive, however, the patient may become completely disabled. Cough, hemoptysis, dyspnea, orthopnea, clubbing of the fingers, and recurrent infections are all features of such cases.

Radiology (Box 9.15)

The changes of radiation pneumonitis on the chest radiograph are generally confined to the field of irradiation (Fig. 9.53). In

---

Box 9.15 Radiologic manifestations of radiation induced lung injury

Early
Hazy opacities, obscured vascular margins
Usually confined to radiation portals
Ground-glass opacities or consolidation on CT

Late
More homogeneous linear or angled opacities
Cicatrial atelectasis and fibrosis
Traction bronchiectasis may be a dominant feature

Time course
Findings typically appear within 6–8 weeks of starting treatment
Findings peak 3–4 months of completing treatment
Findings mature and become quiescent within 12–18 months
Progression or change beyond this time suggests an alternate diagnosis

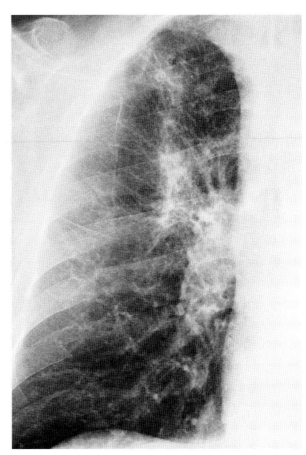

Fig. 9.53 The radiation changes after treatment of lung cancer. The cone down view of a chest radiograph shows a focal right upper lobe opacity with straight lateral margins.

some cases it may be necessary to correlate the chest radiograph with the radiation portals, particularly when tangential beams have been employed. The single most striking feature of radiation pneumonitis is the geometric shape of the resulting pulmonary opacities. The line of demarcation between involved and noninvolved lung is usually linear, and normal anatomic

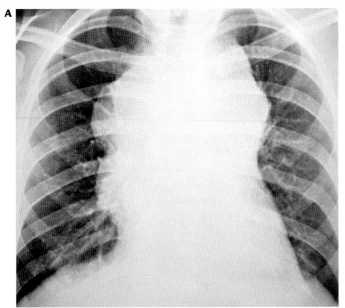

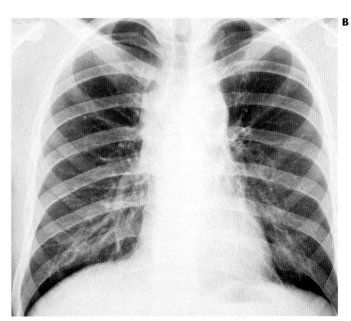

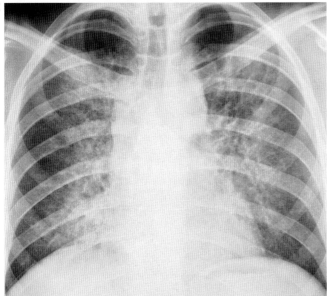

Fig. 9.54 Acute radiation pneumonitis after treatment of lymphoma. **A**, The initial frontal chest radiograph shows bilateral mediastinal adenopathy. **B**, The radiograph obtained at 2 weeks shows marked improvement of adenopathy following irradiation. Lungs remain normal. **C**, The radiograph obtained at 10 weeks shows new, bilateral heterogeneous opacities that conform to radiation port.

boundaries such as fissures are crossed with impunity. On a frontal radiograph of the chest the involved areas may be clearly delineated, but on the lateral radiograph the changes may extend fairly uniformly across the chest in the sagittal plane. To observers accustomed to using the lateral film for segmental or lobar localization, this disregard for anatomic boundaries can be striking. Although radiation induced opacities on the chest radiograph are usually confined to the radiation field, CT or ^{67}Ga-citrate imaging may show opacities in nonirradiated portions of the lungs.[300,301] The cause of opacities outside the field of irradiation has been the subject of speculation. Suggested causes include blockage of lymphatic pathways, errors in dosimetry or placement of portals, scattered radiation, or radiation induced hypersensitivity pneumonitis.[302] As noted above, more recent

evidence suggests that these opacities are foci of OP which may be induced by an immunologically mediated lymphocytic alveolitis.[297]

The first and earliest radiographic finding is a diffuse haze in the irradiated region with obscuration of vascular margins. Scattered consolidations appear, and these areas may coalesce into a nonanatomic but geometric area of pulmonary opacity (Figs 9.53 and 9.54). Pleural effusions are relatively uncommon.[303] Libshitz and Shuman[304] indicate that demonstrable radiographic opacities usually appear at about 8 weeks after treatment with 40 Gy delivered over 4 weeks. For each further increment of 10 Gy, the opacities appear about 1 week earlier. Bell et al[305] have shown that CT (Fig. 9.55) and ventilation perfusion studies, particularly when performed with single photon emission CT

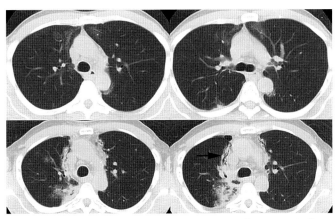

Fig. 9.55   The radiation changes after treatment of lung cancer. The CT (top panels) obtained at 3 months shows subtle paramediastinal ground-glass opacity. The CT (bottom panels) obtained at 6 months shows progressive fibrosis within the paramediastinal lung. Note the traction bronchiectasis (arrow).

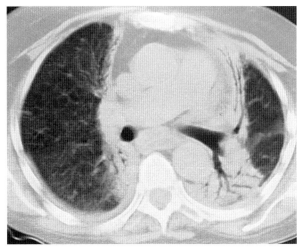

Fig. 9.57   The radiation changes after treatment of lung cancer. The CT shows homogeneous opacities with sharp lateral margins conforming to the radiation ports. Note the extensive air bronchogram.

(SPECT), are more sensitive than chest radiographs in detecting postirradiation changes in the lungs. This applies both to the field of irradiation changes and to the nonirradiated portions of the lungs.

The regenerative fibrotic phase develops almost imperceptibly from the phase of acute pneumonitis. With time the opacities become more linear or reticular, i.e. "more structured". Fibrous contraction condenses the opacities and distorts adjacent structures such as hilar vessels (Figs 9.56 and 9.57). The fibrosis is often not severe, and the changes can easily be overlooked or attributed to granulomatous scarring. The experienced observer, however, instinctively notes the alteration, such as the slight paramediastinal opacity, that may be seen after mediastinal irradiation of patients with lymphoma.

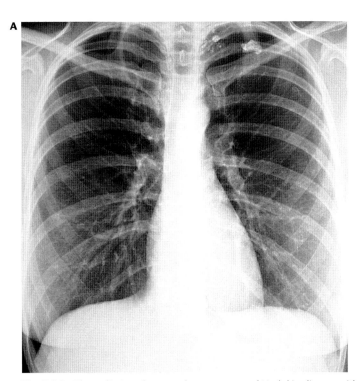

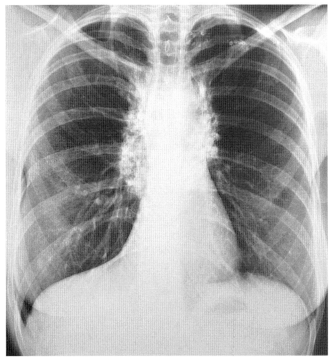

Fig. 9.56   The radiation changes after treatment of Hodgkin disease with a mantle field. **A**, The initial frontal chest radiograph shows lymphangiogram contrast in the left supraclavicular and anterior cervical nodes. **B**, The radiograph obtained 4 months after completion of treatment shows that dense geometric opacities with fibrous contraction have developed in the radiation ports.

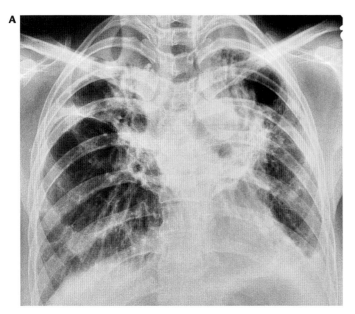

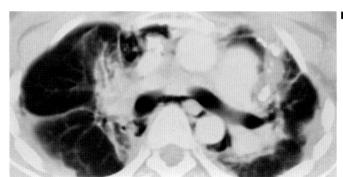

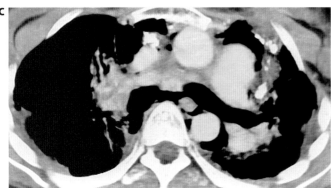

Fig. 9.58 The severe radiation changes after treatment for lymphoma. **A**, The frontal chest radiograph shows bilateral upper lung consolidation with sharp lateral margins and volume loss. Note the radiographically identifiable bronchiectasis. **B** and **C**, CT shows severe central fibrosis, bronchiectasis, and paracicatricial bulla. Note the lymph node calcification.

The earliest radiographic changes appear 6–8 weeks after the beginning of radiation therapy, and the peak reaction occurs usually at 3–4 months. The ensuing fibrosis and contraction continue over a 12–18 month period and then become quiescent. Bronchiectasis may be present within the regions of fibrosis, but this abnormality is usually undetectable on plain films. However, radiation damage to the lung is occasionally severe, and the resultant bronchiectasis may be apparent (Fig. 9.58). Fortunately, such damage is rare with modern radiation therapy.

CT findings of radiation induced lung injury clearly reflect the pathologic changes described above.[304,306] In the phase of acute radiation pneumonitis, scattered and increasingly confluent areas of ground-glass opacity and consolidation appear in the irradiated field (Fig. 9.59). The geographic distribution of the changes may be striking. Transition to the phase of regeneration and fibrosis is gradual. Fibrous stranding that merges smoothly with the pleura becomes apparent, and contraction can be recognized by the distortion of adjacent structures. Bronchiectasis within the contracted portion of lung may be readily apparent on CT (Figs 9.57 and 9.58). CT is more sensitive than chest radiographs in detecting postirradiation changes in the lungs, particularly in peripheral tangential radiation fields (Fig. 9.60).[305]

CT may also show shrinkage of vessels in lung peripheral to a central field of irradiation. This presumably reflects diminished perfusion resulting from radiation induced vascular sclerosis. Bell et al,[305] using scintigraphy, demonstrated significant perfusion abnormalities in the lung beyond the field of irradiation.

Three-dimensional (3D) conformal and intensity modulated radiation therapy (IMRT) are two relatively new approaches to delivering radiotherapy.[307–309] Both techniques use computers to plan and deliver radiotherapy using models derived from 3D image sets, typically spiral CT. These techniques allow higher doses to be delivered to the tumor with maximal sparing of normal tissues. IMRT, in particular, permits dose escalation to levels unattainable with conventional radiotherapy techniques.[308] Because so many overlapping fields are used with these techniques, the appearance of radiation induced lung injury may be quite unusual. Koenig et al[310] reported on the CT features of radiation induced injury in 19 lung cancer patients treated with 3D conformal radiotherapy. Seven patients were imaged in the first 3 months after treatment and all had focal areas of pneumonitis immediately adjacent to the tumor. All 19 patients developed fibrosis in one of three patterns on

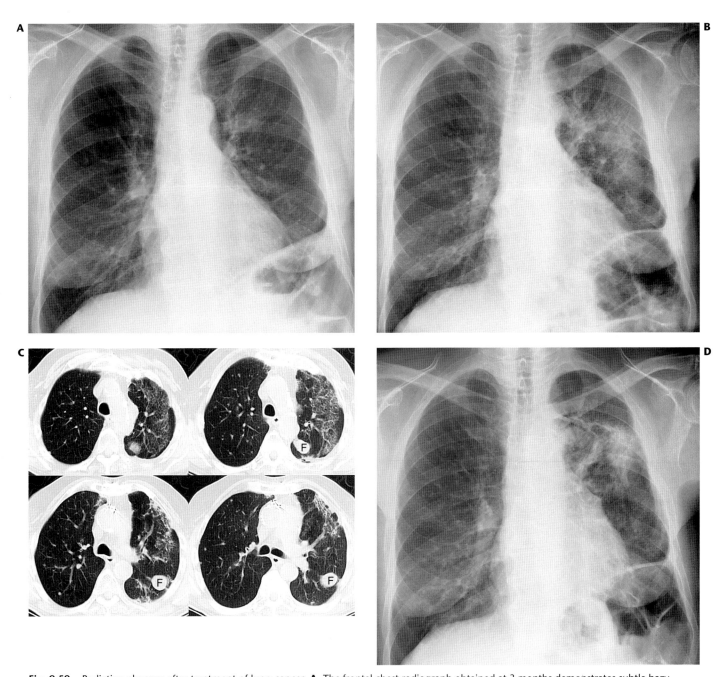

Fig. 9.59 Radiation changes after treatment of lung cancer. **A**, The frontal chest radiograph obtained at 3 months demonstrates subtle hazy opacity in the left upper lobe. **B**, The chest radiograph obtained at 6 months shows progressive homogeneous opacity in the left upper lobe. **C**, The CT obtained at the same time shows ground-glass and reticular opacity in the radiation port with early traction bronchiectasis and bronchiolectasis. Note the loculated fluid (F) within the major fissure. **D**, The radiograph obtained at 1 year shows a more angular opacity in the left upper lobe consistent with mature radiation fibrosis.

follow-up CT. In five patients, fibrosis similar to that seen with conventional radiotherapy was seen. Masslike fibrosis in the area of the original tumor (Fig. 9.61) was seen in eight patients and a linear, scarlike opacity (Fig. 9.62) in the region of the original tumor was seen in six. These authors concluded that the CT appearance of fibrosis due to 3D conformal radiotherapy was often quite different from that of conventional radiotherapy, and

that it could, in some cases, simulate a residual or recurrent tumor mass.

Less common manifestations of radiation induced lung injury[311] include hyperlucency of a lung,[312,313] pleural effusions, and spontaneous pneumothorax.[314,315] Pulmonary hyperlucency presumably results from diminished pulmonary perfusion. Pleural effusions secondary to irradiation are usually small

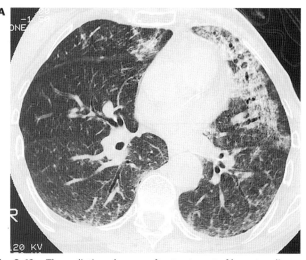

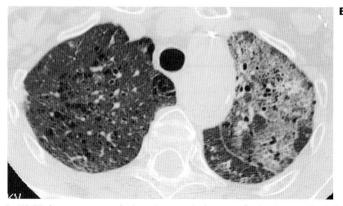

Fig. 9.60 The radiation changes after treatment of breast malignancy. **A**, HRCT demonstrates subpleural ground-glass opacity in the anterior left lung. This finding is consistent with acute radiation pneumonitis in a tangential radiation port. **B**, HRCT through the lung apex demonstrates more diffuse ground-glass opacity due to a more conventional port used to treat supraclavicular adenopathy.

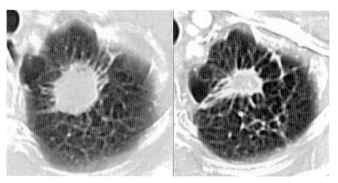

Fig. 9.61 The radiation changes after 3D-conformational treatment of lung malignancy. CT (left panel) shows a spiculated left upper lobe mass. CT (right panel) at 9 months shows a residual masslike opacity, a typical finding after this type of radiation therapy. (Courtesy of Dr. R. Muden, Houston, Texas.)

and coincident with the phase of acute radiation pneumonitis (Fig. 9.62).[316,317] These effusions will spontaneously resolve as the radiation pneumonitis subsides. Failure to do so, or an increasing effusion, is suggestive of metastatic disease.

Second primary tumors can arise either in the radiation field (Fig. 9.63) or, less commonly, in sites remote from the field and may be radiation induced.[318–324] Although there is frequently a long (5–10 year) latent period, risk appears to increase with time thereafter. The most important variables that govern risk of a second primary tumor include the age at treatment (the risk is highest when radiation therapy occurs in childhood[325]), the type of tissue included in the field, and the total dose delivered.[325]

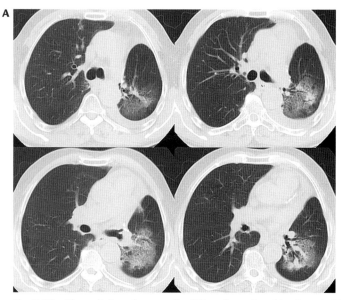

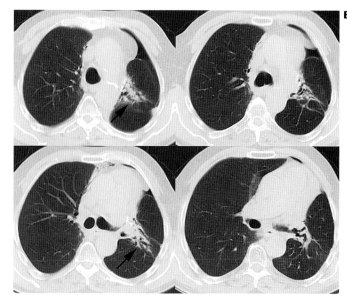

Fig. 9.62 The radiation changes after 3D-conformational treatment of lung malignancy. **A**, CT obtained at 3 months shows focal ground-glass opacity in the left mid lung and a small left pleural effusion. **B**, CT at 9 months shows a linear opacity (arrows) in the radiation field. Note also the small anterior pneumothorax.

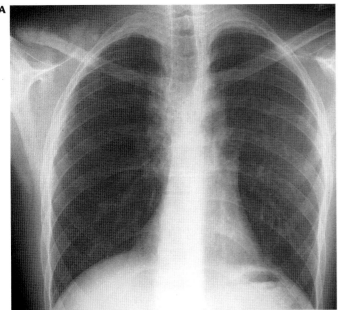

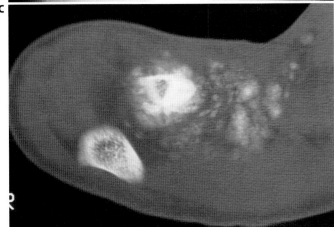

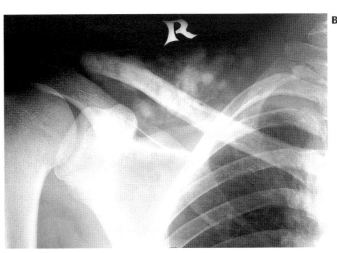

Fig. 9.63   Radiation induced osteosarcoma arising 8 years after treatment of mediastinal and right supraclavicular Hodgkin disease. **A**, The frontal chest radiograph shows typical findings of radiation fibrosis in the paramediastinal lung. Note the amorphous calcification in the right supraclavicular fossa. **B**, The coned down view of the right clavicle shows sclerosis and destruction of the distal clavicle and amorphous ossification in the soft tissues. **C**, CT confirms soft tissue ossification consistent with osteosarcoma.

Low doses (<30 Gy) are associated with an increased risk of thyroid and central nervous system tumors. Higher doses (>30 Gy) are associated with an increased risk of bone and soft tissue tumors. Bone, brain, thyroid, and breast tissue appear to be particularly susceptible when exposed during periods of rapid growth and proliferation.[325] For example, the risk of breast cancer in survivors of childhood Hodgkin disease treated with mediastinal irradiation varies from 10 to 33%.[325] Combined treatment with alkylating agents also seems to increase the risk of a second malignancy. Furthermore, the risk is greater in children with a genetic predisposition to malignancy, e.g. patients with congenital retinoblastoma.[325] Although the greatest risk for cancer induction is in the radiation field, survivors also have an excess risk for second tumors in remote sites.[326]

Differential diagnosis

The two major differential diagnoses to be considered in patients with radiation pneumonitis are infection and tumor recurrence. Infectious pneumonia is not usually confined by the radiotherapy ports and normally runs a less indolent course than radiation pneumonitis. Nevertheless, an area of radiation damage may become secondarily infected, and if it does, the diagnosis cannot be established radiographically. Tumor recurrence may be difficult to discern at the height of the postirradiation change, but as these changes stabilize and contraction develops, a focal mass should become increasingly apparent. A primary bronchogenic carcinoma may develop a lymphangitic pattern of spread initially confined to one lung or even one lobe. Lymphangitic carcinomatosis may initially cause diagnostic problems, but inexorable worsening with the development of septal lines, effusions, and spread to the opposite lung will soon make the diagnosis clear.

CT and MRI have been investigated as means of detecting tumor recurrence. CT, by detecting focal masses or cavitation, may provide some evidence of recurrence. MRI is theoretically capable of differentiating radiation change from tumor. Radiation fibrosis has low signal intensity on both T1- and T2-weighted sequences.[327] Tumors, on the other hand, have high

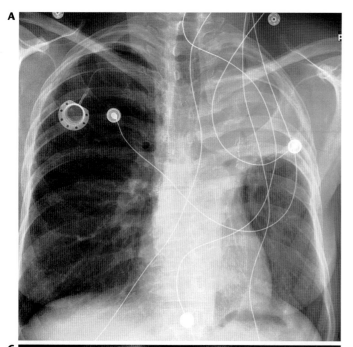

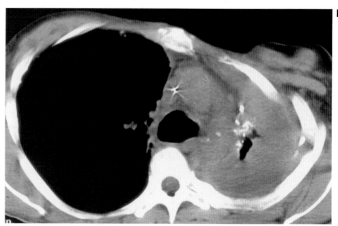

Fig. 9.64 The radiation changes after treatment of lung cancer. **A,** The frontal chest radiograph obtained 2 years after completion of treatment shows a homogeneous opacity in the left upper hemithorax consistent with radiation and postsurgical change. **B,** CT shows fluid and soft tissue in the left upper hemothorax; recurrent tumor cannot be excluded with certainty. **C,** The coronal FDG PET image shows no uptake in the left upper thoracic mass (arrow), consistent with scarring. There is no evidence of residual or recurrent tumor. H = heart.

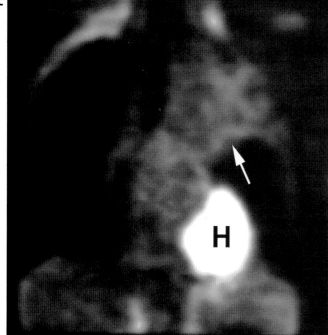

signal intensity on T2-weighted sequences and can therefore be distinguished from pure fibrosis. However, acute radiation pneumonitis, secondary infective pneumonitis, or hemorrhage may have signal intensities similar to tumor and therefore may be confused with recurrent disease. Thus, in practice, MRI has not proven to be very useful for distinguishing radiation change from recurrent tumor. Enhancement with gadolinium-DTPA is also not helpful in distinguishing between radiation fibrosis and tumor recurrence.[328] Magnetic resonance spectroscopy has

been suggested as a possible solution but thus far has not evolved into a clinically accepted method.[329]

Fluoro-dexoxyglucose positron emission tomography (FDG PET) imaging may play an important role in guiding patient care after surgery or radiation therapy. It is more accurate than chest radiographs, CT, or MRI for distinguishing persistent or recurrent tumor from necrotic tumor, posttreatment scarring or fibrosis (accuracy of 78–98%, sensitivity of 97–100%, and specificity of 62–100%) (Figs 9.64 and 9.65).[330–337] False positive

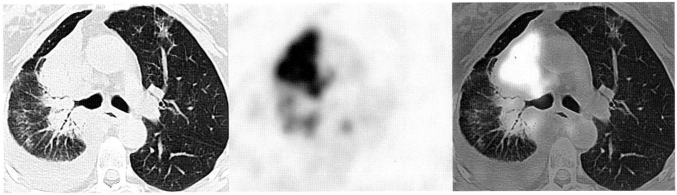

Fig. 9.65 Recurrent lung cancer after radiation treatment for lung cancer. The axial CT image (top left) from a CT PET scan shows a homogeneous opacity in the anterior right lung with a sharp lateral border. More heterogeneous opacity is seen in the posterior perihilar region. Note the moderate right pleural effusion. The axial FDG PET image (top right) shows markedly increased metabolic activity in the anterior opacity, but only moderate activity in the perihilar opacity. The fused image (bottom left) clearly suggests recurrent tumor in the anterior opacity. Moderate activity in the perihilar opacity is consistent with radiation change. (Courtesy of Jeremy Erasmus, MD, Houston, TX)

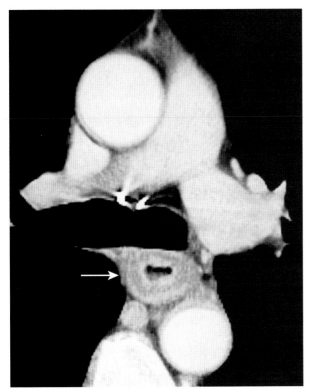

Fig. 9.66 Radiation induced esophagitis after treatment of lung cancer. CT shows marked thickening of the esophagus (arrow) with mucosal hyperemia and submucosal edema. Surgical clips at the carina are from mediastinoscopy.

studies can be caused by acute radiation pneumonitis, however. Thus, follow-up FDG PET studies should not be obtained until at least 4–5 months after completion of radiation therapy.[330]

Radiation effects on other thoracic structures

Radiation may damage other thoracic structures, producing either radiographically visible manifestations or indirect effects on the lungs.[338] Radiation induced abnormalities in the bony thorax are most commonly seen after radiation therapy for carcinoma of the breast. The bones appear atrophic and osteoporotic, fractures are frequent and may fail to unite, and dystrophic calcifications may be seen in the adjacent soft tissues.[339–341] Necrotic bone appears sclerotic. Radiation damage to the heart and the pericardium may cause enlargement of the cardiac silhouette and signs of pulmonary vascular congestion and edema. Pericardial effusion is the most common manifestation of radiation damage to the heart and mediastinum, but myocardial fibrosis and coronary artery damage may occur.[290,342–344] Radiation is known to accelerate coronary atherosclerosis. Radiation damage to the esophagus may cause acute esophagitis (Fig. 9.66), dysmotility, stricture formation, or fistula development, and chronic aspiration may ensue.[345–347]

REFERENCES

1. Rosenow EC, Myers JL, Swensen SJ, et al. Drug-induced pulmonary disease. An update. Chest 1992;102:239–250.
2. Cooper JA Jr, Matthay RA. Drug-induced pulmonary disease. Dis Mon 1987;33: 61–120.
3. Kreisman H, Wolkove N. Pulmonary toxicity of antineoplastic therapy. Semin Oncol 1992;19:508–520.
4. McDonald S, Rubin P, Phillips TL, et al. Injury to the lung from cancer therapy: clinical syndromes, measurable endpoints, and potential scoring systems. Int J Radiat Oncol Biol Phys 1995;31:1187–1203.
5. Libby D, White DA. Pulmonary toxicity of drugs used to treat systemic autoimmune diseases. Clin Chest Med 1998;19:809–821.
6. Shanholtz C. Acute life-threatening toxicity of cancer treatment. Crit Care Clin 2001;17:483–502.
7. Rossi SE, Erasmus JJ, McAdams HP, et al. Pulmonary drug toxicity: radiologic and pathologic manifestations. RadioGraphics 2000;20:1245–1259.
8. Erasmus JJ, McAdams HP, Rossi SE. High-resolution CT of drug-induced lung disease. Radiol Clin North Am 2002;40:61–72.
9. Erasmus JJ, McAdams HP, Rossi SE. Drug-induced lung injury. Semin Roentgenol 2002;37:72–81.
10. Ben-Noun L. Drug-induced respiratory disorders: incidence, prevention and management. Drug Safety 2000;23: 143–164.
11. Dimopoulou I, Galani H, Dafni U, et al. A prospective study of pulmonary function in patients treated with paclitaxel and carboplatin. Cancer 2002;94:452–458.
12. Myers JL, Kennedy JI, Plumb VJ. Amiodarone lung: pathologic findings in clinically toxic patients. Hum Pathol 1987;18:349–354.
13. Kuhlman JE. The role of chest computed tomography in the diagnosis of drug-related reactions. J Thorac Imaging 1991;6:52–61.
14. Lien HH, Brodahl U, Telhaug R, et al. Pulmonary changes at computed tomography in patients with testicular carcinoma treated with cis-platinum, vinblastine and bleomycin. Acta Radiol Diagn (Stockh) 1985;26:507–510.
15. Padley SP, Adler B, Hansell DM, et al. High-resolution computed tomography of drug-induced lung disease. Clin Radiol 1992;46:232–236.
16. Rimmer MJ, Dixon AK, Flower CD, et al. Bleomycin lung: computed tomographic observations. Br J Radiol 1985;58: 1041–1045.
17. Cleverley JR, Screaton NJ, Hiorns MP, et al. Drug-induced lung disease: high-resolution CT and histological findings. Clin Radiol 2002;57:292–299.
18. Akira M, Ishikawa H, Yamamoto S. Drug-induced pneumonitis: thin-section CT findings in 60 patients. Radiology 2002;224:852–860.
19. Kuhlman JE, Scatarige JC, Fishman EK, et al. CT demonstration of high attenuation pleural-parenchymal lesions due to amiodarone therapy. J Comput Assist Tomogr 1987;11:160–162.
20. Nalos PC, Kass RM, Gang ES, et al. Life-threatening postoperative pulmonary complications in patients with previous amiodarone pulmonary toxicity undergoing cardiothoracic operations. J Thorac Cardiovasc Surg 1987;93:904–912.
21. Ren H, Kuhlman JE, Hruban RH, et al. CT-pathology correlation of amiodarone lung. J Comput Assist Tomogr 1990;14: 760–765.
22. Myers JL. Pathology of drug-induced lung disease. In: Katzenstein AA, Askin FB, eds. Surgical pathology of non-neoplastic lung disease, 3rd edn. Philadelphia: WB Saunders, 1997: 81–111.
23. Cooper JA Jr, White DA, Matthay RA. Drug-induced pulmonary disease. Part 1: Cytotoxic drugs. Am Rev Respir Dis 1986;133:321–340.
24. Piguet PF. Cytokines involved in pulmonary fibrosis. Int Rev Exp Pathol 1993;34(Pt B):173–181.
25. Abid SH, Malhotra V, Perry MC. Radiation-induced and chemotherapy-induced pulmonary injury. Curr Opin Oncol 2001;13:242–248.
26. Kay JM. Drug-induced lung disease. In: Hasleton PS, ed. Spencer's pathology of the lung, 5th edn. New York: McGraw-Hill, 1996:551–595.
27. Pietra GG. Pathologic mechanisms of drug-induced lung disorders. J Thorac Imaging 1991;6:1–7.
28. Smith GJ. The histopathology of pulmonary reactions to drugs. Clin Chest Med 1990;11:95–117.
29. Cooper JA Jr, White DA, Matthay RA. Drug-induced pulmonary disease. Part 2: Noncytotoxic drugs. Am Rev Respir Dis 1986;133:488–505.
30. Holoye PY, Jenkins DE, Greenberg SD. Pulmonary toxicity in long-term administration of BCNU. Cancer Treat Rep 1976;60:1691–1694.
31. Kennedy JI, Myers JL, Plumb VJ, et al. Amiodarone pulmonary toxicity. Clinical, radiologic, and pathologic correlations. Arch Intern Med 1987;147:50–55.
32. Kim TS, Lee KS, Chung MP, et al. Nonspecific interstitial pneumonia with fibrosis: high-resolution CT and pathologic findings. AJR Am J Roentgenol 1998;171:1645–1650.
33. Epler GR, Colby TV, McLoud TC, et al. Bronchiolitis obliterans organizing pneumonia. N Engl J Med 1985;312: 152–158.
34. Naisbitt DJ, Pirmohamed M, Park BK. Immunopharmacology of hypersensitivity reactions to drugs. Curr Allergy Asthma Rep 2003;3:22–29.
35. Pirmohamed M, Naisbitt DJ, Gordon F, et al. The danger hypothesis – potential role in idiosyncratic drug reactions. Toxicology 2002;181–182:55–63.
36. Sharma OP, Bethlem EP. The pulmonary infiltration with eosinophilia syndrome. Curr Opin Pulm Med 1996;2:380–389.
37. Parry SD, Barbatzas C, Peel ET, et al. Sulphasalazine and lung toxicity. Eur Respir J 2002;19:756–764.
38. Oh PI, Balter MS. Cocaine induced eosinophilic lung disease. Thorax 1992;47:478–479.
39. Goodwin SD, Glenny RW. Nonsteroidal anti-inflammatory drug-associated pulmonary infiltrates with eosinophilia. Review of the literature and Food and Drug Administration Adverse Drug Reaction reports. Arch Intern Med 1992;152:1521–1524.
40. Khalil H, Molinary E, Stoller JK. Diclofenac (Voltaren)-induced eosinophilic pneumonitis. Case report and review of the literature. Arch Intern Med 1993;153:1649–1652.
41. Pfitzenmeyer P, Meier M, Zuck P, et al. Piroxicam induced pulmonary infiltrates and eosinophilia. J Rheumatol 1994;21: 1573–1577.
42. Yamamoto T, Tanida T, Ueta E, et al. Pulmonary infiltration with eosinophilia (PIE) syndrome induced by antibiotics, PIPC and TFLX during cancer treatment. Oral Oncol 2001;37:471–475.
43. Trojan A, Meier R, Licht A, et al. Eosinophilic pneumonia after administration of fludarabine for the treatment of non-Hodgkin's lymphoma. Ann Hematol 2002;81:535–537.
44. Kim Y, Lee KS, Choi DC, et al. The spectrum of eosinophilic lung disease: radiologic findings. J Comput Assist Tomogr 1997;21:920–930.
45. Holoye PY, Luna MA, MacKay B, et al. Bleomycin hypersensitivity pneumonitis. Ann Intern Med 1978;88:47–49.
46. White DA, Stover DE. Severe bleomycin-induced pneumonitis. Clinical features and response to corticosteroids. Chest 1984;86:723–728.
47. Alkins SA, Byrd JC, Morgan SK, et al. Anaphylactoid reactions to methotrexate. Cancer 1996;77:2123–2126.
48. Goldberg NH, Romolo JL, Austin EH, et al. Anaphylactoid type reactions in two patients receiving high dose intravenous methotrexate. Cancer 1978;41:52–55.

49. Stephan WC, Parks RD, Tempest B. Acute hypersensitivity pneumonitis associated with carbamazepine therapy. Chest 1978;74:463–464.

50. Briasoulis E, Pavlidis N. Noncardiogenic pulmonary edema: an unusual and serious complication of anticancer therapy. Oncologist 2001;6:153–161.

51. Reed CR, Glauser FL. Drug-induced noncardiogenic pulmonary edema. Chest 1991;100:1120–1124.

52. Frand UI, Shim CS, Williams MH Jr. Methadone-induced pulmonary edema. Ann Intern Med 1972;76:975–979.

53. Steinberg AD, Karliner JS. The clinical spectrum of heroin pulmonary edema. Arch Intern Med 1968;122:122–127.

54. MacLennan FM, Thomson MA, Rankin R, et al. Fatal pulmonary oedema associated with the use of ritodrine in pregnancy. Case report. Br J Obstet Gynaecol 1985;92:703–705.

55. Heffner JE, Sahn SA. Salicylate-induced pulmonary edema. Clinical features and prognosis. Ann Intern Med 1981;95:405–409.

56. Rubin RL. Etiology and mechanisms of drug-induced lupus. Curr Opin Rheumatol 1999;11:357–363.

57. Rich MW. Drug-induced lupus. The list of culprits grows. Postgrad Med 1996;100:299–302,307–308.

58. Vergne P, Bertin P, Bonnet C, et al. Drug-induced rheumatic disorders: incidence, prevention and management. Drug Safety 2000;23:279–293.

59. ten Holder SM, Joy MS, Falk RJ. Cutaneous and systemic manifestations of drug-induced vasculitis. Ann Pharmacother 2002;36:130–147.

60. Merkel PA. Drug-induced vasculitis. Rheum Dis Clin North Am 2001;27:849–862.

61. Robertson CH Jr, Reynolds RC, Wilson JE 3rd. Pulmonary hypertension and foreign body granulomas in intravenous drug abusers. Documentation by cardiac catheterization and lung biopsy. Am J Med 1976;61:657–664.

62. Schwartz IS, Bosken C. Pulmonary vascular talc granulomatosis. JAMA 1986;256:2584.

63. Crouch E, Churg A. Progressive massive fibrosis of the lung secondary to intravenous injection of talc. A pathologic and mineralogic analysis. Am J Clin Pathol 1983;80:520–526.

64. O'Donnell AE, Selig J, Aravamuthan M, et al. Pulmonary complications associated with illicit drug use. An update. Chest 1995;108:460–463.

65. McCarroll KA, Roszler MH. Lung disorders due to drug abuse. J Thorac Imaging 1991;6:30–35.

66. Pare JP, Cote G, Fraser RS. Long-term follow-up of drug abusers with intravenous talcosis. Am Rev Respir Dis 1989;139:233–241.

67. Padley SP, Adler BD, Staples CA, et al. Pulmonary talcosis: CT findings in three cases. Radiology 1993;186:125–127.

68. Sieniewicz DJ, Nidecker AC. Conglomerate pulmonary disease: a form of talcosis in intravenous methadone abusers. AJR Am J Roentgenol 1980;135:697–702.

69. Ward S, Heyneman LE, Reittner P, et al. Talcosis associated with IV abuse of oral medications: CT findings. AJR Am J Roentgenol 2000;174:789–793.

70. Gondouin A, Manzoni P, Ranfaing E, et al. Exogenous lipid pneumonia: a retrospective multicentre study of 44 cases in France. Eur Respir J 1996;9:1463–1469.

71. Spickard A 3rd, Hirschmann JV. Exogenous lipoid pneumonia. Arch Intern Med 1994;154:686–692.

72. Lee JS, Im JG, Song KS, et al. Exogenous lipoid pneumonia: high-resolution CT findings. Eur Radiol 1999;9:287–291.

73. Franquet T, Gimenez A, Bordes R, et al. The crazy-paving pattern in exogenous lipoid pneumonia: CT-pathologic correlation. AJR Am J Roentgenol 1998;170:315–317.

74. Hoffmann RM, Jung MC, Motz R, et al. Sarcoidosis associated with interferon-alpha therapy for chronic hepatitis C. J Hepatol 1998;28:1058–1063.

75. Abdi EA, Nguyen GK, Ludwig RN, et al. Pulmonary sarcoidosis following interferon therapy for advanced renal cell carcinoma. Cancer 1987;59:896–900.

76. Nakajima M, Kubota Y, Miyashita N, et al. Recurrence of sarcoidosis following interferon alpha therapy for chronic hepatitis C. Intern Med 1996;35:376–379.

77. Pietropaoli A, Modrak J, Utell M. Interferon-alpha therapy associated with the development of sarcoidosis. Chest 1999;116:569–572.

78. Verdich J, Christensen AL. Pulmonary disease complicating intermittent methotrexate therapy of psoriasis. Acta Derm Venereol 1979;59:471–473.

79. Sybert A, Butler TP. Sarcoidosis following adjuvant high-dose methotrexate therapy for osteosarcoma. Arch Intern Med 1978;138:488–489.

80. Ravenel JG, McAdams HP, Plankeel JF, et al. Sarcoidosis induced by interferon therapy. AJR Am J Roentgenol 2001;177:199–201.

81. Louie S, Gamble CN, Cross CE. Penicillamine associated pulmonary hemorrhage. J Rheumatol 1986;13:963–966.

82. Primack SL, Miller RR, Müller NL. Diffuse pulmonary hemorrhage: clinical, pathologic, and imaging features. AJR Am J Roentgenol 1995;164:295–300.

83. Follath F, Burkart F, Schweizer W. Drug-induced pulmonary hypertension? Br Med J 1971;1:265–266.

84. Abenhaim L, Moride Y, Brenot F, et al. Appetite-suppressant drugs and the risk of primary pulmonary hypertension. International Primary Pulmonary Hypertension Study Group. N Engl J Med 1996;335:609–616.

85. Thomas SH, Butt AY, Corris PA, et al. Appetite suppressants and primary pulmonary hypertension in the United Kingdom. Br Heart J 1995;74:660–663.

86. Vivero LE, Anderson PO, Clark RF. A close look at fenfluramine and dexfenfluramine. J Emerg Med 1998;16:197–205.

87. Connolly HM, Crary JL, McGoon MD, et al. Valvular heart disease associated with fenfluramine-phentermine. N Engl J Med 1997;337:581–588.

88. Girolami A, Spiezia L, Rossi F, et al. Oral contraceptives and venous thromboembolism: which are the safest preparations available? Clin Appl Thromb Hemost 2002;8:157–162.

89. Peverill RE. Hormone therapy and venous thromboembolism. Best Pract Res Clin Endocrinol Metab 2003;17:149–164.

90. Drife J. Oral contraception and the risk of thromboembolism: what does it mean to clinicians and their patients? Drug Safety 2002;25:893–902.

91. MacDonald JS. Lymphography. In: Ansell G, ed. Complications in diagnostic radiology. Oxford: Blackwell, 1976:301–316.

92. Boehler A, Vogt P, Speich R, et al. Bronchiolitis obliterans in a patient with localized scleroderma treated with D-penicillamine. Eur Respir J 1996;9:1317–1319.

93. Renier JC, Bontoux-Carre E, Racineux JL. [Three cases of obliterating bronchiolitis during treatment of rheumatoid polyarthritis with D-penicillamine]. Rev Rhum Mal Osteoartic 1986;53:25–26.

94. Murphy KC, Atkins CJ, Offer RC, et al. Obliterative bronchiolitis in two rheumatoid arthritis patients treated with penicillamine. Arthritis Rheum 1981;24:557–560.

95. Yang CF, Wu MT, Chiang AA, et al. Correlation of high-resolution CT and pulmonary function in bronchiolitis obliterans: a study based on 24 patients associated with consumption of Sauropus androgynus. AJR Am J Roentgenol 1997;168:1045–1050.

96. Padley SP, Adler BD, Hansell DM, et al. Bronchiolitis obliterans: high resolution CT findings and correlation with pulmonary function tests. Clin Radiol 1993;47:236–240.

97. Eber CD, Stark P, Bertozzi P. Bronchiolitis obliterans on high-resolution CT: a pattern of mosaic oligemia. J Comput Assist Tomogr 1993;17:853–856.

98. Hansell DM. HRCT of obliterative bronchiolitis and other small airways diseases. Semin Roentgenol 2001;36:51–65.

99. Copley SJ, Wells AU, Müller NL, et al. Thin-section CT in obstructive pulmonary disease: discriminatory value. Radiology 2002;223:812–819.

100. Johkoh T, Ikezoe J, Nagareda T, et al. Metastatic pulmonary calcification: early detection by high-resolution CT. J Comput Assist Tomogr 1993;17:471–473.

101. Hartman TE, Müller NL, Primack SL, et al. Metastatic pulmonary calcification in patients with hypercalcemia: findings on chest radiographs and CT scans. AJR Am J Roentgenol 1994;162:799–802.

102. Greenberg S, Suster B. Metastatic pulmonary calcification: appearance on high resolution CT. J Comput Assist Tomogr 1994;18:497–499.

103. Brodeur FJ Jr, Kazerooni EA. Metastatic pulmonary calcification mimicking air-space disease. Technetium-99m-MDP SPECT imaging. Chest 1994;106:620–622.

104. de Graaf P, Schicht IM, Pauwels EK, et al. Bone scintigraphy in renal osteodystrophy. J Nucl Med 1978;19:1289–1296.

105. Rosenthal DI, Chandler HL, Azizi F, et al. Uptake of bone imaging agents by diffuse pulmonary metastatic calcification. AJR Am J Roentgenol 1977;129:871–874.

106. Taguchi Y, Fuyuno G, Shioya S, et al. MR appearance of pulmonary metastatic calcification. J Comput Assist Tomogr 1996;20:38–41.

107. Antony VB. Drug-induced pleural disease. Clin Chest Med 1998;19:331–340.

108. Selroos O, Edgren J. Lupus-like syndrome associated with pulmonary reaction to nitrofurantoin. Report of three cases. Acta Med Scand 1975;197:125–129.

109. Chudnofsky CR, Otten EJ. Acute pulmonary toxicity to nitrofurantoin. J Emerg Med 1989;7:15–19.

110. Danoff SK, Grasso ME, Terry PB, et al. Pleuropulmonary disease due to pergolide use for restless legs syndrome. Chest 2001;120:313–316.

111. Jones SE, Moore M, Blank N, et al. Hypersensitivity to procarbazine (Matulane) manifested by fever and pleuropulmonary reaction. Cancer 1972;29:498–500.

112. Gefter WB, Epstein DM, Bonavita JA, et al. Pleural thickening caused by Sansert and Ergotrate in the treatment of migraine. AJR Am J Roentgenol 1980;135:375–377.

113. Gonzalez-Rothi RJ, Hannan SE, Hood CI, et al. Amiodarone pulmonary toxicity presenting as bilateral exudative pleural effusions. Chest 1987;92:179–182.

114. Shaunak S, Wilkins A, Pilling JB, et al. Pericardial, retroperitoneal, and pleural fibrosis induced by pergolide. J Neurol Neurosurg Psychiatry 1999;66:79–81.

115. Varsano S, Gershman M, Hamaoui E. Pergolide-induced dyspnea, bilateral pleural effusion and peripheral edema. Respiration 2000;67:580–582.

116. Abbondazo SL, Irey NS, Frizzera G. Dilantin-associated lymphadenopathy. Spectrum of histopathologic patterns. Am J Surg Pathol 1995;19:675–686.

117. Zisman DA, McCune WJ, Tino G, et al. Drug-induced pneumonitis: the role of methotrexate. Sarcoidosis Vasc Diffuse Lung Dis 2001;18:243–252.

118. Rosenow EC 3rd, Limper AH. Drug-induced pulmonary disease. Semin Respir Infect 1995;10:86–95.

119. Malik SW, Myers JL, DeRemee RA, et al. Lung toxicity associated with cyclophosphamide use. Two distinct patterns. Am J Respir Crit Care Med 1996;154:1851–1856.

120. Frankel S, Weiss M, Worrell RP Jr. A "retinoic acid syndrome" in acute promyelocytic leukemia: reversal by corticosteroids. Blood 1991;78:380a.

121. Vahdat L, Maslak P, Miller WH Jr, et al. Early mortality and the retinoic acid syndrome in acute promyelocytic leukemia: impact of leukocytosis, low-dose chemotherapy, PMN/RAR-alpha isoform, and CD13 expression in patients treated with all-*trans* retinoic acid. Blood 1994;84:3843–3849.

122. Vosburgh E. Pulmonary leukostasis secondary to all-*trans* retinoic acid in the treatment of acute promyelocytic leukemia in first relapse. Leukemia 1992;6:608–610.

123. Suzuki S, Shinohara N, Harabayashi T, et al. Complications of bacillus Calmette-Guerin therapy in superficial urothelial cancer: clinical analysis and implications. Int J Clin Oncol 2002;7:289–293.

124. Grange JM. Complications of bacille Calmette-Guerin (BCG) vaccination and immunotherapy and their management. Commun Dis Public Health 1998;1:84–88.

125. Gonzalez OY, Musher DM, Brar I, et al. Spectrum of bacille Calmette-Guerin (BCG) infection after intravesical BCG immunotherapy. Clin Infect Dis 2003;36:140–148.

126. Bellman GC, Sweetser P, Smith AD. Complications of intracavitary bacillus Calmette-Guerin after percutaneous resection of upper tract transitional cell carcinoma. J Urol 1994;151:13–15.

127. Smith RL, Alexander RF, Aranda CP. Pulmonary granulomata. A complication of intravesical administration of bacillus Calmette-Guerin for superficial bladder carcinoma. Cancer 1993;71:1846–1847.

128. Molina JM, Rabian C, D'Agay MF, et al. Hypersensitivity systemic reaction following intravesical bacillus Calmette-Guerin: successful treatment with steroids. J Urol 1992;147:695–697.

129. Lyons D, Miller I, Jeffers A. Systemic hypersensitivity reaction to intravesical BCG. Scott Med J 1994;39:49–50.

130. Leebeek FW, Ouwendijk RJ, Kolk AH, et al. Granulomatous hepatitis caused by bacillus Calmette-Guerin (BCG) infection after BCG bladder instillation. Gut 1996;38:616–618.

131. Iantorno R, Nicolai M, Storto ML, et al. Miliary tuberculosis of the lung in a patient treated with bacillus Calmette-Guerin for superficial bladder cancer. J Urol 1998;159:1639–1640.

132. Rabe J, Neff KW, Lehmann KJ, et al. Miliary tuberculosis after intravesical bacille Calmette-Guerin immunotherapy for carcinoma of the bladder. AJR Am J Roentgenol 1999;172:748–750.

133. Jasmer RM, McCowin MJ, Webb WR. Miliary lung disease after intravesical bacillus Calmette-Guerin immunotherapy. Radiology 1996;201:43–44.

134. Gupta RC, Lavengood R Jr, Smith JP. Miliary tuberculosis due to intravesical bacillus Calmette-Guerin therapy. Chest 1988;94:1296–1298.

135. LeMense GP, Strange C. Granulomatous pneumonitis following intravesical BCG. What therapy is needed? Chest 1994;106:1624–1626.

136. Kamphuis JT, Buiting AG, Misere JF, et al. BCG immunotherapy: be cautious of granulomas. Disseminated BCG infection and mycotic aneurysm as late complications of intravesical BCG instillations. Neth J Med 2001;58:71–75.

137. Geldmacher H, Taube C, Markert U, et al. Nearly fatal complications of cervical lymphadenitis following BCG immunotherapy for superficial bladder cancer. Respiration 2001;68:420–421.

138. Izes JK, Bihrle W 3rd, Thomas CB. Corticosteroid-associated fatal mycobacterial sepsis occurring 3 years after instillation of intravesical bacillus Calmette-Guerin. J Urol 1993;150:1498–1500.

139. Deresiewicz RL, Stone RM, Aster JC. Fatal disseminated mycobacterial infection following intravesical bacillus Calmette-Guerin. J Urol 1990;144:1331–1333, discussion 1333–1334.

140. Tan L, Testa G, Yung T. Diffuse alveolar damage in BCGosis: a rare complication of intravesical bacillus Calmette-Guerin therapy for transitional cell carcinoma. Pathology 1999;31:55–56.

141. Moseley PL, Shasby DM, Brady M, et al. Lung parenchymal injury induced by bleomycin. Am Rev Respir Dis 1984;130:1082–1086.

142. Wolkowicz J, Sturgeon J, Rawji M, et al. Bleomycin-induced pulmonary function abnormalities. Chest 1992;101:97–101.

143. Copper JA Jr. Drug-induced lung disease. Adv Intern Med 1997;42:231–268.

144. Bellamy EA, Husband JE, Blaquiere RM, et al. Bleomycin-related lung damage:

CT evidence. Radiology 1985;156:155–158.

145. Richman SD, Levenson SM, Bunn PA, et al. [67]Ga accumulation in pulmonary lesions associated with bleomycin toxicity. Cancer 1975;36:1966–1972.

146. Aronchick JM, Gefter WB. Drug-induced pulmonary disorders. Semin Roentgenol 1995;30:18–34.

147. Balikian JP, Jochelson MS, Bauer KA, et al. Pulmonary complications of chemotherapy regimens containing bleomycin. AJR Am J Roentgenol 1982;139:455–461.

148. Cohen MB, Austin JH, Smith-Vaniz A, et al. Nodular bleomycin toxicity. Am J Clin Pathol 1989;92:101–104.

149. Santrach PJ, Askin FB, Wells RJ, et al. Nodular form of bleomycin-related pulmonary injury in patients with osteogenic sarcoma. Cancer 1989;64:806–811.

150. Glasier CM, Siegel MJ. Multiple pulmonary nodules: unusual manifestation of bleomycin toxicity. AJR Am J Roentgenol 1981;137:155–156.

151. Ginsberg SJ, Comis RL. The pulmonary toxicity of antineoplastic agents. Semin Oncol 1982;9:34–51.

152. Ben Arush MW, Roguin A, Zamir E, et al. Bleomycin and cyclophosphamide toxicity simulating metastatic nodules to the lungs in childhood cancer. Pediatr Hematol Oncol 1997;14:381–386.

153. Zucker PK, Khouri NF, Rosenshein NB. Bleomycin-induced pulmonary nodules: a variant of bleomycin pulmonary toxicity. Gynecol Oncol 1987;28:284–291.

154. McCrea ES, Diaconis JN, Wade JC, et al. Bleomycin toxicity simulating metastatic nodules to the lungs. Cancer 1981;48:1096–1100.

155. Galton DAG. Myleran in chronic myeloid leukemia. Lancet 1953;i:208–213.

156. Schallier D, Impens N, Warson F, et al. Additive pulmonary toxicity with melphalan and busulfan therapy. Chest 1983;84:492–493.

157. Heard BE, Cooke RA. Busulphan lung. Thorax 1968;23:187–193.

158. Kirschner RH, Esterly JR. Pulmonary lesions associated with busulfan therapy of chronic myelogenous leukemia. Cancer 1971;27:1074–1080.

159. Feingold ML, Koss LG. Effects of long-term administration of busulfan. Report of a patient with generalized nuclear abnormalities, carcinoma of vulva, and pulmonary fibrosis. Arch Intern Med 1969;124:66–71.

160. Spector JI, Zimbler H, Ross JS. Early-onset cyclophosphamide-induced interstitial pneumonitis. JAMA 1979;242:2852–2854.

161. Burke DA, Stoddart JC, Ward MK, Simpson CG. Fatal pulmonary fibrosis occurring during treatment with cyclophosphamide. Br Med J (Clin Res Ed) 1982;285:696.

162. Andersson BS, Cogan BM, Keating MJ, et al. Subacute pulmonary failure complicating therapy with high-dose Ara-C in acute leukemia. Cancer 1985;56:2181–2184.

163. Haupt HM, Hutchins GM, Moore GW. Ara-C lung: noncardiogenic pulmonary edema complicating cytosine arabinoside therapy of leukemia. Am J Med 1981;70:256–261.

164. Twohig KJ, Matthay RA. Pulmonary effects of cytotoxic agents other than bleomycin. Clin Chest Med 1990;11:31–54.

165. Jehn U, Goldel N, Rienmuller R, et al. Non-cardiogenic pulmonary edema complicating intermediate and high-dose Ara C treatment for relapsed acute leukemia. Med Oncol Tumor Pharmacother 1988;5:41–47.

166. Tham RT, Peters WG, de Bruine FT, et al. Pulmonary complications of cytosine-arabinoside therapy: radiographic findings. AJR Am J Roentgenol 1987;149:23–27.

167. Rosenstein M, Ettinghausen SE, Rosenberg SA. Extravasation of intravascular fluid mediated by the systemic administration of recombinant interleukin 2. J Immunol 1986;137:1735–1742.

168. Ognibene FP, Rosenberg SA, Lotze M, et al. Interleukin-2 administration causes reversible hemodynamic changes and left ventricular dysfunction similar to those seen in septic shock. Chest 1988;94:750–754.

169. Gaynor ER, Vitek L, Sticklin L, et al. The hemodynamic effects of treatment with interleukin-2 and lymphokine-activated killer cells. Ann Intern Med 1988;109:953–958.

170. Conant EF, Fox KR, Miller WT. Pulmonary edema as a complication of interleukin-2 therapy. AJR Am J Roentgenol 1989;152:749–752.

171. Davis SD, Berkmen YM, Wang JC. Interleukin-2 therapy for advanced renal cell carcinoma: radiographic evaluation of response and complications. Radiology 1990;177:127–131.

172. Mann H, Ward JH, Samlowski WE. Vascular leak syndrome associated with interleukin-2: chest radiographic manifestations. Radiology 1990;176:191–194.

173. Saxon RR, Klein JS, Bar MH, et al. Pathogenesis of pulmonary edema during interleukin-2 therapy: correlation of chest radiographic and clinical findings in 54 patients. AJR Am J Roentgenol 1991;156:281–285.

174. White RL Jr, Schwartzentruber DJ, Guleria A, et al. Cardiopulmonary toxicity of treatment with high dose interleukin-2 in 199 consecutive patients with metastatic melanoma or renal cell carcinoma. Cancer 1994;74:3212–3222.

175. Snydman DR, Sullivan B, Gill M, et al. Nosocomial sepsis associated with interleukin-2. Ann Intern Med 1990;112:102–107.

176. Rosenberg SA, Lotze MT, Muul LM, et al. A progress report on the treatment of 157 patients with advanced cancer using lymphokine-activated killer cells and interleukin-2 or high-dose interleukin-2 alone. N Engl J Med 1987;316:889–897.

177. Sostman HD, Matthay RA, Putman CE, et al. Methotrexate-induced pneumonitis. Medicine (Baltimore) 1976;55:371–388.

178. Gockerman JP. Drug-induced interstitial lung diseases. Clin Chest Med 1982;3:521–536.

179. Sharma A, Provenzale D, McKusick A, et al. Interstitial pneumonitis after low-dose methotrexate therapy in primary biliary cirrhosis. Gastroenterology 1994;107:266–270.

180. Dawson JK, Graham DR, Desmond J, et al. Investigation of the chronic pulmonary effects of low-dose oral methotrexate in patients with rheumatoid arthritis: a prospective study incorporating HRCT scanning and pulmonary function tests. Rheumatology (Oxford) 2002;41:262–267.

181. Everts CS, Westcott JL, Bragg DG. Methotrexate therapy and pulmonary disease. Radiology 1973;107:539–543.

182. Cannon GW. Methotrexate pulmonary toxicity. Rheum Dis Clin North Am 1997;23:917–937.

183. Urban C, Nirenberg A, Caparros B, et al. Chemical pleuritis as the cause of acute chest pain following high-dose methotrexate treatment. Cancer 1983;51:34–37.

184. Walden PA, Mitchell-Weggs PF, Coppin C, et al. Pleurisy and methotrexate treatment. Br Med J 1977;2:867.

185. Bernstein ML, Sobel DB, Wimmer RS. Noncardiogenic pulmonary edema following injection of methotrexate into the cerebrospinal fluid. Cancer 1982;50:866–868.

186. Verweij J, van Zanten T, Souren T, et al. Prospective study on the dose relationship of mitomycin C-induced interstitial pneumonitis. Cancer 1987;60:756–761.

187. Ozols RF, Hogan WM, Ostchega Y, et al. MVP (mitomycin, vinblastine, and progesterone): a second-line regimen in ovarian cancer with a high incidence of pulmonary toxicity. Cancer Treat Rep 1983;67:721–722.

188. Cantrell JE Jr, Phillips TM, Schein PS. Carcinoma-associated hemolytic-uremic syndrome: a complication of mitomycin C chemotherapy. J Clin Oncol 1985;3:723–734.

189. McCarthy JT, Staats BA. Pulmonary hypertension, hemolytic anemia, and renal failure. A mitomycin-associated syndrome. Chest 1986;89:608–611.

190. Sheldon R, Slaughter D. A syndrome of microangiopathic hemolytic anemia, renal impairment, and pulmonary edema in chemotherapy-treated patients with adenocarcinoma. Cancer 1986;58: 1428–1436.

191. Litam JP, Dail DH, Spitzer G, et al. Early pulmonary toxicity after administration of high-dose BCNU. Cancer Treat Rep 1981;65:39–44.

192. Weinstein AS, Diener-West M, Nelson DF, Pakuris E. Pulmonary toxicity of carmustine in patients treated for malignant glioma. Cancer Treat Rep 1986;70:943–946.

193. O'Driscoll BR, Kalra S, Gattamaneni HR, et al. Late carmustine lung fibrosis. Age at treatment may influence severity and survival. Chest 1995;107:1355–1357.

194. Iacovino JR, Leitner J, Abbas AK, et al. Fatal pulmonary reaction from low doses of bleomycin. An idiosyncratic tissue response. JAMA 1976;235:1253–1255.

195. Wilson KS, Brigden ML, Alexander S, et al. Fatal pneumothorax in "BCNU lung". Med Pediatr Oncol 1982;10: 195–199.

196. Parish JM, Muhm JR, Leslie KO. Upper lobe pulmonary fibrosis associated with high-dose chemotherapy containing BCNU for bone marrow transplantation. Mayo Clin Proc 2003;78:630–634.

197. Vetter N, Berger E, Otupal I, et al. [Recurrent bilateral pneumothorax in progressive lung fibrosis following combination therapy with BCNU]. Prax Klin Pneumol 1985;39:102–105.

198. O'Driscoll BR, Hasleton PS, Taylor PM, et al. Active lung fibrosis up to 17 years after chemotherapy with carmustine (BCNU) in childhood. N Engl J Med 1990;323:378–382.

199. Taylor PM, O'Driscoll BR, Gattamaneni HR, et al. Chronic lung fibrosis following carmustine (BCNU) chemotherapy: radiological features. Clin Radiol 1991;44:299–301.

200. Chen YM, Perng RP, Lin WC, et al. Phase II study of docetaxel and gemcitabine combination chemotherapy in non-small-cell lung cancer patients failing previous chemotherapy. Am J Clin Oncol 2002;25:509–12.

201. Dunsford ML, Mead GM, Bateman AC, et al. Severe pulmonary toxicity in patients treated with a combination of docetaxel and gemcitabine for metastatic transitional cell carcinoma. Ann Oncol 1999;10:943–947.

202. Read WL, Mortimer JE, Picus J. Severe interstitial pneumonitis associated with docetaxel administration. Cancer 2002;94:847–853.

203. Helman DL Jr, Byrd JC, Ales NC, et al. Fludarabine-related pulmonary toxicity: a distinct clinical entity in chronic lymphoproliferative syndromes. Chest 2002;122:785–790.

204. Sabria-Trias J, Bonnaud F, Sioniac M. [Severe interstitial pneumonitis related to Gemcitabine]. Rev Mal Respir 2002;19:645–647.

205. Roychowdhury DF, Cassidy CA, Peterson P, et al. A report on serious pulmonary toxicity associated with gemcitabine-based therapy. Invest New Drugs 2002;20:311–315.

206. Kirkbride P, Hatton M, Lorigan P, et al. Fatal pulmonary fibrosis associated with induction chemotherapy with carboplatin and vinorelbine followed by CHART radiotherapy for locally advanced non-small cell lung cancer. Clin Oncol 2002;14:361–366.

207. Inoue A, Saijo Y, Maemondo M, et al. Severe acute interstitial pneumonia and gefitinib. Lancet 2003;361:137–139.

208. Huisman C, Postmus PE, Giaccone G, et al. A phase I study of sequential intravenous topotecan and etoposide in lung cancer patients. Ann Oncol 2001;12:1567–1573.

209. Ramanathan RK, Reddy VV, Holbert JM, et al. Pulmonary infiltrates following administration of paclitaxel. Chest 1996;110:289–292.

210. Eisenhauer EA, Vermorken JB. The taxoids. Comparative clinical pharmacology and therapeutic potential. Drugs 1998;55:5–30.

211. Pavlakis N, Bell DR, Millward MJ, et al. Fatal pulmonary toxicity resulting from treatment with gemcitabine. Cancer 1997;80:286–291.

212. Ash-Bernal R, Browner I, Erlich R. Early detection and successful treatment of drug-induced pneumonitis with corticosteroids. Cancer Invest 2002;20:876–879.

213. Gefter WB, Epstein DM, Pietra GG, et al. Lung disease caused by amiodarone, a new antiarrythmic agent. Radiology 1983;147:339–344.

214. Kennedy JI Jr. Clinical aspects of amiodarone pulmonary toxicity. Clin Chest Med 1990;11:119–129.

215. Kay GN, Epstein AE, Kirklin JK, et al. Fatal postoperative amiodarone pulmonary toxicity. Am J Cardiol 1988;62:490–492.

216. Ashrafian H, Davey P. Is amiodarone an underrecognized cause of acute respiratory failure in the ICU? Chest 2001;120:275–282.

217. Jessurun GA, Hoogenberg K, Crijns HJ. Bronchiolitis obliterans organizing pneumonia during low-dose amiodarone therapy. Clin Cardiol 1997;20:300–302.

218. Jessurun GA, Boersma WG, Crijns HJ. Amiodarone-induced pulmonary toxicity. Predisposing factors, clinical symptoms and treatment. Drug Safety 1998;18:339–344.

219. Poll LW, May P, Koch JA, et al. HRCT findings of amiodarone pulmonary toxicity: clinical and radiologic regression. J Cardiovasc Pharmacol Ther 2001;6:307–311.

220. Fraire AE, Guntupalli KK, Greenberg SD, et al. Amiodarone pulmonary toxicity: a multidisciplinary review of current status. South Med J 1993;86:67–77.

221. Nicholson AA, Hayward C. The value of computed tomography in the diagnosis of amiodarone-induced pulmonary toxicity. Clin Radiol 1989;40:564–567.

222. Sunderji R, Kanji Z, Gin K. Pulmonary effects of low dose amiodarone: a review of the risks and recommendations for surveillance. Can J Cardiol 2000;16: 1435–1440.

223. Vorperian VR, Havighurst TC, Miller S, et al. Adverse effects of low dose amiodarone: a meta-analysis. J Am Coll Cardiol 1997;30:791–798.

224. Ott MC, Khoor A, Leventhal JP, et al. Pulmonary toxicity in patients receiving low-dose amiodarone. Chest 2003;123:646–651.

225. Kaushik S, Hussain A, Clarke P, et al. Acute pulmonary toxicity after low-dose amiodarone therapy. Ann Thorac Surg 2001;72:1760–1761.

226. Kinnunen E, Viljanen A. Pleuropulmonary involvement during bromocriptine treatment. Chest 1988;94:1034–1036.

227. McElvaney NG, Wilcox PG, Churg A, et al. Pleuropulmonary disease during bromocriptine treatment of Parkinson's disease. Arch Intern Med 1988;148:2231–2236.

228. Daly AL, Velazquez LA, Bradley SF, et al. Mucormycosis: association with deferoxamine therapy. Am J Med 1989;87:468–471.

229. Boelaert JR, Fenves AZ, Coburn JW. Deferoxamine therapy and mucormycosis in dialysis patients: report of an international registry. Am J Kidney Dis 1991;18:660–667.

230. Jeng YM, Tien HF, Su IJ. Phenytoin-induced pseudolymphoma: reevaluation using modern molecular biology techniques. Epilepsia 1996;37:104–107.

231. Gungor E, Alli N, Comoglu S, et al. Phenytoin hypersensitivity syndrome. Neurol Sci 2001;22:261–265.

232. Kaur S, Sarkar R, Thami GP, et al. Anticonvulsant hypersensitivity syndrome. Pediatr Dermatol 2002; 19:142–145.

233. Knowles SR, Shapiro LE, Shear NH. Anticonvulsant hypersensitivity syndrome: incidence, prevention and management. Drug Safety 1999;21:489–501.

234. Gross SB, Lepor NE. Anorexigen-related cardiopulmonary toxicity. Rev Cardiovasc Med 2000;1:80–89, 102.

235. Rothman RB, Ayestas MA, Dersch CM, et al. Aminorex, fenfluramine, and chlorphentermine are serotonin transporter substrates. Implications for primary pulmonary hypertension. Circulation 1999;100:869–875.

236. Zitnik RJ, Cooper JA Jr. Pulmonary disease due to antirheumatic agents. Clin Chest Med 1990;11:139–150.

237. Evans RB, Ettensohn DB, Fawaz-Estrup F, et al. Gold lung: recent developments in pathogenesis, diagnosis, and therapy. Semin Arthritis Rheum 1987;16:196–205.

238. Weaver LT, Law JS. Lung changes after gold salts. Br J Dis Chest 1978;72:247–250.

239. Biron P, Dessureault J, Napke E. Acute allergic interstitial pneumonitis induced by hydrochlorothiazide. Cmaj 1991;145:28–34.

240. Pfitzenmeyer P, Foucher P, Dennewald G, et al. Pleuropulmonary changes induced by ergoline drugs. Eur Respir J 1996;9:1013–1019.

241. Fibrosis due to ergot derivatives: exposure to risk should be weighed up. Prescrire Int 2002;11:186–189.

242. Taal BG, Spierings EL, Hilvering C. Pleuropulmonary fibrosis associated with chronic and excessive intake of ergotamine. Thorax 1983;38:396–398.

243. Smith WR, Wells ID, Glauser FL. Immunologic abnormalities in heroin lung. Chest 1975;68:651–653.

244. Gotway MB, Marder SR, Hanks DK, et al. Thoracic complications of illicit drug use: an organ system approach. RadioGraphics 2002;22(Suppl):S119–135.

245. Alcantara AL, Tucker RB, McCarroll KA. Radiologic study of injection drug use complications. Infect Dis Clin North Am 2002;16:713–743.

246. VanDette JM, Cornish LA. Medical complications of illicit cocaine use. Clin Pharm 1989;8:401–411.

247. Loper KA. Clinical toxicology of cocaine. Med Toxicol Adverse Drug Exp 1989;4:174–185.

248. Perper JA, Van Thiel DH. Cardiovascular complications of cocaine abuse. Recent Dev Alcohol 1992;10:343–361.

249. Williams RG, Kavanagh KM, Teo KK. Pathophysiology and treatment of cocaine toxicity: implications for the heart and cardiovascular system. Can J Cardiol 1996;12:1295–1301.

250. Isner JM, Estes NA 3rd, Thompson PD, et al. Acute cardiac events temporally related to cocaine abuse. N Engl J Med 1986;315:1438–1443.

251. Murray RJ, Albin RJ, Mergner W, et al. Diffuse alveolar hemorrhage temporally related to cocaine smoking. Chest 1988;93:427–429.

252. Allred RJ, Ewer S. Fatal pulmonary edema following intravenous "freebase" cocaine use. Ann Emerg Med 1981;10:441–442.

253. Cucco RA, Yoo OH, Cregler L, et al. Nonfatal pulmonary edema after "freebase" cocaine smoking. Am Rev Respir Dis 1987;136:179–181.

254. Hoffman CK, Goodman PC. Pulmonary edema in cocaine smokers. Radiology 1989;172:463–465.

255. Eurman DW, Potash HI, Eyler WR, et al. Chest pain and dyspnea related to "crack" cocaine smoking: value of chest radiography. Radiology 1989;172:459–462.

256. Brody SL, Anderson GV Jr, Gutman JB. Pneumomediastinum as a complication of "crack" smoking. Am J Emerg Med 1988;6:241–243.

257. Shesser R, Davis C, Edelstein S. Pneumomediastinum and pneumothorax after inhaling alkaloidal cocaine. Ann Emerg Med 1981;10:213–215.

258. Savader SJ, Omori M, Martinez CR. Pneumothorax, pneumomediastinum, and pneumopericardium: complications of cocaine smoking. J Fla Med Assoc 1988;75:151–152.

259. Seaman ME. Barotrauma related to inhalational drug abuse. J Emerg Med 1990;8:141–149.

260. Kissner DG, Lawrence WD, Selis JE, et al. Crack lung: pulmonary disease caused by cocaine abuse. Am Rev Respir Dis 1987;136:1250–1252.

261. Holmberg L, Boman G. Pulmonary reactions to nitrofurantoin. 447 cases reported to the Swedish Adverse Drug Reaction Committee 1966–1976. Eur J Respir Dis 1981;62:180–189.

262. Cohen AJ, King TE Jr, Downey GP. Rapidly progressive bronchiolitis obliterans with organizing pneumonia. Am J Respir Crit Care Med 1994;149:1670–1675.

263. Sheehan RE, Wells AU, Milne DG, et al. Nitrofurantoin-induced lung disease: two cases demonstrating resolution of apparently irreversible CT abnormalities. J Comput Assist Tomogr 2000;24:259–261.

264. Rowe PA, Rocker GM, Morgan AG, et al. OKT3 and pulmonary capillary permeability. Br Med J (Clin Res Ed) 1987;295:1099–1100.

265. Lee CW, Logan JL, Zukoski CF. Cardiovascular collapse following orthoclone OKT3 administration: a case report. Am J Kidney Dis 1991;17:73–75.

266. Costanzo-Nordin MR. Cardiopulmonary effects of OKT3: determinants of hypotension, pulmonary edema, and cardiac dysfunction. Transplant Proc 1993;25:21–24.

267. Jackson RM. Pulmonary oxygen toxicity. Chest 1985;88:900–905.

268. Griscom NT. Caldwell Lecture. Respiratory problems of early life now allowing survival into adulthood: concepts for radiologists. AJR Am J Roentgenol 1992;158:1–8.

269. Fitzgerald P, Donoghue V, Gorman W. Bronchopulmonary dysplasia: a radiographic and clinical review of 20 patients. Br J Radiol 1990;63:444–447.

270. Lanning P, Tammela O, Koivisto M. Radiological incidence and course of bronchopulmonary dysplasia in 100 consecutive low birth weight neonates. Acta Radiol 1995;36:353–357.

271. Mortensson W, Lindroth M. The course of bronchopulmonary dysplasia. A radiographic follow-up. Acta Radiol Diagn (Stockh) 1986;27:19–22.

272. Griscom NT, Wheeler WB, Sweezey NB, et al. Bronchopulmonary dysplasia: radiographic appearance in middle childhood. Radiology 1989;171:811–814.

273. Oppenheim C, Mamou-Mani T, Sayegh N, et al. Bronchopulmonary dysplasia: value of CT in identifying pulmonary sequelae. AJR Am J Roentgenol 1994;163:169–172.

274. Howling SJ, Northway WH Jr, Hansell DM, et al. Pulmonary sequelae of bronchopulmonary dysplasia survivors: high-resolution CT findings. AJR Am J Roentgenol 2000;174:1323–1326.

275. Aquino SL, Schechter MS, Chiles C, et al. High-resolution inspiratory and expiratory CT in older children and adults with bronchopulmonary dysplasia. AJR Am J Roentgenol 1999;173:963–967.

276. Sternlieb I, Bennett B, Scheinberg IH. D-penicillamine induced Goodpasture's syndrome in Wilson's disease. Ann Intern Med 1975;82:673–676.

277. Niehoff JM, Baltatzis PA. Adult respiratory distress syndrome induced by salicylate toxicity. Postgrad Med 1985;78:117–119,123.

278. Fisher CJ Jr, Albertson TE, Foulke GE. Salicylate-induced pulmonary edema: clinical characteristics in children. Am J Emerg Med 1985;3:33–37.

279. Leatherman JW, Schmitz PG. Fever, hyperdynamic shock, and multiple-system organ failure. A pseudo-sepsis syndrome associated with chronic salicylate intoxication. Chest 1991;100:1391–1396.

280. Chalasani N, Roman J, Jurado RL. Systemic inflammatory response syndrome caused by chronic salicylate intoxication. South Med J 1996;89:479–482.

281. Roy TM, Ossorio MA, Cipolla LM, et al. Pulmonary complications after tricyclic antidepressant overdose. Chest 1989;96:852–856.

282. Varnell RM, Godwin JD, Richardson ML, et al. Adult respiratory distress syndrome from overdose of tricyclic antidepressants. Radiology 1989;170:667–670.

283. Dahlin KL, Lastbom L, Blomgren B, et al. Acute lung failure induced by tricyclic antidepressants. Toxicol Appl Pharmacol 1997;146:309–316.

284. Dahlin KL, Mortberg A, Lastbom L, et al. Amitriptyline-induced release of endothelin-1 in isolated perfused and ventilated rat lungs. Pharmacol Toxicol 1999;85:288–293.

285. Liu X, Emery CJ, Laude E, et al. Adverse pulmonary vascular effects of high dose tricyclic antidepressants: acute and chronic animal studies. Eur Respir J 2002;20:344–352.

286. Libshitz HI. Thoracic radiotherapy changes. In: Herman PG, ed. Iatrogenic thoracic complications. New York: Springer-Verlag, 1983:141–160.

287. Abratt RP, Morgan GW. Lung toxicity following chest irradiation in patients with lung cancer. Lung Cancer 2002;35:103–109.

288. Hill RP, Rodemann HP, Hendry JH, et al. Normal tissue radiobiology: from the laboratory to the clinic. Int J Radiat Oncol Biol Phys 2001;49:353–365.

289. Vujaskovic Z, Marks LB, Anscher MS. The physical parameters and molecular events associated with radiation-induced lung toxicity. Semin Radiat Oncol 2000;10:296–307.

290. Vallebona A. Cardiac damage following therapeutic chest irradiation. Importance, evaluation and treatment. Minerva Cardioangiol 2000;48:79–87.

291. Lamoureux K. Increased clinically symptomatic pulmonary radiation reactions with adjuvant chemotherapy. Cancer Chemother Res (part I) 1975;35:1322–1324.

292. Cassady JR, Richter MP, Piro AJ, et al. Radiation-adriamycin interactions: preliminary clinical observations. Cancer 1975;36:946–949.

293. Ma LD, Taylor GA, Wharam MD, et al. "Recall" pneumonitis: adriamycin potentiation of radiation pneumonitis in two children. Radiology 1993;187:465–467.

294. Parris TM, Knight JG, Hess CE. Severe radiation pneumonitis precipitated by withdrawal of steroids: a diagnostic and therapeutic dilemma. AJR Am J Roentgenol 1970;132:284–286.

295. Crestani B, Valeyre D, Roden S, et al. Bronchiolitis obliterans organizing pneumonia syndrome primed by radiation therapy to the breast. The Groupe d'Etudes et de Recherche sur les Maladies Orphelines Pulmonaires (GERM"O"P). Am J Respir Crit Care Med 1998;158:1929–1935.

296. Stover DE, Milite F, Zakowski M. A newly recognized syndrome—radiation-related bronchiolitis obliterans and organizing pneumonia. A case report and literature review. Respiration 2001;68:540–544.

297. Arbetter KR, Prakash UB, Tazelaar HD, et al. Radiation-induced pneumonitis in the "nonirradiated" lung. Mayo Clin Proc 1999;74:27–36.

298. Cox JB, Ang KK. In: Radiation oncology: rationale, technique, results, 8th edn. St Louis: Mosby, 2002.

299. Slavin JD Jr, Friedman NC, Spencer RP. Radiation effects on pulmonary ventilation and perfusion. Clin Nucl Med 1993;18:81–82.

300. Ikezoe J, Takashima S, Morimoto S, et al. CT appearance of acute radiation-induced injury in the lung. AJR Am J Roentgenol 1988;150:765–770.

301. Kataoka M, Kawamura M, Ueda N, et al. Diffuse gallium-67 uptake in radiation pneumonitis. Clin Nucl Med 1990;15:707–711.

302. Davis SD, Yankelevitz DF, Henschke CI. Radiation effects on the lung: clinical features, pathology, and imaging findings. AJR Am J Roentgenol 1992;159:1157–1164.

303. Bachman AL, Macken K. Pleural effusions following supervoltage radiation for breast carcinoma. Radiology 1959;72:699–709.

304. Libshitz HI, Shuman LS. Radiation-induced pulmonary change: CT findings. J Comput Assist Tomogr 1984;8:15–19.

305. Bell J, McGivern D, Bullimore J, et al. Diagnostic imaging of post-irradiation changes in the chest. Clin Radiol 1988;39:109–119.

306. Bluemke DA, Fishman EK, Kuhlman JE, et al. Complications of radiation therapy: CT evaluation. RadioGraphics 1991;11:581–600.

307. Glatstein E. Intensity-modulated radiation therapy: the inverse, the converse, and the perverse. Semin Radiat Oncol 2002;12:272–281.

308. Leibel SA, Fuks Z, Zelefsky MJ, et al. Intensity-modulated radiotherapy. Cancer J 2002;8:164–176.

309. Patel RR, Mehta M. Three-dimensional conformal radiotherapy for lung cancer: promises and pitfalls. Curr Oncol Rep 2002;4:347–353.

310. Koenig TR, Munden RF, Erasmus JJ, et al. Radiation injury of the lung after three-dimensional conformal radiation therapy. AJR Am J Roentgenol 2002;178:1383–1388.

311. Mesurolle B, Qanadli SD, Merad M, et al. Unusual radiologic findings in the thorax after radiation therapy. RadioGraphics 2000;20:67–81.

312. Farmer W, Ravin C, Schachter EN. Hyperlucent lung after radiation therapy. Am Rev Respir Dis 1975;112:255–258.

313. Wencel ML, Sitrin RG. Unilateral lung hyperlucency after mediastinal irradiation. Am Rev Respir Dis 1988;137:955–957.

314. Blane CE, Silberstein RJ, Sue JY. Radiation therapy and spontaneous pneumothorax. J Can Assoc Radiol 1981;32:153–154.

315. Rowinsky EK, Abeloff MD, Wharam MD. Spontaneous pneumothorax following thoracic irradiation. Chest 1985;88:703–708.

316. Fentanes de Torres E, Guevara E. Pleuritis by radiation: reports of two cases. Acta Cytol 1981;25:427–429.

317. Whitcomb ME, Schwarz MI. Pleural effusion complicating intensive mediastinal radiation therapy. Am Rev Respir Dis 1971;103:100–107.

318. Hill CA, North LB, Osborne BM. Bronchogenic carcinoma in breast carcinoma patients. AJR Am J Roentgenol 1983;140:259–264.

319. Huvos AG, Woodard HQ, Cahan WG, et al. Postradiation osteogenic sarcoma of bone and soft tissues. A clinicopathologic study of 66 patients. Cancer 1985;55:1244–1255.

320. Little MP. Cancer after exposure to radiation in the course of treatment for benign and malignant disease. Lancet Oncol 2001;2:212–220.

321. Patel SR. Radiation-induced sarcoma. Curr Treat Options Oncol 2000;1:258–261.

322. Travis LB. Therapy-associated solid tumors. Acta Oncol 2002;41:323–333.

323. Harrison JD, Muirhead CR. Quantitative comparisons of cancer induction in humans by internally deposited radionuclides and external radiation. Int J Radiat Biol 2003;79:1–13.

324. Jenkin D, Greenberg M, Fitzgerald A. Second malignant tumours in childhood Hodgkin's disease. Med Pediatr Oncol 1996;26:373–379.

325. Meadows AT. Second tumours. Eur J Cancer 2001;37:2074–2079; discussion 2079–2081.

326. Hall EJ, Wuu CS. Radiation-induced second cancers: the impact of 3D-CRT and IMRT. Int J Radiat Oncol Biol Phys 2003;56:83–88.

327. Glazer HS, Lee JK, Levitt RG, et al. Radiation fibrosis: differentiation from recurrent tumor by MR imaging. Radiology 1985;156:721–726.

328. Werthmuller WC, Schiebler ML, Whaley RA, et al. Gadolinium-DTPA enhancement of lung radiation fibrosis. J Comput Assist Tomogr 1989;13:946–948.

329. Charles HC, Baker ME, Hathorn JW, et al. Differentiation of radiation fibrosis from recurrent neoplasia: a role for 31P MR spectroscopy? AJR Am J Roentgenol 1990;154:67–68.

330. Frank A, Lefkowitz D, Jaeger S, et al. Decision logic for retreatment of asymptomatic lung cancer recurrence based on positron emission tomography findings. Int J Radiat Oncol Biol Phys 1995;32:1495–1512.

331. Ichiya Y, Kuwabara Y, Otsuka M, et al. Assessment of response to cancer therapy using fluorine-18-fluorodeoxyglucose and positron emission tomography. J Nucl Med 1991;32:1655–1660.

332. Inoue T, Kim EE, Komaki R, et al. Detecting recurrent or residual lung cancer with FDG-PET. J Nucl Med 1995;36:788–793.

333. Kim EE, Chung SK, Haynie TP, et al. Differentiation of residual or recurrent tumors from post-treatment changes with F-18 FDG PET. RadioGraphics 1992;12:269–279.

334. Patz EF, Jr., Lowe VJ, Hoffman JM, et al. Persistent or recurrent bronchogenic carcinoma: detection with PET and 2-[F-18]-2-deoxy-D-glucose. Radiology 1994;191:379–382.

335. Duhaylongsod FG, Lowe VJ, Patz EF Jr, et al. Detection of primary and recurrent lung cancer by means of F-18 fluorodeoxyglucose positron emission tomography (FDG PET). J Thorac Cardiovasc Surg 1995;110:130–139; discussion 139–140.

336. Kubota K, Yamada S, Ishiwata K, et al. Positron emission tomography for treatment evaluation and recurrence detection compared with CT in long-term follow-up cases of lung cancer. Clin Nucl Med 1992;17:877–881.

337. Kubota K, Yamada S, Ishiwata K, et al. Evaluation of the treatment response of lung cancer with positron emission tomography and L-[methyl-11C]methionine: a preliminary study. Eur J Nucl Med 1993;20:495–501.

338. Dalinka MK, Mazzeo VP Jr. Complications of radiation therapy. Crit Rev Diagn Imaging 1985;23:235–267.

339. Rouanet P, Fabre JM, Tica V, et al. Chest wall reconstruction for radionecrosis after breast carcinoma therapy. Ann Plast Surg 1995;34:465–470.

340. Delanian S, Lefaix JL. [Mature bone radionecrosis: from recent physiopathological knowledge to an innovative therapeutic action]. Cancer Radiother 2002;6:1–9.

341. Howland WJ, Loeffler RK, Starchman DE, et al. Postirradiation atrophic changes of bone and related complications. Radiology 1975;117:677–685.

342. Gutierrez CA, Just-Viera JO. Clinical spectrum of radiation induced pericarditis. Am Surg 1983;49:113–115.

343. Annest LS, Anderson RP, Li W, et al. Coronary artery disease following mediastinal radiation therapy. J Thorac Cardiovasc Surg 1983;85:257–263.

344. Corn BW, Trock BJ, Goodman RL. Irradiation-related ischemic heart disease. J Clin Oncol 1990;8:741–750.

345. Zimmermann FB, Geinitz H, Feldmann HJ. Therapy and prophylaxis of acute and late radiation-induced sequelae of the esophagus. Strahlenther Onkol 1998;174 (Suppl 3):78–81.

346. Trowers E, Thomas C Jr, Silverstein FE. Chemical- and radiation-induced esophageal injury. Gastrointest Endosc Clin N Am 1994;4:657–675.

347. Chowhan NM. Injurious effects of radiation on the esophagus. Am J Gastroenterol 1990;85:115–120.

CHAPTER 10

Idiopathic pneumonias and immunologic diseases of the lungs

IDIOPATHIC INTERSTITIAL PNEUMONIAS

The term idiopathic interstitial pneumonia (IIP) is applied to a group of disorders with distinct histologic and radiologic appearances, and without a known cause. The concept of interstitial pneumonia was first propounded by Liebow and Carrington, and the first comprehensive and critical attempt to subdivide IIP based on histologic changes was made by Liebow,[1] dividing these cases into five groups (Box 10.1). Over time, this list has been repeatedly revised.[2–4] Giant cell interstitial pneumonia is no longer included as it is usually a manifestation of hard metal pneumoconiosis.[5,6] Bronchiolitis interstitial pneumonia was renamed (in the United Kingdom) as cryptogenic organizing pneumonia (COP),[7] and (in the United States) as bronchiolitis obliterans organizing pneumonia (BOOP).[8] Despite the attractions of the mellifluous acronym BOOP, COP is now the recommended term.[4] Although it is now recognized that most cases of lymphoid interstitial pneumonia (LIP) are secondary to other underlying conditions such as acquired immune deficiency syndrome (AIDS) or Sjögren syndrome,[9,10] LIP is still included. The newly recognized entities of acute interstitial pneumonia (AIP) and nonspecific interstitial pneumonia (NSIP) have been added.

Box 10.1 Liebow classification of idiopathic interstitial pneumonias[1]

Usual interstitial pneumonia (UIP)
Desquamative interstitial pneumonia (DIP)
Bronchiolitis obliterans with interstitial pneumonia (BIP)
Lymphoid interstitial pneumonia (LIP)
Giant cell interstitial pneumonia (GIP)

None of the previous classifications of the IIPs[1–3] has clearly delineated the complementary roles of the pathologist, radiologist, and clinician in diagnosing these conditions. Because of this, and because of substantial variation in definition and terminology of the IIPs, the American Thoracic Society (ATS) and the European Respiratory Society (ERS) convened an international committee of pulmonologists, thoracic radiologists, and pulmonary pathologists to clarify the nomenclature and typical patterns of these conditions. The classification is published in full in the American Journal of Respiratory and Critical Care Medicine.[4] The classification includes the following interstitial pneumonias: usual interstitial pneumonia (UIP), NSIP, AIP, desquamative interstitial pneumonia (DIP) and its related entity respiratory bronchiolitis-interstitial lung disease (RB-ILD), LIP, and COP (Table 10.1, Box 10.2). The key concepts underlying the classification are as follows (Box 10.3):

1. The classification is based on histologic criteria, but there is a clear recognition that the CT pattern is important in delineating the macroscopic morphology of the IIPs.
2. Each pattern of interstitial pneumonia may be idiopathic or may be secondary to some identifiable cause such as collagen vascular disease, drugs, or inhalation exposure. Careful clinical evaluation is required to identify an underlying cause for the interstitial pneumonia. The classification clearly separates the morphologic pattern identified by the pathologist and radiologist (which may or may not be idiopathic), from the idiopathic clinical syndrome identified by the clinician. For example, the term idiopathic pulmonary fibrosis (IPF) is reserved for the idiopathic clinical syndrome associated with the morphologic pattern of UIP. The pathologist and radiologist are encouraged to use the term "pattern" when referring to morphologic findings, to emphasize the fact that these morphologic patterns may be due to a variety of types of lung injury.
3. The clinician, radiologist, and pathologist have complementary roles in the diagnosis of the interstitial pneumonias. The final diagnosis is made by integration of the clinical, imaging, and pathologic features.

Histologically, UIP is the most common of the IIPs.[11–14] NSIP and COP are also relatively common, while AIP, DIP, RB-ILD, and LIP are relatively rare.

The 5 year survival in patients with histologic UIP ranges from 15 to 40%, compared with 60–100% for NSIP, and 100% for DIP.[11,13–15] Because of these substantial differences in survival, it is important to clearly separate those patients who have the UIP pattern on histology or imaging from those with other patterns. In those patients who do not undergo biopsy, the CT pattern becomes central in making this distinction.

The emergence of the current classification has depended critically on examination of sizeable specimens of lung (obtained by thoracoscopy or thoracotomy), allowing assessment not only of the nature of the inflammation and fibrosis but also the spatial and temporal distribution of lesions.[3] Nevertheless, it needs to be recognized that a biopsy specimen, however generous, may not be wholly representative, and that different histopathologic subtypes can coexist in a given patient.[16] For these reasons, evaluation by CT is important to determine whether the dominant imaging pattern is consistent with the histologic diagnosis.

Before the publication of the ATS statement on IPF,[17] and the ATS/ERS classification of IIPs,[4] the terms "idiopathic pulmonary fibrosis" (in the United States),[18–21] "cryptogenic fibrosing alveolitis" (in the United Kingdom and Canada),[22–30] or "idiopathic interstitial pneumonia" were generally used to refer to patients who presented with an idiopathic clinical syndrome of progressive shortness of breath associated with physiologic and imaging evidence of interstitial lung disease. On review of the biopsies of such patients using current criteria, the histologic diagnosis is UIP in 50–60% of cases, NSIP in 15–35%, and DIP or RB-ILD in 10–15%.[11–15] Previously published case series of such patients therefore comprise variable and undefined proportions of UIP, NSIP, DIP, and RB-ILD. For this reason, previous descriptions of the imaging appearances of these patients are very difficult to interpret.

The term cryptogenic fibrosing alveolitis (CFA) is applied to patients presenting with a clinical syndrome of IIP. However, it has become clear that understanding of the morphologic pattern of the interstitial pneumonia is of critical importance in determining the likelihood of response to treatment and the likely survival. The use of an umbrella term like CFA, though useful in describing the common clinical presentation of UIP, DIP, and NSIP, obscures the importance of a more precise morphologic description based on histology and/or CT. In this chapter, the term CFA will be used only to describe the clinical presentation of patients with IIP, and the more specific morphologic descriptors of UIP, NSIP, etc, will be used in discussing the imaging appearances.

Despite the importance of morphologic characterization, biopsy has been relatively uncommon in patients presenting

Table 10.1 Current classification of idiopathic interstitial pneumonias.[4]

Morphologic entity	Associated clinical syndrome	Histologic findings	CT features and distribution	Radiologic differential diagnosis
Usual interstitial pneumonia	Idiopathic pulmonary fibrosis	Heterogeneous areas of young connective tissue, scarring, honeycombing, and normal lung Fibroblastic foci Patchy, often subpleural	Reticular abnormality Honeycombing Often patchy Basal, peripheral predominance	Collagen vascular disease Asbestosis Chronic hypersensitivity pneumonitis Nonspecific interstitial pneumonia
Nonspecific interstitial pneumonia/fibrosis	Nonspecific interstitial pneumonia	Alveolar septal thickening by inflammation or fibrosis Spatially and temporally homogeneous	Ground-glass abnormality Reticular abnormality Basal, peripheral/ peribronchovascular predominance	Collagen vascular disease Asbestosis Chronic hypersensitivity pneumonitis Desquamative interstitial pneumonia, organizing pneumonia
Organizing pneumonia	Cryptogenic organizing pneumonia	Intraluminal organizing fibrosis in bronchioles, alveolar ducts, and alveoli Temporally homogeneous Patchy distribution	Consolidation, ground-glass abnormality Patchy Basal, peripheral/ peribronchovascular predominance	Infection Vasculitis Sarcoidosis Lymphoma Bronchioloalveolar carcinoma Nonspecific interstitial pneumonia
Desquamative interstitial pneumonia	Desquamative interstitial pneumonia	Diffuse macrophage accumulation within alveolar spaces Mild interstitial thickening Homogeneous involvement	Ground-glass attenuation Cysts ± Basal, peripheral predominance	Hypersensitivity pneumonitis Nonspecific interstitial pneumonia Lymphoid interstitial pneumonia
Respiratory bronchiolitis-interstitial lung disease	Respiratory bronchiolitis-interstitial lung disease	Bronchiolocentric accumulation of alveolar macrophages Mild bronchiolar fibrosis	Centrilobular nodules Ground-glass attenuation Diffuse or upper lung predominance	Hypersensitivity pneumonitis
Acute interstitial pneumonia	Acute interstitial pneumonia	Alveolar septal thickening by inflammation or fibrosis, with uniform temporal appearance Airspace organization Hyaline membranes	Ground-glass attenuation, consolidation Diffuse	Hydrostatic edema Pneumonia Acute eosinophilic pneumonia
Lymphoid interstitial pneumonia	Lymphoid interstitial pneumonia	Diffuse alveolar infiltration by lymphocytes Frequent lymphoid hyperplasia	Centrilobular nodules, ground-glass attenuation, septal thickening Cysts Diffuse	Sarcoidosis Langerhans cell histiocytosis Nonspecific interstitial pneumonia Desquamative interstitial pneumonia

Box 10.2 Glossary of commonly used abbreviations

AIP: acute interstitial pneumonia
CFA: cryptogenic fibrosing alveolitis
COP: cryptogenic organizing pneumonia
DIP: desquamative interstitial pneumonia
IPF: idiopathic pulmonary fibrosis
LIP: lymphoid interstitial pneumonia
NSIP: nonspecific interstitial pneumonia
OP: organizing pneumonia
RB: respiratory bronchiolitis
RB-ILD: respiratory bronchiolitis-interstitial lung disease
UIP: usual interstitial pneumonia

Box 10.3 Idiopathic interstitial pneumonias (IIPs)

Patterns of IIP are defined on the basis of their histologic features
Each IIP has an associated prototypic CT appearance
Each pattern of pneumonia can be associated with other causes, particularly collagen vascular disease

with the clinical syndrome of CFA. In recent surveys of clinical practice in the United Kingdom, <12% of patients diagnosed as having CFA were submitted for open lung biopsy,[22,24] and it seems unlikely that this figure is much higher outside tertiary referral centers in other countries.[31] Furthermore, in a survey of published studies, Katzenstein and Myers[3] found that open lung biopsy confirmation of the diagnosis of IPF was obtained in only 38% of a total of 1022 cases.[3] Therefore, community based studies will often include patients with CFA who do not have a lung biopsy.[31] Reasons for failure to obtain a biopsy may include medical frailty, lack of access to thoracic surgical services, lack of availability of trained lung pathologists, or lack of appreciation of the importance of histology in determining treatment and prognosis.[4] Increasing awareness of the influence of histology on prognosis, and wide availability of video-assisted thoracoscopy for biopsy, may in future increase the biopsy rate in patients without a definitive diagnosis on CT. In patients who do not undergo biopsy, high-resolution CT (HRCT) assumes a central role in defining the morphologic pattern, and may serve as a surrogate for biopsy.[15]

Clinical presentation

The term CFA is used to refer to patients presenting with a clinical syndrome of IIP in whom no specific histologic diagnosis has been made. As discussed above, UIP will be the histologic diagnosis in the majority of these cases, but 40–50% will have other, more benign, diagnoses, including NSIP, DIP, and RB-ILD.[11–15] Organizing pneumonia (OP) and AIP usually have a more acute presentation. Although LIP may have a similar presentation, it is usually associated with collagen vascular disease.

The most frequent presenting symptoms are progressive exertional dyspnea and cough, which is usually nonproductive but in one series was productive in just over half the patients.[32] Less common symptoms include nonspecific chest pain,[33] and constitutional symptoms such as fever, weight loss, and fatigue.[34] A nonerosive arthropathy that is not part of a recognized connective tissue disorder is quite common in patients with lone CFA. Some patients date the onset to an influenzalike illness.[34] A small proportion of patients present because of an abnormal "routine radiograph". In one series, 47% of patients presented in this manner, an unusually high frequency for this form of presentation.[35] Late, fine inspiratory crackles at the lung bases are an almost universal finding,[32] and two-thirds to three-fourths of patients show clubbing of the fingers.[32,33,35] Occasionally, there is full blown hypertrophic osteoarthropathy.[33] In advanced disease cor pulmonale and cyanosis may develop.[34]

About 40–50% of patients die of a cause directly related to the CFA, e.g. respiratory failure.[37] The second most common cause of death is cardiovascular disease,[38] which occurs four times more commonly than expected.[32]

Changes in respiratory function tests[32,34] are those that might be expected from a diffuse interstitial process: reduced compliance and lung volumes, particularly vital capacity and total lung capacity with relatively normal residual volume. Reduction in gas diffusing capacity is a particularly early and characteristic change. In patients with coexisting emphysema, lung volumes may appear preserved, and in such individuals lung diffusing capacity is usually precipitously decreased.[40–42]

As discussed below, all the patterns of interstitial pneumonia are strongly associated with collagen vascular disease. Features suggestive of collagen vascular disease, such as an isolated arthropathy, Raynaud syndrome, or autoantibodies, are seen in many patients with interstitial pneumonia who do not meet criteria for collagen vascular disease. Some of these patients will later develop a fullblown collagen vascular disease. Overall, more than half the patients with CFA will have autoantibodies, with antinuclear antibody (ANA) positive in 15–45%, and rheumatoid factor present in up to a third.[32,43,44] Available evidence suggests that most patients with interstitial pneumonia related to collagen vascular disease have a better prognosis than those with IIP,[45] but much of this difference is likely due to the fact that NSIP is the predominant histology in patients with collagen vascular disease, particularly in scleroderma.[46–48]

Cigarette smoking confers an increased risk for the subsequent development of CFA.[49] Epidemiologic studies have suggested that prolonged metal or wood dust exposure might account for up to 20% of cases of CFA,[50] and that certain prescribed drugs (particularly antidepressants) may be responsible for approximately 11% of cases.[51]

The clinical and imaging evaluation of the patient with a syndrome of fibrosing alveolitis, as outlined above, should focus on two questions:

1. *Is it idiopathic?* Interstitial pneumonia related to a recognizable cause, such as hypersensitivity pneumonitis, asbestos exposure, drugs, or collagen vascular disease, may be managed differently and may have a different prognosis from IIP. While clinical and laboratory evaluation is important in making this distinction, CT can yield important clues, particularly in raising the suspicion of hypersensitivity pneumonitis or collagen vascular disease (see Figs 10.28 and 10.31).
2. *Does the patient have a morphologic pattern of UIP?* The morphologic pattern of UIP is usually refractory to standard antiinflammatory treatments, and is associated with a significantly worse prognosis than the other interstitial pneumonias. Imaging is often pivotal in making this distinction (Table 10.2).

Table 10.2 CT diagnosis of usual interstitial pneumonia (UIP)

CT features suggestive of UIP	CT features suggesting that the diagnosis is likely not UIP
Lower lung predominance, with tendency to "creep" up the lateral lungs	Mid or upper lung predominance
Peripheral predominance	Peribronchovascular predominance
Honeycombing	Extensive ground-glass abnormality Centrilobular nodules Marked septal thickening Non-honeycomb cysts Air-trapping

Usual interstitial pneumonia/idiopathic pulmonary fibrosis

UIP is the most common histopathologic pattern seen in patients who present with the clinical syndrome of CFA.[3,11–14] Under the new classification, the term IPF is applied exclusively to the idiopathic clinical syndrome associated with the morphologic pattern of UIP.[4,17] The key histopathologic features of UIP (Box 10.4) are: (1) patchy and variable distribution of areas of fibrosis at different stages of maturity; and (2) presence of small areas of young connective tissue (fibroblastic foci). The variation in types of lung fibrosis is most obvious at low magnification, with alternating areas, from one field to another, of young connective tissue, interstitial fibrosis, honeycomb destruction and normal lung. Within areas of honeycomb lung, the enlarged airspaces are lined by bronchiolar epithelium and hyperplastic alveolar pneumocytes; within the airspaces there may be mucus and inflammatory cells (most frequently neutrophils). Other pathologic features encountered in UIP are endarteritis obliterans and smooth muscle hypertrophy, but these are not specific to UIP and are probably secondary phenomena.

Box 10.4 Histologic features of usual interstitial pneumonia

Fibroblastic foci
Dense fibrosis
Honeycombing
Paucity of inflammatory cells
Temporal and spatial nonuniformity

The areas of young connective tissue seen on biopsy in UIP consist of small foci of actively proliferating fibroblasts and myofibroblasts.[53,54] These fibroblastic foci, representing ongoing sites of lung injury and repair, are thought to represent the earliest lesion of UIP, and are very important for the histologic diagnosis of UIP.[4] They may represent areas of lung response to an injury that is as yet undefined.[55,56] They often occur at the interface between fibrotic and normal lung. The number of fibroblastic foci on lung biopsy is an important predictor of survival in patients with UIP.[57]

The recognition of fibroblastic foci as the important pathogenic lesions of UIP represents an important shift from the previous concept of alveolar inflammation or alveolitis as the precursor of UIP.[52] A chronic inflammatory cell infiltrate may indeed be seen in UIP, but is usually mild and consists mainly of lymphocytes with occasional plasma cells and eosinophils. If extensive cellularity is found, the diagnosis is probably not UIP. The extent of alveolar cellularity does not predict survival.[57] The paucity of inflammatory infiltration of the lung, in contrast to the other idiopathic pneumonias, may explain the lack of steroid responsiveness in UIP/IPF.

Causes of a UIP pattern on histology (Box 10.5) include chronic hypersensitivity pneumonitis, collagen vascular disease, familial pulmonary fibrosis, and asbestos exposure.[4,58] Drug toxicity is a rare cause of a UIP pattern, best described with nitrofurantoin.[59]

The pathogenesis of UIP remains unclear. The fibroblastic foci are thought to represent an abnormal wound healing response to lung injury, resulting from release of multiple fibrogenic cytokines.[52] The inciting agent remains unclear. There has been much speculation about the possible role of viruses, particularly

---

Box 10.5 Causes and associations of usual interstitial pneumonia pattern

Idiopathic pulmonary fibrosis
Hypersensitivity pneumonitis
Asbestosis
Collagen vascular disease
Drugs (rare)
Familial (rare)

---

the Epstein–Barr virus, in the initiation of fibrosing alveolitis, but no specific relationship has been proved.[29,60–63] Recently, herpes virus DNA has been identified in patients with UIP.[61]

From the clinical series, it seems that UIP is more common in men than in women (1.5–1.7:1).[22,49,64] Most patients are over 50 years at the time of diagnosis, and about two-thirds are over 60,[64] but the disease may occur in people as young as 30.[3] There have been descriptions of UIP occurring in children and adolescents, but it is not clear whether these entities would meet the current criteria for diagnosis of UIP,[3] and no cases of UIP were recorded in two series of 51 and 38 pediatric patients with diffuse lung disease that used current diagnostic criteria.[65,66]

Patients with UIP usually complain of a dry cough and progressive exertional dyspnea of insidious onset. Systemic symptoms, such as fever, weight loss, and arthralgia, occur with variable frequency,[39] though fever itself is unusual and probably occurs in <15% of patients.[53,67] Finger clubbing is frequent, probably occurring in well over one-half of patients; inspiratory crackles on auscultation of the lung bases are an almost invariable finding.[32,39]

It is generally accepted that the prognosis of patients with biopsy proven UIP is poor, with mean survival after presentation ranging from 2.8 to 9 years,[11,32,68,69] and 5 year survival ranging from 15 to 43%.[13] Lower mortality rates were reported in earlier series,[19,35,66] but it is likely that these included other IIP subtypes such as NSIP. The survival of patients with UIP is clearly worse in recent series which have excluded patients with NSIP and DIP.[13–15,71] At 5 years after diagnosis, only 12[14]–45% of patients with UIP survive.[11,72] Objective evidence that immuno-suppressive therapy, usually steroids, is effective is lacking. It has been suggested that the historical observations of a 15–30% objective response rate to steroid therapy in patients with fibrosing alveolitis[28,32,35,38,73] may have been due to the inclusion of patients with NSIP, and may not apply to patients with histopathologically defined UIP.[11]

Almost all patients with the UIP pattern due to IPF have abnormal chest radiographs when they present with symptoms. Indeed, when prior chest radiographs are available, basal reticular opacities are usually visible in retrospect for several years prior to the development of symptoms (Fig. 10.1). These presymptomatic opacities are commonly reported by the radiologist but, in the absence of symptoms or other abnormalities, disregarded by the clinician. Since early detection of IPF may be of value in treatment, the radiologist should emphasize the significance of these abnormalities, and ensure that they are investigated by careful review of the patient's symptoms and signs, and if appropriate, physiologic and HRCT evaluation. The classic chest radiographic appearance in patients with UIP is of basal reticulonodular shadowing which becomes a coarser reticular, or honeycomb, pattern as the disease progresses (Fig. 10.2). The characteristic subpleural distribution of the abnormality may

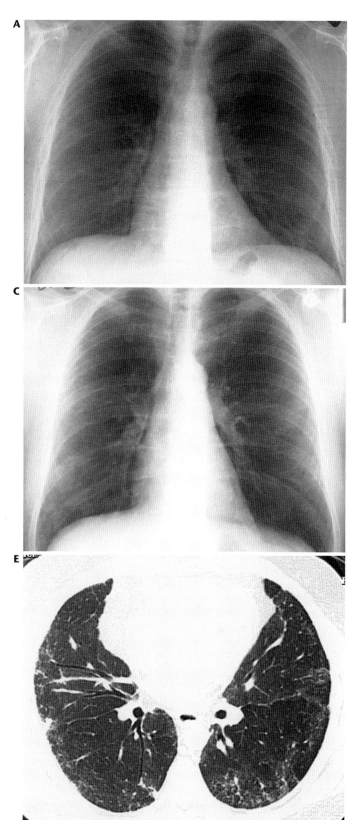

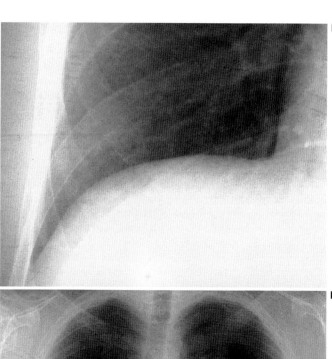

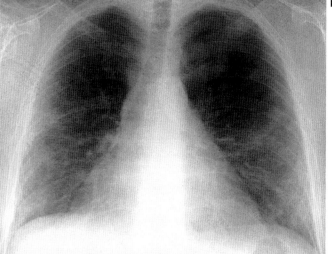

Fig. 10.1 Progressive idiopathic pulmonary fibrosis in a 55-year-old man. **A** and **B,** Initial chest radiograph with detailed view shows minimal basal linear abnormality. **C,** Four years later the abnormality has progressed to involve most of the lungs with a reticular pattern. **D,** Two years later the abnormality shows further progression, with significant decrease in lung volumes. **E,** CT at the time of the latest radiograph shows the typical peripheral distribution of reticular abnormality.

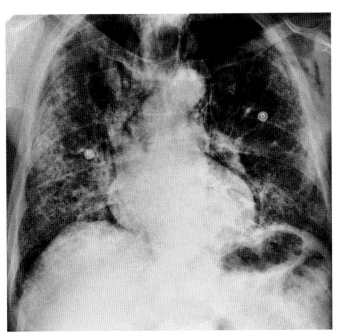

Fig. 10.2 Pneumomediastinum and idiopathic pulmonary fibrosis (usual interstitial pneumonia pattern). This patient has long-standing reticular abnormality with aggregated, small, thick walled, ring opacities (honeycombing), best seen on the right. A pneumomediastinum is visible.

often be recognized in the mid and upper lungs, along the lateral chest wall. The lung volumes usually decrease with time, particularly in the lower lobes, but in patients with associated emphysema, the radiographic lung volumes may be normal or even increased (Fig. 10.3).

Pneumomediastinum is quite common in patients with UIP, and is often asymptomatic. Pneumothorax may be seen; while this may be small and asymptomatic, it may also be associated with a significant air leak if there is rupture of a honeycomb cyst. In patients with advanced UIP who develop pneumothorax, the stiffness of the lung often prevents significant lung collapse.

UIP has a very characteristic appearance on CT. The predominant CT pattern is usually either reticular or honeycombing, or a combination of both (Figs 10.1 to 10.5).[74] Traction bronchiectasis and/or bronchiolectasis is often seen. Although ground-glass abnormality is commonly present,[74] it is usually associated with reticular abnormality and traction bronchiectasis, suggesting that it represents lung fibrosis rather than inflammation. Isolated ground-glass attenuation, if present, in usually sparse. The abnormalities are basal predominant in most, but may be diffuse. Peripheral predominance is present in about 90%. In contrast to the homogeneous appearance of NSIP, the abnormalities of UIP often have a patchy distribution. As the disease progresses, it often appears to "creep" up the periphery of the lung, causing subpleural reticular abnormality in the

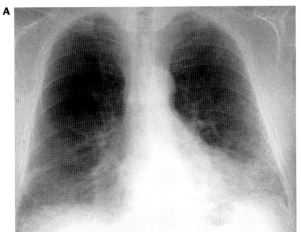

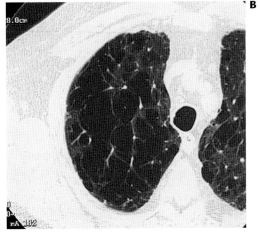

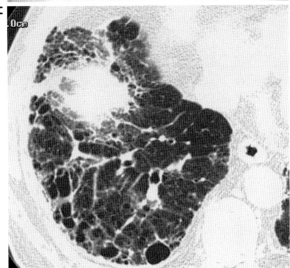

Fig. 10.3 A 67-year-old man with emphysema and idiopathic pulmonary fibrosis. **A**, Chest radiograph shows emphysema in the upper lobes, with basal reticular abnormality, and honeycombing on the left. **B** and **C**, HRCT defines the relative extent of emphysema and lung fibrosis.

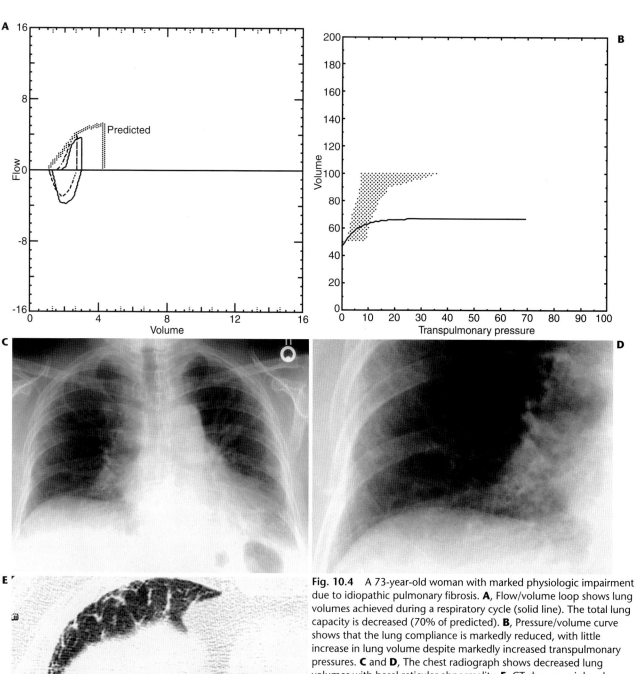

Fig. 10.4 A 73-year-old woman with marked physiologic impairment due to idiopathic pulmonary fibrosis. **A**, Flow/volume loop shows lung volumes achieved during a respiratory cycle (solid line). The total lung capacity is decreased (70% of predicted). **B**, Pressure/volume curve shows that the lung compliance is markedly reduced, with little increase in lung volume despite markedly increased transpulmonary pressures. **C** and **D**, The chest radiograph shows decreased lung volumes with basal reticular abnormality. **E**, CT shows peripheral reticular abnormality, with minor subpleural honeycombing, compatible with usual interstitial pneumonia.

A

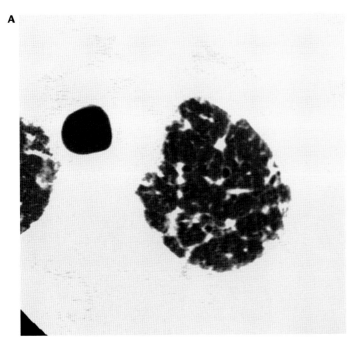

B

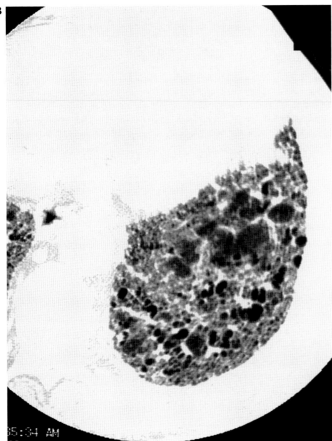

Fig. 10.5   A and **B**, CT in a 66-year-old patient with usual interstitial pneumonia shows lower lobe honeycombing and peripheral irregular lines in the upper lobes.

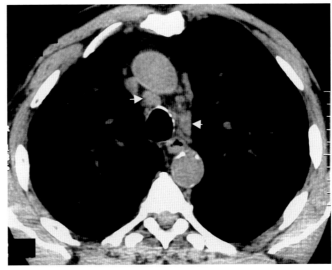

Fig. 10.6   A 73-year-old man with idiopathic pulmonary fibrosis. There are multiple enlarged mediastinal lymph nodes measuring between 1 and 2 cm in diameter (arrows).

upper lungs (Fig. 10.5). In a study by Hunninghake et al,[75] this finding of subpleural lines in the upper lungs was a common and important distinghuising feature of UIP.

As with many other interstitial lung diseases, mediastinal adenopathy may be seen (Fig. 10.6). Usually the enlarged lymph nodes measure between 1 and 2 cm in maximum diameter, and the adenopathy is thought to be reactive.[76] It is never visible on the chest radiograph. There is some evidence that the number of enlarged lymph nodes correlates with the severity of the lung fibrosis.[77] Pulmonary ossification may occur in areas of advanced fibrosis (Fig. 10.7), and will be better seen if the CT images are viewed or photographed at mediastinal windows.[78]

Numerous prospective and retrospective studies have shown that a confident or highly confident diagnosis of UIP, based on the CT features outlined above, has a specificity of >90% for the pathologic diagnosis of UIP.[27,74,79–82] Honeycombing in the lower lobes, and linear abnormality in the upper lobes, are the most reliable features for differentiating between UIP and its clinical mimics (Fig. 10.5).[75] In a study by Flaherty et al,[15] the observation of honeycombing on HRCT indicated the presence of UIP with a sensitivity of 90% and specificity of 86%.

Because of the high degree of accuracy of HRCT in many cases of UIP, the diagnosis of UIP is commonly based on clinical and imaging features, without the need for surgical biopsy. The ATS has published criteria for diagnosis of UIP in the absence of a surgical biopsy (Box 10.6).[17] These criteria indicate that "bibasilar reticular abnormalities with minimal ground-glass opacities on HRCT scans" are a major criterion for diagnosis of IPF. However, since publication of these criteria, the importance of honeycombing in the diagnosis of IPF has become more apparent,[15,75] and a confident CT diagnosis of UIP is not usually made unless honeycombing is present. However, there is a substantial minority (30–50%) of cases of histologic UIP in whom a confident diagnosis of UIP cannot be made based on the CT appearances (Fig. 10.8).[80,82–84] In these patients, the diagnosis of UIP can only be made by lung biopsy. A recent study by Flaherty et al[71] suggested that patients with histologic UIP who had definite or probable UIP by HRCT criteria had a

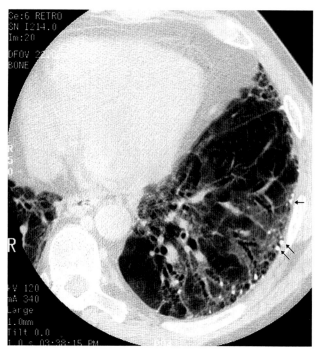

Fig. 10.7 A 45-year-old man with idopathic pulmonary fibrosis and pulmonary ossification. The HRCT image shows ground-glass attenuation, reticular abnormality, traction bronchiectasis, and honeycombing typical for usual interstitial pneumonia. The areas of honeycombing are associated with multiple areas of punctate calcification (arrows).

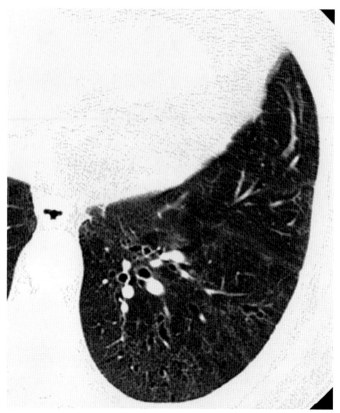

Fig. 10.8 A 58-year-old female with histologic usual interstitial pneumonia. The thin collimation HRCT imaging features in this case of histologic usual interstitial pneumonia more closely resemble nonspecific interstitial pneumonia. The predominant pattern is ground-glass and fine reticular opacities with traction bronchiectasis, but no honeycombing.

Box 10.6 American Thoracic Society criteria for diagnosis of idiopathic pulmonary fibrosis in the absence of a surgical biopsy[17]

Major criteria

Exclusion of other known causes of interstitial lung disease, e.g. certain drug toxicities, environmental exposures, and connective tissue diseases

Abnormal pulmonary function studies that include evidence of restriction (reduced ventilatory capacity often with an increased FEV_1/FVC ratio) and impaired gas exchange (increased $P(A-a)O_2$ with rest or exercise or decreased DLco)

Bibasilar reticular abnormalities with minimal ground-glass opacities on HRCT scans

Transbronchial lung biopsy or bronchoalveolar lavage showing no features to support an alternate diagnosis

Minor criteria

Age >50 years

Insidious onset of otherwise unexplained dyspnea on exertion

Duration of illness 3 months

Bibasilar, inspiratory crackles (dry or "Velcro" type in quality)

---

shorter survival than those who had indeterminate HRCT findings. This is most likely because the typical HRCT criteria for diagnosis of UIP include the presence of honeycombing, and may therefore select patients with more advanced or more severe disease. This study reemphasizes the importance of seeking lung biopsy in patients in whom CT is not diagnostic of

UIP. An equivocal, atypical, or nonspecific CT appearance should always prompt biopsy. Most importantly, the CT features must be interpreted in conjunction with a complete clinical evaluation.

Initial reports of the CT features of IPF or fibrosing alveolitis suggested that the finding of ground-glass attenuation was associated with "alveolitis" on biopsy.[85] Subsequent studies suggested that areas of ground-glass abnormality in IPF or fibrosing alveolitis were reversible on steroids and were associated with a favorable prognosis.[23,86] However, the patients in those studies who had a large amount of ground-glass abnormality probably had NSIP or DIP rather than UIP. HRCT studies of "IPF", "fibrosing alveolitis", or "UIP" published before 1995 are very difficult to interpret, because it is unclear how many cases of NSIP or DIP were included in these papers. As discussed above, under the current definition of UIP, alveolitis is not regarded as an important histologic component of the disease, and therefore ground-glass attenuation in UIP cannot be regarded as reflecting alveolitis. In contrast to DIP[87] and NSIP,[88] true UIP shows inexorable progression and rarely, if ever, reverses in response to steroid treatment (Fig. 10.9).[87] When extensive ground-glass attenuation is present in patients with known UIP, the possibility of an acute exacerbation or accelerated deterioration should be considered.

Several studies have evaluated sequential changes in IPF.[26,30,89,90] Comparison of serial scans in patients with IPF is dependent on identifying comparable scan levels, by matching anatomic features such as vessels and bronchi. In untreated

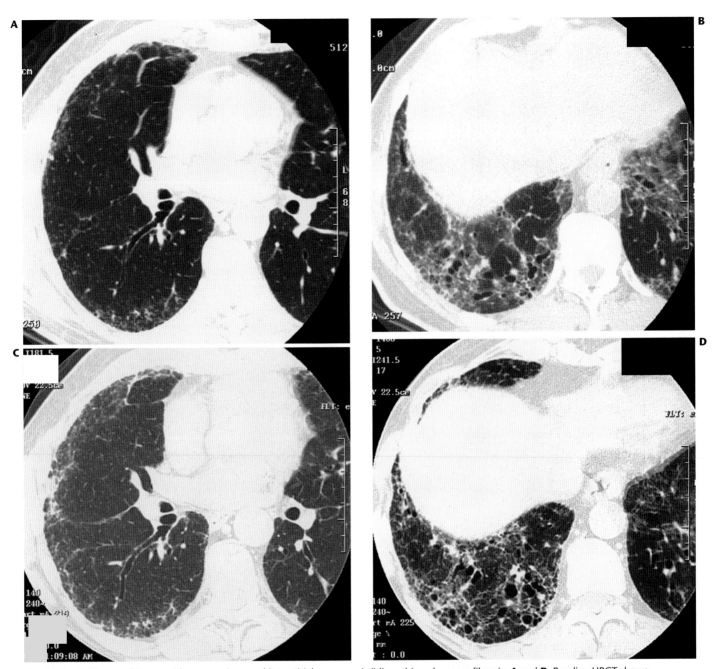

Fig. 10.9 A 65-year-old man with progressive usual interstitial pneumonia/idiopathic pulmonary fibrosis. **A** and **B**, Baseline HRCT shows peripheral ground-glass opacity and mild reticular abnormality in the right mid zone, with more marked reticular abnormality, traction bronchiectasis, and mild honeycombing at the lung base. **C** and **D**, HRCT scan 20 months later shows substantial progression of ground-glass and reticular abnormality, with marked enlargement of the basal honeycomb cysts and associated traction bronchiectasis. Comparison of **A** and **C** shows that ground-glass attenuation has been replaced by reticular abnormality with traction bronchiolectasis.

Box 10.7 Complications of usual interstitial pneumonia

Infection
Lung cancer
Acute exacerbation/accelerated deterioration

---

patients scanned at intervals of >6 months, the extent of IPF increases progressively (Fig. 10.9). In patients who are treated, some areas of ground-glass attenuation progress to reticular abnormality and honeycombing, but some areas regress. Reticular abnormality usually progresses to honeycombing.[26] Areas of honeycombing increase inexorably in extent, and the size of the honeycomb cysts also increases.[89] The appropriate interval for detecting change in patients with IPF would appear to be about 1 year, though some patients may show clear evidence of change in 3–4 months. Of course, sequential scanning is indicated only if it will change management.

Important complications of IPF include infection, lung cancer, and accelerated deterioration (Box 10.7).[37] A variety of opportunistic infectious organisms may occur in treated patients with IPF, including *Pneumocystis jerovici* (Fig. 10.10), *Mycobacterium avium* complex (Fig. 10.11), and mycetoma due to *Aspergillus* species or other organisms (Fig. 10.12).

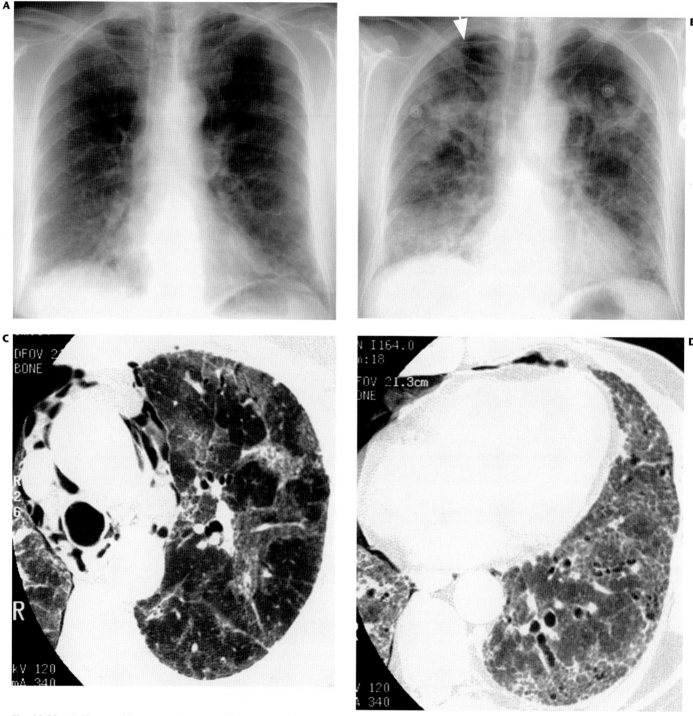

Fig. 10.10 A 67-year-old woman with idiopathic pulmonary fibrosis (IPF), complicated by *Pneumocystis jiroveci pneumonia* (PCP). **A**, Baseline chest radiograph shows basal predominant reticular abnormality and depression of the right hilum compatible with moderate lung fibrosis. **B**, Chest radiograph 4 months later shows patchy bilateral consolidation and ground-glass opacity superimposed on the previously evident fibrosis. There is a small right pneumothorax (arrow). **C** and **D**, HRCT images obtained 4 days after the chest radiograph show patchy ground-glass opacity superimposed on the basal reticular abnormality. A pneumomediastinum has developed. These appearances are indistinguishable from those seen in the acute exacerbation of IPF. Despite treatment for PCP, the patient developed progressive consolidation and subsequently died.

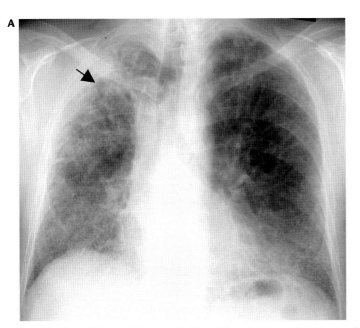

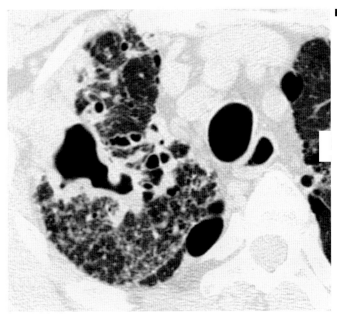

Fig. 10.11 A 54-year-old man with idiopathic pulmonary fibrosis, complicated by *M. avium–intracellulare* infection. **A**, Chest radiograph shows extensive basal fibrosis with honeycombing. There is marked right apical pleural thickening and a subtle peripheral right upper lobe cavity (arrow). **B**, HRCT confirms the irregular cavity with adjacent pleural thickening.

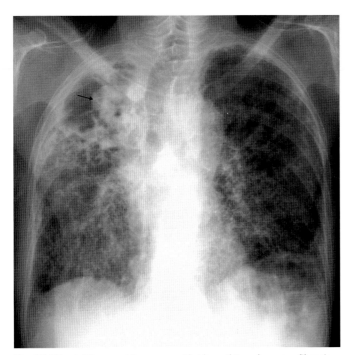

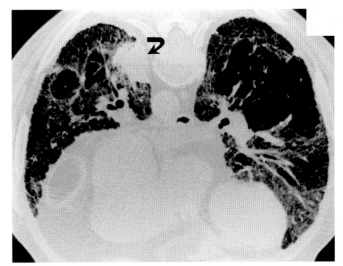

Fig. 10.13 A supervening lung cancer (squamous cell type) in a patient with cryptogenic fibrosing alveolitis, usual interstitial pneumonia (UIP) pattern (arrow). The lung cancers that develop in patients with UIP are usually located in the lung periphery.

Fig. 10.12 A 74-year-old woman with idiopathic pulmonary fibrosis complicated by right upper lobe mycetoma. Chest radiograph shows diffuse bilateral lung fibrosis with basal predominant honeycombing. A large cavity is present in the right upper lobe, containing an intracavitary mass (arrow).

Carcinoma of the lung (Fig. 10.13) develops 14 times more frequently in patients with IIP than in the general population.[91] Lung cancer appears to be primarily associated with UIP, rather than with the other IIPs. The prevalence of carcinoma in various series has ranged between 5 and 13%.[37,38,91] Synchronous multiple lung cancers occur in up to 15% of patients with fibrosing alveolitis. A review of 62 cases found squamous carcinomas in 35%, alveolar cell carcinomas in 27%, adenocarcinomas in 21%, and undifferentiated carcinoma in 11%.[94] This preponderance of adenocarcinoma, particularly bronchioloalveolar cell type, is not a universal finding and in some series the pattern of cell types is no different from the usual experience.[91] Lee et al[92] found lung cancer in 32 (13%) of 244 cases of IPF seen over a 7.5 year period. In this study, just over half of the lung cancers were squamous cell carcinomas, approximating the prevalence of this histopathologic type in patients without pulmonary fibrosis. Unlike smoking related lung cancer, fibrosis related lung cancer is most often located peripherally in the lower lobes, where the fibrosis is most intense (Box 10.8, Fig. 10.13).[92,93] In the majority of cases described by Lee et al,[92] the lung cancer appeared on CT as an area of poorly defined consolidation. Nineteen (60%) of the cancers were peripheral, and 21 (66%) were in the lower lobes. Meticulous comparison of serial radiographs is important for detection of lung cancer. If cancer is detected, careful evaluation by CT is indicated since multiple synchronous cancers are relatively common.[93] Although surgical resection of lung cancer in patients with lung fibrosis is associated with high morbidity, particularly from postoperative respiratory distress syndrome, longterm survival may be achieved in carefully selected patients.[95]

> **Box 10.8 Characteristics of lung cancer in usual interstitial pneumonia**
>
> Lower lung predominant
> Often multifocal
> Usually in patients with moderate or advanced lung fibrosis

Ten to 20% of patients with IPF develop accelerated deterioration, or acute exacerbations, progressing to acute respiratory failure.[96–99] Acute exacerbation is more acute than accelerated deterioration, but the precise distinction between these entities is unclear, and the terms are sometimes used interchangeably. The lungs of most of these patients have a histologic appearance of diffuse alveolar damage (DAD), similar to that of AIP, though OP may also be seen.

Accelerated deterioration or acute exacerbation of IPF presents with a relatively short onset of progressive dyspnea or cough, occasionally associated with systemic symptoms. There is usually a short prodrome of 4–8 weeks duration. The chest radiograph usually shows ground-glass abnormality or consol- idation superimposed on a background reticular abnormality (Fig. 10.14). On CT it is characterized by diffuse or peripheral ground-glass attenuation (Fig. 10.15),[96] which must be distin- guished clinically from opportunistic viral or pneumocystis infection. Consolidation may also be seen. In 17 patients with accelerated IPF, Akira[96] classified the CT distribution of ground- glass attenuation as peripheral (adjacent to preexisting fibrosis), diffuse, or multifocal. They found that all six patients with peripheral opacities improved over 1–3 months with corti- costeroid treatment, compared with three of six patients with a multifocal pattern, and none of five with diffuse opacity. On biopsy, the peripheral pattern of abnormality correlated with the presence of active fibroblastic foci in two patients, while the multifocal and diffuse patterns correlated with acute DAD superimposed on UIP. On sequential evaluation of patients with acute exacerbation or accelerated deterioration, ground- glass attenuation was seen to evolve into consolidation with architectural distortion, and cystic lesions often developed.[97]

Nonspecific interstitial pneumonia

Nonspecific interstitial pneumonia/fibrosis (now called NSIP) was first described in 1994 in response to recognition of a histologic pattern of lung disease which did not fit any of the existing descriptions of interstitial pneumonia.[100] In a retro- spective review of open lung biopsies in cases of IIP, 64 cases were identified that did not fulfill, on histologic grounds, the diagnostic criteria for UIP, DIP, or AIP. It seems highly likely that in the past NSIP was categorized as IPF, UIP, or cellular interstitial pneumonia. The histologic pattern of NSIP does not appear to be associated with a specific clinical syndrome, and presents in a similar fashion to UIP,[3] even though there is a certain clinical, radiologic, and pathologic consistency among cases.[101] Forty-six percent of the cases in the defining series had clear associations with collagen vascular disease, hypersensitivity

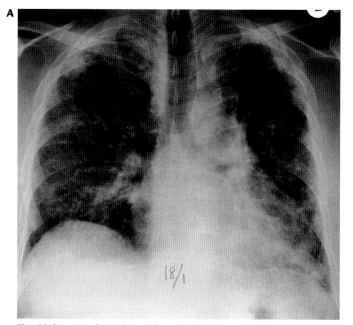
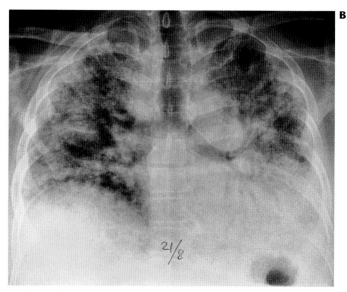

Fig. 10.14   Accelerated usual interstitial pneumonia (UIP). **A** and **B**, These two chest radiographs were taken 7 months apart. In the 5 weeks preceding the second radiograph (**B**), the patient had become increasingly short of breath and subsequently died despite aggressive immunosuppressive treatment. The rapid onset of widespread ground-glass opacification and consolidation is typical of the accelerated phase of UIP.

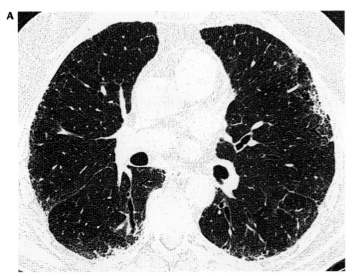
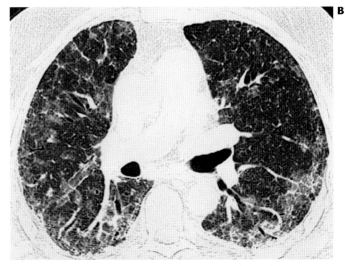

Fig. 10.15 Accelerated usual interstitial pneumonia (UIP) in a 78-year-old man. **A**, Baseline CT shows relatively mild subpleural reticular abnormality. **B**, CT obtained 5 months later, after 4 weeks of progressive breathlessness, shows some progression of reticular abnormality, and extensive patchy ground-glass abnormality. Biopsy showed an organizing pneumonia pattern superimposed on background UIP.

pneumonitis, or drug exposure.[100] The most important clinical finding regarding NSIP is that it is associated with a significantly better prognosis than UIP.[11,13–15,102]

The main pathologic finding is the presence of varying degrees of inflammation and fibrosis within alveolar walls (Box 10.9).[3,4] In contrast to UIP, these changes are spatially and temporally uniform in all sections. In the original series, cases were divided into three groups depending on the relative amounts of inflammation and fibrosis:[100] in 48% interstitial inflammation with lymphocytes and plasma cells was predominant (Type 1); in 38% there was an approximately equal mix of inflammation and fibrosis with mature collagen and few fibroblasts (Type 2); and in 14% there was predominant interstitial collagen with little inflammation and few fibroblasts (Type 3). More recent studies have shown a lower prevalence (5–25%) of the Type 1 pattern of NSIP, and a higher prevalence of Types 2 and 3.[13,14,103] Minor histologic findings included small areas of OP (50%), small fibroblastic foci (20%), macrophage accumulation in alveoli, and occasional lymphoid aggregates and granulomas.[3]

Box 10.9 Histologic features of nonspecific interstitial pneumonia

Alveolar septal thickening by variable amounts of
 inflammation and fibrosis
Temporal and spatial uniformity

At presentation, patients with NSIP have a mean age of 45–55 years with a range of 9–81 years.[11,100,101,104] The mean age at presentation is about 10 years younger than in UIP.[4] All series show a slight excess of females except for one in which 95% were female.[101] The relationship between cigarette smoking and NSIP has not been well evaluated, but some authors suggest that NSIP can be a subtype of smoking related interstitial lung disease.[105]

Clinical features of NSIP resemble those of other IIPs, with progressive dyspnea and nonproductive cough preceding diagnosis by 6–12 months on average,[14,100,101] but ranging from weeks to years.[100] Occasionally there are systemic symptoms

such as weight loss and fever, and in one series 21% of patients had clubbing.[11] NSIP usually responds to steroid treatment and the prognosis is considerably better than that of UIP. The 10 year survival rate in NSIP was 60% versus 10% in UIP in one series,[11] and this relatively favorable prognosis is confirmed by numerous other studies.[13–15,107] In the original series reported by Katzenstein and Fiorelli after an unspecified duration of follow up (mean ranges of various subgroups 8–61 months), 45% were alive, well and disease free; 38% were alive with persisting disease (stable or improved); and 11% had died of NSIP.[100] Histologic changes correlate with outcome, a predominant cellular pattern having a better prognosis than a pattern that is largely fibrotic.[100,101] Indeed, the longterm survival of patients with purely cellular NSIP is close to 100% in several series.[13,14] However, the survival of patients with predominantly fibrotic NSIP is much poorer, with a 5 year survival as low as 45%,[14] and a 10 year survival as low as 35%.[13]

Since NSIP only became an established diagnosis as recently as 1994, radiographic descriptions are limited. The chest radiograph is abnormal in >90% of patients,[11,100,106,107] but changes are not well characterized in the literature. Abnormalities are usually bilateral with a basal predominance. They may be consolidative and patchy, reticulonodular, or mixed. Lower lobe volume loss is common, and traction bronchiectasis is frequently present (Fig. 10.16).

Detailed HRCT descriptions are available in 240 patients (Box 10.10).[12,74,88,103,106,108–111] The prevalence of reported CT findings, particularly consolidation and honeycombing, varies widely from series to series.[112] The most likely reason for this variability is the heterogeneity of histologic diagnostic criteria for NSIP at different sites, since pathologists have been slow to agree on the features that distinguish NSIP from UIP, OP, and DIP, and most papers have used only one pathologist to establish the diagnosis, without determining inter- or intra-observer variability. In a study by Flaherty et al,[16] three expert pathologists agreed on histologic diagnoses of NSIP or UIP in only 67% of cases, while a study by Nicholson et al[14] found that the kappa coefficient of agreement between two pathologists for distinguishing UIP from fibrotic NSIP was only 0.26. In the study

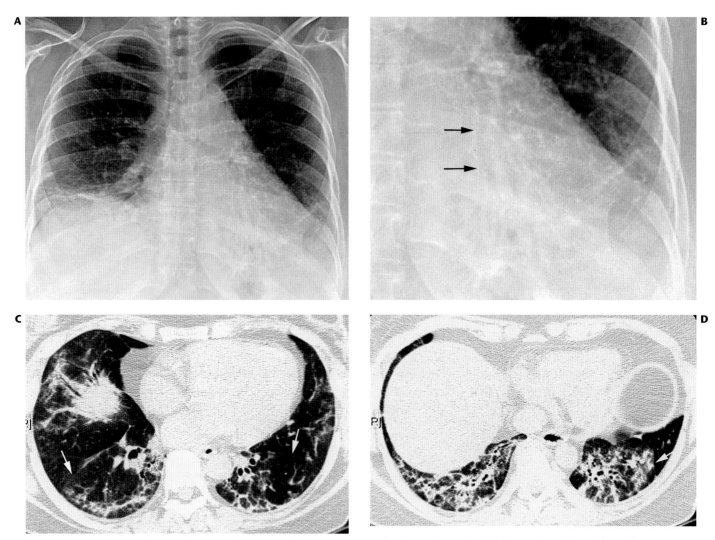

Fig. 10.16 A 50-year-old man with nonspecific interstitial pneumonia. **A** and **B**, Chest radiograph with detailed view shows bilateral lower lobe reticular abnormality, with lobar volume loss and traction bronchiectasis (arrows, **B**). The heart is moderately enlarged. Mediastinal widening is due to fat. **C** and **D**, HRCT shows lower lobe predominant reticular abnormality with traction bronchiectasis, and lobar volume loss evident from posterior displacement of the interlobar fissures (arrows). Note the peribronchovascular distribution of the reticular abnormality.

Box 10.10 CT features of nonspecific interstitial pneumonia

Lower lung predominance
Peripheral and/or peribronchovascular distribution
Ground-glass abnormality
Reticular abnormality with traction bronchiectasis
Honeycombing sparse or absent
Lower lobe volume loss
Consolidation ±

by Flaherty et al[16] of 109 patients who had biopsies of multiple sites showed that discordant diagnoses of UIP and NSIP were obtained from different lobes in 28 (26%). The prevalence of consolidation in series of patients with NSIP reported from Asia[12,74,101,106,111] appears to be greater than in series from Europe or North America[103,104,110]; this may be due to differing thresholds for inclusion of patients with OP.

A ground-glass pattern is the most common CT abnormality in all series of patients with NSIP, being found in 91% of patients.[112] It is usually bilateral and symmetric, with basal predominance (Fig. 10.16). It is most commonly peribronchovascular and/or subpleural in predominant distribution.[108] The peribronchovascular distribution may be helpful in distinguishing NSIP from UIP (Fig. 10.17). Ground-glass opacity occurs as an isolated finding in about one-third of patients, but is more commonly associated with other findings such as reticular abnormality or consolidation. Consolidation is seen in 0[103]–98%[111] of patients, almost always combined with ground-glass opacity. The wide variation in prevalence of consolidation is probably due to the fact that some patients with NSIP have significant amounts of histologic OP, so that it can be difficult to decide whether to classify an individual case as NSIP or OP.[4] Criteria for distinguishing NSIP from OP remain poorly defined. Like ground-glass opacity, consolidation is bilateral, basal, and subpleurally predominant or peribronchovascular. Irregular linear or reticular opacities (Figs 10.16 and 10.17) occur in about 75% of cases (range 29–87%).[106,108,109,112] Traction bronchiectasis

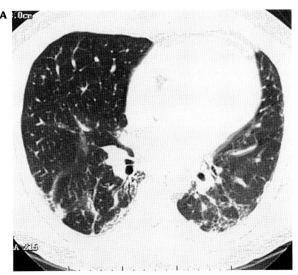
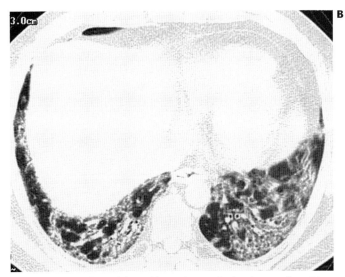

Fig. 10.17 A 40-year-old man with nonspecific interstitial pneumonia. **A** and **B**, HRCT shows bilateral lower lung reticular abnormality with traction bronchiectasis and lower lobe volume loss. Although there is some subpleural abnormality, the reticular pattern also extends along the bronchovascular structures.

is present in areas of ground-glass attenuation or reticular abnormality in 67% of cases.[112] Honeycomb changes were recorded in 20–30% of patients in some series,[12,74,104,109,111] but were absent in others.[88,106,108] This apparent discrepancy may be accounted for by interobserver variability in diagnosis of NSIP and UIP, and by the fact that histologic changes of UIP may coexist with those of NSIP. In general, it is true to say that honeycombing, if present at all in NSIP, is sparse. Other findings occasionally described include nodules (poorly defined and centrilobular with a subpleural and lower zone predominance),[109] pleural effusion (4%),[109] and enlarged hilar or mediastinal nodes (~5%). Pathologic/HRCT correlation[108] has shown that ground-glass opacity is caused by cellular or fibrotic interstitial thickening, bronchial dilatation, and irregular linear opacity indicates predominant fibrosis, and some areas of consolidation are caused by areas of OP.

Since the prognosis of cellular NSIP is known to be better than that of the fibrotic type, it would be very useful if CT were able to reliably discriminate between these entities. However, a paper by MacDonald et al[103] suggested that there was substantial overlap between the CT findings of these subtypes, though cellular NSIP was less likely to be subpleural in distribution, and had a higher proportion of ground-glass type abnormality. More recently, a study by Johkoh et al[111] found that the extent of reticular abnormality and traction bronchiectasis correlated with increasing amounts of fibrosis on histologic grading. Honeycombing was seen mainly in patients with purely fibrotic NSIP. While traction bronchiectasis was present in almost all cases, it tended to involve more proximal airways (lobar and segmental bronchi) in patients with fibrotic NSIP. Patients with cellular NSIP were more likely to have pure ground-glass abnormality without reticular abnormality. However, analysis of this issue is difficult because the proportion of patients with purely cellular NSIP is relatively small (six of 55 patients in the paper by Johkoh et al,[111] and five of 21 patients in the paper by MacDonald et al[103]).

Nishiyama et al[88] evaluated the CT changes on follow up of patients with NSIP after treatment. Parenchymal abnormalities showed improvement or resolution in 12 of 14 patients.

Reticular abnormality, traction bronchiectasis, and ground-glass abnormality were all completely or partially reversible. One patient progressed, with ground-glass abnormality being replaced by honeycombing. In a similar study by Kim et al,[108] the extent of ground-glass abnormality decreased substantially on follow up, but the extent of reticular abnormality decreased only slightly.

In the original series of patients with NSIP,[100] 46% had possible precipitating events or associated disorders, judged to be significant (Box 10.11). These consisted of: (1) connective tissue disorders in 16% (rheumatoid arthritis, dermatomyositis/polymyositis, systemic lupus erythematosus, systemic sclerosis, Sjögren syndrome); (2) other autoimmune disorders in 5%, including primary biliary cirrhosis and Hashimoto thyroiditis; (3) recent surgery, pneumonia, or acute respiratory distress syndrome in 8%; and (4) inhalation of organic antigens in 17%. These disorders must always be considered in the differential diagnosis of NSIP. Connective tissue disease should be suspected on CT if the patient has associated findings, such as enlarged pulmonary arteries or dilated esophagus. Hypersensitivity pneumonitis should be considered if there are micronodules or areas of air-trapping.

Box 10.11 Causes of nonspecific interstitial pneumonia pattern

Collagen vascular disease and other autoimmune diseases
Hypersensitivity pneumonitis
Drugs
Inhalational exposures

Desquamative interstitial pneumonia and respiratory bronchiolitis-interstitial lung disease

DIP and RB-ILD are important differential diagnostic considerations in patients who smoke cigarettes and present with the clinical syndrome of IIP. Because they are almost invariably smoking related, they are considered in Chapter 8.

Organizing pneumonia

Histologically, the OP pattern is characterized by the presence of intraluminal organizing fibrosis in the distal airspaces (bronchioles, alveolar ducts, and alveoli).[4] The distribution is usually patchy, and lung architecture is usually preserved. The connective tissue is characteristically all of the same age. There may be mild interstitial chronic inflammation. This pattern may be seen as the lung recovers from a variety of types of injury (Box 10.12). If a nonrepresentative biopsy (e.g. transbronchial biopsy) is obtained in patients with an OP response, then OP may be the major lesion seen.

Box 10.12 Conditions associated with histologic organizing pneumonia

Organizing pneumonia as a major finding
Cryptogenic organizing pneumonia
Secondary organizing pneumonia (collagen vascular disease, drugs)
Focal organizing pneumonia
Organizing pneumonia as a component of other pathologic entities
Nonspecific organizing pneumonia
Hypersensitivity pneumonitis
Eosinophilic lung disease
Organizing diffuse alveolar damage
Organizing infections
Postobstructive pneumonia
Aspiration pneumonia
Fume and toxic exposures
Radiation pneumonitis
Organizing pneumonia as a reparative reaction around other processes
Wegener granulomatosis
Neoplasms
Infarcts

The recognition of COP as a distinct clinicopathologic entity came with three reports in the early to mid 1980s,[7,8,113] though there had been sporadic earlier descriptions. Understanding of this entity is made more difficult by the fact that it has been called by a variety of names during the past 20 years. In the United States and Canada, it was called bronchiolitis obliterans organizing pneumonia,[8,114–116] because of the tendency of plugs of OP to occlude the smaller bronchioles. The term proliferative bronchiolitis was also used to describe this finding.[117] For this reason, it was often misleadingly classified as a small airways disease. However, its clinical, imaging, and pathologic features are distinctly different from those of small airways disease. There is some controversy about its inclusion as an IIP, because the areas of OP involve the pulmonary airspaces rather than the interstitium, its clinical presentation is more subacute than UIP, DIP or NSIP, and its imaging features are those of airspace disease. However, it is included in the new ATS/ERS classification of IIPs[4] because of its idiopathic nature, its association with collagen vascular diseases, and its tendency to overlap with the other interstitial pneumonias, particularly NSIP.

COP is a rare condition, with a prevalence of 12 per 100,000 hospital admissions in a Canadian series.[118] A striking clinical similarity has been seen among cases of COP reported from various centers.[118–121] Mean patient age is about 58 years (range 20–80 years),[122,123] and the sex incidence is equal.[118] Twenty-five to 50% of patients give a history of an influenzalike prodrome followed by an illness lasting between a week and several months, characterized by cough (persistent and commonly nonproductive), exertional dyspnea, malaise, fever, and weight loss. Less common complaints include pleuritic pain[124,125] and hemoptysis.[125–127] Given these symptoms, coupled with the radiographic findings of airspace opacity, it is not surprising that 50% of patients are initially diagnosed as having infective pneumonia.[118] On clinical examination of the lungs, fine, dry crepitations occur in 70–90% of patients; clubbing is rare.[120] The erythrocyte sedimentation rate is usually raised and may be very high,[128] as is the C-reactive protein level.[126]

Respiratory function tests show a restrictive abnormality, commonly with a diffusion defect and hypoxemia at rest or on exertion.[128,129] Occasionally there are obstructive features.[118] Bronchoalveolar lavage is nonspecific and shows mixed cellularity, usually with predominant lymphocytes accompanied by neutrophils and eosinophils with or without foam cells, mast cells, and plasma cells.[129] Neutrophil/eosinophil predominance indicates an unfavorable prognosis.[130]

The histologic diagnosis may be made by transbronchial biopsy[131] in up to two-thirds of patients,[118,132] especially if a step sectioning technique is used.[128] CT may be helpful in identifying a suitable site for transbronchial biopsy. Bronchoscopy may also be important to exclude other causes of consolidation such as infection, aspiration, or bronchoalveolar carcinoma. In cases where there is diagnostic doubt, thoracoscopic biopsy will be necessary.

The radiographic hallmark of COP is bilateral, patchy, airspace opacity (Fig. 10.18), with a density which ranges from consolidation to ground-glass opacity. Consolidation is nonsegmental and commonly 2–6 cm in diameter. It generally shows no craniocaudal predilection, though some series have shown a basal predominance.[8,120,133] On CT, the consolidation often has a peribronchial (Fig. 10.19)[2] or subpleural distribution and the latter may be apparent on the chest radiograph.[118,125,131,134] In about 10% of cases, opacities are unilateral or focal.[67,126,134,135] Consolidation tends to migrate (Fig. 10.18, Box 10.13) and to come and go even without treatment.[7,125,128,133,136–138] Although cavitation has been reported to occur in COP,[126,139,140] this may be due to unrecognized associated infection or vasculitis.

Box 10.13 Conditions associated with migratory lung opacities

Organizing pneumonia
Eosinophilic lung disease
Simple eosinophilic pneumonia (Löffler syndrome)
Chronic eosinophilic pneumonia
Drug/parasite hypersensitivity
Allergic bronchopulmonary aspergillosis
Churg–Strauss syndrome
Diffuse alveolar hemorrhage
Recurrent pulmonary infarction
Recurrent aspiration
Vasculitis

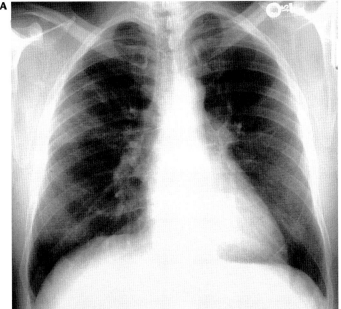

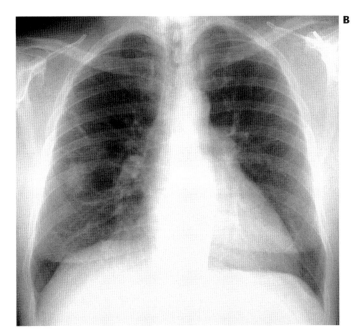

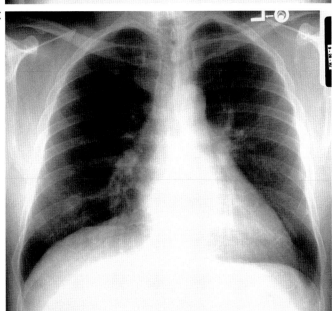

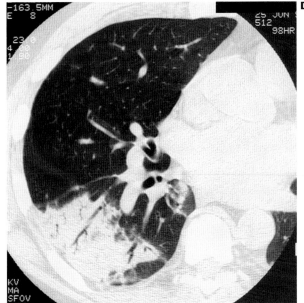

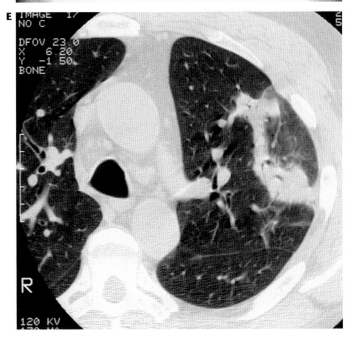

Fig. 10.18 A 62-year-old man with recurrent migratory opacities due to cryptogenic organizing pneumonia (COP). **A–C**, Chest radiographs show migratory poorly defined lung opacities of COP. **D** and **E**, HRCT during another exacerbation shows bilateral patchy lung consolidation typical of COP.

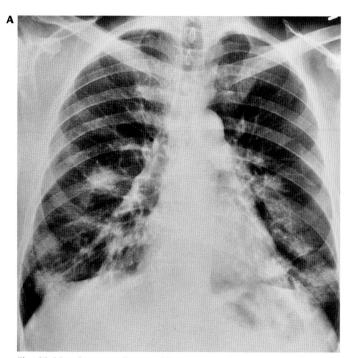

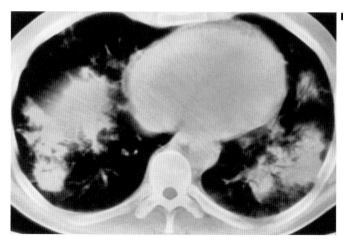

Fig. 10.19 Cryptogenic organizing pneumonia. A 55-year-old man who had a flulike syndrome during the previous 3 months and complained of increasing tiredness and dyspnea. **A,** Posteroanterior radiograph shows multiple poorly defined areas of consolidation. **B,** CT through the lung bases shows multiple peribronchovascular areas of consolidation, some of which have nodular configuration. Air bronchograms are present.

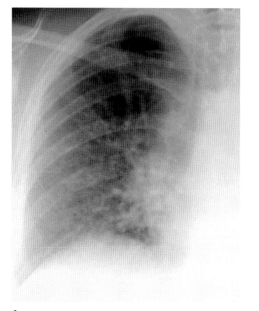

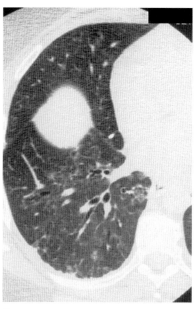

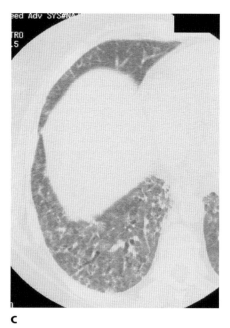

A   **B**   **C**

Fig. 10.20 A 54-year-old woman with organizing pneumonia, showing predominant reticular abnormality. **A,** Chest radiograph shows reticular abnormality. **B,** CT confirms predominantly peribronchovascular reticular abnormality. **C,** Three years later, the reticular abnormality has progressed on CT.

"Atypical" radiologic findings occur in 10–50% of patients with COP, either on their own or in association with consolidation. Such "atypical" findings include multiple large nodules[114]; 1–2 cm ill-defined nodules[114,125,134]; smaller rounded or irregular nodules, ranging from 1 to 10 mm in diameter[67,118,126,134,142,143]; and a basal predominant reticulonodular or irregular linear pattern (Fig. 10.20).[8,118,133,135] A nodular pattern as the sole or major manifestation of COP occurs in about 10–20% of patients.[118,143] Unilateral or bilateral pleural effusions occur occasionally with an overall frequency of about 5–10%.[114,118,128,144]

The CT and HRCT changes in COP are recorded in a number of papers (Box 10.14).[2,114,118,125,134,143,145–147] On CT, as on the chest radiograph, the most common finding is multifocal consolidation, seen in about 80% of patients (Figs 10.21 and 10.22).[148] In up to two-thirds of these patients consolidation is predominantly subpleural (Fig. 10.22), and commonly contains air bronchograms (Fig. 10.21) with dilated airways. Other areas of consolidation show a peribronchovascular distribution (Fig. 10.21).[146] Airspace opacity is usually bilateral (70–90%), asymmetric, and shows no apical/basal predominance. Individual areas of consolidation range in size from 1.5 cm to a segment or more. This characteristic pattern of airspace opacity is commonly accompanied by other signs on HRCT, typically ground-glass or nodular opacities. These associated findings were found in 74% of patients in one series.[146] About 60% of patients[148] have ground-glass opacity on HRCT (Fig. 10.22), often with a lobular, mosaic distribution.[145,149] About 30–50% of patients demonstrate nodules either as an isolated finding or, more commonly, as part of a mixed pattern with consolidation. Nodules show a great range in size but are most commonly in the 1–10 mm range, smooth, well defined and sometimes with a centrilobular or peribronchovascular distribution.[134] They are usually bilateral and grossly distributed in a random fashion. In a small number of patients, some nodules are larger (10–20 mm) and may have ill-defined margins ("airspace" nodules). Other findings described in a minority of patients include: peripheral reticulation and subpleural lines[114]; irregular lines, particularly in the lower zones (Fig. 10.20)[118,150]; perilobular thickening,[147] bronchial dilatation, and wall thickening (Fig. 10.22)[134]; large nodular or masslike peripheral opacities which sometimes have "feeder" airways or vessels[114]; nodules with air bronchograms (45%) and occasional satellite lesions[141]; multiple cavitary nodules[151–153]; mild lymph node enlargement in 14–42% of patients[76,114,134]; and small pleural effusions, either bilateral or unilateral, in about 20–30% of patients.[118,119,134,146] The finding of reticular abnormality on the chest radiograph or CT in a patient with biopsy proven OP merits attention, as it suggests that the patient will not respond to treatment, and may develop progressive fibrosis.[126,150]

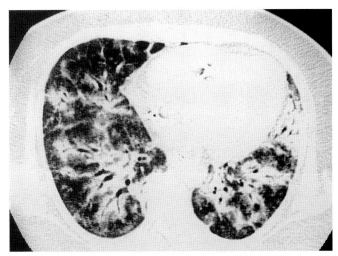

Fig. 10.21 Cryptogenic organizing pneumonia (COP). HRCT through the lower zones shows multifocal consolidation – the most common sign of COP. The consolidation has a strongly peribronchovascular distribution. Airways within the consolidation are dilated.

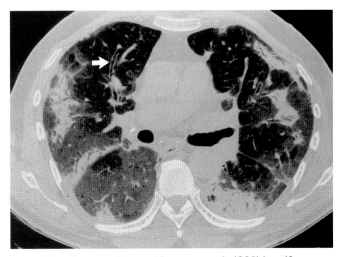

Fig. 10.22 Cryptogenic organizing pneumonia (COP) in a 63-year-old man with a 1 month history of cough, fever, and weight loss. Opacity consists of consolidation and ground-glass attenuation – the most common findings in COP. A few airways remote from the consolidative areas show mild dilatation and wall thickening (arrow).

> **Box 10.14 CT features of organizing pneumonia**
>
> Lower lung predominance
> Peripheral and/or peribronchovascular distribution
> Patchy consolidation
> Ground-glass abnormality

COP occasionally resolves spontaneously[8,121,129] but usually needs treatment with steroids. With therapy, clinical and radiographic signs clear in weeks in 30–60% of patients, but there is a 15% relapse rate,[119] and up to one-third of patients are left with persistent radiographic abnormality,[123] a minority of of patients with COP progress, despite treatment, to lung fibrosis with honeycombing.[126,139] Progression is more common in those with longer duration of symptoms and those who have linear radiographic abnormalities on initial chest radiograph.[126] It is possible that some of these patients may have NSIP or UIP, with a nonrepresentative biopsy sample showing predominant OP. In a recent study of 26 patients with biopsy proven OP, this author found that the presence of a reticular pattern on CT at presentation (Fig. 10.20) was associated with persistent or progressive abnormality on follow-up radiographs,[150] suggesting that CT may have prognostic value in patients with OP.

There is a 3–13% mortality in various series, many of which combine cases of primary and secondary OP,[53,130] and generally the prognosis is less good in OP associated with connective tissue disorders.[119,123,130]

A subgroup of patients with COP is described with high mortality and a fulminant course.[144,154] Histologic examination of biopsies in these cases has shown OP together with UIP and DAD.[130] The poor prognosis in these "hybrid" cases would appear to be due to these latter changes, and at necropsy the OP lesions themselves have often resolved.

Secondary organizing pneumonia

OP is commonly associated with a recognized precipitating cause, and in the Mayo Clinic series of 74 patients, 36% were classified as secondary, compared with 50% as cryptogenic

---

Box 10.15 Conditions associated with organizing pneumonia[119]

Infection[129]
Strep. pneumoniae, Legionella
Mycoplasma
Coxiella
Nocardia
Chlamydia pneumoniae
Influenza and parinfluenza 3 viruses
Adenovirus
HIV[158,159]
Cryptococcus
Malaria[160]

Connective tissue disorder/vasculitis[119,129]
Rheumatoid arthritis[161,162]
Systemic lupus erythematosus[163]
Polyarteritis nodosa[164]
Systemic vasculitis[118]
Polymyositis/dermatomyositis[165]
Systemic sclerosis[166]
CREST syndrome[167]
Mixed connective tissue disease[135]
Sjögren syndrome[168]
Polymyalgia rheumatica[169]
Essential mixed cryoglobulinemia[140]

Immune disorders
Leukemia[170]
Lymphoma[171]
Myelodysplastic syndrome
Mycosis fungoides
Myeloma
Bone marrow transplant[172,173]
Renal transplant[174]
Lung transplant[175]
Common variable immune deficiency[175]

Inflammatory bowel disease[176,177]

Hypothyroidism/chronic thyroiditis[121]

Liver disease[121,178]

Nephropathy[179,180]

Aspiration[129]

Radiation[155,156]

Drug toxicity (see Box 10.16)

Box 10.16 Drugs causing organizing pneumonia

Antiinflammatory
Gold[818]
5-aminosalicylic acid[177]
Nonsteroidal antiinflammatory agents[182]
Sulfasalazine[183]
Mesalazine[119]

Cytotoxic[129]
Cyclophosphamide, busulfan[129]
Bleomycin,[184] mitomycin[185]
Methotrexate[185]
Chlorozotocin (a nitrosourea)[185]

Antibiotic
Nitrofurantoin[119]
Amphotericin B[130]
Cephalosporin[130]
Chloroquine/primaquine[119]

Antiarrhythmic[185]
Amiodarone[129]
Tocainide

Anticonvulsant
Phenytoin[185]

Miscellaneous[185]
Nilutamide
Interferon
Sodium cromoglycate
Cocaine[129,130]
Tryptophan[130]

---

cases.[119] No distinguishing clinical, radiologic, or pathologic features were found between COP and secondary OP apart from a worse overall prognosis in the secondary group,[119] as noted by others.[144] The poorer prognosis includes a slower and less complete resolution and a higher respiratory mortality.

Associations and causes of secondary OP are listed in Box 10.15.[4,118,129,130] In clinical practice, the common causes of an OP pattern are collagen vascular disease (particularly polymyositis/dermatomyositis and rheumatoid arthritis), drugs, and lung or bone marrow transplantation (Box 10.16). One interesting clinical entity is the occurrence in women of migratory OP within a year following radiation therapy for breast cancer (Fig. 10.23).[138,155–157] These patients present with typical symptoms of COP, and show typical migratory pulmonary opacities, both within and outside the radiation port. They usually respond well to steroids, though with a high prevalence of relapse on withdrawal of steroids. It is thought that the radiation treatment in some way "primes" the immune system of the lung for the development of OP.[156]

Focal organizing pneumonia

Focal OP is an uncommon presentation of OP, unrelated to the clinical entity of COP. In the Mayo Clinic series, Lohr et al[119] described 10 cases, nine of which were manifest on the chest radiograph as a single nodule (4–35 mm diameter). Unlike most patients with cryptogenic or secondary OP, acute symptoms were absent and nodules were generally an incidental radiographic finding. Lesions were nonprogressive, carried a good prognosis, and did not necessitate steroid therapy.[119] Typically, the nodules were resected or biopsied because they were suspicious for lung cancer. Similar cases have been reported by other workers, often as single case reports.[126,127,139,184,186] Lesions are described either as nodules or as focal consolidations and a number of the lesions have shown cavitation.[139,186] Many of the lesions have been of obscure origin but in some there has been a clear cause, as in the case of a bleomycin related nodule.[142] HRCT data are essentially limited to one series of 18 patients.[187] Although 83% of these patients were asymptomatic at the time of presentation, 39% gave a clear history of antecedent infective pneumonia 2–4 months

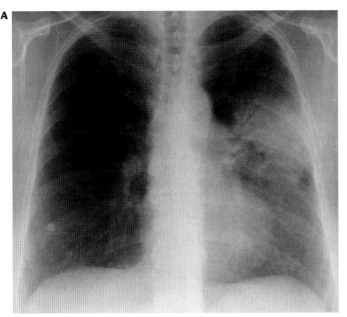
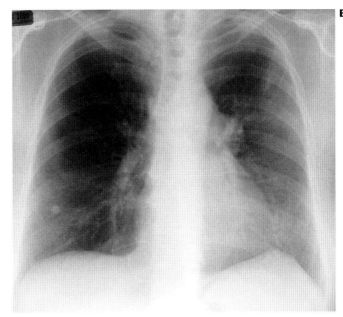

Fig. 10.23 Organizing pneumonia in a 60-year-old woman who had just completed radiation for breast cancer. **A** and **B**, Chest radiographs obtained 5 weeks apart show migratory airspace opacities.

earlier, which is likely to have been etiologically significant. The authors subdivided the HRCT appearances into three types: (1) small irregular masses often with pleural tags, all <2 cm diameter; (2) larger oval lesions with broad pleural contact, some with satellites and air bronchograms, and peripheral lung vessels converged towards the main opacity; and (3) oval lesions lying along bronchovascular bundles, again sometimes accompanied by pleural tags and satellites. Overall 94% of lesions had irregular margins and about 50% had air bronchograms, satellites, or pleural tags. Follow-up CT examinations showed partial or complete resolution and the authors stressed the usefulness of such examinations in management.

Acute interstitial pneumonia

AIP was first described by Hamman and Rich in 1944.[188] They called the condition, which they saw in four adults, acute diffuse interstitial fibrosis of the lungs. It proved fatal in all four subjects and the paper provides detailed postmortem findings. Despite this early description, AIP was not identified as a histologically (and clinically) distinct form of IIP until the histopathologic description of cases in 1986 by Katzenstein et al.[189] The pathology is that of organizing DAD and the condition resembles adult respiratory distress syndrome (ARDS) in all respects save for the lack of an identifiable precipitating event. Synonyms include Hamman-Rich syndrome, accelerated interstitial pneumonitis, and idiopathic ARDS.

Key features of the condition are: (1) fulminant respiratory failure in a previously healthy individual, without an identifiable precipitating event: (2) pathologic changes of DAD; (3) imaging changes of ARDS; and (4) a high mortality, in the order of 80–90%.

AIP may be differentiated histologically into acute, organizing, and fibrotic phases. In the acute exudative phase, there is diffuse alveolar interstitial thickening due to edema, and associated hyaline membranes. The histologic lung changes of organizing DAD[189,191] consist of fibroblast proliferation in the alveolar interstitium. Collagen production is also usually mild.[189,191] Hyaline membranes are usually more sparse.[123] Changes are diffuse and temporally uniform.[189] Other findings include hyaline membranes, intraalveolar organization, type II pneumocyte proliferation, and thrombi in small vessels.[192] In the fibrotic phase, alveolar wall collapse and apposition occurs.[123] Known causes of DAD (Box 10.17) must, of course, be excluded.

Box 10.17 Causes of histologic diffuse alveolar damage pattern[4]

Infection
Collagen vascular disease
Drug toxicity
Toxic inhalation
Uremia
Sepsis
Transfusion related acute lung injury
Shock
Trauma

Clinically, previously healthy patients develop rapidly increasing dyspnea with fever over a few days, often following a short influenzalike prodrome. Males and females are equally affected, with a wide age range (13–83 years); mean ages also vary widely in various series from 28 to 65 years.[193,194] Fulminant respiratory failure rapidly follows, necessitating ventilatory support. Steroid treatment is usually tried but its efficacy is unclear. In five early series comprising 64 patients,[188,189,191,193,194] mortality was 78%.

It is generally accepted that the radiographic appearances of AIP are similar to those of ARDS, but the radiographic changes of AIP have not been systematically described and are frequently simply recorded as "bilateral infiltrates". The chest radiograph

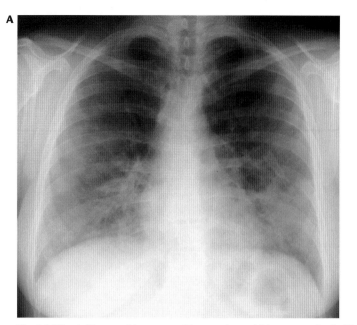
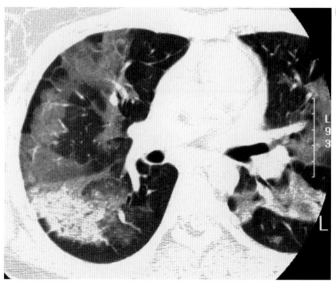

Fig. 10.24 A 31-year-old woman with acute interstitial pneumonia. **A**, Chest radiograph shows basal predominant ground-glass abnormality. **B**, HRCT shows a geographic (mosaic) distribution of ground-glass abnormality, with sparing of some secondary lobules. Consolidation is seen in the more dependent lung.

shows diffuse consolidation, sometimes with a zonal predominance and often with air bronchograms.[193] The distribution is often patchy (Fig. 10.24), sparing the costophrenic sulci. Lung volumes are usually low. As the disease progresses, pulmonary consolidation increases. As the DAD moves from the exudative to the organizing stage, the radiograph tends to show less consolidation, evolving to a ground-glass appearance with irregular linear opacities. The radiographic appearances of AIP, like those of ARDS, may be substantially affected by the ventilator settings, with increasing airway pressures resulting in apparent decrease in consolidation and increase in ground-glass abnormality.

HRCT changes have been described in several series.[97,193–199] On HRCT (Fig. 10.24), ground-glass opacity is a universal finding. It is commonly diffuse and patchy, sometimes with a geographic pattern. The second most common HRCT finding, in 70–90% of patients, is consolidation, often most evident in the dependent lung. In 30–70% of patients, septal thickening is found in areas of ground-glass opacity, perhaps corresponding to alveolar collapse adjacent to septa. Honeycombing is seen in 12–26% of cases. Most series do not systematically record the presence or absence of pleural effusions, but pleural effusions were found in 38% of patients in one series of patients with AIP.[198]

The CT features of AIP are similar but not identical to those of ARDS (Box 10.18). When Tomiyama et al[199] compared the CT features of AIP with those of ARDS, the main differences were a higher prevalence of honeycombing and lower prevalence of septal thickening in AIP. The abnormalities of AIP were more likely to be symmetric, and to have a lower lung predominance, than those of ARDS.

Ichikado et al[194] described a close correlation between the CT findings and the phase of AIP. The acute phase is characterized by ground-glass attenuation and consolidation. The presence of traction bronchiectasis suggests that the disease is in the organizing phase, while honeycombing is seen in the fibrotic phase. When the CT features of patients with AIP who survived were compared with those who died, architectural distortion was more commonly seen in the nonsurvivors.[195] However, because of overlap in CT findings between survivors and nonsurvivors, this observation is of limited value in individual cases.[200]

Lymphoid interstitial pneumonia

LIP is histologically characterized by marked infiltration of the interstitial space, as well as to a lesser extent the alveolar space, by monotonous sheets of lymphocytes. LIP can lead to progressive pulmonary fibrosis, and can resolve with corticosteroid and immunosuppressive therapy. Diseases associated with LIP include dysproteinemias (e.g. common variable immunodeficiency), autoimmune disorders (particularly Sjögren syndrome), autologous bone marrow transplantation, and viral, mycobacterial and HIV infections. HIV related LIP occurs much more commonly in children than in adults.[201] Intrathoracic Castleman disease is commonly associated with LIP.[202] There are also familial and idiopathic forms of LIP.

In the classification of interstitial lung disease, LIP has been classified either as an interstitial pneumonia or as a lymphoproliferative disorder. It is thought to represent a reactive lymphoid hyperplasia rather than a true lymphoproliferative disease, and evolution to frank lymphoproliferative disease, though described in case reports, is quite rare.[4,203] Though not usually idiopathic, it was included in the ATS/ERS classification

---

Box 10.18 **CT features of acute interstitial pneumonia**

Consolidation
Ground-glass abnormality
Traction bronchiectasis (organizing phase)
Honeycombing ±

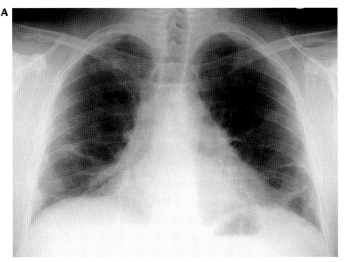

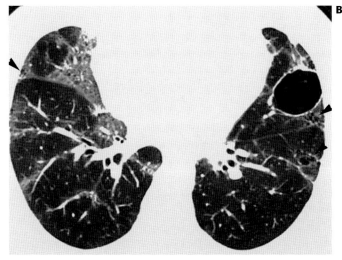

Fig. 10.25 A 44-year-old man with lymphoid interstitial pneumonia (LIP). **A,** Chest radiograph shows lower lobe volume loss, with ground-glass abnormality and linear scarring. **B,** CT through the lower lobes shows scattered areas of ground-glass abnormality. The large cyst in the lingula, and the scattered smaller cysts (arrowheads) are important clues to the diagnosis of LIP, though similar cysts may be seen in desquamative interstitial pneumonia.

of IIPs,[4] largely because it is important in the histologic differential diagnosis of interstitial pneumonia.

LIP is substantially more common in women, and most commonly presents in the 4th–7th decade. Dyspnea and a non-productive cough are common and may be present for months to years. Constitutional symptoms of fever, weight loss, and arthralgia may occur. There may be symptoms of a well defined or evolving connective tissue disease. On examination inspiratory dry crackles are common, while clubbing occasionally occurs. Adenopathy and hepatosplenomegaly may be seen, and may portend a greater likelihood of progression to lymphoma. Laboratory evaluation is nonspecific. Dysproteinemia should be specifically sought. On physiology, a restrictive ventilatory defect, with preserved airflow, is found. The diagnosis of LIP requires histologic confirmation, usually by a surgical biopsy. Special staining techniques are often required to separate LIP from a well differentiated pulmonary lymphoma.

On chest radiograph LIP is generally characterized by basal predominant ground-glass or reticular abnormality (Fig. 10.25).[201] In a study of the radiographs of 16 patients with LIP related to HIV infection, Oldham et al[169] found a fine reticular or reticu-lonodular pattern in five patients, coarse reticulonodular infiltrates in two, and reticular or reticulonodular opacities with superimposed patchy alveolar infiltrates in nine.[204]

Johkoh et al[205] described the CT features of LIP in a series of 22 patients (Box 10.19). Ten of these patients had Sjögren syndrome, seven had multicentric Castleman disease with hypergammaglobulinemia, two had AIDS, and three had no underlying disease. In this series the dominant CT findings, present in all patients, were ground-glass opacity (Fig. 10.25) and poorly defined centrilobular nodules. These findings were usually diffuse in distribution. Subpleural nodules, and bronchovascular and septal thickening were also common, seen in 19 of 22 patients. Discrete cystic airspaces ranging from 1 to 30 mm were found in 15 patients, and have also been described in other series (Fig. 10.26).[206–208] They differ from honeycomb cysts in that they are not clustered. Mediastinal or hilar lymphadenopathy was seen in 15 patients, particularly in those

> **Box 10.19 CT features of lymphoid interstitial pneumonia**
>
> Ground-glass abnormality
> Nodules (centrilobular or subpleural)
> Cysts

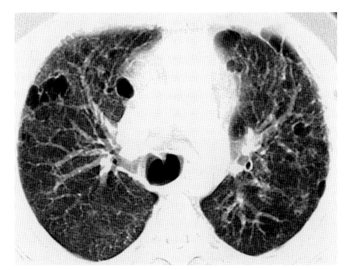

Fig. 10.26 A 48-year-old man with lymphoid interstitial pneumonia (LIP). A 10 mm CT image shows ground-glass abnormality and thin walled cysts as the predominant manifestations of LIP in this patient.

with intrathoracic Castleman syndrome. Areas of consolidation were found in nine patients. Other, smaller series have confirmed that ground-glass abnormality and nodules are the salient CT features of LIP.[209,210] The centrilobular nodules appear to correlate with peribronchiolar lymphocytic infiltration, while the ground-glass abnormality and consolidation presumably correlate with more diffuse infiltration of the alveolar interstitium by lymphocytes. The pathogenesis of the cysts is unclear, but they may be related to check-valve obstruction of bronchioles by adjacent lymphoid tissue.[206] On follow-up CT, the ground-glass abnormality and centrilobular nodules of LIP generally improve on treatment, but new cysts may develop in areas previously occupied by centrilobular nodules, while areas of consolidation may evolve into honeycombing.[211]

Honda et al[208] compared the CT features of LIP with those of lymphoma, and found that large nodules (11–30 mm in diameter), consolidation, and pleural effusions were significantly more common in lymphoma, while cysts were significantly more common in LIP.

Familial lung fibrosis

About 5% of cases of lung fibrosis have a family history of fibrosis in a family member.[212] The histologic appearance of familial lung fibrosis varies, but most cases show either a UIP or NSIP pattern.[213] The CT spectrum is correspondingly varied. Familial DIP may occur in children.[214] Surfactant protein C deficiency may account for some cases of familial fibrosis in both children and adults (Fig. 10.27).[215]

Diagnostic accuracy of CT

Usual interstitial pneumonia

Because of significant differences in prognosis and in management, the most important diagnostic decision is the distinction between UIP and other entities. In a study of 91 patients presenting with a clinical syndrome suggestive of IPF, 60% had UIP on biopsy, 13% had respiratory bronchiolitis, 8% had hypersensitivity pneumonitis, 7% had NSIP, 3% had sarcoidosis, and the remaining patients had a variety of diagnoses including emphysema, bronchioloalveolar carcinoma, OP, eosinophilic pneumonia, pulmonary hypertension, silicosis, and Langerhans histiocytosis.[75] In this series of patients,[82] as in many

others,[27,74,79–81] a confident CT diagnosis of UIP was correct in >90% of cases. It is clear that honeycombing is the most important diagnostic feature of UIP, particularly in making the distinction between UIP and NSIP.[15,75] The presence of upper lobe irregular linear abnormality has been found to be another independent discriminator between UIP and nonUIP.[75] Table 10.2 indicates the CT features which help make this distinction.

Chronic hypersensitivity pneumonitis (CHP) is an important aspect of the differential diagnosis of NSIP and UIP (Fig. 10.28, see p. 561). Features that favor CHP over NSIP or UIP include upper- or mid-lung predominance, and the presence of poorly defined centrilobular nodules.[216] Air-trapping may also be an important indicator of CHP (Fig 10.28).[217,218] However, CHP may present with a histologic pattern identical to that of NSIP[100] or UIP.[219] Therefore, a thorough clinical evaluation for possible sources of hypersensitivity pneumonitis is important in all patients presenting with CT features suggestive of UIP or NSIP.

Pulmonary sarcoidosis, in keeping with its reputation as a great mimic, may rarely simulate the basal and peripheral pattern of UIP, with subpleural cysts being found in a small number of cases.[220] However, the cysts of sarcoidosis are often larger than those of UIP, and are not concentrated in the subpleural lung. Furthermore, in cases of sarcoidosis masquerading as fibrosing alveolitis, septal lines are often a prominent feature – not the case in UIP.

Nonspecific interstitial pneumonia, desquamative interstitial pneumonia, and organizing pneumonia

Early studies of the CT differential diagnosis of NSIP noted difficulty in distinguishing it from other interstitial lung diseases.[74,104] However, since then, understanding of the CT findings of NSIP has evolved, and the typical pattern of basal predominant ground-glass attenuation and reticular abnormality with traction bronchiectasis has been recognized. Two recent studies have evaluated the ability to differentiate between UIP and NSIP using HRCT. In a study by McDonald et al,[103] of

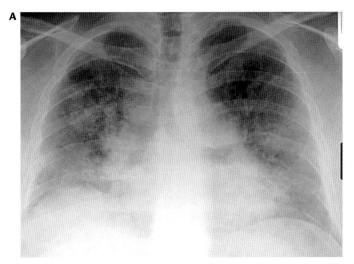
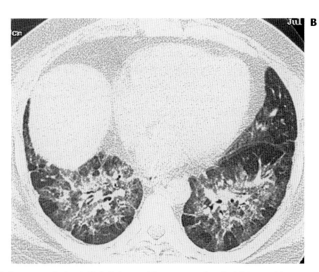

Fig. 10.27 A 36-year-old man with nonspecific interstitial pneumonia (NSIP) due to surfactant C deficiency. There was a family history of lung fibrosis. **A**, Chest radiograph shows marked decrease in lung volumes, with a predominantly central distribution of reticular abnormality. **B**, CT through the lower lungs shows typical appearance of NSIP, with peribronchovascular reticular abnormality, traction bronchiectasis, and fissural displacement, indicating lower lobe volume loss.

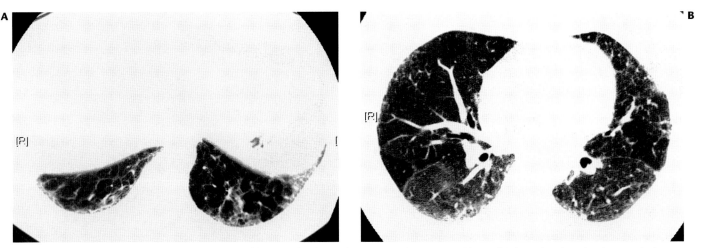

Fig. 10.28   Nonspecific interstitial pneumonia (NSIP) pattern in chronic hypersensitivity pneumonitis. **A**, CT shows basal predominant reticular abnormality with traction bronchiectasis. **B**, CT at a higher level shows geographic areas of decrease in lung attenuation suggesting air-trapping (confirmed on expiratory CT). This finding suggests that the NSIP pattern is due either to hypersensitivity pneumonitis or to collagen vascular disease with bronchiolar involvement.

21 patients with NSIP and 32 with UIP, the sensitivity, specificity, and accuracy of a CT diagnosis of NSIP were 70, 63, and 66%, respectively. UIP was falsely diagnosed in 21 (33%) of 64 readings of patients with fibrotic NSIP. Conversely, NSIP was falsely diagnosed in 48 (38%) of 128 readings in patients with histologic UIP. In a study by Eliot et al (unpublished data), of 29 patients with NSIP and 24 with UIP, a predominant pattern of ground-glass attenuation and/or reticular opacity, with minimal to no honeycombing, was demonstrated in 57 (98%) of 58 readings in patients with NSIP, and in 21 (43%) of 48 readings in patients with UIP. Conversely, the presence of honeycombing as a predominant feature had a specificity of 98% and positive predictive value of 96% for UIP. The positive predictive value of a confident diagnosis of NSIP was 77%, while for UIP it was 91%. These studies suggest that it is possible to confidently identify UIP when honeycombing is present, but a minority of patients with UIP have CT findings similar to those of NSIP, and can only be distinguished by biopsy. As indicated above, pathologists show substantial variation in differentiating between UIP and NSIP, so the gold standard for this diagnosis is not established, and the most accurate assessment requires correlation of CT and biopsy.

At the other end of the spectrum, it may be difficult to distinguish histologic NSIP from OP. Focal areas of OP are seen histologically in about 50% of cases of NSIP.[100] As with UIP, the amount of OP present on an individual biopsy specimen may vary with the site of biopsy. On CT, OP characteristically presents with patchy consolidation and ground-glass attenuation, often with subpleural and peribronchovascular predominance. The main distinguishing features between OP and NSIP are that the consolidation of OP is more patchy and that reticular abnormality and traction bronchiectasis are less common. No clear borderline exists to delineate the extent of consolidation in OP from NSIP, and indeed there are cases where OP appears to evolve into NSIP. OP should be favored in patients with patchy consolidation, while NSIP is favored in patients with basal predominant confluent abnormality associated with evidence of fibrosis.

The imaging features of NSIP may overlap with those of DIP. A subpleural distribution, and the presence of small cysts, should favor the diagnosis of DIP. However, the distinction between NSIP and DIP is not critical, since the treatment of these entities is similar. The longterm survival in DIP is excellent, and similar to that of cellular NSIP.[52]

Acute interstitial pneumonia

In patients presenting with the syndrome of AIP, the other IIPs are not usually considered in the differential diagnosis. However, the differential diagnosis must include infectious pneumonia, acute hypersensitivity pneumonitis, acute eosinophilic pneumonia, pulmonary hemorrhage, drug or transfusion reaction, and cardiac or noncardiac edema. Tomiyama et al[198] compared the CT features of AIP with some other conditions causing acute diffuse lung opacity, including bacterial or mycoplasma pneumonia, acute hypersensitivity pneumonitis, acute eosinophilic pneumonia, and pulmonary hemorrhage. In their study, the combination of airspace consolidation, centrilobular nodules, and segmental distribution was found in most cases of infectious pneumonia, but was not seen in AIP. In particular, the finding of centrilobular nodules or tree-in-bud pattern was very suggestive of infection. Traction bronchiectasis and honeycombing, rarely seen in the other acute pneumonias, should suggest AIP. The presence of septal thickening or pleural effusion as predominant findings should suggest acute eosinophilic pneumonia (see p. 654). In the study by Tomiyama et al,[198] a correct first choice diagnosis of AIP was made in 90% of cases of AIP, based on the findings described above.

Correlation between structure and function

A reliable, objective method for determining the extent of lung parenchymal abnormality would be clinically helpful for staging and follow up of patients with lung fibrosis. Early investigations attempted to quantify the extent of lung disease based on the chest radiographic appearances, either by using a scoring system,[221] or by comparison with standard radiographs.[222] A combined clinical, radiographic, and physiologic (CRP) scoring system has been devised which attempts to improve the accuracy of estimating disease extent (or severity).[221]

The functional deficit in patients with lung fibrosis is typically restrictive, with reduced compliance, lung volume, and decreased gas diffusing capacity. The pulmonary function indices that reflect these abnormalities are routinely used in clinical practice to assess the extent of disease and monitor progress. The value of these tests is limited by the fact that they do not account for the regional inhomogeneity of fibrosing lung disease. However, the severity of physiologic impairment,[20] and the change in physiologic parameters over a 1 year interval, are good predictors of longterm survival.[223,224] Most studies show substantial correlations between pulmonary function test data and visual assessment of disease extent by CT.[42,225] However, there is no widely accepted, reproducible, standardized scoring system for describing the visual extent of lung disease on CT.

Compared with chest radiographs, interobserver variation decreases substantially when the extent of parenchymal abnormality is estimated by CT.[226,227] The most commonly used technique for the quantitation of disease extent is subjective visual estimation.[21,42,227,228] However, some of the more subtle abnormalities caused by interstitial fibrosis may escape visual detection, and more sophisticated approaches to the quantification of interstitial lung disease include analysis of CT density values[229–231] and texture of the lung parenchyma.[232] In patients with pulmonary fibrosis, the density histogram is characteristically more peaked (kurtotic) and skewed to the left than the normal distribution.[230,231] The degree of kurtosis correlates moderately well with the severity of restrictive pulmonary impairment.[231] An operator independent technique which relies on fractal analysis of CT sections has been reported to have good accuracy for the quantification of fibrosing alveolitis.[233] Techniques for image analysis allow estimation of lung volumes, and simultaneous calculation of the relative amounts of soft tissue and air present in the lung.[229] Lung surface area may also be calculated.[234] Textural analysis of images may use multiple image features to differentiate between features of lung fibrosis and ground-glass attenuation,[235] or to distinguish different types of lung disease, such as emphysema, sarcoidosis and IPF.[236] Factors which limit the wide application of quantitative CT include the lack of spirometric gating, and substantial variation in reconstruction algorithms among manufacturers.[231]

Many patients with CFA (usually UIP) are cigarette smokers,[49] and thus emphysema is a common accompaniment. This combination has long been recognized as being responsible for spuriously preserved lung volumes on chest radiography (see Fig. 10.3) and pulmonary function testing.[40,41] On HRCT the morphologic differences between emphysematous and fibrotic lung can usually be readily made: smoker's centrilobular emphysema is predominantly upper zone in distribution compared with the basal predilection of fibrosing alveolitis. Nevertheless, the distinction between the two processes in the mid zones becomes difficult, or impossible (Fig. 10.29). In addition to the confounding effect of coexisting emphysema, variable ventilation of fibrotic lung composed of cystic airspaces is also likely to weaken the relationship between disease extent and pulmonary function test measures of lung volume. Although it seems likely that the majority of such cystic "dead spaces" are ventilated,[237] others may air trap.[238] For a given extent of fibrotic lung on CT, total gas diffusing capacity (DLco) is depressed, reflecting its lack of perfusion (irrespective of whether or not the affected lung is ventilated). Wells et al[239] have developed a

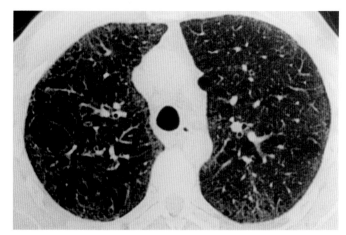

Fig. 10.29 Combination of centrilobular emphysema (more obvious in the right upper lobe) and reticular abnormality in the upper zones.

composite physiologic index based on the DLco, forced expired volume in 1 s (FEV$_1$) and forced vital capacity (FVC), which is a better predictor of extent of lung fibrosis on CT than any one of these tests alone, even in patients with concomitant emphysema.

Prediction of reversibility and survival based on CT appearances

Many studies of CT in patients with IIP performed in the 1990s found that ground-glass abnormality was an important predictor of treatment responsiveness and/or survival.[21,23,30,85,86] With the new understanding of the pathologic subsets of IIP, it seems clear that much of this effect was driven by the fact that ground-glass abnormality is the salient CT finding in NSIP and DIP, but is sparse or absent in patients with UIP. In patients with true UIP, ground-glass abnormality usually indicates lung fibrosis, and commonly progresses to honeycombing. In recent studies of patients with UIP, the extent of honeycombing on CT correlates with poorer survival,[15,240] suggesting that this may be used as a surrogate for histology in patients unable to undergo biopsy.

Given the prognostic importance of the histologic pattern, an important question is whether CT can perform as effectively as histology in predicting outcome. A recent study by Flaherty et al[71] evaluated this issue in 168 patients presenting with suspected IIP. Of these, 106 had histologic UIP, 33 had NSIP, and 22 had RB-ILD/DIP. The presence of honeycombing was strongly predictive of UIP, but its absence did not exclude UIP. The survival of patients with honeycombing on CT was significantly poorer than those without honeycombing. However, with regard to survival, the predictive value of honeycombing was less strong than that of histologic diagnosis.

End-stage lung

Most types of diffuse interstitial lung disease may progress to a final nonspecific pattern termed end-stage lung.[241] The term, as used by radiologists, describes the morphologic appearances and does not imply functional respiratory insufficiency, though this may well be present, and patients with end-stage lung populate waiting lists for lung transplantation. Findings consist principally of honeycomb and cystic changes with or without conglomerate fibrosis. A large number of conditions can evolve into this pattern (Box 10.20).[241–243] Imaging features of each of these disorders are discussed in detail elsewhere in this book.

Pathologically, distal airspaces are restructured, remaining walls becoming thick and fibrotic, and airways are obliterated. This results in the macroscopic appearance of honeycomb lung in which multiple cysts are separated by dense interstitial fibrosis.[241] Grossly, the most characteristic feature of end-stage lung is the presence of small cystic spaces, which give the surface of the lung a bosselated appearance.[241] These cysts vary in size from 1 mm to 2 cm, but the typical size is of the order of 5–10 mm. Three mechanisms account for the formation of cysts: (1) alveolar simplification secondary to septal dissolution; (2) bronchiolectasis; and (3) obstructive emphysema. Just as the cysts are the most characteristic gross morphologic finding in pathologic specimens, so too are they the most characteristic imaging feature. They appear as aggregated, small, ring opacities that are termed honeycomb shadows when they have a diameter of 3–10 mm with walls 2–3 mm thick (Fig. 10.25).[244] There may be additional small rounded and irregular opacities, but these lack the specificity of honeycomb opacities in the diagnosis of end-stage lung. The radiographic changes are usually diffuse, bilateral, and asymmetric. Lung volume may be normal, increased, or decreased – depending on the mix of pathologic processes. There will be features of cor pulmonale in advanced disease and, in long-standing cases, there may be small calcified pulmonary nodules[245] as a result of metaplastic ossification.[78] Scar carcinoma is a recognized complication and may appear radiologically as a mass or as consolidation, either unifocal or multifocal carcinomas may occur.

On CT evaluation, the pattern of end-stage lung can be classified into honeycombing (clustered cysts, usually most extensive subpleurally) (see Figs 10.5 and 10.12), diffuse cystic disease, and conglomerate fibrosis (Fig. 10.30).[246] The honeycomb pattern is usually due to UIP, either from IPF, inhalational exposures, collagen vascular disease, or less frequently sarcoidosis. The diffuse cystic pattern is most commonly due to either lymphangioleiomyomatosis or Langerhans cell histiocytosis. The conglomerate fibrotic pattern may be due to pneumoconiosis or sarcoidosis; this pattern is often associated with peripheral cysts or emphysema. CT diagnosis of these entities is facilitated by evaluation of the more normal lung for findings that reflect the antecedent disorder.[246] The distribution of the abnormality is also helpful. In patients with end-stage

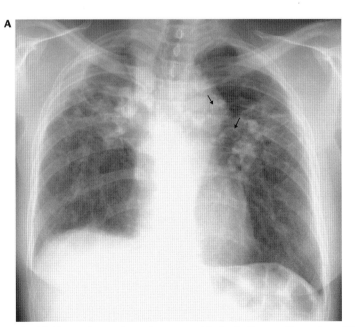
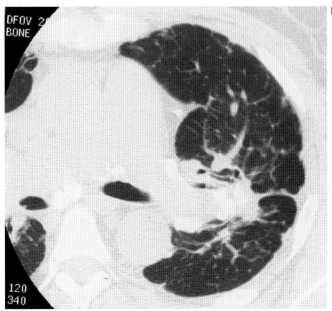

Fig. 10.30 End-stage lung due to sarcoidosis. **A**, Chest radiograph and **B**, chest CT show marked bilateral upper lobe volume loss, with conglomerate perihilar masses and eggshell calcification in mediastinal and hilar nodes (arrows, **A**). This contrasts with the lower lobe predominant honeycombing seen in cases of interstitial pulmonary fibrosis (see Fig. 10.12).

lung, CT diagnoses have a remarkably high specificity of 80–100% in Langerhans cell histiocytosis, silicosis, asbestosis, fibrosing alveolitis, extrinsic allergic alveolitis, hypersensitivity pneumonitis, and sarcoidosis.[246]

COLLAGEN VASCULAR DISEASE

Involvement of the respiratory system in rheumatologic or collagen vascular diseases is common and can result in significant morbidity and mortality. The autoimmune mediated inflammation and fibrosis that characterize these diseases in other organs can easily and irreversibly disrupt the normal functioning of the lung (Table 10.3). Many of these diseases are characterized by the presence of a specific type of autoantibody, which may greatly assist specific diagnosis. The underlying mechanisms that account for the tissue changes encountered in this group of illnesses are unknown. As a group they can affect each portion of the lung: the pleura, alveoli, interstitium, vasculature, lymphatic tissue, and airways, both large and small (Table 10.4). Commonly, more than one compartment is involved (Fig. 10.31). Most of the parenchymal manifestations of collagen vascular disease are similar to those found in IIPs (see p. 537),[4] and can be classified using the same system.[247] While Table 10.4 attempts to show that certain patterns of pulmonary involvement

Table 10.3 Autoantibodies associated with specific collagen vascular diseases

Disease	Associated autoantibodies
Rheumatoid arthritis	Rheumatoid factor
Progressive systemic sclerosis (PSS)	Anticentromere antibody (limited PSS) Anti-SCL-70
Mixed connective tissue disease	Antiribonuclear protein
Dermatomyositis/polymyositis	Anti-Jo-1
Systemic lupus erythematosis	Anti-double-stranded DNA and anti-Sm Antinuclear factor (less specific) Antiphospholipid antibodies
Sjögren syndrome	Anti-SS-A (Ro) Anti-SS-B (La)

Table 10.4 Pulmonary complications of collagen vascular diseases[247,248]

Pattern	RA	SLE	MCTD	PSS	PM/DM	SjS
UIP pattern	++	+	+	++	+	+
NSIP pattern	+	+	++	++++	++	+
Organizing pneumonia	++	+	+	+	+++	
Diffuse alveolar damage	+	++		+	++	
Lymphoproliferative disease (including LIP)	+					++
Alveolar hemorrhage	+	+++	+	+	+	
Upper lobe fibrosis	+					
Aspiration pneumonia			+	+	++	
Pulmonary hypertension	+	+	+	++		+
Bronchiectasis	++					++
Obliterative bronchiolitis	++	+				
Necrobiotic nodules	++					
Pleural effusion	++	++		+		
Muscle weakness/diaphragm dysfunction		+	+		++	

++++ = indicates a frequent clinical association; + = indicates that the entity is relatively uncommon. Empty cells indicate that the entity is not described or rare.
RA = rheumatoid arthritis; SLE = systemic lupus erythematosis; MCTD = mixed connective tissue disease; PSS = progressive systemic sclerosis; PM/DM = polymyositis/dermatomyositis; SjS = Sjögren syndrome; UIP = usual interstitial pneumonia; NSIP = nonspecific interstitial pneumonia; LIP = lymphoid interstitial pneumonia.

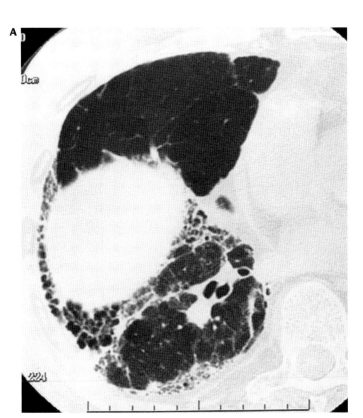

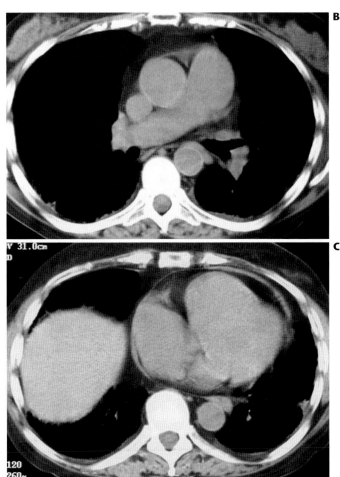

Fig. 10.31 Multicompartment involvement due to rheumatoid arthritis. **A**, CT images (lung windows) show peripheral reticular abnormality and honeycombing compatible with usual interstitial pneumonia. In the anterior right lung there is a marked decrease in attenuation with decreased size of pulmonary vessels, indicating constrictive bronchiolitis. **B** and **C**, Mediastinal windows show pleural and pericardial thickening, and enlargement of the main pulmonary artery and right ventricle due to pulmonary hypertension. These images demonstrate involvement of pulmonary vasculature, bronchioles, interstitium, pleura, and pericardium. Such multicompartment involvement is strongly suggestive of collagen vascular disease.

are more characteristic of particular autoimmune diseases, it is prudent to consider all compartments of the lung at risk in patients with collagen vascular disease. The lung disease associated with collagen vascular disease may precede the clinical presentation of the collagen disease by 5 years or more.

Careful evaluation of the chest radiograph and chest CT in patients with parenchymal abnormalities can yield some useful clues to the presence of collagen vascular disease:

- Joint abnormalities (shoulder or acromioclavicular) suggest rheumatoid arthritis (RA) (see Fig. 10.36).
- A dilated esophagus suggests scleroderma or one of its variants (see Fig. 10.49).
- An enlarged pulmonary artery (out of proportion to extent of lung parenchymal abnormality), reflecting a vasculopathy, may be seen in many types of collagen vascular disease, particularly scleroderma (see Fig. 10.53).
- Soft tissue calcifications may be seen in dermatomyositis or scleroderma (see Fig. 10.57).
- Involvement of multiple compartments of the lung may be seen on CT, particularly in rheumatoid arthritis (see Fig. 10.31).

Rheumatoid arthritis

Rheumatoid arthritis is a subacute or chronic inflammatory polyarthropathy of unknown cause that particularly affects peripheral joints. It is about three times more common in females than males and usually has an insidious onset, pursuing a variable course that is typically one of relapses and remissions. The diagnosis of rheumatoid arthritis is based on the presence of certain clinical and laboratory features.[249]

In addition to an arthropathy many patients have one or more extraarticular manifestations, such as subcutaneous nodules, ocular inflammation, pericarditis, splenomegaly, Felty syndrome, skin ulceration, and a variety of pleuropulmonary disorders.[248] The prevalence of these complications, particularly the pulmonary complications, depends on the diligence with which they are sought. Complications are more common in subjects who are seropositive, particularly with high rheumatoid factor titers, active erosive disease, and in patients with rheumatoid nodules. Smoking may also be a risk factor for extraarticular abnormality.[250] The 5 year mortality of patients with extraarticular manifestations of rheumatoid arthritis is about twice that of those without any extraarticular manifestation.[248]

Box 10.21 **Pleuropulmonary lesions in rheumatoid disease**

Pleural
Pleuritis
Effusion
Pleural thickening
Necrobiotic nodule
Empyema
Pneumothorax/bronchopleural fistula
Interstitial pneumonia
Nonspecific interstitial pneumonia
Usual interstitial pneumonia
Organizing pneumonia
Lymphoid interstitial pneumonia
Upper lobe fibrosis
Nodules
Necrobiotic nodules
Caplan syndrome
Lymphoid hyperplasia
Pulmonary hypertension
Airway disease
Bronchitis
Bronchiectasis
Bronchiolitis
Obliterative bronchiolitis
Follicular bronchiolitis
Miscellaneous
Drug related disease
Methotrexate: pneumonitis or pneumocystis infection
Steroids: opportunistic infections
Gold: pneumonitis/fibrosis
Amyloidosis
Pulmonary neoplasm

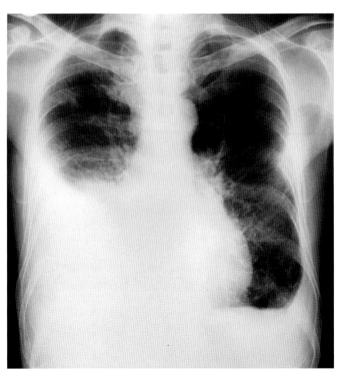

Fig. 10.32 Pleural effusion in rheumatoid disease. Bilateral pleural effusions are present together with mild basal reticular abnormality. Effusions were painless, and the right effusion had been present, more or less unchanged, for 5 months.

The possibility that rheumatoid disease might manifest as chest disease was suggested as early as 1948,[251] and though some large early surveys failed to confirm a positive relationship, it is now accepted that there are a number of manifestations and associations of rheumatoid disease.[252–256] Definite and probable manifestations and associations are listed in Box 10.21.

Pleural disease

Pleural involvement is probably the most common thoracic manifestation of rheumatoid disease.[257] At postmortem examination, there are pleural changes in some 50% of cases,[257] and on the chest radiograph there is pleural thickening in 20% of patients.[254] However, clinical pleural effusion is much less common, with a 3.3% prevalence in one large series,[258] and an annual incidence of effusion of about 1% in patients with rheumatoid disease.[259] Unlike rheumatoid disease in general, but in common with other pulmonary manifestations of the disease, pleural effusion shows a striking preponderance of male patients,[260] and some quite sizeable series have recorded virtually no females.[261] Patients are usually middle aged, with a mean age of about 50 years.[260] The effusions in rheumatoid disease, unlike those seen in systemic lupus erythematosus, are commonly asymptomatic.[252]

Pleural effusions most commonly occur in the setting of established disease and may develop >20 years after its onset. They may, however, develop simultaneously with the onset of arthritis or even antedate the arthritis by several months.[260,261] In one series, 4% of effusions developed several months before the arthritis and 20% developed simultaneously with the onset of joint disease.[258] The arthritis in established disease sometimes undergoes an exacerbation as the pleural effusion develops.[259,261,262] Effusions are associated with the presence of cutaneous nodules in some 50% of patients[260,261] and with pericarditis,[258] but not with the clinical or radiographic severity of the arthritis.[258] In about one-third of patients there will be other rheumatoid related abnormalities on the chest radiograph, such as interstitial pneumonia and fibrosis or parenchymal nodules.[260]

Effusions are most commonly small to moderate in size (Fig. 10.32),[260] though they can be large.[263,264] About one-fifth are bilateral.[260] Once formed, the effusions behave in a variable fashion, and though some resolve within weeks, more characteristically they persist for months and indeed sometimes for several years.[260] Effusions may recur on the same or the opposite side of the chest.[265] Effusions may be associated with a pneumothorax.[266,267] Once the effusion has cleared, it commonly leaves residual pleural thickening.[259,261] Fibrothorax and round atelectasis are recognized complications of rheumatoid pleural disease[257] that may, on occasion, be severe enough to warrant decortication.[258,268]

The diagnosis may be strongly suspected or established by the findings in the pleural fluid,[257,261,269] and sometimes by pleural biopsy which, though frequently nonspecific, may show rheumatoid nodules. The pleural fluid is usually rich in protein and lymphocytes, pale yellow to yellow green, and occasionally milky and pseudochylous. Sometimes, in the acute stage, it is polymorph predominant and, occasionally, eosinophilic.[270] Highly suggestive cytologic findings include large slender or elongated macrophages, round, or oval giant multinucleated cells, and a background of amorphous granular material.[271] Its most characteristic features are its low sugar, low pH, and raised lactic dehydrogenase level. Rheumatoid factor is often present but is a nonspecific finding.[269]

Rheumatoid patients are generally at risk from infection and may develop an empyema either de novo or on top of an established effusion.[272,273] There are isolated reports of pneumothorax and pyopneumothorax in rheumatoid disease,[265,274] some associated with diffuse pulmonary fibrosis and others with cavitary nodules and bronchopleural fistula.[273,275–277]

Interstitial pneumonia and fibrosis

Lung fibrosis was first associated with rheumatoid arthritis by Ellman and Ball in 1948.[251] After the initial case reports, several large series failed to show an increased prevalence of fibrosis in rheumatoid disease.[278,279] Nevertheless, in studies of patients with lung fibrosis, the prevalence of rheumatoid arthritis was in the order of 10–20%.[32,280,281] In a large series of patients with rheumatoid arthritis, eight of the 516 patients (1.6%) had radiographic pulmonary fibrosis.[260] A more recent study found that patients with rheumatoid arthritis had a 30 year cumulative incidence of lung fibrosis of 6.8%.[250] Abnormal pulmonary function tests consistent with interstitial lung disease are much more common[282] with a 40% prevalence in one series.[283]

The two most common histologic patterns of lung fibrosis in rheumatoid arthritis are UIP (see p. 539) and NSIP (see p. 548).[46] OP may also be seen.[127,163,256,284,285] A few cases of DIP have been described.[46,281,285] Lymphoid aggregates with germinal centers are a frequent histologic finding[256] and, though nonspecific, are suggestive of rheumatoid lung. Follicular bronchiolitis is the histologic label given when lymphoid aggregates are seen ranged along bronchioles.

Since most patients with lung fibrosis related to rheumatoid arthritis do not undergo lung biopsy, and since most series of patients with rheumatoid lung have not used the current histologic criteria for diagnosis of interstitial pneumonia, it is difficult to determine the precise prevalence of the histologic subtypes of interstitial pneumonia in these patients. Katzenstein et al[100] suggested that UIP was more common than NSIP in patients with rheumatoid disease. In a recent study of 63 patients with rheumatoid lung, 17 of whom had undergone lung biopsy, histologic NSIP was identified in 10 cases, UIP in two, OP in two, DAD in one, DIP in one, and lymphocytic bronchiolitis in one.[46] However, in patients who did not undergo biopsy, a CT pattern of UIP (n = 22) was more common than NSIP (n = 11) or OP (n = 3), probably reflecting a lower threshold for performing lung biopsy in patients with an imaging pattern of NSIP as compared with UIP.

Rheumatoid lung fibrosis is twice as common in men as in women,[281] with a mean age of onset of about 50 years.[260] Most cases occur after the onset of the arthritis, though some 15–30% occur before or coincident with the initial joint manifestations.[260,281] In general, whichever develops first, the interval between the onset of arthritis and lung disease is not more than 5 years.[260] Respiratory symptoms can be absent despite radiographic changes,[260,286] but, if present, consist chiefly of exertional dyspnea and cough. The severity and pattern of joint involvement does not differ from that seen generally in rheumatoid arthritis,[260,286] but an exacerbation of joint symptoms may occur with the onset of lung fibrosis. The principal physical signs are basal crackles and finger clubbing. It is generally stated that there is a high prevalence of associated subcutaneous nodules,[252] but figures from various series vary considerably from 75%,[260,286] to 15%,[281] and some consider that the prevalence of subcutaneous nodules is no different from that seen in the general rheumatoid population.[287] Pulmonary function tests usually show restriction with impaired carbon monoxide transfer and evidence of hypoxemia at rest or on exercise.[252,282] Rheumatoid factor is elevated in more than two-thirds of patients with IPF.[260,281,288]

The prognosis of interstitial pneumonia in rheumatoid disease varies from series to series. Some studies show that the survival is as poor as that seen in idiopathic forms of lung fibrosis,[281,289] while other authors have suggested that it is less severe.[25,252] The difference between these series is probably related to the clinical and histologic heterogeneity of rheumatoid lung fibrosis. In one series, the mean duration of lung disease to death was 5 years, with a range of 1–17 years.[281] A subset of patients has a fulminant course, dying within months of the initial diagnosis, presumably because of superimposed DAD.[98,290] Treatment with steroids or immunosuppressants helps improve physiologic and radiographic findings of disease in a proportion of the patients, at least in the short term.[281,290]

The chest radiograph shows nonspecific changes consistent with interstitial disease (Fig. 10.33). The abnormalities are largely symmetric and basally predominant,[291] though eventually they can involve all zones,[281] often then displaying a peripheral predominance. Opacities are usually reticular. A ground-glass pattern may also be seen.[291] Sometimes in the early stages there is also evidence of airspace opacity, presumably due to OP. Later on, the reticulonodular pattern becomes coarser and more widespread, and honeycombing may appear (Fig. 10.33).[291] Septal lines are not a prominent feature.[291] As fibrosis advances, the lung volumes decrease, particularly in the lower lobes, with progressive elevation of the diaphragm.[292] Pleural effusion or thickening may coexist with interstitial changes in about 5–15% of cases.[260,281] Necrobiotic nodules may infrequently be seen in association with lung fibrosis.[293]

Early CT and HRCT studies of the interstitial pneumonia associated with rheumatoid arthritis (Figs 10.33 and 10.34) generally considered the findings to be nonspecific.[294–296] However, comprehensive CT/histopathologic correlation in rheumatoid arthritis is lacking and, since lung biopsies in rheumatoid lung disease show a wide range of abnormalities in addition to interstitial pneumonia, including lymphoid hyperplasia, OP, and DAD,[256] it seems likely that HRCT changes reflect more than just interstitial pneumonia. In a recent study of 63 patients with rheumatoid lung disease,[46] 26 had a CT pattern suggestive of UIP, 19 of NSIP, 11 of bronchiolitis, and five of OP (Fig. 10.35). These CT patterns were in agreement with the histology in 13 of the 17 who underwent biopsy. Two patients who were classified as UIP by CT received a pathologic diagnosis of NSIP, one who was classified as NSIP was given a pathologic diagnosis of DIP, and one with a CT diagnosis of LIP was classified pathologically as NSIP.

OP occurring in patients with rheumatoid arthritis is characterized on chest radiograph and chest CT by patchy parenchymal opacities which may be migratory.[127,284] If the patient is on gold therapy, or nonsteroidal antiinflammatory drugs, these should be considered as a possible cause.

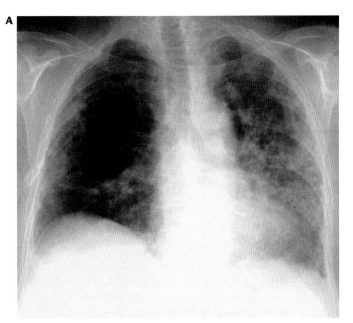
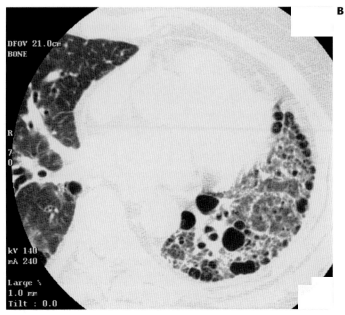

Fig. 10.33 A 64-year-old woman with rheumatoid arthritis. **A**, Chest radiograph shows bilateral reticular abnormality and honeycombing. **B**, HRCT through the left lung confirms reticular abnormality and honeycombing.

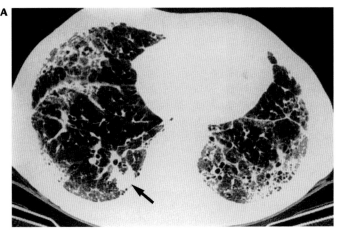
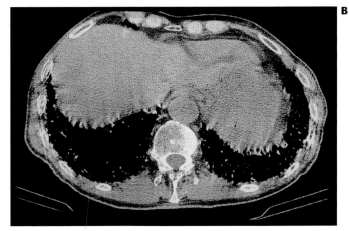

Fig. 10.34 Rheumatoid arthritis – usual intestinal pneumonia (UIP pattern). **A**, HRCT of the lower zones shows typical appearances of usual interstitial pneumonia, with patchy but predominantly peripheral reticular abnormality and honeycombing. There is also ground-glass opacity at the right base. The focal lesion is a bronchogenic carcinoma (arrow). **B**, Mediastinal window settings show that the fibrotic areas are diffusely calcified in a punctate fashion – an uncommon but recognized feature of UIP.

There are several case reports of patients with rheumatoid disease who develop upper lobe fibrosis, sometimes associated with cavitation, giving rise to a radiologic appearance that resembles tuberculosis.[297–301] In some of these patients the pathologic finding has been that of confluent necrobiotic nodules.[301]

Necrobiotic nodules

Necrobiotic nodules occurring in the lung are pathologically identical to subcutaneous rheumatoid nodules,[281] and consist of a necrotic center bounded by palisading histiocytes (epithelioid cells) and surrounded by plasma cells and lymphocytes. Peripherally there may be a moderate, non-necrotizing vasculitis.[302]

Intrapulmonary nodules are rare findings on the chest radiographs of patients with rheumatoid disease; two large series of 955 patients contained no examples[278,279]; and another contained only two cases in 516 patients.[260] Nodules, like pleural effusions and IPF, are more common in men than women, with about a twofold excess. Mean patient age at presentation is 51 years (range 24–64 years). Nodules usually occur in patients with established disease but may occur with or before the onset of arthritis,[281,303] as did some 27% of nodules reported by Eraut et al.[304] Should nodules antedate arthritis, the gap is often less than a year,[270,304,305] but intervals of up to 11 years are reported.[304] Some patients with histologically proven nodules remain seronegative and never develop arthritis.[304,306]

Nodules are usually asymptomatic, but there may be cough or hemoptysis, particularly if a lesion should cavitate.[307]

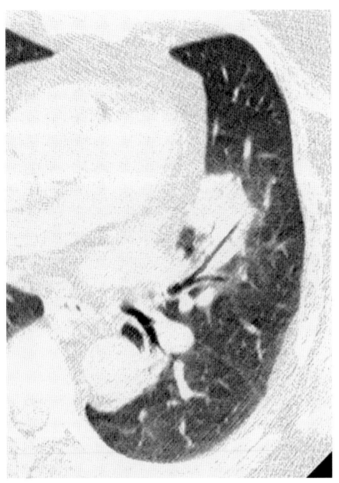

Fig. 10.35 Organizing pneumonia pattern in rheumatoid arthritis. The CT shows focal peribronchovascular consolidation in the lingula.

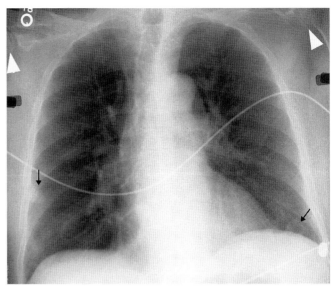

Fig. 10.36 A 62-year-old man with rheumatoid arthritis and multiple rheumatoid nodules. Portable chest radiograph shows a noncavitary lung nodule in the right lower lung and a cavitary nodule in the left lower lobe, just above the diaphragm (arrows). Note the significant joint space loss in both shoulders (arrowheads).

Occasionally, symptoms result from superadded infection,[308] bronchopleural fistula formation, or pneumothorax.[270] Discounting cases in which nodules antedate arthritis, pulmonary necrobiotic nodules usually occur in the context of established and advanced disease,[292] and there are subcutaneous nodules in 80%.[260,265,307] Serum rheumatoid factor is found in nearly 90% of patients with nodules,[265,307] though early on it may be absent or present in low titer.[307] Blood eosinophilia is reported in some cases.[270,309]

The nodules (Fig. 10.36) are usually radiographically discrete, rounded, or lobulated and subpleural.[295] They may be single or, in about three-quarters of patients, multiple,[281] sometimes coalescing,[295] and show some mid/upper zone predilection.[304] They range in size from a few millimeters[281] to 7 cm. Occasionally, when the nodules are small and widely disseminated, a miliary pattern is produced.[265] In about 50% of cases, the nodules cavitate (Fig. 10.36),[265,281] producing ring opacities often with relatively smooth thick walls.[265,291,292] Cavitation is more easily appreciated on CT.[295] Occasionally, nodules calcify.[291,297] Subpleural nodules may erode through the pleura and cause a bronchopleural fistula and hydropneumothorax.[265,275] Rib erosion by a nodule is rare, but has been described as giving an appearance that resembles an invasive carcinoma.[310] Pleural thickening or effusion is present in 40–50% of cases with intrapulmonary nodules.[265,281] Likewise, interstitial

pneumonia and pulmonary nodules can occasionally coexist.[265] Nodular lesions may increase in size and number, resolve completely, or remain stable for many years[281]; at other times, they wax and wane with the activity of subcutaneous nodules and arthritis.[270,311] Unless nodules are indolent or resolve, they are radiographically indistinguishable from pulmonary neoplasms and need either careful follow up for increasing size, or histologic confirmation.[312] Cytologic evaluation of fine needle aspiration can be diagnostic.[313]

Small rheumatoid nodules have also been described in the trachea[314] and pleura.

CT is clearly a more sensitive way of assessing lung nodules than chest radiography. Considering nodules of all sizes from micronodules to exceeding a centimeter, the prevalence of nodules has been recorded in various HRCT studies as 0, 6, 10, 22[235] and 28%.[274,296,315–317] The larger figures contain a high proportion of micronodules. Most nodules identified by HRCT have not been examined pathologically, and it should not be assumed that all or even the majority represent necrobiotic nodules; scars and lymphoid hyperplasia have been suggested as alternative pathologies.[274]

Airways disease

The increasing use of CT in evaluation of patients with rheumatoid arthritis has made it clear that airways disease is one of the most common patterns of abnormality seen in these patients. Both *bronchitis* and *bronchiectasis* are more frequent in patients with rheumatoid disease than in matched controls.[269,279,318] Thus, in a controlled study in 1967, bronchiectasis was 10 times more common in patients with rheumatoid disease than in controls with degenerative joint disease.[318] Bronchiectasis may precede or follow the onset of rheumatoid disease.[319,320] In the past, bronchiectasis has been diagnosed on clinical, plain radiographic, and sometimes bronchographic criteria, favoring the detection of moderate to severe disease. However, more

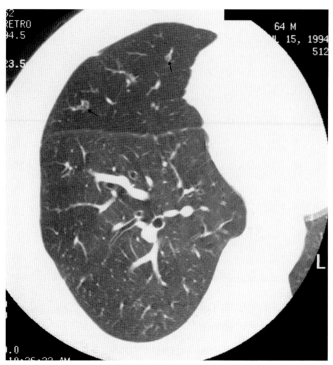

Fig. 10.37 A 64-year-old man with constrictive bronchiolitis and cylindric bronchiectasis due to rheumatoid arthritis. HRCT scan through the right lung base shows a decrease in lung attenuation in the right middle lobe, associated with mild cylindric bronchiectasis (arrows).

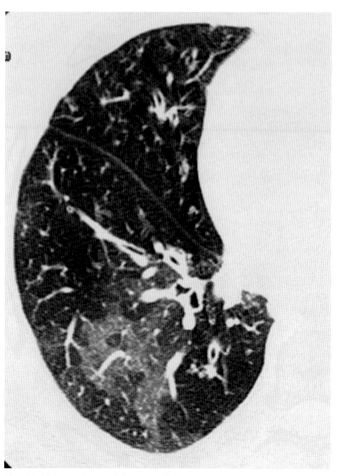

Fig. 10.38 A 56-year-old man with constrictive bronchiolitis related to rheumatoid arthritis. CT through the right lower lung shows mosaic pattern. The decreased caliber of vessels in the areas of low attenuation indicates underperfusion secondary to air-trapping. The bronchi in the areas of air-trapping are thick walled and mildly dilated.

recently a number of studies have looked at the frequency of bronchiectasis as assessed by HRCT (Fig. 10.37). The studies are not homogeneous, particularly with regard to respiratory symptoms, drug treatment, and smoking history. In CT based studies, an overall frequency of bronchiectasis of about 20% is recorded, with a range of 6–31%.[274,315–317,321] It is of interest that in one series there was a 25% prevalence of bronchiectasis in nonsmoking subjects without respiratory symptoms.[321] In rheumatoid arthritis patients with chronic suppurative airways disease, there was no evidence that the bronchiectasis affected the course of the arthritis.[322] Bronchiectasis is usually cylindric in type, and is commonly associated with CT and physiologic evidence of small airways disease (Fig. 10.37).[323]

There is a recognized association between rheumatoid disease and *obliterative bronchiolitis (constrictive bronchiolitis)*[162,297,324–326] in which bronchioles are destroyed and replaced by scar tissue. This condition must be distinguished from OP (see p. 552). In at least half of these patients treatment with penicillamine or gold has been implicated,[327–329] but obliterative bronchiolitis also occurs in patients taking neither drug.[269] Clinically there is progressive dyspnea and evidence of irreversible airflow obstruction. The chest radiograph is either normal or shows hyperinflation, with or without areas of oligemia. The characteristic HRCT finding is a mosaic pattern (Fig. 10.38) with air-trapping,[330–333] often associated with evidence of mild bronchiectasis, which is occasionally severe.

Follicular bronchiolitis is a second type of small airway disorder recognized in rheumatoid lung disease.[256,285,334,336] It is characterized by lymphoid aggregates, with or without germinal centers, lying in the walls of bronchioles and possibly compressing their lumens.[337] Radiographic descriptions of follicular bronchiolitis are lacking but it probably produces a reticular or reticulonodular pattern on the chest radiograph.[256] The major CT finding is centrilobular nodules, often associated with peribronchial nodules, and with areas of ground-glass abnormality.[334,337] HRCT may sometimes be normal.[335] Should lymphoid hyperplasia in rheumatoid lung disease be more concentrated along septa and subpleural areas than in airways, the term *lymphoid hyperplasia* is used.[285] Radiographically it gives rise to reticular or reticulonodular opacities[256] but its HRCT features are not described, though Remy-Jardin et al[274] suggest that it may account for subpleural micronodulation, a common finding in rheumatoid lung disease.

Diffuse panbronchiolitis has been described in patients with rheumatoid arthritis,[338] but this could well be a chance association. A handful of patients with rheumatoid disease have had biopsy proved *bronchocentric granulomatosis* (see p. 670).[339–341] Radiographically there are bilateral nodules and focal consolidations ranging in size from 2 to 15 cm, some of which cavitate.

HRCT findings in rheumatoid lung disease

A number of papers have recorded the HRCT changes in rheumatoid lung disease,[274,296,315,316,321,334,342,343] but data are difficult to interpret, because of patient selection and inadequate assessment and description of the imaging findings. The most comprehensive investigation is by Remy-Jardin et al.[274] The first study[309] comprised 84 patients (female:male ratio 1.9:1) with a mean age of 57 years and a mean duration of articular disease of 12 years. Ninety percent of patients had never smoked. Some patients were selected because of suspected pulmonary disease (56%) and others were selected consecutively from a rheumatology clinic (44%). The most common findings were bronchial abnormalities (30%) (see below), nodules (22%), nonseptal lines (18%), pleural opacity (16%), ground-glass opacity (14%), honeycombing (10%), and consolidation (6%). Bronchiectasis with bronchial wall thickening was the commonest abnormality, either as an isolated finding (Fig. 10.37) or, in about one-third of patients, associated with honeycombing. Bronchiolectasis was also seen. Nodular opacities, the second most common finding, were of three types: (1) parenchymal micronodules (7%) connected to branching bronchovascular structures and associated with small airway dilatation and wall thickening (it seems likely that these changes were caused by follicular or constrictive bronchiolitis);[274] (2) 3–30 mm peripheral lung nodules (4%), most likely due to necrobiotic nodules or lymphoid hyperplasia; and (3) in 17% of patients there were widely distributed subpleural micronodules (rounded, hemispheric, or triangular, and <3 mm in diameter), which sometimes coalesced into plaquelike lesions. The pathology of these lesions is unclear, with necrobiotic nodules, focal scars, and lymphoid hyperplasia being possibilities. The third most common finding (18%) was nonseptal linear opacities, usually peripheral and lower zone, and presumably representing scars. Pleural changes were seen in 16% and ground-glass opacity in 14%, the latter usually being bilateral and symmetric. Honeycomb opacity was seen in 10% of patients and tended to be bilateral and asymmetric with a peripheral predilection (Figs 10.33 and 10.34). It generally affected all vertical lung zones and was associated with lung distortion, traction bronchiectasis and bronchiolectasis, ground-glass opacity, and nonseptal linear opacities. Less common findings overall included consolidation, lung distortion, emphysema, and mediastinal node enlargement.

Caplan syndrome

The original description of Caplan syndrome was of multiple, large (0.5–5.0 cm in diameter) rounded nodules seen on the chest radiographs of coal miners with rheumatoid arthritis.[344] Radiographic evidence of simple coal miner's pneumoconiosis was often absent. Since this time the features of the syndrome have been extended to include: (1) individuals exposed to inorganic agents other than silica or coal; (2) those with serologic but not clinical rheumatoid disease; and (3) patients with radiographic patterns other than large nodules.[345] In affected patients, clinical rheumatoid disease may occur before, with, or after the pulmonary changes.[344] Caplan syndrome – based on broad criteria – has been described with exposure to asbestos,[346,347] aluminum,[348] dolomite,[349] silica,[350–353] and carbon.[354]

Caplan nodules are pathologically similar to necrobiotic rheumatoid nodules: a necrotic center surrounded by a cuff of cellular infiltrate consisting of macrophages and polymorphonuclear leukocytes, fibroblasts, and giant cells.[355] Some of the macrophages contain dust, and on macroscopic section these give the characteristic annular ring pattern that distinguishes the

Caplan nodules from ordinary rheumatoid nodules. Fibroblasts adjacent to the necrotic area show palisading, which is also a striking feature of subcutaneous rheumatoid nodules. Although the pathogenesis of Caplan syndrome is incompletely understood, it is apparent that the development of rheumatoid factor seems to be associated with a modified tissue response in coal dust induced lung disease.[281]

The prevalence rate of Caplan syndrome in a population of >21,000 miners in the United Kingdom, according to the broad criteria,[353] was about 2.5 cases per 1000 subjects without pneumoconiosis, and between 22 and 62 cases per 1000 subjects with pneumoconiosis. For an unexplained reason, the prevalence in the United States appears to be low,[356] and no cases were found in a series of 100 Pennsylvania miners with rheumatoid arthritis.[357]

The classic radiographic finding in Caplan syndrome is bilateral pulmonary nodules (Fig. 10.39), usually 1–2 cm in diameter, but ranging from 0.5 to 5 cm.[344] Nodules are typically situated at the junction of the outer and middle thirds of the lung and tend to appear in crops of lesions having a similar size and rate of growth. Nodules are not necessarily bilateral, and in one series one-fifth were unilateral.[353] Nodules tend to develop rapidly and grow over a period of months. They then often remain stable or grow slowly for several years. Established nodules occasionally heal by fibrosis and give a stellate scarlike shadow. In the East Midlands of England, 10% of coal miners with Caplan syndrome developed calcification (7 of 55) or cavitation (4 of 55) in the nodules.[353] Radiographic changes of coal worker's pneumoconiosis may or may not be present and are not a striking feature. In the original series, the radiographic

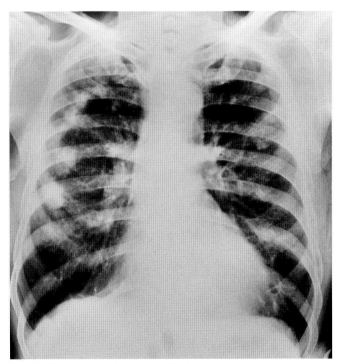

Fig. 10.39 Rheumatoid disease with Caplan syndrome. This 61-year-old coal miner has multiple peripheral nodules, mostly on the right. They range between 1 and 2 cm in diameter. Changes of coal worker's pneumoconiosis are characteristically mild. (Courtesy of Dr PM Hacking, Newcastle upon Tyne, UK)

changes of coal worker's pneumoconiosis were category I or less in 45% of patients.[344]

Other radiographic findings are now included in the wider concept of Caplan syndrome. The most common are: (1) 0.3–1.0 cm rounded opacities ranging from just a few confined to one lung zone to a "snowstorm" appearance[345]; and (2) mixed nodular and irregular opacities with no background of simple pneumoconiosis.[345] CT findings have been reported in one patient with Caplan syndrome, who had two well-defined 2.5 cm and 3 cm nodules, with adjacent small nodules consistent with pneumoconiosis. One of the nodules was calcified, and one cavitated.

Pulmonary vasculopathy

Systemic vasculitis in rheumatoid disease is usually of the small vessel type and affects chiefly the skin with a lifetime risk for males and females with rheumatoid arthritis in a rural United Kingdom population of 9:1 and 38:1.[314] The lung, however, is uncommonly involved in a rheumatoid vasculitis,[358] and there are only a few reported cases,[359–361] some with and some without clinical evidence of a systemic vasculitis. Prognosis is poor and most patients die within a year of diagnosis.[361] In most of these cases the only radiographic finding is enlargement of the heart and proximal pulmonary arteries. Pulmonary hypertension may be out of proportion to the visible extent of lung disease, suggesting the presence of an independent pulmonary vasculopathy. It should be suggested when the pulmonary arteries appear enlarged on chest radiograph or chest CT (see Fig. 10.31). There are also a few case reports of pulmonary consolidation either proved[362] or assumed to be the result of vasculitis,[297,363] and of diffuse pulmonary hemorrhage due to vasculitis.[364]

Other associations

Many of the available treatments for rheumatoid arthritis, including gold, methotrexate and D-penicillamine have been implicated in the development of infiltrative lung disease (Box 10.22).[365] On the chest radiograph, gold-induced lung disease differs radiographically from rheumatoid lung because the infiltrates are most commonly diffuse, though about 30% of cases have basal predominance.[181] On chest CT scans, gold-induced lung disease was characterized in 12 of 20 reported cases by alveolar opacities extending along bronchovascular bundles. This CT finding, when present, is suggestive of gold lung,[181] though OP can cause a similar finding. Administration of low dose methotrexate may be associated with subacute hypersensitivity pneumonitis in 2–5% of cases (Fig. 10.40).[366,367] Preexisting radiographic evidence of interstitial lung disease

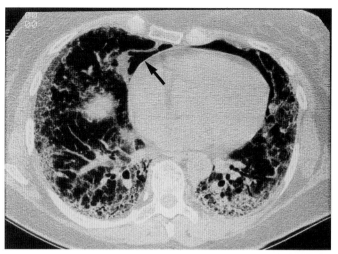

Fig. 10.40 Rheumatoid disease – methotrexate pneumonitis. HRCT through the lower lung zones of a 60-year-old female with an 8 year history of nodular, seropositive rheumatoid disease. Four months after starting methotrexate 7.5 mg weekly, the patient developed cough and rapidly progressive dyspnea. HRCT a month later shows consolidation, ground-glass opacity, reticular abnormality, and traction bronchiolectasis, distributed in a predominantly peripheral fashion. Note the additional pneumomediastinum (arrow). Following cessation of methotrexate therapy and steroid administration the patient improved but has been left with residual dyspnea and lung opacity.

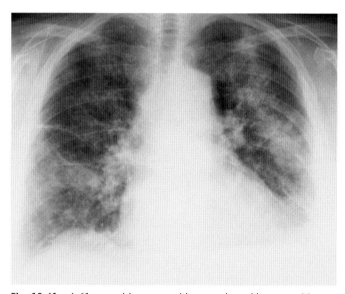

Fig. 10.41 A 61-year-old woman with parenchymal lung opacities related to nonsteroidal antiinflammatory medication. Chest radiograph shows bilateral airspace opacities.

Box 10.22 Pulmonary drug toxicity in rheumatoid arthritis

Aspirin (excessive use) – lung edema
Nonsteroidal antiinflammatory drugs – organizing pneumonia pattern
Gold – organizing pneumonia pattern
Methotrexate – nonspecific interstitial pneumonia pattern
Penicillamine – constrictive bronchiolitis
Cytotoxic drugs – opportunistic infection

probably predisposes to the development of methotrexate pneumonitis in patients with rheumatoid arthritis.[368] Treatment with D-penicillamine is associated with the development of constrictive bronchiolitis. Nonsteroidal antiinflammatory drugs may be associated with hypersensitivity reactions (Fig. 10.41),[369,370] while unintentional therapeutic overdoses of salicylate may result in pulmonary edema. Furthermore, many patients with rheumatoid disease will be immunosuppressed, with increased risk of opportunistic infection.

Most studies show that rheumatoid arthritis is associated with an increased incidence of lymphoma, and of lung cancer (see Fig. 10.34).[371]

Systemic lupus erythematosus

Systemic lupus erythematosus (SLE) is a multisystem collagen vascular disorder that particularly affects vessels, serosa, joints, kidneys, the central nervous system (CNS), skin, and blood elements. Its manifestations are extremely variable both as regards organs involved and severity. A characteristic feature is autoantibody production against a wide variety of cellular constituents, including nuclear material, particularly DNA. In a series of 1000 patients, the five most common autoantibodies were ANA in 96% of cases, anti-double-stranded DNA (anti-dsDNA) (78%), anti-Ro (25%), anti-La (19%) and anti-Sm (10%).[372] Two autoantibodies – anti-dsDNA and anti-Sm, are considered diagnostic, with high specificity but only moderate sensitivity. Because the manifestations of the disease are so variable, diagnostic criteria have been drawn up (Box 10.23). Should any four of the criteria be present simultaneously or serially during a period of observation, then SLE can be diagnosed.[373]

> **Box 10.23 Criteria for diagnosis of systemic lupus erythematosus[373]**
>
> Malar rash
> Discoid lupus erythematosus
> Photosensitivity
> Ulceration of mouth and oropharynx
> Arthropathy (nonerosive, nondeforming)
> Serositis
> Renal disorder (proteinuria or cellular casts)
> Neurologic disorder (epilepsy or psychosis)
> Hematologic disorder (hemolytic anemia, leukopenia, lymphopenia, thrombocytopenia)
> Autoantibodies
> Antinuclear factor (less specific)
> Anti-Sm
> Anti-double-stranded DNA
> Antiphospholipid antibody

The overall prevalence rate of SLE is about 20–50 cases per 10^5 population and it is 10 times as common in women as in men,[374] with an increased prevalence among relatives and blacks. The illness characteristically shows relapses and remissions, with a tendency to progression and eventual multiorgan dysfunction.[375] It presents typically in women of childbearing age, with a wide variety of manifestations, particularly those of joint, skin (malar rash, photosensitivity, livedo reticularis), and systemic disorders.[376] The prevalence of the various clinical manifestations in four series was arthropathy 85%, skin lesions 80%, nephritis 53%, pleurisy 52%, neuropsychiatric disorders 44%, lymphadenopathy 43%, pericarditis 39%, and mucosal ulceration 15%.[375] About 10% of patients present beyond the age of 50 years, with features that resemble Sjögren syndrome or polymyalgia rheumatica.[372] These patients are less likely to present with the typical malar rash or arthritis. There is usually an anemia, leukopenia, and thrombocytopenia – a combination that is unusual in other inflammatory conditions.[377] The reported

Table 10.5 Thoracic manifestations of systemic lupus erythematosus

Pleural	Effusion
Acute parenchymal abnormality	Diffuse alveolar damage
	Acute lupus pneumonitis
	Diffuse pulmonary hemorrhage
Subacute or chronic interstitial pneumonia	Nonspecific interstitial pneumonia
	Organizing pneumonia
	Usual interstitial pneumonia
Pulmonary vascular	Pulmonary arterial hypertension
	Vasculitis/capillaritis
	Antiphospholipid syndrome with pulmonary embolism
	Pulmonary venoocclusive disease
Miscellaneous	Diaphragmatic dysfunction
	Opportunistic infection
	Atelectasis

prognosis has greatly improved over the years, in part due to better therapy but also because less severe or subclinical cases have been included in the various studies. In a recent series, the 5 year survival was 98%, and 10 year survival was 89%.[378]

Thoracic involvement is common in SLE, and the lungs, pleura, heart, diaphragm, and intercostal muscles may all be affected.[379] Thoracic manifestations (Table 10.5) can be divided into primary changes or secondary complications, but this distinction is by no means always clear-cut. Cardiac involvement may include pericarditis, endocarditis, myocarditis, coronary artery disease, and vasculitis.[380] Fifty to 70% of patients with lupus develop pleuropulmonary manifestations in the course of the disease.[252,257,378,381] However, only 5% will have such changes at presentation.[382–384] Pleuropulmonary involvement in SLE may be asymptomatic and it is quite frequently not associated with significant morbidity.

Pleural disease

Pleuritis is found in 40–60% of patients with SLE and it is the most common pleuropulmonary manifestation.[382,383,385] It may be a presenting feature[386] but occurs more commonly during an exacerbation of established disease.[252]

The pleuritis is dry 50% of the time,[387] but in the other 50% it is accompanied by a pleural effusion and sometimes also by a pericardial effusion (Fig. 10.42).[379] Aspirated pleural fluid is usually a clear exudate with white blood cells (neutrophils early on and lymphocytes later) and normal levels of glucose; it often contains antinuclear antibodies.[388] The pleural effusions are usually small or moderate in size,[388] but are, on rare occasions, large.[389] Unilateral and bilateral effusions are found with equal frequency.[386,388] Sometimes the pleural effusions resolve spontaneously, but many require treatment with steroids or immunosuppressive drugs. Clearing may be complete or incomplete, leaving minor pleural thickening.[386,390] It is important to exclude other causes of pleural effusion in SLE, including the nephrotic syndrome, cardiac and renal failure, pulmonary embolism, and infective pneumonia.[257,391] The fact that primary pleural effusions in SLE are almost always painful[387,388] can be a helpful differentiating feature.

Pleural thickening[392] is a common finding at autopsy, but in life is underreported as a radiographic finding. It was, however,

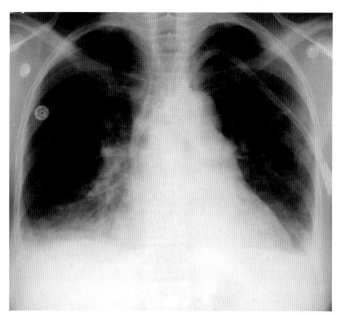

Fig. 10.42 A 31-year-old woman with lupus. Chest radiograph shows bilateral pleural effusions and basal atelectasis. The cardiomegaly was due to a pericardial effusion.

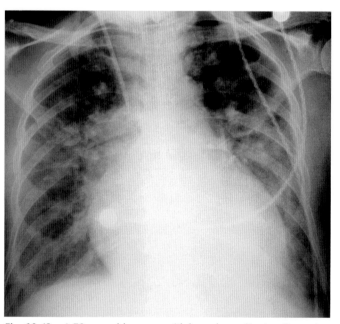

> ### Box 10.24 Differential diagnosis of consolidation in patients with systemic lupus erythematosus
>
> Infection
> Hemorrhage
> Lupus pneumonitis
> Pulmonary infarction

Fig. 10.43 A 72-year-old woman with lupus lung. Chest radiograph shows cardiomegaly and diffuse parenchymal opacity, shown histologically to represent lupus pneumonitis, without hemorrhage. These appearances cannot be distinguished radiographically from edema, diffuse infection, or drug toxicity.

seen in 12% of patients in one series.[378] Pneumothorax is not a feature of pleuropulmonary SLE.

Acute lupus pneumonitis

Acute lupus pneumonitis is characterized histologically by changes of DAD. The histologic and clinical findings of acute lupus pneumonitis may overlap with those of diffuse pulmonary hemorrhage. The alveolar damage is most likely mediated by immune complex deposition,[381] and immunostaining of capillary basement membranes for immunoglobulin and complement commonly shows a granular pattern.[302] Histologically, there is an acute, exudative stage with interstitial and intraalveolar edema, exudates, and hemorrhage; hyaline membrane formation; and sloughing of alveolar lining cells. The later organizing stage is characterized by alveolar lining cell proliferation and interstitial, and to a lesser extent intraalveolar fibrosis.[302]

Acute lupus pneumonitis is an unusual life-threatening condition characterized by acute onset of fever, cough, tachypnea, hypoxia, and radiologic consolidation. Clinically, it resembles infective pneumonia, pulmonary infarction, or hemorrhage and is a diagnosis of exclusion. Rarely it may be a presenting feature of SLE,[393] and an increased frequency postpartum has been noted.[381] The true prevalence is uncertain and is probably in the order of 4% (range 1–12%).[376,378,383,387,393] In a selected group of 30 patients seen in a tertiary center with pleuropulmonary SLE, about one-fifth had probable acute pneumonitis.[394] It carries a mortality of about 50%.[385]

The chest radiograph most commonly shows one or more areas of consolidation, usually bilateral and basal, but sometimes unilateral (Box 10.24; Fig. 10.43).[378,387,393] A mixed alveolar and interstitial pattern with nodules has also been described.[387] The consolidation is often accompanied by pleural effusions,[393] which are sometimes migratory. Cavitation is rare and suggests pneumonia or infarction rather than lupus pneumonitis. Some patients respond dramatically to steroids

with complete or partial clearance,[252] but others have needed additional cyclophosphamide.[381] Residual radiographic shadowing caused by the organizing stage often has an interstitial pattern[393] and may be accompanied by a diffusion defect and restrictive abnormality on pulmonary function testing.

Pulmonary hemorrhage

Pulmonary hemorrhage is common in the lungs at post mortem examination in patients with SLE,[395] but is not often recognized clinically. Lung hemorrhage ranges from a mild, chronic, subclinical process to one that is acute and life threatening.[381] In a large series of >400 patients with SLE at the National Institutes of Health, the prevalence of acute hemorrhage was only about 1.5%,[396] occurring typically in young (mean age ~30 years) adult females. In 10–20% of patients with hemorrhage, it is the first manifestation of SLE.[397,398] Acute pulmonary hemorrhage carries a mortality of 50–60%,[397] and is an important diagnosis to make since urgent treatment is needed. The pathologic findings are diffuse alveolar hemorrhage with acute necrotizing capillaritis.[302,397] A minority of cases may be associated with DAD.[397] Bland pulmonary hemorrhage appears to be rare. Clinically, in acute hemorrhage, there is rapid onset of severe dyspnea, fever, and hemoptysis. However, hemoptysis is absent in 33% of cases on admission. Pulmonary hemorrhage is typically accompanied by signs of active disease elsewhere; fever, arthropathy, and particularly nephritis (14 of 15 patients in one series).[397,399] Helpful clinical pointers include hemoptysis and a drop in blood hemoglobin level. Confirmation can be obtained by finding hemosiderin laden macrophages in the sputum,[400] or a rise in carbon monoxide uptake in the lung.[401]

The radiographic appearances are nonspecific. They resemble those of Goodpasture syndrome (see p. 575) and consist of airspace opacity that is usually bilateral and diffuse (Fig. 10.44). This results in a variety of patterns: multiple acinar nodules; homogeneous, ill-defined, coalescent patchy shadows; ground-glass opacity; and lobar or segmental consolidations with air bronchograms.[399,402] The opacities usually clear within days.[403] CT shows patchy or diffuse parenchymal opacity. MRI findings (intermediate signal on proton density and low signal on T2-weighted images) may be characteristic of pulmonary hemorrhage, but MRI is not usually necessary to make this diagnosis.[404] Acute pulmonary hemorrhage must be differentiated clinically from infection, and from lung edema due to renal or cardiac failure.

Pulmonary fibrosis

Fibrotic interstitial lung disease (Fig. 10.45) is generally regarded as an unusual manifestation of SLE. However, in four autopsy series, chronic interstitial infiltrates were present in just over one-third of cases.[395] In a selected clinical series of 30 patients with pleuropulmonary SLE there was a 13% frequency of lung fibrosis judged radiologically (with biopsy confirmation in two),[394] and in an unselected outpatient series assessed radiographically there was a 3% prevalence of lung fibrosis.[405] A number of patients with lung fibrosis have had preceding acute pneumonitis,[393] and the interstitial changes presumably represent the organizing phase of DAD. The histology of other forms of lung fibrosis is that of interstitial pneumonia, which is likely to be a mixture of UIP and NSIP, the latter probably being more frequent.[302] Although NSIP was only characterized in 1994,[100] autopsy findings of Haupt et al,[391] in which there was a 9% frequency of interstitial pneumonitis and a 4% frequency of interstitial fibrosis, would support the contention that NSIP is more common than UIP. In general, interstitial disease in SLE pursues an indolent course, but there are exceptions and it may cause death.

There is limited information on HRCT changes in SLE. In a study of patients with SLE who did not have previously diagnosed lung disease, Bankier et al[406] found that 17 of 45 patients with a normal chest radiograph had an abnormal HRCT. Interlobular and intralobular lines were the most common type of abnormality, being seen in 15 patients. Airspace nodules, architectural distortion, bronchial wall thickening, bronchial dilatation, pleural irregularity, ground-glass attenuation, and airspace consolidation were less common. Middle and lower lung zone involvement was predominant. The extent of abnormality on CT correlated with the length of the clinical history, and with impaired pulmonary function (decreased FEV_1/FVC ratio and DLco). Fenlon et al[407] studied 34 consecutive patients with SLE, 56% of whom had never smoked and 23% of whom had respiratory symptoms. The most common signs were thickened interlobar septa (44%), parenchymal bands (44%) (Fig. 10.46), subpleural bands (21%), and pleural tags and thickening (15%). Only 6% had ground-glass opacity, con-

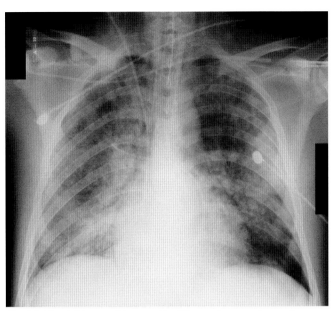

Fig. 10.44 A 24-year-old man with diffuse pulmonary hemorrhage related to systemic lupus erythematosus. Chest radiograph following admission and intubation shows bilateral diffuse parenchymal consolidation, indistinguishable from diffuse edema, infection, or aspiration.

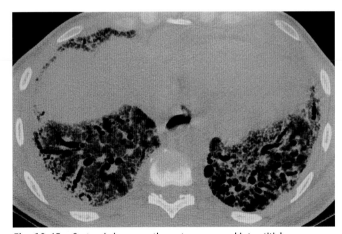

Fig. 10.45 Systemic lupus erythematosus – usual interstitial pneumonitis (UIP). HRCT through the lung bases in a 41-year-old female with a history of respiratory failure. The main findings are ground-glass opacity, honeycombing, and striking traction bronchiectasis and bronchiolectasis, together with pleural thickening and lung shrinkage. Open lung biopsy was characteristic of UIP with a patchy and variable distribution of inflammation and established fibrosis.

solidation, and honeycombing (Fig. 10.45). These interstitial changes were usually mild in degree, less commonly moderate and rarely severe. Overall, 33% of patients were judged to have mild or moderate interstitial lung disease. In 21% of patients there was bronchiectasis and bronchial wall thickening – a compatible figure to the 30% prevalence seen on HRCT in rheumatoid disease.[274] Pleural thickening was surprisingly infrequent, seen in just 15% of patients. Fifteen percent of patients had mediastinal and/or axillary adenopathy with nodes measuring >1 cm in short axis. In contrast to the study by Bankier et al,[406] Fenlon et al[407] did not confirm a relationship between the presence or extent of lung abnormality and pulmonary

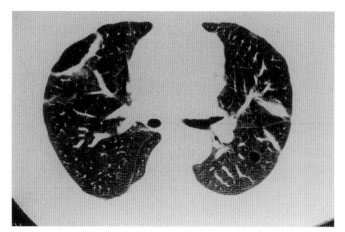

Fig. 10.46 Systemic lupus erythematosus (SLE). HRCT through the mid zones of a 62-year-old female with long-standing SLE and some features of Sjögren syndrome. There are several irregular, broad parenchymal bands, almost certainly representing scars, since they were long standing.

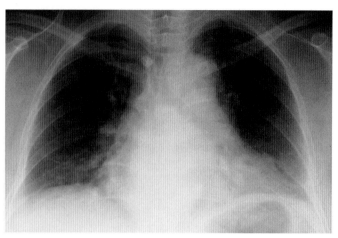

Fig. 10.47 Shrinking lungs in a 47-year-old woman with lupus. Chest radiograph shows marked decrease in lung volumes, with cardiomegaly and basal atelectasis.

physiology or duration of disease. Because the extent of disease on CT in patients with SLE is usually relatively minor, the clinical value of CT in asymptomatic patients is questionable.

Diaphragm dysfunction

Diaphragm dysfunction in SLE may manifest as elevation of one or both hemidiaphragms (Fig. 10.47) and is a cause of dyspnea. Bilateral elevation is a common finding and, in some series, has been the most common radiologic pleuropulmonary abnormality in SLE, being seen in as many as 18% of patients.[378] As the diaphragm rises, the lungs lose volume, hence the term "shrinking lungs",[408] a finding first noted in 1954.[382] The loss of lung volume was initially ascribed to reduction in lung compliance, but recent evidence suggests it is due to diaphragmatic weakness,[409] presumably caused by a myopathy,[410,411] for which there is some pathologic evidence.[412] However, not all authorities agree.[413,414] Pleuritic pain with splinting may be a contributory factor.[410,415] In a few cases, lower lobe interstitial fibrosis may contribute to the volume loss.[416] Steroid treatment has given inconsistent results,[381,403] and treatment with β-agonists or theophylline may be helpful. Most patients stabilize or improve over time.[415] Chest radiograph and chest CT scan show normal lung parenchyma,[415] though basal linear atelectasis is a frequent accompaniment. On fluoroscopy, diaphragmatic motion may be sluggish, or paradoxical upward movement of the diaphragm may be seen with inspiration or sniffing.

Pulmonary vasculopathy

A variety of changes are described pathologically in the pulmonary vessels.[302,417] Chronic lesions consist of intimal thickening, subintimal fibrosis, medial hypertrophy, and periadventitial fibrosis. Plexogenic lesions similar to those of primary pulmonary hypertension, and organizing thrombi may also be seen.[418] Acute lesions of vasculitis and fibrinoid necrosis are generally regarded as unusual.[391] Significant pulmonary arterial hypertension is unusual,[379] many reports consisting of small numbers of cases.[403,418–420] It may be, however, that mild pulmonary artery hypertension is quite common,[421] and in one

study with echocardiographic assessment on two occasions, separated by 5 years, there was, respectively, a 14 and 43% frequency of pulmonary artery hypertension with relatively modest mean pressures of 23 and 28 mmHg, respectively.[422] Pulmonary artery hypertension is associated with digital ischemia, livedo,[423] and in 75% of patients Raynaud phenomenon,[420] findings that are consistent with a vasospastic mechanism.[424] Some cases of pulmonary arterial hypertension have been associated with the presence of lupus anticoagulant, which predisposes to thrombosis and may be pathogenetically important.[420] In these cases, it is very important to exclude central pulmonary thromboembolic disease. A number of cases (~10) have been indistinguishable from primary pulmonary hypertension,[381,418] while others have had interstitial lung disease[419] or features of mixed connective tissue disease.[379]

Miscellaneous manifestations

A sizeable proportion of patients with SLE test positive for *antiphospholipid antibodies*, and in a literature review of >1000 patients, 34% had lupus anticoagulant and 44% anticardiolipin antibodies.[425] The presence of antiphospholipid antibodies is an important risk factor for thrombosis (venous and arterial), neurologic disease, thrombocytopenia, and fetal loss. There is a two- to threefold increase in the frequency of thrombosis,[425] some of which will be manifest as pulmonary embolism. A review of the thoracic imaging features of 88 patients with antiphospholipid antibodies found that pulmonary embolism was the primary intrathoracic manifestation, being seen in nine patients, usually associated with thrombosis of lower extremity veins.[426] Thrombosis of the superior vena cava or its tributaries may also occur.[426] The antiphospholipid antibody syndrome may cause thromboembolic pulmonary hypertension,[427,428] and antiphospholipid antibodies may also be found in patients with primary pulmonary hypertension.[429] Pulmonary arterial aneurysms, presumably due to vasculitis, have also been described in this syndrome.[430] The antiphospholipid antibody syndrome may be found in other collagen vascular diseases,[431] and may also be seen in the absence of other evidence of collagen vascular disease (primary antiphospholipid syndrome). The primary antiphospholipid syndrome can be associated with lung fibrosis.[432] Antiphospholipid syndrome should be suspected in patients with pulmonary embolism or pulmonary hypertension in whom there is no evident predisposing factor, and particularly in those with thrombosis at unusual sites, such as central veins or dural sinuses.[433] MR angiography may be helpful in visualizing the entire vascular system to document the extent of venous and arterial thrombi.[434]

OP has been recorded in a handful of patients.[163,435]

Only a few cases of *lymphocytic interstitial pneumonia/pseudolymphoma* have been reported.[403,436] It is possible that some of these cases may have represented a cellular NSIP.

Acute reversible hypoxemia is thought to be caused by polymorph aggregation in the pulmonary circulation following activation by complement split products. The chest radiograph is normal and the condition resolves with steroid therapy.[437]

Pulmonary venoocclusive disease has been recorded.[438]

Secondary manifestations

Atelectasis
Elevation of the diaphragm with resultant lower zone underinflation may be associated with basal line or band shadows that are usually horizontal, several millimeters wide, and up to 5 cm long. These shadows are often transient, and it seems most likely that they represent discoid or plate atelectasis,[292,378,387,394,416] though some could be due to pulmonary infarcts.[379]

Pneumonia
Pneumonia is probably the single most common pulmonary abnormality in SLE,[252] occurring in about 50% of patients.[391,395,439] Most cases are simple bacterial pneumonias, including tuberculosis,[438] but some are opportunistic infections.[391] These latter are an increasingly important cause of death.[381,440] The responsible organisms include *Candida, Cytomegalovirus, Legionella, Pneumocystis, Cryptococcus, Aspergillus,* and *Nocardia.*[379,387,391,395,396,340] Cavitary lesions, which are uncommon in SLE, are most often the result of infections.[441]

Pericarditis, myocarditis, and renal disease
Twenty to 30% of all SLE patients develop pericarditis at some time.[380] A reliable figure for myocarditis is not available but is probably in the order of 8%.[383] Myocarditis, however, rarely gives rise to cardiac failure. There is an 18–74% prevalence of valve disease (thickening, stenosis/regurgitation, and verrucose endocarditis), the frequency depending on the mode of diagnosis.[442] There is also increased risk of infective endocarditis. Renal failure and the nephrotic syndrome may cause pulmonary edema (Fig. 10.48) and pleural effusion. The pleural effusions, unlike those due to lupus pleuritis, are pain-free.

Drug induced systemic lupus erythematosus

This is considered in Chapter 9 (p. 492).

Progressive systemic sclerosis

Systemic sclerosis is a generalized connective tissue disorder characterized by: (1) tightening, induration, and thickening of the skin (scleroderma); (2) Raynaud phenomenon and other vascular abnormalities; (3) musculoskeletal manifestations; and (4) visceral involvement, especially of the gastrointestinal tract, lungs, heart, and kidneys.[443–446] The lung is the fourth most

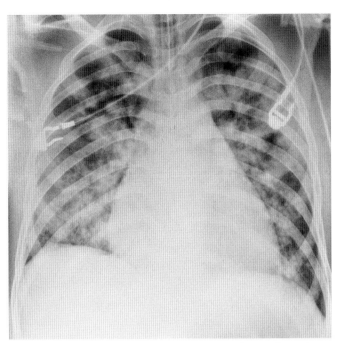

Fig. 10.48 Systemic lupus erythematosus (SLE). Chest radiograph shows diffuse patchy airspace opacity consistent with edema in a patient with acute glomerulonephritis secondary to SLE.

commonly affected structure after skin, vessel, and esophageal involvement.[447] In general, the extent of extrapulmonary involvement does not correlate with the severity of pulmonary fibrosis.[448] The diagnosis can be made with a high degree of certainty if the single major criterion of proximal scleroderma is present (proximal to metacarpophalyngeal joints) or if there are two or more minor criteria (sclerodactyly, pitting scars, or loss of substance of the finger tips, or bilateral basal pulmonary fibrosis).[449] Nailfold capillaroscopy can be very helpful in identifying the microcirculatory disturbance of scleroderma, and may be added to the diagnostic criteria.[450] Antinuclear antibodies are present in virtually every patient. The presence of antitopoisomerase I antibody (found in one-third of patients) is associated with interstitial lung disease,[451] though not all studies have confirmed this.[452] Kane et al[452] found that the presence of anticentromere antibodies was highly associated with the absence of interstitial lung disease.

The pathogenesis is complex and incompletely understood, the fundamental abnormality being persistent overproduction and tissue deposition of collagen and related macromolecules.[453] Factors that contribute to this are fibroblast proliferation, capillary endothelial damage causing increased vascular permeability, and an alveolitis.[447,454–456] There are two types of histopathologic change in the lungs which are independent of each other[457]: (1) interstitial fibrosis[47,48]; and (2) vascular changes in small vessels (intimal proliferation, medial hypertrophy, and myxomatous change).[302] In two recent series of patients with scleroderma who underwent lung biopsy, the prevalence of NSIP was about 75%, with UIP being found in 10–20%.[47,48] At autopsy, the lungs are abnormal in at least 80% of cases.[458] The interstitial fibrosis may affect all lobes, but is particularly marked peripherally and in lower zones.[302,459] Although pleural fibrosis and adhesions are commonly identified at autopsy, clinically significant pleural effusions during life are infrequent.[447,459]

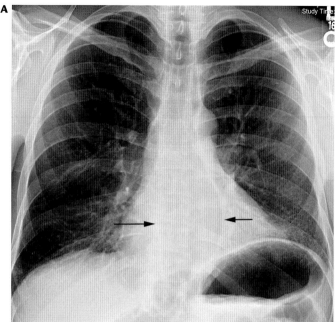

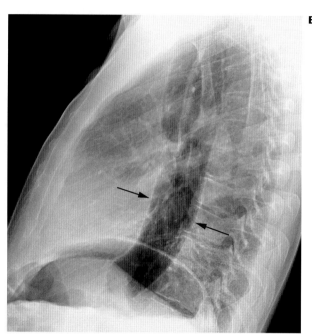

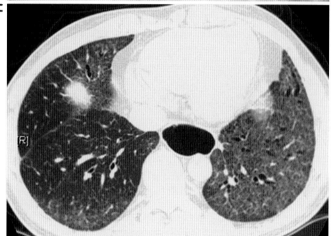

Fig. 10.49 Dilated esophagus and lung fibrosis in a patient with progressive systemic sclerosis. **A**, Posteroanterior and **B**, lateral chest radiographs show marked esophageal dilation (arrows), and basal reticular abnormality with lower lobe volume loss, evident from caudal displacement of the hila and minor fissure. **C**, HRCT confirms esophageal dilation and parenchymal abnormality, with a fine reticular and ground-glass pattern, associated with traction bronchiectasis, consistent with a nonspecific interstitial pneumonia pattern.

Systemic sclerosis has a 3:1 female to male distribution and presents most commonly in the third to fifth decade of life, though there is a wide range from childhood upwards.[449] The clinical syndrome of scleroderma may rarely occur in relationship to silicosis (Erasmus syndrome).[460] In children, a localized cutaneous form of the disease is the most common manifestation, but pulmonary involvement does occur.[461,462] The most frequent presentation in adults is with Raynaud phenomenon (80–90% of cases), which may precede skin changes by several years. Other early manifestations include tendinitis, arthralgia, and arthritis. Various treatments have been tried but none is particularly effective,[463–466] and prognosis is very variable depending on the degree of visceral involvement, particularly of the heart, kidneys, and lungs.[467] The 5 year survival is 70–80%,[445,468] and pulmonary disease has now replaced renal disease as the major cause of death.[468,469]

Less than 1% of patients present initially with respiratory symptoms.[443] However, in established disease respiratory symptoms are common, with dyspnea in >60% and less commonly cough and pleuritic pain.[447] Dyspnea may be due to lung fibrosis and/or pulmonary arterial hypertension.[444] Pulmonary function tests are commonly (80–90%) abnormal in

systemic sclerosis, but the defects are often mild.[443] The main abnormalities are reduction in carbon monoxide diffusion and a restrictive ventilatory defect, with hypoxemia and airflow obstruction in some.[443,447] Restrictive lung disease is more frequent in patients with the diffuse form of the disease, whereas pulmonary hypertension and impaired gas exchange appear to be more prevalent in patients with limited scleroderma.[470] There is a poor correlation between pulmonary function tests and radiographic findings[447,471] (by contrast, there is a strong correlation between the extent of disease on HRCT and DLco[472]). About 50% of patients with systemic sclerosis have abnormal findings on bronchoalveolar lavage (BAL) consistent with an alveolitis.[447] Respiratory disease usually follows an indolently progressive course, and adversely affects survival.[469]

The chest radiograph is abnormal in 10–80% of patients with established scleroderma.[469,473] As with other fibrosing lung diseases, the interstitial fibrosis of systemic sclerosis can be present despite a normal chest radiograph.[302] Occasionally, chest radiographic changes consistent with fibrosis antedate the onset of scleroderma, sometimes by many years.[474] The most common radiographic abnormality is a widespread, symmetric, basally predominant reticulonodular pattern (Fig. 10.49)[459,475] that typically starts as a very fine reticular pattern and progresses to coarser reticulation. Sometimes, the nodular shadowing is so fine that it has a ground-glass appearance.[476] The radiographic distribution may be asymmetric or unilateral, and may involve the entire lung.[473,474] Cystic honeycomb lesions commonly develop in the areas of fibrosis and range in size from 1 to 30 mm.[474] Occasionally, the cysts are quite large – >5 cm in diameter.[477] It is presumably the rupture of subpleural cysts that accounts for the occasional pneumothorax seen in systemic sclerosis. Gross fibrosis can cause airway distortion and bronchiectasis.[476] Loss of lung volume with elevation of the diaphragm often occurs and is caused in part by reduced compliance associated with fibrosis. Respiratory muscle abnormalities can occur in systemic sclerosis and may also play a part.[447] Diaphragmatic muscle atrophy and replacement fibrosis have been demonstrated and there may be additional factors contributing to diaphragm weakness and elevation.[478] Pleural changes detected radiographically are infrequent and almost invariably minor,[447,459] even though at autopsy about one-third of cases have pleural inflammation and adhesions.[458] Posterolateral superior rib erosion has been described in scleroderma,[479] but is not specific for this entity, being seen in other collagen vascular diseases.[473,480]

Involvement of the esophagus is present pathologically in three-quarters of patients with scleroderma.[469] The esophagus becomes functionally abnormal and fibrosed, ending up as a dilated, air-filled tube that may be detected on the frontal or lateral chest radiograph (Fig. 10.49).[481–483] An air esophagogram is found in many other conditions that cause esophageal dysmotility, including other collagen vascular diseases and achalasia.[484] In contrast to patients with achalasia, the esophagus does not contain an air–fluid level, as the dilatation is not usually associated with obstruction.[485] Despite the esophageal dysmotility, aspiration pneumonia is remarkably uncommon in patients with systemic sclerosis. Asymptomatic esophageal dilatation is more readily demonstrated (in up to 80% of patients) on CT.[486]

HRCT findings in systemic sclerosis have been described.[486–495] CT may be abnormal in the face of a normal chest radiograph.[490,496] Changes, other than in advanced disease, tend to occur at the lung bases and posterolaterally.[490,493] The prevalence of various abnormalities has varied between series. The main findings have been: (1) ground-glass opacification; (2) a fine reticular pattern, often posterior and subpleural, usually associated with traction bronchiectasis and bronchiolectasis (Figs 10.49 to 10.51); (3) honeycombing, with subpleural cysts (1–3 cm in diameter); (4) lines of various types – septal, subpleural, and long (nonseptal) parenchymal lines; and (5) subpleural micronodules.[490,493] Correlation between HRCT and lung biopsies has shown that ground-glass changes are more commonly associated with a cellular biopsy (presumably NSIP) than are honeycomb appearances.[492] Not surprisingly, the CT findings in most cases of scleroderma are similar to those of NSIP, since this is the histologic lesion in 75% or more of cases.

Several papers have reported an increased prevalence (32–60%) of enlarged reactive mediastinal lymph nodes in patients with systemic sclerosis.[486,488,491,497] This phenomenon does not appear to be related to the extent of skin involvement or disease activity of the pulmonary fibrosis; however, there is some relationship between the extent of pulmonary disease and the presence of mediastinal lymphadenopathy.[488,497]

Pulmonary arterial hypertension, with pulmonary arterial

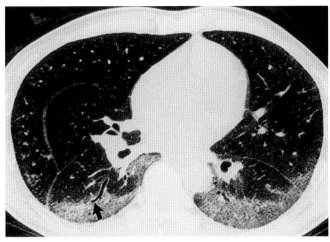

Fig. 10.50 Nonspecific interstitial pneumonia (biopsy proven) in systemic sclerosis. HRCT shows extensive confluent, peripheral ground-glass opacity, mainly affecting the apical/subapical segments of the lower lobes. There is mild airway dilatation (arrow), indicating that the ground-glass opacity is not purely cellular but must have a fibrotic component.

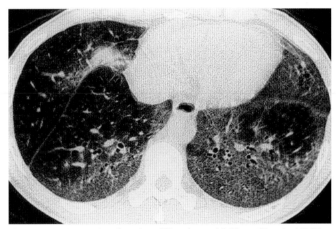

Fig. 10.51 Systemic sclerosis – diffuse interstitial lung fibrosis. HRCT through the lung bases shows characteristic posterobasal distribution of disease, with posterior fissural displacement. The main findings are a mixture of fine reticulation and ground-glass opacity, associated with traction bronchiectasis. These findings are typical of nonspecific interstitial pneumonia.

enlargement, is common in systemic sclerosis,[498,499] and occurs independently of lung fibrosis (Fig. 10.52), though both may occur together (Fig. 10.53).[457,500] The finding of pulmonary arterial enlargement out of proportion to the severity of lung fibrosis is very suggestive of collagen vascular disease, particularly scleroderma. It occurs in one-third to one-half of patients, particularly in anticentromere antibody (ACA)-positive patients with the CREST syndrome (limited cutaneous systemic sclerosis).[457,501,502] Its presence may be signaled by an isolated reduction in diffusing capacity.[501,502] Pulmonary arterial hypertension usually causes enlargement of the main and proximal pulmonary arteries on chest radiograph or CT, and may lead to cor pulmonale with cardiomegaly; however, normal sized

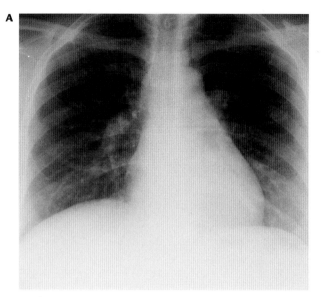 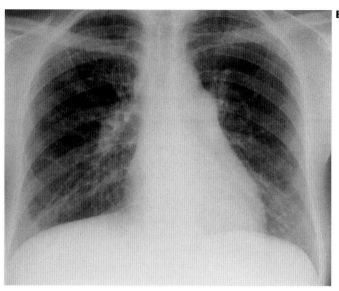

Fig. 10.52 Systemic sclerosis with pulmonary arterial hypertension. A 44-year-old male who developed progressive exertional dyspnea in the 3 year interval between radiographs **A** and **B**. The main and right pulmonary arteries have enlarged progressively between the two radiographs, indicating significant pulmonary arterial hypertension. Because pulmonary vascular changes and hypertension occur independently of interstitial lung disease, the absence of fibrotic opacity is not surprising.

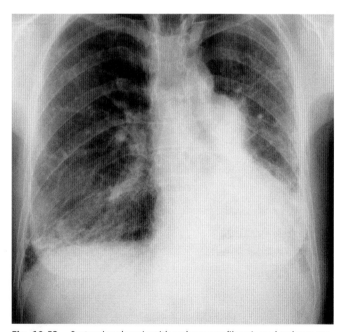

Fig. 10.53 Systemic sclerosis with pulmonary fibrosis and pulmonary arterial hypertension. Unlike the patient illustrated in Fig. 10.52, here interstitial fibrosis and pulmonary arterial hypertension coexist, but the degree of pulmonary arterial enlargement is out of proportion to the degree of fibrosis. Mediastinal air to the left of the trachea and in the region of the left main stem bronchus lies in a dilated dysmotile esophagus.

pulmonary arteries do not exclude the diagnosis.[501] An indirect CT sign of pulmonary hypertension is loss of the gravity dependent density gradient, as judged by measurements of the lung density in the dependent and nondependent parts of the lung.[503]

It is generally accepted that there is an increased prevalence of malignancy in scleroderma, with relative risk of malignancy ranging from 1.8 to 6.5,[469,504] though some studies have not shown an increased risk.[505] Lung cancer (Fig. 10.54) accounts for most of the increased risk, with a relative risk ranging from 5.9[506] to 16.5,[507] and most, though not all, studies have indicated that the presence of lung fibrosis is a risk factor.[504] The relative risk is probably about the same as is seen in patients with IPF (CFA).[371,447] All types of lung cancer may be present, but a slightly higher prevalence of alveolar cell carcinoma and adenocarcinoma has been reported in some series.[506,508] Because lung cancer is usually a late complication of systemic sclerosis,[371] surgical treatment is rarely possible, though it may be feasible in carefully selected cases.[95]

Pneumonia is a recognized complication of systemic sclerosis and, in some cases, may be an aspiration pneumonia related to esophageal dysfunction.[444] Infection is a serious complication of advanced systemic sclerosis, and infection, rather than respiratory failure, is the main cause of respiratory deaths.[443] Because of the esophageal dysmotility, there is a possibility that chronic aspiration contributes to lung fibrosis[509]; however, in a study by Troshinsky et al,[510] which evaluated esophageal manometry, acid reflux (by pH probe), and pulmonary function in 39 patients with scleroderma, no relationship was found between the degree of reflux or motility impairment. An association between esophageal dysmotility and reduced lung volumes in patients with systemic sclerosis has been reported, but the authors suggest that this observation probably reflects simultaneous involvement of the lungs and esophagus, rather than lung

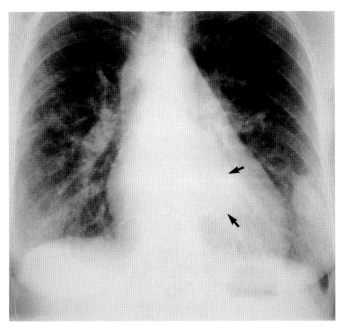

Fig. 10.54 Systemic sclerosis with interstitial fibrosis and carcinoma in a 56-year-old woman with a long history of systemic sclerosis, and a 10 year history of lung fibrosis. The chest radiograph shows fine bibasilar and peripheral reticular abnormality, with a mass in the lateral left lower lung, associated with paraspinal adenopathy (arrows). Histologic examination showed the mass to be an adenocarcinoma.

damage due to aspiration.[511] Furthermore, clinically obvious aspiration is relatively rare in these patients. Most authors consider that aspiration does not play a significant part in the pathogenesis of basal fibrotic changes.[474]

Because of the high prevalence of asymptomatic abnormalities on CT scans in patients with scleroderma, it is important to determine which types of abnormality are likely to progress. Remy-Jardin et al[493] used CT to follow 17 patients with scleroderma. Five patients with initially normal CT scans, but with abnormal BAL, remained normal on follow-up CT. Six of seven patients whose initial CT scans showed some honeycombing progressed on follow-up evaluation, with new honeycombing in areas previously occupied by ground-glass attenuation. Five patients had abnormal initial CT scans without honeycombing: three of these were unchanged on follow up, while two patients had resolution of some of their changes. However, a more recent study suggested that both honeycombing and ground-glass abnormality tended to progress over time.[512] In this author's experience, patients with moderate or extensive parenchymal abnormality, or those with honeycombing, tend to progress over time, while those with relatively mild ground-glass or reticular abnormality show only minor fluctuation. A very few patients show a sudden catastrophic progression of their lung disease with widespread DAD,[513] presumably similar to that seen in accelerated UIP.

The lung fibrosis associated with scleroderma is associated with a much better prognosis than that found in IPF.[45,513,514] This is most likely due in part to the predominant NSIP histology. There may also be a component of lead time bias, since early lung fibrosis is often detected in patients with scleroderma because of increased surveillance. Morphologically, patients with lung fibrosis related to scleroderma differ from those with IPF because

of a lesser degree of upper lobe involvement, and by a firmer reticular pattern, again probably due to the predominance of NSIP in systemic sclerosis.[487]

CREST syndrome (limited cutaneous systemic sclerosis)

The CREST syndrome is a clinical subtype of scleroderma in which (C)alcinosis, (R)aynaud phenomenon, (E)sophageal dysmotility, (S)clerodactyly and (T)elangiectasia are prominent features.[515,516] It is commonly associated with the anticentromere antibody.[452] Although patients with this syndrome often have less severe skin and visceral involvement than in scleroderma, about 60% develop significant pulmonary hypertension.[470] Selection bias in various series makes prevalence difficult to assess, but it is probably similar to that of classic systemic sclerosis.[469] The majority of patients are older females presenting with a long history of Raynaud phenomenon and swollen fingers, but less extensive skin involvement than systemic sclerosis.[469] Between 50 and 80% of patients have anticentromere antibody – an unusual finding in systemic sclerosis.[447,469] It also differs from systemic sclerosis in that life expectancy is greater, and the disease is quite often mild and slowly progressive. Systemic involvement such as of the kidney is less.[517] However, the CREST syndrome is by no means benign, and there are several reports of severe pulmonary hypertension and deaths from cor pulmonale.[517,518] Although earlier reports suggested that the prevalence of pulmonary hypertension in CREST syndrome is about 10%,[518,519] more recent studies have found echocardiographic evidence of pulmonary hypertension in 30–60% of cases.[470,499] The reported prevalence of lung fibrosis in CREST syndrome has ranged from 0 to 72%, depending at least in part on the criteria used for evaluation.[473,517,520,521] In studies using HRCT, the prevalence of parenchymal abnormality is 25–30%,[452,494] but the extent of abnormality is less than that seen in diffuse scleroderma.[494] The anticentromere antibody tends to be associated with the absence of lung fibrosis.[452]

Overlap systemic sclerosis syndrome

This is the other major clinical variant of systemic sclerosis, constituting 10–27% of all cases of systemic sclerosis.[449,473] Overlap occurs with one or more connective tissue disorders: SLE, rheumatoid disease, and dermatomyositis. Pleuropulmonary involvement is more common than in classic systemic sclerosis, with radiographic fibrosis in 25–65%,[449,473] and pleural effusions in 15–36%.[473,514,522]

Polymyositis/dermatomyositis

Polymyositis and dermatomyositis are diffuse inflammatory myopathies of striated muscle. Additionally, in dermatomyositis there are characteristic skin changes. Several subgroups are identified (Box 10.25).[523]

Female patients outnumber males by about 2:1,[252] and most present at between 40 and 60 years of age, with a smaller peak between the ages of 5 and 15.[523] Clinical presentation may be with an acute, subacute, or chronic illness characterized by a progressive, symmetric weakness of the girdle and neck muscles. In the acute disease, muscle pain and tenderness are common,

---

> **Box 10.25 Classification of polymyositis and dermatomyositis (adapted from reference[523])**
>
> Primary idiopathic polymyositis
> Primary idiopathic dermatomyositis
> Amyopathic dermatomyositis
> Polymyositis/dermatomyositis in association with:
> * Neoplasia
> * Other collagen vascular disease (overlap syndromes)
> Polymyositis/dermatomyositis of childhood

> **Box 10.26 Diagnostic criteria for polymyositis and dermatomyositis[523]**
>
> Proximal muscle weakness (symmetric, present for weeks or months)
> Muscle biopsy showing necrobiotic and inflammatory changes
> Raised muscle enzymes (creatine phosphokinase)
> Characteristic electromyography
> Characteristic skin rash

> **Box 10.27 Thoracic manifestations of polymyositis and dermatomyositis**
>
> *Primary*
> Interstitial lung disease
> * Organizing pneumonia
> * Nonspecific interstitial pneumonia
> * Usual interstitial pneumonia
> * Diffuse alveolar damage
> Vascular
> * Vasculitis
> * Capillaritis/hemorrhage
> * Pulmonary hypertension
>
> *Secondary*
> Muscle weakness
> * Respiratory failure
> * Pneumonia/aspiration
> * Atelectasis
> Drug related disorders
> Heart failure
> Lung cancer

and there may also be pharyngeal and respiratory symptoms.[524] In dermatomyositis, additional and characteristic skin changes are present: heliotrope periorbital rash and violaceous/red papular rash over bony prominences. Associated findings, particularly in the subacute form, include systemic symptoms, arthropathy, dysphagia, pulmonary disease, and cardiac disease.[524,525] Anti-Jo-1 antibodies are commonly present, and may precede the onset of clinical myopathy. Five major diagnostic criteria have been suggested (Box 10.26), and all should be present to make a definite diagnosis of dermatomyositis or, if the skin changes are not present, of polymyositis.[523] The term amyopathic dermatomyositis has been used to describe a condition where muscle weakness is absent in patients who have otherwise typical manifestations of dermatomyositis, including lung involvement.[526,527]

Pulmonary involvement is quite common in polymyositis/dermatomyositis and may occur in up to 50% of patients. It is an important determinant of the clinical course and contributes directly to death in some 10% of patients.[528]

The chest manifestations of polymyositis and dermatomyositis take on a variety of forms which are listed in Box 10.27.

Interstitial lung disease

Interstitial fibrosis was first described in dermatomyositis in 1956 by Mills and Matthews.[528] It is now a well recognized association[529] that occurs in 5–10% of patients (Fig. 10.55).[528,530,531] It has been reported slightly more commonly with polymyositis than with dermatomyositis. It may also occur in amyopathic dermatomyositis. The presence of interstitial lung disease (ILD) in polymyositis/dermatomyositis correlates strongly with the presence of anti-Jo-1, a myositis specific autoantibody directed against a cellular enzyme (histidyl-tRNA synthetase),[532] which is found in about 25% of patients with polymyositis/dermatomyositis.[425] Some 50–70% of patients who are anti-Jo-1 positive have ILD,[525] whereas the frequency of ILD falls to

about 10% if antibodies are absent. ILD may antedate myositis in patients with anti-Jo-1 antibodies.[533]

ILD tends to be accompanied by joint involvement,[534] and, as with ILD in other collagen vascular diseases, pulmonary changes on the chest radiograph can be the first clinical manifestation, preceding the skin rash or myositis,[534–536] though the usual pattern is for the ILD to follow soon after the onset of muscle weakness. The clinical manifestations vary greatly. At one extreme is an acute, rapidly fatal illness resistant to therapy,[525,530,537,538] in which the muscle disease can be masked by respiratory involvement. At the other is a benign, indolent, and asymptomatic form.[530,538] It is said that the ILD of polymyositis/dermatomyositis is more steroid responsive than that of systemic sclerosis,[252] perhaps due to a higher prevalence of OP. About half the patients with lung involvement respond with lessening of dyspnea, clearing of the chest radiograph, and improvement in lung function tests.[528,537] The variation in the clinical course of ILD in polymyositis/dermatomyositis and its generally favorable response to steroid therapy reflects the variety of underlying pathologic changes and their relative frequency.

Pathologic findings include: (1) NSIP[100,165,525]; (2) OP[165,302,537,539–541]; (3) UIP[165,525,536,540] (the frequency is less than in other collagen vascular disorders); (4) DAD (which in the organizing phase is probably equivalent to AIP)[165,302,525,538,541,542]; (5) vasculitis (small/medium vessel)[536,540]; (6) primary pulmonary arterial fibroproliferative changes[525,543]; (7) diffuse pulmonary hemorrhage with capillaritis[544]; and (8) chronic eosinophilic pneumonia.[541] Although earlier studies suggested that OP was the most common histologic pattern in this condition, more recent experience indicates that NSIP is more common, though a mixture of the two is frequent.[527,545,546]

Radiographic changes commonly consist of symmetric, basally predominant, reticulonodular opacity (Fig. 10.55).[530,537] The more acute cases may show areas of airspace opacity (Fig. 10.56)[530] or even widespread ground-glass shadowing

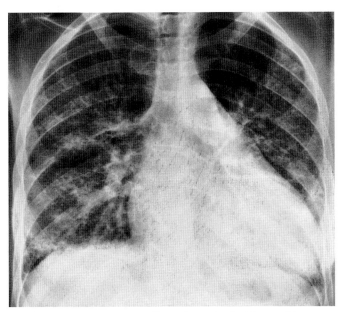

Fig. 10.55 Dermatomyositis. The radiograph of a 21-year-old woman with dermatomyositis shows a large heart secondary to myocarditis and diffuse reticulonodular pattern with apical sparing caused by diffuse interstitial pulmonary fibrosis.

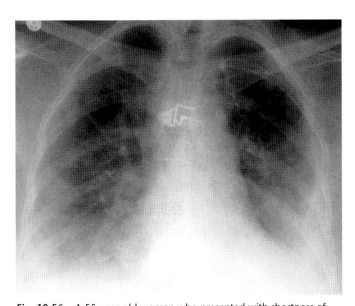

Fig. 10.56 A 55-year-old woman who presented with shortness of breath and mild weakness. The chest radiograph shows bilateral effusions, and bilateral lower lung consolidation and ground-glass abnormality. Lung biopsy showed organizing pneumonia associated with nonspecific interstitial pneumonia. Although muscle enzymes were normal, the anti-Jo-1 antibody confirmed the presence of polymyositis.

superimposed on a reticulonodular background.[528] These various patterns reflect the variety of the underlying pathologic changes. Alveolar opacities tend to occur early in the course of lung disease and are more likely to be steroid responsive. The majority of these are probably caused by OP, with or without a component of NSIP. In time, pulmonary changes can progress to

involve the whole lung (Fig. 10.56), and a fine honeycomb pattern may form.[531,537] As is well recorded in other types of diffuse lung disease, the chest radiograph can be normal with proven disease.[528] Although pleural inflammatory changes and fibrosis together with small effusions are common pathologically,[537] they have not been described radiographically. The same applies to multifocal dystrophic pulmonary ossification, which has also been demonstrated pathologically,[537] but not radiographically. The chest radiograph may rarely show muscle calcifications (Fig. 10.57).

HRCT changes[541,542,547] consist principally of ground-glass opacity, parenchymal bands, and consolidation (Fig. 10.58). Ninety-five percent of patients had diffuse but patchy ground-glass opacity with a peripheral predominance. Unilateral or bilateral multifocal consolidation (Fig. 10.58) was almost as common (75%), tending to occur in the lower zones with a subpleural or peribronchovascular predilection, usually accompanied by linear or ground-glass opacity. Parenchymal band opacities, typically basal and peripheral, occurred in 85% of patients, as did irregular thickening of bronchovascular interfaces (Fig. 10.57). Forty percent had traction bronchiectasis and bronchiolectasis in opacified areas (Fig. 10.59). Honeycombing (Fig. 10.59) is relatively uncommon, with recorded prevalence ranging from 0 to 26%.[539,541,542] Ikezoe et al[542] also recorded micronodules (28%), whilst Mino et al[547] reported pleural thickening and irregularity in all patients.

The imaging findings depend on the type of histologic abnormality. In patients with histologic NSIP, ground-glass abnormality and reticular abnormality with traction bronchiectasis are the most common features, though consolidation may also occur.[546] Pathologic correlation[541,542] showed that patchy consolidation and ground-glass opacity was produced by OP, whereas extensive consolidation and ground-glass opacity indicated DAD. Honeycomb opacity equated with UIP.[541,542] However, as in other collagen vascular diseases, mixed patterns of abnormality are common (Fig. 10.59).

On serial evaluation, the changes of consolidation, ground-glass abnormality, reticular abnormality, and traction bronchiectasis may all be partially reversible with treatment.[541,546,547] Less commonly, consolidation may progress to reticular abnormality,[548] and fatal acute exacerbations of lung disease (presumably DAD) may be associated with CT findings of new consolidation and ground-glass abnormality.[548]

Pulmonary vasculopathy

Pulmonary arterial hypertension produces large main and proximal pulmonary arteries on the chest radiograph or chest CT. Such hypertension may be seen as a complication of ILD (Fig. 10.56),[536] hypoventilation,[549] or vasculitis,[543] but may also be seen in isolation,[525] or may be out of proportion to the extent of parenchymal abnormality, indicating a vasculopathy.

Diaphragmatic myositis

When the diaphragm becomes involved in the myositis,[550] functional and radiographic changes are produced similar to those seen with the diaphragmatic myopathy of SLE. Characteristically, the myopathy produces bilateral hemidiaphragm elevation, reduced lung volume, and discoid basal atelectasis.[528,550]

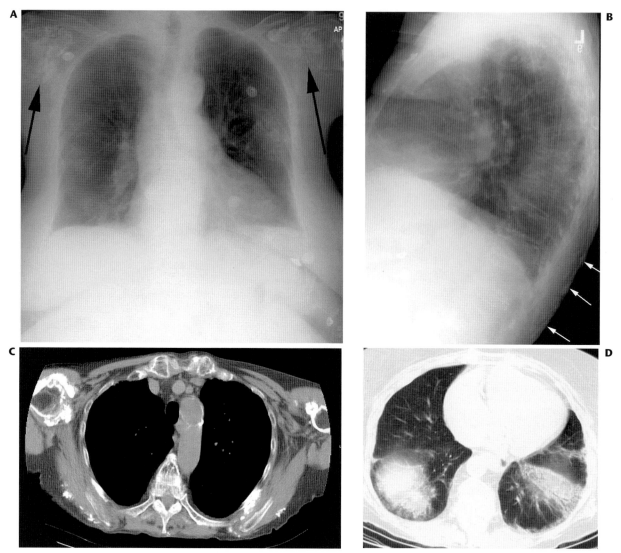

Fig. 10.57 A 69-year-old woman with dermatomyositis. **A** Frontal and **B**, lateral chest radiographs show cardiomegaly, and widespread soft tissue calcifications (arrows). Enlargement of the central pulmonary arteries suggests pulmonary hypertension. **C**, CT (mediastinal windows) shows that the calcifications are primarily in the chest wall muscles. **D**, CT (lung windows) shows that there is basal predominant reticular abnormality with traction bronchiectasis and posterior fissural displacement. The peribronchovascular distribution is seen on the left. Fibrosis in polymyositis/dermatomyositis is often best seen along the diaphragm, as in this case.

Secondary manifestations

Aspiration pneumonia is probably the most common finding on chest radiographs in polymyositis/dermatomyositis. In one series, nearly one-third of patients had radiographic evidence of pneumonia at some stage, and half of these were thought to be due to aspiration.[528] Aspiration is caused by cough impairment, pharyngeal dysfunction, and general weakness of body movements. Pharyngeal dysfunction is probably the most important factor, and most patients who aspirate are dysphagic.[528] Since polymyositis/dermatomyositis affects striated muscle, the upper esophagus and pharynx are selectively involved. These structures are normally closed at rest, but in polymyositis/dermatomyositis they are hypotonic and often contain air on plain radiographs. A barium swallow will demonstrate vallecular and pyriform pooling, defective bolus propulsion, defective pharyngeal emptying, nasopharyngeal reflux, and tracheal aspiration.[551–553]

Other pneumonias may be due to compromised defenses secondary to muscle weakness and impaired cough.[528,554,555] Some pneumonias are opportunistic.[540]

Respiratory muscle weakness coupled with stiff lungs and increased chest wall compliance produce small volume lungs with diaphragmatic elevation and atelectasis, which is often basal and discoid.[528,554,555] Marked weakness of respiratory muscles occasionally produces hypercapnic respiratory failure necessitating mechanical ventilation.[528]

Malignancy and polymyositis/dermatomyositis

There is a two- to sevenfold increase in the frequency of malignant disease in polymyositis/dermatomyositis,[371,556,557] especially in older patients. The average prevalence in various series is 21% for dermatomyositis and 15% for polymyositis.[558] The carcinomas recorded roughly parallel their frequency in the

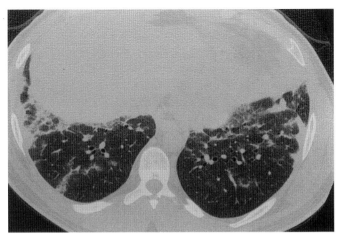

Fig. 10.58 Dermatomyositis – lymphoid interstitial pneumonia (LIP). A 38-year-old male with dermatomyositis who developed bibasal opacity, which, on HRCT, was shown to consist mainly of multifocal areas of consolidation, many of which were pleurally based and wedgelike. These appearances were considered most likely to be caused by organizing pneumonia – the most common form of DILD in polymyositis/dermatomyositis, but thoracoscopic lung biopsy showed LIP.

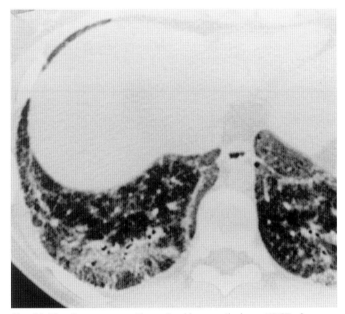

Fig. 10.59 Dermatomyositis – mixed lung pathology. HRCT of the lung bases shows a complex pattern consisting of areas of consolidation/ground-glass opacity, irregular subpleural bands, honeycombing, bronchiolectasis, septal thickening, and irregular bronchovascular interfaces. Open lung biopsy showed a mixture of organizing pneumonia and usual interstitial pneumonia. Such mixed pathology is not uncommon, particularly in collagen vascular disease.

general population,[558] though ovarian cancer may be more common.[559] Polymyositis/dermatomyositis may precede, accompany, or follow the carcinoma, though it is usually found within 1 year of diagnosis.[560] The course of the myopathy often parallels the course of the malignancy, improving when the malignancy is treated, and worsening with relapse, suggesting that it is a true paraneoplastic syndrome.[561] The prevalence of malignancy in most series is higher in patients with dermatomyositis than in those with polymyositis,[560] and

cutaneous necrosis or mucinosis should lead to even higher suspicion for malignancy.[562,563] Using Callen's data,[564] it can be estimated that there is about a 1–2% chance that the chest radiograph will show a previously unrecognized lung carcinoma at the time of diagnosis of polymyositis, and the chance of a preceding or subsequent lung carcinoma is similar. A careful search for malignancy, often including CT of the chest, abdomen, and pelvis, may be indicated in older patients with polymyositis, and particularly in those with dermatomyositis.

Overlap syndrome

Overlap of polymyositis/dermatomyositis with other collagen vascular disorders occurs in 20–40% of patients.[565] It occurs more commonly with polymyositis than dermatomyositis and shows a strong female predilection.[565] Overlap is most common with systemic sclerosis and many of these patients will have the PM-Sc1 autoantiobody which is associated with a 58% frequency of pulmonary disease.[566] Overlap is also seen with SLE, rheumatoid arthritis, and Sjögren syndrome.[567] The chest radiograph will reflect this admixture.

Juvenile dermatomyositis/polymyositis

Juvenile polymyositis/dermatomyositis differs from the adult form in a number of ways.[568,569] In children, dermatomyositis occurs much more frequently (10–20 times) than polymyositis, calcinosis is common, and widespread vasculitis is a feature, though it does not appear to cause pulmonary complications. Diffuse interstitial lung disease is described,[570] particularly if antibodies to histydl-tRNA-synthetase or Jo-1 are present.[569] One-third of patients have soft tissue calcification, particularly over pressure points. When calcinosis affects the chest wall it is detectable on the chest radiograph and may occasionally be a striking finding (Fig. 10.59).

Sjögren syndrome

Sjögren syndrome (sicca syndrome) is an autoimmune disorder characterized by dry eyes (keratoconjunctivitis sicca) and dry mouth (xerostomia), and that particularly affects middle-aged females; only 10% of patients are male. The syndrome is commonly accompanied by features of one or more of the connective tissue diseases. Pathologically, the hallmark of Sjögren syndrome is widespread tissue infiltration by polyclonal B lymphocytes. This infiltration particularly affects various exocrine glands (lacrimal, salivary, airway mucous glands), causing enlargement and later atrophy with impairment of secretion. An agreed standard set of diagnostic criteria has not been established and at least five alternative systems are in use.[571] The European classification criteria[572] are outlined in Box 10.28. The syndrome is divided into primary and secondary forms according to whether there is an associated collagen vascular disease. The most common associated collagen vascular disease is RA, but Sjögren syndrome may also be seen with systemic sclerosis, SLE, or polymyositis. Various autoimmune disorders occur with both primary and secondary forms and include chronic active hepatitis, primary biliary cirrhosis, Hashimoto thyroiditis, myasthenia gravis, and celiac disease. Primary Sjögren syndrome differs from the secondary form in that

---

Box 10.28 European classification criteria for Sjögren syndrome (four or more positive criteria indicate primary Sjögren syndrome)[572]

Dry eyes
Dry mouth
Signs of keratoconjunctivitis sicca (Schirmer test and/or Rose Bengal test positive)
Minor salivary gland positive histopathology (focal mononuclear cell agglomerations)
Objective salivary gland involvement (one or more tests positive)
- Salivary scintigraphy
- Parotid sialography
- Unstimulated salivary flow

Autoantibodies (antibodies to Ro[SS-A] and/or La[SS-B])

Box 10.29 Pleuropulmonary manifestations in Sjögren syndrome

Airway dryness/obstruction: recurrent infection
Xerotrachea (dry cough)
Atelectasis
Bronchitis/pneumonia
Bronchiectasis, bronchiolectasis
Small airway disease
Bullae

Lymphoproliferative
Follicular bronchiolitis
Lymphoid interstitial pneumonia
Lymphomatoid granulomatosis
Malignant lymphoma
Amyloidosis

Manifestations of collagen vascular disease
Pleural thickening, effusion
Interstitial pneumonia/fibrosis
Organizing pneumonia
Vasculitis
Plexogenic pulmonary arterial hypertension
Diaphragm weakness/discoid basal atelectasis

---

exocrine function is more severely disturbed, and extraglandular manifestations are more frequent.[248] These extraglandular features include renal tubular disorders, such as renal tubular acidosis; myopathy and peripheral neuropathy and CNS disorders;[573] vascular disorders, including Raynaud phenomenon, vasculitis, and purpura; and nonerosive polyarthropathy. Finally, both types of Sjögren syndrome may develop a lymphoproliferative disorder. The spectrum of lymphoproliferative disease in Sjögren syndrome includes lymphoid interstitial pneumonia[201,574] (sometimes associated with amyloid deposition[575]), follicular bronchiolitis,[247,576] nodular lymphoid hyperplasia (previously called pseudolymphoma),[201] mucosa associated lymphatic tissue (MALT) lymphoma,[577] and frank lymphoma. Most of the lymphoproliferative disorders are of B-cell origin, and benign or malignant proliferation of MALT tissue is most common.[577,578] Many of the lymphomas originate in the parotid gland, and persistent painless parotid enlargement is an important risk factor or indicator of lymphoma.[578]

Most patients have a polyclonal gammopathy, especially of IgG and IgM. In 90% there is a positive rheumatoid factor, and in 70% there is a positive ANA. Organ specific autoantibodies are also common, and the antibodies to extractable nuclear antigens (SS-A, SS-B) are relatively specific and sensitive for primary Sjögren syndrome.[579]

The pleuropulmonary manifestations of Sjögren syndrome, reviewed by Cain et al,[580] fall into three major groups (Box 10.29). These manifestations give rise to symptoms of hoarseness (dry larynx), cough (xerotrachea), pleuritic pain, and exertional dyspnea. Recurrent infections, particularly bronchitis and pneumonia, are common in some reports,[581,582] though some recent series suggest that this may no longer be so.[583] Factors that predispose to airway infections are complex and include mucus hyposecretion, leading to dry airways,[581] and lymphocytic infiltration of small airway walls, causing obstruction.[584] In general, respiratory disease in Sjögren syndrome follows a relatively benign course.[585] Obstructive, restrictive, and diffusion abnormalities are found on respiratory function tests, with different abnormalities predominating in different series.[584,586,587] Bronchoalveolar lavage shows a lymphocytosis.[588]

The prevalence of pleuropulmonary involvement is difficult to assess. Taking the symptoms and the imaging signs together, the prevalence is probably of the order of 30%, with a range of 9–90%.[579,581,589,590] High rates of involvement are recorded when

assessment is by pulmonary function test,[591,592] HRCT,[593] and bronchoalveolar lavage. Despite these prevalence rates, symptoms of pulmonary involvement are usually mild and often not clinically significant.[589,594] Somewhat surprisingly, the prevalence of pleuropulmonary abnormalities is about the same in primary and secondary Sjögren syndrome.[572,581,587,591,595] Xerotrachea,[596] recurrent tracheobronchitis, and interstitial lung disease (Fig. 10.60) are the most common problems, each occurring in one-third or more of those with chest involvement. Pleuritis with or without effusion and pleural thickening occurs in about a tenth of patients, while most of the other manifestations (Box 10.29) have a prevalence of 5% or less.

On the chest radiograph, most of the common pulmonary manifestations, particularly NSIP, UIP, and LIP[576,597,598] give rise to basally predominant nodular or reticulonodular shadowing (Fig. 10.60).[587,590] In general, the chest radiograph is not specific enough to distinguish among these processes. It is of note that UIP can occur in both primary and secondary Sjögren syndrome.[586,599] Interstitial lung disease is the commonest pulmonary finding in most series and such patients are often asymptomatic.[576,583,600] Pleural effusion is very uncommon in Sjögren syndrome unless Sjögren syndrome is secondary to collagen vascular disease, such as rheumatoid arthritis or SLE.[580] Enlarged mediastinal lymph nodes are usually not visible on the chest radiograph in uncomplicated Sjögren syndrome.[600] Enlargement of mediastinal lymph nodes, or a pattern of multifocal large nodules or alveolar pattern, suggests the development of nodular lymphoid hyperplasia[584,586,590] or malignant lymphoma.[586,590] In Sjögren syndrome there is a twofold increase in malignancy in general and a 44-fold increase in malignant lymphoma. This finding applies to both primary and secondary Sjögren syndrome. Lymphomas tend to occur in patients with extraglandular abnormalities.[579] Pulmonary arterial hypertension is reported in a limited number of cases, all of whom were female and many of whom had Raynaud phenomenon. The

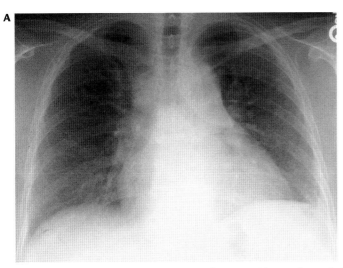
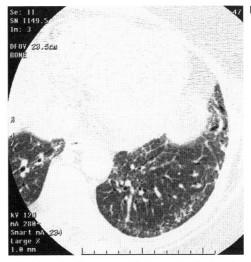

Fig. 10.60 A 47-year-old woman with Sjögren syndrome. **A**, Chest radiograph shows basal predominant ground-glass and reticular abnormality, with significant decrease in lung volumes. **B**, Chest CT shows basal reticular abnormality.

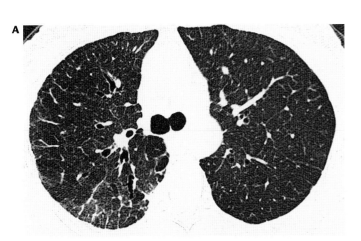
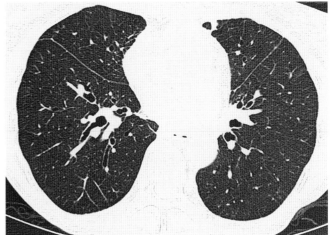

Fig. 10.61 A 65-year-old woman with Sjögren syndrome. **A** and **B**, CT images show ground-glass abnormality with septal thickening in the right upper lung, and cylindric bronchiectasis in the lower lungs. Biopsy of the parenchymal abnormality showed lymphoid interstitial pneumonia.

pathology is that of intimal proliferation, medial hypertrophy, and plexiform lesions rather than a vasculitis.[602]

HRCT provides substantial information regarding the pattern of pulmonary involvement by Sjögren syndrome.[603] The patterns may be divided into airway abnormality, interstitial fibrosis, pulmonary hypertension, and patterns suggestive of LIP.[603] Franquet et al,[593] studied 50 consecutive subjects with primary Sjögren syndrome – 98% were females, with an average age of 63 years. Disease duration was about 12 years, all were nonsmokers, and only 26% had respiratory symptoms. Seventeen (34%) of 50 patients had HRCT abnormalities, compared with 14% on the chest radiograph. Overall, changes were commonest in the lower zones. Airway related abnormalities were common (11 of 17) and consisted of bronchial wall thickening, bronchiectasis (Fig. 10.61), bronchiolectasis, and air-trapping (Fig. 10.62). In three of the 17 patients there was a tree-in-bud pattern. A second common abnormality (11 of 17) was linear opacities (septal and nonseptal). Other findings included patchy ground-glass opacity (seven of 17), nodules (five of 17), honeycombing (four of 17), and consolidation (one of 17). Nodules were of various types; some were associated with the

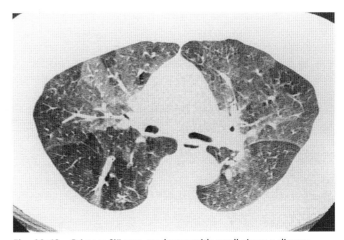

Fig. 10.62 Primary Sjögren syndrome with small airways disease. Expiratory HRCT shows patchy air-trapping, indicating small airways disease.

tree-in-bud appearance, and those >10 mm in diameter were caused by lymphoma. Honeycombing resembled that in UIP. Small airway disease may also be manifest on HRCT by a mosaic attenuation pattern and air-trapping on expiratory scans (Fig. 10.62).[593,604]

LIP occurring in Sjögren syndrome is characterized by ground-glass abnormality due to the homogeneous lymphocytic infiltration (Fig. 10.61).[205] Peribronchovascular, centrilobular, and subpleural nodules may also be seen, and cysts measuring 5–30 mm are often present (see Figs 10.25 and 10.26).[206] Similar cysts may be found in follicular bronchiolitis.[605] These changes are ascribed to bronchiolar obstruction on the basis of lymphocytic wall infiltration. Cysts are helpful in distinguishing LIP from lymphoma.[208] Lymphoma should be suspected if consolidation, large nodules (>1 cm) or effusions are present.[208] LIP is discussed further on page 558.

Overlap syndromes and mixed connective tissue disease

Some patients have an illness with the characteristic features of more than one connective tissue disorder; such patients are said to have an overlap syndrome or undifferentiated connective tissue disorder. The thoracic manifestations in these cases are those of the various connective tissue disorders that make up the overlap, and they are discussed under the individual connective tissue disorders above.

Mixed connective tissue disease (MCTD) is an overlap syndrome that is a distinct clinicopathologic entity.[605] The principal characteristics are the presence of: (1) features of SLE, systemic sclerosis, polymyositis/dermatomyositis, occurring together or evolving sequentially during observation; and (2) antibodies to an extractable nuclear antigen (RNP).[605] Suggested clinical criteria for the diagnosis are: (1) positive anti-RNP; plus (2) three or more clinical features – hand edema, synovitis, myositis, Raynaud phenomenon, acrosclerosis.[606] After several years MCTD may transform into one of the classic collagen vascular diseases, and in one series of 18 patients final diagnoses were SLE (28%), systemic sclerosis (39%), rheumatoid arthritis (17%), and a combination of these disorders (17%).[607] There is also a 10–20% frequency of renal disease. Various antibodies are found in the serum; the presence of anti-snRNP is a prerequisite but others are commonly found, often in high titer, including rheumatoid arthritis, ANA, and extractable nuclear antigen (ENA). Eighty to 90% of patients have been women,[608] with an average age of 37 years (range 4–80 years).[609] Its prevalence is approximately the same as systemic sclerosis,[609] and its overall prognosis similar to SLE and better than systemic sclerosis.

The prevalence of chest disease ranges in various series between 25 and 80%, with the upper figure probably being the closer estimate.[370,610–612] Many affected patients are asymptomatic.[609] In two series the chest radiographs were abnormal in 30%[611] and 63%[610] of cases. The 30% figure represents changes on the initial chest radiograph only and undoubtedly underestimates the longterm chest involvement. The pulmonary abnormalities resemble those seen in SLE, systemic sclerosis, and polymyositis/dermatomyositis.[252] Thus, pleural thickening and pleural and pericardial effusions are described,[610,611,613–615] as is steroid sensitive pneumonitis, manifested as fleeting basal consolidations.[608] The overall prevalence of pleural effusion is probably of the order of 50% and it is more common in patients with systemic sclerosis features.[609] Small irregular interstitial

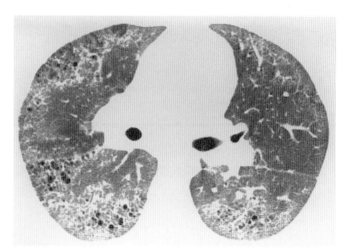

Fig. 10.63 Mixed connective disease. HRCT in an 18-year-old woman with a 6 month history of multisystem complaints and progressive dyspnea. The clinical features suggested a mixture of systemic sclerosis and systemic lupus erythematosus. Lung attenuation is diffusely increased because of widespread ground-glass opacity. In addition, there is peripheral reticular predominant interstitial opacity, associated with small cysts. The small discrete cysts may indicate a component of lymphoid interstitial pneumonia.

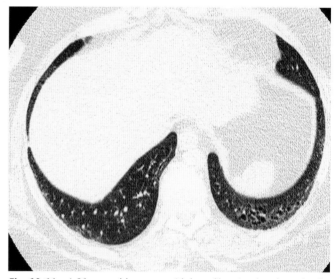

Fig. 10.64 A 31-year-old woman with lung fibrosis related to mixed connective tissue disease. HRCT through the lung bases shows ground-glass abnormality, with marked traction bronchiectasis on the left indicating lung fibrosis.

opacities, most prevalent in the lower half of the lungs, may be seen in 21[370]–85%[611] of patients with MCTD.

In a review of the CT findings in 41 patients with MCTD, Kozuka et al[616] found ground-glass attenuation in all patients (Figs 10.63 and 10.64). Subpleural micronodules, and nonseptal linear and reticular abnormalities were all found in >50% of cases, with a CT pattern corresponding most closely to NSIP (Fig. 10.64). Less common findings (each seen in 20–40% of cases) included honeycombing, consolidation, and poorly defined centrilobular nodules. Bronchiectasis and pulmonary cysts (Fig. 10.63) were seen in a few patients.

Pulmonary arterial hypertension is another important and serious complication of MCTD.[611,617,618] This may be associated with pulmonary arterial enlargement on chest radiographs or CT, and occasionally with poorly defined centrilobular nodules[616]; the latter is a subtle and occasional feature of conditions characterized by very high pulmonary artery pressure (see p. 393). The changes of pulmonary arterial hypertension may or may not be accompanied by an IPF.[608] Other reported associations include pulmonary vasculitis,[618] pulmonary embolism,[619] diffuse pulmonary hemorrhage,[620] and hypoventilatory respiratory failure.[621] There is a high prevalence (74%) of esophageal abnormality, which can lead to aspiration pneumonia.[611] A case has been described with mediastinal adenopathy which was nonspecific on biopsy.[613]

Although early reports suggested that the pulmonary changes responded well to steroids,[610] not all studies bear this out,[618] and in addition pulmonary arterial hypertension is a significant cause of morbidity and mortality.[609]

RELAPSING POLYCHONDRITIS

Relapsing polychondritis is a rare disease of unknown cause characterized by recurrent inflammatory episodes that affect various cartilaginous structures, particularly the pinna, nose, and airways. Other features include nonerosive inflammatory polyarthritis, medium to large vessel arteritis, and recurrent inflammation of the eyes and inner ears.[622] The mean age of onset is in the fifth decade,[622] though all age groups may be affected.[623] Most patients are Caucasian[624] and the overall sex incidence is equal,[622,623] though patients with serious airway involvement are more commonly (3:1) female.[625] About 30% of patients have an associated "autoimmune" disease,[623,626] most commonly rheumatoid arthritis[622] or a systemic vasculitis.[627] The diagnosis is based on characteristic combinations of clinical features[622,626–628] since the pathology is nonspecific.

Pathologically there is marked chondral and perichondral inflammation with loss of basophilic staining, and chondrolysis.

Cartilage is replaced by granulation and fibrous tissue that can calcify. There may be an element of vasculitis. Antibodies to type II collagen are demonstrable in the serum and deposition of complement and immunoglobulin on affected cartilage has been shown.[623]

Fifty percent of patients present with either auricular chondritis or arthropathy, and most of the remainder present with nasal chondritis, ocular inflammation, or respiratory tract involvement.[622,627] Because the affected areas may be inaccessible to biopsy, the diagnosis of relapsing polychondritis must often be made on clinical grounds, particularly in those with disease confined to the tracheobronchial tree. Other causes of long segment tracheobronchial narrowing which should be included in the differential diagnosis are described on page 713. Important differential diagnostic considerations include Wegener granulomatosis, sarcoidosis, amyloidosis, and tracheopathia osteoplastica.

About 20% of patients have respiratory symptoms at presentation,[625] and eventually a third to a half of the patients will develop respiratory tract involvement[622,629] manifested by laryngeal tenderness, hoarseness, dyspnea, and stridor or wheeze. Disease of the respiratory tract is a serious development as it may be immediately life threatening and, in the long term, is associated with a poor prognosis.[627] Airway involvement causes narrowing, primarily of the larynx or trachea, but the major bronchi can also be involved,[625,630,631] including segmental ones.[625,632] Stenoses are usually single and localized,[622] but they can be multiple.[633] Thus, tracheal narrowing is typically subglottic, smooth, and from 1 cm to several centimeters long,[634] but can be diffuse, involving the whole trachea.[630,635] CT (Fig. 10.65) shows tracheal wall thickening, expansion and calcification of cartilage, and luminal narrowing.[636–639] The tracheal lumen may take on a polygonal configuration.[638,640] In a review of patients with relapsing polychondritis, Behar et al[641] emphasized that the most common CT manifestations were

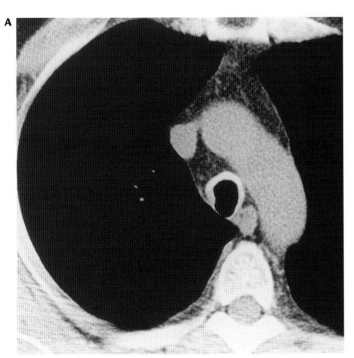

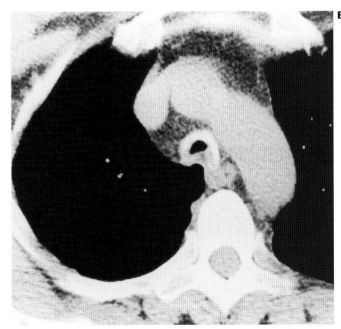

Fig. 10.65 Relapsing polychondritis. **A**, Inspiratory and **B**, expiratory HRCT of the trachea at the level of the aortic arch. On inspiration the tracheal lumen is irregular and mildly stenosed. Its wall is thickened and cartilage expanded and calcified. On expiration the lumen narrows to an abnormal degree.

increased attenuation and smooth thickening of airway walls, with tracheal or bronchial stenosis being less common. Airway collapse and lobar air-trapping were seen in 50% of patients who were examined with expiratory CT. Volumetric CT with multiplanar reconstruction clearly delineates the geometry of stenoses,[642] and may be superior to endoscopy in this respect.[635] Furthermore, stenoses may be fixed or variable (Fig. 10.65). In this latter instance, increased wall compliance predisposes to dynamic collapse.[643] The dynamic behavior of stenoses can be investigated by flow volume loops,[625,633,635] with fluoroscopy and cineradiography,[579,643] or with dynamic CT.[640] Airflow obstruction in lobar and segmental airways can lead to pulmonary oligemia and air-trapping,[631] atelectasis,[633] obstructive pneumonitis, or bronchiectasis.[632,635]

On MRI, acute changes of relapsing polychondritis in the larynx are characterized by decreased signal intensity on T1-weighted images, with increased intensity on T2, and enhancement with gadolinium.[644] These changes resolve with treatment. MRI may therefore be a way of determining the activity of relapsing polychondritis.

Cardiovascular involvement is recorded in 24% of patients,[622] and some of the described lesions such as aortic and mitral regurgitation and aortic aneurysm may produce changes on a chest radiograph. Cardiovascular involvement is an important cause of death in these patients.[622]

The mainstay of treatment is systemic steroids, and tracheostomy may be necessary. Various surgical procedures to maintain airway patency, including stenting, have been tried.[623] The outcome is very variable, and the course may be rapidly fatal or indolent, with about a 75% 5 year survival.[627] The frequency of respiratory involvement as a cause of death has been 50% or more in some series,[622,624] but was only 10% in a more recent major series.[627]

ANKYLOSING SPONDYLITIS

Ankylosing spondylitis is a seronegative spondyloarthritis that affects primarily the axial skeleton, causing pain and progressive stiffness of the spine. Onset is typically between the ages of 15 and 35 years, with males affected three to nine times more commonly than women. There is a strong association with the presence of HLA-B27. The most common and earliest manifestation is sacroiliitis followed by thoracolumbar and lumbosacral spondylitis.[645] The peripheral joints are involved in 35% of patients.[646] Extraarticular features may develop; apart from pleuropulmonary abnormalities these include anterior uveitis (up to 25%), aortic regurgitation (up to 10% in long-standing cases),[647] cardiac conduction defects,[648] and constitutional symptoms. The prognosis is variable but generally benign and not life shortening.[645] Some patients do not progress beyond sacroiliitis, whereas others develop progressive, widespread disease leading in particular to complete fusion of the axial joints and across the intervertebral disks of the spine.

Pleuropulmonary involvement has a late onset and is usually asymptomatic.[649] Two types exist: chest wall restriction and upper lobe fibrobullous disease.[252]

Restrictive disease is caused by dorsal kyphosis and fusion of costovertebral and costotransverse joints.[650] Changes in lung function are less than might be anticipated because the chest becomes fixed at a high resting volume, allowing the diaphragm

to make a greater contribution than usual to inspiration.[252,650] Apical hypoventilation, which might have been expected under these circumstances, is not present.[651] Generally, total lung capacity and vital capacity are mildly or moderately reduced, while functional residual capacity and residual volume are normal or slightly increased.[252,579,650] This contrasts with the marked impairment of respiratory function seen in idiopathic kyphoscoliosis.[579] The extent of restrictive physiologic impairment is related to the extent of lumbar stiffness, but not to the severity of spinal fusion on thoracic radiographs.[652]

Upper zone "fibrobullous" disease was first recorded in 1941,[653] with a further description in 1949.[654] Its recognition as an extraarticular manifestation of ankylosing spondylitis was reinforced by Campbell and MacDonald in 1965.[655] The phenomenon is rare; its frequency, based on a review of 2080 patients at the Mayo Clinic, is 1.25%.[649] A strong male predilection exists, with just three women out of a total of 160 patients in one review.[656] The pathologic findings are nonspecific and consist of fibrosis and a chronic inflammatory cell infiltrate, often lymphocytic, with elastic fragmentation, collagen degeneration, dilated bronchi, thin-walled bullae, and cavities.[657,658] Vasculitic changes are not found.[659]

The radiographic changes consist of nodular and linear opacity and/or pleural thickening that begin in the lung apices (Fig. 10.66).[549,655-658] The early changes are usually symmetric but may be asymmetric (one-third in one series).[660] After a while, opacification tends to become bilateral and symmetric, and the nodules and pleural thickening (Fig. 10.66) become more pronounced and confluent. After a further interval, often several years,[655] one or more rounded transradiancies appear in most cases.[549,658,660] The transradiancies are usually multiple; they may be small or large and have thin or thick walls. These apical changes usually progress slowly,[660] but they can remain stable for many years. At this stage, the process is essentially one of fibrosis; the hila become elevated, producing an appearance that mimics tuberculosis (Fig. 10.67). Tracheobronchomegaly may be seen as a consequence of the intense fibrosis (Fig. 10.66). Apical fibrosis is usually seen only in patients who have long-standing ankylosing spondylitis of 15–20 years average duration,[649,658,660] with marked spinal involvement.[661,662] A few cases are recorded in which the lung changes apparently developed within a few years of the onset of ankylosing spondylitis.[649,655] Patients are also recorded in whom a diagnosis of ankylosing spondylitis was made retrospectively after chest disease developed.[659]

By the time apical changes are visible, the skeletal manifestation of AS[663] are usually obvious on the posteroanterior and lateral chest radiographs. The findings that are most easily seen in frontal view are ossification of costotransverse joints (particularly the first), vertebral syndesmophytes, and interspinous ossification. The diagnosis of ankylosing spondylitis is, however, generally more easily made from a lateral radiograph. The principal changes detected in this projection are kyphosis, syndesmophytes (particularly at the D9–D12 level), and squared or barrel shaped vertebral bodies. The manubriosternal joint is frequently eroded or fused.[664]

The cavities that develop within the fibrotic lung may be colonized by a variety of fungi and nontuberculous mycobacteria,[252,579,649,662,665] most commonly *Aspergillus fumigatus* (Fig. 10.67).[660] Colonization rates with *Aspergillus* vary between 19[649] and 50–60%.[655,660] Hemoptysis is common in patients with mycetoma and may be life threatening. Surgical removal is often attended by complications.[252,579,662]

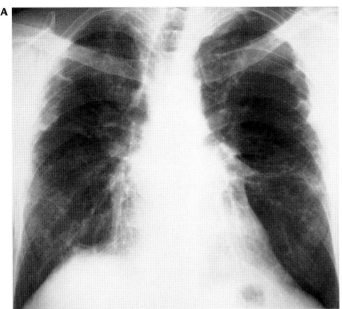

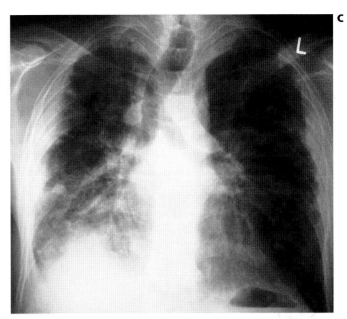

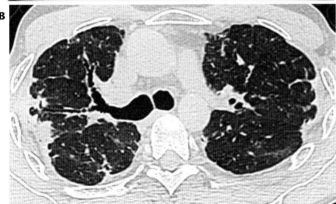

Fig. 10.66 A 47-year-old man with ankylosing spondylitis. **A**, Initial chest radiograph shows mild peripheral reticular abnormality with pleural thickening. **B**, CT shows dense irregular subpleural fibrosis, with traction bronchiectasis. **C**, Two years later, the pleural thickening has progressed dramatically, and lung volumes have decreased.

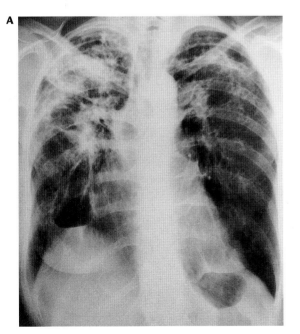

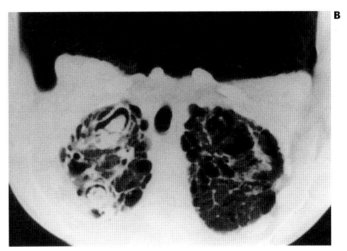

Fig. 10.67 Ankylosing spondylitis. **A**, Chest radiograph shows bilateral mid/upper zone opacity some of which is confluent together with ring and linear elements. The hila are pulled upwards and outwards, indicating marked upper zone volume loss and the lower zones are hyperexpanded. **B**, CT of the apical regions confirms scarring and focal lucencies, many of which are probably bullae. Two ring opacities on the right contain intracavitary bodies caused by aspergillomas.

There have been several descriptions of the CT findings in patients with ankylosing spondylitis.[666–670] Fenlon et al[666] studied 26 consecutive patients attending a rheumatology clinic, with a mean disease duration of 18.5 years. Apical fibrosis was seen in two patients. Four patients were judged to have significant interstitial lung disease as evidenced by predominantly basal subpleural and parenchymal bands, thickened interlobular septa, irregular interfaces, and pleural tags. These interstitial changes were not apparent on the chest radiograph and they were not assessed histologically. However, all four patients with interstitial changes had respiratory symptoms, and three also had physiologic impairment. Three recent series have confirmed a high prevalence (70–90%) of minor CT abnormalities in patients with ankylosing spondylitis.[667,669,670] The most common findings have been subpleural nodules, pleural thickening, and fibrotic bands. Upper lung emphysema has also been described, even in nonsmokers,[670] and mosaic pattern with air-trapping has been seen in patients with early ankylosing spondylitis.[669]

Pleural effusions and pleural thickening remote from the lung apex have been seen in association with ankylosing spondylitis,[671] but the prevalence is so low (only three of 2080 cases in the Mayo Clinic series)[649] that they should be considered incidental findings. The pneumothorax rate, however, is significantly increased, with a prevalence of about 8%.[649] A few reports have documented associations with OP,[672] bronchiectasis (both with and without fibrobullous disease),[666] mild mediastinal adenopathy in 12%,[666] and alveolar/septal amyloidosis (probably incidental).[673]

VASCULITIS/DIFFUSE ALVEOLAR HEMORRHAGE

The noninfectious, systemic, necrotizing vasculitides are a large and varied group of disorders characterized by inflammation and necrosis of blood vessels. Over the last couple of decades a number of classifying schemes have been proposed and the one that is currently most widely used is that resulting from the 1994 Chapel Hill consensus conference (Box 10.30).[674] This scheme is based on the size of vessels involved but this criterion on its own is insufficient to identify entities with confidence because of overlap in size of affected vessels among conditions. For diagnostic certainty, clinical and laboratory findings need to be taken into account as well.[675] Furthermore, overlap features and the evolution of clinical and other findings with time mean that the diagnosis attached to an illness may change as it progresses.[674]

Two recent developments have changed the clinical approach to pulmonary vasculitis. The introduction of the antineutrophil cytoplasmic antibody (ANCA) test has facilitated the diagnosis of vasculitis, and enabled a modified classification of vasculitis based on the pattern of positivity on this test (Table 10.6). Also, there is increased awareness of inflammation of the capillaries (capillaritis) as a manifestation of vasculitis.

The frequency with which various vasculitides affect the chest varies greatly. Wegener granulomatosis is probably the commonest pulmonary vasculitis. Other relatively common vasculitides in the chest are Churg–Strauss vasculitis, Takayasu arteritis, and microscopic polyangiitis. Takayasu arteritis is discussed in Chapter 7.

Box 10.30 Principal noninfectious systemic vasculitides

Large vessel vasculitis
Giant cell (temporal) arteritis
Takayasu arteritis

Medium vessel vasculitis
Polyarteritis nodosa
Kawasaki disease

Small vessel vasculitis
Antineutrophil cytoplasmic antibody associated
- Microscopic polyangiitis
- Wegener granulomatosis
- Churg–Strauss syndrome

Immune complex vasculitis
- Henoch-Schönlein purpura
- Mixed cryoglobulinemia
- Connective tissue disorders
- Hypocomplementemic urticarial vasulitis
- Behçet disease
- Goodpasture syndrome

Serum sickness/drug/infection associated vasculitis

Other
Paraneoplastic
Inflammatory bowel disease

Table 10.6 Frequency (%) of antineutrophil cytoplasmic antibody (ANCA) in ANCA associated vasculitides

	PR3-ANCA	MPO-ANCA
Microscopic polyangiitis	15–45	45–60
Wegener granulomatosis	85	10
Churg–Strauss syndrome	10	60–75

Giant cell (temporal) arteritis

Although giant cell arteritis[676] primarily affects branches of the carotid artery, it may also affect other arteries in up to 10–15% of patients (Fig. 10.68).[677–679] Rarely, the elastic pulmonary arteries are involved[679] and this may cause stenosis and thrombosis.[680] In a series of 146 patients with biopsy proven temporal arteritis, about 10% had respiratory symptoms (cough and hoarseness) either initially or during the course of the disease.[681] Apart from one patient with a pleural effusion, the patients apparently did not have significant chest radiographic findings, though the paper is not explicit about this.[681] Symptoms responded to steroid therapy. There are few descriptions of radiographic changes in the chest and their rarity raises the question that such findings may be purely incidental. Described abnormalities include pleural effusion,[681,682] symmetric basal reticular opacity,[683] a diffuse interstitial pattern affecting the lower and upper zones, with bullae,[684] pulmonary infarction,[685] and multiple nodules up to 3 cm in diameter together with thick walled cavities containing air–fluid levels.[686]

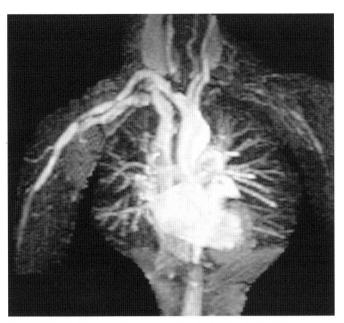

Fig. 10.68 A 68-year-old woman with giant cell arteritis. MR angiography shows occlusion of the left subclavian and axillary arteries, with multiple collateral vessels, and narrowing at the origin of the right common carotid artery. These findings were confirmed at contrast angiography.

Other giant cell arteritides

Patients are described with giant cell arteritis that do not fall into the classic clinicopathologic subgroups of Takayasu or systemic temporal arteritis, some of whom have an idiopathic isolated form of pulmonary arteritis.[687] Described abnormalities in the chest include pulmonary artery stenosis and thrombosis,[688] infarctive middle lobe consolidation with segmental pulmonary artery stenosis,[689] main pulmonary artery aneurysm,[690] and pulmonary capillaritis and hemorrhage.[691]

Medium vessel vasculitis (polyarteritis nodosa)

In classic polyarteritis nodosa there is a necrotizing inflammation of medium sized or small arteries without glomerulonephritis and without vasculitis in arterioles, capillaries, or venules.[692] It is generally accepted that polyarteritis nodosa rarely affects pulmonary arteries. Earlier reports of frequent involvement[693,694] may have been due to inclusion of cases of Churg–Strauss syndrome and microscopic polyangiitis,[695] though the issue is not straightforward.[696] There are, however, just a few isolated case reports of pathologically confirmed involvement of pulmonary arteries.[697] On the other hand, bronchial arteritis is said to be common.[698]

It seems likely that most, if not all, of the pathologic and radiographic pulmonary findings in classic polyarteritis nodosa are secondary and related, for example, to cardiac and renal failure.[699] A number of cases of IPF[698,700] and DAD[698] are recorded in polyarteritis nodosa. The pathogenesis of these lesions and their possible relationship to polyarteritis nodosa remain unclear.[698] OP is described rarely.[164,697]

Small vessel vasculitis

Most lung vasculitides affect small vessels and predominantly involve arterioles, capillaries, and venules. The various types are listed (see Box 10.30) and may conveniently be assigned to one of two subsets: (1) those that are associated with the presence of ANCA, which are also called pauciimmune since, on immunofluorescence, they lack immune complexes; and (2) those that are immune complex mediated.

Pulmonary involvement is common in all the ANCA associated conditions (microscopic polyangiitis, Wegener granulomatosis, Churg–Strauss syndrome). With the exceptions of Goodpasture syndrome and Behçet disease, it is rare for the lung to be affected by other small vessel vasculitides.

ANCA are antibodies directed against granular constituents of neutrophils.[701] The two most important antigens are both enzymes – proteinase 3 and myeloperoxidase, hence PR3-ANCA and MPO-ANCA. The original terms cANCA (for PR3-ANCA) and pANCA (for MPO-ANCA) have been discarded because they lack specificity. Since ANCA testing became widely available in the late 1980s, it has shed considerable light on the small vessel, pauciimmune vasculitides. The prevalence of PR3-ANCA and MPO-ANCA in the three ANCA associated vasculitides is indicated in Table 10.6.

Antineutrophil cytoplasmic antibody associated vasculitis

Wegener granulomatosis

Wegener granulomatosis was first described in the 1930s.[702] It has distinctive clinicopathologic features affecting the upper respiratory tract, lungs, and kidneys and can, therefore, be more easily recognized as a distinct entity than most of the other vasculitides.[699,703] The cause is obscure, but there is accumulating evidence to suggest that the entity is probably an immunologic reaction to a specific antigen.[704]

Wegener granulomatosis is characterized pathologically[302] by three features: (1) a necrotizing granulomatous inflammation of the upper and lower respiratory tracts; (2) a disseminated small vessel necrotizing vasculitis that affects both arteries and veins (inflammation of the vessel wall is commonly granulomatous but may also be acute or chronic. The small vessel vasculitis also commonly affects capillaries, expanding alveolar septa with inflammatory cells and causing their disruption); and (3) a focal, necrotizing glomerulonephritis.[704]

Inflammatory changes in the lung produce large necrotic areas that replace lung parenchyma, together with small microabscesses and small suppurative granulomas.[302] Necrotic areas may be surrounded by consolidation and alveolar hemorrhage. A limited form of the disease has been described as affecting the lung with or without upper respiratory disease but without renal or other systemic involvement.[705,706]

Classic histopathologic changes in the lung are commonly accompanied by other minor findings. Sometimes these minor findings become dominant and in a review of 87 open lung biopsies this was the case in 18% of specimens.[707] Such findings include:

• Diffuse alveolar hemorrhage and capillaritis (with or without acute arteriolitis).[708,709] In one series this was seen in 7% of specimens.[707]

- Diffuse interstitial fibrosis with patchy vasculitis in 7% of specimens.[707] These insidious changes tend to occur in older patients with radiographic appearances like interstitial pneumonitis.[710]
- An eosinophilic variant with eosinophilia confined to the lung.[711]
- A bronchocentric variant, manifest as chronic bronchiolitis,[707] bronchocentric necrosis,[712] and bronchocentric granulomatosis.[707]
- OP.[713] This variant is indistinguishable clinically and radiologically from the classic type.
- Lipoid pneumonia.[707]

A set of four clinical criteria for the diagnosis of Wegener granulomatosis have been proposed:

- An abnormal urine sediment (red blood cells or casts)
- An abnormal chest radiograph (consistent with Wegener granulomatosis)
- Oral ulcers/nasal discharge
- Granulomatous inflammation on biopsy

These criteria are 88% sensitive and 92% specific.[714] In current clinical practice, the diagnosis of Wegener granulomatosis is commonly based on typical clinical and imaging features, associated with PR3-ANCA. In cases in which biopsy is required, lung biopsy is usually preferred, as the renal changes are usually nonspecific, and the specific lesions in the upper airways are often masked by secondary infective changes.

Wegener granulomatosis is an uncommon disease with an estimated prevalence of 3 per 10^5 population in the United States,[715] and an incidence of 8.5 per 10^6 per year in a rural United Kingdom population.[716] The mean age at presentation is in the fifth decade,[703,717–720] with a wide range; 8–75 years in one series.[721] Sex incidence is equal or slightly male predominant. Onset is usually acute or subacute but may be indolent and, when the latter is combined with atypical features, diagnosis is commonly delayed by months or years.[722] At presentation upper airway involvement with sinusitis, rhinitis, and otitis is the most common clinical feature, encountered twice as often as systemic and lung symptoms (cough, hemoptysis, pleurisy). Functional renal impairment is unusual at presentation, being seen in only about 10% of patients.[703] Laboratory examination often shows a normochromic, normocytic anemia; leukocytosis; raised erythrocyte sedimentation ratio (ESR); and a positive rheumatoid factor.[703]

About 85% of patients with active multiorgan Wegener granulomatosis have a positive test for PR3-ANCA.[701,717] With limited disease these figures fall to 60–70% and, in remission, to 30–40%. In a metaanalysis PR3-ANCA was 91% sensitive and 99% specific for active Wegener granulomatosis.[723] However, positive tests are nonspecific for Wegener granulomatosis and are also seen with microscopic polyangiitis (45%), idiopathic crescentic glomerulonephritis (25%), Churg–Strauss syndrome (10%), and polyarteritis nodosa (5%).[701] A small percentage (~10%) have MPO-ANCA. The level of PR3-ANCA correlates with disease activity and increases before clinical relapse.[724]

During the course of the illness 85–90% of patients have lung involvement and all have lung and/or upper respiratory tract disease. The majority (85%) develop renal disease and in about 50% of patients joint, middle ear, skin, and eye disorders become manifest with occasional involvement of the heart and nervous system.[703] In established Wegener granulomatosis,

pulmonary or nonpulmonary infection may precipitate clinical relapse,[724,725] and in some series such infections have accounted for about half of relapses.[726] The chest radiographic pattern of relapse may differ from that seen at presentation.[727] Untreated Wegener granulomatosis carries a poor prognosis, with death in about 5 months from renal failure.[702] The outlook has, however, been transformed by treatment with cyclophosphamide and steroids, which can induce and maintain remission in a high percentage of patients.[703] In a review of 158 patients, 75% had complete remission, often taking a year or more to achieve.[717] Following this, however, 50% had one or more relapses and almost all had serious morbidity from irreversible features of the disease or adverse effects of therapy.[717] Pulmonary infection is a likely factor that precipitates relapse,[724] and there is some evidence that longterm trimethoprim sulfamethoxazole reduces relapse rate.[728] Longterm follow up of the same 158 treated Wegener granulomatosis patients showed a 2.4 times excess incidence of malignancy (see Fig. 10.72).[717]

Wegener granulomatosis was found to be localized to the lung in 9 and 10% of patients in two pulmonary series.[719,720] Localized Wegener granulomatosis is not necessarily benign, and usually becomes systemic after months or years.[719,720] In older patients (>60 years of age) Wegener granulomatosis tends to involve the lungs and kidneys, without involvement of other organs, and carries a worse prognosis.[730]

Radiographic changes in the lungs occur at presentation in 50–75% of patients and are usually due to the primary disease. In established disease the situation is more complicated and radiographic findings may be caused by: (1) relapse or progression; (2) complications of management (drug toxicity, infection, neoplasm);[725,731] or (3) disease of a nonpulmonary organ (e.g. renal failure).

The account that follows concentrates on primary manifestations. These may be accompanied by cough, hemoptysis, pain, or dyspnea, but these symptoms are often not a dominant feature. Not infrequently, the patient is entirely asymptomatic.[676]

The common imaging findings in Wegener granulomatosis are summarized in Table 10.7. The most characteristic pulmonary finding is discrete focal opacities that vary in character from nodular masses (Fig. 10.69) to ill-defined areas of consolidation (Fig. 10.70), either of which may cavitate. Nodular shadows are

Table 10.7 Imaging findings in 198 patients with pulmonary involvement by Wegener granulomatosis[719,725,732–735]

Nodules or masses	88 (44%)
Cavitation in nodules or masses	50 (25%)
Focal or multifocal consolidation	48 (24%)
Cavition in consolidation	9 (5%)
Diffuse consolidation	10 (5%)
Airway abnormalities	19 (9%)
Atelectasis	8 (4%)
Pleural effusion	14 (7%)
Pleural thickening	59 (30%)

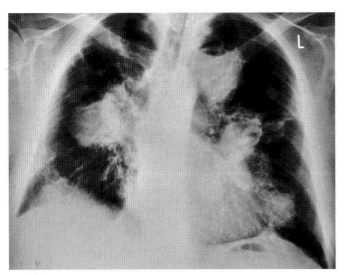

Fig. 10.69 Wegener granulomatosis. There are multiple, well-defined nodules ranging in size from 1 to 7 cm. The lesion in the left upper lung has cavitated and contains a small air–fluid level. (Courtesy of Dr GJ Hunter, London, UK)

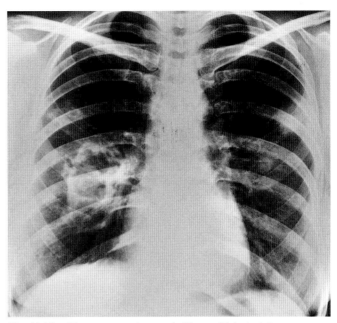

Fig. 10.71 Wegener granulomatosis. The multiple nodules are associated with a large (6 cm) cavitary lesion adjacent to the right hilum. Its walls are thick and irregular on both aspects. (Courtesy of Dr GJ Hunter, London, UK)

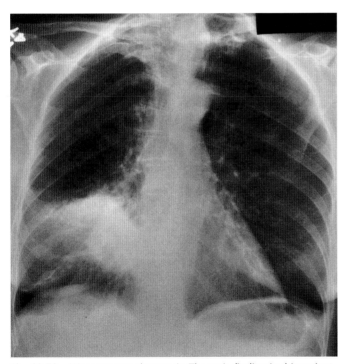

Fig. 10.70 Wegener granulomatosis. The main finding in this patient is a large area of consolidation in the right middle lobe.

visible at presentation in the majority of patients (62% in a combined series).[736] In a fifth to one-third of patients the nodules are single and, in the remaining majority, are multiple (Fig. 10.69). Commonly 2–4 cm in diameter,[737] the nodules may range in size from 3 to 10 cm.[738,739] They are round or oval in shape and may be well or poorly defined, sometimes becoming confluent.[738] The nodules are usually <10 in number but may occasionally be innumerable.[739] There appears to be no strong affinity for any one zone; some series have a preponderance of

nodules in the mid/lower zones,[720,739] while others do not.[740] Nodules commonly resolve with or without treatment over a period of months. They may heal without residual abnormality, or they may leave a visible scar.[739] Focal opacities with the features of pulmonary consolidation occur in some 30% of patients (Fig. 10.69).[736] They may be single or multiple and vary from small inhomogeneous patches[738] to homogeneous segmental or lobar consolidations.[719,736,740] Sometimes there is a mixed pattern of nodules and consolidation, and the radiographic distinction between the two is not always clear-cut.[739] New lung lesions during relapses often appear in areas affected in previous episodes, even though the radiographic appearance of the lesions may be different from that seen originally.[736]

Cavitation of the nodules (Fig. 10.71) and areas of consolidation are common, being seen in ~40% of cases at presentation.[736] Cavities may be unilocular or multilocular, and the outer margins of their walls are more commonly irregular than smooth.[737] Wall width varies greatly. Typically, it is thick with an irregular or smooth inner margin, but when the cavities have been present for some time there is a tendency for the walls to become thinner.[736] Cavities may have air–fluid levels, sometimes indicating secondary infection.[704,725]

Diffuse bilateral consolidation (Fig. 10.72) is likely to be caused by diffuse pulmonary hemorrhage,[707,709,741] which occurs both in established disease[742] and at presentation.[719] In a series of 77 patients with respiratory Wegener granulomatosis, 8% presented with diffuse pulmonary hemorrhage.[719] One case, presenting acutely in respiratory failure, is described in which there was massive consolidation caused by extensive Wegener granulomatosis tissue.[743]

Occasional cases have been described with hilar and mediastinal adenopathy detected on chest radiography[725,740,744] or CT.[719,732,745] In a review of 302 patients with Wegener granulomatosis, some assessed with CT and some with chest radiography, the overall frequency of mediastinal/hilar

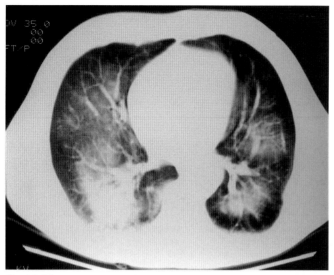
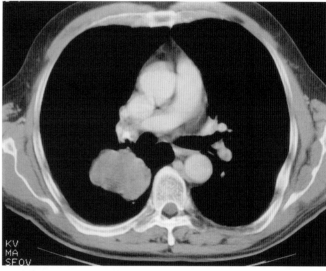

Fig. 10.72 Wegener granulomatosis. **A**, A 56-year-old man who presented with diffuse pulmonary hemorrhage and was PR3-antineutrophil cytoplasmic antibody (ANCA) positive. CT shows ground-glass abnormality and consolidation, consistent with diffuse hemorrhage. About 5–10% of patients with Wegener granulomatosis present in this way. **B**, Following 2 years' treatment with steroids and cyclophosphamide the patient developed a solitary mass. Because ANCA levels were low, it seemed unlikely that this was caused by recurrence of Wegener granulomatosis. Needle biopsy disclosed squamous carcinoma. There is an increased prevalence of malignancy in treated patients with Wegener granulomatosis.

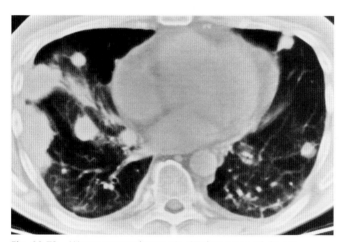

Fig. 10.73 Wegener granulomatosis. CT shows several discrete nodules and confluent subpleural opacities in the right lung.

lymphadenopathy was just under 2%.[746] Nodes were never an isolated finding.

Pleural effusions in Wegener granulomatosis, some of which are quite large, have been reported with a prevalence ranging from 5 to 55%.[720,740,747,748] It seems likely that some of these effusions were only indirectly related to the presence of Wegener granulomatosis, and that, in general, pleural effusions are unusual. Pneumothorax[749] and hydropneumothorax are occasionally seen. In one case they were associated with cavitary lung disease and in another with a bronchopleural fistula, the track of which was lined by Wegener granulomatosis tissue.[747,750]

CT and HRCT findings have confirmed the radiographic changes (Fig. 10.73) and made new observations, particularly in relation to nodule morphology and distal airway disease.[719,732,733,751–753] Nodules are much more commonly multiple than single, and the smallest ones (invisible on the chest radiograph) are of the order of 2–3 mm.[733,751,752] The

frequency of cavitation in nodules is related to size and those that are >2 cm in diameter are usually cavitated,[719,752] with thick irregular walls that later become thinner and smoother. If frank cavitation is not present, CT may show a low density necrotic center to the nodule. Nodules are more commonly irregular in outline[733,751,752] than smooth,[719] and they are frequently spiculated, with tags passing to adjacent pleura.[733,751] Occasionally nodules have a halo of ground-glass opacity and in two cases this CT halo has been shown pathologically to be due to hemorrhage.[754] Some nodules are distributed in a subpleural pattern,[732,733,752,755] but this is generally not a striking finding. "Feeding" vessels entering nodules, described by Kuhlman et al,[751] are not a finding commented on by other authors, though some have noted vessels passing into focal areas of consolidation.[732] Focal consolidation is probably the second most common finding after nodules. Such consolidation is commonly pleural based (Fig. 10.73) and may have a hump- or wedgelike configuration with or without an air bronchogram.

CT has confirmed the impression gained from chest radiographs (see above) that nodal enlargement is very uncommon, with a frequency of 2.5% in a combined total of 121 patients.[719,732,733] Pleural abnormalities – thickening and small effusions – have a frequency of 5 to 20%.[719,732,733,751,752] Other findings infrequently recorded include minor peripheral honeycomb opacity,[732,733] which possibly represents diffuse interstitial fibrosis with vasculitis as described histologically by Travis et al,[707] though the possibility of drug induced fibrosis should also be considered.[732] There has been a report of Wegener granulomatosis presenting as lung fibrosis, similar to NSIP or UIP.[756]

Tracheal narrowing is an important and relatively common manifestation of Wegener granulomatosis, with frequencies of 16% and 23% in two large series.[757,758] There is a female predominance and notably all but one of 17 patients with this complication in a Mayo Clinic series were female.[757] Symptoms may occur early in the course of Wegener granulomatosis and may even be a presenting feature in some patients,[757,758] whilst

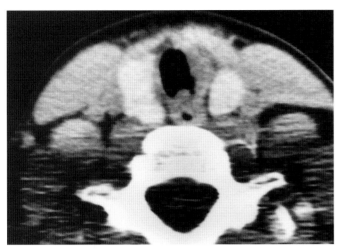

Fig. 10.74 Wegener granulomatosis. CT at the level of the thyroid shows irregular soft tissue thickening of the tracheal wall, posteriorly and on the left, which compromises the lumen. (Courtesy of Dr SC Rankin, London, UK)

in others there is a delay of several years.[757] Symptoms consist of dyspnea, hoarseness, voice change and stridor, and these are usually accompanied by nasal involvement.[757] However, patients with isolated laryngotracheal disease are recorded.[759,760] In the National Institute of Health (NIH) series, about 50% of tracheal stenoses occurred independently of other features of active Wegener granulomatosis.[758] Tracheal stenosis is not particularly responsive to systemic therapy and local intervention is favored.[758] Other tracheobronchial lesions described on bronchoscopy include ulcerating tracheobronchitis and tracheobronchial stenosis without an inflammatory component.[760]

Tracheal stenoses are usually subglottic (Figs 10.74 and 10.75) and usually present as smooth or irregular circumferential stenoses about 2–4 cm long.[745,757,761] In a series of 10 patients studied by CT,[761] 90% of lesions were subglottic, so this area should always be included in the imaging volume in patients with Wegener granulomatosis. CT shows abnormal soft tissue within the tracheal rings (Fig. 10.74), which themselves may be abnormally thickened and calcified,[762] or may be eroded.[761] The mucosal thickening may be irregular or ulcerated, and involvement of adjacent vocal cords may be visible on CT.[761] On MRI the abnormal soft tissue associated with stenoses is of intermediate signal on T1-weighted sequences, high signal on

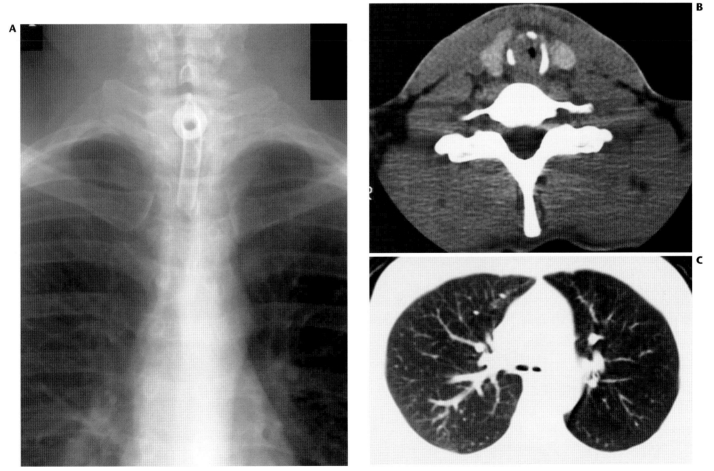

Fig. 10.75 A 29-year-old man with diffuse tracheal narrowing due to Wegener granulomatosis. **A**, Chest radiograph shows tracheostomy, with tracheal narrowing above and below the level of the tracheostomy. **B** and **C**, CT images confirm the marked subglottic mucosal thickening with airway narrowing, and narrowing of both main bronchi.

T2-weighted sequences, and enhances with contrast agents.[763] Stenotic lesions of the more distal airways, usually main or lobar bronchi (Fig. 10.75), are well recognized and in one selected pulmonary series bronchial stenoses had a frequency of 18%.[719] They usually become manifest by causing distal collapse/consolidation of a lobe or lung.[764]

A number of reports have described peribronchovascular thickening and cuffing with soft tissue,[732,733,752,755,765] invariably associated with mild bronchiectasis and bronchial wall thickening. Such airway changes were found in 40% of patients in one series,[733] and a more recent report of 30 patients[766] described bronchial wall thickening in segmental or subsegmental airways as a characteristic finding of Wegener granulomatosis, being found in 73% of patients. These findings presumably relate to bronchocentric lesions described pathologically.[712]

Repeat CT examinations following therapy show that ground-glass abnormality resolves completely, most nodules (<3 cm diameter) resolve, while masses become smaller. Consolidation usually resolves, at least in part.[755,767] Residual linear scarring is common. Airway thickening usually decreases.[766]

An interesting recent report[768] indicated that somatostatin receptor (octreotide) nuclear imaging may be helpful in imaging ANCA-associated vasculitis, including Wegener granulomatosis, Churg–Strauss vasculitis, and microscopic polyangiitis, with reported sensitivity and specificity values of 86 and 96% for active pulmonary disease. If confirmed, this technique might offer a useful method for diagnosis, staging, and follow up of these conditions.

Microscopic polyangiitis

Microscopic polyangiitis is a nongranulomatous, systemic, small vessel vasculitis accompanied by segmental necrotizing glomerulonephritis with no evidence of Wegener granulomatosis or other conditions known to be associated with small vessel vasculitis.[769] Although medium sized vessels may be involved, it is the presence of small vessel disease (arterioles, capillaries, venules) that distinguishes it histologically from classic polyarteritis nodosa.[674] The principal features that distinguish it clinically from polyarteritis nodosa are the presence of glomerulonephritis, absence of renal vasculitis, the frequency of pulmonary hemorrhage, and ANCA positivity (either MPO or, less often, PR3).[770] Microscopic polyangiitis is much more likely than polyarteritis nodosa to be associated with relapses.

The prevalence of diffuse pulmonary hemorrhage in microscopic polyangiitis ranges from 11[771]–33%.[772] It manifests radiographically as airspace opacity (Fig. 10.76). The only other common radiologic findings in the chest are pleural effusion (15%) and pulmonary edema (6%).[772] Uncommon findings in microscopic polyangiitis include lung fibrosis,[710] and obstructive lung disease with features of emphysema or bronchiolitis.[773,774]

Recently, patients have been described with pulmonary hemorrhage and isolated lung capillaritis without any of the multisystem features of microscopic polyangiitis. Some of these patients have been ANCA positive[775] and some ANCA negative.[776]

Churg–Strauss syndrome

Churg–Strauss syndrome is caused by an ANCA-associated small vessel, systemic vasculitis that occurs almost exclusively in patients with asthma, and is characterized by a marked peripheral eosinophilia. Pathologically there is a small vessel (arteries and veins) vasculitis with a prominent eosinophilic

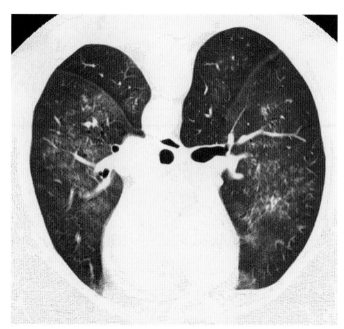

Fig. 10.76 A 74-year-old woman with diffuse pulmonary hemorrhage due to microscopic polyangiitis. Prone HRCT shows patchy ground-glass abnormality consistent with pulmonary hemorrhage.

infiltrate together with vascular and extravascular granulomas.[777] In the lungs there are lesions resembling eosinophilic pneumonia with intraalveolar and interstitial eosinophilic infiltrates. Vasculitic changes are accompanied by necrotizing granulomas both in vessel walls and in the parenchyma.[302] It is very unusual to find all three key histologic elements (vasculitis, granulomas, tissue eosinophilia) together at any one time and it is not entirely satisfactory to base the diagnosis of Churg–Strauss syndrome solely on histologic criteria.[692] A more clinical approach to diagnosis may be adopted and a list of six diagnostic criteria has recently been proposed by the American College of Rheumatology, with 85% sensitivity and 99.7% specificity when four out of six criteria are positive.[778] The criteria are:

- Asthma
- Blood eosinophilia of >10%
- Neuropathy
- Nonfixed pulmonary consolidations
- Paranasal sinus abnormality
- Extravascular eosinophilia on biopsy.

Other workers have suggested alternative criteria.[674,779] Churg–Strauss syndrome has a variety of synonyms including "allergic granulomatosis and angiitis" and "allergic granulomatosis". Since the first description in 1951,[777] several major series have reported the clinical and pathologic features.[779–782] The mean age at onset is 40–50 years in most series,[782] with a range of 17–74 years.[692] The sexes are equally affected, and a significant number of patients are atopic.[779] Definite precipitating factors have not been identified, though hyposensitization therapy,[779,783] drugs,[784,785] cocaine,[786] and inhaled antigens[787] have been implicated. Most recently, there have been numerous reports of Churg–Strauss syndrome occurring in asthmatics treated with leukotriene antagonists (see Fig. 10.78).[788–792] It remains unclear whether this is due to "unmasking" of vasculitis related to decreasing steroid dose, or to a true drug related vasculitis.

In many patients, the disease evolves in three stages: (1) an allergic phase with rhinitis and asthma commonly in a middle-aged, atopic patient; (2) an eosinophilic phase with blood and tissue eosinophilia in the chest, resembling cryptogenic eosinophilic pneumonia or simple eosinophilic pneumonia; and (3) a systemic small vessel vasculitic phase.

Asthma is the first manifestation in virtually all patients and is accompanied in 70% of cases by allergic rhinitis.[780] A forme fruste of Churg–Strauss syndrome is described without asthma.[781,793] There is on average a 3 year gap between the onset of asthma and the development of vasculitis,[779] but this interval has ranged from a few months to as long as 30 years. Occasionally, the illness is so telescoped temporally that asthma and vasculitis are simultaneous in onset.[780] A short interval is associated with a poor prognosis.[780] With the onset of the vasculitic phase, the asthma may increase in severity[779] or it may remit.

An eosinophilic phase commonly follows the asthmatic prodrome. It is characterized by blood eosinophilia and eosinophilic infiltration of tissues, particularly the lungs and gastrointestinal tract. At this stage the disease may relapse and remit for years before transforming into the final vasculitic phase.[779]

Many different tissues and organs may be involved by the vasculitis,[692,782] including the heart (10–40%) (myocardium, pericardium, coronary arteries), and musculoskeletal system (30–50%). The skin (40%) may show palpable purpura, erythema, urticaria, or subcutaneous nodules. Vasculitic involvement of the nervous system may result in a mononeuritis multiplex (70%) and, less commonly, in central lesions. Abdominal pain, diarrhea, or intestinal bleeding occur in 30–60% of patients.[782] The kidneys may show segmental glomerulonephritis similar to that in Wegener granulomatosis; however, such renal involvement rarely causes significant clinical disease,[780] and it is a cause of renal failure in only 7% of patients.[781] The vasculitic phase is accompanied by systemic symptoms such as weight loss and fever. The ESR is raised and there is usually a marked leukocytosis with a striking eosinophilia, which may be as high as $30 \times 10^9/L$. It is possible, however, to have active vasculitis and no peripheral eosinophilia since eosinophil levels in the blood fluctuate rapidly and widely.[779] The serum IgE value is commonly raised.[779,780] Between 60 and 75% of patients are MPO-ANCA positive and this is a most helpful diagnostic finding; PR3-ANCA positivity is very uncommon.[781]

The changes on the chest radiograph in Churg–Strauss syndrome can occur in the eosinophilic or vasculitic phases. The reported frequency of chest radiographic abnormalities varies between 27 and 74%.[779,780] This variation appears to be related to the frequency of obtaining chest radiographs, the higher figure probably being a better reflection of the true frequency of radiographic abnormalities during the course of the disease. The most common finding is transient, multifocal, non-segmental consolidation which shows no zonal predilection (Fig. 10.77),[777,779,794] an appearance which, when combined with blood eosinophilia, may fulfill the criteria for Löffler syndrome (Fig. 10.77; see p. 600). Multifocal consolidation may take on the appearance of multiple fluffy nodules or masses (Fig. 10.78).[795] The pulmonary consolidation can, however, be unifocal,[795] or may even have the pattern of chronic eosinophilic pneumonia.[796–798] Widespread symmetric consolidation is seen with diffuse pulmonary hemorrhage.[779] Cavitation is unusual,[799] and it is noteworthy that both large nodule formation and

cavitation are much less common than in Wegener granulomatosis. Less common findings include a diffuse or basal interstitial pattern,[780] diffuse miliary nodules,[780,800,801] and hilar and mediastinal adenopathy, either unilateral or bilateral.[795,800] Pleural effusions (Fig. 10.77)[802] occurred in 29% of patients in one large review of 154 cases,[779] and in many the effusions were eosinophilic.

CT reports are limited to one series of 17 patients[803] and a few single cases.[801,804,805] In the multicenter series, the most common HRCT finding was multifocal consolidation (59%) with a peripheral (35%) or patchy (24%) pattern.[803] Consolidation occurred in all zones but was basally predominant. Multiple nodules were present in 24% of cases (Fig. 10.79). In 12%, nodules ranged in diameter from 5 to 35 mm with occasional air bronchogram or cavitation. In the other 12% there were scattered centrilobular micronodules – the main opacity being consolidation. Other findings included small pleural effusions (12%), septal lines (6%) related to heart failure, and bronchial dilatation and wall thickening. Airway changes were principally peripheral, mild and diffuse, and were ascribed to asthma. CT scans were normal in two of 17 patients. A single case report with pathologic correlation described HRCT changes in a patient with interstitial opacity on the chest radiograph.[801] The main findings were enlargement with irregularity of outline of peripheral arteries and veins, peribronchial thickening, interlobular septal thickening, and patchy consolidation. Histologically these changes were due to an eosinophilic inflammatory cell infiltrate, granuloma formation, and lymphatic dilatation. In a child with Churg–Strauss there were fluffy, discrete perivascular opacities.[805] Radiographic abnormalities may or may not clear with treatment.[780]

Cardiac involvement causes cardiomegaly resulting from pericarditis, coronary vasculitis (see Fig. 10.78) or myocarditis (see Fig. 10.77), as well as signs of raised pulmonary venous pressure, and these signs may complicate the primary pleuropulmonary changes on the radiograph.[803,806,807]

Churg–Strauss syndrome usually responds to steroid therapy, but a small proportion of patients require adjunctive immunosuppressive agents. The vasculitic phase in most treated patients lasts less than 1 year and late relapses are uncommon.[779] The 5 year survival is in the order of 60–80%,[781,808] 27–47% of deaths being related to cardiac involvement.[809]

Immune complex vasculitis

Anaphylactoid purpura (Henoch-Schönlein purpura)

Though found primarily in children, peaking at 5 years of age,[675] anaphylactoid purpura can occur at any age and frequently follows an upper respiratory tract infection. The virus or bacterium responsible for this infection is the most common source of the inciting antigen. Other antigenic sources include varicella, *Yersinia*, food, drugs, and neoplasms.[810]

Immune complexes containing dominant IgA are found in the walls of blood vessels and distinguish anaphylactoid purpura from other cutaneous vasculitides. The entity is characterized by palpable purpura over the legs and buttocks, abdominal pain, gastrointestinal bleeding, arthralgia and, in 10–25% of cases, renal involvement with glomerulonephritis. Diagnostic criteria have been described.[811] The acute illness may be followed by one or more relapses occurring over weeks or months. The prognosis is generally good, though renal disease can progress to chronic renal failure in about 5% of patients,[675]

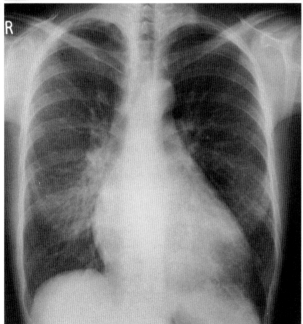

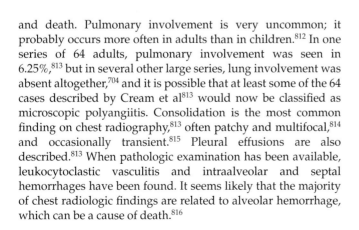

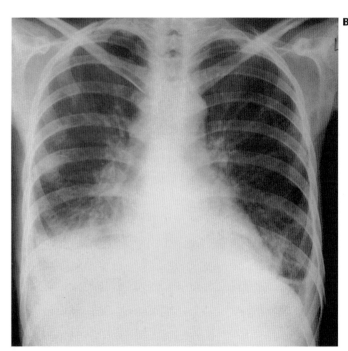

Fig. 10.77 Churg–Strauss syndrome in a 28-year-old asthmatic woman. She presented with colitis, followed by Löffler syndrome with blood eosinophilia (10.3 x 10⁹/L). At this stage a few microaneurysms were demonstrated on hepatic and renal arteries. Within a year cardiomyopathy had developed. **A**, Chest radiograph during Löffler syndrome shows consolidation in the left lower lung. This followed right upper zone consolidation. **B**, Six months later bilateral pleural effusions developed. **C**, One year later cardiomegaly developed, due to cardiomyopathy.

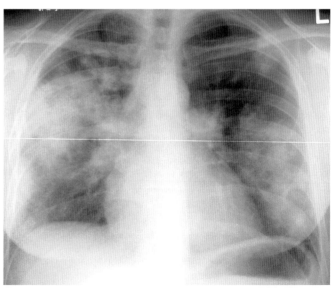

Fig. 10.78 A 34-year-old asthmatic patient, who developed Churg–Strauss syndrome while undergoing treatment with a leukotriene antagonist. Chest radiograph shows multifocal consolidation. Cardiomegaly was due to a myocardial infarct caused by Churg–Strauss syndrome.

and death. Pulmonary involvement is very uncommon; it probably occurs more often in adults than in children.[812] In one series of 64 adults, pulmonary involvement was seen in 6.25%,[813] but in several other large series, lung involvement was absent altogether,[704] and it is possible that at least some of the 64 cases described by Cream et al[813] would now be classified as microscopic polyangiitis. Consolidation is the most common finding on chest radiography,[813] often patchy and multifocal,[814] and occasionally transient.[815] Pleural effusions are also described.[813] When pathologic examination has been available, leukocytoclastic vasculitis and intraalveolar and septal hemorrhages have been found. It seems likely that the majority of chest radiologic findings are related to alveolar hemorrhage, which can be a cause of death.[816]

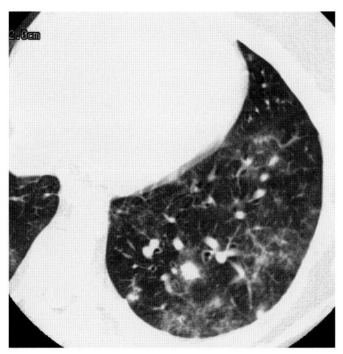

Fig. 10.79 A 16-year-old woman with Churg–Strauss vasculitis. HRCT shows patchy ground-glass attenuation and several nodules. The largest nodule is surrounded by a "halo" of ground-glass attenuation, suggestive of pulmonary hemorrhage.

Mixed cryoglobulinemia

Mixed cryoglobulinemia produces a small vessel vasculitis by virtue of tissue damaging cryoglobulins set down in vessel walls. There is a strong association with hepatitis C infection which is etiologically important.[675] Cryoglobulinemia, however, may also be primary or associated with a wide variety of disorders such as lymphoma, myeloma, collagen vascular disease, Waldenström macroglobulinemia, and various infections.[817] Typically, mixed cryoglobulinemia is seen in middle-aged subjects with a 2:1 female:male ratio. The main manifestations are recurrent palpable purpura, nephritis, polyarthralgia, hepatosplenomegaly, and lymphadenopathy.[684] Lung involvement is unusual.[675] Literature on lung involvement is limited to a few reports of small vessel lung vasculitis[818] interstitial lung disease,[819,820] and pleural effusion.[821] Some reports of series do not mention lung involvement other than pneumonia.[817] However, in one series of 23 patients with mixed cryoglobulinemia there was a high prevalence of small airway disease and impaired gas exchange on respiratory function testing. Nearly 80% of patients had an abnormality on the chest radiograph, with a diffuse fine nodular interstitial pattern.[822] The pathologic basis for these changes is unclear.[684] A case associated with acute respiratory distress syndrome has been reported.[823]

Systemic urticarial vasculitis

Systemic urticarial vasculitis is a syndrome most commonly seen in middle-aged women and characterized by chronic urticaria on the basis of an immune complex mediated vasculitis, invariably accompanied by extradermal features: typically arthralgia, myalgia, and eye disorder. If there is severe multisystem involvement, complement levels fall (hypocomplementemic urticarial

vasculitis syndrome [HUVS]), and the disorder then often closely resembles systemic lupus erythematosus.[824] In view of the latter, an association between HUVS and recurrent pleural effusion is not unexpected.[825] Several studies looking at HUVS patients have recorded a 50–65% prevalence of chronic obstructive pulmonary disease.[826–828] It is progressive, may occur at an early age,[827] and in one series six of 17 patients died of respiratory failure.[828] In four patients from the latter series, lung biopsy showed emphysema but no active pulmonary vasculitis. In the Mayo Clinic series, chest radiography showed hyperinflation and reduced peripheral pulmonary vasculature.[827] The etiology of the pulmonary disease is not clear. Smoking may be a factor, but not all patients have been smokers, and in 15 of 15 subjects serum α_1-antitrypsin levels were normal.[828]

Connective tissue disease and malignancy

An immune complex vasculitis is a recognized finding in some connective tissue diseases and is discussed under the specific disorders above. There is also an established association with various malignancies, particularly lymphoid and reticuloendothelial neoplasms.[699,829]

Behçet disease and Hughes–Stovin syndrome

Behçet disease is a rare, multisystem, chronic relapsing vasculitis considered to be secondary to immune complex deposition.[704] It is characterized by recurrent aphthous ulcerations of the mouth (100% of patients), recurrent genital ulceration (75%), skin lesions (75%) (erythema nodosum, pseudofolliculitis), and ocular lesions (60%) (typically uveitis, but a variety of other lesions are recorded). Almost half of patients have arthropathy, about 20% have thrombophlebitis, and 20% have neurologic manifestations.[830] Lesser degrees of involvement are described in other organs, including the cardiac, renal, and gastrointestinal systems. A set of diagnostic criteria has been proposed consisting of: (1) recurrent oral ulceration; (2) recurrent genital ulceration; (3) eye lesions (specified); (4) skin lesions (specified); and (5) positive pathergy test (pustule formation 24–48 h after skin prick).[831] The diagnosis is considered to be positive if (1) and two other criteria are fulfilled.

Histologically, the affected vessels show a leukocytoclastic vasculitis. Vasculitis leads to thrombosis, obstruction, stenosis, aneurysm formation, and rupture of vessels.[832,833] Arteries, capillaries and veins, both systemic and pulmonary, of various sizes are affected.[834]

Although worldwide in distribution, Behçet disease is most common in the Mediterranean basin, Middle East (prevalence in Turkey ~5 per 10^5 population), and Far East, and particularly Japan (prevalence ~10 per 10^5 population).[835] In Northern Europe and the United States, its prevalence is much lower (~3 per 10^6 population). Behçet disease presents most commonly between the ages of 20 and 35 years,[835] range 6–72 years.[834] In some areas it is a male predominant disease, particularly in the Middle East and Mediterranean basin, but elsewhere, such as in the United States and Japan, it is female predominant.[835] The disease tends to be most severe in young males. About 10% of patients have a family history,[835] and there is an association with HLA B5.

Pleuropulmonary involvement occurs in 1–8% of patients.[830,836–840] Although the incidence is said to be similar in males and females, the disease is usually more severe in males.[836] It is usually heralded by hemoptysis, fever, pleuritic pain, cough, or dyspnea. Hemoptysis is frequently a dominant and life-threatening feature. It may be caused by rupture of a pulmonary artery aneurysm (occasionally via a bronchoarterial fistula), or pulmonary infarct. Rare causes of hemoptysis include airway ulceration[841] or diffuse alveolar hemorrhage secondary to capillaritis. Hemoptysis secondary to aneurysm formation is a serious condition with a poor prognosis, and in a combined series it necessitated transfusion in 40% and led to death in 30%.[839] A review of the literature indicates that 38–75% of patients died within 2 years of the diagnosis of pulmonary artery aneurysm.[842] In two series, totaling 39 patients with pulmonary aneurysms, the mean age at the time of diagnosis of aneurysm was about 30 years and all patients were male. A characteristic feature of patients with pulmonary artery aneurysms is a high prevalence of thrombophlebitis (88%), compared with a prevalence of 18% in Behçet disease in general.[843] A variety of treatments have been tried for pulmonary artery aneurysm, including surgery, immunosuppression, steroids and, in a few cases, embolization.[844–846] Regression and disappearance of pulmonary aneurysms has been reported on several occasions,[834,842–844,847,848] and has been ascribed to resolution of hematoma associated with a false aneurysm.[834]

A series of papers has described the plain radiographic findings in the chest,[830,834,837,839–841,843,849–851] and a limited number describe CT findings.[834,840,851–853] The variety of thoracic imaging abnormalities is best understood in the context of the gross pathologic findings (Box 10.31).

Consolidation not caused by infection is usually due to hemorrhage (Fig. 10.80). It may be focal, multifocal, or diffuse.[839–841,847,851] Sometimes it is fleeting[830] or peripheral and wedge shaped.[840] Some areas of consolidation cavitate (Fig. 10.81), and it seems highly likely that these are infarcts,

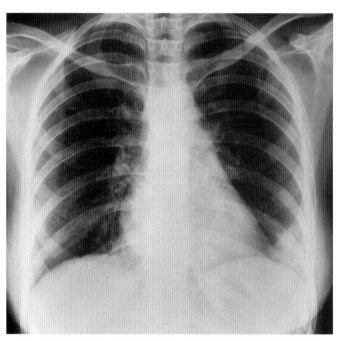

Fig. 10.80 Chest radiography in a 27-year-old woman with known Behçet syndrome and hemoptysis. There is consolidation in the left costophrenic angle, probably caused by pulmonary hemorrhage or infarction. It cleared in 2 months.

Box 10.31 Gross pathologic changes in the thorax in Behçet disease

Pulmonary vascular disease
Pulmonary arterial aneurysm
Pulmonary arterial occlusion (thrombosis/stenosis)
Pulmonary arterial hypertension
Pulmonary infarction
Pulmonary oligemia
Pulmonary hemorrhage (focal/diffuse)
Pulmonary thromboembolism (rare)

Systemic arterial disease
Aortic aneurysm
Coronary artery aneurysm

Systemic venous disease
Superior vena cava thrombosis/narrowing
Mediastinal edema
Venous collaterals (azygos system/chest wall)

Pleural disease
Exudative effusion (infarction/vasculitis/infection)
Hemothorax
Hydropneumothorax
Chylothorax

Airway disease
Ulceration

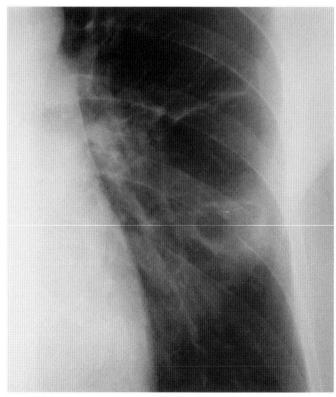

Fig. 10.81 Behçet syndrome. A localized view of the left mid zone in a patient with known Behçet syndrome, complaining of left pleuritic pain and minor hemoptysis. There is a thin walled cavity and a band opacity, most likely due to pulmonary infarcts.

with or without secondary infection and abscess formation.[847] Nodular opacities of several centimeters in diameter are also a common finding. Some of these are caused by pulmonary artery aneurysms, whereas others probably represent focal consolidation rather than a true mass. The nodules may cavitate,[837] and usually resolve over 3–9 months. Basal linear or bandlike opacities (Fig. 10.81), as commonly seen in thromboembolic disease, are described.[840,848]

Pulmonary artery aneurysms, which may be true or false, appear as nodular/masslike lesions on the chest radiograph.[834] Since aneurysms are predominantly of lobar, segmental, or subsegmental branches, they are generally centrally located. There are exceptions, however, and they can be immediately subpleural.[848] Pulmonary artery aneurysms are commonly multiple, bilateral, and up to several centimeters in diameter.[848] They may be sharply marginated or ill defined, the latter appearance being related to acute hemorrhage, inflammation, or fibrosis. Pulmonary artery occlusion caused by thrombus may occur in relation to a pulmonary artery aneurysm or it may occur remotely. Such occlusions are predominantly lobar or segmental,[847] and when widespread can result in pulmonary arterial hypertension.[850] On the plain chest radiograph they produce oligemic areas[847] and, on $\dot{V}/Q$ imaging, areas of mismatch.[840,850] CT scans may show peripheral low attenuation areas, which may be due either to small vessel occlusion or to air-trapping.[834]

A variety of imaging techniques can demonstrate pulmonary artery aneurysms and occlusions (see Fig. 10.82) (pulmonary angiography, CT and MR angiography).[834,848,854,855] The optimal technique is yet to be identified and depends to some extent on the questions being asked, particularly about the state of vessels other than the pulmonary arteries. The different available techniques often provide complementary information. It is stated that procedures involving vessel puncture and contrast injection may initiate thrombosis and aneurysm formation,[834] but the degree of risk involved is unclear. MR angiography[854] or CT angiography are ideal for documenting the extent of pulmonary arterial aneurysms, thoracic aortic or systemic arterial aneurysms, and venous occlusion in patients with Behçet disease. Thrombus may also be shown within the aneurysms.[836]

Mediastinal widening on chest radiography can be due to: (1) aortic or coronary artery aneurysm formation; (2) venous collaterals, particularly those arising from the azygos or hemiazygos system; (3) superior vena cava dilatation caused by a low stenosis; (4) mediastinal edema;[851] or a centrally situated pulmonary artery aneurysm.[834]

Pleural effusions are sometimes present, and these may be serous or bloody. Most are probably secondary to pulmonary infarcts,[847] but some are hemothoraces resulting from rupture of blood vessels,[837] and a few have been chylothoraces secondary to superior vena cava and brachiocephalic vein thrombosis.[856] Pleural effusion with biopsy proven pleural vasculitis is also described.[834] A cavitated infarct in Behçet disease is a reported cause of a hydropneumothorax.[847]

There is limited information on the pulmonary parenchymal changes seen on CT in Behçet disease. Tunaci et al[834] identified small subpleural nodular, linear, and triangular opacities which they ascribed to hemorrhage or infarcts. Enlargement of small vessels with irregularity of outline, stenoses and cut offs on HRCT is described in another study and attributed to vasculitic changes.[840]

The Hughes–Stovin syndrome[857,858] manifests some, but not all, of the features of Behçet disease, and in particular it lacks the pathognomic oral ulceration as well as other characteristic features of Behçet disease, such as genital ulcers and iritis. Some authors consider it to be a variant of Behçet disease.[704] It is a rare condition with probably only about 30 cases in the world literature. Most patients are young adult males in their second

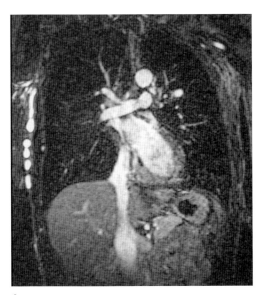

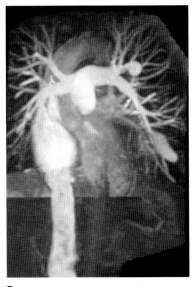

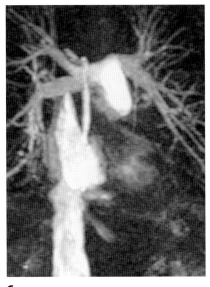

A **B** **C**

Fig. 10.82 A 50-year-old man with Hughes–Stovin syndrome, who presented with multiple venous occlusions and severe hemoptysis. **A**, Coronal image from an MR angiogram shows absence of contrast in the occluded brachiocephalic veins and superior vena cava. A large collateral vein is visible along the right lateral chest wall. A focal arterial dilation in the left lung is due to an aneurysm. **B**, 3D reconstruction of the MR angiogram shows a focal saccular aneurysm in the left upper lung, with a fusiform aneurysm in the left lower lung. **C**, Follow-up MR angiogram after treatment shows resolution of the two aneurysms in the left lung.

to fourth decade (youngest aged 12 years),[859] with at least one reported description of a female patient.[860] The major features are: (1) one or more segmental pulmonary artery aneurysms; (2) pulmonary artery occlusions due to emboli or thrombi; and (3) systemic venous thrombi (limb veins, vena cava, cerebral sinuses).[844] Common presentations are with peripheral venous thromboses, headache, fever, or hemoptysis; the latter is caused by erosion of an aneurysm into an airway[861] and is the major cause of death. Radiographic features are similar to those of Behçet disease. MR angiography[862] or CT angiography are ideal for documenting the extent of proximal aneurysm, and thoracic arterial and venous occlusion in patients with Hughes–Stovin syndrome or Behçet disease (Fig. 10.82). The exact status of patients who present with hemoptysis and have proximal pulmonary artery aneurysms, but no other features of Behçet disease or Hughes–Stovin syndrome (including venous disease), is unclear.[863]

Necrotizing sarcoidal angiitis

Necrotizing sarcoidal angiitis was first described in 1973 by Liebow,[864] and the problem posed then – as to whether the entity was sarcoidosis with necrosis of the granulomas and vessels, or a necrotizing vasculitis with a sarcoid reaction – still remains unsettled. Whilst some workers consider that it is a form of sarcoidosis,[865,866] others think that it may be a heterogeneous condition – a case mix of sarcoidosis, granulomatous infection, and a truly distinct entity.[302] Most recently, Popper et al[867] suggested that it is a variant of nodular sarcoidosis. The pathologic findings include: (1) aggregated sarcoidlike granulomas replacing large areas of lung; (2) infarctlike necrosis[867]; (3) a non-necrotizing vasculitis of arteries and veins that is often granulomatous but which may contain giant cells or chronic inflammatory cells; and (4) small airway obstruction by granulomas, which can cause an endogenous lipoid pneumonia.[302,748,865,867,868]

Much of the information available on this condition comes from several series totaling about 80 cases.[865,869,870] The mean age at presentation is about 45 years (range 12–75 years) with a 2.5:1 predominance of female patients.[865,869,870] At the time of presentation, between one-quarter and two-thirds of patients are asymptomatic,[865,869] the remainder having systemic or respiratory symptoms (cough, chest pain, shortness of breath). Only a few patients have had extrapulmonary lesions that are consistent with sarcoidosis, the chief one being uveitis (9%).[865,870] Other affected sites include the CNS, orbit, and liver.[748,871]

In general, necrotizing sarcoidal angiitis is a benign condition[864] that does not require treatment.[712,872] When treatment is indicated, steroids are used.

Radiographically, the most common pattern is that of bilateral nodules, occurring in about 75% of patients,[865,868] and up to about 4 cm in diameter. Sometimes the nodules are small enough to be considered miliary.[868,873] The nodules tend to show a predilection for the lower zones and occasionally cavitate.[874] When followed over years with repeat chest radiographs, the nodules may show a slow increase in size and number,[873] and may become confluent.[812] Spontaneous disappearance of nodules has been recorded.[865] When the nodules are unilateral, they are often solitary,[873,874] and resemble a bronchial neoplasm.[875] Less common patterns include bilateral consolidations,[868,873] basal interstitial shadowing,[870,872] and pleural effusions, the latter being absent from most series but present in 54% in one study.[870] As with pleural effusions, the

prevalence of hilar adenopathy has varied considerably from series to series, ranging from 10 to 80%.[748,865,870,876]

A limited number of HRCT studies confirm the radiographic findings. They have shown that nodules may be ill- or well-defined, with a tendency for a subpleural or peribronchovascular location.[748,872,876] A few nodules will be cavitated and others will show heterogeneous enhancement with administration of contrast media, indicating necrosis. Rather than large or small nodules, the pattern is occasionally that of consolidation with an air bronchogram.[876] Diffuse pleural thickening, usually due to confluent granulomas, was found on CT in five of seven patients in one series, with pleural effusion in two of seven.[872]

Polyangiitis overlap syndrome

Polyangiitis overlap syndrome is characterized by a systemic vasculitis with features that overlap the well-defined vasculitic syndromes, primarily Churg–Strauss syndrome and polyarteritis nodosa.[704] In one series of 11 such patients there was a pulmonary vasculitis in 54%.[704] Pleuropulmonary radiographic findings are those to be expected from the component conditions. The term is not widely used, and the entity was not included in the Chapel Hill classifications.[674]

DIFFUSE ALVEOLAR HEMORRHAGE

Bleeding into the lung parenchyma is common in a wide variety of disorders, but in this section the discussion will be limited to those conditions in which bleeding is diffuse or multifocal, and contributes significantly to the radiographic changes. A triad of features suggests diffuse pulmonary hemorrhage (DPH): hemoptysis, anemia, and airspace opacities on the chest radiograph.[877] Sometimes, the bleeding is covert and hemoptysis is absent. The diagnosis is often missed, at least initially, particularly when hemoptysis is not present.[878] The pulmonary features of all acute DPH syndromes are the same, and chest radiographs are generally unhelpful in distinguishing among them.[741]

There are over 45 known causes for diffuse pulmonary hemorrhage.[879–882] The underlying lung parenchyma may be normal, or may show capillaritis, DAD, or other miscellaneous abnormalities (Box 10.32).[882] Capillaritis is recognized to be the most common histologic finding in patients with DPH. In patients with bone marrow transplantation or DAD, the pathogenesis of DPH is often multifactorial, commonly a mixture of coagulopathy/thrombocytopenia with pulmonary infection.[881] DPH is rarely seen in the AIDS.[883,884] Other associations with DPH include DAD, mitral stenosis, venoocclusive disease,[885] infectious hemorrhagic/necrotizing pneumonias such as leptospirosis,[886] fat embolism, and hemorrhagic pulmonary edema of renal failure. These disorders can usually be differentiated, taking into account clinical setting, extrapulmonary involvement, serology, and renal biopsy.[879]

Goodpasture syndrome

In 1958, Stanton and Tange[891] were the first to use the term Goodpasture syndrome to describe the combination of pulmonary hemorrhage and glomerulonephritis. With a clearer understanding of the pathogenesis, the term has taken on a restricted meaning that defines a syndrome with: (1) DPH; (2) glomerulonephritis; and (3) antiglomerular basement membrane antibodies in the serum, lung, or kidney.[892] The antibody is directed against an epitope of basement membrane type IV collagen,[893] and it causes injury to glomerular and pulmonary alveolar basement membranes.

Antiglomerular basement membrane (anti-GBM) disease is a common cause of DPH. Sixty to 80% of patients with anti-GBM disease have alveolar hemorrhage and glomerulonephritis (i.e. Goodpasture syndrome),[893] and most of the rest have glomerulonephritis only (i.e. Goodpasture disease). A few patients with anti-GBM disease have alveolar hemorrhage and no kidney disease.[894]

In 1919, Goodpasture[895] described a patient who developed fatal pulmonary hemorrhage and glomerulonephritis 6 weeks after an attack of influenza.

The pathogenesis of alveolar damage is discussed in detail by Ball and Young.[896] Under normal circumstances anti-GBM antibody in the vascular system cannot access the alveolar epithelium because alveolar endothelium lacks the basement membrane fenestrations found in the glomerulus. In anti-GBM disease, however, the antibody is found in contact with the alveolar epithelium, suggesting that additional mechanisms must cause basement membrane injury in order for the patient to develop pulmonary symptoms. In this context, it is interesting that predisposing factors for Goodpasture syndrome include smoking, hydrocarbon exposure, and preceding viral infections (25%).[896]

Goodpasture syndrome is a rare disorder, with an incidence in the order of 0.5 per 10^6 population per year,[893] which is about one-tenth of the rate for Wegener granulomatosis.[896] It is essentially a disease of young adult white males, with a male:female ratio of 2:1–9:1 and an onset between 20 and 30 years of age.[896] It is uncommon in blacks. The entity has been occasionally reported in children.[897] The clinical presentation is usually with respiratory symptoms: hemoptysis (90%), dyspnea (65%), cough (55%), and fatigue (50%),[893] and patients usually have an iron deficient anemia (93%) and an abnormal chest radiograph (80%) (Fig. 10.83). Either at the time of presentation or in the ensuing weeks or months, urinalysis and renal function become abnormal. Occasionally, renal failure takes years to develop.[898] In one series, 55% of patients were anemic on admission, and about 80% had proteinuria or hematuria.[899] Rarely, the order of events is reversed with pulmonary hemorrhage following a nephritic presentation.[877] Demonstrating the presence of antiglomerular basement membrane antibodies in the serum by radioimmunoassay or ELISA is both a sensitive and specific (>95%) indicator of the disease and establishes the diagnosis.[741] There is, however, a general lack of correlation between the level of serum antibody and the severity of the disease,[877] though falling titers usually correlate with improving renal function.[893] It is not uncommon for patients with anti-GBM antibodies to also have ANCA.[900] In this situation renal histology and immunofluorescence show features of both conditions and on the whole these patients have a better response to therapy and shortterm prognosis than those with anti-GBM antibodies alone.[896]

Renal biopsy shows evidence of subacute proliferative glomerulonephritis with linear IgG deposition in the glomeruli. Lung biopsy is not usually performed, but if it were it would show blood and hemosiderin laden macrophages in the alveoli and interstitium, thickened basement membranes, hyperplasia of type I and II pneumocytes, and linear IgG and complement immunofluorescence along alveolar septa. In addition, there is sometimes septal thickening or fibrosis together with linear deposits of IgG on the alveolar capillary membranes.[302,901] A number of studies[902,903] have also shown features of capillaritis.[904] Open lung biopsy is more reliable than transbronchial biopsy, which can be negative.[905] Therapy, apart from supportive measures, is directed at removing anti-GBM antibodies by plasmapheresis and stopping its production with steroids and immunosuppressives.[893] In early series, the reported prognosis was poor, with about half the patients dying of pulmonary complications and almost all the rest of renal disease.[906] The occasional patient went into remission and recovered.[907] In one major study, 96% died, with a mean survival of 15 weeks.[906] The prognosis is currently much better with improved treatment and because milder cases are now included in the various reported series.[877] Thus, short term survival is in the order of 80–85% with 30–55% patients on maintenance dialysis.[893] Relapse is not uncommon, but once antibody production has ceased, recurrence is rare and patients are good transplant subjects.[893] Longterm lung complications are not a feature.

Antineutrophil cytoplasmic antibody associated small vessel vasculitides

The majority of patients presenting with the pulmonary renal syndrome (glomerulonephritis plus lung hemorrhage) are ANCA positive (see p. 592) with, for example, frequencies of 70%[908] and 62.5%.[900] The relative prevalence of the two major types of ANCA (PR3- and MPO-ANCA) in patients with pulmonary hemorrhage has varied among series, with

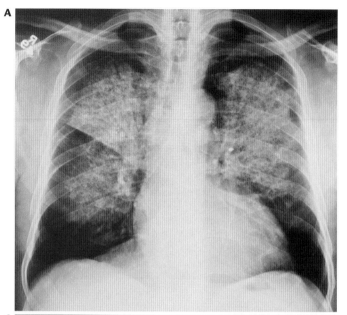

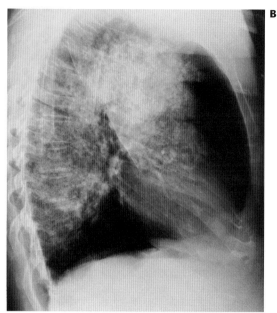

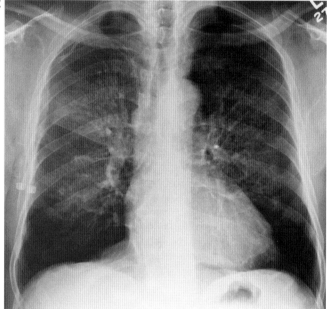

Fig. 10.83 Goodpasture syndrome. **A** and **B**, Radiographs show bilateral perihilar consolidation, some of which is sharply marginated by fissures. Note the bilateral air bronchograms and peripheral acinar nodules. **C**, One week later, there has been considerable, though incomplete, resolution of consolidation. Typically, pulmonary hemorrhage clears in a matter of days.

frequencies of 70, 60 and 33% for MPO-ANCA and 30, 40 and 53 for PR3-ANCA.[900,908,909] MPO-ANCA is associated with microscopic polyangiitis and Churg–Strauss syndrome, whereas PR3-ANCA is more strongly associated with Wegener granulomatosis.

DPH is commonly caused by microscopic polyangiitis (see Fig. 10.76) and Wegener granulomatosis (see Fig. 10.72), but it is rare with Churg–Strauss syndrome. Microscopic polyangiitis as an entity is only recently recognized (see p. 592), and in early series, particularly before ANCA testing, the condition was not identified as such. In a series of 31 open lung and three transbronchial biopsies in patients with diffuse pulmonary hemorrhage, the following entities were identified: (1) Wegener granulomatosis definite/probable 32%; (2) antiglomerular basement membrane disease 12%; (3) collagen vascular disease 12%; (4) immune complex mediated disorder other than collagen vascular disease 12%; (5) idiopathic pulmonary hemorrhage 6%;

and (6) nine of 34 (26%) cases were classified as having systemic necrotizing vasculitis, idiopathic glomerulonephritis without immune complexes, and unclassified pulmonary renal syndrome.[903] It seems highly probable that a significant number of these latter cases would now be classified as microscopic polyangiitis.

Microscopic polyangiitis and Wegener granulomatosis are discussed above in the section Small Vessel Vasculitis.

Immune complex disorders/collagen vascular disease

Several collagen vascular disorders and systemic vasculitides are occasionally associated with DPH, with or uncommonly without a glomerulonephritis. Many, and possibly all, are immune complex mediated. The association is probably most commonly seen with SLE.[397,402]

DPH is well documented in patients with SLE (see Fig. 10.44), usually occurring in the context of established disease with extrapulmonary features including glomerulonephritis.[879] Rarely DPH is a presenting feature.[397,399,910] It carries a poor prognosis, with a mortality of 50–60%.[397] DPH in SLE is frequently associated with other manifestations of SLE, particularly infection, renal failure, and heart failure, and because of this a number of authors recommend lung biopsy to clarify the pathogenesis.[911]

Isolated examples of DPH are reported with rheumatoid disease,[912,913] systemic sclerosis,[904,914,915] polymyositis,[544] and mixed connective tissue disease.[620,916]

DPH may be seen rarely with some immune complex related vasculitides, including Henoch-Schönlein disease[816,888] and the closely related IgA nephropathy,[917] antiphospholipid syndrome,[889,918] Behçet disease,[832,890,893] and mixed cryoglobulinemia.[643,882]

Idiopathic (primary) pulmonary hemosiderosis

Idiopathic pulmonary hemosiderosis (IPH) is a disorder of unknown etiology characterized by episodic alveolar hemorrhage that eventually leads to lung fibrosis.[919] Multisystem involvement and, in particular, glomerulonephritis is not a feature. A case, however, is described that transformed after 8 years into microscopic polyangiitis.[920] An association with celiac disease[921,922] and dermatitis herpetiformis[923] is recognized, and in some of these patients lung disease has responded to a gluten free diet.[921] Autoimmune associations are described as case reports – hyper- and hypo-thyroidism, hemolytic anemia, and IgA gammopathy.[924] Histologically, the light microscopic changes are similar to those of Goodpasture syndrome, namely: alveolar hemorrhage; hemosiderin laden macrophages in the alveoli and, to a lesser extent in the interstitium; and mild interstitial thickening which can become prominent in long-standing cases.[925] Capillaritis is not usually seen.[882] Late in the disease, alveolar septal fibrosis develops.[877] Some workers describe ultrastructural abnormalities of the endothelial cells and capillary basement membranes.[926,927] Immunofluorescent staining is negative.

Unlike Goodpasture syndrome, IPH is a disease of childhood, the onset typically being from 1 to 7 years of age with just a fifth of patients presenting in the late teens and 20s.[928] It is the most common cause of DPH in childhood.[901] The sex incidence in children is equal, but in adults, there is a twofold preponderance in males. Clinically, there is episodic cough, hemoptysis, and the signs and symptoms of anemia (tiredness, pallor, failure to gain weight) and in 20% hepatosplenomegaly.[925] The magnitude of hemoptysis varies greatly. In some patients it is absent altogether, leading to diagnostic difficulties, particularly when swallowed blood gives a positive test for fecal blood,[925] and in others it is massive enough to cause death. Bleeding into the lungs is evidenced by consolidation on the chest radiograph (Fig. 10.84) and the presence of iron deficiency anemia, with low iron stores. With recurrent bleeding, pulmonary hemosiderosis and fibrosis develop (Fig. 10.85). Most of those who survive several years are chronically dyspneic, anemic, and underweight.[928] Diagnosis is by exclusion and has been recently reviewed.[925] Despite the fact that some patients have been followed for 20 years, it is unclear whether the disease ever permanently remits. The outcome is variable with a better prognosis in adults than children.[925] In one series of 68 patients followed for 5 years,

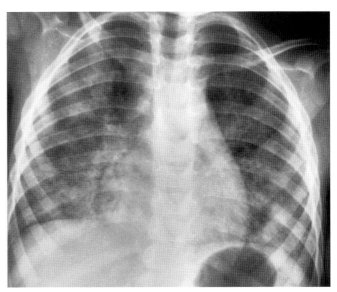

Fig. 10.84 Primary pulmonary hemosiderosis in a 2-year-old boy who had low grade fever, cough, and hemoptysis. Chest radiograph at presentation shows extensive bilateral consolidation.

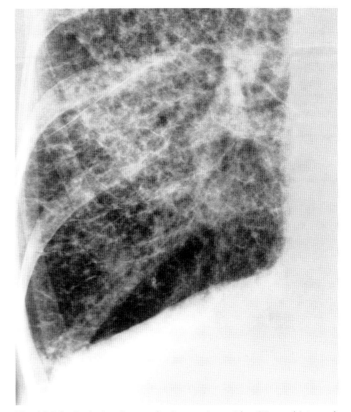

Fig. 10.85 Reticular abnormality in a patient with a 30 year history of primary pulmonary hemosiderosis. The localized view of the right lung base shows a reticulonodular pattern, with a pronounced linear component including septal (Kerley B) lines.

29% died, 25% had active disease, 18% had inactive disease but chronic symptoms, and 28% were well.[928] Deaths are due to pulmonary arterial hypertension and cor pulmonale, respiratory insufficiency, and bleeding. Treatment is supportive. Steroids and immunosuppressive drugs may be used without clear benefit, though there is some evidence that steroid therapy, particularly in adults helps in acute situations.[925]

Coagulopathy

DPH is a surprisingly unusual complication of the various coagulopathies. It has been recorded with thrombocytopenia,[929–931] particularly in the context of leukemia,[932,933] anticoagulation,[934] coronary thrombolysis,[935,936] and diffuse intravascular coagulation.[937]

Drugs/chemicals

A number of exogenous agents cause DPH with or without vasculitis including penicillamine,[741] propythiouracil,[938] diphenylhydantoin,[939] nitrofurantoin,[940] trimellitic anhydride and related agents,[940–942] cocaine,[943] and all-*trans*-retinoic acid (used for acute promyelocytic leukemia) (see Ch. 6).[944]

Imaging of diffuse pulmonary hemorrhage

The radiographic changes of acute alveolar hemorrhage are essentially the same regardless of etiology and consist of airspace consolidation. In some of the conditions under consideration, particularly primary pulmonary hemosiderosis, the bleeding tends to be recurrent over a long period of time and, in these cases, persistent interstitial changes may develop, reflecting interstitial fibrosis. When acute bleeding is superimposed on chronic changes, a mixed alveolar and interstitial pattern will be produced.

The consolidation ranges from acinar shadows (Fig. 10.83),[945] through patchy airspace opacity,[906,945] to widespread confluent consolidation with air bronchograms (Fig. 10.83).[946] At other times the consolidation may be migratory[932] or ground-glass in appearance.[922,946] The consolidation can be widespread or show a perihilar,[880] or mid/lower zone predominance.[932,946] The costophrenic angles and apices are usually spared.[945] The consolidation clears quickly within about 2–3 days, and this rate of resolution, intermediate between that seen with edema and infective consolidation, is very characteristic (Fig. 10.83).[946] Resolution may be complete or partial, leaving a linear/reticular pattern,[946] occasionally with septal lines,[947] or a ground-glass haziness.[946] This interstitial shadowing is also transient and clears completely 10–12 days after the beginning of the episode. There are two reports of associated hilar adenopathy.[948,949] Pleural effusions are not uncommon, but it seems likely that most, if not all, are secondary phenomena related to infection and fluid overload.[946]

With repeated bleeding episodes, seen typically in primary pulmonary hemosiderosis, the interstitial shadowing fails to clear completely, and the patient may be left with a permanent, fine reticulonodular (Fig. 10.85),[928] or nodular (2–3 mm) opacity[922] that tends to increase in profusion with each acute episode. New bleeding episodes superimposed on permanent shadowing will give a mixed alveolar/interstitial pattern. There is one reported case of progressive massive fibrosis in primary pulmonary hemosiderosis, with the masses being of high attenuation (CT number ~360 HU).[950]

In a series of six patients who underwent CT largely in the subacute phase of pulmonary hemorrhage, the striking abnormality was multiple, 1–3 mm nodules (see Fig. 10.76) distributed in a uniform fashion commonly associated with patchy ground-glass opacity (four of six) and interlobular septal thickening (four of six).[922] The centrilobular distribution of these nodules can sometimes mimic hypersensitivity pneumonitis. Similar changes are recorded by Primack et al.[881] In the acute phase CT shows consolidation[880] or ground-glass opacity.[922]

It is worthwhile noting that diffuse pulmonary bleeding can be present when the chest radiograph appears normal.[401,951] In one series, this was found to be the case in 22% of bleeding episodes in patients with DPH of Goodpasture syndrome.[951]

Differential diagnosis of alveolar hemorrhage

Hemoptysis, iron deficient anemia, and a sudden fall in the hematocrit of >2 g without bleeding elsewhere,[946] are obvious pointers to the diagnosis of DPH. It is well recognized that, because alveolar hemorrhage occurs distal to the mucociliary escalator, hemoptysis may be absent. Additionally, blood which does reach the upper airway may be swallowed and produce a misleading positive stool blood test. Hemosiderin laden macrophages in sputum, gastric washings, or alveolar lavage[952] indicate bleeding within the recent past, but can also be positive with pulmonary edema.[946]

Radiographic signs, unfortunately, are not particularly helpful in distinguishing between DPH and the various other causes of consolidation. Nevertheless, airspace opacity that clears over a 2–4 day interval should always raise the possibility of alveolar hemorrhage. The interpretation of the chest radiograph is made particularly difficult by the fact that fluid overload and infection, the two major differential diagnoses, are well recognized precipitators of DPH in Goodpasture syndrome,[946] and may coexist along with hemorrhage.

DPH can be diagnosed by detection of increased carbon monoxide uptake by the blood sequestered in the lungs. This can be demonstrated by the single breath carbon monoxide uptake (K_{co}) test, considering a 40% rise as positive.[951] Bronchoscopy with pulmonary lavage is usually diagnostic, and helps exclude associated infection.

Although some older reports suggest that MRI findings may be relatively specific for DPH,[953,954] the lung parenchyma is notoriously difficult to image by MRI, and the technique is not generally used.

The specific etiology of pulmonary hemorrhage is usually determined by clinical assessment, serologic studies, and biopsy of the kidney or other extrapulmonary organs. Serologic studies should include tests for anti-GMB antibodies, ANCA, antinuclear antibodies ANA, anti-double-stranded DNA antibodies, cryoglobulins, rheumatoid factor, and complement levels. With current methods of serologic diagnosis, lung biopsy is rarely needed, and should it be necessary, open lung biopsy is to be preferred to transbronchial biopsy.

REFERENCES

1. Liebow A. Definition and classification of interstitial pneumonias in human pathology. Prog Respir Res 1975;8:1–33.
2. Müller NL, Colby TV. Idiopathic interstitial pneumonias: high-resolution CT and histologic findings. RadioGraphics 1997;17:1016–1022.
3. Katzenstein AL, Myers JL. Idiopathic pulmonary fibrosis: clinical relevance of pathologic classification. Am J Respir Crit Care Med 1998;157:1301–1315.
4. American Thoracic Society/European Respiratory Society International Multidisciplinary Consensus Classification of the Idiopathic Interstitial Pneumonias. Am J Respir Crit Care Med 2002;165:277–304.
5. Anttila S, Sutinen S, Paananen M, et al. Hard metal lung disease: a clinical, histological, ultrastructural and X-ray microanalytical study. Eur J Respir Dis 1986;69:83–94.
6. Ohori NP, Sciurba FC, Owens GR, et al. Giant-cell interstitial pneumonia and hard-metal pneumoconiosis. A clinicopathologic study of four cases and review of the literature. Am J Surg Pathol 1989;13:581–587.
7. Davison A, Heard B, McAllister W, et al. Cryptogenic organizing pneumonia. Q J Med 1983;52:382–394.
8. Epler GR, Colby TV, McLoud TC, et al. Bronchiolitis obliterans organizing pneumonia. N Engl J Med 1985;312:152–158.
9. Koss MN. Pulmonary lymphoid disorders. Semin Diagn Pathol 1995;12:158–171.
10. Schneider RF. Lymphocytic interstitial pneumonitis and nonspecific interstitial pneumonitis. Clin Chest Med 1996;17:763–766.
11. Bjoraker J, Ryu J, Edwin, et al. Prognostic significance of histopathologic subsets in idiopathic pulmonary fibrosis. Am J Respir Crit Care Med 1998;157:199–203.
12. Nagai S, Kitaichi M, Itoh H, et al. Idiopathic nonspecific interstitial pneumonia/fibrosis: comparison with idiopathic pulmonary fibrosis and BOOP. Eur Respir J 1998;12:1010–1019.
13. Travis WD, Matsui K, Moss J, et al. Idiopathic nonspecific interstitial pneumonia: prognostic significance of cellular and fibrosing patterns: survival comparison with usual interstitial pneumonia and desquamative interstitial pneumonia. Am J Surg Pathol 2000;24:19–33.
14. Nicholson AG, Colby TV, du Bois RM, et al. The prognostic significance of the histologic pattern of interstitial pneumonia in patients presenting with the clinical entity of cryptogenic fibrosing alveolitis. Am J Respir Crit Care Med 2000;162:2213–2217.

15. Flaherty KR, Toews GB, Travis WD, et al. Clinical significance of histological classification of idiopathic interstitial pneumonia. Eur Respir J 2002;19:275–283.
16. Flaherty KR, Travis WD, Colby TV, et al. Histopathologic variability in usual and nonspecific interstitial pneumonias. Am J Respir Crit Care Med 2001;164:1722–1727.
17. American Thoracic Society. Idiopathic pulmonary fibrosis: diagnosis and treatment. International consensus statement. American Thoracic Society (ATS), and the European Respiratory Society (ERS). Am J Respir Crit Care Med 2000;161:646–664.
18. Watters LC, Schwarz MI, Cherniack RM, et al. Idiopathic pulmonary fibrosis. Pretreatment bronchoalveolar lavage cellular constituents and their relationship with lung histopathology and clinical response to therapy. Am Rev Respir Dis 1987;135:696–704.
19. Papiris SA, Vlachoyiannopoulos PG, Maniati MA, et al. Idiopathic pulmonary fibrosis and pulmonary fibrosis in diffuse systemic sclerosis: two fibroses with different prognoses. Respiration 1997;64:81–85.
20. Schwartz DA, Helmers RA, Galvin JR, et al. Determinants of survival in idiopathic pulmonary fibrosis. Am J Respir Crit Care Med 1994;149:450–454.
21. Gay SE, Kazerooni EA, Toews GB, et al. Idiopathic pulmonary fibrosis: predicting response to therapy and survival. Am J Respir Crit Care Med 1998;157:1063–1072.
22. Johnston ID, Prescott RJ, Chalmers JC, et al. British Thoracic Society study of cryptogenic fibrosing alveolitis: current presentation and initial management. Fibrosing Alveolitis Subcommittee of the Research Committee of the British Thoracic Society. Thorax 1997;52:38–44.
23. Lee J, Im J-G, Ahn J, et al. Fibrosing alveolitis: prognostic implication of ground-glass attenuation at high-resolution CT. Radiology 1992;184:451–454.
24. Johnston ID, Gomm SA, Kalra S, et al. The management of cryptogenic fibrosing alveolitis in three regions of the United Kingdom. Eur Respir J 1993;6:891–893.
25. Saravanan V, Kelly CA. Survival in fibrosing alveolitis associated with rheumatoid arthritis is better than cryptogenic fibrosing alveolitis. Rheumatology (Oxford) 2003;42:603–604; author reply 604–605.
26. Terriff B, Kwan S, Chan-Yeung M, et al. Fibrosing alveolitis: chest radiography and CT as predictors of clinical and functional impairment at followup in 26 patients. Radiology 1992;184:445–449.

27. Tung KT, Wells Au, Rubens MB, et al. Accuracy of the typical computed tomographic appearances of fibrosing alveolitis. Thorax 1993;48:334–338.
28. Turner-Warwick M, Burrows B, Johnson A. Cryptogenic fibrosing alveolitis: response to corticosteroid treatment and its effect on survival. Thorax 1980;35:593–599.
29. Turner-Warwick M. In search of a cause of cryptogenic fibrosing alveolitis (CFA): one initiating factor or many? Thorax 1998;53 Suppl 2:S3–9.
30. Wells AU, Rubens MB, du Bois RM, et al. Serial CT in fibrosing alveolitis: prognostic significance of the initial pattern. AJR Am J Roentgenol 1993;161:1159–1165.
31. Mapel DW, Hunt WC, Utton R, et al. Idiopathic pulmonary fibrosis: survival in population based and hospital based cohorts. Thorax 1998;53:469–476.
32. Turner-Warwick M, Burrows B, Johnson A. Cryptogenic fibrosing alveolitis: clinical features and their influence on survival. Thorax 1980;35:171–180.
33. Livingstone JL, Lewis JG, Reid L, et al. Diffuse interstitial pulmonary fibrosis. A clinical, radiological, and pathological study based on 45 patients. Q J Med 1964;33:71–103.
34. Jackson LK. Idiopathic pulmonary fibrosis. Clin Chest Med 1982;3:579–592.
35. Wright PH, Heard BE, Steel SJ, et al. Cryptogenic fibrosing alveolitis: assessment by graded trephine lung biopsy histology compared with clinical, radiographic, and physiological features. Br J Dis Chest 1981;75:61–70.
36. Scadding JG. Diffuse pulmonary alveolar fibrosis. Thorax 1974;29:271–281.
37. Panos RJ, Mortenson RL, Niccoli SA, et al. Clinical deterioration in patients with idiopathic pulmonary fibrosis: causes and assessment. Am J Med 1990;88:396–404.
38. Tukiainen P, Taskinen E, Holsti P, et al. Prognosis of cryptogenic fibrosing alveolitis. Thorax 1983;38:349–355.
39. Crystal RG, Fulmer JD, Roberts WC, et al. Idiopathic pulmonary fibrosis. Clinical, histologic, radiographic, physiologic, scintigraphic, cytologic, and biochemical aspects. Ann Intern Med 1976;85:769–788.
40. Wiggins J, Strickland B, Turner WM. Combined cryptogenic fibrosing alveolitis and emphysema: the value of high resolution computed tomography in assessment. Respir Med 1990;84:365–369.
41. Doherty MJ, Pearson MG, O'Grady EA, et al. Cryptogenic fibrosing alveolitis

with preserved lung volumes. Thorax 1997;52:998–1002.

42. Wells AU, King AD, Rubens MB, et al. Lone cryptogenic fibrosing alveolitis: a functional-morphologic correlation based on extent of disease on thin-section computed tomography Am J Respir Crit Care Med 1997;155:1367–1375.

43. Gottlieb AJ, Spiera H, Teirstein AS, et al. Serologic factors in idiopathic diffuse interstitial pulmonary fibrosis. Am J Med 1965;39:405–410.

44. Winterbauer RH, Hammar SP, Hallman KO, et al. Diffuse interstitial pneumonitis. Clinicopathologic correlations in 20 patients treated with prednisone/azathioprine. Am J Med 1978;65:661–672.

45. Wells AU, Cullinan P, Hansell DM, et al. Fibrosing alveolitis associated with systemic sclerosis has a better prognosis than lone cryptogenic fibrosing alveolitis. Am J Respir Crit Care Med 1994;149:1583–1590.

46. Tanaka N, Kim J, Newell J, et al. CT findings of rheumatoid arthritis-related lung diseases. Radiology 2004; in press.

47. Bouros D, Wells AU, Nicholson AG, et al. Histopathologic subsets of fibrosing alveolitis in patients with systemic sclerosis and their relationship to outcome. Am J Respir Crit Care Med 2002;165:1581–1586.

48. Kim DS, Yoo B, Lee JS, et al. The major histopathologic pattern of pulmonary fibrosis in scleroderma is nonspecific interstitial pneumonia. Sarcoidosis Vasc Diffuse Lung Dis 2002;19:121–127.

49. Baumgartner KB, Samet JM, Stidley CA, et al. Cigarette smoking: a risk factor for idiopathic pulmonary fibrosis. Am J Respir Crit Care Med 1997;155:242–248.

50. Hubbard R, Lewis S, Richards K, et al. Occupational exposure to metal or wood dust and aetiology of cryptogenic fibrosing alveolitis. Lancet 1996;347:284–289.

51. Hubbard R, Venn A, Smith C, et al. Exposure to commonly prescribed drugs and the etiology of cryptogenic fibrosing alveolitis: a case-control study. Am J Respir Crit Care Med 1998;157:743–747.

52. Collard HR, King TE Jr. Demystifying idiopathic interstitial pneumonia. Arch Intern Med 2003;163:17–29.

53. Katzenstein AL, Myers J, Prophet W, et al. Bronchiolitis obliterans and usual interstitial pneumonia: a comparative clinicopathologic study. Am J Surg Pathol 1986;10:373–381.

54. Kuhn C 3rd, Boldt J, King TE Jr, et al. An immunohistochemical study of architectural remodeling and connective tissue synthesis in pulmonary fibrosis. Am Rev Respir Dis 1989;140:1693–1703.

55. Myers JL, Katzenstein AL. Epithelial necrosis and alveolar collapse in the pathogenesis of usual interstitial pneumonia. Chest 1988;94:1309–1311.

56. Fukuda Y, Basset F, Ferrans VJ, et al. Significance of early intra-alveolar fibrotic lesions and integrin expression in lung biopsy specimens from patients with idiopathic pulmonary fibrosis. Hum Pathol 1995;26:53–61.

57. King TE Jr, Schwarz MI, Brown K, et al. Idiopathic pulmonary fibrosis: relationship between histopathologic features and mortality. Am J Respir Crit Care Med 2001;164:1025–1032.

58. Yamamoto S. Histopathological features of pulmonary asbestosis with particular emphasis on the comparison with those of usual interstitial pneumonia. Osaka City Med J 1997;43:225–242.

59. Myers JL, Limper AH, Swensen SJ. Drug-induced lung disease: a pragmatic classification incorporating HRCT appearances. Semin Respir Crit Care Med 2003;24:445–453.

60. Egan JJ, Woodcock AA, Stewart JP. Viruses and idiopathic pulmonary fibrosis. Eur Respir J 1997;10:1433–1437.

61. Tang YW, Johnson JE, Browning PJ, et al. Herpesvirus DNA is consistently detected in lungs of patients with idiopathic pulmonary fibrosis. J Clin Microbiol 2003;41:2633–2640.

62. Tsukamoto K, Hayakawa H, Sato A, et al. Involvement of Epstein-Barr virus latent membrane protein 1 in disease progression in patients with idiopathic pulmonary fibrosis. Thorax 2000;55:958–961.

63. Lok SS, Egan JJ. Viruses and idiopathic pulmonary fibrosis. Monaldi Arch Chest Dis 2000;55:146–150.

64. King TE Jr, Tooze JA, Schwarz MI, et al. Predicting survival in idiopathic pulmonary fibrosis: scoring system and survival model. Am J Respir Crit Care Med 2001;164:1171–1181.

65. Nicholson AG, Kim H, Corrin B, et al. The value of classifying interstitial pneumonitis in childhood according to defined histological patterns. Histopathology 1998;33:203–2111.

66. Fan LL, Kozinetz CA, Deterding RR, et al. Evaluation of a diagnostic approach to pediatric interstitial lung disease. Pediatrics 1998;101:82–85.

67. Guerry-Force M, Müller NL, et al. A comparison of bronchiolitis obliterans with organizing pneumonia, usual interstitial pneumonia, and small airways disease. Am Rev Resp Dis 1987;135:705–712.

68. Carrington CB, Gaensler EA, Coutu RE, et al. Natural history and treated course of usual and desquamative interstitial pneumonia. N Engl J Med 1978;298:801–809.

69. Hubbard R, Johnston I, Britton J. Survival in patients with cryptogenic fibrosing alveolitis: a population-based cohort study. Chest 1998;113:396–400.

70. Hanson D, Winterbauer RH, Kirtland SH, et al. Changes in pulmonary function test results after 1 year of therapy as predictors of survival in patients with idiopathic pulmonary fibrosis. Chest 1995;108:305–310.

71. Flaherty KR, Thwaite EL, Kazerooni EA, et al. Radiological versus histological diagnosis in UIP and NSIP: survival implications. Thorax 2003;58:143–148.

72. Wells AU, Hansell DM, Rubens MB, et al. The predictive value of appearances on thin-section computed tomography in fibrosing alveolitis. Am Rev Respir Dis 1993;148:1076–1082.

73. Stack BH, Choo-Kang YF, Heard BE. The prognosis of cryptogenic fibrosing alveolitis. Thorax 1972;27:535–542.

74. Johkoh T, Müller NL, Cartier Y, et al. Idiopathic interstitial pneumonias: diagnostic accuracy of thin-section CT in 129 patients. Radiology 1999;211:555–560.

75. Hunninghake GW, Lynch DA, Galvin JR, et al. Radiologic findings are strongly associated with a pathologic diagnosis of usual interstitial pneumonia. Chest 2003;124:1215–1223.

76. Niimi H, Kang EY, Kwong JS, et al. CT of chronic infiltrative lung disease: prevalence of mediastinal lymphadenopathy. J Comput Assist Tomogr 1996;20:305–306.

77. Jung JI, Kim HH, Jung YJ, et al. Mediastinal lymphadenopathy in pulmonary fibrosis: correlation with disease severity. J Comput Assist Tomogr 2000;24:706–710.

78. Gevenois PA, Abehsera M, Knoop C, et al. Disseminated pulmonary ossification in end-stage pulmonary fibrosis: CT demonstration. AJR Am J Roentgenol 1994;162:1303–1304.

79. Nishimura K, Izumi T, Kitaichi M, et al. The diagnostic accuracy of high-resolution computed tomography in diffuse infiltrative lung diseases. Chest 1993;104:1149–1155.

80. Swensen S, Aughenbaugh G, Myers J. Diffuse lung disease: Diagnostic accuracy of CT in patients undergoing surgical biopsy of the lung. Radiology 1997;205:229–234.

81. Raghu G, Mageto YN, Lockhart D, et al. The accuracy of the clinical diagnosis of new-onset idiopathic pulmonary fibrosis and other interstitial lung disease: A prospective study. Chest 1999;116:1168–1174.

82. Hunninghake GW, Zimmerman MB, Schwartz DA, et al. Utility of a lung biopsy for the diagnosis of idiopathic pulmonary fibrosis. Am J Respir Crit Care Med 2001;164:193–196.

83. Mathieson JR, Mayo JR, Staples CA, et al. Chronic diffuse infiltrative lung disease:

comparison of diagnostic accuracy of CT and chest radiography. Radiology 1989;171:111–116.

84. Lee KS, Primack SL, Staples CA, et al. Chronic infiltrative lung disease: comparison of diagnostic accuracies of radiography and low- and conventional-dose thin-section CT. Radiology 1994; 191:669–673.

85. Müller NL, Staples CA, Miller RR, et al. Disease activity in idiopathic pulmonary fibrosis: CT and pathologic correlation. Radiology 1987;165:731–734.

86. Wells AU, Hansell DM, Corrin B, et al. High resolution computed tomography as a predictor of lung histology in systemic sclerosis. Thorax 1992;47:508–512.

87. Hartman TE, Primack SL, Kang EY, et al. Disease progression in usual interstitial pneumonia compared with desquamative interstitial pneumonia. Assessment with serial CT. Chest 1996;110:378–382.

88. Nishiyama O, Kondoh Y, Taniguchi H, et al. Serial high resolution CT findings in nonspecific interstitial pneumonia/fibrosis. J Comput Assist Tomogr 2000; 24:41–46.

89. Akira M, Sakatani M, Ueda E. Idiopathic pulmonary fibrosis: progression of honeycombing at thin-section CT. Radiology 1993;189:687–691.

90. Lee JS, Gong G, Song KS, et al. Usual interstitial pneumonia: relationship between disease activity and the progression of honeycombing at thin-section computed tomography. J Thorac Imaging 1998;13:199–203.

91. Turner-Warwick M, Lebowitz M, Burrows B, et al. Cryptogenic fibrosing alveolitis and lung cancer. Thorax 1980;35:496–499.

92. Lee HJ, Im JG, Ahn JM, et al. Lung cancer in patients with idiopathic pulmonary fibrosis: CT findings. J Comput Assist Tomogr 1996;20:979–982.

93. Mizushima Y, Kobayashi M. Clinical characteristics of synchronous multiple lung cancer associated with idiopathic pulmonary fibrosis. A review of Japanese cases. Chest 1995;108:1272–1277.

94. Fraire AE, Greenberg SD. Carcinoma and diffuse interstitial fibrosis of lung. Cancer 1973;31:1078–1086.

95. Kumar P, Goldstraw P, Yamada K, et al. Pulmonary fibrosis and lung cancer: risk and benefit analysis of pulmonary resection. J Thorac Cardiovasc Surg 2003;125:1321–1327.

96. Akira M, Hamada H, Sakatani M, et al. CT findings during phase of accelerated deterioration in patients with idiopathic pulmonary fibrosis. AJR Am J Roentgenol 1997;168:79–83.

97. Akira M. Computed tomography and pathologic findings in fulminant forms of idiopathic interstitial pneumonia. J Thorac Imaging 1999;14:76–84.

98. Pratt DS, Schwartz MI, May JJ, et al. Rapidly fatal pulmonary fibrosis: the accelerated variant of interstitial pneumonitis. Thorax 1979;34:587–593.

99. Kondoh Y, Taniguchi H, Kawabata Y, et al. Acute exacerbation in idiopathic pulmonary fibrosis. Analysis of clinical and pathologic findings in three cases. Chest 1993;103:1808–1812.

100. Katzenstein AL, Fiorelli RF. Nonspecific interstitial pneumonia/fibrosis. Histologic features and clinical significance. Am J Surg Pathol 1994;18:136–147.

101. Kim T, Lee K, Chung M, et al. Nonspecific interstitial pneumonia with fibrosis: high resolution CT and pathologic findings. AJR Am J Roentgenol 1998;171:1645–1650.

102. Riha RL, Duhig EE, Clarke BE, et al. Survival of patients with biopsy-proven usual interstitial pneumonia and nonspecific interstitial pneumonia. Eur Respir J 2002;19:1114–1118.

103. MacDonald SL, Rubens MB, Hansell DM, et al. Nonspecific interstitial pneumonia and usual interstitial pneumonia: comparative appearances and diagnostic accuracy of high-resolution computed tomography. Radiology 2001;221:600–605.

104. Hartman TE, Swensen SJ, Hansell DM, et al. Nonspecific interstitial pneumonia: variable appearance at high-resolution chest CT. Radiology 2000;217:701–705.

105. Hansell DM, Nicholson AG. Smoking-related diffuse parenchymal lung disease. Semin Respir Crit Care Med 2003;24:377–393.

106. Park JS, Lee KS, Kim JS, et al. Nonspecific interstitial pneumonia with fibrosis: radiographic and CT findings in seven patients. Radiology 1995;195:645–648.

107. Nagai S, Kitaichi M, Izumi T. Classification and recent advances in idiopathic interstitial pneumonia. Curr Opin Pulm Med 1998;4:256–260.

108. Kim EY, Lee KS, Chung MP, et al. Nonspecific interstitial pneumonia with fibrosis: serial high-resolution CT findings with functional correlation. AJR Am J Roentgenol 1999;173:949–953.

109. Hartman TE, Primack SL, Swensen SJ, et al. Desquamative interstitial pneumonia: thin-section CT findings in 22 patients. Radiology 1993;187:787–790.

110. Cottin V, Donsbeck A, Revel D, et al. Nonspecific interstitial pneumonia: individualization of a clinicopathologic entity in a series of 12 patients. Am J Respir Crit Care Med 1998;158: 1286–1293.

111. Johkoh T, Müller NL, Colby TV, et al. Nonspecific interstitial pneumonia: correlation between thin-section CT findings and pathologic subgroups in 55 patients. Radiology 2002;225: 199–204.

112. Lynch DA. Fibrotic idiopathic interstitial pneumonia: high-resolution computed tomography considerations. Semin Respir Crit Care Med 2003;24:365–376.

113. Grinblat J, Mechlis S, Lewitus Z. Organizing pneumonia-like process: an unusual observation in steroid responsive cases with features of chronic interstitial pneumonia. Chest 1981;80: 259–263.

114. Bouchardy LM, Kuhlman JE, Ball WJ, et al. CT findings in bronchiolitis obliterans organizing pneumonia (BOOP) with radiographic, clinical, and histologic correlation. J Comput Assist Tomogr 1993;17:352–357.

115. Colby TV. Pathologic aspects of bronchiolitis obliterans organizing pneumonia. Chest 1992;102:38S–43S.

116. Epler GR. *Bronchiolitis obliterans* organizing pneumonia. Semin Resp Infect 1995;10:65–77.

117. Garg K, Lynch DA, Newell JD, et al. Proliferative and constrictive bronchiolitis: classification and radiologic features. AJR Am J Roentgenol 1994;162:803–808.

118. Alasaly K, Müller N, Ostrow DN, et al. Cryptogenic organizing pneumonia. A report of 25 cases and a review of the literature. Medicine 1995;74:201–211.

119. Lohr RH, Boland BJ, Douglas WW, et al. Organizing pneumonia. Features and prognosis of cryptogenic, secondary, and focal variants. Arch Intern Med 1997;157:1323–1329.

120. Costabel U, Teschler H, Schoenfeld B, et al. BOOP in Europe. Chest 1992;102:14S–20S.

121. Yamamoto M, Ina Y, Kitaichi M, et al. Clinical features of BOOP in Japan. Chest 1992;102:21S–25S.

122. King TE Jr, Mortenson RL. Cryptogenic organizing pneumonitis. The North American experience. Chest 1992;102:8S–13S.

123. King T. Idiopathic interstitial pneumonias. In: King T, ed. Interstitial lung disease, 4th edn. Toronto: Brian C Decker, 2003:701–786.

124. Bouchardy LM, Kuhlman JE, Ball WC Jr, et al. CT findings in bronchiolitis obliterans organizing pneumonia (BOOP) with radiographic, clinical, and histologic correlation. J Comput Assist Tomogr 1993;17:352–357.

125. Haddock JA, Hansell DM. The radiology and terminology of cryptogenic organizing pneumonia. Br J Radiol 1992;65:674–680.

126. Cordier JF, Loire R, Brune J. Idiopathic bronchiolitis obliterans organizing pneumonia. Definition of characteristic clinical profiles in a series of 16 patients. Chest 1989;96:999–1004.

127. Mroz BJ, Sexauer WP, Meade A, et al. Hemoptysis as the presenting symptom in

bronchiolitis obliterans organizing pneumonia. Chest 1997;111:1775–1778.

128. Miyagawa Y, Nagata N, Shigematsu N. Clinicopathologic study of migratory lung infiltrates. Thorax 1991;46:233–238.

129. Cordier JF. Cryptogenic organizing pneumonitis. Bronchiolitis obliterans organizing pneumonia. Clin Chest Med 1993;14:677–692.

130. Costabel U, Guzman J, Teschler H. Bronchiolitis obliterans with organising pneumonia: outcome. Thorax 1995;50 Suppl 1:S59–64.

131. Bartter T, Irwin RS, Nash G, et al. Idiopathic bronchiolitis obliterans organizing pneumonia with peripheral infiltrates on chest roentgenogram. Arch Intern Med 1989;149:273–279.

132. Dina R, Sheppard MN. The histological diagnosis of clinically documented cases of cryptogenic organizing pneumonia: diagnostic features in transbronchial biopsies. Histopathology 1993;23: 541–545.

133. Izumi T, Kitaichi M, Nishimura K, et al. Bronchiolitis obliterans organizing pneumonia. Clinical features and differential diagnosis. Chest 1992;102: 715–719.

134. Müller NL, Staples CA, Miller RR. Bronchiolitis obliterans organizing pneumonia: CT features in 14 patients. AJR Am J Roentgenol 1990;154:983–987.

135. Chandler PW, Shin MS, Friedman SE, et al. Radiographic manifestations of bronchiolitis obliterans with organizing pneumonia vs usual interstitial pneumonia. AJR Am J Roentgenol 1986;147:899–906.

136. Epstein DM, Bennett M. Bronchiolitis obliterans organizing pneumonia with migratory pulmonary infiltrates. AJR Am J Roentgenol 1992;158:515–517.

137. King TE Jr. BOOP: an important cause of migratory pulmonary infiltrates? Eur Respir J 1995;8:193–195.

138. Crestani B, Kambouchner M, Soler P, et al. Migratory bronchiolitis obliterans organizing pneumonia after unilateral radiation therapy for breast carcinoma. Eur Respir J 1995;8:318–321.

139. Flowers J, Clunie G, Burke M, et al. Bronchiolitis obliterans organizing pneumonia: the clinical and radiological features of seven cases and a review of the literature. Clin Radiol 1992;45:371–377.

140. Zackrison LH, Katz P. Bronchiolitis obliterans organizing pneumonia associated with essential mixed cryoglobulinemia. Arthritis Rheum 1993;36:1627–1630.

141. Akira M, Yamamoto S, Sakatani M. Bronchiolitis obliterans organizing pneumonia manifesting as multiple large nodules or masses. AJR Am J Roentgenol 1998;170:291–295.

142. Santrach PJ, Askin FB, Wells RJ, et al. Nodular form of bleomycin-related pulmonary injury in patients with osteogenic sarcoma. Cancer 1989;64:806–811.

143. Müller NL, Guerry-Force ML, Staples CA, et al. Differential diagnosis of bronchiolitis obliterans with organizing pneumonia and usual interstitial pneumonia: clinical, functional, and radiologic findings. Radiology 1987;162:151–156.

144. Nizami IY, Kissner DG, Visscher DW, et al. Idiopathic bronchiolitis obliterans with organizing pneumonia. An acute and life-threatening syndrome. Chest 1995;108:271–277.

145. Nishimura K, Itoh H. High-resolution computed tomographic features of bronchiolitis obliterans organizing pneumonia. Chest 1992;102:26S–31S.

146. Lee KS, Kullnic P, Hartman TE, et al. Cryptogenic organizing pneumonia: CT findings in 43 patients. AJR Am J Roentgenol 1994;162:543–546.

147. Oikonomou A, Hansell DM. Organizing pneumonia: the many morphological faces. Eur Radiol 2002;12:1486–1496.

148. McAdams HP, Rosado-de-Christenson ML, Wehunt WD, et al. The alphabet soup revisited: the chronic interstitial pneumonias in the 1990s. RadioGraphics 1996;16:1009–1033; discussion 1033–1034.

149. Worthy SA, Müller NL, Hartman TE, et al. Mosaic attenuation pattern on thin-section CT scans of the lung: differentiation among infiltrative lung, airway, and vascular diseases as a cause. Radiology 1997;205:465–470.

150. Lee J, Lynch D, Sharma S, et al. Organizing pneumonia: prognostic implication of high-resolution CT features. J Comput Assist Tomogr 2003;27:260–265.

151. Haro M, Vizcaya M, Texido A, et al. Idiopathic bronchiolitis obliterans organizing pneumonia with multiple cavitary lung nodules. Eur Respir J 1995;8:1975–1977.

152. Froudarakis M, Bouros D, Loire R, et al. BOOP presenting with haemoptysis and multiple cavitary nodules. Eur Respir J 1995;8:1972–1974.

153. Cordier JF. Cavitary bronchiolitis obliterans organizing pneumonia. Eur Respir J 1995;8:1822–1823.

154. Iannuzzi MC, Farhi DC, Bostrom PD, et al. Fulminant respiratory failure and death in a patient with idiopathic bronchiolitis obliterans. Arch Intern Med 1985;145:733–734.

155. Bayle JY, Nesme P, Bejui-Thivolet F, et al. Migratory organizing pneumonitis "primed" by radiation therapy. Eur Respir J 1995;8:322–326.

156. Crestani B, Valeyre D, Roden S, et al. Bronchiolitis obliterans organizing pneumonia syndrome primed by radiation therapy to the breast. The Groupe d'Etudes et de Recherche sur les Maladies Orphelines Pulmonaires (GERM"O"P). Am J Respir Crit Care Med 1998;158:1929–1935.

157. Takigawa N, Segawa Y, Saeki T, et al. Bronchiolitis obliterans organizing pneumonia syndrome in breast-conserving therapy for early breast cancer: radiation-induced lung toxicity. Int J Radiat Oncol Biol Phys 2000;48: 751–755.

158. Allen JN, Wewers MD. HIV-associated bronchiolitis obliterans organizing pneumonia. Chest 1989;96:197–198.

159. Sanito NJ, Morley TF, Condoluci DV. Bronchiolitis obliterans organizing pneumonia in an AIDS patient. Eur Respir J 1995;8:1021–1024.

160. Yale SH, Adlakha A, Sebo TJ, et al. Bronchiolitis obliterans organizing pneumonia caused by *Plasmodium vivax* malaria. Chest 1993;104:1294–1296.

161. Rees JH, Woodhead MA, Sheppard MN, et al. Rheumatoid arthritis and cryptogenic organising pneumonitis. Respir Med 1991;85:243–246.

162. Herzog CA, Miller RR, Hoidal JR. Bronchiolitis and rheumatoid arthritis. Am Rev Respir Dis 1981;124:636–639.

163. Gammon RB, Bridges TA, al-Nezir H, et al. Bronchiolitis obliterans organizing pneumonia associated with systemic lupus erythematosus. Chest 1992;102: 1171–1174.

164. Robinson BW, Sterrett G. Bronchiolitis obliterans associated with polyarteritis nodosa. Chest 1992;102:309–311.

165. Tazelaar HD, Viggiano RW, Pickersgill J, et al. Interstitial lung disease in polymyositis and dermatomyositis. Clinical features and prognosis as correlated with histologic findings. Am Rev Respir Dis 1990;141:727–733.

166. Bridges AJ, Hsu KC, Dias-Arias AA, et al. Bronchiolitis obliterans organizing pneumonia and scleroderma. J Rheumatol 1992;19:1136–1140.

167. Davison AG, Epstein O. Relapsing organising pneumonitis in a man with primary biliary cirrhosis, CREST syndrome, and chronic pancreatitis. Thorax 1983;38:316–317.

168. Matteson EL, Ike RW. Bronchiolitis obliterans organizing pneumonia and Sjögren's syndrome. J Rheumatol 1990;17:676–679.

169. Anon. Case records of the Massachusetts General Hospital. Weekly clinicopathological exercises. Case 24-1986. A 65-year-old woman with bilateral pulmonary infiltrates. N Engl J Med 1986;314:1627–1635.

170. Stemmelin GR, Bernaciak J, Casas JG. Bronchiolitis with leukemia. Ann Intern Med 1991;114:912–913.

171. Miki Y, Hatabu H, Takahashi M, et al. Computed tomography of bronchiolitis obliterans. J Comput Assist Tomogr 1988;12:512–514.

172. Graham NJ, Müller NL, Miller RR, et al. Intrathoracic complications following allogeneic bone marrow transplantation: CT findings. Radiology 1991;181:153–156.

173. Thirman MJ, Devine SM, O'Toole K, et al. Bronchiolitis obliterans organizing pneumonia as a complication of allogeneic bone marrow transplantation. Bone Marrow Transplant 1992;10: 307–311.

174. Verberckmoes R, Verbeken E, Verschakelen J, et al. BOOP (bronchiolitis obliterans organizing pneumonia) after renal transplantation. Nephrol Dial Transplant 1996;11:1862–1863.

175. Abernathy EC, Hruban RH, Baumgartner WA, et al. The two forms of bronchiolitis obliterans in heart-lung transplant recipients. Hum Pathol 1991;22:1102–1110.

176. Swinburn CR, Jackson GJ, Cobden I, et al. Bronchiolitis obliterans organising pneumonia in a patient with ulcerative colitis. Thorax 1988;43:735–736.

177. Camus P, Piard F, Ashcroft T, et al. The lung in inflammatory bowel disease. Medicine (Baltimore) 1993;72:151–183.

178. Spiteri MA, Klenerman P, Sheppard MN, et al. Seasonal cryptogenic organising pneumonia with biochemical cholestasis: a new clinical entity. Lancet 1992;340:281–284.

179. Rutherford PA, Veale D, Ashcroft T, et al. Mesangiocapillary glomerulonephritis as the presenting feature of cryptogenic organizing pneumonitis. Nephrol Dial Transplant 1992;7:1043–1046.

180. Hernandez JI, Gomez-Roman J, Rodrigo E, et al. Bronchiolitis obliterans and IgA nephropathy. A new cause of pulmonary-renal syndrome. Am J Respir Crit Care Med 1997;156:665–668.

181. Tomioka R, King TE Jr. Gold-induced pulmonary disease: clinical features, outcome, and differentiation from rheumatoid lung disease. Am J Respir Crit Care Med 1997;155:1011–1020.

182. Takimoto C, Lynch D, Stulbarg M. Pulmonary infiltrates associated with sulindac therapy. Chest 1990;97:230–232.

183. Williams T, Eidus L, Thomas P. Fibrosing alveolitis, bronchiolitis obliterans, and sulfasalazine therapy. Chest 1982;81: 766–768.

184. Santrach PJ, Askin FB, Wells RJ, et al. Nodular form of bleomycin-related pulmonary injury in patients with osteogenic sarcoma. Cancer 1989;64: 806–811.

185. Myers J. Pathology of drug-induced lung disease. In: Katzenstein A-L, ed. Katzenstein and Askin's surgical pathology of non-neoplastic lung disease, 3rd edn. Philadelphia: WB Saunders, 1997.

186. Domingo JA, Perez-Calvo JI, Carretero JA, et al. Bronchiolitis obliterans organizing pneumonia. An unusual cause of solitary pulmonary nodule. Chest 1993;103:1621–1623.

187. Kohno N, Ikezoe J, Johkoh T, et al. Focal organizing pneumonia: CT appearance. Radiology 1993;189:119–123.

188. Hamman L, Rich A. Acute diffuse interstitial fibrosis of the lungs. Bull Johns Hopkins Hosp 1944;74:177–212.

189. Katzenstein AL, Myers JL, Mazur MT. Acute interstitial pneumonia. A clinicopathologic, ultrastructural, and cell kinetic study. Am J Surg Pathol 1986;10:256–267.

190. Askin FB. Back to the future: the Hamman-Rich syndrome and acute interstitial pneumonia. Mayo Clin Proc 1990;65:1624–1626.

191. Olson J, Colby TV, Elliott CG. Hamman-Rich syndrome revisited. Mayo Clin Proc 1990;65:1538–1548.

192. Askin RB. Acute interstitial pneumonia: histopathologic patterns of acute lung injury and the Hamman-Rich syndrome revisited. Radiology 1993;188: 620–621.

193. Primack SL, Hartman TE, Ikezoe J, et al. Acute interstitial pneumonia: radiographic and CT findings in nine patients. Radiology 1993;188:817–820.

194. Ichikado K, Johkoh T, Ikezoe J, et al. Acute interstitial pneumonia: high-resolution CT findings correlated with pathology. AJR Am J Roentgenol 1997;168:333–338.

195. Ichikado K, Suga M, Müller NL, et al. Acute interstitial pneumonia: comparison of high-resolution computed tomography findings between survivors and nonsurvivors. Am J Respir Crit Care Med 2002;165:1551–1556.

196. Johkoh T, Müller N, Taniguchi H, et al. Acute interstitial pneumonia: Thin section CT findings in 36 patients. Radiology 1999;211:859–863.

197. Mihara N, Johkoh T, Ichikado K, et al. Can acute interstitial pneumonia be differentiated from bronchiolitis obliterans organizing pneumonia by high-resolution CT? Radiat Med 2000;18:299–304.

198. Tomiyama N, Müller NL, Johkoh T, et al. Acute parenchymal lung disease in immunocompetent patients: diagnostic accuracy of high-resolution CT. AJR Am J Roentgenol 2000;174:1745–1750.

199. Tomiyama N, Müller NL, Johkoh T, et al. Acute respiratory distress syndrome and acute interstitial pneumonia: comparison of thin-section CT findings. J Comput Assist Tomogr 2001;25:28–33.

200. Hansell DM. Acute interstitial pneumonia: clues from the white stuff. Am J Respir Crit Care Med 2002;165: 1465–1466.

201. Swigris JJ, Berry GJ, Raffin TA, et al. Lymphoid interstitial pneumonia: a narrative review. Chest 2002;122: 2150–2164.

202. Johkoh T, Müller NL, Ichikado K, et al. Intrathoracic multicentric Castleman disease: CT findings in 12 patients. Radiology 1998;209:477–481.

203. Cosgrove G, Fessler M, Schwarz MI. Lymphoplasmacytic infiltrations of the lung. In: Schwarz M, King T, eds. Interstitial lung disease, 4th edn. Toronto: Brian C Decker, 2003:825–837.

204. Oldham SA, Castillo M, Jacobson FL, et al. HIV-associated lymphocytic interstitial pneumonia: radiologic manifestations and pathologic correlation. Radiology 1989;170:83–87.

205. Johkoh T, Müller NL, Pickford HA, et al. Lymphocytic interstitial pneumonia: thin-section CT findings in 22 patients. Radiology 1999;212:567–572.

206. Ichikawa Y, Kinoshita M, Koga T, et al. Lung cyst formation in lymphocytic interstitial pneumonitis: CT features. J Comput Assist Tomogr 1994;18:745–748.

207. Koyama M, Johkoh T, Honda O, et al. Chronic cystic lung disease: diagnostic accuracy of high-resolution CT in 92 patients. AJR Am J Roentgenol 2003;180:827–835.

208. Honda O, Johkoh T, Ichikado K, et al. Differential diagnosis of lymphocytic interstitial pneumonia and malignant lymphoma on high-resolution CT. AJR Am J Roentgenol 1999;173:71–74.

209. McGuinness G, Scholes JV, Jagirdar JS, et al. Unusual lymphoproliferative disorders in nine adults with HIV or AIDS: CT and pathologic findings. Radiology 1995;197:59–65.

210. Carignan S, Staples CA, Müller NL. Intrathoracic lymphoproliferative disorders in the immunocompromised patient: CT findings. Radiology 1995;197:53–58.

211. Johkoh T, Ichikado K, Akira M, et al. Lymphocytic interstitial pneumonia: follow-up CT findings in 14 patients. J Thorac Imaging 2000;15:162–167.

212. Hodgson U, Laitinen T, Tukiainen P. Nationwide prevalence of sporadic and familial idiopathic pulmonary fibrosis: evidence of founder effect among multiplex families in Finland. Thorax 2002;57:338–342.

213. Marshall RP, Puddicombe A, Cookson WO, et al. Adult familial cryptogenic fibrosing alveolitis in the United Kingdom. Thorax 2000;55: 143–146.

214. Buchino JJ, Keenan WJ, Algren JT, et al. Familial desquamative interstitial pneumonitis occurring in infants. Am J Med Genet Suppl 1987;3:285–291.

215. Amin RS, Wert SE, Baughman RP, et al. Surfactant protein deficiency in familial interstitial lung disease. J Pediatr 2001;139:85–92.

216. Lynch D, Newell J, Logan P, et al. Can CT distinguish idiopathic pulmonary fibrosis from hypersensitivity

pneumonitis? AJR Am J Roentegenol 1995;165:807–811.

217. Hansell DM, Wells AU, Padley SP, et al. Hypersensitivity pneumonitis: correlation of individual CT patterns with functional abnormalities. Radiology 1996;199:123–128.

218. Chung MH, Edinburgh KJ, Webb EM, et al. Mixed infiltrative and obstructive disease on high-resolution CT: differential diagnosis and functional correlates in a consecutive series. J Thorac Imaging 2001;16:69–75.

219. Perez-Padilla R, Salas J, Chapela R, et al. Mortality in Mexican patients with chronic pigeon breeder's lung compared with those with usual interstitial pneumonia. Am Rev Respir Dis 1993;148:49–53.

220. Padley SP, Padhani AR, Nicholson A, et al. Pulmonary sarcoidosis mimicking cryptogenic fibrosing alveolitis on CT. Clin Radiol 1996;51:807–810.

221. Watters L, King T, Schwarz M, et al. A clinical, radiologic and pathologic scoring system for the longitudinal assessment of patients with idiopathic pulmonary fibrosis. Am Rev Resp Dis 1986;133:97–103.

222. McLoud TC, Carrington CB, Gaensler EA. Diffuse infiltrative lung disease: a new scheme for description. Radiology 1983;149:353–363.

223. Collard HR, King TE Jr, Bartelson BB, et al. Changes in clinical and physiologic variables predict survival in idiopathic pulmonary fibrosis. Am J Respir Crit Care Med 2003;168:538–542.

224. Latsi PI, du Bois RM, Nicholson AG, et al. Fibrotic idiopathic interstitial pneumonia: the prognostic value of longitudinal functional trends. Am J Respir Crit Care Med 2003;168:531–537.

225. Wells AU, Rubens MB, du Bois RM, et al. Functional impairment in fibrosing alveolitis: relationship to reversible disease on thin section computed tomography. Eur Resp J 1997;10:280–285.

226. Grenier P, Valeyre D, Cluzel P, et al. Chronic diffuse interstitial lung disease: diagnostic value of chest radiography and high-resolution CT. Radiology 1991;179:123–132.

227. Collins CD, Wells AU, Hansell DM et al. Observer variation in pattern type and extent of disease in fibrosing alveolitis on thin section computed tomography and chest radiography. Clin Radiol 1994;49:236–240.

228. Gamsu G, Salmon CJ, Warnock ML, et al. CT quantification of interstitial fibrosis in patients with asbestosis: a comparison of two methods. AJR Am J Roentgenol 1995;164:63–64.

229. Coxson HO, Hogg JC, Mayo JR et al. Quantification of idiopathic pulmonary fibrosis using computed tomography and histology. Am J Respir Crit Care Med 1997;155:1649–1656.

230. Hartley PG, Galvin JR, Hunninghake GW, et al. High-resolution CT-derived measures of lung density are valid indexes of interstitial lung disease. J Appl Physiol 1994;76:271–277.

231. Best AC, Lynch AM, Bozic CM, et al. Quantitative CT indexes in idiopathic pulmonary fibrosis: relationship with physiologic impairment. Radiology 2003;228:407–414.

232. Delorme S, Keller-Reichenbecher MA, Zuna I, et al. Usual interstitial pneumonia. Quantitative assessment of high-resolution computed tomography findings by computer-assisted texture-based image analysis. Invest Radiol 1997;32:566–574.

233. Rodriguez LH, Vargas PF, Raff U, et al. Automated discrimination and quantification of idiopathic pulmonary fibrosis from normal lung parenchyma using generalized fractal dimensions in high-resolution computed tomography images. Acad Radiol 1995;2:10–18.

234. Coxson HO, Rogers RM, Whittall KP, et al. A quantification of the lung surface area in emphysema using computed tomography. Am J Respir Crit Care Med 1999;159:851–856.

235. Goldin J. Quantitative CT of the lung. Radiol Clin North Am 2002;40:145–162.

236. Uppaluri R, Hoffman EA, Sonka M, et al. Interstitial lung disease: A quantitative study using the adaptive multiple feature method. Am J Respir Crit Care Med 1999;159:519–525.

237. Strickland NH, Hughes JM, Hart DA, et al. Cause of regional ventilation-perfusion mismatching in patients with idiopathic pulmonary fibrosis: a combined CT and scintigraphic study. AJR Am J Roentgenol 1993;161:719–725.

238. Mino M, Noma S, Kobashi Y, et al. Serial changes of cystic air spaces in fibrosing alveolitis: a CT-pathological study. Clin Radiol 1995;50:357–363.

239. Wells AU, Desai SR, Rubens MB, et al. Idiopathic pulmonary fibrosis: a composite physiologic index derived from disease extent observed by computed tomography. Am J Respir Crit Care Med 2003;167:962–969.

240. Nagao T, Nagai S, Hiramoto Y, et al. Serial evaluation of high-resolution computed tomography findings in patients with idiopathic pulmonary fibrosis in usual interstitial pneumonia. Respiration 2002;69:413–419.

241. Genereux GP. The end-stage lung: pathogenesis, pathology, and radiology. Radiology 1975;116:279–289.

242. Heitzman ER. The lung: radiological and pathologic correlations. St Louis: Mosby, 1984.

243. Hogg JC. Benjamin Felson lecture. Chronic interstitial lung disease of unknown cause: a new classification based on pathogenesis. AJR Am J Roentgenol 1991;156:225–233.

244. Tuddenham WJ. Glossary of terms for thoracic radiology: recommendations of the Nomenclature Committee of the Fleischner Society. AJR Am J Roentgenol 1984;143:509–517.

245. Mendeloff J. Disseminated nodular pulmonary ossification in the Hamman-Rich lung. Am Rev Respir Dis 1971;103:269–274.

246. Primack SL, Hartman TE, Hansell DM, et al. End-stage lung disease: CT findings in 61 patients. Radiology 1993:189:681–686.

247. Kim EA, Lee KS, Johkoh T, et al. Interstitial lung diseases associated with collagen vascular diseases: radiologic and histopathologic findings. RadioGraphics 2002;22:S151–165.

248. Freemer M, King T. Connective tissue diseases. In: Schwarz M, King T, eds. Interstitial lung disease, 4th edn. Toronto: Brian C Decker, 2003:535–598.

249. Arnett FC, Edworthy SM, Bloch DA, et al. The American Rheumatism Association 1987 revised criteria for the classification of rheumatoid arthritis. Arthritis Rheum 1988;31:315–324.

250. Turesson C, O'Fallon WM, Crowson CS, et al. Extra-articular disease manifestations in rheumatoid arthritis: incidence trends and risk factors over 46 years. Ann Rheum Dis 2003;62:722–727.

251. Ellman P, Ball R. "Rheumatoid disease" with joint and pulmonary manifestations. Br Med J 1948;2:816–819.

252. Hunninghake GW, Fauci AS. Pulmonary involvement in the collagen vascular diseases. Am Rev Respir Dis 1979;119:471–503.

253. Tanoue LT. Pulmonary manifestations of rheumatoid arthritis. Clin Chest Med 1998;19:667–685.

254. Jurik AG, Davidsen D, Graudal H. Prevalence of pulmonary involvement in rheumatoid arthritis and its relationship to some characteristics of the patients. A radiological and clinical study. Scand J Rheumatol 1982;11:217–224.

255. Shiel WC Jr, Prete PE. Pleuropulmonary manifestations of rheumatoid arthritis. Semin Arthritis Rheum 1984;13:235–243.

256. Yousem SA, Colby TV, Carrington CB. Lung biopsy in rheumatoid arthritis. Am Rev Respir Dis 1985;131:770–777.

257. Sahn SA. Immunologic diseases of the pleura. Clin Chest Med 1985;6:83–102.

258. Walker WC, Wright V. Rheumatoid pleuritis. Ann Rheum Dis 1967;26:467–474.

259. Jurik AG, Graudal H. Pleurisy in rheumatoid arthritis. Scand J Rheumatol 1983;12:75–80.

260. Walker W, Wright V. Pulmonary lesions and rheumatoid arthritis. Medicine (Baltimore) 1968;47:501–520.

261. Carr D, Mayne J. Pleurisy with effusion in rheumatoid arthritis, with reference to the low concentration of glucose in pleural fluid. Am Rev Respir Dis 1962;85:345–350.

262. Campbell GD, Ferrington E. Rheumatoid pleuritis with effusion. Dis Chest 1968; 53:521–527.

263. Brennan SR, Daly JJ. Large pleural effusions in rheumatoid arthritis. Br J Dis Chest 1979;73:133–140.

264. Pritikin JD, Jensen WA, Yenokida GG, et al. Respiratory failure due to a massive rheumatoid pleural effusion. J Rheumatol 1990;17:673–675.

265. Martel W, Abell MR, Mikkelsen WM, et al. Pulmonary and pleural lesions in rheumatoid disease. Radiology 1968;90: 641–653.

266. Evans WV. Bilateral pneumothoraces and pleural effusions in rheumatoid lung disease. Thorax 1984;39:213–214.

267. Ayzenberg O, Reiff DB, Levin L. Bilateral pneumothoraces and pleural effusions complicating rheumatoid lung disease. Thorax 1983;38:159–160.

268. Brunk JR, Drash EC, Swineford O Jr. Rheumatoid pleuritis successfully treated with decortication. Report of a case and review of the literature. Am J Med Sci 1966;251:545–551.

269. Shannon TM, Gale ME. Noncardiac manifestations of rheumatoid arthritis in the thorax. J Thorac Imaging 1992; 7:19–29.

270. Portner MM, Gracie WA Jr. Rheumatoid lung disease with cavitary nodules, pneumothorax and eosinophilia. N Engl J Med 1966;275:697–700.

271. Chou CW, Chang SC. Pleuritis as a presenting manifestation of rheumatoid arthritis: diagnostic clues in pleural fluid cytology. Am J Med Sci 2002;323: 158–161.

272. Jones FL Jr, Blodgett RC Jr. Empyema in rheumatoid pleuropulmonary disease. Ann Intern Med 1971;74:665–671.

273. Dieppe PA. Empyema in rheumatoid arthritis. Ann Rheum Dis 1975;34: 181–185.

274. Remy-Jardin M, Remy J, Cortet B, et al. Lung changes in rheumatoid arthritis: CT findings. Radiology 1994;193:375–382.

275. Davies D. Pyopneumothorax in rheumatoid lung disease. Thorax 1966;21:230–235.

276. Crisp AJ, Armstrong RD, Grahame R, et al. Rheumatoid lung disease, pneumothorax, and eosinophilia. Ann Rheum Dis 1982;41:137–140.

277. Sharma SS, Reynolds PM. Broncho-pleural fistula complicating rheumatoid lung disease. Postgrad Med J 1982;58: 187–189.

278. Talbott J, Calkins E. Pulmonary involvement in rheumatoid arthritis. JAMA 1964;189:911–913.

279. Aronoff A, Bywaters E, Fearnley G. Lung lesions in rheumatoid arthritis. Br Med J 1955;2:228–232.

280. Doctor L, Snider G. Diffuse interstitial pulmonary fibrosis associated with arthritis. Am Rev Respir Dis 1962;85: 413–422.

281. Turner-Warwick M, Evans R. Pulmonary manifestations of rheumatoid disease. Clin Rheum Dis 1977;3:549–564.

282. Roschmann RA, Rothenberg RJ. Pulmonary fibrosis in rheumatoid arthritis: a review of clinical features and therapy. Semin Arthritis Rheum 1987;16:174–185.

283. Frank ST, Weg JG, Harkleroad LE, et al. Pulmonary dysfunction in rheumatoid disease. Chest 1973; 63:27–34.

284. Pommepuy I, Farny M, Billey T, et al. Bronchiolitis obliterans organizing pneumonia in a patient with rheumatoid arthritis. Revue Du Rhumatisme (English Edn) 1998;65:65–67.

285. Hakala M, Paakko P, Huhti E, et al. Open lung biopsy of patients with rheumatoid arthritis. Clin Rheumatol 1990;9:452–460.

286. Patterson C, Harville W, Pierce J. Rheumatoid lung disease. Ann Intern Med 1965;62:685–697.

287. Popper MS, Bogdonoff ML, Hughes RL. Interstitial rheumatoid lung disease. A reassessment and review of the literature. Chest 1972;62:243–250.

288. Tomasi T, Fudenberg H, Finby N. Possible relationship of rheumatoid factors and pulmonary disease. Am J Med 1962;33:243–248.

289. Hubbard R, Venn A. The impact of coexisting connective tissue disease on survival in patients with fibrosing alveolitis. Rheumatology (Oxford) 2002;41:676–679.

290. Lynch JP 3rd, Hunninghake GW. Pulmonary complications of collagen vascular disease. Annu Rev Med 1992;43:17–35.

291. Locke G. Rheumatoid lung. Clin Radiol 1963;14:43–53.

292. Fraser R, Pare J, Pare P, et al. Diagnosis of diseases of the chest. Philadelphia: WB Saunders, 1989.

293. Thadani U. Rheumatoid lung disease with pulmonary fibrosis necrobiotic nodules and pleural effusion. Br J Dis Chest 1973;67:146–152.

294. Staples C, Müller N, Vedal S, et al. Usual interstitial pneumonia: Correlation of CT with clinical, functional, and radiographic findings. Radiology 1987;162:377–381.

295. Steinberg DL, Webb WR. CT appearances of rheumatoid lung disease. J Comput Assist Tomogr 1984;8:881–884.

296. Fewins HE, McGowan I, Whitehouse GH, et al. High definition computed tomography in rheumatoid arthritis associated pulmonary disease. Br J Rheumatol 1991;30:214–216.

297. Macfarlane JD, Dieppe PA, Rigden BG, et al. Pulmonary and pleural lesions in rheumatoid disease. Br J Dis Chest 1978;72:288–300.

298. Strohl KP, Feldman NT, Ingram RH Jr. Apical fibrobullous disease with rheumatoid arthritis. Chest 1979; 75:739–741.

299. Petrie GR, Bloomfield P, Grant IW, et al. Upper lobe fibrosis and cavitation in rheumatoid disease. Br J Dis Chest 1980;74:263–267.

300. Macfarlane JD, Franken CK, van Leeuwen AW. Progressive cavitating pulmonary changes in rheumatoid arthritis: a case report. Ann Rheum Dis 1984;43:98–101.

301. Yue CC, Park CH, Kushner I. Apical fibrocavitary lesions of the lung in rheumatoid arthritis. Report of two cases and review of the literature. Am J Med 1986;81:741–746.

302. Katzenstein A-L. Katzenstein and Askin's surgical pathology of non-neoplastic lung disease, 3rd edn. Philadelphia: WB Saunders, 1997.

303. Hull S, Mathews JA. Pulmonary necrobiotic nodules as a presenting feature of rheumatoid arthritis. Ann Rheum Dis 1982;41:21–24.

304. Eraut D, Evans J, Caplin M. Pulmonary necrobiotic nodules without rheumatoid arthritis. Br J Dis Chest 1978;72:301–306.

305. Scadding J. The lung in rheumatoid arthritis. Proc Roy Soc Med 1969;62: 227–238.

306. Burke GW, Carrington CB, Grinnan R. Pulmonary nodules and rheumatoid factor in the absence of arthritis. Chest 1977;72:538–540.

307. Panettiere F, Chandler B, Libcke J. Pulmonary cavitation in rheumatoid disease. Am Rev Respir Dis 1968;97:89–95.

308. Burrows FG. Pulmonary nodules in rheumatoid disease: a report of two cases. Br J Radiol 1967;40:256–261.

309. Sieniewicz DJ, Martin JR. Cavitating rheumatoid nodules in the lung: follow-up report. J Can Assoc Radiol 1967;18: 401–403.

310. Hart F. Complicated rheumatoid disease. Br Med J 1966;2:131–135.

311. Morgan WK, Wolfel DA. The lungs and pleura in rheumatoid arthritis. Am J Roentgenol 1966;98:334–342.

312. Jolles H, Moseley PL, Peterson MW. Nodular pulmonary opacities in patients with rheumatoid arthritis. A diagnostic dilemma. Chest 1989;96:1022–1025.

313. Filho JS, Soares MF, Wal R, et al. Fine-needle aspiration cytology of pulmonary rheumatoid nodule: case report and review of the major cytologic features. Diagn Cytopathol 2002;26:150–153.

314. Ip MS, Wong MP, Wong KL. Rheumatoid nodules in the trachea. Chest 1993;103: 301–303.

315. Gabbay E, Tarala R, Will R, et al. Interstitial lung disease in recent onset rheumatoid arthritis. Am J Respir Crit Care Med 1997;156:528–535.

316. McDonagh J, Greaves M, Wright AR, et al. High resolution computed tomography of the lungs in patients with rheumatoid arthritis and interstitial lung disease. Br J Rheumatol 1994;33:118–122.

317. Cortet B, Perez T, Roux N, et al. Pulmonary function tests and high resolution computed tomography of the lungs in patients with rheumatoid arthritis. Ann Rheum Dis 1997;56:596–600.

318. Walker WC. Pulmonary infections and rheumatoid arthritis. Q J Med 1967;36:239–251.

319. Bamji A, Cooke N. Rheumatoid arthritis and chronic bronchial suppuration. Scand J Rheumatol 1985;14:15–21.

320. Shadick NA, Fanta CH, Weinblatt ME, et al. Bronchiectasis. A late feature of severe rheumatoid arthritis. Medicine (Baltimore) 1994;73:161–170.

321. Hassan WU, Keaney NP, Holland CD, et al. High resolution computed tomography of the lung in lifelong non-smoking patients with rheumatoid arthritis. Ann Rheum Dis 1995;54:308–310.

322. McMahon MJ, Swinson DR, Shettar S, et al. Bronchiectasis and rheumatoid arthritis: a clinical study. Ann Rheum Dis 1993;52:776–779.

323. Perez T, Remy-Jardin M, Cortet B. Airways involvement in rheumatoid arthritis: clinical, functional, and HRCT findings. Am J Respir Crit Care Med 1998;157:1658–1665.

324. Geddes DM, Corrin B, Brewerton DA, et al. Progressive airway obliteration in adults and its association with rheumatoid disease. Q J Med 1977;46:427–444.

325. McCann BG, Hart GJ, Stokes TC, et al. Obliterative bronchiolitis and upper-zone pulmonary consolidation in rheumatoid arthritis. Thorax 1983;38:73–74.

326. Hakala M, Paakko P, Sutinen S, et al. Association of bronchiolitis with connective tissue disorders. Ann Rheum Dis 1986;45:656–662.

327. Epler GR, Snider GL, Gaensler EA, et al. Bronchiolitis and bronchitis in connective tissue disease. A possible relationship to the use of penicillamine. JAMA 1979;242:528–532.

328. Murphy KC, Atkins CJ, Offer RC, et al. Obliterative bronchiolitis in two rheumatoid arthritis patients treated with penicillamine. Arthritis Rheum 1981;24:557–560.

329. O'Duffy JD, Luthra HS, Unni KK, et al. Bronchiolitis in a rheumatoid arthritis patient receiving auranofin. Arthritis Rheum 1986;29:556–559.

330. Sweatman MC, Millar AB, Strickland B, et al. Computed tomography in adult obliterative bronchiolitis. Clin Radiol 1990;41:116–119.

331. Aquino SL, Webb WR, Golden J. Bronchiolitis obliterans associated with rheumatoid arthritis: findings on HRCT and dynamic expiratory CT. J Comput Assist Tomogr 1994;18:555–558.

332. Schwarz MI, Lynch DA, Tuder R. Bronchiolitis obliterans: the lone manifestation of rheumatoid arthritis? Eur Respir J 1994;7:817–820.

333. Worthy SA, Müller NL. Small airway diseases. Radiol Clin North Am 1998;36:163–173.

334. Hayakawa H, Sato A, Imokawa S, et al. Bronchiolar disease in rheumatoid arthritis. Am J Respir Crit Care Med 1996;154:1531–1536.

335. Balagopal VP, da Costa P, Greenstone MA. Fatal pulmonary hypertension and rheumatoid vasculitis. Eur Respir J 1995;8:331–333.

336. Kinoshita M, Higashi T, Tanaka C, et al. Follicular bronchiolitis associated with rheumatoid arthritis. Intern Med 1992;31:674–677.

337. Howling SJ, Hansell DM, Wells AU, et al. Follicular bronchiolitis: thin-section CT and histologic findings. Radiology 1999;212:637–642.

338. Homma S, Kawabata M, Kishi K, et al. Diffuse panbronchiolitis in rheumatoid arthritis. Eur Respir J 1998;12:444–452.

339. Hellems SO, Kanner RE, Renzetti AD Jr. Bronchocentric granulomatosis associated with rheumatoid arthritis. Chest 1983;83:831–832.

340. Berendsen HH, Hofstee N, Kapsenberg PD, et al. Bronchocentric granulomatosis associated with seropositive polyarthritis. Thorax 1985;40:396–397.

341. Bonafede RP, Benatar SR. Bronchocentric granulomatosis and rheumatoid arthritis. Br J Dis Chest 1987;81:197–201.

342. Fujii M, Adachi S, Shimizu T, et al. Interstitial lung disease in rheumatoid arthritis: assessment with high-resolution computed tomography. J Thorac Imaging 1993;8:54–62.

343. Cortet B, Flipo RM, Remy-Jardin M, et al. Use of high resolution computed tomography of the lungs in patients with rheumatoid arthritis. Ann Rheum Dis 1995;54:815–819.

344. Caplan A. Certain unusual radiological appearances in the chest of coal-miners suffering from rheumatoid arthritis. Thorax 1953;8:29–37.

345. Caplan A, Payne R, Withey J. A broader concept of Caplan's syndrome related to rheumatoid factors. Thorax 1962;17:205–212.

346. Tellesson WG. Rheumatoid pneumoconiosis (Caplan's syndrome) in an asbestos worker. Thorax 1961;16:372–377.

347. Morgan W. Rheumatoid pneumoconiosis in association with asbestosis. Thorax 1964;19:433–435.

348. Jordan J. Pulmonary fibrosis in a worker using an aluminum powder. Br J Ind Med 1961;18:21–23.

349. Anttila S, Sutinen S, Paakko P, et al. Rheumatoid pneumoconiosis in a dolomite worker: a light and electron microscopic, and X-ray microanalytical study. Br J Dis Chest 1984;78:195–200.

350. Caplan A, Cowen ED, Gough J. Rheumatoid pneumoconiosis in a foundry worker. Thorax 1958;13:181–184.

351. Unge G, Mellner C. Caplan's syndrome – a clinical study of 13 cases. Scand J Respir Dis 1975;56:287–291.

352. Chatgidakis CB, Theron CP. Rheumatoid pneumoconiosis (Caplan's syndrome). A discussion of the disease and a report of a case in a European Witwatersrand gold miner. Arch Environ Health 1961;2:397–408.

353. Cunningham CD, Hugh AE. Pneumoconiosis in women. Clin Radiol 1973;24:491–493.

354. Watson AJ, Black J, Doig AT, et al. Pneumoconiosis in carbon electrode makers. Br J Ind Med 1959;16:274–285.

355. Gough J, Rivers D, Seal R. Pathological studies of modified pneumoconiosis in coal-miners with rheumatoid arthritis (Caplan's syndrome). Thorax 1955;10:9–18.

356. Parkes WR. Occupational lung disorders, 3rd edn. London: Butterworth-Heinemann, 1994.

357. Benedek TG, Zawadzki ZA, Medsger TA Jr. Serum immunoglobulins, rheumatoid factor, and pneumoconiosis in coal miners with rheumatoid arthritis. Arthritis Rheum 1976;19:731–736.

358. Scott DG, Bacon PA, Tribe CR. Systemic rheumatoid vasculitis: a clinical and laboratory study of 50 cases. Medicine (Baltimore) 1981;60:288–297.

359. Kay JM, Banik S. Unexplained pulmonary hypertension with pulmonary arteritis in rheumatoid disease. Br J Dis Chest 1977;71:53–59.

360. Baydur A, Mongan ES, Slager UT. Acute respiratory failure and pulmonary arteritis without parenchymal involvement: demonstration in a patient with rheumatoid arthritis. Chest 1979;75:518–520.

361. Young ID, Ford SE, Ford PM. The association of pulmonary hypertension with rheumatoid arthritis. J Rheumatol 1989;16:1266–1269.

362. Armstrong JG, Steele RH. Localised pulmonary arteritis in rheumatoid disease. Thorax 1982;37:313–314.

363. Beck ER, Hoffbrand BI. Acute lung changes in rheumatoid arthritis. Ann Rheum Dis 1966;25:459–462.

364. Leatherman JW, Sibley RK, Davies SF. Diffuse intrapulmonary hemorrhage and

glomerulonephritis unrelated to anti-glomerular basement membrane antibody. Am J Med 1982;72:401–410.

365. Zitnik R, Cooper J. Pulmonary disease due to antirheumatic agents. Clin Chest Med 1990;11:139–150.

366. Hargreaves MR, Mowat AG, Benson MK. Acute pneumonitis associated with low dose methotrexate treatment for rheumatoid arthritis: report of five cases and review of published reports. Thorax 1992;47:628–633.

367. Hilliquin P, Renoux M, Perrot S, et al. Occurrence of pulmonary complications during methotrexate therapy in rheumatoid arthritis. Br J Rheumatol 1996;35:441–445.

368. Golden MR, Katz RS, Balk RA, et al. The relationship of preexisting lung disease to the development of methotrexate pneumonitis in patients with rheumatoid arthritis. J Rheumatol 1995;22:1043–1047.

369. Goodwin SD, Glenny RW. Nonsteroidal anti-inflammatory drug-associated pulmonary infiltrates with eosinophilia. Review of the literature and Food and Drug Administration Adverse Drug Reaction reports. Arch Intern Med 1992;152:1521–1524.

370. Prakash UB, Luthra HS, Divertie MB. Intrathoracic manifestations in mixed connective tissue disease. Mayo Clin Proc 1985;60:813–821.

371. Bouros D, Hatzakis K, Labrakis H, et al. Association of malignancy with diseases causing interstitial pulmonary changes. Chest 2002;121:1278–1289.

372. Cervera R, Khamashta MA, Font J, et al. Systemic lupus erythematosus: clinical and immunologic patterns of disease expression in a cohort of 1,000 patients. The European Working Party on Systemic Lupus Erythematosus. Medicine (Baltimore) 1993;72: 113–124.

373. Tan EM, Cohen AS, Fries JF, et al. The 1982 revised criteria for the classification of systemic lupus erythematosus. Arthritis Rheum 1982;25:1271–1277.

374. Masi AT, Kaslow RA. Sex effects in systemic lupus erythematosus: a clue to pathogenesis. Arthritis Rheum 1978;21:480–484.

375. Christian CL. Systemic lupus erythematosus: clinical manifestations and prognosis. Arthritis Rheum 1982;25:887–888.

376. Dubois E, Tuffanelli D. Clinical manifestations of systemic lupus erythematosus. Computer analysis of 520 cases. JAMA 1964;190:104–111.

377. Pisetsky DS, Gilkeson G, St Clair EW. Systemic lupus erythematosus. Diagnosis and treatment. Med Clin North Am 1997;81:113–128.

378. Grigor R, Edmonds J, Lewkonia R, et al. Systemic lupus erythematosus.

A prospective analysis. Ann Rheum Dis 1978;37:121–128.

379. Turner-Stokes L, Turner-Warwick M. Intrathoracic manifestations of SLE. Clin Rheum Dis 1982;8:229–242.

380. Chang RW. Cardiac manifestations of SLE. Clin Rheum Dis 1982;8:197–206.

381. Wiedemann HP, Matthay RA. Pulmonary manifestations of systemic lupus erythematosus. J Thorac Imaging 1992;7:1–18.

382. Harvey AM, Shulman LE, Tumulty PA, et al. Systemic lupus erythematosus: review of the literature and clinical analysis of 138 cases. Medicine (Baltimore) 1954;33:291–437.

383. Estes D, Christian CL. The natural history of systemic lupus erythematosus by prospective analysis. Medicine (Baltimore) 1971;50:85–95.

384. Pisetsky DS. Systemic lupus erythematosus. Med Clin North Am 1986;70:337–353.

385. Murin S, Wiedemann HP, Matthay RA. Pulmonary manifestations of systemic lupus erythematosus. Clin Chest Med 1998;19:641–665.

386. Winslow WA, Ploss LN, Loitman B. Pleuritis in systemic lupus erythematosus: its importance as an early manifestation in diagnosis. Ann Intern Med 1958;49:70–88.

387. Levin DC. Proper interpretation of pulmonary roentgen changes in systemic lupus erythematosus. Am J Roentgenol Radium Ther Nucl Med 1971;111: 510–517.

388. Good JT Jr, King TE, Antony VB, et al. Lupus pleuritis. Clinical features and pleural fluid characteristics with special reference to pleural fluid antinuclear antibodies. Chest 1983;84:714–718.

389. Gould D, Daves M. A review of roentgen findings in systemic lupus erythematosus (SLE). Am J Med Sci 1958;235:596–610.

390. Bulgrin J, Dubois E. Chest roentgenographic changes in systemic lupus erythematosus. Radiology 1960;74:42–48.

391. Haupt HM, Moore GW, Hutchins GM. The lung in systemic lupus erythematosus. Analysis of the pathologic changes in 120 patients. Am J Med 1981;71:791–798.

392. Bell R, Lawrence DS. Chronic pleurisy in systemic lupus erythematosus treated with pleurectomy. Br J Dis Chest 1979;73:314–316.

393. Matthay RA, Schwarz MI, Petty TL, et al. Pulmonary manifestations of systemic lupus erythematosus: review of twelve cases of acute lupus pneumonitis. Medicine 1975;54:397–409.

394. Holgate ST, Glass DN, Haslam P, et al. Respiratory involvement in systemic lupus erythematosus. A clinical

and immunological study. Clin Exp Immunol 1976;24:385–395.

395. Miller LR, Greenberg SD, McLarty JW. Lupus lung. Chest 1985;88:265–269.

396. Carette S, Macher AM, Nussbaum A, et al. Severe, acute pulmonary disease in patients with systemic lupus erythematosus: ten years of experience at the National Institutes of Health. Semin Arthritis Rheum 1984;14: 52–59.

397. Zamora MR, Warner ML, Tuder R, et al. Diffuse alveolar hemorrhage and systemic lupus erythematosus. Clinical presentation, histology, survival, and outcome. Medicine (Baltimore) 1997;76:192–202.

398. Wu CY, Chiou YH, Chiu PC, et al. Severe pulmonary hemorrhage as the initial manifestation in systemic lupus erythematosus with active nephritis. Lupus 2001;10:879–882.

399. Eagen JW, Memoli VA, Roberts JL, et al. Pulmonary hemorrhage in systemic lupus erythematosus. Medicine (Baltimore) 1978;57:545–560.

400. Gamsu G, Webb WR. Pulmonary hemorrhage in systemic lupus erythematosus. J Can Assoc Radiol 1978;29:66–68.

401. Ewan PW, Jones HA, Rhodes CG, et al. Detection of intrapulmonary hemorrhage with carbon monoxide uptake. Application in Goodpasture's syndrome. N Engl J Med 1976;295: 1391–1396.

402. Onomura K, Nakata H, Tanaka Y, et al. Pulmonary hemorrhage in patients with systemic lupus erythematosus. J Thorac Imaging 1991;6:57–61.

403. Pines A, Kaplinsky N, Olchovsky D, et al. Pleuro-pulmonary manifestations of systemic lupus erythematosus: clinical features of its subgroups. Prognostic and therapeutic implications. Chest 1985;88: 129–135.

404. Hsu BY, Edwards DK 3rd, Trambert MA. Pulmonary hemorrhage complicating systemic lupus erythematosus: role of MR imaging in diagnosis. AJR Am J Roentgenol 1992;158:519–520.

405. Eisenberg H, Dubois EL, Sherwin RP, et al. Diffuse interstitial lung disease in systemic lupus erythematosus. Ann Intern Med 1973;79:37–45.

406. Bankier AA, Kiener HP, Wiesmayr MN, et al. Discrete lung involvement in systemic lupus erythematosus: CT assessment. Radiology 1995;196: 835–840.

407. Fenlon HM, Doran M, Sant SM, et al. High-resolution chest CT in systemic lupus erythematosus. AJR Am J Roentgenol 1996;166:301–307.

408. Hoffbrand B, Beck E. "Unexplained" dyspnoea and shrinking lungs in systemic lupus erythematosus. Br Med J 1965;1:1273–1277.

409. Gibson GJ. Diaphragmatic paresis: pathophysiology, clinical features, and investigation. Thorax 1989;44:960–970.

410. Gibson CJ, Edmonds JP, Hughes GR. Diaphragm function and lung involvement in systemic lupus erythematosus. Am J Med 1977; 63:926–932.

411. Martens J, Demedts M, Vanmeenen MT, et al. Respiratory muscle dysfunction in systemic lupus erythematosus. Chest 1983;84:170–175.

412. Rubin LA, Urowitz MB. Shrinking lung syndrome in SLE – a clinical pathologic study. J Rheumatol 1983;10:973–976.

413. Hawkins P, Davison AG, Dasgupta B, et al. Diaphragm strength in acute systemic lupus erythematosus in a patient with paradoxical abdominal motion and reduced lung volumes. Thorax 2001;56:329–330.

414. Laroche CM, Mulvey DA, Hawkins PN, et al. Diaphragm strength in the shrinking lung syndrome of systemic lupus erythematosus. Q J Med 1989;71:429–439.

415. Karim MY, Miranda LC, Tench CM, et al. Presentation and prognosis of the shrinking lung syndrome in systemic lupus erythematosus. Semin Arthritis Rheum 2002;31:289–298.

416. Weinrib L, Sharma OP, Quismorio FP Jr. A long-term study of interstitial lung disease in systemic lupus erythematosus. Semin Arthritis Rheum 1990;20:48–56.

417. Fayemi AO. Pulmonary vascular disease in systemic lupus erythematosus. Am J Clin Pathol 1976;65:284–290.

418. Yokoi T, Tomita Y, Fukaya M, et al. Pulmonary hypertension associated with systemic lupus erythematosus: predominantly thrombotic arteriopathy accompanied by plexiform lesions. Arch Pathol Lab Med 1998;122:467–470.

419. Perez HD, Kramer N. Pulmonary hypertension in systemic lupus erythematosus: report of four cases and review of the literature. Semin Arthritis Rheum 1981;11:177–181.

420. Asherson RA, Mackworth-Young CG, Boey ML, et al. Pulmonary hypertension in systemic lupus erythematosus. Br Med J (Clin Res Ed) 1983;287:1024–1025.

421. Simonson JS, Schiller NB, Petri M, et al. Pulmonary hypertension in systemic lupus erythematosus. J Rheumatol 1989;16:918–925.

422. Winslow TM, Ossipov MA, Fazio GP, et al. Five-year follow-up study of the prevalence and progression of pulmonary hypertension in systemic lupus erythematosus. Am Heart J 1995;129:510–515.

423. Rubin LA, Geran A, Rose TH, et al. A fatal pulmonary complication of lupus in pregnancy. Arthritis Rheum 1995;38:710–714.

424. Horn CA. Pulmonary hypertension and autoimmune disease. Chest 1993;104:279–280; discussion 280–282.

425. Love PE, Santoro SA. Antiphospholipid antibodies: anticardiolipin and the lupus anticoagulant in systemic lupus erythematosus (SLE) and in non-SLE disorders. Prevalence and clinical significance. Ann Intern Med 1990;112:682–698.

426. Gilkeson RC, Patz EF Jr, Culhane D, McAdams HP, Provenzale JM. Thoracic imaging features of patients with antiphospholipid antibodies. J Comput Assist Tomogr 1998; 22:241–244.

427. Ando M, Takamoto S, Okita Y, et al. Operation for chronic pulmonary thromboembolism accompanied by thrombophilia in 8 patients. Ann Thorac Surg 1998;66:1919–1924.

428. Sandoval J, Amigo MC, Barragan R, et al. Primary antiphospholipid syndrome presenting as chronic thromboembolic pulmonary hypertension. Treatment with thromboendarterectomy. J Rheumatol 1996;23:772–775.

429. Karmochkine M, Cacoub P, Dorent R, et al. High prevalence of antiphospholipid antibodies in precapillary pulmonary hypertension. J Rheumatol 1996;23: 286–290.

430. Chung MH, Lee HG, Kwon SS, et al. Pulmonary arterial aneurysms in primary antiphospholipid antibody syndrome. J Comput Assist Tomogr 2002;26:608–612.

431. Biyajima S, Osada T, Daidoji H, et al. Pulmonary hypertension and antiphospholipid antibody in a patient with Sjögren's syndrome. Intern Med 1994;33:768–772.

432. Savin H, Huberman M, Kott E, et al. Fibrosing alveolitis associated with primary antiphospholipid syndrome. Br J Rheumatol 1994;33:977–980.

433. Provenzale JM, Ortel TL. Anatomic distribution of venous thrombosis in patients with antiphospholipid antibody: imaging findings. AJR Am J Roentgenol 1995;165:365–368.

434. Bacharach JM, Stanson AW, Lie JT, et al. Imaging spectrum of thrombo-occlusive vascular disease associated with antiphospholipid antibodies. RadioGraphics 1993;13:417–423.

435. Mana F, Mets T, Vincken W, et al. The association of bronchiolitis obliterans organizing pneumonia, systemic lupus erythematosus, and Hunner's cystitis. Chest 1993;104:642–644.

436. Yum MN, Ziegler JR, Walker PD, et al. Pseudolymphoma of the lung in a patient with systemic lupus erythematosus. Am J Med 1979;66: 172–176.

437. Abramson SB, Dobro J, Eberle MA, et al. Acute reversible hypoxemia in systemic lupus erythematosus. Ann Intern Med 1991;114:941–947.

438. Kishida Y, Kanai Y, Kuramochi S, et al. Pulmonary venoocclusive disease in a patient with systemic lupus erythematosus. J Rheumatol 1993;20: 2161–2162.

439. Gross M, Esterly JR, Earle RH. Pulmonary alterations in systemic lupus erythematosus. Am Rev Respir Dis 1972;105:572–577.

440. Hellmann DB, Petri M, Whiting-O'Keefe Q. Fatal infections in systemic lupus erythematosus: the role of opportunistic organisms. Medicine (Baltimore) 1987;66:341–348.

441. Webb WR, Gamsu G. Cavitary pulmonary nodules with systemic lupus erythematosus: differential diagnosis. AJR Am J Roentgenol 1981;136:27–31.

442. Boumpas DT, Austin HA 3rd, Fessler BJ, et al. Systemic lupus erythematosus: emerging concepts. Part 1: Renal, neuropsychiatric, cardiovascular, pulmonary, and hematologic disease. Ann Intern Med 1995;122:940–950.

443. Owens GR, Follansbee WP. Cardiopulmonary manifestations of systemic sclerosis. Chest 1987;91: 118–127.

444. Silver RM, Miller KS. Lung involvement in systemic sclerosis. Rheum Dis Clin North Am 1990;16:199–216.

445. Mayes MD. Classification and epidemiology of scleroderma. Semin Cutan Med Surg 1998;17:22–26.

446. Steen VD. Clinical manifestations of systemic sclerosis. Semin Cutan Med Surg 1998;17:48–54.

447. Minai OA, Dweik RA, Arroliga AC. Manifestations of scleroderma pulmonary disease. Clin Chest Med 1998;19:713–731, viii–ix.

448. Tashkin DP, Clements PJ, Wright RS, et al. Interrelationships between pulmonary and extrapulmonary involvement in systemic sclerosis. A longitudinal analysis. Chest 1994;105:489–495.

449. Preliminary criteria for the classification of systemic sclerosis (scleroderma). Subcommittee for scleroderma criteria of the American Rheumatism Association Diagnostic and Therapeutic Criteria Committee. Arthritis Rheum 1980; 23:581–590.

450. Lonzetti LS, Joyal F, Raynauld JP, et al. Updating the American College of Rheumatology preliminary classification criteria for systemic sclerosis: addition of severe nailfold capillaroscopy abnormalities markedly increases the sensitivity for limited scleroderma. Arthritis Rheum 2001;44:735–738.

451. Steen VD, Powell DL, Medsger TA Jr. Clinical correlations and prognosis based on serum autoantibodies in

patients with systemic sclerosis. Arthritis Rheum 1988;31:196–203.

452. Kane GC, Varga J, Conant EF, et al. Lung involvement in systemic sclerosis (scleroderma): relation to classification based on extent of skin involvement or autoantibody status. Respir Med 1996;90:223–230.

453. LeRoy EC. A brief overview of the pathogenesis of scleroderma (systemic sclerosis). Ann Rheum Dis 1992;51: 286–288.

454. Behr J, Adelmann-Grill BC, Hein R, et al. Pathogenetic and clinical significance of fibroblast activation in scleroderma lung disease. Respiration 1995;62:209–216.

455. Jimenez SA, Hitraya E, Varga J. Pathogenesis of scleroderma. Collagen. Rheum Dis Clin North Am 1996;22: 647–674.

456. White B. Immunopathogenesis of systemic sclerosis. Rheum Dis Clin North Am 1996;22:695–708.

457. Young RH, Mark GJ. Pulmonary vascular changes in scleroderma. Am J Med 1978;64:998–1004.

458. D'Angelo WA, Fries JF, Masi AT, et al. Pathologic observations in systemic sclerosis (scleroderma). A study of fifty-eight autopsy cases and fifty-eight matched controls. Am J Med 1969;46:428–440.

459. Weaver AL, Divertie MB, Titus JL. Pulmonary scleroderma. Dis Chest 1968;54:490–498.

460. Cointrel C, Tillie-Leblond I, Lamblin C, et al. [Erasmus syndrome: clinical, tomographic, respiratory function and bronchoalveolar lavage characteristics]. Revue Maladies Respiratoires 1997;14:21–26.

461. Vancheeswaran R, Black CM, David J, et al. Childhood-onset scleroderma: is it different from adult-onset disease. Arthritis Rheum 1996;39:1041–1049.

462. Emery H. Pediatric scleroderma. Semin Cutan Med Surg 1998;17:41–47.

463. Pope JE. Treatment of systemic sclerosis. Rheum Dis Clin North Am 1996;22: 893–907.

464. van den Hoogen FH, Boerbooms AM, Swaak AJ, et al. Comparison of methotrexate with placebo in the treatment of systemic sclerosis: a 24 week randomized double-blind trial, followed by a 24 week observational trial. Br J Rheumatol 1996;35:364–372.

465. Hunzelmann N, Anders S, Fierlbeck G, et al. Systemic scleroderma. Multicenter trial of 1 year of treatment with recombinant interferon gamma. Arch Dermatol 1997;133:609–613.

466. Wigley FM, Korn JH, Csuka ME, et al. Oral iloprost treatment in patients with Raynaud's phenomenon secondary to systemic sclerosis: a multicenter, placebo-controlled, double-blind study. Arthritis Rheum 1998;41:670–677.

467. Medsger TA Jr, Masi AT. Survival with scleroderma. II. A life-table analysis of clinical and demographic factors in 358 male U.S. veteran patients. J Chronic Dis 1973;26:647–660.

468. Lee P, Langevitz P, Alderdice CA, et al. Mortality in systemic sclerosis (scleroderma). Q J Med 1992;82:139–148.

469. Arroliga AC, Podell DN, Matthay RA. Pulmonary manifestations of scleroderma. J Thorac Imaging 1992;7:30–45.

470. Morelli S, Barbieri C, Sgreccia A, et al. Relationship between cutaneous and pulmonary involvement in systemic sclerosis. J Rheumatol 1997;24:81–85.

471. Steen VD, Owens GR, Fino GJ, et al. Pulmonary involvement in systemic sclerosis (scleroderma). Arthritis Rheum 1985;28:759–767.

472. Wells AU, Hansell DM, Rubens MB, et al. Fibrosing alveolitis in systemic sclerosis: indices of lung function in relation to extent of disease on computed tomography. Arthritis Rheum 1997; 40:1229–1236.

473. Taormina VJ, Miller WT, Gefter WB, et al. Progressive systemic sclerosis subgroups: variable pulmonary features. AJR Am J Roentgenol 1981;137:277–285.

474. Lomeo RM, Cornella RJ, Schabel SI, et al. Progressive systemic sclerosis sine scleroderma presenting as pulmonary interstitial fibrosis. Am J Med 1989;87:525–527.

475. Gondos B. Roentgen manifestations in progressive systemic sclerosis (diffuse scleroderma). Am J Roentgenol Radium Ther Nucl Med 1960;84:235–247.

476. Ashba JK, Ghanem MH. The lungs in systemic sclerosis. Dis Chest 1965;47: 52–64.

477. Bergemann A, Tikly M. Cystic lung disease in systemic sclerosis: a case report with high resolution computed tomography findings. Rev Rheum (Engl edn) 1996;63:213–215.

478. Iliffe GD, Pettigrew NM. Hypoventilatory respiratory failure in generalised scleroderma. Br Med J (Clin Res Ed) 1983;286:337–338.

479. Subbarao K, Jacobson HG. Systemic disorders affecting the thoracic cage. Radiol Clin North Am 1984;22:497–517.

480. Sargent EN, Turner AF, Jacobson G. Superior marginal rib defects. An etiologic classification. Am J Roentgenol Radium Ther Nucl Med 1969;106: 491–505.

481. Gurtler KF, Erbe W, Kreysel HW, et al. [Radiological observations of the chest in progressive scleroderma]. ROFO Fortschr Geb Rontgenstr Nuklearmed 1977;126:97–101.

482. Dinsmore RE, Goodman D, Dreyfuss JR. The air esophagram: a sign of scleroderma involving the esophagus. Radiology 1966;87:348–349 passim.

483. Olive A, Juncosa S, Evison G, et al. Air in the oesophagus: a sign of oesophageal involvement in systemic sclerosis. Clin Rheumatol 1995;14: 319–321.

484. Proto AV, Lane EJ. Air in the esophagus: a frequent radiographic finding. AJR Am J Roentgenol 1977;129:433–440.

485. Martinez LO. Air in the esophagus as a sign of scleroderma (differential diagnosis with some other entities). J Can Assoc Radiol 1974;25:234–237.

486. Bhalla M, Silver RM, Shepard J, et al. Chest CT in patients with scleroderma: prevalence of asymptomatic esophageal dilatation and mediastinal lymphadenopathy. Am J Roentgenol 1993;161:269–272.

487. Chan TY, Hansell DM, Rubens MB, et al. Cryptogenic fibrosing alveolitis and the fibrosing alveolitis of systemic sclerosis: morphological differences on computed tomographic scans. Thorax 1997;52:265–270.

488. Garber SJ, Wells AU, duBois RM, et al. Enlarged mediastinal lymph nodes in the fibrosing alveolitis of systemic sclerosis. Br J Radiol 1992;65:983–986.

489. Wechsler RJ, Ayyangar K, Steiner RM, et al. The development of distant pulmonary infiltrates following thoracic irradiation: the role of computed tomography with dosimetric reconstruction in diagnosis. Comput Med Imaging Graph 1990;14:43–51.

490. Schurawitzki H, Stiglbauer R, Graninger W, et al. Interstitial lung disease in progressive systemic sclerosis: high-resolution CT versus radiography. Radiology 1990;176:755–759.

491. Warrick JH, Bhalla M, Schabel SI, et al. High resolution computed tomography in early scleroderma lung disease. J Rheumatol 1991;18:1520–1528.

492. Wells AU, Hansell DM, Corrin B, et al. High resolution computed tomography as a predictor of lung histology in systemic sclerosis. Thorax 1992;47: 738–742.

493. Remy-Jardin M, Remy J, Wallaert B, et al. Pulmonary involvement in progressive systemic sclerosis: sequential evaluation with CT, pulmonary function tests, and bronchoalveolar lavage. Radiology 1993;188:499–506.

494. Devenyi K, Czirjak L. High resolution computed tomography for the evaluation of lung involvement in 101 patients with scleroderma. Clin Rheumatol 1995;14:633–640.

495. Seely JM, Jones LT, Wallace C, et al. Systemic sclerosis: using high-resolution CT to detect lung disease in children. AJR Am J Roentgenol 1998;170:691–697.

496. Harrison NK, Myers AR, Corrin B, et al. Structural features of interstitial lung disease in systemic sclerosis. Am Rev Respir Dis 1991;144:706–713.

497. Wechsler RJ, Steiner RM, Spirn PW, et al. The relationship of thoracic lymphadenopathy to pulmonary interstitial disease in diffuse and limited systemic sclerosis: CT findings. AJR Am J Roentgenol 1996;167:101–104.

498. Eisenberg H. The interstitial lung diseases associated with the collagen-vascular disorders. Clin Chest Med 1982;3:565–578.

499. Battle RW, Davitt MA, Cooper SM, et al. Prevalence of pulmonary hypertension in limited and diffuse scleroderma. Chest 1996;110:1515–1519.

500. Trell E, Lindstrom C. Pulmonary hypertension in systemic sclerosis. Ann Rheum Dis 1971;30:390–400.

501. Ungerer RG, Tashkin DP, Furst D, et al. Prevalence and clinical correlates of pulmonary arterial hypertension in progressive systemic sclerosis. Am J Med 1983;75:65–74.

502. Stupi AM, Steen VD, Owens GR, et al. Pulmonary hypertension in the CREST syndrome variant of systemic sclerosis. Arthritis Rheum 1986;29:515–524.

503. Cailes JB, du Bois RM, Hansell DM. Density gradient of the lung parenchyma at computed tomographic scanning in patients with pulmonary hypertension and systemic sclerosis. Acad Radiol 1996;3:724–730.

504. Pearson JE, Silman AJ. Risk of cancer in patients with scleroderma. Ann Rheum Dis 2003;62:697–699.

505. Duncan SC, Winkelmann RK. Cancer and scleroderma. Arch Dermatol 1979;115:950–955.

506. Hill CL, Nguyen AM, Roder D, et al. Risk of cancer in patients with scleroderma: a population based cohort study. Ann Rheum Dis 2003;62:728–731.

507. Peters-Golden M, Wise RA, Hochberg M, et al. Incidence of lung cancer in systemic sclerosis. J Rheumatol 1985;12:1136–1139.

508. Guttadauria M, Ellman H, Kaplan D. Progressive systemic sclerosis: pulmonary involvement. Clin Rheum Dis 1979;5:151–166.

509. Johnson DA, Drane WE, Curran J, et al. Pulmonary disease in progressive systemic sclerosis. A complication of gastroesophageal reflux and occult aspiration? Arch Intern Med 1989;149:589–593.

510. Troshinsky MB, Kane GC, Varga J, et al. Pulmonary function and gastroesophageal reflux in systemic sclerosis. Ann Intern Med 1994;121:6–10.

511. Lock G, Pfeifer M, Straub RH, et al. Association of esophageal dysfunction and pulmonary function impairment in systemic sclerosis. Am J Gastroenterol 1998;93:341–345.

512. Kim EA, Johkoh T, Lee KS, et al. Interstitial pneumonia in progressive systemic sclerosis: serial high-resolution CT findings with functional correlation. J Comput Assist Tomogr 2001;25:757–763.

513. Muir TE, Tazelaar HD, Colby TV, et al. Organizing diffuse alveolar damage associated with progressive systemic sclerosis. Mayo Clin Proc 1997;72:639–642.

514. Renzoni E, Rottoli P, Coviello G, et al. Clinical, laboratory and radiological findings in pulmonary fibrosis with and without connective tissue disease. Clin Rheumatol 1997;16:570–577.

515. Schimke RN, Kirkpatrick CH, Delp MH. Calcinosis, Raynaud's phenomenon, sclerodactyly, and telangiectasia. The CRST syndrome. Arch Intern Med 1967;119:365–370.

516. Winterbauer RH. Multiple telangiectasia, Raynaud's phenomenon, sclerodactyly, and subcutaneous calcinosis: a syndrome mimicking hereditary hemorrhagic telangiectasia. Bull Johns Hopkins Hosp 1964;114:361–383.

517. Fritzler MJ, Kinsella TD. The CREST syndrome: a distinct serologic entity with anticentromere antibodies. Am J Med 1980;69:520–526.

518. Salerni R, Rodnan GP, Leon DF, et al. Pulmonary hypertension in the CREST syndrome variant of progressive systemic sclerosis (scleroderma). Ann Intern Med 1977;86:394–399.

519. Yousem SA. The pulmonary pathologic manifestations of the CREST syndrome. Hum Pathol 1990;21:467–474.

520. Velayos EE, Masi AT, Stevens MB, et al. The 'CREST' syndrome. Comparison with systemic sclerosis (scleroderma). Arch Intern Med 1979;139:1240–1244.

521. Owens GR, Fino GJ, Herbert DL, et al. Pulmonary function in progressive systemic sclerosis. Comparison of CREST syndrome variant with diffuse scleroderma. Chest 1983;84:546–550.

522. Dubois EL, Chandor S, Friou GJ, et al. Progressive systemic sclerosis (PSS) and localized scleroderma (morphea) with positive LE cell test and unusual systemic manifestations compatible with systemic lupus erythematous (SLE): presentation of 14 cases including one set of identical twins, one with scleroderma and the other with SLE. Review of the literature. Medicine (Baltimore) 1971;50:199–222.

523. Bohan A, Peter JB. Polymyositis and dermatomyositis (first of two parts). N Engl J Med 1975;292:344–347.

524. Schwarz MI. The lung in polymyositis. Clin Chest Med 1998;19:701–712, viii.

525. Schwarz MI. Pulmonary and cardiac manifestations of polymyositis-dermatomyositis. J Thorac Imaging 1992;7:46–54.

526. el-Azhary RA, Pakzad SY. Amyopathic dermatomyositis: retrospective review of 37 cases. J Am Acad Dermatol 2002; 46:560–565.

527. Cottin V, Thivolet-Bejui F, Reynaud-Gaubert M, et al. Interstitial lung disease in amyopathic dermatomyositis, dermatomyositis and polymyositis. Eur Respir J 2003;22:245–250.

528. Dickey BF, Myers AR. Pulmonary disease in polymyositis/dermatomyositis. Semin Arthritis Rheum 1984;14:60–76.

529. Thompson PL, Mackay IR. Fibrosing alveolitis and polymyositis. Thorax 1970;25:504–507.

530. Frazier AR, Miller RD. Interstitial pneumonitis in association with polymyositis and dermatomyositis. Chest 1974;65:403–407.

531. Salmeron G, Greenberg SD, Lidsky MD. Polymyositis and diffuse interstitial lung disease. A review of the pulmonary histopathologic findings. Arch Intern Med 1981;141:1005–1010.

532. Friedman AW, Targoff IN, Arnett FC. Interstitial lung disease with autoantibodies against aminoacyl-tRNA synthetases in the absence of clinically apparent myositis. Semin Arthritis Rheum 1996;26:459–467.

533. Bernstein RM, Morgan SH, Chapman J, et al. Anti-Jo-1 antibody: a marker for myositis with interstitial lung disease. Br Med J (Clin Res Ed) 1984;289:151–152.

534. Schumacher HR, Schimmer B, Gordon GV, et al. Articular manifestations of polymyositis and dermatomyositis. Am J Med 1979;67:287–292.

535. Olsen GN, Swenson EW. Polymyositis and interstitial lung disease. Am Rev Respir Dis 1972;105:611–617.

536. Duncan PE, Griffin JP, Garcia A, et al. Fibrosing alveolitis in polymyositis. A review of histologically confirmed cases. Am J Med 1974;57:621–626.

537. Schwarz MI, Matthay RA, Sahn SA, et al. Interstitial lung disease in polymyositis and dermatomyositis: analysis of six cases and review of the literature. Medicine (Baltimore) 1976;55:89–104.

538. Fergusson RJ, Davidson NM, Nuki G, et al. Dermatomyositis and rapidly progressive fibrosing alveolitis. Thorax 1983;38:71–72.

539. Johkoh T, Ikezoe J, Kohno N, et al. High-resolution CT and pulmonary function tests in collagen vascular disease: comparison with idiopathic pulmonary fibrosis. Eur J Radiol 1994;18:113–121.

540. Lakhanpal S, Lie JT, Conn DL, et al. Pulmonary disease in polymyositis/dermatomyositis: a clinicopathological analysis of 65 autopsy cases. Ann Rheum Dis 1987;46:23–29.

541. Akira M, Hara H, Sakatani M. Interstitial lung disease in association with polymyositis-dermatomyositis: long-term follow-up CT evaluation in seven patients. Radiology 1999;210:333–338.

542. Ikezoe J, Johkoh T, Kohno N, et al. High-resolution CT findings of lung disease in patients with polymyositis and dermatomyositis. J Thorac Imaging 1996;11:250–259.

543. Bunch TW, Tancredi RG, Lie JT. Pulmonary hypertension in polymyositis. Chest 1981;79:105–107.

544. Schwarz MI, Sutarik JM, Nick JA, et al. Pulmonary capillaritis and diffuse alveolar hemorrhage. A primary manifestation of polymyositis. Am J Respir Crit Care Med 1995;151: 2037–2040.

545. Douglas WW, Tazelaar HD, Hartman TE, et al. Polymyositis-dermatomyositis-associated interstitial lung disease. Am J Respir Crit Care Med 2001;164: 1182–1185.

546. Arakawa H, Yamada H, Kurihara Y, et al. Nonspecific interstitial pneumonia associated with polymyositis and dermatomyositis: serial high-resolution CT findings and functional correlation. Chest 2003;123:1096–1103.

547. Mino M, Noma S, Taguchi Y, et al. Pulmonary involvement in polymyositis and dermatomyositis: sequential evaluation with CT. AJR Am J Roentgenol 1997;169:83–87.

548. Akira M, Hara H, Sakatani M. Interstitial lung disease in association with polymyositis- dermatomyositis: long-term follow-up CT evaluation in seven patients. Radiology 1999;210:333–338.

549. Fishman AP. State of the art: chronic cor pulmonale. Am Rev Respir Dis 1976;114:775–794.

550. Schiavi EA, Roncoroni AJ, Puy RJ. Isolated bilateral diaphragmatic paresis with interstitial lung disease. An unusual presentation of dermatomyositis. Am Rev Respir Dis 1984;129:337–339.

551. O'Hara JM, Szemes G, Lowman RM. The esophageal lesions in dermatomyositis. A correlation of radiologic and pathologic findings. Radiology 1967;89:27–31.

552. Grunebaum M, Salinger H. Radiologic findings in polymyositis-dermatomyositis involving the pharynx and upper oesophagus. Clin Radiol 1971;22:97–100.

553. Metheny JA. Dermatomyositis: a vocal and swallowing disease entity. Laryngoscope 1978;88:147–161.

554. Braun NM, Arora NS, Rochester DF. Respiratory muscle and pulmonary function in polymyositis and other proximal myopathies. Thorax 1983;38:616–623.

555. Rochester DF, Arora NS. Respiratory muscle failure. Med Clin North Am 1983;67:573–597.

556. Barnes BE, Mawr B. Dermatomyositis and malignancy. A review of the literature. Ann Intern Med 1976;84: 68–76.

557. Sigurgeirsson B, Lindelof B, Edhag O, Allander E. Risk of cancer in patients with dermatomyositis or polymyositis. A population-based study. N Engl J Med 1992;326:363–367.

558. Richardson JB, Callen JP. Dermatomyositis and malignancy. Med Clin North Am 1989;73:1211–1220.

559. Callen JP. When and how should the patient with dermatomyositis or amyopathic dermatomyositis be assessed for possible cancer? Arch Dermatol 2002;138:969–971.

560. Wakata N, Kurihara T, Saito E, et al. Polymyositis and dermatomyositis associated with malignancy: a 30-year retrospective study. Int J Dermatol 2002;41:729–734.

561. Buchbinder R, Hill CL. Malignancy in patients with inflammatory myopathy. Curr Rheumatol Rep 2002;4:415–426.

562. Mahe E, Descamps V, Burnouf M, et al. A helpful clinical sign predictive of cancer in adult dermatomyositis: cutaneous necrosis. Arch Dermatol 2003;139:539.

563. Tan E, Tan SH, Ng SK. Cutaneous mucinosis in dermatomyositis associated with a malignant tumor. J Am Acad Dermatol 2003;48:S41–42.

564. Callen JP. Myositis and malignancy. Clin Rheum Dis 1984;10:117–130.

565. Caro I. Dermatomyositis as a systemic disease. Med Clin North Am 1989;73: 1181–1192.

566. Marguerie C, Bunn CC, Copier J, et al. The clinical and immunogenetic features of patients with autoantibodies to the nucleolar antigen PM-Scl. Medicine (Baltimore) 1992;71:327–336.

567. Bohan A, Peter JB, Bowman RL, et al. Computer-assisted analysis of 153 patients with polymyositis and dermatomyositis. Medicine (Baltimore) 1977;56:255–286.

568. Winkelmann RK. Dermatomyositis in childhood. Clin Rheum Dis 1982;8: 353–368.

569. Pachman LM. Juvenile dermatomyositis. Pathophysiology and disease expression. Pediatr Clin North Am 1995;42: 1071–1098.

570. Park S, Nyhan WL. Fatal pulmonary involvement in dermatomyositis. Am J Dis Child 1975;129:723–726.

571. Fox RI. Sjogren's syndrome. Curr Opin Rheumatol 1995;7:409–416.

572. Vitali C, Bombardieri S, Moutsopoulos HM, et al. Assessment of the European classification criteria for Sjogren's syndrome in a series of clinically defined cases: results of a prospective multicentre study. The European Study Group on Diagnostic Criteria for Sjogren's Syndrome. Ann Rheum Dis 1996;55:116–121.

573. Alexander EL, Provost TT, Stevens MB, et al. Neurologic complications of primary Sjogren's syndrome. Medicine (Baltimore) 1982;61:247–257.

574. Fishback N, Koss M. Update of lymphoid interstitial pneumonia. Curr Opin Pulmonary Med 1996;2:429–433.

575. Desai SR, Nicholson AG, Stewart S, et al. Benign pulmonary lymphocytic infiltration and amyloidosis: computed tomographic and pathologic features in three cases. J Thorac Imaging 1997;12: 215–220.

576. Deheinzelin D, Capelozzi VL, Kairalla RA, et al. Interstitial lung disease in primary Sjogren's syndrome. Clinical-pathological evaluation and response to treatment. Am J Respir Crit Care Med 1996;154:794–799.

577. Tonami H, Matoba M, Yokota H, et al. Mucosa-associated lymphoid tissue lymphoma in Sjogren's syndrome: initial and follow-up imaging features. AJR Am J Roentgenol 2002;179:485–489.

578. Ioannidis JP, Vassiliou VA, Moutsopoulos HM. Long-term risk of mortality and lymphoproliferative disease and predictive classification of primary Sjogren's syndrome. Arthritis Rheum 2002;46:741–747.

579. Tanoue LT. Pulmonary involvement in collagen vascular disease: a review of the pulmonary manifestations of the Marfan syndrome, ankylosing spondylitis, Sjogren's syndrome, and relapsing polychondritis. J Thorac Imaging 1992;7:62–77.

580. Cain HC, Noble PW, Matthay RA. Pulmonary manifestations of Sjogren's syndrome. Clin Chest Med 1998;19: 687–699, viii.

581. Bloch KJ, Buchanan WW, Wohl MJ, et al. Sjogren's syndrome. A clinical, pathological, and serological study of sixty-two cases. Medicine (Baltimore) 1965;44:187–231.

582. Shearn MA. Sjogren's syndrome. Med Clin North Am 1977;61:271–282.

583. Constantopoulos SH, Tsianos EV, Moutsopoulos HM. Pulmonary and gastrointestinal manifestations of Sjogren's syndrome. Rheum Dis Clin North Am 1992;18:617–635.

584. Newball HH, Brahim SA. Chronic obstructive airway disease in patients with Sjogren's syndrome. Am Rev Respir Dis 1977;115:295–304.

585. Kruize AA, Hene RJ, van der Heide A, et al. Long-term followup of patients with Sjogren's syndrome. Arthritis Rheum 1996;39:297–303.

586. Fairfax AJ, Haslam PL, Pavia D, et al. Pulmonary disorders associated with Sjogren's syndrome. Q J Med 1981;50:279–295.

587. Segal I, Fink G, Machtey I, et al. Pulmonary function abnormalities in

Sjögren's syndrome and the sicca complex. Thorax 1981;36:286–289.

588. Wallaert B, Hatron PY, Grosbois JM, et al. Subclinical pulmonary involvement in collagen-vascular diseases assessed by bronchoalveolar lavage. Relationship between alveolitis and subsequent changes in lung function. Am Rev Respir Dis 1986;133:574–580.

589. Cain HC, Noble PW, Matthay RA. Pulmonary manifestations of Sjögren's syndrome. Clin Chest Med 1998;19:687–699.

590. Strimlan CV, Rosenow EC 3rd, Divertie MB, et al. Pulmonary manifestations of Sjögren's syndrome. Chest 1976;70:354–361.

591. Bariffi F, Pesci A, Bertorelli G, et al. Pulmonary involvement in Sjögren's syndrome. Respiration 1984;46:82–87.

592. Constantopoulos SH, Papadimitriou CS, Moutsopoulos HM. Respiratory manifestations in primary Sjögren's syndrome. A clinical, functional, and histologic study. Chest 1985;88:226–229.

593. Franquet T, Gimenez A, Monill JM, et al. Primary Sjögren's syndrome and associated lung disease: CT findings in 50 patients. AJR Am J Roentgenol 1997;169:655–658.

594. Quismorio FP Jr. Pulmonary involvement in primary Sjögren's syndrome. Curr Opin Pulm Med 1996;2:424–428.

595. Papathanasiou MP, Constantopoulos SH, Tsampoulas C, et al. Reappraisal of respiratory abnormalities in primary and secondary Sjögren's syndrome. A controlled study. Chest 1986;90:370–374.

596. Constantopoulos SH, Drosos AA, Maddison PJ, et al. Xerotrachea and interstitial lung disease in primary Sjögren's syndrome. Respiration 1984;46:310–314.

597. Liebow AA, Carrington CB. Diffuse pulmonary lymphoreticular infiltrations associated with dysproteinemia. Med Clin North Am 1973;57:809–843.

598. Alkhayer M, McCann BG, Harrison BD. Lymphocytic interstitial pneumonitis in association with Sjögren's syndrome. Br J Dis Chest 1988;82:305–309.

599. Karlish AJ. Lung changes in Sjögren's syndrome. Proc R Soc Med 1969;62:1042–1043.

600. Gardiner P, Ward C, Allison A, et al. Pleuropulmonary abnormalities in primary Sjögren's syndrome. J Rheumatol 1993;20:831–837.

601. Andonopoulos AP, Karadanas AH, Drosos AA, et al. CT evaluation of mediastinal lymph nodes in primary Sjogren syndrome. J Comput Assist Tomogr 1988;12:199–201.

602. Sato T, Matsubara O, Tanaka Y, et al. Association of Sjögren's syndrome with pulmonary hypertension: report of two cases and review of the literature. Hum Pathol 1993;24:199–205.

603. Taouli B, Brauner MW, Mourey I, Lemouchi D, Grenier PA. Thin-section chest CT findings of primary Sjögren's syndrome: correlation with pulmonary function. Eur Radiol 2002;12:1504–1511.

604. Meyer CA, Pina JS, Taillon D, et al. Inspiratory and expiratory high-resolution CT findings in a patient with Sjögren's syndrome and cystic lung disease. AJR Am J Roentgenol 1997;168:101–103.

605. Sharp GC, Irvin WS, Tan EM, et al. Mixed connective tissue disease – an apparently distinct rheumatic disease syndrome associated with a specific antibody to an extractable nuclear antigen (ENA). Am J Med 1972;52:148–159.

606. Alarcon-Segovia D, Cardiel MH. Comparison between 3 diagnostic criteria for mixed connective tissue disease. Study of 593 patients. J Rheumatol 1989;16:328–334.

607. van den Hoogen FH, Spronk PE, Boerbooms AM, et al. Long-term follow-up of 46 patients with anti-(U1)snRNP antibodies. Br J Rheumatol 1994;33:1117–1120.

608. Bennett RM, O'Connell DJ. Mixed connective tisssue disease: a clinicopathologic study of 20 cases. Semin Arthritis Rheum 1980;10:25–51.

609. Prakash UB. Respiratory complications in mixed connective tissue disease. Clin Chest Med 1998;19:733–746, ix.

610. Harmon C, Wolfe F, Lillard S, et al. Pulmonary involvement in mixed connective tissue disease (MCTD) [abstract]. Arthritis Rheum 1976;19:801.

611. Sullivan WD, Hurst DJ, Harmon CE, et al. A prospective evaluation emphasizing pulmonary involvement in patients with mixed connective tissue disease. Medicine (Baltimore) 1984;63:92–107.

612. Derderian SS, Tellis CJ, Abbrecht PH, et al. Pulmonary involvement in mixed connective tissue disease. Chest 1985;88:45–48.

613. Guit GL, Shaw PC, Ehrlich J, et al. Mediastinal lymphadenopathy and pulmonary arterial hypertension in mixed connective tissue disease. Radiology 1985;154:305–306.

614. Oetgen WJ, Mutter ML, Lawless OJ, et al. Cardiac abnormalities in mixed connective tissue disease. Chest 1983;83:185–188.

615. Prakash UB. Lungs in mixed connective tissue disease. J Thorac Imaging 1992;7:55–61.

616. Kozuka T, Johkoh T, Honda O, et al. Pulmonary involvement in mixed connective tissue disease: high-resolution CT findings in 41 patients. J Thorac Imaging 2001;16:94–98.

617. Fagan KA, Badesch DB. Pulmonary hypertension associated with connective tissue disease. Prog Cardiovasc Dis 2002;45:225–234.

618. Wiener-Kronish JP, Solinger AM, Warnock ML, et al. Severe pulmonary involvement in mixed connective tissue disease. Am Rev Respir Dis 1981;124:499–503.

619. Jones MB, Osterholm RK, Wilson RB, et al. Fatal pulmonary hypertension and resolving immune-complex glomerulonephritis in mixed connective tissue disease. A case report and review of the literature. Am J Med 1978;65:855–863.

620. Sanchez-Guerrero J, Cesarman G, Alarcon-Segovia D. Massive pulmonary hemorrhage in mixed connective tissue diseases. J Rheumatol 1989;16:1132–1134.

621. Martyn JB, Wong MJ, Huang SH. Pulmonary and neuromuscular complications of mixed connective tissue disease: a report and review of the literature. J Rheumatol 1988;15:703–705.

622. McAdam LP, O'Hanlan MA, Bluestone R, et al. Relapsing polychondritis: prospective study of 23 patients and a review of the literature. Medicine (Baltimore) 1976;55:193–215.

623. Lee-Chiong TL Jr. Pulmonary manifestations of ankylosing spondylitis and relapsing polychondritis. Clin Chest Med 1998;19:747–757, ix.

624. Dolan DL, Lemmon GB Jr, Teitelbaum SL. Relapsing polychondritis. Analytical literature review and studies on pathogenesis. Am J Med 1966;41:285–299.

625. Eng J, Sabanathan S. Airway complications in relapsing polychondritis. Ann Thorac Surg 1991;51:686–692.

626. Duke OL. Relapsing polychondritis. Br J Rheumatol 1988;27:423–425.

627. Michet CJ Jr, McKenna CH, Luthra HS, et al. Relapsing polychondritis. Survival and predictive role of early disease manifestations. Ann Intern Med 1986;104:74–78.

628. Damiani JM, Levine HL. Relapsing polychondritis – report of ten cases. Laryngoscope 1979;89:929–946.

629. Chang-Miller A, Okamura M, Torres VE, et al. Renal involvement in relapsing polychondritis. Medicine (Baltimore) 1987;66:202–217.

630. Choplin RH, Wehunt WD, Theros EG. Diffuse lesions of the trachea. Semin Roentgenol 1983;18:38–50.

631. Crockford MP, Kerr IH. Relapsing polychondritis. Clin Radiol 1988;39:386–390.

632. Davis SD, Berkmen YM, King T. Peripheral bronchial involvement in relapsing polychondritis: demonstration by thin-section CT. AJR Am J Roentgenol 1989;153:953–954.

633. Mohsenifar Z, Tashkin DP, Carson SA, et al. Pulmonary function in patients with relapsing polychondritis. Chest 1982;81:711–717.

634. Kilman WJ. Narrowing of the airway in relapsing polychondritis. Radiology 1978;126:373–376.

635. Tillie-Leblond I, Wallaert B, Leblond D, et al. Respiratory involvement in relapsing polychondritis. Clinical, functional, endoscopic, and radiographic evaluations. Medicine (Baltimore) 1998;77:168–176.

636. Mendelson DS, Som PM, Crane R, et al. Relapsing polychondritis studied by computed tomography. Radiology 1985;157:489–490.

637. Casselman JW, Lemahieu SF, Peene P, et al. Polychondritis affecting the laryngeal cartilages: CT findings. AJR Am J Roentgenol 1988;150:355–356.

638. Im JG, Chung JW, Han SK, et al. CT manifestations of tracheobronchial involvement in relapsing polychondritis. J Comput Assist Tomogr 1988;12:792–793.

639. Booth A, Dieppe PA, Goddard PL, et al. The radiological manifestations of relapsing polychondritis. Clin Radiol 1989;40:147–149.

640. Goddard P, Cook P, Laszlo G, et al. Relapsing polychondritis: report of an unusual case and a review of the literature. Br J Radiol 1991;64:1064–1067.

641. Behar JV, Choi YW, Hartman TA, et al. Relapsing polychondritis affecting the lower respiratory tract. AJR Am J Roentgenol 2002;178:173–177.

642. Quint LE, Whyte RI, Kazerooni EA, et al. Stenosis of the central airways: evaluation by using helical CT with multiplanar reconstructions. Radiology 1995;194:871–877.

643. Gibson GJ, Davis P. Respiratory complications of relapsing polychondritis. Thorax 1974;29:726–731.

644. Heman-Ackah YD, Remley KB, Goding GS Jr. A new role for magnetic resonance imaging in the diagnosis of laryngeal relapsing polychondritis. Head Neck 1999;21:484–489.

645. Kettering JM, Towers JD, Rubin DA. The seronegative spondyloarthropathies. Semin Roentgenol 1996;31:220–228.

646. Calin A. Ankylosing spondylitis. Clin Rheum Dis 1985;11:41–60.

647. Graham DC, Smythe HA. The carditis and aortitis of ankylosing spondylitis. Bull Rheum Dis 1958;9:171–174.

648. Bergfeldt L. HLA B27-associated rheumatic diseases with severe cardiac bradyarrhythmias. Clinical features and prevalence in 223 men with permanent pacemakers. Am J Med 1983;75:210–215.

649. Rosenow E, Strimlan CV, Muhm JR, et al. Pleuropulmonary manifestations of ankylosing spondylitis. Mayo Clin Proc 1977;52:641–649.

650. Haslock I. Ankylosing spondylitis. Baillière's Clin Rheumatol 1993;7:99–115.

651. Parkin A, Robinson PJ, Hickling P. Regional lung ventilation in ankylosing spondylitis. Br J Radiol 1982;55:833–836.

652. Cerrahoglu L, Unlu Z, Can M, et al. Lumbar stiffness but not thoracic radiographic changes relate to alteration of lung function tests in ankylosing spondylitis. Clin Rheumatol 2002;21:275–279.

653. Dunham C, Kautz F. Spondylarthritis ankylopoietica. Review and report of 20 cases. Am J Med Sci 1941;201:232–250.

654. Hamilton K. Pulmonary disease manifestations of ankylosing spondylarthritis. Ann Intern Med 1949;31:216–227.

655. Campbell AH, Macdonald CB. Upper lobe fibrosis associated with ankylosing spondylitis. Br J Dis Chest 1965;59:90–101.

656. Hillerdal G. Ankylosing spondylitis lung disease – an underdiagnosed entity? Eur J Respir Dis 1983;64:437–441.

657. Jessamine AG. Upper lung lobe fibrosis in ankylosing spondylitis. Can Med Assoc J 1968;98:25–29.

658. Wolson AH, Rohwedder JJ. Upper lobe fibrosis in ankylosing spondylitis. Am J Roentgenol Radium Ther Nucl Med 1975;124:466–471.

659. Cohen AA, Natelson EA, Fechner RE. Fibrosing interstitial pneumonitis in ankylosing spondylitis. Chest 1971;59:369–371.

660. Davies D. Ankylosing spondylitis and lung fibrosis. Q J Med 1972;41:395–417.

661. Chakera TM, Howarth FH, Kendall MJ, et al. The chest radiograph in ankylosing spondylitis. Clin Radiol 1975;26:455–459.

662. Boushea DK, Sundstrom WR. The pleuropulmonary manifestations of ankylosing spondylitis. Semin Arthritis Rheum 1989;18:277–281.

663. Dihlmann W. Current radiodiagnostic concept of ankylosing spondylitis. Skeletal Radiol 1979;4:179–188.

664. Sebes JI, Salazar JE. The manubriosternal joint in rheumatoid disease. AJR Am J Roentgenol 1983;140:117–121.

665. Levy H, Hurwitz MD, Strimling M, et al. Ankylosing spondylitis lung disease and *Mycobacterium scrofulaceum*. Br J Dis Chest 1988;82:84–87.

666. Fenlon HM, Casserly I, Sant SM, et al. Plain radiographs and thoracic high-resolution CT in patients with ankylosing spondylitis. AJR Am J Roentgenol 1997;168:1067–1072.

667. Turetschek K, Ebner W, Fleischmann D, et al. Early pulmonary involvement in ankylosing spondylitis: assessment with thin-section CT. Clin Radiol 2000;55:632–636.

668. El-Maghraoui A, Chaouir S, Bezza A, et al. Thoracic high resolution computed tomography in patients with ankylosing spondylitis and without respiratory symptoms. Ann Rheum Dis 2003;62:185–186.

669. Kiris A, Ozgocmen S, Kocakoc E, et al. Lung findings on high resolution CT in early ankylosing spondylitis. Eur J Radiol 2003;47:71–76.

670. Senocak O, Manisali M, Ozaksoy D, et al. Lung parenchyma changes in ankylosing spondylitis: demonstration with high resolution CT and correlation with disease duration. Eur J Radiol 2003;45:117–122.

671. Kinnear WJ, Shneerson JM. Acute pleural effusions in inactive ankylosing spondylitis. Thorax 1985;40:150–151.

672. Turner JF, Enzenauer RJ. Bronchiolitis obliterans and organizing pneumonia associated with ankylosing spondylitis. Arthritis Rheum 1994;37:1557–1559.

673. Blavia R, Toda MR, Vidal F, et al. Pulmonary diffuse amyloidosis and ankylosing spondylitis. A rare association. Chest 1992;102:1608–1610.

674. Jennette JC, Falk RJ, Andrassy K, et al. Nomenclature of systemic vasculitides. Proposal of an international consensus conference. Arthritis Rheum 1994;37:187–192.

675. Jennette JC, Falk RJ. Small-vessel vasculitis. N Engl J Med 1997;337:1512–1523.

676. Sullivan EJ, Hoffman GS. Pulmonary vasculitis. Clin Chest Med 1998;19:759–776, ix.

677. Klein RG, Hunder GG, Stanson AW, et al. Large artery involvement in giant cell (temporal) arteritis. Ann Intern Med 1975;83:806–812.

678. Lie JT. Disseminated visceral giant cell arteritis: histopathologic description and differentiation from other granulomatous vasculitides. Am J Clin Pathol 1978;69:299–305.

679. Ladanyi M, Fraser RS. Pulmonary involvement in giant cell arteritis. Arch Pathol Lab Med 1987;111:1178–1180.

680. Glover MU, Muniz J, Bessone L, et al. Pulmonary artery obstruction due to giant cell arteritis. Chest 1987;91:924–925.

681. Larson TS, Hall S, Hepper NG, et al. Respiratory tract symptoms as a clue to giant cell arteritis. Ann Intern Med 1984;101:594–597.

682. Romero S, Vela P, Padilla I, et al. Pleural effusion as manifestation of temporal arteritis. Thorax 1992;47:398–399.

683. Karam GH, Fulmer JD. Giant cell arteritis presenting as interstitial lung disease. Chest 1982;82:781–784.

684. Fulmer JD, Kaltreider HB. The pulmonary vasculitides. Chest 1982;82:615–624.

685. Doyle L, McWilliam L, Hasleton PS. Giant cell arteritis with pulmonary involvement. Br J Dis Chest 1988;82:88–92.

686. Bradley JD, Pinals RS, Blumenfeld HB, et al. Giant cell arteritis with pulmonary nodules. Am J Med 1984;77:135–140.

687. Travis WD. Pathology of pulmonary granulomatous vasculitis. Sarcoidosis Vasc Diffuse Lung Dis 1996;13:14–27.

688. Okubo S, Kunieda T, Ando M, et al. Idiopathic isolated pulmonary arteritis with chronic cor pulmonale. Chest 1988;94:665–666.

689. Wagenaar SS, Westermann CJ, Corrin B. Giant cell arteritis limited to large elastic pulmonary arteries. Thorax 1981;36:876–877.

690. Dennison AR, Watkins RM, Gunning AJ. Simultaneous aortic and pulmonary artery aneurysms due to giant cell arteritis. Thorax 1985;40:156–157.

691. Sieber SC, Cuello B, Gelfman NA, et al. Pulmonary capillaritis and glomerulonephritis in an antineutrophil cytoplasmic antibody-positive patient with prior granulomatous aortitis. Arch Pathol Lab Med 1990;114:1223–1226.

692. Lhote F, Guillevin L. Polyarteritis nodosa, microscopic polyangiitis, and Churg-Strauss syndrome. Clinical aspects and treatment. Rheum Dis Clin North Am 1995;21:911–947.

693. Spencer H. Pulmonary lesions in polyarteritis nodosa. Br J Tuberc Dis Chest 1957;51:123–130.

694. Rose GA, Spencer H. Polyarteritis nodosa. Q J Med 1957;26:43–81.

695. Lie JT. Systemic and isolated vasculitis. A rational approach to classification and pathologic diagnosis. Pathol Annu 1989;24 Pt 1:25–114.

696. Lie JT. Nomenclature and classification of vasculitis: plus ca change, plus c'est la meme chose. Arthritis Rheum 1994;37:181–186.

697. Nick J, Tuder R, May R, et al. Polyarteritis nodosa with pulmonary vasculitis. Am J Respir Crit Care Med 1996;153:450–453.

698. Matsumoto T, Homma S, Okada M, et al. The lung in polyarteritis nodosa: a pathologic study of 10 cases. Hum Pathol 1993;24:717–724.

699. Fauci AS, Haynes B, Katz P. The spectrum of vasculitis: clinical, pathologic, immunologic and therapeutic considerations. Ann Intern Med 1978;89:660–676.

700. Carratala J, Vidaller A, Mana J, et al. Polyarteritis nodosa associated with idiopathic pulmonary fibrosis: report of two cases. Ann Rheum Dis 1989;48:876–877.

701. Kallenberg CG, Brouwer E, Weening JJ, et al. Anti-neutrophil cytoplasmic antibodies: current diagnostic and pathophysiological potential. Kidney Int 1994;46:1–15.

702. Edwards CW. Vasculitis and granulomatosis of the respiratory tract. Thorax 1982;37:81–87.

703. Fauci AS, Haynes BF, Katz P, et al. Wegener's granulomatosis: prospective clinical and therapeutic experience with 85 patients for 21 years. Ann Intern Med 1983;98:76–85.

704. Leavitt RY, Fauci AS. Pulmonary vasculitis. Am Rev Respir Dis 1986;134:149–166.

705. Carrington CB, Liebow A. Limited forms of angiitis and granulomatosis of Wegener's type. Am J Med 1966;41:497–527.

706. Hsu JT. Limited form of Wegener's granulomatosis. Chest 1976;70:384–385.

707. Travis WD, Hoffman GS, Leavitt RY, et al. Surgical pathology of the lung in Wegener's granulomatosis. Review of 87 open lung biopsies from 67 patients. Am J Surg Pathol 1991;15:315–333.

708. Myers JL, Katzenstein AL. Wegener's granulomatosis presenting with massive pulmonary hemorrhage and capillaritis. Am J Surg Pathol 1987;11:895–898.

709. Travis WD, Carpenter HA, Lie JT. Diffuse pulmonary hemorrhage. An uncommon manifestation of Wegener's granulomatosis. Am J Surg Pathol 1987;11:702–708.

710. Nada AK, Torres VE, Ryu JH, et al. Pulmonary fibrosis as an unusual clinical manifestation of a pulmonary-renal vasculitis in elderly patients. Mayo Clin Proc 1990;65:847–856.

711. Yousem SA, Lombard CM. The eosinophilic variant of Wegener's granulomatosis. Hum Pathol 1988;19:682–688.

712. Yousem SA. Bronchocentric injury in Wegener's granulomatosis: a report of five cases. Hum Pathol 1991;22:535–540.

713. Uner AH, Rozum-Slota B, Katzenstein AL. Bronchiolitis obliterans-organizing pneumonia (BOOP)-like variant of Wegener's granulomatosis. A clinicopathologic study of 16 cases. Am J Surg Pathol 1996;20:794–801.

714. Leavitt RY, Fauci AS, Bloch DA, et al. The American College of Rheumatology 1990 criteria for the classification of Wegener's granulomatosis. Arthritis Rheum 1990;33:1101–1107.

715. Cotch MF, Hoffman GS, Yerg DE, et al. The epidemiology of Wegener's granulomatosis. Estimates of the five-year period prevalence, annual mortality, and geographic disease distribution from population-based data sources. Arthritis Rheum 1996;39:87–92.

716. Carruthers DM, Watts RA, Symmons DP, et al. Wegener's granulomatosis – increased incidence or increased recognition? Br J Rheumatol 1996;35:142–145.

717. Hoffman GS, Kerr GS, Leavitt RY, et al. Wegener's granulomatosis: an analysis of 158 patients. Ann Intern Med 1992;15;116:488–498.

718. Bajema IM, Hagen EC, van der Woude FJ, et al. Wegener's granulomatosis: a meta-analysis of 349 literary case reports. J Lab Clin Med 1997;129:17–22.

719. Cordier JF, Valeyre D, Guillevin L, et al. Pulmonary Wegener's granulomatosis. A clinical and imaging study of 77 cases. Chest 1990;97:906–912.

720. Anderson G, Coles ET, Crane M, et al. Wegener's granuloma. A series of 265 British cases seen between 1975 and 1985. A report by a sub-committee of the British Thoracic Society Research Committee. Q J Med 1992;83:427–438.

721. DeRemee RA, Weiland LH, McDonald TJ. Respiratory vasculitis. Mayo Clin Proc 1980;55:492–498.

722. Dreisin RB. New perspectives in Wegener's granulomatosis. Thorax 1993;48:97–99.

723. Rao JK, Weinberger M, Oddone EZ, et al. The role of antineutrophil cytoplasmic antibody (c-ANCA) testing in the diagnosis of Wegener's granulomatosis. A literature review and meta-analysis. Ann Intern Med 1995;123:925–932.

724. George J, Levy Y, Kallenberg CG, et al. Infections and Wegener's granulomatosis – a cause and effect relationship? Q J Med 1997;90:367–373.

725. Aberle DR, Gamsu G, Lynch D. Thoracic manifestations of Wegener's granulomatosis: diagnosis and course. Radiology 1990;174:703–709.

726. Pinching AJ, Rees AJ, Pussell BA, et al. Relapses in Wegener's granulomatosis: the role of infection. Br Med J 1980;281:836–838.

727. Odeh M, Best LA, Kerner H, et al. Localized Wegener's granulomatosis relapsing as diffuse massive intra-alveolar hemorrhage. Chest 1993;104:955–956.

728. Stegeman CA, Tervaert JW, de Jong PE, et al. Trimethoprim-sulfamethoxazole (co-trimoxazole) for the prevention of relapses of Wegener's granulomatosis. Dutch Co-Trimoxazole Wegener's Study Group. N Engl J Med 1996;335:16–20.

729. Katzenstein AL, Locke WK. Solitary lung lesions in Wegener's granulomatosis. Pathologic findings and clinical significance in 25 cases. Am J Surg Pathol 1995;19:545–552.

730. Vassallo M, Shepherd RJ, Iqbal P, et al. Age-related variations in presentation and outcome in Wegener's granulomatosis. J R Coll Physicians (Lond) 1997;31:396–400.

731. Allen NB, Bressler PB. Diagnosis and treatment of the systemic and cutaneous necrotizing vasculitis syndromes. Med Clin North Am 1997;81:243–259.

732. Papiris SA, Manoussakis MN, Drosos AA, et al. Imaging of thoracic Wegener's granulomatosis: the computed tomographic appearance. Am J Med 1992;93:529–536.

733. Maskell GF, Lockwood CM, Flower CD. Computed tomography of the lung in Wegener's granulomatosis. Clin Radiol 1993;48:377–380.

734. Reuter M, Schnabel A, Wesner F, et al. Pulmonary Wegener's granulomatosis: correlation between high-resolution CT findings and clinical scoring of disease activity. Chest 1998;114:500–506.

735. Grotz W, Mundinger A, Wurtemberger G, et al. Radiographic course of pulmonary manifestations in Wegener's granulomatosis under immunosuppressive therapy. Chest 1994;105:509–513.

736. Farrelly CA. Wegener's granulomatosis: a radiological review of the pulmonary manifestations at initial presentation and during relapse. Clin Radiol 1982;33: 545–551.

737. Landman S, Burgener F. Pulmonary manifestations in Wegener's granulomatosis. Am J Roentgenol Radium Ther Nucl Med 1974;122:750–757.

738. Israel HL, Patchefsky AS, Saldana MJ. Wegener's granulomatosis, lymphomatoid granulomatosis, and benign lymphocytic angiitis and granulomatosis of lung. Recognition and treatment. Ann Intern Med 1977;87:691–699.

739. Gonzalez L, Van Ordstrand HS. Wegener's granulomatosis. Review of 11 cases. Radiology 1973;107:295–300.

740. Gohel VK, Dalinka MK, Israel HL, et al. The radiological manifestations of Wegener's granulomatosis. Br J Radiol 1973;46:427–432.

741. Leatherman JW, Davies SF, Hoidal JR. Alveolar hemorrhage syndromes: diffuse microvascular lung hemorrhage in immune and idiopathic disorders. Medicine (Baltimore) 1984;63:343–361.

742. Stokes TC, McCann BG, Rees RT, et al. Acute fulminating intrapulmonary haemorrhage in Wegener's granulomatosis. Thorax 1982; 37:315–316.

743. Lenclud C, De Vuyst P, Dupont E, et al. Wegener's granulomatosis presenting as acute respiratory failure with anti-neutrophil-cytoplasm antibodies. Chest 1989;96:345–347.

744. Gutierrez-Rave VM, Ayerza MA. Hilar and mediastinal lymphadenopathy in the limited form of Wegener's granulomatosis. Thorax 1991;46:219–220.

745. Cohen MI, Gore RM, August CZ, et al. Tracheal and bronchial stenosis associated with mediastinal adenopathy in Wegener's granulomatosis: CT findings. J Comput Assist Tomogr 1984;8:327–329.

746. George TM, Cash JM, Farver C, et al. Mediastinal mass and hilar adenopathy: rare thoracic manifestations of Wegener's granulomatosis. Arthritis Rheum 1997;40:1992–1997.

747. Maguire R, Fauci AS, Doppman JL, et al. Unusual radiographic features of Wegener's granulomatosis. AJR Am J Roentgenol 1978;130:233–238.

748. Frazier AA, Rosada-de-Christensen ML, Galvin JR, et al. Pulmonary angiitis and granulomatosis: radiologic-pathologic correlation. RadioGraphics 1998;18:687–710.

749. Jaspan T, Davison AM, Walker WC. Spontaneous pneumothorax in Wegener's granulomatosis. Thorax 1982;37:774–775.

750. Epstein DM, Gefter WB, Miller WT, et al. Spontaneous pneumothorax: an uncommon manifestation of Wegener's granulomatosis. Radiology 1980;135:327–328.

751. Kuhlman JE, Hruban RH, Fishman EK. Wegener's granulomatosis: CT features of parenchymal lung disease. J Comput Assist Tomogr 1991;15:948–952.

752. Weir IH, Müller NL, Chiles C, et al. Wegener's granulomatosis: findings from computed tomography of the chest in 10 patients. Can Assoc Radiol J 1992;43:31–34.

753. Wadsworth DT, Siegel MJ, Day DL. Wegener's granulomatosis in children: chest radiographic manifestations. AJR Am J Roentgenol 1994;163:901–904.

754. Primack SL, Hartman TE, Lee KS, et al. Pulmonary nodules and the CT halo sign. Radiology 1994;190:513–515.

755. Attali P, Begum R, Ban Romdhane H, et al. Pulmonary Wegener's granulomatosis: changes at follow-up CT. Eur Radiol 1998;8:1009–1113.

756. Bicknell S, Mason A. Wegener's granulomatosis presenting as cryptogenic fibrosing alveolitis on CT. Clin Radiol 2000;55:890–891.

757. McDonald TJ, Neel HB 3rd, DeRemee RA. Wegener's granulomatosis of the subglottis and the upper portion of the trachea. Ann Otol Rhinol Laryngol 1982;91:588–592.

758. Langford CA, Sneller MC, Hallahan CW, et al. Clinical features and therapeutic management of subglottic stenosis in patients with Wegener's granulomatosis. Arthritis Rheum 1996;39:1754–1760.

759. Hellmann D, Laing T, Petri M, et al. Wegener's granulomatosis: isolated involvement of the trachea and larynx. Ann Rheum Dis 1987;46:628–631.

760. Daum TE, Specks U, Colby TV, et al. Tracheobronchial involvement in Wegener's granulomatosis. Am J Respir Crit Care Med 1995;151:522–526.

761. Screaton NJ, Sivasothy P, Flower CD, et al. Tracheal involvement in Wegener's granulomatosis: evaluation using spiral CT. Clin Radiol 1998;53:809–815.

762. Stein MG, Gamsu G, Webb WR, et al. Computed tomography of diffuse tracheal stenosis in Wegener's granulomatosis. J Comput Assist Tomogr 1986;10:868–870.

763. Park KJ, Bergin CJ, Harrell J. MR findings of tracheal involvement in Wegener's granulomatosis. AJR. American Journal of Roentgenology 1998;171:52–525.

764. Farrelly C, Foster DR. Atypical presentation of Wegener's granulomatosis. Br J Radiol 1980;53:721–722.

765. Foo SS, Weisbrod GL, Herman SJ, et al. Wegener's granulomatosis presenting on CT with atypical bronchovasocentric distribution. J Comput Assist Tomogr 1990;14:1004–1006.

766. Lee KS, Kim TS, Fujimoto K, et al. Thoracic manifestation of Wegener's granulomatosis: CT findings in 30 patients. Eur Radiol 2003;13:43–51.

767. Komocsi A, Reuter M, Heller M, et al. Active disease and residual damage in treated Wegener's granulomatosis: an observational study using pulmonary high-resolution computed tomography. Eur Radiol 2003;13:36–42.

768. Neumann I, Mirszaei S, Birck R, et al. Expression of somatostatin receptors in inflammatory lesions and diagnostic value of somatostatin receptor scintigraphy in patients with ANCA-associated small vessel vasculitis. Online. http://rheumatology. oupjournals.org/cgi/reprint/keg479v1 Dec 12 2003.

769. Savage CO, Winearls CG, Evans DJ, et al. Microscopic polyarteritis: presentation, pathology and prognosis. Q J Med 1985;56:467–483.

770. Specks U. Pulmonary vasculitis. In: Schwarz M, King T, eds. Interstitial lung disease, 4th edn. Toronto: Brian C Decker, 2003:599–631.

771. Guillevin L, Durand-Gasselin B, Cevallos R, et al. Microscopic polyangiitis: clinical and laboratory findings in eighty-five patients. Arthritis Rheum 1999;42:421–430.

772. Haworth SJ, Savage CO, Carr D, et al. Pulmonary haemorrhage complicating Wegener's granulomatosis and microscopic polyarteritis. Br Med J (Clin Res Ed) 1985;290:1775–1778.

773. Schwarz MI, Mortenson RL, Colby TV, et al. Pulmonary capillaritis. The association with progressive irreversible airflow limitation and hyperinflation. Am Rev Respir Dis 1993;148:507–511.

774. Brugiere O, Raffy O, Sleiman C, et al. Progressive obstructive lung disease associated with microscopic polyangiitis. Am J Respir Crit Care Med 1997;155: 739–742.

775. Bosch X, Font J, Mirapeix E, et al. Antimyeloperoxidase autoantibody-associated necrotizing alveolar capillaritis. Am Rev Respir Dis 1992;146:1326–1329.

776. Jennings CA, King TE Jr, Tuder R, et al. Diffuse alveolar hemorrhage with

underlying isolated, pauciimmune pulmonary capillaritis. Am J Respir Crit Care Med 1997;155:1101–1109.

777. Churg J, Strauss L. Allergic granulomatosis, allergic angiitis and periarteritis nodosa. Am J Pathol 1951;27:277–301.

778. Masi AT, Hunder GG, Lie JT, et al. The American College of Rheumatology 1990 criteria for the classification of Churg–Strauss syndrome (allergic granulomatosis and angiitis). Arthritis Rheum 1990;33:1094–1100.

779. Lanham JG, Elkon KB, Pusey CD, et al. Systemic vasculitis with asthma and eosinophilia: a clinical approach to the Churg–Strauss syndrome. Medicine (Baltimore) 1984;63:65–81.

780. Chumbley LC, Harrison EG Jr, DeRemee RA. Allergic granulomatosis and angiitis (Churg–Strauss syndrome). Report and analysis of 30 cases. Mayo Clin Proc 1977;52:477–484.

781. Reid AJ, Harrison BD, Watts RA, et al. Churg–Strauss syndrome in a district hospital. Q J Med 1998;91:219–229.

782. Keogh KA, Specks U. Churg–Strauss syndrome. clinical presentation, antineutrophil cytoplasmic antibodies, and leukotriene receptor antagonists. Am J Med 2003;115:284–290.

783. Guillevin L, Guittard T, Bletry O, et al. Systemic necrotizing angiitis with asthma: causes and precipitating factors in 43 cases. Lung 1987;165:165–172.

784. English J, 3rd, Greer KE, McCrone SA, et al. Fluticasone-associated cutaneous allergic granulomatous vasculitis. J Drugs Dermatol 2003;2:326–329.

785. Hubner C, Dietz A, Stremmel W, et al. Macrolide-induced Churg–Strauss syndrome in a patient with atopy. Lancet 1997;350:563.

786. Orriols R, Munoz X, Ferrer J, et al. Cocaine-induced Churg–Strauss vasculitis. Eur Respir J 1996;9:175–177.

787. Guillevin L, Amouroux J, Arbeille B, et al. Churg–Strauss angiitis. Arguments favoring the responsibility of inhaled antigens. Chest 1991;100:1472–1473.

788. Soy M, Ozer H, Canataroglu A, et al. Vasculitis induced by zafirlukast therapy. Clin Rheumatol 2002;21: 328–329.

789. Michael AB, Murphy D. Montelukast-associated Churg–Strauss syndrome. Age Ageing 2003;32:551–552.

790. Katsura T, Yoshida F, Takinishi Y. The Churg–Strauss syndrome after pranlukast treatment in a patient not receiving corticosteroids. Ann Intern Med 2003;139:387.

791. Choi IS, Koh YI, Joo JY, et al. Churg–Strauss syndrome may be induced by leukotriene modifiers in severe asthma. Ann Allergy Asthma Immunol 2003;91:98.

792. Jamaleddine G, Diab K, Tabbarah Z, et al. Leukotriene antagonists and the Churg–Strauss syndrome. Semin Arthritis Rheum 2002;31:218–227.

793. Churg A, Brallas M, Cronin SR, et al. Formes frustes of Churg–Strauss syndrome. Chest 1995;108:320–323.

794. Cooper BJ, Bacal E, Patterson R. Allergic angiitis and granulomatosis. Prolonged remission induced by combined prednisone – azathioprine therapy. Arch Intern Med 1978;138:367–371.

795. Koss MN, Antonovych T, Hochholzer L. Allergic granulomatosis (Churg–Strauss syndrome): pulmonary and renal morphologic findings. Am J Surg Pathol 1981;5:21–28.

796. Cogen FC, Mayock RL, Zweiman B. Chronic eosinophilic pneumonia followed by polyarteritis nodosa complicating the course of bronchial asthma. Report of a case. J Allergy Clin Immunol 1977;60:377–382.

797. Kus J, Bergin C, Miller R, et al. Lymphocyte subpopulations in allergic granulomatosis and angiitis (Churg–Strauss syndrome). Chest 1985;87:826–827.

798. Hueto-Perez-de-Heredia JJ, Dominguez-del-Valle FJ, Garcia E, et al. Chronic eosinophilic pneumonia as a presenting feature of Churg–Strauss syndrome. Eur Respir J 1994;7:1006–1008.

799. Degesys GE, Mintzer RA, Vrla RF. Allergic granulomatosis: Churg–Strauss syndrome. AJR Am J Roentgenol 1980;135:1281–1282.

800. Levin DC. Pulmonary abnormalities in the necrotizing vasculitides and their rapid response to steroids. Radiology 1970;97:521–526.

801. Buschman D, Waldron J, King T. Churg Strauss pulmonary vasculitis: high resolution CT scanning and pathologic findings. Am Rev Respir Dis 1990;142:458–461.

802. Erzurum SC, Underwood GA, Hamilos DL, et al. Pleural effusion in Churg–Strauss syndrome. Chest 1989;95:1357–1359.

803. Worthy SA, Müller NL, Hansell DM, et al. Churg–Strauss syndrome: the spectrum of pulmonary CT findings in 17 patients. AJR Am J Roentgenol 1998;170:297–300.

804. Amato MB, Barbas CS, Delmonte VC, et al. Concurrent Churg–Strauss syndrome and temporal arteritis in a young patient with pulmonary nodules. Am Rev Respir Dis 1989;139:1539–1542.

805. Connolly B, Manson D, Eberhard A, et al. CT appearance of pulmonary vasculitis in children. AJR Am J Roentgenol 1996;167:901–904.

806. Rosenberg TF, Medsger TA Jr, DeCicco FA, et al. Allergic granulomatous angiitis (Churg–Strauss syndrome). J Allergy Clin Immunol 1975;55:56–67.

807. Davison AG, Thompson PJ, Davies J, et al. Prominent pericardial and myocardial lesions in the Churg–Strauss syndrome (allergic granulomatosis and angiitis). Thorax 1983;38:793–795.

808. Guillevin L, Lhote F, Gayraud M, et al. Prognostic factors in polyarteritis nodosa and Churg–Strauss syndrome. A prospective study in 342 patients. Medicine (Baltimore) 1996;75:17–28.

809. Kozak M, Gill EA, Green LS. The Churg–Strauss syndrome. A case report with angiographically documented coronary involvement and a review of the literature. Chest 1995;107:578–580.

810. Heng MC. Henoch-Schönlein purpura. Br J Dermatol 1985;112:235–240.

811. Mills JA, Michel BA, Bloch DA, et al. The American College of Rheumatology 1990 criteria for the classification of Henoch-Schönlein purpura. Arthritis Rheum 1990;33:1114–1121.

812. Dreisin RB. Pulmonary vasculitis. Clin Chest Med 1982;3:607–618.

813. Cream JJ, Gumpel JM, Peachey RD. Schönlein-Henoch purpura in the adult. A study of 77 adults with anaphylactoid or Schönlein-Henoch purpura. Q J Med 1970;39:461–484.

814. Kathuria S, Cheifec G. Fatal pulmonary Henoch-Schonlein syndrome. Chest 1982;82:654–556.

815. Jacome AF. Pulmonary hemorrhage and death complicating anaphylactoid purpura. South Med J 1967;60:1003–1004.

816. Olson JC, Kelly KJ, Pan CG, et al. Pulmonary disease with hemorrhage in Henoch-Schönlein purpura. Pediatrics 1992;89:1177–1181.

817. Gorevic PD, Kassab HJ, Levo Y, et al. Mixed cryoglobulinemia: clinical aspects and long-term follow-up of 40 patients. Am J Med 1980;69:287–308.

818. Clinical conference: Mixed cryoimmunoglobulinemia. Am J Med 1976;61:95–102.

819. Limaye V, Glynn T, Kwiatek R, et al. Cryoglobulinaemia causing systemic vasculitis and interstitial lung disease. Aust N Z J Med 2000;30:102.

820. Ferri C, La Civita L, Longombardo G, et al. Mixed cryoglobulinaemia: a cross-road between autoimmune and lymphoproliferative disorders. Lupus 1998;7:275–279.

821. Anon. Case records of the Massachusetts General Hospital. Weekly clinicopathological exercises. Case 23-1975. N Engl J Med 1975;292: 1285–1290.

822. Bombardieri S, Paoletti P, Ferri C, et al. Lung involvement in essential mixed cryoglobulinemia. Am J Med 1979;66: 748–756.

823. Stagg MP, Lauber J, Michalski JP. Mixed essential cryoglobulinemia and adult respiratory distress syndrome: a case report. Am J Med 1989;87:445–448.

824. Asherson RA, Sontheimer R. Urticarial vasculitis and syndromes in association with connective tissue diseases. Ann Rheum Dis 1991;50:743–744.

825. Knobler H, Admon D, Leibovici V, et al. Urticarial vasculitis and recurrent pleural effusion: a systemic manifestation of urticarial vasculitis. Dermatologica 1986;172:120–122.

826. Zeiss CR, Burch FX, Marder RJ, et al. A hypocomplementemic vasculitic urticarial syndrome. Report of four new cases and definition of the disease. Am J Med 1980;68:867–875.

827. Schwartz HR, McDuffie FC, Black LF, et al. Hypocomplementemic urticarial vasculitis: association with chronic obstructive pulmonary disease. Mayo Clin Proc 1982;57:231–238.

828. Wisnieski JJ, Baer AN, Christensen J, et al. Hypocomplementemic urticarial vasculitis syndrome. Clinical and serologic findings in 18 patients. Medicine (Baltimore) 1995;74:24–41.

829. Mertz LE, Conn DL. Vasculitis associated with malignancy. Curr Opin Rheumatol 1992;4:39–46.

830. Chajek T, Fainaru M. Behçet's disease. Report of 41 cases and a review of the literature. Medicine (Baltimore) 1975;54:179–196.

831. Evaluation of diagnostic ('classification') criteria in Behçet's disease – towards internationally agreed criteria. The International Study Group for Behçet's disease. Br J Rheumatol 1992;31:299–308.

832. Slavin RE, de Groot WJ. Pathology of the lung in Behçet's disease. Case report and review of the literature. Am J Surg Pathol 1981;5:779–788.

833. Lakhanpal S, Tani K, Lie JT, et al. Pathologic features of Behçet's syndrome: a review of Japanese autopsy registry data. Hum Pathol 1985;16:790–795.

834. Tunaci A, Berkmen YM, Gokmen E. Thoracic involvement in Behçet's disease: pathologic, clinical, and imaging features. AJR Am J Roentgenol 1995; 164:51–56.

835. Kaklamani VG, Vaiopoulos G, Kaklamanis PG. Behçet's Disease. Semin Arthritis Rheum 1998;27:197–217.

836. Erkan F, Gul A, Tasali E. Pulmonary manifestations of Behçet's disease. Thorax 2001;56:572–578.

837. Davies JD. Behcet's syndrome with haemoptysis and pulmonary lesions. J Pathol 1973;109:351–356.

838. Shimizu T, Inaba G. [Epidemiology of Behcet's disease; status of Behcet's disease in Japan]. Ryumachi 1976;16:224–233.

839. Raz I, Okon E, Chajek-Shaul T. Pulmonary manifestations in Behçet's syndrome. Chest 1989;95:585–589.

840. Erkan F, Cavdar T. Pulmonary vasculitis in Behçet's disease. Am Rev Respir Dis 1992;146:232–239.

841. Fairley C, Wilson JW, Barraclough D. Pulmonary involvement in Behçet's syndrome. Chest 1989;96:1428–1429.

842. Huong DL, Dolmazon C, De Zuttere D, et al. Complete recovery of right intraventricular thrombus and pulmonary arteritis in Behçet's disease. Br J Rheumatol 1997;36:130–132.

843. Hamuryudan V, Yurdakul S, Moral F, et al. Pulmonary arterial aneurysms in Behçet's syndrome: a report of 24 cases. Br J Rheumatol 1994;33:48–51.

844. Durieux P, Bletry O, Huchon G, et al. Multiple pulmonary arterial aneurysms in Behçet's disease and Hughes-Stovin syndrome. Am J Med 1981;71:736–741.

845. Lacombe P, Frija G, Parlier H, et al. Transcatheter embolization of multiple pulmonary artery aneurysms in Behçet's syndrome. Report of a case. Acta Radiol Diagn (Stockh) 1985;26:251–253.

846. Remy-Jardin M, Wattinne L, Remy J. Transcatheter occlusion of pulmonary arterial circulation and collateral supply: failures, incidents, and complications. Radiology 1991;180:699–705.

847. Grenier P, Bletry O, Cornud F, et al. Pulmonary involvement in Behçet disease. AJR Am J Roentgenol 1981;137:565–569.

848. Numan F, Islak C, Berkmen T, et al. Behçet disease: pulmonary arterial involvement in 15 cases. Radiology 1994;192:465–468.

849. Park JH, Han MC, Bettmann MA. Arterial manifestations of Behçet disease. AJR Am J Roentgenol 1984;143:821–825.

850. Efthimiou J, Johnston C, Spiro SG, et al. Pulmonary disease in Behçet's syndrome. Q J Med 1986;58:259–280.

851. Ahn JM, Im JG, Ryoo JW, et al. Thoracic manifestations of Behçet syndrome: radiographic and CT findings in nine patients. Radiology 1995;194:199–203.

852. Winer-Muram HT, Gavant ML. Pulmonary CT findings in Behçet disease. J Comput Assist Tomogr 1989;13:346–347.

853. Gunen H, Evereklioglu C, Kosar F, et al. Thoracic involvement in Behçet's disease and its correlation with multiple parameters. Lung 2000;178:161–170.

854. Berkmen T. MR angiography of aneurysms in Behçet disease: a report of four cases. J Comput Assist Tomogr 1998;22:202–206.

855. Malik KJ, Weber SL, Sohail S, et al. Hilar mass and papilledema on presentation. Chest 1998;113:227–229.

856. Coplu L, Emri S, Selcuk ZT, et al. Life threatening chylous pleural and pericardial effusion in a patient with Behçet's syndrome. Thorax 1992;47:64–65.

857. Hughes JP, Stovin PG. Segmental pulmonary artery aneurysms with peripheral venous thrombosis. Br J Dis Chest 1959;53:19–27.

858. Herb S, Hetzel M, Hetzel J, et al. An unusual case of Hughes-Stovin syndrome. Eur Respir J 1998;11:1191–1193.

859. Roberts DH, Jimenez JF, Golladay ES. Multiple pulmonary artery aneurysms and peripheral venous thromboses – the Hughes Stovin syndrome. Report of a case in a 12-year-old boy and a review of the literature. Pediatr Radiol 1982;12: 214–216.

860. Teplick JG, Haskin ME, Nedwich A. The Hughes–Stovin syndrome. Case report. Radiology 1974;113:607–608.

861. Wolpert SM, Kahn PC, Farbman K. The radiology of the Hughes–Stovin syndrome. Am J Roentgenol Radium Ther Nucl Med 1971;112:383–388.

862. Balci NC, Semelka RC, Noone TC, et al. Multiple pulmonary aneurysms secondary to Hughes–Stovin syndrome: demonstration by MR angiography. J Magn Reson Imaging 1998;8: 1323–1325.

863. Bowman S, Honey M. Pulmonary arterial occlusions and aneurysms: a forme fruste of Behçet's or Hughes–Stovin syndrome. Br Heart J 1990;63:66–68.

864. Liebow A. Pulmonary angiitis and granulomatosis. Am Rev Respir Dis 1973;108:1–18.

865. Churg A. Pulmonary angiitis and granulomatosis revisited. Hum Pathol 1983;14:868–883.

866. Lynch JP 3rd, Kazerooni EA, Gay SE. Pulmonary sarcoidosis. Clin Chest Med 1997;18:755–785.

867. Popper HH, Klemen H, Colby TV, Churg A. Necrotizing sarcoid granulomatosis – is it different from nodular sarcoidosis? Pneumologie 2003;57:268–271.

868. Liebow AA. The J. Burns Amberson lecture – pulmonary angiitis and granulomatosis. Am Rev Respir Dis 1973;108:1–18.

869. Saldana M. Necrotizing sarcoid granulomatosis: clinicopathologic observations in 24 patients. Lab Invest 1978;38:364.

870. Koss MN, Hochholzer L, Feigin DS, et al. Necrotizing sarcoid-like granulomatosis: clinical, pathologic, and immunopathologic findings. Hum Pathol 1980;11:510–519.

871. Dykhuizen RS, Smith CC, Kennedy MM, et al. Necrotizing sarcoid granulomatosis with extrapulmonary involvement. Eur Respir J 1997;10:245–247.

872. Chittock DR, Joseph MG, Paterson NA, et al. Necrotizing sarcoid granulomatosis with pleural involvement. Clinical and radiographic features. Chest 1994;106: 672–676.

873. Churg A, Carrington CB, Gupta R. Necrotizing sarcoid granulomatosis. Chest 1979;76:406–413.

874. Fisher MR, Christ ML, Bernstein JR. Necrotizing sarcoid-like granulomatosis: radiologic-pathologic correlation. J Can Assoc Radiol 1984;35:313–315.

875. Stephen JG, Braimbridge MV, Corrin B, et al. Necrotizing 'sarcoidal' angiitis and granulomatosis of the lung. Thorax 1976;31:356–360.

876. Niimi H, Hartman TE, Müller NL. Necrotizing sarcoid granulomatosis: computed tomography and pathologic findings. J Comput Assist Tomogr 1995;19:920–923.

877. Bradley JD. The pulmonary hemorrhage syndromes. Clin Chest Med 1982;3: 593–605.

878. Briggs WA, Johnson JP, Teichman S, et al. Antiglomerular basement membrane antibody-mediated glomerulonephritis and Goodpasture's syndrome. Medicine (Baltimore) 1979;58:348–361.

879. Leatherman JW. Immune alveolar hemorrhage. Chest 1987;91:891–897.

880. Müller NL, Miller RR. Diffuse pulmonary hemorrhage. Radiol Clin North Am 1991;29:965–971.

881. Primack SL, Miller RR, Müller NL. Diffuse pulmonary hemorrhage: clinical, pathologic, and imaging features. AJR Am J Roentgenol 1995;164:295–300.

882. Fontenot A, Schwarz MI. Diffuse alveolar hemorrhage. In: Schwarz M, King T, eds. Interstitial lung disease, 4th edn. Toronto: Brian C Decker, 2003:535–598.

883. Koziel H, Haley K, Nasser I, et al. Pulmonary hemorrhage. An uncommon cause of pulmonary infiltrates in patients with AIDS. Chest 1994;106:1891–1894.

884. Gruber BL, Schranz JA, Fuhrer J, et al. Isolated pulmonary microangiitis mimicking pneumonia in a patient infected with human immunodeficiency virus. J Rheumatol 1997;24:759–762.

885. Cohn RC, Wong R, Spohn WA, et al. Death due to diffuse alveolar hemorrhage in a child with pulmonary veno-occlusive disease. Chest 1991;100:1456–1458.

886. Im JG, Yeon KM, Han MC, et al. Leptospirosis of the lung: radiographic findings in 58 patients. AJR Am J Roentgenol 1989;152:955–959.

887. Clutterbuck EJ, Pusey CD. Severe alveolar haemorrhage in Churg–Strauss syndrome. Eur J Respir Dis 1987;71: 158–163.

888. Markus HS, Clark JV. Pulmonary haemorrhage in Henoch-Schönlein purpura. Thorax 1989;44:525–526.

889. Gertner E, Lie JT. Pulmonary capillaritis, alveolar hemorrhage, and recurrent microvascular thrombosis in primary antiphospholipid syndrome. J Rheumatol 1993;20:1224–1228.

890. Gamble CN, Wiesner KB, Shapiro RF, et al. The immune complex pathogenesis of glomerulonephritis and pulmonary vasculitis in Behcet's disease. Am J Med 1979;66:1031–1039.

891. Stanton M, Tange J. Goodpasture's syndrome (pulmonary haemorrhage associated with glomerulonephritis). Aust Ann Med 1958; 7:132–144.

892. Thomas HM 3rd, Irwin RS. Editorial: Classification of diffuse intrapulmonary hemorrhage. Chest 1975;68:483–484.

893. Kelly PT, Haponik EF. Goodpasture syndrome: molecular and clinical advances. Medicine (Baltimore) 1994;73:171–185.

894. Carre P, Lloveras JJ, Didier A, et al. Goodpasture's syndrome with normal renal function. Eur Respir J 1989;2: 911–915.

895. Goodpasture E. The significance of certain pulmonary lesions in relation to the etiology of influenza. Am J Med Sci 1919;158:863–870.

896. Ball JA, Young KR Jr. Pulmonary manifestations of Goodpasture's syndrome. Antiglomerular basement membrane disease and related disorders. Clin Chest Med 1998;19:777–791, ix.

897. Ozsoylu S, Hicsonmez G, Berkel I, et al. Goodpasture's syndrome (pulmonary hemosiderosis with nephritis). Clin Pediatr (Phila) 1976;15:358–360.

898. Scheer R, Grossman M. Immune aspects of the glomerulonephritis associated with pulmonary hemorrhage. Ann Intern Med 1964;60:1009–1021.

899. Teague CA, Doak PB, Simpson IJ, et al. Goodpasture's syndrome: an analysis of 29 cases. Kidney Int 1978;13:492–504.

900. Niles JL, Bottinger EP, Saurina GR, et al. The syndrome of lung hemorrhage and nephritis is usually an ANCA-associated condition. Arch Intern Med 1996;156: 440–445.

901. Morgan PG, Turner-Warwick M. Pulmonary haemosiderosis and pulmonary haemorrhage. Br J Dis Chest 1981;75:225–242.

902. Lombard CM, Colby TV, Elliott CG. Surgical pathology of the lung in anti-basement membrane antibody-associated Goodpasture's syndrome. Hum Pathol 1989;20:445–451.

903. Travis WD, Colby TV, Lombard C, et al. A clinicopathologic study of 34 cases of diffuse pulmonary hemorrhage with lung biopsy confirmation. Am J Surg Pathol 1990;14:1112–1125.

904. Mark EJ, Ramirez JF. Pulmonary capillaritis and hemorrhage in patients with systemic vasculitis. Arch Pathol Lab Med 1985;109:413–418.

905. Johnson JP, Moore J Jr, Austin HA 3rd, et al. Therapy of anti-glomerular basement membrane antibody disease: analysis of prognostic significance of clinical, pathologic and treatment factors. Medicine (Baltimore) 1985;64:219–227.

906. Benoit FL, Rulon DB, Theil GB, et al. Goodpasture's syndrome: A Clinicopathologic Entity. Am J Med 1964;37:424–444.

907. Seaton A, Meland JM, Lapp NL. Remission in Goodpasture's syndrome: report of two patients treated by immunosuppression and review of the literature. Thorax 1971;26:683–688.

908. Saxena R, Bygren P, Arvastson B, et al. Circulating autoantibodies as serological markers in the differential diagnosis of pulmonary renal syndrome. J Intern Med 1995;238:143–152.

909. Bosch X, Lopez-Soto A, Mirapeix E, et al. Antineutrophil cytoplasmic autoantibody-associated alveolar capillaritis in patients presenting with pulmonary haemorrhage. Arch Pathol Lab Med 1994;118:517–522.

910. Byrd RB, Trunk G. Systemic lupus erythematosus presenting as pulmonary hemosiderosis. Chest 1973;64:128–129.

911. Green RJ, Ruoss SJ, Kraft SA, et al. Pulmonary capillaritis and alveolar hemorrhage. Update on diagnosis and management. Chest 1996;110:1305–1316.

912. Ognibene AJ, Dito WR. Rheumatoid disease with unusual pulmonary manifestations. Pulmonary hemosiderosis, fibrosis, and concretions. Arch Intern Med 1965;116:567–572.

913. Torralbo A, Herrero JA, Portoles J, et al. Alveolar hemorrhage associated with antineutrophil cytoplasmic antibodies in rheumatoid arthritis. Chest 1994;105:1590–1592.

914. Griffin MT, Robb JD, Martin JR. Diffuse alveolar haemorrhage associated with progressive systemic sclerosis. Thorax 1990;45:903–904.

915. Kallenbach J, Prinsloo I, Zwi S. Progressive systemic sclerosis complicated by diffuse pulmonary haemorrhage. Thorax 1977;32:767–770.

916. Germain MJ, Davidman M. Pulmonary hemorrhage and acute renal failure in a patient with mixed connective tissue disease. Am J Kidney Dis 1984;3:420–424.

917. Lai FM, Li EK, Suen MW, et al. Pulmonary hemorrhage. A fatal manifestation in IgA nephropathy. Arch Pathol Lab Med 1994;118:542–546.

918. Hillerdal G. The lung physician and the antiphospholipid syndrome. Eur Respir J 1997;10:511–512.

919. Turner-Warwick M, Dewar A. Pulmonary haemorrhage and pulmonary haemosiderosis. Clin Radiol 1982;33:361–370.

920. Leaker B, Cambridge G, du Bois RM, et al. Idiopathic pulmonary haemosiderosis: a form of microscopic polyarteritis? Thorax 1992;47:988–990.

921. Pacheco A, Casanova C, Fogue L, et al. Long-term clinical follow-up of adult idiopathic pulmonary hemosiderosis and celiac disease. Chest 1991;99:1525–1526.

922. Cheah FK, Sheppard MN, Hansell DM. Computed tomography of diffuse pulmonary haemorrhage with pathological correlation. Clin Radiol 1993;48:89–93.

923. Nomura S, Kanoh T. Association of idiopathic pulmonary haemosiderosis with IgA monoclonal gammopathy. Thorax 1987;42:696–697.

924. Bouros D, Panagou P, Arseniou P, et al. Idiopathic pulmonary haemosiderosis and autoimmune hypothyroidism: bronchoalveolar lavage findings after cimetidine treatment. Respir Med 1995;89:307–309.

925. Milman N, Pedersen FM. Idiopathic pulmonary haemosiderosis. Epidemiology, pathogenic aspects and diagnosis. Respir Med 1998;92:902–907.

926. Donald KJ, Edwards RL, McEvoy JD. Alveolar capillary basement membrane lesions in Goodpasture's syndrome and idiopathic pulmonary hemosiderosis. Am J Med 1975;59:642–649.

927. Corrin B, Jagusch M, Dewar A, et al. Fine structural changes in idiopathic pulmonary haemosiderosis. J Pathol 1987;153:249–256.

928. Soergel K, Sommers S. Idiopathic pulmonary hemosiderosis and related syndromes. Am J Med 1962;32:499–511.

929. Golde DW, Drew WL, Klein HZ, et al. Occult pulmonary haemorrhage in leukaemia. Br Med J 1975;2:166–168.

930. Palmer PE, Finley TN, Drew WL, et al. Radiographic aspects of occult pulmonary haemorrhage. Clin Radiol 1978;29:139–143.

931. Fireman Z, Yust I, Abramov AL. Lethal occult pulmonary hemorrhage in drug-induced thrombocytopenia. Chest 1981;79:358–359.

932. Albelda SM, Gefter WB, Epstein DM, et al. Diffuse pulmonary hemorrhage: a review and classification. Radiology 1985;154:289–297.

933. Blank N, Castellino RA, Shah V. Radiographic aspects of pulmonary infection in patients with altered immunity. Radiol Clin North Am 1973;11:175–190.

934. Finley TN, Aronow A, Cosentino AM, et al. Occult pulmonary hemorrhage in anticoagulated patients. Am Rev Respir Dis 1975;112:23–29.

935. Nathan PE, Torres AV, Smith AJ, et al. Spontaneous pulmonary hemorrhage following coronary thrombolysis. Chest 1992;101:1150–1152.

936. Awadh N, Ronco JJ, Bernstein V, et al. Spontaneous pulmonary hemorrhage after thrombolytic therapy for acute myocardial infarction. Chest 1994;106:1622–1624.

937. Robboy SJ, Minna JD, Colman RW, et al. Pulmonary hemorrhage syndrome as a manifestation of disseminated intravascular coagulation: analysis of ten cases. Chest 1973;63:718–721.

938. Stankus SJ, Johnson NT. Propylthiouracil-induced hypersensitivity vasculitis presenting as respiratory failure. Chest 1992;102:1595–1596.

939. Yermakov VM, Hitti IF, Sutton AL. Necrotizing vasculitis associated with diphenylhydantoin: two fatal cases. Hum Pathol 1983;14:182–184.

940. Bucknall CE, Adamson MR, Banham SW. Non fatal pulmonary haemorrhage associated with nitrofurantoin. Thorax 1987;42:475–476.

941. Herbert FA, Orford R. Pulmonary hemorrhage and edema due to inhalation of resins containing tri-mellitic anhydride. Chest 1979;76:546–551.

942. Kaplan V, Baur X, Czuppon A, et al. Pulmonary hemorrhage due to inhalation of vapor containing pyromellitic dianhydride. Chest 1993;104:644–645.

943. Murray RJ, Albin RJ, Mergner W, et al. Diffuse alveolar hemorrhage temporally related to cocaine smoking. Chest 1988;93:427–429.

944. Nicolls MR, Terada LS, Tuder RM, et al. Diffuse alveolar hemorrhage with underlying pulmonary capillaritis in the retinoic acid syndrome. Am J Respir Crit Care Med 1998;158:1302–1305.

945. Slonim L. Goodpasture's syndrome and its radiological features. Aust Radiol 1969;13:164–172.

946. Bowley NB, Steiner RE, Chin WS. The chest X-ray in antiglomerular basement membrane antibody disease (Goodpasture's syndrome). Clin Radiol 1979;30:419–429.

947. Herman PG, Balikian JP, Seltzer SE, et al. The pulmonary-renal syndrome. AJR Am J Roentgenol 1978;130:1141–1148.

948. Bruwer A, Kennedy R, Edwards J. Recurrent pulmonary hemorrhage with hemosiderosis: so-called idiopathic pulmonary hemosiderosis. AJR Am J Roentgenol 1956;76:98–107.

949. Ditto W, Ognibene A. Idiopathic pulmonary hemosiderosis without anemia. Report of two cases. Arch Intern Med 1964;114:490–493.

950. Buschman DL, Ballard R. Progressive massive fibrosis associated with idiopathic pulmonary hemosiderosis. Chest 1993;104:293–295.

951. Bowley NB, Hughes JM, Steiner RE. The chest X-ray in pulmonary capillary haemorrhage: correlation with carbon monoxide uptake. Clin Radiol 1979;30:413–417.

952. Drew WL, Finley TN, Golde DW. Diagnostic lavage and occult pulmonary hemorrhage in thrombocytopenic immunocompromised patients. Am Rev Respir Dis 1977;116:215–221.

953. Huber DJ, Kobzik L, Solorzano C, et al. Nuclear magnetic resonance spectroscopy of acute and evolving pulmonary hemorrhage. An in vitro study. Invest Radiol 1987;22:632–637.

954. Rubin GD, Edwards DK 3rd, Reicher MA, et al. Diagnosis of pulmonary hemosiderosis by MR imaging. AJR Am J Roentgenol 1989;152:573–574.

CHAPTER 11

Miscellaneous diffuse lung diseases

SARCOIDOSIS

Sarcoidosis is a common systemic disease characterized by widespread development of noncaseating epithelioid cell granulomas that eventually either resolve or become fibrotic. The clinical manifestations of sarcoidosis are often widespread (Box 11.1), but may be restricted to a single organ. However, the lung and its associated lymph nodes are almost universally involved. In the chest, the lymphatics, airway, and parenchyma of the lung can all be involved, with resultant symptoms and physiologic impairment. Although the cause and pathogenesis of sarcoidosis are obscure, it is thought to be the result of a disordered, immunologically mediated response to one or more unidentified, possibly inhaled, agents. Various agents have been

suggested, including *Mycobacterium* species (either alone or with viruses), other infectious organisms, organic antigens (e.g. pollen), and inorganic dusts.[1-3] However, despite intensive investigation, an etiologic agent has not been identified.[4] It seems most likely that sarcoidosis results from the complex interaction of multiple genes with environmental exposures or infection.[5] The inciting antigen or antigens then trigger a T-lymphocyte response that is characterized by chronic inflammation, monocyte recruitment, and granuloma formation. The HLA allele DRB1*1101 appears to be a risk factor for sarcoidosis, but the mechanism for this increased risk is not known.[6] About 1–3% of patients with sarcoidosis have a family history of the disease.[7]

Pathology and clinical features

Although previous concepts of the pathogenesis of sarcoidosis emphasized the role of a mononuclear alveolitis,[8] it is now generally accepted that the granuloma is the earliest lesion of sarcoidosis.[9] Early loose granulomas evolve into mature ones that consist of a tightly packed central collection of epithelioid histiocytes, and occasional multinucleate giant cells surrounded by lymphocytes (activated T cells), monocytes, and fibroblasts.[1] Epithelioid cells secrete 40 or more different enzymes, cytokines, and other mediators, including angiotensin converting enzyme (ACE) and calcitriol.[10] Necrosis is rare and when it does occur is minimal and confined to the center of granulomas.[11] Granulomas are predominantly interstitial and are distributed along lymphatic pathways, being characteristically found along bronchovascular bundles, interlobular septa, and pleura,[12] with or without interstitial pneumonia in the adjacent lung. Granulomas, once formed, may remain stable for months or years. They may resolve spontaneously or in response to treatment. In a minority of cases (perhaps 20%) the granulomas become obliterated by centripetal fibrosis that may develop into extensive interstitial fibrosis, with destruction and distortion of the lung architecture and eventual end-stage lung.

A wide range of disorders can cause granulomatous lung disease (Box 11.2).[13] The distinguishing features of granulomas caused by sarcoid, or beryllium, include their tendency to conglomerate along lymphatic pathways, and the presence of surrounding dense, eosinophilic lamellar collagen, which often contains granulomas.[14] Sarcoid granulomas differ from infective granulomas because of the absence of caseous necrosis. The granulomas of hypersensitivity pneumonitis tend to be small,

poorly defined, and bronchiolocentric. Intravenous talcosis is characterized by perivascular clusters of giant cells containing birefringent particles. Sarcoid granulomas, however, are not confined to the lung and are found in all organs and tissues, although some, like the adrenal gland, are not commonly involved.[15] The generalized nature of the sarcoid response is an important feature that distinguishes sarcoidosis from various lung limited granulomatous disorders. For example, berylliosis is generally confined to the lungs. The systemic occurrence of granulomas also helps distinguish sarcoidosis from local sarcoidlike responses associated with neoplastic conditions.[16] Such distinctions, however, are not always easy to make and overlap patterns can be encountered.[17] The localized granulomas related to neoplasms can sometimes be suspected by their occurrence in the drainage pathway of a malignant appearing lesion.

Reported incidence rates for sarcoidosis vary greatly from country to country and depend, among other factors, on race, the sophistication of medical care, and use of screening programs. Quoted figures for incidence of clinical disease are of the order of 1–10 cases per 100 000 population per year, but this is almost certainly an underestimate because many cases are subclinical.[18] Studies performed using mass radiographic screening for tuberculosis have yielded a prevalence of 10–30 per 100 000; many of these cases were asymptomatic and might never have been detected clinically.[19,20] Although previous studies suggested that sarcoidosis occurred with about a tenfold greater frequency in blacks than in whites,[21,22] a more recent study suggests that the annual incidence is three- to four-fold greater in blacks than in whites.[23] Some of the highest incidences have been reported in individuals of Irish, West Indian, and Nordic origin.[19,24] In individual cases, therefore, the ethnic origin of the patient is relatively unhelpful in determining the likelihood of sarcoidosis. The prevalence of sarcoidosis is probably lower in cigarette smokers than in non-smokers.[25]

A number of conditions have been reported to show an association with sarcoidosis; the relationship is best established for tuberculosis.[26] In a series of 425 patients with sarcoidosis, tuberculosis immediately preceded sarcoidosis in 1.6% and sarcoidosis developed into overt tuberculosis in 1.9%.[27] More recently, a sarcoidlike reaction has been shown to occur in patients treated with highly active retroviral treatment for AIDS.[28–30]

Sarcoidosis most commonly presents between 20 and 40 years of age,[23,31,32] but the range is wide – from the first year of life[33] to the eighth decade. It is very uncommon in childhood and adolescence. There is a variable, usually slight, female predominance.[19,20,23,24,31,34,35] The mode of presentation varies greatly among series, depending particularly on racial mix and the use of screening radiography. In white dominated series, presentation as an incidental radiographic finding occurs in about 50% of cases.[36,37] Respiratory illness (21%), erythema nodosum (16%), ocular symptoms (7%), and other skin lesions (4%)[36] represent the other common presentations. In blacks, respiratory and systemic symptoms, such as fatigue, malaise, weakness, weight loss, and fever, are the most common.[38] There is a striking difference between blacks and whites at presentation in the frequency of erythema nodosum. This finding is uncommon in blacks but very common in whites, particularly in the United Kingdom, where 30–40% of patients present with the condition,[21,36,39] often as part of Lofgren syndrome (erythema nodosum, fever, and hilar adenopathy[40,41]). In general, sarcoidosis occurring in blacks is later in onset, is more likely to involve peripheral nodes, skin, and eyes, and to become chronic and disseminated. Because of the lower incidence of the benign Lofgren syndrome and the higher incidence of chronic, disseminated disease, the prognosis of sarcoidosis is worse in blacks than in whites.[21,39,42,43]

Investigation

Laboratory investigations may show anemia, leukopenia, or a raised erythrocyte sedimentation rate (ESR). Differential blood count may show lymphopenia or neutropenia. A significant blood eosinophilia has been reported in up to one-quarter of patients.[15,44,45] Sarcoidosis should therefore be considered in the differential diagnosis of pulmonary eosinophilia, though patients with sarcoidosis do not usually have eosinophilia of the lung tissues. Hypercalciuria and hypercalcemia may be prominent features.[1] The former is often transient and occurs in about 11% of patients.[36] It may lead to renal calculi. Hypercalcemia can cause metastatic calcification and renal failure.[31] Hypercalciuria is two- to three-fold more common than hypercalcemia.[46] Disordered calcium homeostasis is caused by synthesis of 1,25-dihydroxyvitamin D3 (calcitriol) by activated sarcoid macrophages,[47] and is rapidly responsive to steroids.[48]

Serum levels of ACE, produced by activated macrophages, are raised in about 50–60% of patients.[49–51] Serum ACE levels correlate with the total body granuloma burden[52] and the activity of clinical disease as a whole,[37] but not convincingly with the degree and activity of pulmonary disease.[1,53] The presence of raised levels of serum ACE is not specific for sarcoidosis, occurring also in other granulomatous conditions, and in Hodgkin lymphoma; the false positive rate is approximately 10%.[39,54] Other biochemical changes may include abnormal liver function (particularly alkaline phosphatase).[52]

Various immunologic derangements are seen with sarcoidosis. Cutaneous anergy is well recognized. About two-thirds of patients have a negative tuberculin test, and in many of the remainder it is only weakly positive.[36,38] Cutaneous anergy is probably related to the relative abundance of suppressor T cells (CD4 cells) in the peripheral blood following sequestration of helper T cells (CD8 cells) in active sarcoid lesions. Activated helper T cells stimulate nonspecific antibody production by B cells,[1] producing a whole range of antibodies and resulting in hypergammaglobulinemia[1] in about 50% of patients, particularly in blacks.[36] In the acute disease about half the patients have circulating immune complexes, the presence of which correlates with various clinical features such as erythema nodosum.[55]

In active sarcoidosis bronchoalveolar lavage (BAL) shows a T-cell lymphocytosis with an increase in activated helper cells manifest as an increase in the CD4/CD8 ratio,[38,56] and to a lesser extent activated alveolar macrophages. Such a lymphocytic alveolitis can even be seen in sarcoidosis manifest as stage I disease with negative transbronchial biopsy or in patients with evidence of only extrathoracic disease.[56] This "sarcoidosis" pattern of BAL is nonspecific and may be seen with other conditions such as chronic beryllium disease and hypersensitivity pneumonitis.[56] Although a high CD4/CD8 ratio in BAL is associated with other measures of disease "activity", its usefulness in predicting outcome and monitoring treatment is debatable,[1] and most clinicians believe it has no role in the routine management of the patient with sarcoidosis.[57]

Another investigation that has previously been used to monitor disease "activity" is ^{67}Ga scintigraphy.[58] In normal individuals imaged 48 h after intravenous administration of this isotope, a little uptake is seen in bone but none in the lung or mediastinum.[59] However, in sarcoidosis, uptake is seen in the lung and in hilar and mediastinal nodes (Fig. 11.1).[60–62] Change in capillary permeability in inflamed tissue probably accounts in part for this local gallium accumulation.[63] The agent seems to be taken up predominantly by activated macrophages,[63,64] and to a lesser extent by activated T lymphocytes.[63] Irrespective of which cell is involved, it seems possible that gallium uptake may reflect the degree of "activity" of the sarcoid process. Unfortunately, there is no consensus regarding the criteria for activity (see below) and no clear-cut way of using gallium scanning has emerged; its clinical value therefore remains undefined.[65–67] Current opinion suggests that it has no place in the assessment of sarcoidosis except in selected clinical settings, e.g. when there is diagnostic difficulty (particularly with apparently isolated extrathoracic disease), or a need to distinguish active from fibrotic disease in the chest.[63]

Recent studies have demonstrated uptake of ^{18}F-fluorodeoxyglucose (^{18}F-FDG) in both affected lung parenchyma[68] and nodes[69] using positron emission tomography (PET) (Fig. 11.2). However, the clinical relevance of this finding is unclear.

Typical physiologic findings in patients with sarcoidosis are restrictive, with decreased total lung capacity, a reduced diffusing capacity, and reduced compliance.[70,71] However, airway obstruction may also be present, either as a manifestation of early disease with small airway involvement,[72–74] or in later disease when there is reticular abnormality and bronchovascular distortion.[75] A loose relationship exists between pulmonary function tests and chest radiographic changes.[71,76] The mean values for pulmonary function tests correlate with the radiographic stage, becoming worse from stage I to III. However, individual exceptions to this correlation are common.

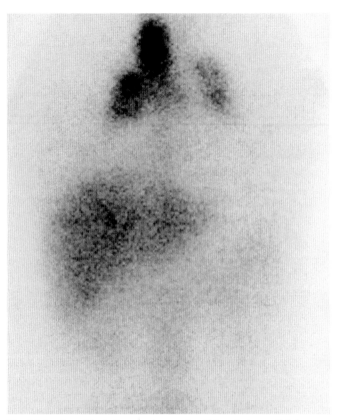

Fig. 11.1 Sarcoidosis, lymphadenopathy; ^{67}Ga scintiscan. This image, taken 72 h after the intravenous administration of ^{67}Ga-citrate, shows abnormal uptake in both hila and right upper mediastinum. Liver uptake is normal. (Courtesy of Dr G Cook, London, UK)

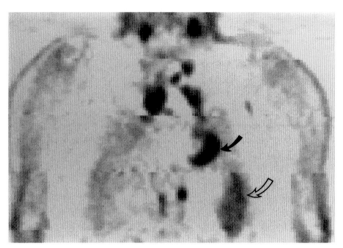

Fig. 11.2 Sarcoidosis, lymphadenopathy; [18]fluoro-deoxyglucose (^{18}F-FDG) positron emission tomogram. The nodes in sarcoidosis show increased activity with ^{18}F-FDG administered 30 min previously. Most nodes are in the upper mediastinum but there are two in the neck and abdomen and possibly one in the left axilla. Left ventricular activity (black arrow) and splenic activity (open arrow) are normal. (With permission from Lewis PJ, Salama A. Uptake of fluorine-18-fluorodeoxyglucose in sarcoidosis. J Nucl Med 1994;35:1647–1649.)

For example, several studies have shown that about 50% of patients in stage I have a diffusion defect.[71,77] Also, pulmonary function tests can give results in the normal range in stage II and III disease. Discrepancies between radiographs and function are most likely to arise when patients are treated with steroids, which may improve function in the face of an unchanging chest radiograph.[71]

Diagnosis and prognosis

The definitive diagnosis of sarcoidosis requires clinical and imaging features compatible with the diagnosis, and the identification of noncaseating granulomas in at least one organ.[78] In clinical practice the organs most commonly sampled are lymph nodes, liver, and lung. Transbronchial biopsy has a diagnostic yield of about 90%, provided that enough tissue samples are obtained.[43,59,79–81] Even in patients with hilar adenopathy who have normal lung parenchyma on chest radiographs, the yield from biopsy is >80%.[82] The high yield of transbronchial biopsy in this condition is due to the predominantly peribronchovascular distribution of the granulomas.

As mentioned above, a large number of conditions can produce granulomatous lesions (Box 11.2), and if the diagnosis of sarcoidosis rests on histologic appearances, these other conditions must be excluded as far as possible by history, special histologic stains, and microbiologic culture. Establishing

the widespread nature of the granulomatous process is also important, since local sarcoidlike reactions can be produced by a number of primary processes, including lymphoma and carcinoma.[17,83] In clinical practice, the diagnosis of sarcoidosis is sometimes accepted without biopsy, provided that clinical, laboratory, and radiologic features are typical. In particular, biopsy is usually unnecessary when the patient presents with Lofgren syndrome, and the resolution is rapid and spontaneous.[78] When the clinical diagnosis is less firmly based, histologic proof is essential. The Kveim test, in which skin biopsy is performed 4–6 weeks after intracutaneous injection of a saline suspension of human sarcoid tissue,[84] is now almost obsolete, largely because the injected material is poorly standardized and is not widely available. It may still have utility in cases where sarcoid is suspected in hard to biopsy sites such as the central nervous system or eye.[78]

The term "activity" is frequently used in relation to sarcoidosis but it is not exactly defined and its clinical relevance is unproven. Under current understanding of the pathogenesis of sarcoidosis, an initiating event (antigen exposure) sets in train a three-phase response: (1) T-lymphocyte/macrophage inflammation; (2) granuloma formation; and (3) active fibrosis; any or all of which can be active, i.e. changing or evolving.[85] Different markers of activity reflect different elements of this process. A great variety of markers have been proposed, including clinical parameters, imaging techniques (chest radiography, high-resolution CT [HRCT], ^{67}Ga scanning), serum levels (e.g. calcium, ACE), and BAL markers. Despite this great variety the consensus view is that the clinical activity of sarcoidosis is best assessed on the basis of symptoms.[78] In general, tests to stage activity are limited to clinical investigation, chest radiography, and lung function testing.[85] The basic problem with all markers of disease "activity" is that they do not necessarily predict outcome or the necessity to start corticosteroid therapy.[85]

Indications for treating chest disease are not firmly established but most patients with symptomatic or progressive stage II or

III disease will be on treatment. The clinician will usually base treatment decisions on the patient's symptoms, physiologic impairment, or evidence of extrathoracic involvement, rather than on the chest radiographic appearance. If treatment of sarcoidosis is indicated, then corticosteroids are the agents of first choice.[9,57,86] There is no doubting the shortterm efficacy of steroids but their longterm value is less clear and a number of controlled studies have shown no longterm difference between treated and untreated patients,[87] and symptoms will commonly recur when treatment is reduced or stopped.[78] Other agents have been tried in steroid resistant sarcoidosis, including immunosuppressive, cytotoxic, and antimalarial drugs.[57]

Lung transplantation has been successfully employed in end-stage sarcoidosis with survival rates at 1 year that are slightly less than in other forms of diffuse lung disease.[88] Recurrence of sarcoidosis has been described in the transplanted lung,[89,90] but is not usually a significant clinical problem because it can be controlled with augmented immunosuppression. In a multiinstitutional study, sarcoidosis was found to have recurred in nine (35%) of 26 patients transplanted for this disease, and was the most common disease to recur in this study.[91] Recurrent sarcoidosis was identifiable on CT in only three of the nine cases identified histologically. In those with an abnormal CT, recurrence was manifest as either miliary nodules ($n = 2$) or a solitary pulmonary nodule ($n = 1$).[91]

The majority of deaths from sarcoidosis are related to pulmonary, cardiac, or neurologic disease. In three series of 113 sarcoid related deaths, 69 (61%) resulted from pulmonary involvement – overwhelming granulomatous disease, pulmonary fibrosis, cor pulmonale, mycetoma formation, and respiratory failure.[92–94] In several large series, overall mortality ranged between 2.2 and 7.6%.[36,78,95]

Staging

Sarcoidosis is commonly staged according to its appearance on the chest radiograph. Several different classifications have been proposed.[32,96,97] A widely used classification is the following:[32,97]

- Stage 0 – normal chest radiograph
- Stage I – nodal enlargement only
- Stage II – nodal enlargement and parenchymal opacity
- Stage III – parenchymal opacity without adenopathy or evidence of fibrosis
- Stage IV – lung fibrosis (parenchymal distortion, lobar volume loss, bullae).

Other classifications[96] use a three-stage system, with fibrotic and non-fibrotic opacities grouped together as stage III. The use of the term "stage" should not be taken to mean that sarcoidosis always begins as stage 0, with orderly progression through the higher stages. For example, stage 0 may be seen in patients with advanced extrathoracic sarcoidosis, and cases are seen in which it seems unlikely that stages III or IV were preceded by stages I or II. Nevertheless, patients commonly pass sequentially from stages I to III, and the system is so hallowed by use that it is unlikely to be changed. At the time of presentation the percentages of patients in each stage are:

- Stage 0 – 5–15%
- Stage I – 45–65%
- Stage II – 30–40%
- Stage III – 10–15%
- Stage IV – 5%.

The stage at presentation is generally considered to correlate with prognosis. Untreated patients with stage I disease experience resolution of symptoms and radiographic abnormalities in 50–90% of cases, compared with 30–70% for stage II, 10–20% for stage III, and 0% for stage IV.[57]

Radiographic patterns

Normal chest radiograph (radiographic stage 0)

A normal chest radiograph, without adenopathy or parenchymal abnormality, is seen in about 10% of patients with sarcoidosis, depending on the population being studied.[76] Patients with this presentation of sarcoidosis usually have significant extrathoracic disease such as uveitis or skin abnormalities. However, 20–30% of those with normal chest radiographs will have decreased vital capacity and/or decreased lung diffusing capacity.[76] CT may be helpful in clarifying the presence or absence of lung disease in these patients. Of 69 patients with sarcoidosis described in three papers,[98–100] 14 had normal chest radiographs at the time of CT. Of these, seven patients had pulmonary parenchymal disease demonstrable on CT scanning, while the remainder had normal parenchyma on CT. As with other interstitial diseases, a normal chest radiograph or chest CT does not exclude pulmonary sarcoidosis. As discussed below, ^{67}Ga scanning may identify occult lymphadenopathy in those with normal or nonspecific chest radiographs.

Mediastinal and hilar lymphadenopathy (radiographic stage 1)

Lymphadenopathy is the most common intrathoracic manifestation of sarcoidosis, occurring in 75–80% of patients at some point in their illness.[31,36,95] Lymph node enlargement is usually seen in the right paratracheal, aortopulmonary window, hilar and tracheobronchial regions (Fig. 11.3, Box 11.3). In one series of 150 patients with sarcoidosis and an abnormal chest radiograph, about 30% had bilateral hilar lymphadenopathy (BHL) alone, 30% had BHL with right paratracheal adenopathy, and 30% had BHL with bilateral paratracheal adenopathy.[31] This series and earlier ones probably underestimate the prevalence of left paratracheal adenopathy, which is not as easy to detect as right-sided adenopathy.[101] However, the aortopulmonary nodes are enlarged in most patients, producing a characteristic local convexity in the aortopulmonary window (Fig. 11.3).[102]

***Box 11.3* Common sites of adenopathy in sarcoidosis**

Common
Hila
Right paratracheal
Aortopulmonary
Subcarinal

Uncommon
Anterior mediastinal
Posterior mediastinal
Paracardiac
Retrocrural
Axillary

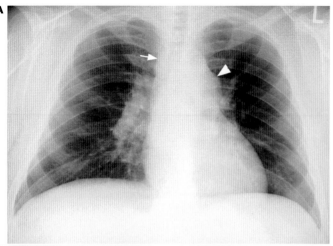

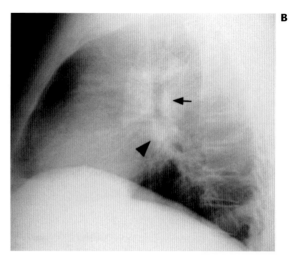

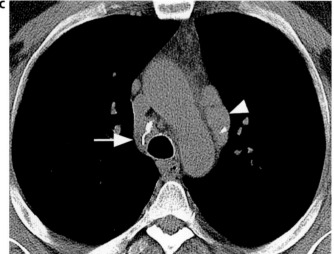

Fig. 11.3 Stage I sarcoidosis showing characteristic distribution of lymphadenopathy. **A**, On the frontal radiograph the right hilar nodes are markedly enlarged, with involvement of both proximal tracheobronchial and more distal bronchopulmonary nodes. Right paratracheal widening is present (arrow) and there is convexity of the aortopulmonary window indicating adenopathy (arrowhead). The lung parenchyma is normal. **B**, On the lateral radiograph there is thickening of the posterior wall of the bronchus intermedius (arrow). Adenopathy is also evident below the hila, in the "inferior hilar window" (arrowhead). **C**, CT confirms right paratracheal adenopathy (arrow), and paraaortic adenopathy (arrowhead). The nodes are partially calcified.

The degree of hilar node enlargement ranges from barely detectable to massive, in which case nodes may reach halfway to the chest wall. The outer margins of the hila are usually lobulated and well demarcated except when there is adjacent parenchymal opacity.[103] Both the more proximal tracheo-bronchial and the more distal bronchopulmonary nodes are involved in sarcoidosis, and enlargement of the latter is characteristic.[104] These more peripheral nodes may have lung or lower lobe bronchus on their medial aspect, and thus when enlarged they typically have a clearly demarcated inner border (Fig. 11.3).[104] Symmetry is an important diagnostic feature of the hilar adenopathy associated with sarcoidosis because symmetric adenopathy is unusual in the major diagnostic alternatives (Box 11.4), such as lymphoma, tuberculosis, and metastatic disease (Fig. 11.4). Sometimes the adenopathy appears more marked on the right on a frontal radiograph simply because the right hilum is more clearly separated from the mediastinum than the left.

Unilateral hilar adenopathy occurs in 3–5% of cases of sarcoidosis (Fig. 11.5).[31,35,103] In one series of 135 patients, an exceptionally high proportion of patients (9.6%) showed unilateral hilar adenopathy,[105] and adenopathy was found to be

Box 11.4 Causes of bilateral hilar lymphadenopathy

Sarcoidosis

Infection
Tuberculosis (especially HIV positive)
Brucellosis
Tularemia
Plague
Anthrax
Infectious mononucleosis
Cat scratch disease
Viral or mycoplasma pneumonia (mainly in children)

Neoplasm
Lymphoma
Metastases
Leukemia

Occupational
Silicosis
Berylliosis

Other
Amyloidosis
Drugs (phenytoin)

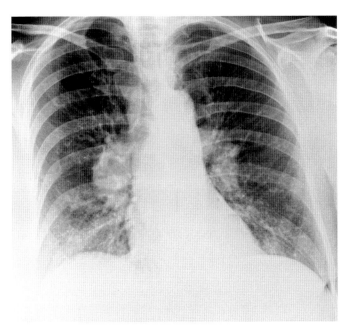

Fig. 11.4 Chronic lymphatic leukemia. Symmetric bilateral hilar and right paratracheal adenopathy simulates sarcoidosis. Adenopathy in tuberculosis, histoplasmosis, and lymphoma is usually asymmetric, but in leukemia, metastatic disease, and silicosis, symmetric nodal enlargement is well recognized.

unilateral in 29% of 21 patients aged 50 years or older.[106] Unilateral hilar adenopathy is about twice as common on the right as on the left, and can occur either alone or with right paratracheal adenopathy.[105,107] In these patients, more aggressive investigation is required, because the differential diagnosis includes not only malignancy but primary or AIDS related tuberculosis or fungal infection.

Other nodes in the chest may be involved with a recorded frequency that reflects the imaging modality used and the diligence with which they are sought. In general, involvement of these other nodal groups accompanies the more classic adenopathy, and the degree of enlargement is usually less marked. Mediastinal adenopathy as a predominant or sole finding in patients with sarcoidosis is uncommon and should prompt consideration of alternative diagnoses. Although CT commonly demonstrates adenopathy in "atypical" locations, such as the anterior or posterior mediastinum, axilla, retroperitoneum, or internal mammary chain, such adenopathy is almost invariably associated with extensive middle mediastinal and hilar adenopathy.[12] Anterior mediastinal nodes are difficult to appreciate on plain radiographs, unless they are calcified (see Fig. 11.10), but CT shows involvement in 25–66% of patients (Fig. 11.6).[108,109] Isolated anterior mediastinal adenopathy, however, is rare,[103,110–112] and should strongly suggest a diagnosis other than sarcoidosis, particularly lymphoma.

Subcarinal adenopathy occasionally may be marked and can cause airway compression[113] or dysphagia.[114] The prevalence of

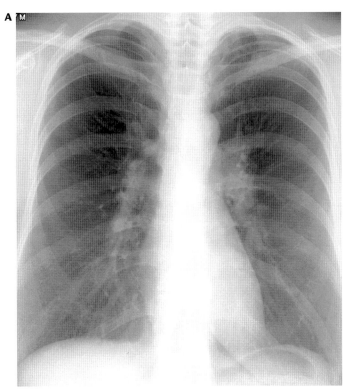

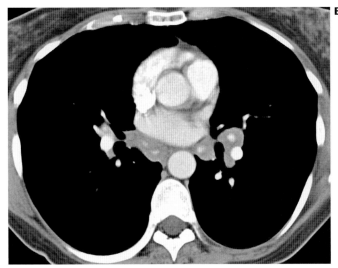

Fig. 11.5 Unilateral sarcoidosis. **A**, Chest radiograph shows pronounced left hilar adenopathy, with convexity of the aortopulmonary window indicating lymph node enlargement. **B**, Contrast-enhanced CT shows a large left hilar node containing central amorphous calcification. There are also several enlarged, partially calcified, subcarinal nodes. This pattern of amorphous calcification is quite suggestive of sarcoidosis.

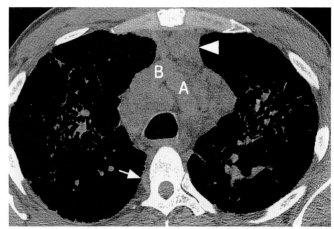

Fig. 11.6 Mediastinal adenopathy in a 40-year-old man with fibrotic sarcoidosis. CT shows extensive adenopathy in the pretracheal and paraaortic locations, moderate enlargement of anterior mediastinal nodes (arrowhead), and mild enlargement of a right paraspinal node (arrow). "A" indicates the top of the aortic arch. "B" indicates the left brachiocephalic vein, uniting with the right brachiocephalic vein. All of the other soft tissue density material in the mediastinum represents adenopathy.

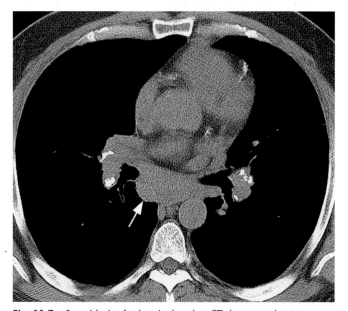

Fig. 11.7 Sarcoidosis of subcarinal nodes. CT shows moderate subcarinal nodal enlargement (arrow). There is punctate nodal calcification in both hila.

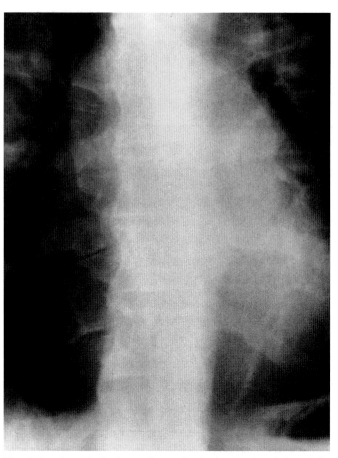

Fig. 11.8 Sarcoidosis of posterior mediastinal nodes. Local view of the lower mediastinum shows a focal convexity of the paraaortic interface, caused by posterior mediastinal, paraaortic node enlargement.

Natural history of stage I sarcoidosis

The enlarged nodes of sarcoidosis are usually at their maximum size when first seen; they decrease in size over the next 3–6 months so that two-thirds are no longer visible after 1 year,[104] and very few are visible after 2 years.[97] In one review only 6% persisted at 2 years, and most of these were smaller than when first examined.[97] If nodes are still present at 2 years, they commonly remain unchanged for many years,[104,118] and probably indefinitely. Given this fact and the commonness of sarcoidosis, the possibility that mediastinal lymphadenopathy is caused by sarcoidosis must always be considered, even in the context of malignant disease.[119,120]

Of patients with stage I disease at initial examination, about 60% go on to complete resolution,[35,97,104,105] with resolution being more common in those with erythema nodosum and arthropathy.[97] In the remaining 30–40% of patients presenting with adenopathy, parenchymal opacity develops,[97,104] usually within the first year, though longer intervals are not uncommon[104] and gaps of 10 years or more are recorded.[118] The adenopathy commonly begins to shrink at the time that parenchymal abnormality appears,[31,97] a feature that can be helpful in distinguishing sarcoidosis from lymphoma or carcinoma, in which the nodes would usually enlarge in parallel with progressive pulmonary involvement.[105]

Fluctuation of nodal enlargement during intermittent steroid therapy is well recognized,[121] but once the nodes have completely

subcarinal adenopathy in a study using chest radiographs was 21%,[102] but with CT (Fig. 11.7) the frequency is of the order of 50%.[108] Involvement of subcarinal nodes in the absence of hilar adenopathy is rare but has been recorded.[115]

Posterior mediastinal adenopathy (Figs 11.6 and 11.8) is one of the least common patterns in sarcoidosis, ranging in frequency from 2 to 20%,[102,109,116] the higher figure being atypical. Only one case report exists of sarcoidosis presenting with isolated posterior mediastinal adenopathy.[117]

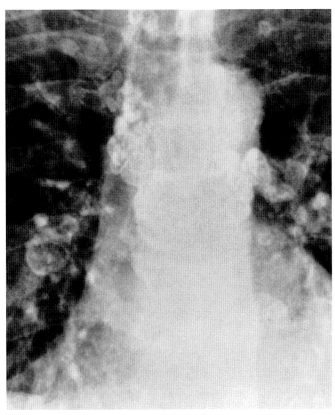

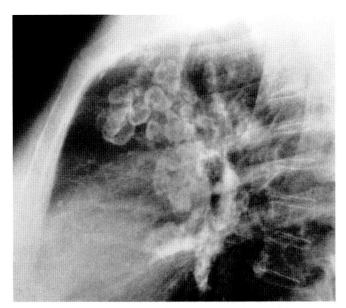

Fig. 11.10 Sarcoidosis, nodal calcification. Lateral view of the upper chest shows extensive nodal calcification, much of which has an eggshell pattern. Many nodes are in the anterior mediastinum.

Fig. 11.9 Sarcoidosis, nodal calcification. Local view of the middle and lower mediastinum shows extensive calcification affecting the hilar, paratracheal, subcarinal, posterior mediastinal, and anterior mediastinal lymph nodes.

resolved radiologically they probably will not enlarge again spontaneously. Such a train of events should raise the possibility of malignant adenopathy.[122] Only about 10 cases of nodal recurrence are reported, and these spanned periods of up to 20 years.[123] Nodal recurrence developed either alone[40,121] or with other features of sarcoidosis.[124] Recurrences may be multiple, and as many as three or four episodes have been recorded.[97] Different nodal groups may be involved in separate episodes, as in one patient in whom first one hilum and then the other was involved.[125]

Nodal calcification

The frequency of detection of nodal calcification in sarcoidosis (Figs 11.9 and 11.10) relates to the mode of detection and the duration of disease.[126] In shortterm studies using chest radiography, nodal calcification is seen in about 1–3% of cases,[31,97] but in a longer term study of 111 patients observed for 10 years or more the prevalence was 20%,[127] leading to the suggestion that sarcoid is probably the most common cause of mediastinal nodal calcification in regions where the prevalence of tuberculosis or fungal infection is low.

Calcification is thought to develop only in diseased nodes, occurring in a dystrophic fashion in fibrous tissue. Its occurrence is unrelated to either hypercalcemia or coincident tuberculosis. Most descriptions are of paratracheal and hilar involvement, but any nodal group may be involved.[101] The morphology of the

calcification on chest radiographs is variable and nonspecific. However, in a number of patients peripheral, eggshell calcification develops (Fig. 11.10).[101,103,111,128,129] This is of diagnostic value because its occurrence is largely limited to sarcoidosis and silicosis.[129] Spontaneous resolution of eggshell calcification has been reported.[27]

CT allows a more detailed analysis of the frequency and morphology of nodal calcification than the chest radiograph. The prevalence of nodal calcification detected by CT in patients with sarcoidosis is 45[130]–55%.[128] Gawne-Cain and Hansell[128] compared findings in 28 patients with tuberculosis and 49 with sarcoidosis, selected on the basis that they had had mediastinal CT. In sarcoidosis there were more calcified nodes (20 versus eight), calcified nodes were larger (12 versus 7 mm mean diameter), calcification was more commonly focal than complete, and hilar calcification when present was more commonly bilateral (65 versus 8%). Nine percent of sarcoid nodes showed an eggshell pattern and in two of 49 patients it was the predominant pattern. One tuberculous patient showed a predominant eggshell pattern as well. In other patients with sarcoidosis, an amorphous, cloudlike pattern of nodal calcification is seen (Fig. 11.5), differing from the punctate dense calcification typically seen in tuberculosis or fungal infection.

Parenchymal sarcoidosis (stages II, III, or IV)

Parenchymal disease is seen radiographically at the time of presentation in a little under half of patients with sarcoidosis.[31,35,36,76,105,131] In addition, about one-third of patients presenting with stage I disease go on to develop parenchymal opacity, with a frequency that shows a marked variation from series to series, ranging from 10 to 43%.[15,35,97,105,131] Such parenchymal abnormality frequently develops within the year and is usually accompanied, at least to some degree, by nodal regression. Parenchymal abnormalities on the chest radiograph or chest CT in sarcoidosis may usefully be classified into reversible and irreversible disease.

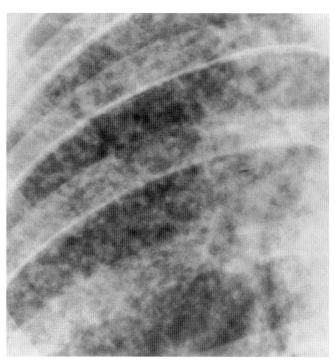

Fig. 11.11 Parenchymal sarcoidosis. Localized view of the right middle zone shows profuse nodules, ranging in size from 2 to 4 mm. Some nodules are rounded, others irregular.

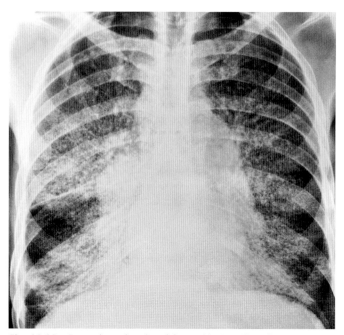

Fig. 11.12 Parenchymal and nodal sarcoidosis. Diffuse fine reticulonodular opacities affect all zones in a symmetric fashion, sparing the apices. The minor fissure is thickened, and there is subpleural thickening in the lateral right lower lung. Adenopathy involves both hila, the right paratracheal region, and the aortopulmonary window.

Reversible changes

Reversible changes on the chest radiograph in sarcoidosis consist of three patterns: reticulonodular opacities; ill-defined opacities with the characteristics of consolidation ("alveolar"); and large nodules. These patterns can occur alone or in varying combinations.[31] They may resolve partially or completely, or they may progress to an irreversible, fibrotic pattern. The approximate frequency of the various patterns of parenchymal abnormality is 75–90% reticulonodular, 10–20% "alveolar", and 2% large nodular.

Reticulonodular and nodular opacities

Small rounded or irregular opacities constitute by far the most frequent pulmonary pattern and are seen in 75–90% of patients with parenchymal abnormalities.[76,132] Reticulonodular opacities are more common than pure nodules. In an attempt to characterize these opacities, a number of workers have used the pneumoconiosis classification of the International Labor Office (ILO)/University of Cincinnati (see Ch. 8), extending it to include x, y, and z opacities to denote small rounded opacities from which irregular linear tentacles arise.[76,133] In the study by McLoud et al,[76] 35% of opacities were classified as "xyz", 33% as "pqr", and 19% as "stu". The nodules range in diameter from just under 1 to >5 mm, with most 2–4 mm (Figs 11.11 to 11.13).[31,132] In addition to discrete interstitial abnormalities such as nodules, more diffuse changes occur and are seen on radiographs as bronchial wall thickening, air bronchograms, and subpleural and fissural thickening (Fig. 11.12).[134] Aggregated subpleural granulomas account for the apparent fissural thickening and these can be well appreciated on HRCT (see Fig. 11.15).

The reticulonodular abnormality is usually bilaterally symmetric (Figs 11.12 and 11.13), with about 15% showing

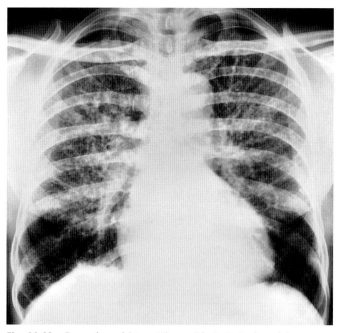

Fig. 11.13 Parenchymal (stage III) sarcoidosis. Reticulonodular opacities measuring 2–4 mm are present in the mid and upper lungs. Adenopathy is not visible.

significant asymmetry.[97] In exceptional cases (<1% of cases),[105,135] parenchymal changes are strictly unilateral. Unilateral change, however, was recorded in 8% in one series.[132] Unilateral parenchymal disease is usually, but not exclusively, of the (reticulo)nodular type and may occur with or without adenopathy.[126,136–138]

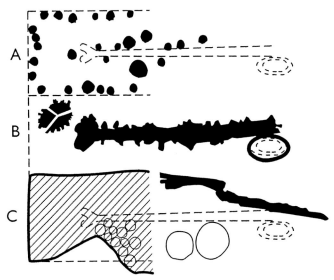

Fig. 11.14 Patterns of sarcoidosis on HRCT. Three peripheral pulmonary lobules with centrilobular artery and accompanying airway are shown. **A** and **B** represent common and **C** less common changes. **A**, Nodules 1–5 mm with predominant distribution along the bronchovascular structures, interlobular septa, and visceral pleura. **B**, Irregular bronchovascular interfaces, widened bronchovascular structures, thick airway walls, acinar nodules with air bronchograms, and prominent centrilobular structures. **C**, Interlobular septal thickening; ground-glass opacity; lobular distortion; long irregular scars; honeycombing, cyst, and bulla formation.

Opacities tend to occur in all zones, often showing a middle zone or middle and upper predominance (Fig. 11.13).[97,131] Isolated lower zone involvement is seen in <4% of patients,[132] mimicking idiopathic pulmonary fibrosis. Occasionally, a strictly upper zone distribution[132] may resemble tuberculosis.[139] Calcification within the lung in parenchymal sarcoidosis is rarely reported. It developed radiographically in five of 136 patients in one series followed for at least 5 years,[140] and in three of 111 cases followed for 10 or more years.[127] Parenchymal calcification is more commonly detected on CT.

On HRCT, the nodular or reticulonodular pattern of sarcoidosis is characterized by peribronchovascular thickening and irregularity with small nodules distributed in a perilymphatic fashion (Figs 11.14 and 11.15).[141] The craniocaudal distribution of this abnormality varies, but it often shows a mid to upper lung predominance. Several studies correlating histology and HRCT appearances have confirmed the predilection for sarcoid granulomas to lie in or adjacent to lymphatic vessels.[12,100,142] Because of this characteristic distribution, the nodules are found along bronchovascular margins (Figs 11.15 to 11.17), along interlobular septa (Fig. 11.17), and subpleurally (Fig. 11.17) (Box 11.5).[143] The subpleural nodules are often particularly well seen along the fissures (Fig. 11.15).

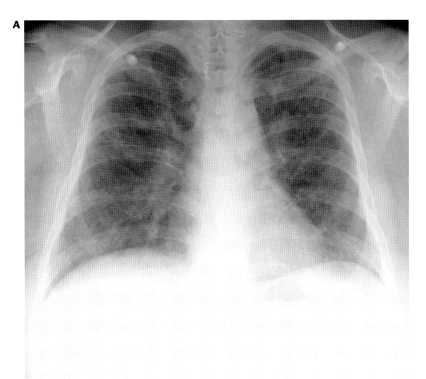

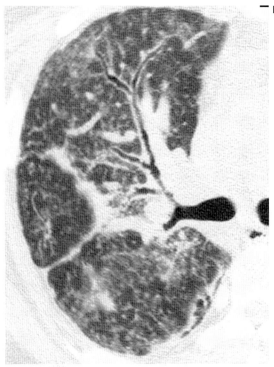

Fig. 11.15 Stage II sarcoidosis. **A**, Chest radiograph shows right hilar enlargement. Obliteration of the aortopulmonary window indicates adenopathy in this region also. Medial deviation of the gastric bubble is due to splenomegaly. **B**, HRCT shows diffuse nodularity, with peribronchial and fissural thickening. Note the irregularity of the bronchial lumen, consistent with submucosal granulomas. The subpleural and peribronchovascular distribution is characteristic of sarcoidosis.

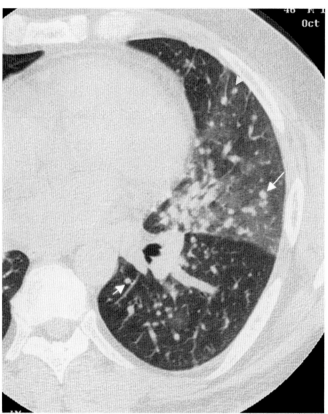

Fig. 11.16 Nodules and ground-glass attenuation in sarcoidosis. HRCT through the left lower lung shows ground-glass attenuation and numerous nodules (arrows), which are predominantly peribronchovascular and centrilobular. A few thickened septa are visible.

Box 11.5 Sites of nodules on HRCT in sarcoidosis

Peribronchovascular
Subpleural
Interlobular septa
Centrilobular

Nodules may also be centrilobular (Figs 11.16 and 11.18).[144] Nodules abutting interfaces make the normally sharp borders of vessels, airways, pleura, and septa irregular and beaded. The overall number of nodules varies greatly, ranging from total lung involvement (often upper and middle zone predominant)[98,145] to a scanty, focal distribution.[100] The nodules typically measure 1–5 mm, but conglomeration into larger irregular nodules or masses is quite common. They are usually sharply defined.

A perilymphatic distribution of nodules may also be seen in lymphangitic carcinoma[146–149] and lymphoproliferative disease.[150,151] Lymphangitic carcinoma can usually be differentiated from sarcoidosis by the presence of dramatic septal thickening, outlining the secondary pulmonary lobule much more markedly than is usually seen in sarcoidosis.[152] Although septal lines are present in about 50% of patients with sarcoidosis, they are not profuse and do not usually form complete polygonal outlines.[12,98,153] Septal thickening in sarcoidosis may be associated with lobular distortion, a finding not seen in lymphangitic carcinoma. Lymphoproliferative disease may also present with predominantly peribronchovascular nodules, usually larger and less profuse than those seen in sarcoidosis.[152]

A purely reticular pattern (Fig. 11.19) is an uncommon manifestation of sarcoidosis, but has been described on CT in two patients who did not have nodules and had an overall appearance suggestive of idiopathic pulmonary fibrosis,[154] quite unlike sarcoidosis. Probably the most common type of linear opacity in sarcoidosis is thick, nonseptal irregular lines caused by scarring. These are reported in about 40% of patients (range 22–72%).[12,130,145,155,156] Occasionally, curvilinear subpleural lines may be identified.[145]

Ground-glass opacity

This is much more easily seen on CT than on the chest radiograph in patients with sarcoidosis. In a large group of patients with sarcoidosis assessed by chest radiograph, Tazi et al[157] described 10 of 1600 with isolated ground-glass parenchymal opacity, all of whom had additional adenopathy. The majority were symptomatic white male smokers. All had active type

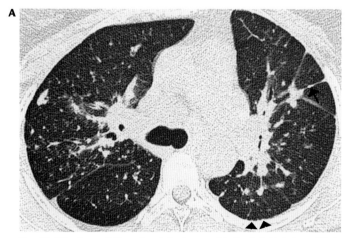
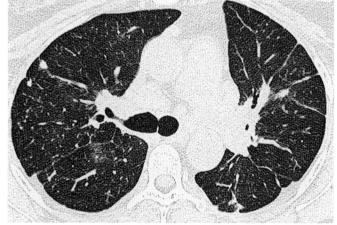

Fig. 11.17 Reversibility of nodules in sarcoidosis. **A**, Initial chest CT shows marked peribronchovascular nodularity due to granuloma deposition. Nodules are also seen along the interlobular septa (arrow) and visceral pleura (arrowheads). **B**, Following 3 months of steroid treatment, the peribronchovascular thickening has decreased significantly, and the subpleural nodules have also decreased. Bronchial distortion persists.

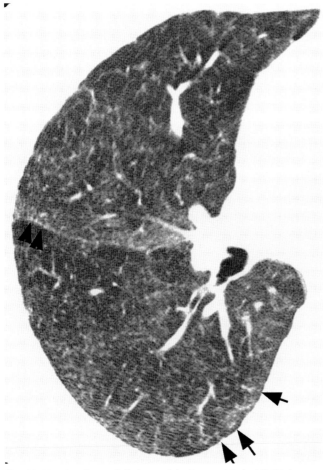

Fig. 11.18 Small centrilobular nodules in sarcoidosis. HRCT shows fine nodules, many of which are centrilobular (arrows). The fissural nodules (arrowheads) are a useful clue to the diagnosis of sarcoidosis.

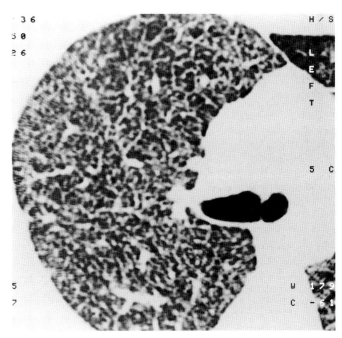

Fig. 11.19 Sarcoidosis, atypical pattern. HRCT shows fine nodular and fine reticular patterns. The reticular pattern is composed of interlobular septal thickening and intralobular lines. There is no traction bronchiectasis to suggest lung fibrosis. There is moderate centrilobular thickening.

disease of recent onset that was steroid sensitive but tended to relapse. When ground-glass opacity is extensive on the chest radiograph it may blur the outer margin of the hilum, giving rise to the "hilar haze" sign.[103]

Ground-glass opacity (Figs 11.16, 11.20, and 11.21) is seen on CT in about 40% of patients with sarcoidosis (range 16–83%).[98,130,145,155,156,158] It is patchy and may have a lobular distribution. In early reports of the CT findings of sarcoidosis, the ground-glass pattern was ascribed to alveolitis,[100] but it is

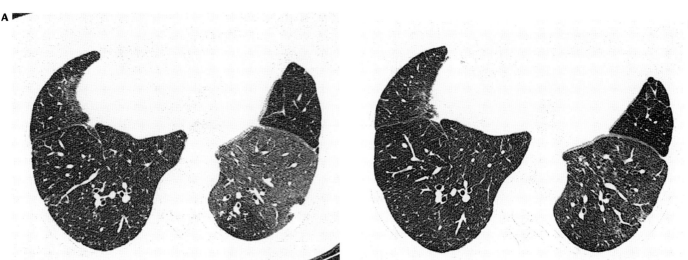

Fig. 11.20 Reversible ground-glass opacity in sarcoidosis. **A**, HRCT shows ground-glass abnormality in the left lower lobe, with a subpleural nodule. **B**, HRCT following 3 months of treatment shows resolution of the ground-glass abnormality. The subpleural nodule has been replaced by linear scars.

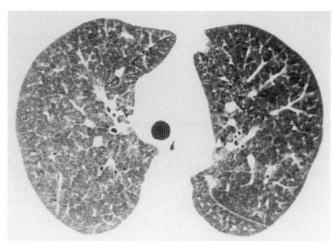

Fig. 11.21 Sarcoidosis – ground-glass opacity. HRCT shows extensive right-sided ground-glass opacity associated with very fine nodules. Other findings include mild interlobular septal thickening, mild bronchial wall thickening, fissural thickening, and a focal subpleural nodule in the anteromedial left upper lung.

now thought to be due to the presence of innumerable small interstitial granulomas, beyond the resolution of CT.[142,159–161] It is usually, but not always, reversible with steroid treatment,[130,159,162] with clearance being more likely if it is of short rather than long duration.[156]

"Alveolar" opacities

In 10–20% of patients with sarcoidosis, opacities with consolidative (airspace) features develop. These opacities form a spectrum ranging from ill-defined, irregular opacities of nondescript shape (Fig. 11.22) to those that are focal, nodular, and quite well defined. In the past, many authors regarded these latter nodules as a separate entity, so-called large nodular sarcoidosis, and though this is an artificial distinction,[126] it is maintained here because it makes consideration of the literature easier. The pathologic basis for the alveolar pattern in sarcoidosis is loss of alveolar air because of compression of the alveoli by coalescent granulomas in the interstitium.[34,103,163] Histologic study may show some of the alveoli to be filled with macrophages[164] or granulomas.[103,165] In a very few cases, alveolar opacities may be produced by airway occlusion by granulomas, causing obstructive pneumonitis.[163]

Alveolar sarcoidosis has been reported to have a prevalence rate of 10–20%, but is rarer in some series.[31,103,165–167] The typical appearance is bilateral, multifocal, poorly defined opacities,[31,113] ranging in size from about 1 to 10 cm.[103] These opacities can occur anywhere, but they show a predilection for the peripheral mid zone,[103,165,166] sparing the costophrenic angles.[166] The peripheral distribution is particularly well seen with CT (Fig. 11.22).[108] An air bronchogram is commonly present.[31,113,166] At the edge the lesions often break up into a nodular pattern that may be very fine, creating an appearance of acinar rosettes. Reticulonodular opacities are also present in about two-thirds of these patients,[31,166] and their detection provides a helpful clue when the principal radiographic finding is multifocal consolidation of obscure

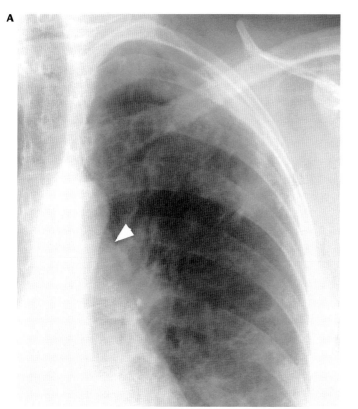

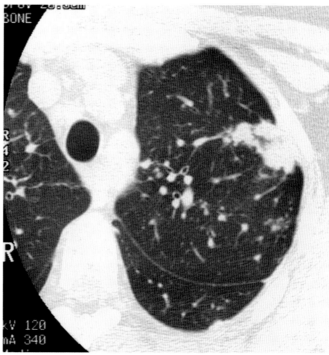

Fig. 11.22 Alveolar sarcoidosis. **A**, Detail view of the left upper lung shows poorly defined opacity. The arrowhead indicates convexity of the aortopulmonary window consistent with adenopathy. **B**, HRCT shows that the "alveolar" opacity is due to a coalescent cluster of nodules.

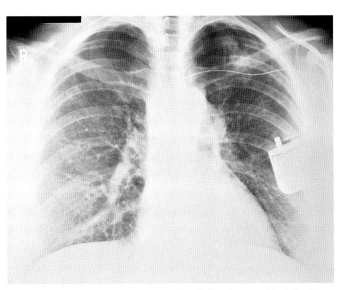

Fig. 11.23 Alveolar sarcoidosis. Localized alveolar sarcoidosis in the left upper zone with ipsilateral hilar adenopathy. This unusual pattern is suggestive of tuberculosis or bronchial carcinoma. Diagnosis in this case was proved at thoracotomy. The patient has a pacemaker for complete heart block, possibly due to cardiac sarcoidosis.

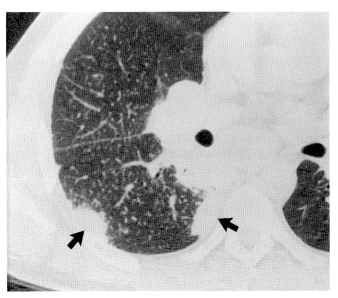

Fig. 11.24 Sarcoidosis – subpleural alveolar opacity. Alveolar opacities in sarcoidosis sometimes have a peripheral, pleural based distribution. Here there are two focal opacities lying posterolaterally and posteromedially (arrows). There are adjacent fine nodules, and close examination suggests that the areas of apparent consolidation are composed of fine nodules. The associated hilar and mediastinal adenopathy, subpleural/fissural nodules, and irregular bronchovascular interfaces are strongly suggestive of sarcoidosis.

origin. Another helpful pointer is mediastinal adenopathy, which is an even more common accompaniment, occurring in >80% of cases.[31,166] Kirks et al[31,168] pointed out that all their patients with alveolar sarcoidosis had mediastinal adenopathy and/or reticulonodular abnormality.

Recognized variants of the alveolar pattern include a unilateral distribution,[26] an upper zone distribution simulating tuberculosis (Fig. 11.23),[138] or a peripheral pattern that resembles cryptogenic eosinophilic pneumonia or crytogenic organizing pneumonia. In one series of 64 patients, 9% showed a pronounced peripheral distribution, some with an alveolar and some with a reticulonodular pattern.[169] Sharma[167] described two confusing cases in which the peripheral alveolar pattern was accompanied by blood eosinophilia, yet lung biopsy showed noncaseating granulomas consistent with sarcoidosis. Peripheral consolidation is usually accompanied by nodal enlargement, but exceptions are recorded.[170] Some authors have stressed the good prognosis and tendency for rapid clearing with alveolar sarcoidosis; in one report the opacity cleared in 21 of 22 patients with or without steroids,[166] and in another clearing occurred in 66% of patients within 9 months.[165] Not all authors agree; in the San Francisco series of 150 patients, clearing occurred in only 31%.[31] Patients with alveolar sarcoidosis usually have relatively minor physiologic impairment, and have a low prevalence of extrathoracic sarcoidosis.[165]

CT of patients with alveolar sarcoidosis usually shows irregular masslike opacities (Figs 11.22 and 11.24), with the characteristic peribronchovascular or subpleural distribution.[171] Air bronchograms are often seen, but the irregular well-defined border of the masses serves to distinguish these opacities from true consolidation.[98,161]

Large nodular sarcoidosis

Focal opacities with the radiologic features of large nodules are an uncommon but well-recognized finding in sarcoidosis (Figs 11.25 and 11.26), and when the various series are

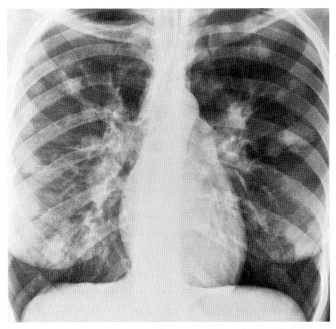

Fig. 11.25 Large nodular sarcoidosis. Note the multiple, relatively well-defined nodules ranging in diameter from 1 to 3 cm. In addition, mild bilateral hilar and right paratracheal adenopathy is evident. Nodal enlargement is an almost universal finding in large nodular sarcoidosis.

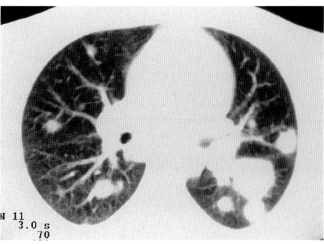

Fig. 11.26 Large nodular sarcoidosis. CT taken several centimeters below the carina shows multiple, bilateral, mid zone nodules ranging in size from 0.5 to 4.0 cm. Nodules, though relatively well defined, are mildly irregular in outline. Two nodules in the left lower lobe are coalescing. Even on the lung window settings it is possible to appreciate bilateral hilar and subcarinal adenopathy.

combined a 2.4% prevalence rate (35 of 1449 cases) is seen.[26,31,35,166,172] The nodules are usually bilateral and multiple, ranging in size from 0.5 to 5 cm.[126] They can occur in any zone, but as with alveolar sarcoid a slight mid zone predilection is evident. The margins of the nodules are occasionally sharp,[126,167] but are much more often ill defined and hazy.[166] Some nodules go on to coalesce.[167] They may contain an air bronchogram, a feature particularly well seen at CT.[98,108] Most are accompanied by mediastinal adenopathy, but a few cases are recorded in which adenopathy was absent.[172,173]

The nodules behave unpredictably over time and may remain static for years,[172] or show partial or complete regression.[172] Occasionally, sarcoid may present with a single large nodule, indistinguishable from bronchogenic carcinoma.[106,126,174–177]

On CT scanning of the large nodular form of sarcoidosis, the nodules may exhibit an irregular outline, with innumerable adjacent small satellite nodules, a finding termed the CT galaxy sign.[178] Patients with the nodular pattern on CT tend to have relatively mild physiologic impairment.[179]

Primary cavitation is rarely seen in either alveolar or large nodular sarcoidosis (Fig. 11.27). It probably occurs because of ischemic necrosis in conglomerate granulomas. Only about 10 cases are recorded.[180–185] Cavitation can be an early or late manifestation and may even be the presenting feature.[183] Cavities can be single or multiple (range one to eight) and may occur with or without adenopathy. The walls of the cavities have a variable appearance: thick or thin, and smooth or irregular. Sarcoid cavities may resolve either with or without steroids.[126] Although cavitation is usually benign, fatal hemoptysis has been recorded.[186] Cavitation is more common in necrotizing sarcoidal angiitis and this diagnosis should be considered particularly if the lesions are peripheral and pleurally based.

Irreversible fibrotic changes

Sarcoid granulomas may resolve completely, or they may heal by fibrosis (Fig. 11.28). Such fibrosis ranges from being minor and radiographically undetectable,[131] to gross, with scarring

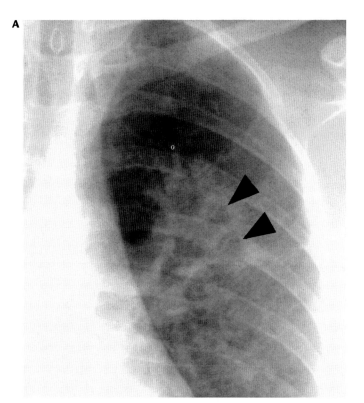

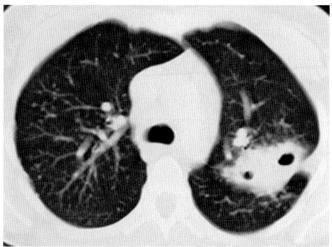

Fig. 11.27 Cavitary sarcoidosis. **A,** Detail view of a chest radiograph shows two cavitary nodules in the left upper lung (arrowheads), with a background of fine nodules. **B,** CT confirms cavitation within a conglomerate mass, along with scattered nodules. Despite intensive investigation, no vasculitis or infection was found to account for the cavitation.

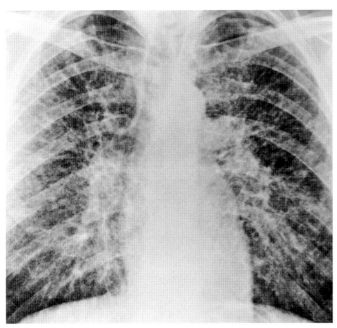

Fig. 11.28 Parenchymal sarcoidosis. Parenchymal shadowing is reticulonodular with a pronounced linear element. Both hila are mildly enlarged.

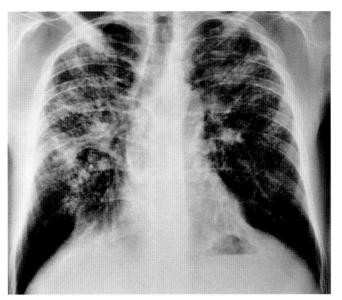

Fig. 11.30 Sarcoidosis with conglomerate fibrosis. Nodules predominate in the upper lungs, with confluent masses in the left upper lung and right mid lung. The hila are elevated, and overexpanded lower zones are transradiant.

and distortion on the chest radiograph (Fig. 11.29). Gross fibrosis is present on the initial chest radiograph in about 5–25% of patients.[31,34] In addition, gross fibrosis develops in 10–15% of patients who, when first examined, have stage 0 to II disease.[113,131] The fibrosis usually takes years to develop,[113] with a range in one series of 2–14 years.[131]

The radiologic changes of gross fibrosis in sarcoidosis are fairly characteristic. Some authors consider them to be almost pathognomonic.[97] The findings classically consist of permanent, coarse, linear opacities radiating laterally from the hilum into the adjacent upper and middle zones (Fig. 11.30).[103] On the lateral view, these changes can be seen to predominate in the lower part of the upper lobes.[97] Coincident with the development of scarring, the extreme upper and lower zones tend to become transradiant (Fig. 11.30). In the upper zones this transradiancy is the result of cyst and bulla formation, whereas in the lower zones it is more commonly the result of compensatory hyperinflation following upper zone volume loss. The hila are generally pulled upward and outward, and vessels and fissures are distorted.[31,105] The fibrosis is occasionally so pronounced that it gives rise to massive parahilar opacities in the mid and upper zones that resemble those seen in progressive massive fibrosis (Figs 11.30 and 11.31).[97,108,131] At the other extreme, minor localized linear scarring may be the only finding.[31] Cor

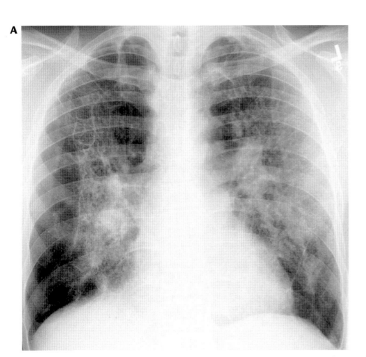

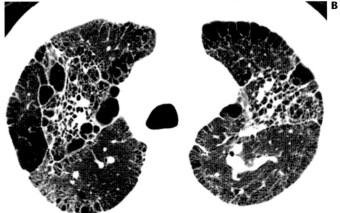

Fig. 11.29 A 40-year-old man with fibrotic, cystic sarcoidosis. **A**, Chest radiograph shows bilateral reticulonodular abnormality, with architectural distortion and thin walled cysts in the right upper lung. **B**, HRCT shows widespread cysts of varying sizes. The central bronchi are distorted. There is bilateral upper lobe volume loss, with anterior displacement of the fissures.

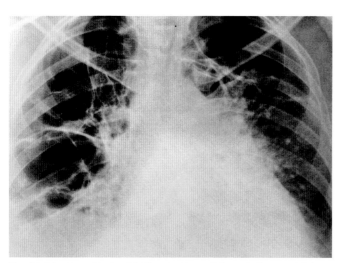

Fig. 11.31 Sarcoidosis with fibrosis. Most of the right lung and left apex are replaced by large cystic spaces.

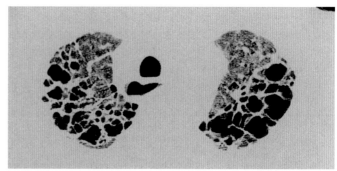

Fig. 11.32 Upper lobe cysts in sarcoidosis. HRCT through the upper lungs shows confluent cysts of varying size and wall thickness replacing normal lung parenchyma. Irregular bandlike opacities separating the ring opacities are caused by scarring. Sarcoid scarring in the mid and upper zones tends, as here, to be posterior.

pulmonale may supervene in the fibrotic stage[187] and may be radiologically recognizable.[188]

Cystic abnormality is particularly common in the upper zones in advanced fibrosis related to sarcoidosis.[34] Thin walled ring opacities may be caused by dilated, distorted bronchi,[108,131] or by cysts (Figs 11.29, 11.32, and 11.33).[34,109] Thick walled ring opacities may be due to an infected bulla, mycetoma, abscess, tuberculous cavity, or necrosis within a mass of conglomerate fibrosis.[34,103] A few cases of "vanishing lung" with marked emphysema and bulla formation have been reported.[189,190]

Irreversible CT findings in sarcoidosis include areas of conglomerate fibrosis, usually centered on the upper lobe bronchi and vessels, and often associated with marked bronchovascular distortion, characterized by posterior displacement of main and upper lobar bronchi.[98] As on the chest radiograph, these lesions (Fig. 11.31) are often difficult to distinguish from progressive massive fibrosis seen in pneumoconiosis. Other signs include lobular distortion, found in about 50% of patients[12,98,130,159]; long, irregular, linear opacities; traction bronchiolectasis; honeycombing; and cyst or bulla formation (Fig. 11.33). Honeycombing tends to be less common in sarcoidosis than in other forms of end-stage lung disease; the honeycomb cysts tend to be larger than in idiopathic pulmonary fibrosis (Fig. 11.34). The honeycombs and cysts of sarcoidosis tend to be distributed subpleurally in the mid and upper zones of the lungs, sparing the bases.[191]

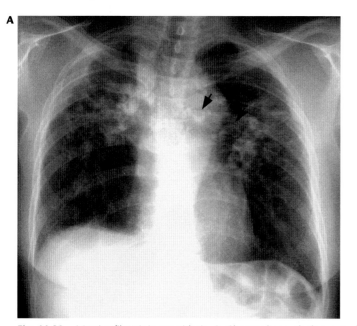

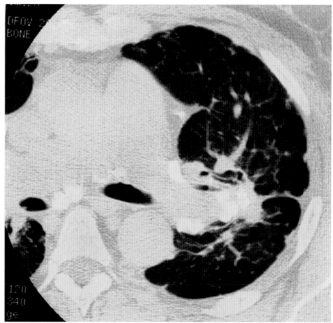

Fig. 11.33 Massive fibrosis in sarcoidosis. **A,** Chest radiograph shows marked bilateral upper lobe volume loss, with bilateral parahilar masses. The mediastinum is widened and distorted. Arrows indicate eggshell nodal calcification. **B,** HRCT of the left upper lung shows a parahilar mass with associated bronchial distortion, and scattered subpleural nodules.

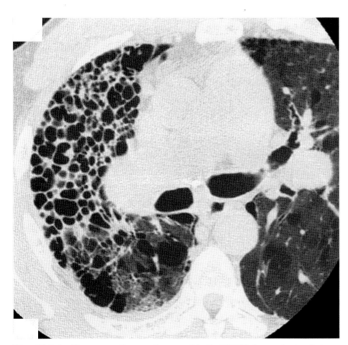

Fig. 11.34 Honeycomb cysts in sarcoidosis. HRCT through the right mid lung shows profuse clustered honeycomb cysts. The cysts are larger than the typical honeycomb cysts seen in usual interstitial pneumonia. Cysts are much less extensive in the left lung.

Airway involvement

Sarcoidosis can affect the trachea, bronchi, or bronchioles (Box 11.6). Tracheal involvement is rare,[192] and in the few reported cases has been associated with laryngeal involvement. Both the proximal and distal trachea may be affected, and the stenosis can be smooth,[193,194] irregular and nodular,[195] or even masslike.[196]

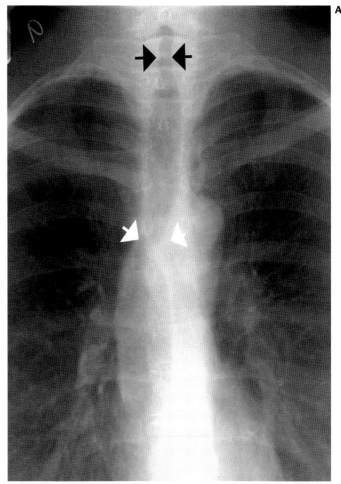

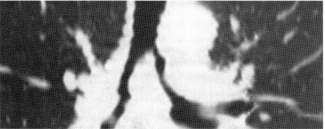

Fig. 11.35 Airway stenoses in sarcoidosis. **A,** Detail view of chest radiograph shows smooth subglottic tracheal narrowing (black arrows), and stenosis of the right and left main bronchi (white arrows). **B,** Coronal CT reconstruction confirms irregular narrowing of the main bronchi.

> **Box 11.6 Airways disease in sarcoidosis**
>
> Tracheal or bronchial granulomas
> Bronchial stenosis
> Bronchial distortion
> Small airways involvement with air-trapping

Bronchial narrowing in sarcoidosis may be due to extrinsic scarring, or to endobronchial granulomas and fibrosis.[126] Despite the sometimes massive enlargement of nodes in sarcoidosis, lymphadenopathy alone is a rare cause of symptomatic airway narrowing,[197] perhaps because the nodal capsules remain intact so that scarring and fixation are rare.[126] However, the parahilar conglomerate fibrosis of sarcoidosis will commonly cause bronchial distortion and narrowing, usually well shown on CT. Although endobronchial stenoses (Figs 11.35 and 11.36) occur most commonly in well-established disease,[97] often with pulmonary fibrosis, they have been recorded early in the course of sarcoidosis and with stage 0 radiographic disease.[198,199] The frequency of large airway narrowing is about 5% (range 2.5–9%).[97,131,199] Patients present with wheeze, stridor, or airflow

limitation,[198,200] or episodes of lobar or segmental collapse and consolidation. Collapse is a well recognized but uncommon manifestation of sarcoidosis, occurring in about 1% of cases.[31,34,35,103,105] Any lobe may be affected, most commonly the middle.[35,126] Collapse of a whole lung has been recorded.

Although the middle lobe is the most common to collapse, stenoses are distributed throughout the lung and show no particular lobar or segmental predilection. The stenoses may be single,[97,199] or multiple,[198–200] and most commonly affect lobar or proximal segmental divisions (Fig. 11.37). At bronchoscopy, depending on the stage of the disease, the mucosa may be

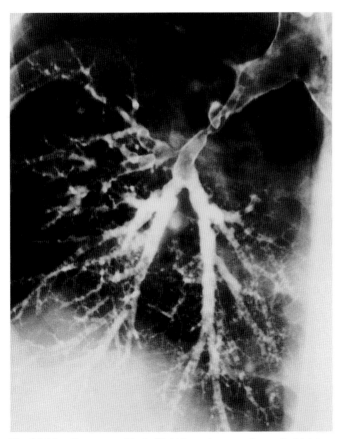

Fig. 11.36 Airway sarcoidosis. Right bronchogram shows cicatricial narrowing of the right upper lobe bronchus and bronchus intermedius. (With permission from Hadfield JW, Page RL, Flower CD, Stark JE. Localised airway narrowing in sarcoidosis. Thorax 1982;37:443–447.)

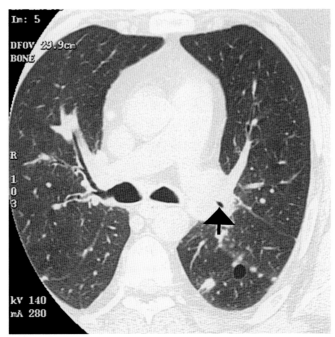

Fig. 11.37 Bronchostenosis due to sarcoidosis. HRCT shows marked narrowing of the apicoposterior left upper lobe bronchus (arrow). Note the endobronchial nodule in the right upper lobe bronchus, and nodules along an interlobular septum in the left lung.

granular and hyperemic or even frankly inflamed and edematous. Granulomas may even give rise to a local obstructing endobronchial mass.[106,201,202] Later, when healing by fibrosis occurs, the mucosa may appear normal.[198] In view of the variable pathogenesis of stenoses, not surprisingly they and their secondary effects show variable behavior, clearing spontaneously or with steroid treatment,[203] or remaining unchanged.[199] Mechanical dilatation or stenting is a therapeutic option.[204,205] When bronchial stenosis is considered, use of thin-section volumetric acquisition through the central bronchi, with multiplanar reconstructions, is likely to be useful (Fig. 11.35).[206]

Obstructive bronchiectasis as a result of endobronchial sarcoidosis is considered rare,[126] though in the context of gross fibrobullous disease it is often difficult to be sure of the exact pathogenesis of bronchiectatic change. Only a few cases have been described.[108,126]

The extent of airway involvement by sarcoidosis is underestimated by the chest radiograph. In an HRCT study of airways in 60 patients with sarcoidosis, 65% had nodular or smooth thickening of the airways from lobar to subsegmental level.[207] Twenty-three percent of patients had luminal narrowing, either smooth or irregular. Most of the patients in this study had stage II disease and the presence of bronchial wall thickening at HRCT correlated with biopsy proven bronchial granulomata. A recent study[208] indicated that there was a high prevalence of airway hyperreactivity in patients with endobronchial sarcoidosis, suggesting that endobronchial disease can cause airway obstruction even when there is no significant airway narrowing.

The occurrence of small airway disease in sarcoid patients was recognized by Carrington in 1976.[133] He described the deposition of peribronchial granulomas which result in air-trapping at the level of the secondary pulmonary lobule. This finding was demonstrated by HRCT 20 years later,[209] and since confirmed by multiple investigators.[72,74,210,211] Small airway obstruction is seen on expiratory HRCT as air-trapping and patchy areas of low attenuation.[209]

Airflow obstruction is common in sarcoidosis.[70,212,213] Potential etiologies include small airway obstruction, endobronchial narrowing,[214] airway hyperreactivity,[208] and bronchial distortion by masslike fibrosis. CT evaluation can be helpful in discriminating among these possibilities. Hansell et al,[75] in a study of 45 patients with airway obstruction in sarcoidosis found that a reticular pattern (presumably associated with bronchial distortion) was the major determinant of airflow limitation, while Davies et al[74] found that the extent of air-trapping on expiratory CT correlated well with physiologic evidence of airway obstruction. These studies confirm that physiologic evidence of airway obstruction is to be expected both in patients with advanced fibrotic sarcoid and in those with earlier disease who have small airway obstruction.

Pulmonary artery involvement

Large vessel involvement is rare in sarcoidosis[215] and is usually the result of compression by large nodes, or bronchovascular distortion by conglomerate masses.[216–220] Typically the lobar divisions, particularly the upper lobe vessels, are involved, and pulmonary arterial hypertension is usually absent. Perfusion scintigraphy shows corresponding large defects.[108,220] A few cases are reported in which stenosis of major pulmonary arteries was attributed to sarcoid induced scarring,[108,187,221,222] and in a single reported case multiple stenoses caused pulmonary arterial hypertension.[221]

Small vessel involvement by granulomas is common and is usually accompanied by widespread parenchymal disease.[82,133] Granulomas can lead to vessel narrowing, but not usually vascular necrosis or thrombosis. These changes probably account for patchy perfusion defects found on scintigraphy[223,224] and for pulmonary arterial hypertension.

Pulmonary artery hypertension in sarcoidosis is most commonly related to advanced lung disease with fibrosis and bullae,[225] but may also be caused by granulomatous vasculitis (Fig. 11.38),[226–228] by fibrobullous disease,[187] or rarely by large vessel disease.[108] When pulmonary hypertension is out of proportion to the visible extent of lung disease, it may respond to corticosteroid therapy.[229]

Pulmonary and systemic vein involvement

Although mediastinal adenopathy can be massive, it rarely causes compression of great veins with subsequent superior vena cava syndrome, a fact that has been ascribed to the lack of perinodal fibrosis in sarcoidosis.[126] A handful of cases are described, some of whom presented with superior vena cava obstruction and others in which it punctuated the course of established disease.[230–232] A single case of subclavian vein obstruction[233] and of innominate vein obstruction, which produced a large exudative pleural effusion, is recorded.[234] The rarity of superior vena cava

syndrome with sarcoidosis is such that other causes of obstruction should be sought.[110,235]

In a case report, granulomatous involvement of small pulmonary veins caused venous obliteration and resultant pulmonary arterial hypertension. The chest radiograph showed dilated proximal pulmonary arteries and a basal "interstitial pattern" resembling venoocclusive disease.[236]

Pleural sarcoidosis

In sarcoidosis, granulomas may be found on both the visceral and parietal pleura. These pleural granulomas uncommonly cause signs or symptoms.[237] On rare occasions, however, they may be associated with a dry pleurisy[238] or a pleural effusion that is usually painless,[239] but may be painful.[240] These effusions are classically lymphocyte rich exudates that in nearly one-fifth of cases are sanguinous or serosanguinous.[241] Eosinophilic effusions are described.[242]

In 1870 cases of sarcoidosis taken from major series in the world literature, 55 had pleural effusions, giving a prevalence of 1.9%.[15,31,34,35,103,105,243,244] Effusions may be present initially, but more often they develop during the course of established disease, a few months to 16 years after onset.[243] Sarcoid effusions are usually seen in the context of extensive pulmonary disease[244] or multisystem involvement.[243] However, pleural effusions with stage I disease are recorded,[31,245] and in rare cases patients have had an otherwise normal chest radiograph.[239,246] In one literature review, 49% were right sided and 28% left sided.[247] About one-

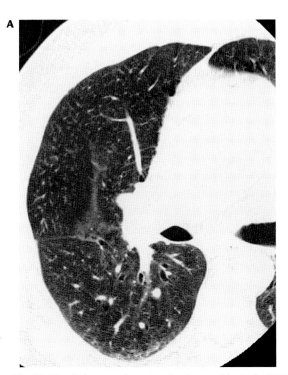
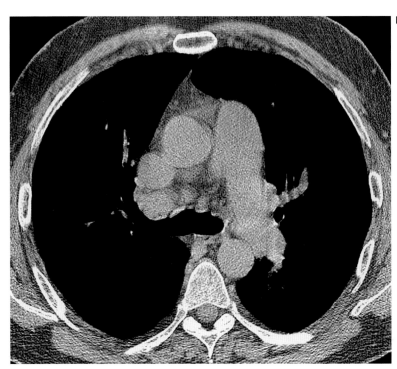

Fig. 11.38 Pulmonary hypertension in sarcoidosis. **A**, HRCT shows mild centrilobular ground-glass abnormality. **B**, CT through the main pulmonary artery shows pulmonary artery enlargement, out of proportion to the extent of parenchymal abnormality. Mediastinal adenopathy is also present.

third of the effusions are bilateral,[243] and while they are usually small, large effusions have been described.[241,248,249] The effusions resolve spontaneously in weeks or months and are almost invariably gone by 6 months.[26] Resolution is usually complete, but about 20% of patients are left with residual pleural thickening.[103,244]

In general, pleural effusion is a relatively minor and incidental finding in the course of sarcoidosis. However, because it is an atypical feature, it may prove a diagnostic puzzle. Several authors stress the importance of excluding other causes, particularly tuberculosis, which may occur concurrently.[250]

Five cases of chylothorax associated with sarcoidosis are recorded,[57] and it may be a presenting feature.[251] Fissural pleural thickening (Figs 11.12 and 11.15) is almost invariably due to subpleural granulomas.

Sarcoidosis is associated with a 2–3% prevalence of pneumothorax in several series, and it is usually seen with advanced fibrocystic disease.[247] Uncommonly pneumothorax can be a presenting manifestation of sarcoidosis, associated with multiple pleural granulomata at thoracotomy or subpleural cavitary nodules and bullae at HRCT.[252] Bilateral pneumothorax is also described.[253]

Bone involvement

Sarcoid bone involvement that is detectable on the chest radiograph is rare; only about 20 cases are reported. The spine is the most common site, and the sternum is the least common. Spinal sarcoidosis is characterized by multiple lower dorsal destructive lesions, often with vertebral body collapse.[126] A few cases have simulated infective spondylitis,[254] and entirely sclerotic lesions are described.[255] In one review, two of eight cases had no radiographic evidence of adenopathy or parenchymal sarcoidosis.[256] Rib lesions have been recorded in five cases[126] and have been lytic or permeative in most cases, one presenting as a rib fracture.[257] One patient had sclerotic lesions.[255] The one reported sternal lesion was lytic and was part of widespread spine and rib involvement.[254]

Mycetoma

Mycetoma formation (Fig. 11.39) is a well-recognized complication of stage IV cystic sarcoidosis.[258,259] Indeed, with the declining incidence of tuberculosis, sarcoidosis is probably now the most common cause of mycetoma. This is particularly so in the United States, where the large black population results in more cases of sarcoidosis who progress to gross fibrobullous disease.[260] In a series of mycetomas reported from Philadelphia, 45% were in patients with sarcoidosis,[261] whereas in a small series of 26 patients in the United Kingdom only 15% were in patients with sarcoidosis.[262] The frequency of mycetoma in sarcoidosis varies from series to series and ranges between 1 and 10% depending on racial mix of the patients and method of detection.[31,34,103,259,263] In the subset of sarcoid patients with stage

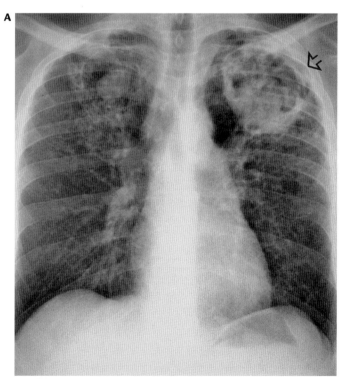

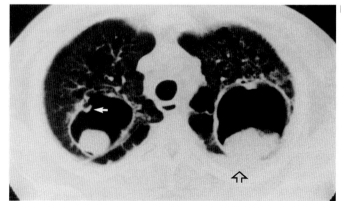

Fig. 11.39 Sarcoidosis – scarring and mycetoma formation. **A,** There are mid to upper zone linear and cystic changes. Focal, rounded masses are seen within the bilateral upper lobe cavities. **B,** CT confirms bilateral intracavitary masses typical of mycetomas. Note, both on the chest radiograph (arrow) and CT (open arrow) the local left-sided pleural thickening – a characteristic finding and pointer to the presence of an underlying mycetoma. Arising from the right cavity wall there is a small frondlike projection (white arrow). Such projections are commonly found in cavities colonized by fungi.

IV fibrocystic disease, the proportion of patients harboring a mycetoma can be as high as 50%.[103,259]

Hemoptysis is the most common and worrisome symptom of mycetoma, and may be life threatening.[259,263] In one small series of patients with sarcoidosis and mycetoma, major hemoptysis occurred every 5 years and minor hemoptysis every 2.5 years.[263] Steroid treatment does not seem to predispose to mycetoma formation.[259] The radiologic features of mycetoma are discussed in Chapter 5. In sarcoidosis, mycetoma formation is worth consideration when new abnormalities, particularly masslike lesions or pleural thickening, develop in patients with grade IV fibrocystic disease.[261] Mycetomas are confined virtually to the upper lobes and are commonly bilateral (Fig. 11.39) in 50% of cases in one series.[263] Serum precipitins against *Aspergillus* spp are almost always strongly positive. CT is the most sensitive imaging modality.[262,264]

Role of CT

A large number of studies have described the CT and HRCT changes in sarcoidosis,[12,98,100,142,145,155,162,265] and evaluated the role of CT in this condition.[99,130,147,156,158,159,266–270]

Follow-up CTs have been used to study the serial change of various opacities identified on HRCT,[98,100,130,156,159,162] giving further insight into the nature of the underlying pathology. Results are not entirely consistent but in general show that nodules, consolidation, ground-glass opacity, and septal lines are potentially reversible (Figs 11.17 and 11.20), while irregular coarse lines, cysts, honeycombing, traction bronchiectasis, and distortion are permanent. A significant proportion of potentially reversible opacities remain stable, e.g. 57 and 39% of nodules did not change in two follow-up studies.[130,156]

Other studies have attempted to correlate HRCT findings with pulmonary function tests and given discrepant results, with a weak overall correlation being the most common finding.[98–100,156,179] However, identification of the predominant pattern of abnormality on CT may be helpful in predicting the degree of physiologic impairment. Patients with focal alveolar abnormality, or masslike opacities, tend to have little or no physiologic impairment, while those with profuse nodules or architectural distortion tend to be significantly impaired.[179] As mentioned above, patients with air-trapping on expiratory imaging will usually have a component of airflow obstruction.

The role of CT scanning in patients with known or suspected pulmonary sarcoidosis remains unclear. Recognition of the characteristic CT pattern of sarcoidosis may help to suggest the diagnosis, and may in some cases be sufficiently specific to obviate the need for biopsy. If a biopsy is desired, CT may provide a "road map", identifying high yield areas for transbronchial biopsy. In patients with unilateral adenopathy, in whom there is concern for the presence of lymphoma or other abnormality, CT may help by identifying bilateral nodal and parenchymal abnormalities suggestive of sarcoidosis. However, CT adds little to the diagnostic evaluation of patients with typical clinical and chest radiographic findings of sarcoidosis. A study by Mana et al[271] of 100 patients with sarcoidosis found that CT added diagnostically useful information in only 1 of 35 patients in whom it was performed. These authors concluded that CT may be helpful in patients with atypical chest radiographic findings, normal chest radiographs, hemoptysis,

or suspicion of a second complicating disease, and in those who are lung transplant candidates. To these indications we would add suspected large or small airway disease, and patients in whom a diagnosis is not made by transbronchial biopsy.

Despite some initial enthusiasm,[272] MRI does not appear to have a role in the evaluation of sarcoidosis. The T2-weighted signal intensity of enlarged nodes shows no characteristic pattern.[273]

EOSINOPHILIC LUNG DISEASE

Despite an explosion of information about the eosinophil, the function of this cell remains unclear. However, it is encountered in a variety of inflammatory processes, and a group of pulmonary disorders is associated with the presence of eosinophils in the lung (Table 11.1). The term *pulmonary eosinophilia* was introduced in 1952 to describe a group of diseases "in which pulmonary infiltration on the radiograph is accompanied by blood eosinophilia but in which pneumonia, hydatid disease of the lung, Hodgkin disease, and sarcoidosis can be excluded".[275] The 16 patients in this study were classified into five groups – simple pulmonary eosinophilia (Löffler syndrome), prolonged pulmonary eosinophilia, tropical eosinophilia, pulmonary eosinophilia with asthma, and polyarteritis nodosa. In the same year, a series of patients with "pulmonary infiltration with eosinophilia" was described.[276] Later authors have widened this concept,[277] using the term *eosinophilic lung disease* to include all disorders associated with blood and/or tissue eosinophilia which affect major airways and/or lung parenchyma.[278] It is important to note that it is not necessary to have a blood eosinophilia to make a diagnosis of eosinophilic lung disease, and indeed BAL has become widely used for the more sensitive and specific diagnosis of eosinophilic pneumonia. In eosinophilic pneumonias, the percentage of eosinophils in BAL fluid is usually >10%.[274] The widely used term *pulmonary infiltration with eosinophilia* is synonymous with the term pulmonary eosinophilia.

Eosinophils are granulocytes that develop in the bone marrow and are carried in the blood to those epithelia that are exposed to the external environment, particularly the mucosa of the respiratory, gastrointestinal, and genitourinary tracts. There is only one eosinophil in the blood compartment for every 100 in the marrow and other tissues, and it is, therefore, not surprising that eosinophilic tissue lesions are not necessarily accompanied by blood eosinophilia.[279] Blood eosinophil counts vary between 0.05 and 0.35×10^9/L and show diurnal variation, with high counts in the night and low ones in the morning.[280] Eosinophilia is generally taken to mean an eosinophil count of $>0.4 \times 10^9$/L, though some set the level at 0.5×10^9/L. Eosinophils contain a range of enzymes which accounts for their ability to damage parasitic worms and cells, including those of man, and to modulate mast cell dependent reactions such as immediate hypersensitivity. Various classifications of eosinophilic lung states have been proposed,[275,277,279–282] but none has proved entirely satisfactory. The conditions considered in detail in this text are only those in which tissue and/or blood eosinophilia are a major feature. The possible causes in a patient under investigation can usually be significantly reduced by taking into account a few key historic, clinical, and laboratory findings, notably work exposure, ethnic background, travel to endemic areas, and a history of asthma, atopy, and any medication. Useful information from first-line investigations include the

Table 11.1 Syndromes of eosinophilic lung disease

Disease	Etiology	Blood eosinophilia	Length of history	Radiologic features
Acute eosinophilic pneumonia	Idiopathic	Uncommon at presentation	1–5 days	Diffuse or basal ground glass/reticular opacities Effusions
Löffler syndrome (simple pulmonary eosinophilia)	May be idiopathic Often due to allergic aspergillosis, drugs, or parasitic infection	Usual		Fleeting airspace opacities
Chronic eosinophilic pneumonia	Idiopathic	95% >1 × 10^9/L	2 weeks to 6 months	Dense, peripheral consolidation, often upper lobe predominant May be migratory
Hypereosinophilic syndrome	Idiopathic	Marked (>1.5 × 10^9/L)	6 months	Heart failure with edema Effusions Rare parenchymal opacities
Churg–Strauss syndrome	Usually idiopathic vasculitis	Usual	Weeks to months	Consolidation (may be migratory), nodules, cavities, bronchiectasis
Allergic bronchopulmonary aspergillosis (ABPA)	Immune response to aspergillus	Usual in acute ABPA	Days to weeks	Migratory opacities Mucoid impaction Central bronchiectasis
Bronchocentric granulomatosis	May be related to aspergillus	Common		Mass lesions, alveolar opacities
Drug reactions	Nonsteroidal antiinflammatory drugs Antibiotics[274]	Usually	Days to weeks	Ground glass/reticular
Tropical eosinophilia	Lymphatic filarial parasites *Wuchereria bancrofti* and *Brugia malayi*	3–60 × 10^9/L	Variable	Reticulonodular basal opacities Migratory opacities Chest radiograph may be normal
Parasitic infection	Many parasites (dirofilaria, ascaris, strongyloides, toxocara)	Usual	Variable	Migratory opacities Chest radiograph may be normal

magnitude of blood eosinophilia, total serum IgE, the presence of skin sensitivity, serum *Aspergillus* precipitins, and cysts, ova, or parasites in the stool.

Eosinophilic pneumonias

The eosinophilic pneumonias are classified on the basis of their severity and chronicity. Simple eosinophilic pneumonia (SEP, Löffler syndrome) has classically been distinguished from chronic eosinophilic pneumonia (CEP) on the basis of duration of symptoms.[275] SEP is defined as lasting <1 month, while CEP lasts >1 month. The 1 month dividing line is rather arbitrary and not universally applied, so that the distinction between the two types is not always clear, and this is particularly true now

that the natural history is commonly modified by steroids. Nevertheless, the division is useful clinically, as the majority of CEPs form a relatively homogeneous group. The more recently recognized acute eosinophilic pneumonia (AEP)[283,284] differs from SEP in that patients often present with respiratory failure.

Acute eosinophilic pneumonia

AEP was first described in 1989[283,284] and is considered to represent a distinct clinical entity with the following diagnostic criteria: (1) acute febrile illness of <5 days' duration; (2) hypoxemic respiratory failure; (3) alveolar or alveolar/interstitial chest radiographic opacity; (4) BAL eosinophil level of >25%; (5) prompt and complete response to steroids without relapse on withdrawal; and (6) absence of parasitic, fungal, and other infection. The etiology of AEP is unknown. It has been suggested that it may represent acute hypersensitivity to an inhaled antigen, and there is one report in which this seems to have been the case following inhalation of the yeast *Trichosporon terrestre*.[285] Several case reports have suggested that this condition may be found in patients who have recently begun to smoke cigarettes,[286–289] and in a series of 22 patients from France, six of eight patients had begun to smoke cigarettes 1 week to 3 months before the onset of AEP.[290] There may also be a relationship to inhalation of other types of materials such as gasoline fumes.[290] A syndrome of AEP has been described with amitryptiline[291] and venlafaxine.[292]

The average age at presentation is about 30 years and there is no gender predilection.[293] Principal symptoms are those of cough, dyspnea, fever, and chest pain coming on over a period of a few days. On examination patients are tachypneic and hypoxic with extensive crepitations on auscultation of the chest. A history of asthma or atopy may or may not be present.[294,295] Respiratory failure, with requirement for mechanical ventilation, develops in most patients.[290] The usual presumptive diagnosis is of a fulminant chest infection. Blood eosinophil levels are elevated in about 35% of cases at presentation, but become abnormal at some point in the course of disease in 70% of patients.[290] The key to diagnosis, however, is provided by BAL which shows a greatly raised eosinophil percentage in the order of 30–80%.[290,293] The other important diagnostic clue lies with chest imaging (Box 11.7). The chest radiograph (Fig. 11.40) commonly shows a mixed alveolar/interstitial pattern with septal lines and pleural effusions in the absence of clinical cardiac failure or overhydration. Such findings would also be unusual for a pneumonia other than one caused by *Mycoplasma* or a virus.[296] AEP responds satisfactorily to steroids with little or no residual functional deficit. The condition does not relapse.[293]

The pathologic changes are those of acute and organizing diffuse alveolar damage with marked numbers of interstitial, and fewer alveolar, eosinophils.[297]

> **Box 11.7 Radiologic features of acute eosinophilic pneumonia**
>
> Pleural effusions
> Septal thickening
> Peribronchovascular thickening
> Ground-glass abnormality
> Consolidation

AEP is one of the few forms of acute interstitial pneumonia in which the diagnosis may be strongly suspected based on chest radiographic and CT features. As stated above, radiographic findings[283,293,295,296,298,299] are usually a mixture of airspace and interstitial opacity, including septal lines.[293,300] These changes are bilateral but range from being diffuse to localized. Either consolidation or septal thickening may be found in isolation.[293] About 70% of patients have pleural effusions (bilateral more commonly than unilateral) at presentation,[301,302] and during the course of the illness most, if not all, patients develop bilateral effusions.[299] In a series of 22 patients studied by Philit et al,[290] pleural effusions were visible on the initial chest radiograph in only two patients, but were seen on CT in 10 of 14 patients who underwent CT. This suggests that the pleural effusions were not seen in some patients on chest radiography, either because of the associated parenchymal abnormality, or because erect frontal and lateral radiographs were not obtained in these ill patients.

HRCT may be very helpful in suggesting the diagnosis, with typical findings of septal lines, pleural effusions, and areas of consolidative and ground-glass opacity (Fig. 11.40).[296,299] Areas of ground-glass abnormality and/or consolidation are found in almost all patients.[301,302] Thickened interlobular septa are seen in about 75%, with thickening of bronchovascular structures in about the same number, and pleural effusions in 70%. Pleural effusions may be small or large. About 30% of cases have an upper lung predominance of parenchymal abnormalities.[302]

In patients with acute respiratory failure, the demonstration by chest radiography or CT of prominent interlobular septal thickening, thickening of bronchovascular bundles, or pleural effusions, should prompt the recommendation of BAL to identify the presence of eosinophilia and make the diagnosis of AEP. If eosinophilia is demonstrated, lung biopsy is probably not indicated.[303] This is an important diagnosis to make, because survival with appropriate management is close to 100%,[290] much better than in most other forms of acute respiratory failure.

Simple eosinophilic pneumonia (Löffler syndrome)

The characteristic features of simple pulmonary eosinophilia or Löffler syndrome are: (1) blood eosinophilia; (2) absent or mild symptoms and signs (cough, fever, dyspnea); (3) one or more nonsegmental pulmonary consolidations that are transitory and/or migratory; and (4) spontaneous clearing of consolidations. Originally, opacities were described as disappearing within 6–12 days,[304] but this interval is now generally extended to a month.[275] Its incidence has been noted to vary seasonally.[305] The prognosis is excellent.[305]

Löffler syndrome may be idiopathic (cryptogenic), or it may result from a variety of inciting agents, particularly allergic bronchopulmonary mycosis, drugs, parasites, and miscellaneous agents such as nickel carbonyl.[306] It seems likely that some, if not all, of Löffler's original cases were related to ascariasis.[305] In developed countries, the most common cause of Löffler syndrome is probably allergic bronchopulmonary aspergillosis (see Fig. 11.46).[274] Careful evaluation will lead to identification of a cause in most cases of Löffler syndrome, and indeed, there is some doubt as to whether this syndrome is ever truly idiopathic.[274]

Pathologically, there is an eosinophilic pneumonia with edema and an eosinophilic infiltrate in both alveoli and interstitium. Radiographically the findings are of one or more fairly homogeneous, nonsegmental consolidations that can be small or so large as to occupy much of a lobe. They are transitory and may be migratory, disappearing from one area and appearing in another. They have a tendency to be peripherally located. Pleural effusions, mediastinal adenopathy, and cavitation are not described.

Chronic eosinophilic pneumonia

CEP is a cryptogenic form of eosinophilic lung disease with consistent and characteristic clinicopathologic features. Pathologically, there is an eosinophil rich exudate in the alveoli and interstitium.[307,308] Angiitis is mild, fibrosis sparse, and necrosis

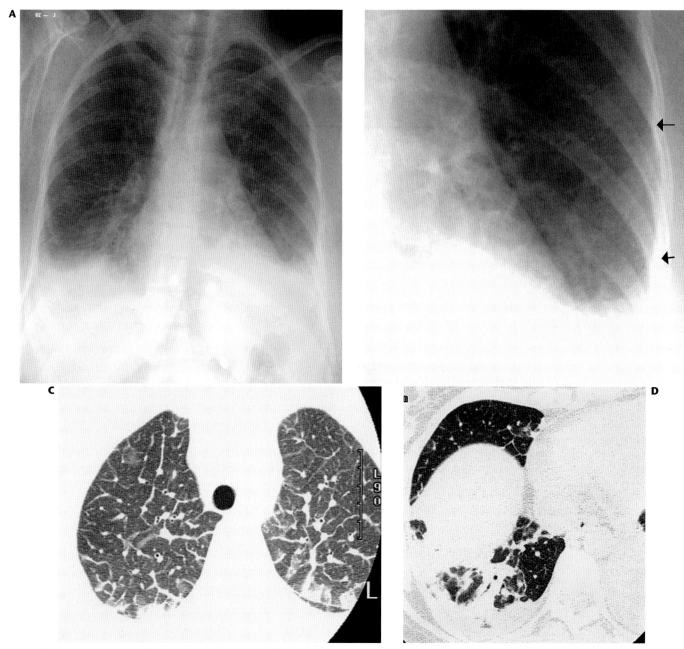

Fig. 11.40 Acute eosinophilic pneumonia. **A**, Chest radiograph with **B**, detail view shows bilateral effusions, with septal thickening (arrows), and basal consolidation. **C** and **D**, HRCT confirms septal thickening, patchy ground-glass abnormality, and basal consolidation.

very rare.[307] Since the condition was first identified in 1969,[307] several series have been published.[281,308–313] Many patients present in middle life but prevalence remains high from the third to seventh decade,[312] range 7–77 years; women outnumber men by 2:1[308]; 50% of patients are atopic, 40% asthmatic, and 5–10% have allergic rhinitis and nasal polyps.[312] Asthma can antedate the condition by many years[281] or can develop with the onset of CEP. The symptoms are usually highly characteristic, ranging from mild to severe, and have often been present for several months. Typical symptoms are cough with mucoid sputum; high fever, particularly in the evenings, often accompanied by

drenching night sweats; dyspnea; wheeze; malaise; and marked weight loss (8–12 kg). Occasionally there is chest pain and hemoptysis. Given this combination of symptoms it is not surprising that patients are often believed initially to have tuberculosis – an impression that may be reinforced by the chest radiograph. Blood eosinophilia is common, but not universal, occurring in nearly 90% of patients,[312] ranging from mild to marked.[308] There is sputum eosinophilia in <50% of patients.[312] Total white blood cell count and the ESR are raised. Serum IgE, which is normal or only minimally elevated,[308] is a particularly helpful finding, allowing distinction from those conditions such as allergic bronchopulmonary aspergillosis and tropical and parasitic pulmonary eosinophilias in which serum IgE levels are markedly elevated. However, there have been a number of reports of significantly raised IgE levels.[314] BAL demonstrates high eosinophil percentages – of the order of 25% of more.

The principal pathologic findings are filling of alveoli with eosinophils and macrophages, sometimes with necrosis and the formation of small eosinophilic abscesses. Foci of organizing pneumonia may be seen. Changes are not confined to alveolar spaces and there is typically an interstitial pneumonia as well, but fibrosis is minimal or absent.[274]

Many patients with CEP have a characteristic radiologic pattern that is virtually pathognomonic (Box 11.8). Its most classic pattern, seen in two-thirds of patients,[312] consists of peripheral, nonsegmental, homogeneous consolidation sometimes with an air bronchogram, the so-called "photographic negative of pulmonary edema" (Fig. 11.41).[310] These opacities lie against the chest wall and may surround the lung or just occupy one or two zones, particularly the apices (Fig. 11.42). In one series the zonal distribution was 46% upper, 40% mid and 14% lower.[309] About half the patients have bilateral consolidation which may cloak the upper and outer aspects of the lung in a very characteristic fashion (Fig. 11.41).[275,310] Opacities may

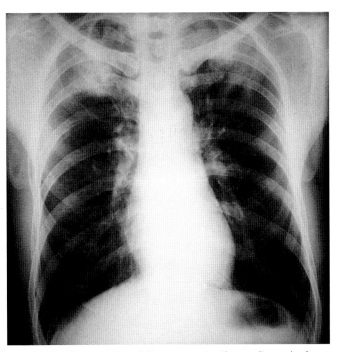

Fig. 11.42 Chronic eosinophilic pneumonia. Chest radiograph of a 52-year-old man who presented with a 2 month history of fever, weight loss, and cough. He had blood eosinophilia (2×10^9/L) and had had nasal polypectomies in the past. The radiographic findings of bilateral apical consolidation coupled with the history were considered very suggestive of tuberculosis, and the patient was inappropriately treated for 1 month despite the lack of firm evidence.

> **Box 11.8 Radiologic features of chronic eosinophilic pneumonia**
>
> Consolidation
> Ground-glass abnormality
> Peripheral predominance
> Upper lung predominance

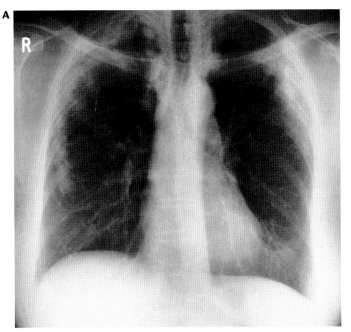

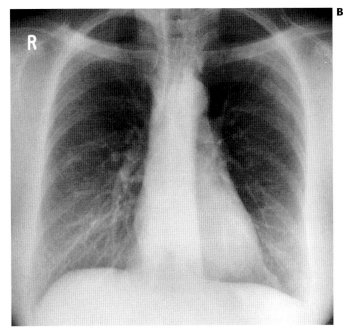

Fig. 11.41 Chronic eosinophilic pneumonia. A 65-year-old woman with a 1 month history of fever, night sweats, cough, and weight loss. The patient did not have asthma but had blood eosinophilia (1.6×10^9/L). **A,** Posteroanterior radiograph shows bilateral, confluent, peripheral opacity in the middle and upper zones. **B,** Radiograph 2 weeks later shows complete resolution following steroid therapy.

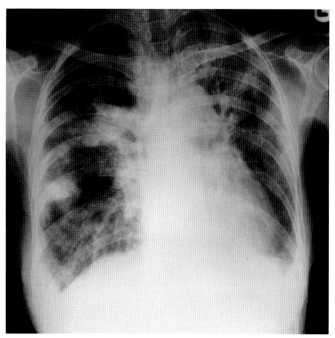

Fig. 11.43 Chronic eosinophilic pneumonia (CEP). Radiograph shows multifocal peripheral and central consolidation. This is a recognized pattern but less common than that shown in Fig. 11.41. Both costophrenic angles are blunted in this patient. On the right, blunting may be a result of peripheral consolidation, but on the left a small pleural effusion cannot be excluded. Pleural effusions are very unusual in CEP.

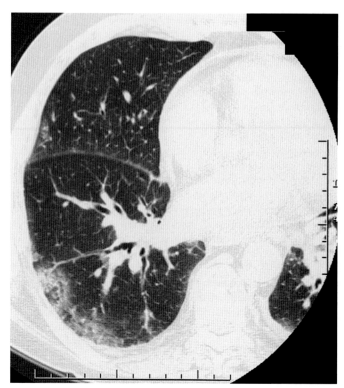

Fig. 11.44 Chronic eosinophilic pneumonia. HRCT shows peripheral predominant consolidation and ground-glass abnormality.

appear in one lung to be followed by others on the opposite side, or they may disappear spontaneously. They are rarely truly migratory; if they resolve they usually recur in the same place.[309,310] Some 30% of patients with CEP do not show the classic peripheral pattern described here (Fig. 11.43).[308–311] The consolidation may even be predominantly perihilar in distribution.[309] A common pattern is mixed peripheral and central consolidation (Fig. 11.43)[309] that can progress to opacify totally one lung.[308] Isolated lesions in the upper zone may closely mimic those of tuberculosis. Other features that are infrequently seen include pleural effusions (2%), cavitation (5%),[312] and occasional mediastinal lymphadenopathy, best appreciated on CT.[315–317]

CT confirms the chest radiographic findings, showing strikingly peripheral, multifocal consolidation or ground-glass abnormality (Fig. 11.44), though there may also be areas of nonperipheral consolidation.[316,318] In one study, ground-glass opacity was as common a finding as consolidation (Fig. 11.44).[318] However, it was infrequently the only finding (12% of patients) and was usually close to the margins of consolidated areas.[318] The bilateral subpleural distribution is universal in patients who are scanned within 1 month of the onset of symptoms.[318] Patients with CEP who are imaged >1 month after the onset of symptoms have a different pattern on CT. The consolidation tends to be more patchy, and though the opacities remain peripheral, the subpleural zone is often relatively clear. A characteristic feature in these more chronic cases is the presence of a dense bandlike structure parallel and about 1–2 cm deep to the chest wall, which may traverse the fissures.[315,318] In chronic

cases of CEP, dense fibrosis and lung distortion may rarely be seen.

The disease occasionally remits spontaneously[310]; however, treatment is usually required, and CEP is remarkably sensitive to steroid therapy (Fig. 11.41). Rapid clearing is usually seen within a few days, with complete clearing by 1 month.[307] In fact, some authors recommend a therapeutic trial of steroids in previously well patients with classic clinical and radiologic features.[312] Radiographic resolution is usually complete. The characteristic bandlike opacities parallel to the chest wall may be seen during the resolving phase (Fig. 11.45).[310,312,318] Clinical relapse is common and in a review of 62 patients 21% relapsed during reduction of steroid dose and 58% after discontinuation.[312] The majority of patients need longterm low dose steroids,[313] and a proportion develop late onset asthma.[310] In rare instances, patients who initially have all the features of CEP go on to develop the Churg-Strauss syndrome[319] or a diffuse vasculitis.[310,320]

Allergic bronchopulmonary mycosis

Allergic bronchopulmonary mycosis (ABPM) is almost certainly the most common cause of eosinophilic lung disease in developed countries. The term ABPM is used in place of the more specific term allergic bronchopulmonary aspergillosis (ABPA) to indicate that other fungi may also cause this clinical syndrome. ABPA accounted for 78% of 143 patients with a diagnosis of pulmonary eosinophilia and who were admitted to a tertiary referral center in the United Kingdom.[321] First described in 1952,[322] the disease is characterized by asthma, radiographic pulmonary opacities,

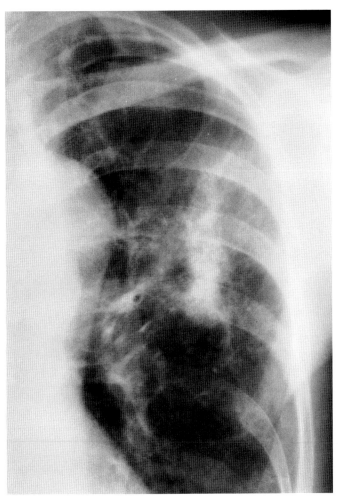

Fig. 11.45 Chronic eosinophilic pneumonia (CEP). Local view of left middle and upper zone. Partial resolution of classic peripheral consolidation has resulted in band opacity parallel to the chest wall.

blood eosinophilia, and evidence of allergy to antigens of *Aspergillus* spp. Its importance lies in the fact that recurrent acute episodes cause progressive lung damage that can be controlled by steroid administration.[323]

Although it may be due to a wide variety of organisms, *Aspergillus* spp are by far the most common causative agent, resulting in ABPA. *Aspergillus* fungi are ubiquitous worldwide. In >90% of patients, the species involved is *A. fumigatus*, but occasionally other species are implicated, including *A. flavus*, *A. niger*, *A. nidulans*,[324] *A. terreus*,[325] *A. oryzae*,[326] and *A. ochraceus*.[327] In addition, there are isolated case reports of an ABPA-like syndrome caused by fungi other than *Aspergillus* spp, including *Candida albicans* and at least seven other genera.[328,329] These conditions may be more difficult to diagnose because aspergillus precipitins may be absent.

In ABPA, a hypersensitivity reaction develops to *Aspergillus* spp that grow as a mycelial plug in proximal airways, usually the second or third order bronchi.[330] Tissue invasion is either absent[324] or very limited.[331] The factors that favor the initial airway colonization by *Aspergillus* are unclear,[324] but in part probably relate to the almost universal presence of asthma and atopy in affected patients. Other important factors are the size of the spores (2.5–3.0 μm) which favors inhalation and airway deposition, and their thermotolerance which allows hyphal

growth at body temperature.[328,332] Certainly, once the fungus gets a foothold, local damage promotes further colonization.

Patients characteristically have evidence of both a type I and type III immune reaction,[333] and possibly an element of a type IV (cell mediated) reaction, as well as complement activation.[334] The type I (IgE mediated) reaction is manifest by bronchospasm and is associated with a blood eosinophilia and IgE production that results in high *specific* and *nonspecific* serum levels. The type III (immune complex mediated) reaction causes tissue damage and is associated with serum precipitins (IgG). IgE enhances the tissue damaging effect of IgG.[328] Because antigen production is localized to the mycelial plug in the proximal airway, tissue damage tends to be greatest in this region, giving rise to granulomatous airway inflammation that results in the characteristic proximal bronchiectasis. In addition, however, there appears to be a separate pathologic process centered on the lung parenchyma giving an eosinophilic pneumonia which does not produce permanent damage.[328]

Typically, ABPA occurs in patients who are atopic and long-standing asthmatics. A few patients, particularly older ones, develop asthma concurrently with their first attack of ABPA.[321] Although unusual, the disease is well recognized in non-asthmatics.[321,335] Overall there is a slight female preponderance.[321,336,337] It may occur at any age,[337–339] but typically presents between 20 and 40 years of age. The length of the interval between the onset of asthma and ABPA is inversely related to the age of onset of asthma. McCarthy et al[340] found that with asthma beginning before 10 years of age, there was an average gap of 24 years, but with late onset asthma (30 years of age or more), the mean gap was only 3.5 years. Late onset asthma was associated with more frequent attacks of ABPA and greater lung damage.[340] ABPA also occurs in patients with cystic fibrosis in whom there is an approximately 10% prevalence.[305]

In about 10% of patients ABPM may be associated with allergic fungal sinusitis.[341] This condition is characterized by accumulation of mucin in the sinuses, associated with polyposis in the sinuses and nose. It is associated with a wider range of organisms than ABPM, including *Curvularia* and *Bipolaris* species.[342–345] On imaging, it is characterized by mucosal thickening and hyperattenuating sinus contents or CT, often associated with bony erosions.[346,347]

ABPA runs a relapsing and remitting course and an acute attack may be indistinguishable from an uncomplicated exacerbation of asthma.[328] Patterson et al[348] described five clinical stages of ABPA; acute, remission, exacerbation, steroid dependent asthma, and fibrosis. These must not be regarded as phases of disease, as patients need not pass from one stage to the next in orderly progression. Characteristic symptoms in the acute stage are wheeze, dyspnea, and a cough that is often productive and associated with minor hemoptysis. Systemic symptoms such as fever, malaise, and weight loss are common. About 50% of patients have pleuritic pain, and about the same percentage give a history of coughing up sputum plugs.[321] These contain fungal mycelia and are important pointers to the diagnosis.[321] Plugs are about 1–2 cm long, firm, friable, and pelletlike.[321] An abnormal chest radiograph, blood eosinophilia, and an immediate skin "wheal and flare" reaction to *Aspergillus* antigens are characteristic of the acute phase. Eosinophilia is usually mild to moderate, with 74% of patients having counts between 1 and 3×10^9/L.[321] The eosinophil level may be depressed by steroid treatment. Serum precipitins against *Aspergillus* antigens are detected in about 90% of patients in the acute phase, particularly if the serum is concentrated.[321,328,333,336] It must be remembered, however, that this test is nonspecific in that 12–25% of patients with extrinsic asthma will have a positive precipitin test.[349] Both nonspecific and *Aspergillus* antigen specific IgE are greatly raised, perhaps 20 times normal.[333] Smaller elevations may be found in simple asthma. As with the finding of positive precipitins, elevation of IgE per se is not diagnostic of ABPA. Nevertheless, the IgE level is probably the single most useful laboratory test in ABPA since levels correlate with disease activity and a normal level virtually excludes the diagnosis.[305,333] Criteria for the diagnosis of ABPA have changed over time as knowledge about the disease has become more sophisticated; yet even now there are no universally accepted diagnostic criteria. Rosenberg et al[333] set out the major and minor criteria (Box 11.9) and suggest that if the first six of the major criteria are satisfied, the diagnosis of ABPA can be made with reasonable certainty.

Box 11.9 Major and minor criteria for the diagnosis of allergic bronchopulmonary mycosis[333]

Major criteria
Asthma
Blood eosinophilia
Immediate skin reactivity to *Aspergillus* antigen
Precipitin antibodies to *Aspergillus* antigen
Raised serum IgE (nonspecific/specific)
History of radiographic pulmonary opacities
Central bronchiectasis

Minor criteria
Aspergillus fumigatus in sputum
History of expectorating brown plugs
Late skin reactivity to *Aspergillus* antigen

Rosenberg et al[333] considered that the presence of central bronchiectasis makes the diagnosis of ABPA certain. However, ABPA can be present without bronchiectasis,[305,350,351] and ABPA without bronchiectasis appears to carry a better prognosis, with fewer exacerbations.[352,353] In a recent study, 11 of 31 patients with serologically diagnosed ABPA did not have bronchiectasis; these patients had less severe disease than those with bronchiectasis.[353] Patients with ABPA without central bronchiectasis do not progress to develop bronchiectasis over a 2 year interval.[354]

In a prospective study of 255 patients with asthma, Eaton et al[355] found that 47 had positive skin prick tests for *A. fumigatus*, of whom 35 underwent CT. Central bronchiectasis was found on CT in 12 of these patients, eight of whom met all the criteria for ABPA. These investigators found that performing CT in patients with skin prick positivity who had histories of sputum plugs, eczema, or steroid dependency identified all cases of ABPA with bronchiectasis. These authors proposed the following minimal criteria for ABPA: asthma, skin prick test positivity, and central bronchiectasis.

A great variety of radiologic change is found in ABPA, and may be related to the phase of the disease.[336,337,339,340,356–358] In the

Table 11.2 Radiographic findings in allergic bronchopulmonary aspergillosis (% = prevalence of finding)

Major	Minor
Acute (transient)	
Consolidation (80%)	Airway wall thickening
Mucoid impaction (bronchocele) (30%)	Small nodules
Atelectasis (20%)	Pleural effusions
Chronic (permanent)	
Bronchiectasis	Pleural thickening
Mid/upper zone volume loss and scarring	Mycetoma
	Small nodules
	Linear scars

acute stage, there is mycelial plugging of segmental airways and an intense local inflammatory response that leads to bronchial wall thickening. Resultant airway obstruction may cause lobar or segmental collapse, a mucoid impaction pattern, or consolidation. Some areas of consolidation are probably eosinophilic pneumonias independent of airway involvement (see above). Secondary infection may also result from airway obstruction.[336] In the chronic phase, the plugs usually disappear, leaving damaged and bronchiectatic airways, while the more distal changes have healed, often with a major fibrotic element.

The radiologic findings are best considered as acute and transient, or chronic and permanent (Table 11.2).[340]

Despite some discrepancies among series, there is no doubt that consolidation is the most common type of *transient* opacity (Figs 11.46 and 11.47). Consolidation ranges from being massive and homogeneous (occupying a whole lobe) to subsegmental and smaller opacities (of the order of 1 cm). The smaller opacities are the more common. Areas of consolidation show little if any zonal predilection and are often multiple. Larger opacities are often segmental or lobar in configuration, as might be expected with airway obstruction (Fig. 11.48). This appearance contrasts with the nonsegmental consolidation seen in other eosinophilic states. Apparent cavitation in areas of consolidation has been described on chest radiographs with a frequency of 3–20%[337,340]; this may be due to bronchiectasis, cavitary bacterial infection, or mycetoma formation. Although consolidation is usually transient, it can last for 6 weeks or more. Phelan and Kerr[337] described some patients with apparently permanent consolidation. When consolidation clears, it often leaves residual bronchiectasis (Fig. 11.48). Such bronchiectasis creates favorable conditions for fungal recolonization, a finding that accounts for the fact that 25–50% of consolidation recurs later in the same area. It is notable that 20–30% of patients with radiographic consolidation are asymptomatic[323,339] and ABPA is one of those conditions in which gross radiographic changes may be accompanied by little in the way of symptoms.[340]

The second most common acute change is probably that of bronchocele formation (mucoid impaction). In this condition, an airway becomes obstructed and distended by retained secretions; yet, at the same time, the subtended lung remains aerated by

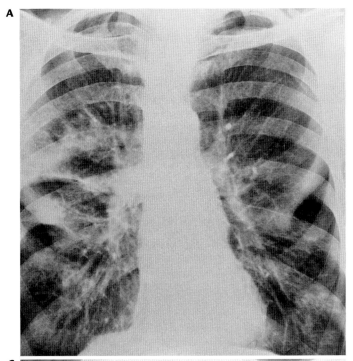

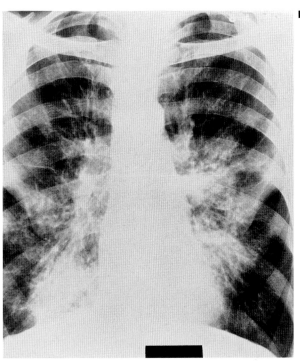

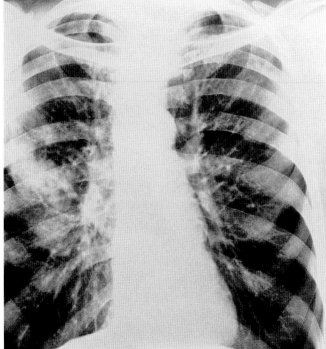

Fig. 11.46   Consolidation in allergic bronchopulmonary aspergillosis. **A–C**, Three radiographs taken at approximately yearly intervals show recurring, multifocal areas of consolidation. Some of the opacities contain air bronchograms. There is associated airway wall thickening, best seen in **B**.

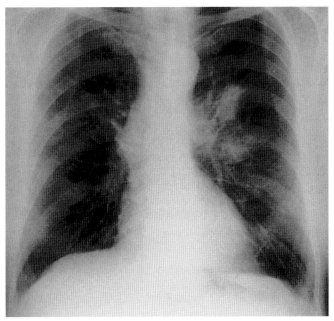

Fig. 11.47   Allergic bronchopulmonary aspergillosis. Chest radiograph shows patchy subsegmental consolidation in the left lung.

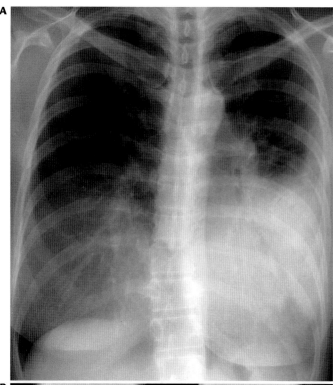

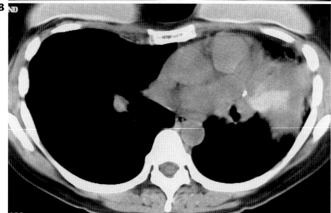

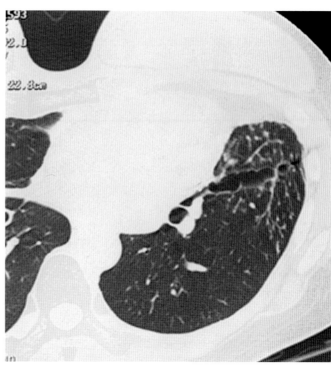

Fig. 11.48 Segmental consolidation in allergic bronchopulmonary mycosis. **A**, Chest radiograph shows dense lingular consolidation. **B**, CT shows consolidation, with central hyperattenuating material representing mucoid impaction. **C**, HRCT following bronchoscopy and removal of the mucus plug shows varicose bronchiectasis and the tree-in-bud pattern. Examination of the plug showed that the responsible fungal species was *Curvularia* rather than *Aspergillus*.

collateral air drift, allowing direct visualization of the impacted airway. Bronchoceles take on a wide variety of shapes depending on the extent and degree of airway filling. The basic opacity is a linear, sharply demarcated, branched or unbranched bandlike shadow that points to the hilum (Fig. 11.49) – the so-called toothpaste shadow – a band about 2–3 cm long and 5–8 mm wide. Variants include V- and Y-shaped opacities. Sometimes bronchoceles are more rounded than linear and can simulate a mass, if single, or a cluster of masses, if multiple ("bunch of grapes"). Similarly, rounded opacities will be produced by linear bronchoceles seen end on. Impacted airways are usually proximal (typically segmental). They are often inseparable from the hilum and may simulate lymphadenopathy[358] or a mass.

Another variant is produced by distal bronchiectatic airways which, when impacted, give a band shadow with a club shaped end; the "gloved finger shadow". Bronchoceles show a strong upper zone predilection (Figs 11.50 and 11.51).[339] They disappear once their contents have been coughed up, leaving ring or parallel line opacities (Fig. 11.51). Like consolidation in ABPA they may recur at the same site. Occasionally they persist for many months and are recorded as remaining for at least 18 months. On CT scanning, the bronchoceles are seen as bandlike abnormalities in the expected position of the bronchi (Fig. 11.49). Their attenuation may be similar to that of water or soft tissue, or they may be hyperattenuating (Figs 11.48 and 11.49).[359] The hyperattenuation is presumed to be due to calcium or metallic

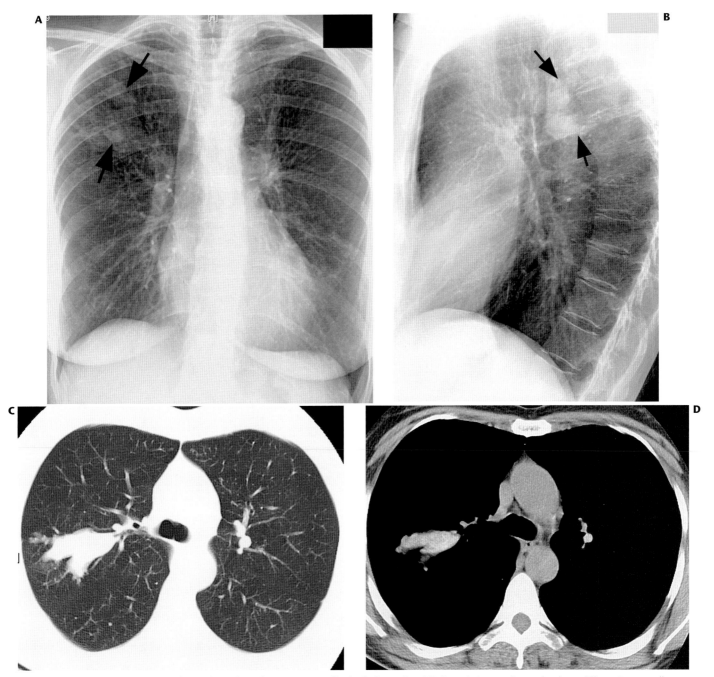

Fig. 11.49 Mucoid impaction in allergic bronchopulmonary aspergillosis. **A**, Frontal and **B**, lateral chest radiographs show diffuse airway wall thickening and bandlike opacities in the right upper lobe (arrows). **C**, CT confirms a branching opacity in the posterior right upper lobe. **D**, Mediastinal window shows that the attenuation of the opacity is greater than that of soft tissue.

ions within the mucus, and was found in 28% of cases in one series.[360]

The third major acute manifestation of ABPA is atelectasis (Fig. 11.52), which ranges in frequency from 3[339] to 46%.[330] It may be subsegmental, segmental, lobar, or even affect a whole lung.[337,357,361] Like consolidation and mucoid impaction, collapse has a tendency to recur in the same area. Atelectasis is not specific for ABPA, since it may occur as a complication of simple asthma.[362] On CT scanning, mucus plugs may be seen within the areas of atelectasis if they are hyperattenuating or of water attenuation.

A variety of other, less important, acute opacities has been described. They include parallel line opacities caused by bronchial wall thickening, presumably from inflammation and edema

(Fig. 11.46). McCarthy et al[340] distinguish between two types of parallel linear abnormalities: (1) tubular opacities, where the walls are inappropriately wide apart, consistent with bronchiectasis; and (2) tramline opacities where wall separation is consistent with a normal airway caliber. Bronchial wall thickening is most commonly seen in patients under 15 years old, an age group in which asthma alone may be associated with such changes. Small, ill-defined, rounded or irregular opacities (miliary opacities) are described as both transient and permanent findings. It is possible that they represent granulomas formed as a result of an extrinsic allergic alveolitis. There have been a few reports of pleural effusion.[339,363]

Permanent changes (Table 11.2) are of importance because: (1) they indicate irreversible lung damage; and (2) they may be the only clue that an asthmatic has ABPA when he/she is in remission. Bronchiectasis is responsible for most of the permanent radiographic changes. Bronchography historically[333,340,358] and HRCT currently (Figs 11.53 and 11.54)[341,350,364,365] have clarified the distribution and type of bronchiectasis. The characteristic finding is proximal bronchiectasis, affecting lobar bronchi and first and second order segmental bronchi (Box 11.10, Figs 11.53

Box 11.10 Characteristic CT features of bronchiectasis in allergic bronchopulmonary aspergillosis

Involves segmental and subsegmental bronchi
Varicose or cystic pattern
Thin walled bronchiectatic airways
Associated mucoid impaction (which may be
  hyperattenuating)
Associated centrilobular nodularity/tree-in-bud pattern

Fig. 11.50 Bronchoceles in allergic bronchopulmonary aspergillosis. Several fingerlike bronchoceles are seen in the left upper lung. In the right lung, several bronchoceles are seen en face overlying the hilum and giving it a lobulated appearance.

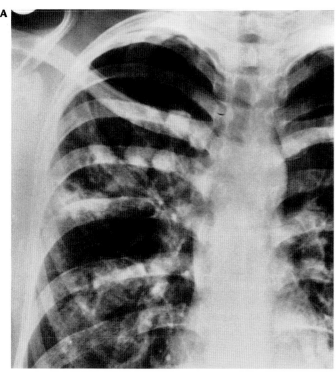
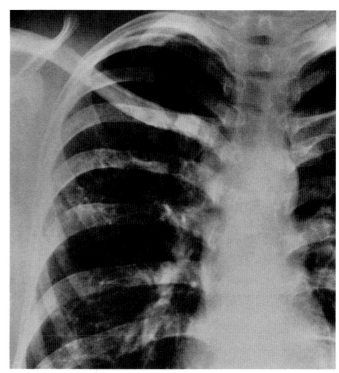

Fig. 11.51 Bronchoceles in allergic bronchopulmonary aspergillosis. **A,** Local view of the right upper and middle lung shows multiple rounded bronchoceles. **B,** When these clear, they leave a collection of delicate curvilinear and ring opacities, which represent the walls of the bronchiectatic airways. Such opacities close to the hilum in the middle and upper zones are a characteristic interval finding in allergic aspergillosis.

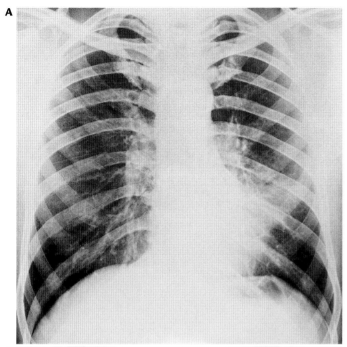

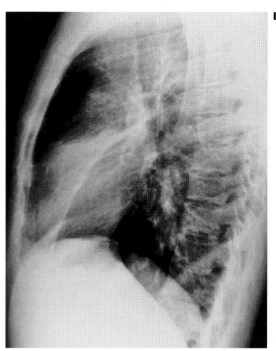

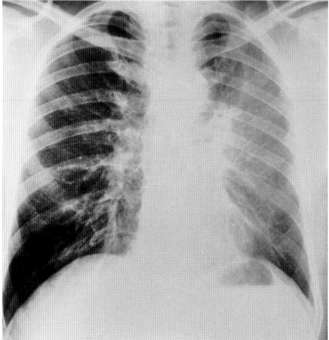

Fig. 11.52 Atelectasis in allergic bronchopulmonary aspergillosis. **A**, Frontal and **B**, lateral chest radiographs show lingular consolidation associated with minor volume loss. **C**, Subsequent radiograph shows complete collapse of the upper lobe.

and 11.54). Beyond the proximal bronchiectasis, more distal airways remain normal and patent, though a tree-in-bud pattern of abnormality is common on HRCT. Proximal bronchiectasis has been considered highly specific for ABPA,[333] and in a selected patient population of asthmatics with skin tests positive for *A. fumigatus* this is probably so.[366] However, in a population of symptomatic patients with bronchiectasis, proximal bronchiectasis does not necessarily separate those with ABPA from those with other conditions. In an HRCT study of 146 such patients with chronic sputum production due to conditions such as ABPA, ciliary dysmotility, hypogammaglobulinemia and cystic fibrosis, and idiopathic bronchiectasis, the distribution

and morphology of the bronchiectasis was analyzed and related to cause.[365] Compared with other diseases, bronchiectasis in ABPA was more commonly widespread and central, and more likely to contain cystic or varicose elements (Fig. 11.53).[365] However, the 37% frequency of central bronchiectasis in ABPA must be compared with a frequency of 20% in primary ciliary dyskinesia and 15% in idiopathic bronchiectasis. The authors considered that CT in an individual patient had limited value in discriminating among the various etiologic types of bronchiectasis. In a similar study, Cartier et al[367] found that CT features suggested the diagnosis of ABPA in only five (56%) of nine patients.

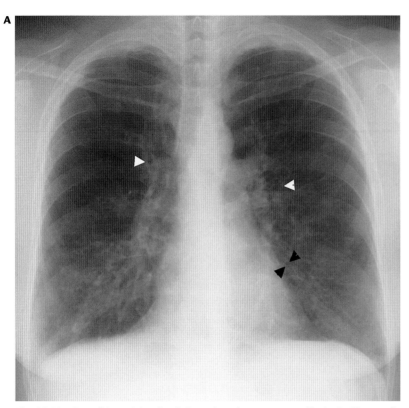
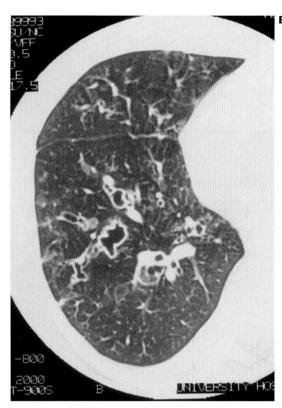

Fig. 11.53 Bronchiectasis in allergic bronchopulmonary aspergillosis. **A,** Chest radiograph shows extensive airway wall thickening, seen both en face (white arrowheads) and in profile as a tubular shadow (black arrowheads). **B,** HRCT shows varicose thick walled bronchiectasis involving subsegmental bronchi.

Several papers have compared the CT features of ABPA with those of uncomplicated asthma.[364,368,369] The prevalence of bronchial dilation in patients with severe or chronic asthma ranges from 17 to 30%, compared with 90% or more in ABPA.[368,369] However, the bronchial dilation in asthma is usually mild, cylindric, and distal, in contrast to the more severe proximal varicose or cystic bronchiectasis of ABPA.[368] Other distinguishing features on CT include a higher prevalence of centrilobular nodules and mucoid impaction.[368,369] The presence of bronchiectasis in three or more lobes is highly suggestive of ABPA.[369]

Parenchymal scarring representing the fibrotic stage of ABPA commonly follows bronchiectasis, and manifests by linear abnormality and lobar shrinkage (Figs 11.54 and 11.55). Mirroring the distribution of bronchiectasis, these features have a strong upper zone predilection, with 78% being so distributed in one series.[340] Such lobar shrinkage is accompanied by a variety of ring and linear opacities. Lower lobe shrinkage, though described, is very unusual.[337] Although there is often chronic lobar shrinkage, the overall lung volume is frequently increased, reflecting airflow limitation, compensatory overinflation of the lower lobes, and bulla formation. Between 30 and 40% of patients in one series showed overinflation.[370] Pleural thickening is not a major feature, having a prevalence of 18% in the same series,[370] though pleural thickening was seen on CT in 14 of 17 cases of ABPA in another series.[366]

Mycetomas may form in the bronchiectatic cavities. In one series of 111 patients with ABPA, eight had mycetomas, predominantly mid zonal.[340] Since mid zone mycetomas are

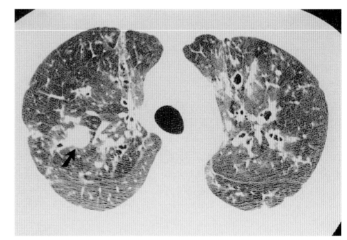

Fig. 11.54 Allergic bronchopulmonary aspergillosis – bronchial disease with scarring. HRCT through the upper zones shows dilated thick walled bronchi and a 1.5 cm rounded opacity (arrow) caused by a bronchocele. Linear opacities seen anteriorly are caused by scarring.

unusual in other conditions, it has been suggested that a mycetoma found in this position should raise the possibility of underlying ABPA.[340] It might be expected that patients with ABPA and mycetoma would be particularly symptomatic because of their immune status coupled with massive antigen

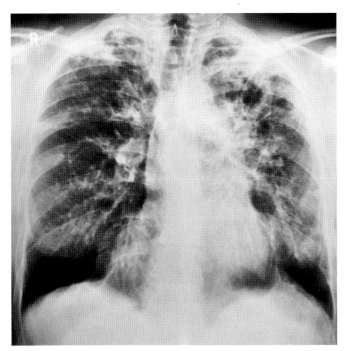

Fig. 11.55 Bilateral middle and upper zone fibrosis following multiple acute attacks of allergic bronchopulmonary aspergillosis. Chest radiograph shows marked bilateral upper lobe volume loss, with linear, ring, and conglomerate opacities in the upper lungs, reflecting underlying bronchiectasis, scarring, and bulla formation.

> **Box 11.11** Criteria for the diagnosis of allergic bronchopulmonary aspergillosis in cystic fibrosis[373]
>
> Classic case
> 1. Acute or subacute clinical deterioration not attributable to another etiology
> 2. Serum total IgE concentration of >1000 IU/ml
> 3. Skin test positivity to *Aspergillus*
> 4. Precipitating antibodies or IgG antibody to *A. fumigatus*
> 5. New or recent abnormalities on chest radiography (infiltrates or mucus plugging) or CT (bronchiectasis) that have not cleared with antibiotics and standard physiotherapy
>
> Minimal diagnostic criteria: 1, 2, 3, and either 4 or 5

bronchiectasis without peripheral bronchiectasis was seen in 11 (37%) of 30 patients with ABPA and in only one (7%) with mild cystic fibrosis.[365] Although varicose or cystic bronchiectasis is quite common in cystic fibrosis, it appears to be more common in ABPA.[373] High-attenuation mucus plugs have been reported in ABPA,[360] but not in cystic fibrosis, so these might be suggestive of ABPA in the correct clinical context.

Drug induced eosinophilic lung disease

A large number of drugs are recorded as producing radiographic abnormalities as part of a hypersensitivity response together with blood eosinophilia (Box 11.12; see also p. 489). Patients generally develop symptoms within days or a few weeks of starting the drug and some develop an associated rash and pyrexia, which provide helpful clues as to the nature of the radiographic opacity. A variety of chest radiographic patterns are produced:

- *Airspace opacity* (Fig. 11.56), which may be localized or diffuse. In some instances the pattern is that of Löffler syndrome. Illnesses vary from a mild, simple eosinophilic pneumonia to a fulminant AEP.[305] Drugs that are particularly associated with a consolidative pattern include penicillin, sulfonamides, paraaminosalicylic acid, chlorpropamide, nitrofurantoin, methotrexate, carbamazepine, mephenesin, imipramine, trimipramine, and hydrochlorothiazide.
- *Hilar lymphadenopathy*. This is recorded with the antiepileptic drugs phenytoin and trimethadione.[380]
- *Pleural effusions*. These are occasionally seen with nitrofurantoin (see Ch. 1048).
- *Reticulonodular opacity*. An interstitial pulmonary fibrosis type of pattern is produced in particular by nitrofurantoin and methotrexate (see Ch. 9). With nitrofurantoin the chronic interstitial pattern is associated with a blood eosinophilia in about 40% of patients.[375] Other drugs that produce an interstitial pattern include gold[380] and clofibrate.[391]
- As mentioned in the section Acute Eosinophilic Pneumonia (p. 654), imaging features of AEP may be seen with drugs such as venlafaxine and amitriptyline.[291,292]

A distinctive syndrome has been described in association with L-tryptophan ingestion (L-tryptophan eosinophilia myalgia

production, but this does not appear to be so. It is of interest that an ABPA type of syndrome has been recorded as developing as a result of a mycetoma lodged in a tuberculous cavity.[371]

In summary, a chest radiograph or CT of an asthmatic individual showing consolidation, collapse, upper zone fibrosis, mucoid impaction, or perihilar and upper zone bronchiectasis should prompt consideration of ABPA.

Allergic bronchopulmonary aspergillosis in cystic fibrosis

The reported prevalence of ABPA in patients with cystic fibrosis varies from 1 to 15%, depending on diagnostic criteria and the aggressiveness of screening for ABPA.[372,373] The prevalence of ABPA in patients with cystic fibrosis in the United States appears to be about 2%,[372] compared with 7.8% in Europe.[373,374] Box 11.11 shows criteria for the diagnosis of ABPA in this condition, based on a recent consensus statement.[373] The diagnosis of ABPA in cystic fibrosis is difficult, and may often be delayed, because many of the diagnostic criteria overlap with common manifestations of the disease.[373]

From an imaging viewpoint, the problem with diagnosis of ABPA in cystic fibrosis is that bronchiectasis and pulmonary opacities are common in uncomplicated cystic fibrosis. The published criteria for diagnosis of ABPA in cystic fibrosis (Box 11.11) suggest that such abnormalities may support the diagnosis of ABPA if they are new and have not responded to standard treatment. The type and distribution of the bronchiectasis may assist in the diagnosis, since central bronchiectasis is relatively uncommon in cystic fibrosis, though common in ABPA. In a study of patients with bronchiectasis, central

Box 11.12 Drugs associated with eosinophilic lung disease

Antibiotics
Ampicillin[375]
Capreomycin[376]
Dapsone[377]
Ethambutol[378]
Isoniazid[375]
Minocycline[379]
Nitrofurantoin[279,375,376,380]
Paraaminosalicylic acid[279,375,376,380]
Penicillin[279,375,376,380]
Pentamidine (inhaled)[381]
Pyrimethamine[382]
Rifampicin[376]
Sulfonamides[279,375,376,380]
Tetracycline[279]

Analgesics and antiinflammatory drugs
Acetaminophen[383]
Aspirin[279,376]
Diclofenac[384]
Fenbufen[305]
Gold[380]
Ibuprofen[385]
Nabumetone[386]
Naproxen[387]
Phenybulazone[386]
Sulindac[305]
Tolfenamic acid[305]

Cytotoxics
Azathioprine[388]
Bleomycin[376,388]
Methotrexate[279,375,376,380]
Procarbazine[388]

Sulfonylureas
Chlorpropamide[279,375,380]
Tolazamide[389]
Tolbutamide[376]

Neuropsychiatric drugs
Amytriptyline[291]
Carbamazepine[279,375,376,390]
Chlorpromazine[279]
Dantrolene[375]
Desipramine[305]
Imipramine[279,375]
Mephenesin[279,375,376]
Phenytoin[375]
Trimethadione[380]
Venlafaxine[292]

Miscellaneous drugs
Beclomethasone[279]
Clofibrate[391]
Cocaine[392]
Cromoglycate[279]
Granulocyte macrophage-colony stimulating factor (GM-CSF)[393]
Heroin[286]
Hydralazine[388]

Box 11.12 cont'd

Interleukin[305]
Methylphenidate[279,375]
Penicillamine[394]
Progesterone in oil[395]
L-tryptophan[396,397]

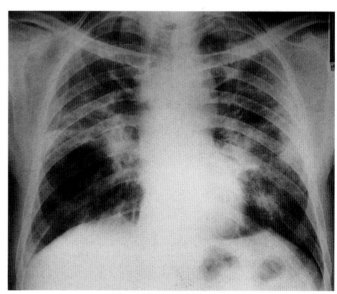

Fig. 11.56 Drug related eosinophilic lung disease. Multifocal nonsegmental consolidations in a 66-year-old man who developed a nonproductive cough and dyspnea after starting a nonsteroidal antiinflammatory drug (naproxen). There was blood eosinophilia (6.4 × 10^9/L). Opacities cleared after naproxen was discontinued and systemic steroids were begun. (Courtesy of Dr JD Stevenson, Poole, Dorset, UK)

syndrome). Principal features include peripheral eosinophilia, myopathy, peripheral neuropathy, eosinophilic fasciitis, and respiratory disorder. This latter is characterized radiologically by bilateral, often basally predominant, opacity with mixed alveolar and interstitial features, and pleural effusions.[396,397] Pathologically there is chronic interstitial pneumonia, tissue eosinophilia, and vasculitis.[396]

Tropical pulmonary eosinophilia

This is a specific systemic disease caused by hypersensitivity to microfilariae – the early larval forms of various filarial nematodes, the most important being *Brugia malayi* and *Wuchereria bancrofti*.[398,399] Transmission is by mosquito. Tropical pulmonary eosinophilia (TPE) is found in all parts of the world where filariasis is endemic, particularly the Indian subcontinent, Southeast Asia, the South Pacific, North Africa, and South America. It occurs chiefly in the indigenous residents (particularly in the Indian subcontinent),[400,401] and is very uncommon in visitors unless they have resided in the area for many months.[402] In nonendemic areas the disease is seen in immigrants and, because of persistence of the parasite in the host, may present as long as 3 years after returning from an endemic area.[403] Occurrence is extremely rare in Caucasians.[404]

The disease is more common in males, in some series by as much as 4:1,[405] but this is not a universal finding.[404] The usual age at presentation is between 5 and 40 years,[405] though the range can be larger; in one series of 350 individuals it varied from 1.5 to 74 years.[401] The principal features of the illness are a systemic disturbance marked by fatigue, weight loss, and low grade fever together with respiratory symptoms. The main respiratory symptoms are chronic cough, which is particularly troublesome at night and may be productive of mucoid or mucopurulent sputum with occasional hemoptysis, dyspnea, and wheeze. Even without treatment, symptoms tend to remit after several weeks or months only to recur later.[402] Patients who have not had treatment or who have responded inadequately may go on to develop progressive dyspnea secondary to interstitial fibrosis.[399] In the acute phase there are crackles and wheezes in the chest. Hepatosplenomegaly and nodal enlargement are rarely seen except in children.[405] There is a gross blood eosinophilia of $>3 \times 10^9/L$, characteristically between 5 and $60 \times 10^9/L$. IgE levels are greatly elevated, usually $>1000\,IU/ml$, and there is a high titer of antifilarial antibody. BAL shows a high percentage of eosinophils, of the order of 50%.

Pathologic changes are initially those of an eosinophilic alveolitis with bronchopneumonia, microabscesses, and granulomas. Bronchioles show mural eosinophilic infiltration. Within a year or so the eosinophilic element decreases, the exudate becomes mononuclear, and interstitial fibrosis develops.[399]

Radiologic findings in the chest[401,404,406,407] may be caused by active alveolitis and/or interstitial scarring. The chest radiograph has a normal appearance in 2–13% of cases. The most common abnormalities, seen in one- to two-thirds of patients, are fine linear opacities distributed diffusely and symmetrically, accompanied by hilar haziness and blurring of vessels. Some authors[404] describe a basal predominance, and others stress a diffuse ground-glass type of pattern.[401] Small nodules are a slightly less common finding, seen in about 30–50% of patients. The nodules range in size from 1 to 5 mm and may occur alone or with the linear opacities described above.[404] Though generally bilateral and symmetric, nodulation may be asymmetric or even unilateral. Other patterns are much less common and consist of areas of consolidation that are generally small and single. They can, however, be large[408] and multifocal,[404,407] a pattern that is now rarely encountered.[399] Cavitation may occur within consolidation,[409] but it seems unlikely that this is directly related to TPE.[399] Diffuse ground-glass opacification[401] and small pleural effusions are also recorded. Many accounts describe bilateral hilar enlargement or prominence.[401,406,407] Enlargement is almost always mild and has been ascribed to vessels rather than nodes,[401] though there was pathologic evidence of slight hilar adenopathy in one study.[410] In a study of 10 patients with TPE,[411] CT was found to be superior for the depiction of reticulonodular abnormality, bronchiectasis, air-trapping and lymphadenopathy.

TPE characteristically responds rapidly to diethylcarbamazine therapy and this is an important diagnostic criterion. However, 5% of patients, even early on in the natural history of the disease, fail to respond adequately and this figure rises to 20–40% in patients who have had long-standing symptoms.[399] A 5 year follow up of a large series of patients showed a 20% relapse rate[399] and a significant number of patients develop chronic, progressive dyspnea on the basis of interstitial fibrosis.

Eosinophilic lung disease from other worm infestations

The larval stages of a number of worms other than filarial nematodes pass through the lung and may, in the process, induce an allergic response. This most commonly takes the form of simple eosinophilic pneumonia/Löffler syndrome with transient, migratory, nonsegmental areas of consolidation associated with a blood eosinophilia (Fig. 11.57).[412] Nearly all the worms that cause this response are nematodes: *Ascaris lumbricoides*,[413] *Ascaris suum*,[414] *Strongyloides stercoralis*,[412] *Toxocara canis* (visceral larva migrans),[415] *Toxocara cati*,[412] *Ancylostoma braziliense* ("creeping eruption"),[416] *Ancylostoma duodenale, Necator americanus*,[278] and *Trichuris trichiura*.[275] Exceptions are *Taenia saginata* and *Echinococcus alveolaris*,[275] both cestodes, and *Schistosoma* spp which are trematodes.[417] It is possible that, in at least some of these infestations, the pulmonary reaction is not related to local larvae but rather is a remote response to a soluble antigen.[416] Thus, in 26 patients with eosinophilic lung disease due to *Ankylostoma braziliense* (Fig. 11.57), it was not possible to demonstrate larvae in the sputum.[418] Some idea of the possible frequency of eosinophilic lung disease caused by nematode infestations may be gained from these authors, who found lung parenchymal abnormality in 34% of 76 patients with cutaneous larva migrans (hookworm infestation).

In the United States, the most common parasites to consider are *Strongyloides, Ascaris, Toxocara,* and *Ankylostoma*.[305] The last three organisms usually give rise to simple eosinophilic pneumonia/Löffler type changes on the chest radiograph. With

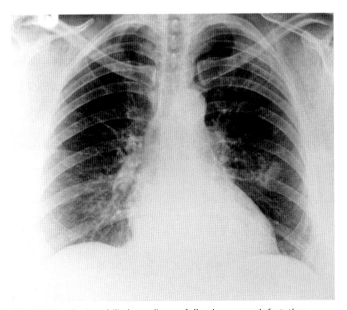

Fig. 11.57 Eosinophilic lung disease following worm infestation. This 52-year-old woman had a buttock rash caused by cutaneous larva migrans (*Ancylostoma braziliense*) acquired on vacation in the West Indies. She had blood eosinophilia and a dry cough. Chest radiograph shows two areas of consolidation: one in the left mid zone and the other peripherally in the left upper zone. Both cleared in 2 weeks.

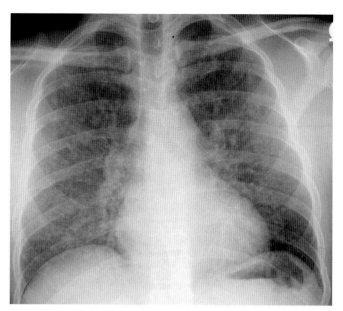

Fig. 11.58 Pulmonary eosinophilia due to *Strongyloides*. Chest radiograph shows bilateral nodules and patches of consolidation.

Strongyloides the lung pathology is more complicated and in the autoinfection stage there is a pulmonary foreign body reaction with inflammatory pneumonitis, bronchopneumonia, and hemorrhage. The chest radiograph (Fig. 11.58) reflects this and shows mixed opacity – miliary nodules, reticular opacities, and airspace opacities, ranging from multifocal and patchy to lobar.[419] About 90% of patients will have a blood eosinophilia. Should the hyperinfection syndrome supervene, the chest radiograph manifests widespread consolidation, at which stage peripheral eosinophilia may be absent.[419]

It is important to know that for a variety of reasons acute eosinophilic lung disease induced by the above four agents is usually not accompanied by ova in the stool.[274,305] Ascariasis and strongyloides may be diagnosed by finding larvae in the sputum, BAL, or gastric aspirates, but ova may not be found in the stool until females are mature, which in ascariasis may be delayed up to 3 months after initial pulmonary manifestations.[274] *Toxocara* and *Ankylostoma* do not replicate in the gut, so ova are not usually found in the stool. Both conditions may be suspected on the basis of a skin rash; toxocariasis may be confirmed by serology.[274]

Bronchocentric granulomatosis

This form of pulmonary granulomatosis, first described by Liebow in 1973,[420] differs from other lung granulomatoses, such as Wegener granulomatosis, in that it is localized to the lung, and centered around airways (bronchocentric) rather than vessels

(angiocentric). Pathologically, small airways and bronchioles are filled and replaced by cellular debris and necrotic granulomas surrounded by palisaded epithelioid cells. In asthmatics the major part of the cellular infiltrate is made up of eosinophils, whereas in nonasthmatics the plasma cell is dominant.[421] Large airways may show bronchocele formation, and distal lung is often consolidated by an eosinophilic or obstructive pneumonitis. Vasculitic changes appear to be minor and incidental.

Only four series of patients with bronchocentric granulomatosis have been recorded,[421-424] representing a total of 60 cases. However, there have been many additional case reports.

Patients commonly present in their 40s, but there is a wide age range (9–76 years) and a tendency for asthmatics to present at a younger age (mean age 22 years) than nonasthmatics (mean age 50 years).[421] The incidence in both sexes is equal. In the combined series, 16 (29%) of 55 patients were asthmatic, and some patients had associated disorders, though the significance of this observation is unclear. These disorders include rheumatoid disease,[425] ankylosing spondylitis,[426] glomerulonephritis,[427] and echinococcosis.[428] Symptoms may be absent or minor and, when present, are not particularly characteristic. They consist of fever, cough, chest pain, wheeze, and hemoptysis. About 50% of patients have a blood eosinophilia, a finding that appears to be limited to asthmatics.[421,423]

Radiographically[421-423,429] two major patterns are seen: consolidation, or masslike lesions (Box 11.13). Consolidation may be lobar or sublobar and may be accompanied by volume loss (Fig. 11.59). The consolidation may either represent eosinophilic or obstructive pneumonitis,[421] tends to be more common in the upper zones,[421,429] and is unilateral in about 75% of patients. Sublobar consolidation was the most common finding (16 of 22) in one large series.[421] Masslike lesions (Fig. 11.60) are commonly solitary, but can be multiple. They are considered to represent a mass of necrotic tissue with surrounding granulomatous or organizing pneumonia. They vary in size from 2 to 15 cm,[425] and are often not particularly well defined. Occasionally they cavitate.[421,425,430] Less common radiologic patterns include mucoid impaction (Fig. 11.61),[420,421,430,431] and reticulonodular opacities.[430] On some occasions the reticulonodular abnormality has evolved from antecedent consolidation. Adenopathy and pleural disease are not features.[430] In a study of five patients with bronchocentric granulomatosis,[424] CT showed spiculated mass lesions in three cases and consolidation in two. Extensive mucoid impaction was seen in two patients. The imaging findings were felt to be due to granuloma formation with or without proximal airway obstruction.

Box 11.13 **Radiologic features of bronchocentric granulomatosis**

Consolidation
Masses or nodules, often spiculated, resembling neoplasm

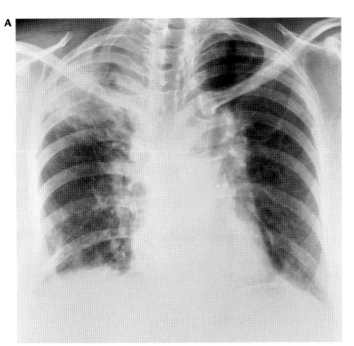

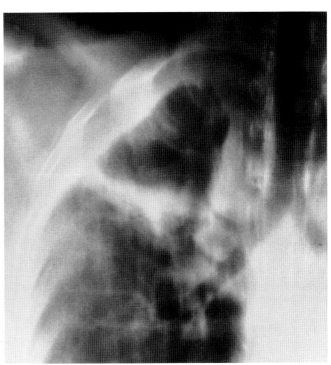

Fig. 11.59 Bronchocentric granulomatosis. This 52-year-old woman presented with weight loss and cough. **A**, Chest radiograph shows right upper zone consolidation with some volume loss and scattered linear and nodular opacities in the left upper zone, these latter changes being ascribed to old granulomatous disease. The patient was treated with antituberculous therapy without an established diagnosis. **B**, Localized tomogram of the right upper zone 1 month later. Consolidation has been replaced by a thick walled, 5 cm diameter cavity. Following right upper lobectomy, asthma and blood eosinophilia developed. Hyphae of *Aspergillus* were found in the pathologic specimen.

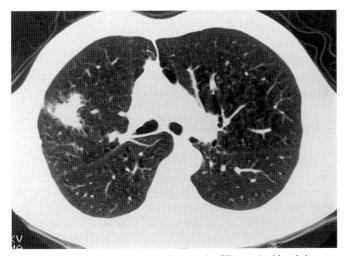

Fig. 11.60 Bronchocentric granulomatosis. CT at carinal level shows an irregular, lobulated and spiculated 3 cm mass lesion in the right upper lobe. Marginal irregularity and spiculation, suggestive of a malignancy, is not uncommon in bronchocentric granulomatosis.

There is evidence that bronchocentric granulomatosis in asthmatics is different etiologically from that seen in non-asthmatics. In many asthmatics there is histologic, serologic, and microbiologic evidence that bronchocentric granulomatosis is caused by *Aspergillus* and forms part of the spectrum of ABPA.[432,433] It is also possible that there is sensitivity to other fungi such as *Candida* spp.[421] In nonasthmatics the cause is generally obscure, though cases have been reported associated with tuberculosis and a variety of fungi.[432]

Prognosis is good. Lesions may clear spontaneously or with steroids and generally do not recur following surgical removal. If this should happen, recurrences can usually be controlled with steroid treatment.

Hypereosinophilic syndrome

Hypereosinophilic syndrome is an uncommon heterogeneous group of disorders in which the eosinophilia may be neoplastic (e.g. an eosinophilic leukemia) or reactive, and in the latter

A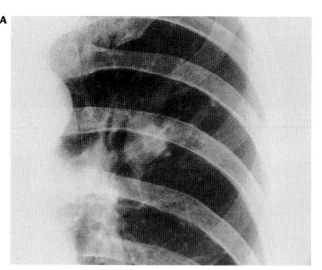
B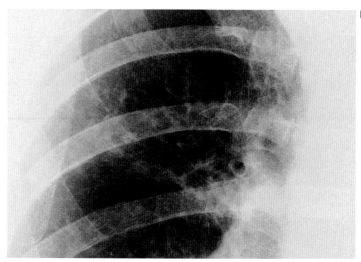

Fig. 11.61 Bronchocentric granulomatosis. **A**, Localized view of left middle zone in a 50-year-old woman shows a 2 x 3 cm lobulated well-demarcated masslike lesion with two fingerlike projections that strongly suggest a bronchocele. **B**, Localized view of the right mid zone shows thin curvilinear and ring opacities caused by bronchiectasis resulting from allergic bronchopulmonary aspergillosis. (Courtesy of Dr JD Stevenson, Poole, Dorset, UK)

instance some appear to be truly idiopathic in that a cause is not established even at death.[434] It is characterized by: (1) prolonged and marked eosinophilia (a blood count of >1.5 × 10⁹/L for >6 months); (2) no recognizable cause for the eosinophilia, such as parasitic infestation or allergy; and (3) signs or symptoms of organ dysfunction.[435] The sustained hypereosinophilia causes tissue damage, particularly cardiac, and this is a key element to the syndrome. The illness varies in severity from mild to fatal, involving in particular the cardiovascular and nervous systems. The cardiac abnormality consists primarily of endocardial thickening and fibrosis. In the past it has been given a variety of other names, including Löffler syndrome with cardiac involvement, Löffler fibroplastic endocarditis, and disseminated eosinophilic collagen disease.[436] Pathologically there is widespread tissue infiltration with mature eosinophils that cause tissue damage,[437] particularly endocardial damage leading to endocardial fibrosis, restrictive cardiomyopathy, and thrombosis. Almost all patients have been men, typically young or middle-aged adults, who present with progressive cardiopulmonary symptoms, skin rash, or myalgia together with systemic symptoms such as weight loss, weakness, fatigue, and fever. The peripheral blood shows a marked eosinophilia, often in the order of 30–70% of the total white blood cell count (10–50 × 10⁹/L), some of the eosinophils being degranulated and vacuolated. Some patients have a mild increase in IgE. The organ systems most commonly affected are the nervous and cardiovascular systems and the skin. Cardiovascular involvement is usually the dominant feature and is a major cause of morbidity, with signs of restrictive cardiomyopathy and pump failure, mitral, and tricuspid regurgitation, and endocardial thrombosis. This latter leads to systemic emboli in about 5% of patients[438] or pulmonary emboli if the thrombus is right sided.[437]

Clinical pulmonary involvement has been recorded in about 40% of patients (Box 11.14).[435,437] In most, these are findings related to heart failure,[436] and include pulmonary edema and pleural effusions.[435] Because the cardiomyopathy is restrictive in type, any accompanying cardiomegaly is often mild.[438]

Box 11.14 Clinical manifestations of hypereosinophilic syndrome

Cardiac
- Endocardial thickening
- Restrictive cardiomyopathy

Skin rash
Ground-glass opacity

Pulmonary emboli were recorded in 9% of 57 patients reviewed from the literature.[435] Other less common pulmonary manifestations include transient consolidations, which are presumably eosinophilic pneumonias, and diffuse interstitial fibrosis.[435,438] HRCT findings in five patients in whom chest radiographs were normal (three of five) or showed nonspecific focal opacities (two of five) consisted of scattered nodules (about 2–10 mm) with ground-glass halos (five of five) and focal areas of ground-glass attenuation (three of five) (Fig. 11.62). There was no pathologic correlation, but the authors considered that the lesions probably represented areas of eosinophilic infiltration.[439] In three patients studied by Johkoh et al,[302] the common imaging features were ground-glass attenuation and nodules, with septal thickening and thickening of bronchovascular bundles. The challenge in these cases is to distinguish findings due to heart failure from those due to pulmonary involvement.[302]

Before the use of steroids and cytotoxic drugs the prognosis of hypereosinophilic syndrome was poor, with a 25% 2 year survival rate,[435] but this figure has now improved considerably, and the 3 year mortality is reduced to 4%.[440]

Other conditions associated with eosinophilia

There is often a mild to moderate eosinophilia in patients with asthma.[441] The radiology of asthma is discussed elsewhere

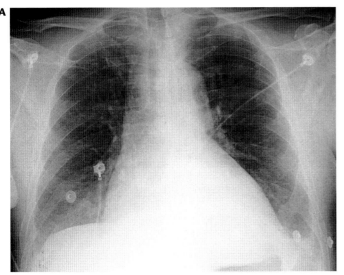

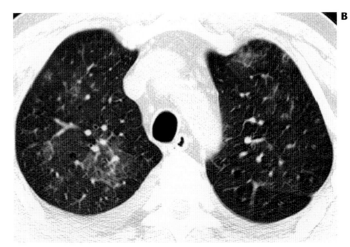

Fig. 11.62 A 55-year-old man with hypereosinophilic syndrome. **A**, Chest radiograph shows cardiomegaly and bilateral effusions. **B**, HRCT shows patchy ground-glass abnormality.

(p. 748). In addition, asthma is often a prominent symptom in a number of specific eosinophilic lung states such as ABPA and the Churg–Strauss syndrome. Other pulmonary conditions associated with blood eosinophilia, and often with tissue eosinophilia, are listed in Box 11.15. The degree of eosinophilia in these conditions is generally relatively slight ($<1 \times 10^9/L$). Box 11.15 emphasizes the importance of considering infection and neoplasm (Fig. 11.63) in patients presenting with eosinophilia and pulmonary parenchymal abnormalities.

Hyperimmunoglobulin E syndrome

This rare primary immunodeficiency syndrome was first described in 1966[442] and is characterized by recurrent bacterial infections of the lungs, sinuses, and skin dating from birth or early childhood, and a more than tenfold elevation of serum IgE.[443] The immunologic derangement is complex and only partly understood.[444] It includes a high titer of IgE antibodies to staphylococcal antigens, reduced numbers of suppressor T cells, and a neutrophil chemotactic defect. Recurrent bronchitis and pneumonia is a major feature, often due to *Staphylococcus aureus* though other bacteria and fungi may also be responsible. There is commonly an eczematous dermatitis, mucocutaneous candidiasis, recurrent furunculosis, and cutaneous cold abscesses. The lack of the usual systemic and local inflammatory findings with the abscesses is a striking feature, particularly because most are due to *Staph. aureus*. Other features include dysmorphism with retarded growth and coarse facies and osteoporosis.[445] A mild or moderate eosinophilia occurs in 77–100% of patients.[443,444] Occasionally, however, eosinophilia is marked.[446] Radiologic findings in the chest have been well described[444,447,448] and consist of recurrent infective consolidations (beginning before the age of 3 years) and cyst formation. All patients in the series of Merten et al,[444] in which the average age was 18 years, had lung cysts. Some cysts disappeared after a few years while others were recurrent or persistent. About a third of cysts were multiple and could be very large, occupying much of a

Box 11.15 Other pulmonary conditions which may be associated with eosinophilia

Asthma

Hyperimmunoglobulin E syndrome

Langerhans cell histiocytosis

Infections
Bacterial (*Brucella*, *Mycobacterium*)
Chlamydia
Viral (adenovirus)
Protozoal (*Pneumocystis*, *Triomonas*)
Fungal (*Coccidioides*, *Histoplasma*)

Neoplasms
Bronchogenic carcinoma, bronchial carcinoid
Metastases
Irradiated neoplasms
Lymphoma (Hodgkin and non-Hodgkin, lymphomatoid granulomatosis)

"Immunologic" conditions
Wegener granulomatosis
Rheumatoid disease
Hypersensitivity pneumonitis
Sarcoidosis
Idiopathic pulmonary fibrosis
Cryptogenic organizing pneumonia

Miscellaneous
Hemodialysis

hemithorax, while their walls were usually smooth but of varying thickness. The pathogenesis of these cysts is not definitely established. Some are probably pneumatoceles and others arise in a cavitating consolidation. In a number of cases, however, their development could not be related to an infective

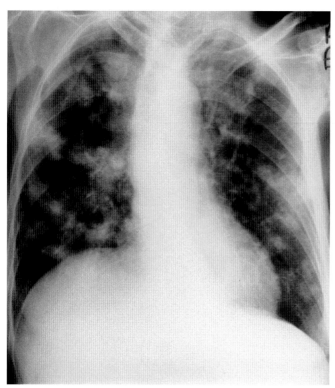

Fig. 11.63 Metastases associated with blood eosinophilia. Frontal radiograph of an 82-year-old woman who presented with a subacute history of malaise, weight loss, and cough. There was a peripheral blood eosinophilia of 8.6×10^9/L. Chest radiograph shows numerous well-defined and poorly defined nodules. The liver was enlarged and contained multiple focal lesions revealing adenocarcinoma on biopsy.

episode.[444] Other pulmonary findings include empyema, fungal superinfection of pneumatocele,[449] bronchopleural fistula,[445] bronchiectasis,[444,449] and pneumothorax.[449,450] Eighty percent of patients in the series of Merten et al[444] had chronic sinusitis.

PULMONARY ALVEOLAR PROTEINOSIS

Pulmonary alveolar proteinosis (PAP) is a rare disorder first described in 1958[451] and characterized pathologically by alveolar filling with a lipid rich, proteinaceous material (positive to periodic acid-Schiff stain), while the lung interstitium remains relatively normal. PAP probably represents a nonspecific response of the type II pneumocyte, alveolar macrophage, or both to a variety of injuries.[452] PAP may be divided into primary and secondary forms (Box 11.16).

Secondary forms are seen in association with:

- *Dust and chemical exposure.*[453,454] Inhalation of silica as in acute silicosis[455] – especially caused by sandblasting,[456,457] aluminum dust,[458] and particulate titanium.[459]
- *Infections.* The association is complicated and some infections (see below) are undoubtedly secondary to primary PAP, whereas others are themselves probably the primary process that precipitates the proteinosis. An example of the latter is pneumocystis infection, both HIV and nonHIV related.[460]

Box 11.16 Types of pulmonary alveolar proteinosis

Primary

Secondary
Dust/chemical exposure
Silica
Aluminum
Titanium
Infection related
Pneumocystis pneumonia
Immunocompromise
Lymphoma
Myeloid leukemia
Severe combined immune deficiency
Lung transplant
Congenital
Surfactant apoprotein deficiency

- *Immunocompromise.* An association with hematologic malignancies (lymphoma, myeloid leukemia) is described,[461] particularly in children, and was present in 8.5 and 15% of PAP patients in two series.[452,462] In another review, 30% of children with PAP had thymic alymphoplasia.[463] PAP is also described with severe combined immune deficiency in mice[464] and humans,[465] and in mice deficient in granulocyte macrophage-colony stimulating factor (GM-CSF),[466] a deficiency leading to macrophage dysfunction. Three cases of PAP developing in lung allograft recipients performed for conditions other than PAP have been recorded.[467]
- *Surfactant apoprotein deficiency.* This is a rare autosomal recessive form of PAP seen in neonates and associated with deficiency of one of the four apoproteins (SP-D) found in surfactant.[468]

The alveolar material in PAP is partly phospholipid derived from type II pneumocytes and it resembles surfactant. The rest is cellular debris and protein from plasma including four apoproteins (SP-A to SP-D) which are critical to surfactant metabolism.[468] Whether phospholipid accumulation is the result of overproduction (proliferation and desquamation of type II pneumocytes), reduced clearance (defective macrophage function), or both is not clear.[452] Recently, it has been discovered that knockout mice with deficiencies of GM-CSF or the β-GM-CSF receptor all develop PAP.[469] GM-CSF appears to have an important role in surfactant clearance. Defects in GM-CSF production and receptor signaling have been found in humans with PAP, and anti-GM-CSF antibodies have been found in serum and BAL specimens of 100% of such patients.[470,471]

PAP is most common in adults, particularly aged 30–50 years, though cases are seen in children (including neonates) and up to the age of 72 years.[453,469] Sixty to 80% of patients are male.[452,453,469] About 70% are cigarette smokers, and it is thought that the male predominance might be due to the higher frequency of cigarette smoking in males.[469] Children with PAP are usually compromised hosts, and the disease is progressive and often fatal, whereas adults generally have no underlying disorder. In about one-fifth of cases the onset is acute, with fever, weight loss, and dyspnea, either with or without a superadded opportunistic infection.[453] Most of the other cases have an insidious onset with progressive dyspnea and cough. Median duration of symptoms prior to presentation is 7 months.[469] Cough is usually dry but is sometimes productive of white sticky sputum. Other early features include pleuritic chest pain, hemoptysis,[452] and pneumothorax.[453] Occasionally the disease is discovered by chest radiography in asymptomatic individuals.[472] The clinical signs consist of crepitations, sometimes hypoxemia, and clubbing. PAP is one of the conditions in which the radiologic signs are often striking even when the symptoms and clinical signs are mild.[473] Seventy percent of patients have a mild to moderate elevation of serum lactate dehydrogenase. The serum levels of surfactant apoproteins A and D (SP-A, SP-D) are markedly elevated, though nonspecific.[474] Antibodies to GM-CSF are universally present in patients with PAP, and may be diagnostically useful. Pulmonary function tests show a restrictive defect with hypoxemia and impaired diffusion.[452]

Diagnosis is established by BAL which shows the characteristic eosinophilic, granular, PAS positive lipoproteinaceous material in the washings.[474] A report suggests that elevated levels of the apoprotein SP-D in the washings may be specific for PAP.[475] In problematic patients it may occasionally be necessary to obtain a transbronchial lung biopsy for histologic study.[474]

On the chest radiograph, the main finding is consolidation or ground-glass abnormality, since the pathologic changes are almost entirely the result of alveolar filling.[451] In some cases, however, mild interstitial fibrosis and septal cellular infiltration and edema are present (Fig. 11.64),[451,453,472,476] and probably account for occasional "interstitial" features on the chest radiograph. The classic radiologic finding is bilateral, symmetric consolidation or ground-glass abnormality, particularly in a perihilar or hilar and basal distribution (Fig. 11.65).[451,453,477] This opacity often has a fine granularity and air bronchograms are surprisingly infrequent. At other times the pattern consists of rather coarse (5 mm), ill-defined acinar nodules, which are sometimes confluent.[478] The nodules may be particularly obvious toward the edge of confluent areas of consolidation,[472] and at times the pattern may even be reticulonodular.[452,472,476,478] Although usually symmetric, the consolidation can be asymmetric,[472] unilateral,[451,452] or lobar.[451,461] Sometimes the consolidation is basally predominant,[461] peripheral rather than central,[473] and multifocal rather than diffuse.[452] A thin zone of clear lung immediately above the diaphragm is sometimes present; this may be due to the action of the diaphragm in pumping proteinaceous material out of the adjacent airspaces. Simultaneous evolution and regression, producing a shifting pattern similar to that found in Löffler syndrome, has been described.[479] Occasional features include Kerley B lines,[452,477] and small rounded transradiances,[477,480] probably produced by obstructive overinflation of distal respiratory units, partly

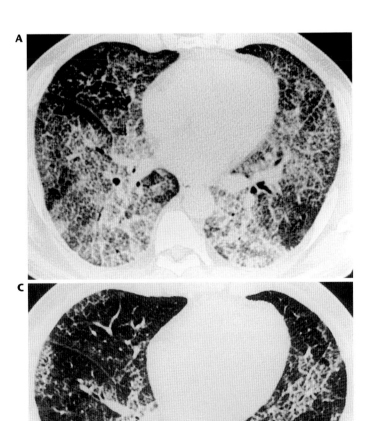

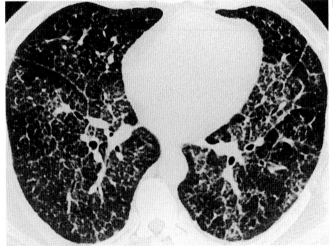

Fig. 11.64 Pulmonary alveolar proteinosis (PAP). **A**, HRCT of the mid/lower zones shows extensive bilateral opacity with a geographic distribution. There is both consolidation and ground-glass opacity. A fine reticular pattern with interlobular septal thickening superimposed on the ground-glass abnormality produces the crazy-paving pattern. **B**, HRCT 2 months later at the same level as **A** and following bilateral saline bronchoalveolar lavage. Consolidative and ground-glass opacity have essentially cleared. There is residual reticular opacity but it is much improved. **C**, HRCT 2 years later shows recurrence. The geographic nature of the opacity in PAP is well shown.

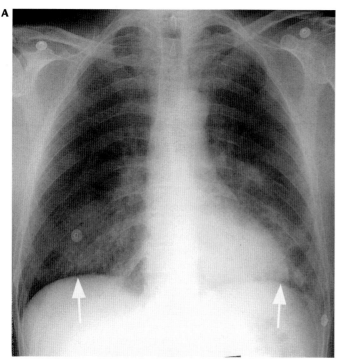

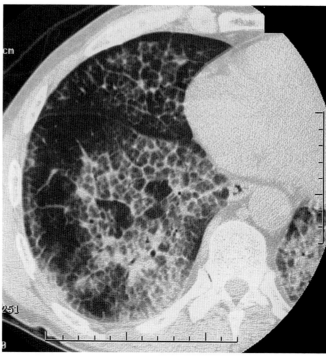

Fig. 11.65   Pulmonary alveolar proteinosis in a 54-year-old man with mild dyspnea on exertion. **A**, Chest radiograph shows bibasilar ground-glass abnormality with reticular abnormality. Note the characteristic thin rim of spared lung above the diaphragm (arrows). **B**, HRCT shows the typical crazy-paving pattern, with septal thickening and intralobular lines superimposed on ground-glass abnormality, without architectural distortion.

blocked by proteinaceous material. Rupture of a subpleural cyst has given rise to a pneumothorax.[473] Obstruction may also give rise to areas of collapse.[452,477,480]

On HRCT, PAP is characterized by the following features[481–486]:

- Geographic ground-glass abnormality
- Lines perpendicular to the pleura and forming polygonal structures, representing thickened interlobular septa
- A finer network of intralobular lines
- Absence of architectural distortion or traction bronchiectasis.

The superimposition of the reticular pattern formed by thickened interlobular septa and intralobular lines on a background of ground-glass abnormality produces the characteristic "crazy-paving" pattern (Figs 11.64 and 11.65). Involved areas are bordered by normal lung and have a sharp, geographic margin reflecting lobular boundaries. Imaging changes tend to be diffuse,[482,485] but some cases show a lower lung predominance.[485] Other airspace opacities that may be found include acinar nodules, limited air bronchograms, and areas of consolidation where the density of the opacity obscures underlying vessels. If consolidation is present, the possibility of superimposed infective consolidation should be considered. The ground-glass abnormality is due to accumulation of protein within the alveoli, but the pathologic correlate of the inter- and intra-lobular lines remains quite unclear. They could be due to inter- and intra-lobular lymphatics stuffed with proteinaceous fluid, but there are few pathologic descriptions of this finding.[453,472,476] Following lavage the ground-glass opacity decreases (Fig. 11.64),[485] and the reticulation may become more prominent.[482] The crazy-paving pattern has been described in a wide variety of lung diseases,[486,487] including exogenous lipoid pneumonia,[488] bronchioloalveolar cell carcinoma,[489] drug toxicity, sarcoidosis, nonspecific interstitial pneumonia,[490] organizing pneumonia, pulmonary hemorrhage, *Pneumocystis carinii* pneumonia, and acute respiratory distress syndrome. The crazy-paving pattern of PAP may distinguished from these other entities in the following ways: (1) clinical presentation is relatively indolent; (2) extent of radiologic abnormality is out of proportion to clinical symptoms and physiologic impairment; (3) architectural distortion and traction bronchiectasis are absent: (4) distribution is geographic; and (5) thickened interlobular septa are more prominent than in the other conditions mentioned above. Where PAP is the working radiologic diagnosis, it is appropriate to recommend BAL to confirm the diagnosis and exclude other entities such as infection, bronchioloalveolar cell carcinoma, and lipoid pneumonia.

Because of the functional macrophage impairment, complicating infections by pathogenic bacteria[477] or opportunistic bacterial, fungal, and viral[461] agents are common. In one review,[462] 15% of 160 patients had such infections, and they were a major cause of death[453] before therapeutic lavage was introduced.[452] Agents most commonly recorded are *Nocardia*,[453,461,472] *Mycobacterium tuberculosis* and nontuberculous mycobacteria,[491,492] and *Cryptococcus*.[491] It seems likely that cardial infections have become less frequent following the adoption of therapeutic lavage.[474] Radiographic pointers to such an opportunistic infection include the development of focal consolidation, cavitation, and pleural effusion.[453] CT may identify focal pneumonia not apparent on chest radiographs.[481]

PAP improves spontaneously in about 10% of patients.[452,453,469] Most of the remaining patients will require treatment, and the standard treatment has been saline whole-lung lavage.[493] Lavage has dramatically reduced mortality[494] and results in complete remission in 75% of patients.[452] When patients are treated with lavage, the chest radiograph is used to decide which side should be treated and to detect any complications.[495] Recurrence of PAP has been documented in a patient who had a double lung transplant for progressive disease.[496] Recently, small scale clinical trials of GM-CSF have resulted in clinical improvement in 35–70% of cases, but the value of this treatment remains unclear.[469] Clinical trials of treatment in PAP are limited by its relative rarity and by the frequency of spontaneous improvement.

PULMONARY ALVEOLAR MICROLITHIASIS

Pulmonary alveolar microlithiasis (PAM) was first described in 1918.[497] It is a rare disorder, with 225 cases recorded in the world literature.[498] Its cause is unknown and, like PAP, gross radiographic changes are often present in the face of minor clinical symptoms.

Alveolar microlithiasis is characterized pathologically by the accumulation of numerous, largely intraalveolar, calcified bodies (calcispherites or microliths). Microliths have a mean diameter of about 200 μm[499] and contain calcium phosphate.[432] Dystrophic ossification occasionally develops around microliths.[499] There have been rare descriptions of extrapulmonary microliths in the testes or kidneys.[500–502] Alveolar walls are commonly normal[503] but later in the disease interstitial fibrosis may develop together with bullae and blebs.[502,504]

Although alveolar microlithiasis occurs worldwide, nearly one-quarter of recorded patients are from Turkey.[498] About 40% of cases are sporadic, while the remainder show a strong familial association,[504] consistent with an autosomal recessive transmission.[505,506] Other congenital disorders are very occasionally associated, such as Waardenburg–anopthalmia syndrome[506] and diaphyseal aclasia.[507] The sex incidence is approximately equal.[503] The disease is commonly first detected in the third and fourth decades,[503] but the range is large, with the disorder recorded in premature neonates[508] and in an 80-year-old woman.[502]

In three of four major series 60–80% of patients have been symptomless at the time of diagnosis.[503,504,509] The exception is a Turkish series in which 80% were symptomatic.[498] The interval between radiographic diagnosis and onset of symptoms may be from 5 to 40 years.[505] Later in the course of the disease cough may appear, and in a small proportion of patients hemoptysis, clubbing, hypertrophic osteoarthropathy,[498] pneumothorax, dyspnea, and cor pulmonale develop.[503,504] Pulmonary function tests are abnormal in about one-third of reported cases and most commonly show a restrictive defect or a decreased carbon monoxide diffusing capacity.[503] Identification of microliths in expectorated sputum or BAL can be diagnostic,[510,511] and whole-lung lavage has been used to relieve symptoms of dyspnea.[510]

The chest radiograph is characteristic,[504] with innumerable, widespread, pinpoint nodules of calcific density. Nodules are <1 mm in diameter, but they may summate in areas to give a ground-glass, reticular, or more coarsely nodular (up to 5 mm) pattern (Fig. 11.66).[512] The radiographic opacity, which tends to be greatest at the bases, sometimes shows subpleural[504,512–514] or peribronchovascular accentuation.[512] In advanced disease the radiographic opacity is so great that anatomic landmarks become completely obscured. Thus, the heart may "vanish"[512] or even

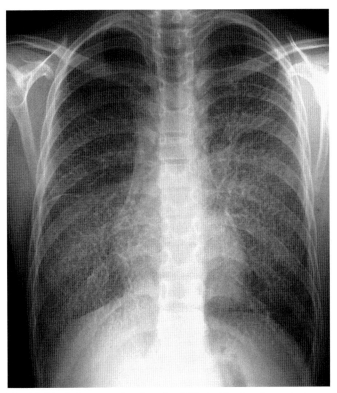

Fig. 11.66 Pulmonary alveolar microlithiasis. Chest radiograph shows extensive coarse reticular abnormality, with polygonal structures formed by thickened interlobular septa. The minor fissure is thickened. A black pleural line is visible in the right lower chest.

appear as a transradiant area on a penetrated radiograph. The parietal pleural region may appear as a thin dark band (Fig. 11.66)[504] which has been variously attributed to artifact related to the adjacent dense pulmonary calcification,[515] subpleural cysts,[516,517] and extrapleural fat.[512,518] Pleural fissures can appear dense, thickened (Fig. 11.66), and beaded,[519] and septal lines are occasionally seen.[512,520] Bullae and blebs develop with late fibrosis,[502–504] and these are particularly well seen on CT.[499,521] Such blebs and bullae probably predispose patients to pneumothorax and pneumomediastinum, which are recognized complications.[502,521]

CT data on microlithiasis are limited.[499,506,513,516–518,521–523] The predominant distribution of abnormality is usually posterobasal (Fig. 11.67). Because of the volume averaging of the tiny microliths, their calcific density may not be apparent, resulting in a micronodular or ground-glass pattern, even on HRCT. With larger nodules, the calcification may be visible. The occasional 5 mm nodule presumably represents dystrophic ossification seen histopathologically. Calcification may be uniform or may show some macroscopic structure with accentuation along pleural margins and fissures, adjacent to interlobular septa (giving polygonal structures), and bronchovascular bundles,[506,513,516,521,523] explaining the coarsely linear nodulations, reticulation, and septal lines occasionally seen on the chest radiograph.[512,520] All CT studies have shown airspaces (blebs or bullae) apically,[516,518,521] throughout the lung, or subpleurally.[513,518] In one study a striking subpleural peel of paraseptal emphysema was seen.[517]

There is a single case report of MRI findings in alveolar microlithiasis.[518] This surprisingly shows the calcific regions as

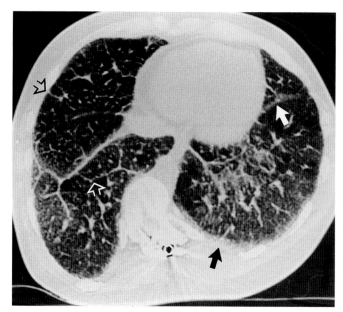

Fig. 11.67 Pulmonary alveolar microlithiasis. A basal HRCT shows predominantly posterior micronodular opacity. Nodules are apparently of calcific density because of the wide window setting. Selective accumulation of calcific deposits accentuates various structures, including superficial and deep interlobular septa (open arrows), some of which are nodular and irregular; major fissures (white arrow); and subpleural parenchyma peripherally (black arrow). A Harrington rod is present.

Box 11.17 Differential diagnosis of diffuse pulmonary calcification

Metastatic pulmonary calcification
Renal failure
Previous infection
- Varicella
- Histoplasmosis
Pulmonary ossification in lung fibrosis
Amyloidosis
Sarcoidosis
Pneumoconiosis

chest radiograph has been documented.[525,526] The micronodular opacities in microlithiasis usually appear to be of calcific density from the beginning. A few patients, however, have been described with nodulation that was initially of soft tissue density and that later became definitely calcific.[525] Bone-seeking agents, such as ^{99m}Tc-diphosphonate, are taken up by microliths, and this may be shown scintigraphically.[527]

The prognosis is variable. Many patients remain asymptomatic with stable chest radiographs for many years.[527] Others, sometimes after many years of stability, go on to experience pulmonary fibrosis or cor pulmonale and ultimately die of the disease.[499,502,528]

The radiologic differential diagnosis of PAM includes several other conditions which cause diffuse pulmonary calcification (Box 11.17).[511] Metastatic pulmonary calcification, due to elevated blood calcium and phosphate levels, is usually upper lung predominant, in contrast to the lower lung predominance of PAM, and is commonly associated with widespread vascular calcification (Fig. 11.68).[529] On CT,[530–532] the calcification may be too fine to cause calcific attenuation values, and may appear as centrilobular ground-glass abnormality, quite similar to that

high signal on T1-weighted images (and low on T2-weighted images) – an appearance also described in metastatic pulmonary calcification[524] and ascribed to a surface effect of diamagnetic calcific particles in shortening T1 relaxation. Very few patients with microlithiasis are recorded in whom a preceding normal

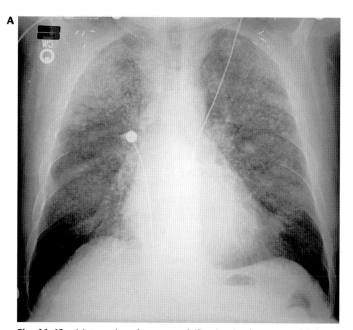

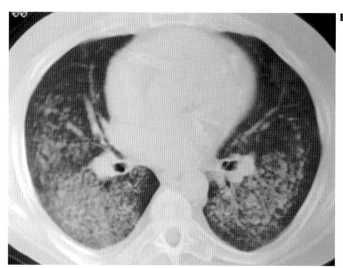

Fig. 11.68 Metastatic pulmonary calcification in chronic renal failure. **A**, Chest radiograph shows upper lung predominant confluent dense nodules. **B**, CT shows poorly defined, confluent centrilobular nodules, some of which are calcified. Marked coronary artery calcification is visible.

seen in hypersensitivity pneumonitis. Other CT findings may include diffuse ground-glass attenuation, and patchy consolidation. The nodules may show ring calcification.[530] The presence of vascular calcifications in the soft tissues and mediastinum may provide an important clue to this diagnosis. Calcifications due to previous infection are usually less profuse and more punctate than in PAM. Dystrophic pulmonary ossification in patients with lung fibrosis[533] is usually quite localized, and associated with typical features of pulmonary fibrosis. Calcification in lesions of sarcoidosis,[534] pneumoconiosis, or amyloidosis are usually associated with other typical features of these disorders.

NEUROCUTANEOUS SYNDROMES

Five conditions are included in the neurocutaneous syndromes: neurofibromatosis, tuberous sclerosis, ataxia telangiectasia, Sturge–Weber syndrome, and von Hippel–Lindau syndrome. In these conditions aberrant development of neuroectodermal tissue causes neurologic abnormalities associated with skin and eye lesions. In some cases there are additional mesodermal and endodermal abnormalities.[535]

Neurofibromatosis and tuberous sclerosis are considered in this section. Pulmonary lymphangioleiomyomatosis (LAM) is also discussed below because, though it is not a neurocutaneous disorder, it has many features in common with pulmonary tuberous sclerosis.

Neurofibromatosis type I

Neurofibromatosis type I (von Recklinghausen disease) is an autosomal dominant neurocutaneous syndrome with a prevalence rate of about 1 per 3000 births,[536] one-half being mutations. The abnormal gene (nf 1) has been identified on chromosome 17.[537] No sex or racial predominance has been found. The principal features are café au lait spots, peripheral nerve tumors (neurofibromas and schwannomas) that particularly affect the skin (fibroma molluscum), and Lisch nodules (pigmented hamartomas of the iris). However, there are a multitude of other possible findings and virtually any organ can be affected.[538] There is marked phenotypic variability of neurofibromatosis I. A set of diagnostic criteria has been proposed (Box 11.18).[537]

Neurofibromatosis has a variety of manifestations in the chest (Table 11.3).

Chest wall involvement

Cutaneous tumors, especially if they are polypoid, appear as nodules on the chest radiograph. If they are peripheral and unequivocally cutaneous in position, they establish the diagnosis of neurofibromatosis. If, however, they project over the lungs, they may resemble intrapulmonary nodules. It should not be assumed that because some nodules are unequivocally cutaneous they all are[540]; to do so runs the risk of missing a primary or secondary pulmonary neoplasm. The latter consideration is particularly important, since in about 5% of patients with generalized neurofibromatosis, neurofibrosarcomas develop,[541] often metastasizing to the lungs.[542]

A neural tumor arising from intercostal nerves away from the spine, if large enough, will give rise to the signs of an extrapleural soft tissue mass,[543] possibly with pressure remodeling (notching) of adjacent upper or lower rib borders (see Figs 15.15 and 15.16). The resulting well-marginated defect is usually relatively wide and shallow compared with the notches seen in coarctation of the aorta. A primary defect in bone formation may also give rise to rib notching,[544] as well as the characteristic "twisted ribbon" deformity.[545,546] Another described pattern of rib abnormality is altered architecture with cyst formation.[547]

Bony thoracic abnormality, particularly kyphoscoliosis, is common and, though a prevalence of about 10% is usually quoted for kyphoscoliosis,[546] some series have recorded it in up to 60% of patients.[545] Kyphosis occurs only in the presence of scoliosis.[548] Although the appearance of the scoliosis may be nonspecific, some patterns are characteristic, in particular low thoracic, short segment, angular scolioses involving five vertebrae or fewer in the primary curve.[546,548,549]

Vertebral lesions include the following modeling and developmental abnormalities: vertebral body scalloping (posterior, lateral, or anterior)[550]; hypoplastic or pressure remodeled pedicles, particularly medial flattening; intervertebral foramen enlargement; and transverse process hypoplasia. The most common and best known of these abnormalities is posterior vertebral scalloping, which is typically sharply marginated and smooth and extends over several segments.[545,549] It is usually associated with, and probably causally related to, dural ectasia,

---

Box 11.18 Diagnostic criteria for neurofibromatosis I (based on the Neurofibromatosis Conference Statement[539])

Positive if two or more of the following are present in an adult:
Café au lait macules: six or more >15 mm in maximum diameter
Neurofibromas: more than two or one plexiform neurofibroma
Freckling in axillary or inguinal regions
Optic glioma
Lisch nodules (iris hamartomas): two or more
Distinctive osseous lesions (e.g. splenoid dysplasia)
First degree relative affected

Table 11.3 Thoracic lesions of neurofibromatosis

Location		Lesion
Chest wall	Skin	Cutaneous tumors (fibroma molluscum)
	Nerves	Intercostal nerve tumors
	Spine	Kyphoscoliosis, vertebral body modeling abnormality
	Ribs	Modeling and architecture abnormality, notching
Mediastinum	Middle	Neural tumor
	Posterior	Lateral meningocele, neural tumor, pheochromcytoma
Lungs		Interstitial fibrosis, cysts, airway tumors

though it will occasionally result from pressure by a tumor or simply be caused by developmental hypoplasia.

Mediastinal masses

Posterior mediastinal masses are usually caused by neural tumor (neurofibroma or neurilemmoma and their malignant counterparts) or a lateral thoracic meningocele. Lateral thoracic meningoceles are produced by protrusion of dura and arachnoid through an exit foramen, and the majority occur at the apex of a scoliosis on its convex aspect, particularly between T3 and T7.[538] Right-sided lesions predominate,[551] and about 10% are multiple.[552] They are often, but not invariably, associated with vertebral scalloping, increased interpedicular distance, pedicle thinning, expansion of intervertebral foramina, and rib erosion.[552] Sometimes, the associated ribs and vertebrae are fused and hypoplastic.[551] Affected patients are commonly middle aged (30–60 years old) and more often than not asymptomatic.[552] Some consider that lateral thoracic meningoceles are the most common posterior mediastinal mass in neurofibromatosis,[538,551] but this is not borne out in all series.[545] The radiologic features of lateral thoracic meningocele are discussed on page 911.

Neural tumors are usually benign and cause well-demarcated, rounded paraspinal masses (discussed in detail in the section Posterior Mediastinal Masses on p. 680). Neural tumors can become malignant with a transformation rate that is probably of the order of 5%.[535]

The third type of associated posterior mediastinal mass is the pheochromocytoma, with a 1% prevalence in neurofibromatosis.[538] It should be considered a possible explanation for hypertension in neurofibromatosis.

Two types of middle mediastinal masses are recognized in neurofibromatosis: one localized and the other diffuse. Discrete masses are the result of solitary neurofibromas, neurilemmomas, or their malignant counterparts affecting the vagus or phrenic nerves. They are more commonly left sided and usually asymptomatic, but they may cause hoarseness if the recurrent laryngeal nerve is affected.[553] In a review of 29 such tumors arising from the vagus, one-third were associated with neurofibromatosis I and only one lesion was sarcomatous.[553] Diffuse masses often involve adjacent mediastinal compartments, extending down from the thoracic inlet to the hilar level, and may be bilateral. They are the result of plexiform neurofibromas, normal nerve elements bizarrely arranged in a network of fusiform swellings that often infiltrate and incorporate adjacent fat and muscle.[535] On CT they appear as low-attenuation masses, often in all compartments of the upper mediastinum, surrounding vessels in an infiltrative fashion.[554] Although usually slow growing and asymptomatic, they can cause tracheal and bronchial compression.[555]

Lung involvement

Parenchymal lung involvement in neurofibromatosis mainly takes the form of an interstitial fibrosis that was first recognized in 1963.[556] Its prevalence increases with age: the youngest patient recorded was 28 years old.[557] The prevalence rate of lung fibrosis in adults with neurofibromatosis was recorded at about 20%,[558,559] but review of the literature for examples of this entity over the past 20 years reveals only scattered case reports,[268,560–565] and two recent reviews[566,567] do not even mention its occurrence, suggesting that neurofibromatosis is in fact a very uncommon

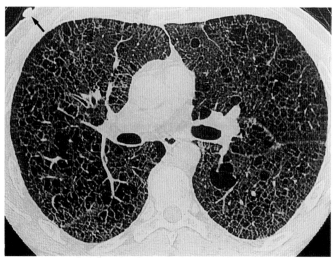

Fig. 11.69 Neurofibromatosis. Mid zone HRCT shows extensive cyst formation from 2 to 25 mm in diameter. Scattered among the cysts are numerous linear opacities indicating inter- and intra-lobular septal thickening. In the right mid zone, airspaces are beginning to coalesce, giving the appearance of panacinar emphysema. Other airspaces appear to contain preserved centrilobular vessels. There is a skin nodule (arrow). (Courtesy of Dr H Massouh, Surrey, UK)

cause of lung disease. Lung involvement in neurofibromatosis is rather benign, in contrast to tuberous sclerosis, and symptoms are often mild, though some patients have progressed to respiratory failure and cor pulmonale.[547] Pulmonary function tests show a mixed obstructive and restrictive pattern with impaired diffusion.[559]

The radiologic findings reflect interstitial and bullous disease.[268] Interstitial abnormality is initially finely linear, with or without a nodular element, and is usually basally predominant.[557,568] Septal (Kerley B) lines are sometimes present.[559] In time the linear element becomes more marked and widespread, and a honeycomb pattern may develop.[559] The other principal findings are thin walled bullae,[268,558,559,568] usually predominantly middle to upper zonal, often asymmetric, and sometimes large (occupying at least one lung zone). Bullae are sometimes an isolated radiologic finding,[558] but lung biopsy in these circumstances always shows an occult interstitial pneumonia.[559] CT data are limited but confirm the findings of bullae, cysts, and reticular abnormality (Fig. 11.69).[268,568]

Rarely, a neurofibroma or neurilemmoma produces a parenchymal mass that appears as a peripheral well-demarcated, lobulated nodule.[569] Just as rarely these lesions may arise endobronchially and cause obstructive bronchiectasis.[559] A patient is also described in whom there were multiple 2 mm intramural schwannomas involving the airways of a single lung subsegment.[570]

Tuberous sclerosis complex

The tuberous sclerosis complex (TSC) is a neurocutaneous syndrome and also one of the most important inherited tumor syndromes. It has a prevalence of 6–10 per 100,000 population[571] (about half that of neurofibromatosis) and is autosomal dominant with an equal sex incidence. The majority of cases are sporadic and arise by mutation.[571] Linkage mapping has identified two separate gene loci on chromosomes 9 (TSC1) and 16 (TSC2), the latter encoding for the protein tuberin which probably acts as a tumor suppressor.[572] Penetrance is high but expression is variable, giving rise to various phenotypes and difficulty in defining the condition for diagnostic purposes.

The classic clinical features make up a triad (Vogt) of mental retardation, epilepsy, and dermal angiofibromas (adenoma sebaceum). However, only about one-third of patients with tuberous sclerosis have all the features of this classic triad.[573] Additional major manifestations include other skin lesions (ungual fibromas, shagreen patches, fibrous forehead plaques, achromic patches), cerebral and paraventricular hamartomas, renal angiomyolipomas, retinal phakomas, bone lesions including calvarial sclerosis, and rhabdomyomas of the heart. Currently the diagnosis is established clinically and considered to be definite, presumptive (probable), or suspect depending on the mix of signs present in an individual.[574,575] According to Gomez[574] the following are definitive features, even when present in isolation: cortical tuber, subependymal nodules, giant cell astrocytoma, retinal hamartomas, facial angiofibromas, ungual fibroma, fibrous forehead plaque, and multiple angiomyolipomas.

In TSC, CT has proved particularly useful in the detection of the highly prevalent intracranial calcifications[576] and renal angiomyolipomas and cysts,[577] whilst MRI has been highly successful in identifying soft tissue central nervous system lesions.[578]

Although previous reports have indicated that clinical pulmonary involvement is unusual in TSC, occurring in 1–2.3% of cases,[579–581] more recent series using CT have indicated that 25–35% of women with TSC have pulmonary cysts.[582,583] As indicated above, considerable clinical, radiologic, and pathologic similarities exist between pulmonary involvement in tuberous sclerosis and that found in LAM (Table 11.4), some of which are touched on here.

On pathologic study the lungs in PTS show perivascular smooth muscle proliferation and small adenomatoid nodules,[584] some of which have been identified as type II pneumocyte hyperplasia.[585–587] Although micronodular type II pneumocyte hyperplasia is characteristic of PTS, it is not specific and is also seen in LAM and occasionally in patients without either condition.[588] The adenomatoid proliferations are a few millimeters in diameter and are scattered throughout the lung.[580] Proliferating smooth muscle spreads into the walls of airspaces, bronchioles, lymphatics, arterioles, and venules and causes obstruction of these structures.

The clinical and imaging manifestations of pulmonary involvement in TSC are produced by obstruction of airways by LAM tissue, producing cysts. Venular obstruction by LAM may cause hemoptysis. Some workers consider that smooth muscle proliferation tends to spare lymphatics,[584,589] but this is not a universal view.[590] The prevalence of chylothorax in PTS is unclear. Some reports have suggested that it is rare,[581,590–593] but tuberous sclerosis accounted for four of eight cases with chylothorax related to LAM in a report by Ryu et al.[594]

The clinical features of patients with PTS[579] differ from those of tuberous sclerosis in general. Almost all patients with TSC who develop LAM are women, with rare case reports of this entity developing in males.[595] Other manifestations of TSC, such as pneumocyte hyperplasia[588] or intrapleural cysts,[596] may develop in males. Patients with PTS are older than the general population with tuberous sclerosis (the mean age of presentation with respiratory symptoms is about 34 years), and with a lower

Table 11.4 Comparison of pulmonary lymphangioleiomyomatosis (PLAM) and tuberous sclerosis (PTS)

Factor	PLAM	PTS
Familial	No	Some
Female sex	All	Almost all
Age	Reproductive	Reproductive
Adenoma sebaceum	No	85%
Epilepsy	No	20%
Intelligence (IQ)	Normal	Low (46%)
Dyspnea	Yes	Yes
Pneumothorax	Yes	Yes
Lymph node involvement	Common	Unusual
Chylous pleural effusions, ascites	Yes	Uncommon
Hemoptysis	Yes	Yes
Chest radiograph	Interstitial opacities, cysts Pleural effusion	Interstitial opacities, cysts
HRCT	Cysts	Cysts, nodules
Renal angiomyolipoma	Common	Very common

prevalence of mental retardation (46%) and epilepsy (20%). However, most patients have adenoma sebaceum,[597] and 60% have renal angiomyolipomas. Once respiratory symptoms develop, they tend to dominate the clinical picture, with progressive dyspnea, recurrent pneumothoraces (in 50%) and, less seriously, cough and hemoptysis.

The radiologic findings in the chest consist of an interstitial process with symmetric nodular, reticular, or reticulonodular opacities. The nodules are small, about 1–2 mm,[580,598] and are often overshadowed by a more dominant, linear element.[580] The changes may be diffuse or basally predominant.[598] With progression of the disease the linear and reticular element becomes more marked, and honeycomb and cystic changes develop.[580,598,599] The cysts tend to be <1 cm in diameter. Large cysts are uncommon.[599] Unlike most other interstitial processes the lung volume tends to be increased because of small airway obstruction, focal emphysema, air-trapping,[600] and cyst formation. Pulmonary function tests support this observation and show airflow obstruction, increased static compliance, and increased total lung volume, together with impaired carbon monoxide diffusion.[580,581]

HRCT findings are essentially the same as those in LAM (see below) (Figs 11.70 and 11.71).[581,601,602] However, a number of case reports have described small (several millimeter) nodular opacities in addition to cysts[587,603] on HRCT. In a study by Moss et al,[583] nodules were found in 25 of 59 females and two of 10 males with TSC. Nodules were seen with or without the presence of LAM cysts. These nodules probably represent areas of adenomatoid pneumocyte hyperplasia, as described by pathologists[588] (see above). On dynamic expiratory HRCT, the cysts of PTS demonstrate air-trapping.[600] Pneumothorax is common,[597] frequently recurrent, and sometimes bilateral.[598] Late in the disease, pulmonary arterial hypertension and cor pulmonale may develop. Chylothorax may be seen.[594] Bone changes are described and may be visible on the chest radiograph, notably an expanded dense rib resembling fibrous

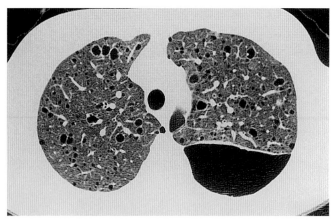

Fig. 11.70 Tuberous sclerosis. HRCT of the upper zones in a 29-year-old woman with tuberous sclerosis. There are numerous well-defined 2–12 mm cysts scattered evenly throughout the lung. The intervening parenchyma is normal. Posteriorly on the left there is a large bulla.

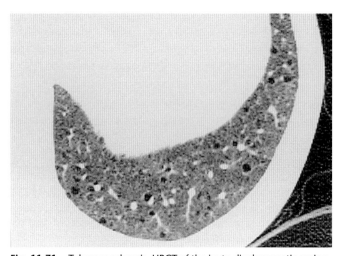

Fig. 11.71 Tuberous sclerosis. HRCT of the juxta-diaphragmatic region in the same patient as in Fig. 11.69. As in lymphangioleiomyomatosis and unlike Langerhans cell histiocytosis, the cysts extend into the costophrenic angles.

dysplasia or Paget disease.[535] Sclerotic lesions within the spine are also described.[604]

Treatment is symptomatic with or without hormonal manipulations as used in pulmonary LAM (PLAM, see below). Part of the rationale for the latter is the finding of estrogen and progesterone receptors on the proliferating muscle in PTS, as in PLAM.[592] In one series, 85% of patients with PTS died within 5 years from either cor pulmonale (59%) or pneumothorax (41%).[579] The prognosis was better in the Mayo Clinic series followed for an average of 17 years – a 78% survival.[581] There was no difference in prognosis between TSC patients with and without pulmonary involvement.

LYMPHANGIOLEIOMYOMATOSIS

LAM (sometimes called lymphangiomyomatosis) is a rare disorder seen in females of childbearing age, characterized by smooth muscle proliferation occurring both in the lungs (related to lymphatics, airways, vessels, and alveolar septa), and also in the mediastinum and retroperitoneum (related to lymphatics). It causes recurrent pneumothoraces, chylous effusions, hemoptysis, and cystic lung disease with eventual respiratory failure.

Although not a neurocutaneous disorder, LAM shares many pulmonary features with PTS. It differs from PTS in that it is not heredofamilial and lacks the neuroectodermal features of TSC, such as adenoma sebaceum, epilepsy, and mental retardation. Furthermore, some findings, such as lymph node enlargement and chylothorax, that are unusual in PTS, are common in LAM. The features of LAM and PTS are compared in Table 11.4. When the lungs are involved in TSC the pathology is that of PLAM.

LAM is commonly associated with mutations in the TSC1 gene, but not in the TSC2 gene.[605] Genetic and protein alterations characteristic of TSC are commonly found in the lung tissue of patients with LAM, and also in angiomyolipomas.[605,606] Although some writers have suggested that LAM should be considered a presumptive feature of TSC,[574,575] the vast majority of women with LAM do not have any manifestations of intracranial TSC, even in the 50% of patients who have associated renal angiomyolipomas.[607–609] Also, there is no recorded case of a woman with PLAM and renal angiomyolipomas having had a child with TSC. Pacheco-Rodriguez et al[605] provides an up-to-date review of the genetic relationship between TSC and LAM.

There have been several major reviews of LAM.[584,610–619]

In the lungs LAM is characterized pathologically by a benign, disorderly proliferation of smooth muscle in the interstitium in relation to vessels, airways, lymphatics, alveolar septa, and pleura.[432,620] Scattered air-filled cysts lined by flattened epithelial and ciliated bronchiolar elements[617] are distributed throughout the lungs and have smooth muscle bundles which may form nodules (myoblastic foci) in their walls.[584] Other small nodules are produced by microcronodular type II pneumocyte hyperplasia.[588] Cysts are thought to arise from air-trapping produced by muscle proliferation in small airways.[432] Some workers, however, consider there is an element of collagen/elastin destruction as well,[621] possibly metalloproteinase induced.[622] Scattered hemosiderin deposits with or without an associated foreign body granulomatous reaction may also be seen,[584] the hemosiderin being derived from small hemorrhages secondary to muscular obstruction of venules. The muscle cells in LAM stain with HMB-45 (a monoclonal antibody derived from melanoma hybridomas) and, in the context of examining lung smooth muscle, this finding is highly sensitive and specific for LAM.[623]

The pathologic changes in the lung described above are similar to those in pulmonary tuberous sclerosis (PTS), but in LAM muscle proliferation is also found in relation to the lymphatic ducts and nodes in the mediastinum and retroperitoneum,[589,611,624–626] findings that are very unusual in PTS. Chylothorax and chyloperitoneum produced by such lymphangiomyomas is thus a common feature of LAM,[627] but unusual in PTS. In one series of patients with LAM, 69% had mediastinal and 53% retroperitoneal node involvement pathologically.[611] Lymphangiomyomas of the mediastinum and retroperitoneum, associated with chylothorax and chylous ascites, may occur in the absence of lung involvement by LAM.[611] Some of these latter patients have been reported to develop lung disease many years later.[611]

Renal angiomyolipomas, which are a characteristic finding in TSC, are also found in LAM, with a recorded prevalence of about 50% when screening abdominal CT is performed.[607,608]

The prevalence of angiomyolipoma in TSC may be up to 80%.[628] The abnormal smooth muscle in angiomyolipomas stains with the HMB-45 antibody, as does the smooth muscle in lung lesions.[629]

The etiology of LAM is unclear. A number of observations suggest that it may be related to female hormone secretion: (1) LAM only occurs in females, usually those of childbearing age; (2) its onset and exacerbations sometimes coincide with pregnancy and parturition; (3) the abnormal smooth muscle commonly has estrogen/progesterone receptors; and (4) LAM may be exacerbated by exogenous estrogens.[630,631] Despite this evidence of the importance of hormones in LAM, hormone manipulations of various sorts have proved at best to be only of modest benefit.

All patients with LAM are female and most are of child-bearing age with a mean age at presentation of 30–35 years.[612] However, at least 14 cases have presented after the menopause,[613,631,632] only some of whom had been taking hormone replacement therapy. The oldest recorded patient at presentation was 72 years of age.[631] The most common initial manifestations are dyspnea, cough, pneumothorax, chest pain, hemoptysis, and chylothorax. Pulmonary function tests, in those who are symptomatic, usually show airflow obstruction, increased total lung capacity, increased compliance, and impaired diffusion.[610]

Pneumothorax occurs as a presenting manifestation of LAM in up to 40–50% of patients (see Fig. 11.72),[613,615,633] while 60–80% develop pneumothorax at some time during the course of their disease.[615,634,635] In patients presenting with pneumothorax, the chest radiograph often shows no other evidence to suggest LAM as the underlying cause,[636] though CT will almost invariably show cysts. Pneumothoraces are commonly recurrent.[634] LAM is a recognized cause of a bilateral pneumothorax[634,635] and should be a primary consideration in a female of reproductive age presenting with bilateral pneumothorax without other radiographic abnormalities.[636]

Chylous pleural effusions are another recognized presenting feature of LAM, and were the initial event in 7% of patients in three series.[584,613,634] Chylous effusions occur during the course of the disease in 10–23% of cases.[594,634,635] Effusions may be unilateral or bilateral and are typically large and often recurrent.[611,624] Hemoptysis occurs in 20% of cases[635] and is occasionally the initial feature.[584,615] Chylous ascites may occur at some stage in the illness but is uncommon (7% of one series)[584] and is usually accompanied by a pleural effusion.[611] Unusual manifestations include chylopericardium, chyluria, and chyloptysis.[611,635] In a group of seven patients, delayed pulmonary parenchymal changes developed up to 5 years after the recognition of lymph node involvement or chylous effusion.[611]

The earliest radiographic signs of LAM consist of fine nodular, reticular, or reticulonodular opacities.[584] These changes are symmetric; they may be generalized[627] or sometimes basally predominant, at least initially.[611] With time the reticular pattern, which may be very delicate and sharp,[584] predominates and tends to become coarser and more irregular (Fig. 11.72). Some of

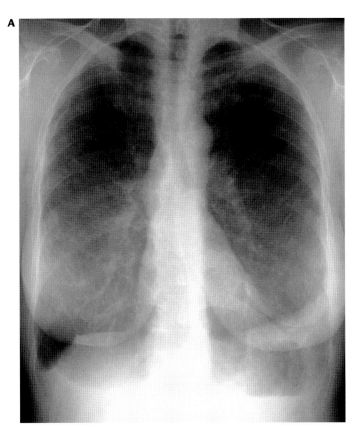

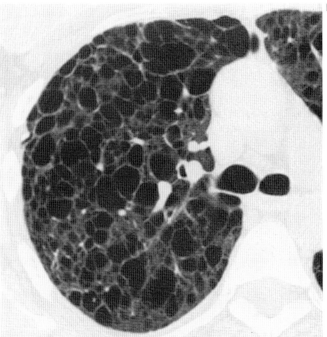

Fig. 11.72 A 54-year-old woman with lymphangioleiomyomatosis. **A**, Chest radiograph shows marked hyperinflation with a diffuse coarse reticular pattern. There is a small left effusion. **B**, HRCT shows profuse round cysts, each with a well-defined thin wall. The cysts are so numerous that they appear to be clustered.

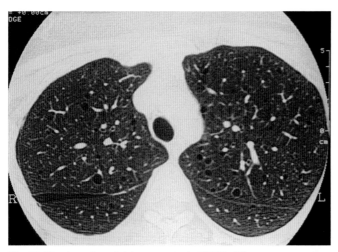

Fig. 11.73 Lymphangioleiomyomatosis. HRCT of the upper zones in a 25-year-old female non-smoker who presented with a pneumothorax. A small pneumothorax is still present in the right oblique fissure. The lung parenchyma is normal apart from a moderate number of well-defined cysts ranging in size from 2 to 8 mm.

the linear elements have features of Kerley B lines and may be transient.[610,627] Cysts, bullae,[627] and thin walled honeycombing eventually develop.[610] During this stage, lung volumes commonly increase.[601,613,615] The combination of a reticular interstitial pattern and increasing lung volume is characteristic of LAM, unlike the progressive loss in volume that accompanies most other interstitial lung disorders (Fig. 11.72).[610] In advanced disease the proximal pulmonary arteries enlarge, with the development of cor pulmonale.[584]

The HRCT features of LAM may be diagnostic in the correct clinical context. Cysts are the pathognomonic feature (Figs 11.72 and 11.73).[267,601,637–641] The cysts are usually multiple, thin walled, and distributed in a uniform fashion in lung that is otherwise essentially normal (Fig. 11.73). Cysts are clearly demarcated by a thin, even wall (1–2 mm thick, Fig. 11.73) and are usually rounded, though larger ones are occasionally polygonal or bizarrely shaped, possibly as a result of cyst coalescence.[601] Vessels are typically seen at the margins of the cysts, rather than at their centers, as is characteristically seen with centrilobular emphysema. The cysts range in size from 2 to 50 mm, with most in the 5–15 mm range. Cyst size increases as the disease becomes more widespread.[638] In general, cysts show no preferential distribution of any type, though two studies record relative apical sparing.[637,639] Cystic involvement of the juxtaphrenic lung and costophrenic sulci (Fig. 11.71) can be helpful in distinguishing LAM from pulmonary Langerhans cell histiocytosis, as this area is usually relatively spared in Langerhans cell histiocytosis (see p. 161 and 432).

The number of cysts varies widely, depending on the clinical presentation; cysts are usually extensive in those who present with symptoms of pulmonary impairment (Fig. 11.72), but often quite sparse in those who present with complications such as pneumothorax and pleural effusion (Fig. 11.73). Cyst size usually decreases on expiration.[642,643] Crausman et al[644] have described a "density mask" HRCT technique to identify and quantitate the

cysts. Values obtained correlated closely with respiratory function tests. Using a similar technique, Avila et al[645] showed that the correlation between quantitative CT measures of disease extent and pulmonary physiology was stronger than that found with qualitative measures. Patients with a history of pleurodesis had greater impairment of physiology (forced expiratory volume in 1 s [FEV_1], diffusing capacity for carbon monoxide [DLco], and total lung capacity) than those without.

HRCT is more sensitive at detecting cysts than standard CT or chest radiographs, and HRCT commonly shows abnormalities in patients with normal radiographs.[601,625,638,640] There has been one report of LAM occurring with a normal HRCT but a positive biopsy.[638]

In addition to cysts, other HRCT abnormalities are occasionally seen in LAM. Small centrilobular nodules have (exceptionally) been described,[646] perhaps representing nodules of hyperplastic muscle or pneumocyte hyperplasia. Occasionally septal thickening may be seen, presumed to be due to lymphatic obstruction.[639,641] Small focal areas of ground-glass opacity were found in 59% of patients in one series, and ascribed to hemosiderosis or muscle cell proliferation.[613,646] In the absence of pathologic correlation the significance of this must be open to question. Localized consolidation may occur,[638] presumed to be due to pulmonary hemorrhage.

Chylous pleural effusions (see p. 1055) were recorded in 75% of cases in an early series,[610] but more recently have been documented in only about 10–20% of cases.[594,634,635] They may be unilateral or bilateral[627] and are typically large and recurrent.[611] Pleural effusion and pneumothorax may coexist.[627] On pathologic grounds[611,647] lymphadenopathy might be expected as a radiologic finding, but it is not usually visible on the chest radiograph.[627,640] On CT, lymphadenopathy is seen in 13–50% of cases.[640,648]

CT has enhanced awareness of the intraabdominal manifestations of LAM. In addition to renal angiomyolipomas (found in about 50% of patients) (Fig. 11.74), other manifestations include hepatic angiomyolipomas, lymphangiomyomas, enlarged retroperitoneal lymph nodes, chylous ascites, and dilation of the thoracic duct or cisterna chyli.[607] Lymphangiomyomas in the pelvis or elsewhere may present with painful swelling as the first manifestation of LAM.[635,649] On CT, they usually are shown to contain material of water density, and they may exhibit diurnal variation in size.[650] Other features may include retroperitoneal hemorrhage[630] and lymphedema of the legs.[630]

Early reports suggested a poor prognosis.[584,611] The prognosis has, however, improved following the introduction of antiestrogen therapy (progesterone administration or oophorectomy),[651] and in a recent series 78% of patients were still alive 8.5 years after the onset of disease.[615] Early diagnosis is important. Lung transplantation is a therapeutic option and, up to 1996, 34 patients had been treated with a 58% 2 year survival.[648] Several cases of recurrence of LAM in the transplanted lung (Fig. 11.75) are reported,[652–654] but the CT findings in these cases have not been described.

Although LAM is a rarity, it should be considered in women of childbearing age with chylous effusion or repeated pneumothoraces, particularly if there is airflow obstruction, large volume lungs, and/or interstitial opacity on the chest radiograph.[610]

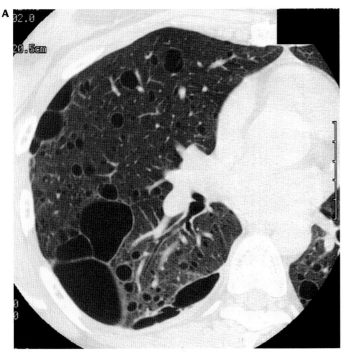

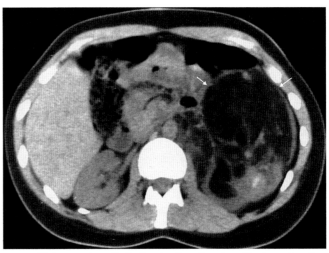

Fig. 11.74 Lymphangioleiomyomatosis with angiomyolipoma. **A,** HRCT shows multiple round or elliptical cysts of varying sizes. The largest cysts are grouped along the major fissure. **B,** Abdominal CT shows a large left renal angiomyolipoma (arrows).

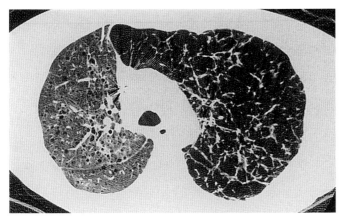

Fig. 11.75 Lymphangioleiomyomatosis (LAM). A 49-year-old woman with LAM who 2 years before had had a right lung transplant. HRCT shows a hyperexpanded, grossly cystic end-stage lung on the left. The transplanted lung on the right shows numerous small (1–5 mm) cysts, proven by biopsy to be caused by LAM.

> **Box 11.19 Respiratory disease associated with inflammatory bowel disease**
>
> Tracheobronchitis[655–657]
> Tracheal or bronchial stenosis[655–658]
> Bronchiectasis[655–657]
> Bronchiolitis
> - Panbronchiolitis pattern[659]
> - Constrictive bronchiolitis pattern[660]
> - Granulomatous bronchiolitis[661]
> Organizing pneumonia[662–664]
> Lung fibrosis[665,666]
> Pulmonary hemorrhage[667]
> Granulomatous lung disease (Crohn disease only)[661,668–670]
> Amyloidosis[671]
> Drug induced disease
> - Sulfasalazine[672–674]

LUNG DISEASE ASSOCIATED WITH INFLAMMATORY BOWEL DISEASE

Ulcerative colitis and Crohn disease are associated with a wide variety of uncommon pulmonary complications (Box 11.19). These complications may precede the diagnosis of inflam-matory bowel disease, or may occur years after the initial diagnosis, and even after complete colectomy for ulcerative colitis. Both conditions can be associated with an intense tracheobronchitis, sometimes associated with subglottic, tracheal, or bronchial stenosis.[655,656] Bronchiectasis may also occur (Fig. 11.76). Small airway involvement can have a pattern of panbronchiolitis,[659] or in Crohn disease, of granulomatous bronchiolitis.[661] In a series of seven patients with inflammatory

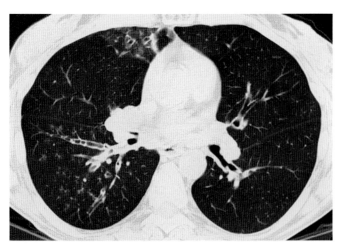

Fig. 11.76 Large and small airways disease in ulcerative colitis. HRCT in a patient with long-standing ulcerative colitis shows marked bronchial wall thickening, right middle and lower lobe bronchiectasis, and a focal tree-in-bud pattern in the right lower lobe.

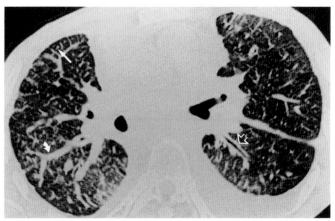

Fig. 11.77 Erdheim–Chester disease. Pathologically this histiocytic disorder has interstitial infiltration that is distributed particularly along the lymphatics. This pattern is reflected in the HRCT which shows: (1) septal lines, some of which are quite thick; (2) subpleural thickening seen as a rind on the right and as fissural thickening on the left (where there is also a pleural effusion); (3) bronchial wall (open arrow) and vascular (curved arrow) thickening; and (4) prominence of centrilobular structures (straight arrow). In this patient the mediastinum is widened and the mediastinal fat was increased in density, indicating infiltration by soft tissue.

airway disease related to ulcerative colitis,[655] all had bronchial wall thickening, six had bronchiectasis, and three had airway stenosis. Four patients had evidence of small airways disease with a pattern similar to that of panbronchiolitis.

Parenchymal abnormalities associated with inflammatory bowel disease include organizing pneumonia,[661–664] pulmonary hemorrhage,[667] and granulomatous infiltration in Crohn disease.[661] In patients presenting with an organizing pneumonia pattern, and in those with eosinophilic pneumonia, it is important to be aware of the treatment history, as sulfasalazine is a common cause of these abnormalities.[672–674]

ERDHEIM–CHESTER DISEASE

Erdheim–Chester disease is a very rare non-Langerhans cell histiocytosis characterized by symmetric lower limb osteosclerosis caused by histiocytic infiltration. At the time of diagnosis about 50% of patients have extraskeletal involvement that mainly affects the skin, retroperitoneum, retroorbital region, heart, hypothalmus/posterior pituitary, and lungs. Age at presentation is about 50 years with a wide range (7–84 years) and no sex predilection.[675] The most common presenting symptom is bone pain and skeletal radiology shows a characteristic symmetric long bone (particular leg) metaphyseal/diaphyseal sclerosis which is very active on radionuclide bone scan.[676] Osteolytic lesions in flat bones are described.

Lungs are involved in about 20–30% of patients[675,677] with about 30 cases in the world literature up to 2003.[678–680] Pulmonary involvement causes progressive shortness of breath and some patients develop end-stage lung and die of respiratory involvement. Histologically there is an interstitial lung infiltrate of foamy histiocytes with additional lymphocytes, giant cells, and fibrosis. These changes are distributed along the lymphatics and affect the visceral pleura, interlobular septa, and bronchovascular bundles.[678] The histiocytes are distinguished from Langerhans cells by the absence of CD1a staining, and by the absence of

Birbeck granules on electron microscopy.[681] Also, the CT features of this condition are quite distinct from those of Langerhans cell histiocytosis.

Chest radiographic appearances are conveniently summarized by Egan et al[678] and consist of diffuse interstitial opacities, usually described as reticular. These changes commonly show a mid to upper zone predominance and may be accompanied by cysts or honeycomb opacity. Septal lines, and thickened fissures and pleura are also described. On HRCT the major finding is widespread smooth thickening of interlobar fissures and interlobular septa (Fig. 11.77).[680] This is usually associated with multifocal ground-glass attenuation, and centrilobular nodules.[680] Intervening lung may be normal[682] or replaced by cystic/emphysematous areas.[677,683] Pleural effusions are seen in about half the patients.[680] Review of the soft tissues showed pericardial thickening or areas of soft tissue infiltration in six of nine patients in the series by Wittenberg et al.[680] Rarely, Erdheim–Chester disease may involve the lung without any evidence of skeletal involvement.[680]

STORAGE DISEASES

Pulmonary involvement may occur in several storage diseases, including Gaucher disease, Niemann–Pick disease, Fabry disease, and Hermansky–Pudlak syndrome (Table 11.5).[681]

Gaucher disease is characterized by hepatosplenomegaly and bone marrow infiltration. Although physiologic abnormalities are quite common in this condition, symptomatic pulmonary involvement is rare. It usually becomes manifest in childhood, but occasionally presents for the first time in adults. It is characterized pathologically by masses of Gaucher cells (alveolar macrophages stuffed with glucocerebroside) in the

Table 11.5 Pulmonary involvement in storage diseases

Disease	Storage metabolite	Site of storage in lungs	Other sites of involvement	Imaging findings
Gaucher disease	Glucocerebroside	Alveolar walls and alveolar interstitium	Liver, spleen, bone marrow	Reticular abnormality, ground-glass abnormality, pulmonary hypertension
Fabry disease	Glycosphingolipid	Not defined	Kidney, heart, skin, brain	Pulmonary hemorrhage
Niemann–Pick disease	Sphingomyelin	Interstitium	Liver, spleen, nodes, brain	Miliary or reticulonodular pattern
Hermansky–Pudlak syndrome	Ceroid	Alveolar macrophages	Albinism, platelet dysfunction	Lung fibrosis

alveoli and interstitium, producing an appearance reminiscent of desquamative interstitial pneumonia.[681] On the chest radiograph, it is characterized by reticular abnormality, or less commonly a miliary pattern. Reported abnormalities on CT have included a reticular pattern, mosaic pattern, ground-glass abnormality, and septal thickening.[684–686] Other intrathoracic manifestations include pulmonary hypertension[681] and extramedullary hematopoiesis.[687]

Niemann–Pick disease is associated with accumulation of sphingomyelin in the reticuloendothelial system and central nervous system.[681] Foamy "sea blue" macrophages may be seen in the lung parenchyma, resulting in a miliary or reticulonodular pattern on chest radiograph or chest CT. CT findings include ground-glass abnormality and septal thickening.[688] A recently reported adult case was characterized by ground-glass and reticular abnormality on chest radiograph.[689] On CT, ground-glass abnormality and consolidation were the predominant findings (Fig. 11.78), reflecting extensive intraalveolar macrophage accumulation, producing an endogenous lipoid pneumonia. Mild reticular abnormality was also present. The extent of abnormality decreased significantly following whole lung lavage.

In *Fabry disease*, glycosphingolipids accumulate in the heart, kidney, skin, and brain.[681] Pulmonary involvement appears to be rare,[690,691] though pulmonary hemorrhage may occur, related to endothelial dysfunction.[681]

Hermansky–Pudlak syndrome is an autosomal recessive syndrome characterized by partial oculocutaneous albinism, platelet dysfunction, and accumulation of ceroid in various tissues including the lung.[681] The syndrome is associated with slowly progressive lung fibrosis occurring in individuals aged between 20 and 40 years. A syndrome of inflammatory bowel disease may also be present.[692] Pulmonary involvement in this syndrome appears to be associated with a mutation on the HPS1 gene.[693] On the chest radiograph, a reticular abnormality is usually seen (Fig. 11.70).[693] In a study of 67 patients with this condition,[693] 31 had normal high-resolution CT, 22 had minimal abnormalities, seven had moderately extensive abnormality, and seven had extensive abnormality on CT. The CT findings varied with the severity of the abnormality. In patients with minimal disease, septal thickening was the most common finding, followed by ground-glass abnormality, and reticular abnormality was the most prominent finding, and subpleural honeycombing was seen in about half the patients (Fig. 11.79).

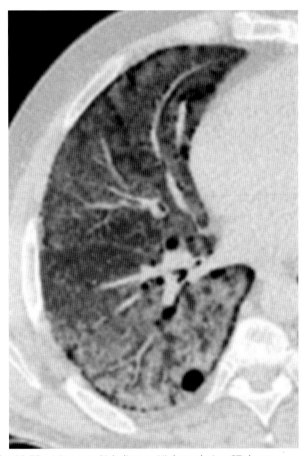

Fig. 11.78 Niemann–Pick disease. High resolution CT shows widespread ground glass opacity and reticular pattern, with posterior consolidation and subpleural cysts.

The abnormality showed subpleural predominance, but was generally diffusely distributed in the craniocaudal plane, with some cases showing predominance in mid or lower lung zones. Five cases showed peribronchovascular thickening. This condition should be considered in the imaging differential diagnosis of nonspecific interstitial pneumonia and usual interstitial pneumonia.

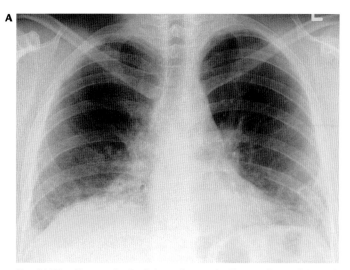

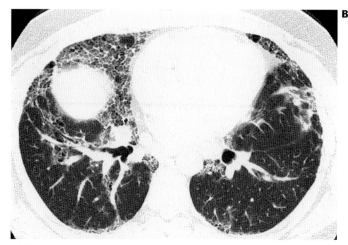

Fig. 11.79 Hermansky–Pudlak syndrome. **A**, Chest radiograph in a 29-year-old man with partial albinism shows basal predominant parenchymal opacity. **B**, HRCT shows basal reticular abnormality compatible with lung fibrosis.

AMYLOIDOSIS

Amyloidosis is a disorder in which amyloid, a substance consisting largely of autologous protein fibrils, is deposited extracellularly in a variety of organs and tissues. Amyloid has a pathognomonic staining reaction because of its unique structure, binding with Congo red and giving a green birefringence in polarized light. In the past the classification of amyloidosis has depended on the identification of various clinicopathologic entities with major subdivisions into primary/secondary amyloidosis and local/systemic disease. However, categorization is usually based on the type of fibrillar protein in the amyloid deposit.[694–696] Important proteins are identified in the following list, with the suffix 'A' being used to indicate amyloid followed by an abbreviation for the protein itself.

- *AL (amyloid light chain)*. AL is made up from the variable fragment of immunoglobulin light chains, γ chains more commonly than *k*. The light chains are manufactured by plasma cells and AL amyloidosis is now considered to be a plasma cell dyscrasia with a monoclonal gammopathy. AL amyloidosis is also seen in association with multiple myeloma and macroglobulinemia. This condition was formerly called primary amyloidosis.
- *AA (amyloid A)*. This is an α globulin derived from serum amyloid A (SAA), which is an acute phase reactant produced particularly in infectious and inflammatory conditions.[697] AA amyloidosis used to be called reactive systemic amyloidosis or secondary amyloidosis. AA amyloidosis is also seen in familial Mediterranean fever.
- *ATTR (amyloid transthyretin)*. Transthyretin is the same as prealbumin, a normal plasma protein that can act as a carrier for thyroxine. Genetically determined mutations substitute amino acids and alter its structure, giving rise to >20 heredofamilial forms of amyloidosis. Rarely, other proteins may be involved in other familial forms of amyloidosis.
- *Aβ₂M (amyloid β-2-microglobulin)*. This normal component of plasma is not cleared and metabolized in patients on chronic

hemodialysis, leading to a form of amyloidosis unique to this clinical situation.
- *Polypeptide hormones*. A number of these can generate amyloid, including atrial naturetic factor (isolated atrial amyloid) and procalcitonin (medullary carcinoma of the thyroid).

At least 25 types of amyloid protein have been described.[698] Some of these predispose to hereditary amyloidosis, which does not usually involve the chest. A classification of the major clinical forms of amyloidosis and amyloid deposition together with the type of chest involvement is given in Table 11.6.

Amyloid is laid down in a number of conditions and as part of the aging process. Organ dysfunction occurs if enough amyloid material accumulates. Broadly speaking the deposition may be generalized (systemic amyloidosis) or localized to a single organ. Local deposition within an organ may itself be diffuse or focal. However, cases with overlap features are not uncommon. Difficulties most commonly occur with so-called localized disease which, although not systemic, is in many instances clearly not limited to a single organ. This occurs, for example, in the chest when lung or airway disease can be accompanied by mediastinal and cervical adenopathy.[700–702]

Systemic amyloidosis

Respiratory involvement is an unimportant part of systemic amyloidosis, and clinical and radiologic findings in the chest are usually incidental or secondary to a complication such as heart failure. Should direct involvement by amyloid deposition occur, it takes the form of interstitial parenchymal disease, lymphadenopathy, or pleural disease.

AL amyloidosis

AL amyloidosis has two main subtypes: one associated with a monoclonal gammopathy (formerly primary amyloidosis), and the other associated with multiple myeloma. They are virtually

Table 11.6 Major clinical forms of amyloidosis and amyloid deposition with type of respiratory involvement. (Pepys M. Amyloidosis: some recent developments. Q J Med 1988; 67(252):283–298 by permission of Association of Physicians of Great Britain.)

Major subdivision	Protein/clinopathogenic entity		Chest involvement
Systemic amyloidosis	AL	AL amyloidosis (immunocyte dyscrasia amyloidosis) Amyloidosis with monoclonal gammography (formerly primary systemic amyloidosis) Multiple myelomatosis Waldenström macroglobulinemia Others	Diffuse parenchymal (usually subclinical) ± Lymph nodes Lymph nodes per se Pleural effusion
	AA	AA amyloidosis (formerly secondary amyloidosis or reactive amyloidosis	Diffuse parenchymal (subclinical)
	ATTR	Heredofamilial amyloidosis (minority not ATTR) Neuropathic Nephropathic Cardiomyopathic	Diffuse parenchymal (rarely)
	ATTR	Senile systemic amyloidosis (formerly senile cardiac amyloidosis)	Diffuse parenchymal
	Aβ$_2$M	Hemodialysis associated	—
Localized amyloidosis	AL	Lung	Tracheobronchial Parenchymal Nodular Diffuse ± Lymph nodes
		Senile (heart, joints) Cerebral amyloid angiopathy Endocrine (thyroid, pancreas, atrium) Skin, bladder, larynx, eye	— — Metastatic medullary carcinoma of thyroid —

identical in their clinical manifestations, save for the fact that the prognosis of amyloidosis associated with myeloma is worse (5 versus 13 month mean survival).[703] In AL amyloidosis, infiltration with amyloid material affects mesenchymal tissues and, to a lesser extent, kidney, liver, and spleen. There is a 2:1 male predominance with a mean age at presentation of about 60 years.[704,705]

The clinical features of AL amyloidosis may be nonspecific, such as weight loss and weakness, or may be part of one or more classic disorders, including nephrotic syndrome, carpal tunnel syndrome, restrictive cardiomyopathy, peripheral neuropathy, orthostatic hypotension, and, occasionally, macroglossia, purpura, papular skin rash, and arthropathy.[703] Some 80% of patients will have proteinuria. Electrophoresis of serum shows a protein spike in 40% and, on immunoelectrophoresis, there is a monoclonal protein in 68%. When urine and blood test results are combined, 89% of patients will have a monoclonal protein.[703] The diagnosis is made by abdominal fat aspiration which is positive in approximately 80% of patients.[706] Bone marrow aspiration is positive in about 50% of patients and allows assessment of plasma cells for the possible presence of myeloma. If both abdominal fat and bone marrow aspiration is negative, rectal biopsy (80% positive) is recommended, followed if necessary by biopsy of a suspect organ.

The median survival in a series of 153 patients with AL amyloidosis was 12 months, with <20% alive at 5 years.[705] Heart failure was associated with a particularly bad prognosis. Patients with cardiac involvement survive 4–6 months, while those without cardiac involvement at the time of diagnosis have a median survival of 30 months.[707]

Involvement of the lungs on pathologic examination is common in AL amyloidosis, with a prevalence ranging between 70 and 92%,[708–712] but it is rarely of clinical importance. For example, in a major clinical review of 229 patients with AL amyloid, there is no mention of the lung being clinically affected,[703] while in a later report of 153 patients with AL amyloidosis just two patients had diffuse interstitial pulmonary involvement.[705] Reports of significant lung involvement occur mostly in individual case reports or in small selected series.[708,713–717] In one such series, five of 12 patients with "primary amyloidosis" developed radiographic and pathologic evidence of diffuse alveolar septal amyloidosis and, in one patient, it contributed to death,[710] as it did in another small series.[717] A further point of importance is that cardiac amyloidosis commonly accompanies lung involvement,[711] and it is well recognized that both the clinical and radiologic signs of pulmonary amyloid infiltration can be obscured by heart failure.[708,711,717,718] In the appropriate context, persistent radiologic changes despite adequate treatment of heart failure should raise the possibility of amyloid infiltration of the lungs.[719] The prevalence of lung involvement in AL amyloidosis is the same in patients with isolated gammopathy or myelomatosis.[711] Isolated massive mediastinal deposition of amyloid, presumably in nodes, has been described in myeloma related AL amyloidosis.[720]

AA amyloidosis

AA amyloidosis (reactive systemic amyloidosis/secondary amyloidosis) is usually secondary to chronic infectious or inflammatory processes (see above).[721,722] Rare cryptogenic cases are described.[722,723] In western societies the most common cause is undoubtedly rheumatoid arthritis[712,722,724] in which the prevalence of amyloidosis is usually quoted as 10%, though this figure seems rather high.[725] In a review of 64 patients with AA amyloidosis from the Mayo Clinic, 48% were secondary to rheumatoid arthritis.[722] Other causes are: (1) chronic rheumatic diseases – ankylosing spondylitis, psoriatic arthritis, juvenile chronic arthritis, Behçet syndrome; (2) chronic infections – tuberculosis, leprosy, osteomyelitis, bronchiectasis, chronically infected decubitus ulcers; (3) chronic inflammations – inflammatory bowel disease, familial Mediterranean fever; and (4) neoplasm – Castleman disease,[726] Hodgkin disease, renal cell carcinoma.[704,721,722] When AA amyloidosis is caused by rheumatic disorders, the underlying disease is usually severe and of long standing with a median duration of 19 years in one series.[724] The organs most commonly affected by amyloid deposition are the kidneys, liver, spleen, and adrenals. AA amyloidosis usually presents with renal disease (proteinuria, nephrotic syndrome, renal insufficiency, hypertension) or hepatosplenomegaly. Gastrointestinal involvement is not uncommon, occurring in about 20% of patients, and is manifest as malabsorption, nausea, and vomiting. A small number of patients (5%) present with goiter.

The prevalence of lung involvement pathologically varies considerably in different series. Two studies give a prevalence rate of 1–5%,[708,711] whereas in others it approaches 100%.[710,727] These discrepancies are probably unimportant as the involvement is usually diffuse within the lung and not severe enough to cause functional or radiologic changes. There have been a few reports of significant clinical lung involvement.[710,723,728] The distribution of amyloid deposition (alveolar septal versus perivascular) differs from patient to patient and affects the type of pathophysiologic disturbance. Predominant perivascular deposits can give pulmonary arterial hypertension.[729]

Treatment in AA amyloidosis is directed at reducing the protein load that provides the amyloid substrate. Prognosis depends on the predisposing condition but is of the order of 50% 2–4 year survival,[730] with renal failure being the most common cause of death.[722]

Radiographic changes

The chest radiograph is normal in the majority of patients with generalized amyloidosis and lung involvement.[731] When abnormalities are seen, the most common finding is that of an interstitial process reflecting the predominantly septal and perivascular nature of amyloid deposition.[711] The radiographic appearances in the AA and AL forms are probably similar, but descriptions in AA amyloidosis are rare.[723] Diffuse parenchymal amyloidosis is also seen in senile systemic and familial amyloidosis, and as a lung limited process (see below). The interstitial infiltration is manifest as a diffuse micronodular, reticulonodular, or linear pattern with accentuation of bronchovascular structures.[708,712,715–717,732,733] Such changes are usually diffuse and symmetric, but they can be segmental.[712] In time the nodules may become conglomerate or calcify.[708] CT descriptions are few.[723,734–736] The main findings are nodules and linear opacities (Fig. 11.80). In general, nodules are in the 2–4 mm range but larger nodules, a centimeter or more in diameter, are described.[736] Nodules range in number from 10 to innumerable with a diffuse or predominantly subpleural distribution. Some nodules are calcified. Linear opacities are mainly basal and peripheral and are produced by thickened interlobular septa or irregular interstitial lines (Fig. 11.80). These linear opacities may also calcify (Fig. 11.80B). Other less common abnormalities include ground-glass opacity, honeycombing, and traction bronchiolectasis.[736] Since septal thickening and ground-glass abnormality can be produced by hydrostatic lung edema,[737] this can be a source of confusion in patients with cardiac amyloidosis.

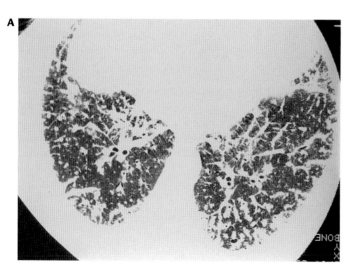
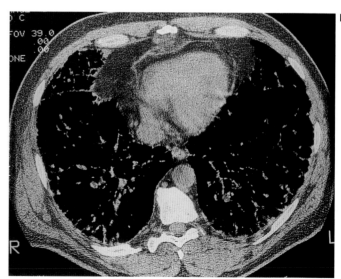

Fig. 11.80 AL alveolar septal amyloidosis in a 53-year-old man. The patient presented with a pneumococcal pneumonia but following successful therapy dyspnea and diffuse interstitial lung opacity persisted in the face of normal cardiac function. Further investigation, including transbronchial lung biopsy, revealed AL amyloidosis secondary to myelomatosis. **A**, Lower zone HRCT shows widespread interstitial opacity consisting of subpleural and parenchymal nodules, enlarged centrilobular structures, irregular thickening of the interlobular septa, and peribronchovascular thickening. **B**, HRCT imaged on mediastinal settings shows calcific densities within the septa. This combination of findings is diagnostic of amyloidosis.

Pleural effusions in amyloidosis are commonly caused by heart failure secondary to myocardial infiltration,[708,710] or by nephrotic syndrome. However, amyloid involvement of the pleura is seen pathologically[738,739] and undoubtedly on occasion causes pleural effusion.[732,736,740–743] In a study of 636 patients with AL amyloidosis, 35 (6%) had persistent effusions requiring three or more thoracenteses[739]; these patients had a very poor prognosis, with median survival of 1.8 months in untreated patients.

Hilar and mediastinal nodal enlargement (Fig. 11.81) is not described in AA amyloidosis, but is seen in proven or presumptive AL amyloidosis, either as the sole radiologic finding in the chest,[712,732,744–746] or with interstitial disease.[708,736,747] In one series of 12 patients with diffuse lung involvement (83% with AL amyloidosis) CT showed that thoracic lymphadenopathy, either alone or with interstitial disease, was the most common finding (in 75% of cases).[736] Both mediastinal and hilar nodes may be involved, often massively, giving a pattern that may resemble sarcoidosis.[732] Nodal calcification is common (Fig. 11.81C).[732,748] The pattern of calcification is usually described as coarse or nonspecific; it may occasionally be of the eggshell type.[744] Nodal enlargement has also been described in AL amyloidosis associated with multiple myeloma[749] and Waldenström macroglobulinemia.[710,744]

When AA amyloidosis is secondary to inflammatory lung disease, the chest radiograph will show major abnormalities, e.g. changes of cystic fibrosis or bronchiectasis.[710,712,744] Heart failure is common in AL amyloidosis and interstitial opacity resulting from raised pulmonary venous pressure may obscure pulmonary lesions of amyloid infiltration.[710,716]

Localized amyloidosis

Localized amyloidosis may affect either the lung parenchyma or the airways (Table 11.7). These structures are usually involved independently,[717] but very occasionally both are affected together.[750] The frequency of airway involvement is about the same as that of parenchymal involvement.[751] A few cases are also recorded in which there is isolated amyloidosis of mediastinal nodes.

Tracheobronchial amyloidosis

Amyloid may occur in the airways as focal or diffuse submucosal deposits of AL amyloid[752]; both are considered together here.[751] The mean age of patients in a large review was 53 years, with a range of 16–76 years.[753] Twice as many men as women experience the disease.[740] Affected patients are often symptomatic[731] for several years before they finally present,[754] an indication that the disease progresses relatively slowly. The major symptoms are cough, dyspnea, hemoptysis, stridor, and

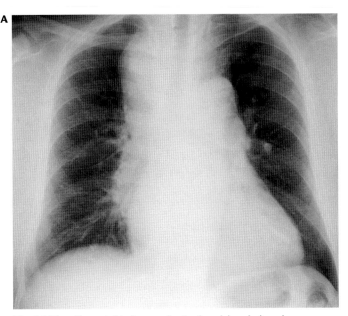

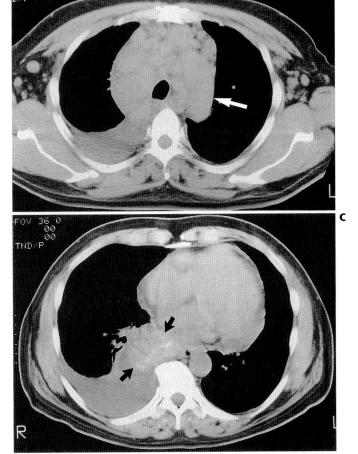

Fig. 11.81 AL amyloidosis – mediastinal nodal and pleural involvement in a 61-year-old man who presented with neck swelling, cough, and weight loss. Initial mediastinal and cervical adenopathy was followed by the development of a large right pleural effusion. There was an IgG gammopathy with biopsy evidence of pleural and nodal amyloidosis but no evidence of disease elsewhere. **A**, Chest radiograph shows massive, mainly right-sided mediastinal adenopoathy. **B**, HRCT at the level of the aortic arch (arrow) demonstrates massive adenopathy and a right pleural effusion. **C**, HRCT at the mid left atrial level shows massive lymphadenopathy in the azygoesophageal recess (arrows) with mild calcification. There is also a right pleural effusion.

Table 11.7 Localized forms of lower respiratory tract amyloidosis with relative percentage prevalence

Classification	Prevalence (%)	Form
Tracheobronchial	45	Multifocal submucosal plaques
	8	Tumorlike masses
Parenchymal	44	Nodular
		Solitary
		Multiple
	4	Diffuse alveolar septal

hoarseness.[740,754] A number of patients are believed initially to have asthma,[755,756] and recurrent pulmonary infections are common.[740]

Airway amyloid is more commonly diffuse than focal.[757,758] When diffuse, it can involve the trachea and main stem, lobar, and proximal segmental bronchi, together or in part. This involvement can be demonstrated by bronchoscopy, spiral CT, preferably with 3D or multiplanar imaging,[759] or MRI.[736] Such examinations show multiple concentric or eccentric strictures and mural nodules (Figs 11.82 and 11.83). Amyloid tissue is commonly partly calcified, and usually spares the posterior membrane[760] (Fig. 11.83). Local as opposed to diffuse lesions give rise to endoluminal masses (amyloidomas) that may be radiologically indistinguishable from neoplasms.[751,761] In the trachea, amyloidomas are usually subglottic and may be calcified or ossified.[762] Localized airway amyloid shows intermediate signal intensity on T1-weighted images and low signal on T2-weighted images.[762] In patients with diffuse or focal airway lesions, the chest radiograph may be normal[755] or may show one of a number of obstructive features, most commonly collapse, which may be seen in >50% of patients.[740] Other manifestations include recurrent infective consolidations, obstructive

hyperinflation, and bronchiectasis (Fig. 11.82).[763] A few patients have had hilar or mediastinal masses on plain chest radiography or CT, usually representing nodal enlargement (Fig. 11.81).[764,765] Such nodes may be calcified (Fig. 11.81).[702]

If treatment is required, the amyloid deposits may be removed by intermittent bronchoscopic resection[766] or laser photoresection.[756] Other treatment options include stenting and radiotherapy.[767,768] Prognosis is not good, and there is a tendency for lesions to recur 6–12 months after treatment.[740] In one review of 39 patients, 21 were well at 4–6 years, but 18 had died, 12 from respiratory causes.[740]

Parenchymal nodular amyloidosis

This form of organ limited amyloidosis produces one or more parenchymal nodules. It is a rare condition, with only 55 reports in a 1983 literature review.[757] Reviews of previous cases have appeared at regular intervals.[738,740,769,770] Pathologically[770] amyloid nodules are discrete and often subpleural, puckering the adjacent pleura to which they may be adherent. They are firm, well demarcated but not encapsulated and, when sectioned, waxy. Microscopically, lung tissue is replaced by eosinophilic amyloid containing nests of plasma cells and lymphocytes surrounded peripherally by a low grade inflammatory infiltrate with giant cells. Calcification, cartilage formation, and ossification within the tumor are common. Bronchioles, alveolar septa, and blood vessels in the region of the tumor often contain amyloid as well. Amyloid is of the AL type[771] and usually polyclonal, though monoclonal cases are reported.[772]

The mean age at presentation in several series was 68 years,[738,769,770] the youngest patient being 38 years old[773]; the sex incidence has been equal. Unless the disease is extensive, the patients are usually asymptomatic, with only occasional reports of cough and hemoptysis.[757] Patients with atelectasis and bronchiectasis secondary to the nodule are described. The nodules may be single or multiple (Fig. 11.84). In some series

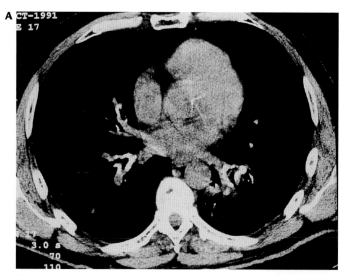
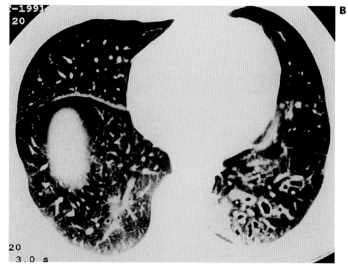

Fig. 11.82 Airway amyloidosis in a 57-year-old man. **A**, HRCT at the level of the inferior pulmonary vein shows mural irregularity and thickening of the segmental bronchi caused by amyloid deposits which are also heavily calcified. **B**, HRCT of the lower zones shows bronchiectasis at the left base secondary to more proximal airway obstruction.

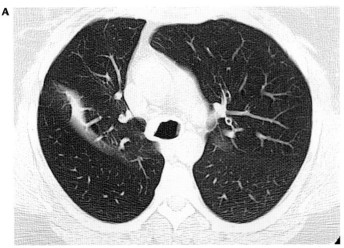

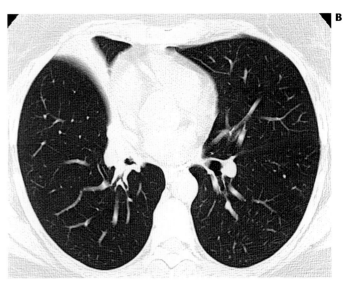

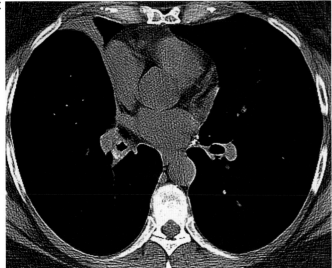

Fig. 11.83 Tracheobronchial stenosis due to amyloid in a 70-year-old woman. **A**, CT through the distal trachea shows irregular narrowing and mural thickening, sparing the posterior tracheal membrane. **B**, CT through the distal bronchus intermedius shows similar findings, with complete obstruction of the right middle lobe bronchus resulting in right middle lobe collapse. **C**, CT with mediastinal window settings shows calcification in the thickened bronchial wall.

both patterns have been equally prevalent,[740] whereas in others multiple nodules have been predominant.[769] When tumors are multiple, the numbers vary from two to innumerable, with two-thirds being bilateral and one-third unilateral.[769] There is no lobar predilection[740,770] but on CT they tend to be peripheral or subpleural.[736] Characteristically, nodules are sharp and round,[731] both radiographically and on CT, but they may also be oval, lobulated,[719,736] irregular,[732,774] or ill defined and speculated, resembling a cancer.[719,736] Marginal irregularity is not a surprising finding given that histologically it is not uncommon to have amyloid infiltration of septa, blood vessels, and airways adjacent to the amyloidoma.[775] Generally, in any one patient, the nodules vary in size and shape. Some authors stress that a radiograph with multiple nodules of different shapes should raise the possibility of amyloidosis.

Nodules are commonly 0.5–5 cm in diameter, but range from micronodular[719,776] to massive – up to 15 cm in diameter. Calcification is quite common in both small[731,770] and large nodules; in the latter it is variously described as irregular, cloudy, flocculant, or stippled. It may occur centrally or throughout the nodule.[719,731,769] Calcification is detected in approximately 30–50% of cases,[740,750] depending on the method of assessment. Although calcification may be seen on the plain radiograph,[731] CT is more sensitive.[777] Calcification is clearly a very helpful finding that may suggest the nature of such lesions.[719] Although cavitation was described in 11% of cases in one review series,[740] this is probably an overestimate.[747] It would seem generally to be a rare complication.[731] An air bronchogram is not a feature, though it has been described in a single case on HRCT.[778] Occasionally, the nodules are locally confluent and mimic consolidation.[779] The nodules tend to behave in a rather indolent fashion, growing slowly and sometimes remaining stable over several years.[750] In rare cases they grow more rapidly, behaving like a neoplasm.[769,774] On MRI, nodules are isointense with muscle on T1-weighted images and hypointense on T2-weighted images.[780] In a few cases, additional mediastinal lymphadenopathy has been described.[712,738,757,781] The unusual association of Sjögren syndrome, multiple amyloid nodules, lung cysts and pulmonary lymphocyte infiltration has been described (Fig. 11.85).[782,783]

The diagnosis is usually established by thoracotomy or percutaneous needle biopsy.[784] In patients with one or a few nodules only, the prognosis is excellent, and recurrence after removal of a nodule, though recorded, is extremely rare.[785] Very occasionally, the disease is so widespread that it contributes to[776] or causes death.[738]

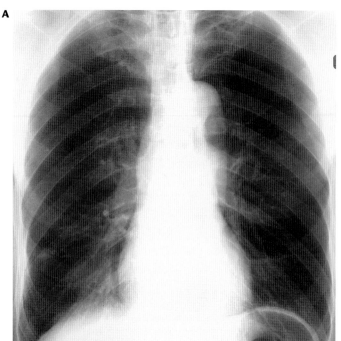

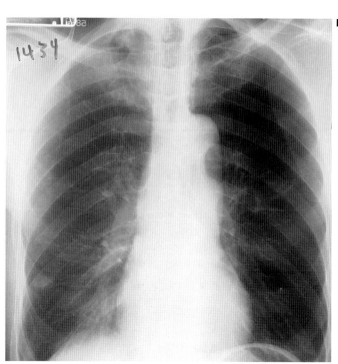

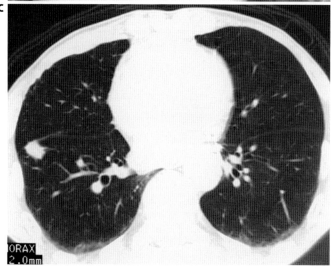

Fig. 11.84 Parenchymal nodular amyloidosis. **A** and **B**, Chest radiographs obtained 4 years apart show a slowly growing oval nodule in the right lower lung. **C**, CT through the right lower lobe shows a noncalcified solitary pulmonary nodule, resected because of concern for malignancy, but proven to be due to amyloidosis.

Parenchymal alveolar septal disease

Although alveolar septal deposition of amyloid is typical of systemic amyloidosis, it is occasionally found in disease that appears to be limited to the lung.[740,758,786,787] Unlike patients with the systemic disorder most patients have symptoms and deaths are recorded.[786] Pathologically, amyloid deposition in the interstitium may be diffuse or micronodular.[758] The radiologic pattern is of an interstitial process with fine linear or reticulonodular opacities that can become confluent. Micronodular calcification and cyst formation are described.[787] On CT scanning, reticular abnormality, septal thickening, and small well-defined 2–4 mm nodules are seen, mainly in the subpleural region.[736,788] The diffuse micronodular pattern may sometimes be accompanied by larger nodules, and they may be considered as one end of the spectrum of parenchymal nodular amyloidosis.[712,719,776,789] These patients are often symptomatic. Alveolar septal, micronodular, and nodular parenchymal amyloidosis may thus be regarded as a continuum.

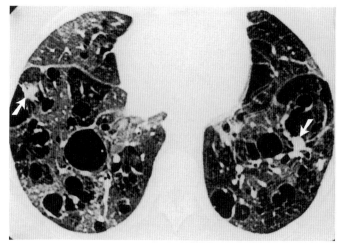

Fig. 11.85 Benign pulmonary lymphocytic infiltration and amyloidosis. Lower zone HRCT in a 44-year-old woman who had dyspnea and lower zone reticulonodular opacity on the chest radiograph. Investigation revealed airflow obstruction and reduced diffusion capacity. Antinuclear antibodies and rheumatoid factor were present in the serum. The HRCT shows multiple thin walled cysts ranging in size from 2 to 50 mm together with a number of irregular nodules (arrows). Histologically there was a lymphocytic infiltrate and widespread amyloid deposition, including cyst wall involvement.

REFERENCES

1. Thomas PD, Hunninghake GW. Current concepts of the pathogenesis of sarcoidosis. Am Rev Respir Dis 1987;135: 747–760.
2. Moller DR. Etiology of sarcoidosis. Clin Chest Med 1997;18:695–706.
3. Kon OM, du Bois RM. Mycobacteria and sarcoidosis. Thorax 1997;52 Suppl 3:S47–51.
4. Judson MA. The etiologic agent of sarcoidosis: what if there isn't one? Chest 2003;124:6–8.
5. Thomas KW, Hunninghake GW. Sarcoidosis. JAMA 2003;289:3300–3303.
6. Rossman MD, Thompson B, Frederick M, et al. HLA-DRB1*1101: A significant risk factor for sarcoidosis in blacks and whites. Am J Hum Genet 2003;73:720–735.
7. Sharma OP, Neville E, Walker AN, et al. Familial sarcoidosis: a possible genetic influence. Ann N Y Acad Sci 1976;278:386–400.
8. Rosen Y, Athanassiades T, Moon S, et al. Nongranulomatous interstitial pneumonitis in sarcoidosis: relationship to development of epithelioid granulomas. Chest 1978;74:122–125.
9. Newman LS, Rose CS, Maier LA. Sarcoidosis. N Engl J Med 1997; 336:1224–1234.
10. Sheffield EA. Pathology of sarcoidosis. Clin Chest Med 1997;18:741–754.
11. Freiman DG. The pathology of sarcoidosis. Semin Roentgenol 1985;20:327–339.
12. Müller NL, Kullnig P, Miller RR. The CT findings of pulmonary sarcoidosis: analysis of 25 patients. Am J Roentgenol 1989;152:1179–1182.
13. Muns G, West WW, Gurney J, et al. Non-sarcoid granulomatous disease with involvement of the lungs. Sarcoidosis 1995;12:99–110.
14. Leslie KO, Colby TV, Swensen SJ. Anatomic distribution and histopathologic patterns of interstitial lung disease. In: Schwarz M, King T, eds. Interstitial lung disease, 4th edn. Toronto: Brian C Decker, 2003:31–54.
15. Mayock RL, Bertrand P, Morrison CE, et al. Manifestations of sarcoidosis. Analysis of 145 patients, with a review of nine series selected from the literature. Am J Med 1963;35:67–89.
16. Gregorie H, Othersen H, Moore M. The significance of sarcoid-like lesions in association with malignant neoplasms. Am J Surg 1962;104:577–586.
17. Hunsaker AR, Munden RF, Pugatch RD, et al. Sarcoidlike reaction in patients with malignancy. Radiology 1996;200:255–261.
18. Levinsky L, Cummiskey J, Romer FK, et al. Sarcoidosis in Europe: a cooperative study. Ann N Y Acad Sci 1976;278:335–346.
19. Milman N, Selroos O. Pulmonary sarcoidosis in the Nordic countries 1950–1982. Epidemiology and clinical picture. Sarcoidosis 1990;7:50–57.
20. Poukkula A, Huhti E, Lilja M, et al. Incidence and clinical picture of sarcoidosis in a circumscribed geographical area. Br J Dis Chest 1986;80:138–147.
21. Edmondstone WM, Wilson AG. Sarcoidosis in caucasians, blacks and Asians in London. Br J Dis Chest 1985;79:27–36.
22. Sartwell PE. Racial differences in sarcoidosis. Ann N Y Acad Sci 1976;278:368–370.
23. Rybicki BA, Major M, Popovich J Jr, et al. Racial differences in sarcoidosis incidence: a 5-year study in a health maintenance organization. Am J Epidemiol 1997;145:234–241.
24. McNicol MW, Luce PJ. Sarcoidosis in a racially mixed community. J R Coll Physicians Lond 1985;19:179–183.
25. Valeyre D, Soler P, Clerici C, et al. Smoking and pulmonary sarcoidosis: effect of cigarette smoking on prevalence, clinical manifestations, alveolitis, and evolution of the disease. Thorax 1988;43:516–524.
26. Littner MR, Schachter EN, Putman CE, et al. The clinical assessment of roentgenographically atypical pulmonary sarcoidosis. Am J Med 1977;62:361–368.
27. Scadding J. Further observations on sarcoidosis associated with M tuberculosis infection. In: Proceedings of 5th International Conference on Sarcoidosis, Prague, 1969: 89–92.
28. Gomez V, Smith PR, Burack J, et al. Sarcoidosis after antiretroviral therapy in a patient with acquired immunodeficiency syndrome. Clin Infect Dis 2000;31:1278–1280.
29. Mirmirani P, Maurer TA, Herndier B, et al. Sarcoidosis in a patient with AIDS: a manifestation of immune restoration syndrome. J Am Acad Dermatol 1999;41:285–286.
30. Lenner R, Bregman Z, Teirstein AS, et al. Recurrent pulmonary sarcoidosis in HIV-infected patients receiving highly active antiretroviral therapy. Chest 2001;119:978–981.
31. Kirks DR, McCormick VD, Greenspan RH. Pulmonary sarcoidosis. Roentgenologic analysis of 150 patients. Am J Roentgenol Radium Ther Nucl Med 1973;117:777–786.
32. Hillerdal G, Nou E, Osterman K, et al. Sarcoidosis: epidemiology and prognosis. A 15-year European study. Am Rev Respir Dis 1984;130:29–32.
33. Hetherington S. Sarcoidosis in young children. Am J Dis Child 1982;136:13–15.
34. Freundlich IM, Libshitz HI, Glassman LM, et al. Sarcoidosis. Typical and atypical thoracic manifestations and complications. Clin Radiol 1970;21: 376–383.
35. Romer FK. Presentation of sarcoidosis and outcome of pulmonary changes. Dan Med Bull 1982;29:27–32.
36. James DG, Neville E, Siltzbach LE. A worldwide review of sarcoidosis. Ann N Y Acad Sci 1976;278:321–334.
37. Rohrbach MS, DeRemee RA. Pulmonary sarcoidosis and serum angiotensin-converting enzyme. Mayo Clin Proc 1982;57:64–66.
38. Sharma OP. Sarcoidosis: clinical, laboratory, and immunologic aspects. Semin Roentgenol 1985;20:340–355.
39. Honeybourne D. Ethnic differences in the clinical features of sarcoidosis in South-East London. Br J Dis Chest 1980;74:63–69.
40. Lofgren S. Primary pulmonary sarcoidosis. Acta Med Scand 1953;145:421–431.
41. Mana J, Gomez-Vaquero C, Montero A, et al. Lofgren's syndrome revisited: a study of 186 patients. Am J Med 1999;107:240–245.
42. Benatar SR. Sarcoidosis in South Africa. A comparative study in whites, blacks and coloureds. S Afr Med J 1977;52: 602–606.
43. Teirstein AS, Chuang M, Miller A, et al. Flexible-bronchoscope biopsy of lung and bronchial wall in intrathoracic sarcoidosis. Ann N Y Acad Sci 1976;278:522–527.
44. Sharma SK, Mohan A, Guleria JS. Clinical characteristics, pulmonary function abnormalities and outcome of prednisolone treatment in 106 patients with sarcoidosis. J Assoc Physicians India 2001;49:697–704.
45. Renston JP, Goldman ES, Hsu RM, et al. Peripheral blood eosinophilia in association with sarcoidosis. Mayo Clin Proc 2000;75:586–590.
46. Meyrier A, Valeyre D, Bouillon R, et al. Resorptive versus absorptive hypercalciuria in sarcoidosis: correlations with 25-hydroxy vitamin D3 and 1,25-dihydroxy vitamin D3 and parameters of disease activity. Q J Med 1985;54: 269–281.
47. Adams JS, Sharma OP, Gacad MA, et al. Metabolism of 25-hydroxyvitamin D3 by cultured pulmonary alveolar macrophages in sarcoidosis. J Clin Invest 1983;72:1856–1860.
48. Sandler LM, Winearls CG, Fraher LJ, et al. Studies of the hypercalcaemia of sarcoidosis: effect of steroids and exogenous vitamin D3 on the circulating concentrations of 1,25-dihydroxy vitamin D3. Q J Med 1984;53:165–180.

49. Shorr AF, Torrington KG, Parker JM. Serum angiotensin converting enzyme does not correlate with radiographic stage at initial diagnosis of sarcoidosis. Respir Med 1997;91:399–401.

50. Lieberman J, Nosal A, Schlessner A, et al. Serum angiotensin-converting enzyme for diagnosis and therapeutic evaluation of sarcoidosis. Am Rev Respir Dis 1979;120:329–335.

51. Lieberman J. Elevation of serum angiotensin-converting-enzyme (ACE) level in sarcoidosis. Am J Med 1975; 59:365–372.

52. Costabel U, Teschler H. Biochemical changes in sarcoidosis. Clin Chest Med 1997;18:827–842.

53. Schoenberger CI, Line BR, Keogh BA, et al. Lung inflammation in sarcoidosis: comparison of serum angiotensin-converting enzyme levels with bronchoalveolar lavage and gallium-67 scanning assessment of the T lymphocyte alveolitis. Thorax 1982;37: 19–25.

54. Studdy P, Bird R, James DG. Serum angiotensin-converting enzyme (SACE) in sarcoidosis and other granulomatous disorders. Lancet 1978;2:1331–1334.

55. Quismorio FP Jr, Sharma OP, Chandor S. Immunopathological studies on the cutaneous lesions in sarcoidosis. Br J Dermatol 1977;97:635–642.

56. Nagai S, Izumi T. Bronchoalveolar lavage. Still useful in diagnosing sarcoidosis? Clin Chest Med 1997;18:787–797.

57. Lynch JP 3rd, Kazerooni EA, Gay SE. Pulmonary sarcoidosis. Clin Chest Med 1997;18:755–785.

58. Line BR, Hunninghake GW, Keogh BA, et al. Gallium-67 scanning to stage the alveolitis of sarcoidosis: correlation with clinical studies, pulmonary function studies, and bronchoalveolar lavage. Am Rev Respir Dis 1981;123:440–446.

59. Gilman MJ, Wang KP. Transbronchial lung biopsy in sarcoidosis. An approach to determine the optimal number of biopsies. Am Rev Respir Dis 1980; 122:721–724.

60. Heshiki A, Schatz SL, McKusick KA, et al. Gallium 67 citrate scanning in patients with pulmonary sarcoidosis. Am J Roentgenol Radium Ther Nucl Med 1974;122:744–749.

61. Israel HL, Park CH, Mansfield CM. Gallium scanning in sarcoidosis. Ann N Y Acad Sci 1976;278:514–516.

62. McKusick KA, Soin JS, Ghiladi A, et al. Gallium 67 accumulation in pulmonary sarcoidosis. JAMA 1973;223:688.

63. Mana J. Nuclear imaging. [67]Gallium, [201]thallium, ^{18}F-labeled fluoro-2-deoxy-D-glucose positron emission tomography. Clin Chest Med 1997;18:799–811.

64. Nakano I, Tsuneta Y, Terai T, et al. [Clinical significance of bronchoalveolar lavage, Ga scintigraphy and serum angiotensin converting enzyme activity in granulomatous lung disease]. Nihon Kyobu Shikkan Gakkai Zasshi 1983;21:615–621.

65. Baughman RP. Sarcoidosis. Usual and unusual manifestations. Chest 1988;94:165–170.

66. Bekerman C, Szidon JP, Pinsky S. The role of gallium-67 in the clinical evaluation of sarcoidosis. Semin Roentgenol 1985;20:400–409.

67. Rizzato G, Blasi A. A European survey on the usefulness of ^{67}Ga lung scans in assessing sarcoidosis. Experience in 14 research centers in seven different countries. Ann N Y Acad Sci 1986;465:463–478

68. Brudin LH, Valind SO, Rhodes CG, et al. Fluorine-18 deoxyglucose uptake in sarcoidosis measured with positron emission tomography. Eur J Nucl Med 1994;21:297–305.

69. Lewis PJ, Salama A. Uptake of fluorine-18-fluorodeoxyglucose in sarcoidosis. J Nucl Med 1994;35:1647–1649.

70. Levinson RS, Metzger LF, Stanley NN, et al. Airway function in sarcoidosis. Am J Med 1977;62:51–59.

71. Winterbauer RH, Hutchinson JF. Use of pulmonary function tests in the management of sarcoidosis. Chest 1980;78:640–647.

72. Fazzi P, Sbragia P, Solfanelli S, et al. Functional significance of the decreased attenuation sign on expiratory CT in pulmonary sarcoidosis : report of four cases. Chest 2001;119:1270–1274.

73. Magkanas E, Voloudaki A, Bouros D, et al. Pulmonary sarcoidosis. Correlation of expiratory high-resolution CT findings with inspiratory patterns and pulmonary function tests. Acta Radiol 2001;42:494–501.

74. Davies CW, Tasker AD, Padley SP, et al. Air trapping in sarcoidosis on computed tomography: correlation with lung function. Clin Radiol 2000;55:217–221.

75. Hansell DM, Milne DG, Wilsher ML, et al. Pulmonary sarcoidosis: morphologic associations of airflow obstruction at thin-section CT. Radiology 1998;209:697–704.

76. McLoud TC, Epler GR, Gaensler EA, et al. A radiographic classification for sarcoidosis: physiologic correlation. Invest Radiol 1982;17:129–138.

77. Miller A, Chuang M, Teirstein AS, et al. Pulmonary function in stage I and II pulmonary sarcoidosis. Ann N Y Acad Sci 1976;278:292–300.

78. Anon. Statement on sarcoidosis. Am J Respir Crit Care Med 1999; 160:736–755.

79. Koerner SK, Sakowitz AJ, Appelman RI, et al. Transbronchinal lung biopsy for the diagnosis of sarcoidosis. N Engl J Med 1975;293:268–270.

80. Mitchell DM, Mitchell DN, Collins JV, et al. Transbronchial lung biopsy through fibreoptic bronchoscope in diagnosis of sarcoidosis. Br Med J 1980;280:679–681.

81. Roethe RA, Fuller PB, Byrd RB, et al. Transbronchoscopic lung biopsy in sarcoidosis. Optimal number and sites for diagnosis. Chest 1980;77:400–402.

82. Rosen Y, Amorosa JK, Moon S, et al. Occurrence of lung granulomas in patients with stage I sarcoidosis. AJR Am J Roentgenol 1977;129:1083–1085.

83. Fossa SD, Abeler V, Marton PF, et al. Sarcoid reaction of hilar and paratracheal lymph nodes in patients treated for testicular cancer. Cancer 1985;56:2212–2216.

84. Munro CS, Mitchell DN. The Kveim response: still useful, still a puzzle. Thorax 1987;42:321–331.

85. Consensus conference: activity of sarcoidosis. Third WASOG meeting, Los Angeles, USA, September 8–11, 1993. Eur Respir J 1994;7:624–627.

86. Sharma OP. Pulmonary sarcoidosis and corticosteroids. Am Rev Respir Dis 1993;147:1598–1600.

87. Selroos O. Glucocorticosteroids and pulmonary sarcoidosis. Thorax 1996;51:229–230.

88. Barbers RG. Role of transplantation (lung, liver, and heart) in sarcoidosis. Clin Chest Med 1997;18:865–874.

89. Martinez FJ, Orens JB, Deeb M, et al. Recurrence of sarcoidosis following bilateral allogeneic lung transplantation. Chest 1994;106:1597–1599.

90. Kazerooni EA, Cascade PN. Recurrent miliary sarcoidosis after lung transplantation. Radiology 1995;194:913.

91. Collins J, Hartman MJ, Warner TF, et al. Frequency and CT findings of recurrent disease after lung transplantation. Radiology 2001;219:503–509.

92. Johns C, MacGregor M, Zachary J, et al. Chronic sarcoidosis: outcome, unusual features and complications. In: Williams W, Davies B, eds. Eighth International Conference on Sarcoidosis and Other Granulomatous Diseases, 1980, Cardiff, Wales. Alpha Omega Publishing, 1980:558–566.

93. Huang C, Heurich A, Rosen Y, et al. Pulmonary sarcoidosis: a radiographic, functional and pathological correlation. In: Williams W, Davies B, eds. Eighth International Conference on Sarcoidosis and Other Granulomatous Diseases, 1980, Cardiff, Wales. Alpha Omega Publishing, 1980:368–377.

94. Perry A, Vuitch F. Causes of death in patients with sarcoidosis. A morphologic study of 38 autopsies with clinicopathologic correlations. Arch Pathol Lab Med 1995;119:167–172.

95. Siltzbach LE, James DG, Neville E, et al. Course and prognosis of sarcoidosis

around the world. Am J Med 1974;57:847–852.

96. DeRemee RA. The roentgenographic staging of sarcoidosis. Historic and contemporary perspectives. Chest 1983;83:128–133.

97. Scadding JG, Mitchell DN. Sarcoidosis. London: Chapman and Hall, 1985.

98. Brauner M, Grenier P, Mompoint D, et al. Pulmonary sarcoidosis: Evaluation with high resolution CT. Radiology 1989;172:467–471.

99. Müller N, Mawson J, Mathieson J, et al. Sarcoidosis: Correlation of extent of disease at CT with clinical, functional, and radiographic findings. Radiology 1989;171:613–618.

100. Lynch D, Webb W, Gamsu G, et al. Computed tomography in sarcoidosis. J Comput Assist Tomogr 1989;13:405–410.

101. Berkmen YM, Javors BR. Anterior mediastinal lymphadenopathy in sarcoidosis. AJR Am J Roentgenol 1976;127:983–987.

102. Bein ME, Putman CE, McLoud TC, et al. A reevaluation of intrathoracic lymphadenopathy in sarcoidosis. AJR Am J Roentgenol 1978;131:409–415.

103. Rabinowitz JG, Ulreich S, Soriano C. The usual unusual manifestations of sarcoidosis and the "hilar haze" – a new diagnostic aid. Am J Roentgenol Radium Ther Nucl Med 1974;120:821–831.

104. Smellie H, Hoyle C. The hilar lymph-nodes in sarcoidosis with special reference to prognosis. Lancet 1957;2:66–70.

105. Ellis K, Renthal G. Pulmonary sarcoidosis. Roentgenographic observations on course of disease. AJR Am J Roentgenol 1962;88:1070–1083.

106. Conant EF, Glickstein MF, Mahar P, et al. Pulmonary sarcoidosis in the older patient: conventional radiographic features. Radiology 1988;169:315–319.

107. Spann RW, Rosenow EC 3rd, DeRemee RA, et al. Unilateral hilar or paratracheal adenopathy in sarcoidosis: a study of 38 cases. Thorax 1971;26:296–299.

108. Hamper UM, Fishman EK, Khouri NF, et al. Typical and atypical CT manifestations of pulmonary sarcoidosis. J Comput Assist Tomogr 1986;10:928–936.

109. Solomon A, Kreel L, McNicol M, et al. Computed tomography in pulmonary sarcoidosis. J Comput Assist Tomogr 1979;3:754–758.

110. Anon. Case records of the Massachusetts General Hospital. Weekly clinicopathological exercises. Case 11-1984. Long-standing sarcoidosis with the recent onset of the superior-vena-cava syndrome. N Engl J Med 1984;310:708–716.

111. McLoud TC, Putman CE, Pascual R. Eggshell calcification with systemic sarcoidosis. Chest 1974;66:515–517.

112. Tsou E, Romano MC, Kerwin DM, et al. Sarcoidosis of anterior mediastinal nodes, pancreas, and uterine cervix: three unusual sites in the same patient. Am Rev Respir Dis 1980;122:333–338.

113. Berkmen YM. Radiologic aspects of intrathoracic sarcoidosis. Semin Roentgenol 1985;20:356–375.

114. Talbot F, Katz S, Matthews M. Bronchopulmonary sarcoidosis. Some unusual manifestations and the serious complications thereof. Am J Med 1959;26:340–355.

115. Karasick SR. Atypical thoracic lymphadenopathy in sarcoidosis. AJR Am J Roentgenol 1979;133:928–929.

116. Schabel SI, Foote GA, McKee KA. Posterior lymphadenopathy in sarcoidosis. Radiology 1978;129:591–593.

117. Kutty CP, Varkey B. Sarcoidosis presenting with posterior mediastinal lymphadenopathy. Postgrad Med 1982;71:64–66.

118. Israel HL, Sperber M, Steiner RM. Course of chronic hilar sarcoidosis in relation to markers of granulomatous activity. Invest Radiol 1983;18:1–5.

119. Olliff JF, Eeles R, Williams MP. Mimics of metastases from testicular tumours. Clin Radiol 1990;41:395–399.

120. Parr MJ, Williams MV. Sarcoidosis mimicking metastatic testicular tumour. Br J Radiol 1988;61:516–518.

121. Steiger V, Fanburg BL. Recurrence of thoracic lymphadenopathy in sarcoidosis. N Engl J Med 1986;314:1512.

122. Brincker H, Wilbek E. The incidence of malignant tumours in patients with respiratory sarcoidosis. Br J Cancer 1974;29:247–251.

123. Macfarlane JT. Recurrent erythema nodosum and pulmonary sarcoidosis. Postgrad Med J 1981;57:525.

124. Symmons DP, Woods KL. Recurrent sarcoidosis. Thorax 1980;35:879.

125. Kent D. Recurrent unilateral hilar adenopathy in sarcoidosis. Am Rev Respir Dis 1965;91:272–276.

126. Rockoff SD, Rohatgi PK. Unusual manifestations of thoracic sarcoidosis. AJR Am J Roentgenol 1985;144:513–528.

127. Israel HL, Lenchner G, Steiner RM. Late development of mediastinal calcification in sarcoidosis. Am Rev Respir Dis 1981;124:302–305.

128. Gawne-Cain ML, Hansell DM. The pattern and distribution of calcified mediastinal lymph nodes in sarcoidosis and tuberculosis: a CT study. Clin Radiol 1996;51:263–267.

129. Gross BH, Schneider HJ, Proto AV. Eggshell calcification of lymph nodes: an update. AJR Am J Roentgenol 1980;135:1265–1268.

130. Murdoch J, Müller N. Pulmonary sarcoidosis: changes on followup examination. Am J Roentgenol 1992;159:473–477.

131. Smellie H, Hoyle C. The natural history of pulmonary sarcoidosis. Q J Med 1960;29:539–559.

132. Israel HL, Karlin P, Menduke H, et al. Factors affecting outcome of sarcoidosis. Influence of race, extrathoracic involvement, and initial radiologic lung lesions. Ann N Y Acad Sci 1986;465:609–618.

133. Carrington CB. Structure and function in sarcoidosis. Ann N Y Acad Sci 1976;278:265–283.

134. Putman CE, Hoeck B. Reassessing the standard chest radiograph for intraparenchymal activity. Ann N Y Acad Sci 1986;465:595–608.

135. Israel H, Sones M. Sarcoidosis. Clinical observation on one hundred sixty cases. Arch Intern Med 1958;102:766–776.

136. Mesbahi SJ, Davies P. Unilateral pulmonary changes in the chest X-ray in sarcoidosis. Clin Radiol 1981;32:283–287.

137. Demicco WA, Fanburg BL. Sarcoidosis presenting as a lobar or unilateral lung infiltrate. Clin Radiol 1982;33:663–669.

138. Hafermann DR, Solomon DA, Byrd RB. Sarcoidosis initially occurring as apical infiltrate and pleural reaction. Chest 1978;73:413–414.

139. Teirstein AL, Siltzbach LE. Sarcoidosis of the upper lung fields simulating pulmonary tuberculosis. Chest 1973;64:303–308.

140. Scadding J. Calcification in sarcoidosis. Tubercle 1961;42:121–135.

141. Kuhlman JE, Fishman EK, Hamper UM, et al. The computed tomographic spectrum of thoracic sarcoidosis. Radiographics 1989;9:449–466.

142. Nishimura K, Itoh H, Kitaichi M, et al. Pulmonary sarcoidosis: correlation of CT and histopathologic findings. Radiology 1993;189:105–109.

143. Remy-Jardin M, Beuscart R, Sault MC, et al. Subpleural micronodules in diffuse infiltrative lung diseases: evaluation with thin-section CT scans. Radiology 1990;177:133–139.

144. Gruden JF, Webb WR, Warnock M. Centrilobular opacities in the lung on high-resolution CT: diagnostic considerations and pathologic correlation. AJR Am J Roentgenol 1994;162:569–574.

145. Grenier P, Valeyre D, Cluzel P, et al. Chronic diffuse interstitial lung disease: diagnostic value of chest radiography and high-resolution CT. Radiology 1991;179:123–132.

146. Munk P, Müller N, Miller R, et al. Pulmonary lymphangitic carcinomatosis: CT and pathologic findings. Radiology 1988;166:705–709.

147. Murata K, Khan A, Herman PG. Pulmonary parenchymal disease: evaluation with high-resolution CT. Radiology 1989;170:629–635.

148. Johkoh T, Ikezoe J, Tomiyama N, et al. CT findings in lymphangitic

carcinomatosis of the lung: correlation with histologic findings and pulmonary function tests. AJR Am J Roentgenol 1992;158:1217–1222.

149. Stein M, Mayo J, Müller N, et al. Pulmonary lymphangitic spread of carcinoma: Appearance on CT scans. Radiology 1987;162:371–375.

150. Collins J, Müller NL, Leung AN, et al. Epstein-Barr-virus-associated lymphoproliferative disease of the lung: CT and histologic findings. Radiology 1998;208:749–759.

151. McGuinness G, Scholes JV, Jagirdar JS, et al. Unusual lymphoproliferative disorders in nine adults with HIV or AIDS: CT and pathologic findings. Radiology 1995;197:59–65.

152. Honda O, Johkoh T, Ichikado K, et al. Comparison of high resolution CT findings of sarcoidosis, lymphoma, and lymphangitic carcinoma: is there any difference of involved interstitium? J Comput Assist Tomogr 1999;23:374–379.

153. Bergin C, Roggli V, Coblentz C, et al. The secondary pulmonary lobule: normal and abnormal CT appearances. Ajr Am J Roentgenol 1988;151:21–25.

154. Padley SP, Padhani AR, Nicholson A, et al. Pulmonary sarcoidosis mimicking cryptogenic fibrosing alveolitis on CT. Clin Radiol 1996;51:807–810.

155. Grenier P, Chevret S, Beigelman C, et al. Chronic diffuse infiltrative lung disease: determination of the diagnostic value of clinical data, chest radiography, and CT and Bayesian analysis. Radiology 1994;191:383–390.

156. Remy-Jardin M, Giraud F, Remy J, et al. Pulmonary sarcoidosis: role of CT in the evaluation of disease activity and functional impairment and in prognosis assessment. Radiology 1994;191:675–680.

157. Tazi A, Desfemmes-Baleyte T, Soler P, et al. Pulmonary sarcoidosis with a diffuse ground glass pattern on the chest radiograph. Thorax 1994;49:793–797.

158. Leung AN, Brauner MW, Caillat-Vigneron N, et al. Sarcoidosis activity: correlation of HRCT findings with those of 67Ga scanning, bronchoalveolar lavage, and serum angiotensin-converting enzyme assay. J Comput Assist Tomogr 1998;22:229–234.

159. Brauner M, Lenoir S, Grenier P, et al. Pulmonary sarcoidosis: CT assessment of lesion reversibility. Radiology 1992;182:349–354.

160. Müller NL, Miller RR. Ground-glass attenuation, nodules, alveolitis, and sarcoid granulomas. Radiology 1993;189:31–32.

161. Traill ZC, Maskell GF, Gleeson FV. High-resolution CT findings of pulmonary sarcoidosis. AJR Am J Roentgenol 1997;168:1557–1560.

162. Nishimura K, Itoh H, Kitaichi M, et al. CT and pathological correlation of pulmonary sarcoidosis. Semin Ultrasound CT MR 1995;16:361–370.

163. Reed JC, Madewell JE. The air bronchogram in interstitial disease of the lungs. A radiological–pathological correlation. Radiology 1975;116:1–9.

164. Sahn SA, Schwarz MI, Lakshminarayan S. Sarcoidosis: the significance of an acinar pattern on chest roentgenogram. Chest 1974;65:684–687.

165. Shigematsu N, Emori K, Matsuba K, et al. Clinicopathologic characteristics of pulmonary acinar sarcoidosis. Chest 1978;73:186–188.

166. Battesti JP, Saumon G, Valeyre D, et al. Pulmonary sarcoidosis with an alveolar radiographic pattern. Thorax 1982;37: 448–452.

167. Sharma OP. Sarcoidosis: unusual pulmonary manifestations. Postgrad Med 1977;61:67–73.

168. Kirks DR, Greenspan RH. Sarcoid. Radiol Clin North Am 1973;11:279–294.

169. Glazer HS, Levitt RG, Shackelford GD. Peripheral pulmonary infiltrates in sarcoidosis. Chest 1984;86:741–744.

170. Judson MA, Ghent S, Close TP. Sarcoidosis manifested as peripheral pulmonary infiltrates. AJR Am J Roentgenol 1993;160:1359–1360.

171. Johkoh T, Ikezoe J, Takeuchi N, et al. CT findings in "pseudoalveolar" sarcoidosis. J Comput Assist Tomogr 1992;16:904–907.

172. Sharma OP, Hewlett R, Gordonson J. Nodular sarcoidosis: an unusual radiographic appearance. Chest 1973;64:189–192.

173. Onal E, Lopata M, Lourenco RV. Nodular pulmonary sarcoidosis. Clinical, roentgenographic, and physiologic course in five patients. Chest 1977;72:296–300.

174. Rose RM, Lee RG, Costello P. Solitary nodular sarcoidosis. Clin Radiol 1985;36:589–592.

175. Chrisholm JC, Lang GR. Solitary circumscribed pulmonary nodule. An unusual manifestation of sarcoidosis. Arch Intern Med 1966;118:376–378.

176. Nutting S, Carr I, Cole FM, et al. Solitary pulmonary nodules due to sarcoidosis. Can J Surg 1979;22:584–586.

177. Pinsker KL. Solitary pulmonary nodule in sarcoidosis. JAMA 1978;240:1379–1380.

178. Nakatsu M, Hatabu H, Morikawa K, et al. Large coalescent parenchymal nodules in pulmonary sarcoidosis: "sarcoid galaxy" sign. AJR Am J Roentgenol 2002;178:1389–1393.

179. Bergin CJ, Bell DY, Coblentz CL, et al. Sarcoidosis: correlation of pulmonary parenchymal pattern at CT with results of pulmonary function tests. Radiology 1989;171:619–624.

180. Bistrong HW, Tenney RD, Sheffer AL. Asymptomatic cavitary sarcoidosis. JAMA 1970;213:1030–1032.

181. Hamilton R, Petty T, Haiby G. Cavitary sarcoidosis of the lung. Arch Intern Med 1965;116:428–430.

182. Tada H, Yasumizu R, Yuasa S, et al. Annular lesion of the lung in sarcoidosis. Thorax 1989;44:756–757.

183. Jones DK, Dent RG, Rimmer MJ, et al. Thin-walled ring shadows in early pulmonary sarcoidosis. Clin Radiol 1984;35:307–310.

184. Rohatgi PK, Schwab LE. Primary acute pulmonary cavitation in sarcoidosis. AJR Am J Roentgenol 1980;134:1199–1203.

185. Tellis CJ, Putnam JS. Cavitation in large multinodular pulmonary disease: a rare manifestation of sarcoidosis. Chest 1977;71:792–793.

186. Edelman RR, Johnson TS, Jhaveri HS, et al. Fatal hemoptysis resulting from erosion of a pulmonary artery in cavitary sarcoidosis. AJR Am J Roentgenol 1985;145:37–38.

187. Battesti JP, Georges R, Basset F, et al. Chronic cor pulmonale in pulmonary sarcoidosis. Thorax 1978;33:76–84.

188. McCort J, Pare P. Pulmonary fibrosis and cor pulmonale in sarcoidosis. Radiology 1954;62:496–504.

189. Miller A. The vanishing lung syndrome associated with pulmonary sarcoidosis. Br J Dis Chest 1981;75:209–214.

190. Packe GE, Ayres JG, Citron KM, et al. Large lung bullae in sarcoidosis. Thorax 1986;41:792–797.

191. Primack SL, Hartman TE, Hansell DM, et al. End-stage lung disease: CT findings in 61 patients. Radiology 1993;189:681–686.

192. Brandstetter RD, Messina MS, Sprince NL, et al. Tracheal stenosis due to sarcoidosis. Chest 1981;80:656.

193. Lefrak S, Di Benedetto R. Systematic sarcoidosis with severe involvement of the upper respiratory tract. Am Rev Respir Dis 1970;102:801–807.

194. Henry DA, Cho SR. Tracheal stenosis in sarcoidosis. South Med J 1983; 76:1323–1324.

195. Kirschner BS, Holinger PH. Laryngeal obstruction in children sarcoidosis. J Pediatr 1976;88:263–265.

196. Weisman RA, Canalis RF, Powell WJ. Laryngeal sarcoidosis with airway obstruction. Ann Otol Rhinol Laryngol 1980;89:58–61.

197. Mendelson DS, Norton K, Cohen BA, et al. Bronchial compression: an unusual manifestation of sarcoidosis. J Comput Assist Tomogr 1983;7:892–894.

198. Hadfield JW, Page RL, Flower CD, et al. Localised airway narrowing in sarcoidosis. Thorax 1982;37:443–447.

199. Olsson T, Bjornstad-Pettersen H, Stjernberg NL. Bronchostenosis due to sarcoidosis: a cause of atelectasis and airway obstruction simulating pulmonary neoplasm and chronic obstructive pulmonary disease. Chest 1979;75:663–666.

200. Udwadia ZF, Pilling JR, Jenkins PF, et al. Bronchoscopic and bronchographic findings in 12 patients with sarcoidosis and severe or progressive airways obstruction. Thorax 1990;45:272–275.

201. Dorman RL Jr, Whitman GJ, Chew FS. Thoracic sarcoidosis. AJR Am J Roentgenol 1995;164:1368.

202. Corsello BF, Lohaus GH, Funahashi A. Endobronchial mass lesion due to sarcoidosis: complete resolution with corticosteroids. Thorax 1983;38:157–158.

203. Munt PW. Middle lobe atelectasis in sarcoidosis. Report of a case with prompt resolution concomitant with corticosteroid administration. Am Rev Respir Dis 1973;108:357–360.

204. Fouty BW, Pomeranz M, Thigpen TP, et al. Dilatation of bronchial stenoses due to sarcoidosis using a flexible fiberoptic bronchoscope. Chest 1994;106:677–680.

205. Iles PB. Multiple bronchial stenoses: treatment by mechanical dilatation. Thorax 1981;36:784–786.

206. Curtin JJ, Innes NJ, Harrison BD. Thin-section spiral volumetric CT for the assessment of lobar and segmental bronchial stenoses. Clin Radiol 1998;53:110–115.

207. Lenique F, Brauner MW, Grenier P, et al. CT assessment of bronchi in sarcoidosis: endoscopic and pathologic correlations. Radiology 1995;194:419–423.

208. Shorr AF, Torrington KG, Hnatiuk OW. Endobronchial involvement and airway hyperreactivity in patients with sarcoidosis. Chest 2001;120:881–886.

209. Gleeson FV, Traill ZC, Hansell DM. Evidence on expiratory CT scans of small-airway obstruction in sarcoidosis. AJR Am J Roentgenol 1996;166:1052–1054.

210. Ng CS, Desai SR, Rubens MB, et al. Visual quantitation and observer variation of signs of small airways disease at inspiratory and expiratory CT. J Thorac Imaging 1999;14:279–285.

211. Bartz RR, Stern EJ. Airways obstruction in patients with sarcoidosis: expiratory CT scan findings. J Thorac Imaging 2000;15:285–289.

212. Miller A, Teirstein AS, Jackler I, et al. Airway function in chronic pulmonary sarcoidosis with fibrosis. Am Rev Respir Dis 1974;109:179–189.

213. Sharma OP. Airway obstruction in sarcoidosis. Chest 1978;73:6–7.

214. Mixides G, Guy E. Sarcoidosis confined to the airway masquerading as asthma. Can Respir J 2003;10:114–116.

215. Schermuly W, Behrend H. [Angiography of pulmonary sarcoidosis]. Radiologe 1968;8:116–123.

216. Faunce HF, Ramsay GC, Sy W. Protracted yet variable major pulmonary artery compression in sarcoidosis. Radiology 1976;119:313–314.

217. Goffman TE, Bloom RL, Dvorak VC. Topics in radiology/case of the month. Acute dyspnea in a young woman taking birth control pills. JAMA 1984;251:1465–1466.

218. Hietala SO, Stinnett RG, Faunce HF 3rd, et al. Pulmonary artery narrowing in sarcoidosis. JAMA 1977;237:572–573.

219. Khan MM, Gill DS, McConkey B. Myopathy and external pulmonary artery compression caused by sarcoidosis. Thorax 1981;36:703–704.

220. Westcott JL, DeGraff AC Jr. Sarcoidosis, hilar adenopathy, and pulmonary artery narrowing. Radiology 1973;108:585–586.

221. Damuth TE, Bower JS, Cho K, et al. Major pulmonary artery stenosis causing pulmonary hypertension in sarcoidosis. Chest 1980;78:888–891.

222. Schowengerdt CG, Suyemoto R, Main FB. Granulomatous and fibrous mediastinitis. A review and analysis of 180 cases. J Thorac Cardiovasc Surg 1969;57:365–379.

223. O'Brien LE, Forsman PJ, Wiltse HE. Early onset sarcoidosis with pulmonary function abnormalities. Chest 1974;65:472–474.

224. Shibel EM, Tisi GM, Moser KM. Pulmonary photoscan – roentgenographic comparisons in sarcoidosis. Am J Roentgenol Radium Ther Nucl Med 1969;106:770–777.

225. Preston IR, Klinger JR, Landzberg MJ, et al. Vasoresponsiveness of sarcoidosis-associated pulmonary hypertension. Chest 2001;120:866–872.

226. Anon. Case records of the Massachusetts General Hospital. Weekly clinicopathological exercises. Case 51-1974. N Engl J Med 1974;291:1402–1408.

227. Davies J, Nellen M, Goodwin JF. Reversible pulmonary hypertension in sarcoidosis. Postgrad Med J 1982;58:282–285.

228. Smith LJ, Lawrence JB, Katzenstein AA. Vascular sarcoidosis: a rare cause of pulmonary hypertension. Am J Med Sci 1983;285:38–44.

229. Rodman DM, Lindenfeld J. Successful treatment of sarcoidosis-associated pulmonary hypertension with corticosteroids. Chest 1990;97:500–502.

230. Brandstetter RD, Hansen DE, Jarowski CI, et al. Superior vena cava syndrome as the initial clinical manifestation of sarcoidosis. Heart Lung 1981;10:101–104.

231. Kinney EL, Murthy R, Ascunce G, et al. Sarcoidosis: rare cause of superior vena caval obstruction. Pa Med 1980;83:31.

232. Morgans WE, Al-Jilahawi AN, Mbatha PB. Superior vena caval obstruction caused by sarcoidosis. Thorax 1980;35:397–398.

233. Simpson JC, Callaway MP, Taylor PM, et al. Recurrent venous obstruction caused by sarcoidosis. Respir Med 1998;92:785–786.

234. Javaheri S, Hales CA. Sarcoidosis: a cause of innominate vein obstruction and massive pleural effusion. Lung 1980;157:81–85.

235. Radke JR, Kaplan H, Conway WA. The significance of superior vena cava syndrome developing in a patient with sarcoidosis. Radiology 1980;134:311–312.

236. Hoffstein V, Ranganathan N, Mullen JB. Sarcoidosis simulating pulmonary veno-occlusive disease. Am Rev Respir Dis 1986;134:809–811.

237. Da Costa JL, Chiang SC. Pleural sarcoidosis. Singapore Med J 1975;16:224–226.

238. Gardiner IT, Uff JS. Acute pleurisy in sarcoidosis. Thorax 1978;33:124–127.

239. Beekman JF, Zimmet SM, Chun BK, et al. Spectrum of pleural involvement in sarcoidosis. Arch Intern Med 1976;136:323–330.

240. Johnson NM, Martin ND, McNicol MW. Sarcoidosis presenting with pleurisy and bilateral pleural effusions. Postgrad Med J 1980;56:266–267.

241. Nicholls AJ, Friend JA, Legge JS. Sarcoid pleural effusion: three cases and review of the literature. Thorax 1980;35:277–281.

242. Durand DV, Dellinger A, Guerin C, et al. Pleural sarcoidosis: one case presenting with an eosinophilic effusion. Thorax 1984;39:468–469.

243. Chusid EL, Siltzbach LE. Sarcoidosis of the pleura. Ann Intern Med 1974;81:190–194.

244. Wilen SB, Rabinowitz JG, Ulreich S, et al. Pleural involvement in sarcoidosis. Am J Med 1974;57:200–209.

245. Selroos O. Exudative pleurisy and sarcoidosis. Br J Dis Chest 1966;60:191–196.

246. Mikhail JR, Lovell D, McGhee KJ. Sarcoidosis presenting with a pleural effusion. Tubercle 1976;57:226–228.

247. Soskel NT, Sharma OP. Pleural involvement in sarcoidosis. Curr Opin Pulm Med 2000;6:455–468.

248. Kanada DJ, Scott D, Sharma OP. Unusual presentations of pleural sarcoidosis. Br J Dis Chest 1980;74:203–205.

249. Watts R Jr, Thompson JR, Jasuja ML. Sarcoidosis presenting with massive pleural effusion. IMJ Ill Med J 1983;163:57–58.

250. Knox AJ, Wardman AG, Page RL. Tuberculous pleural effusion occurring during corticosteroid treatment of sarcoidosis. Thorax 1986;41:651.

251. Jarman PR, Whyte MK, Sabroe I, et al. Sarcoidosis presenting with chylothorax. Thorax 1995;50:1324–1325.

252. Froudarakis ME, Bouros D, Voloudaki A, et al. Pneumothorax as a first manifestation of sarcoidosis. Chest 1997;112:278–280.

253. Akelsson IG, Eklund A, Skold CM, et al. Bilateral spontaneous pneumothorax and sarcoidosis. Sarcoidosis 1990;7:136–138.

254. Stump D, Spock A, Grossman H. Vertebral sarcoidosis in adolescents. Radiology 1976;121:153–155.

255. Young DA, Laman ML. Radiodense skeletal lesions in Boeck's sarcoid. Am J Roentgenol Radium Ther Nucl Med 1972;114:553–558.

256. Brodey PA, Pripstein S, Strange G, et al. Vertebral sarcoidosis. A case report and review of the literature. Am J Roentgenol 1976;126:900–902.

257. Guilford WB, Mentz WM, Kopelman HA, et al. Sarcoidosis presenting as a rib fracture. AJR Am J Roentgenol 1982;139:608–609.

258. Gorske KJ, Fleming RJ. Mycetoma formation in cavitary pulmonary sarcoidosis. Radiology 1970;95:279–285.

259. Wollschlager C, Khan F. Aspergillomas complicating sarcoidosis. A prospective study in 100 patients. Chest 1984;86:585–588.

260. Israel HL, Lenchner GS, Atkinson GW. Sarcoidosis and aspergilloma. The role of surgery. Chest 1982;82:430–432.

261. Libshitz HI, Atkinson GW, Israel HL. Pleural thickening as a manifestation of aspergillus superinfection. Am J Roentgenol Radium Ther Nucl Med 1974;120:883–886.

262. Roberts CM, Citron KM, Strickland B. Intrathoracic aspergilloma: role of CT in diagnosis and treatment. Radiology 1987;165:123–128.

263. Kaplan J, Johns CJ. Mycetomas in pulmonary sarcoidosis: non-surgical management. Johns Hopkins Med J 1979;145:157–161.

264. Breuer R, Baigelman W, Pugatch RD. Occult mycetoma. J Comput Assist Tomogr 1982;6:166–168.

265. Drent M, Vries JD, Lenters M, et al. Sarcoidosis: assessment of disease severity using HRCT. Eur Radiol 2003;13:2462–2471.

266. Bergin C, Bell D, Coblentz C, et al. Sarcoidosis: Correlation of pulmonary parenchymal pattern at CT with results of pulmonary function tests. Radiology 1989;171:619–624.

267. Bergin CJ, Coblentz CL, Chiles C, et al. Chronic lung diseases: specific diagnosis by using CT. AJR Am J Roentgenol 1989;152:1183–1188.

268. Bergin CJ, Müller NL. CT in the diagnosis of interstitial lung disease. AJR Am J Roentgenol 1985;145:505–510.

269. Mathieson JR, Mayo JR, Staples CA, et al. Chronic diffuse infiltrative lung disease: comparison of diagnostic accuracy of CT and chest radiography. Radiology 1989;171:111–116.

270. Müller NL. Differential diagnosis of chronic diffuse infiltrative lung disease on high-resolution computed tomography. Semin Roentgenol 1991;26:132–142.

271. Mana J, Teirstein AS, Mendelson DS, et al. Excessive thoracic computed tomographic scanning in sarcoidosis. Thorax 1995;50:1264–1266.

272. McFadden RG, Carr TJ, Wood TE. Proton magnetic resonance imaging to stage activity of interstitial lung disease. Chest 1987;92:31–39.

273. Mendelson DS, Gray CE, Teirstein AS. Magnetic resonance findings in sarcoidosis of the thorax. Magn Reson Imaging 1992;10:523–529.

274. Cordier JF. Eosinophilic pneumonias. In: Schwarz M, King T, eds. Interstitial lung disease, 4th edn. Toronto: Brian C Decker, 2003:657–700.

275. Crofton J, Livingstone J, Oswald N, et al. Pulmonary eosinophilia. Thorax 1952;7:1–35.

276. Reeder W, Goodrich B. Pulmonary infiltrates with eosinophilia (PIE syndrome). Ann Intern Med 1952;36:1217–1240.

277. Citro LA, Gordon ME, Miller WT. Eosinophilic lung disease (or how to slice P.I.E.). Am J Roentgenol Radium Ther Nucl Med 1973;117:787–797.

278. Fraser R, Pare J, Pare P, et al. Diagnosis of diseases of the chest. Philadelphia: WB Saunders, 1989.

279. Schatz M, Wasserman S, Patterson R. The eosinophil and the lung. Arch Intern Med 1982;142:1515–1519.

280. Geddes DM. Pulmonary eosinophilia. J R Coll Physicians Lond 1986;20:139–145.

281. Liebow AA, Carrington CB. The eosinophilic pneumonias. Medicine (Baltimore) 1969;48:251–285.

282. Patterson R, Irons JS, Kelly JF, et al. Pulmonary infiltrates with eosinophilia. J Allergy Clin Immunol 1974;53:245–255.

283. Allen JN, Pacht ER, Gadek JE, et al. Acute eosinophilic pneumonia as a reversible cause of noninfectious respiratory failure. N Engl J Med 1989;321:569–574.

284. Badesch DB, King TE Jr, Schwarz MI. Acute eosinophilic pneumonia: a hypersensitivity phenomenon? Am Rev Respir Dis 1989;139:249–252.

285. Miyazaki E, Sugisaki K, Shigenaga T, et al. A case of acute eosinophilic pneumonia caused by inhalation of Trichosporon terrestre. Am J Respir Crit Care Med 1995;151:541–543.

286. Brander PE, Tukiainen P. Acute eosinophilic pneumonia in a heroin smoker. Eur Respir J 1993;6:750–752.

287. Miki K, Miki M, Okano Y, et al. Cigarette smoke-induced acute eosinophilic pneumonia accompanied with neutrophilia in the blood. Intern Med 2002;41:993–996.

288. Nakajima M, Manabe T, Sasaki T, et al. Acute eosinophilic pneumonia caused by cigarette smoking. Intern Med 2000;39:1131–1132.

289. Watanabe K, Fujimura M, Kasahara K, et al. Acute eosinophilic pneumonia following cigarette smoking: a case report including cigarette-smoking challenge test. Intern Med 2002;41:1016–1020.

290. Philit F, Etienne-Mastroianni B, Parrot A, et al. Idiopathic acute eosinophilic pneumonia: a study of 22 patients. Am J Respir Crit Care Med 2002;166:1235–1239.

291. Noh H, Lee YK, Kan SW, et al. Acute eosinophilic pneumonia associated with amitriptyline in a hemodialysis patient. Yonsei Med J 2001;42:357–359.

292. Fleisch MC, Blauer F, Gubler JG, et al. Eosinophilic pneumonia and respiratory failure associated with venlafaxine treatment. Eur Respir J 2000;15:205–208.

293. Pope-Harman AL, Davis WB, Allen ED, et al. Acute eosinophilic pneumonia. A summary of 15 cases and review of the literature. Medicine (Baltimore) 1996;75:334–342.

294. Hayakawa H, Sato A, Toyoshima M, et al. A clinical study of idiopathic eosinophilic pneumonia. Chest 1994;105:1462–1466.

295. Ogawa H, Fujimura M, Matsuda T, et al. Transient wheeze. Eosinophilic bronchobronchiolitis in acute eosinophilic pneumonia. Chest 1993;104:493–496.

296. Cheon JE, Lee KS, Jung GS, et al. Acute eosinophilic pneumonia: radiographic and CT findings in six patients. AJR Am J Roentgenol 1996;167:1195–1199.

297. Tazelaar H, Linz L, Colby T, et al. Acute eosinophilic pneumonia: histopathologic findings in nine patients. Am J Respir Crit Care Med 1997;155:296–302.

298. Buchheit J, Eid N, Rodgers G Jr, et al. Acute eosinophilic pneumonia with respiratory failure: a new syndrome? Am Rev Respir Dis 1992;145:716–718.

299. King MA, Pope-Harman AL, Allen JN, et al. Acute eosinophilic pneumonia: radiologic and clinical features. Radiology 1997;203:715–719.

300. Okubo Y, Hossain M, Kai R, et al. Adhesion molecules on eosinophils in acute eosinophilic pneumonia. Am J Respir Crit Care Med 1995;151:1259–1262.

301. Tomiyama N, Müller NL, Johkoh T, et al. Acute parenchymal lung disease in immunocompetent patients: diagnostic accuracy of high-resolution CT. AJR Am J Roentgenol 2000;174:1745–1750.

302. Johkoh T, Müller NL, Akira M, et al. Eosinophilic lung diseases: diagnostic accuracy of thin-section CT in 111 patients. Radiology 2000;216:773–780.

303. du Bois R. Rare lung diseases: orphans no more? Am J Respir Crit Care Med 2002;166:1157–1158.

304. Löffler W. Zur Differential-Diagnose der Lungen Infiltreierunger: III Uber fluchtige Succedan - Infiltrate (mit Eosinophilia). Beitr Klin Tuberk 1932;79:368–392.

305. Allen JN, Davis WB. Eosinophilic lung diseases. Am J Respir Crit Care Med 1994;150:1423–1438.

306. Sunderman F, Sunderman F Jr. Loffler's syndrome associated with nickel sensitivity. Arch Intern Med 1961; 107:405–408.

307. Carrington CB, Addington WW, Goff AM, et al. Chronic eosinophilic pneumonia. N Engl J Med 1969;280:787–798.

308. Turner-Warwick M, Assem ES, Lockwood M. Cryptogenic pulmonary eosinophilia. Clin Allergy 1976;6:135–145.

309. McCarthy DS, Pepys J. Cryptogenic pulmonary eosinophilias. Clin Allergy 1973;3:339–351.

310. Gaensler EA, Carrington CB. Peripheral opacities in chronic eosinophilic pneumonia: the photographic negative of pulmonary edema. AJR Am J Roentgenol 1977;128:1–13.

311. Fox B, Seed WA. Chronic eosinophilic pneumonia. Thorax 1980;35:570–580.

312. Jederlinic PJ, Sicilian L, Gaensler EA. Chronic eosinophilic pneumonia. A report of 19 cases and a review of the literature. Medicine (Baltimore) 1988;67:154–162.

313. Naughton M, Fahy J, FitzGerald MX. Chronic eosinophilic pneumonia. A long-term follow-up of 12 patients. Chest 1993;103:162–165.

314. Gonzalez EB, Hayes D, Weedn VW. Chronic eosinophilic pneumonia (Carrington's) with increased serum IgE levels. A distinct subset? Arch Intern Med 1988;148:2622–2624.

315. Onitsuka H, Onitsuka S, Yokomizo Y, et al. Computed tomography of chronic eosinophilic pneumonia. J Comput Assist Tomogr 1983;7:1092–1094.

316. Mayo JR, Müller NL, Road J, et al. Chronic eosinophilic pneumonia: CT findings in six cases. AJR Am J Roentgenol 1989;153:727–730.

317. Zaki I, Wears R, Parnell A, et al. Case report: mediastinal lymphadenopathy in eosinophilic pneumonia. Clin Radiol 1993;48:61–62.

318. Ebara H, Ikezoe J, Johkoh T, et al. Chronic eosinophilic pneumonia: evolution of chest radiograms and CT features. J Comput Assist Tomogr 1994;18:737–744.

319. Hueto-Perez-de-Heredia JJ, Dominguez-del-Valle FJ, Garcia E, et al. Chronic eosinophilic pneumonia as a presenting feature of Churg-Strauss syndrome. Eur Respir J 1994;7:1006–1008.

320. Cogen FC, Mayock RL, Zweiman B. Chronic eosinophilic pneumonia followed by polyarteritis nodosa complicating the course of bronchial asthma. Report of a case. J Allergy Clin Immunol 1977;60:377–382.

321. McCarthy DS, Pepys J. Allergic broncho-pulmonary aspergillosis. Clinical immunology. 2. Skin, nasal and bronchial tests. Clin Allergy 1971;1:415–432.

322. Hinson K, Moon A, Plummer N. Bronchopulmonary aspergillosis: a review and a report of eight new cases. Thorax 1952;7:317–333.

323. Safirstein BH, D'Souza MF, Simon G, et al. Five-year follow-up of allergic bronchopulmonary aspergillosis. Am Rev Respir Dis 1973;108:450–459.

324. Glimp RA, Bayer AS. Fungal pneumonias. Part 3. Allergic bronchopulmonary aspergillosis. Chest 1981;80:85–94.

325. Laham MN, Carpenter JL. Aspergillus terreus, a pathogen capable of causing infective endocarditis, pulmonary mycetoma, and allergic bronchopulmonary aspergillosis. Am Rev Respir Dis 1982;125:769–772.

326. Akiyama K, Takizawa H, Suzuki M, et al. Allergic bronchopulmonary aspergillosis due to *Aspergillus oryzae*. Chest 1987;91:285–286.

327. Novey HS, Wells ID. Allergic bronchopulmonary aspergillosis caused by Aspergillus ochraceus. Am J Clin Pathol 1978;70:840–843.

328. Elliott MW, Newman Taylor AJ. Allergic bronchopulmonary aspergillosis. Clin Exp Allergy 1997;27 Suppl 1:55–59.

329. Thompson PJ. Allergic bronchopulmonary fungal disease. Postgrad Med J 1988;64 Suppl 4: 96–102.

330. Gefter W, Epstein D, Miller W. Allergic bronchopulmonary aspergillosis: less common patterns. Radiology 1981;140: 307–312.

331. Greene R. The pulmonary aspergilloses: three distinct entities or a spectrum of disease. Radiology 1981;140:527–530.

332. Bateman ED. A new look at the natural history of Aspergillus hypersensitivity in asthmatics. Respir Med 1994;88:325–327.

333. Rosenberg M, Patterson R, Mintzer R, et al. Clinical and immunologic criteria for the diagnosis of allergic bronchopulmonary aspergillosis. Ann Intern Med 1977;86:405–414.

334. Greenberger PA, Patterson R. Allergic bronchopulmonary aspergillosis. Model of bronchopulmonary disease with defined serologic, radiologic, pathologic and clinical findings from asthma to fatal destructive lung disease. Chest 1987;91: 165S–171S.

335. Glancy JJ, Elder JL, McAleer R. Allergic bronchopulmonary fungal disease without clinical asthma. Thorax 1981;36:345–349.

336. Henderson AH. Allergic aspergillosis: review of 32 cases. Thorax 1968;23: 501–512.

337. Phelan MS, Kerr IH. Allergic broncho-pulmonary aspergillosis: the radiological appearance during long-term follow-up. Clin Radiol 1984;35:385–392.

338. Imbeau SA, Cohen M, Reed CE. Allergic bronchopulmonary aspergillosis in infants. Am J Dis Child 1977;131: 1127–1130.

339. Malo JL, Pepys J, Simon G. Studies in chronic allergic bronchopulmonary aspergillosis. 2. Radiological findings. Thorax 1977;32:262–268.

340. McCarthy DS, Simon G, Hargreave FE. The radiological appearances in allergic broncho-pulmonary aspergillosis. Clin Radiol 1970;21:366–375.

341. Panchal N, Bhagat R, Pant C, et al. Allergic bronchopulmonary aspergillosis: the spectrum of computed tomography appearances. Respir Med 1997;91:213–219.

342. Huchton DM. Allergic fungal sinusitis: an otorhinolaryngologic perspective. Allergy Asthma Proc 2003;24:307–311.

343. Willard CC, Eusterman VD, Massengil PL. Allergic fungal sinusitis: Report of 3 cases and review of the literature. Oral Surg Oral Med Oral Pathol Oral Radiol Endod 2003;96:550–560.

344. Venarske DL, deShazo RD. Sinobronchial allergic mycosis: the SAM syndrome. Chest 2002;121:1670–1676.

345. Schubert MS, Goetz DW. Evaluation and treatment of allergic fungal sinusitis. I. Demographics and diagnosis. J Allergy Clin Immunol 1998;102:387–394.

346. deShazo RD, Swain RE. Diagnostic criteria for allergic fungal sinusitis. J Allergy Clin Immunol 1995;96:24–35.

347. Manning S, Merkel M, Kriesel K, et al. Computed tomography and magnetic resonance imaging diagnosis of allergic fungal sinusitis. Laryngoscope 1997;107:170–176.

348. Patterson R, Greenberger PA, Radin RC, et al. Allergic bronchopulmonary aspergillosis: staging as an aid to management. Ann Intern Med 1982;96:286–291.

349. Hoehne JH, Reed CE, Dickie HA. Allergic bronchopulmonary aspergillosis is not rare. With a note on preparation of antigen for immunologic tests. Chest 1973;63:177–181.

350. Currie DC, Goldman JM, Cole PJ, et al. Comparison of narrow section computed tomography and plain chest radiography in chronic allergic bronchopulmonary aspergillosis. Clin Radiol 1987;38:593–596.

351. Greenberger PA. Allergic bronchopulmonary aspergillosis and fungoses. Clin Chest Med 1988;9:599–608.

352. Greenberger PA, Miller TP, Roberts M, et al. Allergic bronchopulmonary aspergillosis in patients with and without evidence of bronchiectasis. Ann Allergy Asthma Immunol 1993;70:333–338.

353. Kumar R, Chopra D. Evaluation of allergic bronchopulmonary aspergillosis in patients with and without central bronchiectasis. J Asthma 2002;39: 473–477.

354. Kumar R. Mild, moderate, and severe forms of allergic bronchopulmonary aspergillosis: a clinical and serologic evaluation. Chest 2003;124:890–892.

355. Eaton T, Garrett J, Milne D, et al. Allergic bronchopulmonary aspergillosis in the asthma clinic. A prospective evaluation of CT in the diagnostic algorithm. Chest 2000;118:66–72.

356. Zimmerman RA, Miller WT. Pulmonary aspergillosis. Am J Roentgenol Radium Ther Nucl Med 1970;109:505–517.

357. Lipinski JK, Weisbrod GL, Sanders DE. Unusual manifestations of pulmonary aspergillosis. J Can Assoc Radiol 1978;29:216–220.

358. Mintzer RA, Rogers LF, Kruglik GD, et al. The spectrum of radiologic findings in allergic bronchopulmonary aspergillosis. Radiology 1978;127:301–307.

359. Goyal R, White CS, Templeton PA, et al. High attenuation mucous plugs in allergic bronchopulmonary aspergillosis: CT appearance. J Comput Assist Tomogr 1992;16:649–650.

360. Logan PM, Müller NL. High-attenuation mucous plugging in allergic bronchopulmonary aspergillosis. Can Assoc Radiol J 1996;47:374–377.

361. Berkin KE, Vernon DR, Kerr JW. Lung collapse caused by allergic bronchopulmonary aspergillosis in non-asthmatic patients. Br Med J (Clin Res Ed) 1982;285:552–553.

362. Hopkirk JA, Stark JE. Unilateral pulmonary collapse in asthmatics. Thorax 1978;33:207–210.

363. Murphy D, Lane DJ. Pleural effusion in allergic bronchopulmonary aspergillosis: two case reports. Br J Dis Chest 1981;75:91–95.

364. Neeld DA, Goodman LR, Gurney JW, et al. Computerized tomography in the evaluation of allergic bronchopulmonary aspergillosis. Am Rev Respir Dis 1990;142:1200–1205.

365. Reiff DB, Wells AU, Carr DH, et al. CT findings in bronchiectasis: limited value in distinguishing between idiopathic and specific types. AJR Am J Roentgenol 1995;165:261–267.

366. Angus RM, Davies ML, Cowan MD, et al. Computed tomographic scanning of the lung in patients with allergic bronchopulmonary aspergillosis and in asthmatic patients with a positive skin test to *Aspergillus fumigatus*. Thorax 1994;49:586–589.

367. Cartier Y, Kavanagh PV, Johkoh T, et al. Bronchiectasis: accuracy of high-resolution CT in the differentiation of specific diseases. AJR Am J Roentgenol 1999;173:47–52.

368. Mitchell TA, Hamilos DL, Lynch DA, et al. Distribution and severity of bronchiectasis in allergic bronchopulmonary aspergillosis (ABPA). J Asthma 2000;37:65–72.

369. Ward S, Heyneman L, Lee MJ, et al. Accuracy of CT in the diagnosis of allergic bronchopulmonary aspergillosis in asthmatic patients. AJR Am J Roentgenol 1999;173:937–942.

370. Phelan M, Kerr I. Allergic bronchopulmonary aspergillosis: the radiologic appearance during long-term follow-up. Clin Radiol 1984;35:385–392.

371. Ein ME, Wallace RJ Jr, Williams TW Jr. Allergic bronchopulmonary aspergillosis-like syndrome consequent to aspergilloma. Am Rev Respir Dis 1979;119:811–820.

372. Geller DE, Kaplowitz H, Light MJ, et al. Allergic bronchopulmonary aspergillosis in cystic fibrosis: reported prevalence, regional distribution, and patient characteristics. Scientific Advisory Group, Investigators, and Coordinators of the Epidemiologic Study of Cystic Fibrosis. Chest 1999;116:639–646.

373. Stevens DA, Moss RB, Kurup VP, et al. Allergic bronchopulmonary aspergillosis in cystic fibrosis – state of the art: Cystic Fibrosis Foundation Consensus Conference. Clin Infect Dis 2003;37 Suppl 3:S225–264.

374. Mastella G, Rainisio M, Harms HK, et al. Allergic bronchopulmonary aspergillosis in cystic fibrosis. A European epidemiological study. Epidemiologic Registry of Cystic Fibrosis. Eur Respir J 2000;16:464–471.

375. Cooper JA Jr, White DA, Matthay RA. Drug-induced pulmonary disease. Part 2: Noncytotoxic drugs. Am Rev Respir Dis 1986;133:488–505.

376. Spry C. Eosinophils: a comprehensive review, and guide to the scientific and medical literature. Oxford: Oxford University Press, 1988.

377. Janier M, Guillevin L, Badillet G. Pulmonary eosinophilia associated with dapsone. Lancet 1994;343:860–861.

378. Wong PC, Yew WW, Wong CF, et al. Ethambutol-induced pulmonary infiltrates with eosinophilia and skin involvement. Eur Respir J 1995;8:866–868.

379. Dykhuizen RS, Zaidi AM, Godden DJ, et al. Minocycline and pulmonary eosinophilia. Br Med J 1995;310:1520–1521.

380. Morrison DA, Goldman AL. Radiographic patterns of drug-induced lung diseases. Radiology 1979;131:299–304.

381. Dupon M, Malou M, Rogues AM, et al. Acute eosinophilic pneumonia induced by inhaled pentamidine isethionate. Br Med J 1993;306:109.

382. Begbie S, Burgess KR. Maloprim-induced pulmonary eosinophilia. Chest 1993;103:305–306.

383. Kondo K, Inoue Y, Hamada H, et al. Acetaminophen-induced eosinophilic pneumonia. Chest 1993;104:291–292.

384. Khalil H, Molinary E, Stoller JK. Diclofenac (Voltaren)-induced eosinophilic pneumonitis. Case report and review of the literature. Arch Intern Med 1993;153:1649–1652.

385. Goodwin SD, Glenny RW. Nonsteroidal anti-inflammatory drug-associated pulmonary infiltrates with eosinophilia. Review of the literature and Food and Drug Administration Adverse Drug Reaction reports. Arch Intern Med 1992;152:1521–1524.

386. Myers J. Pathology of drug-induced lung disease. In: Katzenstein A-L, ed. Katzenstein and Askin's surgical pathology of non-neoplastic lung disease, 3rd edn. Philadelphia: WB Saunders, 1997.

387. Nader DA, Schillaci RF. Pulmonary infiltrates with eosinophilia due to naproxen. Chest 1983;83:280–282.

388. Cooper JA Jr, White DA, Matthay RA. Drug-induced pulmonary disease. Part 1: Cytotoxic drugs. Am Rev Respir Dis 1986;133:321–340.

389. Bondi E, Slater S. Tolazamide-induced chronic eosinophilic pneumonia. Chest 1981;80:652.

390. Cullinan SA, Bower GC. Acute pulmonary hypersensitivity to carbamazepine. Chest 1975;68:580–581.

391. Hendrickson RM, Simpson F. Clofibrate and eosinophilic pneumonia. JAMA 1982;247:3082.

392. Nadeem S, Nasir N, Israel RH. Loffler's syndrome secondary to crack cocaine. Chest 1994;105:1599–1600.

393. Seebach J, Speich R, Fehr J, et al. GM-CSF-induced acute eosinophilic pneumonia. Br J Haematol 1995;90:963–965.

394. Davies D, Jones JK. Pulmonary eosinophilia caused by penicillamine. Thorax 1980;35:957–958.

395. Phy JL, Weiss WT, Weiler CR, et al. Hypersensitivity to progesterone-in-oil after in vitro fertilization and embryo transfer. Fertil Steril 2003;80:1272–1275.

396. Tazelaar HD, Myers JL, Drage CW, et al. Pulmonary disease associated with L-tryptophan-induced eosinophilic myalgia syndrome. Clinical and pathologic features. Chest 1990;97:1032–1036.

397. Strumpf IJ, Drucker RD, Anders KH, et al. Acute eosinophilic pulmonary disease associated with the ingestion of L-tryptophan-containing products. Chest 1991;99:8–13.

398. Ottesen EA, Nutman TB. Tropical pulmonary eosinophilia. Annu Rev Med 1992;43:417–424.

399. Udwadia FE. Tropical eosinophilia: a review. Respir Med 1993;87:17–21.

400. Donohugh D. Tropical eosinophilia. An etiologic inquiry. N Engl J Med 1963;269:1357–1364.

401. Herlinger H. Pulmonary changes in tropical eosinophilia. Br J Radiol 1963;36:889–901.

402. Neva FA, Ottesen EA. Tropical (filarial) eosinophilia. N Engl J Med 1978;298:1129–1131.

403. Dalrymple W. Tropical eosinophilia. Report of two cases occurring more than a year after departure from India. N Engl J Med 1955;252:585–586.

404. Khoo F, Danaraj T. The roentgenographic appearance of eosinophilic lung (tropical eosinophilia). AJR Am J Roentgenol 1960;83:251–259.

405. Spry CJ, Kumaraswami V. Tropical eosinophilia. Semin Hematol 1982;19:107–115.

406. Ball J. Tropical pulmonary eosinophilia. Trans Roy Soc Trop Med Hyg 1950;44:237–258.

407. Basu S. X-ray appearances in the lung fields in tropical eosinophilia. Indian Med Gaz 1954;89:212–217.

408. Jain VK, Beniwal OP. Unusual presentation of tropical pulmonary eosinophilia. Thorax 1984;39:634–635.

409. Islam N, Haq A. Eosinophilic lung abscess – a new entity. Br Med J 1962;1:1810–1811.

410. Webb J, Job C, Gault E. Tropical eosinophilia. Demonstration of microfilariae in lung, liver, and lymph-nodes. Lancet 1960;i:835–842.

411. Sandhu M, Mukhopadhyay S, Sharma SK. Tropical pulmonary eosinophilia: a comparative evaluation of plain chest radiography and computed tomography. Australas Radiol 1996;40:32–37.

412. Reeder MM, Palmer PE. Acute tropical pneumonias. Semin Roentgenol 1980;15:35–49.

413. Gelpi AP, Mustafa A. Ascaris pneumonia. Am J Med 1968;44:377–389.

414. Phills JA, Harrold AJ, Whiteman GV, et al. Pulmonary infiltrates, asthma and eosinophilia due to *Ascaris suum* infestation in man. N Engl J Med 1972;286:965–970.

415. Roig J, Romeu J, Riera C, et al. Acute eosinophilic pneumonia due to toxocariasis with bronchoalveolar lavage findings. Chest 1992;102:294–296.

416. Butland RJ, Coulson IH. Pulmonary eosinophilia associated with cutaneous larva migrans. Thorax 1985;40:76–77.

417. De Leon EP, Pardo de Tavera M. Pulmonary schistosomiasis in the Philippines. Dis Chest 1968;53:154–161.

418. Wright D, Gold E. Loeffler's syndrome associated with creeping eruption (cutaneous helminthiasis). Arch Intern Med 1946;78:303–312.

419. Woodring JH, Halfhill H 2nd, Reed JC. Pulmonary strongyloidiasis: clinical and imaging features. AJR Am J Roentgenol 1994;162:537–542.

420. Liebow AA. The J. Burns Amberson lecture – pulmonary angiitis and granulomatosis. Am Rev Respir Dis 1973;108:1–18.

421. Katzenstein AL, Liebow AA, Friedman PJ. Bronchocentric granulomatosis, mucoid impaction, and hypersensitivity reactions to fungi. Am Rev Respir Dis 1975;111:497–537.

422. Saldana M. Bronchocentric granulomatosis: Clinicopathologic observations in 17 patients. Lab Invest 1979;40:281–282.

423. Koss MN, Robinson RG, Hochholzer L. Bronchocentric granulomatosis. Hum Pathol 1981;12:632–638.

424. Ward S, Heyneman LE, Flint JD, et al. Bronchocentric granulomatosis: computed tomographic findings in five patients. Clin Radiol 2000;55:296–300.

425. Berendsen HH, Hofstee N, Kapsenberg PD, et al. Bronchocentric granulomatosis associated with seropositive polyarthritis. Thorax 1985;40:396–397.

426. Rohatgi PK, Turrisi BC. Bronchocentric granulomatosis and ankylosing spondylitis. Thorax 1984;39:317–318.

427. Warren J, Pitchenik AE, Saldana MJ. Bronchocentric granulomatosis with glomerulonephritis. Chest 1985;87:832–834.

428. Den Hertog RW, Wagenaar SS, Wastermann CJ. Bronchocentric granulomatosis and pulmonary echinococcosis. Am Rev Respir Dis 1982;126:344–347.

429. Robinson RG, Wehunt WD, Tsou E, et al. Bronchocentric granulomatosis: roentgenographic manifestations. Am Rev Respir Dis 1982;125:751–756.

430. Frazier AA, Rosado-de-Christenson ML, Galvin JR, et al. Pulmonary angiitis and granulomatosis: radiologic-pathologic correlation. RadioGraphics 1998;18:687–710.

431. Clee MD, Lamb D, Urbaniak SJ, et al. Progressive bronchocentric granulomatosis: case report. Thorax 1982;37:947–949.

432. Katzenstein A-L. Katzenstein and Askin's Surgical pathology of non-neoplastic lung disease, 3 edn. Philadelphia: WB Saunders, 1997.

433. Hanson G, Flor N, Wells I, et al. Bronchocentric granulomatosis: a complication of allergic bronchopulmonary aspergillosis. J Allergy Clin Immunol 1977;59:83–90.

434. Bain BJ. Eosinophilic leukaemias and the idiopathic hypereosinophilic syndrome. Br J Haematol 1996;95:2–9.

435. Chusid MJ, Dale DC, West BC, et al. The hypereosinophilic syndrome: analysis of fourteen cases with review of the literature. Medicine (Baltimore) 1975;54:1–27.

436. Epstein DM, Taormina V, Gefter WB, et al. The hypereosinophilic syndrome. Radiology 1981;140:59–62.

437. Fauci AS, Harley JB, Roberts WC, et al. NIH conference. The idiopathic hypereosinophilic syndrome. Clinical, pathophysiologic, and therapeutic considerations. Ann Intern Med 1982;97:78–92.

438. Parrillo JE, Borer JS, Henry WL, Wolff SM, Fauci AS. The cardiovascular manifestations of the hypereosinophilic syndrome. Prospective study of 26 patients, with review of the literature. Am J Med 1979;67:572–582.

439. Kang EY, Shim JJ, Kim JS, et al. Pulmonary involvement of idiopathic hypereosinophilic syndrome: CT findings in five patients. J Comput Assist Tomogr 1997;21:612–615.

440. Parrillo JE, Fauci AS, Wolff SM. Therapy of the hypereosinophilic syndrome. Ann Intern Med 1978;89:167–172.

441. Luksza AR, Jones DK. Comparison of whole-blood eosinophil counts in extrinsic asthmatics with acute and chronic asthma. Br Med J (Clin Res Ed) 1982;285:1229–1231.

442. Davis SD, Schaller J, Wedgwood RJ. Job's Syndrome. Recurrent, "cold", staphylococcal abscesses. Lancet 1966;1:1013–1015.

443. Donabedian H, Gallin JI. The hyperimmunoglobulin E recurrent-infection (Job's) syndrome. A review of the NIH experience and the literature. Medicine (Baltimore) 1983;62:195–208.

444. Merten DF, Buckley RH, Pratt PC, et al. Hyperimmunoglobulinemia E syndrome: radiographic observations. Radiology 1979;132:71–78.

445. Kirchner SG, Sivit CJ, Wright PF. Hyperimmunoglobulinemia E syndrome: association with osteoporosis and recurrent fractures. Radiology 1985;156:362.

446. Buckley RH, Wray BB, Belmaker EZ. Extreme hyperimmunoglobulinemia E and undue susceptibility to infection. Pediatrics 1972;49:59–70.

447. Manson DE, Sikka S, Reid B, et al. Primary immunodeficiencies: a pictorial immunology primer for radiologists. Pediatr Radiol 2000;30:501–510.

448. Jhaveri KS, Sahani DV, Shetty PG, et al. Hyperimmunoglobulinaemia E syndrome: pulmonary imaging features. Australas Radiol 2000;44:328–330.

449. Santambrogio L, Nosotti M, Pavoni G, et al. Pneumatocele complicated by fungal lung abscess in Job's syndrome. Successful lobectomy with the aid of videothoracoscopy. Scand Cardiovasc J 1997;31:177–179.

450. Fitch SJ, Magill HL, Herrod HG, et al. Hyperimmunoglobulinemia E syndrome: pulmonary imaging considerations. Pediatr Radiol 1986;16:285–288.

451. Rosen S, Castleman B, Liebow A. Pulmonary alveolar proteinosis. N Engl J Med 1958;258:1123–1142.

452. Prakash UB, Barham SS, Carpenter HA, et al. Pulmonary alveolar phospholipoproteinosis: experience with 34 cases and a review. Mayo Clin Proc 1987;62:499–518.

453. Davidson JM, Macleod WM. Pulmonary alveolar proteinosis. Br J Dis Chest 1969;63:13–28.

454. McEuen DD, Abraham JL. Particulate concentrations in pulmonary alveolar proteinosis. Environ Res 1978;17:334–339.

455. Heppleston AG, Wright NA, Stewart JA. Experimental alveolar lipo-proteinosis following the inhalation of silica. J Pathol 1970;101:293–307.

456. Buechner HA, Ansari A. Acute silico-proteinosis. A new pathologic variant of acute silicosis in sandblasters, characterized by histologic features resembling alveolar proteinosis. Dis Chest 1969;55:274–278.

457. Suratt PM, Winn WC Jr, Brody AR, et al. Acute silicosis in tombstone sandblasters. Am Rev Respir Dis 1977;115:521–539.

458. Miller RR, Churg AM, Hutcheon M, et al. Pulmonary alveolar proteinosis and aluminum dust exposure. Am Rev Respir Dis 1984;130:312–315.

459. Keller CA, Frost A, Cagle PT, et al. Pulmonary alveolar proteinosis in a painter with elevated pulmonary concentrations of titanium. Chest 1995;108:277–280.

460. Tran Van Nhieu J, Vojtek AM, Bernaudin JF, et al. Pulmonary alveolar proteinosis associated with *Pneumocystis carinii*. Ultrastructural identification in bronchoalveolar lavage in AIDS and immunocompromised non-AIDS patients. Chest 1990;98:801–805.

461. Carnovale R, Zornoza J, Goldman AM, et al. Pulmonary alveolar proteinosis: its association with hematologic malignancy and lymphoma. Radiology 1977;122:303–306.

462. Bedrossian CW, Luna MA, Conklin RH, et al. Alveolar proteinosis as a consequence of immunosuppression. A hypothesis based on clinical and pathologic observations. Hum Pathol 1980;11:527–535.

463. Colon AR Jr, Lawrence RD, Mills SD, et al. Childhood pulmonary alveolar proteinosis (PAP). Report of a case and review of the literature. Am J Dis Child 1971;121:481–485.

464. Jennings VM, Dillehay DL, Webb SK, et al. Pulmonary alveolar proteinosis in SCID mice. Am J Respir Cell Mol Biol 1995;13:297–306.

465. Mahut B, Delacourt C, Scheinmann P, et al. Pulmonary alveolar proteinosis: experience with eight pediatric cases and a review. Pediatrics 1996;97:117–122.

466. Stanley E, Lieschke GJ, Grail D, et al. Granulocyte/macrophage colony-stimulating factor-deficient mice show no major perturbation of hematopoiesis but develop a characteristic pulmonary pathology. Proc Natl Acad Sci USA 1994;91:5592–5596.

467. Yousem SA. Alveolar lipoproteinosis in lung allograft recipients. Hum Pathol 1997;28:1383–1386.

468. Chetcuti PA, Ball RJ. Surfactant apoprotein B deficiency. Arch Dis Child Fetal Neonatal Edn 1995;73:F125–127.

469. Seymour JF, Presneill JJ. Pulmonary alveolar proteinosis: progress in the first 44 years. Am J Respir Crit Care Med 2002;166:215–235.

470. Bonfield TL, Russell D, Burgess S, et al. Autoantibodies against granulocyte macrophage colony-stimulating factor are diagnostic for pulmonary alveolar proteinosis. Am J Respir Cell Mol Biol 2002;27:481–486.

471. Kitamura T, Uchida K, Tanaka N, et al. Serological diagnosis of idiopathic pulmonary alveolar proteinosis. Am J Respir Crit Care Med 2000;162:658–662.

472. Rubin E, Weisbrod GL, Sanders DE. Pulmonary alveolar proteinosis: relationship to silicosis and pulmonary infection. Radiology 1980;135:35–41.

473. Anton HC, Gray B. Pulmonary alveolar proteinosis presenting with pneumothorax. Clin Radiol 1967;18:428–431.

474. Wang BM, Stern EJ, Schmidt RA, et al. Diagnosing pulmonary alveolar proteinosis. A review and an update. Chest 1997;111:460–466.

475. Honda Y, Kuroki Y, Matsuura E, et al. Pulmonary surfactant protein D in sera and bronchoalveolar lavage fluids. Am J Respir Crit Care Med 1995;152:1860–1866.

476. Miller PA, Ravin CE, Smith GJ, et al. Pulmonary alveolar proteinosis with interstitial involvement. AJR Am J Roentgenol 1981;137:1069–1071.

477. Ramirez R. Pulmonary alveolar proteinosis. A roentgenologic analysis. AJR Am J Roentgenol 1964;92:571–577.

478. McCook TA, Kirks DR, Merten DF, et al. Pulmonary alveolar proteinosis in children. AJR Am J Roentgenol 1981;137:1023–1027.

479. Phillips W, Constance T. Pulmonary alveolar proteinosis. Med J Aust 1963;2:357–359.

480. Preger L. Pulmonary alveolar proteinosis. Radiology 1969;92:1291–1295.

481. Godwin J, Müller N, Takasugi J. Pulmonary alveolar proteinosis: CT findings. Radiology 1988;169:609–613.

482. Lee KN, Levin DL, Webb WR, et al. Pulmonary alveolar proteinosis: high-resolution CT, chest radiographic, and functional correlations. Chest 1997;111:989–995.

483. Murch CR, Carr DH. Computed tomography appearances of pulmonary alveolar proteinosis. Clin Radiol 1989;40:240–243.

484. Newell JD, Underwood GH, Russo DJ, et al. Computed tomographic appearance of pulmonary alveolar proteinosis in adults. CT 1984;8:21–29.

485. Holbert JM, Costello P, Li W, et al. CT features of pulmonary alveolar proteinosis. AJR Am J Roentgenol 2001;176:1287–1294.

486. Rossi SE, Erasmus JJ, Volpacchio M, et al. "Crazy-paving" pattern at thin-section CT of the lungs: radiologic–pathologic overview. Radiographics 2003;23:1509–1519.

487. Murayama S, Murakami J, Yabuuchi H, et al. "Crazy paving appearance" on high resolution CT in various diseases. J Comput Assist Tomogr 1999;23:749–752.

488. Franquet T, Gimenez A, Bordes R, et al. The crazy-paving pattern in exogenous lipoid pneumonia: CT-pathologic correlation. AJR. Am J Roentgenol 1998;170:315–317.

489. Tan RT, Kuzo RS. High-resolution CT findings of mucinous bronchioloalveolar carcinoma: a case of pseudopulmonary alveolar proteinosis. AJR Am J Roentgenol 1997;168:99–100.

490. Coche E, Weynand B, Noirhomme P, et al. Non-specific interstitial pneumonia showing a "crazy paving" pattern on high resolution CT. Br J Radiol 2001;74:189–191.

491. Witty LA, Tapson VF, Piantadosi CA. Isolation of mycobacteria in patients with pulmonary alveolar proteinosis. Medicine (Baltimore) 1994;73:103–109.

492. Goldschmidt N, Nusair S, Gural A, et al. Disseminated *Mycobacterium kansasii* infection with pulmonary alveolar proteinosis in a patient with chronic myelogenous leukemia. Am J Hematol 2003;74:221–223.

493. Ramirez J. Bronchopulmonary lavage. New techniques and observations. Dis Chest 1966;50:581–588.

494. Rogers RM, Levin DC, Gray BA, et al. Physiologic effects of bronchopulmonary lavage in alveolar proteinosis. Am Rev Respir Dis 1978;118:255–264.

495. Gale ME, Karlinsky JB, Robins AG. Bronchopulmonary lavage in pulmonary alveolar proteinosis: chest radiograph observations. AJR Am J Roentgenol 1986;146:981–985.

496. Parker LA, Novotny DB. Recurrent alveolar proteinosis following double lung transplantation. Chest 1997;111:1457–1458.

497. Harbitz F. Extensive calcification of the lungs as a distinct disease. Arch Intern Med 1918;21:139–146.

498. Ucan ES, Keyf AI, Aydilek R, et al. Pulmonary alveolar microlithiasis:

review of Turkish reports. Thorax 1993;48:171–173.

499. Chalmers AG, Wyatt J, Robinson PJ. Computed tomographic and pathological findings in pulmonary alveolar microlithiasis. Br J Radiol 1986;59:408–411.

500. Pant K, Shah A, Mathur RK, et al. Pulmonary alveolar microlithiasis with pleural calcification and nephrolithiasis. Chest 1990;98:245–246.

501. Coetzee T. Pulmonary alveolar microlithiasis with involvement of the sympathetic nervous system and gonads. Thorax 1970;25:637–642.

502. Sears MR, Chang AR, Taylor AJ. Pulmonary alveolar microlithiasis. Thorax 1971;26:704–711.

503. Prakash UB, Barham SS, Rosenow EC, et al. Pulmonary alveolar microlithiasis. A review including ultrastructural and pulmonary function studies. Mayo Clin Proc 1983;58:290–300.

504. Sosman MC, Dodd GD, Jones WD, et al. The familial occurrence of pulmonary alveolar microlithiasis. Am J Roentgenol Radium Ther Nucl Med 1957;77:947–1012.

505. Castellana G, Gentile M, Castellana R, et al. Pulmonary alveolar microlithiasis: clinical features, evolution of the phenotype, and review of the literature. Am J Med Genet 2002;111:220–224.

506. Schmidt H, Lorcher U, Kitz R, et al. Pulmonary alveolar microlithiasis in children. Ped Radiol 1996;26:33–36.

507. Ritchie DA, O'Connor SA, McGivern D. An unusual presentation of pulmonary alveolar microlithiasis and diaphyseal aclasia. Br J Radiol 1992;65:178–181.

508. Caffrey P, Altman R. Pulmonary alveolar microlithiasis occurring in premature twins. J Pediatr 1965;66:758–763.

509. Mascie-Taylor BH, Wardman AG, Madden CA, et al. A case of alveolar microlithiasis: observation over 22 years and recovery of material by lavage. Thorax 1985;40:952–953.

510. Pracyk JB, Simonson SG, Young SL, et al. Composition of lung lavage in pulmonary alveolar microlithiasis. Respiration 1996;63:254–260.

511. Chan ED, Morales DV, Welsh CH, et al. Calcium deposition with or without bone formation in the lung. Am J Respir Crit Care Med 2002;165:1654–1669.

512. Balikian JP, Fuleihan FJ, Nucho CN. Pulmonary alveolar microlithiasis. Report of five cases with special reference to roentgen manifestations. AJR Am J Roentgenol 1968;103:509–518.

513. Helbich TH, Wojnarovsky C, Wunderbaldinger P, et al. Pulmonary alveolar microlithiasis in children: radiographic and high-resolution CT findings. AJR Am J Roentgenol 1997;168:63–65.

514. Volle E, Kaufmann HJ. Pulmonary alveolar microlithiasis in pediatric patients – review of the world literature and two new observations. Ped Radiol 1987;17:439–442.

515. Felson B. Chest roentgenology. Philadelphia: WB Saunders, 1973.

516. Cluzel P, Grenier P, Bernadac P, et al. Pulmonary alveolar microlithiasis: CT findings. J Comput Assist Tomogr 1991;15:938–942.

517. Korn MA, Schurawitzki H, Klepetko W, et al. Pulmonary alveolar microlithiasis: findings on high-resolution CT. AJR Am J Roentgenol 1992;158:981–982.

518. Hoshino H, Koba H, Inomata S, et al. Pulmonary alveolar microlithiasis: high-resolution CT and MR findings. J Comput Assist Tomogr 1998;22:245–248.

519. Thurairajasingam S, Dharmasena BD, Kasthuriratna T. Pulmonary alveolar microlithiasis. Australas Radiol 1975;19:175–180.

520. Miro JM, Moreno A, Coca A, et al. Pulmonary alveolar microlithiasis with an unusual radiological pattern. Br J Dis Chest 1982;76:91–96.

521. Winzelberg GG, Boller M, Sachs M, et al. CT evaluation of pulmonary alveolar microlithiasis. J Comput Assist Tomogr 1984;8:1029–1031.

522. Chang YC, Yang PC, Luh KT, et al. High-resolution computed tomography of pulmonary alveolar microlithiasis. J Formos Med Assoc 1999;98:440–443.

523. Chai JL, Patz EF Jr. CT of the lung: patterns of calcification and other high-attenuation abnormalities. AJR Am J Roentgenol 1994;162:1063–1066.

524. Taguchi Y, Fuyuno G, Shioya S, et al. MR appearance of pulmonary metastatic calcification. J Comput Assist Tomogr 1996;20:38–41.

525. Kino T, Kohara Y, Tsuji S. Pulmonary alveolar microlithiasis. A report of two young sisters. Am Rev Respir Dis 1972;105:105–110.

526. Thind GS, Bhatia JL. Pulmonary alveolar microlithiasis. Br J Dis Chest 1978;72: 151–154.

527. Brown ML, Swee RG, Olson RJ, et al. Pulmonary uptake of ^{99m}Tc diphosphonate in alveolar microlithiasis. AJR Am J Roentgenol 1978;131:703–704.

528. Moran CA, Hochholzer L, Hasleton PS, et al. Pulmonary alveolar microlithiasis. A clinicopathologic and chemical analysis of seven cases. Arch Pathol Lab Med 1997;121:607–611.

529. Hartman TE, Müller NL, Primack SL, et al. Metastatic pulmonary calcification in patients with hypercalcemia: findings on chest radiographs and CT scans. AJR Am J Roentgenol 1994;162:799–802.

530. Lingam RK, Teh J, Sharma A, et al. Case report. Metastatic pulmonary calcification in renal failure: a new HRCT pattern. Br J Radiol 2002;75:74–77.

531. Ullmer E, Borer H, Sandoz P, et al. Diffuse pulmonary nodular infiltrates in a renal transplant recipient. Metastatic pulmonary calcification. Chest 2001;120:1394–1398.

532. Johkoh T, Ikezoe J, Nagareda T, et al. Metastatic pulmonary calcification: early detection by high-resolution CT. J Comput Assist Tomogr 1993;17: 471–473.

533. Gevenois PA, Abehsera M, Knoop C, et al. Disseminated pulmonary ossification in end-stage pulmonary fibrosis: CT demonstration. AJR Am J Roentgenol 1994;162:1303–1304.

534. Weinstein DS. Pulmonary sarcoidosis: calcified micronodular pattern simulating pulmonary alveolar microlithiasis. J Thorac Imaging 1999;14:218–220.

535. Aughenbaugh GL. Thoracic manifestations of neurocutaneous diseases. Radiol Clin North Am 1984;22:741–756.

536. Riccardi VM. Von Recklinghausen neurofibromatosis. N Engl J Med 1981;305:1617–1627.

537. Mulvihill JJ, Parry DM, Sherman JL, et al. NIH conference. Neurofibromatosis 1 (Recklinghausen disease) and neurofibromatosis 2 (bilateral acoustic neurofibromatosis). An update. Ann Intern Med 1990;113:39–52.

538. Klatte EC, Franken EA, Smith JA. The radiographic spectrum in neurofibromatosis. Semin Roentgenol 1976;11:17–33.

539. Neurofibromatosis. Conference statement. National Institutes of Health Consensus Development Conference. Arch Neurol 1988;45:575–578.

540. Schabel SI, Schmidt GE, Vujic I. Overlooked pulmonary malignancy in neurofibromatosis. J Can Assoc Radiol 1980;31:135–136.

541. Patel YD, Morehouse HT. Neurofibrosarcomas in neurofibromatosis: role of CT scanning and angiography. Clin Radiol 1982;33:555–560.

542. Kumar AJ, Kuhajda FP, Martinez CR, et al. Computed tomography of extracranial nerve sheath tumors with pathological correlation. J Comput Assist Tomogr 1983;7:857–865.

543. Felson B. The extrapleural space. Semin Roentgenol 1977;12:327–333.

544. Klaas VE. A diagnostic approach to asbestosis, utilizing clinical criteria, high resolution computed tomography, and gallium scanning. Am J Ind Med 1993;23:801–809.

545. Casselman ES, Miller WT, Shu Ren L, et al. Von Recklinghausen's disease: incidence of roentgenographic findings with a clinical review of the literature. CRC Crit Rev Diagn Imaging 1977;9:387–419.

546. Hunt J, Pugh D. Skeletal lesions in neurofibromatosis. Radiology 1961;76:1–20.

547. Rosenberg DM. Inherited forms of interstitial lung disease. Clin Chest Med 1982;3:635–641.

548. Holt JF. 1977 Edward B. D. Neuhauser lecture: neurofibromatosis in children. AJR Am J Roentgenol 1978;130:615–639.

549. Meszaros WT, Guzzo F, Schorsch H. Neurofibromatosis. Am J Roentgenol Radium Ther Nucl Med 1966;98:557–569.

550. Salerno NR, Edeiken J. Vertebral scalloping in neurofibromatosis. Radiology 1970;97:509–510.

551. Gibbens DT, Argy N. Chest case of the day. Lateral thoracic meningocele in a patient with neurofibromatosis. AJR Am J Roentgenol 1991;156:1299–1300.

552. Miles J, Pennybacker J, Sheldon P. Intrathoracic meningocele. Its development and association with neurofibromatosis. J Neurol Neurosurg Psychiatry 1969;32:99–110.

553. Dabir RR, Piccione W Jr, Kittle CF. Intrathoracic tumors of the vagus nerve. Ann Thorac Surg 1990;50:494–497.

554. Bourgouin PM, Shepard JO, Moore EH, et al. Plexiform neurofibromatosis of the mediastinum: CT appearance. AJR Am J Roentgenol 1988;151:461–463.

555. Chalmers AH, Armstrong P. Plexiform mediastinal neurofibromas. A report of two cases. Br J Radiol 1977;50:215–217.

556. Davies P. Diffuse pulmonary involvement in von Recklinghausen's disease. A new syndrome. Thorax 1963;18:198.

557. Patchefsky AS, Atkinson WG, Hoch WS, et al. Interstitial pulmonary fibrosis and von Recklinghausen's disease. An ultrastructural and immunofluorescent study. Chest 1973;64:459–464.

558. Massaro D, Katz S. Fibrosing alveolitis: its occurrence, roentgenographic, and pathologic features in von Recklinghausen's neurofibromatosis. Am Rev Respir Dis 1966;93:934–942.

559. Webb WR, Goodman PC. Fibrosing alveolitis in patients with neurofibromatosis. Radiology 1977;122:289–293.

560. De Scheerder I, Elinck W, Van Renterghem D, et al. Desquamative interstitial pneumonia and scar cancer of the lung complicating generalised neurofibromatosis. Eur J Respir Dis 1984;65:623–626.

561. Hardcastle SW, Hendricks ML. Neurofibromatosis (von Recklinghausen's disease) – an unusual cause of parenchymal lung disease. A case report. S Afr Med J 1984;66:959–960.

562. Stark P, Cheng GJ, Hildebrandt-Stark HE. [Pulmonary parenchymal and pleural fibrosis as an expression of Recklinghausen's neurofibromatosis]. Radiologe 1988;28:231–232.

563. Shimizu Y, Tsuchiya S, Watanabe S, et al. von Recklinghausen's disease with lung cancer derived from the wall of emphysematous bullae. Intern Med 1994;33:167–171.

564. Yokoyama A, Kohno N, Sakai K, et al. Distal acinar emphysema and interstitial pneumonia in a patient with von Recklinghausen's disease: five-year observation following quitting smoking. Intern Med 1997;36:413–416.

565. Miyamoto K. Pulmonary manifestations in von Recklinghausen's disease. Intern Med 1997;36:381.

566. North K. Neurofibromatosis type 1. Am J Med Genet 2000;97:119–127.

567. Reynolds RM, Browning GG, Nawroz I, et al. Von Recklinghausen's neurofibromatosis: neurofibromatosis type 1. Lancet 2003;361:1552–1554.

568. White JE, Greaves M, Mohan M, et al. Breathlessness with bumps, lumps, and humps. Chest 1994;105:589–590.

569. Madewell J, Feigin D. Benign tumors of the lung. Semin Roentgenol 1977;12:175–186.

570. Unger PD, Geller GA, Anderson PJ. Pulmonary lesions in a patient with neurofibromatosis. Arch Pathol Lab Med 1984;108:654–657.

571. Osborne JP, Fryer A, Webb D. Epidemiology of tuberous sclerosis. Ann N Y Acad Sci 1991;615:125–127.

572. Wienecke R, Maize JC Jr, Reed JA, et al. Expression of the TSC2 product tuberin and its target Rap1 in normal human tissues. Am J Pathol 1997;150:43–50.

573. Bell DG, King BF, Hattery RR, et al. Imaging characteristics of tuberous sclerosis. AJR Am J Roentgenol 1991;156:1081–1086.

574. Gomez MR. Phenotypes of the tuberous sclerosis complex with a revision of diagnostic criteria. Ann N Y Acad Sci 1991;615:1–7.

575. Roach ES, Smith M, Huttenlocher P, et al. Diagnostic criteria: tuberous sclerosis complex. Report of the Diagnostic Criteria Committee of the National Tuberous Sclerosis Association. J Child Neurol 1992;7:221–224.

576. Fleury P, de Groot WP, Delleman JW, et al. Tuberous sclerosis: the incidence of sporadic cases versus familial cases. Brain Dev 1980;2:107–117.

577. Mitnick JS, Bosniak MA, Hilton S, et al. Cystic renal disease in tuberous sclerosis. Radiology 1983;147:85–87.

578. Braffman BH, Bilaniuk LT, Naidich TP, et al. MR imaging of tuberous sclerosis: pathogenesis of this phakomatosis, use of gadopentetate dimeglumine, and literature review. Radiology 1992;183:227–238.

579. Dwyer JM, Hickie JB, Garvan J. Pulmonary tuberous sclerosis. Report of three patients and a review of the literature. Q J Med 1971;40:115–125.

580. Lie JT, Miller RD, Williams DE. Cystic disease of the lungs in tuberous sclerosis: clinicopathologic correlation, including body plethysmographic lung function tests. Mayo Clin Proc 1980;55:547–553.

581. Castro M, Shepherd CW, Gomez MR, et al. Pulmonary tuberous sclerosis. Chest 1995;107:189–195.

582. Costello LC, Hartman TE, Ryu JH. High frequency of pulmonary lymphangioleiomyomatosis in women with tuberous sclerosis complex. Mayo Clin Proc 2000;75:591–594.

583. Moss J, Avila NA, Barnes PM, et al. Prevalence and clinical characteristics of lymphangioleiomyomatosis (LAM) in patients with tuberous sclerosis complex. Am J Respir Crit Care Med 2001;164:669–671.

584. Corrin B, Liebow AA, Friedman PJ. Pulmonary lymphangiomyomatosis. A review. Am J Pathol 1975;79:348–382.

585. Maruyama H, Seyama K, Sobajima J, et al. Multifocal micronodular pneumocyte hyperplasia and lymphangioleiomyomatosis in tuberous sclerosis with a TSC2 gene. Mod Pathol 2001;14:609–614.

586. Popper HH, Juettner-Smolle FM, Pongratz MG. Micronodular hyperplasia of type II pneumocytes – a new lung lesion associated with tuberous sclerosis. Histopathology 1991;18:347–354.

587. Lantuejoul S, Ferretti G, Negoescu A, et al. Multifocal alveolar hyperplasia associated with lymphangioleiomyomatosis in tuberous sclerosis. Histopathology 1997;30:570–575.

588. Muir TE, Leslie KO, Popper H, et al. Micronodular pneumocyte hyperplasia. Am J Surg Pathol 1998;22:465–472.

589. Stovin PG, Lum LC, Flower CD, et al. The lungs in lymphangiomyomatosis and in tuberous sclerosis. Thorax 1975;30:497–509.

590. Valensi QJ. Pulmonary lymphangiomyoma, a probable forme fruste of tuberous sclerosis. A case report and survey of the literature. Am Rev Respir Dis 1973;108:1411–1415.

591. Foresti V, Casati O, Zubani R, et al. Chylous pleural effusion in tuberous sclerosis. Respiration 1990;57:398–401.

592. Jounieaux V, Druelle S, Mayeux I, et al. Progesterone treatment in chylothorax associated with pulmonary tuberous sclerosis. Eur Respir J 1996;9:2423–2425.

593. Luna CM, Gene R, Jolly EC, et al. Pulmonary lymphangiomyomatosis associated with tuberous sclerosis. Treatment with tamoxifen and tetracycline-pleurodesis. Chest 1985;88:473–475.

594. Ryu JH, Doerr CH, Fisher SD, et al. Chylothorax in lymphangioleiomyomatosis. Chest 2003;123:623–627.

595. Aubry MC, Myers JL, Ryu JH, et al. Pulmonary lymphangioleiomyomatosis in a man. Am J Respir Crit Care Med 2000;162:749–752.

596. Bowen J, Beasley SW. Rare pulmonary manifestations of tuberous sclerosis in children. Pediatr Pulmonol 1997;23: 114–116.

597. Harris JO, Waltuck BL, Swenson EW. The pathophysiology of the lungs in tuberous sclerosis. A case report and literature review. Am Rev Respir Dis 1969;100:379–387.

598. Green GJ. The radiology of tuberose sclerosis. Clin Radiol 1968;19:135–147.

599. Medley BE, McLeod RA, Houser OW. Tuberous sclerosis. Semin Roentgenol 1976;11:35–54.

600. Stern EJ, Webb WR, Golden JA, et al. Cystic lung disease associated with eosinophilic granuloma and tuberous sclerosis: air trapping at dynamic ultrafast high-resolution CT. Radiology 1992;182:325–329.

601. Lenoir S, Grenier P, Brauner MW, et al. Pulmonary lymphangiomyomatosis and tuberous sclerosis: comparison of radiographic and thin-section CT findings. Radiology 1990;175:329–334.

602. Polosa R, Magnano M, Crimi N, et al. Pulmonary tuberous sclerosis in a woman of child-bearing age with no mental retardation. Respir Med 1995;89:227–231.

603. Hanna RM, Dahniya MH, al-Marzouk N, et al. Extrarenal angiomyolipomas of the perinephric space in tuberose sclerosis. Australas Radiol 1997;41:339–341.

604. Pui MH, Kong HL, Choo HF. Bone changes in tuberous sclerosis mimicking metastases. Australas Radiol 1996;40: 77–79.

605. Pacheco-Rodriguez G, Kristof AS, Stevens LA, et al. Filley Lecture. Genetics and gene expression in lymphangioleiomyomatosis. Chest 2002;121:56S–60S.

606. Johnson SR, Clelland CA, Ronan J, et al. The TSC-2 product tuberin is expressed in lymphangioleiomyomatosis and angiomyolipoma. Histopathology 2002;40:458–463.

607. Avila NA, Kelly JA, Chu SC, et al. Lymphangioleiomyomatosis: abdominopelvic CT and US findings. Radiology 2000;216:147–153.

608. Bernstein S, Newell J, Adamczyk D, et al. How common are renal angiomyolipomas in patients with pulmonary lymphangiomyomatosis? Am J Respir Crit Care Med 1995;152:2138–2143.

609. Kerr L, Blute M, Ryu J, et al. Renal angiomyolipoma in association with pulmonary lymphangioleiomyomatosis: forme fruste of tuberous sclerosis? Urology 1993;41:440–444.

610. Carrington CB, Cugell DW, Gaensler EA, et al. Lymphangioleiomyomatosis. Physiologic–pathologic–radiologic correlations. Am Rev Respir Dis 1977;116:977–995.

611. Silverstein EF, Ellis K, Wolff M, et al. Pulmonary lymphangiomyomatosis. Am J Roentgenol Radium Ther Nucl Med 1974;120:832–850.

612. Kitaichi M, Izumi T. Lymphangioleiomyomatosis. Curr Opin Pulm Med 1995;1:417–424.

613. Kitaichi M, Nishimura K, Itoh H, et al. Pulmonary lymphangioleiomyomatosis: a report of 46 patients including a clinicopathologic study of prognostic factors. Am J Respir Crit Care Med 1995;151:527–533.

614. Wahedna I, Cooper S, Williams J, et al. Relation of pulmonary lymphangioleiomyomatosis to use of the oral contraceptive pill and fertility in the UK: a national case control study. Thorax 1994;49:910–914.

615. Taylor JR, Ryu J, Colby TV, et al. Lymphangioleiomyomatosis. Clinical course in 32 patients. N Engl J Med 1990;323:1254–1260.

616. Kalassian KG, Doyle R, Kao P, et al. Lymphangioleiomyomatosis: new insights. Am J Respir Crit Care Med 1997;155:1183–1186.

617. Johnson S. Rare diseases. 1. Lymphangioleiomyomatosis: clinical features, management and basic mechanisms. Thorax 1999;54:254–264.

618. Kelly J, Moss J. Lymphangioleiomyomatosis. Am J Med Sci 2001;321:17–25.

619. Hancock E, Osborne J. Lymphangioleiomyomatosis: a review of the literature. Respir Med 2002;96:1–6.

620. Kristof AS, Moss J. Lymphangioleiomyomatosis. In: Schwarz M, King T, eds. Interstitial lung disease, 4th edn. Toronto: Brian C Decker; 2003:851–864.

621. Fukuda Y, Kawamoto M, Yamamoto A, et al. Role of elastic fiber degradation in emphysema-like lesions of pulmonary lymphangiomyomatosis. Hum Pathol 1990;21:1252–1261.

622. Hayashi T, Fleming MV, Stetler-Stevenson WG, et al. Immunohistochemical study of matrix metalloproteinases (MMPs) and their tissue inhibitors (TIMPs) in pulmonary lymphangioleiomyomatosis (LAM). Hum Pathol 1997;28:1071–1078.

623. Bonetti F, Chiodera PL, Pea M, et al. Transbronchial biopsy in lymphangiomyomatosis of the lung. HMB45 for diagnosis. Am J Surg Pathol 1993;17:1092–1102.

624. Kruglik GD, Reed JC, Daroca PJ. Radiologic–pathologic correlation from the Armed Forces Institute of Pathology. Lymphangiomyomatosis. Radiology 1976;120:583–588.

625. Ernst JC, Sohaey R, Cary JM. Pelvic lymphangioleiomyomatosis. Atypical precursor to pulmonary disease. Chest 1994;106:1267–1269.

626. Guinee DG Jr, Feuerstein I, Koss MN, et al. Pulmonary lymphangioleiomyomatosis. Diagnosis based on results of transbronchial biopsy and immunohistochemical studies and correlation with high-resolution computed tomography findings. Arch Pathol Lab Med 1994;118:846–849.

627. Miller WT, Cornog JL Jr, Sullivan MA. Lymphangiomyomatosis. A clinical-roentgenologic-pathologic syndrome. Am J Roentgenol Radium Ther Nucl Med 1971;111:565–572.

628. Casper KA, Donnelly LF, Chen B, et al. Tuberous sclerosis complex: renal imaging findings. Radiology 2002;225:451–456.

629. Hoon V, Thung SN, Kaneko M, et al. HMB-45 reactivity in renal angiomyolipoma and lymphangioleiomyomatosis. Arch Pathol Lab Med 1994;118:732–734.

630. King TE Jr. Restrictive lung disease in pregnancy. Clin Chest Med 1992;13: 607–622.

631. Baldi S, Papotti M, Valente ML, et al. Pulmonary lymphangioleiomyomatosis in postmenopausal women: report of two cases and review of the literature. Eur Respir J 1994;7:1013–1016.

632. Maziak DE, Kesten S, Rappaport DC, et al. Extrathoracic angiomyolipomas in lymphangioleiomyomatosis. Eur Respir J 1996;9:402–405.

633. Urban T, Kuttenn F, Gompel A, et al. Pulmonary lymphangioleiomyomatosis. Follow-up and long-term outcome with antiestrogen therapy; a report of eight cases. Chest 1992;102:472–476.

634. Johnson SR, Tattersfield AE. Clinical experience of lymphangioleiomyomatosis in the UK. Thorax 2000;55:1052–1057.

635. Chu SC, Horiba K, Usuki J, et al. Comprehensive evaluation of 35 patients with lymphangioleiomyomatosis. Chest 1999;115:1041–1052.

636. Berkman N, Bloom A, Cohen P, et al. Bilateral spontaneous pneumothorax as the presenting feature in lymphangioleiomyomatosis. Respir Med 1995;89: 381–383.

637. Aberle DR, Hansell DM, Brown K, et al. Lymphangiomyomatosis: CT, chest radiographic, and functional correlations. Radiology 1990;176: 381–387.

638. Müller NL, Chiles C, Kullnig P. Pulmonary lymphangiomyomatosis: correlation of CT with radiographic and functional findings. Radiology 1990;175:335–339.

639. Rappaport D, Weisbrod G, Herman S, et al. Pulmonary lymphangioleiomyomatosis: High-resolution CT findings in four cases. AJR Am J Roentgenol 1989;152:961–964.

640. Sherrier RH, Chiles C, Roggli V. Pulmonary lymphangioleiomyomatosis: CT findings. AJR Am J Roentgenol 1989;153:937–940.

641. Templeton PA, McLoud TC, Müller NL, et al. Pulmonary lymphangioleiomyomatosis: CT and pathologic findings. J Comput Assist Tomogr 1989;13:54–57.

642. Lee KN, Yoon SK, Choi SJ, et al. Cystic lung disease: a comparison of cystic size, as seen on expiratory and inspiratory HRCT scans. Korean J Radiol 2000;1:84–90.

643. Worthy SA, Brown MJ, Müller NL. Technical report: Cystic air spaces in the lung: change in size on expiratory high-resolution CT in 23 patients. Clin Radiol 1998;53:515–519.

644. Crausman R, Lynch D, Mortenson R, et al. Quantitative CT predicts the severity of physiologic dysfunction in patients with lymphangioleiomyomatosis. Chest 1996;109:131–137.

645. Avila NA, Kelly JA, Dwyer AJ, et al. Lymphangioleiomyomatosis: correlation of qualitative and quantitative thin-section CT with pulmonary function tests and assessment of dependence on pleurodesis. Radiology 2002;223:189–197.

646. Pallisa E, Sanz P, Roman A, et al. Lymphangioleiomyomatosis: pulmonary and abdominal findings with pathologic correlation. RadioGraphics 2002;22 Spec No:S185–198.

647. Monteforte WJ Jr, Kohnen PW. Angiomyolipomas in a case of lymphangiomyomatosis syndrome: relationships to tuberous sclerosis. Cancer 1974;34:317–321.

648. Boehler A, Speich R, Russi EW, et al. Lung transplantation for lymphangioleiomyomatosis. N Engl J Med 1996;335:1275–1280.

649. Wong YY, Yeung TK, Chu WC. Atypical presentation of lymphangioleiomyomatosis as acute abdomen: CT diagnosis. AJR Am J Roentgenol 2003;181:284–285.

650. Avila NA, Bechtle J, Dwyer AJ, et al. Lymphangioleiomyomatosis: CT of diurnal variation of lymphangioleiomyomas. Radiology 2001;221:415–421.

651. Eliasson AH, Phillips YY, Tenholder MF. Treatment of lymphangioleiomyomatosis. A meta-analysis. Chest 1989;96:1352–1355.

652. Karbowniczek M, Astrinidis A, Balsara BR, et al. Recurrent lymphangiomyomatosis after transplantation: genetic analyses reveal a metastatic mechanism. Am J Respir Crit Care Med 2003;167:976–982.

653. O'Brien JD, Lium JH, Parosa JF, et al. Lymphangiomyomatosis recurrence in the allograft after single-lung transplantation. Am J Respir Crit Care Med 1995;151:2033–2036.

654. Bittmann I, Rolf B, Amann G, et al. Recurrence of lymphangioleiomyomatosis after single lung transplantation: new insights into pathogenesis. Hum Pathol 2003;34:95–98.

655. Garg K, Lynch DA, Newell JD. Inflammatory airways disease in ulcerative colitis: CT and high-resolution CT features. J Thorac Imaging 1993;8:159–163.

656. Camus P, Piard F, Ashcroft T, et al. The lung in inflammatory bowel disease. Medicine (Baltimore) 1993;72:151–183.

657. Prince JS, Duhamel DR, Levin DL, et al. Nonneoplastic lesions of the tracheobronchial wall: radiologic findings with bronchoscopic correlation. RadioGraphics 2002;22 Spec No:S215–230.

658. Kuzniar T, Sleiman C, Brugiere O, et al. Severe tracheobronchial stenosis in a patient with Crohn's disease. Eur Respir J 2000;15:209–212.

659. Desai SJ, Gephardt GN, Stoller JK. Diffuse panbronchiolitis preceding ulcerative colitis. Chest 1989;95:1342–1344.

660. Wilcox P, Miller R, Miller G, et al. Airway involvement in ulcerative colitis. Chest 1987;92:18–22.

661. Casey MB, Tazelaar HD, Myers JL, et al. Noninfectious lung pathology in patients with Crohn's disease. Am J Surg Pathol 2003;27:213–219.

662. Haralambou G, Teirstein AS, Gil J, et al. Bronchiolitis obliterans in a patient with ulcerative colitis receiving mesalamine. Mt Sinai J Med 2001;68:384–388.

663. Mahajan L, Kay M, Wyllie R, et al. Ulcerative colitis presenting with bronchiolitis obliterans organizing pneumonia in a pediatric patient. Am J Gastroenterol 1997;92:2123–2124.

664. Swinburn CR, Jackson GJ, Cobden I, et al. Bronchiolitis obliterans organising pneumonia in a patient with ulcerative colitis. Thorax 1988;43:735–736.

665. Mahadeva R, Walsh G, Flower CD, et al. Clinical and radiological characteristics of lung disease in inflammatory bowel disease. Eur Respir J 2000;15:41–48.

666. Chikano S, Sawada K, Ohnishi K, et al. Interstitial pneumonia accompanying ulcerative colitis. Intern Med 2001;40:883–886.

667. Bar-Dayan Y, Ben-Zikrie S, Fraser G, et al. Pulmonary alveolar hemorrhage in a patient with ulcerative colitis and primary sclerosing cholangitis. Isr Med Assoc J 2002;4:464–465.

668. Al-Binali AM, Scott B, Al-Garni A, et al. Granulomatous pulmonary disease in a child: an unusual presentation of Crohn's disease. Pediatr Pulmonol 2003;36:76–80.

669. Lucero PF, Frey WC, Shaffer RT, et al. Granulomatous lung masses in an elderly patient with inactive Crohn's disease. Inflamm Bowel Dis 2001;7:256–259.

670. Vandenplas O, Casel S, Delos M, et al. Granulomatous bronchiolitis associated with Crohn's disease. Am J Respir Crit Care Med 1998;158:1676–1679.

671. Beer TW, Edwards CW. Pulmonary nodules due to reactive systemic amyloidosis (AA) in Crohn's disease. Thorax 1993;48:1287–1288.

672. Boyd O, Gibbs AR, Smith AP. Fibrosing alveolitis due to sulphasalazine in a patient with rheumatoid arthritis. Br J Rheumatol 1990;29:222–224.

673. Leino R, Liippo K, Ekfors T. Sulphasalazine-induced reversible hypersensitivity pneumonitis and fatal fibrosing alveolitis: report of two cases. J Intern Med 1991;229:553–556.

674. Parry SD, Barbatzas C, Peel ET, et al. Sulphasalazine and lung toxicity. Eur Respir J 2002;19:756–764.

675. Veyssier-Belot C, Cacoub P, Caparros-Lefebvre D, et al. Erdheim-Chester disease. Clinical and radiologic characteristics of 59 cases. Medicine (Baltimore) 1996;75:157–169.

676. Martin W 3rd, Klein A, Buss D. Case report 213. Skeletal Radiol 1982;9:69–71.

677. Devouassoux G, Lantuejoul S, Chatelain P, et al. Erdheim-Chester disease: a primary macrophage cell disorder. Am J Respir Crit Care Med 1998;157:650–653.

678. Egan AJ, Boardman LA, Tazelaar HD, et al. Erdheim-Chester disease: clinical, radiologic, and histopathologic findings in five patients with interstitial lung disease. Am J Surg Pathol 1999;23:17–26.

679. Bourke SC, Nicholson AG, Gibson GJ. Erdheim-Chester disease: pulmonary infiltration responding to cyclophosphamide and prednisolone. Thorax 2003;58:1004–1005.

680. Wittenberg KH, Swensen SJ, Myers JL. Pulmonary involvement with Erdheim-Chester disease: radiographic and CT findings. AJR Am J Roentgenol 2000;174:1327–1331.

681. Schwarz MI. Miscellaneous interstitial lung disease. In: Schwarz M, King T, eds. Interstitial lung disease, 4th edn. Toronto: Brian C Decker, 2003:877–916.

682. Kambouchner M, Colby TV, Domenge C, et al. Erdheim-Chester disease with prominent pulmonary involvement associated with eosinophilic granuloma of mandibular bone. Histopathology 1997;30:353–358.

683. Farre I, Copin MC, Boulanger E, et al. [Erdheim-Chester disease. Clinico-pathologic study of two cases]. Annales de Pathologie 1995;15:59–62.

684. Santamaria F, Parenti G, Guidi G, et al. Pulmonary manifestations of Gaucher disease: an increased risk for L444P homozygotes? Am J Respir Crit Care Med 1998;157:985–989.

685. Yassa NA, Wilcox AG. High-resolution CT pulmonary findings in adults with Gaucher's disease. Clin Imaging 1998;22:339–342.

686. Aydin K, Karabulut N, Demirkazik F, et al. Pulmonary involvement in adult Gaucher's disease: high resolution CT appearance. Br J Radiol 1997;70:93–95.

687. Ch'en IY, Lynch D, Shroyer K, et al. Gaucher disease: An unusual cause of intrathoracic extramedullary hematopoiesis. Chest 1993;104:1923–1924.

688. Duchateau F, Dechambre S, Coche E. Imaging of pulmonary manifestations in subtype B of Niemann-Pick disease. Br J Radiol 2001;74:1059–1061.

689. Nicholson AG, Wells AU, Hooper J, et al. Successful treatment of endogenous lipoid pneumonia due to Niemann-Pick Type B disease with whole-lung lavage. Am J Respir Crit Care Med 2002;165:128–131.

690. Kariman K, Singletary WV Jr, Sieker HO. Pulmonary involvement in Fabry's disease. Am J Med 1978;64:911–912.

691. Brown LK, Miller A, Bhuptani A, et al. Pulmonary involvement in Fabry disease. Am J Respir Crit Care Med 1997;155:1004–1010.

692. Garay SM, Gardella JE, Fazzini EP, et al. Hermansky-Pudlak syndrome. Pulmonary manifestations of a ceroid storage disorder. Am J Med 1979;66:737–747.

693. Avila NA, Brantly M, Premkumar A, et al. Hermansky-Pudlak syndrome: radiography and CT of the chest compared with pulmonary function tests and genetic studies. AJR Am J Roentgenol 2002;179:887–892.

694. Husby G. Nomenclature and classification of amyloid and amyloidoses. J Intern Med 1992;232:511–512.

695. Kyle R. Amyloidosis minisymposium. Introduction and overview. J Intern Med 1992;232:507–508.

696. Goldman AB, Bansal M. Amyloidosis and silicone synovitis: updated classification, updated pathophysiology, and synovial articular abnormalities. Radiol Clin North Am 1996;34:375–394.

697. Skinner M. Protein AA/SAA. J Intern Med 1992;232:513–514.

698. Rocken C, Sletten K. Amyloid in surgical pathology. Virchows Arch 2003;443:3–16.

699. Pepys M. Amyloidosis: some recent developments. Q J Med 1988;67:283–298.

700. Garcia Gallego F, Calleja Canelas JL. Letter: Hilar enlargement in amyloidosis. N Engl J Med 1974;291:531.

701. Desai RA, Mahajan VK, Benjamin S, et al. Pulmonary amyloidoma and hilar adenopathy. Rare manifestations of primary amyloidosis. Chest 1979;76:170–173.

702. Crestani B, Monnier A, Kambouchner M, et al. Tracheobronchial amyloidosis with hilar lymphadenopathy associated with a serum monoclonal immunoglobulin. Eur Respir J 1993;6:1569–1571.

703. Kyle RA, Greipp PR. Amyloidosis (AL). Clinical and laboratory features in 229 cases. Mayo Clin Proc 1983;58:665–683.

704. Glenner G. Amyloid deposits and amyloidosis. The ß fibrilloses. N Engl J Med 1980;302:1283–1292, 1333–1343.

705. Gertz MA, Kyle RA. Primary systemic amyloidosis – a diagnostic primer. Mayo Clin Proc 1989;64:1505–1519.

706. Kyle R. Primary systemic amyloidosis. J Intern Med 1992;232:523–524.

707. Gertz MA, Lacy MQ, Dispenzieri A. Amyloidosis: recognition, confirmation, prognosis, and therapy. Mayo Clin Proc 1999;74:490–494.

708. Wang C, Robbins L. Amyloid disease. Its roentgen manifestations. Radiology 1956;66:489–501.

709. Cohen AS. Amyloidosis. N Engl J Med 1967;277:522–530.

710. Celli BR, Rubinow A, Cohen AS, et al. Patterns of pulmonary involvement in systemic amyloidosis. Chest 1978;74:543–547.

711. Smith RR, Hutchins GM, Moore GW, et al. Type and distribution of pulmonary parenchymal and vascular amyloid. Correlation with cardiac amyloid. Am J Med 1979;66:96–104.

712. Browning MJ, Banks RA, Tribe CR, et al. Ten years' experience of an amyloid clinic – a clinicopathological survey. Q J Med 1985;54:213–227.

713. Brown J. Primary amyloidosis. Clin Radiol 1964;15:358–367.

714. Crosbie WA, Lewis ML, Ramsay ID, et al. Pulmonary amyloidosis with impaired gas transfer. Thorax 1972;27:625–630.

715. Road J, Jacques J, Sparling J. Diffuse alveolar septal amyloidosis presenting with recurrent hemoptysis and medial dissection of pulmonary arteries. Am Rev Respir Dis 1985;132:1368–1370.

716. Kanada D, Sharma O. Long-term survival with diffuse interstitial pulmonary amyloidosis. Am J Med 1979;67:879–882.

717. Cordier JF, Loire R, Brune J. Amyloidosis of the lower respiratory tract. Clinical and pathologic features in a series of 21 patients. Chest 1986;90:827–831.

718. Poh S, Tjia T, Seah H. Primary diffuse alveolar septal amyloidosis. Thorax 1975;30:186–191.

719. Himmelfarb E, Wells S, Rabinowitz JG. The radiologic spectrum of cardiopulmonary amyloidosis. Chest 1977;72:327–332.

720. Jenkins MC, Potter M. Calcified pseudotumoural mediastinal amyloidosis. Thorax 1991;46:686–687.

721. Kyle RA, Bayrd ED. Amyloidosis: review of 236 cases. Medicine (Baltimore) 1975;54:271–299.

722. Gertz MA, Kyle RA. Secondary systemic amyloidosis: response and survival in 64 patients. Medicine (Baltimore) 1991;70:246–256.

723. Planes C, Kleinknecht D, Brauner M, et al. Diffuse interstitial lung disease due to AA amyloidosis. Thorax 1992;47:323–324.

724. Gertz MA. Secondary amyloidosis (AA). J Intern Med 1992;232:517–518.

725. Wright PH, Heard BE, Steel SJ, et al. Cryptogenic fibrosing alveolitis: assessment by graded trephine lung biopsy histology compared with clinical, radiographic, and physiological features. Br J Dis Chest 1981;75:61–70.

726. Ordi J, Grau JM, Junque A, et al. Secondary (AA) amyloidosis associated with Castleman's disease. Report of two cases and review of the literature. Am J Clin Pathol 1993;100:394–397.

727. Wright JR, Calkins E. Clinical-pathologic differentiation of common amyloid syndromes. Medicine (Baltimore) 1981;60:429–448.

728. Monreal F. Pulmonary amyloidosis: ultrastructural study of early alveolar septal deposits. Hum Pathol 1984;15:388–390.

729. Shiue ST, McNally DP. Pulmonary hypertension from prominent vascular involvement in diffuse amyloidosis. Arch Intern Med 1988;148:687–689.

730. Hazenberg BP, van Rijswijk MH. Clinical and therapeutic aspects of AA amyloidosis. Baillières Clin Rheumatol 1994;8:661–690.

731. Gross BH, Felson B, Birnberg FA. The respiratory tract in amyloidosis and the plasma cell dyscrasias. Semin Roentgenol 1986;21:113–127.

732. Wilson SR, Sanders DE, Delarue NC. Intrathoracic manifestations of amyloid disease. Radiology 1976;120:283–289.

733. Morgan RA, Ring NJ, Marshall AJ. Pulmonary alveolar-septal amyloidosis – an unusual radiographic presentation. Respir Med 1992;86:345–347.

734. Graham CM, Stern EJ, Finkbeiner WE, et al. High-resolution CT appearance of diffuse alveolar septal amyloidosis. AJR Am J Roentgenol 1992;158:265–267.

735. Geusens EA, Verschakelen JA, Bogaert JG. Primary pulmonary amyloidosis as a cause of interlobular septal thickening. AJR Am J Roentgenol 1997;168:1116–1117.

736. Pickford HA, Swensen SJ, Utz JP. Thoracic cross-sectional imaging of amyloidosis. AJR Am J Roentgenol 1997;168:351–355.

737. Storto ML, Kee ST, Golden JA, et al. Hydrostatic pulmonary edema: high-resolution CT findings. AJR Am J Roentgenol 1995;165:817–820.

738. Laden SA, Cohen ML, Harley RA. Nodular pulmonary amyloidosis with extrapulmonary involvement. Hum Pathol 1984;15:594–597.

739. Berk JL, Keane J, Seldin DC, et al. Persistent pleural effusions in primary systemic amyloidosis: etiology and prognosis. Chest 2003;124:969–977.

740. Rubinow A, Celli BR, Cohen AS, et al. Localized amyloidosis of the lower respiratory tract. Am Rev Respir Dis 1978;118:603–611.

741. Kavuru MS, Adamo JP, Ahmad M, et al. Amyloidosis and pleural disease. Chest 1990;98:20–23.

742. Romero Candeira S, Martin Serrano C, Hernandez Blasco L. Amyloidosis and pleural disease. Chest 1991;100:292–293.

743. Bontemps F, Tillie-Leblond I, Coppin MC, et al. Pleural amyloidosis: thoracoscopic aspects. Eur Respir J 1995;8:1025–1027.

744. Gross BH. Radiographic manifestations of lymph node involvement in amyloidosis. Radiology 1981;138:11–14.

745. Borge MA, Parker LA, Mauro MA. Amyloidosis: CT appearance of calcified, enlarged periaortic lymph nodes. J Comput Assist Tomogr 1991; 15:855–857.

746. Hiller N, Fisher D, Shmesh O, et al. Primary amyloidosis presenting as an isolated mediastinal mass: diagnosis by fine needle biopsy. Thorax 1995;50:908–909.

747. Weiss L. Isolated multiple nodular pulmonary amyloidosis. Am J Clin Pathol 1960;33:318–329.

748. Shaw P, Grossman R, Fernandes BJ. Nodular mediastinal amyloidosis. Hum Pathol 1984;15:1183–1185.

749. Melato M, Antonutto G, Falconieri G, et al. Massive amyloidosis of mediastinal lymph nodes in a patient with multiple myeloma. Thorax 1983;38:151–152.

750. Teixidor HS, Bachman AL. Multiple amyloid tumors of the lung. A case report. Am J Roentgenol Radium Ther Nucl Med 1971;111:525–529.

751. Thompson P, Citron K. Amyloid and the lower respiratory tract. Thorax 1983;38:84–87.

752. Toyoda M, Ebihara Y, Kato H, et al. Tracheobronchial AL amyloidosis: histologic, immunohistochemical, ultrastructural, and immunoelectron microscopic observations. Hum Pathol 1993;24:970–976.

753. Gottlieb LS, Gold WM. Primary tracheobronchial amyloidosis. Am Rev Respir Dis 1972;105:425–429.

754. Prowse C. Amyloidosis of the lower respiratory tract. Thorax 1958;13: 308–320.

755. Naef AP, Savary M, Gruneck JM, et al. Amyloid pseudotumor treated by tracheal resection. Ann Thorac Surg 1977;23:578–581.

756. Breuer R, Simpson GT, Rubinow A, et al. Tracheobronchial amyloidosis: treatment by carbon dioxide laser photoresection. Thorax 1985;40:870–871.

757. Thompson PJ, Citron KM. Amyloid and the lower respiratory tract. Thorax 1983;38:84–87.

758. Hui AN, Koss MN, Hochholzer L, et al. Amyloidosis presenting in the lower respiratory tract. Clinicopathologic, radiologic, immunohistochemical, and histochemical studies on 48 cases. Arch Pathol Lab Med 1986;110:212–218.

759. Remy-Jardin M, Remy J, Artaud D, et al. Volume rendering of the tracheobronchial tree: clinical evaluation of bronchographic images. Radiology 1998;208:761–770.

760. O'Regan A, Fenlon HM, Beamis JF Jr, et al. Tracheobronchial amyloidosis. The Boston University experience from 1984 to 1999. Medicine (Baltimore) 2000;79:69–79.

761. Cotton R, Jackson J. Localized amyloid 'tumours' of the lung simulating malignant neoplasms. Thorax 1964;19:97–103.

762. Weissman B, Wong M, DN S. Image interpretation session: 1996. RadioGraphics 1997;17:244–245.

763. Dood A, Manan J. Primary diffuse amyloidosis of the respiratory tract. Arch Pathol 1959;67:39–42.

764. Dalton H, Featherstone T, Athanasou N. Organ limited amyloidosis with lymphodenopathy. Postgrad Med J 1992;68:47–50.

765. Schmidt H, McDonald J, Clagett O. Amyloid tumours of the lower respiratory tract and mediastinum. Ann Otol Rhinol Laryngol 1953;62:880–893.

766. Flemming AF, Fairfax AJ, Arnold AG, et al. Treatment of endobronchial amyloidosis by intermittent bronchoscopic resection. Br J Dis Chest 1980;74:183–188.

767. Yang S, Chia SY, Chuah KL, et al. Tracheobronchial amyloidosis treated with rigid bronchoscopy and stenting. Surg Endosc 2003;17:658–659.

768. Kalra S, Utz JP, Edell ES, et al. External-beam radiation therapy in the treatment of diffuse tracheobronchial amyloidosis. Mayo Clin Proc 2001;76:853–856.

769. Firestone FN, Joison J. Amyloidosis. A cause of primary tumors of the lung. J Thorac Cardiovasc Surg 1966;51:292–299.

770. Saab SB, Burke J, Hopeman A, et al. Primary pulmonary amyloidosis. Report of two cases. J Thorac Cardiovasc Surg 1974;67:301–307.

771. Miura K, Shirasawa H. Lambda III subgroup immunoglobulin light chains are precursor proteins of nodular pulmonary amyloidosis. Am J Clin Pathol 1993;100:561–566.

772. Davis CJ, Butchart EG, Gibbs AR. Nodular pulmonary amyloidosis occurring in association with pulmonary lymphoma. Thorax 1991;46:217–218.

773. Condon R, Pinkham R, Hames G. Primary isolated nodular pulmonary amyloidosis. Report of a case. J Thorac Cardiovasc Surg 1964;48:498–505.

774. Matsumoto K, Ueno M, Matsuo Y, et al. Primary solitary amyloidoma of the lung: findings on CT and MRI. Eur Radiol 1997;7:586–588.

775. Leu CY, Lynch DA, Chan ED. The case of the torpid thoracic tumor. Chest 1997;112:535–537.

776. Fenoglio C, Pascal RR. Nodular amyloidosis of the lungs. An unusual case associated with chronic lung disease and carcinoma of the bladder. Arch Pathol 1970;90:577–582.

777. Ayuso MC, Gilabert R, Bombi JA, et al. CT appearance of localized pulmonary amyloidosis. J Comput Assist Tomogr 1987;11:197–199.

778. Sumimoto H, Yamada K, Nomura I, et al. Primary pulmonary amyloidosis mimicking primary lung cancer. J Comput Assist Tomogr 1993;17: 826–827.

779. Moldow RE, Bearman S, Edelman MH. Pulmonary amyloidosis simulating tuberculosis. Am Rev Respir Dis 1972;105:114–117.

780. Matsunaga N, Hayashi K, Sakamoto I, et al. Takayasu arteritis: protean radiologic manifestations and diagnosis. RadioGraphics 1997;17:579–594.

781. Mata JM, Caceres J, Senac JP, et al. General case of the day. Nodular amyloidosis of the lung. RadioGraphics 1991;11:716–718.

782. Kobayashi H, Matsuoka R, Kitamura S, et al. Sjogren's syndrome with multiple bullae and pulmonary nodular amyloidosis. Chest 1988;94:438–440.

783. Desai SR, Nicholson AG, Stewart S, et al. Benign pulmonary lymphocytic infiltration and amyloidosis: computed tomographic and pathologic features in three cases. J Thorac Imaging 1997;12: 215–220.

784. Radiology Ltd, Tucson, Arizona. Multinodular primary amyloidosis of the lung; diagnosis by needle biopsy. AJR Am J Roentgenol 1978;131:1082–1083.

785. Dyke PC, Demaray MJ, Delavan JW, et al. Pulmonary amyloidoma. Am J Clin Pathol 1974;61:301–305.

786. Zundel WE, Prior AP. An amyloid lung. Thorax 1971;26:357–363.

787. Ohdama S, Akagawa S, Matsubara O, et al. Primary diffuse alveolar septal amyloidosis with multiple cysts and calcification. Eur Respir J 1996;9: 1569–1571.

788. Kim HY, Im JG, Song KS, et al. Localized amyloidosis of the respiratory system: CT features. J Comput Assist Tomogr 1999;23:627–631.

789. Gordonson JS, Sargent EN, Jacobson G, et al. Roentgenographic manifestations of pulmonary amyloidosis (classification and case illustrations). J Can Assoc Radiol 1972;23:269–272.

CHAPTER 12

Airways diseases

TRACHEAL DISORDERS

Tracheal lesions that are part of a generalized pulmonary or systemic disorder, together with congenital, traumatic, and neoplastic processes, are discussed in the relevant chapters. With a few exceptions, consideration in this section is given only to conditions in adults that are essentially confined to the trachea. Given that the trachea is rightly regarded as something of a blind spot on chest radiographs,[1] CT has become the imaging examination of choice for investigating tracheal disorders (Fig. 12.1),[2–6] with MRI providing additional information in some specific situations,[7–10] and three-dimensional (3D) reconstructions of volumetric CT data clarifying tracheobronchial anatomy in some situations.[11–20]

The trachea may be affected by a wide variety of extrinsic or intrinsic processes. Extrinsic processes, particularly masses, displace and distort the trachea, while intrinsic ones cause narrowing, widening, or a mass effect. Tracheal diseases can be further conveniently divided into those that show focal[5] or diffuse[6] involvement.

Tracheal narrowing may affect a long or short segment, and since the distinction is not always clear, both types are considered together. The important causes of tracheal narrowing are listed in Box 12.1.

Tracheal narrowing

Tuberculosis (Box 12.2)

Although common in the past,[68] tracheal tuberculosis is now rare. It may be associated with cavitary lung disease and grossly infected sputum.[40] Pathologic study shows mucosal thickening and ulceration and subsequent healing by fibrosis with stricture formation.[40] Very occasionally the trachea is involved by direct spread from adjacent nodes and fistula formation subsequent to this is described.[23] On CT the extent of irregular and circumferential tracheobronchial narrowing is clearly demonstrated (Fig. 12.2),[24,69] and in some patients an accompanying mediastinitis (opacification of the mediastinal fat) is evident. CT shows differences between active disease in which the narrowed trachea (and frequently one or other main bronchus) has an irregularly thickened wall; by contrast, in the fibrotic or healed phase the trachea is narrowed but has a smooth and normal thickness wall.[69]

Scleroma

Scleroma is a chronic progressive granulomatous infection that affects primarily the nose but may also involve the nasopharynx,

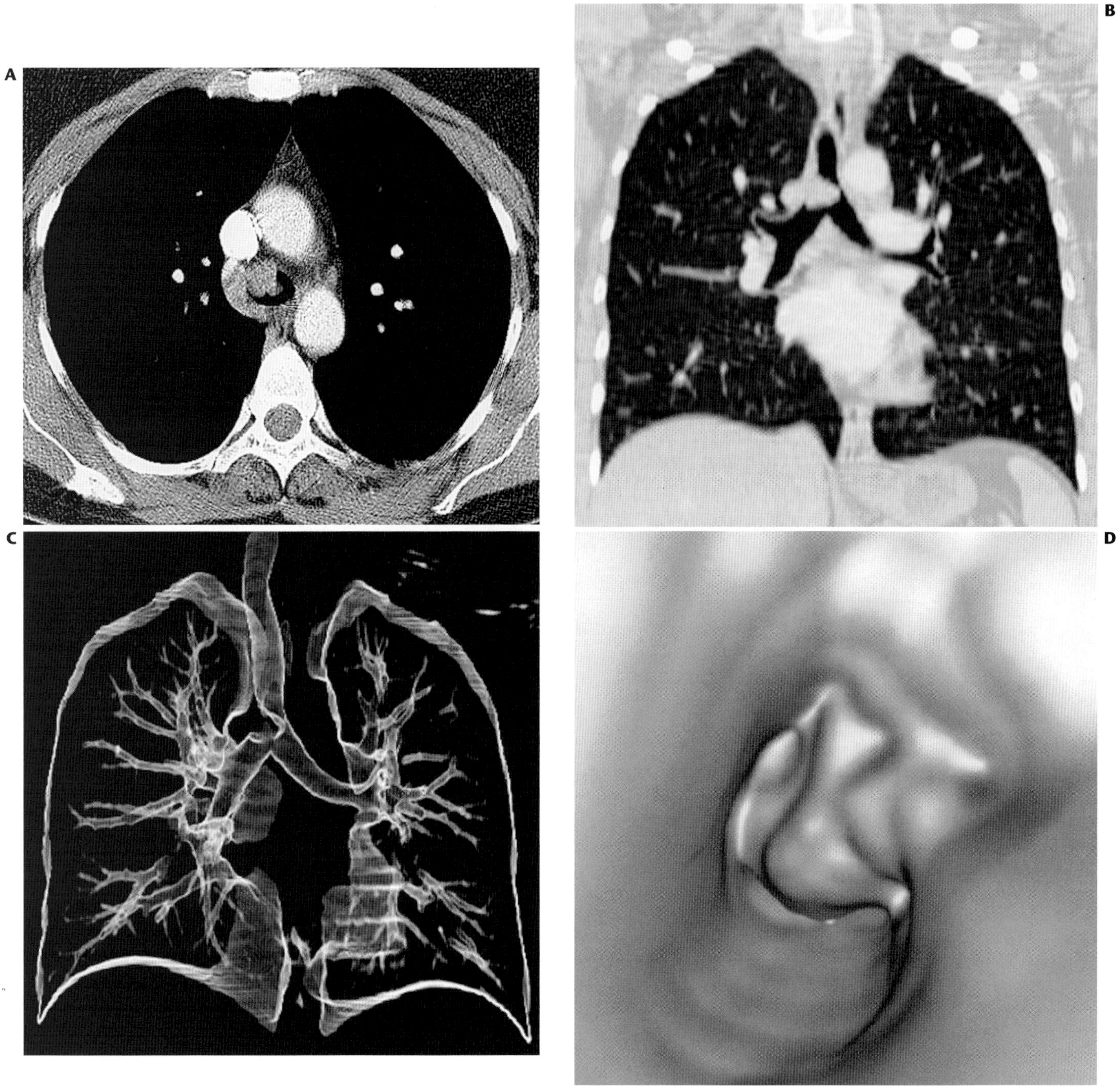

Fig. 12.1 Adenoid cystic tumor in distal trachea images reconstructed from volumetric CT data. **A**, Standard CT section at the level of the azygos vein showing the tumor arising from the thickened right anterolateral tracheal wall, protruding into the lumen. **B**, Coronal reformation through the central airways. **C**, Volume rendered display showing luminal indentation by the tumor. **D**, Virtual bronchoscopic rendition showing the endoluminal component of the tumor.

Box 12.1 Causes of tracheal narrowing

Extrinsic
Mass lesions
Thyroid[21]
Lymph nodes
Vessels[22]
Mediastinal mass
Invading tumors
Thyroid or esophageal carcinoma
Mediastinal fibrosis
Tuberculosis[23,24]
Histoplasmosis[25]

Intrinsic
Congenital[26–29]
Tracheal narrowing[30]
Complete tracheal rings[31]
Down syndrome[32]
Infective
Laryngotracheobronchitis[33]
Papillomatosis[34]
Tuberculosis[24,35]
Bacillary angiomatosis[36]
Scleroma[37]
Fungal[38]
Histoplasmosis
Coccidioidomycosis[39]
Mucormycosis
Candidiasis[40]
Necrotizing tracheobronchial aspergillosis[41,42]
Granulomatous
Necrotizing cytomegalovirus tracheitis[43]
Wegener granulomatosis[44,45]
Sarcoidosis[46]
Crohn disease[47]
Neoplastic[48]
Benign or malignant neoplasm[49]
Lymphoma[50]
Sinus histiocytosis[51]
Traumatic
Tracheostomy or endotracheal intubation[52–54]
Right pneumonectomy syndrome[55]
Blunt or penetrating trauma[56]
Foreign body[57]
Postinflammatory[58]
Epidermolysis bullosa[59]
Deposition or dysplastic
Mucopolysaccharidoses[60]
Chrondrodysplasia punctata[61]
Immunologic
Amyloidosis[62,63]
Relapsing polychondritis[64,65]
Cryptogenic
Tracheopathia osteoplastica[66]
Saber-sheath trachea
Idiopathic[67]

Box 12.2 Tracheal tuberculosis

Tuberculosis confined to tracheal wall involvement is rare
Often accompanied by involvement of one or other main bronchus
Pronounced tracheal wall thickening in active disease
Normal wall thickness of narrowed trachea in healed phase

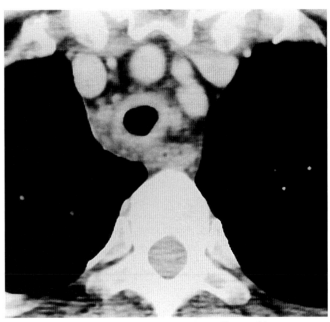

Fig. 12.2 Diffuse thickening of the tracheal wall caused by tuberculosis. The interface between the trachea and the surrounding mediastinal fat is indistinct and there is some opacification of the adjacent fat, presumably due to inflammation and edema.

larynx, trachea, and bronchi. It is caused by the gram-negative bacterium *Klebsiella rhinoscleromatis*. Scleroma is uncommon in the West, occurring mainly in Asia, North Africa, Central and South America, and Eastern Europe. It affects principally rural people from low socioeconomic groups.[40] The disease passes through three phases: catarrhal, granulomatous and proliferative, and scarring.[70] Patients usually present with symptoms related to the nose and paranasal sinuses, and the majority have radiographic signs of sinusitis.[70] Occasionally there is a soft tissue mass or bone destruction suggesting a nasal carcinoma, although MRI appearances may suggest the diagnosis of rhinoscleroma.[71] Laryngeal involvement is usually manifest as glottic or subglottic narrowing and vocal cord thickening.[72,73] About 5% of patients have tracheal involvement, which is nearly always accompanied by laryngeal disease and often, though not necessarily, by paranasal sinus disease.[40]

All, or more commonly part, of the trachea is involved (bronchial involvement is rare), typically the proximal rather than the distal segment.[37] Stenoses are usually concentric and may be nodular or smooth.[74] Less commonly there is diffuse uniform narrowing or multiple masses.[75]

Tracheo(broncho)pathia osteo(chondro)plastica
(Box 12.3)

Tracheopathia osteoplastica was first described more than 100 years ago,[76] yet it remains a curiosity of obscure etiology. Although rare, it is more common than airway amyloidosis, a closely allied condition that some consider identical.[77] Pathologic characteristics include the development of cartilaginous and bony submucosal nodules[40] in the trachea and proximal airways. The nodules are typically found in the lower two-thirds of the trachea and in the main, lobar, and segmental bronchi.[78] The disorder, however, sometimes starts more proximally and affects the first tracheal ring region.[66] The osteochondral nodules develop adjacent to the airway cartilages and only occasionally involve the posterior membranous part of the trachea.[79] The nodules give rise to sessile and polypoidal elevations of the mucosa, which produce airway narrowing,[66] and sometimes lobar collapse.[80] The cause of the condition is obscure. One theory considers the nodules to be a form of ecchondrosis of the airway cartilage because of their distribution in the airways and because they have bony, cartilaginous, and fibrous connections to the cartilage rings themselves.[66] A second theory is that the disorder is due to amyloidosis, a condition in which cartilage and bone formation is known to occur. Several workers have in fact found evidence of amyloid in pathologic specimens from patients with tracheopathia.[77,81]

Most patients are male, and the disease usually develops in middle age (sixth decade), though the age range is wide, from 11 to 78 years.[40] The common early symptoms are dyspnea, hoarseness, cough that is often productive, hemoptysis, and recurrent pulmonary infections.[78] The disease progresses very slowly.

Box 12.3 Tracheo(broncho)pathia osteo(chondro)plastica

Very rare, slowly progressive disease characterized by nodular thickening of the tracheal cartilage
Usually involves the lower trachea and may extend out as far as the segmental bronchi
Calcification within nodular thickening is conspicuous on CT

The chest radiograph may be normal[78] or may demonstrate evidence of collapse or infective consolidation. Airway calcification has diagnostic value but can be difficult to detect on chest radiography.[40] Tracheal calcification is manifest as irregular or scalloped opacities lying inside the cartilage rings.[66] Although this calcification may be seen on a well-penetrated posteroanterior chest radiograph, it is better appreciated on a lateral view.[66] If the tracheal air column is clearly seen, the irregular nodularity of the tracheal wall and the encroachment of these nodules on the lumen can be appreciated. CT descriptions of the condition are sparse but confirm the expected finding of strikingly nodular thickening of the tracheal wall, with calcification in some of the nodules (Fig. 12.3).[80,82–84] The definitive diagnosis is made with bronchoscopy, during which the passage of the instrument may generate a grating sensation. However, the diagnosis may be missed even on bronchoscopy, and some patients have needed several examinations before the diagnosis was eventually made.[78]

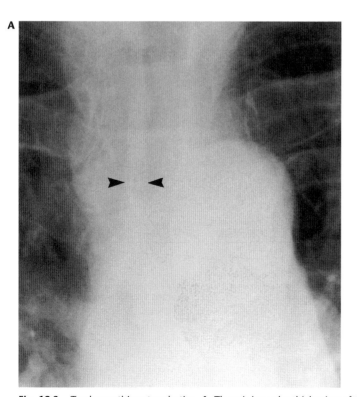
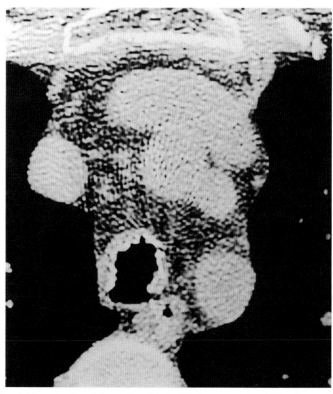

Fig. 12.3 Tracheopathia osteoplastica. **A,** There is irregular thickening of the right tracheal wall (arrowheads). **B,** CT shows nodular thickening and calcific densities in the tracheal wall, with sparing of the posterior membrane.

Saber-sheath trachea (Box 12.4)

The saber-sheath deformity is limited to the intrathoracic part of the trachea, which is flattened from side to side so that the coronal diameter is two-thirds or less of the sagittal diameter at the same level.[85] The condition is virtually confined to men, who are usually >50 years of age; the youngest recorded patient was 37 years.[86] Saber-sheath trachea is strongly associated with the presence of chronic obstructive pulmonary disease (COPD), and in one series COPD was present in 93% of patients with the deformity compared with 18% of control subjects.[86] The pathogenesis of the lesion is obscure, but probably it is an acquired deformity related to the abnormal pattern and magnitude of intrathoracic pressure changes in COPD. In a study of 40 patients, 20 of whom had a saber-sheath trachea, there was a significant relationship between the ratio of the coronal:sagittal tracheal diameter on CT and functional residual capacity ($r = 0.61$, $p<0.00001$), supporting the view that saber-sheath trachea is a consequence of hyperinflation.[87] A reduction in coronal diameter of the trachea, short of the *forme complète* of saber-sheath deformity, correlates significantly with forced expiratory volume in 1 s (FEV_1)/forced vital capacity (FVC).[88]

Saber-sheath trachea can be detected on chest radiography (Fig. 12.4), but is better demonstrated on CT (Fig. 12.5).

The narrowing usually affects the whole of the intrathoracic trachea, with an abrupt return to normal caliber at the thoracic inlet.[85] In Greene's series[86] of 60 patients with saber-sheath trachea and 60 control subjects, the mean coronal diameter of

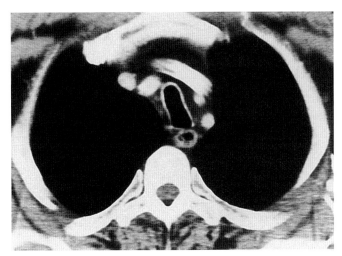

Fig. 12.5 Saber-sheath trachea. CT showing the coronal diameter of the trachea at the level of the left brachiocephalic vein to be 1 cm, whereas the sagittal diameter is 2.6 cm. This represents about 50% coronal reduction and 15% sagittal increase from normal dimensions.

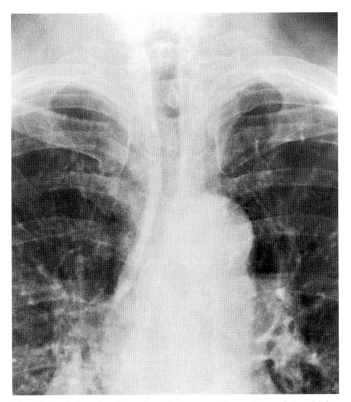

Fig. 12.4 Saber-sheath trachea. Posteroanterior radiograph in which the coronal diameter of the trachea in the cervical region is 19 mm, decreasing to 9 mm in the intrathoracic portion. The transitional zone is at level of the thoracic inlet, and narrowing affects the whole of the intrathoracic trachea. The patient had chronic bronchitis.

the deformed trachea was reduced to 61% and the sagittal diameter increased to 115%, giving a mean tracheal area of 75% compared with control subjects. Cartilage rings are commonly calcified or ossified (but not thickened) both pathologically and radiographically.[85,89]

The inner wall of the trachea is usually smooth (Fig. 12.5) but exceptional examples with nodular irregularity have been described.[90] Patients with both saber-sheath trachea and mediastinal lipomatosis are described in whom the appearance on the plain radiograph therefore strongly resembles a mediastinal mass.[91] The original studies described the trachea as displaying the usual changes in configuration in relation to respiration and considered the trachea to be normally compliant (Fig. 12.6).[86] Other workers, however, have described an abnormal degree of narrowing on forced expiration[89] and have noted that the cross-sectional area was reduced mainly by apposition of the lateral walls with slight invagination of the posterior membrane.[75]

Cryptogenic stenosis

Intrinsic, fibrotic, tracheal stenoses of obscure origin have been described, but truly idiopathic cases are extremely rare.[92,93] These may occur at any site and be multiple.[40] In a series of 15 cases of idiopathic laryngotracheal stenoses, patients were predominantly female (94%) and middle aged (30–60 years).[67]

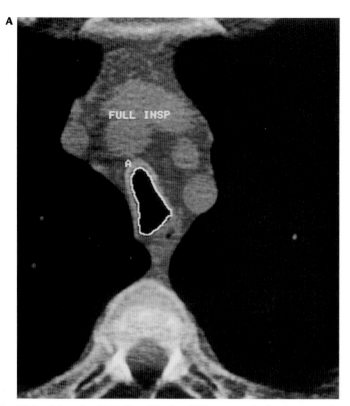
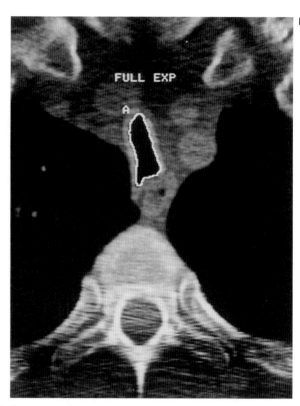

Fig. 12.6 Saber-sheath trachea. Ultrafast CT images at the beginning and end of a rapid expiratory maneuver. **A**, At maximum inspiration. **B**, At maximum expiration. The cross-sectional area (A) of the trachea is essentially the same in **A** and **B**, but its configuration has changed with development of coronal narrowing and sagittal widening on expiration. The trachea is not hypercompliant.

One-third of the stenoses were tracheal, and these were hourglass or eccentric in configuration with smooth or less commonly irregular lobulated margins. Stenoses were 2–4 cm long and 3–5 mm wide. The histologic changes were nonspecific, consisting of scarring of the adventitia and lamina propria.

Some patients with cryptogenic stenoses have positive titers of antineutrophil cytoplasmic antibodies.[94] In these patients stenoses have been recurrent and the histologic features either granulomatous or nonspecific. It seems likely that these cases are part of the Wegener granulomatosis spectrum.

Tracheal widening

A number of studies[86,95–98] have assessed the normal tracheal dimensions in adults using plain radiographs, bronchography, and CT. The most useful study using plain chest radiographs is that of Breatnach et al,[95] who studied 808 subjects. Measurements were made 2 cm above the aortic arch and were subject to 8% magnification. Tracheal diameter increased slightly with age, and taking the largest measurements (between 60 and 80 years of age) the coronal diameter (mean ± SD) was 19.7 ± 2.2 mm in males and 16.8 ± 2.0 mm in females. In light of this data a coronal diameter on a chest radiograph of 26 mm in males and 23 mm in females may be considered abnormal. The CT coronal diameter is smaller, since it is not subject to magnification; values are 3–4 mm less.

A limited number of disorders cause tracheal widening, in some the widening is generalized, and in others it is local, as with a tracheocele or following endotracheal tube cuff damage. In some forms of diffuse disease, widening is mild and confined to one diameter. Thus, in cystic fibrosis the sagittal diameter may be mildly (about 3–5 mm) increased while the coronal dimension remains normal.[99] However, in a small study that investigated the distensibility and CT dimensions of the trachea in five patients with cystic fibrosis compared with five healthy volunteers, no significant differences were found.[100] In day-to-day clinical practice the most common cause of mild enlargement of the trachea is upper zone or diffuse lung fibrosis, as seen in sarcoidosis or tuberculosis.[101] Causes of local and generalized tracheal widening are listed below in Box 12.5.

Tracheobronchomegaly (Mounier–Kuhn syndrome, Box 12.6)

The most striking diffuse increase in tracheal diameter is seen in tracheobronchomegaly (Mounier–Kuhn syndrome). This is a rare abnormality of the trachea and large airways that is associated with recurrent respiratory tract infection and was first described in 1932.[107] Atrophy affects the elastic and muscular elements of both the cartilaginous and membranous parts of the trachea.[97,108–110] In the past the condition was considered to be acquired and to be caused by recurrent infections weakening the airway walls. However, evidence strongly suggests that this is

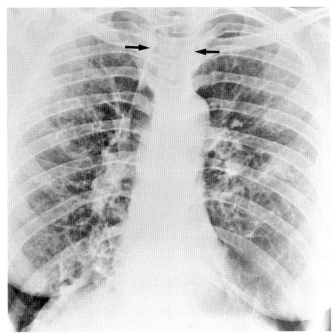

Fig. 12.7 Tracheobronchomegaly on posteroanterior radiograph. The trachea (arrows) is just over 3 cm wide. There is evidence of airflow obstruction with a low, flat right hemidiaphragm. Throughout the lungs, but particularly in the left middle and lower zones, are line and ring opacities consistent with bronchiectasis.

a primary process.[110] Thus, in some patients the condition is familial with an autosomal recessive pattern of transmission.[111] There is a recognized association with anatomic variants of the lungs, ribs, and bronchial tree (including a double tracheal lumen, tracheal trifurcation, and a short left main bronchus).[110,112] Many patients have a history of disease dating back to childhood; presentation at as early as 18 months of age is recorded.[113] Furthermore, pathologic findings of tracheobronchomegaly without inflammation of the tracheal wall are described.[97] The probable chance association of tracheobronchomegaly and ankylosing spondylitis is recorded.[114]

No reliable data on prevalence is available, but in 1800 bronchograms the frequency was about 1%.[109] However, it seems likely that the condition is underdiagnosed, since some patients are asymptomatic or have only minor symptoms.[110] It is markedly male predominant (only about 5% of patients are female) and has a possible racial predisposition for blacks.[112] In a recent review of 27 patients 52% were black,[110] indicating a significant excess of blacks if, as seems likely, most of the populations from which cases were derived were predominantly white. The condition most commonly presents in the third or fourth decade and more than three-quarters of patients have presented by the age of 40 years.[112] Symptoms, however, often date back a decade or even into childhood.[97,109,115] Ineffective cough, because of widened central airways, and diverticula predispose the patient to pulmonary infections. The typical history is of chronic cough that is characteristically loud and productive. Other clinical features include recurrent chest infections and occasionally hoarseness, hemoptysis, and dyspnea. Symptoms therefore closely resemble those of chronic bronchitis or bronchiectasis. A minority of patients have no or surprisingly

mild symptoms.[102,110,111,116] Pulmonary function tests usually show increased dead space, airflow obstruction, and increased total lung capacity and residual volume,[109,111,112] but occasionally findings are normal.[110] Airway compliance is increased, and dynamic airway collapse on expiration and cough can be demonstrated.[97,108–110,113,117,118] The prognosis is variable; some patients have recurrent infections leading to progressive lung damage, bronchiectasis, scarring, and eventual respiratory failure, whereas others survive into old age with relatively mild, nonprogressive disease.[110]

The diagnosis is based on radiologic findings. The immediately subglottic trachea has a normal diameter, but it expands as it passes to the carina (Figs 12.7 and 12.8) and this dilatation often continues into the major bronchi.[109,112,119] The dilatation may vary from segment to segment but overall tends to be relatively even. Atrophic mucosa prolapses between cartilage rings and gives the trachea a characteristically corrugated outline that on a plain radiograph is best appreciated in the lateral view.[102,111,120] Corrugations may become exaggerated to form sacculations or diverticula.[112,121,122] Tracheal changes are well shown on CT (Fig. 12.9)[75,116,121,123] and MRI.[124] Large vessels may indent the compliant trachea.[121]

The dilated proximal airways in the lung show changes of bronchiectasis (Fig. 12.10)[109,112,123] and this affects particularly first- to fourth-order branches.[111] Characteristically there is an abrupt transition from large central airways to normal peripheral ones.[109,121] Small branches that arise from bronchiectatic segments tend to remain patent; this is atypical of bronchiectasis in general, in which they are usually obliterated. This characteristic feature[109] is said to be shared only by allergic bronchopulmonary

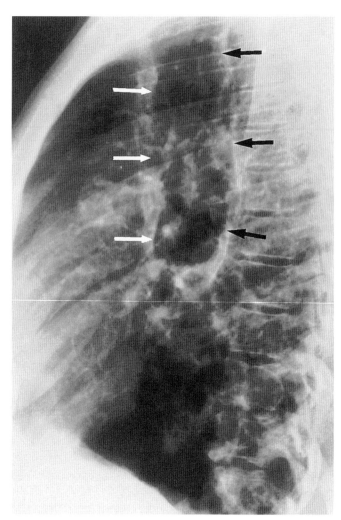

Fig. 12.8 Tracheobronchomegaly. A lateral view of the trachea of the same patient as in Fig. 12.7 shows a grossly dilated trachea (arrows).

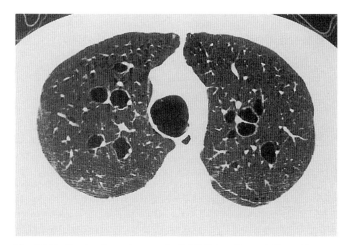

Fig. 12.9 Tracheobronchomegaly. HRCT taken through the mid thoracic trachea of a 39-year-old man with slowly resolving pneumonia. He had had a previous episode of pneumonia but was otherwise well and symptom free despite being a physical training instructor. The tracheal diameter is considerably widened at 30 mm. Fourth- and fifth-order airways show marked varicose bronchiectasis.

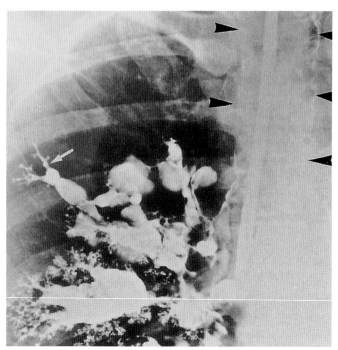

Fig. 12.10 Tracheobronchomegaly in a 53-year-old woman with recurrent lower respiratory tract infections. The bronchogram with contrast medium outlines the dilated trachea (3.3 cm coronal diameter; arrowheads). There is varicose and cystic bronchiectasis with filling of distal bronchi (arrow).

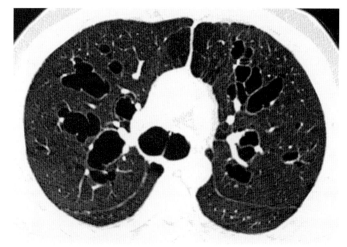

Fig. 12.11 Dramatic thin walled bronchiectasis in the upper lobes of a patient with tracheobronchomegaly (Mounier–Kuhn syndrome).

aspergillosis (ABPA).[125] The dramatic but delicate nature of the typical cystic bronchiectasis is well shown on high-resolution CT (HRCT) (Fig. 12.11). Dynamic collapse of the trachea and central airways on expiration and cough can be demonstrated by a variety of imaging techniques, including CT.[118,121,126,127]

Dilatation of the trachea is generalized in tracheobronchomegaly. Occasionally in other conditions the trachea is locally dilated. This may be seen with a tracheocele, a localized ballooning of the membranous posterior tracheal wall of obscure etiology.[106,128] Tracheoceles tend to arise from the right posterior tracheal wall, and their size varies with transmural tracheal pressure.[120] They may affect the cervical[106] or thoracic trachea and in the latter instance may be seen as a paratracheal, thin walled ring opacity with or without an air–fluid level.[129] Smaller, frequently multiple outpouchings (diverticula) may arise from the trachea and mainstem airways.[130] They are a feature of tracheobronchomegaly[122] but are also described as occurring with cystic dilatation of mucous gland ducts.[120]

Tracheomalacia

Tracheomalacia is present when tracheal compliance is increased. It is usually a localized rather than a generalized process and may be congenital or acquired. Important causes of tracheomalacia are listed in Box 12.7.

Box 12.7 Causes of tracheomalacia

Congenital[27]
Cartilage deficiency[103,131,132]
Generalized tracheomalacia[104,133]
Tracheoesophageal fistula[27]
Compression by anomalous artery[134]

Acquired
Associated with endotracheal tubes and tracheostomy[135,136]
After closed chest trauma[105]
After lung resection[55,105]
After radical neck dissection[137]
After radiation therapy[137]
Chronic obstructive pulmonary disease[138]
Relapsing polychondritis[137]
Lunate trachea[117,139,140]

The increase in compliance is due to the loss of integrity of the wall's structural components and is particularly associated with damage to the cartilage rings.

Tracheomalacia is diagnosed when changes in the transmural pressure gradient produce undue tracheal wall movements. The pressure outside the intrathoracic trachea approximates to pleural pressure and outside the cervical trachea it is atmospheric. When the glottis is open, the luminal pressure is atmospheric. Thus, imaging the intrathoracic trachea at full inspiration and expiration permits observation of the effect of a modest change in transmural pressure (~25 cmH_2O). Static maneuvers such as the Valsalva or Müller can produce bigger pressure gradients across the cervical trachea. Cervical tracheal compliance has been measured using this method with CT imaging.[141] For a 40 cmH_2O change in transmural pressure the cross-sectional area of the cervical trachea changed by about one-third.[141] During dynamic maneuvers such as cough, forced expiration, and forced inspiration the luminal pressure of the intrathoracic trachea is modestly increased or decreased. At the same time large excursions in pleural pressure are generated, and with suitable imaging intrathoracic tracheal compliance can be assessed under more stressful conditions than are produced by static maneuvers.

Until recently the most common cause of tracheomalacia in adults was damage following placement of tracheostomy and endotracheal tubes. However, since the introduction of wide,

low pressure cuffs the problem has largely disappeared. Tracheostomy related compliant segments may develop at the site of the stoma, at the level of the cuff, or in between; in the last instance the pathogenesis is thought to be damage caused by infection associated with stagnant secretions.[135] A compliant tracheal segment may or may not be accompanied by a stenosis.[142] An endotracheal tube cuff lying in a hypercompliant segment appears overinflated, and this may provide an early clue to the presence of tracheomalacia.[136]

Normally the intrathoracic trachea is slightly oval with coronal diameters shorter than sagittal. Occasionally, however, coronal diameters become significantly larger than sagittal ones, producing a lunate configuration to the trachea. A lunate trachea is easily deformed in a sagittal direction, giving rise to a form of tracheomalacia. In a number of patients a lunate trachea has been associated with COPD,[117] but in others it has been cryptogenic,[139] and in one case radiation therapy may have been contributory.[140] Collapse of the affected segment has been observed bronchoscopically.[117]

During forced expiration or coughing a normal trachea shows narrowing both coronally and sagittally, the latter caused by invagination of the membranous posterior wall. Reliable data on the degree of narrowing to be expected is not available, and most studies have been performed in ignorance of the transmural pressure gradient generated. Some authors consider that caliber changes of >50% indicate increased wall compliance.[117,138] In patients who have COPD with high downstream resistance, particularly high dynamic pressure gradients can be generated across the tracheal wall, and it is likely that caliber changes of >50% can occur with normal tracheal compliance.[143] Changes in cross-sectional area, sagittal and coronal diameters in patients with acquired tracheomalacia have been studied by static inspiratory and expiratory CT.[144] Patients with tracheomalacia showed a significantly greater diminution in sagittal (not coronal) diameter and cross-sectional area (Fig. 12.12); more specifically, there was a >89% chance of tracheomalacia if the tracheal cross-sectional change was >18% (upper trachea) or 28% (mid trachea), particularly if the sagittal diameter decreased by >28%.[144]

With the advent of rapid acquisition CT it has become possible to image the trachea during quiet breathing[145] and forced dynamic maneuvers[126,146]; similar information can be acquired with MRI.[147] During forced inspiration and expiration the intrathoracic tracheal cross-sectional area varies by 35% ± 18% (SD),[146] and in view of this data Stern et al[146] suggest that changes in area >70% indicate tracheomalacia (Fig. 12.13). Dynamic studies with CT may be particularly effective in identifying tracheomalacic segments.[126,145,146]

In infants and children most cases occur *secondary* to external compression of the trachea (aberrant subclavian arteries, vascular rings, etc). *Primary* tracheomalacia, caused by defects in the supporting cartilaginous structures, is rare,[148] and is usually associated with more severe congenital malformations such as esophageal atresia.[133,149,150] The trachea in such cases is usually elliptical in shape. The cartilage is deficient and the membranous portion of the trachea is widened.[151] The entire airway, or just short segments, may be affected. Affected infants may not manifest symptoms for several months after birth.[152] The diagnosis is made by observing marked expiratory collapse of the trachea in the anteroposterior dimension.[152] Bronchoscopy is probably the mainstay for diagnosis of tracheomalacia, but as it usually requires general anesthesia in neonates, it is thus

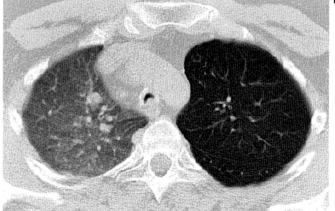
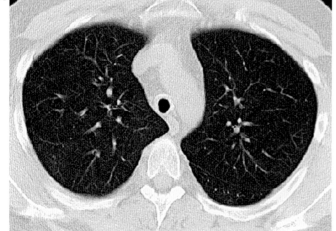

Fig. 12.12 Patient with relapsing polychondritis and hypercompliant trachea. **A**, CT at near total lung capacity showing the caliber reduced by the thick walled trachea. **B**, CT performed at near residual volume with marked decrease in sagittal diameter of the trachea (and air-trapping in the left lung, reflecting collapse of the left main stem bronchus).

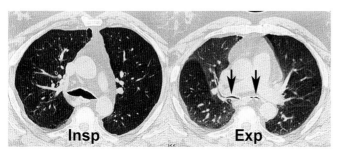

Fig. 12.13 Tracheomalacia in an elderly woman with a history of recurrent pneumonia and "asthma". Inspiratory (Insp) and expiratory (Exp) CT images show marked expiratory collapse of the proximal main bronchi (arrows) and some air-trapping in the right lower lobe and left lung.

> **Box 12.8 Causes of tracheal filling defects**
>
> *Neoplasm*[48,154]
> Benign (epithelial and mesenchymal)
> Malignant
> Carcinoma (squamous, adenoid cystic [Fig. 12.1],
>   adenocarcinoma)
> Sarcoma
> Plasmacytoma
> Lymphoma
> Malignant invasion from without
>
> *Infection or granuloma*
> Viral papilloma
> Membranous croup
> Fungal infection
> Tuberculosis
> Rhinoscleroma
> Wegener granulomatosis
> Bacillary angiomatosis
>
> *Trauma*
> Hematoma
>
> *Miscellaneous*[155]
> Ectopic thyroid and thymus
> Amyloidosis
> Tracheopathia osteoplastica
> Foreign body
> Mucoid pseudotumor
> Cyst or mucocele

a last resort. Less invasive approaches to diagnosis include fluoroscopy, dynamic helical or electron-beam CT,[13,126,152] or MRI.[134,153]

Tracheal filling defects

In adults tracheal filling defects are most commonly produced by neoplasms (see Ch. 13), but there are a number of other causes (Box 12.8).

Ectopic thyroid

Ectopic thyroid is a rare cause of an intratracheal filling defect[156,157] with about 150 cases reported in the literature,[154] mostly from endemic goitrous areas.[49] Females outnumber males by about 3:1.[156] The ectopic thyroid may be histologically normal, though it is usually goitrous. Occasionally it is malignant.[49,156] Three-quarters of intratracheal thyroid nodules are associated with extratracheal goiter. Sometimes they declare themselves years after the removal of an extratracheal goiter because of compensatory hypertrophy. Tumors may occur anywhere between the subglottis and main carina,[154] but typically they are a few centimeters below the vocal cords,

arising as smooth, sessile nodules from the posterolateral wall of the trachea.[156] Ectopic thymus has also been described as causing a submucosal intratracheal mass.[158]

Tracheal papilloma

Squamous papillomas of the trachea in children are usually multiple and a manifestation of laryngeal papillomatosis with

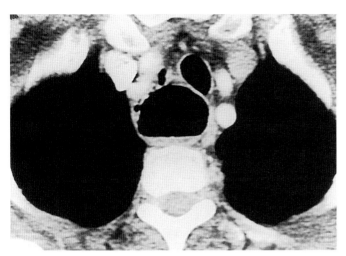

Fig. 12.14 Paratracheal cyst displacing the trachea anteriorly and the esophagus to the left. The cyst contains a fluid level (the patient complained of a gurgling sensation). There are a few adjacent locules of gas within the mediastinum, possibly arising from the paratracheal cyst.

tracheobronchial dissemination (see p. 840)[34,49,159–161] Similar cases are rarely reported in adults.[34,162,163] Solitary squamous cell papillomas of the trachea are also recognized in adults and may undergo malignant transformation.[49,164]

Paratracheal cysts

Small air-filled cysts (ranging in size from 1 to a few cm) arising from the mid or upper trachea are rare and are usually an incidental radiographic or CT finding (Fig. 12.14).[165] They usually occur on the right side and on thin-section CT a communicating channel between the cyst and trachea may occasionally be identified. Although usually considered rare, a Korean study has characterized right paratracheal cysts in 65 individuals.[166] In all but one patient the cysts arose from the

right posterolateral aspect of the trachea. Most cysts were approximately 1 cm in diameter and the majority of patients had functional evidence of obstructive lung disease.[166] Nevertheless, it is not entirely clear whether these cysts are congenital or acquired.[165] Surgical resection is usually undertaken because of the potential for infection within the cyst.

Tracheoesophageal fistula

In the pediatric age group tracheoesophageal fistula is almost invariably congenital.[28] Occasionally such congenital fistulas are first manifested in adults.[167,168] Malignant neoplasia, particularly esophageal, is the most common cause in adults. Infection and trauma are the most frequent nonmalignant causes (Fig. 12.15).[169] The etiology of bronchoesophageal fistulas is similar to that of tracheoesophageal fistula. Causes of tracheoesophageal fistula in adults are listed in Box 12.9.

Box 12.9 Causes of tracheoesophageal fistula

Congenital[167,168]
Neoplasm[170]
Carcinoma of esophagus[171] or trachea
Lymphoma[170,172]
Trauma
Closed chest[173,174]
Penetrating[169]
Postendoscopy or postoperative
Endotracheal intubation[53,175]
Corrosive esophagitis[176,177]
Esophageal foreign body[178]
Postirradiation[179]
Infection
Histoplasmosis[180]
Actinomycosis[169]
Tuberculosis

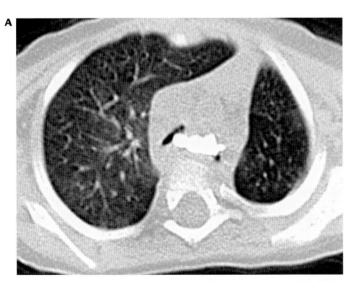
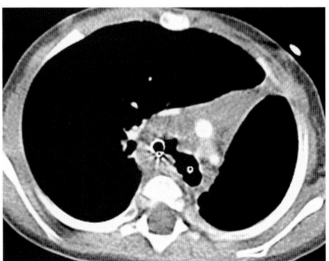

Fig. 12.15 Acquired tracheoesophagheal fistula in a 2-year-old child who swallowed a model soldier. **A**, The hyperdense object has eroded through the esophageal wall and impinges on the trachea (slightly to the right of the midline). **B**, Following thoracotomy and removal of the foreign body there is a large tracheoesophageal fistula. There is an endotracheal tube in place (midline and a nasogastric tube in the dilated esophagus). The fistula subsequently healed.

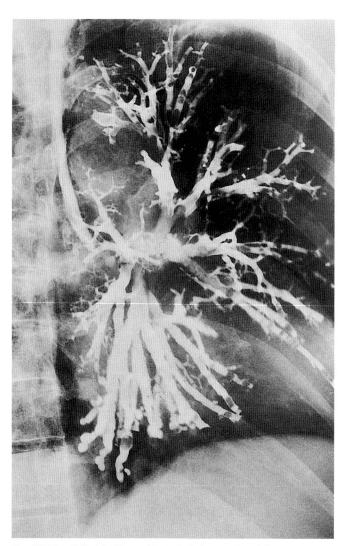

Fig. 12.16 Cylindrical bronchiectasis. Left posterior oblique projection of a left bronchogram showing cylindrical bronchiectasis affecting the whole of the lower lobe except for the superior segment. Few side branches fill. The basal airways are crowded together, indicating volume loss of the lower lobe, a common feature in bronchiectasis.

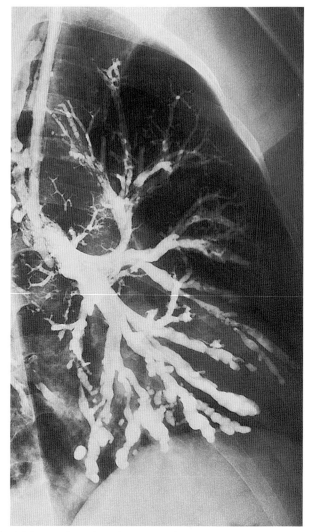

Fig. 12.17 Varicose bronchiectasis. Left posterior oblique projection of a left bronchogram in a patient with ciliary dyskinesia. All the basal bronchi are affected by varicose bronchiectasis.

BRONCHIECTASIS

Bronchiectasis is a chronic condition characterized by local, irreversible dilatation of bronchi, usually associated with inflammation.[181] The qualification "irreversible" is included in the definition to exclude the transient airway dilatation that has been observed in pneumonia and atelectasis.[182–185] Dilatation of the airway in these circumstances is probably partly related to inflammatory changes in the wall, altering compliance, and to exaggerated lung stresses after collapse. On rare occasions some patients show some reversibility of what would otherwise be considered typical idiopathic bronchiectasis.[186]

On macrosopic study, bronchiectatic airways are dilated in a variety of patterns that were historically classified into two[181] or three subtypes.[187] The three-part Reid classification is applicable to gross pathologic, bronchographic, and CT appearances. However, the clinical utility of designating bronchiectasis as cylindrical, varicose or cystic is not obvious, though it is generally agreed that cystic bronchiectasis represents the most advanced disease. The Reid classification, most elegantly shown by bronchography, is as follows:

- *Cylindrical bronchiectasis.* Bronchial dilatation is mild, and the bronchi retain their regular and relatively straight outline (Fig. 12.16).
- *Varicose bronchiectasis.* Bronchial dilatation is greater than in cylindrical bronchiectasis and is accompanied by local constrictions that give the airway an irregular outline (Fig. 12.17). Obstruction and obliteration of small airways is more pronounced.
- *Cystic (saccular) bronchiectasis.* This is the most severe form of bronchiectasis (Fig. 12.18). The airway takes on a ballooned appearance and the number of bronchial divisions is greatly reduced.

Histologic study of bronchiectatic airways shows the walls to be thickened and chronically inflamed with chronic granulation

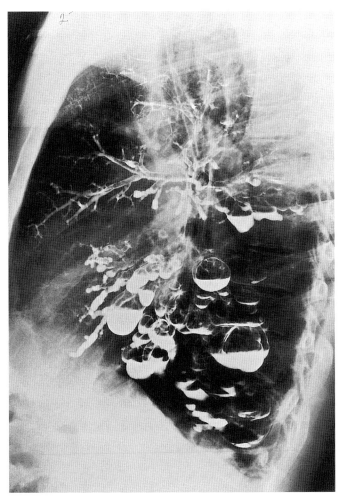

Fig. 12.18 Cystic bronchiectasis. Right lateral bronchogram showing cystic bronchiectasis affecting mainly the lower lobe and posterior segment of the upper lobe.

tissue, and the bronchial arteries to be hypertrophied[188,189] (and these may be conspicuous at CT[190]). Ciliated epithelium is largely replaced by squamous epithelium or areas of squamous metaplasia. The mucosa is sometimes ulcerated or thrown into transverse ridges by circular muscle hypertrophy. Airways are surrounded by fibrosis with acute and organizing pneumonia in the adjacent parenchyma,[189] leading to volume loss and distortion.

The pathogenesis of bronchiectasis is complex, as shown by the large number of recognized causes and associations.[188,191–193] The most important and commonly implicated pathogenic factors are bronchial wall weakness, often brought about by infective inflammatory damage. It seems probable that such damage is self-perpetuating and this has led to the "vicious circle" hypothesis which proposes that colonizing microbes impair normal host clearance mechanisms, thereby modifying the environment within the airways and so allowing microbial growth. The host immune response is ineffective in dealing with the microbial colonization and, paradoxically, the immune response further damages mucociliary clearance, thus setting up a vicious circle of host damage and further microbial growth.[194] Recognized associations and causes[188,192] are listed in Box 12.10.

Box 12.10 Causes and associations of bronchiectasis

Congenital
Cartilage deficiency[103,132,195–197]
Cystic bronchiectasis[198]
Pulmonary sequestration

Postinfection
Childhood pneumonia, measles, pertussis, *Mycoplasma pneumonia*,[199,200] tuberculosis[201]
Swyer–James/McLeod syndrome[202]

Obstruction
Neoplasm
Lymph nodes (including "middle lobe syndrome")[203,204]
Broncholith[205]
Foreign body[206]
Bronchostenosis, including sarcoidosis[207]

Inhalation and aspiration
Ammonia[208,209]
Riley–Day syndrome[210]
Gastric aspiration[211]
Heroin overdose[212]

Impaired host defense and immunologic
Primary ciliary dyskinesia
Cystic fibrosis[213,214]
Primary impaired humoral or cell immunity[215,216]
Infantile X-linked agammaglobulinemia (Bruton disease)[217,218]
Variable immunodeficiency[200,217,219,220]
Good syndrome[221]
Acute and chronic leukemia (with or without IgM deficiency)
Ataxia telangiectasia (Louis–Bar syndrome)
Chédiak–Higashi syndrome
HIV associated[222–224]
Lung transplant[225,226]
Ulcerative colitis[227–230]
Crohn disease[231]
Celiac disease[232]

Allergy
Allergic bronchopulmonary aspergillosis[233,234]

Pulmonary fibrosis
End-stage lung[235]
Radiation[236,237]

Miscellaneous
Purulent rhinosinusitis
Tracheobronchomegaly (Mounier–Kuhn syndrome)
α_1-Antitrypsin deficiency[238–241]
Obstructive azoospermia (Young syndrome)[242,243]
Anhidrotic ectodermal dysplasia[244]
Rheumatoid disease, Sjögren syndrome[245–247]
Marfan syndrome[248,249]
Yellow nail syndrome[250]
Idiopathic

Gross bronchiectasis is characterized by persistent cough, with copious purulent sputum and recurrent pulmonary infections. Symptoms frequently date from childhood, when a precipitating pneumonic event may have occurred. With widespread disease there may be dyspnea and, ultimately, cor pulmonale. Such severe bronchiectasis is becoming unusual and is largely limited to patients with impaired defense mechanisms. A recognized presentation of mild bronchiectasis is recurrent hemoptysis,[251] but mild bronchiectasis may be asymptomatic. This is particularly true of some forms such as that following granulomatous disease of the upper zones.

The classic description of the plain radiographic changes in bronchiectasis is that of Gudbjerg.[252] In this old series 93% of radiographs were said to be abnormal. Although this might seem a high figure as judged by some clinical reports,[253,254] recent studies have reiterated that careful analysis of chest radiographs of patients with bronchiectasis will reveal abnormalities in the majority of cases.[255,256] Some varieties of bronchiectasis such as occur in cystic fibrosis and the ciliary dyskinesia syndrome[257] almost invariably show plain radiographic changes:

- *Bronchial walls* are visible either as single thin lines or as parallel line opacities (Fig. 12.19).
- *Ring and curvilinear opacities* are generated by thickened airway walls seen end on. Ring opacities range in size from 5 to 20 mm and can have very thin (hairline) walls (Fig. 12.20). They may contain air–fluid levels.

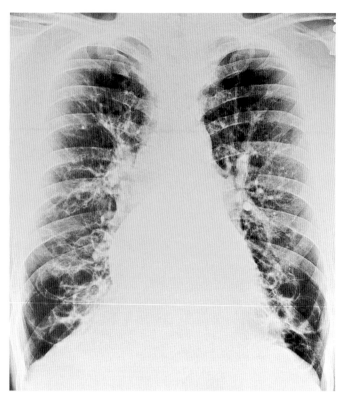

Fig. 12.20 Gross cystic bronchiectasis. Posteroanterior chest radiograph showing overinflated lungs. There are multiple ring opacities, most obvious at the lung bases, ranging from 3 to 15 mm in diameter.

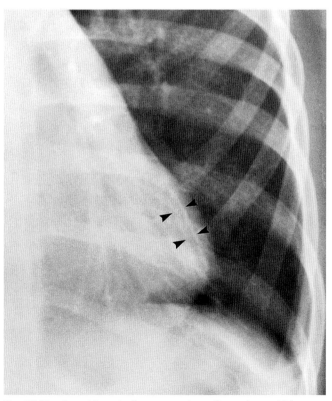

Fig. 12.19 Bronchiectasis. Posteroanterior radiograph on which thickened bronchial walls are seen as line opacities through the heart. Some lines appear paired (arrowheads) and probably represent the opposite walls of a single airway. Separation of these lines is such that the airway must be dilated. Note crowding of the bronchi and obscuration of the medial part of the hemidiaphragm.

- *Plugged airways* give rise to band shadows of variable size (Figs 12.21 and 12.22). Band shadows may branch, giving V, Y, or more complex shaped opacities.
- *Vascular structures* may appear increased in size and may be indistinct because of adjacent peribronchial inflammation and fibrosis.
- *Volume change.* In generalized bronchiectasis, such as that associated with cystic fibrosis, there is often generalized overinflation (Fig. 12.20).[257] Localized forms, however, are frequently accompanied by atelectasis (Fig. 12.23), which may be mild and detected only because of vascular crowding, fissural displacement, or obscuration of part of the diaphragm (Fig. 12.19).
- *Other signs* include evidence of scarring, bulla formation, and pleural thickening. Areas of pulmonary consolidation may be due to infection, e.g. *Pseudomonas aeruginosa*, but can also be a manifestation of ABPA which may be superimposed on other bronchiectatic conditions (e.g. cystic fibrosis[258]).

HRCT signs

By pathologic definition, dilatation of the airways is a prerequisite for the diagnosis of bronchiectasis. Thus, the major sign of HRCT bronchiectasis is dilatation of the bronchi (with or without bronchial wall thickening). The characteristics of bronchiectatic airways on CT first described over 20 years ago[259] have withstood the test of time, with subsequent minor refinements

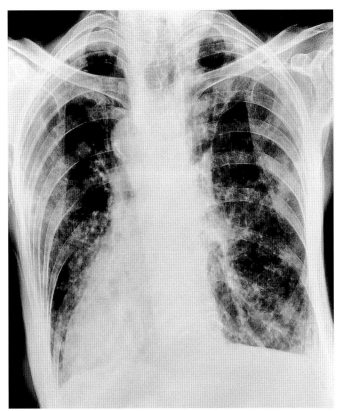

Fig. 12.21 Ciliary dyskinesia syndrome – Kartagener syndrome. This 62-year-old woman gave a 40 year history consistent with bronchiectasis. The aortic arch, descending aorta, heart, and gastric air bubble are all on the right. There is diffuse complex pulmonary shadowing with many ring opacities. Broad-branching band shadows can just be seen through heart and represent dilated fluid-filled airways.

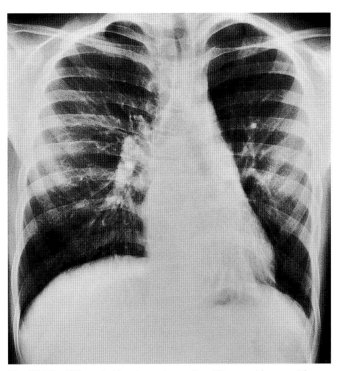

Fig. 12.22 Ciliary dyskinesia syndrome in a 20-year-old man with recurrent pneumonia, otitis, and sinusitis. In the paracardiac region there are bilateral broad linear shadows caused by dilated, fluid-filled bronchi. As with half of patients with ciliary dyskinesia, this patient does not have dextrocardia.

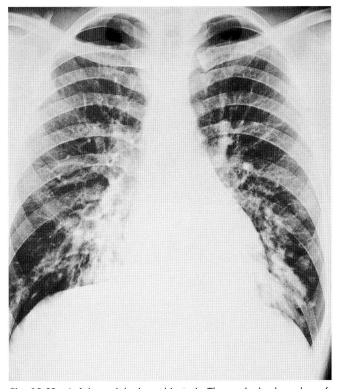

Fig. 12.23 Left lower lobe bronchiectasis. The marked volume loss of left lower lobe is indicated by a depressed hilum, vertical left mainstem bronchus, mediastinal shift, and left-sided transradiancy. Just visible through the heart are parallel line opacities ("tubular" or "tramline" shadows).

and additions.[260–265] Absolute measurements for the diameter of all generations of the bronchi are not available for normal individuals, and relating the size of a bronchus to its immediately adjacent (homologous) pulmonary artery has been the most widely used criterion for the detection of abnormal dilatation.[266] In normal individuals the overall diameter of a bronchus is approximately the same, at any given level, as that of its accompanying pulmonary artery. The ratio of diameter of the bronchus (internal lumen) to pulmonary artery diameter for subjects at sea level has been estimated to be 0.62 ± 0.13 (mean $\pm$ standard deviation).[267] Recognition of abnormal dilatation of a bronchus by comparison with its accompanying pulmonary artery can be readily made for airways running perpendicular to the CT section. When bronchial dilatation is marked, the cross-sectional appearance of the combined bronchus and artery resembles a pearl or signet ring (Fig. 12.24).[268]

In healthy individuals minor discrepancies in the bronchoarterial diameter ratio may occasionally be encountered.[266,269] Furthermore, there are many factors that can cause transient or permanent changes in diameter of the relatively compliant pulmonary arteries, so invalidating this sign. For example, a left-to-right cardiac shunt will result in generalized increase in perfusion and caliber of the pulmonary arterial tree, conversely any cause of underventilation of a region of lung will result in hypoxic vasoconstriction.

Thus, bronchial dilatation in isolation, in the absence of bronchial wall thickening, cannot always be regarded as

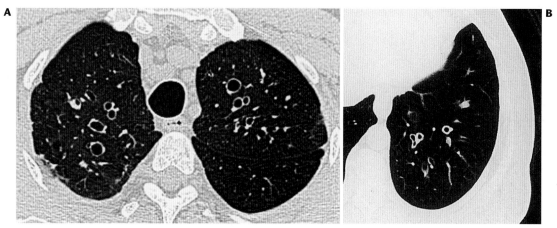

Fig. 12.24 Signet ring sign. Patients with **A**, cystic fibrosis and **B**, idiopathic bronchiectasis, showing several thick walled bronchi which are dilated by comparison with the accompanying pulmonary artery.

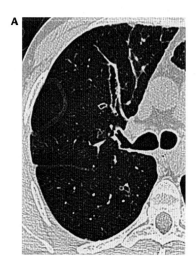
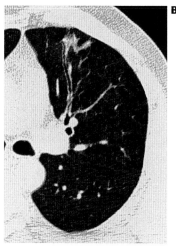

Fig. 12.25 Cylindrical bronchiectasis. **A** and **B**, Examples from two patients. Airways parallel to the plane of section in the anterior segment of an upper lobe show changes of cylindrical bronchiectasis; bronchi are wider than normal and fail to taper, as they proceed towards the lung periphery.

diagnostic of bronchiectasis. This caveat has been reiterated in a study by Lynch et al,[269] which showed that 59% of normal individuals had at least one bronchus with a diameter greater than that of the homologous pulmonary artery. However, in these healthy subjects, bronchial wall thickening was not a common association. One of the factors that appears to have contributed to the apparently high frequency of a decreased bronchoarterial ratio in normal individuals in the study by Lynch et al,[269] was hypoxic vasoconstriction: the study group investigated were all examined in Colorado, at approximately 1600 m above sea level. Kim et al[267] subsequently performed a detailed study which compared the bronchoarterial ratios of normal individuals at sea level with normal individuals at high altitude (1600 m above sea level).[267] The bronchoarterial ratio of individuals at altitude was 0.76 ± 0.14 SD compared with 0.62 ± 0.13 SD at sea level (p<0.001).

When airways lie parallel to the plane of section, abnormal dilatation is recognized by a lack of normal tapering, producing a tramline or even flared appearance (Fig. 12.25). These airways are conspicuous in the lung periphery because of associated bronchial wall thickening. The cylindrical and varicose patterns of bronchiectasis, described by Reid,[187] can be appreciated only for bronchi that lie within the plane of CT section. Cylindrical bronchiectasis is by far the most common morphologic

pattern of bronchiectasis identified on CT.[270] Bronchoarterial ratios >1 has been reported in 95% of patients with cylindrical bronchiectasis.[265] Varicose bronchiectasis is characterized by a beaded appearance (Fig. 12.26) and cystic (or saccular) bronchiectasis is seen as thin walled cystic spaces which may contain fluid levels. In cystic bronchiectasis, recognition that large cystic airspaces represent massively dilated bronchi may sometimes be difficult or impossible (Fig. 12.27). In this type of severe bronchiectasis the accompanying pulmonary artery may be obliterated. When varicose bronchiectatic airways are imaged in cross section, they may appear as either cystic or cylindrical bronchiectatic airways because the characteristic corrugation of the bronchial walls cannot be identified in this orientation. Sections obtained at end-expiration have been advocated to differentiate cystic bronchiectasis from other cystic lung diseases[271]; bronchiectatic airways usually decrease in size on expiratory scans in contrast to other cystic lesions. A more recent study has reported that most cystic lesions in the lungs, whether bronchiectatic or otherwise, decrease in size,[272] rendering this sign of doubtful discriminatory value.

Bronchial wall thickening is a usual, but inconstant, feature of bronchiectasis (Fig. 12.28). Problems with this variable feature have been widely debated and the definition of what constitutes abnormal bronchial wall thickening remains

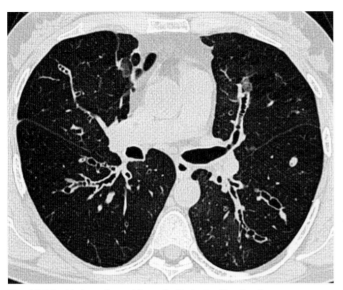

Fig. 12.26 Varicose bronchiectasis. Patient with allergic bronchopulmonary aspergillosis and cystic fibrosis. The bronchiectatic airways have a corrugated, or beaded, appearance.

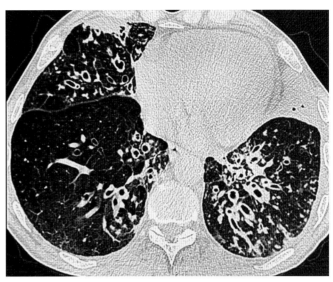

Fig. 12.28 Bronchial wall thickening of variable severity in a patient with idiopathic bronchiectasis. It is likely that at least part of the apparent wall thickening is due to retained secretions. There is a tree-in-bud pattern most conspicuous in the periphery of the left lower lobe.

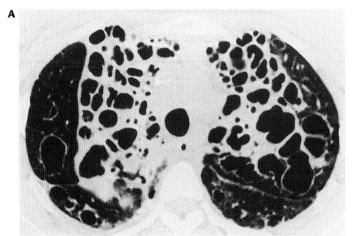

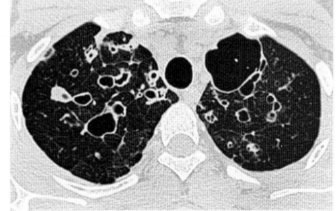

Fig. 12.27 Cystic bronchiectasis in the upper lobes in two patients. In such advanced disease, it is often impossible to distinguish between markedly dilated bronchi and cystic airspaces in destroyed lung. **A,** Etiology of the bronchiectasis was unknown in this patient. **B,** Patient had cystic fibrosis.

unresolved.[264] Minor to mild degrees of bronchial wall thickening are seen in normal subjects, asthmatics, individuals with lower respiratory tract viral infections and asymptomatic smokers.[269,273] There is no simple and robust criterion for the identification of abnormal bronchial wall thickening: Remy-Jardin et al[273] defined a bronchus as being thick walled when the bronchial wall was at least double the thickness of a normal bronchus. However, such a judgment is only possible when comparable "normal" bronchi can be identified. An assessment can also be made by relating the bronchial wall thickness to the diameter of the accompanying pulmonary artery,[270,274] but in practice this does not overcome the difficulties of identifying subtle bronchial wall thickening.[275] Diederich et al[276] defined abnormal bronchial wall thickening as being present if the internal diameter of the bronchus was <80%

of the external diameter.[276] While this sign was associated with good interobserver agreement it cannot be applied to conditions in which there is any significant bronchial dilatation.

Normal airways within 2 cm of the visceral pleural surface are not usually visible because their walls are below the spatial resolution of HRCT.[277] More recently, perhaps as a result of improved CT technology, it has been pointed out that bronchi may be identified within 1 cm of the mediastinal pleura in normal subjects, but that airways seen within 1 cm of the costal pleura or paravertebral pleura should be regarded as abnormal.[265] Secretions within bronchiectatic airways will generally be easily recognizable as such. The larger plugged bronchi will be visible as lobulated or branching opacities. Such airways are usually seen in the presence of nonfluid-filled, obviously bronchiectatic

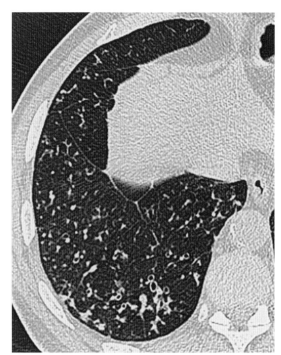

Fig. 12.29 Patient with mild cylindrical bronchiectasis. The numerous peripheral nodular and branching opacities (tree-in-bud pattern) represent exudate in and around the small airways.

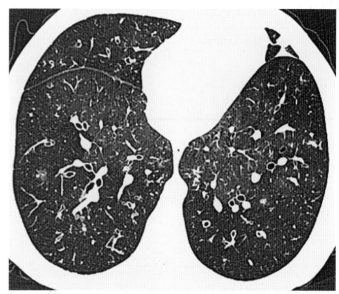

Fig. 12.30 Cylindrical bronchiectasis in the lower lobes. There is regional inhomogeneity of the attenuation of the lung parenchyma (mosaic pattern) reflecting coexisting small airways obliteration.

airways. A less frequent pattern is plugging and thickening of the smaller peripheral centrilobular airways, producing V- and Y-shaped opacities, the so-called "tree-in-bud" appearance (Fig. 12.29).[278–280]

In many patients with bronchiectasis, areas of decreased attenuation of the lung parenchyma can be identified (Fig. 12.30); this mosaic pattern reflects accompanying obliteration of small airways disease.[261,281] Sections taken at end-expiration enhance the feature of decreased attenuation, the extent of which correlates with functional indices of airways obstruction.[281,282] This finding is most prevalent in lobes with severe bronchiectasis but may be seen in some lobes in which there are no CT features of bronchiectasis. In a study by Kang et al,[261] the CT finding of mosaic perfusion was identified in just over half of bronchiectatic lobes subsequently resected, and there was pathologic evidence of obliterative bronchiolitis in 85% of these resected lobes.[261] Areas of decreased attenuation on CT representing constrictive obliterative bronchiolitis may sometimes be confused with the features of emphysema.[283] Nevertheless, the rare association of bronchiectasis and true panacinar emphysema, concentrated in the lower lobes, is encountered in some patients with α_x-antitrypsin deficiency.[284,285] Fluctuations in pulmonary function measures of airflow obstruction most closely correlate with alterations in the degree of mucus plugging on serial HRCTs, rather than other morphologic abnormalities.[286]

Subtle degrees of volume loss may be seen in lobes in relatively early bronchiectasis; this is most evident in the lower lobes where crowding of the mildly bronchiectatic airways and posterior displacement of the oblique fissure may be an early sign of bronchiectasis (Fig. 12.31). CT will readily show completely collapsed lobes containing bronchiectatic airways, though the

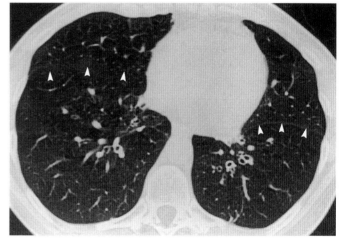

Fig. 12.31 Mild cylindrical bronchiectasis in the left lower lobe. Note the crowding of the affected bronchi and loss of volume of the left lower lobe, as judged by the relative positions of the oblique fissures (arrowheads).

diagnosis of bronchiectasis in acutely collapsed or consolidated lobes may be uncertain because of the reversibility of bronchial dilatation in these situations.[183,184]

Distortion and dilatation of segmental and subsegmental bronchi is a predictable and frequent feature of patients with retractile interstitial fibrosis, of whatever cause, and has been termed (not particularly usefully) "traction bronchiectasis". Many of the HRCT signs of bronchiectasis coexist, particularly in long-standing disease. The signs of bronchiectasis, discussed above, are summarized below in the approximate sequence in which they occur:

- Bronchial wall thickening (nonspecific and not invariable)
- Lobar volume loss (may be minimal; most conspicuous in the lower lobes)
- Bronchial dilatation – signet ring sign or nontapering bronchi (the cardinal sign of bronchiectasis)
- Mosaic attenuation pattern (reflecting coexistent constrictive bronchiolitis, possibly an early feature)
- Tree-in-bud pattern (representing exudate in and around the small airways)
- Mucus plugging of large airways (a late stage sign)

There are several situations in which the signs of bronchiectasis may be obscured by technical artifacts, or mimicked by other lung pathologies,[262,263] and these are summarized in Chapter 4, page 165.

Accuracy of HRCT for diagnosis

In the absence of a true gold standard, the accuracy of HRCT in confirming or excluding bronchiectasis is difficult to ascertain. Evidence from early studies which compared CT (using widely different technical parameters, particularly section collimation)[253,287–289] do not allow any definite conclusions to be drawn, particularly as bronchography cannot be regarded as a wholly reliable or reproducible technique.[290,291] In one study in which thin-section CT findings were compared with pathologic features (from surgically resected bronchiectatic lobes), Kang et al[261] showed that CT identified bronchiectasis in 41 (87%) of 47 lobes with pathologically proven bronchiectasis. Because the patients selected for this study had relatively severe disease, the authors suggested that the detection rate of CT may be less in patients with mild bronchiectasis. In the lobes considered to have bronchiectasis on CT, the most frequently identified sign was a lack of tapering of the bronchial lumens (37 of 41), followed by bronchial wall thickening (32 of 41), bronchial dilatation (28 of 41), identification of bronchi in the lung periphery (21 of 41) and mucus-filled dilated bronchi (three of 41). The causes of the six of 47 (13%) false negatives were due to either mass lesions or areas of pulmonary consolidation in which dilated bronchi were not identifiable. In a further study which compared the CT features of patients with surgically proven or CT diagnosed bronchiectasis with normal subjects, lack of tapering of the bronchi was identified in 95% of patients with bronchiectasis, compared with 10% of healthy subjects.[265] The results of these studies reiterate the observation of Lynch et al[269] that lack of bronchial tapering should be regarded as the most reliable CT feature of bronchiectasis.

In some patients, the cause for bronchiectasis may be evident from other CT features. For example, diagnosis of Swyer–James/McLeod syndrome can be readily made from the additional features of decreased attenuation and reduced pulmonary vasculature of the ipsilateral lung.[292,293] Similarly, the diagnosis of α_1-antitrypsin deficiency may be suggested by the combination of widespread cylindrical or cystic bronchiectasis and panacinar emphysema in the lower zones.[284,285] However, an underlying cause for bronchiectasis is found in fewer than half of patients,[191,193] and CT features alone do not usually allow a confident distinction between idiopathic bronchiectasis versus known cause of bronchiectasis.[270,294] Nevertheless, in some cases the pattern and lobar distribution of bronchiectasis may be sufficiently characteristic for a specific underlying cause to be

diagnosed.[295–297] The bronchiectasis of ABPA is typically upper zone and central in distribution, with more normal distal bronchi. These features may be helpful in distinguishing this condition from other causes or idiopathic bronchiectasis.[298–301]

Several other distinctive, if not diagnostic, patterns have been described in patients with a known cause of bronchiectasis. A lower and middle lobe distribution of cylindrical bronchiectasis with particularly marked bronchial wall thickening is typical in patients with hypogammaglobulinemia.[200,219] A single report suggests a predilection for the middle lobe in patients with immotile cilia syndrome,[257] and an upper lobe distribution of cylindrical bronchiectasis in patients with cystic fibrosis.[213,302,303] In patients with bronchiectasis due to nontuberculous mycobacterial infection, there is often an accompanying nodular pattern[304]; indeed, there appear to be some difference in patterns of disease between the subspecies of nontuberculous tuberculosis.[305] Idiopathic bronchiectasis has been reported to be predominantly basal in distribution.[296] However, studies that have sought to determine whether observers can reliably distinguish between idiopathic bronchiectasis and bronchiectasis of known cause have not been conclusive and suggest that, though several CT features occur more frequently in certain groups of patients with an identifiable underlying cause, none of the CT features evaluated can be regarded as pathognomonic.[270,294,297]

Some conditions with more or less distinctive features on HRCT (including the distribution of disease, pattern of bronchiectasis, and ancillary features) are listed in Box 12.11.

> **Box 12.11 Bronchiectatic conditions with distinctive features on HRCT**
>
> Allergic bronchopulmonary aspergillosis
> Swyer–James/McLeod syndrome
> Tracheobronchomegaly (Mounier–Kuhn syndrome)
> α_1-Antitrypsin deficiency
> Cystic fibrosis
> *Mycobacterium avium–intracellulare* complex

Cystic fibrosis

Cystic fibrosis (CF), also known as cystic fibrosis of the pancreas, fibrocystic disease, and mucoviscidosis, is the most common autosomal recessive disorder in the caucasian population, with a frequency of about 1 in 2500 live births.[306,307] The disease is uncommon in African–Americans and rare in Asians and Native Americans. Worldwide, 60,000 people are affected.[308] CF is caused by a mutation in a gene on chromosome 7 that codes for the cystic fibrosis transmembrane conductance regulator (CTFR).[309,310] Although >800 mutations have been identified,[311] the most common mutation that causes CF is known as $\Delta F508$.[309] CFTR functions primarily as a chloride ion channel and the defective protein affects pancreatic function and the consistency of mucosal secretions. Although the defective gene has been identified, gene replacement therapy is still far from clinical realization.[306,312]

The primary manifestations of CF include abnormal sweat electrolytes, sinus and pulmonary disease, exocrine pancreatic insufficiency, and male infertility.[313] However, virtually any organ system can be affected because of the wide tissue distribution of CFTR. The main clinical consequences of CF are listed in Box 12.12.

Despite major advances in treatment, pulmonary infection remains the major cause of morbidity and mortality. *Staphylococcus aureus* and *Haemophilus influenza* are the most common infecting organisms in the first decade of life, but infections caused by *Pseudomonas* and *Burkholderia* species dominate thereafter. By adulthood, 80% of patients are colonized with *P. aeruginosa* and 3.5% with *B. cepacia*. *Stenotrophomonas maltophilia*, *Achromobacter xylosoxidans*, and nontuberculous mycobacteria are emerging as important pathogens in patients with CF.[308]

Although the disease is present at birth, radiographic abnormalities may not become apparent for months or years, but thereafter are progressive (Fig. 12.32). The earliest findings are nonspecific and include focal atelectasis, recurrent pneumonia, and diffuse bronchial wall thickening. At this stage, the clinical features of the disease, not the chest radiographic findings, suggest the diagnosis. Progression of disease with worsening radiographic abnormalities is unfortunately inexorable despite treatment, but the rate of deterioration varies among patients. Patients with early manifestations of the disease tend to deteriorate the most rapidly.[314] In the fully developed form of the disease the radiographic findings are remarkably uniform and include the following[315–319]:

- *Bronchial wall thickening and bronchiectasis*, which result from chronic inspissation of mucus and airway infection, are the hallmarks of the disease (Fig. 12.33). These findings manifest on chest radiographs with peribronchial cuffing, tram-tracking and ring shadows. Associated mucoid impactions that manifest as "finger-in-glove", "toothpaste" or nodular opacities are also common. Bronchiectasis may be cylindrical or cystic depending upon the severity and chronicity of the disease. Cystic bronchiectasis is often an impressive feature of the disease (Fig. 12.34). The cysts may be up to 2 cm in diameter and often have thin walls. The walls may be thickened by associated infection and the cysts may contain variable quantities of fluid. In advanced disease it may be impossible to distinguish between cystic lung destruction and grossly dilated airways, particularly in the upper lobes.
- *Atelectasis and focal consolidation* are also common and may wax and wane in association with acute infection. Extensive cicatricial atelectasis in the upper lobes may result from chronic or recurrent infection (Fig. 12.35). Large areas of consolidation are uncommon but are seen in overwhelming, usually *P. aeruginosa*, infection or ABPA.[258]
- *Enlarged hila and diffuse perihilar opacities*. Enlargement of the hila is caused by lymphadenopathy, dilatation of the pulmonary arteries (reflecting pulmonary hypertension), and inflammatory changes adjacent to the hila (Fig. 12.36). Lymphadenopathy, presumably due to reactive hyperplasia, is a common finding in patients with CF.[319] Diffuse perihilar opacities are due to peribronchial inflammation and central bronchiectasis (Fig. 12.36).
- Progressive airway obstruction results in *pulmonary hyperinflation*. The thorax becomes barrel shaped with an increased anteroposterior diameter (Fig. 12.32). The diaphragms are usually low and flattened.

Box 12.12   Clinical consequences of cystic fibrosis

End-organ effects of cystic fibrosis, related to viscous secretions

Pancreas
Pancreatitis
Pancreatic insufficiency
Diabetes mellitus

Liver
Cirrhosis
Portal hypertension
Varices
Hypersplenism

Intestines
Meconium ileus
Atresia
Constipation leading to rectal prolapse and inguinal hernias

Upper respiratory tract
Abnormal salivary secretions
Nasal polyps
Sinusitis

Lower respiratory tract
Bronchiectasis
Bronchitis
Bronchopneumonia
Atelectasis
Emphysema
Hilar adenopathy
Pulmonary hypertension
Cor pulmonale
Hemoptysis
Respiratory failure

Female genital tract
Reduced fertility

Male genital tract
Secondary aplasia (vas deferens, epididymis, seminal vesicles)
Sterility

Exocrine gland abnormality
Salt depletion
Heat stroke

Parenchymal findings seen on chest radiographs of patients with cystic fibrosis are often more severe in the upper than lower lungs. This has led to the assumption that the upper lobes are affected first and most severely. However, Marchant et al[320] studied young CF patients with thin-section CT and found that the lower lobes were affected most uniformly and severely; it may be that the obvious upper lobe predominance develops over the years (Figs 12.32 and 12.37).

Chest radiographs over a number of years generally reflect the patient's deteriorating status, but shortterm clinical fluctuations are not necessarily accompanied by any readily detectable radiographic changes. Greene et al[321] studied 14 specific

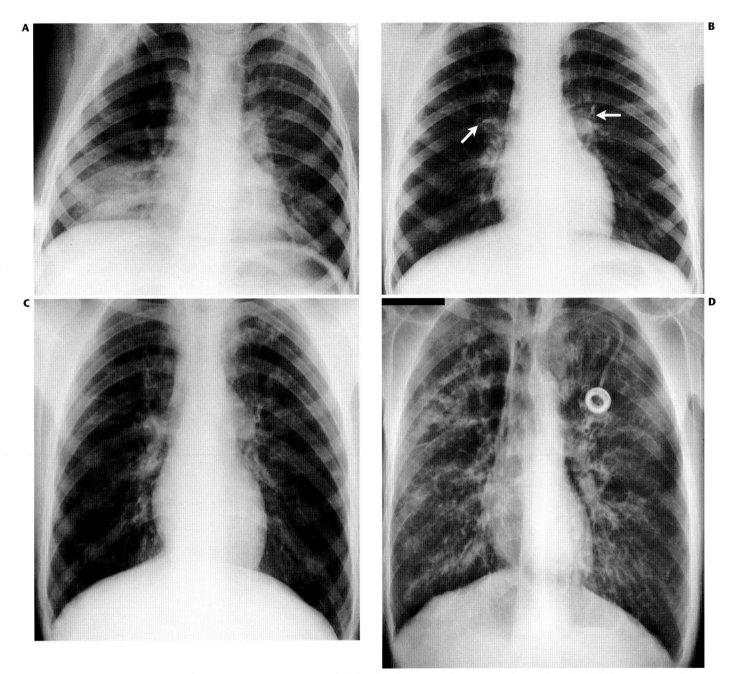

Fig. 12.32 Cystic fibrosis. Serial chest imaging over a 26 year period showing the progressive changes of cystic fibrosis. **A**, At 3 years of age, the patient presented with right middle lobe pneumonia. **B**, There is mild hyperinflation and bronchial wall thickening (arrows) by age 7 years. **C**, At age 15 years, the chest radiograph shows progressive hyperinflation, bronchiectasis and enlargement of the hila. **D**, Frontal (*cont'd*)

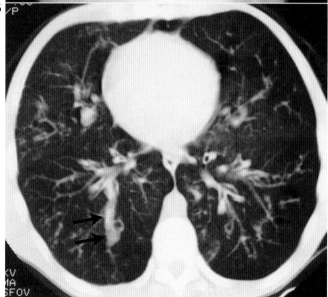

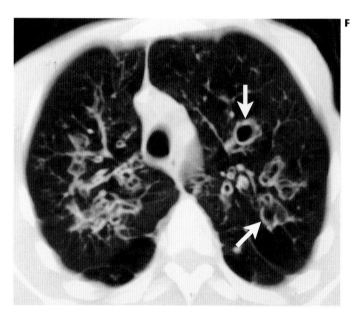

Fig. 12.32 (*cont'd*) **E**, lateral chest radiographs at 29 years show typical findings of end-stage cystic fibrosis. Note marked hyperinflation and "barrel chest" deformity, severe bronchiectasis, and tubular opacities consistent with mucus plugs. **F** and **G**, Standard CT images at 29 years show extensive bronchiectasis (white arrows), which are more severe in the upper (**F**) than the lower (**G**) lobes, mucoid impaction (black arrows) and mosaic attenuation due to small airways obstruction.

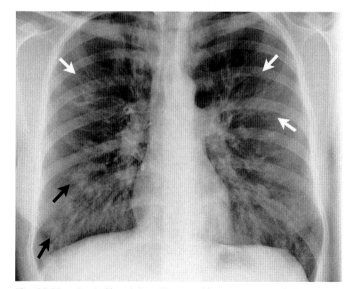

Fig. 12.33 Cystic fibrosis in a 23-year-old woman. Frontal chest radiograph shows extensive perihilar ring shadows (white arrows, bronchiectasis) and tubular opacities (black arrows) in the right lower lobe consistent with mucoid impaction.

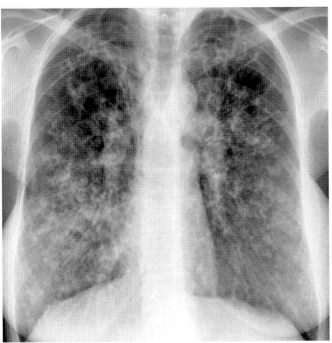

Fig. 12.34 Cystic fibrosis in a 24-year-old woman. Frontal chest radiograph shows marked hyperinflation, and diffuse cystic bronchiectasis.

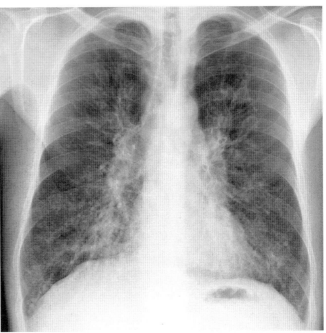

Fig. 12.36 Cystic fibrosis in a 24-year-old man. Frontal chest radiograph shows extensive bronchiectasis, central perihilar opacities, and enlarged hila due to reactive lymphadenopathy or pulmonary artery hypertension or both.

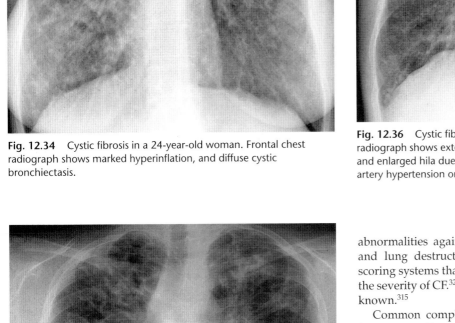

Fig. 12.35 Cystic fibrosis in a 27-year-old woman. Frontal chest radiograph shows extensive bronchiectasis with bilateral upper lobe volume loss and retraction of both hila.

radiographic findings in a group of adults with and without acute exacerbations of cystic fibrosis. They were unable to find a statistically significant association between any of the findings and the presence or absence of acute symptoms. These authors concluded that the value of the chest radiograph in the setting of an acute CF exacerbation lay more in excluding a major complication such as pneumothorax. In part, this must reflect the inherent difficulties in detecting small focal radiographic

abnormalities against a background of diffuse bronchiectasis and lung destruction. Nevertheless, there are a number of scoring systems that use findings on chest radiographs to grade the severity of CF.[322] The Brasfield system remains the most well known.[315]

Common complications of CF include pneumothorax and hemoptysis. Pneumothorax is caused by rupture of emphysematous blebs or bullae.[323] Hemoptysis is usually caused by hypertrophied bronchial arteries and varies in severity from minor blood streaked sputum to massive hemoptysis (>240 ml/24 h).[324] Affected patients tend to have very severe lung disease and a high incidence of infection by multidrug resistant bacteria.[324] Bronchial artery embolization (BAE) is an effective treatment for CF patients with pulmonary bleeding.[324–326] Brinson et al[324] reviewed their experience with BAE in 18 patients treated over a 10 year period. They found that the overall efficacy of BAE for initial control of bleeding was 75% after one, 89% after two, and 93% after three treatments. Unfortunately, they also found that the rate of recurrent bleeding was high (46%); the mean time to recurrence was approximately 12 months. They also found a high incidence (75%) of bleeding from nonbronchial systemic collateral vessels in patients who had undergone previous BAE, indicating the necessity of evaluating all potential systemic collateral vessels. Lung abscess and empyema are surprisingly uncommon complications of CF.

The CT findings of CF on conventional[327] and thin-section CT have been well described.[213,214,302,328–333] As might be expected, CT delineates the morphologic changes of CF with much greater accuracy and detail than chest radiographs. However, as is the case with chest radiography, CT has only limited utility in the investigation of patients with acute exacerbations of CF. The only finding in the study of Shah et al,[331] that had a limited

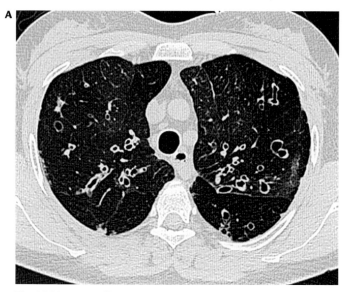
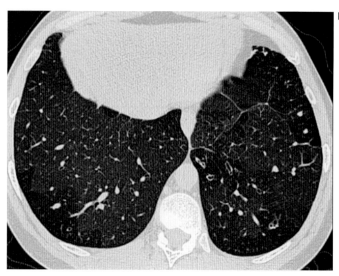

Fig. 12.37 Cystic fibrosis. **A**, Typical upper lobe predominant distribution of bronchiectasis in a 14-year-old patient, with **B**, relative sparing of the lower lobes.

correlation with acute exacerbation, was the presence of air–fluid levels. A more recent study has confirmed that changes in mucus plugging on HRCT are the most labile abnormality in an acute exacerbation.[334] Perhaps not surprisingly, while certain HRCT features have some relationship with functional measures of airflow limitation, they do not correlate with markers of airway inflammation such as sputum cytokine levels.[335]

While CT may not be particularly useful in patients with advanced disease, many investigators have found that thin-section CT could be useful in the identification of early lung disease in patients with minimal respiratory complaints.[302] Scoring systems have also been developed for CT; the best known is the Bhalla system.[336] Numerous investigators have found good correlation between functional impairment and CT findings using this or similar CT scoring methods.[214,320,328,332,336,337] While these methods may be useful from a research standpoint, their utility in everyday clinical practice is limited.

The CT findings of CF vary with duration and severity of disease.[214,320,328,332,333,336–338] Bronchiectasis is the predominant abnormality. Cylindrical bronchiectasis appears to be more common than cystic bronchiectasis, particularly in patients with mild lung disease.[213,302] Cystic bronchiectasis may, therefore, be an expression of more advanced disease. In advanced cases, both forms of bronchiectasis tend to be more severe in the upper lungs. Bronchial and peribronchial thickening is also a common finding on CT that reflects the chronic inflammatory changes in the bronchial wall. Mucus plugs, a very common finding, are seen to advantage with CT. Abscesses may be difficult to distinguish from cystic bronchiectasis, particularly as both may contain air–fluid levels. Other CT findings include emphysema and bulla formation, focal areas of collapse or consolidation, mosaic attenuation, hilar and mediastinal adenopathy, and pleural thickening. Bullae may also be difficult to distinguish from cystic bronchiectasis, particularly in fibrotic upper lobes.[213] Mosaic attenuation presumably reflects obstruction of small airways. Pleural thickening is often apparent on chest radiographs and is demonstrated to advantage by CT. The extent of such thickening may have a bearing on the selection of patients

for lung transplantation, though it has been convincingly shown that pretransplantation CT in this context is of little value.[339] In some patients who develop a pneumothorax, CT may usefully identify the optimal site for chest drain insertion because the visceral pleura is often tethered to the chest wall because of pleural adhesions.[340]

MRI has been used for investigation of patients with CF.[341,342] It can demonstrate many of the salient features of CF, but lacks the spatial resolution of CT. Donnelly et al[311] used hyperpolarized ^{3}He-enhanced MRI to image patients with CF.[311] Because this technique is quite sensitive for small airway obstruction, it may provide a means for evaluating progression of disease in patients with CF without use of ionizing radiation.

Ciliary dyskinesia syndrome (immobile cilia syndrome)

The ciliary dyskinesia syndrome (CDS) is an example of one of many specific causes of bronchiectasis, and with changing patterns of etiology it is becoming relatively more important. In this condition, first identified in 1976,[343] a variety of genetically determined defects in ciliary structure and function[344] interfere with mucociliary clearance.[345] This impaired clearance is associated with recurrent upper and lower respiratory tract infections.[346] Another factor contributing to recurrent infection is defective neutrophil chemotaxis, a common association.[344] CDS shares many features with cystic fibrosis but is less disabling and carries a better prognosis.[257] Kartagener syndrome[347] – situs inversus, paranasal sinusitis, and bronchiectasis – is a subset of CDS, and about 50% of patients with CDS have Kartagener syndrome.[257,346,348] About one-fifth of subjects with dextrocardia have Kartagener syndrome.[349] CDS has autosomal recessive transmission[350] with an equal sex incidence. In Europe and the United States, CDS has a prevalence of about 1:20,000 individuals.[344]

Ciliary function is abnormal throughout the body, and sperm are immotile; thus males are infertile. Fertility in females is generally unaffected, though there are exceptions.[348] Respiratory symptoms may be delayed in onset but can generally be traced back to childhood, and CDS is even described as causing neonatal respiratory distress.[351] Symptoms are those of bronchitis, rhinitis, and sinusitis, which are universal, and otitis, which is less common. Bronchiectasis develops in childhood and adolescence (Figs 12.21 and 12.22)[257] and is associated with recurrent pneumonia. Prognosis is generally good, and the diagnosis is compatible with a full life span.[349] The diagnosis is regarded as established in the following circumstances: (1) complete Kartagener syndrome; (2) men with normal situs but a classic history and immotile sperm; (3) women and children with normal situs but typical history and an affected sibling; and (4) subjects with normal situs but with a classic history and ultrastructural defects of nasal or bronchial cilia on biopsy.[346] Patients with Kartagener syndrome and morphologically normal cilia have been described.[344,352] Findings on the chest radiograph and CT are of bronchiectasis with a predilection for involvement of the anatomic middle lobe.

Young syndrome[242,243] clinically resembles CDS. However, in Young syndrome ciliary function is normal and infertility is due to obstructive azoospermia. Obstruction occurs at the level of the epididymis, which is palpably enlarged. The pathogenesis of increased sinopulmonary infection in these patients is obscure.

BRONCHOLITHIASIS

The term "broncholithiasis" is generally interpreted more widely than meaning simply the condition resulting from endobronchial calcified material.[353] Most authors include, in addition, the effects of airway distortion or inflammation caused by calcified peribronchial nodes[354] or other rarer causes focal calcific endoluminal lesions.[355] Nearly all cases are due to infective nodes, particularly following histoplasmosis.[356,357] Other causal infections include tuberculosis, actinomycosis, coccidioidomycosis, and cryptococcosis. A few cases have been reported with silicosis.[358] Calcified material in an airway or luminal distortion caused by peribronchial disease results in airway obstruction. This in turn leads to collapse, obstructive pneumonitis, mucoid impaction, or bronchiectasis. Rarely, fistulas can form from the airway to the esophagus,[359] pleural space, or aorta,[356] and mediastinal abscess formation has been reported.[360] Symptoms commonly include cough, hemoptysis, and recurrent episodes of fever and purulent sputum.[205,356] The classic symptom of lithoptysis is uncommon, with a reported frequency of between 13 and 16%.[205,356]

In a review of plain radiographic findings, three major types of change were distinguished[353]: (1) disappearance of a previously identified calcified nidus; (2) change in position of a calcified nidus; and (3) evidence of airway obstruction, including segmental or lobar atelectasis, mucoid impaction, obstructive pneumonitis, and obstructive overinflation with air-trapping. There may be signs of bronchiectasis.[356] Calcified hilar or mediastinal nodes are a key feature of the radiograph, and it is important to inspect all calcifications, assessing their position and looking for evidence of movement on serial films. Movement can be difficult to detect and may just be a relatively subtle rotation.[353] Broncholithiasis is more common on the right,[356] and obstructive changes particularly affect the right middle lobe.

The diagnosis may not be suspected on plain radiographs. CT and fiberoptic bronchoscopy complement each other in this

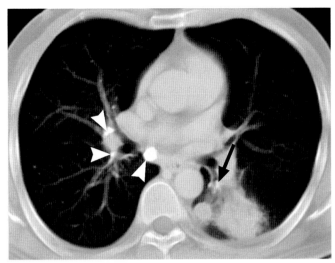

Fig. 12.38 Broncholithiasis in a 50-year-old man who had been treated with pulmonary tuberculosis 10 years earlier. CT shows several calcified lymph nodes in the subcarinal region and adjacent to segmental bronchi of the right middle and lower lobes (arrowheads). There is also a small irregular calcified nodule in the superior segmental bronchus of the left lower lobe (arrow) with distal consolidation. Bronchoscopy revealed a broncholith, which was removed. (With permission from Seo JB, Song KS, Lee JS, et al. Broncholithiasis: review of the causes with radiologic–pathologic correlation. RadioGraphics 2002;22:S199–S213.)

condition, neither on its own being necessarily diagnostic. Principal findings on CT[205,355,361,362] are a calcified lymph node within an airway or immediately adjacent to a distorted airway, distal changes secondary to bronchial obstruction, and absence of an associated soft tissue mass (Fig. 12.38). CT is not always correct in accurately localizing calcification because of partial volume effects, and in one series 40% of truly endobronchial lesions were interpreted on CT as extrabronchial.[205] Reconstruction of volumetric CT data, including 3D depictions, can be used to overcome this problem.[355] The CT appearance of broncholithiasis can be mimicked by calcifying endobronchial hamartomas or carcinoid tumors.[363]

SMALL AIRWAYS DISEASES

Bronchiolitis includes a spectrum of inflammatory and fibrosing disorders that predominantly affect the small airways (membranous and respiratory bronchioles). These disorders show great variability as regards cause, clinical features, and histopathologic changes. A number of attempts to classify these conditions have been made,[364–367] and one of the more comprehensive schemes, described by Myers and Colby,[366] is:

1. Constrictive bronchiolitis (obliterative bronchiolitis, bronchiolitis obliterans)
2. Cryptogenic organizing pneumonia (bronchiolitis obliterans organizing pneumonia, proliferative bronchiolitis)
3. Acute bronchiolitis (infectious bronchiolitis)
4. Small airways disease (adult bronchiolitis)
5. Respiratory bronchiolitis (smoker's bronchiolitis, respiratory bronchiolitis-interstitial lung disease)

6. Mineral dust airways disease (early pneumoconiosis)
7. Follicular bronchiolitis
8. Diffuse panbronchiolitis

The terminology used to classify diseases of the small airways is confusing but can, for imaging purposes, be greatly simplified. Diseases affecting the small airways are difficult to detect by conventional radiographic and physiologic tests; widespread involvement occurs before symptoms or abnormalities on pulmonary function testing become apparent. An understanding of the distribution of disease in relation to the airways at a pathologic level allows some prediction of the likely CT appearances in this wide spectrum of conditions, and thus helps to refine differential diagnosis.

The detection and understanding of various small airways diseases has increased in recent years thanks largely to HRCT appearances of the various pathologic types of small airways disease. The difficulty in detecting small airways dysfunction on pulmonary function testing can be readily appreciated by considering the fact that the summed cross-sectional area of the small airways luminal diameters is much greater than that of the central airways and so accounts for less than one-quarter of total airflow resistance. Thus, an extraordinary number of small airways need to be affected before there is a measurable physiologic deficit.

Features of small airways disease on HRCT can be broadly categorized into direct and indirect signs: considerable thickening of the bronchiolar walls by inflammatory infiltrate and/or luminal and surrounding exudate render affected airways directly visible (tree-in-bud pattern). By contrast, cicatricial scarring of many bronchioles results in the indirect sign of patchy density differences of the lung parenchyma, reflecting areas of under-ventilated, and consequently under-perfused, lung (mosaic attenuation pattern); these two basic patterns are more fully discussed in Chapter 4.

Pathologic classification and clinical background

Inflammation of the bronchioles (bronchiolitis) with or without subsequent scarring and obliteration is a very common lesion in the lungs.[368] However, the extent of such lesions is rarely extensive enough to cause clinical symptoms. Pathologic studies have repeatedly emphasized the frequent involvement of the bronchioles in diverse diffuse lung diseases. Because of the wide diversity of conditions which are characterized by an element of bronchiolar damage, the generic term "small airways disease" is widely used.

The specific and classic term obliterative bronchiolitis (synonymous with bronchiolitis obliterans) has, until recently, been the subject of confusion, primarily because of its use in the context of bronchiolitis obliterans organizing pneumonia (BOOP). The clinicopathologic entity of BOOP, more usefully termed cryptogenic organizing pneumonia (COP),[369,370] is now regarded as quite distinct from obliterative bronchiolitis (Fig. 12.39). There are numerous reports in the literature describing cases of "bronchiolitis obliterans" whose pathologic descriptions contain all the hallmarks of an organizing pneumonia, characterized by buds of loose granulation tissue occupying the airspaces and respiratory bronchioles, without any obliteration of the small airways.[371–373] It is now generally accepted that there is no direct connection between obliterative bronchiolitis and BOOP,[374] such that in the interests of clarity it has been suggested that the bronchiolitis obliterans part of BOOP should be discarded. In those patients in whom no causative agent for the organizing pneumonia can be found, the term COP is more appropriate.[370]

The various conditions included within the term "small airways diseases" are usually classified into pathologic subtypes or by less precise clinical criteria (usually by presumed cause or association). The latter approach has become increasingly unsatisfactory because of the increasing number of new causes and associations reported in the literature. While pathologists categorize small airways diseases according to their histopathologic subtypes,[375] the difficulty with this classical approach is that there are not always obvious clinical (or HRCT) correlates with the pathologic subtypes (see above classification of Myers and Colby[366]).

A simple approach relies on the fundamental difference between the *indirect* HRCT signs of constrictive bronchiolitis and the *direct* visualization on HRCT of exudative forms of bronchiolitis (typified by diffuse panbronchiolitis).[376] These two patterns of small airways disease account for the majority encountered in clinical practice. Other miscellaneous forms of small airways disease with more or less distinctive pathologic and imaging features, if not clinical presentations, are dealt with separately.

Constrictive obliterative bronchiolitis

Constrictive obliterative bronchiolitis is, as its name implies, a condition characterized by bronchiolar and peribronchiolar inflammation and fibrosis that ultimately leads to luminal obliteration.[364,366,375] The early change is a cellular inflammation that is intraluminal, mural, and peribronchial, affecting membranous and respiratory bronchioles. Inflammatory cells

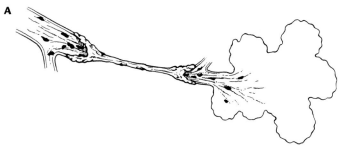

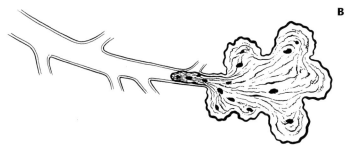

Fig. 12.39 Schematic representation of the pathology of **A**, constrictive obliterative bronchiolitis and **B**, organizing pneumonia (formerly referred to as BOOP); in the latter, the dominant process is plugging of the airspaces and small airways with loose granulation tissue rather than peribronchiolar fibrosis and luminal obliteration.

Box 12.13 Causes of and associations with constrictive obliterative bronchiolitis

Postinfection
Viral[380] (adenovirus,[381] respiratory syncytial virus, influenza,[382,383] and parainfluenza[382])
Mycoplasma[384]

Postinhalation (toxic fumes and gases)[385,386]
Nitrogen dioxide (silo filler's disease), sulfur dioxide, ammonia, chlorine, phosgene[387]
Gastric aspiration[382]
Hot gases[388]

Connective tissue disorders[379]
Rheumatoid arthritis[389,390]
Sjögren syndrome[391,392]
Others very rarely

Allograft recipients
Bone marrow transplant[393,394]
Heart–lung or lung transplant[395–398]

Drugs
Penicillamine[399]
Lomustine

Ulcerative colitis[400,401]

Cryptogenic[377] (truly idiopathic cases are very rare)

Other conditions
Bronchiectasis[261,281]
Chronic bronchitis[402]
Cystic fibrosis[403]
Hypersensitivity pneumonitis
Sarcoidosis
Microcarcinoid tumorlets[404,405]
Sauropus androgynus ingestion[406]

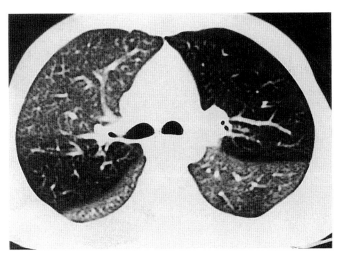

Fig. 12.40 Sequel of mycoplasma pneumonia in a 6-year-old child. CT obtained during breath holding at full inspiration. There are dramatic segmental differences in attenuation of the lung parenchyma, reflecting severe constrictive bronchiolitis. There is a marked reduction in the caliber of the pulmonary vasculature in the affected (decreased attenuation) parts of the lung.

are a mixture of neutrophils, lymphocytes, and plasma cells. The mature lesion is a peribronchiolar fibrosis, encroaching on the lumen, and narrowing and eventually occluding the airway.[366] Other features include smooth muscle hyperplasia and bronchiolectasis with mucoid impaction.[364]

Clinical findings are extremely variable in severity and vary according to cause, but do have common features: symptoms consist of progressive dyspnea and nonproductive cough unaccompanied by significant wheezing. On auscultation of the chest, crackles and, apparently characteristic, inspiratory squeaks and squawks are heard. Pulmonary function tests show airflow obstruction, sometimes with restriction, with a normal gas transfer adjusted for alveolar volume (Kco).[377,378] There is evidence of gas trapping with a low FVC and a high residual volume. Airflow limitation is volume dependent and may be demonstrated using flow volume loops that allow calculation of maximum mid expiratory flow rates (MMEFR). However, a reduced MMEFR is not specific for small airways disease.[379]

Constrictive obliterative bronchiolitis is a relatively uncommon disorder that in most cases is associated with a recognized predisposing condition but rarely is truly cryptogenic. Reported causes and associations are listed in Box 12.13.

Viral infections, particularly by respiratory syncytial virus and adenovirus,[381,407] are a common cause of constrictive

bronchiolitis in children. Nonviral agents are much less commonly implicated, though *Mycoplasma pneumoniae* is a particulary potent cause of constrictive bronchiolitis (Fig. 12.40).[380,382,384] Caution is needed in interpreting reports that suggest bacterial infections, e.g. *Nocardia asteroides* and *Legionella pneumophila*, may be responsible for an obliterative bronchiolitis[373,408]: the pathology described in these particular reports is of an organizing pneumonia rather than constrictive bronchiolitis (highlighting the historical confusion surrounding the terminology of "bronchiolitis obliterans"). Postinfectious constrictive obliterative bronchiolitis is largely confined to children; though repeated viral lower respiratory tract infections are a usual fact of adult life, clinically significant constrictive bronchiolitis as a consequence is fortunately rare (Fig. 12.41).[409] Swyer–James/McLeod syndrome is a particular form of constrictive bronchiolitis that occurs following an insult, usually a viral infection, to the developing lung (see p. 746).

Constrictive bronchiolitis is a predictable consequence of the inhalation of many toxic fumes and gases which reach the small airways.[386] It has been most frequently described following nitrogen dioxide inhalation (silo filler's disease).[410,411]

Among the connective tissue diseases, constrictive bronchiolitis is most strongly associated with rheumatoid arthritis.[379,389,412,413] Constrictive bronchiolitis associated with rheumatoid arthritis may be rapidly progressive with refractory airflow obstruction unresponsive to any treatment.[389] Nevertheless, minor degrees of constrictive bronchiolitis are probably present and subclinical in many patients with rheumatoid arthritis.[414,415] About 50% of patients with rheumatoid arthritis and constrictive obliterative bronchiolitis take penicillamine,[377,389] and a cause and effect relationship has been proposed.[416,417] This is supported by a study of 602 patients with rheumatoid arthritis in which there was a 3% prevalence of constrictive obliterative bronchiolitis in patients receiving penicillamine, but no cases of constrictive obliterative bronchiolitis in those not taking the drug.[399] Furthermore, a close temporal relationship often exists between starting penicillamine and the onset of symptoms.[379]

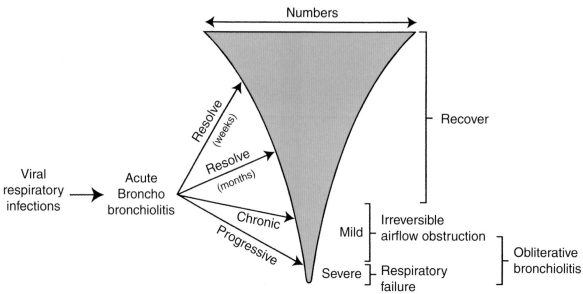

Fig. 12.41 Natural history and potential outcomes of lower respiratory tract viral infections. (Modified with permission from Green M, Turton CW. Bronchiolitis and its manifestations. Eur J Respir Dis Suppl 1982;121:63:36–42. Copyright remains with European Respiratory Society Journals Ltd.)

Nevertheless, it remains possible that penicillamine treatment is merely a "marker" of those patients with more severe rheumatoid arthritis, and who are thus more likely to develop complications of the disease, including constrictive obliterative bronchiolitis. Studies using indirect measures, such as pulmonary function testing and HRCT, suggest that small airways disease is generally more prevalent than earlier studies indicated.[413,415] Patients with Sjögren syndrome may have a combination of interstitial disease (usually lymphocytic interstitial pneumonitis) and small airways disease but, unlike rheumatoid arthritis, constrictive bronchiolitis is rarely the dominant presenting feature.[391,418]

Constrictive bronchiolitis is an important and frequent cause of morbidity and mortality in patients receiving heart and lung transplants.[394,398,419–421] It has a prevalence of between 25 and 50% and usually manifests itself between 9 and 15 months (range 60 days to 5.6 years) after transplantation.[421] It is probable that subclinical damage to small airways epithelium occurs earlier, within the first few weeks following transplantation, and that subtle abnormalities on HRCT may predate the functional abnormalities of supervening small airways obliteration[422]; nevertheless, the sensitivity of HRCT for the early detection of constrictive obliterative bronchiolitis in transplant patients has been questioned,[423] and the correlation between the functional severity of the so-called bronchiolitis obliterans syndrome and extent of CT abnormalities is not strong.[424] Frequent and severe episodes of acute rejection, potentiated by cytomegalovirus and other infective agents, increase the risk of development of constrictive bronchiolitis. Modification of the immunosuppressive regimen may be successful in delaying the development of constrictive obliterative bronchiolitis, but relapses are common.[421] Constrictive bronchiolitis is also a well recognized complication of bone marrow transplantation.[393,394,425] The disorder develops usually within 18 months of transplantation and is also variably responsive to increased immunosuppression.[426]

Constrictive obliterative bronchiolitis is rarely truly cryptogenic.[377,427] Most reported cases probably have an undisclosed precipitating cause or association, such as a connective tissue disease which subsequently declares itself.[428]

The radiographic features of constrictive bronchiolitis can be summarized as diminished pulmonary vasculature and over-inflation of the lungs with or without bronchial wall thickening[429] (Fig. 12.42)[429]; these nonspecific abnormalities, seen in any form of chronic obstructive pulmonary disease, are prone to considerable observer variation. Furthermore, these features are not present in all patients finally diagnosed as having constrictive bronchiolitis.[269,430]

In an early CT study of constrictive bronchiolitis, 15 patients who fulfilled the criteria of Turton et al[377] were examined with conventional (contiguous 10 mm sections) and thin-section CT (interspaced 3 mm sections).[427] Chest radiographs were normal in five of 15 patients; the remaining 10 patients showed "limited vascular attenuation and hyperinflation". In 13 of 15 patients a pattern of "patchy irregular areas of high and low attenuation in variable proportions, accentuated in expiration" was recorded; this, and a report of two cases by Eber et al,[431] were the first studies to identify regional inhomogeneity of the density of the lung parenchyma as the indirect, but key, CT feature of constrictive bronchiolitis.

Subsequent descriptions have confirmed and refined the HRCT features of constrictive bronchiolitis.[378,432–437] The HRCT signs comprise patchy areas of reduced parenchymal density (the "mosaic attenuation pattern"), attenuation of the pulmonary vessels within areas of decreased lung density, bronchial abnormalities (Fig. 12.43), and a relative lack of change of cross-sectional area of affected parts of the lung on sections obtained at end-expiration (Fig. 12.44).[292,438] The individual HRCT signs of constrictive bronchiolitis (Box 12.14) are considered in more detail in Chapter 4.

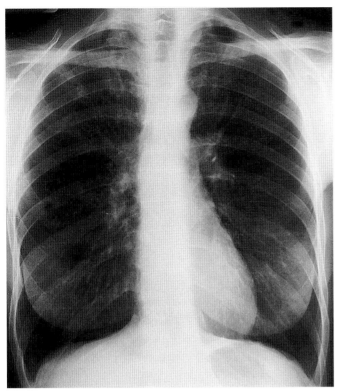

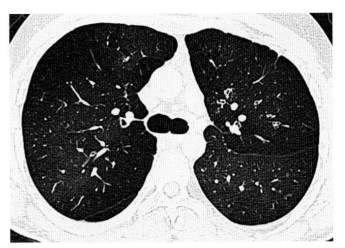

Fig. 12.43 Constrictive bronchiolitis in a patient with rheumatoid arthritis. There is a mosaic attenuation pattern and within the areas of decreased attenuation, the pulmonary vasculature is of reduced caliber. Several of the subsegmental bronchi are thick walled and dilated.

Fig. 12.42 Chest radiograph of a patient with advanced constrictive bronchiolitis awaiting lung transplantation. The lungs are of large volume and there is flattening of the hemidiaphragms. There are subtle and nonspecific features of a reduction of the pulmonary vasculature in the upper zones and mild peribronchial thickening in the lower zones.

The sensitivity and specificity of the sign of decreased attenuation for the diagnosis of constrictive obliterative bronchiolitis depend largely upon the clinical context in which it is sought: e.g. in postlung transplant patients, one series has reported a sensitivity of 40%, and specificity of 78%, for the mosaic pattern. This increased to 80 and 94%, respectively, for the expiratory CT sections.[439] If the other HRCT features associated with constrictive obliterative bronchiolitis are also included (bronchial dilatation, bronchial wall thickening[440]), specificity,

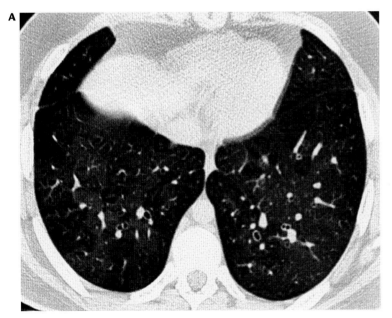

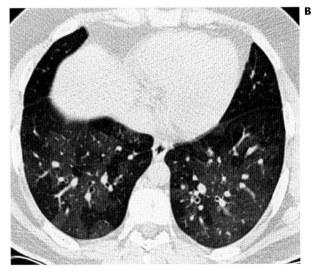

Fig. 12.44 Constrictive bronchiolitis of unknown etiology. **A**, Patchy attenuation differences and mild bronchial abnormalities on CT obtained at near total lung capacity. **B**, End-expiratory CT accentuating the mosaic attenuation pattern and showing relative lack of change in area of the decreased attenuation of the lung.

and to a lesser extent sensitivity, of HRCT is increased.[439] Abnormalities of the macroscopic bronchi are a variable feature on HRCT, but are not unexpected given their anatomic continuity with the small airways; it seems that bronchial dilatation and bronchial wall thickening are relatively late features of constrictive obliterative bronchiolitis, and are more frequent in immunologically driven disease, such as rheumatoid arthritis[441] or postlung transplantation (Fig. 12.45).[442] The regional inhomogeneity of the lung attenuation may be extremely subtle in constrictive bronchiolitis, and is sometimes invisible on inspiratory CTs, but the attenuation differences may be enhanced on CTs obtained at end-expiration (Fig. 12.46)[420,438,443–445] or by postprocessing of the inspiratory CT sections.[446–448] However, in the few patients with extensive or end-stage constrictive obliterative bronchiolitis, the mosaic attenuation pattern may be absent. Furthermore, CT sections taken at end-expiration will appear remarkably similar to inspiratory sections: there will be no obvious change in cross-section area of the lungs (which normally decreases, at the level of the carina, by approximately 55%[449]) (Fig. 12.47). However, the generalized paucity of vessels and bronchial abnormalities will be present, though these findings may be very similar to those seen in widespread and severe panacinar emphysema.[284,450]

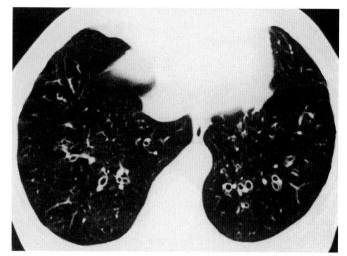

Fig. 12.45 Patient with rheumatoid arthritis and clinical and pulmonary function tests consistent with severe constrictive bronchiolitis. The lung parenchyma is of uniformly decreased attenuation and the pulmonary vessels are of reduced caliber. In this case the bronchial abnormalities are particularly severe with widespread cylindrical bronchiectasis.

The HRCT signs listed above are not, by themselves, specific for constrictive bronchiolitis and may be encountered in other chronic obstructive pulmonary diseases; e.g. the mosaic attenuation pattern may be found in asthmatic patients, albeit usually less extensive than in patients with constrictive bronchiolitis.[451] However, in the context of a known cause or association of constrictive bronchiolitis, an HRCT showing this constellation of features can be regarded as diagnostic. Nevertheless, there are circumstances in which the distinction between constrictive bronchiolitis and other obstructive pulmonary disease, particularly in patients with advanced disease, can be difficult.[452] Areas of decreased attenuation of the

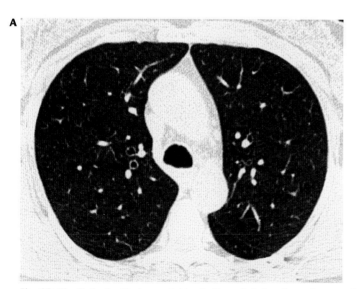
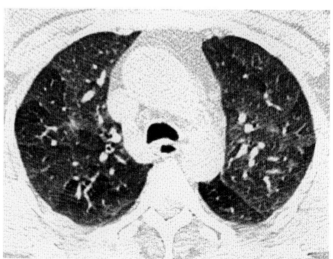

Fig. 12.46 Patient with rheumatoid arthritis and obstructive pulmonary function tests. **A**, Inspiratory CT showing no obvious mosaic attenuation pattern or emphysema. **B**, Expiratory CT revealing extensive patchy air-trapping, consistent with constrictive bronchiolitis.

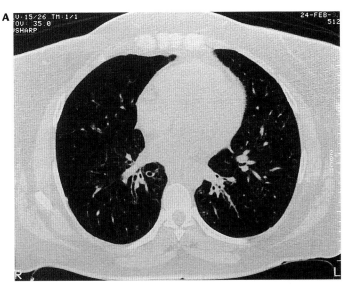
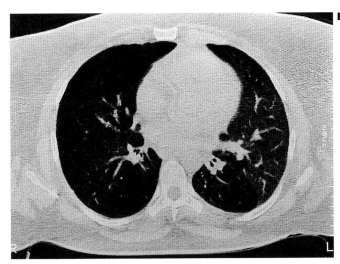

Fig. 12.47   Severe postviral constrictive obliterative bronchiolitis on inspiratory and expiratory CT. **A**, On the inspiratory section the lung is generally of decreased attenuation (most striking in the right middle lobe, which is of increased volume). **B**, On the section taken at end-expiration at approximately the same anatomic level there is virtually no change in the appearance or cross-sectional area of the right lung. There is a moderate increase in the density of the parenchyma in the lingula indicating less severe involvement.

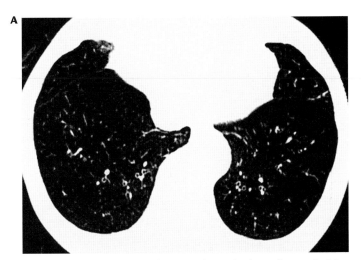
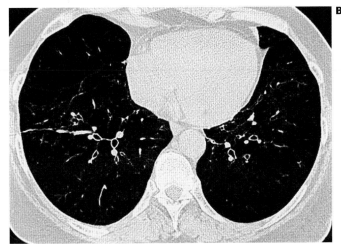

Fig. 12.48   Two patients with severe obstructive lung disease. **A**, Advanced constrictive bronchiolitis. **B**, Panacinar emphysema (α_1-antitrypsin deficiency). Both cases demonstrate nonspecific uniform decreased attenuation of the lung parenchyma and bronchial abnormalities.

lung parenchyma on HRCT in patients with severe obstructive airways disease due to constrictive bronchiolitis may sometimes be interpreted as "emphysema"; in constrictive bronchiolitis, the pulmonary vessels in affected lung are attenuated, but not distorted, as is the case in centrilobular emphysema. Furthermore, the extent of decreased attenuation caused by constrictive bronchiolitis does not correlate with gas diffusing capacity, the functional hallmark of emphysema.[378] The differentiation between panacinar emphysema (typified by patients with α_1-antitrypsin deficiency) and advanced constrictive obliterative bronchiolitis may be less straightforward on HRCT appearances alone (Fig. 12.48). A recent study that tested the ability of observers to distinguish, on the basis of HRCT findings, between cases of constrictive bronchiolitis, asthma, centrilobular emphysema, panacinar emphysema, and normal individuals showed that the first choice diagnosis was correct in 199 of 276 (72%)

observations. Furthermore, agreement on distinguishing between cases of constrictive bronchiolitis and panacinar emphysema was reasonable ($\kappa = 0.63$).[452]

Diffuse panbronchiolitis

Diffuse panbronchiolitis is the exudative small airways disease *par excellence* and is characterized by a tree-in-bud pattern at HRCT. Diffuse (Japanese) panbronchiolitis is a sinobronchial disease and was initially thought to be confined to Asian countries but sporadic cases have been reported in every continent.[453] Symptoms include cough, sputum, chronic sinusitis, and signs of progressive obstructive airways disease; given these clinical features, it has been suggested that the inclusive term "sinobronchial syndrome" would be more appropriate,[454] but the original pathologic term diffuse panbronchiolitis is relatively unambiguous and well established. Some patients respond to longterm low dose erythromycin with subjective and objective improvement,[455] though the mechanism of action of erythromycin is unknown (and is not simply ascribable to its bactericidal properties). The prognosis is surprisingly poor with a reported 10 year survival rate as low as 25%.[456]

Most of the definitive pathologic and imaging studies originate from Japan.[278,457,458] The typical histopathologic features of diffuse panbronchiolitis are chronic inflammatory cell infiltration resulting in bronchiolectasis and striking hyperplasia of lymphoid follicles in the walls of the respiratory bronchioles; profuse foamy macrophages fill the bronchiolar lumens and the immediately adjacent alveoli, though the distal airspaces are not involved. This bronchiolocentric exudate is visible macroscopically as yellow nodules. As the disease progresses, an element of fibrotic bronchiolar constriction supervenes but, in the absence of longitudinal histopathologic studies, the extent to which the basic "exudative" pathology progresses to constrictive bronchiolar obliteration is not clear.

On chest radiography the dominant pattern is of numerous small (<5 mm) ill-defined nodules, such that the radiographic pattern may be interpreted as reflecting an interstitial, rather than airways centered, disease (Fig. 12.49). The nodules are symmetrically distributed and initially most prominent basally. Later, the radiographic features of cylindrical bronchiectasis may become evident. HRCT appearances reflect the pathologic distribution of disease: there is a nodular pattern and small branching opacities (tree-in-bud pattern)[459] can be identified in a predominantly centrilobular distribution, corresponding to the plugged and thickened small airways (Fig. 12.50). Accompanying cylindrical bronchiectasis, usually mild, is an almost invariable feature. Interestingly, though a mosaic attenuation pattern may be present in some cases, it is not usually a major feature; furthermore, air-trapping on expiratory CT is often surprisingly

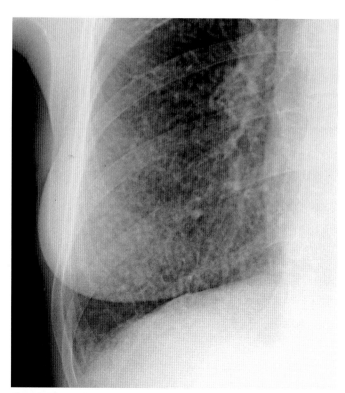

Fig. 12.49 Diffuse panbronchiolitis. The generalized nodular pattern reflects plugging of the small airways, but might be interpreted as representing an interstitial lung disease.

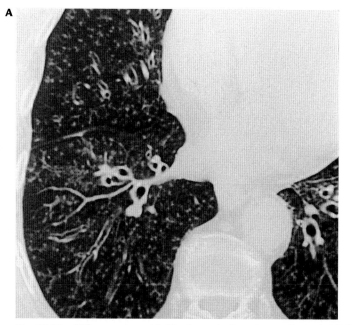

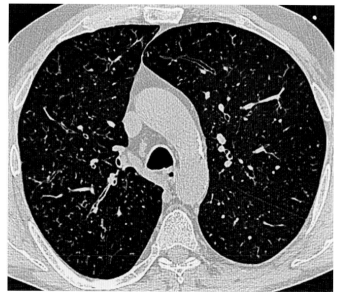

Fig. 12.50 Diffuse panbronchiolitis. Examples from two patients: **A,** HRCT section through the right middle and lower lobes showing a myriad of small nodules and branching structures (tree-in-bud pattern) and accompanying cylindrical bronchiectasis. **B,** Similar combination of findings in another case of diffuse panbronchiolitis.

unimpressive. Nevertheless, functional studies have shown that the peripheral zone of lung is less dense than normal because of air-trapping.[460] The individual HRCT signs of panbronchiolitis are summarized in Box 12.15.

The HRCT features of diffuse panbronchiolitis, in the appropriate clinical setting, are virtually pathognomonic. However, other conditions may cause a similar (primarily tree-in-bud) pattern on HRCT, including infections such as tuberculosis[461,462] and invasive aspergillosis[463]; other causes of a tree-in-bud pattern are listed on page 168.

Miscellaneous conditions with small airways involvement

Hypersensitivity pneumonitis

Inhalation of organic dusts and deposition in the terminal and respiratory bronchioles causes an inflammatory (or cellular) bronchiolitis of variable severity in susceptible individuals. The potential for varying degrees of involvement of the airways and interstitium, and the coexistence of subacute and more chronic changes, explains the sometimes complex abnormalities found on pulmonary function testing.[464] The HRCT features of subacute hypersensitivity pneumonitis are described in detail elsewhere (p. 438). With regard to the small airways involvement, there is a strong correlation between the extent of the areas of decreased attenuation (a component of the mosaic attenuation pattern) on

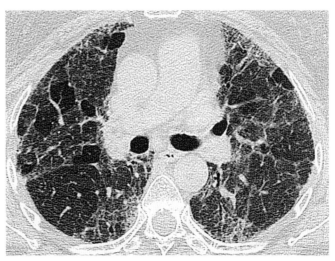

Fig. 12.52 Chronic hypersensitivity pneumonitis. The reticular pattern with distortion of the lung parenchyma indicates established fibrosis in this case of chronic hypersensitivity pneumonitis. There are several secondary pulmonary nodules of decreased attenuation reflecting the coexisting small airways disease.

HRCT and pulmonary function indices of air-trapping.[465,466] The air-trapping, graphically shown on expiratory CT, is present in the majority of patients with subacute disease, and reflects the underlying component of cellular bronchiolitis (Fig. 12.51). Even in patients with chronic fibrotic disease, expiratory CT may show lobular air-trapping amongst the reticular pattern, presumably reflecting fixed constrictive bronchiolitis (Fig. 12.52).

Sarcoidosis

By virtue of their perilymphatic distribution, sarcoid granulomas are concentrated around the airways. Physiologic studies have

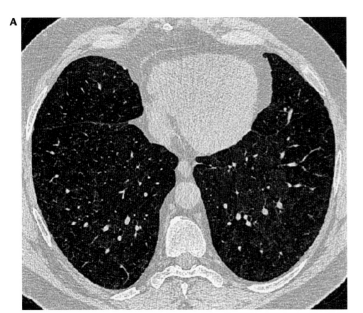
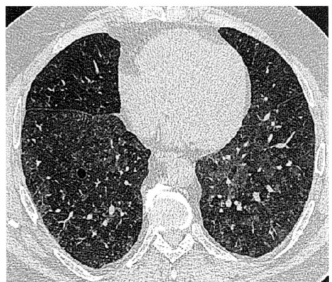

Fig. 12.51 Hypersensitive pneumonitis. **A**, Patchy density differences reflecting both the interstitial infiltrate of subacute hypersensitivity pneumonitis and the coexisting small airways disease. **B**, End-expiratory CT showing enhancement of the patchy density differences, reflecting small airways involvement (note the thin walled cyst in the right lower lobe, an occasional feature of hypersensitivity pneumonitis).

suggested that airflow obstruction located at the level of the small airways may be an early feature of sarcoidosis.[467,468] Supportive evidence, seen as patchy air-trapping on expiratory CT, was first described in three case reports,[469] and later confirmed in larger series (Fig. 12.53).[470,471] In some cases the air-trapping, thought to reflect bronchiolar obstruction, foreshadows the more typical parenchymal manifestations of sarcoidosis. It seems that this phenomenon is common in patients with sarcoidosis at presentation (demonstrated in 20 of 21 patients in one series[470]). However, the prevalence of this phenomenon and its clinical significance have not been established.

Follicular bronchiolitis

Follicular bronchiolitis is primarily a histopathologic diagnosis and is characterized by hyperplastic lymphoid follicles, ranged along bronchioles which are compressed as a consequence; there is also infiltration of the adjacent bronchiolar walls and interstitium by polyclonal lymphocytes.[472,473] The exact relationship between follicular bronchiolitis, lymphocytic interstitial pneumonitis, and constrictive obliterative bronchiolitis, particularly in patients with rheumatoid arthritis in whom these pathologies may coexist, remains controversial.[390] Follicular bronchiolitis is most commonly encountered in patients with rheumatoid arthritis or Sjögren syndrome, but other associations include a familial form with immunodeficiency.[472] The prognostic implication of follicular bronchiolitis (a diagnosis made on the basis of lung biopsy) is uncertain, particularly as it may be identified on a background of other pathology, e.g. usual interstitial pneumonia in association with a connective tissue disease. In some individuals, compression of the bronchioles by the hyperplastic follicles results in severe airflow limitation.[474] Peribronchial lymphoid hyperplasia in children (termed follicular bronchitis) may represent an exaggerated immune response to a viral infection, and results in mild airflow obstruction in the long term.[475]

The plain chest radiograph shows nonspecific small nodular or reticulonodular opacities,[473,476] but may be normal. In an HRCT study of 14 patients (12 with a connective tissue disease) with biopsy proven follicular bronchiolitis, the predominant abnormality was small nodules (3 mm diameter, but up to 12 mm in some cases).[477] In some cases the nodules had a predictably centrilobular bronchocentric distribution, such that the HRCT pattern resembled sarcoidosis (Fig. 12.54). Areas of ground-glass opacification probably reflect the more generalized lymphocytic infiltration, present in just over half of patients.[477] Mild bronchial dilatation with wall thickening occurs in some cases (Fig. 12.54), but whether this is directly related to the presence of follicular bronchiolitis, or is associated with the background autoimmune disease, is unclear.

Respiratory bronchiolitis

The concept of damage to the small airways by cigarette smoke was established by a necropsy study of the lungs of young smokers (who died from an unrelated cause); the characteristic pathologic features were respiratory bronchiolitis, an abundance of pigmented alveolar macrophages within the lumina of the respiratory bronchioles, and associated mild peribronchiolar interstitial fibrosis.[478] The term respiratory bronchiolitis-interstitial lung disease (RB-ILD) has been coined to describe this lesion that is almost unique to cigarette smokers.[479,480] Fuller consideration of this entity is given on page 429. In the very few individuals who develop a full clinicopathologic syndrome with symptoms ascribable to RB-ILD, the dominant pathologic abnormality is profuse intraalveolar macrophages, rather than bronchiolitis. The radiographic and CT appearances are nonspecific.[481–483] The typical constellation of HRCT features includes: patchy ground-glass opacification (reflecting the macrophage accumulation in the airspaces[273,484]); poorly defined centrilobular nodules[482]; a limited reticular pattern with some thickening of the interlobular septa (probably due to minor interstitial fibrosis) (Fig. 12.55); and slight thickening of the macroscopic airways (possibly changes of chronic bronchitis) (Fig. 12.56). Emphysema is generally a minor feature, often no more than a trace of paraseptal emphysema at the lung apices. In

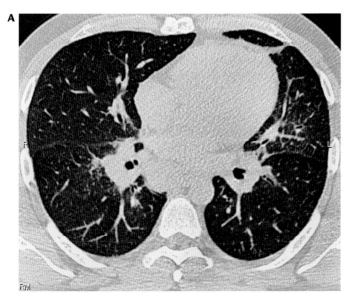
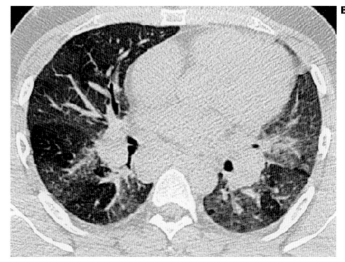

Fig. 12.53 Sarcoidosis. **A,** Bilateral hilar and subcarinal lymphadenopathy and a few pulmonary micronodules on an inspiratory CT. **B,** Expiratory CT showing patchy air-trapping because of small airways obstruction.

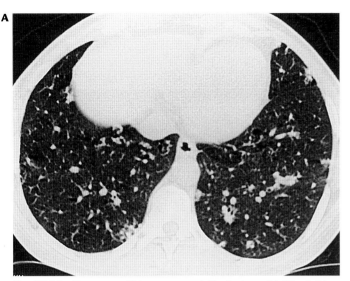
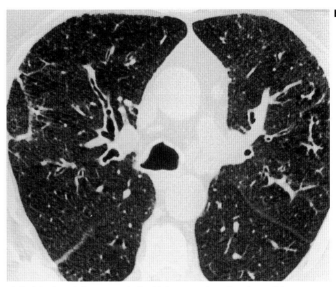

Fig. 12.54 Two cases of biopsy proven follicular bronchiolitis. **A**, Numerous lobulated nodules, several of which are centered on bronchi, presumably representing aggregates of lymphoid hyperplasia. **B**, Mild dilatation of several subsegmental bronchi which have irregularly thickened walls. There is some fibrosis in the upper lobes causing distortion of the pulmonary architecture.

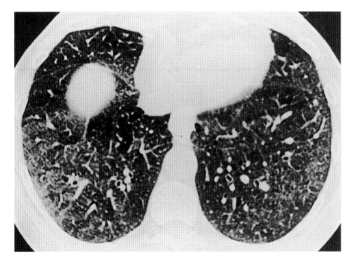
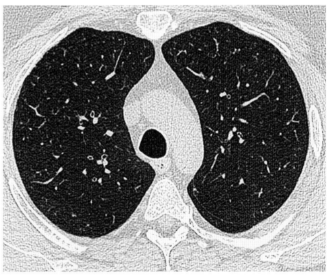

Fig. 12.55 Respiratory bronchiolitis-interstitial lung disease (RB-ILD). Complex combination of ground glass and reticular patterns, as well as some nodular components and a few thickened interlobular septa. In this case of biopsy-proven RB-ILD there was some interstitial fibrosis in addition to the bronchocentric macrophage accumulation.

Fig. 12.56 Mild bronchial wall thickening, particularly in the right upper lobe, in a patient with changes of respiratory bronchiolitis on lung biopsy.

some individuals there is a mosaic attenuation pattern which may reflect the bronchiolitic element of the disease, and/or the patchy desquamative interstitial pneumonia-like component. On expiratory CT, evidence of air-trapping is usually undramatic (Fig. 12.57) and not as extensive as that seen in other mixed interstitial and small airways diseases, such as subacute hypersensitivity pneumonitis.

Microcarcinoid tumorlets

Hyperplastic aggregates of neuroendocrine cells cause an extremely unusual form of obliterative bronchiolitis. Diffuse hyperplasia or more focal carcinoid-like tumorlets are associated with fibrosis and scarring of the bronchioles,[404,405,485] and may be found in association with chronic lung disease, particularly bronchiectasis, or in isolation. The functional consequences of the resulting constrictive obliterative bronchiolitis may be very severe. On HRCT, there are nodules of varying sizes reminiscent of metastatic disease (though the tumorlets are not neoplastic in behavior); close examination of the distribution of the larger nodules may show that they arise at the carinas of adjoining airways (the typical location of "conventional" carcinoid tumors). The nodules are superimposed on a background mosaic

A

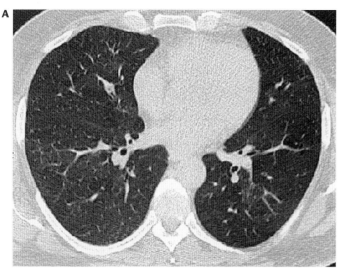

B

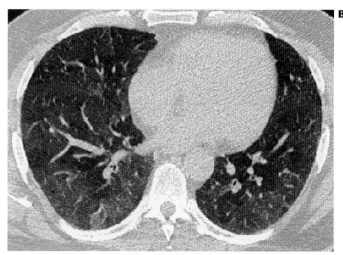

Fig. 12.57 Respiratory bronchiolitis-interstitial lung disease (RB-ILD). **A**, Inspiratory CT section showing minor attenuation differences, but no other features to suggest RB-ILD. **B**, End-expiratory CT showing patchy air-trapping.

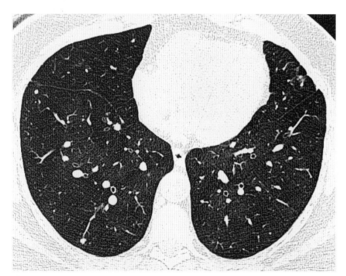

Fig. 12.58 Microcarcinoid tumorlets. A 53-year-old woman with severe airflow obstruction, thought to have emphysema. There are noncalcified nodules scattered throughout the lungs ranging from 3 to 12 mm (see periphery of right lower lobe) on a background mosaic attenuation pattern.

attenuation pattern reflecting the accompanying obliterative bronchiolitis (Fig. 12.58).[485] These two HRCT signs are individually entirely nonspecific but, taken together in the context of a patient with disabling airflow limitation, they are suggestive of this curious and rare condition.

Swyer–James/McLeod syndrome (Box 12.16)

The Swyer–James/McLeod syndrome is a form of obliterative bronchiolitis that has special features: it occurs following an insult to the developing lung, and the lung served by damaged bronchi and bronchioles remains inflated by collateral air drift. As defined in the original descriptions, disease on chest radiography is predominantly unilateral, giving rise to the key finding of unilateral transradiancy.

> **Box 12.16 Swyer–James syndrome**
>
> Sywer–James syndrome results from viral injury to the developing lung (before the age of 8 years)
>
> Unilateral transradiancy on plain chest radiography in Sywer–James syndrome reflects a combination of hypoplasia of the pulmonary vasculature and obliterative bronchiolitis
>
> The affected lung is small or normal in volume
>
> In contrast to the apparently unilateral distribution of Sywer–James syndrome on chest radiography, CT usually reveals bilateral abnormalities (areas of decreased attenuation and cylindrical bronchiectasis) in individuals with Swyer–James syndrome

The condition was first described in the early 1950s, and a variety of noneponymous terms have been used to identify it, particularly unilateral or lobar emphysema. However, these terms may lead to confusion with, for example, congenital lobar emphysema, and the current practice of using eponymous titles seems likely to continue. On some grounds Swyer–James syndrome seems to be the most appropriate (Swyer and James published their report 1 year before McLeod).

The condition is characterized by bronchitis, bronchiolitis, constrictive obliterative bronchiolitis, and probably emphysema.[486,487] Typically the condition is unilateral and a whole lung is affected, but changes may be confined to a lobe or segment.[488] Other recognized patterns are of segmental sparing with the rest of the lung involved[488] and of bilateral lobar or segmental disease. The patchy nature of lung involvement in some patients is particularly well demonstrated on CT examination.[489] Bronchi and bronchioles from the fourth generation to terminal bronchioles have submucosal fibrosis, causing luminal irregularity and occlusion.[486,488] Pulmonary tissue is hypoplastic, including the pulmonary artery and its branches, which are reduced in both size and number. Lung distal to diseased airways is hyperinflated and supplied by collateral air drift. Sometimes panacinar emphysematous changes are present,[490] though the definition of emphysema in the context of developing lung is controversial.

The Swyer–James syndrome is caused by injury of the immature lung. Injury most commonly follows an acute viral infection occurring during the first 8 years of life, before the lung has completed its development.[491] Viruses implicated include adenovirus[60] and measles virus.[492] Nonviral causes include infections such as *Mycoplasma pneumoniae*[493] and pertussis,[492] and noninfectious causes such as hydrocarbon ingestion.[494]

Patients are typically asymptomatic and commonly present as adults with an abnormal radiograph. Less commonly patients have exertional dyspnea,[492] which may be progressive and, exceptionally, quite marked,[487] or repeated respiratory infections.[486,492] When coincidental acute lung disorders occur in the presence of the Swyer–James syndrome, the chest radiograph may show a unilateral distribution of acute abnormality, as is recorded with pulmonary edema[495] and pulmonary hemorrhage.[496] Pulmonary function tests show a reduced vital capacity, airflow obstruction, and a reduced gas diffusing capacity. Lung scintigraphy shows a decrease or absence of perfusion in the affected lung[497] and impaired ventilation.[498] Although a matched perfusion–ventilation defect might raise the possibility of embolic pulmonary artery obstruction, this is rarely a diagnostic problem in the clinical setting.

Findings on the plain chest radiograph are characteristic. Unilateral transradiancy is caused by reduced lung perfusion. Lesser degrees of involvement are not easily detectable on the plain radiograph. On the affected side the size and number of mid lung and peripheral vessels are reduced (Fig. 12.59). Blood flow in the contralateral lung is increased, and frequently this lung looks plethoric, an abnormality that may be more striking than the unilateral transradiance. The hilum of the involved lung is small but lung volumes are normal or only slightly decreased. The mediastinum may show some shift to the affected side at total lung capacity.[487] The fact that the ipsilateral lung volume is not increased is helpful in distinguishing Swyer–James syndrome from emphysema per se.[487] Ipsilateral air-trapping is a key finding and a sine qua non of the condition. It can be demonstrated (Fig. 12.59) on an expiratory radiograph which should be exposed during a forced expiratory maneuver because the short expiratory time maximizes volume differences between the obstructed and nonobstructed lung.[499]

CT shows changes that are often more complex than suspected from the chest radiograph (Fig. 12.60), and while it may confirm that transradiancy is unilateral, it more commonly shows bilateral abnormalities.[292,489,500] Transradiant regions are often inhomogeneous, containing a patchwork of local decreased attenuation and hypovascular areas interspersed with lung of normal density.[489] Such small, low density areas may be poorly or sharply marginated, representing areas of small airways disease and air-trapping.[501] Air-trapping can be confirmed with expiratory CT scans. Other changes on CT include bronchiectasis,[292] which is a frequent but not a universal finding,[489,500] and areas of collapse and scarring.

The described combination of radiographic findings usually allows exclusion of other conditions that may resemble the Swyer–James syndrome. These conditions include congenital hypoplastic lung, congenital lobar emphysema, pulmonary artery hypoplasia, and proximal interruption of the pulmonary artery. The greatest worry is that signs are being produced by a central, large airway obstruction causing lung hypoventilation and a compensatory ipsilateral reduction in perfusion. This is a problem that may be resolved only by bronchoscopy or a tailored CT examination of the central airways.

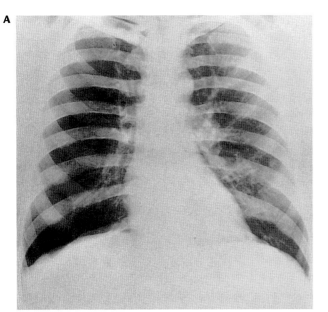
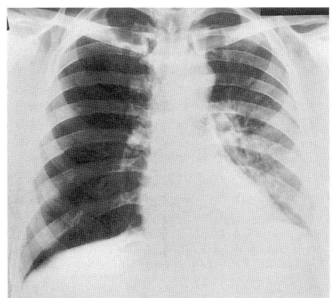

Fig. 12.59 Swyer–James/McLeod syndrome. **A**, Posteroanterior chest radiograph on inspiration shows a transradiant right lung with reduced number and size of vessels and a small right hilum. Lung volume on the right is probably slightly increased. **B**, In the same patient, expiratory radiograph demonstrates air-trapping with relative elevation of the left hemidiaphragm, vascular crowding on the left, and mild mediastinal shift.

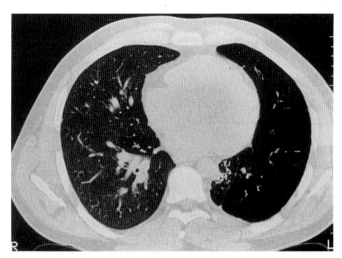

Fig. 12.60 Swyer–James/McLeod syndrome on CT. The left lung shows lower attenuation than the right, and the vessels are reduced in size and number. The left lung volume is reduced, in part because of incomplete collapse of the left lower lobe.

CHRONIC OBSTRUCTIVE PULMONARY DISEASE

COPD (chronic airflow obstruction, chronic obstructive airway disease) encompasses a group of disorders characterized by chronic or recurrent obstruction to airflow.[502] Historically, four principal disorders fall under this heading: asthma, chronic bronchitis, emphysema, and bronchiectasis.[503,504] Although purists object to the use of all-embracing, generic terms such as chronic obstructive airway disease or COPD,[505] they are necessary in clinical practice because the various forms often coexist to a variable extent in the same patient. Nevertheless, the insight that some patients given the label of COPD have "pure" bronchiectasis or emphysema has been provided by HRCT.[506,507] In the round, COPD represents a considerable and underreported burden of morbidity across the world.[508] In industrialized and developing countries, cigarette smoking remains the most important propagator of COPD.[509]

Asthma

Asthma is a recurrent disorder that has been defined functionally as a "disease characterized by wide variations over short periods of time in resistance to air flow in intrapulmonary airways".[510] This definition does not specify the degree of variation, but it is usually taken to be 15–20% of predicted values.

Radiographic findings in uncomplicated asthma are due to both pathologic and pathophysiologic changes. Pathologic changes have been studied largely,[511,512] but not exclusively,[513–515] by postmortem examination of lungs in patients who died of asthma. Such findings represent the severe end of a spectrum of change. On gross examination the lungs are overinflated and fail to deflate because of tenacious mucus plugs in medium sized airways. Bronchial mucosa is damaged or shed, and there is submucosal edema and inflammatory cell infiltrates of eosinophils, sometimes with lymphocytes and plasma cells, causing bronchial wall thickening. Other changes contributing to a general thickening of the bronchial walls include mucus gland hypertrophy, basement membrane thickening, and smooth muscle hyperplasia.[516] The lung parenchyma, in addition to being generally hyperinflated, may show patchy collapse and consolidation.

Routine pulmonary function tests demonstrate pathophysiologic changes in exacerbations but are often normal in remission. Even in remission, however, results of sophisticated tests, particularly of small airway function, may be abnormal.[517] In acute asthma the findings are increased airway resistance, increased total lung capacity (TLC), and increased residual volume and functional residual capacity (FRC) with decreased vital capacity (VC), indicating air-trapping.[518] Changes in TLC and FRC may be at least 20% in an acute attack.[519] With recovery, falls in the TLC and FRC may anticipate increases in the FEV_1. Nonuniform ventilation and perfusion lead to mismatch and hypoxemia in attacks. Diffusing capacity for carbon monoxide, particularly when corrected for accessible alveolar volume, is preserved in nonsmoking asthmatics, even when the condition is severe.[520]

Radiographic findings in simple asthma mirror the pathologic and functional changes of asthma. Hyperinflation may be seen in asthma in both relapse and remission. The prevalence of hyperinflation depends on many factors and is generally higher in children and in patients needing hospital admission. It is also more frequent in patients with an onset of asthma in the first or second decade than in those with a later onset.[521] These latter findings may be related to remodelling of the lungs and thoracic cage induced by airway obstruction during the growing phase.[522] With overinflation, diaphragms become depressed. Although less curved, they rarely become flat or inverted in asthma per se. The frequency of hyperinflation in adults with acute asthma has varied between approximately 20 and 70% in various series, reflecting different patient populations and hyperinflation criteria.[269,523–525] In one series of 117 patients with a mean age of 41 years (range 13–75) admitted to hospital with acute asthma and in whom strict criteria for hyperinflation were applied, the prevalence was 39%.[524] While hyperinflation is often transient, lasting perhaps just 24 h,[526] it may be a permanent change; in the study of 117 patients mentioned previously, 19% showed hyperinflation when in remission.[524] Hyperinflation in such patients is due to a change in lung compliance and is not caused by generalized emphysema, which can be shown to be absent by use of CT.[520,521,527] However, if the patient is a smoker, emphysema may be a contributing factor.[520,528]

In asthmatic patients the walls of end-on segmental airways become thickened (>1 mm) and the normally invisible airways parallel to the radiograph appear as parallel or single line opacities (Fig. 12.61). The most comprehensive study of bronchial wall thickening in asthma was that of Hodson and Trickey[529] in 1960, in which the findings on plain radiographs were assessed in 190 asthmatic patients ranging in age from 3 to 74 years. Bronchial wall thickening was found to be more common in children, and in the small number of children analysed it was a universal finding. Its frequency in adults was less but still surprisingly high, e.g. 50% in the third and fourth decades. Other studies in adults also find that radiographic bronchial wall thickening is common: 71% in 48 asthmatic patients, nearly half of whom were smokers.[269] Bronchial wall thickening was tenfold more common in patients with an infective component to their asthma. In adults bronchial wall thickening, once developed, became a permanent feature. The nontransient nature of bronchial wall thickening has also been shown on CT.[530]

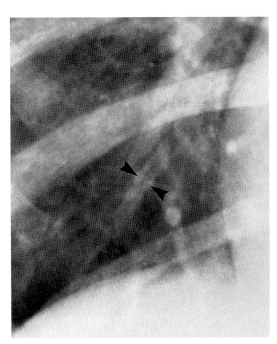

Fig. 12.61 Asthma. Localized view of the right lower zone shows bronchial wall thickening (arrowheads).

Box 12.17 Radiographic features of asthma

Hyperinflation of the lungs (transient or fixed)
Bronchial wall thickening
- More common in children
- Present in up to two-thirds of adult asthmatics
- Usually an irreversible phenomenon

Hilar prominence (uncommon)

About 10% of asthmatic patients show slight prominence of hilar shadows. This is ascribed variously to nodal[531] and vascular enlargement.[524,532,533] Peripheral lung vessels are generally considered normal, but some authors describe diffuse narrowing or subpleural oligemia.[533] The radiographic features directly ascribable to asthma are summarized in Box 12.17.

A number of complications and associations of asthma may be detected on the chest radiograph,[534] including consolidation, atelectasis and mucoid impaction, pneumothorax, pneumomediastinum, and ABPA. Allergic aspergillosis apart, such complications are more common in children than in adults. In one series of 479 hospital patients with a median age of nearly 4 years, 22% had radiographic abnormalities, excluding signs of bronchial wall thickening and hyperinflation.[535] Other pediatric series bear these figures out.[536,537] In adults the prevalence of similar abnormalities is generally <10% even in admissions for acute asthma and is only about 1–2% in series drawn from emergency room patients.[523,524,532,538] Higher figures are reported: in one series of patients with acute asthma, admitted after 12 h of bronchodilator therapy in the emergency room, one-third of chest radiographs were abnormal.[525] A further large retrospective study of 1016 adults who were hospitalized with acute asthma showed that while just over half had normal chest radiographs on admission, 8.2% had significant complications of asthma on chest radiography (e.g. pneumothorax) and 6.7% had important incidental findings (e.g. active tuberculosis).[539]

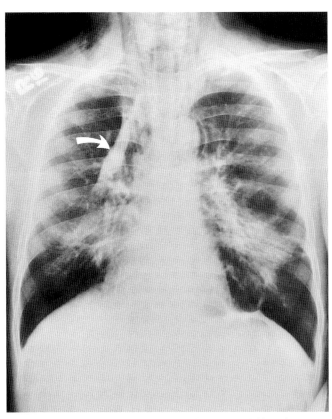

Fig. 12.62 Acute asthma. Radiograph of a 10-year-old boy shows three complications of acute asthma. In the right upper zone, the oblique band shadow is due to segmental collapse (arrow), and in the left lower zone there is infective consolidation. The third complication is a pneumomediastinum with air tracking into the neck.

Consolidation in asthma is commonly infective (Fig. 12.62),[532] but in some cases it is due to eosinophilic consolidation, probably associated with allergic aspergillosis. Collapse (Fig. 12.62) ranges from subsegmental to lobar but occasionally involves a whole lung.[540] Such episodes of collapse are not necessarily associated with an acute illness, a respiratory tract infection, or a worsening of the asthma.[531,541] When segmental or lobar collapse occurs, the middle lobe is commonly affected both in children[535] and adults.[531] Collapse is due to mucoid impaction in large airways or, more commonly, mucus plugging in many small airways. The frequency of occurrence of collapse per se is difficult to determine because in many series consolidation and collapse are considered together.[524] In adults it is probably only a few percent.[523,531]

Pneumothorax is, unexpectedly, an unusual complication of acute asthma in adults, and in combined series consisting largely of adults with acute disease[523,524,533,538] only three pneumothoraces in 566 patients were recorded. In a retrospective survey based on a region of the United Kingdom with >6 million inhabitants, a frequency of pneumothorax in asthma of between 1:300 and 1:1100 was recorded,[542] which was almost identical to figures from a large retrospective study at the Mayo Clinic.[543] In the series reported by Burke[542] it was noted that pneumothorax did not lead to death or morbidity and was usually not suspected clinically. Other workers agree that pneumothorax is not an important factor in mortality except when patients are being treated with positive pressure ventilation.[532,544] A condition that may simulate tension pneumothorax in asthmatic patients receiving mechanical ventilation is described. This is due to a ball valve mucus plug causing localized or unilateral obstructive hyperinflation.[545]

Pneumomediastinum in adults is as uncommon as pneumothorax, and in the combined series of 566 patients discussed above, only two had a pneumomediastinum. Pneumomediastinum is considerably more common in children (Fig. 12.62), with a prevalence of 5.4% in 515 acute asthma admissions.[535] In children it is much more common than pneumothorax, by a factor of 10:1 in one series.[546] Spinal epidural emphysema is a rare complication of mediastinal emphysema in asthma.[547] Radiographically detectable complications in asthmatic patients are listed in Box 12.18.

> **Box 12.19 HRCT findings in asthmatic individuals in approximate order of prevalence (modified from reference[551])**
>
> Bronchial wall thickening
> Cylindrical bronchiectasis
> Thick linear opacities
> Areas of decreased attenuation (part of mosaic pattern)
> Mucoid impaction in the large bronchi
> Small centrilobular opacities
> Airspace consolidation

> **Box 12.18 Radiographically detectable complications of asthma (in approximate order of frequency)**
>
> Complications of airway mucoid impaction
> - Atelectasis, subsegmental through lobar
> - Consolidation (infective or ABPA)
> Features of allergic bronchopulmonary aspergillosis
> - Proximal bronchiectasis
> - Upper zone fibrosis
> Pneumomediastinum or pneumothorax (rare)

The indications for a chest radiograph in adults with asthma are not clearly established. Most authors have recommended chest radiography in all patients who are ill enough to justify admission to a hospital.[523–525,538,547] In the series described by Petheram et al,[524] of 117 patients admitted to the hospital with acute asthma, 9% of chest radiographs showed abnormalities that altered management.[524] White et al[525] recorded an even higher figure, 22%, in 58 patients who were admitted after 12 h of bronchodilator therapy in the emergency ward.

Numerous CT studies have documented the sometimes subtle bronchial and parenchymal abnormalities that occur in asthmatic individuals.[269,530,548–553] Dynamic studies, notably those of Brown et al,[554–557] have made effective use of the ability of HRCT to demonstrate changes in response to pharmacological agents.[554–564] In between exacerbations, the airways and lung parenchyma and bronchi of individuals with early asthma appear normal, explaining the difficulty in discriminating between healthy individuals and mild asthmatics on HRCT.[452]

HRCT has been reported as abnormal (Box 12.19) in between 68 and 90% of patients.[269,530,551] Principal abnormalities involved the airways (Fig. 12.63). Bronchial wall thickening was present in 16%,[530] 82%,[551] and 92%[269] – a discrepancy that cannot be ascribed to the effects of smoking: though nearly half of the subjects in the study of Lynch et al[269] were smokers, only 12 of 50 asthmatic individuals in the study by Grenier et al[551] were current or exsmokers.[551] Comparing bronchial dilatation in the series of Paganin et al[530] with that of Lynch et al[269] is difficult because patients with bronchiectasis (clinically and on CT criteria) were excluded from the latter study.[269] However, if cylindrical bronchiectasis and airway dilatation are taken as roughly equivalent terms, the findings are similar: cylindrical bronchiectasis in 56% of one series[530] and bronchial dilatation in 77% of the other.[269] In the more recent study of Grenier et al,[551] frank bronchiectasis was identified in 29% of asthmatic patients, this lower prevalence perhaps reflecting more stringent criteria for the identification of bronchiectasis. The pathogenesis of these

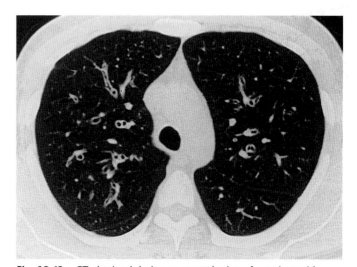

Fig. 12.63 CT obtained during an exacerbation of a patient with severe asthma. The subsegmental bronchi in the upper lobes are thickened and dilated and some of the airways are bronchiectatic by HRCT criteria.

bronchial abnormalities remains controversial. Peribronchial inflammation may be partly responsible for the bronchial wall thickening but this feature is not always steroid responsive.[530] Chronic inflammation of the airways probably leads to some morphologic remodeling with an increase of several components of the bronchial wall, including smooth muscle hypertrophy.[565,566] Explanations for the bronchial dilatation in asthmatics, other than the obvious one of progressive damage by repeated episodes of inflammation, include coexisting subclinical ABPA,[301] or the consequence of severe childhood infection.[567] However, no single explanation is entirely satisfactory, particularly as some reversibility of bronchiectatic changes is possible.[568] Furthermore, it seems surprising that while there is no obvious relationship between the prevalence of bronchiectasis and the severity of asthma,[551] there is some correlation between bronchial wall thickness and the graded severity of asthma.[515,553,562,569] So-called "objective" CT measurement of bronchial dimensions, in particular wall thickness, is prone to many physiologic and technical vagaries, especially changes in window settings.[570] Nevertheless, comparative studies have lent some insights, such as the observation that wall thickening is a more pronounced feature in patients with nonallergic asthma,[549] though this difference has recently been questioned.[571]

The areas of decreased attenuation on HRCT that can be identified in acute or induced asthma almost certainly reflect hypoxic vasoconstriction in parts of the lung that are under-ventilated consequent upon the bronchospasm,[560,564] and such areas of air-trapping are more conspicuous and extensive on expiratory CT scans.[438,443,572] In chronic asthma the significance of areas of "black lung" on HRCT has in the past been controversial. Some studies have implied that emphysema is responsible for the areas of decreased lung attenuation[530,549,552] in non-smoking asthmatics; against this is the striking lack of correlation between the Kco (the functional hallmark of emphysema) and the extent of areas of decreased attenuation in asthma[520,573] and other airways diseases.[378,574] There is increasing evidence in asthmatic individuals that morphologic features of emphysema on HRCT are almost invariably related to cigarette smoking, rather than the asthma per se in which the decreased attenuation merely represents small airways dysfunction.[505,571,573,575–577] In patients with severe asthma a mosaic attenuation pattern, indistinguishable from that of patients with constrictive obliterative bronchiolitis, may be detectable on inspiratory HRCT. However, the decreased attenuation component of the mosaicism is usually not as extensive as that seen in individuals with clinically significant constrictive obliterative bronchiolitis.[451]

Chronic bronchitis

Chronic bronchitis is defined, using clinical criteria, as a chronic or recurrent increase in the volume of mucoid bronchial secretions sufficient to cause expectoration and occurring on most days for 3 months in 2 or more successive years, other causes for expectoration having been excluded.[181,503,578]

Chronic bronchitis is a common disease, affecting up to 20% of the adult population in some studies.[579] It seems to be more common in males than females,[579] but when smoking habits are taken into account the difference is only 2:1.[504] Most studies show an increasing prevalence with age. Cigarette smoking is the most important factor associated with the development of chronic bronchitis. In eight combined series in England there was a sixfold rise in prevalence of chronic bronchitis, from 6.3% in non-smokers to 40% in heavy smokers.[504] In epidemiologic studies a linear relationship exists between the amount smoked and the frequency of chronic bronchitis.[580] Less important factors include occupation, environment, age, and gender.[581] Given the subjective nature of the diagnosis,[582] it is not surprising that there appear to be substantial differences in the prevalence of chronic bronchitis even when there is no obvious difference in risk factors between cities in the same (Baltic) region.[583]

The major pathologic changes are in the mucus glands, which show hypertrophy and hyperplasia and develop enlarged ducts. The enlargement of mucus glands can be quantified histologically using either the proportional mucus gland area or the Reid index, which is the ratio of gland thickness to bronchial wall thickness measured from epithelial basement membrane to perichondrium.[584] However, these indices do not clearly distinguish normal subjects from those with chronic bronchitis, since there is considerable overlap.[585,586] Study of these indexes has shown that mucus glands enlarge with age and in cigarette smokers.[587,588]

Other pathologic changes in chronic bronchitis include goblet cell hyperplasia, squamous metaplasia of the epithelium, and a variable and often mild[584] chronic inflammatory cell infiltrate.[181] Mucus plugs occur in the smaller airways, which themselves

may be stenotic.[504,589,590] Cartilage atrophy probably occurs, but the evidence is conflicting,[591–593] and atrophy seems to be more a feature of emphysema than of chronic bronchitis.[594]

Chronic bronchitis typically occurs as a persistent productive cough following an acute chest infection. Such symptoms may persist for years with normal respiratory function tests and chest radiographs. Indeed, the majority of such patients do not develop chronic airway obstruction, though they are at risk for recurrent episodes of purulent bronchitis.[595] In these patients the annual decrease in FEV$_1$ is within the normal range.[595,596] In some patients with chronic bronchitis, however, particularly those who smoke heavily, there is detectable airflow obstruction with a greater than predicted annual fall in FEV$_1$. These patients become dyspneic, with copious sputum, and tend to become hypoxemic.[597] In such patients pulmonary arterial hypertension and cor pulmonale may develop. The majority of acute exacerbations in chronic bronchitis can be ascribed to a lower respiratory tract infection; up to 30% are viral but other organisms, including atypical bacteria such as *Chlamydia pneumoniae*, may occasionally be responsible.[598] However, doubt has been raised about the role of bacterial infections in causing exacerbations in COPD.[599]

Radiographic signs in pure chronic bronchitis are poorly documented. Nearly all the available information is derived from three series of patients, in whom coexistent emphysema was not excluded.[600–602] Overinflation of the lungs described in these reports is in conflict with the normal TLC usually found in chronic bronchitis,[603] and is now generally ascribed to coexistent emphysema.

The majority of patients with symptoms of chronic bronchitis have a normal chest radiograph.[604] Radiographic signs that can be ascribed to chronic bronchitis include bronchial wall thickening and "increased lung markings". Bronchial wall thickening might be expected in chronic bronchitis because of the known pathologic changes in the airways. However, histologic studies suggest that the magnitude of these changes is small; in one report the absolute increase in gland thickness was only 0.1 mm.[586] Bates et al[600] described parallel line shadows on radiographs representing large airways seen side on (tramline opacities) in 42% of patients with chronic bronchitis. However, this sign was not recorded by Simon[601] and Simon and Garber[602] in earlier studies. Ring shadows vary between 4 and 7 mm in diameter and most commonly represent the end-on anterior or posterior segmental airways of the upper lobes. This is a normal finding, whereas visible side-on airways (tramline opacities) are generally considered abnormal. Fraser et al[594] assessed the frequency of detection of end-on airways and their wall thickness in approximately 150 control subjects and 150 patients with chronic bronchitis. They found end-on airways visible in about 80% of both groups and a slight increase in wall thickness in chronic bronchitis, which was of limited value in distinguishing patients with chronic bronchitis from normal subjects, though the sign was subject to significant interobserver variation. In functional terms, the ratio of wall thickness to external diameter in end-on airways does not appear to correlate with the degree of airflow obstruction.[605] Another radiographic sign described in the series of Bates et al[600] was increased lung markings, detected in 18% (Fig. 12.64). This feature again was rare in other series.[601,602] The sign consists of small, ill-defined linear opacities with or without accentuation of small vascular opacities.[604] It is a subjective sign that in pathologic examination, in one study, was shown to correlate with perivenous edema, inflammatory cell infiltration,

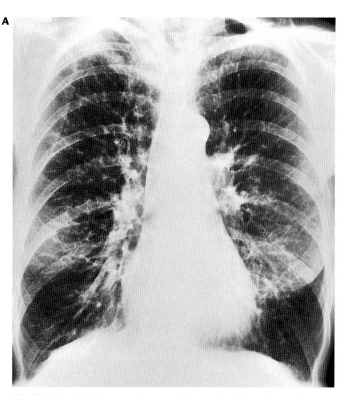 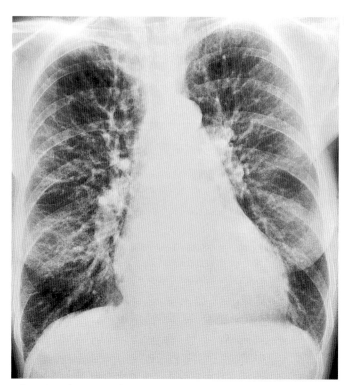

Fig. 12.64 **A,** A 50-year-old man with chronic airflow obstruction. Lungs are large in volume, the diaphragm is flat, and there is vascular attenuation at the lung apices. These features suggest emphysema, and this was supported by a low carbon monoxide diffusion capacity. Lung markings are increased peripherally, particularly in the left mid zone. **B,** Patient became chronically hypoxic and, with respiratory infections, hypercapnic. One of these episodes was associated with cor pulmonale when the patient became edematous, with an enlarged heart and vascular engorgement. The emphysematous right upper zone shows less vascular engorgement and is relatively transradiant. The diaphragm is less depressed and more curved than before.

and fibrosis.[606] It was considered by Fraser et al[607] to be "useful evidence in support of a diagnosis of chronic bronchitis".

Support for the finding of bronchial wall thickening in chronic bronchitis has come from HRCT studies[273,484] in which proximal and distal bronchial wall thickening was present in 33% of smokers (compared with 18% of control subjects).[273] Areas of focal air-trapping can be readily identified in smokers and exsmokers on expiratory CT and this feature may be present in individuals with normal pulmonary function tests.[608] Contrary to expectation, HRCT has not fully elucidated the nature of the increased markings that constitute the "dirty lung" of cigarette smokers,[609] but at least the smoke is beginning to clear thanks largely to the investigations of Remy-Jardin et al.[273,484,610]

Bronchographic findings in chronic bronchitis are of historic interest only. They do, however, illustrate some pathologic features of the disease. Dilated mucus gland ducts in the proximal airways fill with contrast material in >50% of patients.[602,611] However, Gamsu et al[612] recorded this finding in a similar percentage of normal adults, and it cannot be regarded as specific for chronic bronchitis. Other bronchographic findings include incomplete peripheral airway filling,[611] truncated airway ends,[601,613,614] and lack of proximal tapering.[602]

Cor pulmonale is a recognized complication of COPD and is seen almost exclusively in hypoxic patients. With the onset of heart failure the heart and hilar and intermediate lung vessels become enlarged. Enlargement of vessels is present in all zones and affects particularly segmental vessels and a few divisions beyond, giving an appearance of plethora (Fig. 12.64).[615] The

changes of plethora probably reflect two processes: expansion of central blood volume and hypoxic vasoconstriction of small distal pulmonary arteries. The size of the central pulmonary arteries reflects, with some caveats, the degree of pulmonary artery hypertension (see Ch. 7, p. 386).

Emphysema

Emphysema is a major cause of chronic airflow obstruction. It is a diagnosis that has, strictly speaking, relied on pathologic criteria. Thus, emphysema is defined as "a condition of the lung characterized by abnormal, permanent enlargement of airspaces distal to the terminal bronchiole accompanied by the destruction of their (airspace) walls and without obvious fibrosis. The orderly appearance of the acinus and its contents are disturbed and may be lost".[616] This definition, unlike earlier ones,[578] makes destruction of airspace walls a necessary condition, thereby excluding, for example, compensatory "emphysema" and other conditions in which there is only airspace dilatation. The relationship between emphysema and interstitial fibrosis is likely to be more complex than the exclusory definition ("without obvious fibrosis") allows; it seems that at least some patients with "pure" emphysema have a fibrotic component to their cigarette smoking related disease.[617,618]

Pulmonary emphysema has a worldwide distribution but is more frequent in polluted and industrialized societies. It is very common, particularly in its milder forms; some degree of emphysema is recorded in 50–70% of autopsies from various centers around the world.[619] It has maximum prevalence at about 70 years of age and is two- to threefold more common in males.[619] Further information about the epidemiology and prevalence of emphysema in cigarette smokers may be forthcoming from populations screened for lung cancer with CT.[620]

The pathogenesis of emphysema is complex, but two mechanisms are particularly important: (1) structural weakness caused by elastolysis, which itself may be secondary either to a constitutional disorder or to enhanced proteolysis, and (2) airway obstruction caused either by loss of airway support or by inflammatory changes in the walls of small airways. Nevertheless, the relationship between the severity of airflow obstruction and extent of emphysema on HRCT in cigarette smokers: it is not entirely predictable.[621,622]

The most important etiologic factor by far is cigarette smoking, which exerts its effect in a variety of ways.[623,624] Other inhaled pollutants have also been implicated, including gases such as nitrogen oxides and phosgene, as well as particulate smoke.[625] Intravenous injection of ground-up methylphenidate tablets (often containing talc) has been reported to cause severe basal emphysema.[626,627] The pathogenesis of precocious emphysema related to this and other recreational intravenous drug use is unclear.[628] A possible link between severe nutritional deficiency, in a patient with anorexia nervosa, and the development of emphysema has been reported.[629] There is also the suggestion of a casual relationship between HIV infection and the development of early emphysema.[630,631] Various genetic disorders associated with emphysema are described, including α_1-antitrypsin deficiency, heritable diseases of connective tissue such as cutis laxa,[632] osteogenesis imperfecta, Marfan syndrome,[633] and familial emphysema.[634,635]

The pathologic classification of emphysema is traditionally based on the microscopic localization of disease within the acinus or secondary pulmonary lobule. The principal types are:

- *Centriacinar or centrilobular emphysema.* This variety of emphysema is most commonly called centrilobular emphysema. There is selective dilatation of the central elements in the acinus, particularly the respiratory bronchioles and their alveoli. The process tends to be most developed in the upper parts of the upper and lower lobes. It is strongly associated with cigarette smoking. Inflammatory changes in the small airways are common, with plugging, mural infiltration, and fibrosis leading to stenosis, blockage, distortion, and destruction. Focal dust emphysema seen in coal workers may be considered a variety of centriacinar emphysema in which there is little airway inflammation and a more uniform distribution of disease throughout the lung.[616]
- *Paraseptal emphysema.* The name of this type of emphysema emphasizes its main feature, selective expansion of alveoli adjacent to connective tissue septa and bronchovascular bundles, particularly at the margins of the acinus but also subpleurally and adjacent to bronchovascular bundles. It has a tendency to develop where lung margins are sharp. Airspaces in paraseptal emphysema may become confluent and develop into bullae, which may be large. Paraseptal emphysema is thought to be the basic lesion in bullous lung disease.[636] Paraseptal emphysema, seems to be more prevalent in young (<40 years) smokers than centrilobular emphysema.[637] Airway obstruction and physiologic disturbance may be minor in paraseptal emphysema.

- *Panacinar or panlobular emphysema.* In this form the entire acinus is affected by dilatation and destruction. The features differentiating alveoli from alveolar ducts are lost, pores of Kohn enlarge, and fenestrations develop between alveoli. This process has been likened to a diffuse simplification of the lung architecture. With progressive destruction, all that eventually remains are thin strands of deranged tissue surrounding blood vessels. Panacinar emphysema is the most widespread and severe type of emphysema and therefore the most likely to give rise to clinically significant disease. Pathologic changes are distributed throughout the lungs, but they are often basally predominant. Panacinar emphysema is the type occurring in α_1-antitrypsin deficiency, and is described in Swyer–James/McLeod syndrome,[616] and in familial cases. Although generally considered the emphysema of non-smokers, it also coexists with smoking induced centrilobular emphysema.

This type of classification depends on defining microscopic localization of the emphysematous destruction. Given the infrequency with which in vivo biopsies are obtained to confirm the diagnosis and subtype of emphysema, and their frequent coexistence,[452] the utility of histopathologic classification is questionable. At a macroscopic level lesions may be multifocal or uniform, and may show regional predilection, such as upper or lower zone. Regional variation in severity is of particular relevance for patients being considered for lung volume reduction surgery.[638–640]

Patients with limited emphysema are usually asymptomatic.[616] Widespread emphysema, however, causes non-productive cough and progressive exertional dyspnea. With the exception of paraseptal emphysema, the degree of disability is related to the severity of the emphysema rather than to the type.[616] Emphysema tends to be associated with the "pink puffer" clinical picture,[641] characterized by early dyspnea, nonproductive cough, and relatively normal blood gases achieved at the expense of marked dyspnea.[642] There is, however, considerable overlap with the chronic bronchitis ("blue bloater") end of the spectrum. Patients with this latter syndrome have productive cough, episodes of deterioration associated with infection and bronchospasm, hypoxia and hypercapnia, and a tendency to develop pulmonary arterial hypertension and cor pulmonale.[642]

Pulmonary function tests in emphysema reflect the three major pathologic changes: (1) small airway obstruction caused by loss of mural support and inflammatory wall change; (2) loss of lung recoil; and (3) loss of alveolar surface.[642] The work of breathing is increased, and eventually hypoxemia develops, initially during sleep or exercise. Hypercapnia is not a feature, since responsiveness to arterial oxygen levels remains intact. Airflow obstruction in emphysema is contributed to by both the small and large airways. The latter component of resistance is variable and present only in expiration, particularly at low lung volumes.[643–645] Collapse of lobar and segmental airways in emphysematous subjects during forced expiration has been demonstrated,[117,644] and pressure measurements show these to be sites of high resistance.[645] Collapse of large airways is due principally to the large transmural pressures generated in emphysema during forced expiration. In addition, airway walls are probably less able to withstand such pressures because of mural atrophy.[646]

A number of studies have correlated chest radiographic findings and lung function tests in patients with nonspecific chronic airflow obstruction, many of whom have had emphysema. Reich et al[647] found that the length of the right lung and the height of the arc of the right hemidiaphragm correlated well with FEV_1, and the ratio FEV_1/VC. They also found that if the absolute height of the right hemidiaphragm measured against the ribs was corrected for body surface area, this too correlated well with the degree of airflow obstruction. Other workers have not found such corrections to be necessary, and in one study of 189 patients all but 3% of those with the height of the right hemidiaphragm at or below the right seventh rib had airflow obstruction.[605] The sensitivity of this finding, however, was low (30–40%). Similar findings have been reported by others[648,649] and are emphasized in an editorial by Pratt,[650] which concludes that chest radiographs reveal emphysema rather than airflow obstruction per se.

The chest radiographic findings in emphysema may be divided into four types: hyperinflation, vascular change, bullae, and increased markings. Hyperinflation and vascular changes are usually the predominant findings, with hyperinflation reflecting a functional abnormality and vascular change reflecting the pathologic feature of lung destruction.[651] In the early radiologic studies case selection of patients with emphysema lacked certainty because it was based on clinical features and respiratory function changes,[652] and not on morphologic criteria. A number of early studies correlated radiologic and pathologic findings and attempted to assess the accuracy of various signs. However, as Thurlbeck[504] pointed out, these studies were flawed in that they had an excess of patients with chronic airflow obstruction, so that radiologic features of airflow obstruction are given "disproportionate value in recognizing emphysema". Furthermore, it is difficult to give an overview of these studies because of the great variation in the severity of disease studied, the radiographic signs assessed, and the pathologic methods used for quantifying emphysema. Some of the studies have been critically reviewed.[650,653,654]

Hyperinflation on chest radiography is indicated by a number of signs:

- *Low diaphragm* (Fig. 12.65). The right hemidiaphragm is usually assessed because it is not obscured by the heart. The right hemidiaphragm is considered to be low if its border, in the midclavicular line, is at or below the anterior end of the seventh rib.[655] Some workers have taken the sixth rib in pyknic individuals.[656] Occasionally, normal individuals, particularly if young and fit, have a right hemidiaphragm lying at the level of the seventh rib.
- *Flat diaphragm* (Figs 12.65 and 12.66). Flattening of a hemidiaphragm can be assessed subjectively, as well as objectively by drawing a line joining costophrenic and cardiophrenic angles and measuring the maximum perpendicular height from this line to the diaphragm silhouette. A value of <1.5 cm indicates flattening. The combination of depression and flattening is more specific for generalized emphysema, whereas depression on its own is seen with overinflation in other obstructive lung conditions, such as acute asthma. The succeeding signs are less reliable indicators of hyperinflation.
- *Increased retrosternal airspace* (Fig. 12.66). This measurement is taken on the lateral radiograph between the anterior aspect of the ascending aorta and the posterior surface of the sternum at a point 3 cm below the manubriosternal junction.

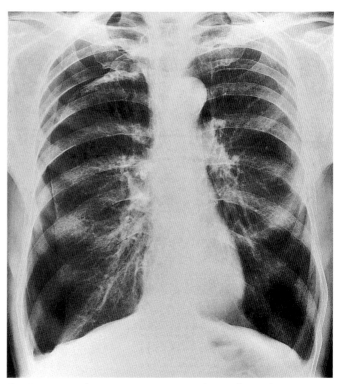

Fig. 12.65 Emphysema. Posteroanterior chest radiograph demonstrates two of the most reliable signs of emphysema: (1) depression of the right hemidiaphragm with its mid point lying on the upper border of the seventh rib anteriorly; and (2) flattening of both hemidiaphragms. Other, less reliable, features include a narrow heart with air density below it. There is a right pneumothorax.

Values indicating hyperinflation have ranged widely from 2.5[657] to 4.5 cm.[652]

- *Obtuse costophrenic angle on the posteroanterior or lateral chest radiograph* (Fig. 12.66).
- *Cardiac diameter <11.5 cm,*[658] with a vertical heart and visible lung beneath the heart (Fig. 12.65).
- *Presence of an infraaortic posterior inferior junction line and the wider stripelike left pleuroesophageal line* occurs more frequently in patients with emphysema but is a relatively insensitive sign.[659]

Several studies have found that signs of overinflation are the best predictors of the presence and severity of emphysema.[656,657,660] Nicklaus et al[657] found that a flat diaphragm on the posteroanterior chest radiograph was the best predictor, detecting 94% of patients with severe emphysema, 76% with moderate, and 21% with mild, with a false positive rate of only 4%.

Several vascular signs have been ascribed to emphysema:

- *Radiographic transradiancy of the lungs* (Figs 12.67 and 12.68). Transradiancy may be a generalized change, which makes reliable assessment difficult, or may be localized, in which case it can be identified with reasonable certainty by comparison with "normal" areas of lung.
- *Reduced number and size of pulmonary vessels and their branches*, particularly in the middle or outer aspect of the lung ("arterial deficiency") (Fig. 12.67).
- *Vessels are distorted and may be unduly straightened or curved and have increased branching angles.*

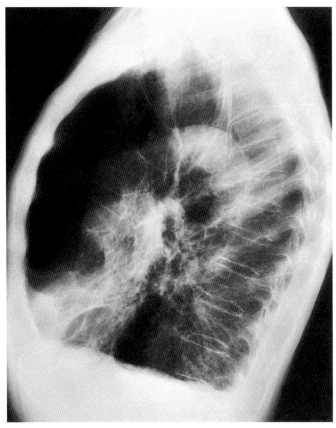

Fig. 12.66   Emphysema. Lateral chest radiograph demonstrates characteristically large retrosternal transradiancy with increased separation of the aorta and sternum measuring 4.6 cm, 3 cm below the angle of Louis and extending to within 3 cm of the diaphragm anteriorly. Both costophrenic angles are obtuse and both hemidiaphragms flat.

- *Transradiant, avascular areas with hairline curvilinear margins* which, at least in part, represent walls of bullae (Fig. 12.68). Several studies have found arterial deficiency to be a more reliable criterion of emphysema than hyperinflation.[202,661,662] Using arterial deficiency alone to detect emphysema, Thurlbeck et al[202] found that its accuracy was similar to that described for hyperinflation criteria by Nicklaus et al.[657] There were no false positive results, and all patients with severe, 66% with moderate, and 35% with mild emphysema were identified.

Thurlbeck et al[202] have described another vascular pattern in emphysema in which increased markings are present peripherally on the chest radiograph (Fig. 12.64). The nature of these markings remains conjectural but they have been interpreted as being caused by an increase in size and number of small vessels, though other factors such as cellular infiltration and scarring may play a part (Fig. 12.64).[606,609] Hyperinflation in such cases is usually absent or mild.[202]

The following conclusions may be drawn from radiographic and pathologic studies in generalized emphysema[202,656,657,660–663]:

- The chest radiograph reliably detects severe emphysema and can be used to exclude severe disease. Mild disease is rarely detected (Box 12.20).[664]

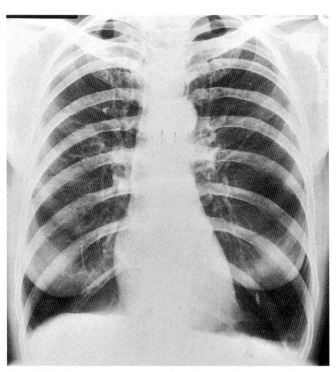

Fig. 12.67   Panacinar emphysema in a 52-year-old woman with α_1-antitrypsin deficiency. Large volume lungs with low flat diaphragms. Both lower zones are hypertransradiant, and vessels within these zones are reduced in size and number, and are pruned. Distribution of these changes is typical of panacinar emphysema.

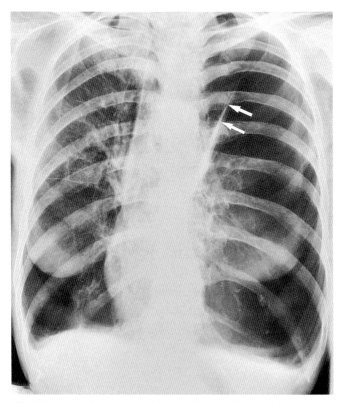

Fig. 12.68   Emphysema in a patient with α_1-antitrypsin deficiency. Both hemidiaphragms are low and flat. The mediastinum is displaced to the right by a large bulla, which occupies much of the left hemithorax, compressing lung tissue medially and inferiorly. Part of wall of the bulla can be identified (arrows). The vasculature is reduced in the right lower zone because of panacinar emphysema. Bulla formation is not a common feature of α_1-antitrypsin deficiency.

Box 12.20 Chest radiography of emphysema

Chest radiography is insensitive for the detection of mild and moderate emphysema

The specificity of chest radiography is higher than its sensitivity but observer variation for the features of emphysema, particularly the vascular signs, is high

The radiographic feature of overinflation of the lungs is probably the most reliable sign of emphysema

---

- The sensitivity of the chest radiograph is not good, ranging from 24%[662] to 80%.[665] The exceptionally low figure of 24% was probably because most subjects had mild or moderate emphysema and only vascular radiologic signs were used. In contrast, specificity is good, between 95 and 100%, giving a low false positive rate. Accuracy of the chest radiograph in diagnosing emphysema is in the order of 65–80%.[665]
- There is a considerable intra- and inter-observer variation in relation to radiographic signs.[657] Vascular signs, not surprisingly, are subject to more variation than signs relating to hyperinflation.[665]
- Most studies have found that the best predictors of generalized emphysema are evidence of hyperinflation (particularly a low diaphragm) and flattening of the diaphragm.[202,656,657,660,663] In general, vascular criteria, in the absence of other signs, should be used with caution in making the radiographic diagnosis of emphysema.

When other chest conditions occur in emphysematous lungs, the radiologic appearances are modified. Thus, with consolidation and centrilobular emphysema the emphysematous spaces produce rounded transradiancies in the airspace opacity (Fig. 12.69). With heart failure, edema may spare emphysematous lung and the diaphragm tends to become more rounded and elevated as lung compliance falls.[666]

In contrast to the chest radiograph, CT has proved very sensitive and specific in assessing emphysema. CT has been used to detect and characterize emphysema and grade its severity since findings were first described >20 years ago.[667]

The signs of emphysema on CT have been extensively reported.[450,667–676] In centrilobular emphysema there are areas of low attenuation with ill-defined margins, usually without visible walls,[677] and this permeative destruction gives the lung parenchyma a "moth eaten" appearance (Figs 12.70 and 12.71). When areas become 1–2 cm in diameter, part of their border may become well defined because of marginating interlobular septa or vessels. In one study assessing various signs of centrilobular emphysema, nonperipheral, low-attenuation areas on in vivo CT correlated best with emphysema assessed postmortem.[671] Other signs of emphysema, mirroring the radiographic features, include bullae (focal air-containing cysts with well-defined, hairline walls), pruning and attenuation of vessels, and vascular distortion. Vessels may be stretched and straightened, and branching angles are widened. Ancillary signs of hyperinflation of the lungs, so readily appreciated on chest radiography, such as the configuration of the diaphragm, may not be as obvious on CT; however, an anterior junction measuring 3 cm or more is a frequent finding in patients with emphysema.[678]

It is possible, especially in patients with mild or mild to moderate disease, to distinguish on HRCT between the various

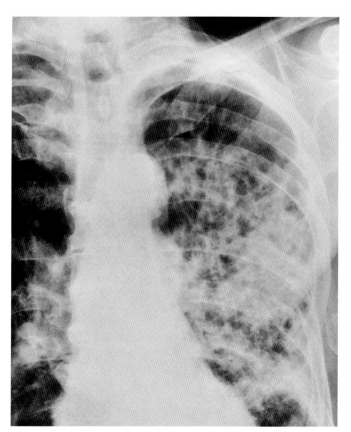

Fig. 12.69 Emphysema. Localized posteroanterior radiograph of the left upper zone of a patient with infective consolidation superimposed on centrilobular emphysema. Emphysematous spaces create round transradiancies within the pneumonia.

types of emphysema.[450,452,669] Centrilobular emphysema, particularly in early disease, has an upper zone predilection[671] and may be confined to this region. Low density areas are typically focal[671] and related to centrilobular arteries.[679] These small discrete areas of emphysematous destruction may resemble small cystic air spaces (Fig. 12.72), but generally without an obvious cyst wall, and sometimes the centrilobular core structure is visible. Lung immediately surrounding the low density lesions appears normal. Very early centrilobular emphysema is readily detected with HRCT in asymptomatic smokers.[680] With progression of disease, centrilobular emphysematous lesions become confluent with more obvious vascular abnormalities.

It should be appreciated that smoking induced infiltrative lung diseases may coexist, particularly in heavy cigarette smokers; thus radiographic appearances may be modulated by components of RB-ILD, Langerhans cell histiocytosis and interstitial fibrosis.[618,681,682]

In panacinar emphysema, lung destruction is much more uniform and gives rise to more generalized, decreased attenuation lung (Fig. 12.48). Small, focal, low density areas, as seen in centrilobular emphysema, are not an expected feature. Mild panacinar emphysema is easily overlooked[683] because it is a diffuse process lacking the juxtaposed contrasting densities of normal lung and focal transradiancies, as seen in centrilobular emphysema. Panacinar emphysema has a predilection for the lower zones. Nevertheless, the HRCT patterns of panacinar and centrilobular emphysema frequently coexist in a given individual.

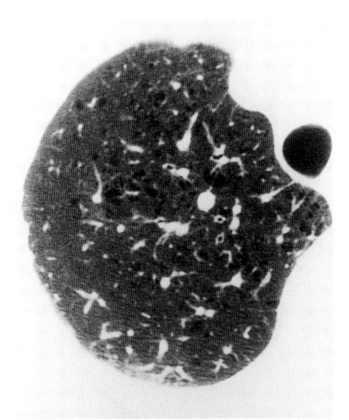

Fig. 12.70 Early centrilobular emphysema. Numerous foci of low attenuation without discernible walls giving a "moth eaten" appearance.

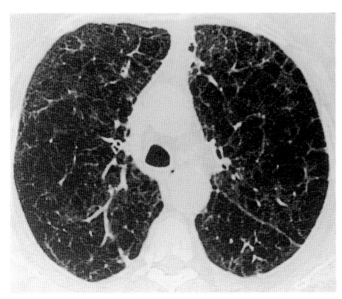

Fig. 12.71 Typical appearances of advanced centrilobular emphysema in the upper lobes. The widespread permeative destruction affects much of the lung parenchyma, throwing into relief the slightly thickened interlobular septa in the lung periphery.

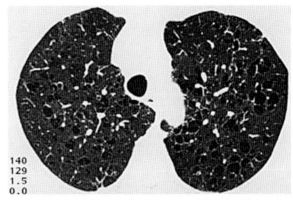

Fig. 12.72 Centrilobular emphysema in an elderly female smoker. The CT appearances of numerous cystic lesions, some of which have an identifiable thin wall, was initially interpreted as lymphangioleiomyomatosis (the lower lobes in this case were near normal).

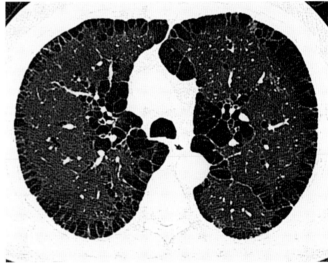

Fig. 12.73 Emphysema highlights the peripheral interlobular septa; most cases do not have such a dramatic "saw-tooth" appearance.

Paraseptal emphysema is easily detected on CT[683] as subpleural well-marginated low density areas with distinct hairline walls (Fig. 12.73). Subpleural cysts are commonly found in the azygoesophageal recess, adjacent to the superior mediastinal border, and along the anterior junctional region.[669,671] This pattern of emphysema whimsically resembles "saw teeth", and occasionally the remaining interlobular septa may appear particularly prominent on chest radiography and, in so doing, mimic lymphangitis carcinomatosis, though HRCT will readily show the true cause.[684]

The distribution and severity of emphysema may be quantitated by CT. CT scans can be assessed by subjective visual methods, density measurements or, more recently, by postprocessing and texture analysis.[668,685–689] Pathologic evaluation in most studies has been of macroscopic emphysema assessed visually by counting lesions or panel matching. The determination of the true macroscopic or microscopic extent of emphysema is fraught and there have been many attempts to define a reproducible method, such as the "destructive index", "mean linear intercept" and "loss of alveolar surface area".[690] It is worth emphasizing that a gold standard for the measurement of the extent of emphysema (whether functional, radiographic or, most particularly, pathologic) does not exist; in the case of pathologic evaluation, many methodologic factors, e.g. the inflation pressure used in the preparation of the lung specimen, conspire to make the quantification of emphysema unique to a particular study. Studies using various CT section thicknesses (between 1 and 10 mm) have shown good correlation between macroscopic pathology scores and visually assessed (HR)CT scores with correlation coefficients ranging from about 0.6 to 0.8.[670,671,683,691] Intra- and inter-observer variation in these early studies is low to moderate.[669,683,691,692] However, Bankier et al[693] have shown that observers, irrespective of experience, tend to overestimate the extent of emphysema on CT by comparison with CT densitometry which correlates better with a morphometric reference.

Emphysematous lesions are more conspicuous and reliably diagnosed on HRCT,[674,694] and CT–pathologic studies comparing sections 1.5 and 10 mm thick have shown improved correlations with pathologic scores: $r = 0.85$ (1.5 mm) versus 0.81 (10 mm) (mixed emphysema),[683] and $r = 0.96$ (1.5 mm) versus 0.90 (10 mm) (panacinar emphysema).[674] However, the difference in visual extent between sections obtained with 2 and 5 mm collimation appears to be insignificant[695]; further correlation between the extent of low-attenuation lung and pulmonary function is very similar for 2 and 5 mm collimation examinations.[696] (HR)CT consistently underestimates the extent of centrilobular and panacinar emphysema,[674] since small lesions (<5 mm in diameter) are not reliably identified.[683] However, the false positive rate for (HR)CT is relatively low,[665] and misdiagnosis may be related, at least in part, to the misinterpretation of low density image artifacts.[674]

Emphysema can also be assessed by measuring lung density. CT lung density is related to the amount of air, tissue, interstitial fluid, and blood within a given voxel, and normal data has been reported.[667,697–699] In one study lung density values in normal subjects at full inspiration varied from –770 to –875 HU.[697] Furthermore, CT densitometry is affected by technical subject variables,[700] including the subject's age and the state of inflation of the lungs.[701,702] Nevertheless, it does not appear that spirometric gating improves the repeatability of quantitative CT measurements of emphysema.[703] In addition, there is a gravitationally induced density gradient in the supine position; posterior values are approximately 20–70 HU greater than anterior ones.[704] The density of emphysematous lung is abnormally low. If a histogram plot is made of frequency against pixel density (HU), the emphysematous curve is shifted to the left compared with normal (Fig. 12.74).[699] Pixels with values below a certain number can be highlighted on a CT image ("density masking"; Fig. 12.75) and expressed as a percentage of the total pixels in a given section. This technique can be automated.[705–709] By choosing an appropriate threshold level the operator can discriminate between "normal" lung and emphysematous lung. Müller et al,[692] in a study comparing macroscopic emphysema as assessed by the "density mask" method and picture graded pathology scores at the same level, found that a density of –910 HU gave the best discrimination between emphysematous and normal lung. More recently, Gevenois et al[706] have shown that a threshold of –950 HU provides an accurate estimation of both macroscopic[706] and, to a slightly lesser degree, microscopic[707] emphysema. Caution is needed in uncritical extrapolation of these findings to other machines because many technical factors can affect CT density measurements.[697,710,711] In particular,

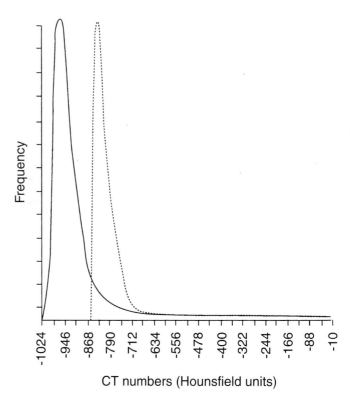

Fig. 12.74 Graph of pixel density numbers derived from CT lung sections, plotted against pixel frequency for a normal subject (interrupted line) and a patient with panacinar emphysema (continuous line). Emphysematous changes in this patient were gross, and there is little overlap with the curve of the normal subject.

reducing the milliAmperage, as in a low dose protocol, may affect the measured extent of low-attenuation lung,[696] though another study has shown little difference between conventional and low dose techniques.[712] It has been recommended that threshold levels be established by experiment for any given scanner.[692] An alternative quantitative method to "density masking" is to calculate the percentage of pixels falling in the lowest fifth percentile of density values.[713] This percentage has been compared with the amount of microscopic emphysema as assessed by an index (airspace wall surface area per unit volume) and a moderately good correlation of $r = 0.77$ was found.[714]

The use of a "density mask" method and both expiratory and inspiratory CT scans has been advocated as a means of distinguishing areas of simple hyperinflation without tissue destruction from areas of emphysema.[715] Expiratory HRCT does not correlate as well as inspiratory HRCT with the morphologic extent of emphysema, but the expiratory HRCT is superior to inspiratory HRCT in reflecting functional air-trapping.[702,716] It has been suggested that a distinction between patients with chronic bronchitis versus those with emphysema may be made based on the larger difference in CT density on scans obtained at 10 and 90% of vital capacity compared with the minor densitometric difference found in normal subjects or patients with chronic bronchitis.[717]

A number of studies have compared the degree of CT determined emphysema and pulmonary function tests.[687,702,718–725] There is an inherent sampling problem that dogs all investigations of the correlation between the extent of emphysema on a limited number of interspaced thin-section CT and

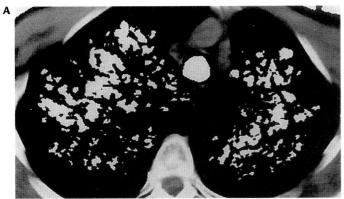

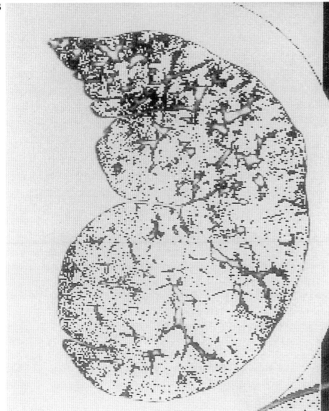

Fig. 12.75 All pixels of −910 HU or less are highlighted (in white), identifying areas of probable emphysema. **A**, Centrilobular emphysema at a level midway between the aortic arch and carina. Highlighting emphasizes the typically focal distribution of the centrilobular distribution. **B**, Panacinar emphysema. Highlighted pixels are distributed in an even, confluent pattern.

pulmonary function tests (the latter, by their very nature, provide a global assessment of disease). This problem has been highlighted in studies that have shown that the extent of emphysema on HRCT in the upper zones correlates with functional abnormalities much less strongly than the extent of emphysema in the lower zones.[723,726] Furthermore, the radial distribution of emphysema may have a functional impact, e.g. emphysema located in the lung periphery has less effect on gas diffusing capacity than more central emphysema.[727] In terms of airflow limitation caused by emphysema, the contribution of (bronchitic) airway wall thickening in smokers should not be overlooked.[728] While most studies report strong correlations

between the extent of emphysema on HRCT (however quantified) and various spirometric and other functional measures, some aspects of pulmonary mechanics, such as the elastic properties of the lung, do not appear to have any relationship with the CT extent of emphysema.[729]

It is possible to extract precise volumetric measurements of abnormally low-attenuation lung parenchyma from 3D reconstructions of spiral CT scans performed in inspiration and expiration; this technique potentially overcomes regional sampling problems and recent studies have shown good correlations with indices of airflow obstruction and air-trapping,[724,730] particularly when a threshold of −900 HU is used.[716]

Perfusion–ventilation lung scintigraphy is abnormal in symptomatic patients with COPD. The agent ^{81m}Kr gives a more accurate estimate of the true ventilation than does ^{133}Xe, but the latter is more widely available. The sensitivity of scintigraphy approaches that of spirometric tests in detecting COPD.[731] In any event, an experimental model suggests that it is possible to detect lesions of approximately the size of a pulmonary acinus.[732]

The characteristic finding on lung scintigraphy in COPD is multiple, patchy, matched defects of both perfusion and ventilation, generally distributed throughout the lungs.[733] Emphysematous defects are due to areas of parenchymal destruction[734] and are therefore nonsegmental and fixed. They may or may not correspond to oligemic or bullous areas on the corresponding chest radiograph.[735] Scintigraphy in emphysema using ^{133}Xe as the ventilation agent shows, in addition to the above findings, a slow wash-in curve so that an equilibrium state may never be achieved.[731] Wash-out is also delayed and prolonged beyond the usual 3 min taken to achieve a background count level.[736]

Lung scintigraphy of patients at the chronic bronchitis end of the COPD spectrum generally resemble those of patients with emphysema, except that defects may be more segmental.[734] Perfusion defects in chronic bronchitis are probably produced by hypoxic vasoconstriction secondary to hypoventilation caused by airway narrowing. Such a mechanism may explain why, in chronic bronchitis, perfusion defects are sometimes smaller than the corresponding ventilation defects.[734] Occasionally hypoxic vasoconstriction fails to occur,[737] and in this situation, typically seen at the lung bases in acute exacerbations of chronic bronchitis, ventilation defects are completely mismatched.[733] With resolution of the acute exacerbation such defects disappear.

Labeled aerosols may be used to study lung ventilation. In normal individuals gases and aerosols produce similar images.[738] In COPD, however, ventilation scintigraphy produced by the two agents gives strikingly different appearances, with focal spots of high and low activity on aerosol scintigraphy.[739–741] Focal deposition tends to be central or mixed in emphysema and peripheral in chronic bronchitis.[739,740,742] Deposition of aerosol is thought to occur in airways at areas of fixed and dynamic narrowing by a variety of complex mechanisms.[739,742,743] In a research context, PET is capable of providing sophisticated physiologic information relating to COPD.[744,745] Using SPECT, 3D quantitation of emphysema by fractal analysis of the deposition of a carbon particle radioaerosol is possible.[746] The value of scintigraphy in evaluating patients for lung volume reduction surgery is not clear,[747,748] but it is probably complementary to CT.[749,750]

Of recent interest is the application of MRI to mapping regional pulmonary ventilation using a variety of gases. Two inert noble gases (^{3}He and ^{129}Xe) have been the most intensively investigated to date.[751–754] The attraction of imaging the airspaces of the lung with hyperpolarized noble gases, over and above a conventional radionuclide ventilation scan, are several. In particular, an apparent diffusion coefficient – which reflects alveolar size (and therefore is modified if there is alveolar disruption, e.g. in the earliest stages of emphysema) – can be derived and displayed as a regional map.[753,755,756] The weak paramagnetic properties of oxygen have also been exploited, such that oxygen enhanced MRI provides information about oxygen dispersion in the airspaces and potentially maps oxygen diffusion into the capillary bed of the lungs.[757–759] In the context of emphysema, early studies suggest that oxygen enhanced MRI shows reasonable correlation with functional and HRCT measures of emphysema.[760] It is not surprising that the perfusion characteristics of emphysematous lung differ from those of normal lung[761] and a recent study suggests that MRI evaluation of pulmonary perfusion in patients with emphysema may be superior to scintigraphy.[762]

α_1-Antitrypsin deficiency

The association between serum α_1-antitrypsin deficiency and COPD was first recognized in 1963,[763] and 6 years later an association with neonatal hepatitis and cirrhosis was recorded.[764]

α_1-Antitrypsin is a serum protein that inhibits a number of lysosomal proteases released during inflammatory reactions, preventing the damaging effects of elastases released by macrophages and particularly neutrophils. Elastase has been shown to produce emphysema in lungs when administered into the airways,[765] and the elastase of neutrophils within the lung has the same potential.[766] Furthermore, the number of macrophages recovered from bronchoalveolar lavage fluid is high in smokers with HRCT evidence of emphysema.[767] It has recently been suggested that the α_1-antitrypsin deficiency may result in the local formation of polymers within the lung which may be a chemoattractant for damaging neutrophils.[768] It is not

surprising therefore that some individuals with reduced levels of α_1-antitrypsin are at risk of developing emphysema, particularly if they are cigarette smokers. At a histologic level the emphysema is predominantly the panacinar type.[202,769,770]

The serum level and type of α_1-antitrypsin depend on two codominant alleles that occupy one locus. Different alleles produce different types and amounts of α_1-antitrypsin. The type of α_1-antitrypsin may be recognized by electrophoresis, and the allele producing it is designated by Pi (protease inhibitor), followed by one of a number of capital letters. By far the most common allele is PiM, and when homozygous (PiMM) it is associated with normal α_1-antitrypsin levels.

Some alleles are associated with low serum levels of α_1-antitrypsin. Although there are a number of these, only a few are important clinically, particularly PiZ but also PiS and Pi–, the last having a silent allele. Homozygous PiZ individuals have about 10–15% of the expected serum α_1-antitrypsin levels, while heterozygotic PiMZ individuals have a level of about 60%.[771] The PiZ allele has a frequency of about 1.2% so that only one to two individuals per 10,000 of the population are homozygous.

A large study of 256 PiZZ patients showed that eventually emphysema developed in nearly every individual and life expectancy was lower.[772] The PiZZ type of emphysema is characterized by an early onset, between 35 and 50 years of age.[772–774] Symptoms develop about 10 years earlier in smokers than in non-smokers, and respiratory function impairment and radiologic change tend to be worse in smokers. Males outnumber females by about 2:1.[774,775]

Opinion is divided over the relationship of the heterozygote state (PiMZ) and respiratory disease. The consensus is that no definite relationship exists between the two but that the heterozygote state may increase susceptibility to emphysema in the presence of other risk factors.[766]

Radiologic changes of emphysema can be seen in about 80% of patients who are homozygous and have COPD.[776] The striking feature of the emphysematous change is its lower zone predominance (Fig. 12.76). In a study of 165 PiZ homozygotes, 98% had lower zone involvement,[775] and in 24% this was the

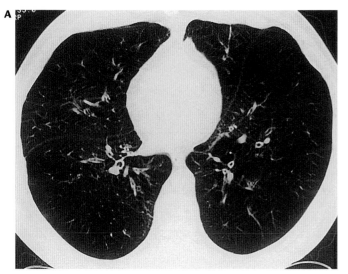
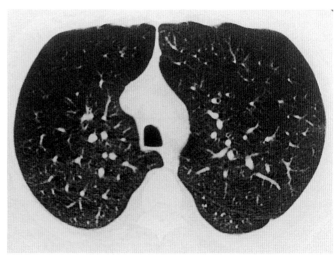

Fig. 12.76 α_1-Antitrypsin deficiency associated panacinar emphysema. **A,** There is generalized decreased attenuation of the lung parenchyma and a striking paucity of the pulmonary vasculature, particularly in the anterior left lower lobe. There is mild cylindrical bronchiectasis which is a frequent finding in this condition. **B,** Upper lobes, particularly the posterior segments in this case, are relatively spared.

only zone involved. In the same series only three of 140 patients with radiologic changes had isolated involvement of the upper or middle and upper zone.[775] Similarly, in a study of 52 PiZZ patients with COPD, 67% showed isolated lower zone emphysema, whereas this pattern was seen in only 8% of PiMM patients.[776] Bullae are not a major feature, but they do occur (Fig. 12.68).[777] The pattern of emphysematous change in heterozygotes, such as PiMZ and PiMS genotypes, is like that in homozygous PiM individuals.

CT findings have been described in several series PiZ.[284,285,778] Emphysematous changes were seen in all zones but had a lower zone predominance in the study of Guest et al,[284] and 41% had bullae, though these were not a major feature; bronchial wall thickening and/or dilatation were present in 41% (Fig. 12.76). Other workers have reported an association between α_1-antitrypsin deficiency and bronchiectasis.[238] A study of 14 patients with α_1-antitrypsin deficiency found that nearly half had CT features of frank bronchiectasis and that these individuals had a higher incidence of lower respiratory tract infections.[285] Serial HRCT, particularly CT densitometry, has been reported to be a sensitive method of monitoring the progress of emphysema in patients with α_1-antitrypsin deficiency.[779–781]

Imaging and lung volume reduction surgery

Lung volume reduction surgery (LVRS) is a palliative treatment for patients with severe emphysema who do not respond to medical management.[782,783] The procedure involves the surgical resection of "target areas" of severely emphysematous lung, the result being a reduction in overall lung volume, thus allowing the thorax to return to a more normal configuration,[784] and thereby improving respiratory mechanics. The mechanisms for the sometimes striking symptomatic and functional improvement seen in patients following LVRS are not fully understood but are likely to include decompression of normal lung with improved elastic recoil and increased efficiency of the repositioned diaphragm,[785–788] the latter having an increased area and an increased zone of apposition following LVRS.[789] Post LVRS pulmonary function tests and imaging convincingly show a reduction in lung volume, however quantified.[790] The immediate symptomatic and functional improvement experienced by patients following LVRS seem to be largely maintained at 2 years

following the operation.[791,792] The main determinant of the immediate and longterm success of LVRS appears to be careful patient selection: approximately 20% of patients initially referred for LVRS are ultimately regarded as suitable for the procedure.[793] Selection criteria vary between centers, but potential patients undergo rigorous investigation including psychologic assessment, pulmonary function testing, arterial blood gas analysis, exercise testing, right heart catheterization, inspiratory and expiratory chest radiographs, CT, and radionuclide perfusion scan. Despite these extensive investigations, the decision to proceed with LVRS is largely subjective and the exact role of imaging investigations in the selection process is still emerging[794–798]; there is certainly some redundancy between the imaging tests bought to bear, e.g. the information about regional blood flow supplied by perfusion scintigraphy can largely be extracted from HRCT images[748]; similarly, visual HRCT and $\dot{V}/Q$ scores of disease severity both provide close predictions of FEV_1.[799]

Patients considered for LVRS have extremely severe emphysema, but the regional distribution of disease has been shown to have a significant effect on the outcome of patients undergoing LVRS.[638,800–802] Several reports have shown that a heterogeneous distribution of emphysema (most commonly the predominantly upper lobe distribution of centrilobular emphysema) (Fig. 12.77) is associated with the greatest improvement in lung function, as judged by the degree of increase in the postoperative FEV_1,[638,792,800,802,803] in contrast to patients with extensive homogeneous (uniform distribution) disease (Fig. 12.78).[638,800,804,805] In one study of 50 patients undergoing LVRS, those with marked heterogeneity on CT showed an improvement in FEV_1 of 81% compared with 34% in patients with a homogeneous distribution[638]; in this study there was no relationship between the zonal predominance of the emphysematous lung (e.g. upper zone centrilobular emphysema versus lower zone panacinar emphysema of α_1-antitrypsin deficiency). Nevertheless, most series that document the heterogeneity of the distribution of emphysema include patients with predominantly upper lobe centrilobular emphysema, and it is this distribution that appears to be associated with the best functional outcome. In one series, the improvement in FEV_1 following bilateral LVRS surgery was 68, 47 and 37%, respectively, for upper lobe predominant, lower lobe

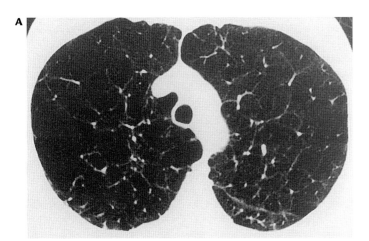
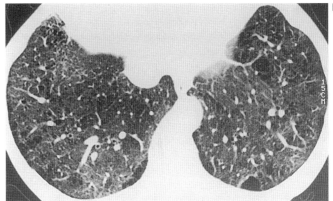

Fig. 12.77 Severe centrilobular emphysema in a patient being assessed for lung volume reduction surgery. The distribution of emphysema is markedly heterogeneous. **A**, Emphysema is concentrated mainly in the upper lobes. **B**, By comparison, the lower lobes are relatively spared.

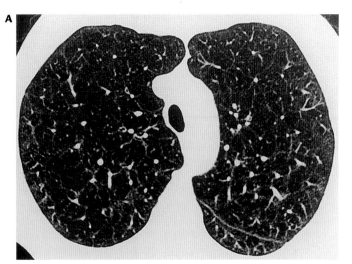
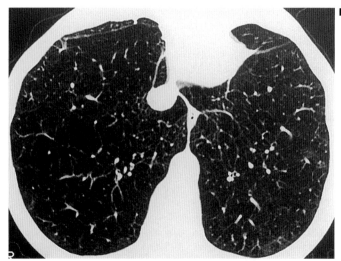

Fig. 12.78 Widespread emphysema in a patient under consideration for lung volume reduction surgery. The disease is of the same severity in **A**, the upper and **B**, lower zones, reflecting a homogeneous distribution (compare with Fig. 12.77).

predominant, and diffuse disease, respectively.[806] Differences in the radial distribution (central versus peripheral) of emphysema may also influence the effects of LVRS: more extensive emphysema in the subpleural lung predicted a better outcome, perhaps in part because the peripherally involved lung was more readily accessible to surgical resection.[807] Several techniques have been described to semiautomate the classification of CT data in terms of the heterogeneity of distribution of emphysema.[639,640,808]

Many studies have evaluated which imaging variables (whether CT,[800,805] MRI,[727,790,809] or radionuclide scanning[793,801,747,810] features) predict a functional improvement following LVRS.[811] There is less information about which imaging features predict a poor outcome, and so exclude patients from LVRS. It seems probable that a combination of parameters – a combined physiologic and imaging assessment – will provide the most accurate means of stratifying patients into those who will, or will not, benefit from LVRS. In one study which has used this approach, patients who were shown to have moderate to severe emphysema on HRCT did not necessarily respond favorably to lung volume reduction surgery despite having heterogeneous disease; in these cases intrinsic small airways disease, as judged by a substantially increased inspiratory resistance, correlated with the poor outcome.[812] Conversely, it is possible to eliminate those patients with severe chronic, obstructive pulmonary disease with a low FEV_1 (<30% predicted) who have mild or negligible emphysema on HRCT, and who are therefore unsuitable for LVRS.[797] It is also possible that HRCT will occasionally reveal an alternative explanation for what appears to be severe and extensive emphysema on plain chest radiography; e.g. severe constrictive obliterative bronchiolitis[813] or end-stage Langerhans cell histiocytosis may sometimes resemble end-stage emphysema radiographically and functionally.

A novel, and as yet unproven, alternative to surgical LVR is the bronchoscopic placement of one-way valves in bronchi supplying emphysematous lobes; the theory being that, since the values allow only the egress of air, there should be progressive collapse of the plugged lobes (Fig. 12.79).[814] The attraction is that bronchoscopic LVR is less invasive than surgical LVR and can be offered to patients deemed unsuitable for surgical LVR.

Nevertheless, judgment about the success of bronchoscopic LVR will require the results of clinical trials.

Several features can be identified on preoperative CT that may change the surgical technique of LVRS, while not necessarily precluding the procedure[796]; these include extensive pleural disease or parenchymal scarring, bronchiectasis, pulmonary nodules (possibly neoplastic), dilated central pulmonary arteries reflecting pulmonary arterial hypertension, and heavily calcified coronary arteries indicating ischemic heart disease. The serendipitous finding of a small pulmonary nodule on a preoperative CT scan is common, and was as high as 40% in one series,[815] but only 5% in another study[816] (Fig. 12.80). The majority of such incidental pulmonary nodules are benign; those that represent small primary lung cancers are usually stage 1 and may be resected at the time of LVRS surgery.[803,816] In some patients with destructive bullous emphysema, chest radiography may reveal masslike lesions, probably representing areas of compressed lung. On CT these pseudomasses are sharply marginated and often have an odd triangular or lenticular shape.[817]

Bullae

A bulla is an emphysematous space within the lungs that has a diameter of >1 cm in the distended state and that causes a local protrusion from the surface of the removed lung.[578,818] Bullae may be single or multiple and may represent a localized abnormality (focal paraseptal emphysema) or, more commonly, be part of widespread panacinar emphysema. Occasionally they are familial.[819] Pathologists recognize three types of bullae, which differ in location, size of neck, and amount of contained residual lung tissue.[818]

Bullae communicate with the bronchial tree, but air enters and leaves slowly and generally bullae do not act as a clinically important dead space,[820] though exceptions have been noted.[821] During tidal breathing pO_2 in bullae is higher than arterial pO_2.[822] Bullae show "paper bag compliance", inflating more easily than lung up to a critical volume, after which they become stiff and much less compliant than lung.[823] The pressure in bullae is normally negative and the same as pleural pressure.[822]

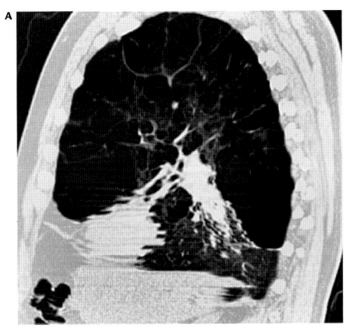

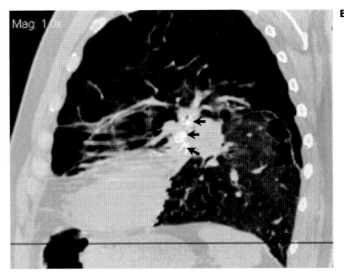

Fig. 12.79 Severe centrilobular emphysema in the upper lobes in a patient undergoing a volume reduction procedure using bronchoscopically placed one-way valves. **A**, Sagittal reformat CT showing severe emphysema in the left upper lobe with consequent volume loss in the left lower lobe. **B**, Following placement of valves within the three segmental bronchi of the left upper lobe (arrows), there is a reduction in volume of the overinflated upper lobe and some reexpansion of the left lower lobe.

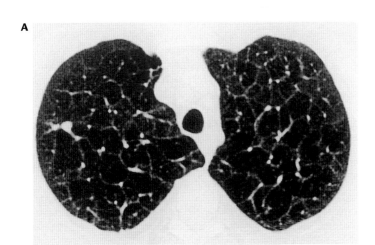

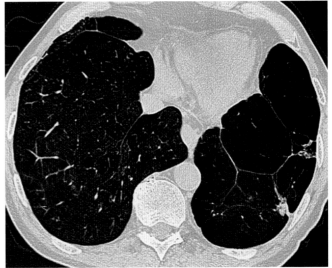

Fig. 12.80 Incidental nodules detected on preoperative CTs of patients under consideration for lung volume reduction surgery. **A**, Resected nodule proved to be a granuloma. **B**, In a different patient, follow-up CT showed that the peripheral opacities in the left lower lobe had resolved, and were presumed to represent infection.

On radiologic examination a bulla produces an avascular transradiant area, usually separated wholly or partly from the remaining lung by a thin curvilinear wall (Fig. 12.81). Occasionally the wall is completely absent, and under these circumstances bullae can be difficult to detect. Plain radiographs markedly underestimate the number of bullae demonstrated at postmortem examination.[661] The wall is usually of hairline thickness. Sometimes segments of the wall are thicker when there are major contributions from redundant pleura or collapsed

adjacent lung. Bullae caused by paraseptal emphysema are much more common in the upper zones,[824] but when they are associated with widespread panacinar emphysema, the distribution is much more even.[818] Bullae may be as small as 1 cm in diameter or may occupy the whole hemithorax, causing marked relaxation collapse of the adjacent lung (Fig. 12.68). They may even extend across into the opposite hemithorax, particularly by way of the anterior junctional area.[825] CT is more sensitive than the chest radiograph in demonstrating bullae (Fig. 12.82).[825–827] CT allows

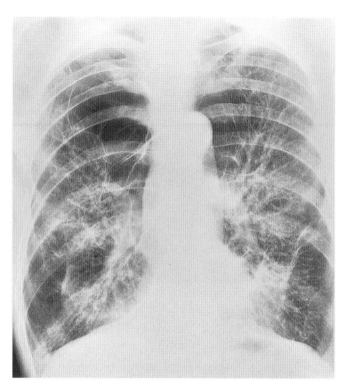

Fig. 12.81 Bullae in a patient with chronic airflow obstruction. In the right upper zone there is a large transradiant area containing thin curvilinear opacities, representing the walls of bullae.

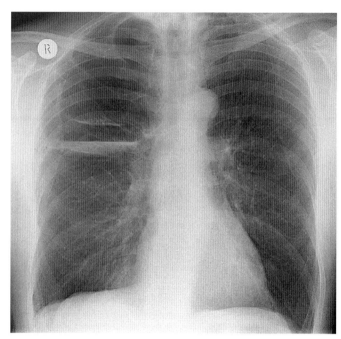

Fig. 12.83 Air–fluid level in a patient with severe chronic obstructive pulmonary disease and symptoms of an infective exacerbation. The fluid level within the bullous space disappeared on follow-up radiographs.

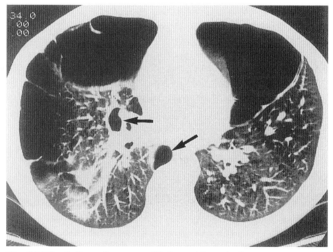

Fig. 12.82 Bullous disease on CT. Several large bullae are situated anterolaterally. Smaller bullae (arrows) are present in the azygoesophageal recess and against major vessels. Intervening lung, well seen paravertebrally, is reduced in volume but is otherwise normal and contains well-preserved vessels.

accurate assessment of the number, size, and position of bullae, and is particularly useful when bullae are obscured by other lung abnormalities, such as diffuse interstitial fibrosis.[826] CT can be helpful in marking the sometimes difficult distinction between bullous disease and a pneumothorax; though the "double-wall" sign (air visible on either side of the wall of the bulla)[828] may be helpful, differentiation may be impossible. Inspiratory and expiratory CT scans indicate the extent to which a bulla is ventilated, and the appearance of the rest of the lung helps in assessing the extent and degree of diffuse lung disease (Fig. 12.82).[826] This capability makes CT useful for identifying patients suitable for treatment with bullectomy.[829]

Bullae usually enlarge over months or years, but the rate is variable and a period of stability may be followed by a sudden expansion. In some patients, often young men, there may be inexorable progression of idiopathic giant bullous disease. The devastating nature of this condition is conveyed by its alternative name "vanishing lung syndrome"; most, but not all, patients are smokers and HRCT usually reveals paraseptal emphysema which merges with the bullae, most of which are 2–8 cm in diameter and in the upper lobes.[830] Marijuana smoking has been incriminated as a cause of large upper zone bullae in some individuals[831]; in these cases the background lung was well preserved with only relatively mild emphysematous changes. It is possible that some patients labeled as having giant bullous disease harbor an unusual condition: pulmonary sarcoidosis and Langerhans cell histiocytosis are both causes of so-called vanishing lung (see Ch. 11 and p. 648). Bullae may disappear either spontaneously[832,833] or following infection or hemorrhage.[824,832,834] The main complications of bullae are pneumothorax,[835] infection, or hemorrhage. When infected, bullae usually contain fluid and develop an air–fluid level (Fig. 12.83).[832,834,836] The hairline wall often becomes thickened, and indeed this may be the only sign of infection. Infected bullae differ from an abscess in that the patient is less ill, the wall of the ring shadow is thinner and has a sharp inner margin, and there is less adjacent pneumonitis.[837] Following infection, bullae often disappear.[832] Hemorrhage into the bulla is a much less common complication,[837,838] that may be accompanied by hemoptysis and a decrease in hemoglobin level. As with infection, the bulla may disappear after bleeding occurs.[839] A few cases of carcinoma arising in or adjacent to bullae are described.[839] Suspicious signs in this context include a mural nodule, mural thickening, a change in diameter of the bulla, pneumothorax, and the accumulation of fluid within the bulla.[840,841] Evidence has not shown that a carcinoma arising in relation to a bulla is any more than a chance association, unlike the situation with a variety of lung cysts, most of which are probably congenital.[842] Nevertheless, small foci of carcinoma are found on microscopic examination in resected lung of up to 5% of patients undergoing surgery for bullous emphysema.[843]

Patients with isolated bullous disease are usually asymptomatic. Occasionally, bullae produce breathlessness, which may be relieved by bullectomy.[821] The greatest benefit from surgery is seen in patients with a large bulla (occupying 50% or more of a hemithorax), a moderate reduction in FEV_1, a rapid onset of dyspnea, and no evidence of generalized emphysema.[820,844] The physiologic basis of the functional improvement following bullectomy is thought to be similar to that following LVRS.[845]

REFERENCES

1. Berkmen YM. The trachea: the blind spot in the chest. Radiol Clin North Am 1984;22:539–562.
2. Kwong JS, Adler BD, Padley SPG, et al. Diagnosis of diseases of the trachea and main bronchi: chest radiography vs CT. AJR Am J Roentgenol 1993;161:519–522.
3. Kwong JS, Müller NL, Miller RR. Diseases of the trachea and main-stem bronchi: correlation of CT with pathologic findings. RadioGraphics 1992;12:645–657.
4. Webb EM, Elicker BM, Webb WR. Using CT to diagnose nonneoplastic tracheal abnormalities: appearance of the tracheal wall. AJR Am J Roentgenol 2000;174:1315–1321.
5. Marom EM, Goodman PC, McAdams HP. Focal abnormalities of the trachea and main bronchi. AJR Am J Roentgenol 2001;176:707–711.
6. Marom EM, Goodman PC, McAdams HP. Diffuse abnormalities of the trachea and main bronchi. AJR Am J Roentgenol 2001;176:713–717.
7. Donnelly LF, Strife JL, Bisset GS. The spectrum of extrinsic lower airway compression in children: MR imaging. AJR Am J Roentgenol 1997;168:59–62.
8. Weber AL. Radiologic evaluation of the trachea. Chest Surg Clin North Am 1996;6:637–673.
9. Freeman SJ, Harvey JE, Goddard PR. Demonstration of supernumerary tracheal bronchus by computed tomographic scanning and magnetic resonance imaging. Thorax 1995;50:426–427.
10. Simoneaux SF, Bank ER, Webber JB, et al. MR imaging of the pediatric airway. RadioGraphics 1995;15:287–298.
11. Ferretti GR, Vining DJ, Knoplioch J, et al. Tracheobronchial tree: three-dimensional spiral CT with bronchoscopic perspective. J Comput Assist Tomogr 1996;20:777–781.
12. Ferretti GR, Knoplioch J, Bricault I, et al. Central airway stenoses: preliminary results of spiral-CT-generated virtual bronchoscopy simulations in 29 patients. Eur Radiol 1997;7:854–859.
13. Kauczor HU, Wolcke B, Fischer B, et al. Three-dimensional helical CT of the tracheobronchial tree: evaluation of imaging protocols and assessment of suspected stenoses with bronchoscopic correlation. AJR Am J Roentgenol 1996;167:419–424.
14. Lee KS, Yoon JH, Kim TK, et al. Evaluation of tracheobronchial disease with helical CT with multiplanar and three-dimensional reconstruction: correlation with bronchoscopy. RadioGraphics 1997;17:555–567.
15. Remy-Jardin M, Remy J, Deschildre F, et al. Obstructive lesions of the central airways: evaluation by using spiral CT with multiplanar and three-dimensional reformations. Eur Radiol 1996;6:807–816.
16. Whyte RI, Quint LE, Kazerooni EA, et al. Helical computed tomography for the evaluation of tracheal stenosis. Ann Thorac Surg 1995;60:27–30.
17. Ferretti GR, Bricault I, Coulomb M. Virtual tools for imaging of the thorax. Eur Respir J 2001;18:381–392.
18. Ferretti GR, Bricault I, Coulomb M. Helical CT with multiplanar and three-dimensional reconstruction of nonneoplastic abnormalities of the trachea. J Comput Assist Tomogr 2001;25:400–406.
19. Salvolini L, Bichi SE, Costarelli L, et al. Clinical applications of 2D and 3D CT imaging of the airways – a review. Eur J Radiol 2000;34:9–25.
20. Hoppe H, Walder B, Sonnenschein M, et al. Multidetector CT virtual bronchoscopy to grade tracheobronchial stenosis. AJR Am J Roentgenol 2002;178:1195–1200.
21. Anders HJ. Compression syndromes caused by substernal goitres. Postgrad Med J 1998;74:327–329.
22. Lincoln JC, Deverall PB, Stark J, et al. Vascular anomalies compressing the oesophagus and trachea. Thorax 1969;24:295–306.
23. Adenis L, Laurent JC, Charle J, et al. [Mediastinal lymph node tuberculosis fistulized into the esophagus in adults]. Lille Med 1976;19:766–769.
24. Kim Y, Lee KS, Yoon JH, et al. Tuberculosis of the trachea and main bronchi: CT findings in 17 patients. AJR Am J Roentgenol 1997;168:1051–1056.
25. Wieder S, Rabinowitz JG. Fibrous mediastinitis: a late manifestation of mediastinal histoplasmosis. Radiology 1977;125:305–312.
26. Benjamin B, Pitkin J, Cohen D. Congenital tracheal stenosis. Ann Otol Rhinol Laryngol 1981;90:364–371.
27. Carpenter BLM, Merten DF. Radiographic manifestations of congenital anomalies affecting the airway. Radiol Clin North Am 1991;29:219–240.
28. Landing BH, Dixon LG. Congenital malformations and genetic disorders of the respiratory tract (larynx, trachea, bronchi, and lungs). Am Rev Respir Dis 1979;120:151–185.
29. Jaffe RB. Balloon dilation of congenital and acquired stenosis of the trachea and bronchi. Radiology 1997;203:405–409.
30. Cantrell J, Guild H. Congenital stenosis of the trachea. Am J Surg 1964;108:297–305.
31. Nagappan R, Parkin G, Wright CA, et al. Adult long-segment tracheal stenosis attributable to complete tracheal rings masquerading as asthma. Crit Care Med 2002;30:238–240.
32. Aboussouan LS, O'Donovan PB, Moodie DS, et al. Hypoplastic trachea in Down's syndrome. Am Rev Respir Dis 1993;147:72–75.
33. Han BK, Dunbar JS, Striker TW. Membranous laryngotracheobronchitis (membranous croup). AJR Am J Roentgenol 1979;133:53–58.
34. Greenfield H, Herman PG. Papillomatosis of the trachea and bronchi. AJR Am J Roentgenol 1963;89:45–50.
35. Mariotta S, Masullo M, Guidi L, et al. Tracheobronchial involvement in 84 cases of pulmonary tuberculosis. Monaldi Arch Chest Dis 1995;50:356–359.
36. Slater LN, Kyung-Whan M. Polypoid endobronchial lesions: a manifestation of

bacillary angiomatosis. Chest 1992;102:972–974.

37. Holinger PH, Gelman HK, Wolfe CK Jr. Rhinoscleroma of the lower respiratory tract. Laryngoscope 1977;87:1–9.

38. Clarke A, Skelton J, Fraser RS. Fungal tracheobronchitis. Report of 9 cases and review of the literature. Medicine Balt 1991;70:1–14.

39. Gardner S, Seilheimer D, Catlin F, et al. Subglottic coccidioidomycosis presenting with persistent stridor. Pediatrics 1980;66:623–625.

40. Choplin RH, Wehunt WD, Theros EG. Diffuse lesions of the trachea. Semin Roentgenol 1983;18:38–50.

41. Edmonds LC, Prakash UB. Lymphoma, neutropenia, and wheezing in a 70-year-old man. Chest 1993;103:585–587.

42. Hines DW, Haber MH, Yaremko L, et al. Pseudomembranous tracheobronchitis caused by Aspergillus. Am Rev Respir Dis 1991;143:1408–1411.

43. Imoto EM, Stein RM, Shellito JE, et al. Central airway obstruction due to cytomegalovirus-induced necrotizing tracheitis in a patient with AIDS. Am Rev Respir Dis 1990;142:884–886.

44. Daum TE, Specks U, Colby TV, et al. Tracheobronchial involvement in Wegener's granulomatosis. Am J Respir Crit Care Med 1995;151:522–526.

45. Screaton NJ, Sivasothy P, Flower CDR, et al. Tracheal involvement in Wegener's granulomatosis: evaluation using spiral CT. Clin Radiol 1998;53:809–815.

46. Brandstetter RD, Messina MS, Sprince NL, et al. Tracheal stenosis due to sarcoidosis. Chest 1981;80:656.

47. Kuzniar T, Sleiman C, Brugiere O, et al. Severe tracheobronchial stenosis in a patient with Crohn's disease. Eur Respir J 2000;15:209–212.

48. McCarthy MJ, Rosado-de-Christenson ML. Tumors of the trachea. J Thorac Imaging 1995;10:180–198.

49. Felson B. Neoplasms of the trachea and main stem bronchi. Semin Roentgenol 1983;18:23–37.

50. Pradhan DJ, Rabuzzi D, Meyer JA. Primary solitary lymphoma of the trachea. J Thorac Cardiovasc Surg 1975;70:938–940.

51. Okada K, Lee MO, Hitomi S, et al. Sinus histiocytosis with massive lymphadenopathy and tracheobronchial lesions: CT and MR findings. J Comput Assist Tomogr 1988;12:1039–1040.

52. Norwood S, Vallina VL, Short K, et al. Incidence of tracheal stenosis and other late complications after percutaneous tracheostomy. Ann Surg 2000;232:233–241.

53. Grillo HC. Surgical treatment of postintubation tracheal injuries. J Thorac Cardiovasc Surg 1979;78:860–875.

54. Zietek E, Matyja G, Kawczynski M. Stenosis of the larynx and trachea: diagnostics and treatment. Otolaryngol Pol 2001;55:515–520.

55. Shepard JA, Grillo HC, McLoud TC, et al. Right-pneumonectomy syndrome: radiologic findings and CT correlation. Radiology 1986;161:661–664.

56. Wiot JF. Tracheobronchial trauma. Semin Roentgenol 1983;18:15–22.

57. Vas L, Sanzgiri S, Patil B, et al. An unusual cause of tracheal stenosis. Can J Anaesth 2000;47:261–264.

58. Holinger P, Johnston K, Basinger C. Benign stenosis of the trachea. Ann Otol Rhinol Laryngol 1950;59:837–859.

59. Thompson JW, Ahmed AR, Dudley JP. Epidermolysis bullosa dystrophica of the larynx and trachea. Acute airway obstruction. Ann Otol Rhinol Laryngol 1980;89:428–429.

60. Peters ME, Dickie HA, Crummy AB, et al. Swyer–James Macleod syndrome: a case with a baseline normal chest radiograph. Pediatr Radiol 1982; 12:211–213.

61. Kaufmann HJ, Mahboubi S, Spackman TJ, et al. Tracheal stenosis as a complication of chondrodysplasia punctata. Ann Radiol (Paris) 1976;19:203–209.

62. Cook AJ, Weinstein M, Powell RD. Diffuse amyloidosis of the tracheobronchial tree. Bronchographic manifestations. Radiology 1973;107:303–304.

63. Kirchner J, Jacobi V, Kardos P, et al. CT findings in extensive tracheobronchial amyloidosis. Eur Radiol 1998;8: 352–354.

64. Tillie-Leblond I, Wallaert B, Leblond D, et al. Respiratory involvement in relapsing polychondritis. Clinical, functional, endoscopic, and radiographic evaluations. Medicine 1998;77:168–176.

65. Tsunezuka Y, Sato H, Shimizu H. Tracheobronchial involvement in relapsing polychondritis. Respiration 2000;67:320–322.

66. Young RH, Sandstrom RE, Mark GJ. Tracheopathia osteoplastica: clinical, radiologic, and pathological correlations. J Thorac Cardiovasc Surg 1980;79: 537–541.

67. Bhalla M, Grillo HC, McLoud TC, et al. Idiopathic laryngotracheal stenosis: radiologic findings. AJR Am J Roentgenol 1993;161:515–517.

68. Silverman G. Tuberculosis of the trachea and major bronchi. Dis Chest 1945; 11:3–17.

69. Im JG, Song KS, Kang HS, et al. Mediastinal tuberculous lymphadenitis: CT manifestations. Radiology 1987;164:115–119.

70. Becker TS, Shum TK, Waller TS, et al. Radiological aspects of rhinoscleroma. Radiology 1981;141:433–438.

71. Razek AA, Elasfour AA. MR appearance of rhinoscleroma. Am J Neuroradiol 1999;20:575–578.

72. Amoils CP, Shindo ML. Laryngotracheal manifestations of rhinoscleroma. Ann Otol Rhinol Laryngol 1996;105:336–340.

73. Fajardo-Dolci G, Chavolla R, Lamadrid-Bautista E, et al. Laryngeal scleroma. J Otolaryngol 1999;28:229–231.

74. Feldman F, Seaman W, Baker D. The roentgen manifestations of scleroma. AJR Am J Roentgenol 1967;101:807–813.

75. Gamsu G, Webb WR. Computed tomography of the trachea and mainstem bronchi. Semin Roentgenol 1983;18:51–60.

76. Wilks S. Ossific deposits on the larynx, trachea and bronchi. Trans Pathol Soc Lond 1857;8:88.

77. Alroy GG, Lichtig C, Kaftori JK. Tracheobronchopathia osteoplastica: end stage of primary lung amyloidosis? Chest 1972;61:465–468.

78. Lundgren R, Stjernberg NL. Tracheobronchopathia osteochondroplastica. A clinical bronchoscopic and spirometric study. Chest 1981;80:706–709.

79. Way SP. Tracheopathia osteoplastica. J Clin Pathol 1967;20:814–820.

80. Manning JE, Goldin JG, Shpiner RB, et al. Case report: tracheobronchopathia osteochondroplastica. Clin Radiol 1998;53:302–309.

81. Sakula A. Tracheobronchopathia osteoplastica: its relationship to primary tracheobronchial amyloidosis. Thorax 1968;23:105–110.

82. Onitsuka H, Hirose N, Watanabe K, et al. Computed tomography of tracheopathia osteoplastica. AJR Am J Roentgenol 1983;140:268–270.

83. Matsuba T, Andoh K, Hirota N, et al. CT diagnosis of tracheobronchopathia osteochondroplastica. Respiration 2001;68:200.

84. Zack JR, Rozenshtein A. Tracheobronchopathia osteochondroplastica: report of three cases. J Comput Assist Tomogr 2002;26:33–36.

85. Greene R, Lechner GL. "Saber-Sheath" trachea: A clinical and functional study of marked coronal narrowing of the intrathoracic trachea. Radiology 1975;115:265–268.

86. Greene R. "Saber-sheath" trachea: relation to chronic obstructive pulmonary disease. AJR Am J Roentgenol 1978;130:441–445.

87. Trigaux JP, Hermes G, Dubois P, et al. CT of saber-sheath trachea. Correlation with clinical, chest radiographic and functional findings. Acta Radiol 1994;35:247–250.

88. Arakawa H, Kurihara Y, Nakajima Y, et al. Computed tomography measurements of overinflation in chronic obstructive pulmonary disease: evaluation of various radiographic signs. J Thorac Imaging 1998;13:188–192.

89. Gamsu G, Webb WR. Computed tomography of the trachea: normal and abnormal. AJR Am J Roentgenol 1982;139:321–326.

90. Rubenstein J, Weisbrod G, Steinhardt MI. Atypical appearances of "saber-sheath" trachea. Radiology 1978;127:41–42.

91. Hoskins MC, Evans RA, King SJ, et al. 'Sabre sheath' trachea with mediastinal lipomatosis mimicking a mediastinal tumour. Clin Radiol 1991;44:417–418.

92. Jazbi B, Goodwin C, Tackett D, et al. Idiopathic subglottic stenosis. Ann Otol Rhinol Laryngol 1977;86:644–648.

93. Yamada S, Kikuchi K, Kosaka A, et al. Surgical management of idiopathic tracheal stenosis. Jpn J Thorac Cardiovasc Surg 1999;47:335–338.

94. Gans R, de Vries N, Donker AJ, et al. Circulating anti-neutrophil cytoplasmic autoantibodies in subglottic stenosis: a useful aid in diagnosing vasculitis in this condition?. Q J Med 1991;80: 565–574.

95. Breatnach E, Abbott GC, Fraser RG. Dimensions of the normal human trachea. AJR Am J Roentgenol 1984;142:903–906.

96. Jesseph JE, Merendino KA. The dimensional interrelationships of the major components of the human tracheobronchial tree. Surg Gynecol Obstet 1957;105:210–214.

97. Katz I, LeVine M, Herman P. Tracheobronchomegaly: the Mounier–Kuhn syndrome. AJR Am J Roentgenol 1962;88:1084–1094.

98. Vock P, Spiegel T, Fram EK, et al. CT assessment of the adult intrathoracic cross section of the trachea. J Comput Assist Tomogr 1984;8:1076–1082.

99. Griscom NT, Vawter GF, Stigol LC. Radiologic and pathologic abnormalities of the trachea in older patients with cystic fibrosis. AJR Am J Roentgenol 1987;148:691–693.

100. Lebecque P, Liistro G, Veriter C, et al. Tracheal distensibility in cystic fibrosis. Eur Respir J 1996;9:770–772.

101. Woodring JH, Barrett PA, Rehm SR, et al. Acquired tracheomegaly in adults as a complication of diffuse pulmonary fibrosis. AJR Am J Roentgenol 1989; 152:743–747.

102. Aaby GV, Blake HA. Tracheobronchomegaly. Ann Thorac Surg 1966;2:64–70.

103. Wanderer AA, Ellis EF, Goltz RW, et al. Tracheobronchomegaly and acquired cutis laxa in a child. Physiologic and immunologic studies. Pediatrics 1969;44:709–715.

104. Lallemand D, Chagnon S, Buriot D, et al. Tracheomegaly and immune deficiency syndromes in childhood. Ann Radiol (Paris) 1981;24:67–72.

105. Feist JH, Johnson TH, Wilson RJ. Acquired tracheomalacia: etiology and differential diagnosis. Chest 1975;68:340–345.

106. Gronner AT, Trevino RJ. Tracheocoele. Br J Radiol 1971;44:979–981.

107. Mounier–Kuhn P. Dilatation de la trachee: constatations radiographiques et bronchoscopiques. Lyon Med 1932;150:106–109.

108. al Mallah Z, Quantock OP. Tracheobronchomegaly. Thorax 1968;23:320–324.

109. Gay S, Dee P. Tracheobronchomegaly – the Mounier–Kuhn syndrome. Br J Radiol 1984;57:640–644.

110. Woodring JH, Howard RS, Rehm SR. Congenital tracheobronchomegaly (Mounier–Kuhn syndrome): a report of 10 cases and review of the literature. J Thorac Imag 1991;6:1–10.

111. Johnston RF, Green RA. Tracheobronchomegaly: report of five cases and demonstration of familial occurrence. Am Rev Respir Dis 1965;91:35–50.

112. Bateson EM, Woo-Ming M. Tracheobronchomegaly. Clin Radiol 1973;24:354–358.

113. Hunter TB, Kuhns LR, Roloff MA et al. Tracheobronchomegaly in an 18 month old child. AJR Am J Roentgenol 1975;123:687–690.

114. Padley S, Varma N, Flower CD. Tracheobronchomegaly in association with ankylosing spondylitis. Clin Radiol 1991;43:139–141.

115. Benesch M, Eber E, Pfleger A, et al. Recurrent lower respiratory tract infections in a 14-year-old boy with tracheobronchomegaly (Mounier–Kuhn syndrome). Pediatr Pulmonol 2000; 29:476–479.

116. Dunne MG, Reiner B. CT features of tracheobronchomegaly. J Comput Assist Tomogr 1988;12:388–391.

117. Campbell AH, Young IF. Tracheobronchial collapse, a variant of obstructive respiratory disease. Br J Dis Chest 1963;57:174–181.

118. Goh RH, Dobranowski J, Kanaha L, et al. Dynamic computed tomography evaluation of tracheobronchomegaly. Can Assoc Radiol J 1995;46:212–215.

119. Rahbar M, Tabatabai D. Tracheobronchomegaly. Br J Dis Chest 1971;65:65–68.

120. Surprenant EL, O'Loughlin BJ. Tracheal diverticula and tracheobronchomegaly. Dis Chest 1966;49:345–351.

121. Doyle AJ. Demonstration on computed tomography of tracheomalacia in tracheobronchomegaly (Mounier–Kuhn syndrome). Br J Radiol 1989;62:176–177.

122. Ettman IK, Keel DT. Tracheal diverticulosis. Radiology 1962;78:187–191.

123. Shin MS, Jackson RM, Ho KJ. Tracheobronchomegaly (Mounier–Kuhn syndrome): CT diagnosis. AJR Am J Roentgenol 1988;150:777–779.

124. Rindsberg S, Friedman AC, Fiel SB, et al. MRI of tracheobronchomegaly. J Can Assoc Rad 1987;38:126–128.

125. Scadding JG. The bronchi in allergic aspergillosis. Scand J Respir Dis 1967;48:372–377.

126. Hein E, Rogalla P, Hentschel C, et al. Dynamic and quantitative assessment of tracheomalacia by electron beam tomography: correlation with clinical symptoms and bronchoscopy. J Comput Assist Tomogr 2000;24:247–252.

127. Heussel CP, Hafner B, Lill J, et al. Paired inspiratory/expiratory spiral CT and continuous respiration cine CT in the diagnosis of tracheal instability. Eur Radiol 2001;11:982–989.

128. Scholl PD. Adult tracheocele. Otolaryngol Head Neck Surg 1994;111:519–521.

129. Grassi R, Rea G, Scaglione M, et al. Imaging of tracheocele: report of three cases and review of the literature. Radiol Med (Torino) 2000;100:285–287.

130. Barbato A, Novello A Jr, Zanolin D, et al. Diverticulosis of the main bronchi: a rare cause of recurrent bronchopneumonia in a child. Thorax 1993;48:187–188.

131. Jones VF, Eid NS, Franco SM, et al. Familial congenital bronchiectasis: Williams-Campbell syndrome. Pediatr Pulmonol 1993;16:263–267.

132. Watanabe Y, Nishiyama Y, Kanayama H, et al. Congenital bronchiectasis due to cartilage deficiency: CT demonstration. J Comput Assist Tomogr 1987;11:701–703.

133. Masters IB, Chang AB, Patterson L, et al. Series of laryngomalacia, tracheomalacia, and bronchomalacia disorders and their associations with other conditions in children. Pediatr Pulmonol 2002;34:189–195.

134. Faust RA, Rimell FL, Remley KB. Cine magnetic resonance imaging for evaluation of focal tracheomalacia: innominate artery compression syndrome. Int J Pediatr Otorhinolaryngol 2002;65:27–33.

135. Weber AL, Grillo HC. Tracheal stenosis: an analysis of 151 cases. Radiol Clin North Am 1978;16:291–308.

136. Ravin CE, Handel DB, Kariman K. Persistent endotracheal tube cuff overdistension: a sign of tracheomalacia. AJR Am J Roentgenol 1981;137: 408–409.

137. Ell SR, Jolles H, Galvin JR. Cine CT demonstration of nonfixed upper airway obstruction. AJR Am J Roentgenol 1986;146:669–677.

138. Johnson TH, Mikita JJ, Wilson RJ, et al. Acquired tracheomalacia. Radiology 1973;109:576–580.

139. Liddelow AG, Campbell AH. Widening of the membranous wall and flattening of the trachea and main bronchi. Br J Dis Chest 1964;58:56–60.

140. Lomasney L, Bergin CJ, Lomasney J, et al. CT appearance of lunate trachea. J Comput Assist Tomogr 1989;13:520–522.

141. Griscom NT, Wohl ME. Tracheal size and shape: effects of change in intraluminal pressure. Radiology 1983;149:27–30.

142. Gamsu G, Borson DB, Webb WR, et al. Structure and function in tracheal stenosis. Am Rev Respir Dis 1980;121:519–531.

143. Holden WS, Ardran GM. Observations on the movements of the trachea and main bronchi in man. J Facul Radiol 1957;8:267–275.

144. Aquino SL, Shepard JA, Ginns LC, et al. Acquired tracheomalacia: detection by expiratory CT scan. J Comput Assist Tomogr 2001;25:394–399.

145. Kao SC, Smith WL, Sato Y, et al. Ultrafast CT of laryngeal and tracheobronchial obstruction in symptomatic postoperative infants with esophageal atresia and tracheoesophageal fistula. AJR Am J Roentgenol 1990;154:345–350.

146. Stern EJ, Graham CM, Webb WR, et al. Normal trachea during forced expiration: dynamic CT measurements. Radiology 1993;187:27–31.

147. Suto Y, Tanabe Y. Evaluation of tracheal collapsibility in patients with tracheomalacia using dynamic MR imaging during coughing. AJR Am J Roentgenol 1998;171:393–394.

148. Landing BH, Wells TR. Tracheobronchial anomalies in children. Perspect Pediatr Pathol 1973;1:1–32.

149. Altman KW, Wetmore RF, Marsh RR. Congenital airway abnormalities in patients requiring hospitalization. Arch Otolaryngol Head Neck Surg 1999;125:525–528.

150. Altman KW, Wetmore RF, Marsh RR. Congenital airway abnormalities requiring tracheotomy: a profile of 56 patients and their diagnoses over a 9 year period. Int J Pediatr Otorhinolaryngol 1997;41:199–206.

151. Chen JC, Holinger LD. Congenital laryngeal lesions: pathology study using serial macrosections and review of the literature. Pediatr Pathol 1994;14:301–325.

152. Filler RM, de Fraga JC. Tracheomalacia. Semin Thorac Cardiovasc Surg 1994;6:211–215.

153. Faust RA, Remley KB, Rimell FL. Real-time, cine magnetic resonance imaging for evaluation of the pediatric airway. Laryngoscope 2001;111:2187–2190.

154. Weber AL, Grillo HC. Tracheal tumors. A radiological, clinical, and pathological evaluation of 84 cases. Radiol Clin North Am 1978;16:227–246.

155. Prince JS, Duhamel DR, Levin DL, et al. Nonneoplastic lesions of the tracheobronchial wall: radiologic findings with bronchoscopic correlation. RadioGraphics 2002;22 Spec No: S215–S230.

156. Dowling EA, Johnson IM, Collier FCD, et al. Intratracheal goitre: a clinicopathologic review. Ann Surg 1962;156:258–267.

157. Randolph J, Grunt JA, Vawter GF. The medical and surgical aspects of intratracheal goitre. N Engl J Med 1963;268:457–461.

158. Martin KW, McAlister WH. Intratracheal thymus: a rare cause of airway obstruction. AJR Am J Roentgenol 1987;149:1217–1218.

159. Caldarola VT, Harrison EG, Clagett OT, et al. Benign tumors and tumorlike conditions of the trachea and bronchi. Ann Otol Rhinol Laryngol 1964;73:1042–1061.

160. Rosenbaum HD, Alavi SM, Bryant LR. Pulmonary parenchymal spread of juvenile laryngeal papillomatosis. Radiology 1968;90:654–660.

161. Singer DB, Greenberg SD, Harrison GM. Papillomatosis of the lung. Am Rev Respir Dis 1966;94:777–783.

162. Glazer G, Webb WR. Laryngeal papillomatosis with pulmonary spread in a 69-year-old man. AJR Am J Roentgenol 1979;132:820–822.

163. Gruden JF, Webb WR, Sides DM. Adult-onset disseminated tracheobronchial papillomatosis: CT features. J Comput Assist Tomogr 1994;18:640–642.

164. Dallimore NS. Squamous bronchial carcinoma arising in a case of multiple juvenile papillomatosis. Thorax 1985;40:797–798.

165. Tanaka H, Mori Y, Kurokawa K, et al. Paratracheal air cysts communicating with the trachea: CT findings. J Thorac Imaging 1997;12:38–40.

166. Goo JM, Im JG, Ahn JM, et al. Right paratracheal air cysts in the thoracic inlet: clinical and radiologic significance. AJR Am J Roentgenol 1999;173:65–70.

167. Black RJ. Congenital tracheo-oesophageal fistula in the adult. Thorax 1982;37:61–63.

168. Stephens RW, Lingeman RE, Lawson LJ. Congenital tracheoesophageal fistulas in adults. Ann Otol Rhinol Laryngol 1976;85:613–617.

169. Wychulis AR, Ellis FH Jr, Andersen HA. Acquired nonmalignant esophagotracheobronchial fistula. Report of 36 cases. JAMA 1966;196:117–122.

170. Martini N, Goodner JT, D'Angio GJ, et al. Tracheoesophageal fistula due to cancer. J Thorac Cardiovasc Surg 1970;59:319–324.

171. Little AG, Ferguson MK, DeMeester TR, et al. Esophageal carcinoma with respiratory tract fistula. Cancer 1984;53:1322–1328.

172. Berkmen YM, Auh YH. CT diagnosis of acquired tracheoesophageal fistula in adults. J Comput Assist Tomogr 1985;9:302–304.

173. Stanbridge RD. Tracheoesophageal fistula and bilateral recurrent laryngeal nerve palsies after blunt chest trauma. Thorax 1982;37:548–549.

174. Sakamoto Y, Seki Y, Tanaka N, et al. Tracheoesophageal fistula after blunt chest trauma: successful diagnosis by computed tomography. Thorac Cardiovasc Surg 2000;48:102–103.

175. Collier KP, Zubarik RS, Lewis JH. Tracheoesophageal fistula from an indwelling endotracheal tube balloon: a report of two cases and review. Gastrointest Endosc 2000;51:231–234.

176. Amoury RA, Hrabovsky EE, Leoidas JC, et al. Tracheoesophageal fistula after lye ingestion. J Paediatr Surg 1975;10:273–276.

177. Singh AK, Kothawla LK, Karlson KE. Tracheoesophageal and aortoesophageal fistulae complicating corrosive esophagitis. Chest 1976;70:549–551.

178. Maruyama Y, Petter JR, Green CR. Acquired esophagotracheal fistula secondary to a foreign body in the esophagus. N Engl J Med 1959;260:126–127.

179. Becker M, Schroth G, Zbaren P, et al. Long-term changes induced by high-dose irradiation of the head and neck region: imaging findings. RadioGraphics 1997;17:5–26.

180. Judd DR, Dubuque T Jr. Acquired benign esophagotracheobronchial fistula. Dis Chest 1968;54:237–240.

181. Heard BE, Khatchatourov V, Otto H, et al. The morphology of emphysema, chronic bronchitis, and bronchiectasis: definition, nomenclature, and classification. J Clin Pathol 1979;32:882–892.

182. Bachman AL, Hewitt WR, Beekley HC. Bronchiectasis: a bronchographic study of 60 cases of pneumonia. Arch Intern Med 1953;91:78–96.

183. Nelson SW, Christoforidis A. Reversible bronchiectasis. Radiology 1958;71:375–382.

184. Pontius JR, Jacobs LG. The reversal of advanced bronchiectasis. Radiology 1957;68:204–208.

185. Smith KR, Morris JF. Reversible bronchial dilatation: a report of a case. Dis Chest 1962;42:652–656.

186. Tsang KW, Lam WK, Sun J, et al. Regression of bilateral bronchiectasis with inhaled steroid therapy. Respirology 2002;7:77–81.

187. Reid LM. Reduction in bronchial subdivision in bronchiectasis. Thorax 1950;5:233–247.

188. Barker AF, Bardana EJ. Bronchiectasis: update of an orphan disease. Am Rev Respir Dis 1988;137:969–978.

189. Katzenstein ALA, Askin FB. Surgical pathology of non-neoplastic lung disease, 2nd edn. Philadelphia: WB Saunders, 1990.

190. Song JW, Im JG, Shim YS, et al. Hypertrophied bronchial artery at thin-

section CT in patients with bronchiectasis: correlation with CT angiographic findings. Radiology 1998;208:187–191.

191. Cole P, Flower CDR, Lavender JP. Clinical and imaging aspects of bronchiectasis. In: Potchen EJ, Grainger RG, Greene R, eds. Pulmonary radiology: The Fleischner Society. Philadelphia: WB Saunders, 1993:242–258.

192. Cohen M, Sahn SA. Bronchiectasis in systemic diseases. Chest 1999;116: 1063–1074.

193. Pasteur MC, Helliwell SM, Houghton SJ, et al. An investigation into causative factors in patients with bronchiectasis. Am J Respir Crit Care Med 2000;162: 1277–1284.

194. Cole PJ. A new look at the pathogenesis and management of persistent bronchial sepsis; a vicious circle hypothesis and its logical therapeutic connotations. In: Davies RJ, ed. Strategies for the management of chronic bronchial sepsis. Oxford: Medical Publishing Foundation, 1984:1–37.

195. Kaneko K, Kudo S, Tashiro M, et al. Case report: computed tomography findings in Williams–Campbell syndrome. J Thorac Imaging 1991;6:11–13.

196. Mitchell RE, Bury RG. Congenital bronchiectasis due to deficiency of bronchial cartilage (Williams–Campbell syndrome): a case report. J Pediatr 1975;87:230–234.

197. Wayne KS, Taussig LM. Probable familial congenital bronchiectasis due to cartilage deficiency (Williams–Campbell syndrome). Am Rev Respir Dis 1976; 114:15–22.

198. Aliabadi P, Shafiepoor H. Bronchography in the recognition of congenital cystic bronchiectasis. AJR Am J Roentgenol 1978;131:255–257.

199. Whyte KF, Williams GR. Bronchiectasis after mycoplasma pneumonia. Thorax 1984;39:390–391.

200. Curtin JJ, Webster ADB, Farrant J, et al. Bronchiectasis in hypogammaglobulinaemia – a computed tomography assessment. Clin Radiol 1991;44:82–84.

201. Nelson SW, Christoforidis AJ. Bronchography in diseases of the adult chest. Radiol Clin North Am 1973;11: 125–152.

202. Thurlbeck WM, Henderson JA, Fraser RG, et al. Chronic obstructive lung disease: a comparison between clinical, roentgenologic, functional and morphologic criteria in chronic bronchitis, emphysema, asthma and bronchiectasis. Medicine 1970;49:82–145.

203. Bertelsen S, Struve-Christensen E, Aasted A, et al. Isolated middle lobe atelectasis: aetiology, pathogenesis, and treatment of the so-called middle lobe syndrome. Thorax 1980;35:449–452.

204. Kwon KY, Myers JL, Swensen SJ, et al. Middle lobe syndrome: a clinicopathological study of 21 patients. Hum Pathol 1995;26:302–307.

205. Conces DJ Jr, Tarver RD, Vix VA. Broncholithiasis: CT features in 15 patients. AJR Am J Roentgenol 1991;157:249–253.

206. Kurklu EU, Williams MA, Le Roux BT. Bronchiectasis consequent upon foreign body retention. Thorax 1973;28:601–602.

207. Udwadia ZF, Pilling JR, Jenkins PF, et al. Bronchoscopic and bronchographic findings in 12 patients with sarcoidosis and severe or progressive airways obstruction. Thorax 1990;45:272–275.

208. Hoeffler HB, Schweppe HI, Greenberg SD. Bronchiectasis following pulmonary ammonia burn. Arch Pathol Lab Med 1982;106:686–687.

209. Kass I, Zamel N, Dobry CA, et al. Bronchiectasis following ammonia burns of the respiratory tract. A review of two cases. Chest 1972;62:282–285.

210. Fishbein D, Grossman RF. Pulmonary manifestations of familial dysautonomia in an adult. Am J Med 1986;80:709–713.

211. Winterbauer RH, Bedon GA, Ball WC Jr. Recurrent pneumonia. Predisposing illness and clinical patterns in 158 patients. Ann Intern Med 1969;70: 689–700.

212. Banner AS, Muthuswamy P, Shah RS, et al. Bronchiectasis following heroin-induced pulmonary edema. Rapid clearing of pulmonary infiltrates. Chest 1976;69:552–555.

213. Hansell DM, Strickland B. High-resolution computed tomography in pulmonary cystic fibrosis. Br J Radiol 1989;62:1–5.

214. Helbich TH, Heinz-Peer G, Eichler I, et al. Cystic fibrosis: CT assessment of lung involvement in children and adults. Radiology 1999;213:537–544.

215. Williams JL, Markowitz RI, Capitanio MA, et al. Immune deficiency syndromes. Semin Roentgenol 1975;10:83–89.

216. Obregon RG, Lynch DA, Kaske T, et al. Radiologic findings of adult primary immunodeficiency disorders. Chest 1994;106:490–495.

217. Kainulainen L, Varpula M, Liippo K, et al. Pulmonary abnormalities in patients with primary hypogammaglobulinemia. J Allergy Clin Immunol 1999;104: 1031–1036.

218. Newson T, Chippindale AJ, Cant AJ. Computed tomography scan assessment of lung disease in primary immunodeficiencies. Eur J Pediatr 1999;158:29–31.

219. Dukes RJ, Rosenow EC, Hermans PE. Pulmonary manifestations of hypogammaglobulinaemia. Thorax 1978;33:603–607.

220. Martinez Garcia MA, de Rojas MD, Nauffal M, et al. Respiratory disorders in common variable immunodeficiency. Respir Med 2001;95:191–195.

221. Fox MA, Lynch DA, Make BJ. Thymoma with hypogammaglobulinemia (Good's syndrome): an unusual cause of bronchiectasis. AJR Am J Roentgenol 1992;158:1229–1230.

222. Holmes AH, Trotman-Dickenson B, Edwards A, et al. Bronchiectasis in HIV disease. Q J Med 1992;85:875–882.

223. McGuinness G, Naidich DP, Garay S, et al. AIDS associated bronchiectasis: CT features. J Comput Assist Tomogr 1993;17:260–266.

224. King MA, Neal DE, St John R, et al. Bronchial dilatation in patients with HIV infection: CT assessment and correlation with pulmonary function tests and findings at bronchoalveolar lavage. AJR Am J Roentgenol 1997;168:1535–1540.

225. Skeens JL, Fuhrman CR, Yousem SA. Bronchiolitis obliterans in heart-lung transplantation patients: radiologic findings in 11 patients. AJR Am J Roentgenol 1989;153:253–256.

226. Loubeyre P, Revel D, Delignette A, et al. Bronchiectasis detected with thin-section CT as a predictor of chronic lung allograft rejection. Radiology 1995;194:213–216.

227. Butland RJ, Cole P, Citron KM, et al. Chronic bronchial suppuration and inflammatory bowel disease. Q J Med 1981;50:63–75.

228. Gibb WR, Dhillon DP, Zilkha KJ, et al. Bronchiectasis with ulcerative colitis and myelopathy. Thorax 1987;42:155–156.

229. Moles KW, Varghese G, Hayes JR. Pulmonary involvement in ulcerative colitis. Br J Dis Chest 1988;82:79–83.

230. Garg K, Lynch DA, Newell JD, et al. Proliferative and constrictive bronchiolitis: classification and radiologic features. AJR Am J Roentgenol 1994;162:803–808.

231. Eaton TE, Lambie M, Wells AU. Bronchiectasis following colectomy for Crohn's disease. Thorax 1998;53:529–531.

232. Mahadeva R, Flower C, Shneerson J. Bronchiectasis in association with coeliac disease. Thorax 1998;53:527–529.

233. Mitchell TA, Hamilos DL, Lynch DA, et al. Distribution and severity of bronchiectasis in allergic bronchopulmonary aspergillosis (ABPA). J Asthma 2000;37:65–72.

234. Eaton T, Garrett J, Milne D, et al. Allergic bronchopulmonary aspergillosis in the asthma clinic. A prospective evaluation of CT in the diagnostic algorithm. Chest 2000;118:66–72.

235. Westcott JL, Cole SR. Traction bronchiectasis in end-stage pulmonary fibrosis. Radiology 1986;161:665–669.

236. Cooper G, Guerrant JL, Harden AG, et al. Some consequences of pulmonary irradiation. AJR Am J Roentgenol 1961;85:865–874.

237. Libshitz HI, Shuman LS. Radiation-induced pulmonary change: CT findings. J Comput Assist Tomogr 1984;8:15–19.

238. Jones DK, Godden D, Cavanagh P. Alpha-1-antitrypsin deficiency presenting as bronchiectasis. Br J Dis Chest 1985;79:301–304.

239. Kagan E, Soskolne CL, Zwi S, et al. Immunologic studies in patients with recurrent bronchopulmonary infections. Am Rev Respir Dis 1975;111:441–451.

240. Longstreth GF, Weitzman SA, Browning RJ, et al. Bronchiectasis and homozygous alpha1-antitrypsin deficiency. Chest 1975;67:233–235.

241. Mahadeva R, Zhao MH, Stewart S, et al. Vasculitis and bronchiectasis in a patient with antibodies to bactericidal/permeability-increasing protein and alpha1-antitrypsin deficiency. Chest 1997;112:1699–1701.

242. Handelsman DJ, Conway AJ, Boylan LM, et al. Young's syndrome. Obstructive azoospermia and chronic sinopulmonary infections. N Engl J Med 1984;310:3–9.

243. Neville E, Brewis R, Yeates WK, et al. Respiratory tract disease and obstructive azoospermia. Thorax 1983;38:929–933.

244. Reed WB, Lopez DA, Landing B. Clinical spectrum of anhidrotic ectodermal dysplasia. Arch Dermatol 1970;102:134–143.

245. Fairfax AJ, Haslam PL, Pavia D, et al. Pulmonary disorders associated with Sjogren's syndrome. Q J Med 1981;50:279–295.

246. Allain J, Saraux A, Guedes C, et al. Prevalence of symptomatic bronchiectasis in patients with rheumatoid arthritis. Revue Du Rheumatisme (English edn) 1997;64:531–537.

247. Koyama M, Johkoh T, Honda O, et al. Pulmonary involvement in primary Sjogren's syndrome: spectrum of pulmonary abnormalities and computed tomography findings in 60 patients. J Thorac Imaging 2001;16:290–296.

248. Foster ME, Foster DR. Bronchiectasis and Marfan's syndrome. Postgrad Med J 1980;56:718–719.

249. Wood JR, Bellamy D, Child AH, et al. Pulmonary disease in patients with Marfan syndrome. Thorax 1984;39:780–784.

250. Wiggins J, Strickland B, Chung KF. Detection of bronchiectasis by high-resolution computed tomography in the yellow nail syndrome. Clin Radiol 1991;43:377–379.

251. Naidich DP, Funt S, Ettenger NA, et al. Hemoptysis: CT-bronchoscopic correlations in 58 cases. Radiology 1990;177:357–362.

252. Gudbjerg CE. Roentgenologic diagnosis of bronchiectasis. An analysis of 112 cases. Acta Radiol 1955;43:209–217.

253. Cooke JC, Currie DC, Morgan AD, et al. Role of computed tomography in diagnosis of bronchiectasis. Thorax 1987;42:272–277.

254. Currie DC, Cooke JC, Morgan AD, et al. Interpretation of bronchograms and chest radiographs in patients with chronic sputum production. Thorax 1987;42:278–284.

255. Woodring JH. Improved plain film criteria for the diagnosis of bronchiectasis. J Kentucky Med Assoc 1994;92:8–13.

256. van der Bruggen-Bogaarts BA, van der Bruggen HM, van Waes PF, et al. Screening for bronchiectasis. A comparative study between chest radiography and high-resolution CT. Chest 1996;109:608–611.

257. Nadel HR, Stringer DA, Levison H, et al. The immotile cilia syndrome: radiological manifestations. Radiology 1985;154:651–655.

258. Simmonds EJ, Littlewood JM, Evans EG. Cystic fibrosis and allergic bronchopulmonary aspergillosis. Arch Dis Child 1990;65:507–511.

259. Naidich DP, McCauley DI, Khouri NF, et al. Computed tomography of bronchiectasis. J Comput Assist Tomogr 1982;6:437–444.

260. Grenier P, Cordeau MP, Beigelman C. High-resolution computed tomography of the airways. J Thorac Imag 1993;8:213–229.

261. Kang EY, Miller RR, Müller NL. Bronchiectasis: comparison of preoperative thin-section CT and pathologic findings in resected specimens. Radiology 1995;195:649–654.

262. McGuinness G, Naidich DP, Leitman BS, et al. Bronchiectasis: CT evaluation. AJR Am J Roentgenol 1993;160:253–259.

263. McGuinness G, Naidich DP. Bronchiectasis: CT/clinical correlations. Semin US CT MRI 1995;16:394–419.

264. Smith IE, Flower CDR. Imaging in bronchiectasis. Br J Radiol 1996;69:589–593.

265. Kim JS, Müller NL, Park CS, et al. Cylindrical bronchiectasis: diagnostic findings on thin-section CT. AJR Am J Roentgenol 1996;168:751–754.

266. Kim SJ, Im JG, Kim IO, et al. Normal bronchial and pulmonary arterial diameters measured by thin section CT. J Comput Assist Tomogr 1995;19:365–369.

267. Kim JS, Müller NL, Park CS, et al. Bronchoarterial ratio on thin section CT: comparison between high altitude and sea level. J Comput Assist Tomogr 1997;21:306–311.

268. Ouellette H. The signet ring sign. Radiology 1999;212:67–68.

269. Lynch DA, Newell JD, Tschomper BA, et al. Uncomplicated asthma in adults: comparison of CT appearance of the lungs in asthmatic and healthy subjects. Radiology 1993;188:829–833.

270. Reiff DB, Wells AU, Carr DH, et al. CT findings in bronchiectasis: limited value in distinguishing between idiopathic and specific types. AJR Am J Roentgenol 1995;2:261–267.

271. Marti-Bonmati L, Catala FJ, Perales FR. Computed tomography differentiation between cystic bronchiectasis and bullae. J Thorac Imag 1991;7:83–85.

272. Worthy SA, Brown MJ, Müller NL. Cystic air spaces in the lung: change in size on expiratory high-resolution CT in 23 patients. Clin Radiol 1998;53:515–519.

273. Remy-Jardin M, Remy J, Boulenguez C, et al. Morphologic effects of cigarette smoking on airways and pulmonary parenchyma in healthy adult volunteers: CT evaluation and correlation with pulmonary function tests. Radiology 1993;186:107–115.

274. Miszkiel KA, Wells AU, Rubens MB, et al. Effects of airway infection by Pseudomonas aeruginosa: a computed tomographic study. Thorax 1997;52:260–264.

275. Bhalla M, Noble ER, Shepard JA, et al. Normal position of trachea and anterior junction line on CT. J Comput Assist Tomogr 1993;17:714–718.

276. Diederich S, Jurriaans E, Flower CDR. Interobserver variation in the diagnosis of bronchiectasis on high-resolution computed tomography. Eur Radiol 1996;6:801–806.

277. Webb WR, Stein MG, Finkbeiner WE, et al. Normal and diseased isolated lungs: High-resolution CT. Radiology 1988;166:81–87.

278. Nishimura K, Kitaichi M, Izumi T, et al. Diffuse panbronchiolitis: correlation of high-resolution CT and pathologic findings. Radiology 1992;184:779–785.

279. Im JG, Itoh H, Shim YS, et al. Pulmonary tuberculosis: CT findings – early active disease and sequential change with antituberculous therapy. Radiology 1993;186:653–660.

280. Gruden JF, Webb WR. Identification and evaluation of centrilobular opacities on high-resolution CT. Semin US CT MRI 1995;16:435–449.

281. Hansell DM, Wells AU, Rubens MB, et al. Bronchiectasis: functional significance of areas of decreased attenuation at expiratory CT. Radiology 1994;193:369–374.

282. Roberts HR, Wells AU, Milne DG, et al. Airflow obstruction in bronchiectasis: correlation between computed tomography features and pulmonary function tests. Thorax 2000;55:198–204.

283. Noble MI, Fox B, Horsfield K, et al. Obliterative bronchiolitis with atypical features: CT scan and necropsy findings. Eur Respir J 1993;6:1221–1225.

284. Guest PJ, Hansell DM. High resolution computed tomography in emphysema

associated with alpha-1-antitrypsin deficiency. Clin Radiol 1992;45:260–266.

285. King MA, Stone JA, Diaz PT, et al. Alpha 1-antitrypsin deficiency: evaluation of bronchiectasis with CT. Radiology 1996;199:137–141.

286. Sheehan RE, Wells AU, Copley SJ, et al. A comparison of serial computed tomography and functional change in bronchiectasis. Eur Respir J 2002;20:581–587.

287. Silverman PM, Godwin JD. CT/bronchographic correlations in bronchiectasis. J Comput Assist Tomogr 1987;11:52–56.

288. Müller NL, Bergin CJ, Ostrow DN, et al. Role of computed tomography in the recognition of bronchiectasis. AJR Am J Roentgenol 1984;143:971–976.

289. Philips MS, Williams MP, Flower CDR. How useful is computed tomography in the diagnosis and assessment of bronchiectasis? Clin Radiol 1986;37:321–325.

290. Munro NC, Cooke JC, Currie DC, et al. Comparison of thin section computed tomography with bronchography for identifying bronchiectatic segments in patients with chronic sputum production. Thorax 1990;45:135–139.

291. Grenier P, Maurice F, Musset D, et al. Bronchiectasis: assessment by thin-section CT. Radiology 1986;161:95–99.

292. Marti-Bonmati L, Ruiz Perales F, Catala F, et al. CT findings in Swyer–James syndrome. Radiology 1989;172:477–480.

293. Ohri SK, Rutty G, Fountain SW. Acquired segmental emphysema: the enlarging spectrum of Swyer–James/Macleod's syndrome. Ann Thorac Surg 1993;56:120–124.

294. Lee PH, Carr DH, Rubens MB, et al. Accuracy of CT in predicting the cause of bronchiectasis. Clin Radiol 1995;50:839–844.

295. Takasugi JE, Godwin JD. The airways. Semin Roentgenol 1991;26:175–190.

296. Westcott JL. Bronchiectasis. Radiol Clin North Am 1991;29:1031–1042.

297. Cartier Y, Kavanagh PV, Johkoh T, et al. Bronchiectasis: accuracy of high-resolution CT in the differentiation of specific diseases. AJR Am J Roentgenol 1999;173:47–52.

298. McCarthy DS, Simon G, Hargreave FE. The radiological appearances in allergic bronchopulmonary aspergillosis. Clin Radiol 1970;21:366–375.

299. Currie DC, Goldman JM, Cole PJ, et al. Comparison of narrow section computed tomography and plain chest radiography in chronic allergic bronchopulmonary aspergillosis. Clin Radiol 1987;38:593–596.

300. Greenberger PA. Allergic bronchopulmonary aspergillosis and fungoses. Clin Chest Med 1988;9:599–608.

301. Neeld DA, Goodman LR, Gurney JW, et al. Computerised tomography in the evaluation of allergic bronchopulmonary aspergillosis. Am Rev Respir Dis 1990;142:1200–1205.

302. Santis G, Hodson ME, Strickland B. High resolution computed tomography in adult cystic fibrosis patients with mild lung disease. Clin Radiol 1991;44:20–22.

303. Gurney JW, Habbe TG, Hicklin J. Distribution of disease in cystic fibrosis: correlation with pulmonary function. Chest 1997;112:357–362.

304. Hartman TE, Swensen SJ, Williams DE. Mycobacterium avium-intracellulare complex: evaluation with CT. Radiology 1993;187:23–26.

305. Hollings NP, Wells AU, Wilson R, et al. Comparative appearances of non-tuberculous mycobacteria species: a CT study. Eur Radiol 2002;12:2211–2217.

306. Ratjen F, Doring G. Cystic fibrosis. Lancet 2003;361:681–689.

307. Wood BP. Cystic fibrosis: 1997. Radiology 1997;204:1–10.

308. Rajan S, Saiman L. Pulmonary infections in patients with cystic fibrosis. Semin Respir Infect 2002;17:47–56.

309. Ko YH, Pedersen PL. Cystic fibrosis: a brief look at some highlights of a decade of research focused on elucidating and correcting the molecular basis of the disease. J Bioenerg Biomembr 2001;33:513–521.

310. Bobadilla JL, Macek M Jr, Fine JP, et al. Cystic fibrosis: a worldwide analysis of CFTR mutations – correlation with incidence data and application to screening. Hum Mutat 2002;19:575–606.

311. Donnelly LF, MacFall JR, McAdams HP, et al. Cystic fibrosis: combined hyperpolarized ^{3}He-enhanced and conventional proton MR imaging in the lung – preliminary observations. Radiology 1999;212:885–889.

312. Griesenbach U, Ferrari S, Geddes DM, et al. Gene therapy progress and prospects: cystic fibrosis. Gene Ther 2002;9:1344–1350.

313. Noone PG, Knowles MR. 'CFTR-opathies': disease phenotypes associated with cystic fibrosis transmembrane regulator gene mutations. Respir Res 2001;2:328–332.

314. Mukhopadhyay S, Kirby ML, Duncan AW, et al. Early focal abnormalities on chest radiographs and respiratory prognosis in children with cystic fibrosis. Br J Radiol 1996;69:122–125.

315. Brasfield D, Hicks G, Soong S, et al. The chest roentgenogram in cystic fibrosis: a new scoring system. Pediatrics 1979;63:24–29.

316. Friedman PJ. Chest radiographic findings in the adult with cystic fibrosis. Semin Roentgenol 1987;22:114–124.

317. Friedman PJ, Harwood IR, Ellenbogen PH. Pulmonary cystic fibrosis in the adult: early and late radiologic findings with pathologic correlations. AJR Am J Roentgenol 1981;136:1131–1144.

318. Grum CM, Lynch JP, III. Chest radiographic findings in cystic fibrosis. Semin Respir Infect 1992;7:193–209.

319. Don CJ, Dales RE, Desmarais RL, et al. The radiographic prevalence of hilar and mediastinal adenopathy in adult cystic fibrosis. Can Assoc Radiol J 1997;48:265–269.

320. Marchant JM, Masel JP, Dickinson FL, et al. Application of chest high-resolution computed tomography in young children with cystic fibrosis. Pediatr Pulmonol 2001;31:24–29.

321. Greene KE, Takasugi JE, Godwin JD, et al. Radiographic changes in acute exacerbations of cystic fibrosis in adults: a pilot study. AJR Am J Roentgenol 1994;163:557–562.

322. Conway SP, Pond MN, Bowler I, et al. The chest radiograph in cystic fibrosis: a new scoring system compared with the Chrispin-Norman and Brasfield scores. Thorax 1994;49:860–862.

323. Flume PA. Pneumothorax in cystic fibrosis. Chest 2003;123:217–221.

324. Brinson GM, Noone PG, Mauro MA, et al. Bronchial artery embolization for the treatment of hemoptysis in patients with cystic fibrosis. Am J Respir Crit Care Med 1998;157:1951–1958.

325. Cipolli M, Perini S, Valletta EA, et al. Bronchial artery embolization in the management of hemoptysis in cystic fibrosis. Pediatr Pulmonol 1995;19:344–347.

326. Tonkin ILD, Hanissian AS, Boulden TF, et al. Bronchial arteriography and embolotherapy for hemoptysis in patients with cystic fibrosis. Cardiovasc Intervent Radiol 1991;14:241–246.

327. Jacobsen LE, Houston CS, Habbick BF, et al. Cystic fibrosis: a comparison of computed tomography and plain chest radiographs. J Can Assoc Radiol 1986;37:17–21.

328. Demirkazik FB, Ariyurek OM, Ozcelik U, et al. High resolution CT in children with cystic fibrosis: correlation with pulmonary functions and radiographic scores. Eur J Radiol 2001;37:54–59.

329. Bhalla M, Turcios N, Aponte V, et al. Cystic fibrosis: scoring system with thin-section CT. Radiology 1991;179:783–788.

330. Maffessanti M, Candusso M, Brizzi F, et al. Cystic fibrosis in children: HRCT findings and distribution of disease. J Thorac Imaging 1996;11:27–38.

331. Shah RM, Sexauer W, Ostrum BJ, et al. High resolution CT in the acute exacerbation of cystic fibrosis: evaluation of acute findings, reversibility of those findings, and clinical correlation. AJR Am J Roentgenol 1997;169:375–380.

332. Helbich TH, Heinz-Peer G, Fleischmann D, et al. Evolution of CT findings in

patients with cystic fibrosis. AJR Am J Roentgenol 1999;173:81–88.

333. Lugo-Olivieri CH, Soyer PA, Fishman EK. Cystic fibrosis: spectrum of thoracic and abdominal CT findings in the adult patient. Clin Imaging 1998;22:346–354.

334. Robinson TE, Leung AN, Northway WH, et al. Spirometer-triggered high-resolution computed tomography and pulmonary function measurements during an acute exacerbation in patients with cystic fibrosis. J Pediatr 2001;138:553–559.

335. Dakin CJ, Pereira JK, Henry RL, et al. Relationship between sputum inflammatory markers, lung function, and lung pathology on high-resolution computed tomography in children with cystic fibrosis. Pediatr Pulmonol 2002;33:475–482.

336. Oikonomou A, Manavis J, Karagianni P, et al. Loss of FEV_1 in cystic fibrosis: correlation with HRCT features. Eur Radiol 2002;12:2229–2235.

337. Santamaria F, Grillo G, Guidi G, et al. Cystic fibrosis: when should high-resolution computed tomography of the chest be obtained? Pediatrics 1998;101:908–913.

338. Donnelly LF, Gelfand MJ, Brody AS, et al. Comparison between morphologic changes seen on high-resolution CT and regional pulmonary perfusion seen on SPECT in patients with cystic fibrosis. Pediatr Radiol 1997;27:920–925.

339. Marom EM, McAdams HP, Palmer SM, et al. Cystic fibrosis: usefulness of thoracic CT in the examination of patients before lung transplantation. Radiology 1999;213:283–288.

340. Phillips GD, Trotman-Dickenson B, Hodson ME, et al. Role of CT in the management of pneumothorax in patients with complex cystic lung disease. Chest 1997;112:275–278.

341. Carr DH, Oades P, Trotman-Dickenson B, et al. Magnetic resonance scanning in cystic fibrosis: comparison with computed tomography. Clin Radiol 1995;50:84–89.

342. Kinsella D, Hamilton A, Goddard P, et al. The role of magnetic resonance imaging in cystic fibrosis. Clin Radiol 1991;44:23–26.

343. Afzelius BA. A human syndrome caused by immotile cilia. Science 1976;193:317–319.

344. Rubin BK. Immotile cilia syndrome (primary ciliary dyskinesia) and inflammatory lung disease. Clin Chest Med 1988;9:657–668.

345. Holzmann D, Ott PM, Felix H. Diagnostic approach to primary ciliary dyskinesia: a review. Eur J Pediatr 2000;159:95–98.

346. Afzelius BA, Mossberg B. Immotile cilia. Thorax 1980;35:401–404.

347. Kartagener M. Zur pathogenese der bronchiektasien: bronchiektasien bei

situs viscerum inversus. Beitr Klin Tuberk 1933;83:489–501.

348. Greenstone M, Rutman A, Dewar A, et al. Primary ciliary dyskinesia: cytological and clinical features. Q J Med 1988;67:405–423.

349. Miller RD, Divertie MB. Kartagener's syndrome. Chest 1972;62:130–135.

350. Rott HD. Kartagener's syndrome and the syndrome of immotile cilia. Hum Genet 1979;46:249–261.

351. Whitelaw A, Evans A, Corrin B. Immotile cilia syndrome: a new cause of neonatal respiratory distress. Arch Dis Child 1981;56:432–435.

352. Greenstone M, Rutman A, Pavia D, et al. Normal axonemal structure and function in Kartagener's syndrome: an explicable paradox. Thorax 1985;40:956–957.

353. Vix VA. Radiographic manifestations of broncholithiasis. Radiology 1978;128:295–299.

354. Arrigoni MG, Bernatz PE, Donoghue FE. Broncholithiasis. J Thorac Cardiovasc Surg 1971;62:231–237.

355. Seo JB, Song KS, Lee JS, et al. Broncholithiasis: review of the causes with radiologic-pathologic correlation. RadioGraphics 2002;22:S199–S213.

356. Dixon GF, Donnerberg RL, Schonfeld SA, et al. Advances in the diagnosis and treatment of broncholithiasis. Am Rev Respir Dis 1984;129:1028–1030.

357. Weed LA, Andersen HA. Etiology of broncholithiasis. Dis Chest 1960;37:270–277.

358. Carasso B, Couropmitree C, Heredia R. Egg-shell silicotic calcification causing bronchoesophageal fistula. Am Rev Respir Dis 1973;108:1384–1387.

359. Davis EW, Katz S, Peabody JW. Broncholithiasis, a neglected cause of bronchoesophageal fistula. JAMA 1956;160:555–557.

360. Studer SM, Heitmiller RF, Terry PB. Mediastinal abscess due to passage of a broncholith. Chest 2002;121:296–297.

361. Kowal LE, Goodman LR, Zarro VJ, et al. CT diagnosis of broncholithiasis. J Comput Assist Tomogr 1983;7:321–323.

362. Shin MS, Ho KJ. Broncholithiasis: its detection by computed tomography in patients with recurrent hemoptysis of unknown etiology. J Comput Tomogr 1983;7:189–193.

363. Shin MS, Berland LL, Myers JL, et al. CT demonstration of an ossifying bronchial carcinoid simulating broncholithiasis. AJR Am J Roentgenol 1989;153:51–52.

364. Colby TV, Myers JL. Clinical and histologic spectrum of bronchiolitis obliterans, including bronchiolitis obliterans organizing pneumonia. Semin Respir Med 1992;13:119–133.

365. Epler GR, Colby TV. The spectrum of bronchiolitis obliterans. Chest 1983;83:161–162.

366. Myers JL, Colby TV. Pathologic manifestations of bronchiolitis, constrictive bronchiolitis, cryptogenic organizing pneumonia, and diffuse panbronchiolitis. Clin Chest Med 1993;14:611–622.

367. Wright JL, Cagle P, Churg A, et al. Diseases of the small airways. Am Rev Respir Dis 1992;146:240–262.

368. Thurlbeck WM. Chronic airflow obstruction. In: Thurlbeck WM, Churg AM, eds. Pathology of the lung. New York: Thieme, 1995:739–825.

369. Geddes DM. BOOP and COP. Thorax 1991;46:545–547.

370. Travis WD, King TE. American Thoracic Society/European Respiratory Society International Multidisciplinary Consensus Classification of the Idiopathic Interstitial Pneumonias. This joint statement of the American Thoracic Society (ATS), and the European Respiratory Society (ERS) was adopted by the ATS board of directors, June 2001 and by the ERS Executive Committee, June 2001. Am J Respir Crit Care Med 2002;165:277–304.

371. Miki Y, Hatabu H, Takahashi M, et al. Computed tomography of bronchiolitis obliterans. J Comput Assist Tomogr 1988;12:512–514.

372. Kargi HA, Kuhn C 3rd. Bronchiolitis obliterans. Unilateral fibrous obliteration of the lumen of bronchi with atelectasis. Chest 1988;93:1107–1108.

373. Camp M, Mehta JB, Whitson M. Bronchiolitis obliterans and Nocardia asteroides infection of the lung. Chest 1987;92:1107–1108.

374. Sulavik SS. The concept of "organizing pneumonia". Chest 1989;96:967–968.

375. Colby TV. Bronchiolar pathology. In: Epler GR, ed. Diseases of the bronchioles. New York: Raven Press, 1994:77–100.

376. Hansell DM. Small airways diseases: detection and insights with computed tomography. Eur Respir J 2001;17:1294–1313.

377. Turton CW, Williams G, Green M. Cryptogenic obliterative bronchiolitis in adults. Thorax 1981;36:805–810.

378. Hansell DM, Rubens MB, Padley SPG, et al. Obliterative bronchiolitis: individual CT signs of small airways disease and functional correlation. Radiology 1997;203:721–726.

379. Wells AU, Du Bois RM. Bronchiolitis in association with connective tissue disorders. Clin Chest Med 1993;14:655–666.

380. Penn CC, Liu C. Bronchiolitis following infection in adults and children. Clin Chest Med 1993;14:645–654.

381. Becroft DMO. Bronchiolitis obliterans, bronchiectasis, and other sequelae of adenovirus type 21 infection in young children. J Clin Pathol 1971;24:72–82.

382. Hardy KA, Schidlow DV, Zaeri N. Obliterative bronchiolitis in children. Chest 1988;93:460–466.

383. Laraya-Cuasay LR, DeForest A, Huff D, et al. Chronic pulmonary complications of early influenza virus infection in children. Am Rev Respir Dis 1977; 116:617–625.

384. Prabhu MB, Barber D, Cockcroft DW. Bronchiolitis obliterans and Mycoplasma pneumonia. Respir Med 1991;85:535–537.

385. Wright JL. Inhalational lung injury causing bronchiolitis. Clin Chest Med 1993;14:635–644.

386. Douglas WW, Colby TV. Fume-related bronchiolitis obliterans. In: Epler GR, ed. Diseases of the bronchioles. New York: Raven Press, 1994:187–213.

387. Bhargava DK, Verma A, Batni G, et al. Early observations on lung function studies in symptomatic gas exposed population of Bhopal. Ind J Med Res 1987;86:1–10.

388. Perez-Guerra F, Walsh RE, Sagel SS. Bronchiolitis obliterans and tracheal stenosis. Late complications of inhalation burn. JAMA 1971;218:1568–1570.

389. Geddes DM, Corrin B, Brewerton DA, et al. Progressive airway obliteration in adults and its association with rheumatoid arthritis. Q J Med 1977;46:427–444.

390. Hayakawa H, Sato A, Imokawa S, et al. Bronchiolar disease in rheumatoid arthritis. Am J Respir Crit Care Med 1996;154:1531–1536.

391. Franquet T, Gimenez A, Monill JM, et al. Primary Sjogren's syndrome and associated lung disease: CT findings in 50 patients. AJR Am J Roentgenol 1997;169:655–658.

392. Meyer CA, Pina JS, Taillon D, et al. Inspiratory and expiratory high-resolution CT findings in a patient with Sjogren's syndrome and cystic lung disease. AJR Am J Roentgenol 1997;168:101–103.

393. Breuer R, Lossos IS, Berkman N, et al. Pulmonary complications of bone marrow transplantation. Respir Med 1993;87:571–579.

394. Worthy SA, Flint JD, Müller NL. Pulmonary complications after bone marrow transplantation: high-resolution CT and pathologic findings. RadioGraphics 1997;17:1359–1371.

395. Worthy SA, Park CS, Kim JS, et al. Bronchiolitis obliterans after lung transplantation: high-resolution CT findings in 15 patients. AJR Am J Roentgenol 1997;169:673–677.

396. Scott JP, Sharples L, Mullins P, et al. Further studies on the natural history of obliterative bronchiolitis following heart-lung transplantation. Transplant Proc 1991;23:1201–1202.

397. Ikonen T, Kivisaari L, Harjula ALJ, et al. Value of high-resolution computed tomography in routine evaluation of lung transplantation recipients during development of bronchiolitis obliterans syndrome. J Heart Lung Transplant 1996;15:587–595.

398. Bankier AA, Van Muylem A, Knoop C, et al. Bronchiolitis obliterans syndrome in heart-lung transplant recipients: diagnosis with expiratory CT. Radiology 2001;218:533–539.

399. Wolfe F, Schurle DR, Lin JJ, et al. Upper and lower airway disease in penicillamine treated patients with rheumatoid arthritis. J Rheumatol 1983;10:406–410.

400. Wilcox P, Miller R, Miller G, et al. Airway involvement in ulcerative colitis. Chest 1987;92:18–22.

401. Karadag F, Ozhan MH, Akcicek E, et al. Is it possible to detect ulcerative colitis-related respiratory syndrome early? Respirology 2001;6:341–346.

402. Hogg JC. Bronchiolitis in asthma and chronic obstructive airways pulmonary disease. Clin Chest Med 1993;14:733–740.

403. Mellins RB. The site of airway obstruction in cystic fibrosis. Pediatrics 1969;44:315–318.

404. Aguayo SM, Miller YE, Waldron JA, et al. Idiopathic diffuse hyperplasia of pulmonary neuroendocrine cells and airways disease. N Engl J Med 1992; 327:1285–1288.

405. Brown MJ, English J, Müller NL. Bronchiolitis obliterans due to neuroendocrine hyperplasia: high resolution CT – pathologic correlation. AJR Am J Roentgenol 1997;168: 1561–1562.

406. Yang CF, Wu MT, Chiang AA, et al. Correlation of high-resolution CT and pulmonary function in bronchiolitis obliterans: a study based on 24 patients associated with consumption of *Sauropus androgynus*. AJR Am J Roentgenol 1997;168:1045–1050.

407. Milner AD, Murray M. Acute bronchiolitis in infancy: treatment and prognosis. Thorax 1989;44:1–5.

408. Sato P, Madtes DK, Thorning D, et al. Bronchiolitis obliterans caused by *Legionella pneumophila*. Chest 1985;87:840–842.

409. Green M, Turton CW. Bronchiolitis and its manifestations. Eur J Respir Dis 1982;63:36–42.

410. Morrissey WL, Gould IA, Carrington CB, et al. Silo-filler's disease. Respiration 1975;32:81–92.

411. Douglas WW, Hepper N, Colby TV. Silo filler's disease. Mayo Clin Proc 1989;64:291–304.

412. Herzog CA, Miller RR, Hoidal JR. Bronchiolitis and rheumatoid arthritis. Am Rev Respir Dis 1979;119:555–560.

413. Remy-Jardin M, Remy J, Cortet B, et al. Lung changes in rheumatoid arthritis: CT findings. Radiology 1994;193: 375–382.

414. Perez T, Remy-Jardin M, Cortet B. Airways involvement in rheumatoid arthritis: clinical, functional, and HRCT findings. Am J Respir Crit Care Med 1998;157:1658–1665.

415. Cortet B, Perez T, Roux N, et al. Pulmonary function tests and high resolution computed tomography of the lungs in patients with rheumatoid arthritis. Ann Rheum Dis 1997;56: 596–600.

416. Epler GR, Snider GL, Gaensler EA, et al. Bronchiolitis and bronchitis in connective tissue disease: a possible relationship to the use of penicillamine. JAMA 1979;242:528–532.

417. Murphy KC, Atkins CJ, Offer RC, et al. Obliterative bronchiolitis in two rheumatoid arthritis patients treated with penicillamine. Arthritis Rheum 1981;24:557–560.

418. Cain HC, Noble PW, Matthay RA. Pulmonary manifestations of Sjogren's syndrome. Clin Chest Med 1998;19: 687–699.

419. Halvorsen RA Jr, DuCret RP, Kuni CC, et al. Obliterative bronchiolitis following lung transplantation. Diagnostic utility of aerosol ventilation lung scanning and high resolution CT. Clin Nuclear Med 1991;16:256–258.

420. Leung AN, Fisher K, Valentine V, et al. Bronchiolitis obliterans after lung transplantation: detection using expiratory HRCT. Chest 1998;113:365–370.

421. Paradis I, Yousem S, Griffith B. Airway obstruction and bronchiolitis obliterans after lung transplantation. Clin Chest Med 1993;14:751–763.

422. Ikonen T, Kivisaari L, Taskinen E, et al. High-resolution CT in long-term follow-up after lung transplantation. Chest 1997;111:370–376.

423. Miller WT Jr, Kotloff RM, Blumenthal NP, et al. Utility of high resolution computed tomography in predicting bronchiolitis obliterans syndrome following lung transplantation: preliminary findings. J Thorac Imaging 2001;16:76–80.

424. Choi YW, Rossi SE, Palmer SM, et al. Bronchiolitis obliterans syndrome in lung transplant recipients: correlation of computed tomography findings with bronchiolitis obliterans syndrome stage. J Thorac Imaging 2003;18:72–79.

425. Trisolini R, Stanzani M, Agli LL, et al. Delayed non-infectious lung disease in allogeneic bone marrow transplant recipients. Sarcoidosis Vasc Diffuse Lung Dis 2001;18:75–84.

426. Crawford SW, Clark JG. Bronchiolitis associated with bone marrow transplantation. Clin Chest Med 1993;14:741–749.

427. Sweatman MC, Millar AB, Strickland B, et al. Computed tomography in adult obliterative bronchiolitis. Clin Radiol 1990;41:116–119.

428. Tukiainen P, Poppius H, Taskinen E. Slowly progressive bronchiolitis obliterans: a case report with detailed pulmonary function studies. Eur J Respir Dis 1980;61:77–83.

429. Breatnach E, Kerr I. The radiology of cryptogenic obliterative bronchiolitis. Clin Radiol 1982;33:657–661.

430. Friedman PJ. Radiology of the airways with emphasis on the small airways. J Thorac Imag 1986;1:7–22.

431. Eber CD, Stark P, Bertozzi P. Bronchiolitis obliterans on high-resolution CT: a pattern of mosaic oligemia. J Comput Assist Tomogr 1993;17:853–856.

432. Hartman TE, Primack SL, Lee KS, et al. CT of bronchial and bronchiolar diseases. RadioGraphics 1994;14:991–1003.

433. Müller NL, Miller RR. Diseases of the bronchioles: CT and histopathologic findings. Radiology 1995;196:3–12.

434. Hwang JH, Kim TS, Lee KS, et al. Bronchiolitis in adults: pathology and imaging. J Comput Assist Tomogr 1997;21:913–919.

435. Padley SP, Adler BD, Hansell DM, et al. Bronchiolitis obliterans: high resolution CT findings and correlation with pulmonary function tests. Clin Radiol 1993;47:236–240.

436. Abernathy EC, Hruban RH, Baumgartner WA, et al. The two forms of bronchiolitis obliterans in heart-lung transplant recipients. Hum Pathol 1991;22:1102–1110.

437. Franquet T, Stern EJ. Bronchiolar inflammatory diseases: high-resolution CT findings with histologic correlation. Eur Radiol 1999;9:1290–1303.

438. Stern EJ, Frank MS. Small-airways disease of the lungs: findings at expiratory CT. AJR Am J Roentgenol 1994;163:37–41.

439. Worthy SA, Müller NL, Hartman TE, et al. Mosaic attenuation pattern on thin-section CT scans of the lung: differentiation among infiltrative lung, airway, and vascular diseases as a cause. Radiology 1997;205:465–470.

440. Lentz D, Bergin CJ, Berry GJ, et al. Diagnosis of bronchiolitis obliterans in heart-lung transplantation patients: importance of bronchial dilatation on CT. AJR Am J Roentgenol 1992;159:463–467.

441. Cortet B, Flipo RM, Remy-Jardin M, et al. Use of high resolution computed tomography of the lungs in patients with rheumatoid arthritis. Ann Rheum Dis 1995;54:815–819.

442. Loubeyre P, Revel D, Delignette A, et al. High-resolution computed tomographic findings associated with histologically diagnosed acute lung rejection in heart-lung transplant recipients. Chest 1995;107:132–138.

443. Arakawa H, Webb WR, McCowin M, et al. Inhomogeneous lung attenuation at thin-section CT: diagnostic value of expiratory scans. Radiology 1998;206:89–94.

444. Arakawa H, Webb WR. Air trapping on expiratory high-resolution CT scans in the absence of inspiratory scan abnormalities: correlation with pulmonary function tests and differential diagnosis. AJR Am J Roentgenol 1998;170:1349–1353.

445. Desai SR, Hansell DM. Small airways disease: expiratory computed tomography comes of age. Clin Radiol 1997;52:332–337.

446. Bhalla M, Naidich DP, McGuinness G, et al. Diffuse lung disease: assessment with helical CT – preliminary observations of the role of maximum and minimum intensity projection images. Radiology 1996;200:341–347.

447. Remy-Jardin M, Remy J, Gosselin B, et al. Sliding thin slab, minimum intensity projection technique in the diagnosis of emphysema: histopathologic-CT correlation. Radiology 1996;200:665–671.

448. Yang GZ, Hansell DM. CT image enhancement with wavelet analysis for the detection of small airways disease. IEEE Transac Med Imag 1997;16:953–961.

449. Mitchell AW, Wells AU, Hansell DM. Changes in cross sectional area of the lungs on end expiratory computed tomography in normal individuals. Clin Radiol 1996;51:804–806.

450. Foster WLJ, Gimenez EI, Roubidoux MA, et al. The emphysemas: radiologic-pathologic correlations. RadioGraphics 1993;13:311–328.

451. Jensen SP, Lynch DA, Brown KK, et al. High-resolution CT features of severe asthma and bronchiolitis obliterans. Clin Radiol 2002;57:1078–1085.

452. Copley SJ, Wells AU, Müller NL, et al. Thin-section CT in obstructive pulmonary disease: discriminatory value. Radiology 2002;223:812–819.

453. Fitzgerald JE, King TE Jr, Lynch DA, et al. Diffuse panbronchiolitis in the United States. Am J Respir Crit Care Med 1996;154:497–503.

454. Koyama H, Geddes DM. Erythromycin and diffuse panbronchiolitis. Thorax 1997;52:915–918.

455. Ichikawa Y, Hotta M, Sumita S, et al. Reversible airway lesions in diffuse panbronchiolitis. Detection by high-resolution computed tomography. Chest 1995;107:120–125.

456. Sugiyama Y. Diffuse panbronchiolitis. Clin Chest Med 1993;14:765–772.

457. Homma H, Yamanaka A, Shinichi T, et al. Diffuse panbronchiolitis: a disease of the transitional zone of the lung. Chest 1983;83:63–69.

458. Akira M, Higashihara S, Sakatani M, et al. Diffuse panbronchiolitis: follow-up CT examination. Radiology 1993;189:559–562.

459. Collins J, Blankenbaker D, Stern EJ. CT patterns of bronchiolar disease: what is "tree-in-bud"? AJR Am J Roentgenol 1998;171:365–370.

460. Murata K, Itoh H, Senda M, et al. Stratified impairment of pulmonary ventilation in "diffuse panbronchiolitis": PET and CT studies. J Comput Assist Tomogr 1989;13:48–53.

461. Aquino SL, Gamsu G, Webb WR, et al. Tree-in-bud pattern: frequency and significance on thin section CT. J Comput Assist Tomogr 1996;20:594–599.

462. Lynch DA, Simone PM, Fox MA, et al. CT features of pulmonary Mycobacterium avium complex infection. J Comput Assist Tomogr 1995;19:353–360.

463. Logan PM, Primack SL, Miller RR, et al. Invasive aspergillosis of the airways: radiographic, CT, and pathologic findings. Radiology 1994;193:383–388.

464. Warren CP, Tse KS, Cherniack RM. Mechanical properties of the lung in extrinsic allergic alveolitis. Thorax 1978;33:315–321.

465. Hansell DM, Wells AU, Padley SPG, et al. Hypersensitivity pneumonitis: correlation of individual CT patterns with functional abnormalities. Radiology 1996;199:123–128.

466. Small JH, Flower CDR, Traill ZC, et al. Air-trapping in extrinsic allergic alveolitis on CT. Clin Radiol 1996;51:684–688.

467. Kaneko K, Sharma OP. Airway obstruction in pulmonary sarcoidosis. Bull Eur Physiopathol Respir 1977;13:231–240.

468. Levinson RS, Metzger LF, Stanley NN, et al. Airway function in sarcoidosis. Am J Med 1977;62:51–59.

469. Gleeson FV, Traill ZC, Hansell DM. Expiratory CT evidence of small airways obstruction in sarcoidosis. AJR Am J Roentgenol 1996;166:1052–1054.

470. Davies CWH, Tasker AD, Padley SPG, et al. Air trapping in sarcoidosis on computed tomography: correlation with lung function. Clin Radiol 2000;55:217–221.

471. Hansell DM, Milne DG, Wilsher ML, et al. Pulmonary sarcoidosis: morphologic associations of airflow obstruction at thin-section CT. Radiology 1998;209:697–704.

472. Yousem SA, Colby TV, Carrington CB. Follicular bronchitis/bronchiolitis. Hum Pathol 1985;16:700–706.

473. Fortoul TI, Cano-Valle F, Oliva E, et al. Follicular bronchiolitis in association with connective tissue diseases. Lung 1985;163:305–314.

474. Oh YW, Effmann EL, Redding GJ, et al. Follicular hyperplasia of bronchus-associated lymphoid tissue causing severe air trapping. AJR Am J Roentgenol 1999;172:745–747.

475. Bramson RT, Cleveland R, Blickman JG, et al. Radiographic appearance of follicular bronchitis in children. AJR Am J Roentgenol 1996;166:1447–1450.

476. Yousem SA, Colby TV, Carrington CB. Lung biopsy in rheumatoid arthritis. Am Rev Respir Dis 1985;131:770–777.

477. Howling SJ, Hansell DM, Wells AU, et al. Follicular bronchiolitis: thin-section CT and histologic findings. Radiology 1999;212:637–642.

478. Niewoehner DE, Kleinerman J, Rice DB. Pathologic changes in the peripheral airways of young cigarette smokers. N Engl J Med 1974;291:775–777.

479. King TE. Respiratory bronchiolitis-associated interstitial lung disease. Clin Chest Med 1993;14:693–698.

480. Fraig M, Shreesha U, Savici D, et al. Respiratory bronchiolitis: a clinicopathologic study in current smokers, ex-smokers, and never-smokers. Am J Surg Pathol 2002; 26:647–653.

481. Holt RM, Schmidt RA, Godwin JD, et al. High resolution CT in respiratory bronchiolitis-associated interstitial lung disease. J Comput Assist Tomogr 1993;17:46–50.

482. Heyneman LE, Ward S, Lynch DA, et al. Respiratory bronchiolitis, respiratory bronchiolitis-associated interstitial lung disease, and desquamative interstitial pneumonia: different entities or part of the spectrum of the same disease process? AJR 1999;173:1617–1622.

483. Park JS, Brown KK, Tuder RM, et al. Respiratory bronchiolitis-associated interstitial lung disease: radiologic features with clinical and pathologic correlation. J Comput Assist Tomogr 2002;26:13–20.

484. Remy-Jardin M, Remy J, Gosselin B, et al. Lung parenchymal changes secondary to cigarette smoking: pathologic-CT correlations. Radiology 1993;186:643–651.

485. Sheerin N, Harrison NK, Sheppard MN, et al. Obliterative bronchiolitis caused by multiple tumourlets and microcarcinoids successfully treated by single lung transplantation. Thorax 1995;50:207–209.

486. Swyer PR, James GCW. A case of unilateral pulmonary emphysema. Thorax 1953;8:133–136.

487. MacLeod WM. Abnormal transradiancy of one lung. Thorax 1954;9:147–153.

488. Reid L, Simon G. Unilateral lung transradiancy. Thorax 1962;17:230–239.

489. Moore ADA, Godwin JD, Dietrich PA, et al. Swyer–James syndrome: CT findings in eight patients. AJR Am J Roentgenol 1992;158:1211–1215.

490. Thurlbeck WM. Pathophysiology of chronic obstructive pulmonary disease. Clin Chest Med 1990;11:389–403.

491. Houk VN, Kent DC, Fosburg RG. Unilateral hyperlucent lung: a study in pathophysiology and etiology. Am J Med Sci 1967;253:406–416.

492. Margolin HN, Rosenberg L, Felson B, et al. Idiopathic unilateral hyperlucent lung: a roentgenologic syndrome. AJR Am J Roentgenol 1959;82:63–75.

493. Stokes D, Sigler A, Khouri NF, et al. Unilateral hyperlucent lung (Swyer–James syndrome) after severe *Mycoplasma pneumoniae* infection. Am Rev Respir Dis 1978;117:145–152.

494. Kogutt MS, Swischuk LE, Goldblum R. Swyer–James syndrome. (Unilateral hyperlucent lung) in children. Am J Dis Child 1973;125:614–618.

495. Saleh M, Miles AI, Lasser RP. Unilateral pulmonary edema in Swyer–James syndrome. Chest 1974;66:594–597.

496. Mont JL, Botey A, Subias R, et al. Unilateral pulmonary hemorrhage in a patient with Goodpasture's and Swyer–James' syndrome. Eur J Respir Dis 1985;67:145–147.

497. White RI, James A, Wagner HN. The significance of unilateral absence of pulmonary artery perfusion by lung scanning. AJR Am J Roentgenol 1971;111:501–509.

498. O'Dell CW, Taylor A, Higgins CB, et al. Ventilation-perfusion lung images in the Swyer–James syndrome. Radiology 1976;121:423–426.

499. Greenspan RH, Sagel S, McMahon J, et al. Timed expiratory chest films in detection of air-trapping. Invest Radiol 1973;8:264–265.

500. Lucaya J, Gartner S, Garcia-Pena P, et al. Spectrum of manifestations of Swyer–James-MacLeod syndrome. J Comput Assist Tomogr 1998;22:592–597.

501. McLoud TC, Bourgouin PM, Greenberg RW, et al. Bronchogenic carcinoma: Analysis of staging in the mediastinum with CT by correlative lymph node mapping and sampling. Radiology 1992;182:319–323.

502. Chitkara RK, Sarinas PS. Recent advances in diagnosis and management of chronic bronchitis and emphysema. Curr Opin Pulm Med 2002;8:126–136.

503. Fletcher CM, Pride NB. Definitions of emphysema, chronic bronchitis, asthma, and airflow obstruction: 25 years on from the Ciba symposium. Thorax 1984;39:81–85.

504. Thurlbeck WM. Chronic airflow obstruction in lung disease. In: Bennington JL, editor. Major problems in pathology. Philadelphia: WB Saunders, 1976.

505. Fabbri LM, Romagnoli M, Corbetta L, et al. Differences in airway inflammation in patients with fixed airflow obstruction due to asthma or COPD. Am J Respir Crit Care Med 2003;167:418–424.

506. O'Brien C, Guest PJ, Hill SL, et al. Physiological and radiological characterisation of patients diagnosed with chronic obstructive pulmonary disease in primary care. Thorax 2000;55:635–642.

507. Flaherty KR, Kazerooni EA, Martinez FJ. Differential diagnosis of chronic airflow obstruction. J Asthma 2000;37:201–223.

508. Rennard S, Decramer M, Calverley PM, et al. Impact of COPD in North America and Europe in 2000: subjects' perspective of Confronting COPD International Survey. Eur Respir J 2002;20:799–805.

509. Rennard SI. Overview of causes of COPD. New understanding of pathogenesis and mechanisms can guide future therapy. Postgrad Med 2002;111:28–34.

510. Scadding JG. Definition of clinical categories of asthma. In: Clark TJH, Godfrey S, eds. Asthma. London: Chapman Hall, 1977:5.

511. Cardell BS. Pathological findings in deaths from asthma. Int Arch Allergy Appl Immunol 1956;9:189–199.

512. Dunnill MS. The pathology of asthma, with special reference to changes in the bronchial mucosa. J Clin Pathol 1960;13:27–33.

513. Glynn AA, Michaels L. Bronchial biopsy in chronic bronchitis and asthma. Thorax 1960;15:142–153.

514. Djukanovic R, Roche WR, Wilson JW, et al. Mucosal inflammation in asthma. Am Rev Respir Dis 1990;142:434–457.

515. Niimi A, Matsumoto H, Amitani R, et al. Airway wall thickness in asthma assessed by computed tomography. Relation to clinical indices. Am J Respir Crit Care Med 2000;162:1518–1523.

516. Hossain S. Quantitative measurement of bronchial muscle in men with asthma. Am Rev Respir Dis 1973;107:99–109.

517. McCarthy D, Milic-Emili J. Closing volume in asymptomatic asthma. Am Rev Respir Dis 1973;107:559–570.

518. Woolcock AJ, Read J. Lung volumes in exacerbations of asthma. Am J Med 1966;41:259–273.

519. Woolcock AJ, Rebuck AS, Cade JF, et al. Lung volume changes in asthma measured concurrently by two methods. Am Rev Respir Dis 1971;104:703–709.

520. Mochizuki T, Nakajima H, Kokubu F, et al. Evaluation of emphysema in patients with reversible airway obstruction using high-resolution CT. Chest 1997;112:1522–1526.

521. Kinsella M, Müller NL, Staples C, et al. Hyperinflation in asthma and emphysema. Assessment by pulmonary function testing and computed tomography. Chest 1988;94:286–289.

522. Blackie SP, al Majed S, Staples CA, et al. Changes in total lung capacity during acute spontaneous asthma. Am Rev Respir Dis 1990;142:79–83.

523. Findley LJ, Sahn SA. The value of chest roentgenograms in acute asthma in adults. Chest 1981;80:535–536.

524. Petheram IS, Kerr IH, Collins JV. Value of chest radiographs in severe acute asthma. Clin Radiol 1981;32:281–282.

525. White CS, Cole RP, Lubetsky HW, et al. Acute asthma. Admission chest radiography in hospitalized adult patients. Chest 1991;100:14–16.

526. Rebuck AS. Radiological aspects of severe asthma. Austr Radiol 1970;14:264–268.

527. Rimondi MR, Zompatori M, Battaglia M, et al. Use of computerized tomography in asthmatic patients. Radiol Med (Torino) 1994;88:758–764.

528. Kondoh Y, Taniguchi H, Yokoyama S, et al. Emphysematous change in chronic asthma in relation to cigarette smoking. Assessment by computed tomography. Chest 1990;97:845–849.

529. Hodson CJ, Trickey SE. Bronchial wall thickening in asthma. Clin Radiol 1960;11:183–191.

530. Paganin F, Trussard V, Senetere E, et al. Chest radiography and high resolution computed tomography of the lungs in asthma. Am Rev Respir Dis 1992;146:1084–1087.

531. Royle H. X-ray appearances in asthma: a study of 200 cases. Br Med J 1952;1:577–580.

532. Blair DN, Coppage L, Shaw C. Medical imaging in asthma. J Thorac Imaging 1986;1:23–35.

533. Genereux GP. Radiology and pulmonary immunopathological disease. In: Steiner RE, ed. Recent advances in radiology and medical imaging. Edinburgh: Churchill Livingstone, 1983:213–240.

534. Lynch DA. Imaging of asthma and allergic bronchopulmonary mycosis. Radiol Clin North Am 1998;36:129–142.

535. Eggleston PA, Ward BH, Pierson WE, et al. Radiographic abnormalities in acute asthma in children. Pediatrics 1974;54:442–449.

536. Brooks LJ, Cloutier MM, Afshani E. Significance of roentgenographic abnormalities in children hospitalized for asthma. Chest 1982;82:315–318.

537. Gillies JD, Reed MH, Simons FE. Radiologic findings in acute childhood asthma. J Can Assoc Radiol 1978;29:28–33.

538. Zieverink SE, Harper AP, Holden RW, et al. Emergency room radiography of asthma: an efficacy study. Radiology 1982;145:27–29.

539. Pickup CM, Nee PA, Randall PE. Radiographic features in 1016 adults admitted to hospital with acute asthma. J Accident Emerg Med 1994;11:234–237.

540. Brashear RE, Meyer SC, Manion MW. Unilateral atelectasis in asthma. Chest 1973;63:847–849.

541. Hopkirk JA, Stark JE. Unilateral pulmonary collapse in asthmatics. Thorax 1978;33:207–210.

542. Burke GJ. Pneumothorax complicating acute asthma. S Afr Med J 1979;55:508–510.

543. Legge DA, Tiede JJ, Peters GA, et al. Death from tension pneumothorax and chlorpromazine cardiorespiratory collapse as separate complications of asthma. Ann Allergy 1969;27:23–29.

544. Karetzky MS. Asthma mortality: an analysis of one years experience, review of the literature and assessment of current modes of therapy. Medicine Balt 1975;54:471–484.

545. Niederman MS, Gambino A, Lichter J, et al. Tension ball valve mucus plug in asthma. Am J Med 1985;79:131–134.

546. Bierman CW. Pneumomediastinum and pneumothorax complicating asthma in children. Am J Dis Child 1967;114:42–50.

547. Sherman S, Skoney JA, Ravikrishnan KP. Routine chest radiographs in exacerbations of chronic obstructive pulmonary disease. Diagnostic value. Arch Intern Med 1989;149:2493–2496.

548. Newman KB, Lynch DA, Newman LS, et al. Quantitative computed tomography detects air trapping due to asthma. Chest 1994;106:105–109.

549. Paganin F, Senetere E, Chanez P, et al. Computed tomography of the lungs in asthma: influence of disease severity and etiology. Am J Respir Crit Care Med 1996;153:110–114.

550. Park CS, Müller NL, Worthy SA, et al. Airway obstruction in asthmatic and healthy individuals: inspiratory and expiratory thin-section CT findings. Radiology 1997;203:361–367.

551. Grenier P, Mourey-Gerosa I, Benali K, et al. Abnormalities of the airways and lung parenchyma in asthmatics: CT observations in 50 patients and inter- and intra-observer variability. Eur Radiol 1996;6:199–206.

552. Biernacki W, Redpath AT, Best JJ, et al. Measurement of CT lung density in patients with chronic asthma. Eur Respir J 1997;10:2455–2459.

553. Awadh N, Müller NL, Park CS, et al. Airway wall thickness in patients with near fatal asthma and control groups: assessment with high resolution computed tomographic scanning. Thorax 1998;53:248–253.

554. Brown RH, Herold CJ, Hirshman CA, et al. In vivo measurements of airway reactivity using high-resolution computed tomography. Am Rev Respir Dis 1991;144:208–212.

555. Brown RH, Herold CJ, Hirshman CA, et al. Individual airway constrictor response heterogeneity to histamine assessed by high-resolution computed tomography. J Appl Physiol 1993;74:2615–2620.

556. Brown RH, Herold C, Zerhouni EA, et al. Spontaneous airways constrict during breath holding studied by high-resolution computed tomography. Chest 1994;106:920–924.

557. Brown RH, Zerhouni EA, Mitzner W. Variability in the size of individual airways over the course of one year. Am J Respir Crit Care Med 1995;151:1159–1164.

558. Amirav I, Kramer SS, Grunstein MM, et al. Assessment of methacholine-induced airway constriction by ultrafast high-resolution computed tomography. J Appl Physiol 1993;75:2239–2250.

559. McNamara AE, Müller NL, Okazawa M, et al. Airway narrowing in excised canine lungs measured by high-resolution computed tomography. J Appl Physiol 1992;73:307–316.

560. Gückel C, Wells AU, Taylor DA, et al. Mechanism of mosaic attenuation of the lungs on computed tomography in induced bronchospasm. J Appl Physiol 1999;86:701–708.

561. Wetzel RC, Herold CJ, Zerhouni EA, et al. Hypoxic bronchodilation. J Appl Physiol 1992;73:1202–1206.

562. Okazawa M, Müller NL, McNamara AE, et al. Human airway narrowing measured using high resolution computed tomography. Am J Respir Crit Care Med 1996;154:1557–1562.

563. Goldin JG, McNitt-Gray MF, Sorenson SM, et al. Airway hyperreactivity: assessment with helical thin-section CT. Radiology 1998;208:321–329.

564. Beigelman-Aubry C, Capderou A, Grenier PA, et al. Mild intermittent asthma: CT assessment of bronchial cross-sectional area and lung attenuation at controlled lung volume. Radiology 2002;223:181–187.

565. Carroll N, Elliot J, Morton A, et al. The structure of large and small airways in nonfatal and fatal asthma. Am Rev Respir Dis 1993;147:405–410.

566. Ketai L, Coutsias C, Williamson S, et al. Thin-section CT evidence of bronchial thickening in children with stable asthma: bronchoconstriction or airway remodeling? Acad Radiol 2001;8:257–264.

567. Gurwitz D, Mindorff C, Levison H. Increased incidence of bronchial reactivity in children with a history of bronchiolitis. J Paediatr 1981;98:551–555.

568. Cukier A, Stelmach R, Kavakama JI, et al. Persistent asthma in adults: comparison of high resolution computed tomography of the lungs after one year of follow-up. Rev Hosp Clin Fac Med Sao Paulo 2001;56:63–68.

569. Little SA, Sproule MW, Cowan MD, et al. High resolution computed tomographic assessment of airway wall thickness in chronic asthma: reproducibility and relationship with lung function and severity. Thorax 2002;57:247–253.

570. Bankier AA, Fleischmann D, Mallek R, et al. Bronchial wall thickness: appropriate window settings for thin-section CT and radiologic-anatomic correlation. Radiology 1996;199:831–836.

571. Harmanci E, Kebapci M, Metintas M, et al. High-resolution computed tomography findings are correlated with disease severity in asthma. Respiration 2002;69:420–426.

572. Lucidarme O, Coche E, Cluzel P, et al. Expiratory CT scans for chronic airway disease: correlation with pulmonary function test results. AJR Am J Roentgenol 1998;170:301–307.

573. Mitsunobu F, Mifune T, Ashida K, et al. Influence of age and disease severity on high resolution CT lung densitometry in asthma. Thorax 2001;56:851–856.

574. Loubeyre P, Paret M, Revel D, et al. Thin-section CT detection of emphysema associated with bronchiectasis and correlation with pulmonary function tests. Chest 1996;109:360–365.

575. Hong KY, Lee JH, Park SW, et al. Evaluation of emphysema in patients with asthma using high-resolution CT. Korean J Intern Med 2002;17:24–30.

576. Laurent F, Latrabe V, Raherison C, et al. Functional significance of air trapping detected in moderate asthma. Eur Radiol 2000;10:1404–1410.

577. Mitsunobu F, Mifune T, Ashida K, et al. Low-attenuation areas of the lungs on high-resolution computed tomography in asthma. J Asthma 2001;38:413–422.

578. Ciba Guest Symposium: terminology, definitions, and classification of chronic pulmonary emphysema and related conditions. Thorax 1959;14:286–299.

579. Mueller RE, Keble DL, Plummer J, et al. The prevalence of chronic bronchitis, chronic airway obstruction, and respiratory symptoms in a Colorado city. Am Rev Respir Dis 1971;103:209–228.

580. Tager IB, Speizer FE. Risk estimates for chronic bronchitis in smokers: a study of male-female differences. Am Rev Respir Dis 1976;113:619–625.

581. Sherrill DL, Lebowitz MD, Burrows B. Epidemiology of chronic obstructive pulmonary disease. Clin Chest Med 1990;11:375–387.

582. Bobadilla A, Guerra S, Sherrill D, et al. How accurate is the self-reported diagnosis of chronic bronchitis? Chest 2002;122:1234–1239.

583. Pallasaho P, Lundback B, Meren M, et al. Prevalence and risk factors for asthma and chronic bronchitis in the capitals Helsinki, Stockholm, and Tallinn. Respir Med 2002;96:759–769.

584. Reid L. Measurement of the bronchial mucous gland layer: a diagnostic yardstick in chronic bronchitis. Thorax 1960;15:132–141.

585. Hayes JA. Distribution of bronchial gland measurements in a Jamaican population. Thorax 1969;24:619–622.

586. Thurlbeck WM, Angus GE. A distribution curve for chronic bronchitis. Thorax 1964;19:436–442.

587. Niewoehner DE. New messages from morphometric studies of chronic obstructive pulmonary disease. Semin Respir Med 1986;8:140–146.

588. Mitchell RS, Ryan SF, Petty TL, et al. The significance of morphologic chronic hyperplastic bronchitis. Am Rev Respir Dis 1966;93:720–729.

589. Esterley JR, Heard BE. Multiple bronchiolar stenoses in a patient with generalized airway obstruction. Thorax 1965;20:309–316.

590. Matsuba K, Thurlbeck WM. Disease of the small airways in chronic bronchitis. Am Rev Respir Dis 1973;107:552–558.

591. Greenberg SD, Boushy SF, Jenkins DE. Chronic bronchitis and emphysema: correlation of pathologic findings. Am Rev Respir Dis 1967;96:918–928.

592. Restrepo GL, Heard BE. Air trapping in chronic bronchitis and emphysema: measurements of the bronchial cartilage. Am Rev Respir Dis 1964;90:395–400.

593. Tandon MK, Campbell AH. Bronchial cartilage in chronic bronchitis. Thorax 1969;24:607–612.

594. Fraser RG, Fraser RS, Renner JW, et al. The roentgenologic diagnosis of chronic bronchitis: a reassessment with emphasis on parahilar bronchi seen end-on. Radiology 1976;120:1–9.

595. Bates DV. The fate of the chronic bronchitic: a report of the ten-year follow-up in the Canadian Department of Veteran's Affairs coordinated study of chronic bronchitis. The J Burns Amberson Lecture of the American Thoracic Society. Am Rev Respir Dis 1973;108:1043–1065.

596. Brinkman GL, Block DL. The prognosis in chronic bronchitis. JAMA 1966;197:1–7.

597. Burrows B, Fletcher CM, Heard BE, et al. The emphysematous and bronchial types of chronic airways obstruction. A clinicopathological study of patients in London and Chicago. Lancet 1966;1:830–835.

598. Sethi S. Infectious etiology of acute exacerbations of chronic bronchitis. Chest 2000;117:380S–385S.

599. Hirschmann JV. Do bacteria cause exacerbations of COPD? Chest 2000;118:193–203.

600. Bates DV, Gordon CA, Paul GI, et al. Chronic bronchitis. Report on the third and fourth stages of the co-ordinated study of chronic bronchitis in the Department of Veterans Affairs, Canada. Med Serv J Can 1966;22:1–59.

601. Simon G. Chronic bronchitis and emphysema: a symposium. III. Pathological findings and radiological changes in chronic bronchitis and emphysema. B. Radiological changes in chronic bronchitis. Br J Radiol 1959;32:292–294.

602. Simon G, Galbraith HJB. Radiology of chronic bronchitis. Lancet 1953;2:850–852.

603. Macklem PT. The pathophysiology of chronic bronchitis and emphysema. Med Clin North Am 1973;57:669–670.

604. Gamsu G, Nadel JA. The roentgenologic manifestations of emphysema and chronic bronchitis. Med Clin North Am 1973;57:719–733.

605. Burki NK, Krumpleman JL. Correlation of pulmonary function with the chest roentgenogram in chronic airway obstruction. Am Rev Respir Dis 1980;121:216–223.

606. Feigin DS, Abraham JL. "Increased pulmonary markings" – a radiologic-pathologic correlation study (abstract). Invest Radiol 1980;15:425.

607. Fraser RS, Müller NL, Colman N, Pare PD, eds. Diagnosis of diseases of the chest, 4th edn. Philadelphia: WB Saunders, 1999.

608. Verschakelen JA, Scheinbaum K, Bogaert J, et al. Expiratory CT in cigarette smokers: correlation between areas of decreased lung attenuation, pulmonary function tests and smoking history. Eur Radiol 1998;8:1391–1399.

609. Gückel C, Hansell DM. Imaging the 'dirty lung' – has high resolution computed tomography cleared the smoke? Clin Radiol 1998;53:717–722.

610. Remy-Jardin M, Edme JL, Boulenguez C, et al. Longitudinal follow-up study of smoker's lung with thin-section CT in correlation with pulmonary function tests. Radiology 2002;222:261–270.

611. Gregg I, Trapnell DH. The bronchographic appearances of early chronic bronchitis. Br J Radiol 1969;42:132–139.

612. Gamsu G, Forbes AR, Ovenfors CO. Bronchographic features of chronic bronchitis in normal men. AJR Am J Roentgenol 1981;136:317–322.

613. Reid L. Chronic bronchitis and emphysema: a symposium III. Pathological findings and radiological changes in chronic bronchitis and emphysema. Pathological finding in chronic bronchitis. Br J Radiol 1959;32:291–292.

614. Reid LM. Correlation of certain bronchographic abnormalities seen in chronic bronchitis with the pathological changes. Thorax 1955;10:199–204.

615. Jefferson K, Rees S. Clinical cardiac radiology, 2nd edn. London: Butterworths, 1980.

616. Snider GL, Kleinerman J, Thurlbeck WM, et al. The definition of emphysema. Report of a National Heart, Lung, and Blood Institute, Division of Lung Diseases workshop. Am Rev Respir Dis 1985;132:182–185.

617. Lang MR, Fiaux GW, Gillooly M, et al. Collagen content of alveolar wall tissue in emphysematous and non-

emphysematous lungs. Thorax 1994;49:319–326.

618. Hansell DM, Nicholson AG. Smoking-related diffuse parenchymal lung disease: HRCT-pathologic correlation. Semin Respir Crit Care Med 2003; 24:377–392.

619. Sobonya RE, Burrows B. The epidemiology of emphysema. Clin Chest Med 1983;4:351–358.

620. Wang Q, Takashima S, Wang JC, et al. Prevalence of emphysema in individuals who underwent screening CT for lung cancer in Nagano prefecture of Japan. Respiration 2001;68:352–356.

621. Clark KD, Wardrobe-Wong N, Elliott JJ, et al. Patterns of lung disease in a "normal" smoking population: are emphysema and airflow obstruction found together? Chest 2001;120:743–747.

622. Reid J, Cockcroft D. Severe centrilobular emphysema in a patient without airflow obstruction. Chest 2002;121:307–308.

623. Gurney JW. Pathophysiology of obstructive airways disease. Radiol Clin North Am 1998;36:15–27.

624. Ekberg-Jansson A, Andersson B, Bake B, et al. Neutrophil-associated activation markers in healthy smokers relates to a fall in DL(CO) and to emphysematous changes on high resolution CT. Respir Med 2001;95:363–373.

625. Ozbay B, Uzun K, Arslan H, et al. Functional and radiological impairment in women highly exposed to indoor biomass fuels. Respirology 2001;6: 255–258.

626. Stern EJ, Frank MS, Schmutz JF, et al. Panlobular pulmonary emphysema caused by i.v. injection of methylphenidate (ritalin): findings on chest radiographs and CT scans. AJR Am J Roentgenol 1994;162:555–560.

627. Ward S, Heyneman LE, Reittner P, et al. Talcosis associated with IV abuse of oral medications: CT findings. AJR Am J Roentgenol 2000;174:789–793.

628. Weisbrod GL, Rahman M, Chamberlain D, et al. Precocious emphysema in intravenous drug abusers. J Thorac Imaging 1993;8:233–240.

629. Cook VJ, Coxson HO, Mason AG, et al. Bullae, bronchiectasis and nutritional emphysema in severe anorexia nervosa. Can Respir J 2001;8:361–365.

630. Diaz PT, King MA, Pacht ER, et al. Increased susceptibility to pulmonary emphysema among HIV-seropositive smokers. Ann Intern Med 2000;132: 369–372.

631. Diaz PT, King MA, Pacht ER, et al. The pathophysiology of pulmonary diffusion impairment in human immunodeficiency virus infection. Am J Respir Crit Care Med 1999;160:272–277.

632. Turner-Stokes L, Turton C, Pope FM, et al. Emphysema and cutis laxa. Thorax 1983;38:790–792.

633. Bolande RP, Tucker AS. Pulmonary emphysema and other cardiorespiratory lesions as part of the Marfan abiotrophy. Pediatrics 1964;33:356–366.

634. Hole BV, Wasserman K. Familial emphysema. Ann Intern Med 1965;63:1009–1017.

635. Bense L, Eklund G, Lewander R. Hereditary pulmonary emphysema. Chest 2002;121:297–300.

636. Snider GL. A perspective on emphysema. Clin Chest Med 1983;4:329–336.

637. Satoh K, Kobayashi T, Misao T, et al. CT assessment of subtypes of pulmonary emphysema in smokers. Chest 2001; 120:725–729.

638. Weder W, Thurnheer R, Stammberger U, et al. Radiologic emphysema morphology is associated with outcome after surgical lung volume reduction. Ann Thorac Surg 1997;64:313–319.

639. Cederlund K, Bergstrand L, Hogberg S, et al. Visual classification of emphysema heterogeneity compared with objective measurements: HRCT vs spiral CT in candidates for lung volume reduction surgery. Eur Radiol 2002;12:1045–1051.

640. Cederlund K, Tylen U, Jorfeldt L, et al. Classification of emphysema in candidates for lung volume reduction surgery: a new objective and surgically oriented model for describing CT severity and heterogeneity. Chest 2002;122:590–596.

641. Dornhorst AC. Respiratory insufficiency, Frederick W Price Memorial Lecture. Lancet 1955;1:1185–1187.

642. Robins AG. Pathophysiology of emphysema. Clin Chest Med 1983;4:413–420.

643. Bowen JH, Woodard BH, Pratt PC. Bronchial collapse in obstructive lung disease. Chest 1981;80:510–513.

644. Fraser RG. The radiologist and obstructive airway disease. AJR Am J Roentgenol 1974;120:737–775.

645. Macklem PT, Fraser RG, Brown WG. Bronchial pressure measurements in emphysema and bronchitis. J Clin Invest 1965;44:897–905.

646. Maisel JC, Silvers GW, George MS, et al. The significance of bronchial atrophy. Am J Pathol 1972;67:371–386.

647. Reich SB, Weinshelbaum A, Yee J. Correlation of radiographic measurements and pulmonary function tests in chronic obstructive pulmonary disease. AJR Am J Roentgenol 1985;144:695–699.

648. Andersen PE Jr, Andersen LH, Jest P. The chest radiograph in chronic obstructive lung disease compared with measurements of single-breath nitrogen washout and spirometry. Clin Radiol 1982;33:51–55.

649. Dull WL, Bohadana AB, Teculescu DB, et al. The standard chest roentgenogram

for determining lung overinflation. Lung 1982;160:311–314.

650. Pratt PC. Conventional chest films can reveal emphysema BUT NOT COPD. Chest 1987;92:8.

651. Pugatch RD. The radiology of emphysema. Clin Chest Med 1983;4:433–442.

652. Simon G, Pride NB, Jones NL, et al. Relation between abnormalities in the chest radiograph and changes in pulmonary function in chronic bronchitis and emphysema. Thorax 1973;28:15–23.

653. Pratt PC. Radiographic appearance of the chest in emphysema. Invest Radiol 1987;22:927–929.

654. Pratt PC. Role of conventional chest radiography in diagnosis and exclusion of emphysema. Am J Med 1987;82: 998–1006.

655. Lennon EA, Simon G. The height of the diaphragm in the chest radiograph of normal adults. Br J Radiol 1965;38: 937–943.

656. Katsura S, Martin CJ. The roentgenologic diagnosis of anatomic emphysema. Am Rev Respir Dis 1967;96:700–706.

657. Nicklaus TM, Stowell DW, Christiansen WR, et al. The accuracy of the roentgenologic diagnosis of chronic pulmonary emphysema. Am Rev Respir Dis 1966;93:889–899.

658. Simon G. Radiology and emphysema. Clin Radiol 1964;15:293–306.

659. Curtis BR, Fisher MS. Posterior inferior junction line and left pleuroesophageal stripe: their association with emphysema. J Thorac Imaging 1998;13:184–187.

660. Sutinen S, Christoforidis AJ, Klugh GA, et al. Roentgenologic criteria for the recognition of nonsymptomatic pulmonary emphysema. Am Rev Respir Dis 1965;91:69–76.

661. Laws JW, Heard BE. Emphysema and the chest film: a retrospective radiological and pathological study. Br J Radiol 1962;35:750–761.

662. Thurlbeck WM, Simon G. Radiographic appearance of the chest in emphysema. AJR Am J Roentgenol 1978;130: 429–440.

663. Reid L, Millard FJC. Correlation between radiological diagnosis and structural lung changes in emphysema. Clin Radiol 1964;15:307–311.

664. Sashidhar K, Gulati M, Gupta D, et al. Emphysema in heavy smokers with normal chest radiography. Detection and quantification by HCRT. Acta Radiol 2002;43:60–65.

665. Sanders C. The radiographic diagnosis of emphysema. Radiol Clin North Am 1991;29:1019–1030.

666. Milne EN, Bass H. Roentgenologic and functional analysis of combined chronic obstructive pulmonary disease and congestive cardiac failure. Invest Radiol 1969;4:129–147.

667. Goddard PR, Nicholson EM, Lazlo G, et al. Computed tomography in pulmonary emphysema. Clin Radiol 1982;33:379–387.

668. Newell JD, Jr. CT of emphysema. Radiol Clin North Am 2002;40:31–42.

669. Bergin CJ, Müller NL, Miller RR. CT in the qualitative assessment of emphysema. J Thorac Imaging 1986;1:94–103.

670. Bergin C, Müller N, Nichols DM, et al. The diagnosis of emphysema. A computed tomographic-pathologic correlation. Am Rev Respir Dis 1986;133:541–546.

671. Foster WL Jr, Pratt PC, Roggli VL, et al. Centrilobular emphysema: CT-pathologic correlation. Radiology 1986;159:27–32.

672. Gevenois PA, Koob MC, Jacobovitz D, et al. Whole lung sections for computed tomographic-pathologic correlations. Modified Gough-Wentworth technique. Invest Radiol 1993;28:242–246.

673. Noma S, Herman PG, Khan A, et al. Sequential morphologic changes of elastase-induced pulmonary emphysema in pig lungs. Evaluation by high-resolution computed tomography. Invest Radiol 1991;26:446–453.

674. Spouge D, Mayo JR, Cardoso W, et al. Panacinar emphysema: CT and pathologic findings. J Comput Assist Tomogr 1993;17:710–713.

675. Webb WR. Radiology of obstructive pulmonary disease. AJR Am J Roentgenol 1997;169:637–647.

676. Takasugi JE, Godwin JD. Radiology of chronic obstructive pulmonary disease. Radiol Clin North Am 1998;36:29–55.

677. Austin JHM, Müller NL, Friedman PJ, et al. Glossary of terms for CT of the lungs: recommendations of the nomenclature committee of the Fleischner Society. Radiology 1996;200:327–331.

678. Hagen G, Kolbenstvedt A. CT measurement of mediastinal anterior junction line in emphysema patients. Acta Radiol 1993;34:194–195.

679. Murata K, Itoh H, Todo G, et al. Centrilobular lesions of the lung: demonstration by high-resolution CT and pathologic correlation. Radiology 1986;161:641–645.

680. Tylen U, Boijsen M, Ekberg-Jansson A, et al. Emphysematous lesions and lung function in healthy smokers 60 years of age. Respir Med 2000;94:38–43.

681. Aubry MC, Wright JL, Myers JL. The pathology of smoking-related lung diseases. Clin Chest Med 2000;21:11–35, vii.

682. Hartman TE, Tazelaar HD, Swensen SJ, et al. Cigarette smoking: CT and pathologic findings of associated pulmonary diseases. RadioGraphics 1997;17:377–390.

683. Miller RR, Müller NL, Vedal S, et al. Limitations of computed tomography in the assessment of emphysema. Am Rev Respir Dis 1989;139:980–983.

684. Zompatori M, Rimondi MR, Gavelli G, et al. Paraseptal emphysema mimicking unilateral lymphangitic carcinomatosis: CT findings. J Comput Assist Tomogr 1993;17:810–812.

685. Uppaluri R, Mitsa T, Sonka M, et al. Quantification of pulmonary emphysema from lung computed tomography images. Am J Respir Crit Care Med 1997;156:248–254.

686. Goldin JG. Quantitative CT of the lung. Radiol Clin North Am 2002;40:145–162.

687. Madani A, Keyzer C, Gevenois PA. Quantitative computed tomography assessment of lung structure and function in pulmonary emphysema. Eur Respir J 2001;18:720–730.

688. Madsen MT, Uppaluri R, Hoffman EA, et al. Pulmonary CT image classification with evolutionary programming. Acad Radiol 1999;6:736–741.

689. Blechschmidt RA, Werthschutzky R, Lorcher U. Automated CT image evaluation of the lung: a morphology-based concept. IEEE Trans Med Imaging 2001;20:434–442.

690. Thurlbeck WM, Müller NL. Emphysema: definition, imaging, and quantification. AJR Am J Roentgenol 1994;163:1017–1025.

691. Kuwano K, Matsuba K, Ikeda T, et al. The diagnosis of mild emphysema. Correlation of computed tomography and pathology scores. Am Rev Respir Dis 1990;141:169–178.

692. Müller NL, Staples CA, Miller RR, et al. "Density mask". An objective method to quantitate emphysema using computed tomography. Chest 1988;94:782–787.

693. Bankier AA, De M, V, Keyzer C, et al. Pulmonary emphysema: subjective visual grading versus objective quantification with macroscopic morphometry and thin-section CT densitometry. Radiology 1999;211:851–858.

694. Müller NL. CT diagnosis of emphysema. It may be accurate, but is it relevant? [editorial, comment]. Chest 1993;103:329–330.

695. Nishimura K, Murata K, Yamagishi M, et al. Comparison of different computed tomography scanning methods for quantifying emphysema. J Thorac Imaging 1998;13:193–198.

696. Mishima M, Itoh H, Sakai H, et al. Optimized scanning conditions of high resolution CT in the follow-up of pulmonary emphysema. J Comput Assist Tomogr 1999;23:380–384.

697. Adams H, Bernard MS, McConnochie K. An appraisal of CT pulmonary density mapping in normal subjects. Clin Radiol 1991;43:238–242.

698. Fromson BH, Denison DM. Quantitative features in the computed tomography of healthy lungs. Thorax 1988;43:120–126.

699. Hayhurst MD, Flenley DC, McLean A, et al. Diagnosis of pulmonary emphysema by computerised tomography. Lancet 1984;2:320–322.

700. Stoel BC, Vrooman HA, Stolk J, et al. Sources of error in lung densitometry with CT. Invest Radiol 1999;34:303–309.

701. Gevenois PA, Scillia P, de MV, et al. The effects of age, sex, lung size, and hyperinflation on CT lung densitometry. AJR Am J Roentgenol 1996;167:1169–1173.

702. Gevenois PA, De Vuyst P, Sy M, et al. Pulmonary emphysema: quantitative CT during expiration. Radiology 1996;199:825–829.

703. Gierada DS, Yusen RD, Pilgram TK, et al. Repeatability of quantitative CT indexes of emphysema in patients evaluated for lung volume reduction surgery. Radiology 2001;220:448–454.

704. Millar AB, Fromson B, Strickland BA, et al. Computed tomography based estimates of regional gas and tissue volume of the lung in supine subjects with chronic airflow limitation or fibrosing alveolitis. Thorax 1986;41:932–939.

705. Archer DC, Coblentz CL, deKemp RA, et al. Automated in vivo quantification of emphysema. Radiology 1993;188:835–838.

706. Gevenois PA, de Maertelaer V, De Vuyst P, et al. Comparison of computed density and macroscopic morphometry in pulmonary emphysema. Am J Respir Crit Care Med 1995;152:653–657.

707. Gevenois PA, De Vuyst P, de Maertelaer V, et al. Comparison of computed density and microscopic morphometry in pulmonary emphysema. Am J Respir Crit Care Med 1996;154:187–192.

708. Sakai N, Mishima M, Nishimura K, et al. An automated method to assess the distribution of low attenuation areas on chest CT scans in chronic pulmonary emphysema patients. Chest 1994;106:1319–1325.

709. Zagers R, Vrooman HA, Aarts NJ, et al. Quantitative analysis of computed tomography scans of the lungs for the diagnosis of pulmonary emphysema. A validation study of a semiautomated contour detection technique. Invest Radiol 1995;30:552–562.

710. Kemerink GJ, Lamers RJ, Thelissen GR, et al. CT densitometry of the lungs: scanner performance. J Comput Assist Tomogr 1996;20:24–33.

711. Kemerink GJ, Kruize HH, Lamers RJ, et al. CT lung densitometry: dependence of CT number histograms on sample volume and consequences for scan protocol comparability. J Comput Assist Tomogr 1997;21:948–954.

712. Zompatori M, Fasano L, Mazzoli M, et al. Spiral CT evaluation of pulmonary

emphysema using a low-dose technique. Radiol Med (Torino) 2002;104:13–24.

713. MacNee W, Gould G, Lamb D. Quantifying emphysema by CT scanning. Clinicopathologic correlates. Ann N Y Acad Sci 1991;624:179–194.

714. Gould GA, MacNee W, McLean A, et al. CT measurements of lung density in life can quantitate distal airspace enlargement – an essential defining feature of human emphysema. Am Rev Respir Dis 1988;137:380–392.

715. Knudson RJ, Standen JR, Kaltenborn WT, et al. Expiratory computed tomography for assessment of suspected pulmonary emphysema. Chest 1991; 99:1357–1366.

716. Arakawa A, Yamashita Y, Nakayama Y, et al. Assessment of lung volumes in pulmonary emphysema using multidetector helical CT: comparison with pulmonary function tests. Comput Med Imaging Graph 2001;25:399–404.

717. Lamers RJ, Thelissen GR, Kessels AG, et al. Chronic obstructive pulmonary disease: evaluation with spirometrically controlled CT lung densitometry. Radiology 1994;193:109–113.

718. Gould GA, Redpath AT, Ryan M, et al. Lung CT density correlates with measurements of airflow limitation and the diffusing capacity. Eur Respir J 1991;4:141–146.

719. Kinsella M, Müller NL, Abboud RT, et al. Quantitation of emphysema by computed tomography using a "density mask" program and correlation with pulmonary function tests. Chest 1990;97:315–321.

720. Sakai F, Gamsu G, Im J, et al. Pulmonary function abnormalities in patients with CT determined emphysema. J Comput Assist Tomogr 1987;11:963–968.

721. Sanders C, Nath PH, Bailey WC. Detection of emphysema with computed tomography. Correlation with pulmonary function tests and chest radiography. Invest Radiol 1988;23: 262–266.

722. Eda S, Kubo K, Fujimoto K, et al. The relations between expiratory chest CT using helical CT and pulmonary function tests in emphysema. Am J Respir Crit Care Med 1997;155:1290–1294.

723. Gurney JW, Jones KK, Robbins RA, et al. Regional distribution of emphysema: correlation of high-resolution CT with pulmonary function tests in unselected smokers. Radiology 1992;183:457–463.

724. Mergo PJ, Williams WF, Gonzalez-Rothi R, et al. Three-dimensional volumetric assessment of abnormally low attenuation of the lung from routine helical CT: inspiratory and expiratory quantification. AJR Am J Roentgenol 1998;170:1355–1360.

725. Crausman RS, Ferguson G, Irvin CG, et al. Quantitative chest computed

tomography as a means of predicting exercise performance in severe emphysema [published erratum appears in Acad Radiol 1995;2:870]. Acad Radiol 1995;2:463–469.

726. Saitoh T, Koba H, Shijubo N, et al. Lobar distribution of emphysema in computed tomographic densitometric analysis. Invest Radiol 2000;35:235–243.

727. Nakano Y, Sakai H, Muro S, et al. Comparison of low attenuation areas on computed tomographic scans between inner and outer segments of the lung in patients with chronic obstructive pulmonary disease: incidence and contribution to lung function. Thorax 1999;54:384–389.

728. Nakano Y, Muro S, Sakai H, et al. Computed tomographic measurements of airway dimensions and emphysema in smokers. Correlation with lung function. Am J Respir Crit Care Med 2000;162:1102–1108.

729. Baldi S, Miniati M, Bellina CR, et al. Relationship between extent of pulmonary emphysema by high-resolution computed tomography and lung elastic recoil in patients with chronic obstructive pulmonary disease. Am J Respir Crit Care Med 2001;164: 585–589.

730. Kauczor HU, Heussel CP, Fischer B, et al. Assessment of lung volumes using helical CT at inspiration and expiration: comparison with pulmonary function tests. AJR Am J Roentgenol 1998;171: 1091–1095.

731. Alderson PO, Line BR. Scintigraphic evaluation of regional pulmonary ventilation. Semin Nucl Med 1980;10:218–242.

732. Chicco P, Magnussen JS, Palmer AW, et al. Threshold of detection of diffuse lung disease. J Nucl Med 1999;40: 85–90.

733. Cunningham DA, Lavender JP. Krypton 81m ventilation scanning in chronic obstructive airways disease. Br J Radiol 1981;54:110–116.

734. Fazio F, Lavender JP, Steiner RE. ^{81m}Kr ventilation and ^{99m}Tc perfusion scans in chest disease: comparison with standard radiographs. AJR Am J Roentgenol 1978;130:421–428.

735. Alderson PO, Secker-Walker RH, Forrest JV. Detection of obstructive pulmonary disease. Relative sensitivity of ventilation-perfusion studies and chest radiography. Radiology 1974;112:643–648.

736. Alderson PO, Lee H, Summer WR, et al. Comparison of Xe-133 washout and single-breath imaging for the detection of ventilation abnormalities. J Nucl Med 1979;20:917–922.

737. Sostman HD, Neumann RD, Gottschalk A, et al. Perfusion of nonventilated lung: failure of hypoxic vasoconstriction? AJR Am J Roentgenol 1983;141:151–156.

738. Chamberlain MJ, Morgan WK, Vinitski S. Factors influencing the regional deposition of inhaled particles in man. Clin Sci (Lond) 1983;64:69–78.

739. Hayes M, Taplin GV. Lung imaging with radioaerosols for the assessment of airway disease. Semin Nucl Med 1980;10:243–251.

740. Lin MS, Goodwin DA. Pulmonary distribution of an inhaled radioaerosol in obstructive pulmonary disease. Radiology 1976;118:645–651.

741. Santolicandro A, Ruschi S, Fornai E, et al. Imaging of ventilation in chronic obstructive pulmonary disease. J Thorac Imaging 1986;1:36–53.

742. Isawa T, Wasserman K, Taplin GV. Lung scintigraphy and pulmonary function studies in obstructive airway disease. Am Rev Respir Dis 1970;102:161–172.

743. Taplin GV, Poe ND, Greenberg A. Lung scanning following radioaerosol inhalation. J Nucl Med 1966;7:77–87.

744. Brudin LH, Rhodes CG, Valind SO, et al. Regional structure-function correlations in chronic obstructive lung disease measured with positron emission tomography. Thorax 1992;47:914–921.

745. Schuster DP. Positron emission tomography: theory and its application to the study of lung disease. Am Rev Respir Dis 1989;139:818–840.

746. Nagao M, Murase K, Yasuhara Y, et al. Quantitative analysis of pulmonary emphysema: three-dimensional fractal analysis of single-photon emission computed tomography images obtained with a carbon particle radioaerosol. AJR Am J Roentgenol 1998;171:1657–1663.

747. Thurnheer R, Engel H, Weder W, et al. Role of lung perfusion scintigraphy in relation to chest computed tomography and pulmonary function in the evaluation of candidates for lung volume reduction surgery. Am J Respir Crit Care Med 1999;159:301–310.

748. Cleverley JR, Desai SR, Wells AU, et al. Evaluation of patients undergoing lung volume reduction surgery: ancillary information available from computed tomography. Clin Radiol 2000;55: 45–50.

749. Sandek K, Bratel T, Lagerstrand L, et al. Relationship between lung function, ventilation-perfusion inequality and extent of emphysema as assessed by high-resolution computed tomography. Respir Med 2002;96:934–943.

750. Todd TR. The preoperative selection of patients for emphysema surgery. Eur J Cardiothorac Surg 1999;16 Suppl 1:S51–S56.

751. Kauczor HU, Hofmann D, Kreitner KF, et al. Normal and abnormal pulmonary ventilation: visualization at hyperpolarized He-3 MR imaging. Radiology 1996;201:564–568.

752. McAdams HP, Hatabu H, Donnelly LF, et al. Novel techniques for MR imaging of pulmonary airspaces. Magn Reson Imaging Clin North Am 2000;8: 205–219.

753. Saam BT, Yablonskiy DA, Kodibagkar VD, et al. MR imaging of diffusion of (3)He gas in healthy and diseased lungs. Magn Reson Med 2000;44:174–179.

754. Gierada DS, Saam B, Yablonskiy D, et al. Dynamic echo planar MR imaging of lung ventilation with hyperpolarized (3)He in normal subjects and patients with severe emphysema. NMR Biomed 2000;13:176–181.

755. Kauczor HU, Chen XJ, van Beek EJ, et al. Pulmonary ventilation imaged by magnetic resonance: at the doorstep of clinical application. Eur Respir J 2001;17:1008–1023.

756. Salerno M, de Lange EE, Altes TA, et al. Emphysema: hyperpolarized helium 3 diffusion MR imaging of the lungs compared with spirometric indexes – initial experience. Radiology 2002; 222:252–260.

757. Edelman RR, Hatabu H, Tadamura E, et al. Noninvasive assessment of regional ventilation in the human lung using oxygen-enhanced magnetic resonance imaging. Nature Med 1996;2:1236–1239.

758. Müller CJ, Schwaiblmair M, Scheidler J, et al. Pulmonary diffusing capacity: assessment with oxygen-enhanced lung MR imaging – preliminary findings. Radiology 2002;222:499–506.

759. Mai VM, Bankier AA, Prasad PV, et al. MR ventilation-perfusion imaging of human lung using oxygen-enhanced and arterial spin labeling techniques. J Magn Reson Imaging 2001;14:574–579.

760. Ohno Y, Hatabu H, Takenaka D, et al. Oxygen-enhanced MR ventilation imaging of the lung: preliminary clinical experience in 25 subjects. AJR Am J Roentgenol 2001;177:185–194.

761. Amundsen T, Torheim G, Waage A, et al. Perfusion magnetic resonance imaging of the lung: characterization of pneumonia and chronic obstructive pulmonary disease. A feasibility study. J Magn Reson Imaging 2000;12:224–231.

762. Johkoh T, Müller NL, Kavanagh PV, et al. Scintigraphic and MR perfusion imaging in preoperative evaluation for lung volume reduction surgery: pilot study results. Radiat Med 2000;18:277–281.

763. Laurell CB, Erickson S. The electrophoretic α_1 globulin pattern of serum in α_1-antitrypsin deficiency. Scand J Clin Invest 1963;15:132–140.

764. Sharp HL, Bridges RA, Krivit W, et al. Cirrhosis associated with alpha-1-antitrypsin deficiency: a previously unrecognized inherited disorder. J Lab Clin Med 1969;73:934–939.

765. Pushpakom R, Hogg JC, Woolcock AJ, et al. Experimental papain-induced emphysema in dogs. Am Rev Respir Dis 1970;102:778–789.

766. Idell S, Cohen AB. Alpha-1-antitrypsin deficiency. Clin Chest Med 1983;4: 359–375.

767. Abboud RT, Ofulue AF, Sansores RH, et al. Relationship of alveolar macrophage plasminogen activator and elastase activities to lung function and CT evidence of emphysema. Chest 1998;113:1257–1263.

768. Parmar JS, Mahadeva R, Reed BJ, et al. Polymers of alpha(1)-antitrypsin are chemotactic for human neutrophils: a new paradigm for the pathogenesis of emphysema. Am J Respir Cell Mol Biol 2002;26:723–730.

769. Greenberg SD, Jenkins DE, Stevens PM, et al. The lungs in homozygous alpha1 antitrypsin deficiency. Am J Clin Pathol 1973;60:581–592.

770. dAlmaine SP, Reid CB, Thompson WD. Widespread panacinar emphysema with alpha-1-antitrypsin deficiency. Br J Dis Chest 1980;74:289–295.

771. Erickson S. Pulmonary emphysema and alpha-1-antitrypsin deficiency Acta Med Scand 1964;175:197–205.

772. Larsson C. Natural history and life expectancy in severe alpha 1-antitrypsin deficiency, Pi Z. Acta Med Scand 1978;204:345–351.

773. Erickson S. Studies in α-1-antitrypsin deficiency. Acta Med Scand 1965;432 Suppl:5–85.

774. Kueppers F, Black LF. Alpha1-antitrypsin and its deficiency. Am Rev Respir Dis 1974;110:176–194.

775. Gishen P, Saunders AJS, Tobins MJ, et al. Alpha-antitrypsin deficiency: The radiological features of pulmonary emphysema in subjects of Pi Type Z and Pi Type SZ: a survey by the British thoracic association. Clin Radiol 1982;33:371–377.

776. Hepper NG, Muhm JR, Sheehan WC, et al. Roentgenographic study of chronic obstructive pulmonary disease by alpha1-antitrypsin phenotype. Mayo Clin Proc 1978;53:166–172.

777. Rosen RA, Dalinka MK, Gralino BJ Jr, et al. The roentgenographic findings in alpha-1 antitrypsin deficiency (AAD). Radiology 1970;95:25–28.

778. Dowson LJ, Guest PJ, Hill SL, et al. High-resolution computed tomography scanning in alpha1-antitrypsin deficiency: relationship to lung function and health status. Eur Respir J 2001;17:1097–1104.

779. Dirksen A, Friis M, Olesen KP, et al. Progress of emphysema in severe alpha 1-antitrypsin deficiency as assessed by annual CT. Acta Radiol 1997;38:826–832.

780. Dowson LJ, Guest PJ, Stockley RA. Longitudinal changes in physiological, radiological, and health status measurements in alpha(1)-antitrypsin deficiency and factors associated with decline. Am J Respir Crit Care Med 2001;164:1805–1809.

781. Stolk J, Dirksen A, van der Lugt AA, et al. Repeatability of lung density measurements with low-dose computed tomography in subjects with alpha-1-antitrypsin deficiency-associated emphysema. Invest Radiol 2001;36: 648–651.

782. Lieberman J, Colp C. A role for intermediate, heterozygous alpha 1-antitrypsin deficiency in obstructive lung disease. Chest 1990;98:522–523.

783. Cooper JD, Patterson GA. Lung volume reduction surgery for severe emphysema. Semin Thorac Cardiovasc Surg 1996;8:52–60.

784. Takasugi JE, Wood DE, Godwin JD, et al. Lung-volume reduction surgery for diffuse emphysema: radiologic assessment of changes in thoracic dimensions. J Thorac Imaging 1998;13:36–41.

785. Sciurba FJ, Rogers RM, Keenan RJ, et al. Improvement in pulmonary function and elastic recoil after lung-reduction surgery for diffuse emphysema. N Engl J Med 1996;334:1095–1099.

786. Martinez FJ, Montes de Oca M, Whyte RI, et al. Lung-volume reduction improves dyspnea, dynamic hyperinflation and respiratory muscle function. Am J Respir Crit Care Med 1997;155:1984–1990.

787. Quint LE, Bland PH, Walker JM, et al. Diaphragmatic shape change after lung volume reduction surgery. J Thorac Imaging 2001;16:149–155.

788. Lando Y, Boiselle P, Shade D, et al. Effect of lung volume reduction surgery on bony thorax configuration in severe COPD. Chest 1999;116:30–39.

789. Cassart M, Hamacher J, Verbandt Y, et al. Effects of lung volume reduction surgery for emphysema on diaphragm dimensions and configuration. Am J Respir Crit Care Med 2001;163:1171–1175.

790. Gierada DS, Hakimian S, Slone RM, et al. MR analysis of lung volume and thoracic dimensions in patients with emphysema before and after lung volume reduction surgery. AJR Am J Roentgenol 1998;170: 707–714.

791. Cooper JD, Patterson GA, Sundaresan RS, et al. Results of 150 consecutive bilateral lung volume reduction procedures in patients with severe emphysema. J Thorac Cardiovasc Surg 1996;112:1319–1329.

792. Flaherty KR, Kazerooni EA, Curtis JL, et al. Short-term and long-term outcomes after bilateral lung volume reduction surgery : prediction by quantitative CT. Chest 2001;119:1337–1346.

793. Yusen RD, Lefrak SS. Evaluation of patients with emphysema for lung volume reduction surgery. Washington University Emphysema Surgery Group. Semin Thorac Cardiovasc Surg 1996;8:83–93.

794. Kazerooni EA. Radiologic evaluation of emphysema for lung volume reduction surgery. Clin Chest Med 1999;20:845–861.

795. Sciurba FC. Preoperative predictors of outcome following lung volume reduction surgery. Thorax 2002;57 Suppl 2:II47–II52.

796. Slone RM, Gierada DS, Yusen RD. Preoperative and postoperative imaging in the surgical management of pulmonary emphysema. Radiol Clin North Am 1998;36:57–89.

797. Hunsaker A, Ingenito E, Topal U, et al. Preoperative screening for lung volume reduction surgery: usefulness of combining thin-section CT with physiologic assessment. AJR Am J Roentgenol 1998;170:309–314.

798. Gierada DS, Yusen RD, Villanueva IA, et al. Patient selection for lung volume reduction surgery: An objective model based on prior clinical decisions and quantitative CT analysis. Chest 2000;117:991–998.

799. Hunsaker AR, Ingenito EP, Reilly JJ, et al. Lung volume reduction surgery for emphysema: correlation of CT and V/Q imaging with physiologic mechanisms of improvement in lung function. Radiology 2002;222:491–498.

800. Slone RM, Pilgram TK, Gierada DS, et al. Lung volume reduction surgery: comparison of preoperative radiologic features and clinical outcome. Radiology 1997;204:685–693.

801. Wang SC, Fischer KC, Slone RM, et al. Perfusion scintigraphy in the evaluation for lung volume reduction surgery: correlation with clinical outcome. Radiology 1997;205:243–248.

802. Gierada DS, Slone RM, Bae KT, et al. Pulmonary emphysema: comparison of preoperative quantitative CT and physiologic index values with clinical outcome after lung-volume reduction surgery. Radiology 1997;205:235–242.

803. McKenna RJJ, Fischel RJ, Brenner M, et al. Combined operations for lung volume reduction surgery and lung cancer. Chest 1996;110:885–888.

804. Slone RM, Gierada DS, Fischer KC, et al. Preoperative radiologic findings in patients with an unfavorable outcome after lung volume reduction surgery. AJR Am J Roentgenol 1996;166:74–75.

805. Wisser W, Klepetko W, Kontrus M, et al. Morphologic grading of the emphysematous lung and its relation to improvement after lung volume reduction surgery. Ann Thorac Surg 1998;65:793–799.

806. McKenna R, Brenner M, Fischel R, et al. Should lung volume reduction surgery for emphysema be unilateral or bilateral? J Thorac Cardiovasc Surg 1996;112:1331–1339.

807. Nakano Y, Coxson HO, Bosan S, et al. Core to rind distribution of severe emphysema predicts outcome of lung volume reduction surgery. Am J Respir Crit Care Med 2001;164:2195–2199.

808. Rogers RM, Coxson HO, Sciurba FC, et al. Preoperative severity of emphysema predictive of improvement after lung volume reduction surgery: use of CT morphometry. Chest 2000;118:1240–1247.

809. Gierada DS, Slone RM, Cooper JD, et al. Dynamic MR imaging to analyse respiratory mechanics in patients having lung volume reduction surgery. AJR Am J Roentgenol 1996;166:210.

810. Jamadar DA, Kazerooni EA, Martinez FJ, et al. Semi-quantitative ventilation/perfusion scintigraphy and single-photon emission tomography for evaluation of lung volume reduction surgery candidates: description and prediction of clinical outcome. Eur J Nuc Med 1999;26:734–742.

811. Gevenois PA, Estenne M. Can computed tomography predict functional benefit from lung volume reduction surgery for emphysema? Am J Respir Crit Care Med 2001;164:2137–2138.

812. Hunsaker A, Ingenito E, Topal U, et al. Preoperative screening for lung volume reduction surgery: usefulness of combining thin-section CT with physiologic assessment. AJR Am J Roentgenol 1998;170:309–314.

813. Gelb AF, Zamel N, Hogg JC, et al. Pseudophysiologic emphysema resulting from severe small-airways disease. Am J Respir Crit Care Med 1998;158:815–819.

814. Toma TP, Hopkinson NS, Hillier J, et al. Bronchoscopic volume reduction with valve implants in patients with severe emphysema. Lancet 2003;361:931–933.

815. Hazelrigg SR, Boley TM, Weber D, et al. Incidence of lung nodules found in patients undergoing lung volume reduction. Ann Thorac Surg 1997;64:303–306.

816. Rozenshtein A, White CS, Austin JH, et al. Incidental lung carcinoma detected at CT in patients selected for lung volume reduction surgery to treat severe pulmonary emphysema. Radiology 1998;207:487–490.

817. Gierada DS, Glazer HS, Slone RM. Pseudomass due to atelectasis in patients with severe bullous emphysema. AJR Am J Roentgenol 1997;168:85–92.

818. Reid L. The pathology of emphysema. London: Lloyd-Luke Ltd, 1967.

819. Gibson GJ. Familial pneumothoraces and bullae. Thorax 1977;32:88–90.

820. Kinnear WJM, Tattersfield AE. Emphysematous bullae: surgery is best for large bullae and moderately impaired lung function. Br Med J 1990;300:208–209.

821. Bateman ED, Westerman DE, Hewitson RP, et al. Pneumonectomy for massive

ventilated lung cysts. Thorax 1981;36:554–556.

822. Morgan MD, Edwards CW, Morris J, et al. Origin and behaviour of emphysematous bullae. Thorax 1989;44:533–538.

823. Ting EY, Klopstock R, Lyons HA. Mechanical properties of pulmonary cysts and bullae. Am Rev Respir Dis 1963;87:538–544.

824. Boushy SF, Kohen R, Billig DM, et al. Bullous emphysema: clinical, roentgenologic and physiologic study of 49 patients. Dis Chest 1968;54:327–334.

825. Fiore D, Biondetti PR, Sartori F, et al. The role of computed tomography in the evaluation of bullous lung disease. J Comput Assist Tomogr 1982;6:105–108.

826. Morgan MD, Strickland B. Computed tomography in the assessment of bullous lung disease. Br J Dis Chest 1984;78:10–25.

827. Putman CE, Godwin JD, Silverman PM, et al. CT of localized lucent lung lesions. Semin Roentgenol 1984;19:173–188.

828. Waitches GM, Stern EJ, Dubinsky TJ. Usefulness of the double-wall sign in detecting pneumothorax in patients with giant bullous emphysema. AJR Am J Roentgenol 2000;174:1765–1768.

829. Morgan MD, Denison DM, Strickland B. Value of computed tomography for selecting patients with bullous lung disease for surgery. Thorax 1986;41:855–862.

830. Stern EJ, Webb WR, Weinacker A, et al. Idiopathic giant bullous emphysema (vanishing lung syndrome): imaging findings in nine patients. AJR Am J Roentgenol 1994;162:279–282.

831. Johnson MK, Smith RP, Morrison D, et al. Large lung bullae in marijuana smokers. Thorax 2000;55:340–342.

832. Douglas AC, Grant IWB. Spontaneous closure of large pulmonary bullae: a report on three cases. Br J Tubercle 1957;51:335–338.

833. Satoh H, Suyama T, Yamashita YT, et al. Spontaneous regression of multiple emphysematous bullae. Can Respir J 1999;6:458–460.

834. Stone DJ, Schwartz A, Feitman JA. Bullous emphysema: a long-term study of the natural history and the effects of therapy. Am Rev Respir Dis 1960;82:493–507.

835. Smit HJ, Wienk MA, Schreurs AJ, et al. Do bullae indicate a predisposition to recurrent pneumothorax? Br J Radiol 2000;73:356–359.

836. Mahler DA, D'Esopo ND. Peri-emphysematous lung infection. Clin Chest Med 1981;2:51–57.

837. Bersack SR. Fluid collection in emphysematous bullae. AJR Am J Roentgenol 1960;83:283–292.

838. Jay SJ, Johanson WG, Jr. Massive intrapulmonary hemorrhage: an uncommon complication of bullous

emphysema. Am Rev Respir Dis 1974;110:497–501.

839. McCluskie RA. Unusual fate of emphysematous bullae. Thorax 1981;36:77.

840. Tsutsui M, Araki Y, Shirakusa T, et al. Characteristic radiographic features of pulmonary carcinoma associated with large bulla. Ann Thorac Surg 1988;46: 679–683.

841. Richardson MS, Reddy VD, Read CA. New air–fluid levels in bullous lung disease: a reevaluation. J Nat Med Assoc 1996;88:185–187.

842. Prichard MG, Brown PJ, Sterrett GF. Bronchioloalveolar carcinoma arising in longstanding lung cysts. Thorax 1984; 39:545–549.

843. Venuta F, Rendina EA, Pescarmona EA, et al. Occult lung cancer in patients with bullous emphysema. Thorax 1997;52:289–290.

844. Gaensler EA, Jederlinic PJ, Fitzgerald MX. Patient work-up for bullectomy. J Thorac Imaging 1986;1:75–93.

845. De Giacomo T, Rendina EA, Venuta F, et al. Bullectomy is comparable to lung volume reduction in patients with end-stage emphysema. Eur J Cardiothorac Surg 2002;22:357–362.

CHAPTER 13

Neoplasms of the lungs, airways, and pleura

BRONCHIAL CARCINOMA

The American Cancer Society estimates that 171,900 new cases of lung cancer and 157,200 deaths from lung cancer will have occurred in 2002 in the US: 88,400 of the deaths will have been in men and 68,800 in women.[1]

Pathology

The most widely accepted histologic classification of bronchial carcinoma is that of the World Health Organization (WHO).[2–4] The common types are (see Box 13.1):

1. *Epidermoid (squamous cell) carcinoma*, which accounts for 30–35% of cases. Its relative incidence appears to be falling, probably because the prevalence of smoking is falling.[5] Squamous cell carcinomas are subdivided into well, moderately, and poorly differentiated varieties.
2. *Adenocarcinoma*, which accounts for up to 35% of cases. Its relative incidence is rising, and it now appears to be the predominant form of lung cancer in the US.[6] Bronchioloalveolar carcinoma (alveolar cell carcinoma) is included under adenocarcinoma. Its relative incidence appears to be rising dramatically as smoking declines and it may now comprise 10–20% of all lung cancers.[5] Adenocarcinomas, like epidermoid tumors, are subdivided into well, moderately, and poorly differentiated varieties. A small proportion of adenocarcinomas show neuroendocrine features, which confer greater aggressiveness to the tumor.[7]
3. *Large cell carcinoma (including the giant cell variety)*, which accounts for 10–15% of cases. These tumors may have some areas of differentiation into squamous or adenocarcinoma. They may show neuroendocrine differentiation, in which case the prognosis is comparable to small cell carcinoma.[8–10]
4. *Small (formerly oat) cell carcinoma*, which accounts for 20–30% of cases. Small cell lung carcinomas grow rapidly and metastasize early. They contain neurosecretory granules and are part of a spectrum of neuroendocrine tumors[11]: the other tumors in the spectrum are typical and atypical carcinoid tumors, carcinoid tumorlets, and large cell neuroendocrine carcinoma.[9,12]

The histologic distinction among the nonsmall cell carcinomas is not always clear-cut: pathologists may differ in their interpretations, and different portions of the same tumor may warrant different classifications. Mixed tumors with features of both adenocarcinoma and epidermoid carcinoma may be classified separately as adenosquamous cancers.[13–15] A very small proportion of tumors are mixed small cell and squamous cell or adenocarcinomas.[16]

Mucoepidermoid carcinomas[17] are usually classified along with other carcinomas that have analogous histology to salivary gland tumors, namely adenoid cystic carcinoma and the very rare acinic cell carcinoma.[18–20]

Primary carcinoma of the lung is usually solitary, but synchronous multiple primary tumors are not uncommon; the precise incidence depends on how carefully further primary tumors are sought, and the rigidity of the criteria used to define whether or not two tumors in the lung are both regarded as primary lesions.[21–27] Difference in cell type is an accepted criterion for synchronous primary neoplasms, but tumors of the same histologic type can be accepted as synchronous provided they are

---

Box 13.1 WHO classification of preinvasive and malignant lung tumors[2]

Preinvasive lesions
Squamous dysplasia
  • Carcinoma in situ
Atypical adenomatous hyperplasia
Diffuse idiopathic pulmonary neuroendocrine cell
  hyperplasia

Malignant
Squamous cell carcinoma
  Variants
  • Papillary
  • Clear cell
  • Small cell
  • Basaloid
Small cell carcinoma
  Variant
  • Combined small cell carcinoma
Adenocarcinoma
  • Acinar
  • Papillary
  • Bronchioloalveolar carcinoma
    — Nonmucinous
    — Mucinous
    — Mixed mucinous and nonmucinous or
      indeterminate cell type
  • Solid adenocarcinoma with mucin
  • Adenocarcinoma with mixed subtypes
    Variants
    — Well-differentiated fetal adenocarcinoma
    — Mucinous ("colloid") adenocarcinoma
    — Mucinous cystadenocarcinoma
    — Signet ring adenocarcinoma
    — Clear cell adenocarcinoma
Large cell carcinoma
  Variants
  • Large cell neuroendocrine carcinoma
    — Combined large cell neuroendocrine carcinoma
  • Basaloid carcinoma
  • Lymphoepithelioma-like carcinoma
  • Clear cell carcinoma
  • Large cell carcinoma with rhabdoid phenotype
Adenosquamous carcinoma
Carcinomas with pleomorphic, sarcomatoid or sarcomatous
  elements
  • Carcinomas with spindle and/or giant cells
    — Pleomorphic carcinoma
    — Spindle cell carcinoma
    — Giant cell carcinoma
  • Carcinosarcoma
  • Pulmonary blastoma
Carcinoid tumor
  • Typical carcinoid
  • Atypical carcinoma
Carcinomas of salivary gland type
  • Mucoepidermoid carcinoma
  • Adenoid cystic carcinoma
  • Others
Unclassified carcinoma

of similar size and physically quite separate. Metachronous lesions are generally regarded as multiple primary lesions only if they show unique histologic features.[28]

Smoking and asbestos exposure are well recognized etiologic factors for lung cancer.[29] A discussion of the epidemiologic and causative factors of lung cancer are beyond the scope of this book, but several reviews suitable for radiologists have been published.[30–32] Three predisposing factors may provide visible radiologic evidence of their presence: evidence of asbestos exposure, interstitial pulmonary fibrosis of many different etiologies, including asbestosis, and lipoid pneumonia.[13,33] In one series, lung cancer was found in 32 of 244 patients with idiopathic pulmonary fibrosis. The carcinomas were often ill-defined lesions mimicking airspace consolidation, corresponding to the location of the most advanced fibrosis.[34] Heart or lung transplantation may also predispose to lung cancer, the resulting tumors showing standard radiographic features.[35,36] It is no longer accepted that lung cancers in general arise from old tuberculous scars. In most so-called focal "scar carcinomas", the fibrous tissue is probably a desmoplastic response to the cancer; i.e. the scar follows, rather than precedes, the development of carcinoma.[37–39] However, the prevalence of bronchioloalveolar carcinoma within preexisting lung scars is striking.[40]

The presence of one lung cancer appears to predispose to the subsequent development of further primary tumors.[41]

Clinical features

Approximately 15–25% of patients with bronchial carcinoma are asymptomatic at the time of diagnosis.[42,43] The symptoms vary with extent of disease.[44] Cough, dyspnea, occasionally associated with wheeze, mild hemoptysis, recurrent pneumonia, and paraneoplastic syndromes (Table 13.1) are the cardinal symptoms of the disease at a stage when the carcinoma is still confined to the lung and major bronchi. Hoarseness, chest wall pain, brachial plexus neuropathy, Horner syndrome, phrenic nerve paresis, superior vena cava obstruction, dysphagia, and the symptoms due to pleural effusion or pericardial tamponade indicate invasion of the mediastinum, pleura, pericardium, or chest wall.[45] Peripheral tumors are clinically silent for a longer period and are more likely to be discovered incidentally on routine chest radiography.

The clinical symptoms and signs vary with cell type.[42] Squamous cell carcinoma is a relatively slow growing, late metastasizing tumor that most often arises centrally within the bronchial tree and, therefore, usually manifests as obstructive atelectasis or pneumonia, hemoptysis, or the signs and symptoms of invasion of adjacent structures, such as recurrent laryngeal nerve paralysis. When squamous cell cancers arise peripherally in the lung, they may grow to a substantial size before symptoms develop.

Adenocarcinoma most often arises as a peripheral pulmonary nodule and is frequently first discovered on a chest radiograph or CT in a patient with no chest symptoms. Nevertheless, hilar and mediastinal node involvement and distant metastases, particularly to the brain and adrenal glands, are frequently present at or soon after presentation. Dyspnea resulting from pleural effusion is a particular feature of adenocarcinoma. Bronchioloalveolar carcinoma when it presents as a solitary pulmonary nodule or mass, unlike other bronchial adenocarcinomas, is often an indolent tumor that metastasizes late.

Table 13.1 Classification of extrapulmonary manifestations of carcinoma of the lung. (Modified from references[42,44].)

Endocrine and metabolic	Cushing syndrome
	Inappropriate secretion of antidiuretic hormone
	Carcinoid syndrome
	Hypercalcemia and ectopic parathyroid hormone secretion
	Hypercalcitonemia
	Ectopic gonadotropin, gynecomastia
	Male gonadal dysfunction
	Hypoglycemia
	Acromegaly
	Hyperthyroidism
	Cachexia of malignancy
	Lactic acidosis
	Hypouricemia
Neurologic and neuromuscular	Eaton–Lambert syndrome
	Polymyositis
	Mononeuritis multiplex
	Subacute cerebellar degeneration
	Encephalomyelopathy
	Retinopathy
Skeletal	Clubbing
	Pulmonary hypertrophic osteoarthropathy
	Osteomalacia
Renal	Glomerulonephritis
	Nephrotic syndrome
Dermatologic	Acanthosis nigricans
	Scleroderma
	Hypertrichosis lanuginosa
	Erythema gyratum repens
	Erythema multiforme
	Tylosis
	Exfoliative dermatitis
	Sweet syndrome
	Other dermatoses
	Urticaria
	Pruritis
Vascular	Migratory thrombophlebitis
	Disseminated intravascular coagulation
	Arterial thrombosis
	Nonbacterial verrucous endocarditis
Hematologic	Anemia
	Red cell aplasia
	Thrombocytopenic/ fibrinolytic purpura
	Nonspecific leukocytosis
	Thrombocytosis
	Polycythemia
	Eosinophilia
	Leukoerythroblastic reaction
Systemic	Anorexia
	Cachexia
	Fever

Large cell anaplastic carcinoma is similar to epidermoid carcinoma in that the tumor may grow to a large size, but dissimilar in that it metastasizes early, particularly to the mediastinum and brain.[46]

Small cell carcinoma also metastasizes early and widely; metastases are usually present at initial diagnosis. Hormone production, notably adrenocorticotrophic hormone, antidiuretic hormone, and melanocyte stimulating hormone, is a feature of small cell tumors.

Imaging features

The imaging appearances of lung cancer are considered in the following framework: (1) peripheral tumors (tumors arising beyond the hilum/segmental bronchi); and (2) central tumors (tumors arising at or close to the hilum/segmental bronchi).

Peripheral tumors (see Box 13.2)

Approximately 40% of bronchial carcinomas arise beyond the segmental bronchi,[5] and in 30% a peripheral mass is the sole radiographic finding.[47–52] The fact that peripheral tumors tend to grow predominantly in the direction of the hilum may explain the variable proportions of peripheral versus central tumors reported in large surveys and the unexpectedly high number of "peripheral" masses visible at bronchoscopy. The mass can be virtually any size, but it is rare for a bronchial carcinoma to be seen on plain chest radiographs unless it is >1 cm in diameter.[53,54] CT, because of its better contrast resolution, detects much smaller lesions (see section Screening for lung cancer using low dose CT later in this chapter).

Shape

In general, peripheral bronchial carcinomas assume an approximately spherical or oval configuration. The major exceptions are tumors at the lung apex (Pancoast tumors, superior sulcus tumors), which may resemble apical pleural thickening, certain

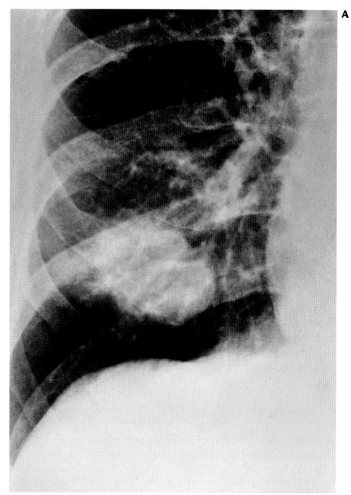

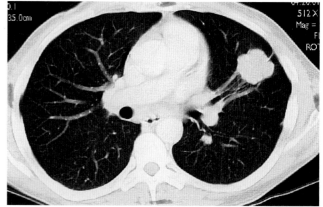

Fig. 13.1 **A** and **B**, Squamous cell bronchial carcinoma occurring as a solitary lobular shaped peripheral mass in two different patients. A pleural tail sign is present in **B**.

> **Box 13.2 Imaging features of peripheral bronchial carcinomas**
>
> Approximately 40% of bronchial carcinomas arise beyond segmental bronchi
>
> Rarely visible on plain chest radiographs when below 1 cm in diameter
>
> Usual shapes are spherical or oval
>
> Edge is usually lobular or irregular, but may, rarely, be ill-defined enough to resemble pneumonia
>
> A "corona radiata" is nearly specific for bronchial carcinoma
>
> May present as mucocele (mucoid impaction, bronchocele)
>
> Cavitation is seen in 16% of cases on plain chest radiographs and more frequently on CT
>
> Air bronchograms and bubble-like lucencies are rarely visible on plain chest radiographs, though they are seen in 25% of cases on HRCT
>
> Visible calcification is virtually never identified on plain chest radiograph but is seen in a small proportion of cases on CT
>
> Volume doubling times are very rarely <1 month or >18 months

---

bronchioloalveolar carcinomas, and carcinomas arising in areas of interstitial fibrosis. Bronchogenic carcinoma is, therefore, one of the major diagnostic considerations in adults with a solitary pulmonary nodule (see Ch. 3, p. 107).

Lobulation, a sign that indicates uneven growth rates for differing portions of the tumor, is common (Fig. 13.1).[52] An equally frequent sign is a notch (umbilication), a sign that is the counterpart of lobulation because it indicates relatively slow growth of a particular portion of the tumor.[55] Occasionally, a

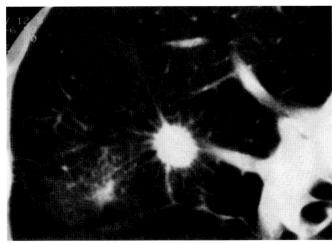

Fig. 13.2 CT of bronchial carcinoma showing irregular infiltrating edge ("corona radiata").

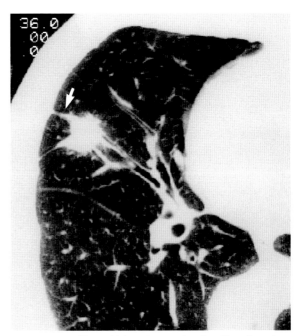

Fig. 13.3 HRCT of bronchial carcinoma showing distortion of adjacent vessels and a "pleural tail" sign (arrow).

dumbbell shape is encountered or two nodules are seen next to each other.

Sometimes the edge of the tumor is irregular, with one or more strands radiating into the surrounding lung, an appearance often described as spiculated (Fig. 13.2). The term "corona radiata"[56] indicates multiple strands extending into the surrounding lung because of either tumor extension or a fibrotic response to the tumor. Such stranding is best seen on CT, particularly thin-section CT (Figs 13.2 and 13.3).[57] Coarse spiculation has been shown, in adenocarcinoma at least, to confer a worse prognosis than a smooth or lobulated outline.[58] A well-developed corona radiata is a useful sign in the differential diagnosis of a solitary pulmonary nodule because it makes the diagnosis of bronchogenic carcinoma highly likely. It is not, however, entirely specific: similar very irregular margins are encountered in a variety of lesions, including benign processes, notably chronic pneumonia and granuloma.

A single linear or bandlike shadow may connect the lesion to the pleura (Figs 13.1 and 13.3). This so-called "pleural tail sign", as discussed on page 117, is seen with both benign and malignant pulmonary nodules.

Careful observation of the pattern of vessels in the neighboring lung parenchyma may show convergence of peripheral blood vessels, leading to and entering the cancerous mass (Fig. 13.3), a sign that is best appreciated with thin-section CT.[57] In one small series using multiplanar reconstruction CT, all 15 bronchial cancers showed direct involvement of a pulmonary vein.[59]

Regardless of the irregularity of the border, the nodules or masses described thus far can be regarded as having a well-defined edge. Some peripheral cancers, 25% in one series,[52] show a very poorly defined edge on chest radiographs, similar to that seen in pneumonia (Figs 13.4 and 13.5). In such cases the spherical shape and relatively slow growth usually allows distinction from infectious processes, which in general change size within a few weeks.

Occasionally, bronchial carcinomas arising in segmental or subsegmental bronchi are seen radiographically as mucoid impaction (bronchial mucocele or bronchocele) (Fig. 13.6),[60–63] in which case the resulting shadow, to a greater or lesser extent, represents dilated bronchi filled with tumor or inspissated

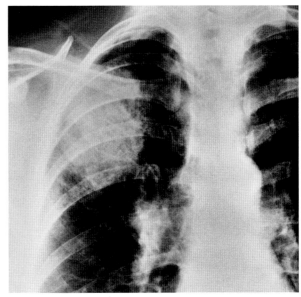

Fig. 13.4 Poorly differentiated squamous cell carcinoma of lung with ill-defined edge resembling pneumonia.

secretions. For a mucoid impaction to be visible on chest radiography, the adjacent lung must be aerated by collateral air drift. Mucoid impactions (see p. 123) result in V shaped, Y shaped, or branching tree densities with their stems pointing towards the hilum.

Another rare pattern is an infarct shadow extending from the primary tumor, giving two contiguous but distinct components to the opacity, the distal one being a pleural based infarct.[64]

Calcification and cavitation

Most lung cancers are of soft tissue density on imaging. Some show partial calcification and some show cavitation.

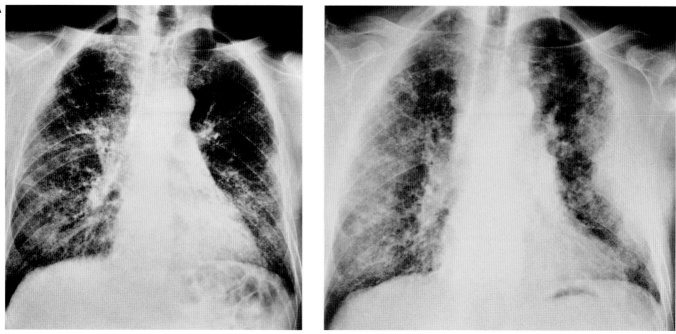

Fig. 13.5 **A** and **B**, Adenocarcinoma in the periphery of the left midzone developing in a patient with diffuse interstitial pulmonary fibrosis (rheumatoid lung). In this case the tumor has a very ill-defined edge resembling pneumonia. The two radiographs were taken 6 months apart.

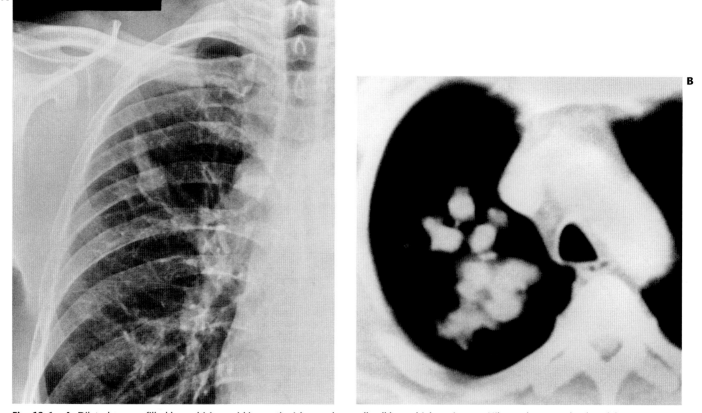

Fig. 13.6 **A**, Dilated mucus-filled bronchi (mucoid impaction) beyond a small cell bronchial carcinoma. Hilar and paratracheal nodal metastases are also present. **B**, CT in another patient showing mucoid impaction beyond a bronchial carcinoma.

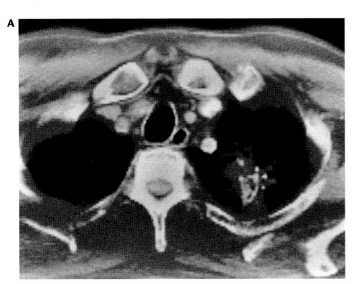

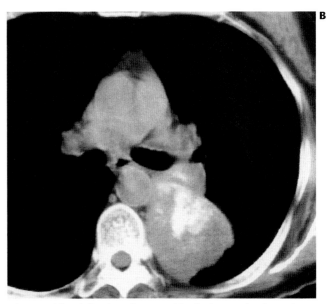

Fig. 13.7 Bronchial carcinoma showing substantial calcification. **A**, Adenocarcinoma with calcification, shown on histologic examination to be dystrophic calcification in necrotic areas of tumor, not preexisting granulomatous calcification. (Courtesy of Dr John Pitman, Williamsburg, VA) **B**, Calcification in a large centrally located carcinoma. The tumor obstructed the left lower lobe bronchus and caused left lower lobe collapse.

Calcification. Pathologists have long recognized that calcification is seen on histologic examination of bronchial carcinomas. Such calcification may be dystrophic in areas of tumor necrosis or may be an intrinsic part of the tumor. Tumor calcification is very rarely demonstrable with conventional radiography, except at specimen radiography.[65] CT demonstrates calcification within 6 to 10% of bronchogenic carcinomas.[66–69] Mostly, the calcifications represent preexisting granulomatous calcifications engulfed by the tumor. However, amorphous or cloudlike calcification, in keeping with dystrophic tumor calcification, is seen in a significant proportion.[69] Both small cell and nonsmall cell carcinomas may calcify, and there does not appear to be a predilection for cancers of any particular cell type.[66,67] Most tumors which show calcification are large with a diameter of 5 cm or more,[66,67] but amorphous or cloudlike calcification can be seen in small peripheral tumors (Fig. 13.7). Granulomatous calcifications engulfed by the tumor are likely to be eccentric in location (Fig. 13.8), but central granulomatous calcifications are occasionally seen.

Cavitation. Cavitation may be seen in tumors of any size and is best demonstrated by CT, which may show air, liquefaction, or a mixture of the two. The cavity is frequently eccentric, the walls are often very irregular, and tumor nodules may be visible (Fig. 13.9). The wall is usually at least 8 mm thick, but on rare occasions it is notably thin, 4 mm or less (Figs 13.10 and 13.11).[70] Cavitating bronchial carcinoma may even have smooth inner and outer margins. It has been suggested that such very thin walled cavities represent tumor cells lining bullae rather than true cavitation.[71] Fluid levels are common, and necrotic tumor fragments may be seen within the cavity. Very rarely, the cavity shows as an air crescent, similar to a mycetoma, caused by air around an intracavitary tumor mass or formed debris.[72]

Approximately 16% of peripheral carcinomas show cavitation on plain chest radiography.[52,71] The incidence is clearly much higher on CT. Squamous cell carcinoma is much more likely

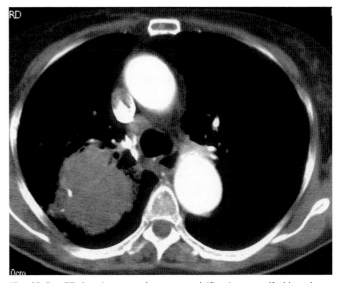

Fig. 13.8 CT showing granulomatous calcification engulfed by a lung carcinoma. A further calcified granuloma is seen in the same lobe.

to cavitate than cancers of other cell types. In one series of 100 cavitating cancers, 82 were squamous cell lesions.[71] Adenocarcinomas and large cell carcinomas cavitate occasionally, whereas small cell carcinomas, for practical purposes, do not cavitate.[48–50,71]

An appearance closely resembling a pulmonary cyst has been described in mucinous cystadenocarcinoma.[73]

Ground-glass density, air bronchograms, and bubble-like lucencies

Ground-glass density. The proportion of the nodule showing ground-glass opacity correlates with both cell type and histologic

A

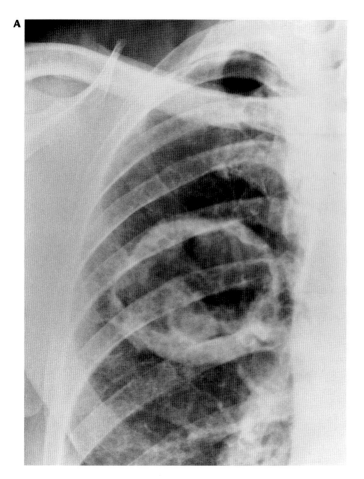

B

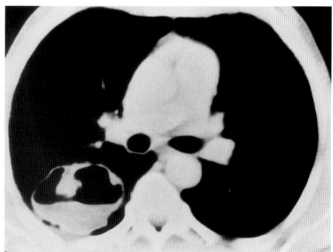

Fig. 13.9 Squamous cell carcinoma of bronchus showing cavitation. The cavity wall is of variable thickness and shows a mural nodule as well as an air-fluid level. **A**, Posteroanterior radiograph. **B**, CT.

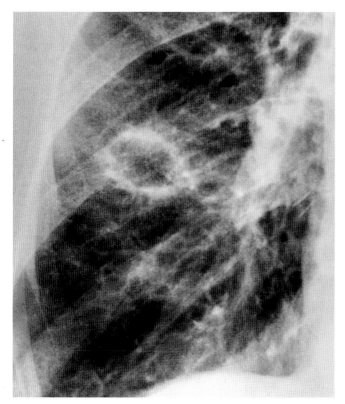

Fig. 13.10 Squamous cell carcinoma of bronchus showing a thin, uniform thickness cavity wall.

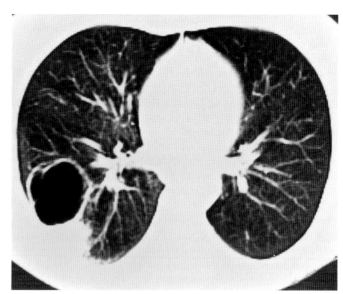

Fig. 13.11 Bronchial adenocarcinoma showing a very thin, uniform thickness cavity wall.

features. Some bronchioloalveolar carcinomas show pure diffuse ground-glass opacity. In an analysis of 124 surgically resected, peripheral adenocarcinomas <2 cm in diameter, the proportion of ground-glass opacity in individual lesions was significantly greater in bronchioloalveolar carcinoma than in other types of adenocarcinoma.[74] Minor degrees of ground-glass opacity are seen in other cell types due to adjacent inflammation, edema or hemorrhage.[75] Aoki et al[58] compared the extent of vessel invasion and regional node metastases with the margin characteristics and extent of ground-glass opacity on high-resolution computed tomography (HRCT) of 127 peripheral adenocarcinomas <3 cm in diameter. They found that both vessel invasion and regional lymph node spread were significantly lower when the ground-glass component of primary tumor was >50%. They also showed that tumors with ground-glass components of >50% had a statistically significantly better prognosis than those whose solid component comprised >50%. The same center[76] also approached the problem of prognosis in a slightly different way by showing that the greater the proportion of ground-glass shadowing in adenocarcinomas, the slower the growth rate.

Air bronchograms and bubble-like lucencies. Lung cancers, particularly adenocarcinomas and bronchioloalveolar carcinomas, may contain air bronchograms or bubble-like lucencies. Air bronchograms are usually thought of as a feature of infective consolidation or other alveolar filling processes. Kuriyama et al,[77] however, found that with HRCT some air-filled bronchi or bronchioles could be identified within the majority of peripherally situated small adenocarcinomas.[77] "Bubble-like" areas of low attenuation are seen fairly frequently: they were identified in 25% of one series of 93 cases of solitary pulmonary nodule caused by lung cancer.[78] These lucencies, which are seen in lung cancers of all cell types, but are most frequently encountered in adenocarcinoma and bronchioloalveolar carcinoma,[78–80] are due either to patent small bronchi or to small cystic spaces within the tumor.

An abruptly obstructed bronchus entering a tumor is highly predictive of squamous cell carcinoma.[79]

Contrast enhancement

Contrast enhancement reflects intratumoral microvessel vascularity (angiogenesis). Tateishi et al[81] correlated dynamic CT contrast enhancement with pathologic findings and the vascular endothelial growth factor (VEGF) expressed by various resected adenocarcinomas and showed that dynamic CT reflects the microvessel density of adenocarcinomas of the lungs.

Peripheral lung cancers enhance following the intravenous injection of contrast agents at both CT and MRI. This phenomenon has been exploited in an attempt to distinguish lung cancer from other causes of solitary pulmonary nodule (see p. 107).

Rate of growth

The volume doubling time for most bronchial carcinomas is between 1 and 18 months[82–87]; a 26% increase in diameter is equivalent to a doubling of volume. The primary tumors that grow more slowly are likely to be bronchioloalveolar carcinoma,[88] mucoepidermoid tumors, or adenoid cystic carcinomas. In one large series, with data from an era prior to the introduction of CT, and therefore based on radiographic rates of growth, the average doubling time was 4.1 months for undifferentiated carcinomas, 4.2 months for squamous cell carcinoma, and 7.3 months for adenocarcinoma.[89]

Central tumors

The cardinal imaging signs of a central tumor are collapse and consolidation of the lung beyond the tumor, and the presence of

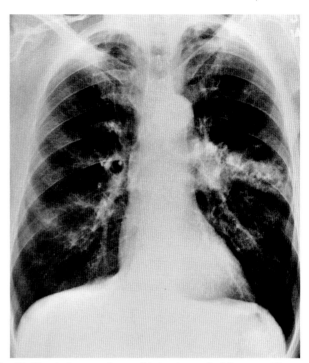

Fig. 13.12 Collapse and consolidation beyond a hilar mass. The mass was a bronchial carcinoma.

hilar enlargement, signs that may be seen in isolation or in conjunction with one another.

Collapse and consolidation in association with central tumors

Obstruction of a major bronchus may lead to a combination of atelectasis and retention of secretions with consequent pulmonary opacity,[90] but collateral air drift may partially or completely prevent these postobstructive changes. Obstructed portions of the lung may become secondarily infected, though this is relatively uncommon, at least in patients whose tumors are still amenable to surgical resection.[90] With time, lipid laden alveolar macrophages accumulate within the airspaces distal to an obstruction, giving rise to an appearance known to pathologists as endogenous lipoid pneumonia ("golden pneumonia"). The interstitium thickens because of chronic inflammatory infiltration and collagen deposition.[90] As might be expected, the cancer most frequently responsible for collapse and consolidation is squamous cell carcinoma, partly because it is a common cell type and partly because a larger proportion of squamous carcinomas originate centrally.

Collapse and consolidation beyond an obstructing bronchial carcinoma are readily recognizable radiographically as patchy (Fig. 13.12) or homogeneous pulmonary opacity. Loss of volume is usual with central tumors, but consolidation without loss of volume may be encountered. Air bronchograms visible on plain chest radiographs are uncommon, particularly before antibiotic therapy, but they are seen fairly frequently at CT (Fig. 13.13). If the tumor regresses with therapy, a previously invisible air bronchogram may become visible on chest radiographs.

Retained mucus may accumulate in and distend the airways. Mucus-filled dilated bronchi are more apparent on the

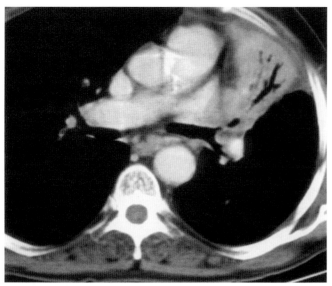

Fig. 13.13 An air bronchogram in a left upper lobe collapse beyond a bronchial carcinoma in the left upper lobe bronchus.

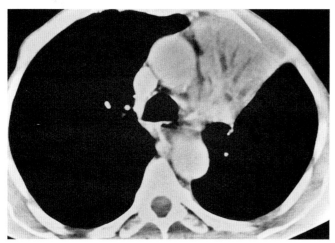

Fig. 13.14 Dilated fluid-filled bronchi in a collapsed left upper lobe beyond a central bronchial carcinoma. (A plain chest radiograph of this patient is shown in Fig. 13.16.)

Golden S sign

Pneumonia confined to one lobe (or more lobes if supplied by a common bronchus)

Expansion of a consolidated lobe

Visible stenosis of supplying bronchus

Visible central mass

Localized pneumonia that is unchanged for >2 weeks or one that recurs in the same lobe after a short interval

Visibly dilated fluid-filled bronchi at CT or MRI

similar in density. After administration of contrast material there is differential enhancement, most obvious if rapid sequential scanning is used: the neoplastic tissue enhances to a minimal degree, whereas distal atelectasis may show substantial enhancement.[94,95] MRI shows a difference in signal between tumor and postobstructive pulmonary changes, particularly on T2-weighted images,[95,96] or gadolinium-enhanced T1-weighted images.[97,98] Based on one small series it appears that cholesterol pneumonitis and distal bronchiectasis are seen as higher signal than tumor on T2-weighted images, whereas organizing pneumonia and atelectasis are isointense with tumors.[99]

The following features suggest that pneumonia is secondary to an obstructing neoplasm (see Box 13.3):

- Alteration in the shape of the collapsed or consolidated lobe due directly to the bulk of the underlying tumor. The fissure in the region of the mass may be unable to move in the usual manner, with the result that the fissure appears bulged ("Golden S" sign) (Fig. 13.15). This sign indicates that the collapse is the result of an underlying mass and predicts that the mass will be sufficiently central that successful bronchoscopic biopsy should be readily achievable.

- The presence of pneumonia confined to one lobe (or more lobes if there is a common bronchus supplying multiple lobes) in patients over the age of 45 years, particularly if the lobe shows loss of volume and no air bronchograms (Fig. 13.16). Occasionally the opacified lobe appears larger than normal because of secretions and infection trapped behind the obstructing carcinoma (Fig. 13.17), an appearance that has been labeled the "drowned lobe". In cases of obstructive pneumonitis or atelectasis, the tumor should be readily visible at bronchoscopy, an investigation that is usually performed without delay.

- The presence of a visible mass or irregular stenosis in a main stem or lobar bronchus. Careful analysis of CT images will demonstrate the presence of an obstructing tumor in virtually every case of postobstructive atelectasis caused by a lung carcinoma.[93]

- The presence of an associated central mass (see Fig. 13.12). Simple pneumonia rarely causes radiographically visible hilar adenopathy, although enlarged central nodes may be seen at CT or MRI. Bacterial lung abscess can, however, be confused with bronchial carcinoma because it may result in hilar or mediastinal adenopathy.[100]

- A localized pneumonia that persists unchanged for >2 weeks or one that recurs in the same lobe. Simple pneumonia often clears or spreads to other segments during

postcontrast CT than they are on the images taken prior to contrast administration,[91–93] and when seen should prompt a search for a centrally obstructing tumor. They may be seen within collapsed lobes on CT or MRI examinations as branching tubular structures (Fig. 13.14) or, when seen in cross section, as round or oval densities.

Defining the presence or extent of the central tumor mass in the presence of postobstructive consolidation and atelectasis can be difficult, even with CT or MRI. This decision can be important in making the initial diagnosis of a central tumor. It is also an important factor in planning radical radiotherapy. Although CT or MRI may allow the tumor to be more accurately measured, the size of the lesion does not in itself affect decisions regarding surgery, since both small and large tumors are surgically excised, provided they have not spread too far. On unenhanced CT the neoplastic and non-neoplastic tissue may be

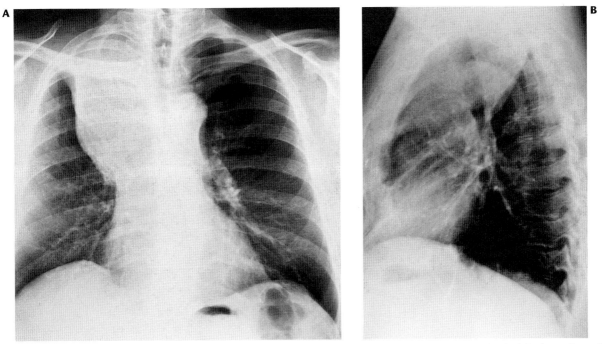

Fig. 13.15   Golden S sign in right upper lobe collapse shown on **A**, posteroanterior and **B**, lateral chest radiograph. The lobe has collapsed around a large obstructing centrally positioned bronchial carcinoma occluding the right upper lobe bronchus.

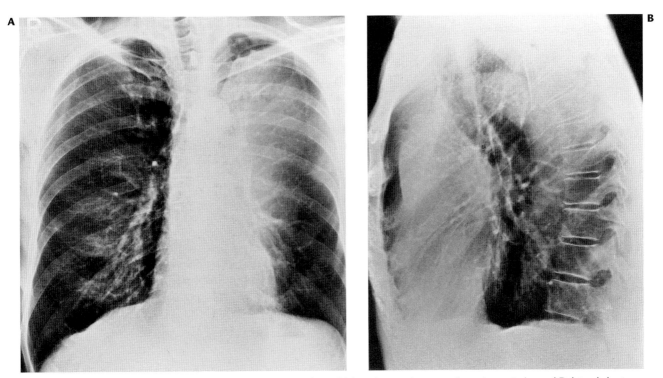

Fig. 13.16   Left upper lobe collapse beyond a centrally obstructing bronchial carcinoma shown on **A**, posteroanterior and **B**, lateral chest radiograph. (A CT of this patient is shown in Fig. 13.14.)

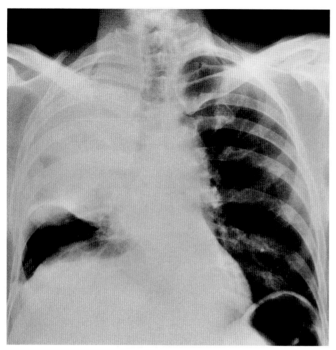

Fig. 13.17 "Drowned lobe" beyond a bronchial carcinoma in the right upper lobe bronchus. The right upper lobe shows extensive consolidation and expansion.

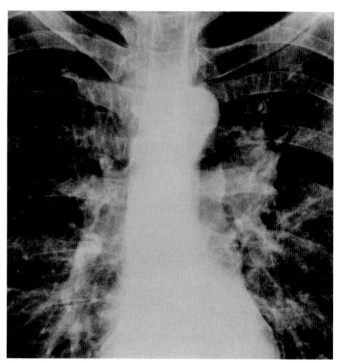

Fig. 13.18 Small cell carcinoma of bronchus occurring as a hilar mass. As is so often the case, it is not possible to tell whether the mass is all tumor, all enlarged nodes, or a mixture of the two.

this time interval. Complete resolution of pneumonia, in practice, excludes an obstructing neoplasm as the cause of infection. Although consolidation may improve partially with appropriate antibiotic therapy, it virtually never resolves completely if it is secondary to an underlying carcinoma.

- Visibly dilated fluid-filled bronchi in the affected lobe on CT or MRI.

Hilar enlargement

Hilar enlargement is a common presenting feature on chest radiographs in patients with bronchial carcinoma. In the Mayo Clinic series, 38% of patients had a hilar or perihilar mass, and in 12% a central mass was the only radiographic abnormality (Fig. 13.18).[47–51] Such masses may result from the tumor itself, from enlargement of hilar nodes containing metastatic tumor, from consolidated lung, or from a combination of these phenomena. Deciding their relative contribution to the tumor mass can be difficult on plain chest radiography. In general, the more lobular the shape, the more likely it is that enlarged lymph nodes are present. CT can be very helpful in this regard.

A mass superimposed on the hilum may lead to increased density of the hilum because of summation of the opacity of the mass added to the density of the normal hilar shadow (Fig. 13.19). Increased hilar density may be the only indication of lung cancer on a frontal chest film; when the sign is suspected, careful inspection of a lateral film or CT is essential.

Air-trapping

Expiration films to detect air-trapping, although occasionally positive,[101] have not proved useful in the diagnosis of bronchial carcinoma. Recognizable overinflation by check valve obstruction appears to be even more unusual; no example was found in the 600 cases reported from the Mayo Clinic.[47–51]

Staging intrathoracic spread of tumor

The International Staging System

For staging purposes, lung carcinoma is classified into nonsmall cell and small cell types, reflecting the marked differences in natural history and response to therapy.

The International Staging System for *nonsmall cell lung cancer* stratifies disease extent in terms of prognosis,[102] and has been adopted by the International Union Against Cancer.[103] It is based on the TNM grading of the primary tumor, regional nodes and distant metastases (Table 13.2). The stages have been devised to produce groups (Tables 13.3 and 13.4) which reflect the management options and survival (Table 13.4).[102,104]

Stage I tumors are divided into A and B according to whether the tumor is T1 or T2. Stage I and II tumors are confined to the lung and investing visceral pleura, without extension to the parietal pleura; when in a major bronchus the tumor is >2 cm beyond the tracheal carina. There is no nodal or distant spread. *Stage II tumors* are divided into A and B. Stage IIA tumors are the same as Stage IA, but with ipsilateral hilar nodal metastasis. Stage IIB tumors can be: (1) either the same as Stage IB, but with ipsilateral hilar nodal metastasis; or (2) tumors without nodal or distant spread which have invaded the adjacent chest wall, mediastinum, or diaphragm, but are potentially surgically resectable. *Stage III tumors* are divided into A and B. Stage IIIA comprises: (1) T3 tumors in which the only spread is to hilar nodes; and (2) T1–T3 tumors without distant metastases which have spread to ipsilateral mediastinal and/or subcarinal nodes (N2). Stage III B tumors are T4 tumors or any tumor that has spread to contralateral nodes. *Stage IV* comprises patients with distant metastatic disease (M1).

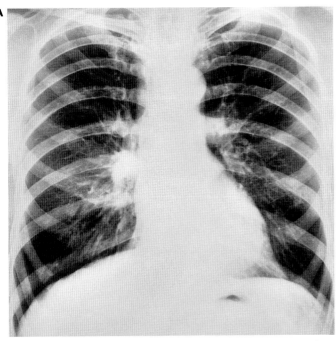
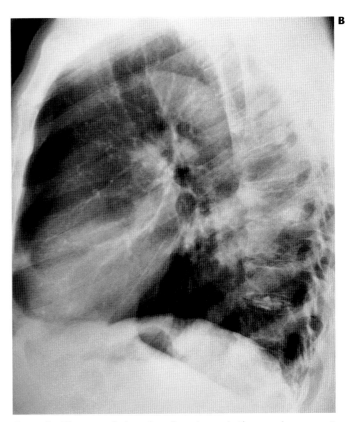

Fig. 13.19 Dense hilum sign shown on **A**, posteroanterior and **B**, lateral radiographs. The most obvious sign of carcinoma in the superior segment of the right lower lobe is an increase in the density of the right hilum caused by superimposition of a mass, distal pneumonia, and hilar structures.

Small cell lung cancer is classified as limited (confined to one hemithorax but may involve contralateral mediastinal and supraclavicular nodes), or extensive, according to the requirements for radiotherapy fields.[105–107] Small cell lung cancer is generally regarded as a systemic disease and is usually disseminated from the outset. The major role for imaging is to determine extrathoracic spread, a topic beyond the scope of this book.

As with most other cancers, the treatment options and outcomes for lung cancer are heavily dependent on the stage and cell type (see Table 13.5). The treatment of choice for *nonsmall cell lung cancer*, in the absence of evidence of dissemination, is surgical resection. The prime issue for the surgeon, therefore, is whether the tumor can be completely removed by surgery. Clear surgical margins in resection specimens and absence of tumor cells in resected lymph nodes are prime determinants of local recurrence and survival.[108]

Stage I and II tumors are treated by lobectomy or pneumonectomy,[109] with selected stage II tumors receiving adjuvant radiotherapy and/or chemotherapy.[110] Tumors that extend along the main bronchi to within 2 cm of the carina, but do not involve it, are included in stage II provided there is no nodal involvement. Such tumors may be resected with bronchoplastic techniques.[111–113] T3 tumors are regarded as operable provided there is no nodal or distant spread (i.e. still stage II), but the results of surgery are less good than for T1 and T2 tumors, even when complete clearance of tumor is possible.

The treatment of Stage IIIA tumors ranges from surgical resection to nonsurgical modes of treatment and varies greatly from center to center.[114] Some patients may benefit from mediastinal lymphadenectomy of involved ipsilateral nodes (N2).

Stage IIIB tumors involve critical mediastinal structures, such as the great vessels, esophagus, and trachea (T4), or have spread to contralateral mediastinal nodes (N3). Patients with stage IIIB tumors are not considered to be surgical candidates, unless preoperative neoadjuvant chemotherapy is given to "downstage" the tumor.[102,115]

In patients with nonsmall cell lung cancers deemed unsuitable for surgery, either due to intrathoracic spread or metastatic disease, treatment options include various chemotherapy and radiotherapy regimens, which in suitable patients in some centers may be followed by surgical resection. Radical radiotherapy requires the tumor volume to be encompassed within a suitable radiation field, in a manner that critical organ and total body doses are not exceeded. The oncologist needs to know the total disease burden and disease quantification is also important when measuring therapeutic response. In addition, imaging can help to guide biopsy and can confirm and characterize metastases.

Small cell lung cancer is almost always treated medically,[107,116] but may, in highly selected cases of early disease, be treated by surgery alone or combined surgery and chemotherapy.[108,117]

Imaging for staging nonsmall cell lung cancer

Currently, the standard imaging techniques used to stage the intrathoracic spread of lung cancer are plain chest radiography

Table 13.2 TNM descriptions of non-small cell bronchial carcinoma[102,103]

Primary tumor (T)

TX	Primary tumor cannot be assessed, or tumor proven by the presence of malignant cells in sputum or bronchial washings but not visualized by imaging or bronchoscopy
T0	No evidence of primary tumor
Tis	Carcinoma in situ
T1	Tumor <3 cm in greatest dimension surrounded by lung or visceral pleura, without bronchoscopic evidence of invasion more proximal than the lobar bronchus* (i.e. not in the main bronchus)
T2	Tumor with any of the following features of size or extent: >3 cm in greatest dimension; involves main bronchus ≥2 cm distal to the carina; invades the visceral pleura; associated with atelectasis or obstructive pneumonitis that extends to the hilar region but does not involve the entire lung
T3	Tumor of any size that directly invades any of the following: chest wall (including superior sulcus tumors), diaphragm, mediastinal pleura, parietal pericardium; or tumor in the main bronchus <2 cm distal to the carina, but without involvement of the carina; or associated atelectasis or obstructive pneumonitis of the entire lung
T4	Tumor of any size that invades any of the following: mediastinum, heart, great vessels, trachea, esophagus, vertebral body, carina; or tumor with a malignant pleural or pericardial effusion,[†] or with satellite tumor nodule(s) within the ipsilateral primary tumor lobe of the lung

Regional lymph nodes (N)

NX	Regional lymph nodes cannot be assessed
N0	No regional lymph node metastasis
N1	Metastasis to ipsilateral peribronchial and/or ipsilateral hilar lymph nodes and intrapulmonary nodes involved by direct extension of the primary tumor
N2	Metastasis to ipsilateral mediastinal and/or subcarinal lymph node(s)
N3	Metastasis to contralateral mediastinal, contralateral hilar, ipsilateral or contralateral scalene, or supraclavicular lymph node(s)

Distant metastasis (M)

MX	Distant metastasis cannot be assessed
M0	No distant metastasis
M1	Distant metastasis present[‡]

*The uncommon superficial tumor of any size with its invasive component limited to the bronchial wall, which may extend proximal to the main bronchus, is also classified T1.

†Most pleural effusions associated with lung cancer are due to tumor. However, there are a few patients in whom multiple cytopathologic examinations of pleural fluid show no tumor. In these cases, the fluid is nonbloody and is not an exudate. When these elements and clinical judgment dictate that the effusion is not related to the tumor, the effusion should be excluded as a staging element and the patient's disease should be staged T1, T2, or T3; pericardial effusion is classified according to the same rules.

‡Separate metastatic tumor nodule(s) in the ipsilateral nonprimary tumor lobe(s) of the lung also are classified M1.

Table 13.3 Stage definitions of nonsmall cell bronchial carcinoma[102]

Stage	Definition
IA	T1 N0 M0
IB	T2 N0 M0
IIA	T1 N1 M0
IIB	T2 N1 M0
	T3 N0 M0
IIIA	T3 N1 M0
	T1 N2 M0
	T2 N2 M0
	T3 N2 M0
IIIB	T4 N0 M0
	T4 N1 M0
	T4 N2 M0
	T1 N3 M0
	T2 N3 M0
	T3 N3 M0
	T4 N3 M0
IV	Any T, any N, M1

Staging is not relevant for occult carcinoma, designated TX N0 M0.
T0 tumors are classified as: stage IIA when N1M0; stage IIIA when N2M0, and stage IIIB when N3M0.[103]

Table 13.4 Summary of descriptions of stage for nonsmall cell bronchial carcinoma

Stage I	No nodal metastases and totally removable by lobectomy or pneumonectomy. Divided into A or B based on tumor size/involvement of major bronchi
Stage II	Adds hilar node involvement or T3 tumor with no node involvement
Stage IIIA	Extensive but resectable disease (T3 N1, T1 N2, T2 N2, T3 N2)
Stage IIIB	Irresectable disease by conventional criteria but still confined to chest, so eligible for radical radiotherapy
Stage IV	Distant metastases

and CT of the chest.[106,118–122] In some centers bronchoscopy is undertaken prior to CT, but in other centers CT is done routinely before bronchoscopy, an approach that can be justified on the grounds that it is cost effective and, on occasion, will obviate the need for bronchoscopy by showing irresectable disease, or by showing benign disease only.[123]

CT is usually performed following intravenous contrast enhancement, but the evidence for the routine use of contrast is relatively weak. In a series of 96 patients with pathologically proven lung cancer, no change in management resulted from

Table 13.5 Five year survival figures (%) for nonsmall cell bronchial carcinoma based on stage

Stage	Clinical staging		Pathologic staging	
	US[102]	Japan[104]	US[102]	Japan[104]
IA	61	71	67	79
IB	38	44	57	60
IIA	34	41	55	56
IIB	22–34	33–39	38–55	44–47
IIIA	9–13	22–23	23–25	22–26
IIIB	1–8	12–24		3–21
IV	1	22		5

the availability of contrast-enhanced CT of the chest and liver compared to nonenhanced CT of the chest down to the adrenal glands.[124] Another study investigated whether more enlarged mediastinal nodes were evident on post- as opposed to noncontrast-enhanced examinations,[125] and found that only in station 2R were significantly more nodes appreciated following contrast. The detection of hilar lymph nodes using CT is, however, significantly better following contrast enhancement.[126,127] (The presence of ipsilateral enlarged hilar nodes – N1 disease – does not alter the decision to operate because N1 disease does not by itself preclude surgical resection for potential cure.)

It should be appreciated that even CT, which is significantly more sensitive than chest radiography, disagrees with the TNM stage found at surgery in a significant proportion of patients.[128] In 40% of cases in one typical series, CT categorized the extent of tumor sufficiently poorly that the overall stage was overestimated or underestimated.[129]

The preoperative decision whether lobectomy or pneumonectomy will be required for centrally situated tumors, or whether conservative bronchoplastic surgery, i.e. sleeve lobectomy or pneumonectomy,[130,131] will be feasible, depends on whether or not the tumor has crossed fissures, invaded central vessels, or spread centrally within the bronchial tree. Chest radiography and CT, particularly multiplanar CT using multidetector machines, and virtual CT bronchoscopy,[132] provide important information, but have not, in general, proved sufficiently accurate in predicting whether or not a pneumonectomy will be required. Currently, therefore, the surgeon still mostly makes this decision based on bronchoscopic findings or on the findings at thoracotomy.[128,133] But imaging advances are being made: spiral CT with multiplanar reformations proved accurate for determining whether or not peripherally located lung cancers had crossed fissures in one recent series,[134] and tilted HRCT can, similarly, show the relationship of a tumor to the adjacent minor fissure better than conventional CT.[135] Multidetector CT is likely to further improve the predictive accuracy.

Even with tumors amenable to surgical resection, a major decision in many patients is whether or not lung function would be adequate once a pneumonectomy has been carried out. Pulmonary perfusion scans have a role to play here. The relative perfusion of each lung can be quantified from the number of radioactive counts in the combined anterior and posterior scans. The percentage contribution of each lung is then multiplied by the overall forced expiratory volume in 1 s (FEV_1) to predict the

FEV_1 of the lung that would remain after surgery.[136] Quantitative regional ventilation and perfusion can also be assessed using nuclear medicine techniques in order to predict postoperative loss of lung function.[137]

Staging the primary tumor

T1 and T2 tumors are confined to the lung and its investing pleura, or to bronchi >2 cm from the carina. T3 tumors have limited extrapulmonary extension, including invasion of the chest wall, mediastinal pleura, pericardium, diaphragm, and thoracic apex, but are mostly considered to be resectable. Tumors that extend to within 2 cm of the carina, but do not involve the carina are also classified as T3. T4 tumors invade the heart, great vessels, trachea, carina, esophagus, or vertebral body. Any tumor associated with a malignant pleural effusion is also designated T4.

The distinction between T3 and T4 tumors is critical because it reflects the dividing line between conventional surgical and nonsurgical management. T4 tumors make the disease at least stage IIIB and are regarded as irresectable by the great majority of surgeons, either because they have invaded the vertebrae or critical mediastinal structures, such as the heart and great vessels, trachea, and carina, and esophagus, or because they have disseminated within the pleura or a lobe. A few surgeons try to resect tumors in the occasional highly selected patient with a T4 tumor, provided complete resection can be performed.[138] Some of the patients will have had a preoperative course of neoadjuvant chemotherapy in order to "downstage" the tumor.[139–143] There are anecdotal reports of 5 year survivors who have undergone reconstruction of the superior vena cava, resection of vertebral bodies, or partial cardiac dissections.[144,145] However, most surgeons believe that such radical surgery is not justified. (Invasion of the diaphragm is classified as T3, but deep invasion of the diaphragm was shown in one large surgical series to be associated with an outcome similar to T4 tumors.[146])

It is easy to assess the size and position of a primary tumor surrounded by aerated lung on plain chest radiography, and even easier with CT. It may, however, be difficult to distinguish the tumor from distal collapsed or consolidated lung on CT and, therefore, overestimate or underestimate tumor size and extent of chest wall or mediastinal contact. At dynamic contrast-enhanced CT, collapsed lung enhances more than central tumor,[94] and may show mucus-filled bronchi, an indicator of collapsed lung. T2-weighted MRI can be useful for separately identifying tumor from distal collapse/consolidation.[99,147] The tumor usually shows much lower T2 signal than the distal changes, and mucus-filled dilated bronchi can be specifically identified as high intensity tubular structures.[95] PET scanning has not proved to be of use in determining the extent of the primary tumor,[148] though combined PET/CT may improve this delineation.

Mediastinal invasion

The chest radiograph is a poor indicator of mediastinal invasion, although involvement of the phrenic nerve is suggested by elevation of the ipsilateral hemidiaphragm, particularly if it is a new finding. Caution is needed before deciding that a high hemidiaphragm is caused by phrenic nerve invasion, because lobar collapse can lead to diaphragm elevation, and subpulmonary effusion may mimic it. Ultrasonography can

---

Box 13.4 Mediastinal invasion

The CT features of limited mediastinal contact or preserved mediastinal fat plane (< 3 cm, <90° of circumferential contact with descending aorta) are reasonably accurate at predicting tumor respectability

MRI is of similar value; its multiplanar capability is advantageous only in specific regions

Both techniques are less accurate at identifying T4 disease and irresectability

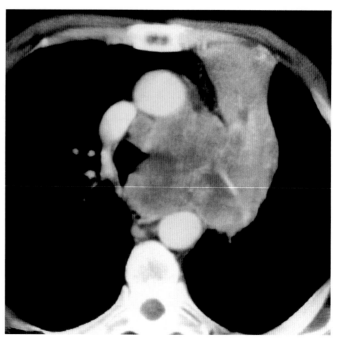

Fig. 13.20 Contrast-enhanced CT showing extensive mediastinal invasion (T4 tumor) encasing the ascending and descending aorta, as well as the right main bronchus and the main, left, and right pulmonary arteries. The bronchial carcinoma has caused collapse of the left upper lobe.

provide information about diaphragmatic movement and, by inference, phrenic nerve involvement.[149] Barium swallow may show esophageal displacement or invasion.

Both CT and MRI (Box 13.4) can show the presence of extensive tumor within the mediastinum. Clear-cut encasement of vital structures such as the esophagus, trachea or major vessels, or deep penetration of tissue planes, is conclusive evidence of a T4 tumor (Figs 13.20 and 13.21). Mere contact with the mediastinum is not enough for the diagnosis of invasion (Fig. 13.22), and apparent interdigitation with mediastinal fat can be a misleading sign on both CT and MRI.[150] Also, associated pneumonia or atelectasis may make it difficult to determine whether mediastinal contact is even present (Fig. 13.23).

CT is reasonably accurate at assessing resectability of nonsmall cell lung cancers which are in contact with the mediastinum. Glazer et al[151] correlated operative findings with three features of tumors: (1) <3 cm of mediastinal contact; (2) maintained fat plane separating the tumor mass from the mediastinum, (3) <90° of circumferential aortic contact.[151] The presence of at least one of these features predicted resectability in 36 of 37 tumors in contact with the mediastinum. However, criteria for irresectability are harder to identify,[152] and this is the crucial information required by the surgeon if unnecessary thoracotomies are to be avoided. In Glazer et al's series almost half the technically resectable tumors showed >3 cm of mediastinal contact, and loss of the fat plane may be due to blurring from motion artifact, fibrosis, or reactive inflammatory change. Similar criteria have been evaluated by other authors, with disappointing results.[150,153–155] In one recent study, >90° of circumferential contact with a mediastinal structure was found to have only 40% sensitivity for mediastinal invasion.[156] In another study, infiltration of the mediastinal fat had a sensitivity of only 27% for irresectable disease, and even structural encasement was an unreliable sign.[157] Obliteration of a superior pulmonary vein within the mediastinum immediately adjacent to the left atrium was reliable evidence of unresectable intra-pericardial extension of tumor in one center,[158] but not in another[159]; whereas obliteration of one of the inferior pulmonary veins is not reliable evidence of intrapericardial extension, unless the tumor can be seen within the left atrium (Fig. 13.24).[158]

Some groups have investigated specialized CT techniques in an attempt to obtain more accurate information. Ultrafast cine CT with respiratory and cardiac gating has been used to show relative movement between the tumor and mediastinal structures, implying lack of invasion.[160,161] CT performed following the induction of a diagnostic pneumothorax can similarly reveal lack of tumor fixation.[162] Although these techniques are effective methods of excluding mediastinal extension, they do not address the important converse problem, namely diagnosing invasion, because benign adhesions, as well as tumor invasion, can cause fixation of lung to the mediastinum.

The advent of volumetric (spiral) CT, particularly the introduction of multidetector CT, has enabled better assessment of mediastinal invasion. Advantages include more reliable contrast opacification of vascular structures, reduced cardiac and respiratory motion artifact, and limitation of partial volume averaging. High quality multiplanar reformations allow detailed assessment of important regions such as the tracheal carina, aortopulmonary window, and aortic arch, although formal analysis of data are awaited. Visualization of the bronchial tree using planar and 3D techniques is now an established technique.

In certain specific situations, MRI may be superior to single detector CT for the assessment of mediastinal invasion,[150,154,163,164] but the case for the routine use of MRI for the diagnosis of mediastinal invasion has not been made; the signs are basically the same and the axial imaging plane is the standard projection for both tests.[150,154] MRI is no more accurate than CT in distinguishing between contiguity of tumor with the mediastinum and mediastinal invasion, largely because invasion of the mediastinal fat can be mimicked by adjacent inflammatory changes.[98,154,165]

MRI can, however, provide useful information in certain circumstances.[147,150,154,163,165–168] Endobronchial tumor extension remains the province of bronchoscopy, but extraluminal encasement is well seen by MRI. Also, the ability to show the superior vena cava in the coronal plane without having to inject contrast medium allows easy, often exquisite, demonstration of the extent of tumor in patients with the superior vena cava syndrome. Similarly, pulmonary vein, pericardial, and cardiac involvement are well demonstrated.[159] Tumor may grow along the pulmonary veins to become intrapericardial or to lie within

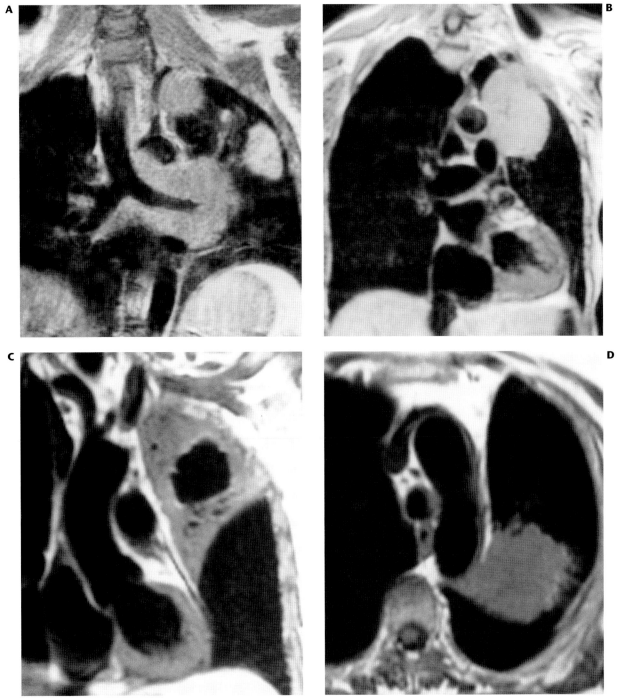

Fig. 13.21 MRI (cardiac gated T1-weighted spin echo) of four patients with bronchial carcinoma. **A**, Coronal image showing deep invasion into the subcarinal and aortopulmonary window regions. **B**, Coronal image showing growth into the aortopulmonary window and chest wall invasion. **C**, Coronal image showing large cavitating tumor which extends close to the main pulmonary artery but with no evidence of mediastinal invasion. **D**, Axial image showing invasion of the mediastinal fat over the posterior portion of the aortic arch.

the left atrium – features that can be well demonstrated by MRI (Fig. 13.24). The normal pericardium is seen as a low signal membrane and disruption of the pericardium can, therefore, be recognized. Contrast enhancement with gadolinium[97,98] does not appear to confer sufficient advantage in distinguishing neoplastic from normal tissue or benign disease for it to be recommended as a routine. Multiple ECG-triggered contrast-

enhanced MR angiography allowed better detection of hilar and mediastinal invasion than nongated MR angiography in one series.[169]

Ultrasound has a limited role in assessing mediastinal invasion. Echocardiography can be used to assess cardiac involvement. Endoscopic transbronchial ultrasound has been shown to be reasonably accurate for determining the depth of

A

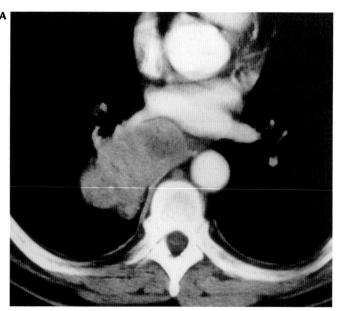

B

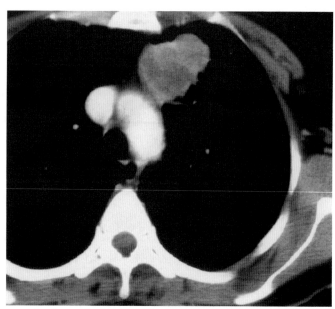

Fig. 13.22 Mediastinal contact by a bronchial carcinoma in two cases that proved to be surgically resectable. **A,** Despite the distortion of the left atrium, the tumor had not invaded the left atrium or adjacent mediastinum. At surgery the tumor was confined to the lung and visceral pleura. **B,** The mediastinal pleura was involved, but the tumor proved to be resectable.

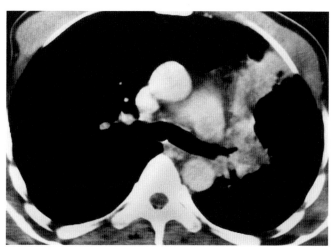

Fig. 13.23 CT of a centrally located bronchial carcinoma in which the distal pneumonia/atelectasis mimics mediastinal contact by the tumor.

tumor within the wall of major bronchi for centrally located tumors,[170] and for distinguishing between invasion and compression of the walls of the airways.[171]

Chest wall invasion

A peripheral lung tumor may cross the parietal pleura and invade ribs and intercostal muscles. Such localized invasion of the chest wall (T3) by nonsmall cell lung cancer need not be a contraindication to surgery, but it adversely affects prognosis and alters the surgical technique, requiring en bloc resection and, in some instances, chest wall reconstruction.[172–178] Five year survivals of up to 40% have been achieved, provided all the tumor has been cleared. The main determinant of outcome is the existence of hilar/mediastinal nodal disease, rather than the presence or depth of chest wall invasion.[179] The value of any radiologic assessment is to predict the extent of surgery required. The value of imaging chest wall invasion depends on

the surgeon's practice.[164,180] Provided the surgeon is prepared to perform a chest wall resection, the surgical technique can be modified according to the operative findings. Also, it should be appreciated that thoracoscopy is more accurate than imaging for determining chest wall invasion.[181]

The chest radiograph can reveal advanced rib or spinal destruction (Fig. 13.25) but does not enable minor degrees of chest wall invasion to be diagnosed.

Several CT signs of parietal pleural invasion have been described, including obtuse angle of contact between the tumor and the chest wall, obliteration of the extrapleural fat plane, pleural thickening, and the presence of extrapleural soft tissue.[175] Tumor tissue clearly destroying bone (Fig. 13.25) or extending through the intercostal muscles beyond the line of the ribs is undoubted evidence of invasion, but lesser degrees of involvement are harder to evaluate.[175,182–184] Contact with the pleura (Fig. 13.26), even if the pleura is thickened, does not necessarily indicate invasion, and increased density of the extrapleural fat adjacent to a lung tumor can be due to inflammatory reaction rather than neoplastic invasion (see Fig. 13.35). However, the greater the degree of contact and the greater the pleural thickening, the more likely it is that the parietal pleura has been invaded, particularly if the extrapleural fat plane is obliterated.[175] A clear extrapleural fat plane adjacent to the mass may be helpful, but again not definitive, in excluding chest wall invasion.[153] Local chest wall pain may still be the most specific indicator of invasion.[182]

Modified CT techniques have been studied. Diagnostically induced pneumothoraces can reveal separation of a pulmonary mass from the chest wall and so exclude invasion.[162,185] CT performed during the respiratory cycle with an electron beam scanner may reveal relative movement between the tumor and chest wall, implying lack of fixation.[160] Conventional CT,[186] and MRI performed during inspiration and expiration can similarly detect relative movement.[187] Manipulation of helically acquired volumetric data may be useful. Multiplanar reformations may help assess lesions adjacent to the diaphragm. One recent study

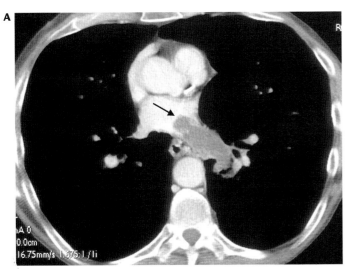
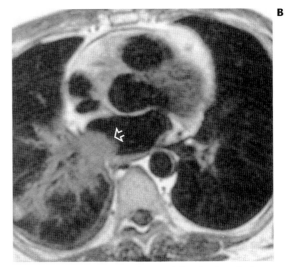

Fig. 13.24 **A**, Contrast-enhanced CT showing tumor extension into the left atrium (arrow). **B**, A cardiac gated T1-weighted spin-echo image showing the ability of MRI to demonstrate left atrial invasion by tumor (arrow).

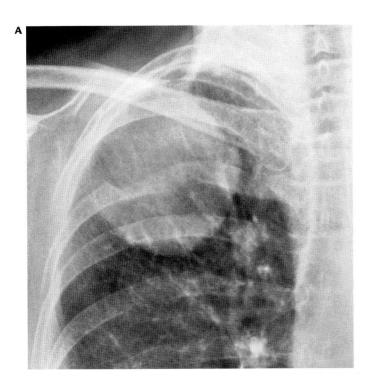
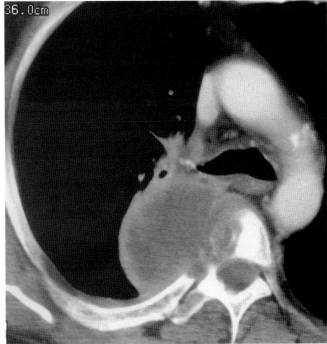

Fig. 13.25 **A**, Bronchial carcinoma showing invasion of the right fifth rib, causing irregular destruction of the rib. In this case there is widening of the adjacent rib interspace. Such widening is unusual in bronchial carcinoma. **B**, Bronchial carcinoma with obvious invasion of the medial end of a posterior rib and the adjacent vertebral body on a contrast-enhanced CT in another patient.

showed that 3D surface-shaded reformations could characterize pleural puckering, and distinguish visceral from parietal pleural invasion with 80% accuracy.[188] However, it remains to be shown whether any technique which evaluates the physical attachment of tumor to the chest wall can reliably differentiate tumor invasion from inflammatory adhesions in a large series of patients.

The early promise of MRI[147,154,189] is unfulfilled, because of overlap in appearances between tumor extension and associated inflammatory changes (Fig. 13.27).[121,165] The use of contrast enhancement has so far not shown to be beneficial.[190] Tumor tissue beyond the line of the ribs, as with CT, is good evidence of chest wall invasion (Fig. 13.28). A key observation is the appearance of the extrapleural fat, which is seen best as a thin high intensity line on T1-weighted images.[190,191] In one prospective study of 34 patients, the presence of material of identical signal to tumor extending into the layer of fat was 85% sensitive and 100% specific for chest wall invasion,[190] but other series did not provide such good results, notably a large prospective multicenter study, which showed no difference between the accuracy of MRI and CT.[168] Dynamic ciné MRI during breathing can, like CT, demonstrate lack of fixity of a tumor to the adjacent chest wall and so exclude parietal pleural and chest wall involvement, but cannot distinguish between

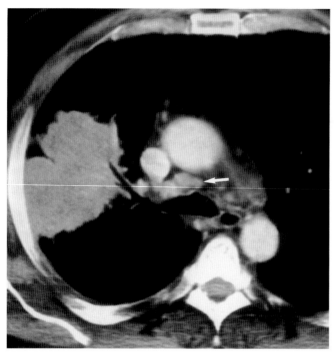

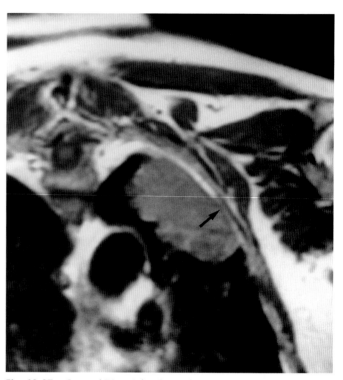

Fig. 13.26 Bronchial carcinoma showing extensive chest wall contact but no rib destruction. At surgery the parietal pleura was not invaded. Note the enlarged mediastinal lymph node (arrow), which on histology showed reactive hyperplasia but no neoplastic involvement. Note also the "bronchus sign" (see p. 118 for a description of the "bronchus sign").

Fig. 13.27 Coronal T1-weighted MRI showing a false positive impression of extrapleural fat invasion (arrow) by tumor. At surgery, this large cell anaplastic bronchial carcinoma had not extended beyond the visceral pleura.

benign adhesions and malignant tumor crossing the pleural cavity.[192]

There have been promising reports from Japan concerning the use of ultrasound for diagnosing chest wall invasion, although these techniques have not become widely used. The pleura can be seen as an echogenic interface, and disruption of the pleural line is a useful sign of chest wall invasion. Lack of movement of the tumor with breathing, implying adherence, can

also be observed. One report found ultrasound to be superior to CT, with >95% sensitivity and specificity for invasion.[193]

Apical (Pancoast, superior sulcus) tumors. Apical, or Pancoast, tumors deserve special mention. The eponym nowadays refers to the symptom complex of pain in the shoulder and arm that results from an apical tumor invading the lower cords of the brachial plexus and the sympathetic chain. Pancoast's original

A

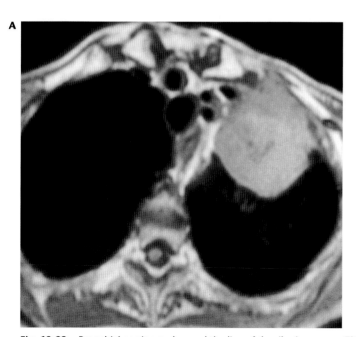

B

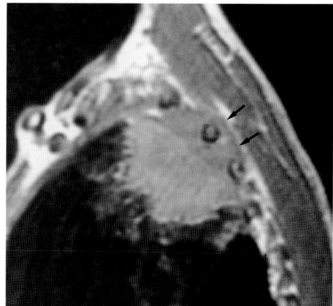

Fig. 13.28 Bronchial carcinoma beyond the line of the ribs (arrows on **B**), shown by **A**, T1-weighted axial MRI, and **B**, T1-weighted sagittal MRI.

description included ipsilateral Horner syndrome from invasion of the sympathetic chain, and local destruction of bone by the tumor.[194] Because these tumors arise adjacent to the groove for the subclavian artery, they are also called superior sulcus tumors. They may be of any cell type,[195–197] and have a propensity to invade the adjacent chest wall, root of neck, brachial plexus, subclavian vessels, and spine. In some centers survival has been significantly increased by preoperative radiotherapy and en bloc resection of the tumor, providing the tumor is technically resectable.[138,198–201] In such centers preoperative CT/MRI is essential.[138]

Radiographically,[196] superior sulcus tumors appear as a mass in approximately one-half to three-quarters of cases, and as an apical cap resembling pleural thickening in the remainder. Bone

destruction of the adjacent ribs or spine is seen on chest radiographs in approximately one-third of cases (Fig. 13.29).[202] These tumors are, however, often difficult to diagnose on chest radiographs because the lung apex is partly hidden by overlying ribs and clavicles. Also, the tumor so often closely resembles a benign apical pleural cap (Figs 13.29 and 13.30) and the cardinal plain film sign of the lesion – bone destruction – is either absent or difficult to diagnose with confidence. Asymmetric pleural thickening, particularly if associated with appropriate symptoms, should be viewed with suspicion. A chronically enlarging unilateral apical cap strongly suggests superior sulcus carcinoma.[203]

CT can be helpful for diagnosing Pancoast tumors (Fig. 13.31).[202,204,205] It may demonstrate an intrapulmonary mass

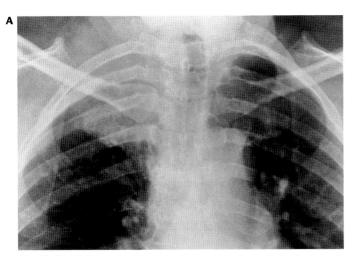
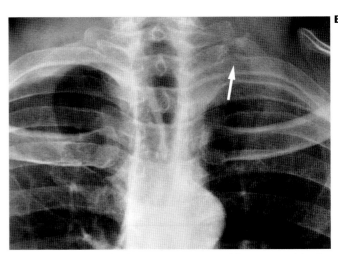

Fig. 13.29   **A,** Superior sulcus carcinoma of the lung destroying a major portion of the right first rib. The patient, a 52-year-old man, complained of chest wall pain and pain in the right arm. **B,** More subtle example of a superior sulcus carcinoma of the lung. The apical cap is thin and the destruction of the neck and head of the first rib (arrow) are not easy to see.

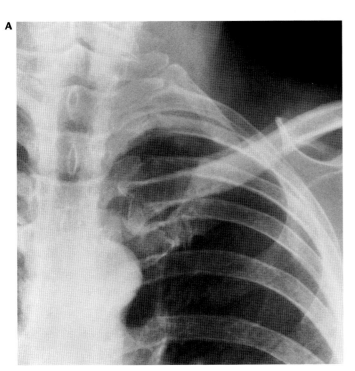
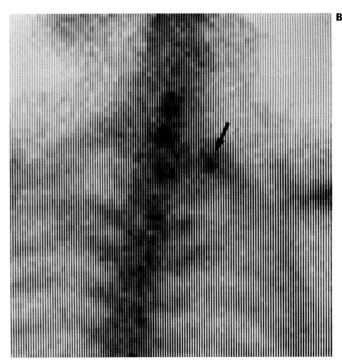

Fig. 13.30   Pancoast tumor. **A,** Plain film showing an appearance resembling an apical pleural cap. **B,** ^{99m}Tc bone scan showing increased activity in the invaded left first rib (arrow).

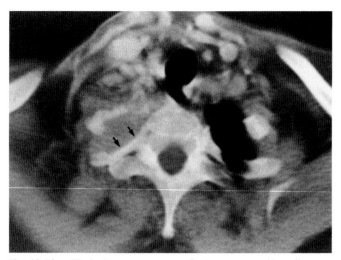

Fig. 13.31 CT of a Pancoast tumor at the lung apex and invading an adjacent rib (arrows).

rather than just pleural thickening, providing extra confidence that the diagnosis is neoplasm rather than inflammatory pleural disease. Also, CT is a sensitive technique with which to diagnose the full extent of tumor, particularly any chest wall invasion.

MRI is currently regarded as the optimal modality for demonstrating the extent of superior sulcus tumors, largely because the coronal and sagittal planes are the optimal imaging planes to demonstrate the cupola shape of the chest wall in the apical regions and to show the brachial plexus, subclavian vessels, neural foramina, and any bone marrow invasion to advantage (Fig. 13.32).[147,166,194,195,206–209] Thin sections (5 mm or less) and surface coils are recommended. T1-weighted and STIR images in coronal and sagittal planes appear to be the optimal sequences. Interruption of the normal extrapleural fat line over the lung apex can be readily shown, as can the relationship of tumor to brachial plexus, subclavian vessels, and spinal canal.

Rib and vertebral body destruction, however, may be less well shown by MRI than by CT.[195,207]

Intrathoracic lymph node staging (Box 13.5)

The most important predictor of outcome in the majority of patients with nonsmall cell lung cancer limited to the chest is the presence or absence of involved mediastinal lymph nodes.[210] Surgery is not a curative option for patients with positive contralateral mediastinal nodes (N3). Surgery is also considered inappropriate in symptomatic N2 disease. The surgical management of lesser degrees of N2 disease is controversial. Conflicting published results are partly due to differences in selection criteria and data analysis. Some surgeons operate with the hope of cure on patients with N2 disease as long as the involved nodes can be completely resected, are few in number, are not bulky, and are not in the high paratracheal region.[108] The prognosis correlates with the method by which N2 disease is established. Positive nodal disease, established only after operative mediastinal dissection, has a better outcome than nodal involvement discovered preoperatively by mediastinal biopsy or CT. Several recent series have confirmed that a 20–32% 5 year

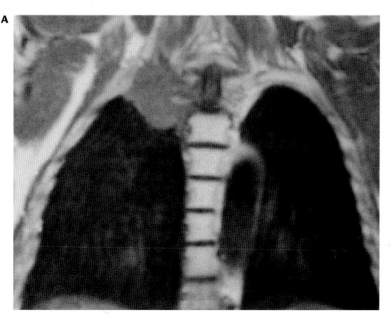

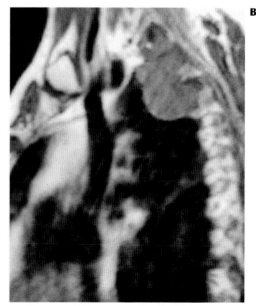

Fig. 13.32 MRI of a Pancoast tumor (T1-weighted images). **A**, The invasion of root of the neck and obliteration of the extrapleural fat line of the right apex are well seen on this coronal view. **B**, The precise size and shape of tumor are well shown in sagittal plane.

survival can be achieved in patients discovered to have N2 disease at operation after negative preoperative CT or mediastinoscopy, provided that complete removal of tumor is possible.[104,211–216] In one series, a 5 year survival of 57% was achieved in a subset of patients with N2 disease in whom the nodes were not enlarged by CT criteria and in whom only single level nodes, which could be completely removed at surgery, were involved.[217] Some authors noted more favorable outcomes with squamous carcinoma when compared with other cell types,[108,172,213,215] but most have not found the cell type for nonsmall cell cancers to be a significant factor.[211,212,218–221]

Mediastinal nodal metastases are often present at the time of initial diagnosis of nonsmall cell lung cancers, particularly with adenocarcinomas[222]. Primary tumors >3 cm in diameter (T2 tumors) have a higher incidence of mediastinal nodal involvement than tumors of smaller diameter.[222] Also, the more central the primary tumor, the more likely it is to be accompanied by nodal metastases.

The position of hilar and mediastinal nodes should be described according to the recently unified American Thoracic Society (ATS) and American Joint Committee on Cancer (AJCC) classification as summarized by Mountain and Dresler,[223–225] which uses fixed anatomic landmarks to localize individual nodal stations (see Fig. 2.44). It is worth noting that there is no division into right and left subcarinal stations, so subcarinal nodal disease is always designated N2.

Distinction between nodal stations may be difficult and subject to interobserver variation.[164,180,226,227] The pleural boundaries cannot be resolved at CT, and even at surgery their location varies with the force of retraction.[228] The differentiation between hilar nodes (station 10), which lie outside the mediastinal pleural reflection, and the adjacent tracheobronchial nodes (station 4, e.g. azygos nodes) or subcarinal nodes (station 7), which are contained within the mediastinal pleura, can therefore be problematic, particularly on the right.[104] The differentiation between these locations is, however, of crucial importance because tracheobronchial or subcarinal node involvement converts N1 to N2 disease.[229] This factor may also influence the interpretation of data on the accuracy of imaging techniques.

Spread is usually sequential, first to the ipsilateral segmental, interlobar or lobar intrapulmonary nodes (N1 nodes), then to ipsilateral hilar nodes (N1 nodes), and thereafter to ipsilateral mediastinal nodes (N2), but skip metastases to mediastinal nodes, with clear hilar nodes, are recognized in up to 33% of cases,[230,231] and skip involvement of contralateral mediastinal nodes (N3) is not infrequent.

CT and MRI staging of nodal metastases

The most extensively validated CT sign of lymph node metastasis is nodal enlargement (Fig. 13.33). CT enhancement characteristics have proved to be unhelpful and low density

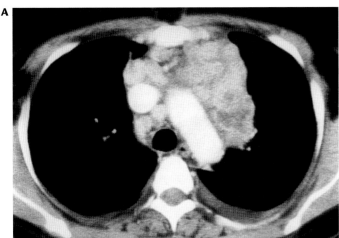

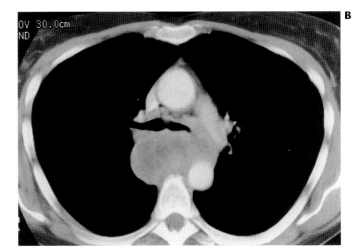

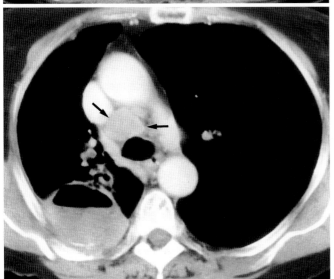

Fig. 13.33 CT of mediastinal lymph node enlargement caused by metastases from a bronchial carcinoma. The enlarged nodes have enhanced to the same degree as muscle following intravenous contrast enhancement. **A**, Massive multifocal lymphadenopathy. **B**, Matted massively enlarged subcarinal, and lower paratracheal nodes. **C**, Greatly enlarged precarinal lymph node (arrows). Note also the chest wall involvement by the primary tumor—a thin walled cavitating carcinoma.

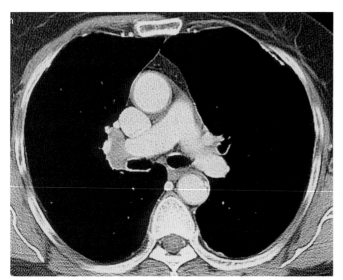

Fig. 13.34 Hilar lymph node metastases from adenocarcinoma of lung shown by contrast-enhanced CT.

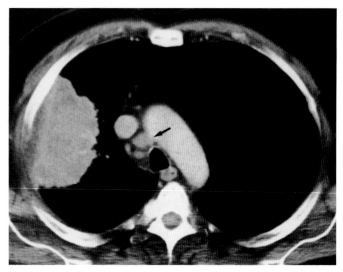

Fig. 13.35 Benign enlargement of mediastinal nodes draining a bronchial carcinoma. The patient had a large squamous cell carcinoma of the lung and enlarged low right paratracheal node (arrow) which measured 1.8 mm in short axis diameter and showed only reactive hyperplasia. (The tumor had not crossed the pleural space despite extensive contact with the chest wall and apparent rib destruction.)

necrotic areas within a node, a good sign of metastatic involvement and one that has proved useful in diagnosing metastases from head and neck tumors in cervical lymph nodes, has proved to be infrequent in mediastinal nodal involvement by lung cancer.

Normal *hilar lymph node size* is below 3 mm in short-axis diameter, except around the left lower lobe artery where they may be up to 7 mm in short axis diameter.[127] Normal nodes show a flat or concave interface with the adjacent lung, whereas nodes which are enlarged due to metastasis show a convex bulge at the pulmonary interface.[232] Metastasis to hilar lymph nodes (N1 disease) (Fig. 13.34), whilst conferring a poorer prognosis, does not preclude potentially curative surgical resection.

Normal *mediastinal lymph node size* at CT varies according to location within the mediastinum[233–237]: normal nodes in the subcarinal and lower paratracheal regions can be up to 11 mm in short axis diameter, with a few reaching 15 mm, whereas normal nodes in the upper paratracheal regions rarely exceed 7 mm. A simple and reasonably accurate rule is that mediastinal nodes smaller than 10 mm in short axis diameter fall within the 95th percentile and should, therefore, be considered normal.

The problem with using size as the only criterion for malignant involvement is that intrathoracic lymph node enlargement has nonmalignant causes, including previous tuberculosis, histoplasmosis, pneumoconiosis, sarcoidosis, and, notably, reactive hyperplasia to the tumor or to associated pneumonia and atelectasis (Figs 13.26 and 13.35). False positive enlargement of mediastinal lymph nodes is more common with centrally located and large primary tumors.[238] One-half to two-thirds of enlarged nodes draining postobstructive pneumonia and atelectasis are free of tumor.[239–241] Indeed these nodes can be remarkably enlarged: in the series by McLoud et al[241] from Boston in the US, 37% of nodes between 2 and 4 cm were hyperplastic and did not contain metastases. Conversely, microscopic involvement by tumor can be present without causing enlargement of affected nodes. The frequency of this phenomenon varies greatly in different series, ranging from 7 to 40%.[212,242–245] It is perhaps worth noting that the frequency of metastatic

involvement in normal sized nodes is significantly higher with central adenocarcinomas than with central squamous cell carcinomas.[246] Therefore, there is no single measurement above which all nodes can be assumed to be malignant and below which all nodes can be considered benign.

The reported sensitivity and specificity of CT for diagnosing mediastinal nodal metastases depends on the nodal diameter used to distinguish normal from abnormal and the thoroughness of mediastinal dissection to provide histologic correlation.[247] Formal mediastinal lymphadenectomy may reveal up to twice the number of positive nodes discovered by limited preoperative sampling.[248–250] Early reports quoted values >85% for sensitivity and specificity, but later studies using complete mediastinal lymphadenectomy and 10 mm short axis diameter as the cut-off measurement for normality obtained figures of the order of 50–65% for both sensitivity and specificity.[168,212,240,241,244,246,251–262] Similar sensitivities but better specificity figures have been obtained from Japan,[255] and some,[263,264] but not all,[265] centers in Europe, probably because the prevalence of coincidental histoplasmosis and other fungal disease is much lower than in the US.

One method of reducing the frequency of false positive interpretations is to ensure that nodes draining the tumor are larger than nodes elsewhere in the mediastinum. By only counting enlarged nodes (>10 mm short axis diameter) that were at least 5 mm greater in diameter than nodes in regions not draining the tumor, Buy et al[263] were able to achieve a 95% positive predictive value for nodal metastatic disease.

Substantial interobserver variation is a further constraint on the performance of CT,[164,180,223] which affects both the measurement of nodal size, and the designation of nodal position.

The utility of chest CT in T1N0M0 cancers, diagnosed on clinical and chest radiographic criteria, is controversial. The prevalence of mediastinal nodal involvement with such small tumors is up to 33%.[266–274,277] A cost-effectiveness analysis

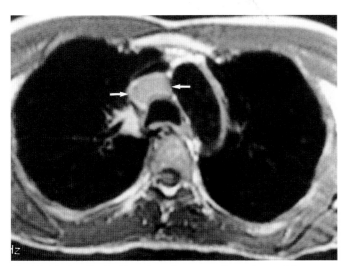

Fig. 13.36 Mediastinal lymph node metastasis causing nodal enlargement (arrows) on axial T1-weighted MRI.

showed that, with current surgical techniques, chest CT would be both clinically useful and cost saving, provided the prevalence of nodal involvement was 12.5% or greater.[275] However, Becker et al[276] showed that routine CT scanning did not correctly alter the stage in any of 38 patients. Daly et al[246] found that the true positive yield in 64 patients with tumors <2 cm in diameter was zero. Others,[268,277] have found evidence for unresectable spread of disease in up to one-third of patients with T1N0M0 nonsmall cell lung cancer based on plain chest films and, therefore, advocate routine preoperative CT. In practice, pre-operative chest CT has become routine in the developed world.

The use of MRI for staging nodal disease relies, like CT, on recognizing nodal enlargement (Fig. 13.36). The considerable overlap of the T1 and T2 relaxation times of benign and malignant lymph nodes prevents the use of unenhanced MR signal intensity for tissue characterization.[154,278] Intravenous gadolinium has not proved useful for distinguishing between chronic inflammation and neoplastic involvement, though one report suggested that enhancement characteristics after intravenous gadolinium could be used to identify nodes infiltrated with squamous cell carcinoma.[279] Newly introduced agents containing ultra small iron particles which are taken up by reticuloendothelial cells in lymph nodes are being investigated. The concept is that nodes replaced by tumor show no signal change, whereas inflammatory nodes take up the agent and show reduced signal on T1-weighted images. Based on early results,[280,281] the problem appears to be that not all the inflammatory nodes in the mediastinum show signal loss, and there are also false negative results. Formal evaluation of sensitivity and specificity is not yet available, because too few cases have been reported.

Potential advantages of MRI over CT are the ability to distinguish lymph nodes from blood vessels owing to the different signal in areas of fast flowing blood, a particular advantage in demonstrating hilar node involvement,[96,154,282] and that coronal, or very occasionally the sagittal imaging plane, may be better than single detector CT images for demonstrating enlargement of aortopulmonary and subcarinal nodes.[147,283] It should be remembered, however, that there are disadvantages to using MRI in order to demonstrate mediastinal nodal enlargement: (1) respiratory or other motion may cause blurring of images and a group of normal sized nodes may, therefore, be misdiagnosed as a single large node (Fig. 13.37)[154]; (2) calcification may be overlooked[167] and, therefore, an enlarged node that would be clearly recognized as benign because of the presence of calcification may be misdiagnosed as metastatic disease; and (3) blood vessels may be misdiagnosed as lymph nodes or masses when they show signal due to slow flow. Several comparisons of single detector CT and MRI have shown similar

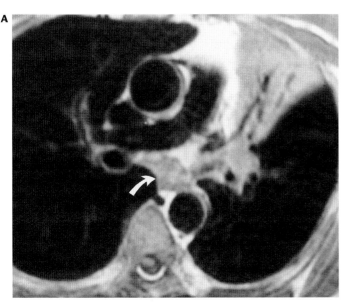

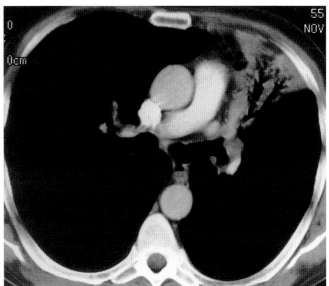

Fig. 13.37 False positive diagnosis of subcarinal lymph node metastasis by MRI. **A**, Axial T1-weighted scan showing a bronchial carcinoma in the left upper lobe bronchus causing atelectasis of the left upper lobe. There appears to be subcarinal lymph node enlargement (arrow), but at surgery the subcarinal nodes were all small and free of tumor. The false positive interpretation is likely to be due to motion artifact which makes several small nodes appear as a single large mass. **B**, CT taken at the same time shows no enlarged subcarinal nodes.

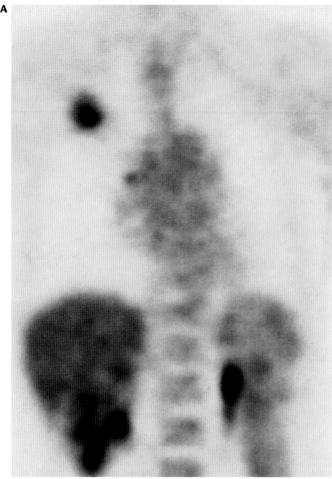

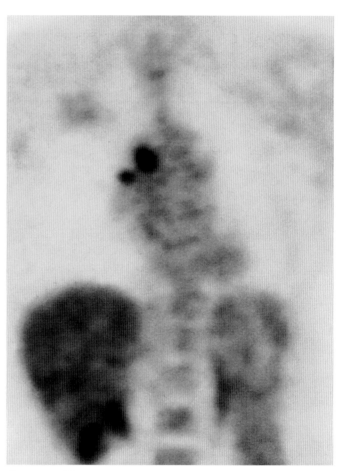

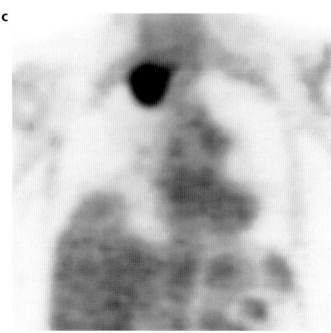

Fig. 13.38 ¹⁸F-FDG PET scan in lung cancer. **A,** Obvious activity in a primary adenocarcinoma in the right upper lobe. **B,** Section slightly anterior to **A,** showing activity in two lower right paratracheal lymph nodes. Surgical biopsy revealed adenocarcinoma in material obtained from the nodes. **C,** Negative scan for hilar and mediastinal nodes in a different patient with a Pancoast tumor at the right apex.

Radionuclide imaging for staging of nodal metastases

Radionuclide imaging techniques, particularly positron emission tomography (PET), are being used increasingly for staging lung carcinoma.

¹⁸F-fluoro-deoxyglucose (FDG), a glucose analog with ¹⁸F substituted for one of the hydroxy groups, is the most widely used PET tracer. It is a marker for glucose metabolism which, after phosphorylation, is not metabolized further but remains trapped within tumor cells. FDG uptake is proportional to the metabolic rate of the cells which take up glucose and correlates with tumor aggressiveness and tumor growth rates.[286,287] The specific criterion for a positive scan (Fig. 13.38) is either greater uptake in the lesion than in the background mediastinum, or a standardized uptake value (SUV) of >2.5 (SUV is quantified as the ratio of the activity per estimated tumor volume compared to the activity administered to the patient, corrected for lean body mass[288]).

The studies published so far have consistently shown significantly greater accuracy of PET compared with CT for the detection or exclusion of mediastinal nodal disease,[148,289–306] and PET has been shown to reduce the rate of futile thoracotomy[307] and to influence patient management decisions.[308] False

accuracies[98,150,154,165,258,284,285] with no difference in interobserver variability. The most thorough study was the Radiologic Diagnostic Oncology Group (RDOG) report, which found sensitivities of 52 and 48%, and specificities of 69 and 64% for CT and MRI, respectively.[168]

positive results are seen less frequently than with CT; the usual cause is inflammation of the lymph nodes due to incidental inflammatory disease or to reactive hyperplasia associated with pneumonia or atelectasis beyond the primary tumor.[309]

In a meta-analysis of 514 patients who had undergone PET and 2226 patients who had undergone CT, the mean sensitivity of PET was 79% and the mean specificity was 91%, compared with 60% and 77% for CT, respectively.[310] FDG PET imaging using a coincidence mode gamma camera has a significantly lower sensitivity and specificity than a dedicated PET scanner.[311,312]

The early reports showed variation in the rigor of nodal sampling and in the spatial resolution of the PET scanners, and further validation of the results will be needed. But several individual studies have been very carefully performed. For example, Steinert et al[293] prospectively compared the accuracy of nodal staging of nonsmall cell lung cancer using FDG PET with that of contrast-enhanced CT in 47 patients suspected of having, or known to have, newly diagnosed nonsmall cell lung cancer. Each nodal station was localized according to the American Thoracic Society mapping system. Extensive lymph node sampling (599 nodes from 191 nodal stations) of the ipsi- and contra-lateral tracheobronchial and mediastinal nodal stations was performed at thoracotomy and/or mediastinoscopy. The results of PET were far superior to CT. The sensitivity of PET was 89% and the specificity was 99%. Importantly, PET correctly assigned the N stage in 96% of cases.

Correlating PET and CT images improves the accuracy of FDG PET compared with viewing the PET images in isolation.[306] For example, Vansteenkiste et al,[296] in a carefully conducted study, compared the accuracy of CT alone and FDG PET plus CT for intrathoracic lymph node staging of 68 patients with potentially operable nonsmall cell lung cancer. The sensitivity of FDG PET plus CT was 93% and the specificity was 95%.

CT and PET image coregistration using computer techniques,[313] or colocation using combined CT and PET scanners, so-called PET/CT machines, will further increase the accuracy of PET scanning.[314,315]

Because of the excellent sensitivity of PET, it has been suggested that invasive mediastinal nodal staging can be substantially reduced when PET is negative for nodal spread (Fig. 13.38),[316,317] particularly when both the PET and CT are normal.[296,318] This recommendation is particularly strong for patients with presumed stage 1 disease.[319] False positive PET images, due to infection, active inflammation, hyperplasia, etc, are sufficiently frequent to justify invasive staging in selected cases when PET is positive.

A decision analysis, using variables based on the literature, showed that a strategy whereby patients with enlarged nodes on chest CT or positive appearances on PET scanning undergo preoperative nodal biopsy, whereas those in whom both the chest CT and the PET scan are normal go direct to thoracotomy, can be cost-effective, compared with basing decisions on CT alone, without denying surgery to patients with resectable disease.[320] The savings come from identifying inoperable patients prior to thoracotomy. A subsequent more detailed analysis from the same center confirmed the cost-effectiveness of adding PET to chest CT over a wide range of variables.[321]

[11]C methionine is an alternative PET agent with better accuracies than CT,[322] and apparently similar to FDG PET.[323] Other PET agents, such as ^{11}C choline, and ^{18}F-deoxy-fluorothymidine (FLT) are also under investigation.[324,325]

Other radionuclide imaging agents have also been tried. [67]Ga has proved to be insensitive and nonspecific in diagnosing the spread of bronchial carcinoma.[256,326–328] [201]Tl, an analog of potassium, and ^{99m}Tc-sestamibi when imaged with single photon emission CT (SPECT), can be used to detect lung cancer metastases in mediastinal lymph nodes.[329–331] These radionuclide tests are reported to have a higher sensitivity and specificity than CT, but lower accuracy than FDG PET.[332] Radiolabeled antibodies that attach to lung cancer cells are also being evaluated with mixed success.[333] NRLU-10 murine antibody has shown promise, with a better sensitivity and specificity than CT in one series,[334] but other agents, such as ^{111}In and ^{99m}Tc labeled monoclonal anti-CEA antibodies have been less accurate.[335–337]

Endoscopic ultrasound for staging nodal metastases

In some centers, transesophageal ultrasound techniques are used to assess both the operability of the primary tumor, and the presence of enlarged nodes.[338–340] The technique is primarily of value in visualizing and sampling the right and left paratracheal (station 2R, 4L and 4R) and subcarinal (station 7) nodes. The information regarding mediastinal lymph node metastases can be significantly more accurate than CT. Endosonographic features of neoplastic involvement of the nodes are rounded rather than oval shape, sharply demarcated border, and inhomogeneous hypoechoic texture, but the major value is to guide trans-esophageal fine needle aspiration of visible nodes.

Spread to distant pulmonary sites

Nonsmall cell lung cancer can metastasize to the lungs.[341] The International Staging System classifies nodules of tumor in the same lobe as T4, whereas tumor nodules in another lobe on the ipsilateral side and all tumor nodules in the contralateral lung are classified as metastases, a distinction that is borne out by evidence that the prognosis of metastases to these different locations corresponds to T4 and M1 respectively.[342]

The likelihood that pulmonary nodules detected by CT during staging for nonsmall cell lung cancer are deposits of tumor is poorly quantified. Keogan et al[343] showed that 16% of 551 patients with potentially operable lung cancer had small noncalcified pulmonary nodules. Adequate follow up was possible in only 25 patients and 70% of the nodules in these 25 patients proved to be benign. Kim et al[344] found that 44% of 141 patients had small (10 mm diameter or less) nodules in lobes other than the lobe containing the primary carcinoma. Only six nodules in these 141 patients were malignant. Yuan et al,[345] in a series of 223 patients with potentially operable lung cancer, over two-thirds of which were adenocarcinomas, found 58 patients with one or two pulmonary nodules <1 cm in diameter, either in the same or another lobe as the lung cancer. In 14 of these 58 patients the additional nodules were malignant, either metastases or synchronous primaries.

Pleural involvement

Lung carcinoma may involve the pleura by direct spread, lymphatic permeation, or tumor emboli.[346]

Visceral pleural invasion carries deleterious prognostic implications compared to tumors that do not invade the pleura.[347] This fact is recognized in the staging system by classifying all tumors that invade the visceral pleura as T2, even those below

3 cm in diameter. A study from Japan found that tumors crossing a fissure to invade the adjacent lobe have the same survival as T3 tumors.[348]

Pleural effusions occur with lung carcinoma of all cell types, but appear to be most frequent with adenocarcinoma.[349] They may be freely mobile or may be loculated. Pleural effusion in association with a primary lung cancer designates the tumor as T4 except in the few patients who have clinical evidence of another cause for the effusion (such as heart failure), and in whom multiple pleural fluid cytologic examinations do not show tumor cells, in which case the effusion can be disregarded as a staging element. The presence of pleural effusion sufficiently large to be recognized at the time of diagnosis on plain chest radiography in patients with lung cancer carries a poor prognosis, however, whether or not malignant cells are identified.[350,351] For example, Decker et al[352] studied 73 patients with bronchogenic carcinoma who had cytologically negative pleural effusions on chest radiography and found that only four had surgically resectable disease. Hemorrhagic effusion on pleural aspiration is a strong indication of direct involvement by tumor.[352]

Attempts to characterize the nature of the pleural fluid based on density measurements at CT or signal intensities at unenhanced MRI have so far not proved useful. There is one report on the use of contrast-enhanced MRI in which all four patients with exudative pleural effusions in association with lung cancer showed significant contrast enhancement of the pleural fluid, whereas no contrast enhancement was seen with the 10 patients with transudative effusions.[353] The authors postulated that the transport of gadolinium DTPA was increased due to the increased permeability of pleural surfaces in the cases with exudative effusion.

FDG PET may be useful in evaluating patients with nonsmall lung cancer and pleural effusion. The examination has proved highly sensitive in two relatively small series,[354,355] but the specificity has yet to be determined because the number of benign effusions in reported series is too small for the results to be meaningful.

The ultrasound demonstration of a pleural mass indicates neoplastic involvement, but other signs, such as echoes or septations within the fluid or sheetlike pleural thickening, are seen in both benign and malignant pleural effusions.[356]

On occasion, bronchial adenocarcinoma takes the form of a sheet of lobular pleural thickening indistinguishable clinically and radiologically from malignant mesothelioma (Fig. 13.39),[357] and may then be designated pseudomesotheliomatous adenocarcinoma of the lung.[358]

Staging lung cancer: a summary

The prime issue for the surgeon is whether the tumor can be completely removed at thoracotomy, whereas the radiotherapist considering radical radiotherapy needs to know that the tumor volume will be encompassed within a suitable radiation field. Disease quantification and therapeutic response are important for radiotherapists and chemotherapists treating patients deemed unsuitable for surgery.

Staging the intrathoracic extent of nonsmall cell lung cancer is a multidisciplinary process employing imaging, bronchoscopy, and biopsy (see Box 13.6). Thoracoscopy can be performed on patients with suspected pleural involvement, and may also play

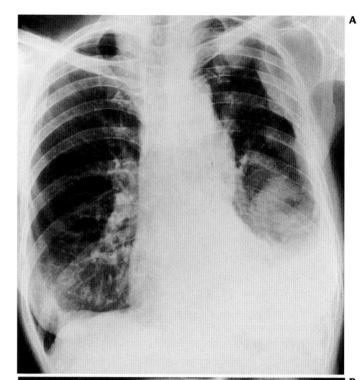

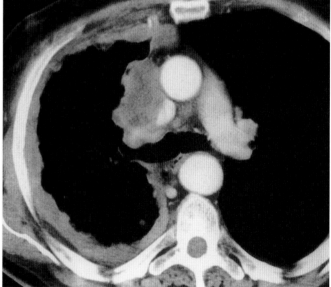

Fig. 13.39 Extensive lobular pleural thickening caused by a bronchial adenocarcinoma in two different patients. Note the resemblance to malignant mesothelioma of pleura. **A,** Chest radiograph shows a sheet of pleural tumor and a left pleural effusion. **B,** CT shows extensive nodular pleural thickening caused by the tumor.

a part in preventing fruitless surgery in patients with no CT evidence of nodal enlargement by enabling inspection of pleural surfaces and access to lower mediastinal nodes.[181] Chest radiography and CT (along with PET scanning in some centers) are currently the routine imaging procedures for assessing intrathoracic spread and determining resectability, with MRI and ultrasound reserved for specific indications. Several reports comparing CT and MRI for staging lung cancer have been published. Based on these, MRI has not demonstrated enough advantages to replace chest CT as a routine staging procedure, though it can, in highly selected patients, be useful as a problem solving technique.

The poor specificity of chest CT for determining nodal involvement must be appreciated. Nodal enlargement, although it may be due to metastatic carcinoma, may also be due to coincidental benign disease or to reactive hyperplasia directly connected to the presence of the tumor. Thus, in practice, CT and MRI examinations for staging nodal involvement are used largely to decide whether to perform mediastinoscopy or mediastinotomy and, equally importantly, to demonstrate which nodes should undergo biopsy. A convenient policy is to consider nodes with a short axis diameter of >10 mm to be abnormal. Nodes above this diameter should be subjected to some form of biopsy. Clearly there are occasions when the chances of a negative biopsy are so slim that a surgeon may decide that the presence of greatly enlarged nodes is sufficient reason not to proceed with surgical resection, but these cases should be the exception to the general rule that the imaging diagnosis of mediastinal nodal metastases should be corroborated by biopsy before a patient is denied potentially curative surgery. Routine mediastinoscopy provides access only to the paratracheal nodes, proximal tracheobronchial nodes, and superior subcarinal nodes. The other nodal sites require alternative approaches such as mediastinotomy. These other sites include nodal stations with a high propensity to early metastases, such as the aortopulmonary and anterior mediastinal nodes.

Some thoracic surgeons believe it appropriate to proceed to thoracotomy without prior mediastinoscopy or mediastinotomy in patients with normal sized mediastinal nodes.[129,212] Others advocate routine mediastinoscopy even in those patients whose CT scans do not show enlarged nodes.[265,359,360] A randomized controlled trial of the use of CT in 685 patients with apparently operable lung cancer (with mediastinoscopy for those patients who showed enlarged nodes and thoracotomy without prior mediastinoscopy for those who showed no enlarged nodes) versus no CT (all patients having mediastinoscopy) showed that the strategy of using CT to determine which patients should have mediastinoscopy is likely to produce the same number or fewer unnecessary thoracotomies in comparison with doing mediastinoscopy on all patients, and is also likely to be as or less expensive.[361] Another argument against routine preoperative mediastinoscopy of patients with normal sized nodes is that, as discussed on page 806, patients with microscopic metastases discovered only at the time of thoracotomy have an improved survival rate if the primary tumor and the affected mediastinal nodes are resected.

PET scanning has proved significantly more accurate than CT for diagnosing or excluding mediastinal nodal metastases, but has not obviated the need for histological confirmation of nodal involvement when the PET scan is positive. Patients with no enlarged nodes on CT and no abnormal uptake of FDG on PET have such a low incidence of nodal involvement that mediastinoscopy is very unlikely indeed to be positive and can be omitted.

For lung cancers that have invaded the mediastinum or chest wall, the important decision is whether the tumor is nevertheless resectable for possible cure, recognizing the poorer prognosis compared with tumors confined to the lung. CT may show definitively that the tumor is too extensive for resective surgery. Alternatively, CT may leave the issue in doubt, and MRI can then be used as a problem solving modality, but the introduction of multiplanar CT has significantly reduced the number of occasions when MRI is needed. In practice, the use of MRI is largely limited to evaluating superior sulcus tumors, to define brachial plexus and subclavian and axillary artery involvement, and for establishing vertebral body involvement.[122]

The most important single message is that patients with primary nonsmall cell lung cancer should not be denied potentially curative surgery based on indeterminate imaging findings.

Imaging extrathoracic metastases from bronchial carcinoma

A reasonable approach for patients with no clinical features to suggest extrathoracic metastases is to extend the staging chest CT to image the liver and adrenals.[362] In most centers no further routine imaging is undertaken, and there is good evidence to support this approach.[122,304,363,364] In centers where FDG PET imaging is readily available, it should be used.

The wider availability of FDG PET imaging will probably change the approach to diagnosing asymptomatic extrathoracic metastases, because it is a single test which can encompass all the organs in the body. The results so far suggest higher accuracy than CT, MRI, ultrasound, or most other radionuclide procedures for all body sites, apart from the brain. In particular, PET has been shown to be highly sensitive.[298,300,303,365,366] Even better results are anticipated with the introduction of PET CT fusion imaging.

Whole body PET alters management in a significant proportion of patients, the proportion ranging from 24 to 65%.[298,367–369] However, few studies have addressed the potential cost-effectiveness of routine preoperative PET screening. A recent randomized prospective trial in 188 patients with suspected operable nonsmall cell lung cancer showed that the addition of PET to the conventional work-up prevented unnecessary thoracotomy in 20%.[369]

Nine studies comprising 837 patients examining the utility of FDG PET were reviewed by Shon et al.[302] FDG PET detected 94% of all metastases, considerably higher than a combination of the other standard tests. PET was the only modality to correctly exclude metastatic disease in 53 patients in whom other imaging had suggested metastases. Put another way,[370] FDG PET has been shown to detect occult extrathoracic metastases in 11–14% of patients selected for curative resection by conventional methods,[299,371] with two studies[365,371] having no false positive results. Higher detection rates are seen with more advanced tumors.[372]

FDG PET is relatively poor at detecting cerebral metastases, probably due to the high background activity of normal brain.[299,302,373] But the accuracy of FDG PET for detecting bone and adrenal metastases has been shown to be good. PET is superior to ^{99m}Tc radionuclide bone scintigraphy for the detection of bone metastases. It had a 92% sensitivity and a 99% specificity compared with 50 and 92% for bone scans, respectively, in one series.[299] Apart from issues of availability and cost, the level of accuracy of PET could potentially eliminate the need for radionuclide bone scans altogether. No specific studies on liver metastases or more unusual metastatic sites have yet been published, but the results from whole body imaging using PET suggest it is much more sensitive than CT and is also more specific.[302]

Liver metastases

The presence of clinical and laboratory features suggestive of liver disease has only a 25% positive predictive value for metastases.[374]

The advent of spiral and multidetector CT provides rapid scanning with several technical advantages, including the optimal use of intravenous contrast medium, the limitation of respiratory misregistration, and the reduction of partial volume averaging by using overlapping image reconstruction or retrospective thin sections. The use of narrow reconstruction intervals can result in an increased detection rate of small lesions. An accepted figure for the accuracy of CT in detecting metastatic disease, extrapolated from studies of colorectal tumors,[375,376] is approximately 85%, and given the appropriate circumstances biopsy confirmation is not usually required. A major diagnostic problem is distinguishing between small metastases and incidental benign lesions, such as simple cysts/hemangiomas.

Ultrasound is also a suitable method to search for liver metastases, although it is less sensitive than CT. Most deposits are hypoechoic, although hyperechoic and targetlike appearances occur.

Recent technical advances mean that body MRI is now comparable, if not superior, to CT for imaging colorectal liver metastases,[377,378] and by extrapolation this is also likely to be true for liver metastases from lung cancer. Greater tissue contrast results in increased sensitivity for the detection of metastases. However, the cost and speed limitations of MRI mean that it is currently reserved to solve specific problems.

Adrenal metastases

The adrenal gland is a common site for metastasis.[374,379] However, incidental nonfunctioning adrenocortical adenomas are relatively common in patients undergoing CT, with a frequency of approximately 1%.[380] A small solitary adrenal nodule in a patient with nonsmall cell lung cancer is more likely to be an incidental benign adenoma than a metastasis.[379] MRI is a useful non-invasive method of diagnosing a benign adenoma. A study of 546 patients with lung cancer found one or more adrenal masses in 22(4%) of patients. On percutaneous biopsy only 5 of the 22 nodules of these proved to be malignant.[381] The relative incidence of benign adenoma and metastasis reverses when an adrenal mass is >2 cm in size.

Given that there is a substantial chance that an adrenal mass of <2 cm will be an incidental adenoma,[379] the diagnosis of metastasis must be confirmed with a high degree of certainty in order to prevent an otherwise operable patient being denied surgery. In some instances image guided percutaneous aspiration biopsy may be performed for definitive diagnosis.[381]

Brain metastases

MRI of the brain is more sensitive and may be more specific for metastases than CT.[382] Yokoi et al[383] showed that MRI was more sensitive than CT and detected smaller metastases.

Cerebral metastases occur commonly in lung cancer, particularly from poorly differentiated tumors and adenocarcinoma.[374,384] MRI with contrast enhancement is the imaging modality of choice.[383] It has particular advantages in the posterior fossa and adjacent to the skull.

The incidence of a truly "silent" brain metastasis is difficult to determine, and may be of the order of 2–4%,[385] though it depends on the thoroughness of clinical examination and method of detection. There is some logic in limiting cerebral imaging to those patients with the more aggressive histologic types of primary tumors.[362]

Bone metastases

Bone metastases are a relatively frequent finding at clinical presentation in patients with lung cancer, although the frequencies vary widely between series.[374,386] Bone scintigraphy is considerably more sensitive than plain radiography for their detection.[387] However, radionuclide bone scans have a high false positive rate because of the presence of coincidental benign skeletal disorders, notably old trauma and degenerative disease, and this limits their value. The prevalence of asymptomatic bone deposits detected by radionuclide bone scan is probably of the order of 3–10%. One study of potentially operable nonsmall cell cancers demonstrated bone metastases in 3.4% of patients on radionuclide bone scans. Ichinose et al[388] studied the bone scans of 196 patients with nonsmall cell lung cancer.[388] Metastatic bone disease was identified in just under 10% and subsequently proven on biopsy or follow up. Of these true positive scans for metastases, 94% of patients were symptomatic or had abnormal biochemistry.[388] Another study similarly showed that all patients with proven skeletal metastases had at least one clinical or biochemical indicator of bone involvement,[389] emphasizing that bone scintigraphy should in general only be performed in patients with symptoms suggesting bone metastases.

MRI is both sensitive and specific for diagnosing skeletal metastases, but it is not a cost-effective approach, because currently in most centers, each region of the body must be imaged as a separate examination.

Imaging patterns of lung cancer according to cell type

The imaging patterns of bronchial carcinoma vary with cell type.[390] Certain generalizations can be made, but clearly the imaging findings are no substitute for histologic examination. Bronchioloalveolar carcinoma is considered separately in the following section, because it shows significant differences from cancers of the other major cell types.[391]

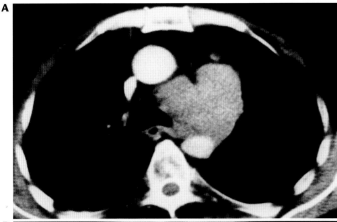

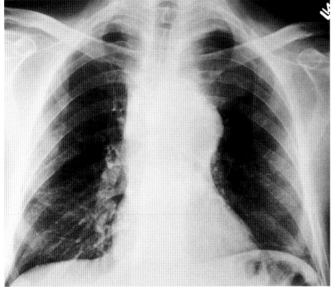

Fig. 13.40 **A**, Chest radiograph and **B**, CT of a small cell carcinoma showing massive mediastinal adenopathy. The primary tumor, which was centrally located in the bronchial tree, is not visible radiographically.

Early, often massive, lymphadenopathy and direct mediastinal invasion are well-recognized phenomena in both small (Fig. 13.40) and large cell carcinoma. Woodring and Stelling[357] have pointed out that adenocarcinoma appears to be changing its pattern and often shows hilar and mediastinal adenopathy,[228] although the nodal enlargement is not as massive as with small and large cell tumors. A mass in, or adjacent to, the hilum is a particular characteristic of small cell carcinoma (Fig. 13.18).

A peripheral nodule is common in adenocarcinoma, adenosquamous carcinoma (76% of cases), and large cell tumors, including large cell neuroendocrine carcinomas[392]; the largest peripheral masses are seen with squamous and large cell tumors, whereas most peripheral adenocarcinomas and small cell carcinomas are <4 cm in diameter.[393,394] Squamous cell cancers may attain great size, and they cavitate much more frequently than cancers of other cell types (Fig. 13.41).[71]

The majority of adenocarcinomas develop in the periphery of the lung and are associated with adjacent pulmonary scarring and indrawing of the pleura. A spiculated outline, which pathologically may correspond to a desmoplastic reaction, lymphangitic response, or direct tumor extension, is a common

finding on CT, particularly on HRCT.[58,76,78] Fine air bronchograms or bubble-like lucencies are fairly frequently present on HRCT.[58,76,78] The tumor itself may be of soft tissue density or may show a core of soft tissue density, the periphery of the nodule being of ground-glass density. (An adenocarcinoma which is of pure ground-glass density is likely to be a bronchioloalveolar carcinoma, a topic discussed immediately below.)

Collapse and consolidation of the lung beyond the tumor are the most frequent features of squamous cell carcinoma, in keeping with the predominantly central origin of this neoplasm.

Bronchioloalveolar carcinoma

The WHO classifies bronchioloalveolar carcinoma, also known as alveolar cell carcinoma or bronchiolar carcinoma, as a subtype of adenocarcinoma.[2] (The somewhat confusingly named intravascular bronchioloalveolar tumor is a separate entity and is discussed on p. 52 Ch. 13.) Some published series contain a mixture of pure bronchioloalveolar carcinoma and adenocarcinoma with bronchioloalveolar features, leading to confusion over imaging findings and survival characteristics.[395] Bronchioloalveolar carcinomas are divided into: (1) nonmucinous; (2) mucinous; and (3) mixed mucinous and nonmucinous (indeterminate cell type) subsets. Cigarette smoking does not appear to play a prominent etiologic role,[396] but the prevalence of this tumor within preexisting lung scars is striking.[40]

Bronchioloalveolar carcinomas account for some 2–5% of all lung cancers, but with smoking on the decline the relative incidence of bronchioloalveolar carcinoma in some series is rising.[5] The tumor occurs equally in both sexes, and the average age at onset is between 55 and 65 years. The characteristic pathologic feature is a peripheral neoplasm showing lepidic growth, the malignant cells using the surrounding alveolar walls as a scaffold. These tumors are believed to arise from type II pneumocytes and probably also from bronchiolar epithelium,[346] or a common stem cell. The cells produce mucus, sometimes in such large amounts that one of the presenting symptoms in the consolidative form of the disease is bronchorrhea, namely the expectoration of large quantities of mucoid sputum.

The tumor presents in two clinically different forms: a discrete solitary pulmonary nodule (sometimes more than one nodule is present), and unifocal or multifocal areas of pulmonary consolidation; the form presenting with a solitary pulmonary nodule being the more common.[396–398] The mucinous type is more likely to be seen as airspace consolidation and the nonmucinous type is more likely to be masslike in configuration and associated with secondary scarring and inflammation, but there is no exact correlation between the cell type and the imaging appearance.[3,399] The scarring may lead to difficulties in determining whether the carcinoma is an invasive adenocarcinoma with a prominent bronchioloalveolar growth pattern or a bronchioloalveolar carcinoma associated with scarring.[400]

Pathologists may find it difficult to distinguish histologically between the nonmucinous form of bronchioloalveolar carcinoma and atypical adenomatous hyperplasia, a benign proliferation of bronchioloalveolar cells that is believed to be a precursor lesion to adenocarcinoma. This difficulty translates to interobserver variability in the diagnosis of these two conditions, a problem discussed further in the section Population screening for bronchial carcinoma later in this chapter.

The prognosis for bronchioloalveolar carcinoma when it occurs as a solitary pulmonary nodule is better than that seen

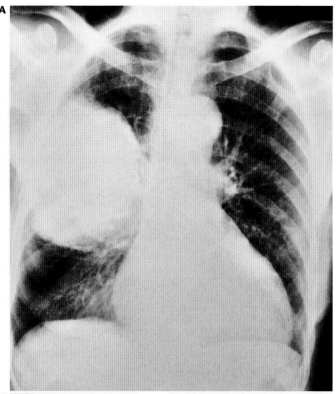

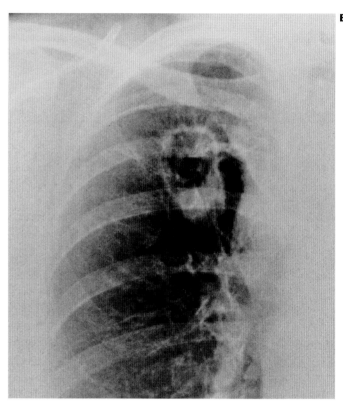

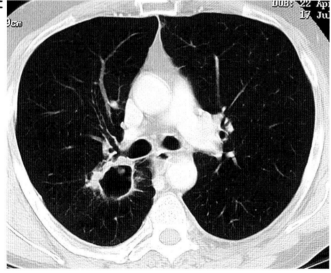

Fig. 13.41 Squamous cell carcinoma of the bronchus **A**, illustrating the huge size these tumors may attain before first discovery and **B**, occurring as cavitating mass. **C**, CT in a similar patient. Part of the wall is very thin and smooth in both **B** and **C**.

with other lung cancer cell types.[401] It is more likely to be stage I and therefore surgically resectable. Also, the tumor is relatively slow growing,[396] so that 5 year survivals are better, regardless of stage.[402] Bronchioloalveolar carcinomas <2 cm in diameter, showing a purely lepidic growth pattern without invasion, had no lymph node metastases and 100% 5 and 10 year survival in one series.[400] The prognosis for the larger, more ill-defined lesion, which radiographically resembles pneumonia, and for the disseminated form are both poor.[398,403]

Imaging[40,88,404]

Because bronchioloalveolar carcinomas arise from the alveoli and the immediately adjacent small airways, they tend to appear as

peripheral pulmonary opacities. The most common appearance is a solitary lobulated or spiculated pulmonary nodule of soft tissue density indistinguishable from other types of carcinoma (Fig. 13.42).[405–407] There is a propensity to a subpleural location and the development of a pleuropulmonary tail; the tail is due to desmoplastic reaction in the peripheral septa of the lung.[88,407]

The nodular form may show a definite air bronchogram, a phenomenon that is best seen with CT,[404,406] particularly HRCT.[405,408] Bubble-like lucencies corresponding to patent small bronchi or air-containing cystic lucencies are a frequent finding.[78,404–406,408] The bubbles, as in the nodular form, correspond pathologically to small patent bronchi or cystic spaces within the tumor.[409] It is a particular feature of the goblet

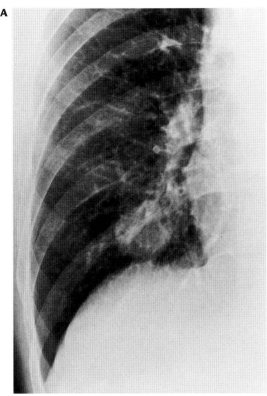

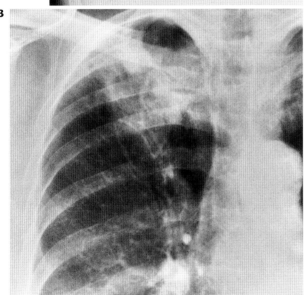

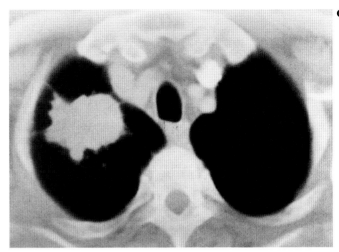

Fig. 13.42 Two examples of a bronchioloalveolar carcinoma occurring as a solitary pulmonary nodule or mass. **A**, Chest radiograph in a 47-year-old asymptomatic man. **B**, In a different patient, an ill-defined tumor that resembles pneumonia is seen, but **C**, on CT the lesion is clearly a lobular mass with irregular edges.

cell subtype of bronchioloalveolar carcinoma.[410] The tumor may be composed entirely of ground-glass density or there may be a halo of ground-glass density, surrounding the central soft tissue density.[74,404,405,411,412] Frank cavitation, however, is unusual, but an appearance resembling cavitation may be produced by paracicatricial emphysema, fibrosis with honeycombing, and localized bronchiectasis.[413]

The radiographic presentation that distinguishes bronchioloalveolar carcinoma from the other types of lung cancer is when the lesion takes the form of single or multiple areas of consolidation or ill-defined opacities. Bronchorrhea is a recognized clinical manifestation. A variety of radiographic, CT, and HRCT appearances are seen with this form of the disease[399,407,414]: (1) ill-defined consolidation, resembling pneumonia (Fig. 13.43); (2) pure ground-glass opacity[404,411,412,415]; (3) ground-glass opacity surrounding a core of soft tissue density; (4) mixed ground-glass opacity and denser consolidation[395]; (5) homogeneous consolidation of one or more lobes (Fig. 13.44)[403]; (6) multifocal patchy consolidation[416]; (7) or multiple ill-defined nodules spread widely through multiple lobes in one or both lungs, which may show a centrilobular distribution on HRCT (Fig. 13.45).[414] More than one of these patterns is often present simultaneously.[414] Extensive, patchy, ground-glass opacity and septal thickening, resembling alveolar proteinosis, has also been described (Fig. 13.45).[417,418] Both atelectasis and expansile consolidation (Fig. 13.46) have been reported.[419]

Cavitation within consolidation is unusual but has been recorded, as have multiple thin walled cystic lesions at CT within or coexistent with the consolidative form of bronchioloalveolar carcinoma.[414,420] In one reported case the wall of a preexisting lung cavity became thickened, presumably by tumor growing around the wall of the cavity.[419]

Air bronchograms may be an obvious feature (Figs 13.43 and 13.45); they are particularly well demonstrated by CT.[408] The bronchi may show uniform narrowing and stretching.[421] CT may show a "bubble-like pattern" (sometimes referred to as "pseudocavitation") (Figs 13.43 and 13.45) in the consolidative as well as the nodular form.[78]

Thickened septal lines caused by lymphatic permeation may also be visible, as may branching tubular densities of mucoid impaction.[419] Mucus within the tumor may be visible as ground-glass opacity at CT.[408]

Differentiating between the consolidative forms of bronchioloalveolar carcinoma and various non-neoplastic conditions, such as pulmonary infection, organizing pneumonia, aspiration, or pulmonary edema, depends on knowing the clinical findings and appreciating the lack of response to treatment. The presence of coexistent nodules along with the consolidation and a

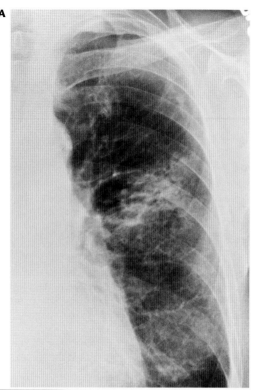

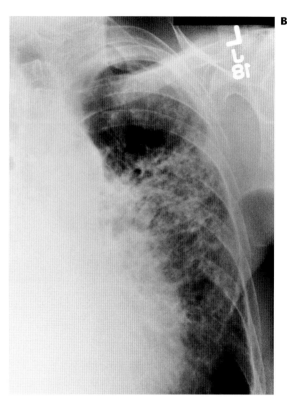

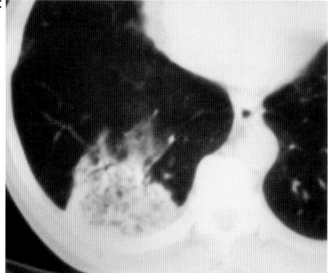

Fig. 13.43 A bronchioloalveolar cell carcinoma appearing as an ill-defined opacity with air bronchograms. **A**, Chest radiograph at initial examination and **B**, 7 months later. Note the resemblance of each individual image to pneumonia. The time course is a major clue to the diagnosis of neoplasm. **C**, CT in another patient showing the "air bronchogram/bubbly pattern" that is often seen with bronchioloalveolar carcinoma.

peripheral distribution proved to be a statistically significant predictor of bronchioloalveolar carcinoma rather than pneumonia.[422] In another study, stretching and squeezing of air bronchograms traversing the consolidated areas, and bulging of fissures, were significantly more frequent in bronchioloalveolar carcinoma than in pneumonia.[423] The appearances have also been compared to tuberculous pneumonia, and it was shown that while both entities had a similar combination of signs, the ground-glass opacity in bronchioloalveolar carcinoma tended to be remote from the consolidation, whereas in tuberculosis it was adjacent.[414]

Also, the pulmonary abnormalities showed a lower lobe predominance in bronchioloalveolar carcinoma, but an upper lung predominance in tuberculosis.

An interesting sign is the CT angiogram sign. It refers to clearly visible vessels coursing through the tumor on contrast-enhanced images, presumably because of the contrast against the background of abundant low density mucus within the neoplasm. This sign was described before the advent of faster injection rates for contrast agent consequent on spiral CT; it was present in a high proportion of patients with lobar consolidation caused by bronchioloalveolar cell carcinoma, but was unusual in

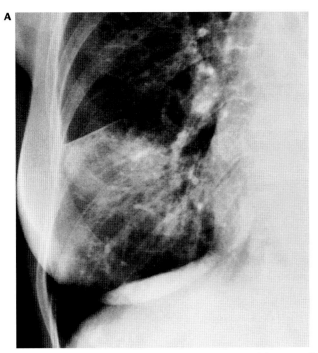

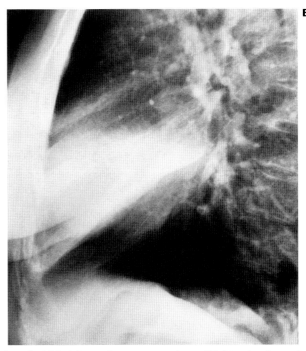

Fig. 13.44 Bronchioloalveolar cell carcinoma occurring as lobar consolidation of middle lobe on **A**, posteroanterior and **B**, lateral radiographs. The patient complained of coughing up copious amounts of mucoid sputum.

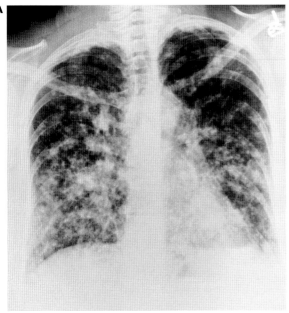

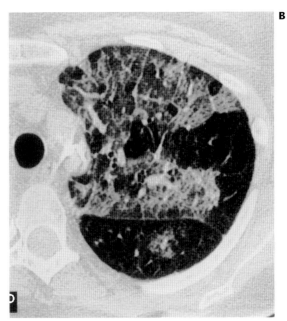

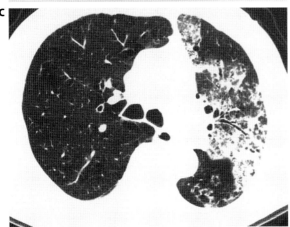

Fig. 13.45 Bronchioloalveolar cell carcinoma presenting as **A**, widespread ill-defined patchy areas of consolidation, **B**, multifocal ground-glass shadowing with intervening thickened interlobular septa, and **C**, focal mixed ground glass and consolidation with air bronchograms and a "bubble-like pattern".

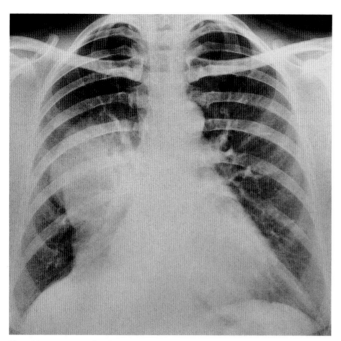

Fig. 13.46 Bronchioloalveolar cell carcinoma presenting as expansile consolidation of the right lower lobe.

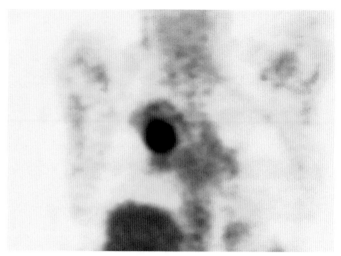

Fig. 13.47 ^{18}F-FDG PET scan showing considerable activity in a recurrent lung cancer following radiotherapy treatment.

consolidation from other causes.[424] The sign is now regarded as nonspecific, since it is seen in many conditions, notably pneumonia and lymphoma.[425,426]

Pleural effusions are seen in up to one-third of patients, and hilar and mediastinal lymphadenopathy is seen in close to one-fifth.

CT scanning is advocated as a routine before surgery in all patients with the consolidative form of disease to make sure that the tumor is confined to one lobe, since CT frequently shows further pulmonary foci that are not appreciated on plain chest radiographs.[427]

MRI provides little extra information compared to CT. Ground-glass shadowing, an important CT feature, is not visible on MRI, but very heavily T2-weighted sequences can show the presence of mucin as high signal.[428] The nodular forms of the tumor show enhancement following gadolinium enhancement.[428]

Bronchioloalveolar carcinomas may grow slowly, with doubling times far greater than the 18 months usually quoted as the upper limit for bronchial carcinoma.[88] Similarly, reflecting the slow growth and hence relatively low metabolic activity, FDG PET shows less uptake in bronchioloalveolar carcinoma than other cell types and may be negative.[417,429]

Recurrence of treated bronchial carcinoma

There are only one or two reports in the literature on imaging local recurrence of the primary tumor following treatment and no generally accepted imaging protocols for follow up of patients who have been, or are undergoing treatment for lung cancer. It needs to be borne in mind that recurrent tumor is rarely amenable to cure; a retrospective survey of the experience at the M D Anderson Hospital in the United States showed that only 3% of patients with recurrent tumor were even offered potentially

curative treatment.[430] Also, the survival benefit of any form of routine imaging follow up has yet to be demonstrated.[431] Routine CT or MRI are not recommended, because they are both insensitive and nonspecific for detecting posttreatment recurrence; the only recommended follow-up modality for asymptomatic patients is chest radiography,[432] and possibly radionuclide imaging, notably FDG PET.

The signs of local recurrence on chest radiography, CT, and MRI are, in general, similar to those used to diagnose the original tumor. CT has been shown to be significantly more sensitive than plain chest radiography.[433] The general principle is recognizing or being able to exclude an abnormal mass, particularly a growing mass, or enlarging mediastinal lymph nodes.[434,435] This is relatively easy to do following segmental resection, or lobectomy, because these two surgical procedures do not, in general, lead to confusing degrees of scar formation. Following pneumonectomy or radiation therapy, however, posttreatment fibrosis can make it very difficult to distinguish benign scar tissue from recurrent tumor. The consolidation and fibrosis of radiation pneumonitis may be impossible to distinguish from neoplastic tissue.[436,437] Libshitz et al[435] made the interesting observation that opacification of previously air-filled dilated bronchi in areas of postradiation fibrosis is a reliable sign of locally recurrent lung cancer.

Radionuclide imaging, notably FDG PET, would appear to be the most accurate technique for diagnosing recurrent tumor.[438–442] Since all forms of radionuclide imaging depend on the altered function of neoplastic cells rather than disordered anatomy, the distorted scarred background is not an impediment to diagnosis (Fig. 13.47). Shon et al[302] in a recent review of the literature stated that FDG PET has been shown to be highly sensitive in the detection of recurrent lung cancer with sensitivities ranging from 97 to 100%, but the false positive rate, whilst not as poor as with CT or MRI, could be as high as 40%. The advice is to wait at least 3 months, and preferably 6 months, after completion of radiotherapy before performing FDG PET imaging in order to avoid false positive results due to radiation fibrosis and glycolysis in macrophages in successfully treated tumors.[302,442] Sequential scans can reduce the false positive observations because uptake in non-neoplastic tissue decreases with time.

Atypical adenomatous hyperplasia

Atypical adenomatous hyperplasia (also called bronchioloalveolar adenoma – there are many other synonyms, including atypical alveolar cuboidal cell hyperplasia, alveolar epithelial hyperplasia, and atypical alveolar hyperplasia) is a relatively recently described pulmonary neoplasm. The lesion is defined by the WHO[2] as "a focal lesion, often 5 mm or less in diameter, in which the involved alveoli and respiratory bronchioles are lined by monotonous, slightly atypical, cuboidal to low columnar epithelial cells with dense nuclear chromatin, inconspicuous nucleoli and scant cytoplasm". Atypical adenomatous hyperplasia was originally reported as an incidental discovery in autopsy patients without lung cancer, and in up to 10% of lobes removed from patients who had had surgery for bronchial carcinoma, notably adenocarcinomas.[443–445]

The precise nature of the lesion is debated. The debate centers on whether the condition is a highly differentiated adenocarcinoma and part of a continuous spectrum with nonmucinous bronchioloalveolar carcinoma, or whether the lesion is a potentially malignant benign neoplasm, i.e. a precursor to bronchioloalveolar carcinoma/adenocarcinoma.[446–456] The lesions are mostly too small and of insufficient density to be seen on chest radiography, but they can be seen on CT as a round area of ground-glass density, usually <10 mm, but sometimes as large as 32 mm in diameter.[446,457,458] There may be a solid portion of soft tissue density in the center of the ground-glass density in up to 27% of cases.[455]

Atypical adenomatous hyperplasia is being reported in a small proportion of patients in lung cancer CT screening programs.

Population screening for bronchial carcinoma

The underlying concept of an early lung cancer detection program is that more cures are achieved when stage I tumors are found in asymptomatic individuals, since the surgical results and 5 year survival figures are much better, compared to patients who first present with symptoms and those who have more advanced tumors. Considerably more than half of all patients currently present with stage III disease or higher and it is well accepted that the overall average 5 year survival is somewhere between 13 and 15%,[459,460] whereas 5 year survival rates for Stage 1A nonsmall cell carcinomas are 67% or better.[102,104]

It is generally held that the measure of success of a lung cancer screening program should be reduced mortality from lung cancer rather than improved 5 year survival, which suffers from leadtime bias (see below). It has, however, been suggested that other outcome measures are more appropriate, notably fatality rate and all cause mortality (see Table 13.6 for definitions). The major problem with using fatality rates is inherent overdiagnosis bias: if lesions that grow too slowly to kill the patient during their natural life expectancy are included in the denominator, the proportionate number of deaths is reduced and the test appears more beneficial than if only truly life-threatening cancers are included. All-cause mortality is a good

Table 13.6 Definition of the terms survival, mortality, fatality, and all-cause mortality with respect to screening

Survival	Number diagnosed with cancer alive/Total number diagnosed with cancer (%)
Mortality	Number of cancer deaths/Total number screened or in control group (deaths per 1000 per year)
Fatality	Number of cancer deaths/Number of cancers detected (%)
All-cause	Number of deaths/Number of patients screened (deaths per 1000 per Mortality year)

measure, but is only a true guide in meticulously randomized trials.

Biases in cancer screening programs

The presumption that earlier diagnosis necessarily equates to a decrease in mortality from lung cancer is simplistic because there are so many variables to take into account.[461–466]

Screening programs which are compared simply to historic or nonrandom controls suffer from three fundamental biases: leadtime bias, length bias, and overdiagnosis bias. Such programs have the following characteristics: earlier stage at diagnosis, improved resectability rates, and improved survival, but no change in the number of late stage tumors and, most importantly, no reduction in mortality from the tumor. The inherent biases can be minimized by comparing disease specific deaths (deaths due to lung cancer) in a randomized controlled trial of a screened versus a nonscreened population with sufficiently long follow up to compensate for leadtime bias. A fourth potential bias operates even in randomized trials, namely selection bias, where conclusions may be based on series of patients in whom the randomization procedures do not result in truly similar groups which may not be representative of the population at large.

The term "leadtime bias" refers to the extra life expectancy that occurs simply from diagnosing a tumor earlier, regardless of whether or not treatment is effective. In other words, moving the time of diagnosis of a lung cancer forward inevitably improves 5 year survival, which is calculated from the time of diagnosis, regardless of the effect on mortality.

The term "length bias" refers to the tendency for tumors with an inherently better prognosis, e.g. slow growing bronchioloalveolar carcinoma, to be discovered by population screening, particularly on the first round (referred to in screening parlance as the "prevalence" round). An indication that length bias can be a highly significant factor is the observation that the volume-doubling times of the lung cancers found in one of the two large Japanese CT screening programs was a mean of 15 months (range 1–40 months)[467]; by way of comparison the vast majority of lung cancers found by means other than CT screening double their volume with median times of between 4 and 7 months.[83–87,468]

The term "overdiagnosis bias" refers to overdiagnosing a benign lesion as a malignant tumor, or diagnosing a very slow growing malignancy that would not kill the patient during his or her natural life expectancy.[469] Overdiagnosis bias is an extreme form of length bias. Atypical adenomatous hyperplasia (believed to be either a benign process or a preinvasive carcinoma – see preceding section) is found in a small but significant proportion of patients in all CT screening programs.[449,457] It resembles the nonmucinous form of bronchioloalveolar carcinoma histologically,[3,453] and histopathologists vary considerably among themselves over whether they designate very small lung lesions as atypical adenomatous hyperplasia, or whether they classify the lesion in question as invasive carcinoma. Another possible pointer to overdiagnosis in CT screening is that in one of the Japanese screening studies the rate of detection of lung cancer was similar among smokers and non-smokers,[470] whereas mortality from lung cancer is heavily slanted to smokers.

The arguments against overdiagnosis being a significant factor center on: (1) the comparatively few lung cancers demonstrated at screening CT of high risk populations (the highest reported prevalence in population screening is 2.7%[471]), and on preoperative CTs of patients undergoing lung volume reduction surgery for emphysema (where the lung cancer detection rate is between 2 and 5%[472–475]); and (2) the low incidence of previously unsuspected indolent cancers at routine autopsy of older individuals.[476] The reply from those who believe that overdiagnosis is a significant factor is that small lung cancers are not looked for carefully enough at routine autopsy, and evidence has been provided to support the claim that the true incidence is higher than reported.[477]

There is conflicting data regarding survival and fatality from the small tumors likely to be found by population screening with CT. Patz et al,[478] rather than ask "does population screening diagnose lung cancer earlier?", investigated whether there was any correlation between survival and precise size in 510 patients with tumors <3 cm in diameter without nodal or distant metastases (T1N0M0 or Stage 1A tumors). Rather unexpectedly, they found no correlation, in other words the patients with lung cancers <1 cm in diameter did not show better survival than patients whose tumors were 2–3 cm in diameter. Their point was that survival following surgical resection from lung cancer is complex and multifactorial, depending not only on tumor size and stage, but also on tumor biology, the ability of body defense systems to cope with micrometastases and a variety of other host factors.[479] Koike at al,[266] on the other hand, found that 5 year survival for patients with tumors <2 cm in diameter was significantly better than for patients with tumors between 2 and 3 cm in diameter, a difference that could be explained by leadtime bias alone, particularly as there was no significant difference in the rate of mediastinal nodal involvement between the two groups. Henschke et al[480] approached the same basic question in yet another way by analyzing the 8 year fatality rate of unresected T1 lung cancers of varying size in the NIH Surveillance, Epidemiology, and End Results (SEER) registry and found that almost all lung cancers, even those <15 mm in diameter, are fatal if not treated.

Screening for lung cancer using plain chest radiography

Two large randomized controlled trials of population screening using chest radiography have been undertaken, the National Cancer Institute (NCI) Mayo Lung Project[481–483] and the Czechoslovakian study,[484] as well as a number of trials of less rigorous design.[485–491] The results have been broadly similar.

The multicenter survey conducted by the NCI between 1971 and 1983 has been extensively analyzed and is the only one that will be discussed in any detail. From a population of approximately 10,000 high risk patients at each of three centers (men over 45 years of age who were chronic, excessive cigarette smokers), 0.73% had lung cancer diagnosed at their initial screening.[481,482,492–496] After excluding nearly 1000 individuals who were ruled ineligible because of serious medical problems, the Mayo Clinic portion of the study randomly assigned half of those who did not have cancer at the initial screening to surveillance by chest radiography and sputum cytology every 4 months, and the remaining half, who served as control subjects, were recommended to have annual chest radiographs and sputum cytology.[482,497] The rate of cancer diagnosis in the screened group was 5.5 per 1000 per year, compared with 4.3 per 1000 per year in the control group. The resectability rate was higher in the study group (46%) than in the control group (32%), and the median survival was at least three times better, but after a median of 20 years the lung cancer deaths were virtually identical in the two groups: 4.4 per 1000 in the screened arm compared to 3.9 per 1000 in the control group.[483] The apparent disparity between the greatly improved survival and the lack of improvement in mortality from lung cancer is believed to be due to overdiagnosis in the screened population.[483,498] Another piece of evidence pointing to biases in the study is that 70% of the cancers that had been overlooked on previous chest radiographs were still stage I when finally diagnosed.[54] Huhti et al[462] also noted that when the diagnosis was previously missed, the survival rates were better (see p. 823 for an explanation of biases in cancer screening).

Two of the three centers investigated the benefit of using sputum cytology as an adjunct to plain chest radiography. Some 15–20% of patients with cancer showed malignant cells in the sputum when the plain chest radiograph was normal. Interestingly, these patients, who all had either centrally situated squamous cell carcinoma or mixed histologic features with squamous cell carcinoma as one element, had a more favorable prognosis than those who had positive radiographic findings.[54,482] However, neither study showed that the addition of sputum cytology reduced mortality from lung cancer.[493,499]

The conclusion was that large scale radiographic and cytologic screening for lung cancer did not result in a mortality benefit. Critics of this conclusion have argued that there might have been a benefit to a subset of patients and that the chest radiography component of the study only had the power to show a reduction in mortality of 50%, rather than a more realistic expectation,[498,500–502] but a subsequent detailed reanalysis of the data has confirmed the initial conclusions of no significant reduction in the death rate: 95% confidence intervals allowed for at most only a tiny improvement in mortality.[483] The initial hope that intensive screening would detect a large proportion of early cases of squamous cell carcinoma, the cell type with the best surgical result, was also not fulfilled.[481]

An ongoing multicenter trial by the NCI Early Detection Branch, which commenced in 1994, will likely provide a definitive answer to the question of whether conventional chest radiography has any role to play in screening for lung cancer. The trial, known as the Prostate, Lung, Colorectal, and Ovarian (PLCO) Cancer Screening Trial,[503] is a randomized controlled trial in which 37,000 men and 37,000 women aged 55–74 years will be screened for the various cancers, with a control arm of 74,000 matched individuals receiving routine medical care. The lung cancer detection portion of the trial will have an 89% power to detect whether annual chest radiography in smokers and non-smokers can effect a 10% reduction in lung cancer mortality. The trial will follow partcipants for at least 13 years.

Screening for lung cancer using low dose CT

Low dose CT has been used in several centers as the primary technique for screening an at risk population for lung cancer. The results from the major published studies are listed in Table 13.7. (By way of comparison, the yield for diagnosing breast carcinoma by large scale mammography is 0.7% at initial screening.)

The points to note from the CT screening programs listed in Table 13.7 are:

- The diagnostic yield of lung cancer from CT is far superior to chest radiography.[471,505,510] At least twice as many small lung cancers are visible on CT as on plain chest radiography. The lesions that are invisible on chest radiographs are either below the threshold for noncalcified nodule detection or, when above this threshold, have infiltrating and, therefore, relatively ill-defined margins.[511]
- A very high proportion of the cancers diagnosed are stage IA (Fig. 13.48) fulfilling one of the primary objectives of screening, namely to diagnose asymptomatic early stage disease.
- The cancer diagnosis rate is highly dependent on risk factors inherent in the inclusion criteria, with a much higher incidence of lung cancer when the age of those screened is above 60 years, and when screening CT is limited to those with a strong smoking history.
- The pickup rate of clinically insignificant benign nodules is very high (Fig. 13.49). Between 90 and 97% of noncalcified nodules proved to be benign. (As discussed below, imaging algorithms have been developed to ensure that, as far as possible, thoracotomy is limited to malignant lesions.)
- As expected, the pickup rate of lung cancers drops considerably in the later rounds of screening. As can be seen from Table 13.7 the proportion of lung cancers diagnosed in the later rounds of screening is between one-half and one-quarter of those diagnosed in the initial round.

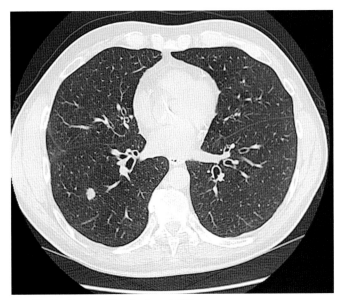

Fig. 13.48   True positive finding at CT lung cancer screening – a bronchial adenocarcinoma. (Courtesy of Dr Mary Roddie, Medicsight, London)

The high false positive rate of screening CT is a major disadvantage.[507] In the ELCAP study,[471] 233 of 1000 (23.3%) patients were found to have at least one noncalcified nodule. Therefore, follow-up protocols to assess interval growth were developed for nodules <10 mm in diameter, with biopsy limited to those nodules whose growth characteristics make lung cancer likely. In the ELCAP study, nodules >10 mm were biopsied. Remarkably, using this algorithm, only 28 of the 233 patients with noncalcified nodules required biopsy. Of these nodules, all but one proved to be malignant.

Table 13.7   Published results of lung cancer CT screening programs

	US[471,504]	Japan[486,505]	Japan[470]	Germany[506,508]	USA[507]	Italy[509]
Number of patients	1000	1369	5483	817	1520	1035
Age	>60	>50	>40	>40	>50	>50
Number of patients with lung cancer in *prevalence* round	27 (2.7%)	3/663 (0.5%)	22 (0.4%)	11 (1.3%)	26 (1.7%)	11 (1.1%)
Stage I (%) *prevalence* round	85	93	88	73	60	77
Number of patients with lung cancer in *incidence* round(s)	7 (0.59%)	7/706 (1.0%) in 1st twice yearly screen	25/4425 (0.56 %) in 1st annual screen	10/792 (1.26%)	10 (0.7%) in two incidence rounds	11 (1.1%)
		5/1111 (0.2%) in 2nd or later twice yearly screen	9/3878 (0.23%) 2nd annual screen			

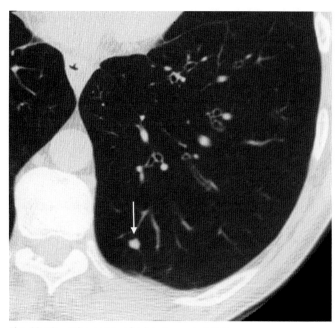

Fig. 13.49 False positive finding (arrow) at CT lung cancer screening – diagnosed as an incidental benign nodule on the basis that it did not grow under observation for 18 months.

False positive rates appear to be even higher in areas, such as the American Mid-West, in which there is a very high prevalence of histoplasmosis, but they are also high in Europe,[506] where histoplasmosis is rare. The CT screening study from the Mayo Clinic, with patients from a region with a high prevalence of granulomatous infection, showed that 51% of 1520 screened patients revealed one or more benign noncalcified nodules.[512] It should be borne in mind, however, that several technical factors may have played a role: multidetector CT scanners, narrower collimation, and ciné rather than film viewing were used and, therefore, the sensitivity for the detection of small nodules would have been higher than in the ELCAP and Japanese studies. Careful assessment of nodules avoids thoracotomy for a substantial proportion of benign nodules, but benign nodules are being removed surgically even in the best surgical centers.[507]

The false positive rate is also surprisingly high in the subsequent rounds of screening. The ELCAP study found 30 new nodules on 1184 rescreens, 22 (73%) of which proved to be benign.[504] The Mayo Clinic program[507] has reported the findings of two annual incidence screens showing a 12–13% frequency of benign nodules first recognized on the incidence screens. Diederich et al[508] found an even higher incidence of new benign nodules, namely 21.6%, on annual rescreen. Therefore, the growth rate of new small nodules must be assessed and shown to be consistent with lung carcinoma prior to surgical removal.[504]

Appearance of lung cancers detected in CT screening programs

Cancers detected by CT screening may be[513]:

- Pure ground-glass opacity
- Central solid nodule (i.e. soft tissue density) surrounded by glass opacity, sometimes referred to as a part solid nodule
- Homogeneously solid (i.e. wholly of soft tissue density)
- Heterogeneous low density and soft tissue density.

The correlations of these CT patterns are:

- The greater the proportion of ground-glass opacity the more likely it is that the lesion will grow relatively slowly,[76] and will be a well-differentiated tumor, such as a bronchioloalveolar carcinoma or atypical adenomatous hyperplasia.[514–516] It has been postulated that these CT patterns may correlate with prognosis, with solitary nodules of pure ground glass showing better prognosis and pure solid nodules being associated with a poorer prognosis.[58]
- Nodules that grow quickly tend mostly to be either homogeneously or predominantly solid at CT.[76,517]
- The less the solid component the less visible the lesion is at plain chest radiography.[518]

Imaging algorithms to determine the nature of a small pulmonary nodule

The basic principles underlying the diagnostic approach to individual nodules detected during a lung cancer CT screening program are similar to those described for a solitary pulmonary nodule first detected on plain chest radiography. There is, however, a very important difference, namely that follow up alone is an accepted approach for nodules <10 mm in diameter. (It is generally regarded as unwise to follow a nodule >1 cm with imaging characteristics compatible with bronchial carcinoma because the delay inherent in follow up would be detrimental to life-expectancy.)

Follow up alone is an accepted approach for nodules <1 cm in diameter, largely because of the much higher probability of any particular nodule being an incidental benign lesion. There is, in reality, no practical alternative: such small lesions are not in general suitable for biopsy, PET or contrast enhancement, and a large majority of patients would be severely disadvantaged by indiscriminate surgical resection. The harm done by the delay inherent in follow up, which may allow tumors to metastasize in the interval, is still not accurately quantified,[519] but there are indications that the outcome may be affected relatively little.[520] It is hoped that the delay required to check that the growth rate is compatible with lung cancer, thereby avoiding unnecessary surgery, will outweigh the disadvantage of delaying treatment for what should still be a small tumor at the time of surgery. A variety of algorithms for following nodules, which differ in points of detail, have been recommended.[506,512,521,522] The approach advocated by us is:

- Follow up at 12 months for individuals with one to six noncalcified nodules <5 mm in diameter. The concept behind this recommendation is that, based on expected growth rates, 90% of nonsmall cell lung cancers <5 mm in diameter will still be no bigger than 10 or 11 mm in diameter at an annual follow up.
- Individuals with more than six nodules, all under 1 cm in diameter, can be assumed to have multiple granulomas (or metastases if there is a known primary which could have metastasized).
- The shape and density of nodules between 5 and 10 mm in diameter should be assessed. If the lesion is clearly linear, Y shaped, or another specifically benign shape, and/or it shows a benign pattern of calcification (see Ch. 3), the lesion can be assumed to be benign.
- If none of these specific benign features is present, and the nodule is of uniform soft tissue density, then follow-up CT after 3 months should be performed. The frequency of

follow up beyond 3 months should be tailored to the estimated range of possible growth rates determined at the first 3 month review. Growth rates are expressed as the time taken for the nodule to double in volume.

- If the nodule is composed of pure ground-glass density, it is reasonable to delay the follow-up CT for 6, or even 12, months, because the chances are strongly in favor of a benign process, notably infection, atypical adenomatous hyperplasia, or a slow growing tumor such as a bronchioloalveolar carcinoma.
- The total follow-up period should be sufficient to establish the growth rate: (1) a nodule that shows no growth over a 2 year period is very unlikely to be malignant, although it is important to emphasize that 2 year stability does not totally rule out lung carcinoma,[523] and in particular does not exclude bronchial carcinoid; and (2) a nodule that shows a volume doubling time compatible with lung cancer, namely between 1 and 18 months should be assumed to be a carcinoma and treated appropriately.
- For those center with ready access to positron emission tomography (PET), it is reasonable to perform PET on nodules above 5 mm in diameter and expedite biopsy for a nodule which shows abnormal uptake of the tracer.[509,524] It is important to recognize, however, that a negative PET for nodules in the 5–10 mm range is unreliable evidence of benignity.
- A cluster of nodules (i.e. two or more nodules, none of which is >1 cm distant from an adjacent nodule), all of which are <1 cm in diameter, should be regarded as being due to tuberculosis or histoplasmosis; there is a very low probability of any individual nodule being lung carcinoma.
- Above 1 cm in diameter, the approach is identical to that described for a solitary pulmonary nodule discovered on plain chest radiography.

It is important not to underestimate the difficulty in accurately determining the growth rate of nodules <1 cm in diameter. A nodule only has to increase its diameter by 26% to double its volume. For example, a 5 mm nodule which doubles in volume during a 6 month period will increase by just 1.25 mm, a difference which requires meticulous methods of nodule measurement, preferably using dedicated software.[525] With appropriate software it is possible to achieve accuracies for volume measurement with phantom nodules of within 3%, and it is possible to detect in vivo growth after 30 days, even in cancers growing at average rates.[526,527] Three-dimensional computerized techniques demonstrate asymmetrical growth better than 2D displays, a feature that can be diagnostically useful.[526] There may be a surprising degree of variation between volume measurements of small nodules performed using the same software on different occasions, and different results may be obtained even on a single occasion depending on the region of interest or the starting point for the computer calculation. Measurements are subject to several errors, notably related to computer algorithm, image acquisition and observer variation.[528] To gain widespread application, the various computerized methods will need to become more widely accessible and less labor intensive.

Advances in technology, notably multidetector CT scanners, ciné viewing, computerized nodule detection systems, and 3D reconstruction techniques,[529–538] may improve the ability to detect and accurately characterize lung nodules, but all the available systems overdiagnose nodules compared to human observers and are, therefore, currently used adjunctively along with radiologists.

Radiation dose

All lung cancer CT screening programs use a low dose, by which is meant the lowest dose compatible with diagnosing early lung carcinoma. In practice, all use between 40 and 50 mAs and between 120–140 kVp. Several studies have also been undertaken to determine the optimum low dose,[539–541] and the use of filters to reduce the dose further.[542] These studies confirmed that an mAs in the region 25–50 mAs provides images on which it is just as easy to diagnose malignant pulmonary nodules, as would be the case with much higher exposures (the study populations included both primary and secondary tumors).

Is CT screening for lung cancer beneficial? (Box 13.7)

The central aim of any population screening program is to do more good than harm at an acceptable cost. The potential beneficial effect of a lung cancer CT screening program is that it might extend life by reducing mortality due to the lung cancer. Potential harmful effects include extra radiation from repetitive CT examinations and the consequences of false positive diagnoses, notably anxiety due to leadtime, anxiety, and complications from unnecessary further imaging, biopsy, and even surgery.

There has been considerable debate in the literature regarding the advisability of introducing large scale CT screening for the early diagnosis of lung cancer.[464,500,501,522,543–549] The debate centers on the significance of the various biases outlined on

---

Box 13.7 CT screening for lung cancer: a summary

The central aim of any population screening program is to do more good than harm at an acceptable financial cost

The major potential beneficial effect of introducing a chest CT screening program for lung cancer would be a reduction in mortality from the tumor. Potential harmful effects include: extra radiation from repetitive CT examinations; and the consequences of false positive diagnoses, notably anxiety due to leadtime, anxiety, and complications from unnecessary further imaging, biopsy, and even unnecessary surgery

CT can detect lung cancers <1 cm in size at a time when the tumor is still stage IA

There is no conclusive evidence that population screening using CT saves lives in patients with lung cancer

The debate regarding the advisability of introducing chest CT screening for the early diagnosis of lung cancer centers on how important the various biases are in the face of the clearly demonstrated ability of CT to detect stage IA lung cancers

It will take a randomized controlled trial with many years of follow up to determine the answer to the following important questions: does early detection using up-to-date CT techniques result in a measurable reduction in the mortality of lung cancer?; can thoracotomy be largely limited to those patients with life-threatening malignancies?; and can mass screening with helical CT be performed in a cost-effective manner?

page 821 in the face of the clearly demonstrated ability of CT to detect lung cancers under a centimeter in size at a time when the tumor is still stage IA. Two biases, in particular, may be pivotal: length bias and overdiagnosis.

Currently, cost-effectiveness studies have to make assumptions regarding mortality reduction. When such assumptions are made, the cost per year of life in the United States healthcare system is estimated at somewhere between $2500 and $62,000 per year of life saved, depending on the screening round being analyzed, the frequency of screening, and the prevalence of lung cancer in the population being screened.[550–554]

It will take a randomized controlled trial with many years of follow up to determine any mortality reduction and until this vital piece of information is known it will not be possible to calculate the cost in any meaningful way.[548] The three vital questions to answer in future large scale studies are: does early detection using up-to-date CT techniques result in a measurable reduction in the mortality of lung cancer?; can thoracotomy be limited largely to those patients with life-threatening malignancies?; and can mass screening with CT be performed in a cost-effective manner (perhaps in the future combined with molecular or biochemical markers for lung cancer)?

"Missed" lung cancers

The problem of "missed" lung cancers on chest radiography has been highlighted by several series. The miss rate was particularly high in the plain chest radiography lung cancer screening programs, a particular setting involving the opportunity to undertake meticulous review of recent previous films. In the Mayo chest radiography lung cancer screening project,[54] 45 of the eventually diagnosed 50 primary peripheral cancers were visible in retrospect but had been overlooked at the first opportunity. The equivalent figure for central lesions was 12 of 16. Similarly, Heelan et al[496] found that 65% of cancers in a yearly screening program had been overlooked on the previous film. Many of the overlooked cancers were very difficult to see even in retrospect.

Austin et al[555] analyzed 27 patients in whom a potentially resectable lung cancer had been missed in routine practice, which was visible in retrospect on previous films. The mean diameter of the lesions was 1.6 cm, and almost all had ill-defined edges. As part of the study, six consultants reviewed the chest radiographs of 22 cases of missed lung cancer and failed to detect a mean of 26% of the lesions. Most were in an upper lobe and in women. In another analysis of 17 cancers visible in retrospect, the failure to diagnose the cancers at the first opportunity was partly due to failure to see the lesion and partly due to misinterpreting the shadow as "inflammatory disease".[556] In another recent series of 40 nonsmall cell lung cancers that were overlooked on chest radiography at a time when the tumors were potentially resectable, the mean diameter of the missed lung cancers was 1.9 cm and again the great majority were peripheral in location and in an upper lobe.[557] Quekel et al[558] surveyed chest radiographs of patients with nonsmall cell lung cancer in a typical community setting and found that the diagnosis was missed in 19% of 259 patients with lung cancer presenting as a pulmonary nodule. The mean diameter of the missed cancers was 16 mm and the median delay in diagnosis was 472 days.[558] The miss rate was strongly correlated with the presence of superimposed normal structures and size of nodule. Lesions that contain a large proportion of ground-glass density are also more frequently overlooked compared to solid nodules.[559]

There have also been reports of lung cancers overlooked at initial chest CT[560–563]: the mean diameter of overlooked tumors in one series of 14 patients was 1.2 cm and the maximum 2.0 cm.[562] Most cancers missed at CT are endobronchial in location or are situated in the perihilar region and confused with blood vessels.

Deciding whether the failure to diagnose lung cancer on an initial chest radiograph or chest CT constitutes malpractice is very difficult, since "misses" are inevitable even under the best conditions.[564,565] If failure to diagnose a lung cancer at the first opportunity were to be regarded ipso facto as malpractice, radiologists would be found guilty of malpractice even though their films and interpretation conformed to the same standards as a group of experienced chest radiologists. Many factors contribute to a radiologist's failure to detect a lung cancer on a chest radiograph,[560,565] including the size and shape of the nodule, lesion conspicuity, viewing time,[566] and the visual search patterns used by the radiologist.[567,568] There may also be intentional or unintentional underreporting, driven by the desire to avoid further unnecessary, invasive, or expensive investigation.[53]

A variety of techniques to reduce errors of detection have been recommended or investigated,[565,569] including high kilovoltage technique, the use of wide latitude film, feedback systems,[570,571] and double reporting.[572] Comparison with previous normal radiographs allows greater confidence in the diagnosis of small nodules and permits recognition of smaller lesions.[573]

Clearly the dividing line between negligence and acceptable practice is difficult to define. Since there are no clear-cut criteria, these decisions, as so often in the medicolegal arena, depend on the testimony of expert witnesses and local laws.[564,574] It is worth noting, however, that the legal case sometimes hinges as much on the technical adequacy of the radiographs and appropriate communication of the findings, as on the issue of film interpretation.

BRONCHIAL CARCINOID

Bronchial carcinoids (see Box 13.8) are neuroendocrine tumors.[11] They constitute <5% of all pulmonary tumors.[575,576] The age range is wide, extending from adolescence[577] to old age. They show a spectrum of microscopic appearances and clinical behavior ranging from a slow growing locally invasive tumor to a malignant metastasizing tumor with a moderately fast growth rate, but even widely metastatic carcinoids may grow very slowly.[578]

There are two well-described forms of bronchial carcinoid: typical and atypical carcinoid. Typical carcinoids account for 85–90% of carcinoid tumors, atypical forms accounting for the remaining 10–15%. Atypical carcinoid has cellular and clinical features intermediate between those of typical carcinoid and small cell carcinoma of the lung.[579,580] These three neoplasms,

Box 13.8 Bronchial carcinoids

Constitute <5% of all pulmonary tumors

Age range from adolescence to old age

Believed to be part of a spectrum that includes small cell carcinoma

Two well-described forms: typical carcinoid (85–90%) and atypical carcinoid (10–15%)

Both forms have good prognosis if resected

Cushing syndrome due to ectopic adrenocorticotrophic hormone (ACTH) production by the tumor is more common than the carcinoid syndrome. The responsible tumors may be very small

Most common site of origin is central bronchi

Calcification is fairly common

Somatostatin receptor radionuclide scanning (e.g. with octreotide) is highly sensitive

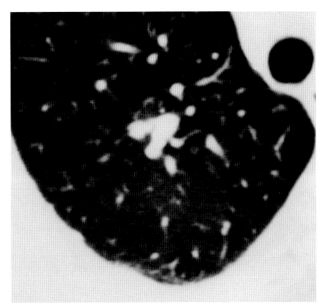

Fig. 13.50   Bronchial carcinoid causing ectopic adrenocorticotropic hormone syndrome. The small bronchial carcinoid measured only 6–7 mm in diameter. It caused a mucocele beyond it. Following surgical removal, the patient's Cushing disease was cured.

along with large cell neuroendocrine tumor, are believed to be a spectrum of tumors of neuroendocrine origin with varying degrees of malignancy.[9,391,576,580–582] Bronchial carcinoids may be difficult to differentiate from small cell carcinoma in small biopsy or needle aspiration samples.[575,583] Also, individual tumors may show different patterns in different portions of a lesion. Bronchial carcinoids are, in general, highly vascular tumors with blood supply from the bronchial arteries.[584]

Typical carcinoids without nodal or other metastases have an excellent outcome following surgical resection.[585,586] Even when spread to hilar or ipsilateral mediastinal lymph nodes has taken place, 5 year survival is 92%.[587–589] Spread is usually first to hilar[575] or mediastinal nodes, and bloodborne metastases at presentation are unusual. The great majority arise centrally in the main, lobar, or segmental bronchi and may cause cough and occasionally wheezing. Repetitive bouts of pneumonia are common, and bronchiectasis and lung abscess may occur beyond the obstruction; hemoptysis and weight loss are also common.[575,586,590,591] Centrally located bronchial carcinoids[391] may be predominantly intraluminal, assuming a polypoid configuration, may grow within the lumen of the bronchus in a "toothpaste-like" fashion, or may be predominantly extraluminal, in which case they are known as "iceberg" lesions. The mucosal surface is usually smooth; only rarely is it ulcerated to any degree.

Atypical carcinoids usually arise peripherally in the lung, and both hemoptysis and pneumonitis are rare. They have a worse outcome than typical carcinoids.[592]

The *carcinoid syndrome* is rare with bronchial carcinoids, unless liver metastases are present.[590,591,593] Bronchial carcinoid tumors may secrete adrenocorticotrophic hormone (ACTH) in sufficient quantities to cause *Cushing syndrome* (ectopic ACTH syndrome), clinically indistinguishable from pituitary dependent Cushing disease.[594–598] ACTH secreting tumors may be more aggressive than the usual typical carcinoid.[599] They are often small, sometimes tiny, and require meticulous searching with chest CT (Fig. 13.50) or radionuclide imaging to reveal their presence.[594,597,598] Some are so small that they cannot be found

until they grow large enough to be visualized with imaging examinations. It is possible to perform needle aspiration of a suspicious pulmonary nodule in a patient with Cushing disease to analyze the sample for ACTH,[600] but analysis of bronchial lavage fluid is unhelpful.[601]

The chest radiograph is abnormal in most cases of bronchial carcinoid,[593] but in approximately 10% the chest radiograph is normal. The majority arise in the larger bronchi and cause partial or complete bronchial obstruction with consequent atelectasis (Fig. 13.51). Collateral air drift may keep segments aerated when the lesion is in a segmental bronchus; even whole lobes can be kept fully aerated despite complete occlusion of a lobar bronchus. The consequent hypoxia of the affected lung may occasionally cause recognizable local vasoconstriction on plain film and perfusion scintigraphy.[602] In about 25% of patients with a central lesion the tumor is visible on plain chest radiographs as a hilar mass (Fig. 13.52).[603,604]

Small tumors in lobar, segmental, or subsegmental bronchi may cause mucus distension of the bronchi beyond the obstruction (Figs 13.50 and 13.53 to 13.55), the surrounding lung remaining aerated by collateral air drift. The resulting bronchocele (mucoid impaction) may then be the dominant feature.[61,605]

Approximately 10–20% of bronchial carcinoids present as a solitary pulmonary nodule (see Fig. 13.56). The nodule is well-defined, round, oval, lobulated, or notched, usually with a smooth edge,[593] although spiculation is reported.[579] Calcification or ossification is occasionally recognizable on chest radiography.[606] Two large series describing the chest radiographic appearances have been reported, both from the Mayo

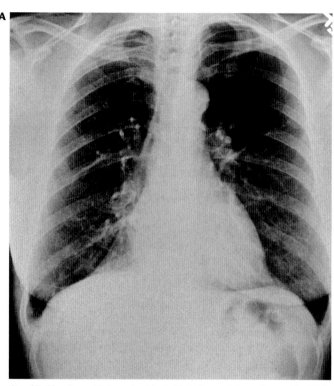

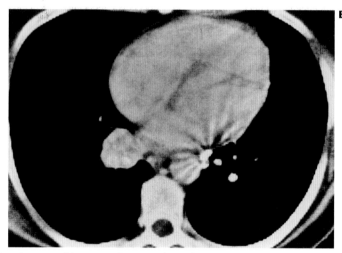

Fig. 13.51 Bronchial carcinoid. **A**, Right lower lobe collapse. **B**, CT showing the tumor lying centrally. Note the uniform contrast-enhancement of the tumor mass.

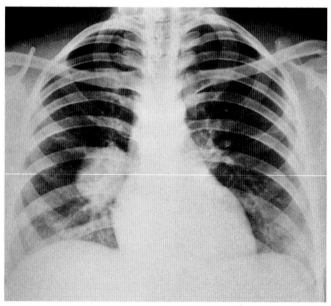

Fig. 13.52 Bronchial carcinoid presenting as a hilar mass without distal atelectasis. (Courtesy of Dr Peter Hacking, Newcastle, UK)

Clinic.[603,607] In the earlier series of 23 cases, the average diameter of the nodule was 4 cm; however, the later report on 20 similarly located tumors showed none with a diameter >4 cm. Multiple lesions are a frequent pathologic finding[346]; but usually they are tiny and are not recognized on plain radiography.

CT provides superb anatomic localization of both the intraluminal and extraluminal components of tumors in the major bronchi and shows all the imaging features to advantage.[391,608–611] CT is excellent for showing the details of a central mass, which may be purely intraluminal, a mixture of intraluminal and extraluminal, or almost entirely extraluminal (Figs 13.51,13.53 and 13.57). The tumor may narrow, deform or obstruct the airway. On occasion the bronchial lumen can be seen to widen as it approaches the tumor, a point of distinction from bronchial carcinoma (Figs 13.54 and 13.57). Even peripheral carcinoids can be shown to lie adjacent to recognizable small airways.[612]

The incidence of calcification detectable by CT appears to be considerable: four of 12 cases in one series[613] and eight of 31 in another.[614] The incidence of calcification is significantly greater in centrally located tumors and more frequent in the larger tumors. A variety of patterns of calcification are seen,[609,614] including multiple nodular and curvilinear configurations (Figs 13.56 and 13.58). Sometimes the calcification takes the form of recognizable ossification and is so extensive that it occupies the whole of the tumor mass (Fig. 13.56).[614,615]

Contrast enhancement, which is sometimes marked, is seen in some cases (Figs 13.51 and 13.58).[616,617] Pronounced and rapid contrast enhancement with gadolinium at MRI has also been reported.[618,619]

Carcinoid tumors cannot in general be distinguished from carcinomas on chest radiography and CT unless the lesion is

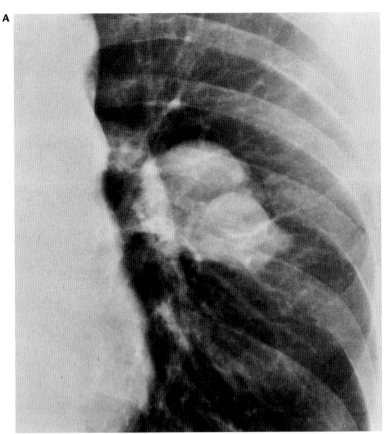

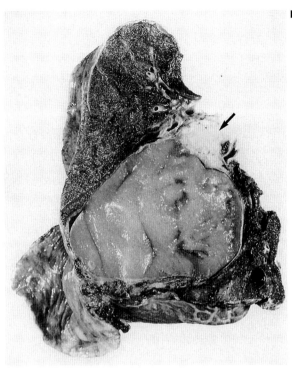

Fig. 13.53 Bronchial carcinoid causing mucoid impaction. **A**, Chest radiograph showing mucus-filled, dilated bronchi (bronchocele) beyond the obstruction resembling a bilobed mass. **B**, Operative specimen from another patient shows a central bronchial carcinoid (arrow) and hugely dilated, mucus-filled bronchi (mucocele) mimicking a large neoplastic mass beyond the true tumor.

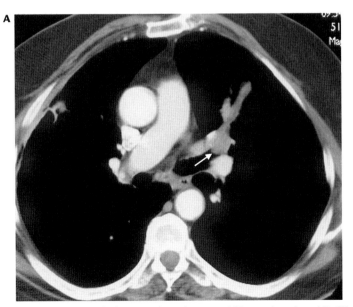

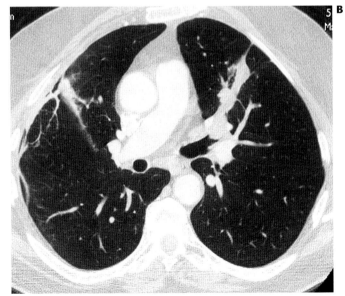

Fig. 13.54 Bronchial carcinoid causing mucoid impaction. **A** and **B**, CT showing a rounded mass (arrow) obstructing the right upper lobe bronchus with mucocele formation beyond the mass. Note that the bronchus widens as it approaches the tumor.

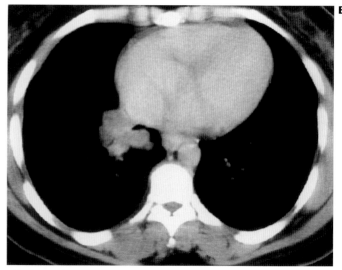

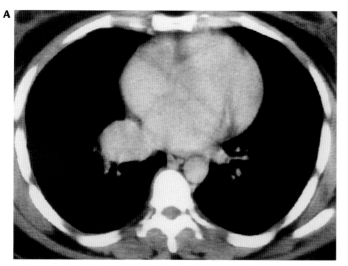

Fig. 13.55 Bronchial carcinoid with **A**, contrast-enhancing central mass, and **B**, lower density mucocele distal to the mass.

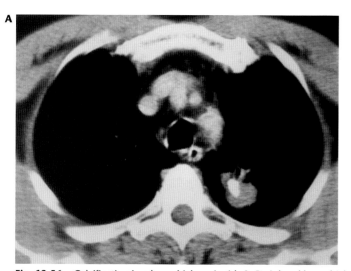

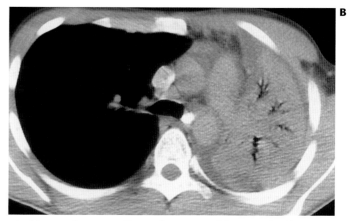

Fig. 13.56 Calcification in a bronchial carcinoid. **A**, Peripheral bronchial carcinoid presenting as a solitary pulmonary nodule containing dense calcification shown on CT (but not visible on standard plain chest radiographs). **B**, Heavily calcified carcinoid tumor in the proximal left main bronchus obstructing the left lung on a nonenhanced CT.

demonstrably heavily calcified, enhances brightly or shows widening of the approaching bronchus.

Small tumors may be difficult to distinguish from the larger blood vessels at CT,[620] and may, on occasion, be shown to advantage by MRI because on appropriate sequences (particularly T2-weighted or STIR sequences) the contrast between high signal from the tumor compared with the low background signal of normal lung and flowing blood in pulmonary vessels may make the lesions more conspicuous than at CT.

Carcinoids have somatostatin receptors and can therefore be imaged with [113]In octreotide, a radiolabeled somatostatin analog.[621-623] Somatostatin receptor scintigraphy, while 96%

sensitive, is also positive in inflammatory conditions as well as in a variety of other tumors. It shows those carcinoids that are visible on chest radiographs or CT scanning,[621] but has not yet been shown to be of proven value for the diagnosis of ACTH producing bronchial carcinoid tumors that are not visible on cross-sectional imaging.[624]

Other radionuclides that have been shown to accumulate in sufficient quantities to demonstrate a bronchial carcinoid include ^{123}I-N-isopropyl-*p*-iodoamphetamine,[625] and PET agents, such as ^{18}F-FDG,[626] 5-hydroxytrytophan (5-HTP) labeled with ^{11}C,[627] and ^{18}F-labeled analogs of octreotide.[628] Currently, however, [113]In octreotide remains the preferred radionuclide in widespread clinical practice for imaging carcinoid tumors.

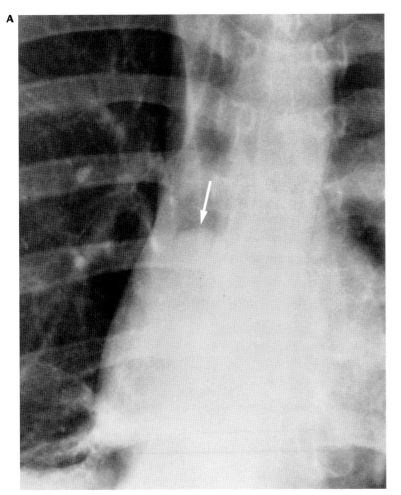

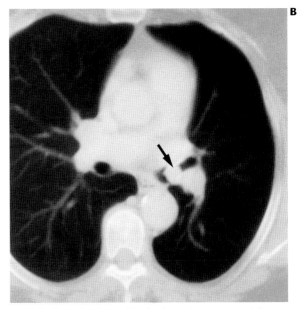

Fig. 13.57 **A**, Bronchial carcinoid in the intermediate stem bronchus showing widening of the bronchus immediately above the tumor and the top of the intraluminal mass (arrow). **B**, Intraluminal bronchial carcinoid tumor (arrow) shown by CT. (Courtesy of Dr Martin Wastie, Nottingham, UK)

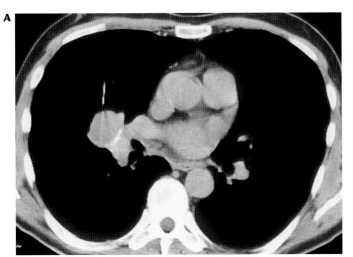

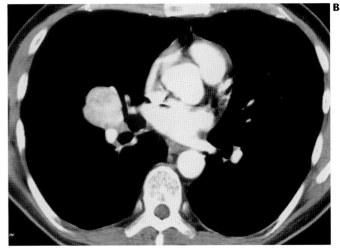

Fig. 13.58 Bronchial carcinoid arising close to the right hilum showing rim calcification and contrast enhancement. **A**, Precontrast image taken as part of needle biopsy procedure, and **B**, previous postcontrast image.

HAMARTOMAS

Hamartomas are defined pathologically as tumorlike malformations composed of an abnormal mixture of the normal constituents of the organ in which they are found. Most pulmonary hamartomas contain masses of cartilage with clefts lined by bronchial epithelium and fibromyxoid stroma; they may also contain fat or cystic collections of fluid.[629–632] Although the precise nature of pulmonary hamartomas is debatable, they are usually regarded as benign neoplasms.[630] They grow slowly and are usually solitary, though there are a few case reports of multiple pulmonary hamartomas.[632,633] Malignant transformation is either nonexistent or extremely rare,[630,634] but there are two series showing a higher than expected incidence of lung carcinoma in patients with pulmonary hamartoma.[635,636] Also, malignant sarcomas arising in the wall of so-called cystic mesenchymal hamartomas have been reported in children, but cystic mesenchymal hamartomas are histologically quite different from the usual hamartoma seen in adults.[637,638] (It has been suggested that cystic mesenchymal hamartoma is part of the spectrum of childhood pulmonary blastoma developing in congenital cystic lung.[639])

The peak age at presentation of pulmonary hamartomas is in the seventh decade of life.[630] They are rarely seen in children. The great majority are situated peripherally, with a few arising in central bronchi.[630,640] In the largest series published to date, only four of 215 patients with hamartomas had symptoms attributable to the hamartoma, the symptoms being cough, hemoptysis, or recurrent pneumonia.[630]

A triad of pulmonary chondroma (often multiple), gastric epithelioid leiomyosarcoma (leiomyoblastoma), and functioning extraadrenal paraganglioma, known as Carney's triad, has been described (see Box 13.9).[641] The importance of the condition, which is seen mostly in women under 35 years of age, is that if multiple slow growing cartilage tumors are found in the lung, the other tumors in the triad should be sought, since the other neoplasms are potentially lethal. Furthermore, patients with a smooth muscle tumor in the wall of the stomach should not automatically be assumed to have pulmonary metastases just because they have multiple pulmonary nodules. An incomplete form of the triad manifesting just the pulmonary chondromata and gastric smooth muscle tumors is also seen.[642,643] In addition to Carney's triad, the association of pulmonary hamartomas with other developmental anomalies and benign tumors has been noted.[644]

On chest radiograph, peripheral hamartomas are seen as a spherical, lobulated, or notched pulmonary nodule with a very well-defined edge surrounded by normal lung (Fig. 13.59).[645] Pulmonary hamartomas can range up to 10 cm in diameter.[646] Large lesions are unusual, however, and most are <4 cm.[640] The larger the lesion, the more likely it will calcify. Definite calcification is seen on plain chest radiographs in up to 15% of patients.[640] The calcification may show the typical popcorn configuration of cartilage calcification, in which case the diagnosis is virtually certain (Figs 13.60 and 13.61). The presence of fat density within the mass is a specific diagnostic feature (Figs 13.60 to 13.62). Radiologically detectable air within the tumors is exceedingly rare,[647] but central lucency caused by fat can be confused with cavitation.

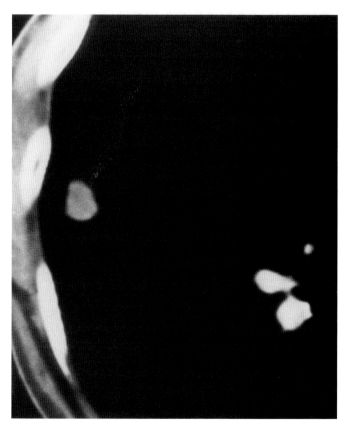

Fig. 13.59 CT of a hamartoma of the lung presenting as a small, noncalcified, very well-defined, slightly lobulated solitary pulmonary nodule of uniform soft tissue density.

The signs at CT are similar to those at chest radiography, but because of the better contrast resolution, calcium and particularly fat are more easy to identify (Fig. 13.62).[648] In a series of 47 patients with pulmonary hamartomas it was possible to identify fat (CT numbers in the range −80 HU to −120 HU) or calcium plus fat within the nodule in 28 patients by use of thin-section CT; this combination appears to be specific for hamartoma, at least in nodules <2.5 cm in diameter.[648] In 17 of the cases the hamartomas showed neither calcification nor fat, and in the remaining two there was diffuse calcification throughout the lesion. An air bronchogram may be seen within the nodule on rare occasions.[649]

Hamartomas show enhancement on CT following intravenous contrast injection,[649–651] but usually the only enhancement is in the surrounding capsule or in septa separating nonenhancing

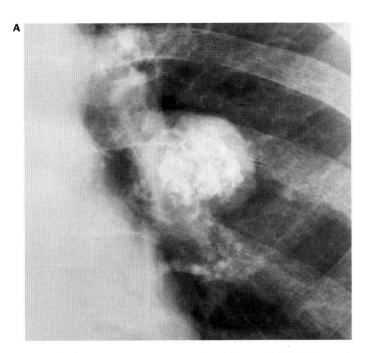

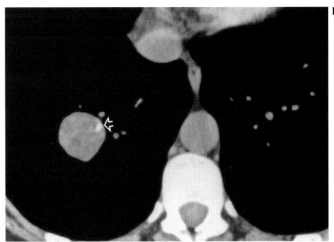

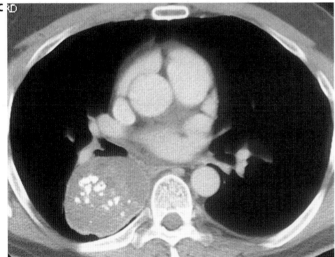

Fig. 13.60 Hamartoma showing a smooth edge and central cartilage calcification. **A,** Extensive popcorn calcification is clearly visible on chest radiography. **B,** CT showing variable density including focal calcification (arrow) and fat density. **C,** CT of an unusually large hamartoma in the right lower lobe showing rounded and popcorn calcifications.

components; on occasion, however, there is nonspecific more generalized enhancement.

At MRI,[652] hamartomas show intermediate signal on T1-weighted and high signal on T2-weighted images. Septa can be seen separating the nodule into lobules. These septa show marked enhancement following intravenous gadolinium.

Endobronchial hamartomas[653,654] can lead to airway obstruction, the radiologic features being similar to centrally located bronchial carcinoid, except that the tumor mass does not enhance to the same degree.

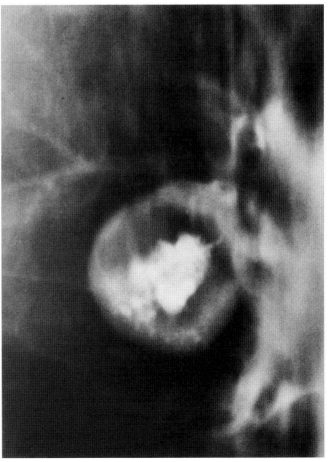

Fig. 13.61 Conventional tomogram of a hamartoma showing central cartilage calcification and surrounding fat density within the lesion.

A

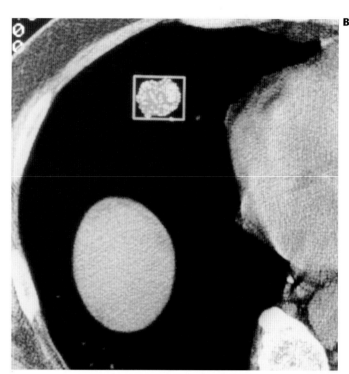

C

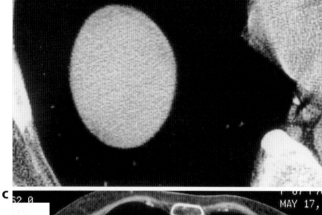

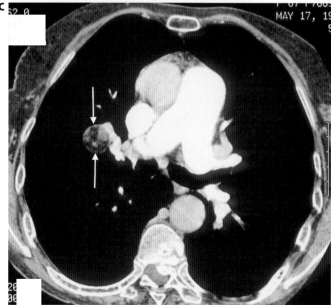

Fig. 13.62 Hamartoma containing fat density on CT. **A**, HRCT with window adjusted to show focal fat density within the hamartoma. **B**, Pixel highlighting in the same case shows fat density as white. **C**, Fat content (arrows) in another case is so extensive that it is difficult to distinguish the mass from lung on mediastinal windows.

TRACHEAL NEOPLASMS

Benign tumors of the trachea are rare. They are most frequent in children, in whom squamous papillomas are the most common.[655] These papillomas are usually part of laryngeal papillomatosis, a condition discussed on page 840. The next most common benign tracheal tumors of childhood are hemangiomas. They are often associated with cutaneous hemangiomas and are frequently in the subglottic region. Stridor may develop in the first year of life. On imaging examinations tracheal hemangiomas are seen as eccentrically situated nodular masses.

A variety of connective tissue, neural, and other benign neoplasms are occasionally encountered in the trachea,[656] including lipoma, fibroma, leiomyoma,[657] hemangioendothelioma, cartilage tumors,[658,659] granular cell myoblastoma (also known as granular cell tumor),[660] laryngeal papillomatosis (Fig.

13.63), and neurilemmoma, neurofibroma and paraganglioma (glomus tumor).[612,661,662] All these lesions produce a nonspecific focal mass in the wall of the trachea.[655]

The most common malignant tumor of the trachea is invasion from an adjacent neoplasm, notably bronchial carcinoma.

Primary malignant tumors of the trachea are rare and are virtually confined to adults.[37,656,661,663,664] The most frequent are adenoid cystic carcinoma (formerly known as cylindroma) and squamous cell carcinoma. Mucoepidermoid tumor is the next most common carcinoma: it is more frequent in the major bronchi than in the trachea.[19,665] Adenoid cystic carcinomas of the trachea present at an earlier age than squamous cell carcinoma, usually between 30 and 50 years. Squamous cell carcinoma is strongly associated with smoking.

These three tumors make up over 90% of primary tracheal tumors. The remaining 10% consist of a wide variety of neoplasms, including sarcomas, lymphoma, adenocarcinoma, adenosquamous carcinoma, carcinoid, chondrosarcoma, plasmacytoma, small cell carcinoma, and metastases.[612,663,666–668]

Primary malignant tracheal tumors grow slowly, tend to involve the posterior wall of the lower two-thirds of the trachea, and infiltrate submucosally for long distances.[37,612] Therefore, stridor and wheezing are common early symptoms. Tracheoesophageal fistula may be the initial feature. By the time of clinical presentation these tumors have often invaded the mediastinum and adjacent esophagus; they are, however, frequently amenable to surgical resection.[663,669]

All three tumors are seen on imaging studies[655,665,670] as an intraluminal nodule or stenosis with lobular or irregular contours (Figs 13.64 and 13.65). The tumors grow within or through the tracheal wall to produce a paratracheal mass

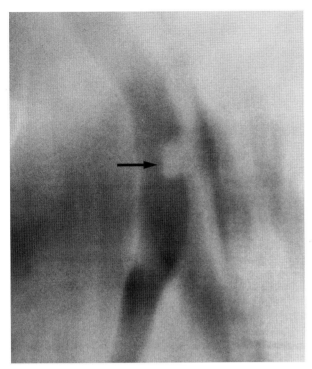

Fig. 13.63 Laryngeal papillomatosis showing a single polypoid lesion (arrow) in the trachea.

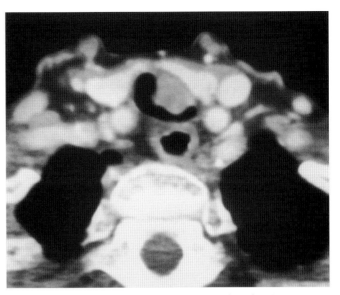

Fig. 13.64 Squamous cell carcinoma of the trachea showing a mass projecting into the lumen.

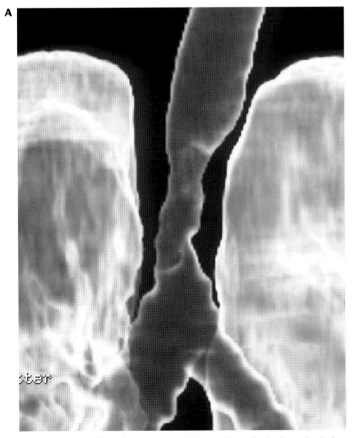

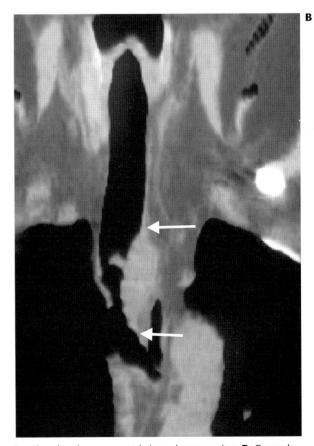

Fig. 13.65 Adenoid cystic carcinoma of the trachea. **A**, Surface shaded reconstruction showing asymmetric irregular narrowing. **B**, Coronal reconstruction in the same patient showing a large extraluminal mass in the paratracheal region (the arrows indicate the upper and lower extent of tumor).

and/or a stenosing mass of variable length (Figs 13.64 and 13.65). Low grade mucoepidermoid carcinomas usually appear as polypoid lesions, a feature most frequently seen with adenoid cystic carcinoma.[670] As with bronchial carcinoid, there may be a relatively large mediastinal mass with a much smaller intratracheal component. Like bronchial carcinoids, mucoepidermoid tumors may travel along bronchi and so adapt their shape to the airways. Like bronchial carcinoid and various benign tumors, adenoid cystic carcinomas may calcify.

The full extent of submucosal spread tends to be underestimated with CT.[671] Although CT shows the extraluminal component of tumors of the trachea, it is poor at indicating whether or not mediastinal structures, such as the esophagus and aorta, are invaded. Obliteration of the fat planes between the tumor and these structures is sometimes caused by invasion, but at other times no invasion is found when surgery is finally performed.[672] Multiplanar MRI can be helpful in assessing the degree of spread.[673]

RARE MALIGNANT PULMONARY NEOPLASMS

Most sarcomas of the lung are metastases from extrathoracic primary tumors. *Primary pulmonary sarcomas* are usually fibrosarcomas, leiomyosarcomas,[674–676] or sarcomas of the pulmonary artery.[677] In a large review from the Armed Forces Institute of Pathology,[678] endobronchial fibrosarcomas and leiomyosarcomas exhibited, for the most part, a relatively benign behavior compared with tumors arising within the lung parenchyma, which showed great variability in their degree of malignancy and a significant incidence of highly aggressive behavior. Chondrosarcomas, fibroleiomyosarcomas, malignant fibrous histiocytoma,[679–682] osteosarcoma,[683,684] rhabdomyosarcomas,[685,686] liposarcomas, which may show fat density on CT,[687] myxosarcomas, neurofibrosarcomas, and angiosarcomas,[688] may also arise primarily in the lung.

All these sarcomas, except angiosarcomas, appear on imaging examinations as a solitary pulmonary nodule or as an endobronchial mass, usually causing atelectasis, indistinguishable from bronchial carcinoma (Fig. 13.66). Angiosarcomas extend or arise intravascularly,[682,689–691] a feature that is well demonstrated on MRI and contrast-enhanced CT, and the tumor itself enhances brightly. A case of pulmonary leiomyosarcoma presenting as a pseudoaneurysm of a peripheral pulmonary artery has been reported.[692]

Hemangiopericytomas, which may be benign or malignant, occasionally arise primarily in the lung. The larger the lesion, the more likely it is to be malignant. These tumors are most common in the fourth and fifth decades with no sex predominance. They are usually asymptomatic but cough, hemoptysis, hypertrophic osteoarthropathy, and chest pain are the more common symptoms in larger lesions, and there may be associated hypoglycemia or coagulopathy.[693] On imaging examinations, the tumors appear as one or more well-defined pulmonary masses of any size. Speckled, eccentric calcification is seen on occasions. MRI shows a heterogeneous signal pattern corresponding to necrosis and hemorrhage with no specific features.[693–695]

Malignant angioendotheliosis is discussed on page 853 since it is now classified as a lymphoma (intravascular large B-cell lymphoma).

Carcinosarcomas are composed of mixed malignant epithelial and connective tissue components. They are usually first found in

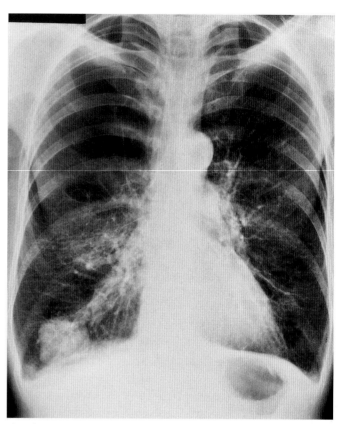

Fig. 13.66 Primary rhabdomyosarcoma of the lung. The right lower lobe mass was surgically resected on the preoperative assumption that it was a bronchial carcinoma.

middle aged to elderly patients. Carcinosarcomas may arise centrally or peripherally and are indistinguishable radiologically from other endobronchial or pulmonary tumors.[696]

Pulmonary blastomas are malignant tumors which histologically show embryonic bronchial structures in a background of abundant immature sarcoma.[346,697] Pulmonary blastomas were originally thought to arise from a multipotential mesodermal cell, but like carcinosarcomas they are now believed to arise from two germ cell layers. They are therefore classified as a form of carcinosarcoma. The peak age of clinical presentation is somewhat younger than carcinoma, a small proportion being found in children.[698,699] Pulmonary blastomas generally arise peripherally in the lung (Fig. 13.67) as a solitary well-defined mass or occasionally as multiple pulmonary masses.[700–703] Blastomas in adults are often of moderate size but range from 2.5 to 26 cm in diameter. Cavitation has been noted on chest radiographs.[700] CT and ultrasound have shown a cystic structure within the mass itself.[704] Calcification has been reported on CT.[699] Pleural effusion may accompany the mass.

Pleuropulmonary blastoma is classified separately.[639,705] It is an aggressive dysontogenic neoplasm of early childhood, characterized histologically by primitive mixed blastomatous and sarcomatous elements.[706] The tumors may arise in preexisting congenital lung lesions, including cystic adenomatoid malformation, extralobar sequestration, bronchogenic cyst and pulmonary hamartoma. There are few reports of the imaging features. Chest radiographs and CT show an appearance

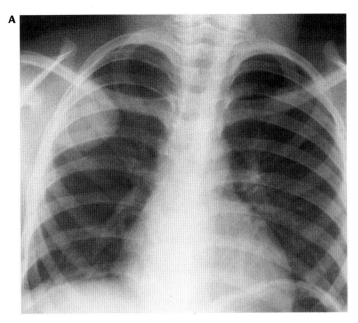

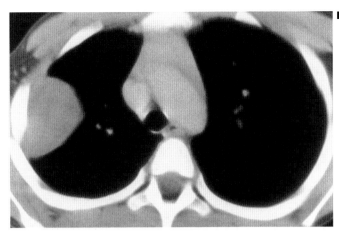

Fig. 13.67 Pulmonary blastoma in a 13-year-old child on **A**, chest radiograph, **B**, CT, and **C**, MRI. Note the peripheral location of this solitary well-defined mass.

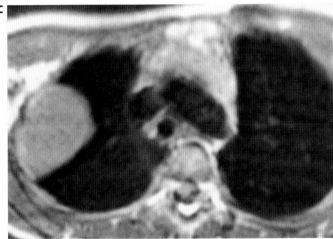

resembling pneumonia, empyema, or lung cyst, which may be air filled; in some cases there is an accompanying pneumothorax which may recur.[706,707] In one report on seven children with "pulmonary blastoma",[639] all the tumors were unilateral and large at initial presentation. The four patients who underwent CT examination showed similar findings: a heterogeneous mass with areas of low attenuation and whorls of high attenuation. In three cases, CT showed a rounded tumor arising within an area of preexisting cystic lung. The association of pulmonary blastomas and developmental cysts of the lung has also been reported by others.[704] In rare instances the childhood tumor resembles empyema both clinically and radiologically.[698]

Primary choriocarcinoma and *primary malignant teratoma* of the lung are both very rare indeed. The few published cases show a nonspecific pulmonary mass.[708–710]

Plasmacytoma of the lungs or major airways is an exceedingly rare tumor, even in patients with multiple myeloma. With solitary lesions the sheets of plasma cells may be difficult to distinguish histologically from a benign plasma cell granuloma, and some of the cases in the literature may have been wrongly categorized. The most common form of intrathoracic plasma-

cytoma is inward extension from a rib. Rarely, plasmacytoma presents radiographically as a tracheal,[711] bronchial, or lung mass,[712,713] or as greatly enlarged intrathoracic lymph nodes.[235] Scattered cases of myeloma involvement of the pulmonary interstitium have also been reported.[714]

Askin tumors are malignant small cell tumors of neuroepithelial origin seen in childhood and adolescence,[715] and, rarely, in adults.[716] The great majority arise in the chest wall;[717,718] a few are almost exclusively in the lung, but even these show pleural involvement. The condition has a poor prognosis, even with combined chemoradiation and surgery, with few longterm survivors, though some are reported.[719] On imaging,[718,720] there is an intrathoracic soft tissue mass, which may show calcification, and can be huge with either no visible rib destruction or only focal rib lysis. Pleural effusions and hilar adenopathy may accompany the mass.

Epithelioid hemangioendothelioma (intravascular bronchioloalveolar tumor) is a rare cause of multiple small pulmonary nodules.[721–725] The tumor is believed to be a neoplasm of blood vessels,[726] related to hemangioendothelioma. There is a strong predilection for females, and the age range is 12–61 with a mean in the 40s. The

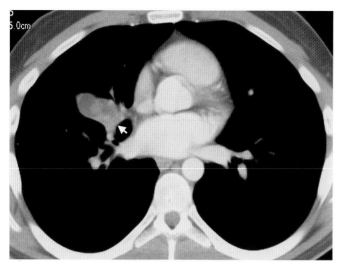

Fig. 13.68 Mucoepidermoid carcinoma (arrow) occluding the middle lobe bronchus and causing middle lobe collapse.

patients are often asymptomatic, or have minor symptoms only, and the diagnosis is established following the discovery of multiple perivascular pulmonary nodules,[687] which may mimic interstitial lung disease,[726] on chest radiography or CT. The nodules, which may be up to 2 cm in diameter, are well defined or slightly ill defined in outline. They may calcify.[722,727] Associated pleural effusion may be seen and metastases to hilar nodes are recorded. The course may be indolent with survivals of up to 15 years.

Until the advent of acquired immune deficiency syndrome (AIDS), *Kaposi sarcoma* was regarded primarily as a skin tumor of the lower extremities. The tumor is now being encountered with increased frequency in the bronchial tree and lungs of patients with AIDS (see Ch. 6, p. 296).

Mucoepidermoid (Fig. 13.68) and *adenoid cystic carcinomas* may occur in the bronchi but are more common in the trachea (see p. 834).

RARE BENIGN LUNG NEOPLASMS

The WHO classification of lung and pleural tumors[2] divides benign epithelial tumors into papillomas and adenomas. The adenomas are divided into alveolar, papillary, mucinous, and salivary gland adenomas. *Bronchioloalveolar adenoma* is now referred to as *atypical adenomatous hyperplasia* and is discussed on page 821.

Alveolar adenomas and *papillary adenomas* are very rare and present as peripheral solitary pulmonary nodules.[670,728,729] *Salivary gland tumors* (notably mucous gland and pleomorphic adenomas) are usually found in the larger bronchi as solitary, predominantly polypoid or exophytic tumors arising from submucosal seromucus glands and ducts, or occasionally from smaller bronchi within lung parenchyma.[670,730,731] They occur in adults and need to be distinguished pathologically from low grade malignant tumors of the bronchus – particularly mucoepidermoid carcinoma.[730] Radiologically they cause postobstructive atelectasis and pneumonia or present as a solitary pulmonary nodule.

Granular cell myoblastoma is a benign tumor most commonly found in subcutaneous tissues, but may rarely occur in the larger bronchi and even more rarely in the lung parenchyma,[660] trachea, or mediastinum.[732–734] It usually presents in adults as postobstructive atelectasis or pneumonia beyond the lesion itself, occasionally as a small solitary pulmonary nodule, or as a polypoid lesion arising in a bronchus.[735,736] Multiple lesions are occasionally encountered and hemoptysis may be a presenting feature.[734]

Fibroma, chondroma, lipoma,[737] hemangioma, neurofibroma, neurilemmoma,[738] chemodectoma, benign clear cell tumor, fibrous tumor of the pleura,[739] meningioma,[740] and *thymoma[741]* may arise in the lung parenchyma or in the walls of the bronchi. Those that arise in the lung parenchyma present as a nonspecific solitary pulmonary nodule; those that arise in the larger bronchi are indistinguishable from the more common bronchial carcinoid, except that it may be possible to diagnose fat in a lipoma by CT (Fig. 13.69).[742,743] Endobronchial lipoma has been reported to contain a focus of dense calcification within the tumor, as well as fat density.[737] Most intrathoracic lipomas arise extrapleurally

A
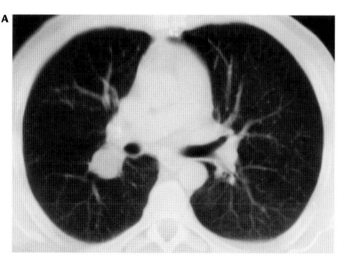

B
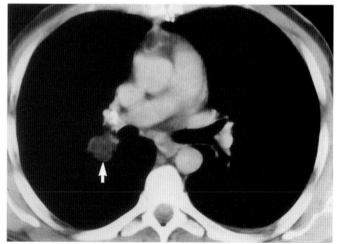

Fig. 13.69 Endobronchial lipoma (arrow on **B**). Fat density of the mass is well shown by CT. **A,** At lung window settings. **B,** Narrow window settings. (Courtesy of Dr Ted A Glass, Fredericksburg, MD)

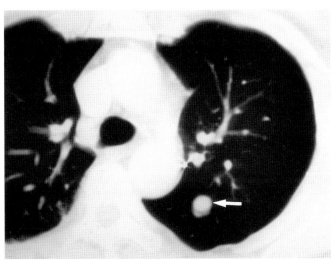

Fig. 13.70 Benign metastasizing leiomyoma. CT showing one of many pulmonary nodules (arrow) that developed over 15 years.

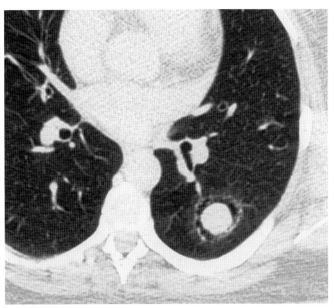

Fig. 13.72 Sclerosing hemangioma. CT showing a nodule surrounded by a halo of air and a ring shadow. (With permission from Nicholson AG, Magkou C, Snead D, et al. Unusual sclerosing hemangiomas and sclerosing hemangioma-like lesions, and the value of TTF-1 in making the diagnosis. Histopathology 2002;41:400–413, Blackwell Publishing Ltd.)

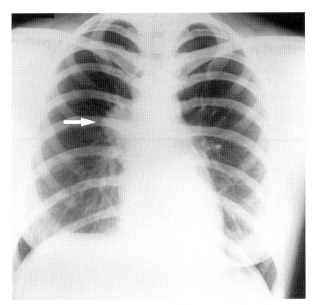

Fig. 13.71 Intrapulmonary teratoma. This teratoma (arrow) was totally within the lung at surgery.

from the chest wall, mediastinum, or diaphragm.[744,745] (Pleural lipoma is discussed on page 863.)

Leiomyoma of the lung may be a solitary lesion, radiographically indistinguishable from the other benign connective tissue neoplasms.

Multiple leiomyomas occur as multiple nodules, of uniform soft tissue density in the lung, up to 7 cm in diameter (Fig. 13.70),[746–749] or very occasionally in the pleura.[750] They are given a wide variety of names, notably *benign metastasizing leiomyoma*. These tumors are probably very slow growing metastases from a uterine leiomyoma; there is often a history of previous hysterectomy for uterine fibroids, which may have been up to 20 years previous.[749] Their behavior varies from a benign lesion to a low grade sarcoma but they are sufficiently indolent that death is commonly from other causes. They are usually asymptomatic and discovered incidentally on chest

imaging.[749] The nodules may cavitate showing air–fluid levels and forming very thin walled, air-filled cavities. A miliary pattern has been described in one case.[751] The lesions may be hormone sensitive.[746]

Pulmonary *endometriosis* also appears as single or multiple pulmonary nodules,[752] which may cavitate.[753] Catamenial hemoptysis (coinciding with menstruation) is a specific diagnostic feature. (Pleural endometriosis is discussed on page 1066.)

Benign intrapulmonary teratomas are unusual. They occur equally in men and women and usually are diagnosed in the second to fourth decade. Chest pain, hemoptysis, and cough are the most frequent initial symptoms; expectoration of hair (trichoptysis) is the most specific feature. On chest radiography and CT, intrapulmonary teratomas appear as lobulated masses that may show calcification or cavitation (Fig. 13.71).[754] Fat, a feature of mediastinal teratomas, has not yet been reported on imaging examinations, but the number of cases examined by CT so far is tiny.[754] The lesions are often large, and there may be bronchiectasis in the neighboring lung.

Sclerosing hemangioma is thought to be an epithelial pulmonary tumor derived from a primitive epithelial cell.[755] It has also been reported in the mediastinum.[756] The tumor may be combined with bronchial carcinoid and metastasis to the mediastinum has been reported.[755] The average age at diagnosis is 42 years with a range from the teenage years upwards. There is a marked female predominance. In almost all reported cases the lesion is a solitary well-defined, round pulmonary nodule, which usually enhances inhomogeneously following intravenous contrast injection.[757–761] The lesion is frequently juxtapleural in location,[759] ranging in diameter from very small to 8 cm, with an average of 3 cm.[762] Calcification may be seen on plain film as well as CT.[759] CT may show-well marginated central liquefaction,[758] and an air meniscus sign has been reported on plain film.[763] A halo of lucency has been reported at CT (Fig. 13.72), corresponding

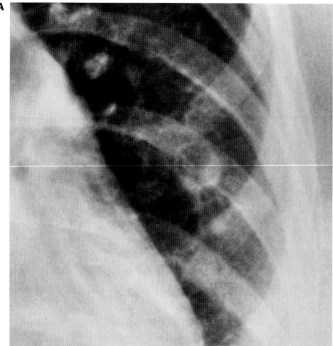

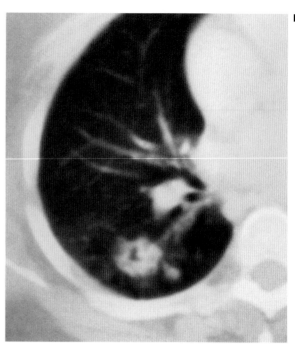

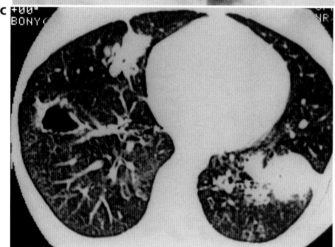

Fig. 13.73 Laryngeal papillomatosis. **A**, Chest radiograph in a 7-year-old child who had multiple small cavitary nodules. **B**, CT in another child with multiple cavitating nodules. **C**, 31 year old woman with unusually large nodules, some of which show cavitation with strikingly thin walls.

pathologically to enlarged alveoli and interstitial septal destruction suggesting bleeding into the lung from this highly vascular tumor and subsequent expectoration of the blood.[760] The number of reported cases subjected to MRI is small[764]: the signal is heterogeneous with hyper- and isointense regions relative to muscle on T1-weighted images and high signal intensity on T2-weighted images. The lesions show marked enhancement on T1-weighted images following intravenous gadolinium injection.

Squamous papillomas of the bronchi and lungs are most commonly associated with *laryngeal papillomatosis*, a disease that usually commences in childhood and is believed to be viral in origin.[765] *Tracheobronchial papillomatosis* occurs in 5–10% of cases of laryngeal papillomatosis, an average of 10 years after the initial diagnosis of the laryngeal disease. Carcinomatous transformation has been reported.[766–768] Papillomatosis is almost invariably confined to the larynx, but in a small minority of patients one or more papillomas are found in the trachea and bronchi, where they may cause atelectasis and bronchiectasis.[769]

Even more rarely, the papillomas are present in the lung and are seen on chest radiographs or CT as multiple small, widely scattered, well-defined round pulmonary nodules, frequently with cavitation (Fig. 13.73).[765,769–772] The cavities, which may become several centimeters in diameter, are often thin walled but may have thick walls. Secondary infection may lead to air–fluid levels. Atelectasis is surprisingly infrequent. Squamous cell papilloma of the trachea without laryngeal papillomatosis has been described in adults.[773]

A single case of multiple small pulmonary nodules due to *intravascular papillary endothelial hyperplasia*, also known as *intravascular endothelial proliferation*, has been reported.[774]

Amyloidoma is a form of amyloidosis in which one or more nodular masses are seen in the lung parenchyma or tracheobronchial tree (Fig. 13.74). The lesions occur in the elderly and are frequently asymptomatic. A fuller discussion of intrathoracic amyloidosis is provided in Chapter 11.

Matsubara et al,[775] based on an analysis of 32 cases, believed that most or possibly all cases of *plasma cell granuloma* originate as

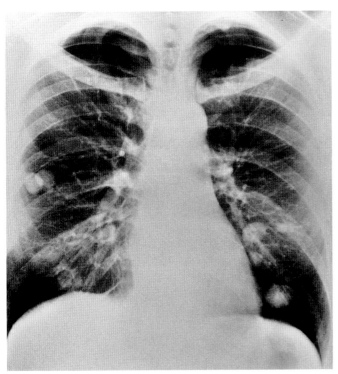

Fig. 13.74 Multiple pulmonary nodules caused by amyloidosis. Several nodules contain a central core of calcification.

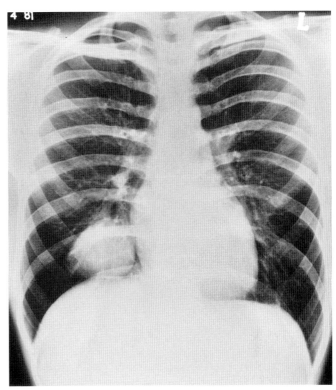

Fig. 13.75 Plasma cell granuloma of the right lower lobe bronchus. The mass shows no distinguishing features.

organizing pneumonia and that these lesions are not neoplasms. The condition may be a heterogeneous group of disorders with similar histologic features,[776] and histologic confusion with plasmacytoma and lymphoma may occur.[777] Numerous other terms have been applied, notably *inflammatory pseudotumor of the lung, inflammatory myofibroblastic tumor, histiocytoma, plasma cell histiocytoma complex, xanthoma, fibrous xanthoma, xanthogranuloma,* and *fibroxanthoma.* The age range is wide and includes particularly children[778,779] and young adults. Macroscopically the lesions are pale, firm, sharply circumscribed masses. Histologic examination shows a localized benign proliferation of plasma cells within a background of granulation or fibrocollagenous tissue. The lesions may be large and locally invasive. Complete resection, when possible, leads to an excellent outcome.[779] Most patients are asymptomatic but cough, fever, chest pain, hemoptysis or wheezing may be the presenting features. Since most lung tumors are uncommon in children, plasma cell granuloma, despite its rarity, is one of the more frequent causes for asymptomatic solitary pulmonary nodule in a child.[780]

Radiographically and at CT, the plasma cell granulomas present as a well-defined solitary pulmonary nodule (Fig. 13.75), which can be a large mass, or as focal ill-defined consolidation.[778,780–784] Multiple pulmonary nodules are seen on occasion.[780,785] Calcification, which may be extensive, and cavitation have both been described.[778,780,786–792] The occasional plasma cell granuloma arises in a central bronchus,[780,784,793,794] and is radiologically indistinguishable from bronchial carcinoid. Bronchial involvement can cause distal atelectasis and pneumonia.[795] A pleural origin has been described.[780,796] Hilar and mediastinal adenopathy are occasionally seen.[780] CT and MRI show all the imaging features to advantage and allow contrast enhancement to be recognized.[781,788,792,797]

Plasma cell granulomas may or may not enhance at CT and MRI, following intravenous contrast administration.[780] MRI shows slightly greater signal intensity than muscle on T1-weighted sequences,[780] and high intensity on T2-weighted sequences. Pleural effusions, which are usually small but can be large, are also reported.[780] A case showing intense uptake on an FDG PET scan has been reported.[798]

MALIGNANT LYMPHOMAS

Classification

Traditionally, the lymphomas have been divided into Hodgkin disease and non-Hodgkin lymphoma. In the most recent iteration of the WHO classification of the Haematopoietic and Lymphoid Tissues,[799] Hodgkin disease has been reincorporated into the schema for lymphomas, in recognition that most Reed-Sternberg cells originate from B lymphocytes. Also, the term Hodgkin lymphoma has been dropped in favor of Hodgkin disease. Despite the nomenclature shuffling the clinical differences and histologic distinctions remain unchanged.

Hodgkin lymphoma is, in the great majority of cases, a lymphoid neoplasm of B lymphocyte lineage. In the WHO classification, it is broadly divided into nodular lymphocyte predominant Hodgkin lymphoma, which in European and N American series comprises approximately 5% of cases, and classic Hodgkin lymphoma, which comprises the remaining 95% (see Box 13.10). Classic Hodgkin lymphoma continues to be classified into four subtypes according to the Rye modification of the Lukes-Butler classification.[800] These subtypes are nodular sclerosing, which comprises some 70% of cases of classic Hodgkin lymphoma, and three further categories based on the relative proportion of reactive elements to Sternberg-Reed cells (and their mononuclear counterparts) – lymphocyte rich (5% of cases), mixed cellularity (20–25% of cases), and lymphocyte depleted (<5% of cases).

The *non-Hodgkin lymphomas* can be regarded as neoplasms of a lymphoreticular cell of a specific lineage, notably, in order of prevalence, B, T, or NK (natural killer) lymphocytes. Immunohistochemical stains can be used to establish the B, T or NK cell origin, and a variety of specialized tests can be used to determine whether or not a lymphoproliferative lesion is monoclonal (i.e. neoplastic). The classification of non-Hodgkin lymphomas, unlike Hodgkin lymphoma, has undergone many changes. Until recently, the Working Formulation for Clinical Usage was the standard classification used in the US.[801] This had only 10 categories and did not require immunophenotyping or genetic studies. It provided simple clinical groupings for determining the approach to treatment (low, intermediate, and high clinical grades). However, advances in understanding the immune system and lymphoid neoplasms have led to the recognition of many new categories of lymphoid neoplasms and the development of better methods for diagnosis and treatment. Therefore, the International Lymphoma Study Group introduced a new classification in 1994, known as the Revised European–American Classification of Lymphoid Neoplasms (REAL).[802] WHO modified the REAL classification, which has now become the standard classification (see Box 13.11).[799,803] The relative importance of morphology, immunophenotype, and genetic features varies among the conditions, and there is no one "gold standard" in the WHO classification. Morphology is the basis for both diagnosis and classification in many typical cases of lymphoma. Immunophenotyping and, particularly, molecular genetic studies are not needed in all cases, but they are very important in some diseases, particularly in difficult cases, and they improve interobserver reproducibility. Regular updating, rather than wholesale modification, is anticipated.

Staging

Hodgkin lymphoma is staged using the Ann Arbor classification (adopted by the WHO), which takes into account the extent of nodal disease, the presence of extranodal disease, and clinical symptoms[804] (Table 13.8). A modification, known as the Cotswold's classification (Table 13.9),[805] takes into account tumor bulk and the increased use of CT for assessing the extent of disease. The great majority of patients are stage I or II at diagnosis. Hodgkin lymphoma spreads predictably from one lymph node group to contiguous groups.[806] In this context the term "contiguous" does not mean physical contiguity, but a directly connected lymphatic pathway.[807] Understanding the pattern of spread is useful when considering imaging procedures for staging and when designing radiation therapy ports. The ports usually include both the areas of known disease and the adjacent node groups. Direct invasion from affected nodes into the lung or bone is another characteristic form of spread.[808] Otherwise, initial presentation with extranodal disease is rare in Hodgkin lymphoma.

The American Joint Committee on Cancer (AJCC) and the Union Internationale Contre le Cancer (UICC) have adopted the Ann Arbor system, originally designed for staging Hodgkin lymphoma (see Table 13.8) for classifying the anatomic extent of disease in adults with non-Hodgkin lymphoma. It has less value, however, because the course of non-Hodgkin lymphoma

---

Box 13.10 WHO classification of Hodgkin lymphoma[799]

Nodular lymphocyte predominance Hodgkin lymphoma (NLPHL)
Classic Hodgkin lymphoma (CHL)
  Nodular sclerosis Hodgkin lymphoma (NSHL)
  Mixed cellularity Hodgkin lymphoma (MCHL)
  Lymphocyte rich classic Hodgkin lymphoma (LRCHL)
  Lymphocyte depletion Hodgkin lymphoma (LDHL)

Box 13.11 WHO classification of lymphoid neoplasms (excluding Hodgkin lymphomas – see Box 13.10)[799]

B-cell neoplasms
Precursor B-cell neoplasm
  • Precursor B-lymphoblastic lymphoma/leukemia
Mature (peripheral) B-cell neoplasms
  • B-cell chronic lymphocytic leukemia/small lymphocytic lymphoma
  • B-cell prolymphocytic leukemia
  • Lymphoplasmacytic lymphoma
  • Splenic marginal zone B-cell lymphoma
  • Hairy cell leukemia
  • Plasma cell myeloma/plasmacytoma
  • Extranodal marginal zone B-cell lymphoma of MALT type
  • Nodal marginal zone B-cell lymphoma
  • Follicular lymphoma
  • Mantle cell lymphoma
  • Diffuse large B-cell lymphoma
  • Mediastinal (thymic) large B-cell lymphoma
  • Intravascular large B-cell lymphoma
  • Primary effusion lymphoma
  • Burkitt lymphoma/leukemia
B-cell proliferations of uncertain malignant potential
  • Lymphomatoid granulomatosis
  • Posttransplant lymphoproliferative disorder, polymorphic

T and NK (natural killer-cell neoplasms)
Precursor T-cell neoplasm
  • Precursor T-lymphoblastic lymphoma/leukemia
  • Blastic NK-cell lymphoma
Mature (peripheral) T/NK-cell neoplasms
  • T-cell prolymphocytic leukemia
  • T-cell large granular lymphocytic leukemia
  • Aggressive NK-cell leukemia
  • Adult T-cell lymphoma/leukemia
  • Extranodal NK/T-cell lymphoma, nasal type
  • Enteropathy type T-cell lymphoma
  • Hepatosplenic T-cell lymphoma
  • Subcutaneous panniculitis-like T-cell lymphoma
  • Mycosis fungoides/Sezary syndrome
  • Primary cutaneous anaplastic large cell lymphoma
  • Peripheral T-cell lymphoma, unspecified
  • Angioimmunoblastic T-cell lymphoma
  • Anaplastic large cell lymphoma
T-cell proliferation of uncertain malignant potential
  • Lymphomatoid papulosis

Table 13.8 Ann Arbor staging classification for Hodgkin lymphoma. (Modified from reference[804].)

Stage*

I	Involvement of a single lymph node region (I) or of a single extralymphatic organ or site (IE)
II	Involvement of two or more lymph node regions on the same side of the diaphragm (II); or localized involvement of a single extralymphatic organ or site in association with regional lymph node involvement with or without involvement of other lymph node regions on the same side of the diaphragm (IIE). The number of regions involved may be indicated by a subscript, as in, for example, II_3
III	Involvement of lymph node regions of both sides of the diaphragm (III), which may also be accompanied by involvement of the spleen (III_S) or by localized involvement of an extralymphatic organ or site (III_E) or both (III_{SE})
IV	Diffuse or disseminated involvement of one or more extralymphatic organs, with or without associated lymph node involvement; or isolated extralymphatic organ involvement in the absence of adjacent regional lymph node involvement, but in conjunction with disease in distant site(s). Any involvement of the liver or bone marrow, or nodular involvement of the lung(s). The location of Stage IV disease is identified further by specifying the site

*The absence or presence of fever, night sweats, or unexplained loss of 10% or more of body weight in the 6 months preceding admission are to be denoted in all cases by the suffix letters A or B, respectively.

Table 13.9 Cotswold's classification of Hodgkin lymphoma[805]

Stage	Area of involvement
I	One lymph node region or extralymphatic site
II	Two or more lymph node regions on the same side of the diaphragm
III	Involvement of lymph node region or structures on both sides of diaphragm, subdivided so that:
III(1*)	With involvement of spleen and/or splenic hilar, celiac and portal nodes
III(2*)	With paraaortic, iliac or mesenteric nodes
IV	Extranodal sites beyond those designated E (see below)

Additional qualifiers

A	No symptoms
B	Fever, sweats, weight loss (to 10% of body weight)
E	Involvement of single extranodal site, contiguous in proximity to a known nodal site
X*	Bulky disease Mass >1/3 thoracic diameter at T5 Mass >10 cm maximum dimension
CE*	Clinical stage
PS*	Pathologic stage (PS) at a given site denoted by a subscript (i.e. M = marrow, H = liver, L = lung, O = bone, P = pleural, D = skin)

* Modifications from Ann Arbor system.

Table 13.10 Murphy staging system for childhood non-Hodgkin lymphoma[816]

Stage	Criteria for extent of disease
I	A single tumor (extranodal) or single anatomic area (nodal) with the exclusion of the mediastinum or abdomen
II	A single tumor (extranodal) with regional nodal involvement Two or more nodal areas on the same side of the diaphragm Two single (extranodal) tumors with or without regional node involvement of the same side of the diaphragm A primary gastrointestinal tract tumor, usually in the ileocecal area, with or without involvement of associated mesenteric nodes only, grossly completely resected
III	Two single tumors (extranodal) on opposite sides of the diaphragm Two or more nodal areas above and below the diaphragm All primary intrathoracic tumors (mediastinal, pleural, thymic) All extensive primary intraabdominal disease, unresected All paraspinal or epidural tumors, regardless of other tumor site(s)
IV	Any of the above with initial central nervous system and/or bone marrow involvement

depends more on histologic grade and parameters such as tumor bulk and specific organ involvement than on stage of disease.

Non-Hodgkin lymphoma in childhood often takes a different form from that seen in adults.[809–812] Almost all children show high grade histologic features and many have extranodal involvement.[813,814] In the series of 80 patients with childhood non-Hodgkin lymphoma reported by Ng et al,[815] only 20% presented with intrathoracic lymph node enlargement as the primary site of disease. The most frequently used staging classification is the Murphy (St Jude's) classification (Table 13.10).[816]

Imaging features of intrathoracic lymphadenopathy in malignant lymphoma

The cardinal feature of malignant lymphoma on chest radiographs and CT is mediastinal and hilar node enlargement, which may be accompanied by pulmonary, pleural, or chest wall involvement. The appearances of intrathoracic lymphadenopathy on imaging examination are similar in Hodgkin and non-Hodgkin lymphoma, but the frequency and distribution differ. Any intrathoracic nodal group may be enlarged and the possible combinations are legion, but the following remarks regarding chest radiography, CT, and MRI may be useful:

- Filly et al[817] reviewed the chest radiographs of patients with untreated malignant lymphomas. Of the 164 patients with Hodgkin lymphoma, 67% had visible intrathoracic disease, and all but one had mediastinal or hilar adenopathy, whereas 43% of the patients with non-Hodgkin lymphoma had visible intrathoracic abnormality, 87% of which showed mediastinal/hilar lymphadenopathy. Similarly, Castellino et al,[818] who studied the prevalence of intrathoracic abnormalities on chest CT and chest radiography in 181 patients with newly diagnosed non-Hodgkin lymphoma, found that 45% of the patients had visible disease within the thorax, 80% of whom showed mediastinal/hilar adenopathy. The anterior mediastinal and paratracheal nodes are the most frequently involved groups (Fig. 13.76). The tracheobronchial and subcarinal nodes are also enlarged in many cases. In most cases the lymphadenopathy is bilateral but asymmetric. Large B-cell non-Hodgkin lymphoma and Hodgkin lymphoma both have a propensity to involve the anterior mediastinal and paratracheal nodes – almost all patients with the nodular sclerosing form of Hodgkin lymphoma have disease in the anterior mediastinum.

- The incidence of visible hilar and mediastinal lymphadenopathy on chest radiographs in younger patients with malignant lymphomas is lower: under 10 years of age, approximately 33% of those with Hodgkin lymphoma and only 20–25% of those with non-Hodgkin lymphoma show mediastinal and hilar node enlargement.[815,819–821]
- The great majority of cases of Hodgkin lymphoma show enlargement of two or more nodal groups, whereas only one nodal group is involved in about half the cases of non-Hodgkin lymphoma.
- Hilar node enlargement is rare without accompanying mediastinal node enlargement, particularly in Hodgkin lymphoma.
- The posterior mediastinum is infrequently involved. The enlarged nodes are often low in the mediastinum, and contiguous retroperitoneal disease is likely (Fig. 13.77).[821]

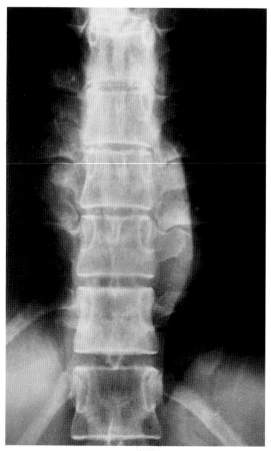

Fig. 13.77 Posterior mediastinal lymph node enlargement in Hodgkin disease. The left paraspinal line is displaced by enlarged nodes. Note the sclerosis of the body of T12 resulting from lymphomatous involvement of bone.

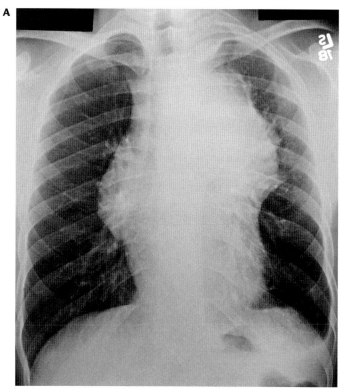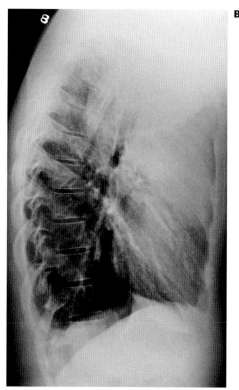

Fig. 13.76 **A**, Posteroanterior and **B**, lateral radiographs of an anterior mediastinal lymph node enlargement in Hodgkin disease.

- The paracardiac nodes are rarely involved but become important as sites of recurrence because they may not be included in the radiation field (Fig. 13.78).[822,823] They may be visibly enlarged on chest radiographs, but frequently CT is needed for their demonstration (Fig. 13.79).[824]
- Compression of the pulmonary arteries,[817] superior vena cava,[825] and major bronchi[826] by enlarged nodes may be seen in both Hodgkin and non-Hodgkin lymphoma.

- CT demonstrates enlarged mediastinal nodes despite normal plain chest radiographs in about 10% of those with both Hodgkin[827] and non-Hodgkin lymphoma.[818]
- At CT, the enlarged lymph nodes in any of the malignant lymphomas may be discrete or matted together, and their edges may be well- or ill-defined (Fig. 13.80).[828] The nodes show minor or moderate enhancement following intravenous contrast material in most instances, but enhancement by >50 HU is seen in a small proportion of cases.[829] Low density

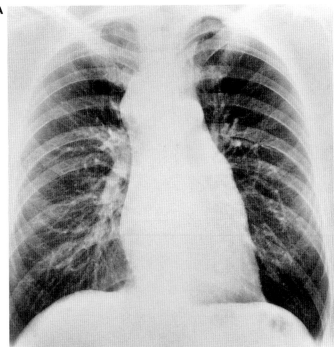

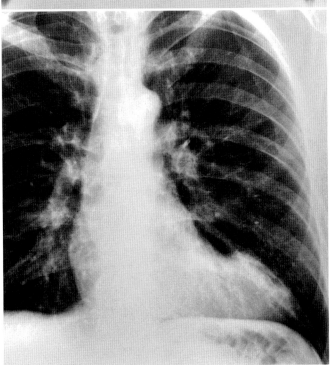

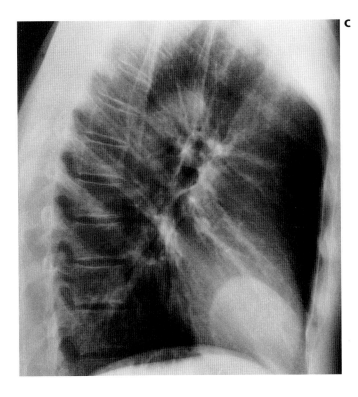

Fig. 13.78 Paracardiac node enlargement in Hodgkin disease. **A**, Plain radiograph before radiotherapy. There is enlargement of the paratracheal nodes bilaterally and of the nodes along the left heart border. Nodes in the left cardiophrenic angle are not enlarged. **B** and **C**, Four years later, at time of recurrence, posteroanterior and lateral radiographs show massive enlargement of the left cardiophrenic angle nodes but no detectable enlargement of mediastinal nodes in the original radiation field.

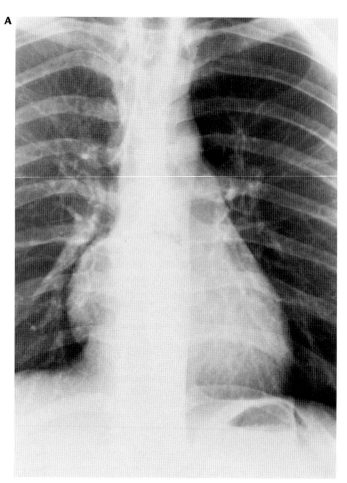

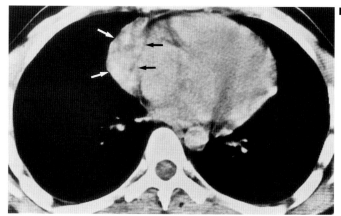

Fig. 13.79 Paracardiac node enlargement in non-Hodgkin lymphoma. **A,** Distortion of the right mediastinal border is difficult to distinguish from right atrial enlargement on plain film (lateral projection was unremarkable). **B,** CT demonstrates enlarged lymph nodes (arrows) to advantage.

areas (Fig. 13.80) resulting from cystic degeneration may be seen in both Hodgkin[830] and non-Hodgkin lymphoma.[825,831] The cystic areas may persist following therapy, when the rest of the nodal mass shrinks away.

- Lymph node calcification before therapy is rare, even at CT,[832,833] but is seen occasionally following therapy. Irregular, eggshell, and diffuse patterns of calcification may be seen.[832]
- MRI shows much the same anatomic features as CT, but MRI allows the demonstration of vascular and cardiac invasion or compression without the use of intravascular contrast agents (Fig. 13.81). The MRI signal intensity of lymphomatous masses is usually homogeneous.[834] On T1-weighted images lymphomatous tissue is slightly hyperintense compared with muscle and well below fat, whereas on T2-weighted images it is of greater signal intensity than muscle and isointense with fat. These findings appear to be independent of the grade of the tumor.[834] Negendank et al[834] found that active tumor with dense fibrous tissue had unexpectedly high signal on T2-weighted images, perhaps explaining the tendency for Hodgkin lymphoma to show higher signal on T2-weighted images than non-Hodgkin lymphoma.

Thymic lymphoma

Thymic enlargement is seen in a high proportion of patients with lymphoma,[835–837] particularly mediastinal large B-cell and Hodgkin lymphoma, in adults and T-cell lymphobastic lymphoma in children. Since the thymus is of lymphatic origin, there is little point in determining radiologically whether an anterior mediastinal mass is of thymic or nodal origin, but it is worth noting that massive thymic enlargement is a highly characteristic presentation of mediastinal large B-cell lymphoma and T-cell lymphobastic lymphoma.

The thymus in children may enlarge following successful treatment of lymphoma or leukemia due to the phenomenon known as rebound thymic hyperplasia (see p. 969).

Post-treatment residual mediastinal masses

Successfully treated lymphomatous nodes often return to normal size and extranodal masses resolve, but bulky mediastinal nodal disease in both Hodgkin and non-Hodgkin lymphoma, particularly nodular sclerosing Hodgkin lymphoma, are often slow to resolve and may leave residual masses of sterilized

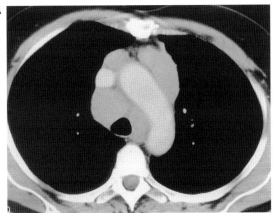

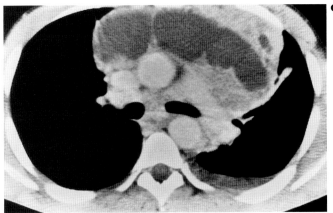

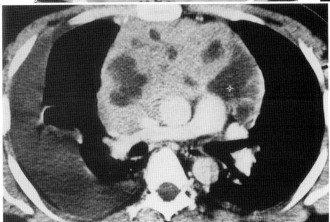

Fig. 13.80 CT of enlarged lymph nodes in malignant lymphoma. **A**, Multifocal, greatly enlarged, moderately discrete nodes. **B**, Hodgkin lymphoma. The nodes are matted together and appear as a conglomerate mass. Fluid density areas caused by necrosis are present. **C**, High grade non-Hodgkin lymphoma showing multiple rounded areas of low density in greatly enlarged nodes. Note the large right pleural effusion.

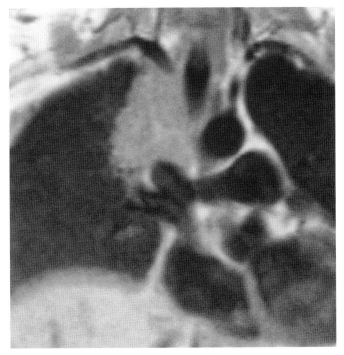

Fig. 13.81 Hodgkin lymphoma (stage II) showing large lymph node masses compressing the right brachiocephalic vein and superior vena cava. MRI (T1-weighted coronal scan) shows venous compression without the need for contrast medium. (Courtesy of Dr William C Black, Washington, DC)

> **Box 13.12 Imaging findings in posttreatment residual mediastinal masses of lymphoma**
>
> CT shows soft tissue density which may calcify
> Cystic change may be demonstrated, which may be degenerative or due to epithelial cyst formation
> ^{67}Ga scanning is helpful in excluding active disease if there is no uptake in a mass that previously showed substantial activity
> PET can be both false positive and false negative for active lymphoma, but a negative scan in a patient with enlarged mediastinal nodes is good evidence against active lymphoma
> MRI findings are uniform low signal on T2- as well T1-weighted images, but this combination does not rule out active disease

fibrous tissue (Fig. 13.82), particularly when the initial tumor mass consists chiefly of fibrous tissue to start with.[838–841] Determining the nature of such residual masses by imaging is difficult (see Box 13.12).

CT shows soft tissue density masses, sometimes partially calcified, but cannot distinguish between tumor and fibrous tissue on density grounds alone.

^{67}Ga scanning can be of help in determining whether or not a posttreatment residual mass contains active disease,[842–844]

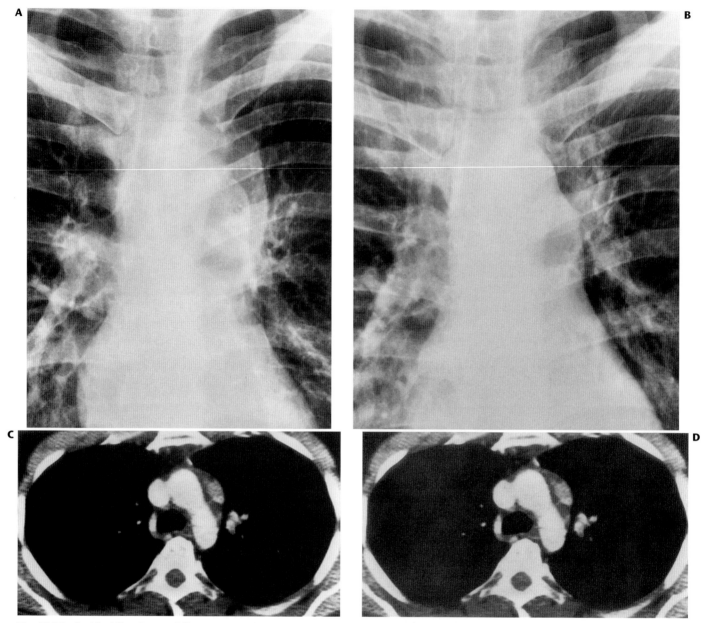

Fig. 13.82 Residual fibrotic mass following successful radiation treatment for Hodgkin lymphoma. **A** and **B**, show enlarged nodes in the aortopulmonary window and left paratracheal area. **C** and **D**, show residual mass of fibrous tissue in the aortopulmonary window. This residual mass remained unchanged over 3 years with no further treatment.

particularly if radionuclide imaging shows no uptake in a mass which previously showed substantial activity.[845–847] The converse conclusion, namely that positive uptake suggests active neoplasm, whilst not totally reliable (false positive results are seen with infection and with thymic hyperplasia),[845] is used in some centers for determining active disease in a residual mass.[847–851]

According to some authors,[852,853] but not all,[854] FDG PET can be helpful in assessing posttreatment residual masses; it can be both false positive and false negative when trying to determine active disease in residual masses, but a negative PET scan in nodes which remain large following treatment is a strong indicator of inactive disease.[853]

At MRI, posttreatment residual masses show lower signal on T2-weighted images than prior to treatment, reflecting a reduction in water content.[855,856] Early studies suggested that residual mediastinal masses which show uniform low signal on

T2- as well as T1-weighted images are likely to consist of mature fibrosis,[857,858] but more recent investigations have shown that MRI on its own is too unreliable to be decision making.[854] Active tumor cannot be excluded on the basis of signal intensity alone, because small foci of active disease within a mass of predominantly mature fibrosis are not detectable. MRI is also unreliable at diagnosing posttreatment active disease. High signal on T2-weighted images is seen within active tumor, but can also be seen with necrosis and inflammation in inactive tumor.[856–858] The interval development of higher T2 signal on sequential scans taken at least 6 months apart is a more reliable finding than the presence of high signal alone.[858]

Spiers et al[836] examined 25 patients with treated lymphoma involving the thymus and showed that relapse was more likely in patients with large volume masses or masses with heterogeneous high signal on T2-weighted images, but relapse did occasionally occur in patients with homogeneous or heterogeneous low signal. Nyman et al[859] found that tumors with low tumor:fat, and low tumor:muscle signal intensity ratios on T2-weighted scans did not decrease in size as much as those with higher signal intensity, possibly, but not necessarily,[860] reflecting the amount of fibrous tissue in the untreated tumor.

Significant reduction in gadolinium enhancement of the lymphomatous tissue on follow-up MRI scans occurs in patients with complete remission, unlike patients with relapse whose residual mass shows the same or greater degree of enhancement as the initial untreated mass.[855,856]

Posttreatment cystic degeneration of the thymus can be confused with active tumor.[861,862] Cysts, which may be degenerative or epithelial in nature, can develop in the thymus after radiation therapy for anterior mediastinal disease; they should not be confused with recurrent lymphoma. Either CT or MRI can be used to confirm the presence of cysts in the thymus.[836,855]

Pulmonary involvement in association with extrapulmonary disease (Box 13.13)

Lymphoma usually involves the lung in association with extrapulmonary lymphomatous disease, notably lymph node involvement, rather than by originating primarily in the lung. Parenchymal involvement of the lung becomes more frequent as the disease takes hold. It is three times more frequent in Hodgkin than in non-Hodgkin lymphoma as a whole, but mediastinal large B-cell lymphoma has a propensity to invade the lung.

The pulmonary opacities on chest radiography and CT in both Hodgkin[817,826,863–869] and non-Hodgkin lymphoma[817,865–867,870,871] are varied and resist easy classification. The most frequent pattern is one or more discrete pulmonary nodules resembling primary or metastatic carcinoma, but usually rather less well defined.[817,865,871] Such nodules may, on rare occasions, cavitate

(Fig. 13.83).[817,826,872] Another common pattern is round or segmental shaped, focal or patchy consolidations (Figs 13.84 and 13.85) which resemble pneumonia. A pattern of peribronchial pulmonary nodules or interstitial infiltration extending from the hila out into the parenchyma is sometimes seen at CT.[869,873] Similarly, focal, streaky shadowing, which at CT can be seen to be peribronchial,[865] may be seen, perhaps reflecting spread by way of the bronchopulmonary lymphatics. Widespread, reticulonodular shadowing (Fig. 13.86) resembling diffuse interstitial lung disease (sometimes called a "lymphangitic pattern") and widespread micronodules are also seen.[869] They are, however, an uncommon pattern in Hodgkin lymphoma.

Hodgkin lymphoma often appears to spread from nodal sites into the adjacent lung parenchyma.[863,869,873] However, peripheral subpleural masses or masses without visible connection to enlarged nodes in the mediastinum and hila (Fig. 13.87) are seen occasionally in Hodgkin lymphoma.[866] If an individual presents with Hodgkin lymphoma and a focal pulmonary shadow, but no evidence of hilar or mediastinal disease, it is likely that the pulmonary process represents something other than Hodgkin lymphoma.[873] A caveat here is that the patient should not previously have received radiation therapy to the mediastinum; when mediastinal and hilar nodes have been previously irradiated, then recurrence confined to the lungs may be seen in both Hodgkin and non-Hodgkin lymphoma (see Fig. 13.84).

Rapid growth of pulmonary lesions may be seen with non-Hodgkin lymphoma.[870,874,875] The development of large opacities or widespread disease in under 4 weeks, even in as little as 7 days, may cause great diagnostic confusion with pneumonia.

Primary pulmonary Hodgkin lymphoma

Primary pulmonary Hodgkin lymphoma is rare. In their review of the literature, Lee et al[876] found <100 cases of Hodgkin

---

> ### Box 13.13 Pulmonary involvement in lymphoma can be divided into three broad categories
>
> *In association with existing (or previously treated) nodal disease*
> Seen in some 10-15% of untreated cases
> Three times more frequent in Hodgkin than non-Hodgkin lymphoma
> Patterns of pulmonary involvement are highly variable
> Pulmonary involvement usually extends from hilum or mediastinum in previously untreated Hodgkin lymphoma
> Pulmonary non-Hodgkin lymphoma may grow very rapidly
>
> *Primary Hodgkin lymphoma of the lung*
> Rare entity
> Pattern is usually solitary or multiple pulmonary nodules and/or consolidations
>
> *Primary non-Hodgkin lymphoma of the lung*
> Lymphomas of mucosa associated lymphoid tissue (MALT) are by far the most common
> Rarely, nonMALT B-cell lymphomas, notably lymphomatoid granulomatosis and intravascular large B-cell lymphoma
> Rarely, peripheral T-cell lymphomas

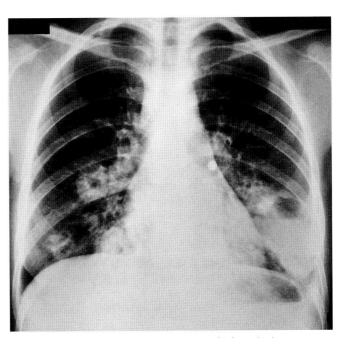

Fig. 13.83   Hodgkin lymphoma showing multiple cavitating pulmonary nodules (and right paratracheal nodal enlargement).

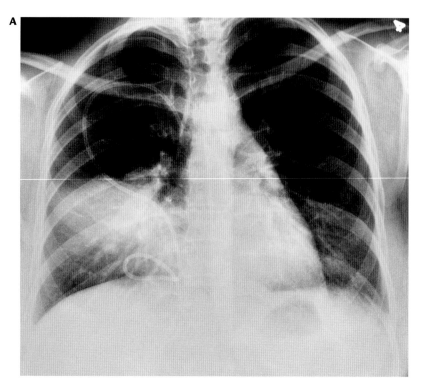
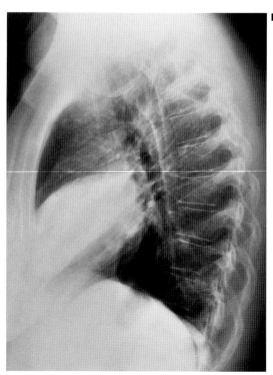

Fig. 13.84 Hodgkin lymphoma of the lung shown on **A**, posteroanterior and **B**, lateral radiographs. The pulmonary involvement has taken the form of lobar consolidation. This young woman previously had radiation therapy to enlarged mediastinal lymph nodes.

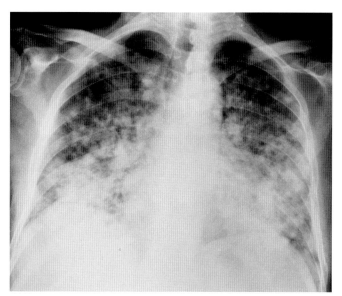

Fig. 13.85 Non-Hodgkin lymphoma of the lung in an elderly man. The multifocal ill-defined pulmonary consolidations were originally thought to be due to pneumonia because of accompanying fever and chills, but at autopsy were shown to be due to lymphoma.

lymphoma restricted to the pulmonary parenchyma at presentation. On imaging,[876–878] the most common feature is upper lobe predominant single or multiple nodules, some of which may be enlarged intrapulmonary lymph nodes. Some masses may be endobronchial in location. Single or multiple focal areas of consolidation may be seen in isolation or combined with pulmonary nodules. Cavitation of the pulmonary lesions may be seen.

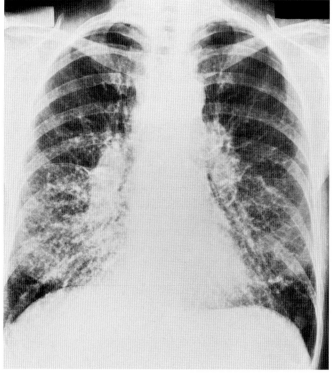

Fig. 13.86 Non-Hodgkin lymphoma showing widespread reticulonodular shadowing in both lungs (and enlargement of hilar and right paratracheal nodes).

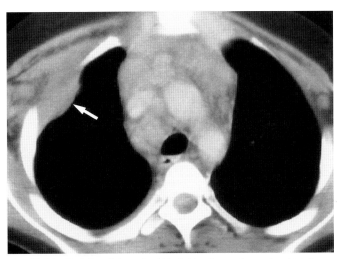

Fig. 13.87 Peripheral deposit of Hodgkin disease (arrow), which has no visible connection with the mediastinal adenopathy.

Primary pulmonary non-Hodgkin lymphoma

Most lymphomas arising primarily in the lung are marginal zone *lymphomas of mucosa associated lymphoid tissue (MALT)*.[879]

The distinct clinicopathologic entity of a "low grade" B-cell lymphoma arising from mucosa associated lymphoid tissue was first described in 1983 in a patient with primary gastrointestinal lymphoma.[880] Since then further reports have been published of similar tumors, of both low and intermediate grade, which have arisen in many other mucosal sites, including in the lungs, salivary glands, thyroid gland, thymus, skin, orbit, bladder, and genitourinary tract.[881–883] This particular form of lymphoma was previously categorized as pseudolymphoma and believed to be an inflammatory disorder with a propensity to convert to lymphoma.

The lymphoid tissue in lung parenchyma comprises lymphoid aggregates called bronchial MALT, sited predominantly in the peribronchial interstitium at the divisions of the respiratory bronchioles and to a lesser extent in the bronchial walls, interlobular septa and subpleural interstitium. When marginal zone non-Hodgkin lymphomas of MALT origin develop in the lung, they may be solitary or multicentric, and the cell of origin is a small B lymphocyte with either plasmacytoid, lymphocyte-like or monocytoid features that is believed to be derived from bronchial MALT. The tumors show dense infiltration of the lung parenchyma by the lymphoid infiltrate, with destruction of alveoli but comparative preservation of airways (correlating with air bronchograms) and pulmonary arteries. At their periphery, lymphomatous spread is typically along the distribution of pulmonary lymphatics. Immunohistochemistry and/or molecular studies may show evidence of clonality to confirm the diagnosis. Spread from marginal zone non-Hodgkin lymphomas of MALT origin tends to be to lymph nodes as well as extranodal sites. Prognosis is generally good. However, a minority of primary pulmonary cases are diffuse large B-cell non-Hodgkin lymphomas, some of which may represent transformation of marginal zone non-Hodgkin lymphomas of MALT origin. These tumors comprise sheets of blastic lymphoid cells, often with necrosis and brisk mitotic activity, and they behave in a more aggressive fashion.

The clinical features of MALT lymphoma are varied. The patients range in age from 11 to 80, the mean age being in the sixth decade. A substantial portion are asymptomatic, the lesions being detected incidentally on chest radiography. Those with symptoms have nonproductive cough, dyspnea, or respiratory infection.[884,885] Systemic symptoms such as fever and weight loss are less common. There may also be extrathoracic sites of extranodal lymphoma, particularly in the stomach, salivary glands, bone marrow, and skin.[885,886] A significant proportion of patients who develop MALT lymphoma have a history of inflammatory or autoimmune disease,[885,887] such as Sjögren syndrome, dysgammaglobulinemia,[888] and various collagen vascular diseases.

On imaging,[870,876,884,885,887,889–895] MALT lymphomas usually show one or more rounded or segmental-shaped consolidations varying in size from small to the size of a lobe (Fig. 13.88). The opacities may be sufficiently well defined to be called nodules or masses. There is no lobar predilection and the consolidations

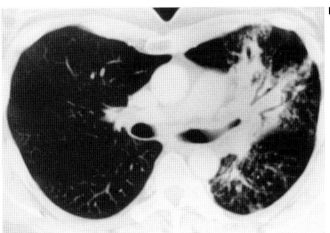

Fig. 13.88 MALT (mucosa associated lymphoid tumor) lymphoma taking the form of focal pulmonary consolidation. **A**, Chest radiograph. **B**, CT showing an obvious air bronchogram. (Courtesy of Dr Leonard King, London)

may be placed centrally or peripherally in the lung parenchyma. A few of the lesions show cavitation, but calcification does not occur. Air bronchograms are common and bubble-like lucencies may be seen within the pulmonary opacities. These two features are well shown by CT (Fig. 13.88),[887,891,893–896] on which it may be apparent that the bronchi within the lymphomatous process are dilated, stretched, or narrowed, similar to the appearances seen with bronchioloalveolar carcinoma.[891] HRCT may show in addition centrilobular micronodules and thickened interlobular septa.[893,894] Areas of ground-glass opacity are common. Diffuse interstitial shadowing closely resembling interstitial fibrosis has also been reported.[887] Pleural effusion is demonstrated in up to 20% of cases. Hilar and/or mediastinal node enlargement may also be present.

Primary pulmonary non-Hodgkin lymphomas other than MALT lymphoma are very rare and include: lymphomatoid granulomatosis, intravascular large B-cell lymphoma, and unspecified peripheral T-cell lymphoma.

Lymphomatoid granulomatosis (also known as angiocentric immunoproliferative lesion) is believed to be an Epstein–Barr virus associated B-cell lymphoproliferative disorder in which T cells predominate over B cells.[897]

The literature on the appearances at chest radiography and CT needs to be interpreted with caution since it is largely based on histologic diagnoses that would now be questioned, because modern immunohistochemical techniques were unavailable at the time.[898,899,899–906] The most frequent appearance, occurring in up to 80% of patients, is multiple pulmonary nodules, which are usually bilateral but may be unilateral; occasionally, only a solitary pulmonary mass is seen (Fig. 13.89). The nodules, which closely resemble metastases, are usually round in shape and have ill-defined margins, though a small proportion have a

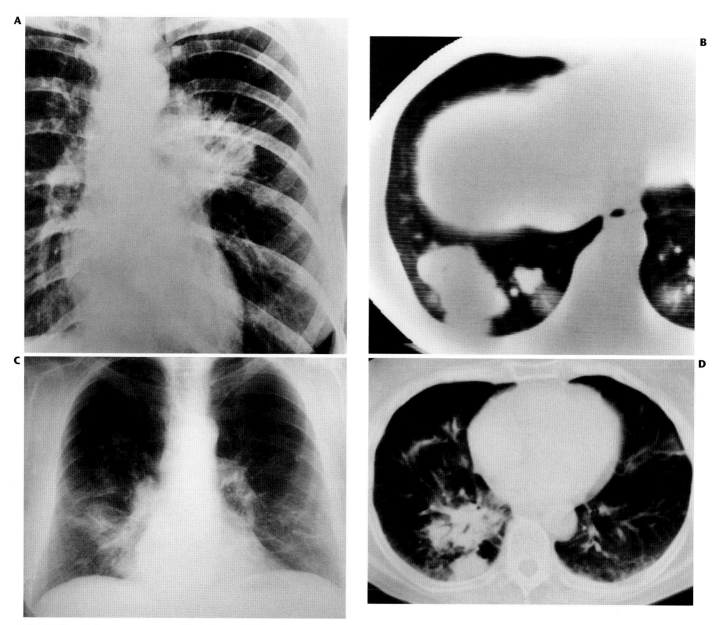

Fig. 13.89 Various appearances of lymphomatoid granulomatosis. **A**, Large irregular, lobular mass adjacent to the left hilum. **B**, Multiple lobular pulmonary masses resembling metastases on CT. **C**, Multiple, ill-defined pulmonary shadows that, **D**, on CT are seen to be masses with very irregular edges and air bronchograms.

well-defined edge. They may be very large: nodules of up to 10 cm in diameter have been reported. Multiple, ill-defined areas of consolidation resembling pneumonia are a less common radiographic manifestation. Coalescence of the nodules or consolidations is a feature that may help in the radiographic differential diagnosis from pulmonary metastases. The lesions show a predisposition for the mid and lower lung zones, with a tendency to spare the apices. A bronchocentric distribution may be noted at CT. Invasion into the lumen of a main pulmonary artery has been reported.[906] At least some of the nodules seen on plain chest radiograph are a result of infarcts related to the angiodestructive nature of the disease.[900,907] Dee et al[900] showed on histologic examination in three cases that the bulk of the lesion was an infarct, the cellular infiltrate of lymphomatoid granulomatosis being confined to the periphery and contributing little to the radiographic shadow. Cavitation was seen in approximately 10% of patients in one review of the literature,[903] but in individual series, the rate of cavitation is as high as 25%.[898,908] The cavities are usually thick walled, but thin walled cystlike cavities have been reported.[906,908] Cavitation appears to be associated with a poor prognosis.[898] Air bronchograms are seen in some cases (Fig. 13.89), the highest reported incidence being 40%.[898] Widely distributed reticulonodular shadowing has been reported in a few cases.[900,908] When examined at biopsy, these lesions proved to result from cellular infiltration without infarction.[900] The few reported cases of MRI of lymphomatoid granulomatosis of the lung reveals no features that permit distinction from other lymphomas.[906,909]

Visible hilar and mediastinal adenopathy are very unusual. Pleural effusion does not appear to be a major feature of the disease, though small pleural effusions are seen on plain chest radiograph in up to one-third of patients. The plain chest radiograph may be normal in patients diagnosed as having lymphomatoid granulomatosis of the sinuses or skin.

Intravascular large B-cell lymphoma[910–912] (also known as *malignant angioendotheliosis or angiotropic lymphoma*) is characterized by proliferation of neoplastic cells in small vessels, which on occasions may present primarily in the lungs.[913] Mostly the disease presents with widespread central nervous system involvement. Chest radiography and CT show widespread, ill-defined or ground-glass pulmonary shadowing which may show air bronchograms.[914,915]

Peripheral T-cell lymphomas represent a diverse, and mostly very aggressive, group of lymphomas derived from mature T cells. They are relatively uncommon in Europe and N America, comprising about 12% of all non-Hodgkin lymphomas, but much more common in Asia. The imaging features are similar to other malignant lymphomas.[916] Mediastinal lymph node enlargement, widespread parenchymal infiltrates, and a reticulonodular pattern with septal lines have been reported.[916] Pulmonary nodules are also encountered and pleural effusions are not uncommon.

Endobronchial disease

Endobronchial disease is rare, particularly in non-Hodgkin lymphoma,[917–920] but so is bronchial occlusion by neighboring lymph node enlargement. Therefore, when atelectasis is encountered, the possibility of endobronchial lymphoma should be seriously considered. Endobronchial lymphoma may be seen as an intramural nodule or irregular tumor mass at CT.[918–921]

Pleural and pericardial disease

Pleural effusions, mostly unilateral, were seen in up to one-quarter of patients with lymphoma on plain chest radiographs in several larger series,[817,827,863,864] and in 50% of patients on CT.[865] Pleural effusion is accompanied by mediastinal lymphadenopathy, sufficiently large to be visible on chest radiographs or CT, in some 80% of patients with Hodgkin lymphoma.[817,827] Pleural and adjacent extrapleural lymphomatous nodules or masses are found in some 25–40% of patients with pleural effusion in both Hodgkin and non-Hodgkin lymphoma.[922] The effusions are usually exudates and may disappear with irradiation of the mediastinal lymph nodes.[923,924] Chylothorax is occasionally encountered.[873] Lymphomatous pleural masses, particularly primary pleural lymphoma, are rare[925,926]; the more usual "pleural" manifestation is lymphomatous pulmonary disease in the subpleural region just beneath the visceral pleura.[866]

A rare pleural based lymphoma is *pyothorax associated diffuse large B-cell lymphoma*, in which lymphoma develops in the walls of an empyema.[927–929]

So-called *"Primary effusion lymphoma"* is a rare and aggressive neoplasm of large B cells, which usually presents initially as serous effusions in the pleural, pericardial, or peritoneal cavities without detectable masses and no lymphadenopathy or organomegaly. It is mostly associated with human immunodeficiency virus infection.[930] Some patients have coexistent Kaposi sarcoma or multicentric Castleman disease.[931]

Pericardial effusions are presumptive evidence of pericardial involvement. For practical purposes, pericardial effusion requires ultrasound, CT, or MRI for its recognition. In Castellino et al's series of 203 patients with Hodgkin lymphoma who had CT on initial presentation, 6% had pericardial effusion, and in all these patients there were coexistent large lymph nodes adjacent to the cardiac margins. A nodular mass within the pericardium was seen in just one case.

Chest wall invasion

Chest wall invasion and rib destruction are seen on occasion (Fig. 13.90).[866] Chest wall invasion is well demonstrated by CT and appears to be even better shown by MRI.[932,933] As with so many neoplasms which invade muscle and fat, it can be difficult to differentiate between tumor and surrounding edema, which means the true extent of tumor may be difficult to determine and the distinction between recurrence of lymphoma and postradiotherapy changes may not be possible.

Role of imaging in staging lymphoma

Chest radiography can accurately demonstrate the extent of lymphomatous involvement in many patients, but chest CT is more informative,[934,935] and may show that suspected lymphomatous involvement is due to an alternative process.[936] In general, chest CT is more useful in the initial staging of Hodgkin than non-Hodgkin lymphoma,[807,818] because radiation therapy is often a vital component of treatment for Hodgkin lymphoma,[827,937] and inadequate radiation portals are a potential cause of treatment failure. Castellino et al[827] found that

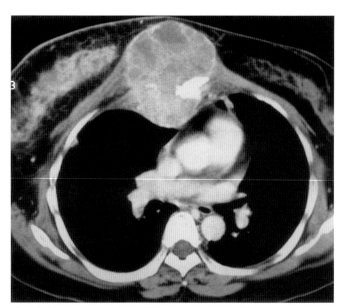

Fig. 13.90 Massive chest wall invasion by non-Hodgkin lymphoma.

the incremental information obtained from chest CT prompted a change in treatment in almost 10% of 203 new patients with Hodgkin lymphoma. As expected, the impact was greatest in the 65 patients being treated with radiation therapy alone. Similarly, in the 107 new cases of Hodgkin lymphoma reported by Hopper et al,[936] chest CT changed the stage of disease in 20 patients. Chest CT is most useful in patients in whom the appearance of the mediastinum on plain chest radiograph is normal or equivocal.

Non-Hodgkin lymphoma is so often disseminated at the time of initial diagnosis that demonstrating the extent of intrathoracic disease may not change management, because the treatment for disseminated disease is chemotherapy rather than radiation therapy. Although the findings on routine chest CT can increase the stage of disease in some patients with non-Hodgkin lymphoma, it had no effect on the initial treatment of newly diagnosed non-Hodgkin lymphoma in one large series.[818]

The role of chest CT may be rather different in children with non-Hodgkin lymphoma. In the series by Ng et al,[814] chest radiography provided the necessary management information in almost all cases; in only one of 34 children who had chest CT did the CT findings increase the stage. Cohen et al,[938] however, found that chest CT altered the stage in three of 11 children with non-Hodgkin lymphoma.

Mediastinal sonography, using a suprasternal and parasternal approach, has been advocated as a method of following the response to treatment of lymphomatous mediastinal lymphadenopathy. Wernecke et al[939] believe that sonography is comparable to CT for monitoring mediastinal lymphomas, claiming it has the advantage that in some cases it can correctly predict residual disease based on the hypoechoic ultrasound texture of the affected nodes when the CT scan is normal. Mediastinal sonography has not, however, become a widely used technique.[940]

So far, MRI has not proved to be of greater value than CT in the routine staging of thoracic lymphoma, but it may answer highly specific questions such as the extent of pericardial, cardiac, chest wall, or spinal involvement.[873,932,941] As discussed

on p. 848, the initial hope that MRI signal characteristics might allow distinction between active disease and posttreatment residual fibrosis has not yet been realized. It has, however, been suggested that it might be possible to predict prognostic grade in certain circumstances: patients with high grade non-Hodgkin lymphoma and a homogeneous signal pattern tend to have a better survival rate than those with an inhomogeneous pattern.[942]

Radionuclide scintigraphy, with agents such as ^{67}Ga, ^{201}Tl, or radiolabeled octreotide, is not generally believed to be of value for initial staging.[806,943–945] ^{67}Ga scanning, however, has its advocates, who argue that with recent technical advances it is becoming sufficiently sensitive to detect active disease, and can be used in follow up,[843,844,850] particularly when SPECT is used.[946] It may also be useful for predicting outcome following treatment,[849,947–949] and can be of help in determining whether or not a posttreatment residual mass contains active disease.[842–844]

FDG PET can achieve the same or greater accuracy as CT for initial staging and is better than CT for finding extranodal lymphoma.[844,950–953] but it does give some false positive results.[852,952] FDG PET imaging can alter management in a substantial proportion of patients with lymphoma, either by excluding active disease or by diagnosing active disease in sites where CT fails to show an abnormality.[852,951,954,955] FDG PET can also predict response to treatment. A negative PET scan, even if there are large residual nodes on CT or MRI, appears to be reasonably reliable for predicting remission, whereas a positive scan is much less accurate for predicting relapse.[843,852–854,956]

NON-NEOPLASTIC LYMPHOID LESIONS OF THE LUNGS

Included under the general heading of pulmonary lymphoid lesions of the lungs are true lymphomatous and leukemic lesions of the lung, as well as several entities that are non-neoplastic (see Box 13.14). The understanding of many of the entities is constantly evolving and has changed significantly over the last two decades. For example:

- Conditions that were previously regarded as non-neoplastic, such as lymphomatoid granulomatosis (see p. 852) and most cases of pseudolymphoma are now classified as lymphomas.
- Lymphocytic interstitial pneumonia (LIP) has changed status frequently, being classified initially as an interstitial pneumonia, before it was recognized that most of the cases were low grade B-cell lymphomas which would now be called marginal zone non-Hodgkin lymphomas of MALT origin. With these lymphomas stripped out, LIP is now once again regarded as a non-neoplastic, inflammatory,

---

Box 13.14 Non-neoplastic pulmonary lymphoid lesions[957]

Intrapulmonary lymph node (see Ch. 2, p. 39)
Follicular bronchiolitis (MALT hyperplasia) (see Ch. 12, p. 744)
Lymphocytic interstitial pneumonia (see Ch. 13, p. 855)
Nodular lymphoid hyperplasia (see p. 855)
Castleman disease (see Ch. 14, p. 929)

interstitial pneumonia. Idiopathic lymphocytic interstitial pneumonia is included in the recent American Thoracic Society/European Respiratory Society classification of the idiopathic interstitial pneumonias, but cases are exceptionally rare.[958] LIP is far more commonly associated with a variety of autoimmune disorders and with HIV infection and AIDS (see p. 300).

- Follicular bronchiolitis is a newly described entity consisting of hyperplasia of bronchial MALT in relation to the airways (see p. 744).
- Hyaline vascular Castleman disease (see p. 929) is regarded as a form of reactive hyperplasia, which predominantly affects lymph nodes, although cases are described within the lung.
- The entity "nodular lymphoid hyperplasia", which refers to the occurrence of one or more pulmonary nodules consisting of reactive lymphoid cells, is a rare condition, cases of which were previously included in series of cases labeled as pulmonary pseudolymphoma. Pseudolymphoma was initially described in the early 1960s, but during the 1980s and early 1990s immunohistochemical and molecular studies showed that most cases were neoplastic from the outset.[890,959–963] But a few cases, generally single localized masses (though they can be multiple), lack evidence of clonality, and the term "nodular lymphoid hyperplasia" has been proposed for these cases.[963] Patients with nodular lymphoid hyperplasia have a wide age range and are usually asymptomatic at presentation. Systemic symptoms (fever) and a high erythrocyte sedimentation ratio (ESR) are observed in a few cases. Usually, recurrence has not been reported after surgical excision. Steroids and cytotoxic drugs can have some benefit in patients with multiple lesions.

Other conditions with proliferation of lymphoid cells include plasma cell granuloma (see p. 840) and posttransplant lymphoproliferative disorder.

LEUKEMIA

Several abnormalities may be seen on chest imaging in leukemic patients:

- Intrathoracic lymph node enlargement, leukemic infiltration of the lungs and pleura, and granulocytic sarcoma.
- Non-neoplastic complications of leukemia or its treatment, notably pulmonary infection, organizing pneumonia, pulmonary hemorrhage (Fig. 13.91), pulmonary edema, and drug reactions.
- Cardiac enlargement and pulmonary venous congestion in patients with severe anemia.

Leukemic infiltration of the lungs (Fig. 13.92) is defined as extravascular leukemic cells in portions of the lung parenchyma not involved by infection, infarction, or hemorrhage. Leukostasis is a separate category that may or may not be accompanied by leukemic infiltration of the lung parenchyma.

Apart from patients with leukostasis (see below), leukemic infiltration of the lungs does not appear to be a cause of pulmonary symptoms. When respiratory impairment is present, the leukemic infiltrates are accompanied by pulmonary infection, edema, or hemorrhage, and these are the likely cause of the patient's symptoms.

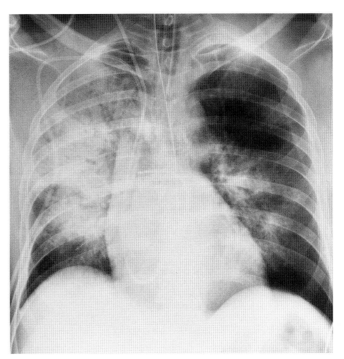

Fig. 13.91 Acute pulmonary shadowing in a 39-year-old man with acute myeloid leukemia. The bilateral airspace shadowing is due to intrapulmonary bleeding.

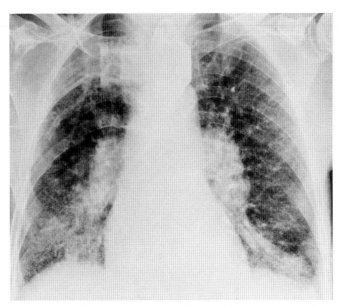

Fig. 13.92 Leukemic infiltrates in the lungs. Note also the bilateral hilar adenopathy caused by leukemic involvement of lymph nodes.

The incidence of leukemic infiltration of the lungs, mediastinal lymph nodes, and pleura varies with the course of the disease. Clearly, the highest incidence is shown in autopsy series,[964–966] but only rarely is this infiltration visible on chest radiography. In one typical series,[965] 41% of the patients showed leukemic infiltrates of the lung histologically, but the leukemic infiltration was almost never visible radiologically. Ninety percent of patients in the study had pulmonary opacities on chest radiographs

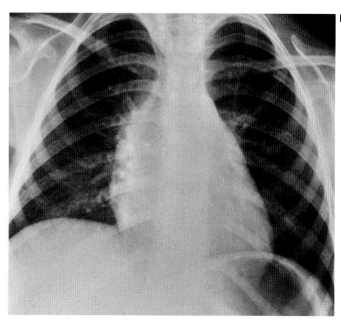

Fig. 13.93 T-cell leukemia/lymphoma in a 4-year-old girl. **A,** Massive mediastinal adenopathy. **B,** Following very rapid response to chemotherapy 9 days later.

immediately prior to death. In all except two, the opacities were the result of a complication of the disease, not leukemic infiltration per se. Focal masses or consolidations are very rare, but are reported.[965–967] In one case multifocal consolidation due to leukemic infiltration showed an air crescent sign,[968] a feature previously only reported in cases complicated by infection.

All 10 patients in one HRCT series[969] with biopsy proven leukemic infiltration, without coexisting pathology, had thickening of interlobular septa and small pulmonary nodules. In some cases the septal thickening was smooth, in others it was nodular and in yet others a mixture of the two. In all but one case there was also thickening of the bronchovascular bundles. The nodules varied in number from numerous to just a few; most were small in size, varying from barely perceptible to 10 mm in diameter. They were either randomly distributed or showed bronchocentric or centrilobular predominance. Ground-glass attenuation and focal consolidation, with or without air bronchograms, were also common. Similarly, another HRCT series of 11 patients, seven of whom underwent pathologic correlation, evaluated the relative frequency of HRCT signs in leukemic infiltration compared with the findings in 22 leukemic patients with other pulmonary complications.[970] The signs seen significantly more frequently with leukemic infiltration were peribronchial thickening and prominence of peripheral pulmonary arteries, which corresponded pathologically to thickening of the interstitium. The other statistically significant differences were multifocal areas of nonlobular, nonsegmental airspace consolidation or ground-glass opacity.

The incidence of leukemic infiltration of the nodes on autopsy examination is very high – 50% in the large series of Klatte et al,[964] but most involved nodes show little or no enlargement on plain chest radiography. The distribution of nodal enlargement closely resembles the lymphomas.

T-cell leukemias may show massive mediastinal adenopathy that responds rapidly to chemotherapy or radiation treatment.

Huge mediastinal masses of T-cell leukemia may disappear within a few days with appropriate treatment (Fig. 13.93).

Pleural effusion is common in leukemia. Subpleural deposits of leukemic cells are often found at autopsy, but pulmonary infection, infarction, hemorrhage, and edema so frequently coexist with these leukemic deposits that it is not possible to state the cause of the effusion with any confidence.

A focal mass of leukemic cells in patients with myeloid leukemia, so-called *granulocytic sarcoma* or *chloroma* (because of its green appearance), may be encountered on rare occasions.[971–976] Granulocytic sarcoma mostly presents before, or at the time of, the initial diagnosis of leukemia, but in approximately one-fifth of reported cases it developed after a previous remission. Granulocytic sarcoma may arise as a focal mediastinal mass or more generalized mediastinal widening. The other presentations include pleural effusion, an airway, hilar, pulmonary, or pleural mass, or cardiac enlargement due to the tumor or to pericardial effusion. Pulmonary masses may cavitate.[977] In one reported case with combined pleural and pulmonary granulocytic sarcoma, the bone marrow was normal.[978]

Leukostasis

Leukostasis is a condition seen in patients with acute myeloid leukemia who have very high white blood cell counts, in the order of 100,000 to 300,000 cells/mm^3, together with accumulations of leukemic cells in small blood vessels, especially of the lungs, heart, brain, and testes. Central nervous system symptoms are frequent, and the patients may be dyspneic due to obliteration of small pulmonary blood vessels by the leukemic cells.[979] The chest radiograph may be normal or may show airspace shadowing (Fig. 13.94). In a report on the radiographic findings in 10 patients who died with leukostasis,

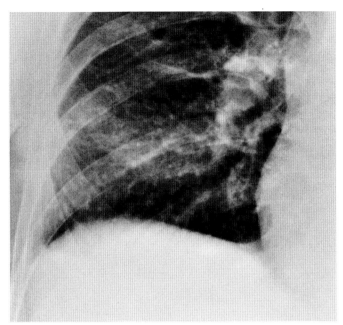

Fig. 13.94 Leukostasis in a 43-year-old man in blast crisis, showing hazy opacity in lungs resembling pulmonary edema. The abnormalities cleared with leukapheresis therapy.

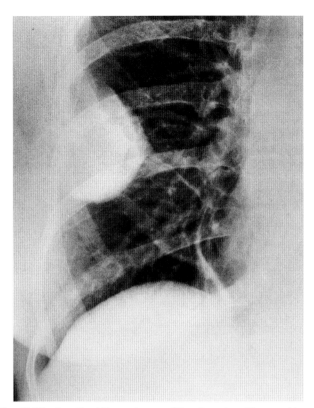

Fig. 13.95 Localized fibrous tumor of the pleura in a 61-year-old woman. At surgery this lesion was found to lie in the major fissure and was benign.

four had a normal appearing chest film, four showed wide airspace disease attributed to superimposed pulmonary edema, and one showed a small area of pulmonary consolidation.[980] The radiographic shadowing in leukostasis appears to be due to pulmonary edema rather than directly due to the accumulation of leukemic cells in the lungs.[979–981]

LOCALIZED FIBROUS TUMOR OF THE PLEURA

This tumor has been given a variety of names, including pleural fibroma, fibrous mesothelioma, localized pleural mesothelioma, and benign mesothelioma. Benign mesothelioma appears to be a particularly inappropriate term since the tumors are not mesotheliomas, nor do they all behave in a benign fashion (see Fig. 13.99). The current term, localized fibrous tumor of the pleura, has been recommended because the lesion is thought to arise from subpleural mesenchymal cells rather than epithelial cells.[982] It is probably best to regard them as a spectrum from benign to malignant.[982,983] Because of the difficulty distinguishing benign from malignant lesions, surgical resection is advised for all fibrous tumors of the pleura. Local recurrence is the major clinical problem with malignant tumors.

Most patients are between 45 and 65 years (range 5–87 years), with no significant sex difference.[982,984,985] Unlike diffuse malignant mesothelioma, the localized tumor is not asbestos related,[982,984,985] though a relationship with previous irradiation has been recorded.[986] Histologically, the lesion consists of spindle shaped cells separated by collagen.[987] It exists in benign and malignant forms, 14–30% being malignant.[982,983,988]

Macroscopically, the tumor is seen as a mass in contact with the pleura, but a small number appear to be totally encased within the lung.[739,989] Up to 87% arise from visceral pleura, the remainder from parietal pleura.[982,984,985] An origin from within a fissure is fairly common.[990] Pedunculation is present in about half the cases[985,991]; the stalk can be up to 9 cm in length.[992]

The benign tumors usually behave in a very indolent fashion and some have been known to be present for 20 years before removal,[993] but rapid growth even of the benign form is encountered occasionally.[988] Synchronous multiple tumors have been reported but are very unusual.[985]

Some 40–50% of patients are asymptomatic, the tumor being detected incidentally at chest radiography.[984,991] The most common symptoms are chest pain and dyspnea.[991] Although hypertrophic osteoarthropathy and finger clubbing were common in earlier series, its prevalence in series reported since 1972 has been much lower, 4–12%[982,984]; the phenomenon appears to be more common in tumors >7 cm in diameter. Other reported symptoms include cough, chills and fevers, weight loss, and debility. Symptomatic hypoglycemia is seen in up to 7% of patients.[982,984,991,994,995]

On chest radiography, the usual finding is a slow growing, rounded or oval, often lobulated, homogeneous mass in contact with a pleural surface, which may invaginate into or arise within a fissure (Fig. 13.95).[982,986,991,996] The lesions vary in diameter from <1 to 30 cm, but are usually large, 7 cm or more at initial presentation (Fig. 13.96). They are slightly more common in the lower half of the chest.[986] When very large, the origin from pleura may not be obvious,[986] and on occasion the tumor may simulate a raised hemidiaphragm (Fig. 13.97). There is usually an obtuse angle at the margin with the chest wall, a finding present in 16 of 17 cases in one chest film series,[990] but lesions with acute angles, resembling an intrapulmonary mass, are not

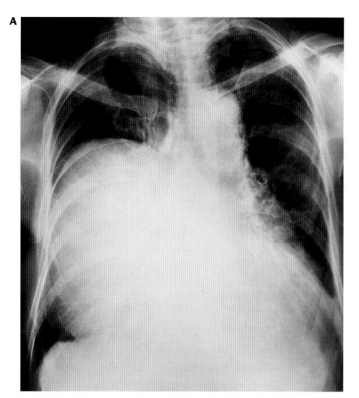

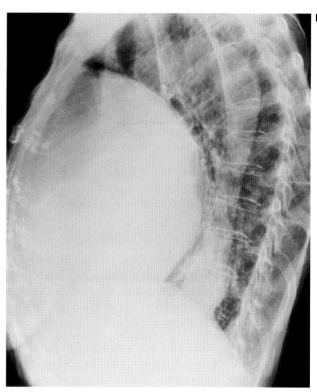

Fig. 13.96 **A**, Posteroanterior and **B**, lateral radiographs of a huge localized fibrous tumor of pleura in an elderly woman. Despite the size of the tumor, the patient had no chest symptoms. It was histologically benign.

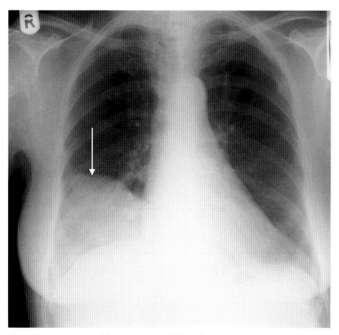

Fig. 13.97 Benign fibrous tumor of the pleura (arrow) mimicking elevation of the right hemidiaphragm (same patient as in Figs 13.98C and D).

uncommon.[986,997,998] Tumors on pedicles may change in shape and position on images taken on different occasions and in different postures.[986,993,996,999–1001] If the lesion is not pedunculated, inspiration/expiration imaging will show whether the mass is in the lung or is attached to the chest wall.[986] Pressure effects on the adjacent ribs are very unusual but have been reported in both benign and malignant tumors.[991]

On CT (Figs 13.98 and 13.99),[991,997,1001–1003] the lesions are usually well marginated and based on a pleural surface, some 95% showing at least one acute angle with the chest wall. In other words they grow outwards from a relatively narrow base or pedicle, and a stalk may be visible at CT. The smaller lesions show uniform soft tissue density whereas a substantial proportion of the larger tumors show low attenuation centrally due to necrosis. The soft tissue elements enhance to a much greater degree than muscle following intravenous contrast administration[998,1002–1004]; inhomogeneous contrast enhancement is a frequent feature in benign tumors and is virtually always seen with malignant tumors.[984,991] Calcification is uncommon, but recorded in benign lesions[986,1002–1006]; it appears to be more common in the localized malignant lesions.[984] Pleural effusions are occasionally present,[986,994,998] and are sometimes large enough to obscure the underlying mass.[983] Ultrasound can be used to characterize the tumors; it shows a hypoechoic mass.[1007]

There are multiple reports of the MRI features of solitary fibrous tumor of the pleura,[994,997,1002,1007–1011] the largest series being those of Rosado-de-Christianson et al[991] and Tateishi et al.[1012] The signal intensity on both T1- and T2-weighted images is usually heterogeneous. On T1-weighted images the

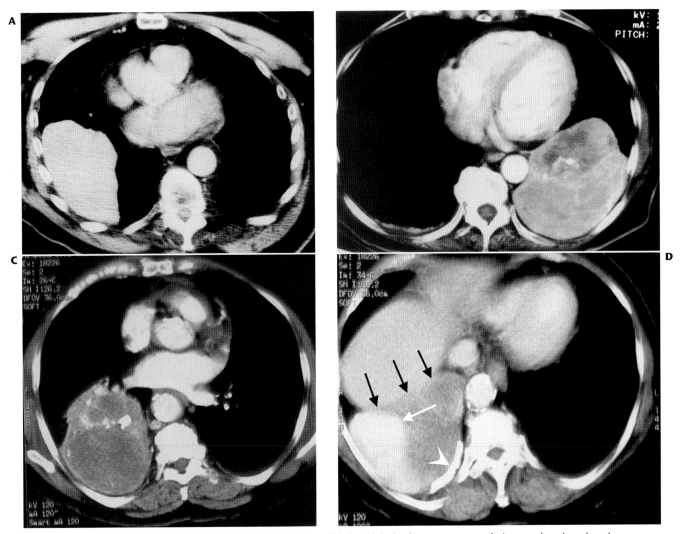

Fig. 13.98 CT of localized benign fibrous tumor of the pleura. **A**, Well-defined lobular, homogeneous, soft tissue, enhancing pleural mass. (Courtesy Dr Pablo Ros, Gainesville, FL) **B**, Large mass showing variable density and focal area of dense calcification. **C**, Well-defined multiple foci of calcification (same case as **D**) **D**, Part of the mass (same case as **C**) has dense uniform contrast enhancement. The black arrows point to the anterior surface of the tumor; the white arrow to the enhancing portion; and the white arrowhead to a curvilinear band of dense calcification.

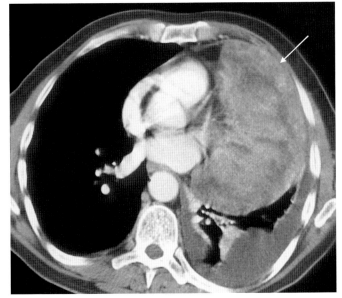

Fig. 13.99 Malignant fibrous tumor of pleura. Note the pleural effusion and the local invasion of the chest wall (arrow).

signal intensity is usually predominantly lower than muscle but may be the same as or higher; on T2-weighted images the signal intensity is usually low, or mixed high and low, though it may occasionally be high. In the majority of reported cases the signal intensity seems to reflect the high fibrous content of the tumor; namely low signal on both T1- and T2-weighted images, though a high intensity rim or more central, small, high intensity foci may be seen on the T2-weighted images. The tumors enhance following intravenous gadolinium and signal void due to the blood vessels within the tumor may be seen. There are no MRI features that allow a distinction between benign and malignant fibrous tumors of the pleura.[991]

DIFFUSE MALIGNANT MESOTHELIOMA

Asbestos exposure is documented in about half the patients with diffuse malignant mesothelioma,[1013,1014] but the incidence in various series ranges from under 25%[1015] to almost 90%.[1016]

The contribution of asbestos in the usual urban environment is unknown. Of the various forms of asbestos, crocidolite appears to be the most carcinogenic form, followed by chrysolite and then by amosite, but because chrysolite is the most widely used form of asbestos, it is believed to account for most cases of diffuse mesothelioma.[1017] The interval between first exposure to asbestos and presentation with the tumor is in the order of 20–40 years.[1018] Inhalation of other substances, such as nonoccupational exposure to erionite, have been etiologically implicated,[1019] and the possibility of an association with AIDS has been questioned.[1020] Prior thoracic irradiation has occasionally been noted,[1014,1015,1021] and may, therefore, play an etiologic role in a few cases.

Pathologically, diffuse malignant mesothelioma appears as plaques and nodules on the visceral or parietal pleura which may form a lobular sheet of tumor up to several centimeters thick encasing the lungs, maximal in the lower thorax, extending through the pleural cavity and growing into the interlobar fissures. Invasion into the adjacent chest wall, diaphragm, and mediastinal structures usually occurs relatively late, but may be seen early.[1016] Lymphatic and hematogenous metastases are usually late manifestations which, though present in 50% of patients at autopsy, are generally clinically silent.[1013] Histologically, malignant mesotheliomas are divided into epithelial, mesenchymal (fibrous or sarcomatous), or mixed tumors; their relative prevalence varies considerably from series to series and also varies according to the diligence with which the entire tumor is examined for mixed cell types. In Legha and Muggia's compilation of 382 cases from the literature,[1022] 54% were epithelial, 21% were fibrosarcomatous, and 25% were mixed, and the proportions were very similar in the Mayo Clinic series.[1023] The pure epithelial type has a better prognosis following surgical treatment.[1024] The epithelial type consists of cuboidal cells in various arrangements, whereas the mesenchymal type shows sheets of parallel spindle shaped cells similar to many soft tissue sarcomas. Immunohistochemical techniques and electron microscopy are often needed to distinguish between malignant mesothelioma and bronchial adenocarcinoma.[1025]

Focal osteosarcoma formation, which may produce a heavily calcified mass, has been reported to arise within malignant pleural mesothelioma.[1026,1027]

Pleural fluid associated with malignant mesothelioma is an exudate, which is serosanguinous in half the cases. With large tumors, the glucose and pH levels are low. On cytologic examination, the fluid may contain malignant mesothelial cells together with varying numbers of lymphocytes and polymorphonuclear leukocytes,[1022] but the cytologic distinction between benign and malignant mesothelial cells is difficult,[1023] and biopsy of the pleura is usually needed to establish the diagnosis.

A TNM staging system (Tables 13.11 and 13.12) has been adopted by the American Joint Committee on Cancer (AJCC).[1028] It is a modification of the staging system proposed by the International Mesothelioma Interest Group (IMIG).[1029–1031]

The peak age at presentation is between 40 and 70 years, with males predominating.[1015,1022,1023] The usual symptoms are chest wall pain, shortness of breath, and cough, followed by dyspnea and weight loss.[1015,1016,1022,1023] There may be intermittent low grade fever. Clubbing of the fingers and hypertrophic pulmonary osteoarthropathy are seen, but are much less common than with localized fibrous tumors of the pleura.[1013]

Table 13.11 IMIG staging system for diffuse malignant pleural mesothelioma[1028]

Primary tumor (T)	
TX	Primary tumor cannot be assessed
T0	No evidence of primary tumor
T1	Tumor involves ipsilateral parietal pleura, with or without focal involvement of visceral pleura
T1a	Tumor involves ipsilateral parietal (mediastinal, diaphragmatic) pleura. No involvement of the visceral pleura
T1b	Tumor involves ipsilateral parietal (mediastinal, diaphragmatic) pleura, with focal involvement of the visceral pleura
T2	Tumor involves any of the ipsilateral pleural surfaces with at least one of the following: confluent visceral pleural tumor (including fissure); invasion of diaphragmatic muscle; invasion of lung parenchyma
T3*	Tumor involves any of the ipsilateral pleural surfaces, with at least one of the following: invasion of the endothoracic fascia; invasion into mediastinal fat; solitary focus of tumor invading the soft tissues of the chest wall; nontransmural involvement of the pericardium
T4**	Tumor involves any of the ipsilateral pleural surfaces, with at least one of the following: diffuse or multifocal invasion of soft tissues of the chest wall; any involvement of the rib; invasion through the diaphragm to the peritoneum; invasion of any mediastinal organ(s); direct extension to the contralateral pleura; invasion into the spine; extension to the internal surfaces of the pericardium; pericardial effusion with positive cytology; invasion of the myocardium; invasion of the brachial plexus

*T3 describes locally advanced but potentially respectable tumor
**T4 describes locally advanced, technically unresectable tumor

Regional lymph nodes (N)	
NX	Regional lymph nodes cannot be assessed
N0	No regional lymph node metastases
N1	Metastases in the ipsilateral bronchopulmonary and/or hilar lymph node(s)
N2	Metastases in the subcarinal lymph node(s) and/or the ipsilateral internal mammary or mediastinal lymph node(s)
N3	Metastases in the contralateral mediastinal, internal mammary, or hilar lymph node(s)

Distant metastasis (M)	
MX	Distant metastases cannot be assessed
M0	NO distant metastases
M1	Distant metastases

Table 13.12 AJCC stage groupings for mesothelioma[1028]

Stage I	T1	N0	M0
Stage IA	T1a	N0	M0
Stage IB	T1b	N0	M0
Stage II	T2	N0	M0
Stage III	T1, T2	N1	M0
	T1, T2	N2	M0
	T3	N0, N1, N2	M0
Stage IV	T4	Any N	M0
	Any T	N3	M0
	Any T	Any N	M1

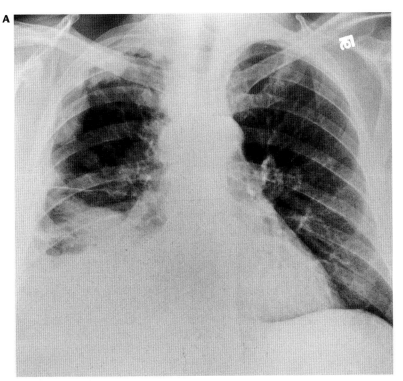

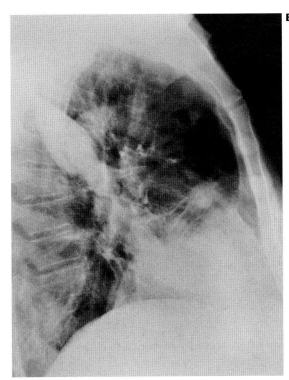

Fig. 13.100 **A**, Anteroposterior and **B**, lateral radiographs of malignant mesothelioma of pleura, showing lobular pleural masses. Note lobular thickening of the major fissures.

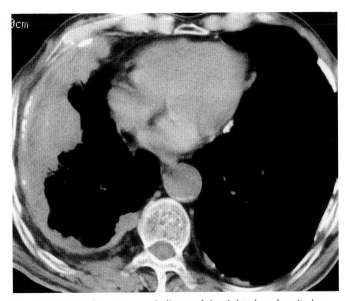

Fig. 13.101 Malignant mesothelioma of the right pleural cavity in a patient with bilateral asbestosis related partially calcified pleural plaques.

The imaging features[1014,1023,1032–1042] are essentially similar on chest radiographs, CT, and MRI (Figs 13.100 to 13.104), but CT and MRI show the extent of the tumor with greater accuracy than chest radiography, and show the accompanying pleural fluid with greater sensitivity. CT is useful for detecting recurrent disease following surgical treatment.[1043] CT and MRI appear to be of similar diagnostic accuracy for surgical staging. MRI is superior to conventional CT for revealing solitary foci of chest

wall involvement and for showing diaphragmatic invasion, but this advantage does not affect surgical treatment. CT is, therefore, considered the standard diagnostic study for pretreatment assessment.[1044] This recommendation will no doubt be even stronger in the era of multidetector CT. Involvement of mediastinal lymph nodes, chest wall invasion, bone destruction and direct extension to the pericardium, other mediastinal structures, or the opposite lung and pleura, and invasion through the diaphragm into the upper abdomen are all usually well seen on CT or MRI,[1014,1015,1032,1033,1035,1036,1038,1039,1041] but CT fails to show chest wall involvement in a proportion of patients.[1041] Extension to the contralateral thoracic cavity may also be seen. Extension beyond the pleural cavity is seen in approximately 11–18% of patients at initial presentation, increasing to 30% or more during the course of the disease. The multiplanar imaging capability of MRI can be advantageous for demonstrating chest wall, diaphragm, and mediastinal invasion. Extrathoracic spread can be diagnosed by FDG PET imaging.[1045]

The imaging findings typically consist of extensive nodular or lobular thickening of the pleura, which may conglomerate to form a circumferential lobular sheet of soft tissue density encasing the lung. The tumor often runs into the fissures, accompanied by varying amounts of pleural fluid, and the adjacent lung may show evidence of invasion. The nodularity/lobulation of the pleural thickening is an important diagnostic feature (Fig. 13.100). Sometimes the accompanying pleural effusion is very large, and obscures the pleural masses on chest radiography (Fig. 13.103). In such cases, the chest radiographic appearances may be indistinguishable from other causes of pleural effusion. One point of distinction from other pleural effusions is that the neoplastic encasement of the lung may fix the position of the mediastinum, so that shift away from the side of the effusion is

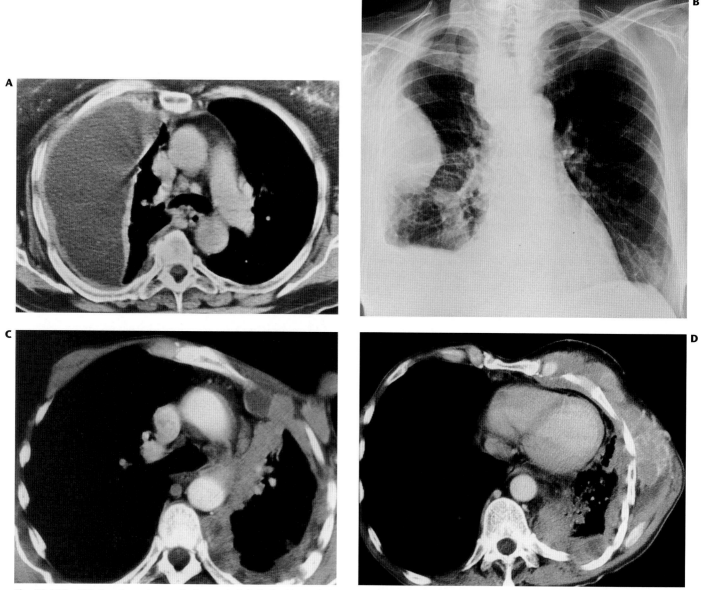

Fig. 13.102 CT of malignant mesothelioma. **A**, Relatively thin rind of nodular pleural thickening and a large loculus of pleural fluid. **B**, Plain radiograph of the same patient for comparison. **C** and **D**, Two images from a single examination showing extensive nodular pleural thickening surrounding the lung and invading through the chest wall. Note the variable degrees of enhancement of various parts of the tumor.

not seen as often in patients with malignant mesothelioma as it is with nonmalignant causes of large pleural effusion.[990] Indeed, the pleural shadowing is often associated with ipsilateral volume loss and a fixed mediastinum[1046]; and the hemithorax is frequently contracted owing to encasement of the lung by pleural tumor.[1014] The tumor nodules may become evident only on plain chest radiographs if air enters the pleural space following thoracentesis. At CT, the soft tissue density of tumor tissue can be readily distinguished from the adjacent pleural effusion (Figs 13.102 and 13.104), but the nodules are not infrequently so tiny that they are unrecognizable and the only CT feature is, therefore, a pleural effusion. Calcification of the

tumor is extremely rare, though reported.[1014,1047] Asbestos related pleural plaques may be seen in either pleural cavity, and calcified plaques may be engulfed by tumor (Fig. 13.101).[1035]

The typical MRI signal intensity is slightly greater than muscle on T1-weighted images and moderately greater than muscle on T2-weighted images. The tumor enhances significantly with gadolinium. MRI can help distinguish benign disease and other neoplasms from malignant mesothelioma, especially if contrast-enhanced T1-weighted sequences with fat saturation are used, by showing the distribution of thickened pleural tissue.[1042]

FDG PET has proved highly sensitive in several small series of malignant mesothelioma,[1045,1048,1049] indicating a possible use

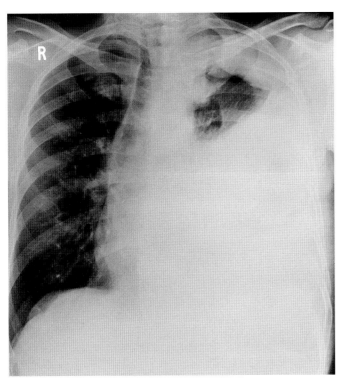

Fig. 13.103 Malignant mesothelioma showing a very large pleural effusion that partially hides lobular neoplastic thickening of pleura.

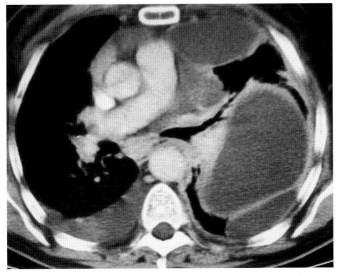

Fig. 13.104 Malignant mesothelioma causing widespread, uniform, mild thickening of pleura and multiple fluid loculations. Note the resemblance to empyema.

of PET for initial diagnosis; the numbers of benign pleural processes included in these studies is, however, far too small to assess the false positive rate.

The differential diagnosis includes pleural involvement by other malignant tumors, notably bronchial adenocarcinoma, breast carcinoma, malignant thymoma, and lymphoma, as well as benign conditions such as asbestos related benign pleural effusion, tuberculous pleural thickening, past or present empyema (Fig. 13.104), and asbestos related pleural plaques. Unless there are other features to indicate the primary tumor, the distinction between adenocarcinoma of the lung and malignant mesothelioma cannot be made radiographically from the appearance of the pleural involvement alone. Although pleural involvement by breast carcinoma can also appear identical, there is usually no diagnostic difficulty because the primary tumor will have been diagnosed previously or will be clinically obvious. Pleural deposits of lymphoma and thymoma usually appear as more discrete localized masses than malignant mesothelioma, and the primary thymoma or other foci of lymphoma are visible or have previously been documented. The distinction from benign pleural thickening[1050] due to conditions such as previous tuberculosis or old hemothorax is usually readily made by noting the smoothness of the pleural shadowing in these disorders.[1023] A helpful feature in distinguishing benign pleural thickening from malignant mesothelioma is that circumferential pleural thickening and thickening extending over the mediastinal pleura are not infrequent in malignant mesothelioma but are rare in benign pleural disease.[1034]

The differentiation of early malignant pleural mesothelioma from noncalcified or partially calcified asbestos related plaques can, on occasion, be difficult: some pleural plaques associated with advanced asbestosis can be large and irregular, and can resemble mesothelioma.[1046]

The uptake of FDG with PET imaging has been shown to correlate with prognosis; the higher the uptake the shorter the survival.[1051]

OTHER TUMORS OF THE PLEURA

Pleural and extrapleural *lipomas* are fairly unusual tumors with liposarcomas being distinctly unusual.[1052] The exact origin of pleural lipomas is not always clear, but they can arise from subpleural adipose tissue and be present as a local pleural mass. The benign lipoma is totally asymptomatic, though if it protrudes through the rib interspaces it may produce a focal swelling and be palpable. On chest radiography, lipomas are seen as well-marginated, oval or lens shaped soft tissue masses based on the pleura (Fig. 13.105). On CT,[745,982,1053,1054] the uniform fat density, containing no more than a few linear strands of soft tissue density, makes the diagnosis straightforward (Fig. 13.105). Punctate calcification is very occasionally visible at CT.[1053] Since they are soft lesions, they may change shape with respiration.[1055] On MRI, lipomas show standard fat signal, namely high signal on T1-weighted images and intermediate signal on T2-weighted images.[1056] Heterogeneity of density with a mixture of fat and soft tissue attenuation is the CT feature of *liposarcoma*.[1057]

The most common *sarcomas* of the pleura are metastatic. Primary pleural *liposarcoma*[1057–1059] and *osteosarcoma*[683,1060] are rare tumors. The fat density within liposarcoma and the extensive calcification in osteosarcoma on CT are of considerable diagnostic value.

Plasmacytoma[1061] and *epitheliod hemangioendothelioma*[1062] are two other very rarely encountered pleural tumors which can appear similar to mesothelioma at imaging.[1063]

A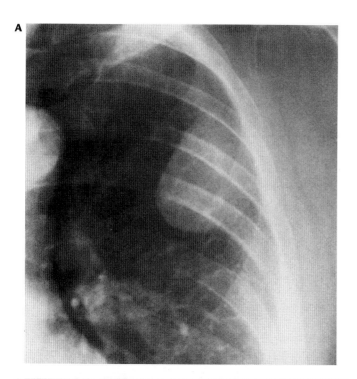

B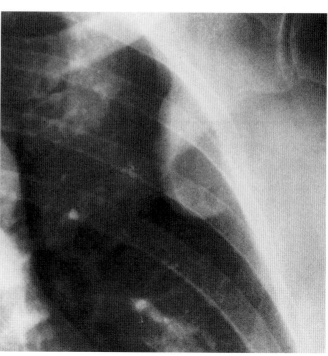

C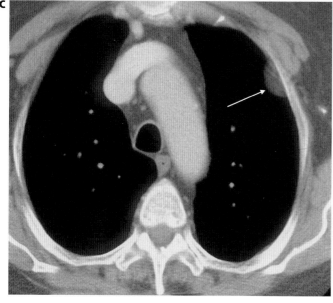

Fig. 13.105 Pleural lipoma. **A** and **B**, Frontal and oblique radiographs showing typical shape of a pleural mass. **C**, CT showing a similar mass composed mostly of fat (arrow), in another patient.

METASTASES

Pulmonary metastases

The incidence of pulmonary metastases varies with the primary tumor and the stage of disease. In autopsy series, the most common sources include tumors of the breast, colon, kidney, uterus, prostate, head, and neck.[1064] Tumors such as choriocarcinoma, osteosarcoma, Ewing sarcoma, testicular tumors, melanoma, and thyroid carcinoma have a high incidence of pulmonary metastases, but because they are not as prevalent in the population, lung deposits from these tumors are encountered less frequently.[1064]

The hallmark of bloodborne metastases to the lungs on imaging studies is one or more oval or spherical, discrete pulmonary nodules, maximal in the outer portions of the lungs (Figs 13.106 and 13.107).[1065–1067] They vary in size from microscopic to many centimeters in diameter, are usually multiple, and have well or moderately well-defined, smooth or irregular outlines.[1068,1069] They are usually of soft tissue density, but may show calcification or conversely be of ground-glass density, if mucin producing, as in gastric carcinoma metastases,[1070] or even lower density.[1071] A variety of other patterns are encountered.[1072] On occasion, particularly when due to metastatic adenocarcinoma, or if the metastases have bled into the surrounding lung,[1068,1073,1074] they show irregular or ill-defined edges (Fig. 13.108) or the features of airspace shadowing.[1075,1076] Metastases from highly vascular primary tumors, such as choriocarcinoma and angiosarcoma, may have a surrounding halo of ground-glass opacity, due to hemorrhage into the

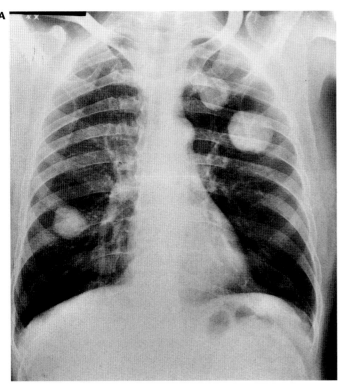

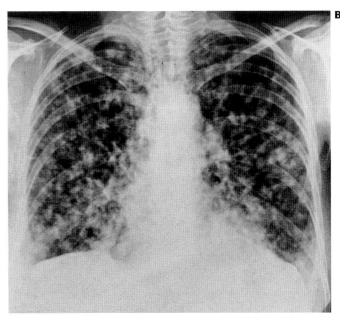

Fig. 13.106 Typical hematogenous metastases. **A**, In a patient with colon carcinoma. **B**, In a patient with rhabdomyosarcoma of the anterior abdominal wall.

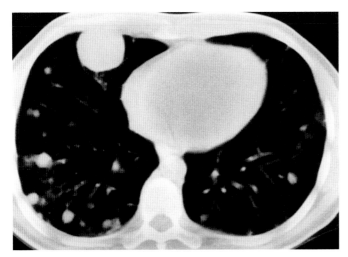

Fig. 13.107 CT showing peripheral distribution of hematogenous metastases, in this case from a germ cell tumor of the testis.

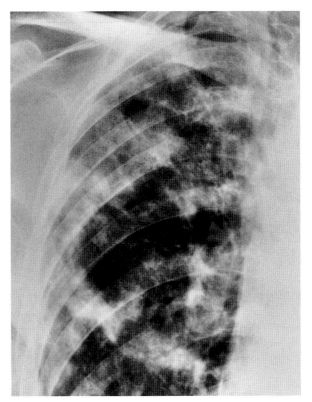

Fig. 13.108 Metastases from adenocarcinoma of the colon showing an irregular outline of pulmonary nodules.

adjacent parenchyma.[1069,1077,1078] Irregular, sometimes frankly nodular, thickening of the interstitial pulmonary septa is a frequent finding on specimen HRCT.[1079] This finding, labeled the "beaded septum sign" is regarded as suggestive of metastatic carcinoma. It corresponds to neoplastic invasion of the interlobular septa, their capillaries and lymphatic vessels, and when widespread would be labeled lymphangitis carcinoma.

Using CT, it is possible to show pulmonary vessels leading directly to individual metastases.[1080] The sign was observed in 30–75% of metastases in one series, the frequency depending on whether the lesion was in the upper, mid or lower zone.[1080] In a CT pathologic correlation, however, the sign was found in <20%.[1081] This variation is probably related to CT section

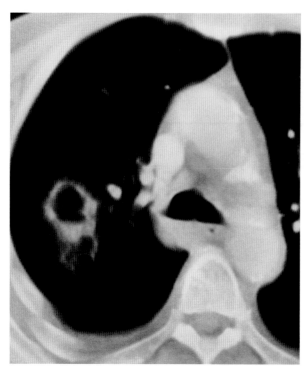

Fig. 13.109 CT of cavitating metastasis (squamous cell carcinoma).

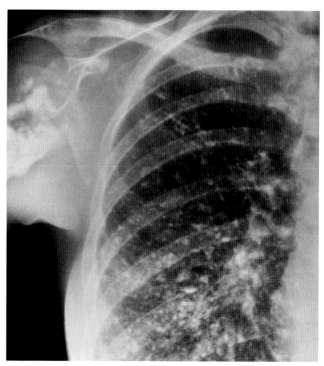

Fig. 13.110 Calcified metastases in a case of osteosarcoma (the primary tumor is visible in the upper right humerus).

thickness, thinner sections more accurately correlating with the macroscopic pathologic findings. The specificity of the sign is uncertain.

Cavitation (Fig. 13.109) is most frequent in metastases from tumors of the uterine cervix, colon, and head and neck; the presence of cavitation is unrelated to the size of the metastasis.[1082,1083] In general, metastases from squamous cell cancers originating in the head and neck undergo cavitation when quite small and may have strikingly thin walls,[1083] though many other cell types also show thin walls.[1084–1086] When multiple, it is usual for cavitary lesions to coexist with solid nodules.[1066] Metastatic sarcoma can also be accompanied by cavitation and pneumothorax is then a relatively frequent complication.[1069]

Detectable calcification in pulmonary metastases is very unusual indeed, except in deposits from sarcomas, notably osteosarcoma and chondrosarcoma, in which the calcification is part of the tumor matrix just as it is in the primary tumor (Figs 13.110 and 13.111). Even in tumors such as breast, ovarian, colon, and thyroid carcinomas, where calcification can be seen in the primary tumor, calcification in pulmonary metastases has only been recognized in a few isolated cases.[1087,1088] Calcification may, however, be seen in successfully treated metastases.[1088,1089]

Miliary nodulation, a pattern of innumerable tiny nodules resembling miliary tuberculosis, is occasionally encountered but is decidedly rare (Fig. 13.112). Miliary metastases are most likely to be due to thyroid or renal carcinoma, bone sarcoma, trophoblastic disease, or melanoma.[1090]

Very occasionally, metastases present radiographically as myriads of tiny shadows which summate to resemble pulmonary consolidation and may then be confused with infection, edema, or drug reaction. This pattern has been seen particularly with melanoma.[1090–1092] One case of metastatic renal cell carcinoma has been reported in which innumerable tiny metastases resembling consolidation were confined to one lobe.[1093]

In general, pulmonary metastases that respond to treatment with chemotherapy disappear and are no longer visible radiographically as nodules. Some may cavitate first. Rarely, however, a residual nodule of sterilized fibrous tissue may remain, and in this case there can be a major dilemma deciding whether treatment should be continued. This phenomenon has been observed particularly with choriocarcinoma[1094,1095] and testicular cancer.[1096]

Thin walled air cysts, also known as pulmonary lacunae, may persist in sites of metastases that have been successfully treated. This phenomenon is most frequently encountered with germ cell tumors of the testes (both seminoma and non-seminomatous germ cell tumors),[1097,1098] though other tumors such as bladder carcinomas may, very rarely, show the phenomenon.[1098] Pulmonary lacunae were encountered in 7% of a series of 59 patients with teratomatous tumors of the testis.[1098] These air cysts seem to be different from cavitating metastases in that they appear to be healed deposits and do not contain viable tumor.[1098] The diagnosis depends on noting uniformly very thin, virtually imperceptible, walls to the cyst and no evidence of a mural nodule.

Metastases from nonseminomatous germ cell tumors may enlarge, despite responding successfully to chemotherapy.[1099] In such cases, they are transforming to a mature form of teratoma. The serum tumor markers are not raised, an important point in differential diagnosis.

Parenchymal metastases from extrathoracic primary tumors occur at least 10 times as often as intrathoracic nodal metastases, and nodal disease alone is quite unusual, except in seminoma of the testis.[1100] McLoud et al[1101] reviewed 1071 cases of extrathoracic malignant neoplasms. Only 2–3% had evidence of hilar or mediastinal lymph node metastases, and concomitant pulmonary metastases were present in almost half

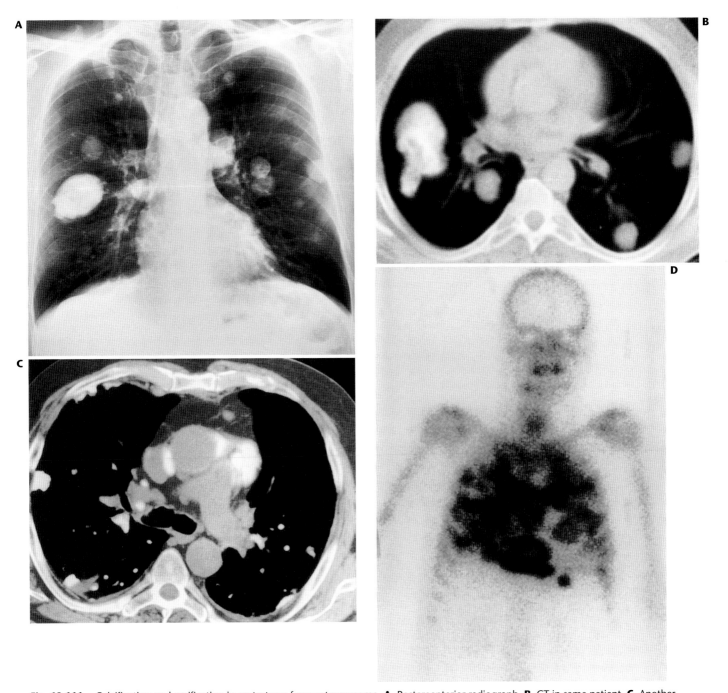

Fig. 13.111 Calcification and ossification in metastases from osteosarcoma. **A**, Posteroanterior radiograph. **B**, CT in same patient. **C**, Another patient showing heavily calcified metastases in the lungs, mediastinum and pleura on CT. (Courtesy of Dr Abram Patterson, Roanoke, VA) **D**, Radionuclide bone scan showing matched uptake in the numerous metastases. (Courtesy of Dr Abram Patterson, Roanoke, VA)

these cases (Fig. 13.113). They found that the primary neoplasms consisted chiefly of tumors of the head and neck, tumors of the genitourinary system, breast cancer, and malignant melanoma.

The subject of lymphangitis carcinomatosa is discussed on p. 870 and tumor emboli are discussed on p. 385.

Detection

The standard initial test for the detection of pulmonary metastases is the plain chest radiograph. A high kilovoltage technique shows more lesions than low kilovoltage films. Digital radiographic techniques, which lend themselves to computer processing,[1102,1103] computer aided diagnosis,[531,1104,1105] and temporal subtraction,[1106] may also improve sensitivity.

Computed tomography

Volumetric multidetector CT is currently the most sensitive technique for the detection of pulmonary metastases. Slice-by-slice CT may not provide truly contiguous sections, because small nodules may be out of section on each image if the patient breathes erratically during the examination. The use of

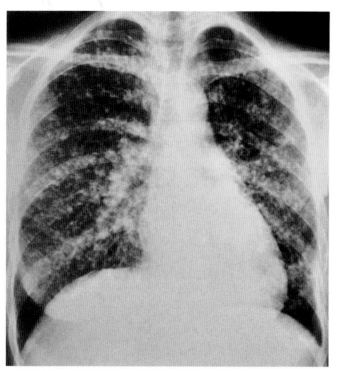

Fig. 13.112 Miliary metastases from breast carcinoma.

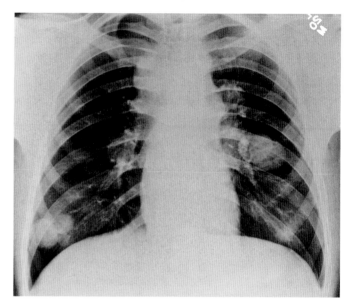

Fig. 13.113 Concomitant pulmonary and mediastinal metastases in a 17 year old boy with a seminoma of the testis.

contiguous sections during a single breath with volumetric CT obviates skipping a portion of the lung and missing a nodule.[1107–1109] Reconstruction of overlapping sections minimizes this risk further,[1110,1111] as does the use of multidetector CT with reconstruction of contiguous 1.25 mm sections,[456] but viewing the large numbers of images then becomes a problem. Viewing the numerous images obtained with multidetector CT is best done at a computer console using ciné (stack) mode. Stack mode viewing improves radiologists' ability to detect small pulmonary nodules, notably by improving the distinction between normal blood vessels and nodules <5 mm in diameter.[530,1112] (Computer aided detection and analysis of growth of pulmonary nodules is under development.[529,533])

The better contrast resolution of CT allows very small nodules to be demonstrated. Individual nodules as small as 2–3 mm in diameter may be visible on CT, whereas the lower limit for uncalcified nodules on plain chest radiographs is somewhere between 7 and 9 mm. But even with the best CT technique, very small metastases are undetectable.[1113] Diederich et al[1109] showed that the sensitivity for conventional spiral CT was only 69% for lesions <6 mm; for metastases of 6 mm or larger the sensitivity was 100%. The use of maximum intensity projection images with stacks of thin sections improves conspicuity.[1114,1115]

The increased sensitivity of CT for detecting metastases carries with it a decrease in specificity, since many of the smaller nodules, even in children,[1116] are benign lesions, notably granulomas, particularly in those parts of the world where fungal granulomas, such as histoplasmomas, are common.[1067] In countries, such as the United Kingdom, where fungal granulomas are virtually nonexistent, the specificity of CT rises, but even in the United Kingdom caution is needed because 6% of noncalcified nodules revealed by CT in a series of 200 patients with seminoma of the testis were nonmetastatic in nature, presumably tuberculous granulomas[1100]; and in another survey

of patients with a variety of extrathoracic primary tumors, the great majority of nodules detected by CT in the presence of a normal chest radiograph surprisingly proved to be benign.[1117]

CT is used only in selected cases because it is rarely necessary to demonstrate further metastases once the presence of definite pulmonary metastatic disease has been established. General indications for CT include:

- *Patients with a normal chest radiograph in whom the presence of pulmonary metastases would significantly alter patient management.* CT scans of the chest are often obtained to find neoplastic deposits not visible on chest radiographs in patients with tumors such as osteosarcoma, choriocarcinoma, and testicular germ cell tumors,[1118] all of which have a significant incidence of pulmonary metastases at presentation, but which may have no detectable metastatic spread to other sites. The incidence of pulmonary metastases from seminoma is low, but since the incidence of mediastinal nodal disease can be as high as 12.5%, chest CT is recommended for initial staging as well as follow up for potential relapse.[1100]
- Locally advanced melanoma is cited as an example of a tumor with high propensity to metastasize to the lungs,[1090,1119] but whether routine chest CT is justified in cases with a normal chest radiograph is far from clear. In one series of 42 patients with locally advanced melanoma and either a solitary pulmonary nodule or no abnormality on chest radiographs, CT scanning showed further nodules believed to be metastases in approximately one-third of patients.[1120] The authors did, however, point out that in only one of the 42 patients did the discovery of an additional nodule by CT alter the management of the patient. In another similar sized series, there was a change in management in 26% of patients following the CT scan.[1121] The incidence of pulmonary metastases in patients with head and neck carcinoma, superficial melanoma, and carcinomas of the kidney, bladder, and female genital tract is relatively low. In patients with these tumors, CT should be reserved for those with advanced local disease

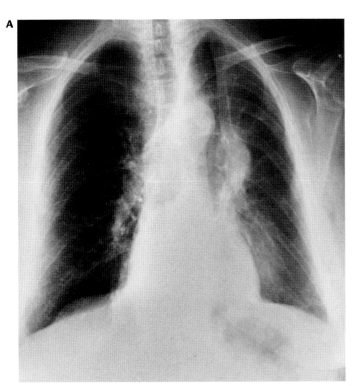
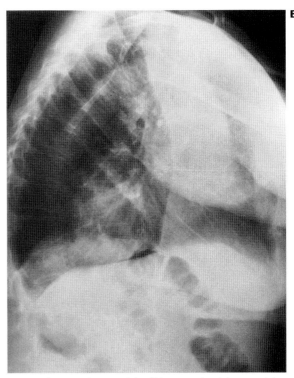

Fig. 13.114   A, Anteroposterior and **B,** lateral radiographs of endobronchial metastases from carcinoma of the kidney causing left upper lobe collapse.

and thoracic symptoms.[1122,1123] Similarly, patients with carcinoma of the gastrointestinal tract, breast, or prostate are unlikely to have pulmonary metastases in the absence of metastases to such organs as the liver and bones, and CT should, therefore, be reserved for those patients in whom thoracic involvement is uncertain on plain chest radiograph and in whom the information would change management.[1122,1124]

- *Patients who are being considered for surgical resection of known pulmonary metastases.* CT is clearly indicated to demonstrate all pulmonary metastases when pulmonary surgical resection is being considered. Currently, such surgery is recommended when the primary tumor has been (or can be) definitively treated and all known metastatic disease can be safely encompassed by the projected pulmonary resection.[1125–1128] Resection of pulmonary metastases can be a safe and potentially curative procedure as shown by the multicenter trial of 5206 patients established by the International Registry of Lung Metastases.[1129] Resection appears most beneficial for tumors of the urinary tract, testicular and uterine neoplasms, colon and rectal carcinoma,[1130–1135] tumors of the head and neck, and various sarcomas,[1136,1137] notably osteogenic sarcoma.[1126] How many other tumors should be added to this list is debatable.[1125,1138–1140]

- *Distinguishing solitary from multiple pulmonary nodules where the diagnostic dilemma is metastasis versus new primary bronchial carcinoma.* A solitary pulmonary nodule may represent a primary bronchogenic carcinoma rather than a metastasis, even in a patient with a known extrathoracic primary tumor.[1141] Clearly, the relative probabilities depend on the likelihood of the specific primary tumor metastasizing to the lungs and such factors as the smoking habits of the patient, the interval between the original diagnosis, and the appearance of the nodule.[1142]

Magnetic resonance imaging

MRI currently has a limited role for detecting metastases. Even though Feuerstein et al,[1143] using a 0.5 T magnet, showed that MRI could be at least as sensitive as CT in detecting metastases, the general view is that CT, particularly using volumetric scanning techniques, is the most cost-effective method.[1144,1145] There are, however, a few potential specific advantages of MRI: (1) the absence of ionizing radiation with MRI is a clear-cut advantage over CT, particularly for young patients undergoing repeated follow-up scans; and (2) MRI can sometimes distinguish between small centrally located metastases and adjacent normal blood vessels, based on the signal of flowing blood in arteries and veins.

Radionuclide imaging

Radionuclide and PET imaging can be useful for demonstrating intrathoracic metastases[1146–1148] when the neoplasms concentrate the chosen radionuclide.

Endobronchial metastases

Metastases to the walls of a large bronchus are unusual. Bramman and Whitcomb[1149] found the incidence to be only 2% in a very large series of patients who had died from solid neoplasms. The most common primary sites appear to be kidney, breast, colon, and rectum,[1150,1151] but endobronchial metastases have been reported from melanoma[1152,1153] and primary neoplasms of the stomach, thyroid, cervix, prostate, and testis. The clinical and radiologic features are indistinguishable from those produced by other central tumors, namely cough, wheezing, hemoptysis, atelectasis, and obstructive pneumonitis (Fig. 13.114).[1150,1154] On chest radiography the lesion itself is not visible and the evidence for an endobronchial metastasis will be obstructive atelectasis. The endobronchial metastasis itself may be visible at CT.[1155]

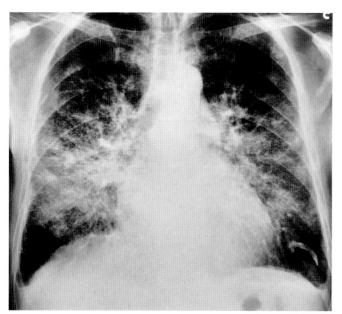

Fig. 13.115 Lymphangitis carcinomatosa from carcinoma of the prostate showing bilateral centrally predominant reticulonodular shadows.

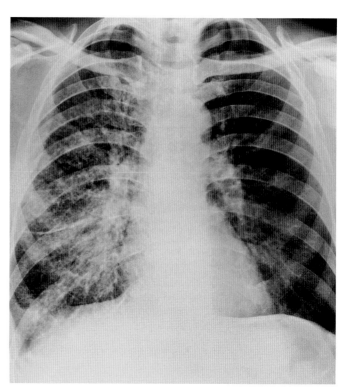

Fig. 13.117 Unilateral lymphangitis carcinomatosa from bronchial carcinoma. Note reticulonodular shadows and subpleural thickening of minor fissure and of the lung in the right cardiophrenic angle. Septal lines are also present.

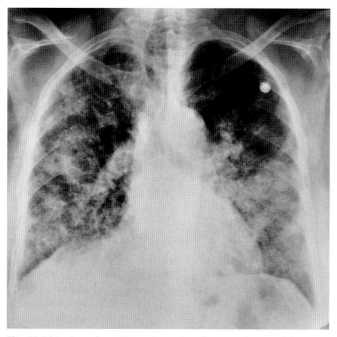

Fig. 13.116 Lymphangitis carcinomatosa from carcinoma of the breast showing randomly distributed reticulonodular shadowing with areas of confluence.

Lymphangitis carcinomatosa

Lymphangitis carcinomatosa is the name given to permeation of pulmonary lymphatics by neoplastic cells. The most common tumors that spread in this manner are carcinomas of the bronchus, breast, pancreas, stomach, colon, and prostate. The route by which tumor cells reach the intrapulmonary lymphatics

is debated. Spencer,[346] when reviewing the subject, concluded that some cases are caused by bloodborne emboli that lodge in smaller pulmonary arteries and subsequently spread through the vessel walls into the lymphatic vessels. Some tumors, notably upper abdominal cancers, appear to spread by way of lymph vessels to hilar nodes and thence in retrograde fashion into the pulmonary lymphatics. Primary carcinoma of the lung can invade the pulmonary lymphatics directly and may give rise to segmental or lobar lymphangitis carcinomatosa, as well as involving one or both lungs diffusely.

Histologically, there is interstitial thickening of the interlobular septa due to a combination of tumor cells, desmoplastic response, and dilated lymphatics. The lymphatic obstruction can lead to interstitial edema. The hilar lymph nodes may, or may not, show histologic evidence of tumor involvement.

The chest radiographic findings are fine reticulonodular shadowing and/or thickened septal lines (Figs 13.115 and 13.116). These signs occur because of a combination of dilated lymphatics and interstitial edema, together with shadows due to the tumor cells themselves and any desmoplastic response.[1156,1157] Another useful sign of lymphangitis carcinomatosa is subpleural edema resulting from lymphatic obstruction by tumor cells, a feature that is most readily visible as thickening of the fissures. The process can be unilateral (Fig. 13.117), particularly in cases resulting from bronchial carcinoma, but the pulmonary shadowing is more often bilateral and symmetrical. Pleural effusion is common.

CT is more sensitive than chest radiography for the detection of lymphangitic spread and may show changes in patients whose chest radiograph is normal. CT, particularly

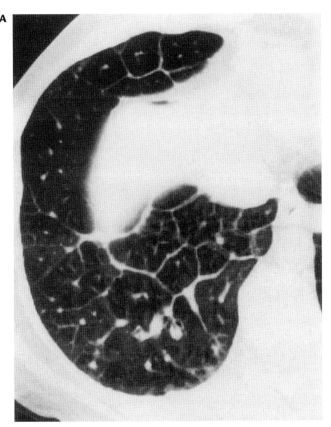

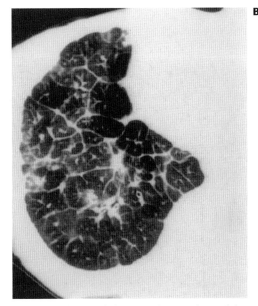

Fig. 13.118 Lymphangitis carcinomatosa. **A,** and **B,** Two examples of HRCT showing thickened interlobular septa. Note polygonal shape of lobule and variable degree of thickening of septa.

HRCT (Fig. 13.118),[1079,1158–1160] shows nonuniform, often nodular, thickening of the interlobular septa and irregular thickening of the bronchovascular bundles.[1159] There is often patchy airspace shadowing. Small, peripherally located, wedge-shaped densities are sometimes seen as well; they may represent volume averaging of thickened septa. Nodular shadows may be seen scattered through the parenchyma. The distribution of the changes varies greatly. The abnormalities may involve all zones of both lungs or they may be centrally or peripherally predominant; sometimes they are confined to a lobe or one lung.

There are no studies which formally report the sensitivity of HRCT for the diagnosis of lymphangitis carcinomatosa, but it is clear from autopsy correlation that in patients with discrete pulmonary metastases, lymphangitis carcinomatosa is often present in areas of the lung which appear normal at HRCT.[1068]

Hilar lymph node enlargement is seen in only some patients, five of the 12 cases in one series, supporting the supposition that lymphangitis carcinomatosa is sometimes the result of hematogenous spread of tumor to the interstitium.[1156]

The major differential diagnosis of lymphangitis carcinomatosa is pulmonary edema. The nodularity of the septal thickening at HRCT is very helpful and an important differential diagnostic feature from pulmonary edema is that many of the acini subtended by thickened interlobular septa are normally aerated. On chest radiographs, at least in those cases without

visible lung cancer or lymphadenopathy, the findings may be so similar to pulmonary edema that distinguishing between the two conditions can be impossible. Clearly, knowledge of the clinical or radiographic progression of disease is very helpful and is frequently decisive.

Malignant pleural effusion and pleural metastases

Carcinomatous metastases to the pleura can originate from almost any organ, but the lung appears to be the most frequent primary site, followed by the breast, pancreas, stomach, and ovary.[349,1161–1163] Carcinoma of the lung and breast, together with lymphoma, accounts for approximately 75% of malignant pleural effusions.[1161] Leukemic deposits and sarcomatous metastases are rare causes of pleural effusion.[350,1164] The responsible neoplasm usually involves both the visceral and parietal pleura.[1165]

A malignant tumor can lead to a pleural effusion in several different ways.[1163,1166] Decreased lymphatic drainage due to blockage of the small lymphatic stomas that drain the pleura is the probable mechanism in many cases, and obstruction to lymphatic drainage through mediastinal nodes which have been infiltrated by tumor is also believed to play a significant role. Another, probably less common, mechanism is increased permeability of the pleural surfaces because of the presence of metastases so that more protein enters the pleural cavity than

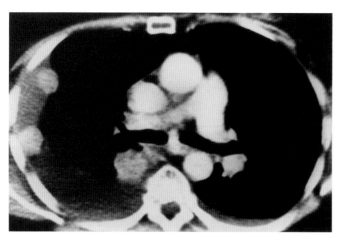

Fig. 13.119   Pleural metastases shown as tumor nodules by CT in a patient with metastatic melanoma. The tumor was widely metastatic, involving not only the pleura bilaterally but also mediastinal lymph nodes.

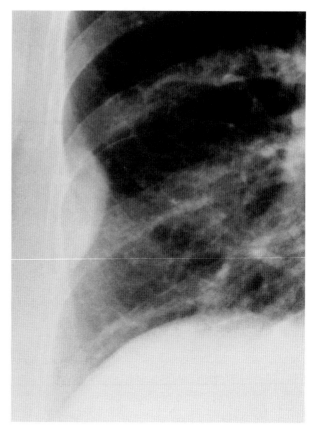

Fig. 13.120   Pleural metastasis from carcinoma of uterus. This case is unusual in that the lesion is solitary and no pleural effusion is present.

can be removed. Malignant tumors can also produce pleural effusions by obstructing the thoracic duct, in which case the resulting pleural effusion will be chylous.

Not all patients with pleural metastases have pleural effusions. Meyer[1165] found that only 60% of autopsy patients with pleural metastases had pleural effusions, and that the presence of a pleural effusion was more closely related to neoplastic invasion of the mediastinal lymph nodes than to the extent of pleural involvement by nodular metastases.

Clinically, the most frequent symptom of pleural effusion resulting from metastases is dyspnea on exertion. Chest pain is relatively uncommon, being seen in less than one-quarter of patients.[349]

Pleural effusions resulting from malignant tumor[349,1167] contain high levels of protein and may show a low pH and glucose level, and a high lactic acid dehydrogenase level. Approximately 10% of patients with malignant pleural effusion have an elevated level of amylase in the pleural fluid, even though the primary tumor is usually not in the pancreas.[1168] Bleeding may occur into the effusion, and typically the fluid contains a large number of lymphocytes. Unlike tuberculous effusions, which are also lymphocyte predominant, malignant effusions often contain mesothelial cells. The presence of definite malignant cells on cytologic examination or pleural biopsy removes all doubt about the diagnosis. The percentage of cases in which cytologic study of the pleural fluid establishes the diagnosis ranges from 40 to 80%. The rate varies with the cell type, the yield being low with squamous tumors.[1166]

Usually the finding on plain chest radiograph, CT, and ultrasound is free or loculated pleural effusion without any specific features to the effusion itself. There may be recognizable tumor nodules in the pleura on CT (Fig. 13.119), particularly on HRCT,[1169] or ultrasound,[1170,1171] MRI or even, occasionally, on chest radiographs (Fig. 13.120). Widespread pleural thickening, resembling mesothelioma, may be seen, particularly with metastases from breast carcinoma and thymoma.

FDG PET is of limited value in determining the malignant nature of a pleural effusion.

REFERENCES

1. Jemal A, Murray T, Samuels A, et al. Cancer statistics, 2003. CA Cancer J Clin 2003;53:5–26.
2. Travis WD, Colby TV, Corrin B, et al. World Health Organization Pathology Panel: World Health Organization. Histological typing of lung and pleural tumors: international histological classification of tumors. New York: Springer Verlag, 1999.
3. Vazquez MF, Yankelevitz DF. The radiologic appearance of solitary pulmonary nodules and their cytologic-histologic correlation. Semin Ultrasound CT MR 2000;21:149–162.
4. Franklin WA. Diagnosis of lung cancer: pathology of invasive and preinvasive neoplasia. Chest 2000;117:80S–89S.
5. Auerbach O, Garfinkel L. The changing pattern of lung carcinoma. Cancer 1991;68:1973–1977.
6. Travis WD, Lubin J, Ries L, et al. US lung carcinoma incidence trends: declining for most histologic types among males, increasing among females. Cancer 1996;77:2464–2470.
7. Hiroshima K, Iyoda A, Shibuya K, et al. Prognostic significance of neuroendocrine differentiation in adenocarcinoma of the lung. Ann Thorac Surg 2002;73:1732–1735.
8. Iyoda A, Hiroshima K, Baba M, et al. Pulmonary large cell carcinomas with neuroendocrine features are high-grade neuroendocrine tumors. Ann Thorac Surg 2002;73:1049–1054.

9. Travis WD, Rush W, Flieder DB, et al. Survival analysis of 200 pulmonary neuroendocrine tumors with clarification of criteria for atypical carcinoid and its separation from typical carcinoid. Am J Surg Pathol 1998;22:934–944.

10. Takei H, Asamura H, Maeshima A, et al. Large cell neuroendocrine carcinoma of the lung: A clinicopathologic study of eighty-seven cases. J Thorac Cardiovasc Surg 2002;124:285–292.

11. Flieder DB, Vazquez MF. Lung tumors with neuroendocrine morphology. A perspective for the new millennium. Radiol Clin North Am 2000;38: 563–577, ix.

12. Franklin WA. Pathology of lung cancer. J Thorac Imaging 2000;15:3–12.

13. Kazerooni EA, Bhalla M, Shepard JA, et al. Adenosquamous carcinoma of the lung: radiologic appearance. AJR Am J Roentgenol 1994;163:301–306.

14. Naunheim KS, Taylor JR, Skosey C, et al. Adenosquamous lung carcinoma: clinical characteristics, treatment, and prognosis. Ann Thorac Surg 1987;44: 462–466.

15. Sridhar KS, Bounassi MJ, Raub W Jr, et al. Clinical features of adenosquamous lung carcinoma in 127 patients. Am Rev Respir Dis 1990;142:19–23.

16. Hage R, Elbers JR, de la Riveira B, et al. Surgery for combined type small cell lung carcinoma. Thorax 1998;53:450–453.

17. Yousem SA, Hochholzer L. Mucoepidermoid tumors of the lung. Cancer 1987;60:1346–1352.

18. Fisher DA, Mond DJ, Fuchs A, et al. Mucoepidermoid tumor of the lung: CT appearance. Comput Med Imaging Graph 1995;19:339–342.

19. Heitmiller RF, Mathisen DJ, Ferry JA, et al. Mucoepidermoid lung tumors. Ann Thorac Surg 1989;47:394–399.

20. Moran CA, Suster S, Koss MN. Acinic cell carcinoma of the lung ("Fechner tumor"). A clinicopathologic, immunohistochemical, and ultrastructural study of five cases. Am J Surg Pathol 1992;16:1039–1050.

21. Stark P. Multiple independent bronchogenic carcinomas. Radiology 1982;145:599–601.

22. Bower SL, Choplin RH, Muss HB. Multiple primary bronchogenic carcinomas of the lung. AJR Am J Roentgenol 1983;140:253–258.

23. Carey FA, Donnelly SC, Walker WS, et al. Synchronous primary lung cancers: prevalence in surgical material and clinical implications. Thorax 1993;48:344–346.

24. McElvaney G, Miller RR, Muller NL, et al. Multicentricity of adenocarcinoma of the lung. Chest 1989;95:151–154.

25. Miller RR, Nelems B, Evans KG, et al. Glandular neoplasia of the lung. A proposed analogy to colonic tumors. Cancer 1988;61:1009–1014.

26. van Bodegom PC, Wagenaar SS, Corrin B, et al. Second primary lung cancer: importance of long term follow up. Thorax 1989;44:788–793.

27. Zwirewich CV, Miller RR, Muller NL. Multicentric adenocarcinoma of the lung: CT-pathologic correlation. Radiology 1990;176:185–190.

28. Antakli T, Schaefer RF, Rutherford JE, et al. Second primary lung cancer. Ann Thorac Surg 1995;59:863–866.

29. Wilkinson P, Hansell DM, Janssens J, et al. Is lung cancer associated with asbestos exposure when there are no small opacities on the chest radiograph? Lancet 1995;345:1074–1078.

30. Alberg AJ, Samet JM. Epidemiology of lung cancer. Chest 2003;123:21S–49S.

31. Bepler G. Lung cancer epidemiology and genetics. J Thorac Imaging 1999;14:228–234.

32. Smith RA, Glynn TJ. Epidemiology of lung cancer. Radiol Clin North Am 2000;38:453–470.

33. Felson B, Ralaisomay G. Carcinoma of the lung complicating lipoid pneumonia. AJR Am J Roentgenol 1983;141:901–907.

34. Lee HJ, Im JG, Ahn JM, et al. Lung cancer in patients with idiopathic pulmonary fibrosis: CT findings. J Comput Assist Tomogr 1996;20: 979–982.

35. Choi YH, Leung AN, Miro S, et al. Primary bronchogenic carcinoma after heart or lung transplantation: radiologic and clinical findings. J Thorac Imaging 2000;15:36–40.

36. Collins J, Kazerooni EA, Lacomis J, et al. Bronchogenic carcinoma after lung transplantation: frequency, clinical characteristics, and imaging findings. Radiology 2002;224:131–138.

37. Haque AK. Pathology of carcinoma of lung: an update on current concepts. J Thorac Imaging 1991;7:9–20.

38. Barsky SH, Huang SJ, Bhuta S. The extracellular matrix of pulmonary scar carcinomas is suggestive of a desmoplastic origin. Am J Pathol 1986;124:412–419.

39. Madri JA, Carter D. Scar cancers of the lung: origin and significance. Hum Pathol 1984;15:625–631.

40. Epstein DM. Bronchioloalveolar carcinoma. Semin Roentgenol 1990;25:105–111.

41. Martini N, Bains MS, Burt ME, et al. Incidence of local recurrence and second primary tumors in resected stage I lung cancer. J Thorac Cardiovasc Surg 1995;109:120–129.

42. Filderman AE, Shaw C, Matthay RA. Lung cancer. Part I: Etiology, pathology, natural history, manifestations, and diagnostic techniques. Invest Radiol 1986;21:80–90.

43. Ferguson MK. Diagnosing and staging of non-small cell lung cancer. Hematol Oncol Clin North Am 1990;4: 1053–1068.

44. Beckles MA, Spiro SG, Colice GL, et al. Initial evaluation of the patient with lung cancer: symptoms, signs, laboratory tests, and paraneoplastic syndromes. Chest 2003;123:97S–104S.

45. Jett JR, Cortese DA, Fontana RS. Lung cancer: current concepts and prospects. CA Cancer J Clin 1983;33:74–86.

46. Shin MS, Jackson LK, Shelton RW Jr, et al. Giant cell carcinoma of the lung. Clinical and roentgenographic manifestations. Chest 1986;89:366–369.

47. Byrd RB, Carr DT, Miller WE, et al. Radiographic abnormalities in carcinoma of the lung as related to histological cell type. Thorax 1969;24:573–575.

48. Byrd RB, Miller WE, Carr DT, et al. The roentgenographic appearance of squamous cell carcinoma of the bronchus. Mayo Clin Proc 1968;43:327–332.

49. Byrd RB, Miller WE, Carr DT, et al. The roentgenographic appearance of large cell carcinoma of the bronchus. Mayo Clin Proc 1968;43:333–336.

50. Byrd RB, Miller WE, Carr DT, et al. The roentgenographic appearance of small cell carcinoma of the bronchus. Mayo Clin Proc 1968;43:337–341.

51. Lehar TJ, Carr DT, Miller WE, et al. Roentgenographic appearance of bronchogenic adenocarcinoma. Am Rev Respir Dis 1967;96:245–248.

52. Theros EG. 1976 Caldwell Lecture: varying manifestation of peripheral pulmonary neoplasms: a radiologic-pathologic correlative study. AJR Am J Roentgenol 1977;128:893–914.

53. Kundel HL. Predictive value and threshold detectability of lung tumors. Radiology 1981;139:25–29.

54. Muhm JR, Miller WE, Fontana RS, et al. Lung cancer detected during a screening program using four-month chest radiographs. Radiology 1983;148:609–615.

55. Rigler LG. The roentgen signs of carcinoma of the lung. AJR Am J Roentgenol 1955;74:415–428.

56. Heitzman ER, Markarian B, Raasch BN, et al. Pathways of tumor spread through the lung: radiologic correlations with anatomy and pathology. Radiology 1982;144:3–14.

57. Kuriyama K, Tateishi R, Doi O, et al. CT-pathologic correlation in small peripheral lung cancers. AJR Am J Roentgenol 1987;149:1139–1143.

58. Aoki T, Tomoda Y, Watanabe H, et al. Peripheral lung adenocarcinoma:

correlation of thin-section CT findings with histologic prognostic factors and survival. Radiology 2001;220:803–809.

59. Mori K, Saitou Y, Tominaga K, et al. Small nodular lesions in the lung periphery: new approach to diagnosis with CT. Radiology 1990;177:843–849.

60. Aronberg DJ, Sagel SS, Jost RG, et al. Oat cell carcinoma manifesting as a bronchocele. AJR Am J Roentgenol 1979;132:23–25.

61. Felson B. Mucoid impaction (inspissated secretions) in segmental bronchial obstruction. Radiology 1979;133:9–16.

62. Woodring JH. Unusual radiographic manifestations of lung cancer. Radiol Clin North Am 1990;28:599–618.

63. Woodring JH, Bernardy MO, Loh FK. Mucoid impaction of the bronchi. Australas Radiol 1985;29:234–239.

64. Marriott AE, Weisbrod G. Bronchogenic carcinoma associated with pulmonary infarction. Radiology 1982;145:593–597.

65. Good CA. The solitary pulmonary nodule: a problem of management. Radiol Clin North Am 1963;1:429–438.

66. Grewal RG, Austin JH. CT demonstration of calcification in carcinoma of the lung. J Comput Assist Tomogr 1994;18:867–871.

67. Mahoney MC, Shipley RT, Corcoran HL, et al. CT demonstration of calcification in carcinoma of the lung. AJR Am J Roentgenol 1990;154:255–258.

68. Stewart JG, MacMahon H, Vyborny CJ, et al. Dystrophic calcification in carcinoma of the lung: demonstration by CT. AJR Am J Roentgenol 1987;148:29–30.

69. Zerhouni EA, Stitik FP, Siegelman SS, et al. CT of the pulmonary nodule: a cooperative study. Radiology 1986;160:319–327.

70. Woodring JH, Fried AM, Chuang VP. Solitary cavities of the lung: diagnostic implications of cavity wall thickness. AJR Am J Roentgenol 1980;135:1269–1271.

71. Chaudhuri MR. Primary pulmonary cavitating carcinomas. Thorax 1973;28:354–366.

72. Felson B, Wiot JF. Some less familiar roentgen manifestations of carcinoma of the lung. Semin Roentgenol 1977;12:187–206.

73. Gaeta M, Blandino A, Scribano E, et al. Mucinous cystadenocarcinoma of the lung: CT-pathologic correlation in three cases. J Comput Assist Tomogr 1999;23:641–643.

74. Kuriyama K, Seto M, Kasugai T, et al. Ground-glass opacity on thin-section CT: value in differentiating subtypes of adenocarcinoma of the lung. AJR Am J Roentgenol 1999;173:465–469.

75. Yabuuchi H, Murayama S, Sakai S, et al. Resected peripheral small cell carcinoma of the lung: computed tomographic-histologic correlation. J Thorac Imaging 1999;14:105–108.

76. Aoki T, Nakata H, Watanabe H, et al. Evolution of peripheral lung adenocarcinomas: CT findings correlated with histology and tumor doubling time. AJR Am J Roentgenol 2000;174:763–768.

77. Kuriyama K, Tateishi R, Doi O, et al. Prevalence of air bronchograms in small peripheral carcinomas of the lung on thin-section CT: comparison with benign tumors. AJR Am J Roentgenol 1991;156:921–924.

78. Zwirewich CV, Vedal S, Miller RR, et al. Solitary pulmonary nodule: high-resolution CT and radiologic-pathologic correlation. Radiology 1991;179:469–476.

79. Choi JA, Kim JH, Hong KT, et al. CT bronchus sign in malignant solitary pulmonary lesions: value in the prediction of cell type. Eur Radiol 2000;10:1304–1309.

80. Nambu A, Miyata K, Ozawa K, et al. Air-containing space in lung adenocarcinoma: high-resolution computed tomography findings. J Comput Assist Tomogr 2002;26:1026–1031.

81. Tateishi U, Nishihara H, Watanabe S, et al. Tumor angiogenesis and dynamic CT in lung adenocarcinoma: radiologic-pathologic correlation. J Comput Assist Tomogr 2001;25:23–27.

82. Geddes DM. The natural history of lung cancer: a review based on rates of tumour growth. Br J Dis Chest 1979;73:1–17.

83. Hayabuchi N, Russell WJ, Murakami J. Slow-growing lung cancer in a fixed population sample. Radiologic assessments. Cancer 1983;52:1098–1104.

84. Nathan MH, Collins VP. Differentiation of benign and malignant pulmonary nodules by growth rate. Radiology 1962;79:221–232.

85. Steele JD, Buell P. Asymptomatic solitary pulmonary nodules. Host survival, tumor size, and growth rate. J Thorac Cardiovasc Surg 1973;65:140–151.

86. Straus MJ. The growth characteristics of lung cancer and its application to treatment design. Semin Oncol 1974;1:167–174.

87. Usuda K, Saito Y, Sagawa M, et al. Tumor doubling time and prognostic assessment of patients with primary lung cancer. Cancer 1994;74:2239–2244.

88. Hill CA. Bronchioloalveolar carcinoma: a review. Radiology 1984;150:15–20.

89. Garland LH. The rate of growth and natural duration of primary bronchial cancer. Am J Roentgenol Radium Ther Nucl Med 1966;96:604–611.

90. Burke M, Fraser R. Obstructive pneumonitis: a pathologic and pathogenetic reappraisal. Radiology 1988;166:699–704.

91. Glazer HS, Anderson DJ, Sagel SS. Bronchial impaction in lobar collapse: CT demonstration and pathologic correlation. AJR Am J Roentgenol 1989;153:485–488.

92. Shin MS, Ho KJ. CT fluid bronchogram: observation in postobstructive pulmonary consolidation. Clin Imaging 1992;16:109–113.

93. Woodring JH. Determining the cause of pulmonary atelectasis: a comparison of plain radiography and CT. AJR Am J Roentgenol 1988;150:757–763.

94. Onitsuka H, Tsukuda M, Araki A, et al. Differentiation of central lung tumor from postobstructive lobar collapse by rapid sequence computed tomography. J Thorac Imaging 1991;6:28–31.

95. Tobler J, Levitt RG, Glazer HS, et al. Differentiation of proximal bronchogenic carcinoma from postobstructive lobar collapse by magnetic resonance imaging. Comparison with computed tomography. Invest Radiol 1987;22:538–543.

96. Kameda K, Adachi S, Kono M. Detection of T-factor in lung cancer using magnetic resonance imaging and computed tomography. J Thorac Imaging 1988;3:73–80.

97. Kono M, Adachi S, Kusumoto M, et al. Clinical utility of Gd-DTPA-enhanced magnetic resonance imaging in lung cancer. J Thorac Imaging 1993;8:18–26.

98. Stiglbauer R, Schurawitzki H, Klepetko W, et al. Contrast-enhanced MRI for the staging of bronchogenic carcinoma: comparison with CT and histopathologic staging—preliminary results. Clin Radiol 1991;44:293–298.

99. Bourgouin PM, McLoud TC, Fitzgibbon JF, et al. Differentiation of bronchogenic carcinoma from postobstructive pneumonitis by magnetic resonance imaging: histopathologic correlation. J Thorac Imaging 1991;6:22–27.

100. Rohlfing BM, White EA, Webb WR, et al. Hilar and mediastinal adenopathy caused by bacterial abscess of the lung. Radiology 1978;128:289–293.

101. Fraser RG, Pare JAP. Diagnosis of diseases of the chest. Philadelphia: WB Saunders, 1999.

102. Mountain CF. Revisions in the International System for Staging Lung Cancer. Chest 1997;111:1710–1717.

103. International Union Against Cancer. TNM classification of malignant

tumors. In: Sobin LH, Wittekind CH, eds. New York: Wiley-Liss, 1997.

104. Naruke T, Tsuchiya R, Kondo H, et al. Prognosis and survival after resection for bronchogenic carcinoma based on the 1997 TNM-staging classification: the Japanese experience. Ann Thorac Surg 2001;71:1759–1764.

105. Johnson BE. Management of small-cell lung cancer. Clin Chest Med 1993;14: 173–187.

106. Stahel RA, Ginsberg R, Havemann K, et al. Staging and prognostic factors in small cell lung cancer: a consensus report. Lung Cancer 1989;5: 119–126.

107. Simon GR, Wagner H. Small cell lung cancer. Chest 2003;123:259S–271S.

108. Park BJ, Louie O, Altorki N. Staging and the surgical management of lung cancer. Radiol Clin North Am 2000; 38:545–561, ix.

109. Smythe WR. Treatment of stage I non-small cell lung carcinoma. Chest 2003;123:181S–187S.

110. Scott WJ, Howington J, Movsas B. Treatment of stage II non-small cell lung cancer. Chest 2003;123: 188S–201S.

111. Kesler KA, Conces DJ Jr, Heimansohn DA, et al. Assessing the feasibility of bronchoplastic surgery with magnetic resonance imaging. Ann Thorac Surg 1991;52:145–147.

112. Mehran RJ, Deslauriers J, Piraux M, et al. Survival related to nodal status after sleeve resection for lung cancer. J Thorac Cardiovasc Surg 1994;107: 576–582.

113. End A, Hollaus P, Pentsch A, et al. Bronchoplastic procedures in malignant and nonmalignant disease: Multivariable analysis of 144 cases. J Thorac Cardiovasc Surg 2000; 120:119–127.

114. Robinson LA, Wagner H Jr, Ruckdeschel JC. Treatment of stage IIIA non-small cell lung cancer. Chest 2003;123:202S–220S.

115. Jett JR, Scott WJ, Rivera MP, et al. Guidelines on treatment of stage IIIB non-small cell lung cancer. Chest 2003;123:221S–225S.

116. Spiro SG, Porter JC. Lung cancer – where are we today? Current advances in staging and nonsurgical treatment. Am J Respir Crit Care Med 2002;166: 1166–1196.

117. Inoue M, Miyoshi S, Yasumitsu T, et al. Surgical results for small cell lung cancer based on the new TNM staging system. Thoracic Surgery Study Group of Osaka University, Osaka, Japan. Ann Thorac Surg 2000;70:1615–1619.

118. Bonomo L, Ciccotosto C, Guidotti A, et al. Lung cancer staging: the role of computed tomography and magnetic resonance imaging. Eur J Radiol 1996;23:35–45.

119. Hanson JA, Armstrong P. Staging intrathoracic non-small-cell lung cancer. Eur Radiol 1997;7:161–172.

120. Romney BM, Austin JH. Plain film evaluation of carcinoma of the lung. Semin Roentgenol 1990;25:45–63.

121. Quint LE, Francis IR. Radiologic staging of lung cancer. J Thorac Imaging 1999;14:235–246.

122. Silvestri GA, Tanoue LT, Margolis ML, et al. The noninvasive staging of non-small cell lung cancer: the guidelines. Chest 2003;123:147S–156S.

123. Laroche C, Fairbairn I, Moss H, et al. Role of computed tomographic scanning of the thorax prior to bronchoscopy in the investigation of suspected lung cancer. Thorax 2000;55:359–363.

124. Patz EF Jr, Erasmus JJ, McAdams HP, et al. Lung cancer staging and management: comparison of contrast-enhanced and nonenhanced helical CT of the thorax. Radiology 1999;212: 56–60.

125. Cascade PN, Gross BH, Kazerooni EA, et al. Variability in the detection of enlarged mediastinal lymph nodes in staging lung cancer: a comparison of contrast-enhanced and unenhanced CT. AJR Am J Roentgenol 1998;170: 927–931.

126. Glazer GM, Francis IR, Shirazi KK, et al. Evaluation of the pulmonary hilum: comparison of conventional radiography, 55° posterior oblique tomography, and dynamic computed tomography. J Comput Assist Tomogr 1983;7:983–989.

127. Remy-Jardin M, Duyck P, Remy J, et al. Hilar lymph nodes: identification with spiral CT and histologic correlation. Radiology 1995;196:387–394.

128. Lahde S, Paivansalo M, Rainio P. CT for predicting the resectability of lung cancer. A prospective study. Acta Radiol 1991;32:449–454.

129. Lewis JW Jr, Pearlberg JL, Beute GH, et al. Can computed tomography of the chest stage lung cancer? Yes and no. Ann Thorac Surg 1990;49:591–595.

130. Mezzetti M, Panigalli T, Giuliani L, et al. Personal experience in lung cancer sleeve lobectomy and sleeve pneumonectomy. Ann Thorac Surg 2002;73:1736–1739.

131. Fadel E, Yildizeli B, Chapelier AR, et al. Sleeve lobectomy for bronchogenic cancers: factors affecting survival. Ann Thorac Surg 2002;74:851–858.

132. Fleiter T, Merkle EM, Aschoff AJ, et al. Comparison of real-time virtual and fiberoptic bronchoscopy in patients with bronchial carcinoma: opportunities and limitations. AJR Am J Roentgenol 1997;169:1591–1595.

133. Quint LE, Glazer GM, Orringer MB. Central lung masses: prediction with CT of need for pneumonectomy versus lobectomy. Radiology 1987;165:735–738.

134. Storto ML, Ciccotosto C, Guidotti A, et al. Neoplastic extension across pulmonary fissures: value of spiral computed tomography and multiplanar reformations. J Thorac Imaging 1998;13:204–210.

135. Uchisako H, Matsumoto T, Kuramitsu T, et al. Thin-section oblique CT with 25 degrees cranially tilted images. Evaluation of pulmonary tumors adjacent to the interlobar fissures. Acta Radiol 1997;38:246–249.

136. Chen CY, Kao CH, Hsu NY, et al. Prediction of probability of pneumonectomy for lung cancer using Tc-99m MAA perfusion lung imaging. Clin Nucl Med 1994;19:1094–1097.

137. Ryo UY. Prediction of postoperative loss of lung function in patients with malignant lung mass. Quantitative regional ventilation-perfusion scanning. Radiol Clin North Am 1990;28:657–663.

138. Detterbeck FC, Jones DR, Kernstine KH, et al. Lung cancer. Special treatment issues. Chest 2003;123: 244S–258S.

139. Ciriaco P, Rendina EA, Venuta F, et al. Preoperative chemotherapy and immunochemotherapy for locally advanced stage IIIA and IIIB non small cell lung cancer. Preliminary results. Eur J Cardiothorac Surg 1995;9: 305–309.

140. Martini N, Yellin A, Ginsberg RJ, et al. Management of non-small cell lung cancer with direct mediastinal involvement. Ann Thorac Surg 1994;58:1447–1451.

141. Grunenwald D, Mazel C, Girard P, et al. Total vertebrectomy for en bloc resection of lung cancer invading the spine. Ann Thorac Surg 1996;61: 723–725.

142. Klepetko W, Wisser W, Birsan T, et al. T4 lung tumors with infiltration of the thoracic aorta: is an operation reasonable? Ann Thorac Surg 1999;67:340–344.

143. Spaggiari L, Regnard JF, Magdeleinat P, et al. Extended resections for bronchogenic carcinoma invading the superior vena cava system. Ann Thorac Surg 2000;69:233–236.

144. Dartevelle P, Chapelier A, Navajas M, et al. Replacement of the superior vena cava with polytetrafluoroethylene grafts combined with resection of mediastinal-pulmonary malignant tumors. Report of thirteen cases. J Thorac Cardiovasc Surg 1987;94:361–366.

145. Grunewald D, Mazel C, Girard P, et al. Radical en bloc resection for lung

cancer invading the spine. J Thorac Cardiovasc Surg 2002;123:271–279.

146. Yokoi K, Tsuchiya R, Mori T, et al. Results of surgical treatment of lung cancer involving the diaphragm. J Thorac Cardiovasc Surg 2000;120: 799–805.

147. Haramati LB, White CS. MR imaging of lung cancer. Magn Reson Imaging Clin North Am 2000;8:43–57, viii.

148. Lowe VJ, Naunheim KS. Positron emission tomography in lung cancer. Ann Thorac Surg 1998;65:1821–1829.

149. Houston JG, Fleet M, McMillan N, et al. Ultrasonic assessment of hemidiaphragmatic movement: an indirect method of evaluating mediastinal invasion in non-small cell lung cancer. Br J Radiol 1995; 68:695–699.

150. Martini N, Heelan R, Westcott J, et al. Comparative merits of conventional, computed tomographic, and magnetic resonance imaging in assessing mediastinal involvement in surgically confirmed lung carcinoma. J Thorac Cardiovasc Surg 1985;90:639–648.

151. Glazer HS, Kaiser LR, Anderson DJ, et al. Indeterminate mediastinal invasion in bronchogenic carcinoma: CT evaluation. Radiology 1989;173: 37–42.

152. McLoud TC. CT of bronchogenic carcinoma: indeterminate mediastinal invasion. Radiology 1989;173:15–16.

153. Scott IR, Müller NL, Miller RR, et al. Resectable stage III lung cancer: CT, surgical, and pathologic correlation. Radiology 1988;166:75–79.

154. Musset D, Grenier P, Carette MF, et al. Primary lung cancer staging: prospective comparative study of MR imaging with CT. Radiology 1986;160:607–611.

155. Izbicki JR, Thetter O, Karg O, et al. Accuracy of computed tomographic scan and surgical assessment for staging of bronchial carcinoma. A prospective study. J Thorac Cardiovasc Surg 1992;104:413–420.

156. Herman SJ, Winton TL, Weisbrod GL, et al. Mediastinal invasion by bronchogenic carcinoma: CT signs. Radiology 1994;190:841–846.

157. White PG, Adams H, Crane MD, et al. Preoperative staging of carcinoma of the bronchus: can computed tomographic scanning reliably identify stage III tumours? Thorax 1994;49:951–957.

158. Choe DH, Lee JH, Lee BH, et al. Obliteration of the pulmonary vein in lung cancer: significance in assessing local extent with CT. J Comput Assist Tomogr 1998;22:587–591.

159. Takahashi K, Furuse M, Hanaoka H, et al. Pulmonary vein and left atrial invasion by lung cancer: assessment by breath-hold gadolinium-enhanced three-dimensional MR angiography. J Comput Assist Tomogr 2000;24: 557–561.

160. Murata K, Takahashi M, Mori M, et al. Chest wall and mediastinal invasion by lung cancer: evaluation with multisection expiratory dynamic CT. Radiology 1994;191:251–255.

161. Ohtsuka T, Minami M, Nakajima J, et al. Ciné computed tomography for evaluation of tumors invasive to the thoracic aorta: seven clinical experiences. J Thorac Cardiovasc Surg 1996;112:190–192.

162. Yokoi K, Mori K, Miyazawa N, et al. Tumor invasion of the chest wall and mediastinum in lung cancer: evaluation with pneumothorax CT. Radiology 1991;181:147–152.

163. Laurent F, Drouillard J, Dorcier F, et al. Bronchogenic carcinoma staging: CT versus MR imaging. Assessment with surgery. Eur J Cardiothorac Surg 1988;2:31–36.

164. Webb WR, Sarin M, Zerhouni EA, et al. Interobserver variability in CT and MR staging of lung cancer. J Comput Assist Tomogr 1993;17:841–846.

165. Mayr B, Lenhard M, Fink U, et al. Preoperative evaluation of bronchogenic carcinoma: value of MR in T- and N-staging. Eur J Radiol 1992;14:245–251.

166. Gefter WB. Magnetic resonance imaging in the evaluation of lung cancer. Semin Roentgenol 1990;25:73–84.

167. Levitt RG, Glazer HS, Roper CL, et al. Magnetic resonance imaging of mediastinal and hilar masses: comparison with CT. AJR Am J Roentgenol 1985;145:9–14.

168. Webb WR, Gatsonis C, Zerhouni EA, et al. CT and MR imaging in staging non-small cell bronchogenic carcinoma: report of the Radiologic Diagnostic Oncology Group. Radiology 1991;178:705–713.

169. Ohno Y, Adachi S, Motoyama A, et al. Multiphase ECG-triggered 3D contrast-enhanced MR angiography: utility for evaluation of hilar and mediastinal invasion of bronchogenic carcinoma. J Magn Reson Imaging 2001;13:215–224.

170. Kurimoto N, Murayama M, Yoshioka S, et al. Assessment of usefulness of endobronchial ultrasonography in determination of depth of tracheobronchial tumor invasion. Chest 1999;115:1500–1506.

171. Herth F, Ernst A, Schulz M, et al. Endobronchial ultrasound reliably differentiates between airway infiltration and compression by tumor. Chest 2003;123:458–462.

172. Cangemi V, Volpino P, D'Andrea N, et al. Results of surgical treatment of stage IIIA non-small cell lung cancer. Eur J Cardiothorac Surg 1995;9: 352–359.

173. Allen MS, Mathisen DJ, Grillo HC, et al. Bronchogenic carcinoma with chest wall invasion. Ann Thorac Surg 1991;51:948–951.

174. Piehler JM, Pairolero PC, Weiland LH, et al. Bronchogenic carcinoma with chest wall invasion: factors affecting survival following en bloc resection. Ann Thorac Surg 1982;34:684–691.

175. Ratto GB, Piacenza G, Frola C, et al. Chest wall involvement by lung cancer: computed tomographic detection and results of operation. Ann Thorac Surg 1991;51:182–188.

176. Magdeleinat P, Alifano M, Benbrahem C, et al. Surgical treatment of lung cancer invading the chest wall: results and prognostic factors. Ann Thorac Surg 2001;71:1094–1099.

177. Facciolo F, Cardillo G, Lopergolo M, et al. Chest wall invasion in non-small cell lung carcinoma: A rationale for en bloc resection. J Thorac Cardiovasc Surg 2001;121:649–656.

178. Burkhart H, Allen M, Nichols F, et al. Results of en bloc resection for bronchogenic carcinoma with chest wall invasion. J Thorac Cardiovasc Surg 2002;123:670–675.

179. McCaughan BC. Primary lung cancer invading the chest wall. Chest Surg Clin North Am 1994;4:17–28.

180. Guyatt GH, Lefcoe M, Walter S, et al. Interobserver variation in the computed tomographic evaluation of mediastinal lymph node size in patients with potentially resectable lung cancer. Canadian Lung Oncology Group. Chest 1995;107:116–119.

181. Roberts JR, Blum MG, Arildsen R, et al. Prospective comparison of radiologic, thoracoscopic, and pathologic staging in patients with early non-small cell lung cancer. Ann Thorac Surg 1999; 68:1154–1158.

182. Glazer HS, Duncan-Meyer J, Aronberg DJ, et al. Pleural and chest wall invasion in bronchogenic carcinoma: CT evaluation. Radiology 1985;157: 191–194.

183. Pearlberg JL, Sandler MA, Beute GH, et al. Limitations of CT in evaluation of neoplasms involving chest wall. J Comput Assist Tomogr 1987;11: 290–293.

184. Pennes DR, Glazer GM, Wimbish KJ, et al. Chest wall invasion by lung cancer: limitations of CT evaluation. AJR Am J Roentgenol 1985;144: 507–511.

185. Watanabe A, Shimokata K, Saka H, et al. Chest CT combined with artificial pneumothorax: value in determining

origin and extent of tumor. AJR Am J Roentgenol 1991;156:707–710.

186. Shirakawa T, Fukuda K, Miyamoto Y, et al. Parietal pleural invasion of lung masses: evaluation with CT performed during deep inspiration and expiration. Radiology 1994; 192:809–811.

187. Kodalli N, Erzen C, Yuksel M. Evaluation of parietal pleural invasion of lung cancers with breathhold inspiration and expiration MRI. Clin Imaging 1999;23:227–235.

188. Kuriyama K, Tateishi R, Kumatani T, et al. Pleural invasion by peripheral bronchogenic carcinoma: assessment with three-dimensional helical CT. Radiology 1994;191:365–369.

189. Haggar AM, Pearlberg JL, Froelich JW, et al. Chest-wall invasion by carcinoma of the lung: detection by MR imaging. AJR Am J Roentgenol 1987;148: 1075–1078.

190. Padovani B, Mouroux J, Seksik L, et al. Chest wall invasion by bronchogenic carcinoma: evaluation with MR imaging. Radiology 1993;187:33–38.

191. Heelan RT, Demas BE, Caravelli JF, et al. Superior sulcus tumors: CT and MR imaging. Radiology 1989;170:637–641.

192. Sakai S, Murayama S, Murakami J, et al. Bronchogenic carcinoma invasion of the chest wall: evaluation with dynamic cine MRI during breathing. J Comput Assist Tomogr 1997;21: 595–600.

193. Suzuki N, Saitoh T, Kitamura S. Tumor invasion of the chest wall in lung cancer: diagnosis with US. Radiology 1993;187:39–42.

194. Pancoast HK. Superior sulcus tumor: tumor characterized bypain, Horner's syndrome, destruction of bone and atropy of hand muscles. JAMA 1932;99:1391–1396.

195. Freundlich IM, Chasen MH, Varma DG. Magnetic resonance imaging of pulmonary apical tumors. J Thorac Imaging 1996;11:210–222.

196. Johnson DH, Hainsworth JD, Greco FA. Pancoast's syndrome and small cell lung cancer. Chest 1982;82:602–606.

197. Paulson DL. Carcinomas in the superior pulmonary sulcus. J Thorac Cardiovasc Surg 1975;70:1095–1104.

198. Paulson DL. Carcinoma in the superior pulmonary sulcus. Ann Thorac Surg 1979;28:3–4.

199. Attar S, Krasna MJ, Sonett JR, et al. Superior sulcus (Pancoast) tumor: experience with 105 patients. Ann Thorac Surg 1998;66:193–198.

200. Martinod E, D'Audiffret A, Thomas P, et al. Management of superior sulcus tumors: experience with 139 cases treated by surgical resection. Ann Thorac Surg 2002;73:1534–1539.

201. Wright CD, Menard MT, Wain JC, et al. Induction chemoradiation compared with induction radiation for lung cancer involving the superior sulcus. Ann Thorac Surg 2002;73:1541–1544.

202. O'Connell RS, McLoud TC, Wilkins EW. Superior sulcus tumor: radiographic diagnosis and workup. AJR Am J Roentgenol 1983;140: 25–30.

203. McLoud TC, Isler RJ, Novelline RA, et al. The apical cap. AJR Am J Roentgenol 1981;137:299–306.

204. Hamlin DJ, Burgener FA. CT, including sagittal and coronal reconstruction, in the evaluation of pancoast tumors. J Comput Tomogr 1982;6:43–50.

205. Webb WR, Jeffrey RB, Godwin JD. Thoracic computed tomography in superior sulcus tumors. J Comput Assist Tomogr 1981;5:361–365.

206. Castagno AA, Shuman WP. MR imaging in clinically suspected brachial plexus tumor. AJR Am J Roentgenol 1987;149:1219–1222.

207. McLoud TC, Filion RB, Edelman RR, et al. MR imaging of superior sulcus carcinoma. J Comput Assist Tomogr 1989;13:233–239.

208. Takasugi JE, Rapoport S, Shaw C. Superior sulcus tumors: the role of imaging. J Thorac Imaging 1989;4: 41–48.

209. Knisely BL, Broderick LS, Kuhlman JE. MR imaging of the pleura and chest wall. Magn Reson Imaging Clin North Am 2000;8:125–141.

210. Myrdal G, Lambe M, Gustafsson G, et al. Survival in primary lung cancer potentially cured by operation: influence of tumor stage and clinical characteristics. Ann Thorac Surg 2003;75:356–363.

211. Mountain CF. Surgery for stage IIIa-N2 non-small cell lung cancer. Cancer 1994;73:2589–2598.

212. Daly BD, Mueller JD, Faling LJ, et al. N2 lung cancer: outcome in patients with false-negative computed tomographic scans of the chest. J Thorac Cardiovasc Surg 1993;105: 904–910.

213. Goldstraw P, Mannam GC, Kaplan DK, et al. Surgical management of non-small-cell lung cancer with ipsilateral mediastinal node metastasis (N2 disease). J Thorac Cardiovasc Surg 1994;107:19–27.

214. Nakanishi R, Osaki T, Nakanishi K, et al. Treatment strategy for patients with surgically discovered N2 stage IIIA non-small cell lung cancer. Ann Thorac Surg 1997;64:342–348.

215. Vansteenkiste JF, De Leyn PR, Deneffe GJ, et al. Survival and prognostic factors in resected N2 non-small cell lung cancer: a study of 140 cases. Leuven Lung Cancer Group. Ann Thorac Surg 1997;63: 1441–1450.

216. Okada M, Tsubota N, Yoshimura M, et al. Prognosis of completely resected N2 non-small cell lung carcinomas: What is the significant node that affects survival? J Thorac Cardiovasc Surg 1999;118:270–275.

217. Suzuki K, Nagai K, Yoshida J, et al. The prognosis of surgically resected N2 non-small cell lung cancer: The importance of clinical N status. J Thorac Cardiovasc Surg 1999; 118:145–153.

218. Cybulsky IJ, Lanza LA, Ryan MB, et al. Prognostic significance of computed tomography in resected N2 lung cancer. Ann Thorac Surg 1992;54:533–537.

219. Martini N, Flehinger BJ, Zaman MB, et al. Results of resection in non-oat cell carcinoma of the lung with mediastinal lymph node metastases. Ann Surg 1983;198:386–397.

220. Naruke T, Goya T, Tsuchiya R, et al. The importance of surgery to non-small cell carcinoma of lung with mediastinal lymph node metastasis. Ann Thorac Surg 1988;46:603–610.

221. Watanabe Y, Shimizu J, Oda M, et al. Aggressive surgical intervention in N2 non-small cell cancer of the lung. Ann Thorac Surg 1991;51:253–261.

222. Suzuki K, Nagai K, Yoshida J, et al. Clinical predictors of N2 disease in the setting of a negative computed tomographic scan in patients with lung cancer. J Thorac Cardiovasc Surg 1999;117:593–598.

223. Mountain CF, Dresler CM. Regional lymph node classification for lung cancer staging. Chest 1997;111: 1718–1723.

224. Cymbalista M, Waysberg A, Zacharias C, et al. CT demonstration of the 1996 AJCC-UICC regional lymph node classification for lung cancer staging. Radiographics 1999;19:899–900.

225. Ko JP, Drucker EA, Shepard JA, et al. CT depiction of regional nodal stations for lung cancer staging. AJR Am J Roentgenol 2000;174:775–782.

226. Bollen EC, Goei R, van 't Hof-Grootenboer BE, et al. Interobserver variability and accuracy of computed tomographic assessment of nodal status in lung cancer. Ann Thorac Surg 1994;58:158–162.

227. Watanabe S, Ladas G, Goldstraw P. Inter-observer variability in systematic nodal dissection: comparison of European and Japanese nodal designation. Ann Thorac Surg 2002;73:245–248.

228. Friedman PJ. Lung cancer: update on staging classifications. AJR Am J Roentgenol 1988;150:261–264.

229. Asamura H, Suzuki K, Kondo H, et al. Where is the boundary between N1

and N2 stations in lung cancer? Ann Thorac Surg 2000;70:1839–1845.

230. Libshitz HI, McKenna RJ Jr, Mountain CF. Patterns of mediastinal metastases in bronchogenic carcinoma. Chest 1986;90:229–232.

231. Tateishi M, Fukuyama Y, Hamatake M, et al. Skip mediastinal lymph node metastasis in non-small cell lung cancer. J Surg Oncol 1994;57:139–142.

232. Shimoyama K, Murata K, Takahashi M, et al. Pulmonary hilar lymph node metastases from lung cancer: evaluation based on morphology at thin-section, incremental, dynamic CT. Radiology 1997;203:187–195.

233. Genereux GP, Howie JL. Normal mediastinal lymph node size and number: CT and anatomic study. AJR Am J Roentgenol 1984;142:1095–1100.

234. Ingram CE, Belli AM, Lewars MD, et al. Normal lymph node size in the mediastinum: a retrospective study in two patient groups. Clin Radiol 1989;40:35–39.

235. Quint LE, Glazer GM, Orringer MB, et al. Mediastinal lymph node detection and sizing at CT and autopsy. AJR Am J Roentgenol 1986;147:469–472.

236. Kiyono K, Sone S, Sakai F, et al. The number and size of normal mediastinal lymph nodes: a postmortem study. AJR Am J Roentgenol 1988;150:771–776.

237. Schnyder PA, Gamsu G. CT of the pretracheal retrocaval space. AJR Am J Roentgenol 1981;136:303–308.

238. Takamochi K, Nagai K, Yoshida J, et al. The role of computed tomographic scanning in diagnosing mediastinal node involvement in non-small cell lung cancer. J Thorac Cardiovasc Surg 2000;119:1135–1140.

239. Kerr KM, Lamb D, Wathen CG, et al. Pathological assessment of mediastinal lymph nodes in lung cancer: implications for non-invasive mediastinal staging. Thorax 1992;47:337–341.

240. Libshitz HI, McKenna RJ Jr. Mediastinal lymph node size in lung cancer. AJR Am J Roentgenol 1984;143:715–718.

241. McLoud TC, Bourgouin PM, Greenberg RW, et al. Bronchogenic carcinoma: analysis of staging in the mediastinum with CT by correlative lymph node mapping and sampling. Radiology 1992;182:319–323.

242. Arita T, Kuramitsu T, Kawamura M, et al. Bronchogenic carcinoma: incidence of metastases to normal sized lymph nodes. Thorax 1995;50:1267–1269.

243. Aronchick JM. CT of mediastinal lymph nodes in patients with non-small cell lung carcinoma. Radiol Clin North Am 1990;28:573–581.

244. Gross BH, Glazer GM, Orringer MB, et al. Bronchogenic carcinoma

metastatic to normal-sized lymph nodes: frequency and significance. Radiology 1988;166:71–74.

245. Asamura H, Nakayama H, Kondo H, et al. Lymph node involvement, recurrence, and prognosis in resected small, peripheral, non-small-cell lung carcinomas: are these carcinomas candidates for video-assisted lobectomy? J Thorac Cardiovasc Surg 1996;111:1125–1134.

246. Daly BD Jr, Faling LJ, Bite G, et al. Mediastinal lymph node evaluation by computed tomography in lung cancer. An analysis of 345 patients grouped by TNM staging, tumor size, and tumor location. J Thorac Cardiovasc Surg 1987;94:664–672.

247. Quint LE, Francis IR, Wahl RL, et al. Preoperative staging of non-small-cell carcinoma of the lung: imaging methods. AJR Am J Roentgenol 1995;164:1349–1359.

248. Bollen EC, van Duin CJ, Theunissen PH, et al. Mediastinal lymph node dissection in resected lung cancer: morbidity and accuracy of staging. Ann Thorac Surg 1993;55:961–966.

249. Izbicki JR, Passlick B, Karg O, et al. Impact of radical systematic mediastinal lymphadenectomy on tumor staging in lung cancer. Ann Thorac Surg 1995;59:209–214.

250. Graham A, Chan K, Pastorino U, et al. Systematic nodal dissection in the intrathoracic staging of patients with non-small cell lung cancer. J Thorac Cardiovasc Surg 1999;117:246–251.

251. Arita T, Matsumoto T, Kuramitsu T, et al. Is it possible to differentiate malignant mediastinal nodes from benign nodes by size? Reevaluation by CT, transesophageal echocardiography, and nodal specimen. Chest 1996;110: 1004–1008.

252. Backer CL, Shields TW, Lockhart CG, et al. Selective preoperative evaluation for possible N2 disease in carcinoma of the lung. J Thorac Cardiovasc Surg 1987;93:337–343.

253. Baron RL, Levitt RG, Sagel SS, et al. Computed tomography in the preoperative evaluation of bronchogenic carcinoma. Radiology 1982;145:727–732.

254. Dales RE, Stark RM, Raman S. Computed tomography to stage lung cancer. Approaching a controversy using meta-analysis. Am Rev Respir Dis 1990;141:1096–1101.

255. Ikezoe J, Kadowaki K, Morimoto S, et al. Mediastinal lymph node metastases from nonsmall cell bronchogenic carcinoma: reevaluation with CT. J Comput Assist Tomogr 1990;14:340–344.

256. Libshitz HI, McKenna RJ Jr, Haynie TP, et al. Mediastinal evaluation in lung cancer. Radiology 1984;151:295–299.

257. Osborne DRKM. Detection of intrathoracic lymph node metastases from lung carcinoma (letter). Radiology 1982;144:187–188.

258. Patterson GA, Ginsberg RJ, Poon PY, et al. A prospective evaluation of magnetic resonance imaging, computed tomography, and mediastinoscopy in the preoperative assessment of mediastinal node status in bronchogenic carcinoma. J Thorac Cardiovasc Surg 1987;94: 679–684.

259. Primack SL, Lee KS, Logan PM, et al. Bronchogenic carcinoma: utility of CT in the evaluation of patients with suspected lesions. Radiology 1994;193:795–800.

260. Rendina EA, Bognolo DA, Mineo TC, et al. Computed tomography for the evaluation of intrathoracic invasion by lung cancer. J Thorac Cardiovasc Surg 1987;94:57–63.

261. Staples CA, Muller NL, Miller RR, et al. Mediastinal nodes in bronchogenic carcinoma: comparison between CT and mediastinoscopy. Radiology 1988;167:367–372.

262. Watanabe Y, Shimizu J, Tsubota M, et al. Mediastinal spread of metastatic lymph nodes in bronchogenic carcinoma. Mediastinal nodal metastases in lung cancer. Chest 1990;97:1059–1065.

263. Buy JN, Ghossain MA, Poirson F, et al. Computed tomography of mediastinal lymph nodes in nonsmall cell lung cancer. A new approach based on the lymphatic pathway of tumor spread. J Comput Assist Tomogr 1988;12: 545–552.

264. Prenzel KL, Monig SP, Sinning JM, et al. Lymph node size and metastatic infiltration in non-small cell lung cancer. Chest 2003;123:463–467.

265. Gdeedo A, Van Schil P, Corthouts B, et al. Prospective evaluation of computed tomography and mediastinoscopy in mediastinal lymph node staging. Eur Respir J 1997;10:1547–1551.

266. Koike T, Terashima M, Takizawa T, et al. Clinical analysis of small-sized peripheral lung cancer. J Thorac Cardiovasc Surg 1998;115:1015–1020.

267. Conces DJ Jr, Klink JF, Tarver RD, et al. T1N0M0 lung cancer: evaluation with CT. Radiology 1989;170:643–646.

268. Duncan KA, Gomersall LN, Weir J. Computed tomography of the chest in T1N0M0 non-small cell bronchial carcinoma. Br J Radiol 1993;66:20–22.

269. Heavey LR, Glazer GM, Gross BH, et al. The role of CT in staging radiographic T1N0M0 lung cancer. AJR Am J Roentgenol 1986;146:285–290.

270. Seely JM, Mayo JR, Miller RR, et al. T1 lung cancer: prevalence of mediastinal

nodal metastases and diagnostic accuracy of CT. Radiology 1993;186:129–132.

271. Pearlberg JL, Sandler MA, Beute GH, et al. T1N0M0 bronchogenic carcinoma: assessment by CT. Radiology 1985;157:187–190.

272. Kawano R, Hata E, Ikeda S, et al. Micrometastasis to lymph nodes in stage I left lung cancer patients. Ann Thorac Surg 2002;73:1558–1562.

273. Okada M, Yoshikawa K, Hatta T, et al. Is segmentectomy with lymph node assessment an alternative to lobectomy for non-small cell lung cancer of 2 cm or smaller? Ann Thorac Surg 2001;71: 956–960.

274. Takizawa T, Terashima M, Koike T, et al. Mediastinal lymph node metastasis in patients with clinical stage I peripheral non-small-cell lung cancer. J Thorac Cardiovasc Surg 1997;113:248–252.

275. Black WC, Armstrong P, Daniel TM. Cost effectiveness of chest CT in T1N0M0 lung cancer. Radiology 1988;167:373–378.

276. Becker GL, Whitlock WL, Schaefer PS, et al. The impact of thoracic computed tomography in clinically staged T1, N0, M0 chest lesions. Arch Intern Med 1990;150:557–559.

277. Parker LA, Mauro MA, Delany DJ, et al. Evaluation of T1N0M0 lung cancer with CT. J Comput Assist Tomogr 1991;15:943–947.

278. Glazer GM, Orringer MB, Chenevert TL, et al. Mediastinal lymph nodes: relaxation time/pathologic correlation and implications in staging of lung cancer with MR imaging. Radiology 1988;168:429–431.

279. Laissy JP, Gay-Depassier P, Soyer P, et al. Enlarged mediastinal lymph nodes in bronchogenic carcinoma: assessment with dynamic contrast-enhanced MR imaging. Work in progress. Radiology 1994;191:263–267.

280. Bluemke DABRNWK. MR lymph node contrast agent (Combidex): use in directing hronchoscopic fine needle aspiration of mediastinal nodes. Radiology 1998;209(P):375.

281. Kernstine KH, Stanford W, Mullan BF, et al. PET, CT, and MRI with Combidex for mediastinal staging in non-small cell lung carcinoma. Ann Thorac Surg 1999;68:1022–1028.

282. Glazer GM, Gross BH, Aisen AM, et al. Imaging of the pulmonary hilum: a prospective comparative study in patients with lung cancer. AJR Am J Roentgenol 1985;145:245–248.

283. Batra P, Brown K, Steckel RJ, et al. MR imaging of the thorax: a comparison of axial, coronal, and sagittal imaging planes. J Comput Assist Tomogr 1988;12:75–81.

284. Poon PY, Bronskill MJ, Henkelman RM, et al. Mediastinal lymph node metastases from bronchogenic carcinoma: detection with MR imaging and CT. Radiology 1987;162:651–656.

285. Heelan RT, Martini N, Westcott JW, et al. Carcinomatous involvement of the hilum and mediastinum: computed tomographic and magnetic resonance evaluation. Radiology 1985;156: 111–115.

286. Duhaylongsod FG, Lowe VJ, Patz EF Jr, et al. Lung tumor growth correlates with glucose metabolism measured by fluoride-18 fluorodeoxyglucose positron emission tomography. Ann Thorac Surg 1995;60:1348–1352.

287. Higashi K, Ueda Y, Yagishita M, et al. FDG PET measurement of the proliferative potential of non-small cell lung cancer. J Nucl Med 2000;41:85–92.

288. Goldsmith SJ, Kostakoglu L. Nuclear medicine imaging of lung cancer. Radiol Clin North Am 2000;38:511–524.

289. Chin R Jr, Ward R, Keyes JW, et al. Mediastinal staging of non-small-cell lung cancer with positron emission tomography. Am J Respir Crit Care Med 1995;152:2090–2096.

290. Patz EF Jr, Lowe VJ, Goodman PC, et al. Thoracic nodal staging with PET imaging with [18]FDG in patients with bronchogenic carcinoma. Chest 1995;108:1617–1621.

291. Sazon DA, Santiago SM, Soo Hoo GW, et al. Fluorodeoxyglucose-positron emission tomography in the detection and staging of lung cancer. Am J Respir Crit Care Med 1996;153:417–421.

292. Scott WJ, Gobar LS, Terry JD, et al. Mediastinal lymph node staging of non-small-cell lung cancer: a prospective comparison of computed tomography and positron emission tomography. J Thorac Cardiovasc Surg 1996;111:642–648.

293. Steinert HC, Hauser M, Allemann F, et al. Non-small cell lung cancer: nodal staging with FDG PET versus CT with correlative lymph node mapping and sampling. Radiology 1997;202:441–446.

294. Wahl RL, Quint LE, Greenough RL, et al. Staging of mediastinal non-small cell lung cancer with FDG PET, CT, and fusion images: preliminary prospective evaluation. Radiology 1994;191: 371–377.

295. Guhlmann A, Storck M, Kotzerke J, et al. Lymph node staging in non-small cell lung cancer: evaluation by [18F]FDG positron emission tomography (PET). Thorax 1997;52:438–441.

296. Vansteenkiste JF, Stroobants SG, De Leyn PR, et al. Lymph node staging in non-small-cell lung cancer with FDG-PET scan: a prospective study on 690 lymph node stations from 68

patients. J Clin Oncol 1998;16: 2142–2149.

297. Vansteenkiste JF, Stroobants SG, De Leyn PR, et al. Mediastinal lymph node staging with FDG-PET scan in patients with potentially operable non-small cell lung cancer: a prospective analysis of 50 cases. Leuven Lung Cancer Group. Chest 1997;112: 1480–1486.

298. Saunders CA, Dussek JE, O'Doherty MJ, et al. Evaluation of fluorine-18-fluorodeoxyglucose whole body positron emission tomography imaging in the staging of lung cancer. Ann Thorac Surg 1999;67:790–797.

299. Marom EM, McAdams HP, Erasmus JJ, et al. Staging non-small cell lung cancer with whole-body PET. Radiology 1999;212:803–809.

300. Bury T, Dowlati A, Paulus P, et al. Whole-body 18FDG positron emission tomography in the staging of non-small cell lung cancer. Eur Respir J 1997;10:2529–2534.

301. Kim S, Park CH, Han M, et al. The clinical usefulness of F-18 FDG coincidence PET without attenuation correction and without whole-body scanning mode in pulmonary lesions comparison with CT, MRI, and clinical findings. Clin Nucl Med 1999;24: 945–949.

302. Shon IH, O'Doherty MJ, Maisey MN. Positron emission tomography in lung cancer. Semin Nucl Med 2002;32: 240–271.

303. Pieterman RM, van Putten JW, Meuzelaar JJ, et al. Preoperative staging of non-small-cell lung cancer with positron-emission tomography. N Engl J Med 2000;343:254–261.

304. Toloza EM, Harpole L, McCrory DC. Noninvasive staging of non-small cell lung cancer: a review of the current evidence. Chest 2003;123:137S–146S.

305. Graeber G, Gupta N, Murray G. Positron emission tomographic imaging with fluorodeoxyglucose is efficacious in evaluating malignant pulmonary disease. J Thorac Cardiovasc Surg 1999;117:719–727.

306. Albes JM, Dohmen BM, Schott U, et al. Value of positron emission tomography for lung cancer staging. Eur J Surg Oncol 2002;28:55–62.

307. van Tinteren H, Hoekstra OS, Smit EF, et al. Effectiveness of positron emission tomography in the preoperative assessment of patients with suspected non-small-cell lung cancer: the PLUS multicentre randomised trial. Lancet 2002;359:1388–1393.

308. Seltzer MA, Yap CS, Silverman DH, et al. The impact of PET on the management of lung cancer: the referring physician's perspective. J Nucl Med 2002;43:752–756.

309. Roberts PF, Follette DM, von Haag D, et al. Factors associated with false-positive staging of lung cancer by positron emission tomography. Ann Thorac Surg 2000;70:1154–1159.

310. Dwamena BA, Sonnad SS, Angobaldo JO, et al. Metastases from non-small cell lung cancer: mediastinal staging in the 1990s – meta-analytic comparison of PET and CT. Radiology 1999;213:530–536.

311. Tatsumi M, Yutani K, Watanabe Y, et al. Feasibility of fluorodeoxyglucose dual-head gamma camera coincidence imaging in the evaluation of lung cancer: comparison with FDG PET. J Nucl Med 1999;40:566–573.

312. Shreve PD, Steventon RS, Deters EC, et al. Oncologic diagnosis with 2-[fluorine-18]fluoro-2-deoxy-D-glucose imaging: dual-head coincidence gamma camera versus positron emission tomographic scanner. Radiology 1998;207:431–437.

313. Aquino SL, Asmuth JC, Alpert NM, et al. Improved radiologic staging of lung cancer with 2-[18F]-fluoro-2-deoxy-D-glucose-positron emission tomography and computed tomography registration. J Comput Assist Tomogr 2003;27:479–484.

314. D'Amico TA, Wong TZ, Harpole DH, et al. Impact of computed tomography-positron emission tomography fusion in staging patients with thoracic malignancies. Ann Thorac Surg 2002;74:160–163.

315. Vansteenkiste JF, Stroobants SG, Dupont PJ, et al. FDG-PET scan in potentially operable non-small cell lung cancer: do anatometabolic PET-CT fusion images improve the localisation of regional lymph node metastases? The Leuven Lung Cancer Group. Eur J Nucl Med 1998;25:1495–1501.

316. Kernstine KH, McLaughlin KA, Menda Y, et al. Can FDG-PET reduce the need for mediastinoscopy in potentially resectable nonsmall cell lung cancer? Ann Thorac Surg 2002;73:394–401.

317. Graeter TP, Hellwig D, Hoffmann K, et al. Mediastinal lymph node staging in suspected lung cancer: comparison of positron emission tomography with F-18-fluorodeoxyglucose and mediastinoscopy. Ann Thorac Surg 2003;75:231–235.

318. Erasmus JJ, McAdams HP, Patz EF, Jr. Non-small cell lung cancer: FDG-PET imaging. J Thorac Imaging 1999;14:247–256.

319. Farrell MA, McAdams HP, Herndon JE, et al. Non-small cell lung cancer: FDG PET for nodal staging in patients with stage I disease. Radiology 2000;215:886–890.

320. Gambhir SS, Hoh CK, Phelps ME, et al. Decision tree sensitivity analysis for cost-effectiveness of FDG-PET in the staging and management of non-small-cell lung carcinoma. J Nucl Med 1996;37:1428–1436.

321. Scott WJ, Shepherd J, Gambhir SS. Cost-effectiveness of FDG-PET for staging non-small cell lung cancer: a decision analysis. Ann Thorac Surg 1998;66:1876–1883.

322. Yasukawa T, Yoshikawa K, Aoyagi H, et al. Usefulness of PET with 11C-methionine for the detection of hilar and mediastinal lymph node metastasis in lung cancer. J Nucl Med 2000;41:283–290.

323. Nettelbladt OS, Sundin AE, Valind SO, et al. Combined fluorine-18-FDG and carbon-11-methionine PET for diagnosis of tumors in lung and mediastinum. J Nucl Med 1998;39:640–647.

324. Hara T, Inagaki K, Kosaka N, et al. Sensitive detection of mediastinal lymph node metastasis of lung cancer with 11C-choline PET. J Nucl Med 2000;41:1507–1513.

325. Rasey JS, Grierson JR, Wiens LW, et al. Validation of FLT uptake as a measure of thymidine kinase-1 activity in A549 carcinoma cells. J Nucl Med 2002;43:1210–1217.

326. McKenna RJ Jr, Haynie TP, Libshitz HI, et al. Critical evaluation of the gallium-67 scan for surgical patients with lung cancer. Chest 1985;87:428–431.

327. Bekerman C, Caride VJ, Hoffer PB, et al. Noninvasive staging of lung cancer. Indications and limitations of gallium-67 citrate imaging. Radiol Clin North Am 1990;28:497–510.

328. Santiago S, Houston D, Ezer J, et al. Gallium scanning and tomography in the preoperative evaluation of lung cancer. Cancer 1986;58:341–343.

329. Chiti A, Maffioli LS, Infante M, et al. Assessment of mediastinal involvement in lung cancer with technetium-99m-sestamibi SPECT. J Nucl Med 1996;37:938–942.

330. Yokoi K, Okuyama A, Mori K, et al. Mediastinal lymph node metastasis from lung cancer: evaluation with Tl-201 SPECT – comparison with CT. Radiology 1994;192:813–817.

331. Wang H, Maurea S, Mainolfi C, et al. Tc-99m MIBI scintigraphy in patients with lung cancer. Comparison with CT and fluorine-18 FDG PET imaging. Clin Nucl Med 1997;22:243–249.

332. Higashi K, Nishikawa T, Seki H, et al. Comparison of fluorine-18-FDG PET and thallium-201 SPECT in evaluation of lung cancer. J Nucl Med 1998;39:9–15.

333. Machac J, Krynyckyi B, Kim C. Peptide and antibody imaging in lung cancer. Semin Nucl Med 2002;32:276–292.

334. Rusch V, Macapinlac H, Heelan R, et al. NR-LU-10 monoclonal antibody scanning. A helpful new adjunct to computed tomography in evaluating non-small-cell lung cancer. J Thorac Cardiovasc Surg 1993;106:200–204.

335. Buccheri G, Biggi A, Ferrigno D, et al. Anti-CEA immunoscintigraphy and computed tomographic scanning in the preoperative evaluation of mediastinal lymph nodes in lung cancer. Thorax 1996;51:359–363.

336. Kairemo KJ, Aronen HJ, Liewendahl K, et al. Radioimmunoimaging of non-small cell lung cancer with 111In- and 99mTc-labeled monoclonal anti-CEA-antibodies. Acta Oncol 1993;32:771–778.

337. Vuillez JP, Moro D, Brichon PY, et al. Two-step immunoscintigraphy for non-small-cell lung cancer staging using a bispecific anti-CEA/anti-indium-DTPA antibody and an indium-111-labeled DTPA dimer. J Nucl Med 1997;38:507–511.

338. Wallace MB, Silvestri GA, Sahai AV, et al. Endoscopic ultrasound-guided fine needle aspiration for staging patients with carcinoma of the lung. Ann Thorac Surg 2001;72:1861–1867.

339. Fritscher-Ravens A, Bohuslavizki KH, Brandt L, et al. Mediastinal lymph node involvement in potentially resectable lung cancer: comparison of CT, positron emission tomography, and endoscopic ultrasonography with and without fine-needle aspiration. Chest 2003;123:442–451.

340. Silvestri GA, Hoffman B, Reed CE. One from column A: choosing between CT, positron emission tomography, endoscopic ultrasound with fine-needle aspiration, transbronchial needle aspiration, thoracoscopy, mediastinoscopy, and mediastinotomy for staging lung cancer. Chest 2003;123:333–335.

341. Marom EM, Patz EF Jr, Swensen SJ. Radiologic findings of bronchogenic carcinoma with pulmonary metastases at presentation. Clin Radiol 1999;54:665–668.

342. Okumura T, Asamura H, Suzuki K, et al. Intrapulmonary metastasis of non-small cell lung cancer: A prognostic assessment. J Thorac Cardiovasc Surg 2001;122:24–28.

343. Keogan MT, Tung KT, Kaplan DK, et al. The significance of pulmonary nodules detected on CT staging for lung cancer. Clin Radiol 1993;48:94–96.

344. Kim YH, Lee KS, Primack SL, et al. Small pulmonary nodules on CT accompanying surgically resectable lung cancer: likelihood of malignancy. J Thorac Imaging 2002;17:40–46.

345. Yuan Y, Matsumoto T, Hiyama A, et al. The probability of malignancy in small

pulmonary nodules coexisting with potentially operable lung cancer detected by CT. Eur Radiol 2003;13: 2447–2453.

346. Spencer H. Pathology of the lung, 4th edn. Philadelphia: WB Saunders, 1985.

347. Manac'h D, Riquet M, Medioni J, et al. Visceral pleura invasion by non-small cell lung cancer: an underrated bad prognostic factor. Ann Thorac Surg 2001;71:1088–1093.

348. Okada M, Tsubota N, Yoshimura M, et al. How should interlobar pleural invasion be classified? Prognosis of resected T3 non-small cell lung cancer. Ann Thorac Surg 1999;68:2049–2052.

349. Chernow B, Sahn SA. Carcinomatous involvement of the pleura: an analysis of 96 patients. Am J Med 1977;63: 695–702.

350. Sahn SA. Malignant pleural effusions. Clin Chest Med 1985;6:113–125.

351. Sahn SA. Pleural effusion in lung cancer. Clin Chest Med 1993;14: 189–200.

352. Decker DA, Dines DE, Payne WS, et al. The significance of a cytologically negative pleural effusion in bronchogenic carcinoma. Chest 1978;74:640–642.

353. Frola C, Cantoni S, Turtulici I, et al. Transudative vs exudative pleural effusions: differentiation using Gd-DTPA-enhanced MRI. Eur Radiol 1997;7:860–864.

354. Erasmus JJ, McAdams HP, Rossi SE, et al. FDG PET of pleural effusions in patients with non-small cell lung cancer. AJR Am J Roentgenol 2000;175:245–249.

355. Bury T, Paulus P, Dowlati A, et al. Evaluation of pleural diseases with FDG-PET imaging: preliminary report. Thorax 1997;52:187–189.

356. Gorg C, Restrepo I, Schwerk WB. Sonography of malignant pleural effusion. Eur Radiol 1997;7: 1195–1198.

357. Woodring JH, Stelling CB. Adenocarcinoma of the lung: a tumor with a changing pleomorphic character. AJR Am J Roentgenol 1983;140:657–664.

358. Oka K, Otani S, Yoshimura T, et al. Mucin-negative pseudomesotheliomatous adenocarcinoma of the lung: report of three cases. Acta Oncol 1999;38:1119–1121.

359. De Leyn P, Vansteenkiste J, Cuypers P, et al. Role of cervical mediastinoscopy in staging of non-small cell lung cancer without enlarged mediastinal lymph nodes on CT scan. Eur J Cardiothorac Surg 1997;12:706–712.

360. Hammoud Z, Anderson R, Meyers B, et al. The current role of mediastinoscopy in the evaluation of

thoracic disease. J Thorac Cardiovasc Surg 1999;118:894–899.

361. Canadian Lung Oncology Group. Investigation for mediastinal disease in patients with apparently operable lung cancer. Ann Thorac Surg 1995;60: 1382–1389.

362. Muers MF. Preoperative screening for metastases in lung cancer. Thorax 1994;49:1–2.

363. The Canadian Lung Oncology Group. Investigating extrathoracic metastatic disease in patients with apparently operable lung cancer. The Canadian Lung Oncology Group. Ann Thorac Surg 2001;71:425–434.

364. Tanaka K, Kubota K, Kodama T, et al. Extrathoracic staging is not necessary for non-small-cell lung cancer with clinical stage T1-2 N0. Ann Thorac Surg 1999;68:1039–1042.

365. Weder W, Schmid RA, Bruchhaus H, et al. Detection of extrathoracic metastases by positron emission tomography in lung cancer. Ann Thorac Surg 1998;66:886–892.

366. Vesselle H, Pugsley J, Vallieres E, et al. The impact of fluorodeoxyglucose F 18 positron-emission tomography on the surgical staging of non-small cell lung cancer. J Thorac Cardiovasc Surg 2002;124:511–519.

367. Weng E, Tran L, Rege S, et al. Accuracy and clinical impact of mediastinal lymph node staging with FDG-PET imaging in potentially resectable lung cancer. Am J Clin Oncol 2000;23:47–52.

368. Kalff V, Hicks RJ, MacManus MP, et al. Clinical impact of (18)F fluorodeoxyglucose positron emission tomography in patients with non-small-cell lung cancer: a prospective study. J Clin Oncol 2001;19:111–118.

369. van Tinteren H, Hoekstra OS, Smit EF, et al. Effectiveness of positron emission tomography in the preoperative assessment of patients with suspected non-small-cell lung cancer: the PLUS multicentre randomised trial. Lancet 2002;359:1388–1393.

370. Pope RJ, Hansell DM. Extra-thoracic staging of lung cancer. Eur J Radiol 2003;45:31–38.

371. Valk PE, Pounds TR, Hopkins DM, et al. Staging non-small cell lung cancer by whole-body positron emission tomographic imaging. Ann Thorac Surg 1995;60: 1573–1581.

372. MacManus MP, Hicks RJ, Matthews JP, et al. High rate of detection of unsuspected distant metastases by pet in apparent stage III non-small-cell lung cancer: implications for radical radiation therapy. Int J Radiat Oncol Biol Phys 2001;50:287–293.

373. Larcos G, Maisey MN. FDG-PET screening for cerebral metastases in

patients with suspected malignancy. Nucl Med Commun 1996;17:197–198.

374. Salvatierra A, Baamonde C, Llamas JM, et al. Extrathoracic staging of bronchogenic carcinoma. Chest 1990;97:1052–1058.

375. Charnley RM, Morris DL, Dennison AR, et al. Detection of colorectal liver metastases using intraoperative ultrasonography. Br J Surg 1991;78: 45–48.

376. Leen E, Angerson WJ, Wotherspoon H, et al. Detection of colorectal liver metastases: comparison of laparotomy, CT, US, and Doppler perfusion index and evaluation of postoperative follow-up results. Radiology 1995; 195:113–116.

377. Hagspiel KD, Neidl KF, Eichenberger AC, et al. Detection of liver metastases: comparison of superparamagnetic iron oxide-enhanced and unenhanced MR imaging at 1.5 T with dynamic CT, intraoperative US, and percutaneous US. Radiology 1995;196:471–478.

378. Soyer P. Will ferumoxides-enhanced MR imaging replace CT during arterial portography in the detection of hepatic metastases? Prologue to a promising future. Radiology 1996; 200:610–611.

379. Oliver TW Jr, Bernardino ME, Miller JI, et al. Isolated adrenal masses in nonsmall-cell bronchogenic carcinoma. Radiology 1984;153:217–218.

380. Glazer HS, Weyman PJ, Sagel SS, et al. Nonfunctioning adrenal masses: incidental discovery on computed tomography. AJR Am J Roentgenol 1982;139:81–85.

381. Gillams A, Roberts CM, Shaw P, et al. The value of CT scanning and percutaneous fine needle aspiration of adrenal masses in biopsy-proven lung cancer. Clin Radiol 1992;46:18–22.

382. Sze G, Shin J, Krol G, et al. Intraparenchymal brain metastases: MR imaging versus contrast-enhanced CT. Radiology 1988;168:187–194.

383. Yokoi K, Kamiya N, Matsuguma H, et al. Detection of brain metastasis in potentially operable non-small cell lung cancer: a comparison of CT and MRI. Chest 1999;115:714–719.

384. Newman SJ, Hansen HH. Proceedings: Frequency, diagnosis, and treatment of brain metastases in 247 consecutive patients with bronchogenic carcinoma. Cancer 1974;33:492–496.

385. Hillers TK, Sauve MD, Guyatt GH. Analysis of published studies on the detection of extrathoracic metastases in patients presumed to have operable non-small cell lung cancer. Thorax 1994;49:14–19.

386. Napoli LD, Hansen HH, Muggia FM, et al. The incidence of osseous involvement in lung cancer, with

special reference to the development of osteoblastic changes. Radiology 1973;108:17–21.

387. Donato AT, Ammerman EG, Sullesta O. Bone scanning in the evaluation of patients with lung cancer. Ann Thorac Surg 1979;27:300–304.

388. Ichinose Y, Hara N, Ohta M, et al. Preoperative examination to detect distant metastasis is not advocated for asymptomatic patients with stages 1 and 2 non-small cell lung cancer. Preoperative examination for lung cancer. Chest 1989;96:1104–1109.

389. Michel F, Soler M, Imhof E, et al. Initial staging of non-small cell lung cancer: value of routine radioisotope bone scanning. Thorax 1991;46:469–473.

390. Sider L. Radiographic manifestations of primary bronchogenic carcinoma. Radiol Clin North Am 1990;28:583–597.

391. Schraufnagel D, Peloquin A, Pare JA, et al. Differentiating bronchioloalveolar carcinoma from adenocarcinoma. Am Rev Respir Dis 1982;125:74–79.

392. Jung KJ, Lee KS, Han J, et al. Large cell neuroendocrine carcinoma of the lung: clinical, CT, and pathologic findings in 11 patients. J Thorac Imaging 2001;16:156–162.

393. Shin AR, Shin BK, Choi JA, et al. Large cell neuroendocrine carcinoma of the lung: radiologic and pathologic findings. J Comput Assist Tomogr 2000;24:567–573.

394. Ooi C, Ho M, Khong L, et al. Computed tomography characteristics of advanced primary pulmonary lymphoepithelioma-like carcinoma. Eur Radiol 2003;13:522–526.

395. Mirtcheva RM, Vazquez M, Yankelevitz DF, et al. Bronchioloalveolar carcinoma and adenocarcinoma with bronchioloalveolar features presenting as ground-glass opacities on CT. Clin Imaging 2002;26:95–100.

396. Greco RJ, Steiner RM, Goldman S, et al. Bronchoalveolar cell carcinoma of the lung. Ann Thorac Surg 1986;41:652–656.

397. Harpole DH, Bigelow C, Young WG, Jr., et al. Alveolar cell carcinoma of the lung: a retrospective analysis of 205 patients. Ann Thorac Surg 1988;46:502–507.

398. Hsu CP, Chen CY, Hsu NY. Bronchioloalveolar carcinoma. J Thorac Cardiovasc Surg 1995;110:374–381.

399. Shah RM, Balsara G, Webster M, et al. Bronchioloalveolar cell carcinoma: impact of histology on dominant CT pattern. J Thorac Imaging 2000;15:180–186.

400. Noguchi M, Morikawa A, Kawasaki M, et al. Small adenocarcinoma of the lung. Histologic characteristics and prognosis. Cancer 1995;75:2844–2852.

401. Okubo K, Mark E, Flieder D, et al. Bronchoalveolar carcinoma: Clinical, radiologic, and pathologic factors and survival. J Thorac Cardiovasc Surg 1999;118:702–709.

402. Daly RC, Trastek VF, Pairolero PC, et al. Bronchoalveolar carcinoma: factors affecting survival. Ann Thorac Surg 1991;51:368–376.

403. Epstein DM, Gefter WB, Miller WT. Lobar bronchioloalveolar cell carcinoma. AJR Am J Roentgenol 1982;139:463–468.

404. Lee KS, Kim Y, Han J, et al. Bronchioloalveolar carcinoma: clinical, histopathologic, and radiologic findings. Radiographics 1997;17:1345–1357.

405. Gaeta M, Barone M, Caruso R, et al. CT-pathologic correlation in nodular bronchioloalveolar carcinoma. J Comput Assist Tomogr 1994;18:229–232.

406. Kuhlman JE, Fishman EK, Kuhajda FP, et al. Solitary bronchioloalveolar carcinoma: CT criteria. Radiology 1988;167:379–382.

407. Bonomo L, Storto ML, Ciccotosto C, et al. Bronchioloalveolar carcinoma of the lung. Eur Radiol 1998;8:996–1001.

408. Adler B, Padley S, Miller RR, et al. High-resolution CT of bronchioloalveolar carcinoma. AJR Am J Roentgenol 1992;159:275–277.

409. Gaeta M, Caruso R, Blandino A, et al. Radiolucencies and cavitation in bronchioloalveolar carcinoma: CT-pathologic correlation. Eur Radiol 1999;9:55–59.

410. Mihara N, Ichikado K, Johkoh T, et al. The subtypes of localized bronchioloalveolar carcinoma: CT-pathologic correlation in 18 cases. AJR Am J Roentgenol 1999;173:75–79.

411. Jang HJ, Lee KS, Kwon OJ, et al. Bronchioloalveolar carcinoma: focal area of ground-glass attenuation at thin-section CT as an early sign. Radiology 1996;199:485–488.

412. Gaeta M, Caruso R, Barone M, et al. Ground-glass attenuation in nodular bronchioloalveolar carcinoma: CT patterns and prognostic value. J Comput Assist Tomogr 1998;22:215–219.

413. Weisbrod GL, Chamberlain D, Herman SJ. Cystic change (pseudocavitation) associated with bronchioloalveolar carcinoma: a report of four patients. J Thorac Imaging 1995;10:106–111.

414. Akira M, Atagi S, Kawahara M, et al. High-resolution CT findings of diffuse bronchioloalveolar carcinoma in 38 patients. AJR Am J Roentgenol 1999;173:1623–1629.

415. Kobayashi T, Satoh K, Sasaki M, et al. Bronchioloalveolar carcinoma with widespread ground-glass shadow on CT in two cases. J Comput Assist Tomogr 1997;21:133–135.

416. Schulze ES, Mattia AR, Chew FS. Bronchioloalveolar carcinoma. AJR Am J Roentgenol 1994;162:1294.

417. Kim BT, Kim Y, Lee KS, et al. Localized form of bronchioloalveolar carcinoma: FDG PET findings. AJR Am J Roentgenol 1998;170:935–939.

418. Tan RT, Kuzo RS. High-resolution CT findings of mucinous bronchioloalveolar carcinoma: a case of pseudopulmonary alveolar proteinosis. AJR Am J Roentgenol 1997;168:99–100.

419. Huang D, Weisbrod GL, Chamberlain DW. Unusual radiologic presentations of bronchioloalveolar carcinoma. Can Assoc Radiol J 1986;37:94–99.

420. Weisbrod GL, Towers MJ, Chamberlain DW, et al. Thin-walled cystic lesions in bronchioalveolar carcinoma. Radiology 1992;185:401–405.

421. Im JG, Choi BI, Park JH, et al. CT findings of lobar bronchioloalveolar carcinoma. J Comput Assist Tomogr 1986;10:320–322.

422. Aquino SL, Chiles C, Halford P. Distinction of consolidative bronchioloalveolar carcinoma from pneumonia: do CT criteria work? AJR Am J Roentgenol 1998;171:359–363.

423. Jung JI, Kim H, Park SH, et al. CT differentiation of pneumonic-type bronchoalveolar cell carcinoma and infectious pneumonia. Br J Radiol 2001;74:490–494.

424. Im JG, Han MC, Yu EJ, et al. Lobar bronchioloalveolar carcinoma: "angiogram sign" on CT scans. Radiology 1990;176:749–753.

425. Vincent JM, Ng YY, Norton AJ, et al. CT "angiogram sign" in primary pulmonary lymphoma. J Comput Assist Tomogr 1992;16:829–831.

426. Shah RM, Friedman AC. CT angiogram sign: incidence and significance in lobar consolidations evaluated by contrast-enhanced CT. AJR Am J Roentgenol 1998;170:719–721.

427. Metzger RA, Mulhern CB Jr, Arger PH, et al. CT differentiation of solitary from diffuse bronchioloalveolar carcinoma. J Comput Assist Tomogr 1981;5:830–833.

428. Gaeta M, Blandino A, Scribano E, et al. Magnetic resonance imaging of bronchioloalveolar carcinoma. J Thorac Imaging 2000;15:41–47.

429. Higashi K, Ueda Y, Seki H, et al. Fluorine-18-FDG PET imaging is negative in bronchioloalveolar lung carcinoma. J Nucl Med 1998;39:1016–1020.

430. Walsh GL, O'Connor M, Willis KM, et al. Is follow-up of lung cancer patients after resection medically indicated and cost-effective? Ann Thorac Surg 1995;60:1563–1570.

431. Younes RN, Gross JL, Deheinzelin D. Follow-up in lung cancer: how often and for what purpose? Chest 1999;115:1494–1499.

432. Downey RJ. Follow-up of patients with completely resected lung cancer. Chest 1999;115:1487–1488.

433. Gorich J, Beyer-Enke SA, Flentje M, et al. Evaluation of recurrent bronchogenic carcinoma by computed tomography. Clin Imaging 1990;14:131–137.

434. Bourgouin P, Cousineau G, Lemire P, et al. Differentiation of radiation-induced fibrosis from recurrent pulmonary neoplasm by CT. Can Assoc Radiol J 1987;38:23–26.

435. Libshitz HI, Sheppard DG. Filling in of radiation therapy-induced bronchiectatic change: a reliable sign of locally recurrent lung cancer. Radiology 1999;210:25–27.

436. Lever AM, Henderson D, Ellis DA, et al. Radiation fibrosis mimicking local recurrence in small cell carcinoma of the bronchus. Br J Radiol 1984;57:178–180.

437. Glazer HS, Lee JK, Levitt RG, et al. Radiation fibrosis: differentiation from recurrent tumor by MR imaging. Radiology 1985;156:721–726.

438. Patz EF Jr, Lowe VJ, Hoffman JM, et al. Persistent or recurrent bronchogenic carcinoma: detection with PET and 2-[F-18]-2-deoxy-D-glucose. Radiology 1994;191:379–382.

439. Frank A, Lefkowitz D, Jaeger S, et al. Decision logic for retreatment of asymptomatic lung cancer recurrence based on positron emission tomography findings. Int J Radiat Oncol Biol Phys 1995;32:1495–1512.

440. Hicks RJ, Kalff V, MacManus MP, et al. The utility of (18)F-FDG PET for suspected recurrent non-small cell lung cancer after potentially curative therapy: impact on management and prognostic stratification. J Nucl Med 2001;42:1605–1613.

441. Inoue T, Kim EE, Komaki R, et al. Detecting recurrent or residual lung cancer with FDG-PET. J Nucl Med 1995;36:788–793.

442. Marom EM, Erasmus JJ, Patz EF. Lung cancer and positron emission tomography with fluorodeoxyglucose. Lung Cancer 2000;28:187–202.

443. Miller RR. Bronchioloalveolar cell adenomas. Am J Surg Pathol 1990;14:904–912.

444. Yokose T, Ito Y, Ochiai A. High prevalence of atypical adenomatous hyperplasia of the lung in autopsy specimens from elderly patients with malignant neoplasms. Lung Cancer 2000;29:125–130.

445. Yokose T, Doi M, Tanno K, et al. Atypical adenomatous hyperplasia of the lung in autopsy cases. Lung Cancer 2001;33:155–161.

446. Kushihashi T, Munechika H, Ri K, et al. Bronchioloalveolar adenoma of the lung: CT-pathologic correlation. Radiology 1994;193:789–793.

447. Chapman AD, Kerr KM. The association between atypical adenomatous hyperplasia and primary lung cancer. Br J Cancer 2000;83:632–636.

448. Kitamura H, Kameda Y, Ito T, et al. Atypical adenomatous hyperplasia of the lung. Implications for the pathogenesis of peripheral lung adenocarcinoma. Am J Clin Pathol 1999;111:610–622.

449. Vazquez MF, Flieder DB. Small peripheral glandular lesions detected by screening CT for lung cancer. A diagnostic dilemma for the pathologist. Radiol Clin North Am 2000;38:579–589.

450. Colby TV, Wistuba II, Gazdar A. Precursors to pulmonary neoplasia. Adv Anat Pathol 1998;5:205–215.

451. Mori M, Rao SK, Popper HH, et al. Atypical adenomatous hyperplasia of the lung: a probable forerunner in the development of adenocarcinoma of the lung. Med Pathol 2001;14:72–84.

452. Nakahara R, Yokose T, Nagai K, et al. Atypical adenomatous hyperplasia of the lung: a clinicopathological study of 118 cases including cases with multiple atypical adenomatous hyperplasia. Thorax 2001;56:302–305.

453. Ritter JH. Pulmonary atypical adenomatous hyperplasia. A histologic lesion in search of usable criteria and clinical significance. Am J Clin Pathol 1999;111:587–589.

454. Slebos RJ, Baas IO, Clement MJ, et al. p53 alterations in atypical alveolar hyperplasia of the human lung. Hum Pathol 1998;29:801–808.

455. Takashima S, Maruyama Y, Hasegawa M, et al. CT findings and progression of small peripheral lung neoplasms having a replacement growth pattern. AJR Am J Roentgenol 2003;180:817–826.

456. Greenberg AK, Yee H, Rom WN. Preneoplastic lesions of the lung. Respir Res 2002;3:20.

457. Kawakami S, Sone S, Takashima S, et al. Atypical adenomatous hyperplasia of the lung: correlation between high-resolution CT findings and histopathologic features. Eur Radiol 2001;11:811–814.

458. Logan PM, Miller RR, Evans K, et al. Bronchogenic carcinoma and coexistent bronchioloalveolar cell adenomas. Assessment of radiologic detection and follow-up in 28 patients. Chest 1996;109:713–717.

459. Jemal A, Thomas A, Murray T, et al. Cancer statistics, 2002. CA Cancer J Clin 2002;52:23–47.

460. Fry WA, Phillips JL, Menck HR. Ten-year survey of lung cancer treatment and survival in hospitals in the United States: a national cancer data base report. Cancer 1999;86:1867–1876.

461. Black WC, Welch HG. Screening for disease. AJR Am J Roentgenol 1997;168:3–11.

462. Huhti E, Saloheimo M, Sutinen S. The value of roentgenologic screening in lung cancer. Am Rev Respir Dis 1983;128:395–398.

463. Strauss GM. Measuring effectiveness of lung cancer screening: from consensus to controversy and back. Chest 1997;112:216S–228S.

464. Patz EF Jr, Goodman PC, Bepler G. Screening for lung cancer. N Engl J Med 2000;343:1627–1633.

465. Ellis JR, Gleeson FV. Lung cancer screening. Br J Radiol 2001;74:478–485.

466. Ellis SM, Husband JE, Armstrong P, et al. Computed tomography screening for lung cancer: back to basics. Clin Radiol 2001;56:691–699.

467. Hasegawa M, Sone S, Takashima S, et al. Growth rate of small lung cancers detected on mass CT screening. Br J Radiol 2000;73:1252–1259.

468. Winer-Muram HT, Jennings SG, Tarver RD, et al. Volumetric growth rate of stage I lung cancer prior to treatment: serial CT scanning. Radiology 2002;223:798–805.

469. Black WC. Overdiagnosis: An underrecognized cause of confusion and harm in cancer screening. J Natl Cancer Inst 2000;92:1280–1282.

470. Sone S, Li F, Yang ZG, et al. Results of three-year mass screening programme for lung cancer using mobile low-dose spiral computed tomography scanner. Br J Cancer 2001;84:25–32.

471. Henschke CI, McCauley DI, Yankelevitz DF, et al. Early Lung Cancer Action Project: overall design and findings from baseline screening. Lancet 1999;354:99–105.

472. Rozenshtein A, White CS, Austin JH, et al. Incidental lung carcinoma detected at CT in patients selected for lung volume reduction surgery to treat severe pulmonary emphysema. Radiology 1998;207:487–490.

473. Pigula FA, Keenan RJ, Ferson PF, et al. Unsuspected lung cancer found in work-up for lung reduction operation. Ann Thorac Surg 1996;61:174–176.

474. McKenna RJ Jr, Fischel RJ, Brenner M, et al. Combined operations for lung volume reduction surgery and lung cancer. Chest 1996;110:885–888.

475. Hazelrigg SR, Boley TM, Weber D, et al. Incidence of lung nodules found in patients undergoing lung volume reduction. Ann Thorac Surg 1997;64: 303–306.

476. McFarlane MJ, Feinstein AR, Wells CK. Clinical features of lung cancers discovered as a postmortem "surprise". Chest 1986;90:520–523.

477. Dammas S, Patz EF Jr, Goodman PC. Identification of small lung nodules at autopsy: implications for lung cancer screening and overdiagnosis bias. Lung Cancer 2001;33:11–16.

478. Patz EF Jr, Rossi S, Harpole DH Jr, et al. Correlation of tumor size and survival in patients with stage IA non-small cell lung cancer. Chest 2000;117:1568–1571.

479. Black WC. Unexpected observations on tumor size and survival in stage IA non-small cell lung cancer. Chest 2000;117:1532–1534.

480. Henschke CI, Wisnivesky JP, Yankelevitz DF, et al. Small stage I cancers of the lung: genuineness and curability. Lung Cancer 2003;39: 327–330.

481. Fontana RS, Sanderson DR, Taylor WF, et al. Early lung cancer detection: results of the initial (prevalence) radiologic and cytologic screening in the Mayo Clinic study. Am Rev Respir Dis 1984;130:561–565.

482. Fontana RS, Sanderson DR, Woolner LB, et al. Lung cancer screening: the Mayo program. J Occup Med 1986;28:746–750.

483. Marcus PM, Bergstralh EJ, Fagerstrom RM, et al. Lung cancer mortality in the Mayo Lung Project: impact of extended follow-up. J Natl Cancer Inst 2000;92: 1308–1316.

484. Kubik AK, Parkin DM, Zatloukal P. Czech Study on Lung Cancer Screening: post-trial follow-up of lung cancer deaths up to year 15 since enrollment. Cancer 2000;89:2363–2368.

485. Nash FA, Morgan JM, Tomkins JG. South London Lung Cancer Study. Br Med J 1968;2:715–721.

486. Kaneko M, Eguchi K, Ohmatsu H, et al. Peripheral lung cancer: screening and detection with low-dose spiral CT versus radiography. Radiology 1996;201:798–802.

487. Hutchinson E. Caution over use of lung-cancer screening as standard practice. Lancet 2000;356:742.

488. Flehinger BJ, Kimmel M, Melamed MR. The effect of surgical treatment on survival from early lung cancer. Implications for screening. Chest 1992;101:1013–1018.

489. Brett GZ. The value of lung cancer detection by six-monthly chest radiographs. Thorax 1968;23:414–420.

490. Wilde J. A 10 year follow-up of semi-annual screening for early detection of lung cancer in the Erfurt County, GDR. Eur Respir J 1989;2:656–662.

491. Lilienfield A, Archer PG, Burnett CH, et al. An evaluation of radiologic and cytologic screening for the early detection of lung cancer: a cooperative pilot study of the American Cancer Society and the Veterans Administration. Cancer Res 1966;26:2083–2121.

492. Sanderson DR. Lung cancer screening. The Mayo Study. Chest 1986;89 (Suppl):324S.

493. Tockman MS. Survival and mortality from lung cancer in a screened population. The John Hopkins Study. Chest 1986;89(Suppl): 324S–325S.

494. Flehinger BJ, Melamed MR, Zaman MB, et al. Early lung cancer detection: results of the initial (prevalence) radiologic and cytologic screening in the Memorial Sloan-Kettering study. Am Rev Respir Dis 1984;130:555–560.

495. Frost JK, Ball WC Jr, Levin ML, et al. Early lung cancer detection: results of the initial (prevalence) radiologic and cytologic screening in the Johns Hopkins study. Am Rev Respir Dis 1984;130:549–554.

496. Heelan RT, Flehinger BJ, Melamed MR, et al. Non-small-cell lung cancer: results of the New York screening program. Radiology 1984;151:289–293.

497. Fontana RS, Sanderson DR, Woolner LB, et al. Screening for lung cancer. A critique of the Mayo Lung Project. Cancer 1991;67:1155–1164.

498. Eddy DM. Screening for lung cancer. Ann Intern Med 1989;111:232–237.

499. Melamed MR, Flehinger BJ, Zaman MB, et al. Screening for early lung cancer. Results of the Memorial Sloan-Kettering study in New York. Chest 1984;86:44–53.

500. Miettinen OS. Screening for lung cancer. Radiol Clin North Am 2000;38:479–486.

501. Henschke CI, Yankelevitz DF. CT screening for lung cancer. Radiol Clin North Am 2000;38:487–495.

502. Rubin SA. Lung cancer: past, present, and future. J Thorac Imaging 1991;7:1–8.

503. Prorok PC, Andriole GL, Bresalier RS, et al. Design of the Prostate, Lung, Colorectal and Ovarian (PLCO) Cancer Screening Trial. Control Clin Trials 2000;21:273S–309S.

504. Henschke CI, Naidich DP, Yankelevitz DF, et al. Early lung cancer action project: initial findings on repeat screenings. Cancer 2001;92:153–159.

505. Kaneko M, Kusumoto M, Kobayashi T, et al. Computed tomography screening for lung carcinoma in Japan. Cancer 2000;89:2485–2488.

506. Diederich S, Wormanns D, Semik M, et al. Screening for early lung cancer with low-dose spiral CT: prevalence in 817 asymptomatic smokers. Radiology 2002;222:773–781.

507. Swensen SJ, Jett JR, Hartman TE, et al. Lung cancer screening with CT: Mayo Clinic experience. Radiology 2003; 226:756–761.

508. Diederich S, Thomas M, Semik M, et al. Screening for early lung cancer with low-dose spiral computed tomography: results of annual follow-up examinations in asymptomatic smokers. Eur Radiol 2004;14:691–702.

509. Pastorini U, Bellomi M, Landoni C, De Fiori E et al. Early lung-cancer detection with spiral CT and positron emission tomography in heavy smokers: 2-year results. Lancet 2003;362:588–589.

510. Sone S, Li F, Yang ZG, et al. Characteristics of small lung cancers invisible on conventional chest radiography and detected by population based screening using spiral CT. Br J Radiol 2000;73:137–145.

511. Yang ZG, Sone S, Li F, et al. Visibility of small peripheral lung cancers on chest radiographs: influence of densitometric parameters, CT values and tumour type. Br J Radiol 2001;74:32–41.

512. Swensen SJ, Jett JR, Sloan JA, et al. Screening for lung cancer with low-dose spiral computed tomography. Am J Respir Crit Care Med 2002;165:508–513.

513. Henschke CI, Yankelevitz DF, Mirtcheva R, et al. CT screening for lung cancer: frequency and significance of part-solid and nonsolid nodules. AJR Am J Roentgenol 2002;178:1053–1057.

514. Yang ZG, Sone S, Takashima S, et al. Small peripheral carcinomas of the lung: thin-section CT and pathologic correlation. Eur Radiol 1999;9: 1819–1825.

515. Kodama K, Higashiyama M, Yokouchi H, et al. Natural history of pure ground-glass opacity after long-term follow-up of more than 2 years. Ann Thorac Surg 2002;73:386–392.

516. Suzuki K, Asamura H, Kusumoto M, et al. "Early" peripheral lung cancer: prognostic significance of ground glass opacity on thin-section computed tomographic scan. Ann Thorac Surg 2002;74:1635–1639.

517. Wang JC, Sone S, Feng L, et al. Rapidly growing small peripheral lung cancers detected by screening CT: correlation between radiological appearance and pathological features. Br J Radiol 2000;73:930–937.

518. Yang ZG, Sone S, Takashima S, et al. High-resolution CT analysis of small peripheral lung adenocarcinomas revealed on screening helical CT. AJR Am J Roentgenol 2001;176:1399–1407.

519. Ginsberg RJ. The solitary pulmonary nodule: can we afford to watch and wait? J Thorac Cardiovasc Surg 2003;125:25–26.

520. Quarterman RL, McMillan A, Ratcliffe MB, et al. Effect of preoperative delay on prognosis for patients with early stage non-small cell lung cancer. J Thorac Cardiovasc Surg 2003;125:108–113.

521. Yankelevitz DF, Henschke CI. Small solitary pulmonary nodules. Radiol Clin North Am 2000;38:471–478.

522. Aberle DR, Gamsu G, Henschke CI, et al. A consensus statement of the Society of Thoracic Radiology: screening for lung cancer with helical computed tomography. J Thorac Imaging 2001;16:65–68.

523. Yankelevitz DF, Henschke CI. Does 2-year stability imply that pulmonary nodules are benign? AJR Am J Roentgenol 1997;168:325–328.

524. Marom EM, Sarvis S, Herndon JE, et al. T1 lung cancers: sensitivity of diagnosis with fluorodeoxyglucose PET. Radiology 2002;223:453–459.

525. Zhao B, Yankelevitz D, Reeves A, et al. Two-dimensional multi-criterion segmentation of pulmonary nodules on helical CT images. Med Phys 1999;26:889–895.

526. Yankelevitz DF, Gupta R, Zhao B, et al. Small pulmonary nodules: evaluation with repeat CT – preliminary experience. Radiology 1999;212:561–566.

527. Yankelevitz DF, Reeves AP, Kostis WJ, et al. Small pulmonary nodules: volumetrically determined growth rates based on CT evaluation. Radiology 2000;217:251–256.

528. Wormanns D, Diederich S, Lentschig MG, et al. Spiral CT of pulmonary nodules: interobserver variation in assessment of lesion size. Eur Radiol 2000;10:710–713.

529. Armato SG, III, Giger ML, Moran CJ, et al. Computerized detection of pulmonary nodules on CT scans. Radiographics 1999;19:1303–1311.

530. Tillich M, Kammerhuber F, Reittner P, et al. Detection of pulmonary nodules with helical CT: comparison of cine and film-based viewing. AJR Am J Roentgenol 1997;169:1611–1614.

531. MacMahon H, Engelmann R, Behlen FM, et al. Computer-aided diagnosis of pulmonary nodules: results of a large-scale observer test. Radiology 1999;213:723–726.

532. Armato SG, III, Giger ML, MacMahon H. Automated detection of lung nodules in CT scans: preliminary results. Med Phys 2001;28:1552–1561.

533. Ko JP, Betke M. Chest CT: automated nodule detection and assessment of change over time – preliminary experience. Radiology 2001;218:267–273.

534. Wormanns D, Fiebich M, Saidi M, et al. Automatic detection of pulmonary nodules at spiral CT: clinical application of a computer-aided diagnosis system. Eur Radiol 2002;12:1052–1057.

535. Reeves AP, Kostis WJ. Computer-aided diagnosis for lung cancer. Radiol Clin North Am 2000;38:497–509.

536. Armato SG, III, Li F, Giger ML, et al. Lung cancer: performance of automated lung nodule detection applied to cancers missed in a CT screening program. Radiology 2002;225:685–692.

537. Brown MS, Goldin JG, Suh RD, et al. Lung micronodules: automated method for detection at thin-section CT – initial experience. Radiology 2003;226:256–262.

538. Ko JP, Naidich DP. Lung nodule detection and characterization with multislice CT. Radiol Clin North Am 2003;41:575–597, vi.

539. Oguchi K, Sone S, Kiyono K, et al. Optimal tube current for lung cancer screening with low-dose spiral CT. Acta Radiol 2000;41:352–356.

540. Rusinek H, Naidich DP, McGuinness G, et al. Pulmonary nodule detection: low-dose versus conventional CT. Radiology 1998;209:243–249.

541. Itoh S, Ikeda M, Arahata S, et al. Lung cancer screening: minimum tube current required for helical CT. Radiology 2000;215:175–183.

542. Itoh S, Koyama S, Ikeda M, et al. Further reduction of radiation dose in helical CT for lung cancer screening using small tube current and a newly designed filter. J Thorac Imaging 2001;16:81–88.

543. Patz EF Jr, Black WC, Goodman PC. CT screening for lung cancer: not ready for routine practice. Radiology 2001;221:587–591.

544. Miettinen OS, Henschke CI. CT screening for lung cancer: coping with nihilistic recommendations. Radiology 2001;221:592–596.

545. Smith IE. Screening for lung cancer: time to think positive. Lancet 1999;354:86–87.

546. Heffner JE, Silvestri G. CT screening for lung cancer: is smaller better? Am J Respir Crit Care Med 2002;165:433–434.

547. Jett JR. Spiral computed tomography screening for lung cancer is ready for prime time. Am J Respir Crit Care Med 2001;163:812–815.

548. Patz EF Jr, Goodman PC. Low-dose spiral computed tomography screening for lung cancer: not ready for prime time. Am J Respir Crit Care Med 2001;163:813–814.

549. Bach PB, Niewoehner DE, Black WC. Screening for lung cancer: the guidelines. Chest 2003;123:83S–88S.

550. Chirikos TN, Hazelton T, Tockman M, et al. Screening for lung cancer with CT: a preliminary cost-effectiveness analysis. Chest 2002;121:1507–1514.

551. Marshall D, Simpson KN, Earle CC, et al. Economic decision analysis model of screening for lung cancer. Eur J Cancer 2001;37:1759–1767.

552. Marshall D, Simpson KN, Earle CC, et al. Potential cost-effectiveness of one-time screening for lung cancer (LC) in a high risk cohort. Lung Cancer 2001;32:227–236.

553. Wisnivesky JP, Braz-Parente D, Smith JP, et al. Cost-effectiveness evaluation of low-dose computed tomography screening for non-small cell lung cancer. Radiology 2000;217(Suppl):244.

554. Wisnivesky JP, Mushlin AI, Sicherman N, et al. The cost-effectiveness of low-dose CT screening for lung cancer: preliminary results of baseline screening. Chest 2003;124:614–621.

555. Austin JH, Romney BM, Goldsmith LS. Missed bronchogenic carcinoma: radiographic findings in 27 patients with a potentially resectable lesion evident in retrospect. Radiology 1992;182:115–122.

556. Hayabuchi N, Russell WJ, Murakami J. Problems in radiographic detection and diagnosis of lung cancer. Acta Radiol 1989;30:163–167.

557. Shah PK, Austin JH, White CS, et al. Missed non-small cell lung cancer: radiographic findings of potentially resectable lesions evident only in retrospect. Radiology 2003;226:235–241.

558. Quekel LG, Kessels AG, Goei R, et al. Miss rate of lung cancer on the chest radiograph in clinical practice. Chest 1999;115:720–724.

559. Tsubamoto M, Kuriyama K, Kido S, et al. Detection of lung cancer on chest radiographs: analysis on the basis of size and extent of ground-glass opacity at thin-section CT. Radiology 2002;224:139–144.

560. Davis SD. Through the "retrospectoscope": a glimpse of missed lung cancer at CT. Radiology 1996;199:23–24.

561. Gurney JW. Missed lung cancer at CT: imaging findings in nine patients. Radiology 1996;199:117–122.

562. White CS, Romney BM, Mason AC, et al. Primary carcinoma of the lung overlooked at CT: analysis of findings in 14 patients. Radiology 1996;199:109–115.

563. Li F, Sone S, Abe H, et al. Lung cancers missed at low-dose helical CT screening in a general population:

comparison of clinical, histopathologic, and imaging findings. Radiology 2002;225:673–683.

564. Potchen EJ, Bisesi MA. When is it malpractice to miss lung cancer on chest radiographs? Radiology 1990;175:29–32.

565. Woodring JH. Pitfalls in the radiologic diagnosis of lung cancer. AJR Am J Roentgenol 1990;154:1165–1175.

566. Oestmann JW, Greene R, Kushner DC, et al. Lung lesions: correlation between viewing time and detection. Radiology 1988;166:451–453.

567. Kundel HL, Nodine CF, Carmody D. Visual scanning, pattern recognition and decision-making in pulmonary nodule detection. Invest Radiol 1978;13:175–181.

568. Oestmann JW, Greene R, Bourgouin PM, et al. Chest "gestalt" and detectability of lung lesions. Eur J Radiol 1993;16:154–157.

569. Vincent JM, Armstrong P. Detection and diagnosis of the primary tumor in lung cancer. Curr Opin Radiol 1991;3:341–350.

570. Krupinski EA, Nodine CF, Kundel HL. A perceptually based method for enhancing pulmonary nodule recognition. Invest Radiol 1993;28:289–294.

571. Kundel HL, Nodine CF, Krupinski EA. Computer-displayed eye position as a visual aid to pulmonary nodule interpretation. Invest Radiol 1990;25:890–896.

572. Swensson RG, Theodore GH. Search and nonsearch protocols for radiographic consultation. Radiology 1990;177:851–856.

573. Brogdon BG, Kelsey CA, Moseley RD Jr. Factors affecting perception of pulmonary lesions. Radiol Clin North Am 1983;21:633–654.

574. White CS, Salis AI, Meyer CA. Missed lung cancer on chest radiography and computed tomography: imaging and medicolegal issues. J Thorac Imaging 1999;14:63–68.

575. Hallgrimsson JG, Jonsson T, Johannsson JH. Bronchopulmonary carcinoids in Iceland 1955–1984. A retrospective clinical and histopathologic study. Scand J Thorac Cardiovasc Surg 1989;23:275–278.

576. Paladugu RR, Benfield JR, Pak HY, et al. Bronchopulmonary Kulchitzky cell carcinomas. A new classification scheme for typical and atypical carcinoids. Cancer 1985;55:1303–1311.

577. Wang LT, Wilkins EW Jr, Bode HH. Bronchial carcinoid tumors in pediatric patients. Chest 1993;103:1426–1428.

578. Davila DG, Dunn WF, Tazelaar HD, et al. Bronchial carcinoid tumors. Mayo Clin Proc 1993;68:795–803.

579. Choplin RH, Kawamoto EH, Dyer RB,

et al. Atypical carcinoid of the lung: radiographic features. AJR Am J Roentgenol 1986;146:665–668.

580. Mills SE, Cooper PH, Walker AN, et al. Atypical carcinoid tumor of the lung. A clinicopathologic study of 17 cases. Am J Surg Pathol 1982;6:643–654.

581. Müller NL, Miller RR. Neuroendocrine carcinomas of the lung. Semin Roentgenol 1990;25:96–104.

582. Warren WH, Gould VE, Faber LP, et al. Neuroendocrine neoplasms of the bronchopulmonary tract. A classification of the spectrum of carcinoid to small cell carcinoma and intervening variants. J Thorac Cardiovasc Surg 1985;89:819–825.

583. Hurt R, Bates M. Carcinoid tumours of the bronchus: a 33 year experience. Thorax 1984;39:617–623.

584. Eustace S, Valentine S, Murray J. Acquired intralobar bronchopulmonary sequestration secondary to occluding endobronchial carcinoid tumor. Clin Imaging 1996;20:178–180.

585. Schreurs AJ, Westermann CJ, van den Bosch JM, et al. A twenty-five-year follow-up of ninety-three resected typical carcinoid tumors of the lung. J Thorac Cardiovasc Surg 1992;104:1470–1475.

586. Harpole DH Jr, Feldman JM, Buchanan S, et al. Bronchial carcinoid tumors: a retrospective analysis of 126 patients. Ann Thorac Surg 1992;54:50–54.

587. Ducrocq X, Thomas P, Massard G, et al. Operative risk and prognostic factors of typical bronchial carcinoid tumors. Ann Thorac Surg 1998;65:1410–1414.

588. Martini N, Zaman MB, Bains MS, et al. Treatment and prognosis in bronchial carcinoids involving regional lymph nodes. J Thorac Cardiovasc Surg 1994;107:1–6.

589. Marty-Ane CH, Costes V, Pujol JL, et al. Carcinoid tumors of the lung: do atypical features require aggressive management? Ann Thorac Surg 1995;59:78–83.

590. Travis WD, Linnoila RI, Tsokos MG, et al. Neuroendocrine tumors of the lung with proposed criteria for large-cell neuroendocrine carcinoma. An ultrastructural, immunohistochemical, and flow cytometric study of 35 cases. Am J Surg Pathol 1991;15:529–553.

591. McCaughan BC, Martini N, Bains MS. Bronchial carcinoids. Review of 124 cases. J Thorac Cardiovasc Surg 1985;89:8–17.

592. Gould PM, Bonner JA, Sawyer TE, et al. Bronchial carcinoid tumors: importance of prognostic factors that influence patterns of recurrence and overall survival. Radiology 1998;208: 181–185.

593. Nessi R, Basso RP, Basso RS, et al. Bronchial carcinoid tumors: radiologic observations in 49 cases. J Thorac Imaging 1991;6:47–53.

594. Doppman JL, Nieman L, Miller DL, et al. Ectopic adrenocorticotropic hormone syndrome: localization studies in 28 patients. Radiology 1989;172:115–124.

595. Findling JW, Tyrrell JB. Occult ectopic secretion of corticotropin. Arch Intern Med 1986;146:929–933.

596. Howlett TA, Drury PL, Perry L, et al. Diagnosis and management of ACTH-dependent Cushing's syndrome: comparison of the features in ectopic and pituitary ACTH production. Clin Endocrinol (Oxf) 1986;24:699–713.

597. Vincent JM, Trainer PJ, Reznek RH, et al. The radiological investigation of occult ectopic ACTH-dependent Cushing's syndrome. Clin Radiol 1993;48:11–17.

598. Horton KM, Fishman EK. Cushing syndrome due to a pulmonary carcinoid tumor: multimodality imaging and diagnosis. J Comput Assist Tomogr 1998;22:804–806.

599. Shrager JB, Wright CD, Wain JC, et al. Bronchopulmonary carcinoid tumors associated with Cushing's syndrome: a more aggressive variant of typical carcinoid. J Thorac Cardiovasc Surg 1997;114:367–375.

600. Doppman JL, Loughlin T, Miller DL, et al. Identification of ACTH-producing intrathoracic tumors by measuring ACTH levels in aspirated specimens. Radiology 1987;163 501–503.

601. Doppman JL, Pass HI, Nieman L, et al. Failure of bronchial lavage to detect elevated levels of adrenocorticotropin (ACTH) in patients with ACTH-producing bronchial carcinoids. J Clin Endocrinol Metab 1989;69:1302–1304.

602. McGuinnis EJ, Lull RJ. Bronchial adenoma causing unilateral absence of pulmonary perfusion. Radiology 1976;120:367–368.

603. Altman RL, Miller WE, Carr DT, et al. Radiographic appearance of bronchial carcinoid. Thorax 1973;28:433–434.

604. Giustra PE, Stassa G. The multiple presentations of bronchial adenomas. Radiology 1969;93:1013–1019.

605. Pugatch RD, Gale ME. Obscure pulmonary masses: bronchial impaction revealed by CT. AJR Am J Roentgenol 1983;141:909–914.

606. Bateson EM, Whimster WF, Woo-Ming M. Ossified bronchial adenoma. Br J Radiol 1970;43:570–573.

607. Good CA. Asymptomatic bronchial adenoma. Mayo Clin Proc 1953;28: 577–586.

608. Naidich DP, McCauley DI, Siegelman SS. Computed

tomography of bronchial adenomas. J Comput Assist Tomogr 1982;6: 725–732.

609. Rosado de Christenson ML, Abbott GF, Kirejczyk WM, et al. Thoracic carcinoids: radiologic-pathologic correlation. Radiographics 1999;19: 707–736.

610. Jeung MY, Gasser B, Gangi A, et al. Bronchial carcinoid tumors of the thorax: spectrum of radiologic findings. Radiographics 2002;22: 351–365.

611. Ferretti GR, Thony F, Bosson JL, et al. Benign abnormalities and carcinoid tumors of the central airways: diagnostic impact of CT bronchography. AJR Am J Roentgenol 2000;174:1307–1313.

612. Naidich DP. CT/MR correlation in the evaluation of tracheobronchial neoplasia. Radiol Clin North Am 1990;28:555–571.

613. Magid D, Siegelman SS, Eggleston JC, et al. Pulmonary carcinoid tumors: CT assessment. J Comput Assist Tomogr 1989;13:244–247.

614. Zwiebel BR, Austin JH, Grimes MM. Bronchial carcinoid tumors: assessment with CT of location and intratumoral calcification in 31 patients. Radiology 1991;179:483–486.

615. Shin MS, Berland LL, Myers JL, et al. CT demonstration of an ossifying bronchial carcinoid simulating broncholithiasis. AJR Am J Roentgenol 1989;153:51–52.

616. Aronchick JM, Wexler JA, Christen B, et al. Computed tomography of bronchial carcinoid. J Comput Assist Tomogr 1986;10:71–74.

617. Davis SD, Zirn JR, Govoni AF, et al. Peripheral carcinoid tumor of the lung: CT diagnosis. AJR Am J Roentgenol 1990;155:1185–1187.

618. Douek PC, Simoni L, Revel D, et al. Diagnosis of bronchial carcinoid tumor by ultrafast contrast-enhanced MR imaging. AJR Am J Roentgenol 1994;163:563–564.

619. Marcilly MC, Howarth NR, Berthezene Y. Bronchial carcinoid tumor: demonstration by dynamic inversion recovery turbo-flash MR imaging. Eur Radiol 1998;8:1400–1402.

620. Doppman JL, Pass HI, Nieman LK, et al. Detection of ACTH-producing bronchial carcinoid tumors: MR imaging vs CT. AJR Am J Roentgenol 1991;156:39–43.

621. de Herder WW, Krenning EP, Malchoff CD, et al. Somatostatin receptor scintigraphy: its value in tumor localization in patients with Cushing's syndrome caused by ectopic corticotropin or corticotropin-releasing hormone secretion. Am J Med 1994;96:305–312.

622. Krenning EP, Kwekkeboom DJ, Bakker WH, et al. Somatostatin receptor scintigraphy with [^{111}In-DTPA-D-Phe1]- and [123I-Tyr3]-octreotide: the Rotterdam experience with more than 1000 patients. Eur J Nucl Med 1993;20: 716–731.

623. Westlin JE, Janson ET, Arnberg H, et al. Somatostatin receptor scintigraphy of carcinoid tumours using the [111In-DTPA-D-Phe1]-octreotide. Acta Oncol 1993;32:783–786.

624. Doppman JL. Somatostatin receptor scintigraphy and the ectopic ACTH syndrome – the solution or just another test? Am J Med 1994;96:303–304.

625. Nishizawa S, Higa T, Kuroda Y, et al. Increased accumulation of N-isopropyl-(I-123)p-iodoamphetamine in bronchial carcinoid tumor. J Nucl Med 1990;31:240–242.

626. Erasmus JJ, McAdams HP, Patz EF Jr, et al. Evaluation of primary pulmonary carcinoid tumors using FDG PET. AJR Am J Roentgenol 1998;170:1369–1373.

627. Eriksson B, Bergstrom M, Sundin A, et al. The role of PET in localization of neuroendocrine and adrenocortical tumors. Ann N Y Acad Sci 2002;970: 159–169.

628. Wester HJ, Schottelius M, Scheidhauer K, et al. PET imaging of somatostatin receptors: design, synthesis and preclinical evaluation of a novel 18F-labelled, carbohydrated analogue of octreotide. Eur J Nucl Med Mol Imaging 2003;30:117–122.

629. Bateson EM. Relationship between intrapulmonary and endobronchial cartilage containing tumours, so called hamartomata. Thorax 1965;29:447–461.

630. Gjevre JA, Myers JL, Prakash UB. Pulmonary hamartomas. Mayo Clin Proc 1996;71:14–20.

631. Miura K, Hori T, Yoshizawa K, et al. Cystic pulmonary hamartoma. Ann Thorac Surg 1990;49:828–829.

632. Mushtaq M, Ward SP, Hutchison JT, et al. Multiple cystic pulmonary hamartomas. Thorax 1992;47 1076–1077.

633. Bennett LL, Lesar MS, Tellis CJ. Multiple calcified chondrohamartomas of the lung: CT appearance. J Comput Assist Tomogr 1985;9:180–182.

634. Poulsen JT, Jacobsen M, Francis D. Probable malignant transformation of a pulmonary hamartoma. Thorax 1979;34:557–558.

635. Karasik A, Modan M, Jacob CO, et al. Increased risk of lung cancer in patients with chondromatous hamartoma. J Thorac Cardiovasc Surg 1980;80:217–220.

636. Ribet M, Jaillard-Thery S, Nuttens MC. Pulmonary hamartoma and malignancy. J Thorac Cardiovasc Surg 1994;107:611–614.

637. Hedlund GL, Bisset GS, III, Bove KE. Malignant neoplasms arising in cystic hamartomas of the lung in childhood. Radiology 1989;173:77–79.

638. Mark EJ. Mesenchymal cystic hamartoma of the lung. N Engl J Med 1986;315:1255–1259.

639. Senac MO Jr, Wood BP, Isaacs H, et al. Pulmonary blastoma: a rare childhood malignancy. Radiology 1991;179: 743–746.

640. Poirier TJ, Van Ordstrand HS. Pulmonary chondromatous hamartomas. Report of seventeen cases and review of the literature. Chest 1971;59:50–55.

641. Carney JA. The triad of gastric epithelioid leiomyosarcoma, pulmonary chondroma, and functioning extra-adrenal paraganglioma: a five-year review. Medicine (Baltimore) 1983;62:159–169.

642. Evans RA, Salisbury JR, Gimson A, et al. Indolent gastric epithelioid leiomyosarcoma in Carney's triad. Clin Radiol 1990;42:437–439.

643. Mazas-Artasona L, Romeo M, Felices R, et al. Gastro-oesophageal leiomyoblastomas and multiple pulmonary chondromas: an incomplete variant of Carney's triad. Br J Radiol 1988;61:1181–1184.

644. Gabrail NY, Zara BY. Pulmonary hamartoma syndrome. Chest 1990;97:962–965.

645. Schmutz GR, Fisch-Ponsot C, Sylvestre J. Carney syndrome: radiologic features. Can Assoc Radiol J 1994;45:148–150.

646. Darke CS, Day P, Grainger RG, et al. The bronchial circulation in a case of giant hamartoma of the lung. Br J Radiol 1972;45:147–150.

647. Doppman JL, Wilson G. Cystic pulmonary hamartoma. Br J Radiol 1965;38:629–631.

648. Siegelman SS, Khouri NF, Scott WW Jr, et al. Pulmonary hamartoma: CT findings. Radiology 1986;160:313–317.

649. Potente G, Macori F, Caimi M, et al. Noncalcified pulmonary hamartomas: computed tomography enhancement patterns with histologic correlation. J Thorac Imaging 1999;14:101–104.

650. Swensen SJ, Brown LR, Colby TV, et al. Pulmonary nodules: CT evaluation of enhancement with iodinated contrast material. Radiology 1995;194:393–398.

651. Swensen SJ, Brown LR, Colby TV, et al. Lung nodule enhancement at CT: prospective findings. Radiology 1996;201:447–455.

652. Sakai F, Sone S, Kiyono K, et al. MR of pulmonary hamartoma: pathologic correlation. J Thorac Imaging 1994;9: 51–55.

653. Ahn JM, Im JG, Seo JW, et al. Endobronchial hamartoma: CT

findings in three patients. AJR Am J Roentgenol 1994;163:49–50.

654. Stey CA, Vogt P, Russi EW. Endobronchial lipomatous hamartoma: a rare cause of bronchial occlusion. Chest 1998;113:254–255.

655. McCarthy MJ, Rosado-de-Christenson ML. Tumors of the trachea. J Thorac Imaging 1995;10:180–198.

656. Regnard JF, Fourquier P, Levasseur P. Results and prognostic factors in resections of primary tracheal tumors: a multicenter retrospective study. The French Society of Cardiovascular Surgery. J Thorac Cardiovasc Surg 1996;111:808–813.

657. Allen HA, Angell F, Hankins J, et al. Leiomyoma of the trachea. AJR Am J Roentgenol 1983;141:683–684.

658. Davis WK, Roberts L Jr, Foster WL Jr, et al. Computed tomographic diagnosis of an endobronchial hamartoma. Invest Radiol 1988;23:941–944.

659. Swain ME, Coblentz CL. Tracheal chondroma: CT appearance. J Comput Assist Tomogr 1988;12:1085–1086.

660. Raymond GS, Murray SK, Logan PM. Granular cell tumour of the trachea: case report. Can Assoc Radiol J 1997;48:48–50.

661. Dennie CJ, Coblentz CL. The trachea: pathologic conditions and trauma. Can Assoc Radiol J 1993;44:157–167.

662. Koskinen SK, Niemi PT, Ekfors TO, et al. Glomus tumor of the trachea. Eur Radiol 1998;8:364–366.

663. Allen MS. Malignant tracheal tumors. Mayo Clin Proc 1993;68:680–684.

664. Gelder CM, Hetzel MR. Primary tracheal tumours: a national survey. Thorax 1993;48:688–692.

665. Kim TS, Lee KS, Han J, et al. Mucoepidermoid carcinoma of the tracheobronchial tree: radiographic and CT findings in 12 patients. Radiology 1999;212:643–648.

666. Kairalla RA, Carvalho CR, Parada AA, et al. Solitary plasmacytoma of the trachea treated by loop resection and laser therapy. Thorax 1988;43:1011–1012.

667. Logan PM, Miller RR, Muller NL. Solitary tracheal plasmacytoma: computed tomography and pathological findings. Can Assoc Radiol J 1995;46:125–126.

668. Chen JS, Chang YL, Shu HS, et al. Surgical treatment of a primary tracheal angiosarcoma. J Thorac Cardiovasc Surg 2003;125:191–193.

669. Maziak DE, Todd TR, Keshavjee SH, et al. Adenoid cystic carcinoma of the airway: thirty-two-year experience. J Thorac Cardiovasc Surg 1996;112:1522–1531.

670. Kim TS, Lee KS, Han J, et al. Sialadenoid tumors of the respiratory tract: radiologic-pathologic correlation. AJR Am J Roentgenol 2001;177:1145–1150.

671. Kwong JS, Muller NL, Miller RR. Diseases of the trachea and main-stem bronchi: correlation of CT with pathologic findings. Radiographics 1992;12:645–657.

672. Spizarny DL, Shepard JA, McLoud TC, et al. CT of adenoid cystic carcinoma of the trachea. AJR Am J Roentgenol 1986;146:1129–1132.

673. Akata S, Ohkubo Y, Park J, et al. Multiplanar reconstruction MR image of primary adenoid cystic carcinoma of the central airway: (MPR of central airway adenoid cystic carcinoma). Clin Imaging 2001;25:332–336.

674. Beluffi G, Bertolotti P, Mietta A, et al. Primary leiomyosarcoma of the lung in a girl. Pediatr Radiol 1986;16:240–244.

675. Yellin A, Rosenman Y, Lieberman Y. Review of smooth muscle tumours of the lower respiratory tract. Br J Dis Chest 1984;78:337–351.

676. Fitoz S, Atasoy C, Kizilkaya E, et al. Radiologic findings in primary pulmonary leiomyosarcoma. J Thorac Imaging 2000;15:151–152.

677. Delany SG, Doyle TC, Bunton RW, et al. Pulmonary artery sarcoma mimicking pulmonary embolism. Chest 1993;103:1631–1633.

678. Guccion JG, Rosen SH. Bronchopulmonary leiomyosarcoma and fibrosarcoma. A study of 32 cases and review of the literature. Cancer 1972;30:836–847.

679. McDonnell T, Kyriakos M, Roper C, et al. Malignant fibrous histiocytoma of the lung. Cancer 1988;61:137–145.

680. Reifsnyder AC, Smith HJ, Mullhollan TJ, et al. Malignant fibrous histiocytoma of the lung in a patient with a history of asbestos exposure. AJR Am J Roentgenol 1990;154:65–66.

681. Yousem SA, Hochholzer L. Malignant fibrous histiocytoma of the lung. Cancer 1987;60:2532–2541.

682. Pui MH, Yu SP, Chen JD. Primary intrathoracic malignant fibrous histiocytoma and angiosarcoma. Australas Radiol 1999;43:3–6.

683. Petersen M. Radionuclide detection of primary pulmonary osteogenic sarcoma: a case report and review of the literature. J Nucl Med 1990;31:1110–1114.

684. Stark P, Smith DC, Watkins GE, et al. Primary intrathoracic extraosseous osteogenic sarcoma: report of three cases. Radiology 1990;174:725–726.

685. Doval DC, Kannan V, Acharya R, et al. Bronchial embryonal rhabdomyosarcoma – a case report. Acta Oncol 1994;33:832–833.

686. Shariff S, Thomas JA, Shetty N, et al. Primary pulmonary rhabdomyosarcoma in a child, with a review of literature. J Surg Oncol 1988;38:261–264.

687. Gimenez A, Franquet T, Prats R, et al. Unusual primary lung tumors: a radiologic-pathologic overview. Radiographics 2002;22:601–619.

688. Sheppard MN, Hansell DM, Du Bois RM, et al. Primary epithelioid angiosarcoma of the lung presenting as pulmonary hemorrhage. Hum Pathol 1997;28:383–385.

689. Simpson WL Jr, Mendelson DS. Pulmonary artery and aortic sarcomas: cross-sectional imaging. J Thorac Imaging 2000;15:290–294.

690. Kacl GM, Bruder E, Pfammatter T, et al. Primary angiosarcoma of the pulmonary arteries: dynamic contrast-enhanced MRI. J Comput Assist Tomogr 1998;22:687–691.

691. Cox JE, Chiles C, Aquino SL, et al. Pulmonary artery sarcomas: a review of clinical and radiologic features. J Comput Assist Tomogr 1997;21:750–755.

692. Ablett MJ, Elliott ST, Mitchell L. Case report: Pulmonary leiomyosarcoma presenting as a pseudoaneurysm. Clin Radiol 1998;53:851–852.

693. Wu YC, Wang LS, Chen W, et al. Primary pulmonary malignant hemangiopericytoma associated with coagulopathy. Ann Thorac Surg 1997;64:841–843.

694. Halle M, Blum U, Dinkel E, et al. CT and MR features of primary pulmonary hemangiopericytomas. J Comput Assist Tomogr 1993;17:51–55.

695. Katz DS, Lane MJ, Leung AN, et al. Primary malignant pulmonary hemangiopericytoma. Clin Imaging 1998;22:192–195.

696. Kim KI, Flint JD, Muller NL. Pulmonary carcinosarcoma: radiologic and pathologic findings in three patients. AJR Am J Roentgenol 1997;169:691–694.

697. Koss MN, Hochholzer L, O'Leary T. Pulmonary blastomas. Cancer 1991;67:2368–2381.

698. Katz DS, Scalzetti EM, Groskin SA, et al. Pleuropulmonary blastoma simulating an empyema in a young child. J Thorac Imaging 1995;10:112–116.

699. Solomon A, Rubinstein ZJ, Rogoff M, et al. Pulmonary blastoma. Pediatr Radiol 1982;12:148–149.

700. Han SS, Wills JS, Allen OS. Pulmonary blastoma: case report and literature review. Am J Roentgenol 1976;127:1048–1049.

701. Herzog KA, Putman CE. Pulmonary blastoma. Br J Radiol 1974;47:286–288.

702. Peacock MJ, Whitwell F. Pulmonary blastoma. Thorax 1976;31:197–204.

703. Weisbrod GL, Chamberlain DW, Tao LC. Pulmonary blastoma, report of three cases and a review of the literature. Can Assoc Radiol J 1988;39:130–136.

704. Manivel JC, Priest JR, Watterson J, et al. Pleuropulmonary blastoma. The so-called pulmonary blastoma of childhood. Cancer 1988;62:1516–1526.

705. Kovanlikaya A, Pirnar T, Olgun N. Pulmonary blastoma: a rare case of childhood malignancy. Pediatr Radiol 1992;22:155.

706. Priest JR, McDermott MB, Bhatia S, et al. Pleuropulmonary blastoma: a clinicopathologic study of 50 cases. Cancer 1997;80:147–161.

707. Kiziltepe TT, Patrick E, Alvarado C, et al. Pleuropulmonary blastoma and ovarian teratoma. Pediatr Radiol 1999;29:901–903.

708. Kayser K, Gabius HJ, Hagemeyer O. Malignant teratoma of the lung with lymph node metastasis of the ectodermal compartment: a case report. Anal Cell Pathol 1993;5:31–37.

709. Maasilta PK, Salminen US, Taskinen EI. Malignant teratoma of the lung. Acta Oncol 1999;38:1113–1115.

710. Arslanian A, Pischedda F, Filosso PL, et al. Primary choriocarcinoma of the lung. J Thorac Cardiovasc Surg 2003;125:193–196.

711. Dines DE, Lillie JC, Henderson LL, et al. Solitary plasmacytoma of the trachea. Am Rev Respir Dis 1965;92:949–951.

712. Egashira K, Hirakata K, Nakata H, et al. CT and MRI manifestations of primary pulmonary plasmacytoma. Clin Imaging 1995;19:17–19.

713. Joseph G, Pandit M, Korfhage L. Primary pulmonary plasmacytoma. Cancer 1993;71:721–724.

714. Shin MS, Carcelen MF, Ho KJ. Diverse roentgenographic manifestations of the rare pulmonary involvement in myeloma. Chest 1992;102:946–948.

715. Askin FB, Rosai J, Sibley RK, et al. Malignant small cell tumor of the thoracopulmonary region in childhood: a distinctive clinicopathologic entity of uncertain histogenesis. Cancer 1979;43:2438–2451.

716. Cabezali R, Lozano R, Bustamante E, et al. Askin's tumor of the chest wall: a case report in an adult. J Thorac Cardiovasc Surg 1994;107:960–962.

717. Howman-Giles R, Uren RF, Kellie SJ. Gallium and thallium scintigraphy in pediatric peripheral primitive neuroectodermal tumor (Askin tumor) of the chest wall. J Nucl Med 1995;36:814–816.

718. Saifuddin A, Robertson RJ, Smith SE. The radiology of Askin tumours. Clin Radiol 1991;43:19–23.

719. Takanami I, Imamura T. The treatment of Askin tumor: results of two cases. J Thorac Cardiovasc Surg 2002;123:391–392.

720. Sabate JM, Franquet T, Parellada JA, et al. Malignant neuroectodermal tumour of the chest wall (Askin tumour): CT and MR findings in eight patients. Clin Radiol 1994;49:634–638.

721. Dail DH, Liebow AA, Gmelich JT, et al. Intravascular, bronchiolar, and alveolar tumor of the lung (IVBAT). An analysis of twenty cases of a peculiar sclerosing endothelial tumor. Cancer 1983;51:452–464.

722. Luburich P, Ayuso MC, Picado C, et al. CT of pulmonary epithelioid hemangioendothelioma. J Comput Assist Tomogr 1994;18:562–565.

723. Ross GJ, Violi L, Friedman AC, et al. Intravascular bronchioloalveolar tumor: CT and pathologic correlation. J Comput Assist Tomogr 1989;13:240–243.

724. Sherman JL, Rykwalder PJ, Tashkin DP. Intravascular bronchioloalveolar tumor. Am Rev Respir Dis 1981;123:468–470.

725. Erasmus JJ, McAdams HP, Carraway MS. A 63-year-old woman with weight loss and multiple lung nodules. Chest 1997;111:236–238.

726. Mukundan G, Urban BA, Askin FB, et al. Pulmonary epithelioid hemangioendothelioma: atypical radiologic findings of a rare tumor with pathologic correlation. J Comput Assist Tomogr 2000;24:719–720.

727. Ledson MJ, Convery R, Carty A, et al. Epithelioid haemangioendothelioma. Thorax 1999;54:560–561.

728. Yoon YC, Lee KS, Kim TS, et al. Benign bronchopulmonary tumors: radiologic and pathologic findings. J Comput Assist Tomogr 2002;26:784–796.

729. Bohm J, Fellbaum C, Bautz W, et al. Pulmonary nodule caused by an alveolar adenoma of the lung. Virchows Arch 1997;430:181–184.

730. England DM, Hochholzer L. Truly benign "bronchial adenoma". Report of 10 cases of mucous gland adenoma with immunohistochemical and ultrastructural findings. Am J Surg Pathol 1995;19:887–899.

731. Kwon JW, Goo JM, Seo JB, et al. Mucous gland adenoma of the bronchus: CT findings in two patients. J Comput Assist Tomogr 1999;23:758–760.

732. Aisner SC, Chakravarthy AK, Joslyn JN, et al. Bilateral granular cell tumors of the posterior mediastinum. Ann Thorac Surg 1988;46:688–689.

733. Coleman BG, Arger PH, Stephenson LW. CT features of endobronchial granular cell myoblastoma. J Comput Assist Tomogr 1984;8:998–1000.

734. Deavers M, Guinee D, Koss MN, et al. Granular cell tumors of the lung. Clinicopathologic study of 20 cases. Am J Surg Pathol 1995;19:627–635.

735. Butchart EG, Urquhart W, Porteous IB, et al. Granular cell myoblastoma of the bronchus. Br J Radiol 1976;49:87–90.

736. Teplick JG, Teplick SK, Haskin ME. Granular cell myoblastoma of the lung. Am J Roentgenol Radium Ther Nucl Med 1975;125:890–894.

737. Mata JM, Caceres J, Ferrer J, et al. Endobronchial lipoma: CT diagnosis. J Comput Assist Tomogr 1991;15:750–751.

738. Feldhaus RJ, Anene C, Bogard P. A rare endobronchial neurilemmoma (Schwannoma). Chest 1989;95:461–462.

739. Aufiero TX, McGary SA, Campbell DB, et al. Intrapulmonary benign fibrous tumor of the pleura. J Thorac Cardiovasc Surg 1995;110:549–551.

740. Moran CA, Hochholzer L, Rush W, et al. Primary intrapulmonary meningiomas. A clinicopathologic and immunohistochemical study of ten cases. Cancer 1996;78:2328–2333.

741. Veynovich B, Masetti P, Kaplan PD, et al. Primary pulmonary thymoma. Ann Thorac Surg 1997;64:1471–1473.

742. Child SD, Staples CA, Chan N, et al. Lingular opacity with an endobronchial mass. Can Assoc Radiol J 1991;42:435–437.

743. Mendelsohn SL, Fagelman D, Zwanger-Mendelsohn S. Endobronchial lipoma demonstrated by CT. Radiology 1983;148:790.

744. Storey TF, Narla LD. Pleural lipoma in a child—CT evaluation. Pediatr Radiol 1991;21:141–142.

745. Trigaux JP, van Beers B, Weynants P. Hour-glass lipoma. Br J Radiol 1990;63:497–498.

746. Martin E. Leiomyomatous lung lesions: a proposed classification. AJR Am J Roentgenol 1983;141:269–272.

747. Shin MS, Fulmer JD, Ho KJ. Unusual computed tomographic manifestations of benign metastasizing leiomyomas as cavitary nodular lesions or interstitial lung disease. Clin Imaging 1996;20:45–49.

748. Maredia R, Snyder BJ, Harvey LA, et al. Benign metastasizing leiomyoma in the lung. Radiographics 1998;18:779–782.

749. Abramson S, Gilkeson RC, Goldstein JD, et al. Benign metastasizing leiomyoma: clinical, imaging, and pathologic correlation. AJR Am J Roentgenol 2001;176:1409–1413.

750. Budde RB, Jr., Yankura JA. Leiomyomatosis with a solitary pleural metastasis. Clin Imaging 1989;13:228–230.

751. Lipton JH, Fong TC, Burgess KR. Miliary pattern as presentation of

leiomyomatosis of the lung. Chest 1987;91:781–782.

752. Hertzanu Y, Heimer D, Hirsch M. Computed tomography of pulmonary endometriosis. Comput Radiol 1987;11:81–84.

753. Volkart JR. CT findings in pulmonary endometriosis. J Comput Assist Tomogr 1995;19:156–157.

754. Morgan DE, Sanders C, McElvein RB, et al. Intrapulmonary teratoma: a case report and review of the literature. J Thorac Imaging 1992;7:70–77.

755. Nicholson AG, Magkou C, Snead D, et al. Unusual sclerosing haemangiomas and sclerosing haemangioma-like lesions, and the value of TTF-1 in making the diagnosis. Histopathology 2002;41:404–413.

756. Sakamoto K, Okita M, Kumagiri H, et al. Sclerosing hemangioma isolated to the mediastinum. Ann Thorac Surg 2003;75:1021–1023.

757. Dawson WB, Müller NL, Miller RR. Pulmonary sclerosing hemangioma: unusual cause of a solitary pulmonary nodule. Can Assoc Radiol J 1990;41: 372–374.

758. Sugio K, Yokoyama H, Kaneko S, et al. Sclerosing hemangioma of the lung: radiographic and pathological study. Ann Thorac Surg 1992;53:295–300.

759. Im JG, Kim WH, Han MC, et al. Sclerosing hemangiomas of the lung and interlobar fissures: CT findings. J Comput Assist Tomogr 1994;18:34–38.

760. Nam JE, Ryu YH, Cho SH, et al. Air-trapping zone surrounding sclerosing hemangioma of the lung. J Comput Assist Tomogr 2002;26:358–361.

761. Cheung YC, Ng SH, Chang JW, et al. Histopathological and CT features of pulmonary sclerosing haemangiomas. Clin Radiol 2003;58:630–635.

762. Katzenstein AL, Gmelich JT, Carrington CB. Sclerosing hemangioma of the lung: a clinicopathologic study of 51 cases. Am J Surg Pathol 1980;4: 343–356.

763. Bahk YW, Shinn KS, Choi BS. The air meniscus sign in sclerosing hemangioma of the lung. Radiology 1978;128:27–29.

764. Fujiyoshi F, Ichinari N, Fukukura Y, et al. Sclerosing hemangioma of the lung: MR findings and correlation with pathological features. J Comput Assist Tomogr 1998;22:1006–1008.

765. Kramer SS, Wehunt WD, Stocker JT, et al. Pulmonary manifestations of juvenile laryngotracheal papillomatosis. AJR Am J Roentgenol 1985;144:687–694.

766. Clements R, Gravelle IH. Laryngeal papillomatosis. Clin Radiol 1986;37: 547–550.

767. Lui D, Kumar A, Aggarwal S, et al. CT findings of malignant change in recurrent respiratory papillomatosis. J Comput Assist Tomogr 1995;19: 804–807.

768. Kawanami T, Bowen A. Juvenile laryngeal papillomatosis with pulmonary parenchymal spread. Case report and review of the literature. Pediatr Radiol 1985;15:102–104.

769. Gruden JF, Webb WR, Sides DM. Adult-onset disseminated tracheobronchial papillomatosis: CT features. J Comput Assist Tomogr 1994;18:640–642.

770. Glazer G, Webb WR. Laryngeal papillomatosis with pulmonary spread in a 69-year-old man. AJR Am J Roentgenol 1979;132:820–822.

771. Oleszczuk-Raszke K, Cremin BJ. Computed tomography in pulmonary papillomatosis. Br J Radiol 1988;61: 160–161.

772. Ravin CE, Bergin D, Bisset GS, III, et al. Image interpretation session: 2000. Radiographics 2001;21:267–287.

773. Naka Y, Nakao K, Hamaji Y, et al. Solitary squamous cell papilloma of the trachea. Ann Thorac Surg 1993;55:189–193.

774. Hong SS, Lee JS, Lee KH, et al. Intravascular papillary endothelial hyperplasia of the lung. J Comput Assist Tomogr 2002;26:362–364.

775. Matsubara O, Tan-Liu NS, Kenney RM, et al. Inflammatory pseudotumors of the lung: progression from organizing pneumonia to fibrous histiocytoma or to plasma cell granuloma in 32 cases. Hum Pathol 1988;19:807–814.

776. Bragg DG, Chor PJ, Murray KA, et al. Lymphoproliferative disorders of the lung: histopathology, clinical manifestations, and imaging features. AJR Am J Roentgenol 1994;163:273–281.

777. Copin MC, Gosselin BH, Ribet ME. Plasma cell granuloma of the lung: difficulties in diagnosis and prognosis. Ann Thorac Surg 1996;61:1477–1482.

778. Laufer L, Cohen Z, Mares AJ, et al. Pulmonary plasma-cell granuloma. Pediatr Radiol 1990;20:289–290.

779. Cerfolio RJ, Allen MS, Nascimento AG, et al. Inflammatory pseudotumors of the lung. Ann Thorac Surg 1999;67: 933–936.

780. Agrons GA, Rosado-de-Christenson ML, Kirejczyk WM, et al. Pulmonary inflammatory pseudotumor: radiologic features. Radiology 1998;206:511–518.

781. Mas EF, Andres V, Vallcanera A, et al. Plasma cell granuloma of the lung in childhood: atypical radiologic findings and association with hypertrophic osteoarthropathy. Pediatr Radiol 1995;25:369–372.

782. Urschel JD, Horan TA, Unruh HW. Plasma cell granuloma of the lung. J Thorac Cardiovasc Surg 1992;104: 870–875.

783. Alexiou C, Obuszko Z, Beggs D, et al. Inflammatory pseudotumors of the lung. Ann Thorac Surg 1998;66: 948–950.

784. Narla LD, Newman B, Spottswood SS, et al. Inflammatory pseudotumor. Radiographics 2003;23:719–729.

785. Kundu S, Weiser WJ, Chiu B. Inflammatory pseudotumour of the lung presenting as multiple pulmonary nodules: case report. Can Assoc Radiol J 1997;48:44–47.

786. Cruz JF, Garcia AG, Casas PE, et al. Pulmonary lymphoproliferative disorders with affinity to lymphoma: a clinicopathoradiologic study of 16 cases. Eur Radiol 1993;3:106–114.

787. Doyle AJ. Plasma cell granuloma of the lung. Australas Radiol 1988;32:144–146.

788. Hadimeri U, Hadimeri H, Resjo M. Inflammatory pseudotumour of the lung. A case report. Pediatr Radiol 1993;23:624–625.

789. Kaufman RA. Calcified postinflammatory pseudotumor of the lung: CT features. J Comput Assist Tomogr 1988;12:653–655.

790. Monzon CM, Gilchrist GS, Burgert EO Jr, et al. Plasma cell granuloma of the lung in children. Pediatrics 1982;70:268–274.

791. Schwartz EE, Katz SM, Mandell GA. Postinflammatory pseudotumors of the lung: fibrous histiocytoma and related lesions. Radiology 1980;136: 609–613.

792. Shapiro MP, Gale ME, Carter BL. Variable CT appearance of plasma cell granuloma of the lung. J Comput Assist Tomogr 1987;11:49–51.

793. Ahn JM, Kim WS, Yeon KM, et al. Plasma cell granuloma involving the tracheobronchial angle in a child: a case report. Pediatr Radiol 1995;25: 204–205.

794. Armstrong P, Elston C, Sanderson M. Endobronchial histiocytoma. Br J Radiol 1975;48:221–222.

795. Verbeke JI, Verberne AA, Den Hollander JC, et al. Inflammatory myofibroblastic tumour of the lung manifesting as progressive atelectasis. Pediatr Radiol 1999;29:816–819.

796. Erasmus JJ, McAdams HP, Patz EF Jr, et al. Calcifying fibrous pseudotumor of pleura: radiologic features in three cases. J Comput Assist Tomogr 1996;20:763–765.

797. Zennaro H, Laurent F, Vergier B, et al. Inflammatory myofibroblastic tumor of the lung (inflammatory pseudotumor): uncommon cause of solitary pulmonary nodule. Eur Radiol 1999;9:1205–1207.

798. Slosman DO, Spiliopoulos A, Keller A, et al. Quantitative metabolic PET imaging of a plasma cell granuloma. J Thorac Imaging 1994;9:116–119.

799. World Health Organization Classification of Tumours. Pathology and genetics of tumours of haematopoietic and lymphoid tissues. Lyon: IARC Press, 2001.

800. Lukes RJ, Craver LF, Hall TC, et al. Report of the nomenclature committee. Cancer Res 1966;26:1311.

801. Anonymous. National Cancer Institute sponsored study of classifiction of non-Hodgkin's lymphomas: summary and description of a working formulation for clinical usage. The Non-Hodgkin's Lymphoma Pathologic Classification Project. Cancer 1982;49:2112–2135.

802. Chan JK, Banks PM, Cleary ML, et al. A revised European-American classification of lymphoid neoplasms proposed by the International Lymphoma Study Group. A summary version. Am J Clin Pathol 1995;103:543–560.

803. Harris NL, Jaffe ES, Diebold J, et al. World Health Organization classification of neoplastic diseases of the hematopoietic and lymphoid tissues: report of the Clinical Advisory Committee meeting-Airlie House, Virginia, November 1997. J Clin Oncol 1999;17:3835–3849.

804. Carbone PP, Kaplan HS, Musshoff K, et al. Report of the Committee on Hodgkin's Disease Staging Classification. Cancer Res 1971;31:1860–1861.

805. Lister TA, Crowther D, Sutcliffe SB, et al. Report of a committee convened to discuss the evaluation and staging of patients with Hodgkin's disease: Cotswolds meeting. J Clin Oncol 1989;7:1630–1636.

806. Urba WJ, Longo DL. Hodgkin's disease. N Engl J Med 1992;326:678–687.

807. Marglin SI, Castellino RA. Selection of imaging studies for the initial staging of patients with Hodgkin's disease. Semin US CT MR 1985;6:380–393.

808. Castellino RA. Hodgkin disease: practical concepts for the diagnostic radiologist. Radiology 1986;159:305–310.

809. Carty H, Martin J. Staging of lymphoma in childhood. Clin Radiol 1993;48:151–159.

810. Hamrick-Turner JE, Saif MF, Powers CI, et al. Imaging of childhood non-Hodgkin lymphoma: assessment by histologic subtype. Radiographics 1994;14:11–28.

811. Parker BR. Leukemia and lymphoma in childhood. Radiol Clin North Am 1997;35:1495–1516.

812. White KS. Thoracic imaging of pediatric lymphomas. J Thorac Imaging 2001;16:224–237.

813. Magrath IT. Malignant non-Hodgkin's lymphomas in children. Hematol Oncol Clin North Am 1987;1:577–602.

814. Smith SD, Rubin CM, Horvath A, et al. Non-Hodgkin's lymphoma in children. Semin Oncol 1990;17:113–119.

815. Ng YY, Healy JC, Vincent JM, et al. The radiology of non-Hodgkin's lymphoma in childhood: a review of 80 cases. Clin Radiol 1994;49:594–600.

816. Murphy SB. Childhood non-Hodgkin's lymphoma. N Engl J Med 1978;299:1446–1448.

817. Filly R, Bland N, Castellino RA. Radiographic distribution of intrathoracic disease in previously untreated patients with Hodgkin's disease and non-Hodgkin's lymphoma. Radiology 1976;120:277–281.

818. Castellino RA, Hilton S, O'Brien JP, et al. Non-Hodgkin lymphoma: contribution of chest CT in the initial staging evaluation. Radiology 1996;199:129–132.

819. Parker BR, Castellino RA, Kaplan HS. Pediatric Hodgkin's disease. I. Radiographic evaluation. Cancer 1976;37:2430–2435.

820. Castellino RA, Bellani FF, Gasparini M, et al. Radiographic findings in previously untreated children with non-Hodgkin's lymphoma. Radiology 1975;117:657–663.

821. Grossman H, Winchester PH, Bragg DG, et al. Roentgenographic changes in childhood Hodgkin's disease. Am J Roentgenol Radium Ther Nucl Med 1970;108:354–364.

822. Castellino RA, Blank N. Adenopathy of the cardiophrenic angle (diaphragmatic) lymph nodes. Am J Roentgenol Radium Ther Nucl Med 1972;114:509–515.

823. Jochelson MS, Balikian JP, Mauch P, et al. Peri- and paracardial involvement in lymphoma: a radiographic study of 11 cases. AJR Am J Roentgenol 1983;140:483–488.

824. Cho CS, Blank N, Castellino RA. CT evaluation of cardiophrenic angle lymph nodes in patients with malignant lymphoma. AJR Am J Roentgenol 1984;143:719–721.

825. Samuels TH, Margolis M, Hamilton PA, et al. Mediastinal large-cell lymphoma. Can Assoc Radiol J 1992;43:120–126.

826. Simon G. Intra-thoracic Hodgkin's disease. Part 1. Less common intra-thoracic manifestations of Hodgkin's disease. Br J Radiol 1967;40:926–929.

827. Castellino RA, Blank N, Hoppe RT, et al. Hodgkin disease: contributions of chest CT in the initial staging evaluation. Radiology 1986;160:603–605.

828. Blank N, Castellino RA. The mediastinum in Hodgkin's and non-Hodgkin's lymphomas. J Thorac Imaging 1987;2:66–71.

829. Pombo F, Rodriguez E, Caruncho MV, et al. CT attenuation values and enhancing characteristics of thoracoabdominal lymphomatous adenopathies. J Comput Assist Tomogr 1994;18:59–62.

830. Hopper KD, Diehl LF, Cole BA, et al. The significance of necrotic mediastinal lymph nodes on CT in patients with newly diagnosed Hodgkin disease. AJR Am J Roentgenol 1990;155:267–270.

831. Shaffer K, Smith D, Kirn D, et al. Primary mediastinal large-B-cell lymphoma: radiologic findings at presentation. AJR Am J Roentgenol 1996;167:425–430.

832. Strijk SP. Lymph node calcification in malignant lymphoma. Presentation of nine cases and a review of the literature. Acta Radiol Diagn (Stockh) 1985;26:427–431.

833. Wycoco D, Raval B. An unusual presentation of mediastinal Hodgkin's lymphoma on computed tomography. J Comput Tomogr 1983;7:187–188.

834. Negendank WG, al Katib AM, Karanes C, et al. Lymphomas: MR imaging contrast characteristics with clinical-pathologic correlations. Radiology 1990;177:209–216.

835. Heron CW, Husband JE, Williams MP. Hodgkin disease: CT of the thymus. Radiology 1988;167:647–651.

836. Spiers AS, Husband JE, MacVicar AD. Treated thymic lymphoma: comparison of MR imaging with CT. Radiology 1997;203:369–376.

837. Wernecke K, Vassallo P, Rutsch F, et al. Thymic involvement in Hodgkin disease: CT and sonographic findings. Radiology 1991;181:375–383.

838. Chen JL, Osborne BM, Butler JJ. Residual fibrous masses in treated Hodgkin's disease. Cancer 1987;60:407–413.

839. Jochelson M, Mauch P, Balikian J, et al. The significance of the residual mediastinal mass in treated Hodgkin's disease. J Clin Oncol 1985;3:637–640.

840. Uematsu M, Kondo M, Tsutsui T, et al. Residual masses on follow-up computed tomography in patients with mediastinal non-Hodgkin's lymphoma. Clin Radiol 1989;40:244–247.

841. Radford JA, Cowan RA, Flanagan M, et al. The significance of residual mediastinal abnormality on the chest radiograph following treatment for Hodgkin's disease. J Clin Oncol 1988;6:940–946.

842. Fletcher BD, Xiong X, Kauffman WM, et al. Hodgkin disease: use of Tl-201 to monitor mediastinal involvement after treatment. Radiology 1998;209:471–475.

843. Bar-Shalom R, Mor M, Yefremov N, et al. The value of Ga-67 scintigraphy

and F-18 fluorodeoxyglucose positron emission tomography in staging and monitoring the response of lymphoma to treatment. Semin Nucl Med 2001;31:177–190.

844. Rehm PK. Radionuclide evaluation of patients with lymphoma. Radiol Clin North Am 2001;39:957–978.

845. Drossman SR, Schiff RG, Kronfeld GD, et al. Lymphoma of the mediastinum and neck: evaluation with Ga-67 imaging and CT correlation. Radiology 1990;174:171–175.

846. Israel O, Front D, Epelbaum R, et al. Residual mass and negative gallium scintigraphy in treated lymphoma. J Nucl Med 1990;31:365–368.

847. Weiner M, Leventhal B, Cantor A, et al. Gallium-67 scans as an adjunct to computed tomography scans for the assessment of a residual mediastinal mass in pediatric patients with Hodgkin's disease. A Pediatric Oncology Group study. Cancer 1991;68:2478–2480.

848. Front D, Bar-Shalom R, Epelbaum R, et al. Early detection of lymphoma recurrence with gallium-67 scintigraphy. J Nucl Med 1993;34:2101–2104.

849. Front D, Ben Haim S, Israel O, et al. Lymphoma: predictive value of Ga-67 scintigraphy after treatment. Radiology 1992;182:359–363.

850. McLaughlin AF, Magee MA, Greenough R, et al. Current role of gallium scanning in the management of lymphoma. Eur J Nucl Med 1990;16:755–771.

851. Front D, Bar-Shalom R, Israel O. The continuing clinical role of gallium 67 scintigraphy in the age of receptor imaging. Semin Nucl Med 1997;27:68–74.

852. Shah N, Hoskin P, McMillan A, et al. The impact of FDG positron emission tomography imaging on the management of lymphomas. Br J Radiol 2000;73:482–487.

853. Naumann R, Vaic A, Beuthien-Baumann B, et al. Prognostic value of positron emission tomography in the evaluation of post-treatment residual mass in patients with Hodgkin's disease and non-Hodgkin's lymphoma. B.J.Haematol 2001;115:793–800.

854. Maisey NR, Hill ME, Webb A, et al. Are [18]fluorodeoxyglucose positron emission tomography and magnetic resonance imaging useful in the prediction of relapse in lymphoma residual masses? Eur J Cancer 2000;36:200–206.

855. Forsgren G, Nyman R, Glimelius B, et al. Gd-DTPA-enhanced MR imaging in mediastinal Hodgkin's disease. Acta Radiol 1994;35:564–569.

856. Rahmouni A, Divine M, Lepage E, et al. Mediastinal lymphoma: quantitative changes in gadolinium enhancement at MR imaging after treatment. Radiology 2001;219:621–628.

857. Nyman R, Forsgren G, Glimelius B. Long-term follow-up of residual mediastinal masses in treated Hodgkin's disease using MR imaging. Acta Radiol 1996;37:323–326.

858. Rahmouni A, Tempany C, Jones R, et al. Lymphoma: monitoring tumor size and signal intensity with MR imaging. Radiology 1993;188:445–451.

859. Nyman RS, Rehn SM, Glimelius BL, et al. Residual mediastinal masses in Hodgkin disease: prediction of size with MR imaging. Radiology 1989;170:435–440.

860. Webb WR. MR imaging of treated mediastinal Hodgkin disease. Radiology 1989;170:315–316.

861. Baron RL, Sagel SS, Baglan RJ. Thymic cysts following radiation therapy for Hodgkin disease. Radiology 1981;141:593–597.

862. Kim HC, Nosher J, Haas A, et al. Cystic degeneration of thymic Hodgkin's disease following radiation therapy. Cancer 1985;55:354–356.

863. MacDonald JB. Lung involvement in Hodgkin's disease. Thorax 1977;32:664–667.

864. Whitcomb ME, Schwarz MI, Keller AR, et al. Hodgkin's disease of the lung. Am Rev Respir Dis 1972;106:79–85.

865. Lewis ER, Caskey CI, Fishman EK. Lymphoma of the lung: CT findings in 31 patients. AJR Am J Roentgenol 1991;156:711–714.

866. Shuman LS, Libshitz HI. Solid pleural manifestations of lymphoma. AJR Am J Roentgenol 1984;142:269–273.

867. Au V, Leung AN. Radiologic manifestations of lymphoma in the thorax. AJR Am J Roentgenol 1997;168:93–98.

868. Fisher AM, Kendal B, Van Leuven BD. Hodgkin's disease: a radiological survey. Clin Radiol 1962;13:115–127.

869. Diederich S, Link TM, Zuhlsdorf H, et al. Pulmonary manifestations of Hodgkin's disease: radiographic and CT findings. Eur Radiol 2001;11:2295–2305.

870. Balikian JP, Herman PG. Non-Hodgkin lymphoma of the lungs. Radiology 1979;132:569–576.

871. Burgener FA, Hamlin DJ. Intrathoracic histiocytic lymphoma. AJR Am J Roentgenol 1981;136:499–504.

872. Jackson SA, Tung KT, Mead GM. Multiple cavitating pulmonary lesions in non-Hodgkin's lymphoma. Clin Radiol 1994;49:883–885.

873. North LB, Libshitz HI, Lorigan JG. Thoracic lymphoma. Radiol Clin North Am 1990;28:745–762.

874. Cathcart-Rake W, Bone RC, Sobonya RE, et al. Rapid development of diffuse pulmonary infiltrates in histiocytic lymphoma. Am Rev Respir Dis 1978;117:587–593.

875. Dunnick NR, Parker BR, Castellino RA. Rapid onset of pulmonary infiltration due to histiocytic lymphoma. Radiology 1976;118:281–285.

876. Lee KS, Kim Y, Primack SL. Imaging of pulmonary lymphomas. AJR Am J Roentgenol 1997;168:339–345.

877. Yousem SA, Weiss LM, Colby TV. Primary pulmonary Hodgkin's disease. A clinicopathologic study of 15 cases. Cancer 1986;57:1217–1224.

878. Cartier Y, Johkoh T, Honda O, et al. Primary pulmonary Hodgkin's disease: CT findings in three patients. Clin Radiol 1999;54:182–184.

879. Ferraro P, Trastek VF, Adlakha H, et al. Primary non-Hodgkin's lymphoma of the lung. Ann Thorac Surg 2000;69:993–997.

880. Isaacson P, Wright DH. Malignant lymphoma of mucosa-associated lymphoid tissue. A distinctive type of B-cell lymphoma. Cancer 1983;52:1410–1416.

881. Isaacson PG, Spencer J. Malignant lymphoma of mucosa-associated lymphoid tissue. Histopathology 1987;11:445–462.

882. Isaacson PG. Lymphomas of mucosa-associated lymphoid tissue (MALT). Histopathology 1990;16:617–619.

883. Pelstring RJ, Essell JH, Kurtin PJ, et al. Diversity of organ site involvement among malignant lymphomas of mucosa-associated tissues. Am J Clin Pathol 1991;96:738–745.

884. Holland EA, Ghahremani GG, Fry WA, et al. Evolution of pulmonary pseudolymphomas: clinical and radiologic manifestations. J Thorac Imaging 1991;6:74–80.

885. O'Donnell PG, Jackson SA, Tung KT, et al. Radiological appearances of lymphomas arising from mucosa-associated lymphoid tissue (MALT) in the lung. Clin Radiol 1998;53:258–263.

886. Kennedy JL, Nathwani BN, Burke JS, et al. Pulmonary lymphomas and other pulmonary lymphoid lesions. A clinicopathologic and immunologic study of 64 patients. Cancer 1985;56:539–552.

887. King LJ, Padley SP, Wotherspoon AC, et al. Pulmonary MALT lymphoma: imaging findings in 24 cases. Eur Radiol 2000;10:1932–1938.

888. Kradin RL, Mark EJ. Benign lymphoid disorders of the lung, with a theory regarding their development. Hum Pathol 1983;14:857–867.

889. Bolton-Maggs PH, Colman A, Dixon GR, et al. Mucosa associated

lymphoma of the lung. Thorax 1993;48:670–672.

890. Cordier JF, Chailleux E, Lauque D, et al. Primary pulmonary lymphomas. A clinical study of 70 cases in nonimmunocompromised patients. Chest 1993;103:201–208.

891. Knisely BL, Mastey LA, Mergo PJ, et al. Pulmonary mucosa-associated lymphoid tissue lymphoma: CT and pathologic findings. AJR Am J Roentgenol 1999;172:1321–1326.

892. Lazar EB, Whitman GJ, Chew FS. Lymphoma of bronchus-associated lymphoid tissue. AJR Am J Roentgenol 1996;167:116.

893. McCulloch GL, Sinnatamby R, Stewart S, et al. High-resolution computed tomographic appearance of MALToma of the lung. Eur Radiol 1998;8: 1669–1673.

894. Bosanko CM, Korobkin M, Fantone JC, et al. Lobar primary pulmonary lymphoma: CT findings. J Comput Assist Tomogr 1991;15:679–682.

895. Lee DK, Im JG, Lee KS, et al. B-cell lymphoma of bronchus-associated lymphoid tissue (BALT): CT features in 10 patients. J Comput Assist Tomogr 2000;24:30–34.

896. Takamori M, Noma S, Kobashi Y, et al. CT findings of BALTOMA. Radiat Med 1999;17:349–354.

897. Guinee DG Jr, Perkins SL, Travis WD, et al. Proliferation and cellular phenotype in lymphomatoid granulomatosis: implications of a higher proliferation index in B cells. Am J Surg Pathol 1998;22:1093–1100.

898. Liebow AA, Carrington CR, Friedman PJ. Lymphomatoid granulomatosis. Hum Pathol 1972;3:457–558.

899. Pisani RJ, DeRemee RA. Clinical implications of the histopathologic diagnosis of pulmonary lymphomatoid granulomatosis. Mayo Clin Proc 1990;65:151–163.

900. Dee PM, Arora NS, Innes DJ Jr. The pulmonary manifestations of lymphomatoid granulomatosis. Radiology 1982;143:613–618.

901. Doyle TC. Lymphomatoid granulomatosis – the varying lung appearances in four cases. Australas Radiol 1983;27:139–142.

902. Glickstein M, Kornstein MJ, Pietra GG, et al. Nonlymphomatous lymphoid disorders of the lung. AJR Am J Roentgenol 1986;147:227–237.

903. Hicken P, Dobie JC, Frew E. The radiology of lymphomatoid granulomatosis in the lung. Clin Radiol 1979;30:661–664.

904. Prenovault JM, Weisbrod GL, Herman SJ. Lymphomatoid granulomatosis: a review of 12 cases. Can Assoc Radiol J 1988;39:263–266.

905. Voyvodic F, Whyte A. Lymphomatoid granulomatosis. Australas Radiol 1992;36:163–164.

906. Lee JS, Tuder R, Lynch DA. Lymphomatoid granulomatosis: radiologic features and pathologic correlations. AJR Am J Roentgenol 2000;175:1335–1339.

907. Israel HL, Patchefsky AS, Saldana MJ. Wegener's granulomatosis, lymphomatoid granulomatosis, and benign lymphocytic angiitis and granulomatosis of lung. Recognition and treatment. Ann Intern Med 1977;87:691–699.

908. Wechsler RJ, Steiner RM, Israel HL, et al. Chest radiograph in lymphomatoid granulomatosis: comparison with Wegener granulomatosis. AJR Am J Roentgenol 1984;142:79–83.

909. Mendelson DS, Apter S, Kirschner PA, et al. Magnetic resonance imaging and computed tomography findings in a patient with lymphomatoid granulomatosis. Clin Imaging 1989;13:130–133.

910. Mori S, Itoyama S, Mohri N, et al. Cellular characteristics of neoplastic angioendotheliosis. An immunohistological marker study of 6 cases. Virchows Arch A Pathol Anat Histopathol 1985;407:167–175.

911. Stroup RM, Sheibani K, Moncada A, et al. Angiotropic (intravascular) large cell lymphoma. A clinicopathologic study of seven cases with unique clinical presentations. Cancer 1990;66:1781–1788.

912. Yousem SA, Colby TV. Intravascular lymphomatosis presenting in the lung. Cancer 1990;65:349–353.

913. Honda N, Machida K, Kamano T, et al. Gallium scintigraphy in neoplastic angioendotheliosis of the lung. Clin Nucl Med 1991;16:43–46.

914. Nambu A, Kurihara Y, Ichikawa T, et al. Lung involvement in angiotropic lymphoma: CT findings. AJR Am J Roentgenol 1998;170:940–942.

915. Jang HJ, Lee KS, Han J. Intravascular lymphomatosis of the lung: radiologic findings. J Comput Assist Tomogr 1998;22:427–429.

916. Lee HJ, Im JG, Goo JM, et al. Peripheral T-cell lymphoma: spectrum of imaging findings with clinical and pathologic features. Radiographics 2003;23:7–26.

917. Gallagher CJ, Knowles GK, Habeshaw JA, et al. Early involvement of the bronchi in patients with malignant lymphoma. Br J Cancer 1983;48: 777–781.

918. Gollub MJ, Castellino RA. Diffuse endobronchial non-Hodgkin's lymphoma: CT demonstration. AJR Am J Roentgenol 1995;164: 1093–1094.

919. Kilgore TL, Chasen MH. Endobronchial non-Hodgkin's lymphoma. Chest 1983;84:58–61.

920. Mason AC, White CS. CT appearance of endobronchial non-Hodgkin lymphoma. J Comput Assist Tomogr 1994;18:559–561.

921. Kim KI, Lee JW, Lee MK, et al. Polypoid endobronchial Hodgkin's disease with pneumomediastinum. Br J Radiol 1999;72:392–394.

922. Aquino SL, Chen MY, Kuo WT, et al. The CT appearance of pleural and extrapleural disease in lymphoma. Clin Radiol 1999;54:647–650.

923. Carmel RJ, Kaplan HS. Mantle irradiation in Hodgkin's disease. An analysis of technique, tumor eradication, and complications. Cancer 1976;37:2813–2825.

924. Weick JK, Kiely JM, Harrison EG Jr, et al. Pleural effusion in lymphoma. Cancer 1973;31:848–853.

925. Dynes MC, White EM, Fry WA, et al. Imaging manifestations of pleural tumors. Radiographics 1992;12: 1191–1201.

926. Malatskey A, Fields S, Libson E. CT appearance of primary pleural lymphoma. Comput Med Imaging Graph 1989;13:165–167.

927. Nakatsuka S, Yao M, Hoshida Y, et al. Pyothorax-associated lymphoma: a review of 106 cases. J Clin Oncol 2002;20:4255–4260.

928. Kim Y, Lee SW, Choi HY, et al. A case of pyothorax-associated lymphoma simulating empyema necessitatis. Clin Imaging 2003;27:162–165.

929. Brun V, Revel MP, Danel C, et al. Case report. Pyothorax-associated lymphoma: Diagnosis at percutaneous core biopsy with CT guidance. AJR Am J Roentgenol 2003;180:969–971.

930. Ansari MQ, Dawson DB, Nador R, et al. Primary body cavity-based AIDS-related lymphomas. Am J Clin Pathol 1996;105:221–229.

931. Nador RG, Cesarman E, Chadburn A, et al. Primary effusion lymphoma: a distinct clinicopathologic entity associated with the Kaposi's sarcoma-associated herpes virus. Blood 1996;88:645–656.

932. Bergin CJ, Healy MV, Zincone GE, et al. MR evaluation of chest wall involvement in malignant lymphoma. J Comput Assist Tomogr 1990;14:928–932.

933. Carlsen SE, Bergin CJ, Hoppe RT. MR imaging to detect chest wall and pleural involvement in patients with lymphoma: effect on radiation therapy planning. AJR Am J Roentgenol 1993;160:1191–1195.

934. Khoury MB, Godwin JD, Halvorsen R, et al. Role of chest CT in non-Hodgkin lymphoma. Radiology 1986;158: 659–662.

935. Salonen O, Kivisaari L, Standertskjold-Nordenstam CG, et al. Chest radiography and computed tomography in the evaluation of mediastinal adenopathy in lymphoma. Acta Radiol 1987;28:747–750.

936. Hopper KD, Diehl LF, Lesar M, et al. Hodgkin disease: clinical utility of CT in initial staging and treatment. Radiology 1988;169:17–22.

937. Meyer JE, Linggood RM, Lindfors KK, et al. Impact of thoracic computed tomography on radiation therapy planning in Hodgkin disease. J Comput Assist Tomogr 1984;8:892–894.

938. Cohen MD, Siddiqui A, Weetman R, et al. Hodgkin disease and non-Hodgkin lymphomas in children: utilization of radiological modalities. Radiology 1986;158:499–505.

939. Wernecke K, Vassallo P, Hoffmann G, et al. Value of sonography in monitoring the therapeutic response of mediastinal lymphoma: comparison with chest radiography and CT. AJR Am J Roentgenol 1991;156:265–272.

940. Marglin SI, Laing FC, Castellino RA. Current status of mediastinal sonography in the posttreatment evaluation of patients with lymphoma. AJR Am J Roentgenol 1991;157:469–470.

941. Tesoro-Tess JD, Balzarini L, Ceglia E, et al. Magnetic resonance imaging in the initial staging of Hodgkin's disease and non-Hodgkin lymphoma. Eur J Radiol 1991;12:81–90.

942. Rehn SM, Nyman RS, Glimelius BL, et al. Non-Hodgkin lymphoma: predicting prognostic grade with MR imaging. Radiology 1990;176:249–253.

943. Fletcher BD, Kauffman WM, Kaste SC, et al. Use of Tl-201 to detect untreated pediatric Hodgkin disease. Radiology 1995;196:851–855.

944. Fox K, Silfen D, Alavi A. Applications of gallium-67 scintigraphy in the management of patients with malignant lymphoma. J Nucl Med 1991;32:2299–2305.

945. Lipp RW, Silly H, Ranner G, et al. Radiolabeled octreotide for the demonstration of somatostatin receptors in malignant lymphoma and lymphadenopathy. J Nucl Med 1995;36:13–18.

946. Tumeh SS, Rosenthal DS, Kaplan WD, et al. Lymphoma: evaluation with Ga-67 SPECT. Radiology 1987;164:111–114.

947. Kaplan WD, Jochelson MS, Herman TS, et al. Gallium-67 imaging: a predictor of residual tumor viability and clinical outcome in patients with diffuse large-cell lymphoma. J Clin Oncol 1990;8:1966–1970.

948. Front D, Bar-Shalom R, Mor M, et al. Hodgkin disease: prediction of outcome with 67Ga scintigraphy after one cycle of chemotherapy. Radiology 1999;210:487–491.

949. Front D, Bar-Shalom R, Mor M, et al. Aggressive non-Hodgkin lymphoma: early prediction of outcome with 67Ga scintigraphy. Radiology 2000;214:253–257.

950. Bangerter M, Kotzerke J, Griesshammer M, et al. Positron emission tomography with 18-fluorodeoxyglucose in the staging and follow-up of lymphoma in the chest. Acta Oncol 1999;38:799–804.

951. Moog F, Bangerter M, Diederichs CG, et al. Lymphoma: role of whole-body 2-deoxy-2-[F-18]fluoro-D-glucose (FDG) PET in nodal staging. Radiology 1997;203:795–800.

952. Moog F, Bangerter M, Diederichs CG, et al. Extranodal malignant lymphoma: detection with FDG PET versus CT. Radiology 1998;206:475–481.

953. Partridge S, Timothy A, O'Doherty MJ, et al. 2-Fluorine-18-fluoro-2-deoxy-D glucose positron emission tomography in the pretreatment staging of Hodgkin's disease: influence on patient management in a single institution. Ann Oncol 2000;11:1273–1279.

954. Cremerius U, Fabry U, Neuerburg J, et al. Positron emission tomography with 18F-FDG to detect residual disease after therapy for malignant lymphoma. Nucl Med Commun 1998;19:1055–1063.

955. Naumann R, Beuthien-Baumann B, Reiss A, et al. Substantial impact of FDG PET imaging on the therapy decision in patients with early stage Hodgkin's lymphoma. Br J Cancer 2004;90:620–625.

956. Jerusalem G, Beguin Y, Fassotte MF, et al. Whole-body positron emission tomography using ^{18}F-fluorodeoxyglucose for posttreatment evaluation in Hodgkin's disease and non-Hodgkin's lymphoma has higher diagnostic and prognostic value than classical computed tomography scan imaging. Blood 1999;94:429–433.

957. Travis WD, Galvin JR. Non-neoplastic pulmonary lymphoid lesions. Thorax 2001;56:964–971.

958. American Thoracic Society/European Respiratory Society International Multidisciplinary Consensus Classification of the Idiopathic Interstitial Pneumonias. This joint statement of the American Thoracic Society (ATS), and the European Respiratory Society (ERS) was adopted by the ATS board of directors, June 2001 and by the ERS Executive Committee, June 2001 Am J Respir Crit Care Med 2002;165:277–304.

959. Addis BJ, Hyjek E, Isaacson PG. Primary pulmonary lymphoma: a re-appraisal of its histogenesis and its relationship to pseudolymphoma and lymphoid interstitial pneumonia. Histopathology 1988;13:1–17.

960. Li G, Hansmann ML, Zwingers T, et al. Primary lymphomas of the lung: morphological, immunohistochemical and clinical features. Histopathology 1990;16:519–531.

961. Nicholson AG, Wotherspoon AC, Diss TC, et al. Pulmonary B-cell non-Hodgkin's lymphomas. The value of immunohistochemistry and gene analysis in diagnosis. Histopathology 1995;26:395–403.

962. Fiche M, Caprons F, Berger F, et al. Primary pulmonary non-Hodgkin's lymphomas. Histopathology 1995;26:529–537.

963. Abbondanzo SL, Rush W, Bijwaard KE, et al. Nodular lymphoid hyperplasia of the lung: a clinicopathologic study of 14 cases. Am J Surg Pathol 2000;24:587–597.

964. Klatte EC, Yardley J, Smith EB, et al. The pulmonary manifestations and complications of leukemia. AJR Am J Roentgenol 1963;89:598–609.

965. Maile CW, Moore AV, Ulreich S, et al. Chest radiographic-pathologic correlation in adult leukemia patients. Invest Radiol 1983;18:495–499.

966. Winer-Muram HT, Rubin SA, Fletcher BD, et al. Childhood leukemia: diagnostic accuracy of bedside chest radiography for severe pulmonary complications. Radiology 1994;193:127–133.

967. Kovalski R, Hansen-Flaschen J, Lodato RF, et al. Localized leukemic pulmonary infiltrates. Diagnosis by bronchoscopy and resolution with therapy. Chest 1990;97:674–678.

968. Seynaeve P, Mathijs R, Kockx M, et al. Case report: the air crescent sign in pulmonary leukaemic infiltrate. Clin Radiol 1992;45:40–41.

969. Heyneman LE, Johkoh T, Ward S, et al. Pulmonary leukemic infiltrates: high-resolution CT findings in 10 patients. AJR Am J Roentgenol 2000;174:517–521.

970. Tanaka N, Matsumoto T, Miura G, et al. CT findings of leukemic pulmonary infiltration with pathologic correlation. Eur Radiol 2002;12:166–174.

971. Desjardins A, Ostiguy G, Cousineau S, et al. Recurrent localised pneumonia due to bronchial infiltration in a patient with chronic lymphocytic leukaemia. Thorax 1990;45:570.

972. Lee MJ, Grogan L, Meehan S, et al. Pleural granulocytic sarcoma: CT characteristics. Clin Radiol 1991;43:57–59.

973. Neiman RS, Barcos M, Berard C, et al. Granulocytic sarcoma: a

clinicopathologic study of 61 biopsied cases. Cancer 1981;48:1426–1437.

974. Siegel MJ, Shackelford GD, McAlister WH. Pleural thickening. An unusual feature of childhood leukemia. Radiology 1981;138:367–369.

975. Kim FM, Fennessy JJ. Pleural thickening caused by leukemic infiltration: CT findings. AJR Am J Roentgenol 1994;162:293–294.

976. Takasugi JE, Godwin JD, Marglin SI, et al. Intrathoracic granulocytic sarcomas. J Thorac Imaging 1996;11:223–230.

977. Ooi GC, Chim CS, Khong PL, et al. Radiologic manifestations of granulocytic sarcoma in adult leukemia. AJR Am J Roentgenol 2001;176:1427–1431.

978. Hicklin GA, Drevyanko TF. Primary granulocytic sarcoma presenting with pleural and pulmonary involvement. Chest 1988;94:655–656.

979. Vernant JP, Brun B, Mannoni P, et al. Respiratory distress of hyperleukocytic granulocytic leukemias. Cancer 1979;44:264–268.

980. van Buchem MA, Wondergem JH, Kool LJ, et al. Pulmonary leukostasis: radiologic-pathologic study. Radiology 1987;165:739–741.

981. Myers TJ, Cole SR, Klatsky AU, et al. Respiratory failure due to pulmonary leukostasis following chemotherapy of acute nonlymphocytic leukemia. Cancer 1983;51:1808–1813.

982. England DM, Hochholzer L, McCarthy MJ. Localized benign and malignant fibrous tumors of the pleura. A clinicopathologic review of 223 cases. Am J Surg Pathol 1989;13:640–658.

983. Saifuddin A, Da Costa P, Chalmers AG, et al. Primary malignant localized fibrous tumours of the pleura: clinical, radiological and pathological features. Clin Radiol 1992;45:13–17.

984. Briselli M, Mark EJ, Dickersin GR. Solitary fibrous tumors of the pleura: eight new cases and review of 360 cases in the literature. Cancer 1981;47:2678–2689.

985. Cardillo G, Facciolo F, Cavazzana AO, et al. Localized (solitary) fibrous tumors of the pleura: an analysis of 55 patients. Ann Thorac Surg 2000;70:1808–1812.

986. Hill JK, Heitmiller RF, Askin FB, et al. Localized benign pleural mesothelioma arising in a radiation field. Clin Imaging 1997;21:189–194.

987. Ellis K, Wolff M. Mesotheliomas and secondary tumors of the pleura. Semin Roentgenol 1977;12:303–311.

988. de Perrot M, Kurt AM, Robert JH, et al. Clinical behavior of solitary fibrous tumors of the pleura. Ann Thorac Surg 1999;67:1456–1459.

989. Okike N, Bernatz PE, Woolner LB. Localized mesothelioma of the pleura: benign and malignant variants. J Thorac Cardiovasc Surg 1978;75:363–372.

990. Spizarny DL, Gross BH, Shepard JA. CT findings in localized fibrous mesothelioma of the pleural fissure. J Comput Assist Tomogr 1986;10:942–944.

991. Rosado-de-Christenson ML, Abbott GF, McAdams HP, et al. From the Archives of the AFIP: Localized Fibrous Tumors of the Pleura. Radiographics 2003;23:759–783.

992. Hahn PF, Novelline RA, Mark EJ. Arteriography in the localization of massive pleural tumors. AJR Am J Roentgenol 1982;139:814–817.

993. Scharifker D, Kaneko M. Localized fibrous "mesothelioma" of pleura (submesothelial fibroma): a clinicopathologic study of 18 cases. Cancer 1979;43:627–635.

994. Kinoshita T, Ishii K, Miyasato S. Localized pleural mesothelioma: CT and MR findings. Magn Reson Imaging 1997;15:377–379.

995. Chamberlain MH, Taggart DP. Solitary fibrous tumor associated with hypoglycemia: an example of the Doege-Potter syndrome. J Thorac Cardiovasc Surg 2000;119:185–187.

996. Karabulut N, Goodman LR. Pedunculated solitary fibrous tumor of the interlobar fissure: a wandering chest mass. AJR Am J Roentgenol 1999;173:476–477.

997. Desser TS, Stark P. Pictorial essay: solitary fibrous tumor of the pleura. J Thorac Imaging 1998;13:27–35.

998. Dedrick CG, McLoud TC, Shepard JA, et al. Computed tomography of localized pleural mesothelioma. AJR Am J Roentgenol 1985;144:275–280.

999. Lewis MI, Horak DA, Yellin A, et al. The case of the moving intrathoracic mass. Pedunculated benign localized pleural mesothelioma. Chest 1985;88:897–898.

1000. Weisbrod GL, Yee AC. Computed tomographic diagnosis of a pedunculated fibrous mesothelioma. J Can Assoc Radiol 1983;34:147–148.

1001. Soulen MC, Greco-Hunt VT, Templeton P. Cases from A3CR2. Migratory chest mass. Invest Radiol 1990;25:209–211.

1002. Ferretti GR, Chiles C, Choplin RH, et al. Localized benign fibrous tumors of the pleura. AJR Am J Roentgenol 1997;169:683–686.

1003. Lee KS, Im JG, Choe KO, et al. CT findings in benign fibrous mesothelioma of the pleura: pathologic correlation in nine patients. AJR Am J Roentgenol 1992;158:983–986.

1004. Mendelson DS, Meary E, Buy JN, et al. Localized fibrous pleural mesothelioma: CT findings. Clin Imaging 1991;15:105–108.

1005. Phillips CJ, Muller NL, Miller RR, et al. Large calcified pleural-based mass in the left hemithorax. Can Assoc Radiol J 1990;41:232–235.

1006. Truong M, Munden RF, Kemp BL. Localized fibrous tumor of the pleura. AJR Am J Roentgenol 2000;174:42.

1007. Tublin ME, Tessler FN, Rifkin MD. US case of the day. Solitary fibrous tumor of the pleura (SFTP). Radiographics 1998;18:523–525.

1008. Harris GN, Rozenshtein A, Schiff MJ. Benign fibrous mesothelioma of the pleura: MR imaging findings. AJR Am J Roentgenol 1995;165:1143–1144.

1009. Lee KS, Im JG. Benign fibrous mesothelioma of the pleura: MR findings (letter). AJR Am J Roentgenol 1993;160:205.

1010. George JC. Benign fibrous mesothelioma of the pleura: MR findings. AJR Am J Roentgenol 1993;160:204–205.

1011. Padovani B, Mouroux J, Raffaelli C, et al. Benign fibrous mesothelioma of the pleura: MR study and pathologic correlation. Eur Radiol 1996;6:425–428.

1012. Tateishi U, Nishihara H, Morikawa T, et al. Solitary fibrous tumor of the pleura: MR appearance and enhancement pattern. J Comput Assist Tomogr 2002;26:174–179.

1013. Antman KH. Clinical presentation and natural history of benign and malignant mesothelioma. Semin Oncol 1981;8:313–320.

1014. Kawashima A, Libshitz HI. Malignant pleural mesothelioma: CT manifestations in 50 cases. AJR Am J Roentgenol 1990;155:965–969.

1015. Brenner J, Sordillo PP, Magill GB, et al. Malignant mesothelioma of the pleura: review of 123 patients. Cancer 1982;49:2431–2435.

1016. Antman KH, Corson JM. Benign and malignant pleural mesothelioma. Clin Chest Med 1985;6:127–140.

1017. Hillerdal G. Malignant mesothelioma 1982: review of 4710 published cases. Br J Dis Chest 1983;77:321–343.

1018. Aisner J, Wiernik PH. Malignant mesothelioma. Current status and future prospects. Chest 1978;74:438–444.

1019. Erzen C, Eryilmaz M, Kalyoncu F, et al. CT findings in malignant pleural mesothelioma related to nonoccupational exposure to asbestos and fibrous zeolite (erionite). J Comput Assist Tomogr 1991;15:256–260.

1020. Behling CA, Wolf PL, Haghighi P. AIDS and malignant mesothelioma —is there a connection? Chest 1993;103:1268–1269.

1021. Anderson KA, Hurley WC, Hurley BT, et al. Malignant pleural mesothelioma following radiotherapy in a 16-year-old boy. Cancer 1985;56:273–276.

1022. Legha SS, Muggia FM. Pleural mesothelioma: clinical features and therapeutic implications. Ann Intern Med 1977;87:613–621.

1023. Adams VI, Unni KK, Muhm JR, et al. Diffuse malignant mesothelioma of pleura. Diagnosis and survival in 92 cases. Cancer 1986;58:1540–1551.

1024. Sugarbaker DJ, Garcia JP, Richards WG, et al. Extrapleural pneumonectomy in the multimodality therapy of malignant pleural mesothelioma. Results in 120 consecutive patients. Ann Surg 1996;224:288–294.

1025. Otis CN, Carter D, Cole S, et al. Immunohistochemical evaluation of pleural mesothelioma and pulmonary adenocarcinoma. A bi-institutional study of 47 cases. Am J Surg Pathol 1987;11:445–456.

1026. Andrion A, Mazzucco G, Bernardi P, et al. Sarcomatous tumor of the chest wall with osteochondroid differentiation. Evidence of mesothelial origin. Am J Surg Pathol 1989;13:707–712.

1027. Raizon A, Schwartz A, Hix W, et al. Calcification as a sign of sarcomatous degeneration of malignant pleural mesotheliomas: a new CT finding. J Comput Assist Tomogr 1996;20:42–44.

1028. AJCC. AJCC Cancer Staging Handbook. New York: Springer, 2002.

1029. Rusch VW. A proposed new international TNM staging system for malignant pleural mesothelioma. From the International Mesothelioma Interest Group. Chest 1995;108:1122–1128.

1030. Rusch VW, Venkatraman E. The importance of surgical staging in the treatment of malignant pleural mesothelioma. J Thorac Cardiovasc Surg 1996;111:815–825.

1031. Patz EF Jr, Rusch VW, Heelan R. The proposed new international TNM staging system for malignant pleural mesothelioma: application to imaging. AJR Am J Roentgenol 1996;166:323–327.

1032. Grant DC, Seltzer SE, Antman KH, et al. Computed tomography of malignant pleural mesothelioma. J Comput Assist Tomogr 1983;7:626–632.

1033. Law MR, Gregor A, Husband JE, et al. Computed tomography in the assessment of malignant mesothelioma of the pleura. Clin Radiol 1982;33:67–70.

1034. Leung AN, Müller NL, Miller RR. CT in differential diagnosis of diffuse pleural disease. AJR Am J Roentgenol 1990;154:487–492.

1035. Libshitz HI. Malignant pleural mesothelioma: the role of computed tomography. J Comput Tomogr 1984;8:15–20.

1036. Lorigan JG, Libshitz HI. MR imaging of malignant pleural mesothelioma. J Comput Assist Tomogr 1989;13:617–620.

1037. Miller BH, Rosado-de-Christenson ML, Mason AC, et al. From the archives of the AFIP. Malignant pleural mesothelioma: radiologic-pathologic correlation. Radiographics 1996;16:613–644.

1038. Mirvis S, Dutcher JP, Haney PJ, et al. CT of malignant pleural mesothelioma. AJR Am J Roentgenol 1983;140:665–670.

1039. Patz EF Jr, Shaffer K, Piwnica-Worms DR, et al. Malignant pleural mesothelioma: value of CT and MR imaging in predicting resectability. AJR Am J Roentgenol 1992;159:961–966.

1040. Wechsler RJ, Rao VM, Steiner RM. The radiology of thoracic malignant mesothelioma. Crit Rev Diagn Imaging 1984;20:283–310.

1041. Ng CS, Munden RF, Libshitz HI. Malignant pleural mesothelioma: the spectrum of manifestations on CT in 70 cases. Clin Radiol 1999;54:415–421.

1042. Knuuttila A, Kivisaari L, Kivisaari A, et al. Evaluation of pleural disease using MR and CT. With special reference to malignant pleural mesothelioma. Acta Radiol 2001;42:502–507.

1043. Rusch VW, Godwin JD, Shuman WP. The role of computed tomography scanning in the initial assessment and the follow-up of malignant pleural mesothelioma. J Thorac Cardiovasc Surg 1988;96:171–177.

1044. Heelan RT, Rusch VW, Begg CB, et al. Staging of malignant pleural mesothelioma: comparison of CT and MR imaging. AJR Am J Roentgenol 1999;172:1039–1047.

1045. Gerbaudo VH, Sugarbaker DJ, Britz-Cunningham S, et al. Assessment of malignant pleural mesothelioma with (18)F-FDG dual-head gamma-camera coincidence imaging: comparison with histopathology. J Nucl Med 2002;43:1144–1149.

1046. Rabinowitz JG, Efremidis SC, Cohen B, et al. A comparative study of mesothelioma and asbestosis using computed tomography and conventional chest radiography. Radiology 1982;144:453–460.

1047. Nichols DM, Johnson MA. Calcification in a pleural mesothelioma. J Can Assoc Radiol 1983;34:311–313.

1048. Carretta A, Landoni C, Melloni G, et al. 18-FDG positron emission tomography in the evaluation of malignant pleural diseases – a pilot study. Eur J Cardiothorac Surg 2000;17:377–383.

1049. Benard F, Sterman D, Smith RJ, et al. Metabolic imaging of malignant pleural mesothelioma with fluorodeoxyglucose positron emission tomography. Chest 1998;114:713–722.

1050. Muller NL. Imaging of the pleura. Radiology 1993;186:297–309.

1051. Benard F, Sterman D, Smith RJ, et al. Prognostic value of FDG PET imaging in malignant pleural mesothelioma. J Nucl Med 1999;40:1241–1245.

1052. Evans AR, Wolstenholme RJ, Shettar SP, et al. Primary pleural liposarcoma. Thorax 1985;40:554–555.

1053. Buxton RC, Tan CS, Khine NM, et al. Atypical transmural thoracic lipoma: CT diagnosis. J Comput Assist Tomogr 1988;12:196–198.

1054. Epler GR, McLoud TC, Munn CS, et al. Pleural lipoma. Diagnosis by computed tomography. Chest 1986;90:265–268.

1055. Gramiak R, Koerner HJ. A roentgen diagnostic observation in subpleural lipoma. Am J Roentgenol Radium Ther Nucl Med 1966;98:465–467.

1056. McLoud TC, Flower CD. Imaging the pleura: sonography, CT, and MR imaging. AJR Am J Roentgenol 1991;156:1145–1153.

1057. Munk PL, Müller NL. Pleural liposarcoma: CT diagnosis. J Comput Assist Tomogr 1988;12:709–710.

1058. Wong WW, Pluth JR, Grado GL, et al. Liposarcoma of the pleura. Mayo Clin Proc 1994;69:882–885.

1059. Iqbal M, Posen J, Bhuiya TA, et al. Lymphocyte-rich pleural liposarcoma mimicking pericardial cyst. J Thorac Cardiovasc Surg 2000;120:610–612.

1060. Shanley DJ, Mulligan ME. Osteosarcoma with isolated metastases to the pleura. Pediatr Radiol 1991;21:226.

1061. Kravis MM, Hutton LC. Solitary plasma cell tumor of the pleura manifested as massive hemothorax. AJR Am J Roentgenol 1993;161:543–544.

1062. Lin BT, Colby T, Gown AM, et al. Malignant vascular tumors of the serous membranes mimicking mesothelioma. A report of 14 cases. Am J Surg Pathol 1996;20:1431–1439.

1063. Crotty EJ, McAdams HP, Erasmus JJ, et al. Epithelioid hemangioendothelioma of the pleura: clinical and radiologic features. AJR Am J Roentgenol 2000;175:1545–1549.

1064. Coppage L, Shaw C, Curtis AM. Metastatic disease to the chest in patients with extrathoracic malignancy. J Thorac Imaging 1987;2:24–37.

1065. Crow J, Slavin G, Kreel L. Pulmonary metastasis: a pathologic and radiologic study. Cancer 1981;47:2595–2602.

1066. Davis SD. CT evaluation for pulmonary metastases in patients with extrathoracic malignancy. Radiology 1991;180:1–12.

1067. Gross BH, Glazer GM, Bookstein FL. Multiple pulmonary nodules detected by computed tomography: diagnostic implications. J Comput Assist Tomogr 1985;9:880–885.

1068. Hirakata K, Nakata H, Haratake J. Appearance of pulmonary metastases on high-resolution CT scans: comparison with histopathologic findings from autopsy specimens. AJR Am J Roentgenol 1993;161:37–43.

1069. Hirakata K, Nakata H, Nakagawa T. CT of pulmonary metastases with pathological correlation. Semin Ultrasound CT MR 1995;16:379–394.

1070. Kundu S, Murphy J, Towers M, et al. Computed tomographic demonstration of very-low-density pulmonary nodules in metastatic gastric carcinoma: case report. Can Assoc Radiol J 1999;50:198–201.

1071. Yousem DM, Scatarige JC, Fishman EK, et al. Low-attenuation thoracic metastases in testicular malignancy. AJR Am J Roentgenol 1986;146:291–293.

1072. Seo JB, Im JG, Goo JM, et al. Atypical pulmonary metastases: spectrum of radiologic findings. Radiographics 2001;21:403–417.

1073. Benditt JO, Farber HW, Wright J, et al. Pulmonary hemorrhage with diffuse alveolar infiltrates in men with high-volume choriocarcinoma. Ann Intern Med 1988;109:674–675.

1074. Nirenberg A, Meikle GR, Goldstein D, et al. Metastatic carcinoma infiltrating lung mimicking BOOP. Australas Radiol 1995;39:405–407.

1075. Gaeta M, Volta S, Scribano E, et al. Air-space pattern in lung metastasis from adenocarcinoma of the GI tract. J Comput Assist Tomogr 1996;20:300–304.

1076. Herold CJ, Bankier AA, Fleischmann D. Lung metastases. Eur Radiol 1996;6:596–606.

1077. Libshitz HI, North LB. Pulmonary metastases. Radiol Clin North Am 1982;20:437–451.

1078. Patel AM, Ryu JH. Angiosarcoma in the lung. Chest 1993;103:1531–1535.

1079. Ren H, Hruban RH, Kuhlman JE, et al. Computed tomography of inflation-fixed lungs: the beaded septum sign of pulmonary metastases. J Comput Assist Tomogr 1989;13:411–416.

1080. Milne EN, Zerhouni EA. Blood supply of pulmonary metastases. J Thorac Imaging 1987;2:15–23.

1081. Murata K, Takahashi M, Mori M, et al. Pulmonary metastatic nodules: CT-pathologic correlation. Radiology 1992;182:331–335.

1082. Chaudhuri MR. Cavitary pulmonary metastases. Thorax 1970;25:375–381.

1083. Dodd GD, Bozeman PM. Excavating pulmonary metastases. AJR Am J Roentgenol 1961;85:277–293.

1084. Alexander PW, Sanders C, Nath H. Cavitary pulmonary metastases in transitional cell carcinoma of urinary bladder. AJR Am J Roentgenol 1990;154:493–494.

1085. Godwin JD, Webb WR, Savoca CJ, et al. Multiple, thin-walled cystic lesions of the lung. AJR Am J Roentgenol 1980;135:593–604.

1086. Chan DP, Griffith JF, Lee TW, et al. Cystic pulmonary metastases from epithelioid cell sarcoma. Ann Thorac Surg 2003;75:1652–1654.

1087. Jimenez JM, Casey SO, Citron M, et al. Calcified pulmonary metastases from medullary carcinoma of the thyroid. Comput Med Imaging Graph 1995;19:325–328.

1088. Maile CW, Rodan BA, Godwin JD, et al. Calcification in pulmonary metastases. Br J Radiol 1982;55:108–113.

1089. Cockshott WP, Hendrickse JP. Pulmonary calcification at the site of trophoblastic metastases. Br J Radiol 1969;42:17–20.

1090. Webb WR, Gamsu G. Thoracic metastasis in malignant melanoma. A radiographic survey of 65 patients. Chest 1977;71:176–181.

1091. Dwyer AJ, Reichert CM, Woltering EA, et al. Diffuse pulmonary metastasis in melanoma: radiographic-pathologic correlation. AJR Am J Roentgenol 1984;143:983–984.

1092. Chen JT, Dahmash NS, Ravin CE, et al. Metastatic melanoma in the thorax: report of 130 patients. AJR Am J Roentgenol 1981;137:293–298.

1093. Toye R, Jones DK, Armstrong P, et al. Numerous pulmonary metastases from renal cell carcinoma confined to the middle lobe. Clin Radiol 1990;42:443–444.

1094. Libshitz HI, Jing BS, Wallace S, et al. Sterilized metastases: a diagnostic and therapeutic dilemma. AJR Am J Roentgenol 1983;140:15–19.

1095. Swett HA, Westcott JL. Residual nonmalignant pulmonary nodules in choriocarcinoma. Chest 1974;65:560–562.

1096. Vogelzang NJ, Stenlund R. Residual pulmonary nodules after combination chemotherapy of testicular cancer. Radiology 1983;146:195–197.

1097. Sella A, Logothetis CJ, Dexeus FH, et al. Pulmonary air cyst associated with combination chemotherapy containing bleomycin. AJR Am J Roentgenol 1989;153:191.

1098. Charig MJ, Williams MP. Pulmonary lacunae: sequelae of metastases following chemotherapy. Clin Radiol 1990;42:93–96.

1099. Panicek DM, Toner GC, Heelan RT, et al. Nonseminomatous germ cell tumors: enlarging masses despite chemotherapy. Radiology 1990;175:499–502.

1100. Williams MP, Husband JE, Heron CW. Intrathoracic manifestations of metastatic testicular seminoma: a comparison of chest radiographic and CT findings. AJR Am J Roentgenol 1987;149:473–475.

1101. McLoud TC, Kalisher L, Stark P, et al. Intrathoracic lymph node metastases from extrathoracic neoplasms. AJR Am J Roentgenol 1978;131:403–407.

1102. Correa J, Souto M, Tahoces PG, et al. Digital chest radiography: comparison of unprocessed and processed images in the detection of solitary pulmonary nodules. Radiology 1995;195:253–258.

1103. Croisille P, Souto M, Cova M, et al. Pulmonary nodules: improved detection with vascular segmentation and extraction with spiral CT. Work in progress. Radiology 1995;197:397–401.

1104. Kobayashi T, Xu XW, MacMahon H, et al. Effect of a computer-aided diagnosis scheme on radiologists' performance in detection of lung nodules on radiographs. Radiology 1996;199:843–848.

1105. MacMahon H. Improvement in detection of pulmonary nodules: digital image processing and computer-aided diagnosis. Radiographics 2000;20:1169–1177.

1106. Difazio MC, MacMahon H, Xu XW, et al. Digital chest radiography: effect of temporal subtraction images on detection accuracy. Radiology 1997;202:447–452.

1107. Remy-Jardin M, Remy J, Giraud F, et al. Pulmonary nodules: detection with thick-section spiral CT versus conventional CT. Radiology 1993;187:513–520.

1108. Costello P, Anderson W, Blume D. Pulmonary nodule: evaluation with spiral volumetric CT. Radiology 1991;179:875–876.

1109. Diederich S, Semik M, Lentschig MG, et al. Helical CT of pulmonary nodules in patients with extrathoracic malignancy: CT-surgical correlation. AJR Am J Roentgenol 1999;172:353–360.

1110. Buckley JA, Scott WW Jr, Siegelman SS, et al. Pulmonary nodules: effect of increased data sampling on detection with spiral CT and confidence in diagnosis. Radiology 1995;196:395–400.

1111. Diederich S, Lentschig MG, Winter F, et al. Detection of pulmonary nodules with overlapping vs non-overlapping image reconstruction at spiral CT. Eur Radiol 1999;9:281–286.

1112. Seltzer SE, Judy PF, Adams DF, et al. Spiral CT of the chest: comparison of cine and film-based viewing. Radiology 1995;197:73–78.

1113. Waters DJ, Coakley FV, Cohen MD, et al. The detection of pulmonary metastases by helical CT: a clinicopathologic study in dogs. J Comput Assist Tomogr 1998; 22:235–240.

1114. Coakley FV, Cohen MD, Johnson MS, et al. Maximum intensity projection images in the detection of simulated pulmonary nodules by spiral CT. Br J Radiol 1998;71:135–140.

1115. Gruden JF, Ouanounou S, Tigges S, et al. Incremental benefit of maximum-intensity-projection images on observer detection of small pulmonary nodules revealed by multidetector CT. AJR Am J Roentgenol 2002;179: 149–157.

1116. Grampp S, Bankier AA, Zoubek A, et al. Spiral CT of the lung in children with malignant extra-thoracic tumors: distribution of benign vs malignant pulmonary nodules. Eur Radiol 2000;10:1318–1322.

1117. Chalmers N, Best JJ. The significance of pulmonary nodules detected by CT but not by chest radiography in tumour staging. Clin Radiol 1991;44:410–412.

1118. Husband JE, Barrett A, Peckham MJ. Evaluation of computed tomography in the management of testicular teratoma. Br J Urol 1981;53:179–183.

1119. Fishman EK, Kuhlman JE, Schuchter LM, et al. CT of malignant melanoma in the chest, abdomen, and musculoskeletal system. Radiographics 1990;10:603–620.

1120. Heaston DK, Putman CE, Rodan BA, et al. Solitary pulmonary metastases in high-risk melanoma patients: a prospective comparison of conventional and computed tomography. AJR Am J Roentgenol 1983;141:169–174.

1121. Kostrubiak I, Whitley NO, Aisner J, et al. The use of computed body tomography in malignant melanoma. JAMA 1988;259:2896–2897.

1122. Chiles C, Ravin CE. Intrathoracic metastasis from an extrathoracic malignancy: a radiographic approach to patient evaluation. Radiol Clin North Am 1985;23:427–438.

1123. Lim DJ, Carter MF. Computerized tomography in the preoperative staging for pulmonary metastases in patients with renal cell carcinoma. J Urol 1993;150:1112–1114.

1124. Curtis AM, Ravin CE, Collier PE, et al. Detection of metastatic disease from carcinoma of the breast: limited value of full lung tomography. AJR Am J Roentgenol 1980;134:253–255.

1125. Matthay RA, Arroliga AC. Resection of pulmonary metastases. Am Rev Respir Dis 1993;148:1691–1696.

1126. Mountain CF, McMurtrey MJ, Hermes KE. Surgery for pulmonary metastasis: a 20-year experience. Ann Thorac Surg 1984;38:323–330.

1127. Kandioler D, Kromer E, Tuchler H, et al. Long-term results after repeated surgical removal of pulmonary metastases. Ann Thorac Surg 1998;65:909–912.

1128. Groeger AM, Kandioler D, Mueller MR, et al. Survival after surgical treatment of recurrent pulmonary metastases. Eur J Cardiothorac Surg 1997;12:703–705.

1129. Pastorino U, Buyse M, Friedel G, et al. Long-term results of lung metastasectomy: prognostic analyses based on 5206 cases. The International Registry of Lung Metastases. J Thorac Cardiovasc Surg 1997;113:37–49.

1130. Cerfolio RJ, Allen MS, Deschamps C, et al. Pulmonary resection of metastatic renal cell carcinoma. Ann Thorac Surg 1994;57:339–344.

1131. McCormack PM, Burt ME, Bains MS, et al. Lung resection for colorectal metastases. 10-year results. Arch Surg 1992;127:1403–1406.

1132. McAfee MK, Allen MS, Trastek VF, et al. Colorectal lung metastases: results of surgical excision. Ann Thorac Surg 1992;53:780–785.

1133. Okumura S, Kondo H, Tsuboi M, et al. Pulmonary resection for metastatic colorectal cancer: experiences with 159 patients. J Thorac Cardiovasc Surg 1996;112:867–874.

1134. Robert JH, Ambrogi V, Mermillod B, et al. Factors influencing long-term survival after lung metastasectomy. Ann Thorac Surg 1997;63:777–784.

1135. Saito Y, Omiya H, Kohno K, et al. Pulmonary metastasectomy for 165 patients with colorectal carcinoma: A prognostic assessment. J Thorac Cardiovasc Surg 2002;124:1007–1013.

1136. Pogrebniak HW, Roth JA, Steinberg SM, et al. Reoperative pulmonary resection in patients with metastatic soft tissue sarcoma. Ann Thorac Surg 1991;52:197–203.

1137. Robinson MH, Sheppard M, Moskovic E, et al. Lung metastasectomy in patients with soft tissue sarcoma. Br J Radiol 1994;67:129–135.

1138. Gorenstein LA, Putnam JB, Natarajan G, et al. Improved survival after resection of pulmonary metastases from malignant melanoma. Ann Thorac Surg 1991;52:204–210.

1139. Moores DW. Pulmonary metastases revisited. Ann Thorac Surg 1991;52: 178–179.

1140. Tafra L, Dale PS, Wanek LA, et al. Resection and adjuvant immunotherapy for melanoma metastatic to the lung and thorax.

J Thorac Cardiovasc Surg 1995; 110:119–128.

1141. Lefor AT, Bredenberg CE, Kellman RM, et al. Multiple malignancies of the lung and head and neck. Second primary tumor or metastasis? Arch Surg 1986;121:265–270.

1142. Cahan WG, Castro EB, Hajdu SI. Proceedings: The significance of a solitary lung shadow in patients with colon carcinoma. Cancer 1974;33: 414–421.

1143. Feuerstein IM, Jicha DL, Pass HI, et al. Pulmonary metastases: MR imaging with surgical correlation – a prospective study. Radiology 1992;182:123–129.

1144. Panicek DM. MR imaging for pulmonary metastases? Radiology 1992;182:10–11.

1145. Kersjes W, Mayer E, Buchenroth M, et al. Diagnosis of pulmonary metastases with turbo-SE MR imaging. Eur Radiol 1997;7:1190–1194.

1146. Bohdiewicz PJ, Juni JE, Ball D, et al. Krukenberg tumor and lung metastases from colon carcinoma diagnosed with F-18 FDG PET. Clin Nucl Med 1995;20:419–420.

1147. Connolly LP, Bloom DA, Kozakewich H, et al. Localization of Tc-99m MDP in neuroblastoma metastases to the liver and lung. Clin Nucl Med 1996;21: 629–633.

1148. Pevarski DJ, Drane WE, Scarborough MT. The usefulness of bone scintigraphy with SPECT images for detection of pulmonary metastases from osteosarcoma. AJR Am J Roentgenol 1998;170:319–322.

1149. Braman SS, Whitcomb ME. Endobronchial metastasis. Arch Intern Med 1975;135:543–547.

1150. Baumgartner WA, Mark JB. Metastatic malignancies from distant sites to the tracheobronchial tree. J Thorac Cardiovasc Surg 1980;79:499–503.

1151. Carlin BW, Harrell JH, Olson LK, et al. Endobronchial metastases due to colorectal carcinoma. Chest 1989;96: 1110–1114.

1152. Heitmiller RF, Marasco WJ, Hruban RH, et al. Endobronchial metastasis. J Thorac Cardiovasc Surg 1993;106: 537–542.

1153. Plavsic BM, Robinson AE, Freundlich IM, et al. Melanoma metastatic to the bronchus: radiologic features in two patients. J Thorac Imaging 1994;9: 67–70.

1154. Albertini RE, Ekberg NL. Endobronchial metastasis in breast cancer. Thorax 1980;35:435–440.

1155. Ikezoe J, Johkoh T, Takeuchi N, et al. CT findings of endobronchial metastasis. Acta Radiol 1991;32:455–460.

1156. Janower ML, Blennerhassett JB. Lymphangitic spread of metastatic cancer to the lung. A radiologic-pathologic classification. Radiology 1971;101:267–273.

1157. Trapnell DH. The radiological appearances of lymphangitis carcinomatosa of the lung. Thorax 1964;19:251–260.

1158. Johkoh T, Ikezoe J, Tomiyama N, et al. CT findings in lymphangitic carcinomatosis of the lung: correlation with histologic findings and pulmonary function tests. AJR Am J Roentgenol 1992;158:1217–1222.

1159. Munk PL, Müller NL, Miller RR, et al. Pulmonary lymphangitic carcinomatosis: CT and pathologic findings. Radiology 1988;166:705–709.

1160. Stein MG, Mayo J, Muller N, et al. Pulmonary lymphangitic spread of carcinoma: appearance on CT scans. Radiology 1987;162:371–375.

1161. Anderson CB, Philpott GW, Ferguson TB. The treatment of malignant pleural effusions. Cancer 1974;33:916–922.

1162. Fentiman IS, Millis R, Sexton S, et al. Pleural effusion in breast cancer: a review of 105 cases. Cancer 1981;47:2087–2092.

1163. Matthay RA, Coppage L, Shaw C, et al. Malignancies metastatic to the pleura. Invest Radiol 1990;25:601–619.

1164. Hough DM. Multifocal osteosarcoma with extensive pleural metastatic disease. Australas Radiol 1992;36:147–149.

1165. Meyer PC. Metastatic carcinoma of the pleura. Thorax 1966;21:437–443.

1166. Light RW. Pleural disease. Philadelphia: Lippincott, Williams and Wilkins, 1995.

1167. Berger HW, Maher G. Decreased glucose concentration in malignant pleural effusions. Am Rev Respir Dis 1971;103:427–429.

1168. Light RW, Ball WC Jr. Glucose and amylase in pleural effusions. JAMA 1973;225:257–259.

1169. Mori K, Hirose T, Machida S, et al. Helical computed tomography diagnosis of pleural dissemination in lung cancer: comparison of thick-section and thin-section helical computed tomography. J Thorac Imaging 1998;13:211–218.

1170. Goerg C, Schwerk WB, Goerg K, et al. Pleural effusion: an "acoustic window" for sonography of pleural metastases. J Clin Ultrasound 1991;19:93–97.

1171. Steinberg HV, Erwin BC. Metastases to the pleura: sonographic detection. J Clin Ultrasound 1987;15:276–279.

CHAPTER 14

Mediastinal and aortic disease

MEDIASTINAL DISEASES

Imaging techniques

The chest radiograph is usually the first imaging study obtained in a patient with a known or suspected mediastinal or hilar mass. Furthermore, mediastinal or hilar abnormalities are often discovered serendipitously on chest radiographs obtained for other purposes. Thus, the role of chest radiography for detection of hilar and mediastinal abnormalities remains essential and thorough knowledge of the relevant radiographic anatomy is of utmost importance to the practising radiologist.

Despite the advent of cross-sectional imaging techniques, such as CT or MRI, the chest radiograph remains important for localization of the mass (useful for formulating an appropriate differential diagnosis) and, in some instances, for characterization of the lesion. Some abnormalities, such as vascular lesions or mediastinal lipomatosis, may have a sufficiently characteristic appearance on the chest radiograph to obviate further evaluation. Findings of calcification within the mass on chest radiography can also be a clue to the correct diagnosis.

However, in the great majority of cases, once a mediastinal or hilar abnormality is detected, or at least suspected, on the chest radiograph, cross-sectional imaging is performed. CT or MRI are used to assess the location and extent of the abnormality and, because of their superior contrast resolution when compared to radiography, are also used to characterize the tissue components of the mass. CT or MRI are also quite useful for distinguishing vascular lesions or benign processes of the mediastinum, such as lipomatosis, from true pathologic conditions that warrant further investigation.

Ultrasound can also be useful for imaging mediastinal abnormalities in selected patients. Because it does not use ionizing radiation, ultrasound may be preferred to CT for evaluation of some mediastinal masses in children, such as mediastinal cysts.[1] If the lesion is believed to be related to the heart or great vessels, either transthoracic or endoscopic ultrasound may be the first line of investigation. Furthermore, ultrasound can be useful for guiding biopsy of mediastinal masses.[2]

Although cross-sectional imaging is primarily used to evaluate abnormalities detected by radiography, it may also be performed in certain situations when the chest radiograph is normal. For example, CT may be performed in patients with myasthenia gravis even if the chest radiograph is normal, because of the strong association between myasthenia gravis and thymoma. Furthermore, malignancies such as lung cancer have a predilection to metastasize to mediastinal lymph nodes. These metastases may not be visible on the chest radiograph and CT is used to further assess the mediastinal nodes in such patients.

In most centers, CT is the mainstay for the evaluation of known or suspected mediastinal or hilar abnormalities. However, because of its multiplanar capabilities and high contrast resolution compared to CT, MRI is sometimes used to further evaluate the location and extent of mediastinal or hilar disease. Further, MRI is probably the modality of choice for imaging suspected neurogenic tumors because it not only shows the size, location, and internal features of the lesions, but because it also clearly depicts spinal involvement.[3] MRI is also useful for confirming the cystic nature of mediastinal lesions that appear solid on CT, such as bronchogenic cysts, and for demonstrating

vascular structures in patients for whom administration of iodinated intravenous contrast is contraindicated.[3] Two potential disadvantages of MRI compared to CT are its poor demonstration of calcification and comparatively poorer spatial resolution.

Recent advances in CT imaging, e.g. single- and multi-detector spiral CT, have further improved the ability of CT to image the mediastinum.[3] By significantly shortening scan time, respiratory motion artifacts are limited and, in some instances, the total dose of iodinated contrast can be reduced.[4] Spiral CT data sets can also be effectively reconstructed in a variety of nonaxial planes, often facilitating interpretation of mediastinal abnormalities. The application of nonaxial two- and three-dimensional (2D and 3D) reconstruction techniques has proved most useful for imaging abnormalities of the central airways and great vessels.[5,6] By presenting anatomic information in a context more familiar to referring clinicians, these reconstructed images may show the location and extent of an abnormality in a way that radiologic reports and axial CT images do not.

Positron emission tomography (PET) is a physiologic imaging technique that uses metabolic markers labeled with positron emitting radionuclides, such as ^{18}F, ^{11}C, or ^{15}O.[7] ^{18}F-2-deoxy-D-glucose (^{18}F-FDG), a D-glucose analog labeled with ^{18}F, is ideally suited for tumor imaging.[8] PET performed with this agent (^{18}F-FDG PET) exploits the differences in glucose metabolism between normal and neoplastic cells. After intravenous administration, ^{18}F-FDG preferentially accumulates in neoplastic cells, allowing accurate, noninvasive differentiation of benign from malignant abnormalities by PET imaging.[9] ^{18}F-FDG PET imaging has proved quite useful for staging patients with a variety of systemic malignancies that affect the mediastinum, including lymphoma and lung cancer.[10,11] Thus far, ^{18}F-FDG PET imaging has only had a limited role in the evaluation of more localized mediastinal processes, such as thymoma.[12] In these tumors, accurate information about the location and anatomic extent of disease, as provided by MRI or CT, may be of greater importance than the assessment of metabolic activity of the tumor.

CT PET imaging is the latest advance.[13] These scanners combine both a PET and a high speed spiral CT machine and provide images that accurately show both the anatomic extent and location of the abnormalities, as well as their metabolic activity. Whether this type of imaging represents a significant improvement over available techniques for imaging mediastinal and hilar disorders is not known yet.

Incidence of mediastinal masses

The relative incidence of various mediastinal lesions is difficult to ascertain because most published series are biased toward patients whose lesions undergo biopsy or resection. Some common mediastinal masses, such as thyroid goiter, aortic aneurysms, or lymphadenopathy, and patients with previously established diagnoses such as lymphoma or sarcoidosis may be underrepresented in many surgical reviews. The relative incidence of lesions in several large series is shown in Table 14.1. In the Mayo Clinic series,[14] about 75% of mediastinal masses in both adults and children were benign and completely respectable, and 25% were malignant. The authors highlighted the significant differences in the relative frequencies of mediastinal lesions in children and adults. Neurogenic tumors, germ cell neoplasms, and foregut cysts accounted for almost 80% of the masses seen in children. Conversely, primary thymic

Table 14.1 Incidence (%) of mediastinal masses

Series	Wychulis et al[14]	Benjamin et al[18]	Cohen et al[19]	Azarow et al[15]		Whooley et al[20]	Temes et al[16†]		Takeda et al[17]	
Population	All	All	All	Pediatric	Adult	All	Adult	Pediatric	Adult	Pediatric
Number	1064	214	230	62	195	124	197	22	676	130
Neurogenic	20	23	17	32	12	12	1	23	11	46
Thymic	19	21	24	33	26	33	16	0	36	4
Lymphoma	10	15	16	6	21	19	55	55	12	13
Germ cell	9	13	10	6	12	23	15	18	16	19
Benign cyst	18	7	20	23	16	4	NA	NA	14	10
Thyroid	5	11	2	0	*	0	NA	NA	4	*
Granuloma	6	*	0	0	*	0	NA	NA	*	*
Mesenchymal	6	3	4	0	*	5	6	4	*	*
Primary carcinoma	2	*	*	0	*	0	0	0	*	*
Vascular tumor/ malformation	*	7	2	0	*	0	NA	NA	*	b
Miscellaneous	5	*	5	0	13	4	7	0	7	8

†Only mediastinal malignancies were included.
*Not reported as a separate category.

neoplasms, pericardial cysts, and thoracic goiters were rare in childhood.[14] Azarow et al[15] found that the only significant differences between the adult and pediatric populations were a higher incidence of lymphoma in adults and of neurogenic tumors in children. Surprisingly, the frequency of thymic tumors in adults and children was not significantly different.[15] Temes et al[16] and Takeda et al,[17] however, reported a significantly lower incidence of thymic tumors and a higher incidence of neurogenic tumors in children. Although all of these series were limited by the biases inherent in retrospective, single institution, surgical studies, a few trends emerge. Neurogenic tumors are more frequent in children than adults, perhaps reflecting the prevalence of neuroblastoma in that population. Thymic and thyroid tumors are more common in adults. Lymphoma tends to occur as a mediastinal mass with roughly equal frequency in adults and children, as do benign cysts of the mediastinum.

Differential diagnosis of mediastinal masses

Mediastinal masses are classically defined and discussed according to their location in the anterior, middle, or posterior mediastinal compartments. This classification is primarily a matter of descriptive convenience because there are no anatomic boundaries that limit growth between these various compartments. Indeed, many radiologists do not use these terms in the manner defined by anatomy textbooks. As Heitzman[21] has pointed out, apart from being useful for remembering that thymic, thyroid, and teratomatous masses are found in the anterior mediastinum and that most neurogenic tumors are posteriorly situated, this simple classification "tends to constrict thinking and minimizes more detailed anatomic analysis". Much more important is the accurate assessment of the location of the mass, together with a description of its size, shape, and characteristics, such as CT attenuation and MR signal intensity. Cross-sectional imaging techniques, notably CT,[22] provide the best information with which to refine the differential diagnosis and, on occasion, to suggest a specific diagnosis.

The differential diagnosis of a mediastinal mass depends on the age of the patient, the location of the mass, the imaging technique used to evaluate the mass, and findings on that imaging examination. For example, Ahn et al[23] analyzed chest radiographs and CT of 128 patients with anterior mediastinal masses and showed that, using chest radiograph, the first choice diagnosis was correct in 36% of cases; using CT, it was correct in 48%. Using chest radiographs, the correct diagnosis was included among the top three choices in 59% of cases; using CT, the correct diagnosis was included among the top three choices in 73% for CT. This serves to emphasize that CT can help narrow the differential diagnosis, but may also reflect the rather limited range of pathologies encountered in the anterior mediastinum.

The first step in the differential diagnosis of a mediastinal mass is to be sure that the mass arises from the mediastinum rather than from contiguous lung, pleura, spine, or sternum. Masses that lie deep to mediastinal vessels are certainly mediastinal in origin and those that arise from the sternum or spine should be obvious at CT. The interface with the adjacent lung is a most useful sign, particularly at CT. With few exceptions, a mass with spiculated, nodular, or irregular borders arises in the lung; likewise, a well-marginated mass with a broad base against the mediastinum arises either from the mediastinum or the mediastinal pleura.[24] Masses arising from the mediastinal pleura project into the lung and usually have obtuse rather than acute angles at their margins. Using these criteria, Woodring and Johnson[24] were able correctly to localize 99% of masses to the lung, pleura, or mediastinum.

Some general comments regarding patient age, CT attenuation, or MR signal intensity and multiplicity are made here, since all three features are relevant, whatever the location of the mass:

- Lymphoma, benign thymic enlargement, germ cell tumors, foregut cysts, and neurogenic tumors of ganglion cell origin make up 80% of mediastinal masses in children.[25] In adults, lymphoma, metastatic carcinoma to lymph nodes, intrathoracic goiter, thymoma, neurogenic tumors of nerve sheath origin, aortic aneurysms, germ cell tumors and foregut cysts are the prime considerations.

- Lesions that are of higher attenuation than muscle on noncontrast CT scans are usually calcified, have high iodine content (indicating thyroid tissue), or contain areas of acute hemorrhage.[26] Furthermore: (1) irregular, granular or eggshell calcification within *multiple* small mediastinal masses limits the differential diagnosis, for practical purposes, to lymphadenopathy due to such benign conditions as granulomatous infection, coal worker's pneumoconiosis, silicosis, and sarcoidosis. Amyloidosis, treated lymphoma, metastasis, and Castleman disease may be an occasional cause; (2) calcification in a *solitary* mass has a broader differential diagnosis. Neurogenic tumors may calcify, as may thymoma and germ cell tumors; (3) curvilinear calcification is seen in the walls of foregut cysts, mature teratoma, and, occasionally, pericardial cysts. Untreated lymphoma almost never calcifies. Aneurysms of the aorta or its major branches frequently have curvilinear calcification in their walls or in thrombus lining the aneurysm. This pattern of calcification, along with the observation that the mass arises from, or is in intimate contact with, the aorta or branch vessels, suggests the correct diagnosis.
- Lesions that are of homogeneous water attenuation on CT or have characteristics of water on MRI, and have a thin wall of uniform thickness are most likely congenital cysts, pericardial recesses, meningoceles, or lymphangiomas. Necrotic malignant or benign neoplasms are usually heterogeneous and have thick or irregular walls.[27] Some neurogenic tumors may be of low attenuation on CT; however, they are typically of higher attenuation than water, occur in characteristic locations, and enhance after administration of contrast material.
- Lesions that contain fat on CT or MRI include collections of normal fat (epicardial fat pads, lipomatosis, and herniated abdominal fat), lipomas, lipoblastomas, liposarcomas, extramedullary hematopoiesis, teratomas, thymolipoma, and fat-replaced lymph nodes.[28] A fat–fluid level within a cystic mass is pathognomonic of mature teratoma. Benign lipomas and thymolipomas are composed almost entirely of fat and should contain but a few thin strands of soft tissue. Liposarcomas are rare and usually manifest as mixed fat and soft tissue masses.
- Contrast enhancement, either by iodinated contrast material at CT or by gadolinium based contrast material at MRI, is an important feature and can be diagnostic of a vascular lesion such as an aneurysm. A minor degree of enhancement of the soft tissue component of a mass is a nonspecific finding. However, marked enhancement suggests thyroid tissue, vascular tumors such as paragangliomas, and Castleman disease.[29]
- The finding of multiple small masses within the mediastinum is suggestive of lymphadenopathy. The nodes may be separated by fat or may conglomerate into multiple larger lobulated masses.
- At MRI, most mediastinal masses are of low to intermediate signal on T1-weighted images and relatively high signal on T2-weighted images. (1) Those that contain water, or fluid similar to water, have uniformly low signal on T1-weighted images and uniformly very high signal on T2-weighted or

STIR images. (2) Lesions that contain fat or subacute hemorrhage have substantially higher signal intensity compared to muscle on T1-weighted images.[30] The differential diagnosis of masses with areas of high signal intensity on T1-weighted images is extensive, because many primary and secondary mediastinal tumors occasionally contain such foci even in the absence of fat or recent hemorrhage. Furthermore, cysts that contain proteinaceous debris may be of high signal intensity on T1-weighted images. Thus, mediastinal masses that may have signal intensity similar to or near that of fat on T1-weighted images include neurogenic tumors, lipomas, teratomas, foregut cysts, lymphangioma, pheochromocytoma, carcinoid tumors, and a variety of primary and secondary carcinomas.[30,31]

Finally, location is clearly of great importance for differentiating mediastinal masses. Cross-sectional imaging, particularly CT, has become the mainstay for evaluation of known or suspected mediastinal masses. Thus, the differential diagnosis is best discussed by location on cross-sectional imaging:

Prevascular masses (Box 14.1)

Prevascular masses are located anterior to the ascending aorta and branch vessels. Almost all masses in this location[32] are thyroid or thymic masses, germ cell tumors, or lymphadenopathy. Thyroid masses can usually be specifically diagnosed or excluded based on their contiguity with the thyroid gland in the neck and their high CT attenuation on both pre- and post-contrast scans. In addition, most thyroid lesions are heterogeneous and have focal cysts as well as one or more areas of discrete calcification. A mass located superiorly in the anterior mediastinum that causes lateral deviation of the trachea is likely to be of thyroid origin.

Box 14.1 Prevascular masses

Common
Thyroid masses
Thymic lesions
Germ cell tumors
Lymphadenopathy

Uncommon
Parathyroid adenoma
Lymphangioma (cystic hygroma)
Pericardial cyst
Aortic body paraganglioma
Mesenchymal tumor
Aneurysm

Thymic masses and germ cell tumors can have a similar appearance on cross-sectional imaging. Clinical and laboratory features may help distinguish between the two. For example, myasthenia gravis, red cell aplasia, and hypogammaglobulinemia are associated with thymoma, whereas high α-fetoprotein or human chorionic gonadotropin levels are associated with malignant germ cell tumors. If there is an associated pleural mass, then lymphoma or transpleural spread of thymoma becomes a strong possibility. If fat, cartilaginous calcification, or likely teeth are present in the mass, then teratoma is the diagnosis.

More unusual causes of masses anterior to the aorta and branch vessels are parathyroid adenoma, lymphangioma (cystic hygroma), pericardial cyst, aortic body paraganglioma, lipoma, liposarcoma or other mesenchymal tumors, or aneurysms. Aneurysms are extremely rare in this location and, when seen, are likely to be congenital or mycotic in origin. Many of these masses have features that permit a specific diagnosis to be made. Parathyroid adenomas are usually associated with hyperparathyroidism and are discovered in the quest for an ectopic parathyroid gland. Lymphangiomas, because they are composed largely of lymph-filled spaces, show numerous cysts on CT. Cystic hygroma should be a serious consideration for a prevascular mass that extends into the neck in a child. Lipomas may be indistinguishable from normal fat collections but are readily distinguished from more significant fat-containing mediastinal masses. Liposarcomas show a mixture of fat and irregular strands or masses of soft tissue. Pericardial cysts are, in general, of uniform water density with a thin, uniform thickness wall, and they need only be considered when the mass in question is in contact with the pericardium. It should be remembered, however, that the pericardium extends to the level of the junction between the proximal and middle thirds of the ascending aorta. Mesenchymal tumors, such as fibrosarcomas, or blood vessel tumors have no distinguishing features.

Paracardiac masses (Box 14.2)

The likely diagnoses for paracardiac masses that contact the diaphragm are pericardial cyst, diaphragmatic hernia, fat pad, lymphadenopathy, or, in patients with portal hypertension, cardiophrenic varices.[33] Most pericardial cysts are diagnosable by their uniform water attenuation on CT and their thin walls. Morgagni hernias are recognized by the omental fat within the hernia and sometimes by opacified bowel either within the mass or leading into it. If the mass is not in contact with the diaphragm, the differential diagnosis broadens to include germ cell tumors, mesenchymal and pericardial tumors, and thymic masses. Approximately 20% of thymomas are found in a paracardiac location, though contact with the diaphragm is very unusual. Lack of contact with the diaphragm excludes the possibility of a diaphragmatic hernia.

Box 14.2 Paracardiac masses

Pericardial cyst
Diaphragmatic hernia
Epicardial fat pad
Lymphadenopathy
Varices

Paratracheal, subcarinal, and paraesophageal masses (Box 14.3)

These sites are considered together because the trachea, central bronchi, and esophagus are contained within a common fascial sheath. This compartment continues into the neck around the airway, the esophagus, and the pharynx. Prime considerations for nonvascular masses in these locations are lymphadenopathy, intrathoracic thyroid mass, foregut cysts, esophageal lesions,

---

Box 14.3 Paratracheal, subcarinal, and paraesophageal masses

Lymphadenopathy
Foregut malformations/cysts
Esophageal lesions
Thyroid lesions
Hiatal hernia
Aneurysms
Vascular anomalies

---

hiatal hernias, and paraspinal masses encroaching on the middle mediastinum. In terms of incidence, lymphadenopathy is by far the most frequent. Masses deep to the azygos vein in either the right paratracheal area or in the pretracheal or precarinal space are almost invariably enlarged lymph nodes. For masses arising in the aortopulmonary window, the only other alternative is aortic aneurysm – a diagnosis that can be readily confirmed or excluded with contrast-enhanced CT or MRI. As mentioned earlier, lymphadenopathy is frequently multifocal and, in the case of metastatic carcinoma, the primary tumor is usually already known. Bronchogenic cyst can be diagnosed with confidence if the criteria of a simple cyst are met. But many bronchogenic cysts do not meet these criteria and these, therefore, are included in the differential diagnosis of a solid mediastinal mass. Thyroid masses that pass lateral to or posterior to the trachea are distinctive, partly because of the signs discussed below, but also because thyroid masses show far greater contact, displacement, and compression of the trachea than do lymph nodes. Separation of the trachea from the esophagus is a characteristic shared only by thyroid masses, bronchogenic cysts, esophageal tumors, and an aberrant origin of the left pulmonary artery. Aortic arch anomalies, though they deform the trachea and esophagus in various ways, do not pass between these two structures.

Esophageal lesions very rarely present as unexpected mediastinal masses. Patients with esophageal carcinoma, the most common esophageal tumor, nearly always present with dysphagia at a time when the tumor mass is relatively small. Although the tumor can sometimes be seen as a mass on plain chest radiographs and may be recognized at CT, the diagnosis of esophageal carcinoma is usually made at endoscopy or barium swallow examination. Leiomyoma or other mesenchymal tumors of the esophagus may grow to a considerable size without causing dysphagia and may, on occasion, present as a mediastinal mass on chest radiography or CT. Hiatal hernia is an exceedingly common cause of a mediastinal mass in the region of the lower esophagus. The diagnosis from chest radiographs is so straightforward and reliable that barium swallow or CT should rarely be required for diagnosis.

As discussed below, a number of vascular anomalies may mimic a paratracheal mass on chest radiographs and sometimes even on CT.

Paravertebral masses (Box 14.4)

Strictly speaking, masses situated on either side of the vertebral column are outside the mediastinum since, according to anatomists' definitions, the mediastinum lies anterior to the spine. However, it is standard practice among radiologists and thoracic surgeons to label masses against the spine as posterior mediastinal masses.

Neurogenic lesions and neoplastic lymphadenopathy dominate the differential diagnosis for paraspinal masses. Lymphadenopathy is rarely confined to the paraspinal areas; usually it is accompanied by enlarged lymph nodes in adjacent mediastinal or retroperitoneal areas. The most common causes of posterior mediastinal lymph node enlargement are lymphoma and metastatic carcinoma from genitourinary primary tumors. Other, less common, causes of paraspinal masses include metastases from other sites, extramedullary hematopoiesis, pancreatic pseudocyst, mesenchymal tumors such as lipoma, fibroma, chordoma and hemangioma, and lesions arising from the esophagus, pharynx, spine, or aorta. The esophageal or pharyngeal lesions that may project posteriorly include leiomyoma, foregut cyst, and congenital or acquired diverticula of the esophagus. The spinal origin of lesions such as paraspinal abscess, tumors of the vertebral body that have spread into the adjacent paravertebral space, or hematomas from trauma to the spine, are usually readily diagnosed by observing corresponding changes in the spine.

Aneurysms of the descending aorta that truly mimic mediastinal masses are uncommon. Most large aneurysms in this location are obvious. Saccular aneurysms that could be confused with a mass show a broad base on the aorta and almost always have curvilinear calcification in their walls. The diagnosis is readily made on CT or MRI when opacification of the lumen can be demonstrated.

Specific mediastinal lesions

Cysts or cystlike lesions (Box 14.5)

Most true mediastinal cysts or cystlike lesions are usually developmental in origin and include bronchogenic cysts, esophageal duplication cysts, neurenteric cysts, and pericardial cysts. Takeda et al[34] reviewed their experience with 105 patients with cysts of the mediastinum. In their series, the majority of cysts were bronchogenic (45%), thymic (28%) or pericardial (11%) cysts. The remainder were esophageal duplication cysts, meningoceles or thoracic duct cysts. Bronchogenic cysts are discussed on page 1114 in Chapter 16; parathyroid cysts, thymic cysts, and lymphangioma are discussed on pages 960, 975, and 904, respectively.

Distinguishing between the various cysts and cystlike lesions of the mediastinum is not always straightforward. For example, a cyst deep in the wall in the esophagus, and unquestionably by

all anatomic criteria an esophageal duplication cyst, may contain respiratory epithelium. In order to emphasize their origin from the embryological foregut, bronchogenic, esophageal, and neurenteric cysts are often collectively referred to as foregut duplication cysts.[35,36] Foregut duplication cysts account for approximately 20% of all mediastinal masses.[34,37,38] Bronchogenic cysts are the most common mediastinal foregut cysts; esophageal duplication and neurenteric cysts are less common. Mediastinal cysts that contain cartilage are classified as bronchogenic cysts and those that contain gastric epithelium are classified as enteric duplication cysts. Those cysts with seromucinous glands are considered as probably, although not definitely, respiratory in origin. Most congenital mediastinal cysts are lined by respiratory epithelium and these are usually labeled bronchogenic cysts even though their precise origin can only be conjectured.[36]

Esophageal duplication cysts

Esophageal duplication cysts are uncommon. They may present in adults or children.[39] The cysts are located in the middle or posterior mediastinum, have muscular coats, and contain mucosa that resembles esophagus, stomach, or small intestine. Esophageal duplication cysts usually occur within the wall, or are adherent to the wall, of the esophagus, are either spherical or tubular in shape, and are usually located along the lateral aspect of the distal esophagus.[40,41] Many cysts are clinically silent and are first discovered as asymptomatic masses on chest imaging examinations. The remainder manifest with symptoms of dysphagia or chest pain, or symptoms due to compression of adjacent structures.[39] Ectopic gastric mucosa in the cyst may cause bleeding into the cyst or perforation of the cyst and the cyst may become infected.

On chest radiographs, esophageal duplication cysts manifest as well-defined round or lobular masses in the middle or posterior mediastinum (Figs 14.1 and 14.2).[40,41] The masses are usually solid, unless they are infected and contain air. Calcification is rarely detected in the cyst walls. On CT, the cysts manifest as round or tubular water attenuation masses, usually in close proximity to the esophageal wall. These features are similar to those seen in cases of bronchogenic cysts, except that the wall of the esophageal duplication cyst may appear thicker and the mass may have more of a tubular shape than the typical bronchogenic cyst (Fig. 14.2).[39,42–44] On barium swallow examination, the cyst may manifest as either an intramural or an extrinsic mass.[39] Although esophageal duplication cysts are usually of water attenuation on CT (Fig. 14.1), some contain

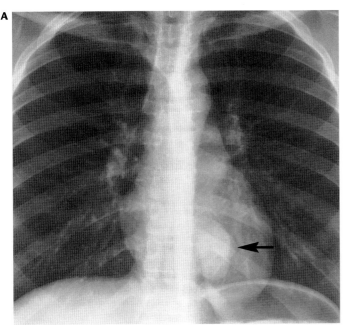

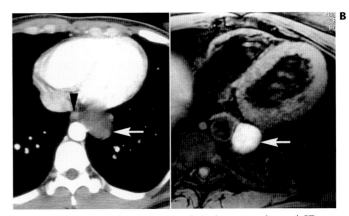

Fig. 14.1 Esophageal duplication cyst. **A**, Frontal chest radiograph shows a lobulated left retrocardiac mass (arrow). **B**, Contrast-enhanced CT (left panel) shows a well-marginated water attenuation mass (arrow) that is closely associated with the distal esophagus (arrowhead). Note that the lesion is homogeneous and of high signal intensity on T2-weighted MRI (right panel).

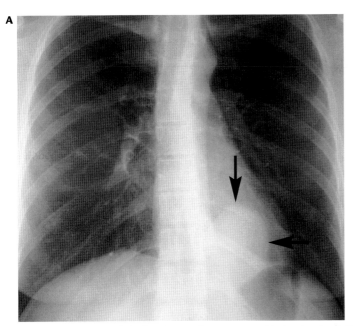

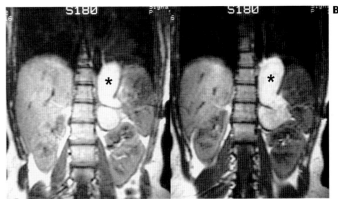

Fig. 14.2 Esophageal duplication cyst in a woman with dysphagia. **A**, Frontal chest radiograph shows a well-marginated left retrocardiac mass (arrows). **B**, Coronal T1-weighted MRI shows a tubular mass (*) extending into the abdomen. The mass is of high signal intensity consistent with proteinaceous fluid. (Courtesy of Jeffrey Galvin, Washington, DC)

proteinaceous fluid or blood and thus appear as soft tissue masses.[40,41] On MRI, the cysts have similar signal intensity characteristics to bronchogenic cysts, being of variable signal intensity on T1-weighted images, depending upon intracystic content, and of markedly increased signal intensity on T2-weighted images (Figs 14.1 and 14.2).[45]

Pericardial cysts

Pericardial cysts are anomalous outpouchings of parietal pericardium, but only rarely have an identifiable communication

with the pericardial sac. Pericardial diverticula are related anomalies of the visceral pericardium that communicate with the pericardial space.[46] Rapid change in size, particularly a decrease in size, suggests a pericardial diverticulum rather than a pericardial cyst.[47] The cysts contain clear yellow fluid. The interior is usually unilocular but can be trabeculated. In one series, 20% of cases examined pathologically were multilocular,[48] though in another large series of 72 patients, only one pericardial cyst was truly loculated.[49] The wall of the cyst is composed of collagen and scattered elastic fibers lined by a single layer of mesothelial cells.[48] Most affected patients are asymptomatic at presentation, but in series derived from surgical case material, symptoms such as chest pain, cough and dyspnea are reported in up to one-third of patients.[35,48,49]

There is a strong predilection for the anterior cardiophrenic angles and the cysts typically contact the heart, the diaphragm and the anterior chest wall. They are more frequent on the right than the left. In one large series, 37 of 72 pericardial cysts were in the right cardiophrenic angle, and 17 were in the left.[49] The remaining 18 arose higher in the mediastinum, and 11 extended into the superior mediastinum. In a review of the chest radiographs of 41 cases at the Armed Forces Institute of Pathology, the right:left ratio was 4:3.[48]

On radiologic studies, the cysts are seen as smooth round or oval well-defined masses in contact with the heart (Figs 14.3 to 14.6). An oval shape coming to a point has been observed in some cases.[48,50,51] Calcification is exceptional on chest radiographs. On CT, the cysts are usually homogeneous water attenuation masses with thin or imperceptible walls (Figs 14.4 and 14.5). The cyst contents should not enhance after administration of intravenous contrast.[52] Soft tissue attenuation pericardial cysts are quite rare.[52] The size of the cysts is quite variable, with very large cysts occasionally reported (Figs 14.3 and 14.4).[48,49] Ultrasonography can be used to demonstrate the cystic nature of these lesions. MRI shows the mass to be homogeneous and of low signal intensity on T1-weighted images and of high signal intensity on T2-weighted images (Fig. 14.6), similar to water.[31] Cyst puncture and aspiration can be diagnostic in difficult cases or therapeutic in symptomatic patients (Fig. 14.4).[53]

Neurenteric cysts

Neurenteric cysts result from incomplete separation of endoderm from notochord, resulting in a diverticulum of endoderm. Neurenteric cysts are pathologically identical to esophageal

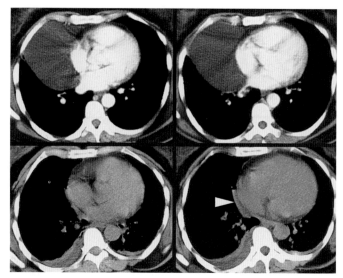

Fig. 14.4 Pericardial cyst in a patient with chest pain. Contrast-enhanced CT (upper panels) shows a large water attenuation mass along the right heart border. Noncontrast CT obtained after percutaneous aspiration and drainage (bottom panels) shows only minimal residual fluid in the cyst (arrowhead) and a new small right pleural effusion.

duplication cysts and usually have either a fibrous connection to the spine or an intraspinal component.[54] These cysts are typically associated with vertebral body anomalies, such as hemivertebra, butterfly vertebra, or spina bifida that occur at or above the level of the cyst. Most neurenteric cysts occur in the posterior, rather than middle mediastinum, and usually above the level of the carina.[35] Neurenteric cysts are relatively rare,

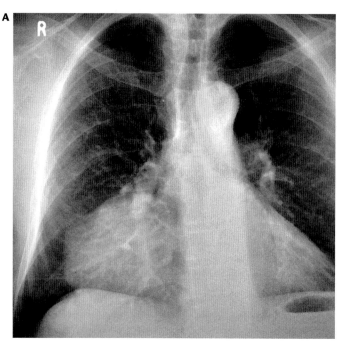

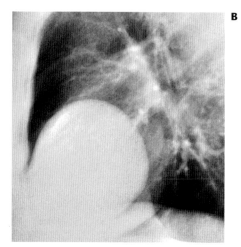

Fig. 14.3 Pericardial cyst. **A**, Frontal and **B**, lateral chest radiographs show a large well-marginated mass in the right cardiophrenic angle.

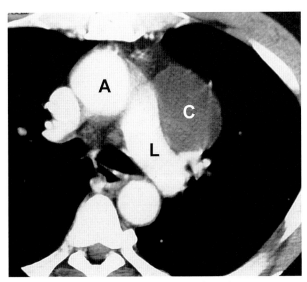

Fig. 14.5 Pericardial cyst. Contrast-enhanced CT shows a homogeneous water attenuation mass (C) along the left pulmonary artery (L). A = ascending aorta.

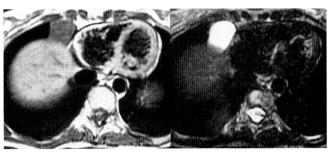

Fig. 14.6 Pericardial cyst in an asymptomatic patient. T1- (left panel) and T2-weighted (right panel) MRI shows a small right sided cyst with signal characteristics of water. Note that the cyst wall is imperceptible.

forming either a small minority of mediastinal cysts, or not being encountered at all in the larger surgical series.[14,35,55]

Radiographically (Figs 14.7 and 14.8)[56,57] neurenteric cysts are round, oval, or lobulated masses of water density situated in the posterior mediastinum or paravertebral region. Their cystic nature can be demonstrated by ultrasonography (Fig. 14.7). The CT and MRI appearance of these lesions (Fig. 14.8) is similar to that of other foregut cysts.[41] MRI is useful for optimally demonstrating the extent of spinal abnormality and degree of intraspinal involvement. Because the cysts may communicate with the subarachnoid space, CT myelography can also be diagnostic.

Mediastinal pancreatic pseudocysts

On rare occasions, a pancreatic pseudocyst extends into the mediastinum.[58,59] Most affected patients are adults and have clinical features of chronic pancreatitis. In children, the usual etiology is trauma.[60] Radiographically, most patients have either bilateral or left sided pleural effusions.[61] The mediastinal component of the pseudocyst is almost always in the middle and posterior mediastinum, having gained access to the chest via the esophageal or aortic hiatus. The pseudocyst in many instances therefore, deforms the esophagus. CT is the optimum method of demonstrating the full extent of these pseudocysts.[62] CT shows a thin walled cyst containing fluid within the mediastinum in continuity with the pancreas (Fig. 14.9), as well as any peripancreatic fluid collections.[63] Magnetic resonance cholangiopancreaticography has been used to successfully diagnose a mediastinal pancreatic pseudocyst.[64] The cyst may, on rare occasion, rupture into the pericardium, resulting in tamponade.[65] Hemothorax and esophagobronchial fistula have also been reported as complications of mediastinal pseudocyst.[66]

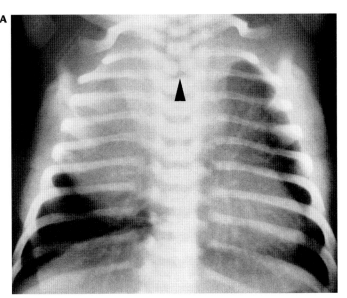

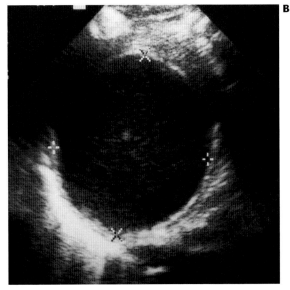

Fig. 14.7 Neurenteric cyst in an infant. **A**, Frontal chest radiograph shows a large right sided mediastinal mass. Note the butterfly vertebral body (arrowhead). **B**, Transthoracic ultrasound shows typical findings of a cyst. (Courtesy of Helen Carty, Liverpool, UK)

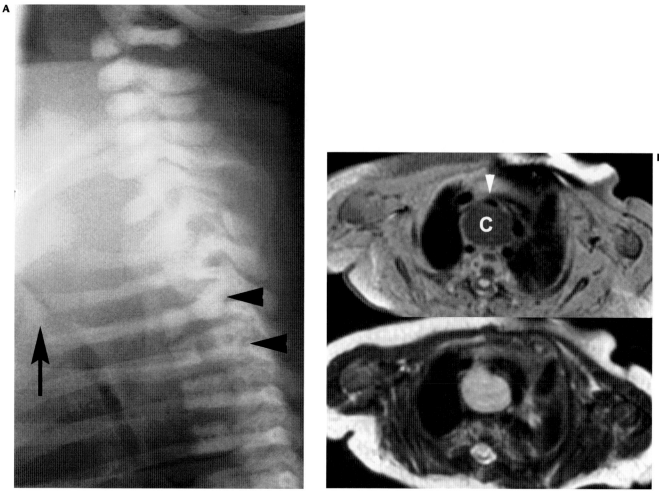

Fig. 14.8 Neuroenteric cyst in an infant with stridor. **A**, Lateral chest radiograph shows a large retrotracheal mass that anteriorly displaces and narrows the trachea (arrow). Note also the vertebral body clefts (arrowheads). **B**, Axial T1- (upper panel) and T2-weighted (lower panel) MRI shows the cyst (C) between the vertebral body and trachea. Note the anterior displacement and narrowing of the trachea (arrowhead). (Courtesy of Lane Donnelly, Cincinnati, OH)

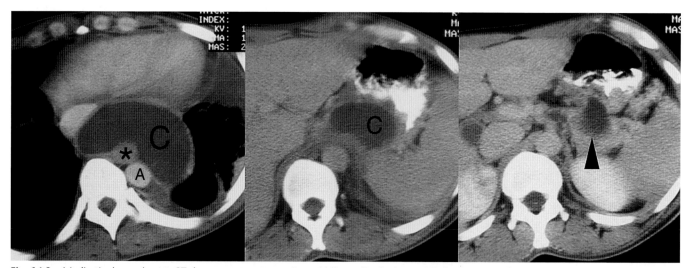

Fig. 14.9 Mediastinal pseudocyst. CT shows a water attenuation middle mediastinal mass (C) that traverses the esophageal hiatus and is associated with a pseudocyst in the tail of the pancreas (arrowhead). Note the close association with the intrathoracic esophagus (*) and descending thoracic aorta (A). (Courtesy of May Lesar, Bethesda, MD)

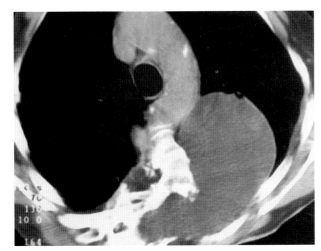

Fig. 14.10 Lateral thoracic meningocele. Noncontrast CT shows a well-marginated water attenuation mass arising from the spinal canal. Note the marked widening of the neural foramen.

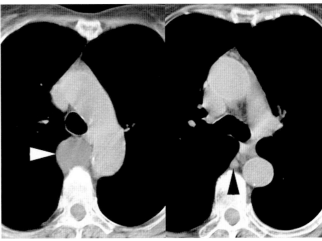

Fig. 14.12 Thoracic duct cyst. Noncontrast CT shows a water attenuation mass (white arrowhead) anterior to the thoracic vertebral body. The inferior aspect of the lesion (black arrowhead) is closely associated with the thoracic duct. Aspiration showed chylous fluid.

Lateral thoracic meningocele

Intrathoracic meningoceles are protrusions of spinal meninges through the intervertebral foramina.[67] They are usually detected in patients between 30 and 60 years of age as asymptomatic masses on chest radiograph. They are rarely associated with pain or neurologic abnormalities.[68] Approximately two-thirds of cases occur in association with neurofibromatosis.[68] On rare occasions, multiple or bilateral intrathoracic meningoceles are encountered.[69]

On chest radiographs,[70] they manifest as well-defined paravertebral masses, usually associated with scalloping and deformity of the adjacent ribs, pedicles, or vertebral bodies. Enlargement of the adjacent intervertebral foramen is an important diagnostic feature. Kyphoscoliosis is often present. These findings are identical to those seen in patients with so-called "dumbbell" nerve sheath tumors – a diagnostic problem that is complicated by the fact that both conditions are so frequently associated with neurofibromatosis. CT[71,72] better demonstrates these features and also shows that the "mass" is of water attenuation, since the bulk of the lesion consists of

cerebrospinal fluid (CSF) (Fig. 14.10). If CT is performed with intrathecal contrast medium, the contrast will enter the meningocele, confirming the diagnosis. Similarly, uniform CSF signal is seen throughout the lesion on MRI (Fig. 14.11).[71]

Lymphoceles and thoracic duct cysts

Thoracic lymphoceles are usually due to trauma and are discussed on page 1166. Mediastinal thoracic duct cysts are extremely rare lesions that may be due to either congenital or degenerative weaknesses in the wall of the thoracic duct. In the series of Takeda et al,[34] only one of 105 mediastinal cysts proved to be a thoracic duct cyst. The cysts can occur anywhere along the course of the thoracic duct, but have also been reported in the neck.[73] Very large cysts are reported.[74] In the review of Mattila et al,[75] approximately half of affected patients were asymptomatic. The remainder presented with symptoms such as chest pain, dysphagia, and dyspnea due to compression of adjacent structures.[75,76] CT usually shows a homogeneous mass of water attenuation along the course of the thoracic duct (Fig. 14.12).[75]

A

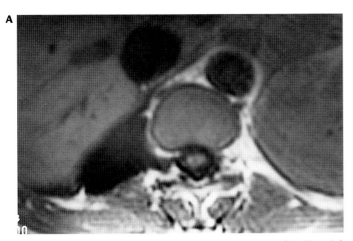

B

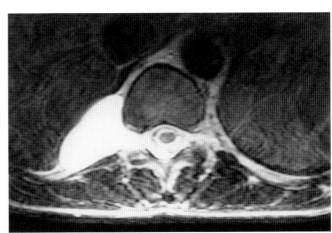

Fig. 14.11 Lateral thoracic meningocele. **A**, Axial T1- and **B**, T2-weighted MRI shows a homogeneous right sided mass with signal characteristics of water. Note that the MRI clearly shows that the mass communicates with the subarachnoid space.

Desmoid tumor (fibromatosis) of the mediastinum

Desmoid tumors, also known as aggressive fibromatosis, are locally invasive tumors of fibrous origin that primarily involve the soft tissues of the extremities, neck, and trunk. The mediastinum and chest wall are rarely involved.[77–83] Desmoid tumors may arise in areas of previous trauma or surgery.[77] Although the tumors frequently show extensive local invasion, distant metastases are rare.[84]

On chest radiographs, desmoid tumors manifest as soft tissue masses (Fig. 14.13) that may cause a localized periosteal reaction or cortical erosion of adjacent bone. On noncontrast CT, the mass is usually homogeneous and of the same attenuation as skeletal muscle.[82] On enhanced CT, the lesions are often more heterogeneous and may become hyperattenuating to muscle or show areas of necrosis.[81] Desmoids are usually heterogeneous and of variable signal intensity compared to muscle on both T1- and T2-weighted MRI.[85] As such, there are no particular imaging features to distinguish desmoid tumors from other soft tissue masses in the mediastinum or chest wall.[86,87] The lesions may be quite invasive, however, infiltrating in and around the great vessels,[88] or extending through the diaphragm to involve the abdomen.[89] Thus, complete resection may be impossible. The lesions are frequently hypervascular at angiography.[90]

Diaphragmatic hernia

Herniation of mesenteric fat or abdominal viscera through congenital or acquired defects in the diaphragm is a common cause of a mediastinal abnormality on chest radiographs or CT. Only hernias through the esophageal hiatus are discussed here. Hernias through the foramina of Bochdalek and Morgagni are discussed in Chapter 16.

Hiatal hernia

Hiatal (hiatus) hernias are frequent incidental findings on chest radiographs and CT. They may be responsible for pain as a result of gastroesophageal reflux and for anemia or upper gastrointestinal bleeding. On chest radiography, they produce a smooth, focal widening of the posterior junction anatomy extending down to the diaphragm. Varying amounts of fat surround the hernia itself, and in most instances some air can be appreciated within the hernia and there is often a visible air–fluid level (Fig. 14.14). At CT, the esophagus can be traced down into the hernia, and air (and contrast material) within the lumen usually enables the diagnosis to be made without difficulty (Fig. 14.14). The fat surrounding the hernia may be a striking feature. Hiatal hernias can be huge and may contain a major portion of the stomach. With large paraesophageal

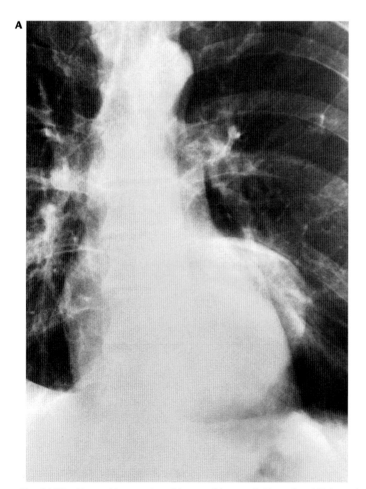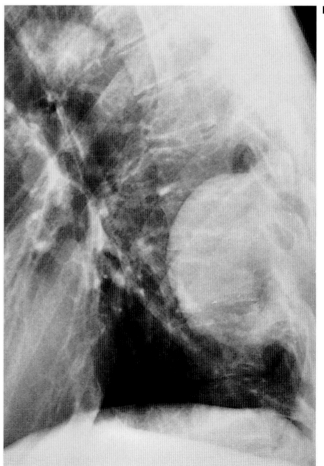

Fig. 14.13 Desmoid tumor in a 34-year-old man. **A**, Frontal and **B**, lateral chest radiographs show a well-circumscribed posterior mediastinal mass.

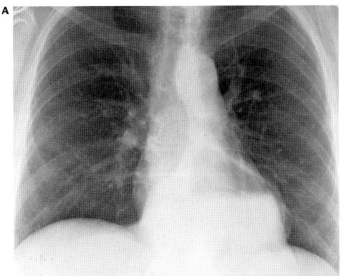

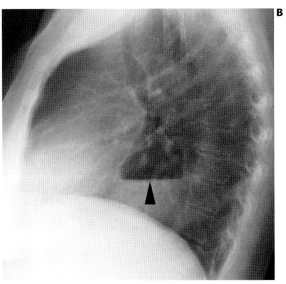

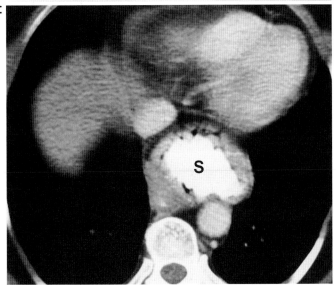

Fig. 14.14 Hiatal hernia. **A**, Frontal and **B**, lateral chest radiographs show a retrocardiac mass with an air–fluid level (arrowhead). **C**, CT shows the contrast-filled stomach (S) in the middle mediastinum.

hernias, the stomach not infrequently undergoes organoaxial rotation.[91]

On occasion, ascitic fluid under tension may herniate into the mediastinum at the gastroesophageal junction, usually contained by the parietal peritoneum.[92] This so-called "communicating thoracic hydrocele" can occur in the absence of a hiatal hernia and manifests as a mass on chest radiographs.[92] Because the fluid freely communicates with the abdominal cavity, the "mass" may spontaneously disappear. CT shows a water attenuation middle mediastinal mass closely associated with the esophageal hiatus in a patient with ascites (Fig. 14.15).[93]

Esophageal lesions (Box 14.6)

Various lesions of the esophagus can manifest as mediastinal masses, including esophageal dilation, esophageal duplication cysts (see above), esophageal diverticula, and esophageal neoplasms.[94,95]

Diffuse dilation of the esophagus can occur as a result of motility disorders, or distal obstruction or destruction of the myenteric plexus by tumor at the esophagogastric junction.[95]

Massive, radiographically evident, esophageal dilation is most often caused by achalasia or, in the developing world, Chaga disease.[96] Achalasia is caused by failure of relaxation of the lower esophageal sphincter. The esophagus can dilate to enormous size in severely affected patients. Esophageal dilation is usually best appreciated on the lateral view where the fluid-filled, dilated esophagus displaces the trachea and carina forward (Fig. 14.16).[97] In healthy individuals, the lung usually invaginates posterior to the right half of the trachea, resulting in a thin stripe of soft tissue along the posterior tracheal wall (the posterior tracheal stripe, see Ch. 2). When the esophagus is dilated, the esophagus displaces this lung, and the posterior tracheal stripe may appear thickened on the lateral radiograph (Fig. 14.17). This thickened stripe is due to the combined thickness of the trachea and esophageal walls, contained fluid in the dilated esophagus, and, sometimes, periesophageal lymphatic involvement by tumor.[98] The specificity of this finding in isolation is poor, as the stripe can appear thickened in normal patients due to interposition of collapsed normal esophagus between lung and trachea. However, if this sign is seen in association with anterior bowing of the trachea and

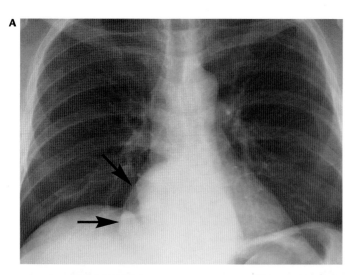

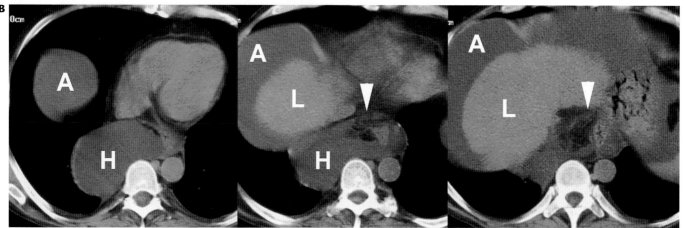

Fig. 14.15 Communicating thoracic hydrocele in a patient with cirrhosis. **A**, Frontal chest radiograph shows a well-marginated right retrocardiac mass (arrows). **B**, CT shows a water attenuation mass (H) in the mediastinum that communicates with the ascitic fluid (A) in the abdomen through the esophageal hiatus (arrowhead). L = liver.

Box 14.6 Esophageal lesions that can manifest as mediastinal masses

Diffuse dilation
Motility disorder
- Achalasia
- Postvagotomy syndrome
- Chaga disease
- Scleroderma
- Systemic lupus erythematosus
- Presbyesophagus
- Diabetic neuropathy
- Esophagitis
Distal obstruction
- Carcinoma
- Stricture
- Extrinsic compression
- Destruction of the myenteric plexus by tumor (pseudoachalasia)

Esophageal duplication cysts

Esophageal diverticula

Esophageal neoplasms
Carcinoma
Stromal tumors

---

anterior displacement of the carina, then esophageal dilation can be confidently diagnosed. The diagnosis of achalasia is further suggested by absence of air in the expected location of the stomach bubble on the frontal radiograph and an air–fluid level within the dilated esophagus.

Carcinoma of the esophagus, the most common neoplasm of the esophagus, is only occasionally detected as a focal mediastinal mass on chest radiographs (Fig. 14.18). Instead, the most frequent finding in affected patients is proximal dilation of the esophagus (Fig. 14.19), which may be accompanied by recognizable thickening of the esophageal wall. Esophageal dilation due to an obstructing lesion such as carcinoma is rarely as severe as that seen in patients with achalasia.

Submucosal esophageal neoplasms (gastrointestinal stromal tumors, leiomyomas, leiomyosarcomas) may grow to substantial size without causing dysphagia and may, therefore, present first as an asymptomatic mediastinal mass.[99] Leiomyomas are the most common esophageal stromal tumor (Fig. 14.20).[100] The esophagus is an uncommon location for gastrointestinal stromal tumors; <10% of gastrointestinal stromal tumors are found in the esophagus.[100–103] The diagnosis of an esophageal stromal tumor is suggested at barium swallow examination by observing the characteristic signs of an intramural extramucosal mass. On CT, esophageal leiomyomas manifest as smooth, round or ovoid, homogeneous masses that enhance following administration of intravenous contrast material (Fig. 14.20). The mass is typically inseparable from the esophagus. The esophagus is usually not

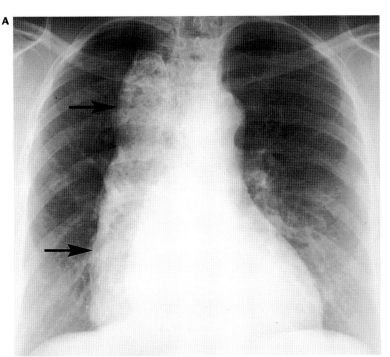

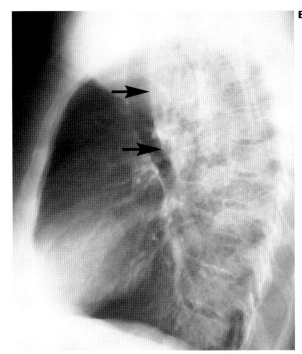

Fig. 14.16 Achalasia. **A**, Frontal and **B**, lateral chest radiographs show massive esophageal dilation (arrows on **A**). Note the anterior bowing of the trachea (arrows on **B**). **C**, Barium swallow examination shows typical findings of achalasia with smooth esophageal narrowing at the esophagogastric junction.

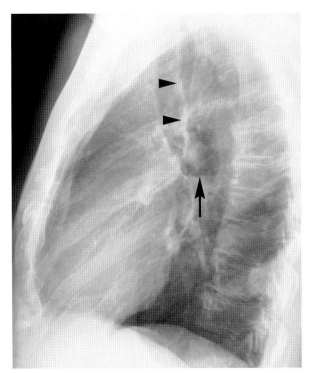

Fig. 14.17 Achalasia. Lateral chest radiograph shows an air–fluid level in the mid esophagus (arrow) and thickening of the posterior tracheal stripe (arrowheads).

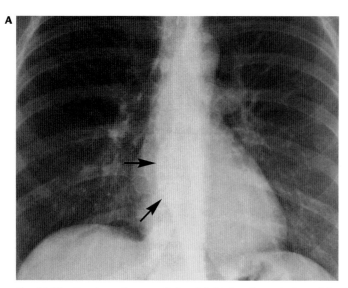

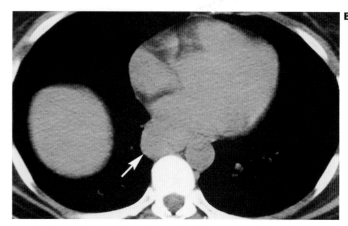

Fig. 14.18 Esophageal cancer. **A**, Frontal chest radiograph shows lateral convexity (arrows) along the mid aspect of the azygoesophageal interface. **B**, CT shows a soft tissue attenuation mass (arrow) in the middle mediastinum. Biopsy revealed squamous cell carcinoma of the esophagus.

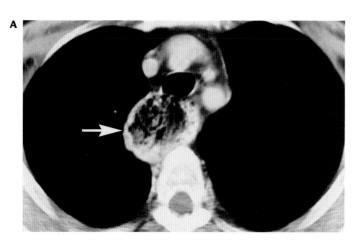

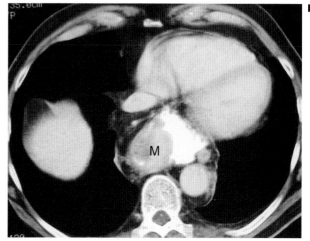

Fig. 14.19 Esophageal cancer. Chest radiographs (not shown) showed diffuse esophageal dilation. Contrast-enhanced CT confirms **A**, marked proximal esophageal dilation (arrow) and **B**, a mass (M) at the gastroesophageal junction.

dilated above the level of the tumor. The absence of proximal esophageal dilation is an important feature that helps differentiate a stromal tumor such as a leiomyoma from esophageal carcinoma. Leiomyosarcomas and large gastrointestinal stromal tumors (Fig. 14.21) tend to be more heterogeneous on CT.[104]

Fat-containing lesions of the mediastinum (Box 14.7)

There are many fat-containing lesions that can manifest as mediastinal masses on chest radiography or cross-sectional imaging, including lipomatosis, mature teratoma (see the section Germ cell tumors of the mediastinum), thymolipoma (see the section Thymic lesions), fatty neoplasms, hernias, and extramedullary hematopoesis.[105]

Mediastinal lipomatosis
Excessive deposition of fat may result in mediastinal widening, a condition sometimes known as mediastinal lipomatosis.[106,107]

Box 14.7 Fat-containing lesions of the mediastinum

Mediastinal lipomatosis
- Obesity
- Cushing disease
- Corticosteroid therapy

Neoplasms of fat tissue
- Lipoma
- Lipoblastoma
- Hibernoma
- Liposarcoma

Fat-containing tumors
- Teratoma
- Thymolipoma

Herniation of abdominal fat
Extramedullary hematopoiesis

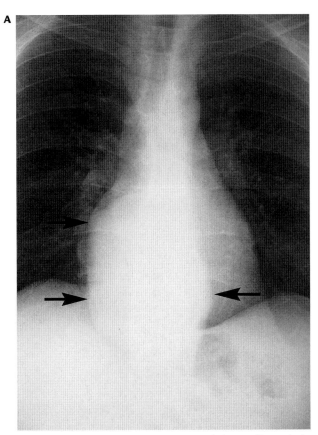

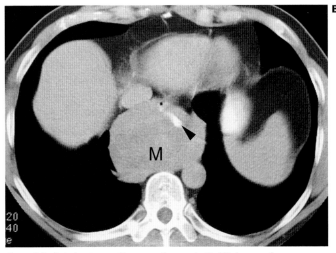

Fig. 14.20 Esophageal leiomyoma. **A,** Frontal chest radiograph shows a large lobulated retrocardiac mass (arrows). **B,** CT shows a homogeneous, soft tissue attenuation mass (M). Note the eccentric contrast-filled esophageal lumen (arrowhead).

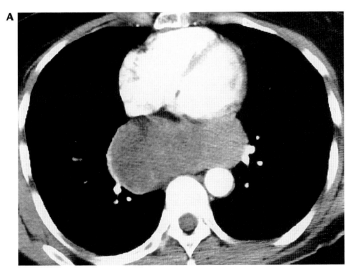

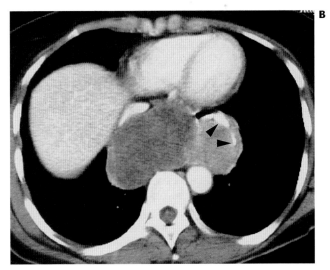

Fig. 14.21 Gastrointestinal stomal tumor of the esophagus. **A,** Contrast-enhanced CT shows a large soft tissue attenuation mediastinal mass. **B,** CT at a lower level shows that the mass encases and distorts the distal esophagus (arrowheads). Note that the mass is quite heterogeneous with a large low-attenuation region.

When associated with generalized obesity, mediastinal lipomatosis does not usually pose a diagnostic problem. However, in patients on steroid therapy or in those with Cushing disease, focal collections of histologically normal, but unencapsulated, fat can deposit in many sites, including the mediastinum, and simulate mass lesions on chest radiographs.[108–110] Furthermore, a similar phenomenon is occasionally encountered in patients with normal steroid hormone levels.[111,112] On chest radiographs, mediastinal lipomatosis usually manifests as smooth, diffuse widening of the superior mediastinum (Fig. 14.22). There is usually no mass effect upon the trachea or other mediastinal structures. In addition to findings of mediastinal fat deposition,

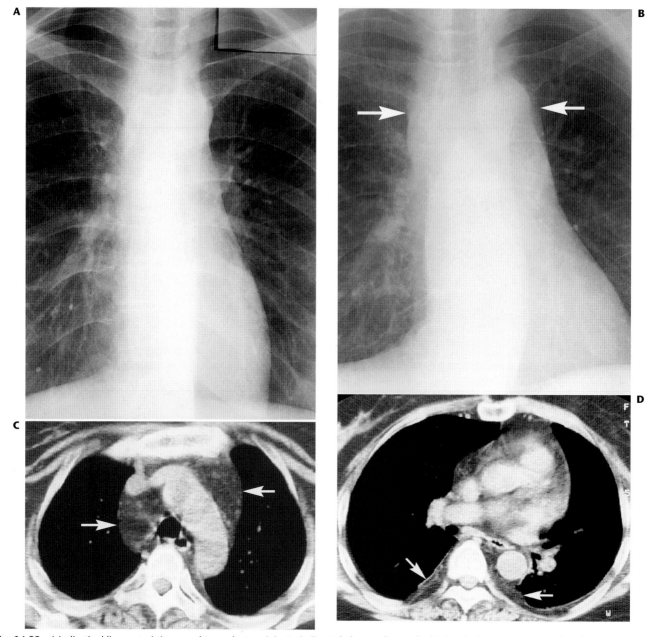

Fig. 14.22 Mediastinal lipomatosis in a renal transplant recipient. **A**, Frontal chest radiograph obtained prior to transplantation demonstrates a normal mediastinum. **B**, Radiograph obtained 2 years after transplantation now shows bilateral upper mediastinal widening (arrows). CT shows **C**, diffuse deposition of fat in the mediastinum (arrows) and **D**, extrapleural fat in the paravertebral regions (arrows).

chest radiographs in affected patients also usually show a symmetric increase in extrapleural fat and the costophrenic angle fat pads may be enlarged as well. When mediastinal fat deposition is symmetric and diffuse, the radiographic appearance is characteristic enough to pose no significant diagnostic difficulty. On the other hand, when deposition is asymmetric or more focal, CT may be required to exclude a soft tissue mass. This may be the case in patients with lymphoma who are being treated with corticosteroids. At CT, the uniform low attenuation of fat (−70 to −130 HU) is diagnostic (Fig. 14.22).[111,113,114]

There is a very rare condition termed *multiple symmetric lipomatosis*, also known as Madelung disease, that radiographically resembles mediastinal lipomatosis, but is the result of a specific biochemical abnormality.[115,116] In this condition,

multiple masses of benign fat tissue proliferate at various sites including the mediastinum. Unlike mediastinal lipomatosis, however, these masses occasionally compress mediastinal structures, such as the trachea[117] or larynx.[118]

Fatty tumors of the mediastinum

True mediastinal tumors of fatty origin are uncommon, accounting for <1% of 1064 surgically proved mediastinal masses.[14] On chest radiographs, both benign and malignant fat-containing tumors manifest as well-defined round or oval mediastinal masses.[119] Benign lipomas usually do not compress surrounding structures unless they are very large. Quinn et al[120] reported one unusual case where a mediastinal lipoma extended into the spinal canal and caused pressure deformity of the

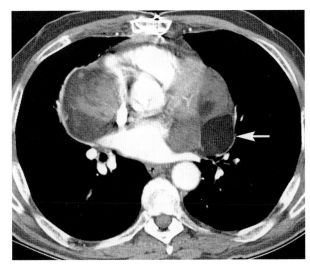

Fig. 14.23 Liposarcoma. Contrast-enhanced CT shows a large heterogeneous mediastinal mass with a significant fat component (arrow). (Courtesy of Jeremy Erasmus, Houston, TX)

adjacent bones. Large mediastinal lipomas may mold so completely to mediastinal contours as to simulate the appearance of an enlarged heart.[121] CT of mediastinal lipomas reveals any homogeneous mass of fat attenuation that may contain a few strands of soft tissue.[120,122] Lipoblastomas are benign fat-containing tumors that usually occur in childhood.[123] On CT, both fat and soft tissue components are seen.[28,124,125] Occasionally, the amount of fat seen on CT is relatively small and the mass is primarily of soft tissue attenuation.[126] Hibernomas are rare benign tumors that contain brown fat. Mediastinal hibernomas are quite rare. The CT features of mediastinal hibernomas are the subject of case reports only.[127] Based upon these reports, the masses appear as mixed fat and soft tissue attenuation. The amount of fat that is identifiable seems to be variable.[128]

Angiolipoma and myelolipomas are also very rare benign tumors that can occur in the mediastinum. They also manifest as masses of mixed soft tissue and fat attenuation on CT, and are thus indistinguishable from liposarcoma.[129,130]

Liposarcomas are malignant fat-containing tumors that usually occur in the anterior mediastinum (when they occur in the mediastinum).[131] Most affected patients are middle aged and present with symptoms of chest pain and dyspnea. The masses are typically large and diffusely infiltrate the mediastinum. Low grade liposarcomas may have large amounts of fat admixed with a significant soft tissue component on CT or MRI (Fig. 14.23).[105] Rarely, the lesion may be almost completely fatty with only a minimal soft tissue component.[132] High grade tumors usually do not have significant amounts of fat demonstrable on CT or MRI; instead, these lesions manifest as infiltrative masses of heterogeneous soft tissue attenuation or signal intensity.[131] Mxyoid liposarcomas of the mediastinum may contain regions of near water attenuation on CT (Fig. 14.24) and may have calcified stroma.[133]

Herniation of abdominal fat

Herniation of omental or perigastric fat is a common cause of a localized fatty mass in the mediastinum. The fat may herniate through the esophageal hiatus, the foramen of Morgagni, or the foramen of Bochdalek. Such herniations are usually readily diagnosed on chest radiographs because of their characteristic locations. The masses are of fat attenuation (–70 to –130 HU) or signal intensity on CT[28] or MRI,[134] and may contain linear or nodular foci due to contained omental vessels (Fig. 14.25).

Extramedullary hematopoiesis

Extramedullary hematopoiesis in potential blood-forming organs such as the liver, spleen, and lymph nodes is common in patients with severe anemia. Thoracic manifestations are rare and usually consist of paravertebral soft tissue masses, although pulmonary parenchymal involvement has been described.[135] The

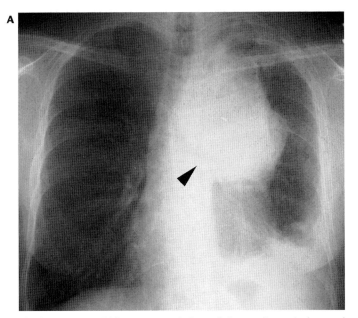

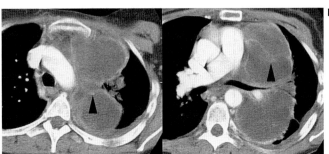

Fig. 14.24 Myxoid liposarcoma. **A,** Frontal chest radiograph shows a large, ill-defined, left sided mediastinal mass and left pleural effusion. Note the mass effect upon the left main bronchus (arrowhead). **B,** Contrast-enhanced CT shows a large heterogeneous mass that diffusely infiltrates the left mediastinum. Note the enhancing septa (arrowheads).

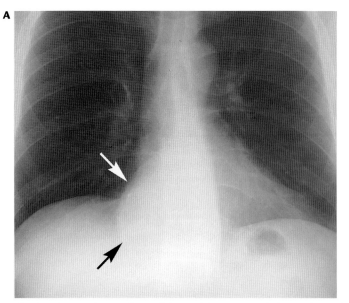

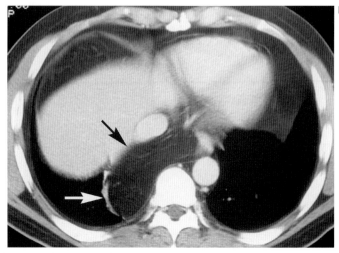

Fig. 14.25 Herniation of intraabdominal fat. **A**, Frontal chest radiograph shows a well-marginated retrocardiac mass (arrows). **B**, Contrast-enhanced CT shows a well-circumscribed fatty mass (arrows) in the posterior mediastinum. Note the thin wisps of soft tissue that likely represent mesenteric blood vessels.

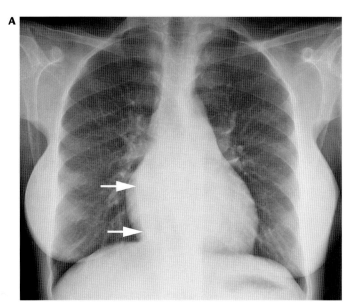

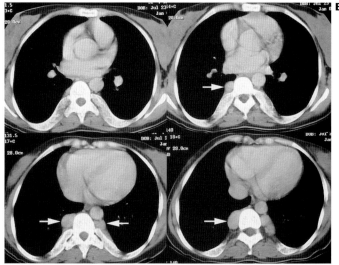

Fig. 14.26 Extramedullary hematopoiesis in a patient with thalassemia. **A**, Frontal chest radiograph shows a well-marginated right paravertebral mass (arrows). **B**, CT shows bilateral soft tissue masses (arrows) in the posterior mediastinum. Note the typical osseous changes in the posterior ribs.

masses are caused by extrusion of the marrow through the thinned cortex of the posterior ribs. Histologically the masses resemble splenic tissue with hematopoetic elements mixed with fat. The masses themselves are usually asymptomatic, though paraplegia from cord compression may occur.[136,137] The most common anemias that result in extramedullary hematopoiesis are the congenital hemolytic anemias, notably thalassemia, hereditary spherocytosis, and sickle cell disease.[138] However, it may rarely occur in other anemias and even in patients without anemia.[139]

Thoracic extramedullary hematopoesis manifests on chest radiographs,[137,139,140] CT,[140,141] and MRI,[142] as focal paravertebral masses, usually in the lower half of the thorax (Fig. 14.26). The masses are usually well marginated because they are covered by pleura, bilateral in distribution, contain no calcification, and show no rib destruction. Further foci of extramedullary hematopoiesis can also be seen as subpleural masses adjacent to ribs. These subpleural masses may be continuous or discontinuous with the paravertebral masses. The adjacent bone is usually normal or shows findings of marrow expansion; pressure erosions or bone destruction do not occur.[139] CT is particularly useful for demonstrating the lacelike marrow expansion in the adjacent bones (Fig. 14.26).[140] On CT, the lesions manifest as heterogeneous or homogeneous soft tissue attenuation masses (Figs 14.26 and 14.27). There may be some fat within the mass (Fig. 14.27),[143] but calcification is uncommon.[144] On MRI, the masses are usually heterogeneous with increased signal intensity on T1-weighted images because of contained fat.[142] Radionuclide studies using agents that show erythropoiesis or the reticuloendothelial system may demonstrate activity in the mass,[140,145,146] but can be negative.[140,147]

Germ cell tumors of the mediastinum (Boxes 14.8 and 14.9)

Germ cell tumors account for 10–15% of anterior mediastinal masses and are thought to arise from mediastinal remnants left behind after embryonal cell migration.[148–151] The mediastinum is the most common primary extragonadal site for germ cell tumors and mediastinal lesions account for about 60% of all germ cell tumors in adults. Germ cell tumors usually occur in young adults; the mean age at presentation is 27 years.[148–150] Most malignant germ cell tumors (>90%) occur in men. Benign lesions (typically mature teratoma) occur with equal frequency in men and women. Histopathologic types of germ cell tumors that occur in the mediastinum include teratoma, seminoma, embryonal carcinoma, endodermal sinus tumor, chorio-carcinoma, and mixed tumors.[152] Malignant germ cell tumors frequently secrete tumor markers such as human chorionic gonadotropin (HCG), α-fetoprotein (AFP), or lactic dehy-drogenase. These serum markers can be used to diagnose and monitor the progress of the disease.[153]

Mediastinal teratoma

Teratomas are the most common mediastinal germ cell tumors and are derived from more than one embryonic germ layer. Most mediastinal teratomas arise in cell rests within, or in

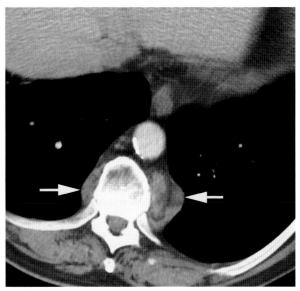

Fig. 14.27 Extramedullary hematopoiesis in a patient with sickle cell anemia. CT shows bilateral paraspinal masses (arrows). Note that the masses are of mixed attenuation and contain punctate areas of fat.

Box 14.8 Germ cell tumors of the mediastinum

Location
Usually anterior
Rarely middle or posterior

Demographics
Young adults
15% of anterior mediastinal masses
90% of malignant tumors occur in men
Benign tumors occur with equal frequency in men and
    women

Histopathology
Benign
 • Mature teratoma
Malignant
 • Seminoma – most common pure histology
 • Malignant teratoma
 • Embryonal carcinoma
 • Choriocarcinoma
 • Mixed tumors – most common malignancy

Clinical
May be asymptomatic
Malignant more likely to present with symptoms
Malignant associated with serologic markers
 • α-fetoprotein
 • Human chorionic gonadotropin

Box 14.9 Germ cell tumors of the mediastinum: imaging features

Mature teratoma
Chest radiography
 • Well-circumscribed mediastinal mass
 • Typically unilateral
 • May contain calcification
CT
 • Appear as uni- or multi-locular cystic mass
 • Fat
   – Seen in 75%
   – Predominant feature in 15%
   – Fat–fluid level rare, but diagnostic
 • Calcification common
   – Rimlike
   – Internal coarse
 • Rupture
   – Lesions are more heterogeneous
   – Fat in pleural space, pericardium, lung
MRI
 • Complex signal patterns depending on proportion of water, soft tissue, fat, and calcification

Malignant germ cell tumors
Seminoma
 • Large, lobulated, homogeneous
 • May have prominent cystic component
 • Fat or calcification rare
 • Often indistinguishable from lymphoma
Nonseminomatous
 • Larger and more ill-defined borders
 • May be bilateral
 • Frequently invasive
 • Very heterogeneous with areas of necrosis or cysts
 • Fat or calcification rare

intimate contact with, the thymus.[154,155] Teratomas are classified histopathologically as mature, immature, or malignant. Mature or benign teratomas are composed of different tissue types (ectoderm, endoderm, mesoderm), with ectodermal derivatives predominating.[156] The term dermoid cyst is commonly used when the tumor contains primarily ectodermal components such as skin, sebaceous material, hair, and calcification.[152,157] Such lesions are typically unilocular; multilocular lesions with intervening solid portions are less common.[14] These tumors may grow to a large size and occupy much of one hemithorax.

Mature teratomas account for 70% of germ cell tumors in childhood and 60% of mediastinal germ cell tumors in adults. Mature teratomas occur most frequently in children and young adults.[14,148,158] About half of affected patients are asymptomatic at presentation, with the lesion being detected on chest radiographs obtained for other purposes. In the remainder, symptoms due to local compression, rupture or infection occur. The most common presenting complaints are chest pain, productive cough, dyspnea or fever.[159] Rarely, affected patients present with pneumonia, hemoptysis, or the superior vena cava syndrome. Trichoptysis (the expectoration of hair) is a dramatic, but extremely rare symptom, that occurs when the lesion ruptures into the airway.[14,152] By definition, patients with mature teratoma have normal serum levels of β-hCG hormone and AFP; elevation of any of these markers implies a malignant component. Complete resection is the treatment for teratomas and usually results in a complete cure. Despite a benign histology, these tumors may be difficult to remove when they are adherent to local structures.

On chest radiographs or CT, mature teratomas manifest as well-defined, rounded or lobulated masses that usually project to one side of the midline (Fig. 14.28).[14] They most commonly occur in the anterior mediastinum, typically in the prevascular space. On occasion, they occur in the posterior mediastinum or the lung parenchyma itself.[14,149,159–162] The lesions tend to grow very slowly, but may increase in size rapidly if intratumoral hemorrhage occurs. On rare occasions, the lesions rupture into the airway, pleural space or pericardium. When the tumor ruptures into the airway, air may enter the cyst and become visible on imaging examinations; severe chemical pneumonitis or

lung abscess can also result.[35] Rupture into the pericardium[163] or pleura can result in the appearance of a fat–fluid level within these spaces on imaging examinations.[164] Calcification, ossification or even teeth[159,160] may be visible on chest radiographs (Fig. 14.29) and, occasionally, sufficient fat is present within the lesion to be detectable radiographically.

The CT appearance of mediastinal teratoma is quite variable because it depends upon the content of the lesion (Figs 14.28 and 14.29).[165,166] Almost all lesions have some areas of water attenuation on CT. Regions of fat attenuation are seen on CT in up to three-quarters of lesions and are the predominant tissue type in 15%.[159] Fat–fluid levels within the lesion, while uncommon, are virtually diagnostic of teratoma (Fig. 14.30).[167,168] More often, however, the fat is interspersed with regions of water and soft tissue attenuation. A definite cyst wall, which may have curvilinear calcification, may be visible on CT (Fig. 14.28), as is characteristic intralesional calcification (Fig. 14.29).[159] Choi et al[169] reported a series of teratomas and noted that the lesions that ruptured were more internally heterogeneous than were those that had not ruptured. Additional findings suggestive of rupture in their series were adjacent consolidation, atelectasis, pleural or pericardial effusion. In two cases, fat was seen in the lung parenchyma.

As is the case with CT, the MRI appearance of mediastinal teratomas is quite variable (Fig. 14.29). Because the contents of the cyst are typically rich in proteinaceous fluid, the cystic component of the lesion may be of high signal intensity on T1-weighted images.[31,159,170] Furthermore, the lesion may be of high signal on T1-weighted images because of fat or hemorrhage. On ultrasonography, the lesions may appear as completely cystic or solid masses, or as mixed cystic and solid masses.[171] The pattern on ultrasonography is often quite complex because of intralesional calcification (densely echogenic), hair (hyperechoic dots), and fat (dense echo pattern).[172] One case that showed echogenic floating spherules in the mass has been described.[173]

Malignant mediastinal germ cell tumors
Histopathologic types of malignant germ cell tumors that occur in the mediastinum include seminoma, embryonal cell carcinoma, endodermal sinus tumor, choriocarcinoma, and mixed germ cell

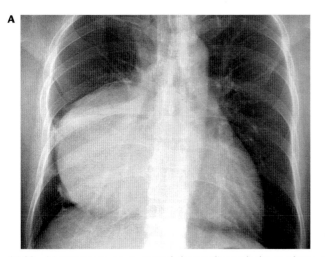
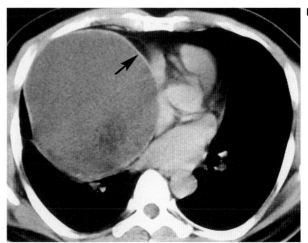

Fig. 14.28 Mature teratoma. **A**, Frontal chest radiograph shows a large, well-circumscribed right anterior mediastinal mass. **B**, CT shows that the mass is predominantly of water attenuation, though there are a few small posterior foci of fat. Note the thin uniform cyst wall (arrow).

A

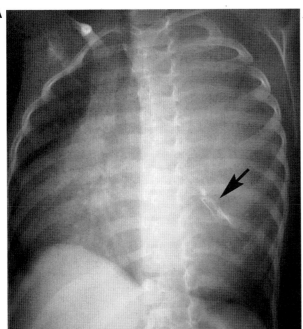

Fig. 14.29   Mediastinal teratoma in an infant with dyspnea.
A, Frontal chest radiograph shows a large left thoracic mass with linear calcification (arrow). **B**, Contrast-enhanced CT (left panel), T1- (center panel) and T2-weighted (right panel) MRI shows that the mass contains fluid, fat, and calcium. Note that the calcification is not easily appreciated on MRI. (Courtesy of Lane Donnelly, Cincinnati, OH)

B

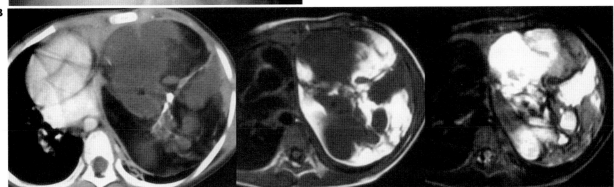

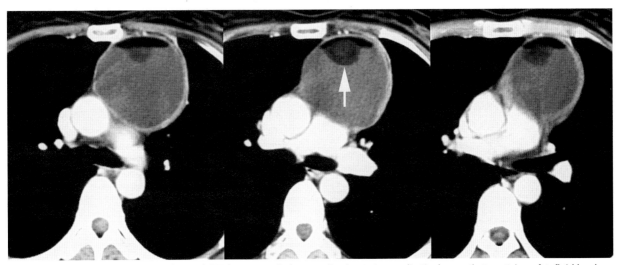

Fig. 14.30   Mature teratoma. Contrast-enhanced CT shows a well-circumscribed anterior mediastinal mass that contains a fat–fluid level, a diagnostic feature. The low-attenuation mass (arrow) at the interface was a hairball. (Courtesy of Jeffrey Galvin, Washington, DC)

tumors.[174,175] Seminoma is the most common pure histologic type in men and accounts for 40% of such tumors.[175] Teratoma with embryonal cell carcinoma (teratocarcinoma) is the next most common subtype, with pure endodermal sinus tumor, choriocarcinoma, and embryonal carcinoma being much less common.[174] Malignant mediastinal germ cell tumors are usually encountered in young adults and are much more common in men than women.[154] Polansky et al[176] reviewed 103 cases of primary mediastinal seminoma and found that only five occurred in women. Even mediastinal choriocarcinoma in adults is more common in men than women; in children, the male:female ratio is more even.[154]

Malignant mediastinal germ cell tumors are more frequently symptomatic than benign teratomas.[150,153,154] Common presenting complaints include cough, dyspnea, and chest pain.[176] Superior vena cava obstruction is reported in up to 10% of affected patients.[176,177] Weight loss may also be a notable feature. However, between 10 and 30% of affected patients are asymptomatic at presentation, with the mass discovered on routine chest radiographs.[152]

Serum levels of human hCG and AFP are useful for diagnosis and monitoring of some mediastinal germ cell malignancies.[150,153] Both hCG and AFP levels are typically normal in cases of pure seminoma; elevation of AFP indicates a nonseminomatous component of the tumor. Up to 80% of patients with non-seminomatous germ cell malignancies have elevated levels of AFP and 54% have elevated levels of hCG.[150,153] There is an association between malignant nonseminomatous germ cell tumors of the mediastinum and hematologic malignancies,[178,179]

and up to 20% of affected patients may have Klinefelter syndrome.[180,181]

On chest radiographs, seminomas manifest as focal, typically unilateral, mediastinal masses (Fig. 14.31). On CT or MRI, they are usually large lobulated masses of homogeneous attenuation or signal intensity, often indistinguishable from lymphoma (Fig. 14.31).[150,153] Cysts or areas of necrosis may also be seen in association with mediastinal seminoma (Fig. 14.32).[150,153] Invasion of adjacent structures is uncommon and calcification is rare. Metastases to regional nodes can occur. hCG and AFP levels are normal; elevation of AFP suggests a nonseminomatous component.[175]

Nonseminomatous germ cell malignancies usually manifest as large lobular or ill-defined anterior mediastinal masses (Fig. 14.33).[153] The mass is typically asymmetric and projects to one side of the thorax.[148,182,183] Calcification is an exceptional finding on chest radiographs. On CT or MRI, the mass may be quite heterogeneous and may contain cysts or areas of necrosis and hemorrhage (Figs 14.33 and 14.34).[184,185] These features may be accentuated following administration of intravenous contrast. Areas of fat attenuation or signal intensity within the masses are uncommon (Fig. 14.34). Coarse tumor calcification is also rarely seen on CT.[184,186] Adjacent mediastinal fat planes are often obliterated and extensive local invasion may be identified.[187] Invasion of the adjacent mediastinal structures, chest wall and lung, as well as metastases to the regional lymph nodes and distant sites, is common.[153]

A residual mediastinal mass is sometime seen on CT after successful treatment of a primary mediastinal nonseminomatous

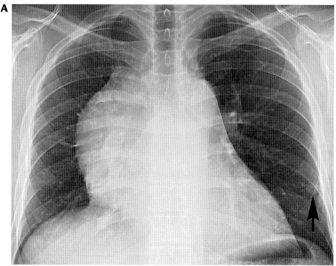

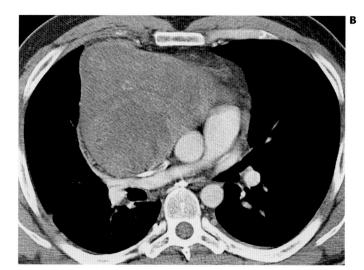

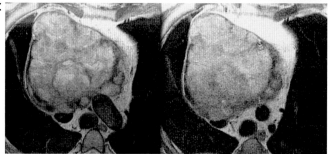

Fig. 14.31 Mediastinal seminoma. **A**, Frontal chest radiograph shows a large, well-marginated right anterior mediastinal mass. Note the small left lower lobe nodule (arrow) consistent with a metastasis. The left central venous catheter is looped in the left subclavian vein. **B**, Contrast-enhanced CT shows that the mass is homogeneous, of soft tissue attenuation, and has ill-defined borders. **C**, Axial MRI shows numerous internal septations. (Courtesy of Jeremy Erasmus, Houston, TX)

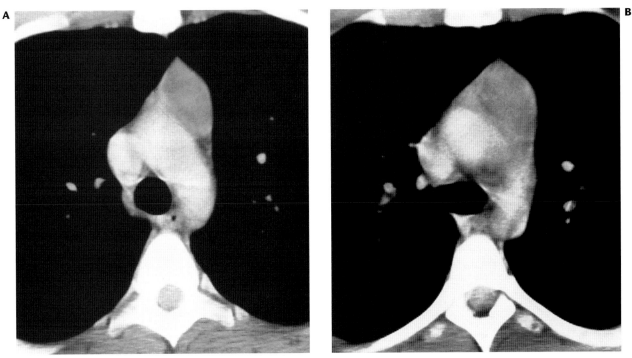

Fig. 14.32   Mediastinal seminoma. **A**, Contrast-enhanced CT shows a predominantly water attenuation prevascular mass with a thin enhancing wall. **B**, CT at a lower level shows a significant soft tissue component along the inferior surface. Resection revealed seminoma with an associated cyst.

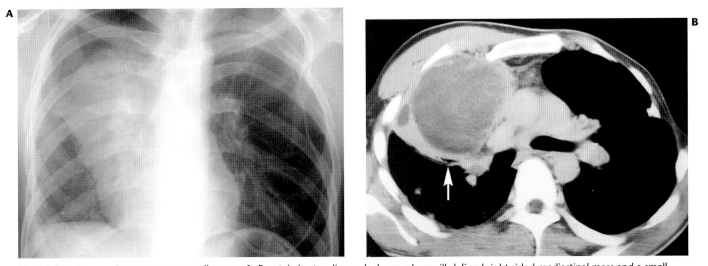

Fig. 14.33   Nonseminomatous germ cell tumor. **A**, Frontal chest radiograph shows a large, ill-defined right sided mediastinal mass and a small right pleural effusion. **B**, CT shows that the mass is heterogeneous with large water attenuation regions. Note compression and possible invasion of the right upper lobe (white arrow).

germ cell malignancy or after treatment of metastatic disease from a gonadal primary (Fig. 14.35). This mass may be cystic in nature, contain residual mature teratoma, and enlarge with time.[188,189] This phenomenon is known as the "growing teratoma" syndrome.[190–193] The benign or malignant nature of the residual mass cannot be confidently determined based upon the CT appearance alone. However, elevation of serum tumor markers suggests a malignant component. Andre et al[191] followed 30 patients with growing teratoma syndrome. All 30 lesions were biopsied or resected and 86% were found to have a mature teratoma component. All but one patient who underwent curative resection survived disease free. Five of the six patients who had only partial resection developed recurrent disease and one died of progressive tumor. Andre et al[191] and others[188] concluded that complete surgical resection was the treatment of choice.

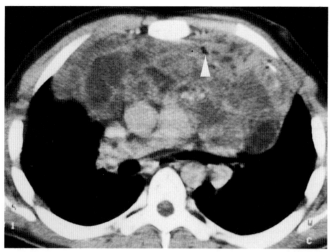

Fig. 14.34 Teratocarcinoma. CT shows a large heterogeneous and infiltrative mass of the anterior mediastinum. There are a few punctuate collections of fat (arrowhead) within the lesion.

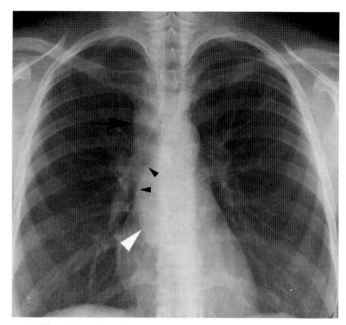

Fig. 14.36 Non-Hodgkin lymphoma. Frontal chest radiograph shows adenopathy in the right paratracheal (arrow) and subcarinal (white arrowhead) regions. Note the mass effect along the medial wall of the bronchus intermedius (black arrowheads).

Lymphadenopathy (Box 14.10)

Lymphadenopathy can be caused by a variety of infectious, inflammatory, and neoplastic conditions. Neoplastic causes include lymphoma (Fig. 14.36), leukemia, and metastatic carcinoma. Lymph node metastases frequently occur in the setting of thoracic malignancies such as lung (Fig. 14.37), esophagus, and breast cancer. Extrathoracic tumors that frequently spread to intrathoracic lymph nodes include renal (Fig. 14.38), testicular, and head and neck malignancies.[194,195] The most common infections that result in intrathoracic

lymphadenopathy are tuberculosis (Fig. 14.39) and fungal disease (particularly histoplasmosis and coccidioidomycosis). Lymph node enlargement is frequent in AIDS patients and can be caused by lymphoma or granulomatous infection. Infections such as tularemia, anthrax, and plague can also cause lymphadenopathy, but these infections are quite uncommon.

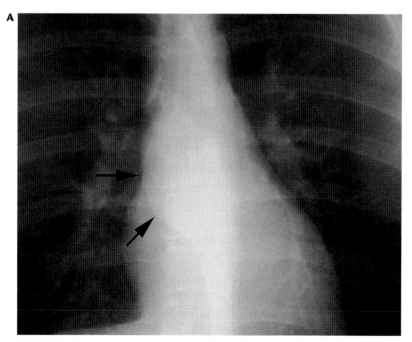

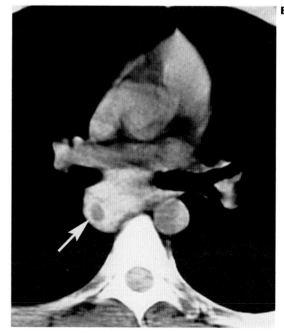

Fig. 14.35 Growing teratoma syndrome in a patient previously treated for a nonseminomatous germ cell malignancy of the testis. **A,** Coned-down view of a frontal chest radiograph shows a new subcarinal mass (arrows). **B,** CT shows that the mass is partially calcified and contains a small cystic region (arrow). Resection showed mature teratoma. (Courtesy of Jeffrey Galvin, Washington, DC)

Box 14.10 Causes of mediastinal and hilar lymph node enlargement

Infection
Common
Primary tuberculosis[204]
Fungal infection (esp. histoplasmosis)[205]
Uncommon
Viral (esp. Epstein–Barr virus)[206]
Parasitic (esp. *Pneumocystis jiroveci*)[207]
Bacterial
- Anthrax[196,208]
- Tularemia[209]
- Pneumonic plague (*Yersinia pestis*)[210]

Inflammatory
Sarcoidosis[211]
Silicosis[212]
Coal worker's pneumoconiosis[213]
Asbestos exposure[203]
Chronic beryllium disease[214–216]
Wegener granulomatosis[217]
Chronic interstitial pneumonia[197,201,202]
Collagen vascular disease[218–220]

Neoplasm
Primary
- Lymphoma
- Leukemia (especially CLL)
- Myeloma[221]
Metastatic[194,195]
- Lung
- Breast
- Melanoma
- Renal
- Testicular
- Unknown primary[222]

Other
Reactive hyperplasia
Castleman disease[223]
Amyloidosis[224–227]
Whipple disease[228–230]
Bronchiectasis (any cause)
Common variable immunodeficiency
Chronic eosinophilic pneumonia
Chronic congestive heart failure[198–200]
Drug induced lymphadenopathy (see Ch. 9)

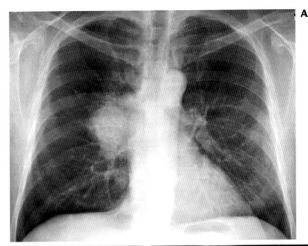

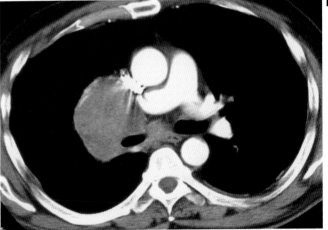

Fig. 14.37 Nonsmall cell lung cancer. **A**, Frontal chest radiograph shows a right hilar mass. Note splaying of the right upper and lower lobe bronchi. **B**, Contrast-enhanced CT confirms metastatic adenopathy.

Enlarged nodes in patients with anthrax are characteristically of high attenuation on CT due to extensive hemorrhage.[196] Significant lymphadenopathy is quite uncommon in other infections, particularly bacterial pneumonia, and, when present, suggests an unusual organism or alternative diagnosis.

Sarcoidosis is a particularly frequent cause of intrathoracic lymph node enlargement in young adults (Fig. 14.40). When multiple lymph node groups in the hila and mediastinum are symmetrically enlarged in a young patient, sarcoid is the most likely diagnosis. Lymphoma is the most important differential diagnosis in such patients, but lymphoma is rarely so symmetrically distributed with equal involvement of the hilar and mediastinal lymph node groups (Fig. 14.36). Isolated paracardiac node enlargement is unusual in cases of sarcoid or infection, and is often due to lymphoma or metastatic carcinoma.[231,232] Lymphoma and sarcoidosis are discussed further in Chapters 13 and 11 respectively.

Reactive hyperplasia is a term used to describe an acute or chronic nonspecific inflammatory response in which both inflammation and hyperplasia are present. Lymph nodes undergo reactive changes whenever challenged by infection, cell debris, or foreign substances. Thus, nodal enlargement due to reactive hyperplasia is seen in nodes draining areas of pulmonary infection, bronchiectasis, and a variety of inflammatory and chronic interstitial lung diseases,[197,233] and also in nodes draining neoplasms. Reactive hyperplasia is a common cause of false positive lymph nodes on ^{18}F-FDG PET scans in patients with nonsmall cell carcinoma.[234]

Chronic left heart failure is an important, and perhaps underrecognized, cause of mediastinal lymphadenopathy.[198–200] Slanetz et al[198] retrospectively reviewed CT scans of 46 patients with congestive heart failure and reported that enlarged mediastinal lymph nodes were present in 55% and that the mediastinal fat was of increased attenuation ("hazy") in 33%.

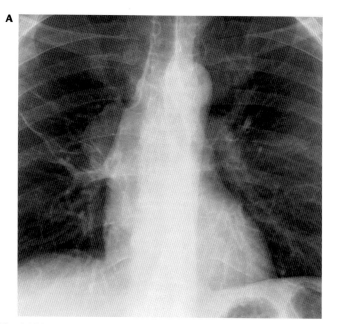

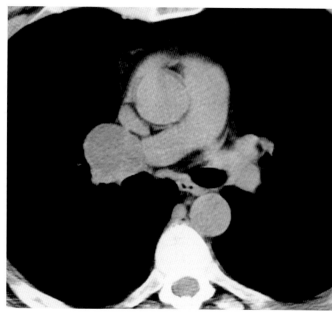

Fig. 14.38 Metastatic renal cell carcinoma. **A,** Frontal chest radiograph shows a well-marginated right hilar mass. **B,** Noncontrast CT shows that the nodal mass is of lower attenuation than the remainder of the mediastinum.

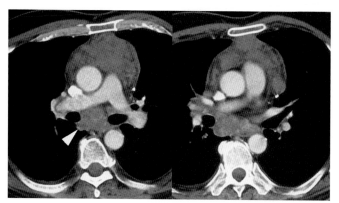

Fig. 14.39 Mediastinal tuberculosis. Contrast-enhanced CT shows a conglomerate mass of enlarged prevascular lymph nodes, as well as subcarinal lymphadenopathy. Note the subtle rim enhancement (arrowhead) of some of the nodes. Biopsy showed *Mycobacterium tuberculosis*.

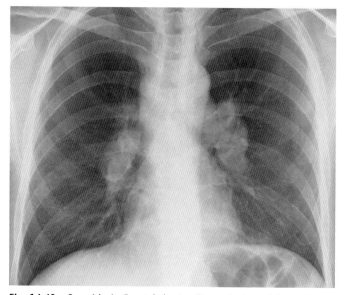

Fig. 14.40 Sarcoidosis. Frontal chest radiograph shows bilateral hilar, right paratracheal, aortopulmonary window and subcarinal lymphadenopathy. This symmetric pattern of lymphadenopathy is typical of sarcoidosis.

Ngom et al[199] reported three patients with congestive heart failure and mediastinal lymphadenopathy who underwent histopathologic sampling that showed sinus histiocytosis but no evidence of malignancy. Lymph nodes in one patient returned to normal when the patient was treated for heart failure. Erly et al[200] retrospectively reviewed CT scans of 44 patients with chronic left heart dysfunction and found that 66% had at least one enlarged mediastinal lymph node (short axis diameter >1 cm, see below). The presence of enlarged nodes was significantly correlated with a decline in left ventricular ejection fraction and enlarged nodes were observed in 81% of patients with an ejection fraction of <35%. Most (63%) of the enlarged nodes were in the pretracheal region and the mean short axis diameter for all enlarged nodes was 1.3 cm.[200] The precise etiology for lymphadenopathy in patients with chronic left heart dysfunction is unknown. It has been speculated, however, that

mediastinal lymph nodes hypertrophy in response to chronic mediastinal edema and lymphatic congestion.[199]

Mediastinal lymph node enlargement is also commonly seen in patients with *pulmonary fibrosis* that occurs idiopathically,[201,202] or in the setting of collagen vascular disease (Fig. 14.41)[199,207,235] or of asbestos exposure.[203] Bergin et al[202] reviewed CT scans of 14 patients with usual interstitial pneumonia and found that 13 (93%) had enlarged mediastinal lymph nodes. Nodes with a short axis diameter of >2 cm were seen in three (21%).[202] Niimi et al[197] reviewed CT scans in 175 patients with diffuse infiltrative lung disease and saw enlarged nodes in 67%. They reported that

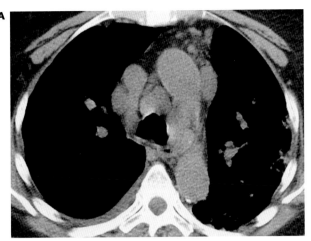
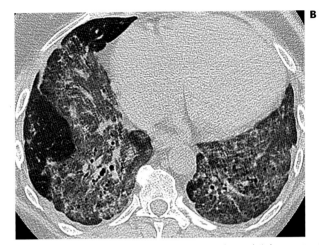

Fig. 14.41 Pulmonary fibrosis in a patient with scleroderma. **A**, CT shows multiple enlarged lymph nodes in the prevascular and right paratracheal regions. The largest node measures 1.5 cm in short axis dimension. **B**, HRCT shows diffuse ground-glass and irregular linear opacities and traction bronchiectasis consistent with nonspecific interstitial pneumonia.

67% of patients with usual interstitial pneumonia and 70% of those with fibrosis due to collagen vascular disease had lymphadenopathy. However, they also noted that the vast majority of patients had only a few enlarged nodes and that they rarely exceeded 15 mm in short axis diameter.[197] Jung et al[201] retrospectively analyzed CT scans in 30 patients with pulmonary fibrosis. They saw enlarged nodes in 86% of patients and also found that the number of enlarged nodes positively correlated with the severity of fibrosis. Histopathologic analysis of enlarged lymph nodes in patients with fibrosis usually shows reactive change or sinus histiocytosis.[197]

Castleman disease (Box 14.11)

Castleman disease[236] (also known as giant lymph node hyperplasia or angiofollicular lymph node hyperplasia) is a rare cause of massive lymph node enlargement.[237] Although intrathoracic lymph nodes are most commonly affected, nodes at any location can be involved.[223,238] There are two important histopathologic variants: hyaline vascular and plasma cell. The hyaline vascular type is the most common (90%) and shows a follicular structure with tumor nodules composed predominantly of small lymphocytes, and a large number of blood vessels in the interfollicular areas. The plasma cell type (10%) shows sheets of interfollicular cells and fewer blood vessels.[239] Surgical excision can be curative if the lesion can be completely excised.[240] The pathogenesis of Castleman disease remains a subject of investigation, but the disease is believed to be mediated by abnormal production of a B lymphocyte growth factor, such as interleukin-6, leading to abnormal lymphoid proliferation.[237]

Patients with Castleman disease have been classically distinguished by histopathologic type (hyaline vascular versus plasma cell). However, more recent research suggests that the more important distinction, particularly in terms of treatment and prognosis, is whether the disease is localized or disseminated (multifocal).[223,237] Furthermore, hyaline vascular and plasma cell lesions may occur concomitantly at separate sites.[237] However, there are important clinical and radiologic differences between patients who have focal hyaline vascular disease and those that have focal or multifocal plasma cell disease.

Box 14.11 Thoracic Castleman disease

Etiology
Unknown
Abnormal production of B lymphocyte growth factor

Histopathology
Hyaline vascular (90%)
Plasma cell (10%)
Both types may coexist

Location
Middle mediastinum (subcarinal or paratracheal)
Hila
Other mediastinal, chest wall, lung parenchyma

Types
Localized – usually hyaline vascular
Multifocal – usually plasma cell or mixed

Clinical features
Localized hyaline vascular
• Asymptomatic or symptoms due to mass effect
• Good prognosis with resection
Multifocal plasma cell
• Constitutional symptoms (fever, weight loss, night sweats)
• Variable prognosis

Imaging
Localized hyaline vascular
• Large solitary mass ± associated lymphadenopathy
• May be locally invasive
• Heterogeneous soft tissue attenuation
• Intense contrast enhancement, large feeding vessels
• Flow voids on MRI
Multifocal plasma cell
• Diffuse lymphadenopathy
• Less intense enhancement

Lung parenchymal Castleman disease
Rare
Usually in setting of multifocal disease
Histopathology: lymphocytic interstitial pneumonia
CT
• Centrilobular nodules
• Septal thickening
• Thin walled cysts

A

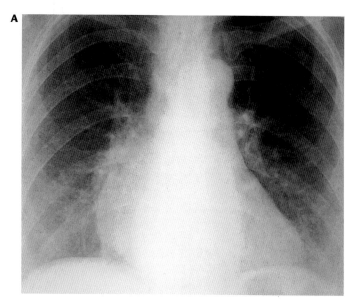

B

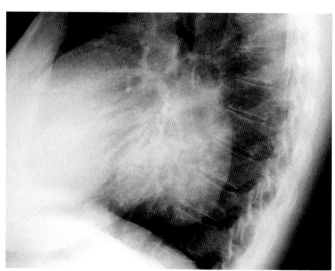

C

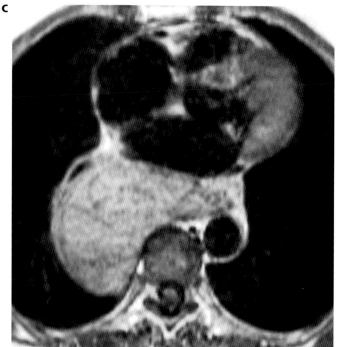

Fig. 14.42 Hyaline vascular Castleman disease. **A**, Frontal and **B**, lateral chest radiographs show a large, well-marginated subcarinal mass. **C**, Axial T1-weighted MRI shows that the mass is of slightly increased signal intensity compared to skeletal muscle. Note low signal internal septations. (With permission from McAdams HP, Rosado-de-Christenson M, Fishback NF, Templeton PA. Castleman disease of the thorax: radiologic features with clinical and histopathologic correlation. Radiology 1998;209:221–228.)

Patients with focal hyaline vascular Castleman disease are often asymptomatic at presentation.[223,238] The remainder present with signs or symptoms related to compression or invasion of adjacent mediastinal structures. Patients with focal or multifocal plasma cell Castleman disease usually present with constitutional signs or symptoms, such as fever, fatigue, anemia, gamma globulin abnormalities and elevated lactic dehydrogenase.[239] Castleman disease of either type may occur at any age, but it most frequently affects young adults.[223] McAdams et al[204] reviewed 30 cases of pathologically proven Castleman disease at the Armed Forces Institute of Pathology. In this series, 80% of patients had focal Castleman disease, but this proportion could reflect the referral bias typical of surgical series. Other authors have reported a higher frequency of multifocal disease.[241,242] Multifocal Castleman disease is almost always due to the plasma

cell variant and pursues a course similar to lymphoma. An association between multifocal Castleman disease and Kaposi sarcoma is reported in AIDS patients.[243,244]

On chest radiographs, localized hyaline vascular Castleman disease usually manifests as a focal, well-defined, smooth or lobular, mediastinal or hilar mass (Fig. 14.42). The mass is typically quite large and most commonly occurs in the middle mediastinum or hila.[203,240,245] Occasionally, the lesion is found in other sites, including the posterior mediastinum and chest wall.[203,238,245] On noncontrast-enhanced CT, the mass is usually homogeneous and of soft tissue attenuation (Fig. 14.43). Calcification is uncommon (5–10%) and, when it occurs, is typically coarse and central in location (Fig. 14.44). Imaging studies show one of three morphologic patterns: (1) solitary mass (50%); (2) dominant infiltrative mass with associated

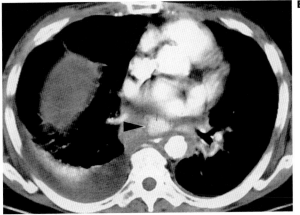

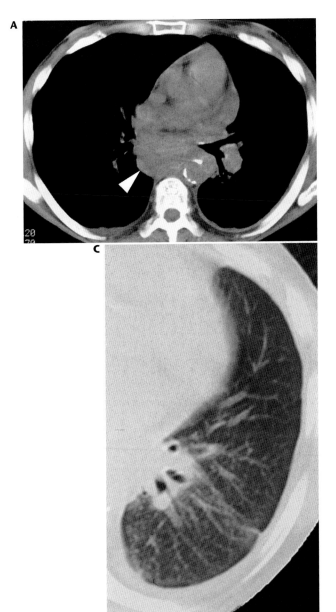

Fig. 14.43   Multifocal hyaline vascular Castleman disease. **A**, Noncontrast CT shows a homogeneous soft tissue mass (arrowhead) in the subcarinal region. **B**, Contrast-enhanced CT shows marked enhancement within the mass (arrowhead). **C**, CT coned to the left lung shows tiny centrilobular nodules in the lower lobe. Biopsy showed lymphocytic interstitial pneumonia.

lymphadenopathy (40%); and (3) diffuse lymphadenopathy confined to a single mediastinal compartment (10%).[204] Identification of the first pattern suggests that complete surgical resection is likely; the second or third pattern suggests that complete excision may be difficult or impossible.[204]

Because of its highly vascular nature, hyaline vascular Castleman disease usually enhances intensely following administration of intravenous contrast material (Fig. 14.43)[223,238,241,246–251] – a distinctive feature that helps differentiate Castleman disease from many other mediastinal lesions including lymphoma. The lesions are also found to be highly vascular at angiography.[240,246,252] Plasma cell Castleman disease is less vascular, and shows less enhancement at contrast-enhanced CT or angiography.[204]

The lesions are typically heterogeneous and have increased signal intensity compared to skeletal muscle on T1-weighted MRI sequences (Figs 14.42 and 14.44).[252–254] They become markedly hyperintense on T2-weighted sequences (Fig. 14.44).

Low signal intensity septa are occasionally visible within the lesions. In larger lesions, flow voids in and around the mass may be identified and are important clues to the hypervascular nature of the mass. Because the lesions are hypervascular, diffuse enhancement following administration of intravenous gadolinium is common (Fig. 14.44).

Multifocal Castleman disease usually manifests on chest radiographs with diffuse mediastinal widening (Fig. 14.45). On CT or MRI, multifocal lymph node enlargement is noted. Because the lesions are usually due to the plasma cell variant, enhancement with iodinated contrast material or gadolinium may not be a prominent finding.

Castleman disease may, very rarely, involve the lung parenchyma (Fig. 14.43). Reported manifestations include a pulmonary mass,[239,255] centrilobular nodules,[256] septal thickening,[256] and thin walled cysts.[256] Most patients with diffuse lung involvement have multifocal disease and the lung findings are usually due to associated lymphocytic interstitial pneumonia.[256]

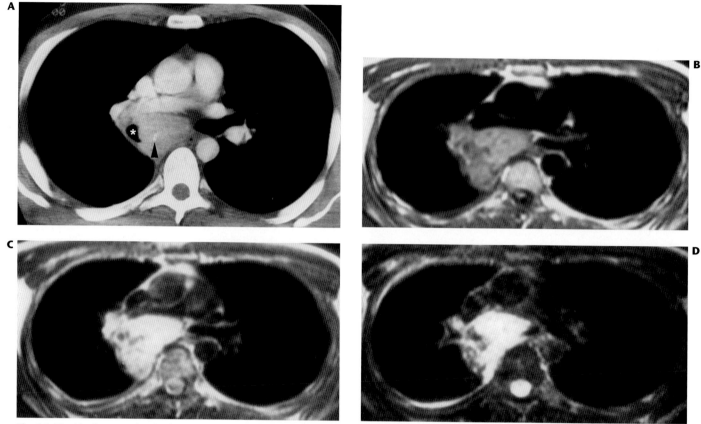

Fig. 14.44 Hyaline vascular Castleman disease. **A**, Contrast-enhanced CT shows an enhancing subcarinal mass. Note the mass effect upon the bronchus intermedius (*) and two small foci of calcification (arrowhead). Axial T1-weighted MRI obtained **B**, before and **C**, after administration of gadolinium based contrast material shows that the mass is heterogeneous and intensely enhances. **D**, T2-weighted MRI shows marked increase signal intensity within the mass. (With permission from McAdams HP, Rosado-de-Christenson M, Fishback NF, Templeton PA. Castleman disease of the thorax: radiologic features with clinical and histopathologic correlation. Radiology 1998;209:221–228.)

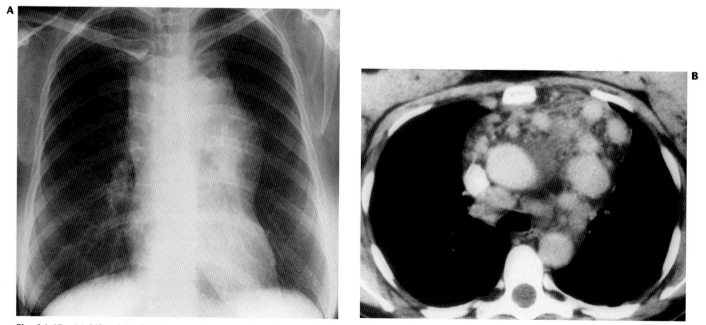

Fig. 14.45 Multifocal Castleman disease in a patient with weight loss and night sweats. **A**, Frontal chest radiograph shows bilateral mediastinal widening. **B**, Contrast-enhanced CT shows multiple enhancing lymph nodes with ill-defined margins. (With permission from McAdams HP, Rosado-de-Christenson M, Fishback NF, Templeton PA. Castleman disease of the thorax: radiologic features with clinical and histopathologic correlation. Radiology 1998;209:221–228.)

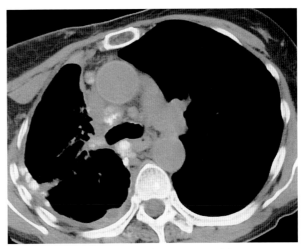

Box 14.12 Causes of lymph node calcification

Benign disease
Tuberculous and fungal disease* (notably histoplasmosis)
Pneumocystis jiroveci infection in patients with AIDS
Sarcoidosis*
Silicosis and coal worker's pneumoconiosis*
Amyloidosis*
Castleman disease

Malignant disease
Treated lymphoma and other neoplasms* (calcification in untreated lymphoma almost never occurs)
Metastases from primary tumor
- Osteosarcoma
- Chondrosarcoma
- Mucinous adenocarcinoma

(*eggshell calcification is reported)

Fig. 14.47 Metastatic mucinous adenocarinoma of the ovary. Noncontrast CT shows multiple calcified lymph nodes within the right mediastinum and hilum. Note also the partially calcified pleural nodules.

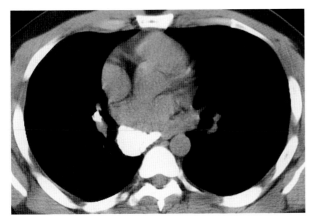

Fig. 14.46 Histoplasmosis. Noncontrast CT shows a densely calcified nodal mass in the subcarinal region as well as a small calcified right hilar node.

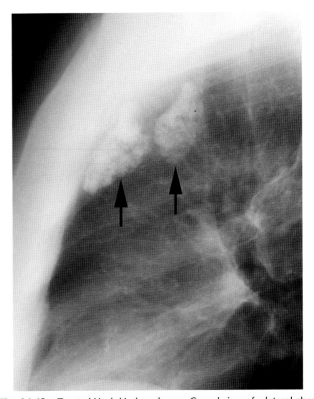

Fig. 14.48 Treated Hodgkin lymphoma. Coned view of a lateral chest radiograph shows calcified nodal masses (arrows) in the anterior mediastinum.

Diagnosis of Lymphadenopathy

Important clues to the presence and sometimes the cause of mediastinal or hilar lymph node disease include enlargement and abnormal density on chest radiographs, attenuation on CT or signal intensity on MRI. It is important to remember, however, that lymph nodes of normal size and attenuation or signal intensity can harbor disease, including malignancy.

Lymph node calcification (Box 14.12)
Calcification of intrathoracic lymph nodes is a common sequela of certain infections, particularly tuberculosis and histoplasmosis (Fig. 14.46). It can also be seen in other benign conditions, such as sarcoidosis, silicosis, coal worker's pneumoconiosis, amyloidosis, and Castleman disease. Lymph node calcification is very rarely due to neoplastic disease. Lymph node metastases from calcifying primary malignancies, such as osteosarcoma, chondrosarcoma, carcinoid tumors, and mucinous colorectal and ovarian carcinomas (Fig. 14.47) may calcify.[257,258] Lymph node calcification can occur after treatment of mediastinal lymphoma (Fig. 14.48), but is quite rare prior to treatment.[259,260] CT clearly demonstrates

lymph node calcification to better advantage than chest radiographs. MRI is limited, however, in its ability to show calcification, a notable disadvantage.[261]

Various patterns of lymph node calcification can be seen. Coarse irregular clumplike calcification of a part of the node and homogeneous calcification of the entire node are the two most common patterns. A strikingly foamy pattern of calcification is described in AIDS patients with disseminated *Pneumocystis jiroveci* infection,[262,263] and in patients with metastatic mucinous

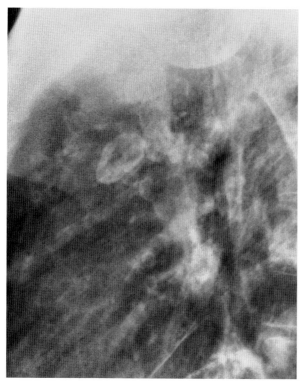

Fig. 14.49 Amyloidosis. Coned view of a lateral chest radiograph shows enlarged, rim calcified ("egg-shell") mediastinal lymph nodes.

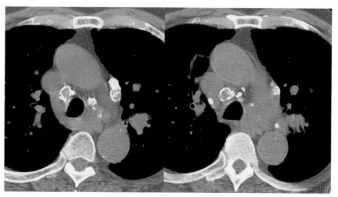

Fig. 14.50 Sarcoidosis. Noncontrast CT shows multiple slightly enlarged mediastinal lymph nodes with thin rim ("egg-shell") calcification.

neoplasms. Thin peripheral calcification – so-called "eggshell calcification" (Figs 14.49 and 14.50) – is seen in patients with coal worker's pneumoconiosis, silicosis and, sometimes, sarcoidosis.[264–266] In one series, eggshell calcification was seen on chest radiographs in 3% of coalworkers with >30 years' experience.[265] Eggshell calcification is rarely seen in other conditions, but has been reported in patients with amyloidosis, histoplasmosis, blastomycosis, and treated lymphoma.[224]

Low attenuation on CT

Areas of low CT attenuation within enlarged nodes, likely due to necrosis (Fig. 14.51), are seen in a variety of conditions, including tuberculosis,[267,268] nontuberculous mycobacterial infection, metastatic disease, particularly testicular tumors,[269,270] and lymphoma. In one series, 16 of 76 patients with Hodgkin disease had low-attenuation lymphadenopathy on CT at presentation.[271] Some nodes have a prominent fatty hilum on CT. This feature is associated with benign disease and is usually thought to be the result of previous inflammation. Low-attenuation or even fatty nodes have also been described in patients with Whipple disease.[230]

Contrast enhancement on CT

Contrast enhancement in enlarged nodes, when moderate in degree, is nonspecific and is seen in patients with tuberculosis,[268,272] fungal infection,[267] sarcoidosis, and metastatic neoplasm. When enhancement is dramatic, however, it suggests metastatic neoplasm from a highly vascular primary tumor, such as melanoma, renal or thyroid carcinoma, carcinoid tumor

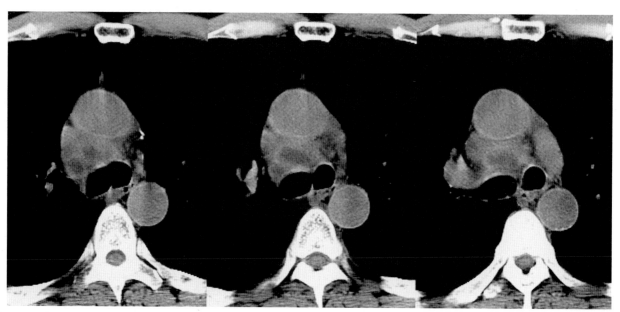

Fig. 14.51 Tuberculosis. Noncontrast CT shows multiple enlarged lymph nodes with low-attenuation centers.

or leiomyosarcoma. Castleman disease is a further, though rare, cause of markedly enhancing lymph nodes (see Fig. 14.45). Peripheral, or rim, enhancement is a feature of tuberculosis (see Fig. 14.39)[268] and can be of diagnostic value in situations where tuberculosis is likely and metastatic carcinoma is not.[272]

Chest radiographic signs of mediastinal lymph node enlargement

How large a mediastinal or hilar node has to be for it to be detectable on chest radiographs cannot easily be established. The size threshold depends largely upon the location of the node in the mediastinum, the presence of other mediastinal abnormalities such as tortuous great vessel or lipomatosis, and radiographic technique. Most nodes with a short axis diameter of 2 cm or greater in the right paratracheal region, the aortopulmonary window, the hilar, or the paravertebral regions should be detected on appropriately exposed posteroanterior chest radiographs. However, nodes in the pretracheal, left paratracheal, subcarinal, and paracardiac regions may be considerably >2 cm in diameter and yet not be identified on chest radiographs.[231,273]

Upper right paratracheal node enlargement (Fig. 14.52) (station 2R of the AJCC/UICC nomenclature,[274] see p. 56) manifests as uniform or lobular widening of the right paratracheal stripe.[275] When the paratracheal nodes become substantially enlarged, the lateral border of the superior vena cava may become convex rather than flat or concave. The apparent density of the superior vena cava may be increased and equal that of the aortic arch (normally the density of the superior vena cava in the right paratracheal area is significantly less than that of the aortic arch). When the lower right paratracheal (azygos) nodes (station 4R) enlarge, they displace the azygos vein laterally so that the diameter of the combined shadow of the azygos node and vein enlarges (the normal diameter on an upright chest film should be 7 mm or less[276]).

Enlargement of the upper left paratracheal nodes (station 2L) is frequently obscured by the shadows of the left carotid and subclavian arteries. These nodes have to be quite large to be detected on chest radiographs. If the aortopulmonary nodes (station 5) are substantially enlarged, they project beyond the aortopulmonary window and appear as a mass in the angle between the aortic arch and the main pulmonary artery (Fig. 14.53).[277] Enlargement of the anterior mediastinal nodes, i.e. nodes anterior to the aorta (station 6), the innominate artery (station 3), and the trachea (stations 2 and 4), must be substantial to be recognizable on chest radiographs. The resulting mediastinal abnormality is frequently bilateral and lobulated in contour (Fig. 14.54). Sometimes, the only finding of lymph node enlargement in these areas is increased opacity of the retrosternal area on the lateral view.

Enlargement of the anterior intercostal, or internal mammary, nodes is best recognized on the lateral chest radiograph as well-marginated, retrosternal soft tissue masses along the course of the internal mammary arteries. Significant enlargement may result in upper parasternal opacities on the frontal radiograph.[278]

The most useful sign of subcarinal node (station 7) enlargement on chest radiographs is a change from the normally concave contour of the superior portion of the azygoesophageal interface (Fig. 14.55) into a convex bulge.[279] Alteration of the contour of the azygoesophageal interface is, unfortunately, a relatively insensitive sign of subcarinal lymphadenopathy. It was noted in only 23% of the patients with subcarinal lymph node enlargement reported by Müller et al.[273] Effacement of the interface, without a bulge, is a less specific finding for subcarinal pathology, particularly in children.[280,281] Other chest radiographic findings of subcarinal node enlargement include increased opacity in the subcarinal region,[282] and obscuration of the medial margin of the bronchus intermedius.[273] Since the esophagus passes immediately behind the carina, subcarinal node enlargement may cause posterior displacement of the esophagus.

Enlarged paraesophageal nodes (station 8) and posterior mediastinal nodes result in displacement of the azygoesophageal and paraspinal interfaces.

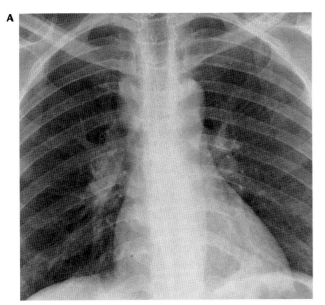
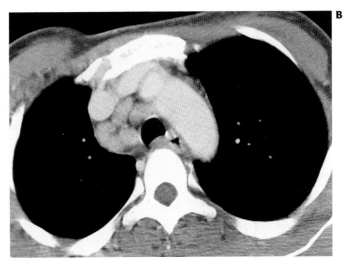

Fig. 14.52 *Mycobacterium avium* complex infection in a patient with AIDS. **A,** Frontal chest radiograph shows right paratracheal and possibly right hilar lymphadenopathy. **B,** Contrast-enhanced CT confirms lymphadenopathy in the right paratracheal region.

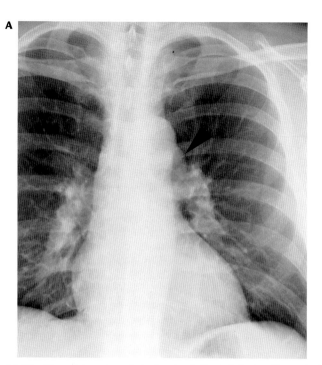

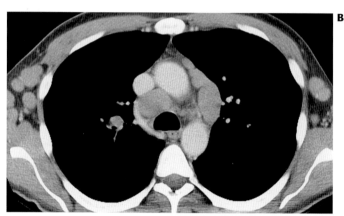

Fig. 14.53 Chronic lymphocytic leukemia. **A,** Frontal chest radiograph shows convexity in the aortopulmonary window (arrowhead). **B,** Contrast-enhanced CT confirms aortopulmonary window lymphadenopathy. Note also the enlarged nodes in the right paratracheal region and both axilla.

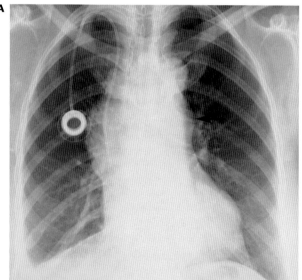

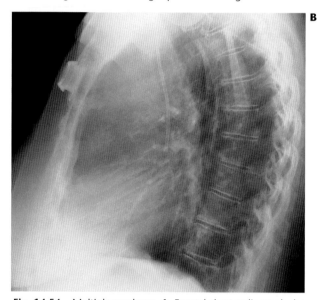

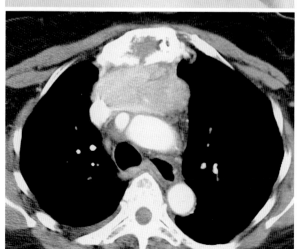

Fig. 14.54 Multiple myeloma. **A,** Frontal chest radiograph shows lateral displacement and convexity of the aortopulmonary reflection (arrow), as well as widening of the right mediastinum. These findings suggest prevascular adenopathy. **B,** Lateral chest radiograph shows increased soft tissue opacity in the retrosternal region. **C,** Contrast-enhanced CT confirms matted lymphadenopathy in the prevascular space. Note also the lytic expansile sternal lesion.

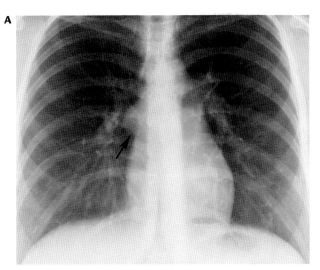
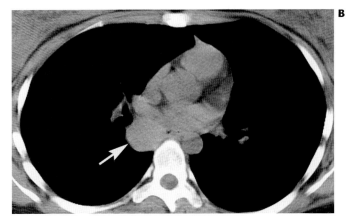

Fig. 14.55 Subcarinal mass. **A,** Frontal chest radiograph shows a smooth subcarinal mass (arrow). Note displacement of the right bronchus. **B,** CT shows that the mass (arrow) is homogeneous and of soft tissue attenuation.

CT of mediastinal lymph node enlargement

CT more readily demonstrates lymph node enlargement than chest radiography. The optimal CT technique for detection of enlarged mediastinal lymph nodes remains a subject of debate and is related to the rapidly changing nature of CT technology. In general, the thinner the slice collimation used, the better individual nodes will be shown.[283] Thin collimation images obtained on a multidetector spiral CT scanner will likely show more nodes than relatively thick collimation images on a single slice spiral or nonspiral scanner. However, whether this improvement in node detection makes a significant clinical difference to the patient is less certain and depends upon the specific clinical circumstances. Furthermore, although CT images are traditionally reviewed in axial format, Kozuka et al[284] has shown that coronal reformat images from multidetector CT data sets obtained using thin slice collimation (0.5 or 2 mm collimation) performed better for the detection of enlarged lymph nodes than conventional 5 mm postcontrast scans.[284] Again, whether this improvement translates into improved patient outcome remains to be seen.

Whether or not intravenous contrast is necessary for detection of mediastinal lymphadenopathy also remains a subject of debate and is, for the most part, a decision that rests upon the experience of the interpreter and individual preference. Cascade et al[285] compared contrast-enhanced to noncontrast CT for staging lung cancer and found that contrast-enhanced CT revealed more enlarged lymph nodes, particularly at the 2R station.[285] However, they also reported excellent overall agreement between the two studies for the presence and total number of enlarged lymph nodes, suggesting that the observed differences might not be clinically relevant. Patz et al[286] compared contrast-enhanced to noncontrast CT for staging lung cancer and found that contrast-enhanced CT rarely changed the tumor stage determined by noncontrast CT.[286] These authors concluded that intravenous contrast was not needed for routine thoracic CT.

CT findings of mediastinal lymphadenopathy (Figs 14.50 to 14.54) include: (1) an increase in size of individual nodes; (2) focal mediastinal contour abnormalities or lobulations of the interface between the mediastinum and lung; (3) invasion of surrounding mediastinal fat; (4) coalescence of adjacent and enlarged nodes to form larger masses; and (5) diffuse soft tissue attenuation throughout the mediastinum obliterating the mediastinal fat. Individually enlarged nodes are seen as round or oval soft tissue lesions in the mediastinum. Distinguishing enlarged nodes from normal vascular structures requires thorough knowledge of the normal arrangement of blood vessels and an understanding of the various anomalies and variations in the arrangement of the mediastinal vessels (see pp. 50 and 999). Intravenous contrast enhancement may be needed to help distinguish vessels from lymph nodes in problematic cases.

Many authors have studied CT scans in normal patients in order to establish normal size criteria for mediastinal or hilar lymph nodes (see p. 56).[287–290] These studies suggest that the upper limit of normal for short axis lymph node diameter is about 1 cm. However, nodes between 10 and 15 mm in short axis diameter may be normally found in certain areas, such as the subcarinal region. Short axis diameter is considered the standard for diagnosis because it is the most reproducible measurement and has the best correlation with lymph node volume at autopsy.[291]

It is easier to identify and measure right sided mediastinal lymph nodes than to evaluate the left sided nodes, because of the more abundant mediastinal fat and less complex vascular anatomy on the right.[291] Subcarinal lymph node enlargement may be difficult to recognize at CT. Important signs include: a soft tissue mass between the esophagus and either the left atrium or the intramediastinal portions of the right or left pulmonary arteries; or a soft tissue mass that extends into the azygoesophageal recess, posterior to the bronchus intermedius and the left lower lobe bronchus.

MRI of mediastinal lymph node enlargement

For the most part, MRI and CT provide comparable information regarding enlarged mediastinal nodes. However, MRI is frequently more time consuming, more difficult for patients, and more limited in availability than CT at most centers. It can also be difficult to distinguish a cluster of small normal nodes from a single enlarged node or to detect intranodal calcification

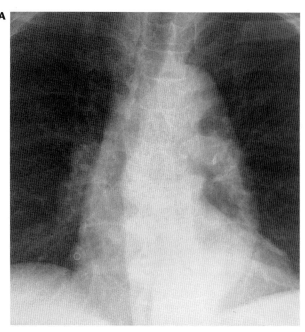

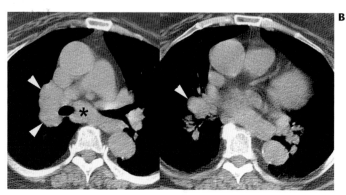

Fig. 14.56 Chronic lymphocytic leukemia. **A**, Frontal chest radiograph shows subtle lobulation of the right hilum. Note the normal appearance of the left hilum and the enlarged descending thoracic aorta. **B**, Noncontrast CT confirms right hilar (arrowheads) and subcarinal (*) lymphadenopathy.

at MRI.[261] Furthermore, differences in signal intensity at MRI have not proved to be a reliable method for differentiating benign from malignant adenopathy. For these reasons, MRI is used primarily for patients for whom the use of iodinated intravenous contrast material is contraindicated.[234,292]

There has been some interest in using contrast agents such as gadolinium DTPA[293,294] and superparamagnetic iron oxide[295,296] to increase sensitivity and specificity of MRI for detection of lymph node metastases. While these agents have shown promise in small series, their utility for staging malignancies such as lung cancer remains unproven, at least in large clinical trials.

Chest radiographic findings of hilar lymph node enlargement

The findings of hilar node enlargement on chest radiographs are enlargement of the hilum, increased lobulation of the hilar contours, a rounded mass in a portion of the hilum that does not contain major vessels (Fig. 14.56, see also Figs 14.37, 14.38 and 14.40), and increased density of the hilum.[297] In certain highly vascular regions of the hila (e.g. the intersection of the right superior pulmonary vein and interlobar artery, and the inferior aspect of the hilum where the inferior pulmonary veins intersect the lower lobe segmental arteries), nodal enlargement must be substantial to be recognized radiographically. Enlarged nodes adjacent to the lower lobe arteries increase the overall diameter of the hilum (the transverse diameter of each lower lobe artery should be no greater than 16 mm) and result in a lobular rather than the normal tubular configuration. Lymph node enlargement in the upper portions of the hila is often easily detected because the vessels in these regions are normally small. Even mild nodal enlargement can be recognized on the lateral view when the enlarged nodes lie posterior to the right main bronchus and bronchus intermedius (Fig. 14.57), because

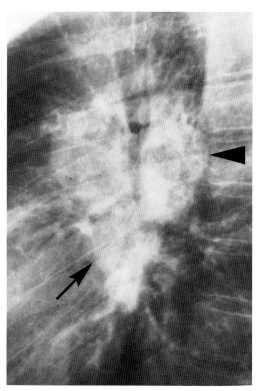

Fig. 14.57 Sarcoidosis. Lateral chest radiograph shows typical finding of hilar lymphadenopathy. Note the abnormal opacity posterior to the bronchus intermedius (arrowhead) and anterior to the lower lobe bronchus (arrow), two areas normally devoid of opacity on the lateral view.

lung normally contacts the posterior wall of the airway in this region. Another important region to evaluate for hilar adenopathy on the lateral view is the angle formed by the lower lobe bronchi and the middle lobe or lingula bronchus (Fig. 14.58) – the so-called inferior hilar window.[298]

It may, at times, be very difficult to distinguish enlarged hilar lymph nodes from enlargement of the hilar arteries due to pulmonary hypertension (Fig. 14.59). Correct diagnosis depends on determining that the abnormality is truly centered on the pulmonary arteries and on evaluating the degree of lobulation.

A hilar mass in a location that is normally devoid of vessels clearly favors nodal enlargement. Enlarged central pulmonary arteries usually retain their tubular configuration. Lobulated hilar enlargement favors lymphadenopathy. If needed, contrast-enhanced CT will answer the question.

CT of hilar node enlargement

The recognition of hilar node enlargement at CT is facilitated by intravenous contrast opacification of the hilar vessels (see Fig. 14.37).[299] Lymph nodes generally do not enhance to the same

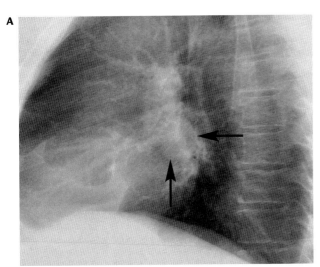
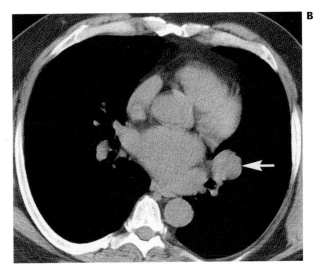

Fig. 14.58 Metastatic adenocarcinoma. **A,** Lateral chest radiograph shows a mass (arrows) in the "inferior hilar window". **B,** Noncontrast CT confirms left hilar lymphadenopathy (arrow).

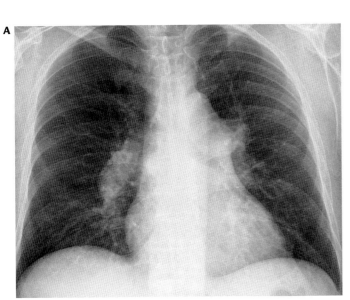
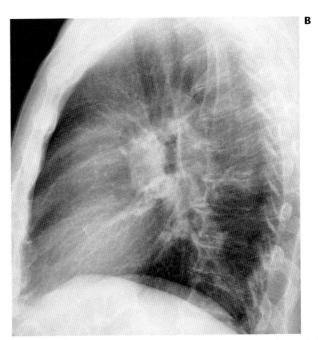

Fig. 14.59 Pulmonary arterial hypertension. **A,** Frontal and **B,** lateral chest radiographs show enlarged central pulmonary arteries. Note the typical tubular configuration of the enlarged pulmonary arteries and the evidence of right heart enlargement on the lateral view, a finding that supports the diagnosis.

degree as blood vessels. The majority of nodes in the hilum, except those around the lower hilum, are normally <3 mm in short axis diameter.[300] However, nonenhancing hilar tissue that is up to 7 mm in short axis diameter is commonly seen in the lower hila.[300] If the examination is performed without contrast, then the recognition of nodal enlargement depends on demonstrating rounded soft tissue densities that are too large to be blood vessels (see Figs 14.38, 14.56 and 14.58).[301–304] The smallest node that can be reliably detected on noncontrast CT varies with location. Some portions of the hilum are normally devoid of vessels >5 mm in diameter and thus relatively small nodes may be detected as contour abnormalities in these regions. In other regions of the hila, however, the vessel diameters may be 15 mm, or greater if there is increased pulmonary blood flow or pulmonary arterial hypertension, limiting detection of all but the largest nodes. Perhaps the most sensitive area for detection of hilar adenopathy on noncontrast CT is the region immediately behind the right main bronchus and its divisions – the right upper lobe bronchus and the bronchus intermedius – because, in these regions, the lung normally contacts the posterior wall of the airway.[305] Increased soft tissue opacity, especially if it is lobulated, in this region is suggestive of adenopathy. The equivalent area in the left hilum is occupied by the descending aorta and left descending pulmonary artery; therefore, only a small portion of lung contacts the posterior wall of the left main bronchus,[306] limiting detection of adenopathy in this region. The most difficult, and therefore the least sensitive, area for detection of hilar adenopathy is the central portion of the right hilum, where the right superior pulmonary vein crosses directly anterior to the right pulmonary artery and its major divisions. Additionally, there are fat pads at the bifurcation of the right pulmonary artery that can resemble lymph node enlargement on axial CT. It can be difficult to recognize the fatty nature of these pads because of partial volume averaging with the adjacent arteries and lung.[307]

MRI of hilar node enlargement

As is the case with imaging mediastinal lymph node enlargement, MRI and CT provides comparable information regarding enlarged hilar nodes. However, hilar node enlargement may be more easily recognized with MRI than with noncontrast CT.[261,267,308,309] For the most part, MRI is used primarily in patients for whom the use of iodinated intravenous contrast material is contraindicated.[234,292]

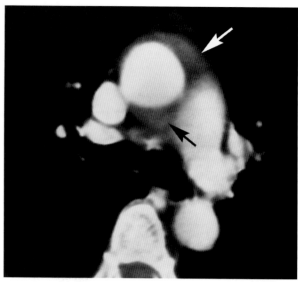

Fig. 14.60 Superior pericardial recesses. Contrast-enhanced CT shows crescent shaped structures anterior (white arrow) and posterior (black arrow) to the proximal ascending aorta. The recesses are differentiated from lymphadenopathy by virtue of their attenuation value (water) and characteristic shape and location.

Pitfalls in the diagnosis of intrathoracic lymph node enlargement

There are a variety of anatomic structures that can be confused with mediastinal lymph node enlargement,[310–312] including enlarged blood vessels and vascular variants such as aortic anomalies (p. 999), azygos continuation of the inferior vena cava, varix of the azygos vein,[313–316] and aneurysmal dilation of the brachiocephalic vein or superior vena cava.[316–318] Fluid in the various pericardial recesses can occasionally mimic lymphadenopathy or other mediastinal masses.[319,320] Choi et al[319] described a series of patients with posterior superior pericardial recesses that extended cephalad to the level of the aortic arch ("high riding") and were misdiagnosed as lymphadenopathy. Some of these pitfalls are illustrated in Figures 14.60 to 14.62.

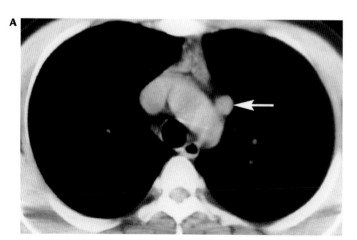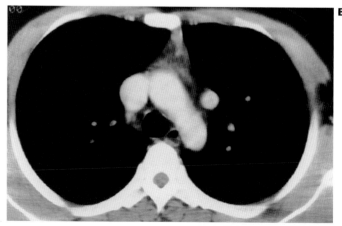

Fig. 14.61 Persistent left superior vena cava. **A**, Noncontrast CT shows a round soft tissue attenuation structure in the left prevascular space (arrow). **B**, The anomalous vein enhances following administration of intravenous contrast.

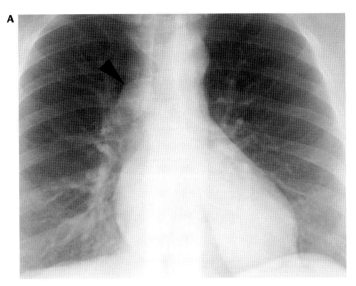

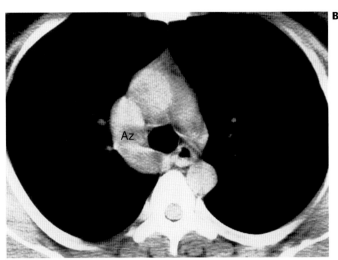

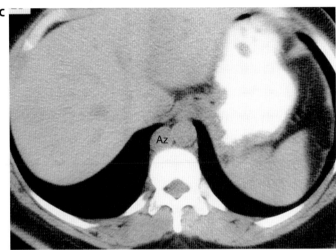

Fig. 14.62 Azygos continuation of the inferior vena cava. **A**, Frontal chest radiograph shows a right tracheobronchial angle mass (arrowhead), concerning for lymphadenopathy. **B** and **C**, CT confirms that the opacity is a dilated azygos vein (Az) due to interruption of the inferior vena cava.

Lymphovascular tumors of the mediastinum

Lymphangioma
Mediastinal lymphangioma (cystic hygroma) is discussed in Chapter 16.

Blood vessel tumors
Blood vessel tumors in the mediastinum are rare and frequently benign. Capillary or cavernous hemangiomas[321] are the most common lesions. Hemangioendothelioma,[322] hemangiosarcoma, hemangiopericytoma,[323] hemangioendothelioma,[324] and mixed lymphatic and blood vessel lesions, such as lymphangiohemangiomas[325–327] are quite rare.

Hemangiomas are rare mediastinal tumors that account for <0.5% of all mediastinal masses.[328] Mediastinal hemangiomas usually occur in the anterior (68%) or posterior mediastinum (22%), though multicompartment involvement is found in up to 14% of cases.[329–332] Most mediastinal lesions are cavernous hemangiomas and are composed of large interconnecting vascular spaces with varying amounts of interposed stromal elements, such as fat and fibrous tissue. Focal areas of organized thrombus can calcify as phleboliths. Affected patients are usually asymptomatic.

On chest radiographs, hemangiomas manifest as sharp, well-marginated mediastinal masses (Fig. 14.63). Phleboliths are seen in <10% of cases but, when present, are diagnostic. CT typically reveals a heterogeneous mass with intense central and peripheral rimlike enhancement after administration of intravenous contrast.[322,328,329,333,334] Hemangiomas typically have heterogeneous signal intensity on T1-weighted images. In lesions with significant stromal fat, linear areas of increased signal intensity on T1-weighted images can occasionally be identified. The central vascular spaces typically become markedly hyperintense on T2-weighted images, a suggestive feature (Fig. 14.63).[335]

Mixed lymphangioma/hemangioma is a variant of hemangioma seen most frequently in children and young adults.[336] The lesion may be localized to the thorax or occur as a more systemic process. When it occurs in the chest, the lesion may involve the mediastinum, pleura, and chest wall as a single process causing widespread lobular soft tissue swelling, bone destruction and chylous pleural effusion. This destructive form of the disease is known as Gorham disease.[337,338] Cystic angiomatosis is another, probably distinct, form of widespread lymphangiomatosis[339] in which lymphangiomas and hemangiomas may coexist. Many different sites in the body are involved, including the mediastinum, pericardium, and pleura.

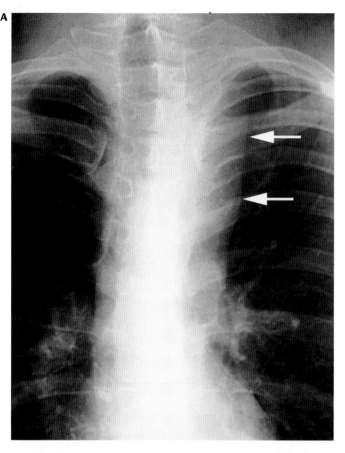

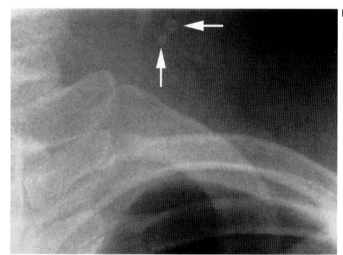

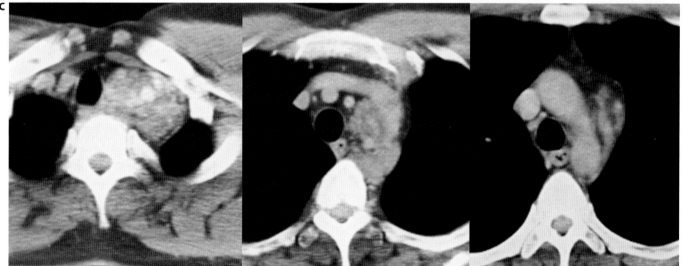

Fig. 14.63 Mediastinal hemangioma. **A,** Frontal chest radiograph shows left mediastinal widening (arrows). **B,** Coned view shows phleboliths (arrows) in the left supraclavicular fossa. **C,** Contrast-enhanced CT shows a heterogeneous enhancing mass extending from the neck into the left upper mediastinum.

Multiple lytic lesions may be seen in the bones.[340] The condition is most frequently seen in children and young adults. Lymphangiomatosis is discussed further in Chapter 16.

Mediastinal hemorrhage

Trauma to the aorta, branch vessels or spine (Fig. 14.64) is a frequent cause of mediastinal hemorrhage (Ch. 17). Common spontaneous causes of mediastinal hemorrhage include aortic dissection (see p. 986), rupture of an aneurysm (see p. 982), malposition of central catheters (Figs 14.65 and 14.66), bleeding disorders or anticoagulant therapy. Other causes of spontaneous mediastinal hemorrhage are extremely unusual and include chronic hemodialysis,[341] bleeding into preexisting mediastinal tumors, such as thymic masses and thyroid goiter, radiation vasculitis,[342,343] and severe vomiting.[344,345]

D

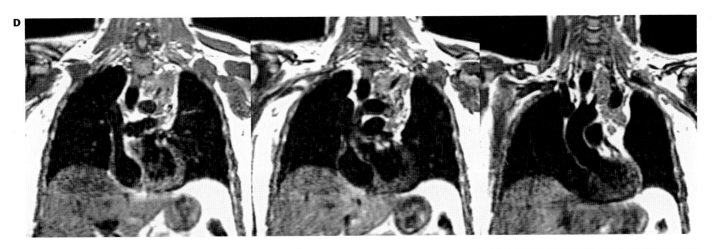

E

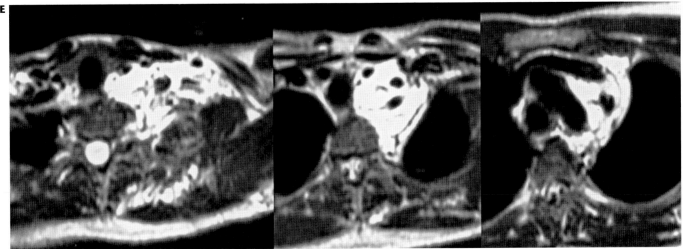

Fig. 14.63 (*cont'd*)   **D**, Coronal T1-weighted MRI shows an infiltrative, heterogeneous mass with signal intensity similar to skeletal muscle. **E**, On T2-weighted MRI, the majority of the mass is of very high signal intensity, consistent with a hemangioma.

Patients with mediastinal hemorrhage can be asymptomatic or present with substernal chest pain that often radiates to the back. Its investigation depends on the probable cause. CT is usually the first line of investigation after chest radiography to confirm the presence of hemorrhage and occasionally to elucidate its cause. The chest radiographic findings of mediastinal hemorrhage depend upon the cause and source of the bleeding. Blood may affect one mediastinal compartment and manifest as a focal mass (Fig. 14.65), or may dissect freely throughout the mediastinum and manifest as diffuse mediastinal widening.[346] Blood may also dissect extrapleurally over the lung apices, giving rise to the important sign of apical capping (Fig. 14.66).[347] When the hemorrhage is severe, blood may rupture into the pleural cavity or dissect into the lung along perivascular and peribronchial sheaths, resulting in opacities that can resemble pulmonary edema.[348]

The appearance of mediastinal hemorrhage on CT can be fairly characteristic (Figs 14.64 and 14.65). Linear bands of soft tissue attenuation are seen interspersed with mediastinal fat in affected regions of the mediastinum. On occasion, it is possible to appreciate the high-attenuation values of fresh thrombus on noncontrast CT images. A focal hematoma may, however, be difficult to distinguish from a solid mediastinal mass on CT. The appearance of hemorrhage on MRI varies with the age of the hemorrhage (Fig. 14.67). In the hyperacute phase, there is low signal on T1-weighted and high signal on T2-weighted images. Over the ensuing days, the signal on the T1-weighted images rises and there is a period during the subacute phase in which high signal is seen on both T1- and T2-weighted images. Thereafter, complex signal patterns are seen in which the signal intensity depends on the amount of water in the area of hemorrhage and the degree of conversion from methemoglobin to ferritin and hemosiderin.[349]

Mediastinitis

Acute mediastinitis

Acute mediastinitis is a potentially life-threatening, but fortunately rare, condition that requires prompt diagnosis and treatment. Spontaneous or iatrogenic esophageal rupture is the most common cause, accounting for up to 90% of cases.[350,351] Other causes of acute mediastinitis include necrosis of neoplasm, extension of infection from the neck, pharynx, teeth,[352,353] retroperitoneum, lungs, pleura, or adjacent bones and joints,[354] and mediastinitis after cardiac surgery. Acute mediastinitis may also be associated with empyema or subphrenic abscess.

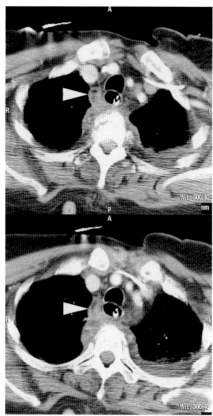

Fig. 14.64 Mediastinal hematoma due to spine trauma. CT shows bilateral paraspinal hemorrhage due to a vertebral body fracture. Note that the hemorrhage infiltrates anteriorly into the right paratracheal region (arrowheads).

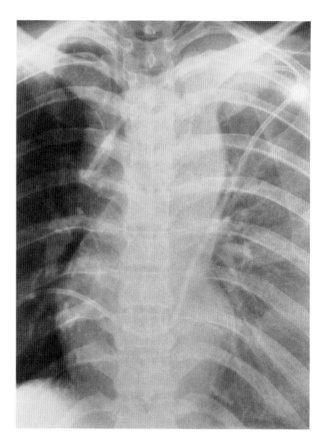

Fig. 14.66 Mediastinal hemorrhage after inadvertent arterial puncture during line placement. Frontal chest radiograph shows widening of the left mediastinum and left apical pleural fluid (apical cap).

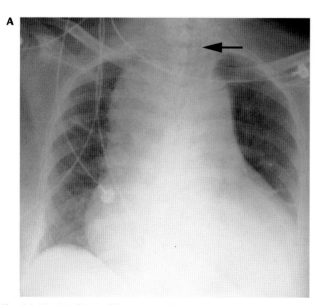

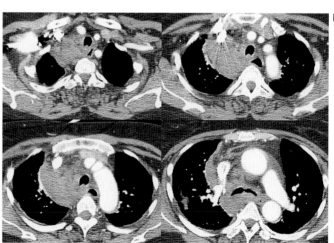

Fig. 14.65 Mediastinal hematoma after inadvertent arterial puncture during line placement. **A,** Frontal chest radiograph shows marked widening of the right mediastinum. Note the shift of the extrathoracic trachea (arrow) to the left. **B,** Contrast-enhanced CT shows that the portions of the hematoma are of high attenuation and that it diffusely infiltrates the right side of the mediastinum. Note the extrinsic narrowing of the right and left main bronchi.

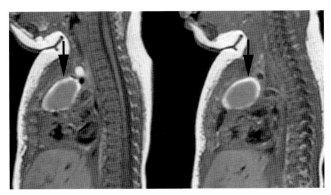

Fig. 14.67 Mediastinal hematoma after cardiac surgery. Coronal T1-weighted MRI shows a large prevascular mass (arrow) that compresses the pulmonary outflow tract. Note the high signal intensity rim and isointense center, consistent with acute hemorrhage.

Clinically, affected patients are often very ill with chills, high fever, tachycardia, and chest pain. Circulatory shock is frequent. Dysphagia is common in those patients in whom the mediastinitis is caused by perforation of the esophagus. Diffuse mediastinitis has a particularly high mortality.

Esophageal perforation is usually caused by penetrating trauma, particularly from surgery, endoscopy, or swallowing sharp objects such as chicken bones. In young children, the possibility of child abuse as a cause of pharyngeal or esophageal perforation must be considered.[355] Spontaneous perforation may occur, as in the Boerhaave syndrome, when forceful vomiting causes a tear in the esophageal wall. The tear in the esophagus is almost invariably just above the gastroesophageal junction. It may be of any depth, but is usually confined to the mucosa, in which case bleeding may occur but there is no immediate danger of mediastinitis. If the tear is complete, however, air, alimentary juices, and food leak into the mediastinum resulting in mediastinitis.

The primary radiologic features of acute mediastinitis are mediastinal widening, pneumomediastinum, obliteration of fat planes, localized fluid collections, and abscess formation (Figs 14.68 to 14.70).[356] Mediastinal widening is the result of inflammatory swelling or abscess formation within the mediastinum. Because so many cases of acute mediastinitis are secondary to esophageal perforation, an important clue to the diagnosis is air within the mediastinum, a feature that may be difficult to appreciate on chest radiographs. The air may be bubbly or streaky and may be localized or widespread in distribution. As with all types of pneumomediastinum, the air may extend into the neck or retroperitoneum. Accompanying pleural effusions in one or both pleural cavities are also common. Pleural effusion tends to be right sided in patients with iatrogenic, mid esophageal perforation and left sided in patients with spontaneous, distal esophageal perforation (Boerhaave syndrome). In patients with Boerhaave syndrome, the effusion is particularly striking on the left and is often accompanied by consolidation of the left lower lobe.[357] All these features are better demonstrated on CT than on chest radiographs.[356,358,359] Findings of esophageal perforation on CT include periesophageal fluid collections (100%), extraluminal mediastinal air (100%), esophageal wall thickening (82%), and pleural effusion (82%).[360] The site of perforation is rarely identifiable on CT (18%).[360] Contrast esophagography can be critical in determining the presence and precise location of esophageal perforation.[357] In cases of acute mediastinitis without discrete abscess formation, CT may show diffuse obliteration of normal fat planes, and gas bubbles may be scattered throughout the mediastinum (Fig. 14.71). When a walled-off abscess develops, the gas may be seen in discrete rounded collections or as air–fluid levels. Mediastinal abscesses may be solitary, but are frequently multiple. CT is an invaluable guide should percutaneous drainage be indicated.[356,361] CT may also show important associated abnormalities such as jugular vein thrombosis, pericardial effusion, or rupture of the hypopharynx or esophagus.

Descending cervical mediastinitis is an uncommon, but potentially life-threatening cause of mediastinitis.[362] These infections begin in the head and neck region and spread via

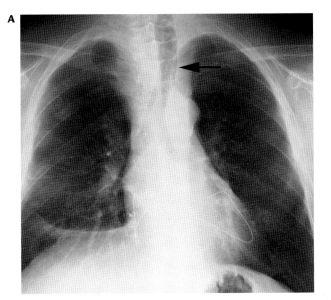
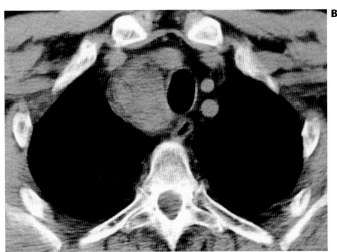

Fig. 14.68 Mediastinal abscess in lung transplant recipient. **A**, Frontal chest radiograph shows a right neck and mediastinal mass with lateral tracheal displacement (arrow). **B**, CT shows that the mass is heterogeneous. Percutaneous aspiration confirmed abscess due to anaerobic, probably odontogenic, organisms.

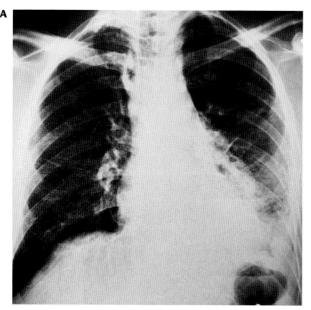

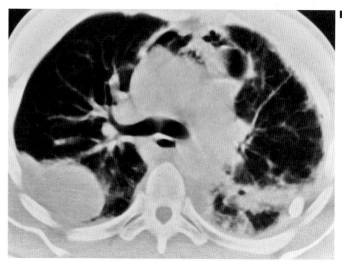

Fig. 14.69 Acute mediastinitis after perforation of the pharynx by a chicken bone. **A,** Frontal chest radiograph shows pneumomediastinum, left lower lobe consolidation, and left pleural effusion. **B,** CT obtained after placement of a left pleural chest tube shows extensive air and fluid in the mediastinum and a loculated right pleural fluid collection.

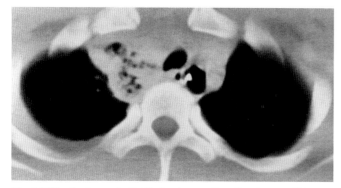

Fig. 14.70 Acute mediastinitis due to a peritonsillar abscess. CT shows fluid and bubbles of air in the right superior mediastinum. The mediastinal abscess required surgical drainage.

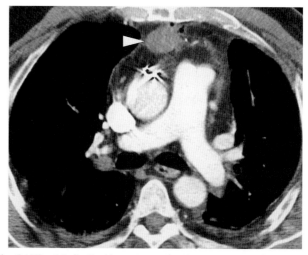

Fig. 14.71 Mediastinal hematoma after bypass surgery. Contrast-enhanced CT shows a well-defined fluid collection (arrowhead) with punctate collections of gas in the prevascular space. Needle aspiration confirmed hematoma; all cultures were negative.

fascial planes (usually in the prevertebral space) into the middle (Fig. 14.70) and posterior mediastinum. Typical causes include odontogenic infection, suppurative tonsillitis, and retropharyngeal abscess. CT in cases of descending cervical mediastinitis shows fluid collections in the mediastinum that may be contiguous with a fluid collection in the cervical region.[362] CT is essential for confirming the diagnosis, assisting in fluid aspiration to confirm infection, and for monitoring response to therapy.

Mediastinitis after cardiac surgery is uncommon, occurring in only 0.5–1% of patients.[356,363–367] CT is frequently performed in patients with clinically suspected mediastinitis but can be difficult to interpret since fluid and air collections, hematomas, pleural effusions, and increased attenuation of anterior mediastinal fat, all potential findings of mediastinitis, are expected findings in the immediate postoperative period (Fig.

14.71). These findings generally resolve, however, in the first days and weeks after median sternotomy. Jolles et al[364] found that mediastinal air or fluid collections on CT were not specific for mediastinitis in the first 2 weeks after sternotomy. However, such findings were highly indicative of mediastinitis after the first 2 weeks. Air or fluid collections that appear de novo or that progressively increase without other explanation are suggestive of mediastinitis (Figs 14.72 and 14.73).[368] Needle aspiration of fluid collections may be necessary to rule out infection when mediastinitis is suspected. CT is most

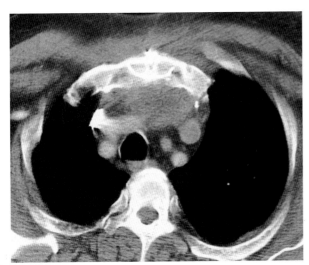

Fig. 14.72 Mediastinitis following bypass surgery. CT shows a heterogeneous soft tissue mass in the prevascular space. At surgery, a phlegmon was identified without focal abscess; however, cultures showed *Staphylococcus aureus*.

useful for distinguishing patients with significant retrosternal fluid collections that require open drainage from those that have only superficial wound infections. CT has limited ability for detecting early changes of sternal osteomyelitis. Minor degrees of sternal separation are common in asymptomatic patients after uncomplicated operations.[363,365] However, gross sternal destruction, indicative of osteomyelitis, is occasionally seen on CT (Fig. 14.73).

Fibrosing (sclerosing) mediastinitis (Box 14.13)

Fibrosing mediastinitis (sclerosing mediastinitis or mediastinal fibrosis) is a rare disorder caused by proliferation of acellular collagen and fibrous tissue within the mediastinum.[369] Most cases in the United States are believed to be caused by an abnormal

---

Box 14.13 Fibrosing mediastinitis

Etiology
Infection
- *H. capsulatum* (in the United States)
- *M. tuberculosis*
- Other fungi
Radiation, autoimmune disease, drug therapy
Idiopathic

Clinical features
Symptoms related to mediastinal structures involved
Airway
- Recurrent pneumonia
- Persistent atelectasis
- Hemoptysis
Pulmonary vein
- Mimics mitral stenosis
- Dyspnea, hemoptysis
Superior vena cava
- Distended neck veins
- Facial swelling and edema

Imaging
When related to infection
- Focal invasive mediastinal mass
- Typically unilateral
- Calcification in two-thirds
When idiopathic
- Diffuse mediastinal soft tissue mass
- Calcification uncommon
Caveats
- Chest radiograph frequently underestimates extent of mediastinal disease
- CT best for showing calcification
- MRI good for showing vascular involvement
Differential diagnosis
- Lymphoma
- Calcifying mediastinal metastases

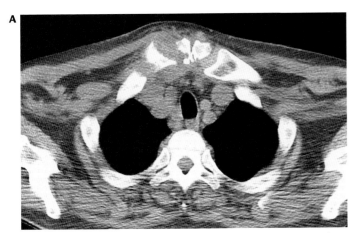
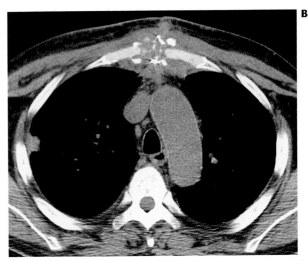

Fig. 14.73 Acute mediastinitis in a heart transplant recipient. **A**, CT shows soft tissue opacity in the prevascular space and destruction of the right clavicular head. **B**, CT at a lower level shows sternal osteomyelitis and substernal phlegmon.

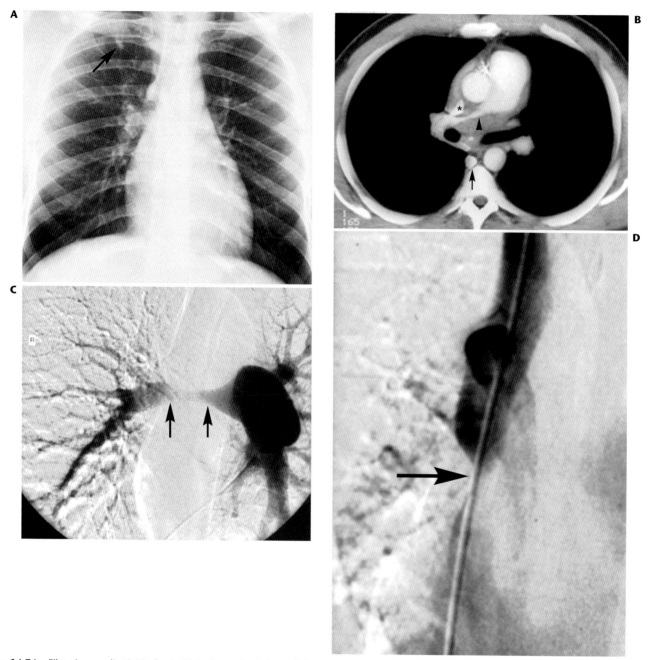

Fig. 14.74 Fibrosing mediastinitis due to histoplasmosis. **A**, Frontal chest radiograph shows a calcified right upper lobe nodule (arrow). **B**, Contrast-enhanced CT shows an infiltrating subcarinal mass with punctate calcification. Note the smooth narrowing of proximal right pulmonary artery (arrowhead), encasement, and narrowing of the distal superior vena cava, and dilation of the azygos vein (arrow). **C**, Arteriogram confirms marked stenosis of the right pulmonary artery (arrows). **D**, Superior vena cavagram confirms near complete occlusion of the distal superior vena cava (arrow). (With permission from Rossi SE, McAdams HP, Rosado-de-Christenson ML, Franks TJ, Galvin JR. Fibrosing mediastinitis. RadioGraphics 2001;21:737–757.)

immunologic response to *H. capsulatum* antigens in genetically susceptible individuals.[370–372] However, fibrosing mediastinitis is rare, even in areas where histoplasmosis is endemic, and recovery of organisms in affected specimens is unusual. Other etiologies that are likely more important in other parts of the world where *H. capsulatum* is rare include *Mycobacterium tuberculosis*, autoimmune disease, radiation therapy, trauma, and drugs such as methysergide.[373,374] A rare familial form associated with

retroperitoneal fibrosis, sclerosing cholangitis, Riedel thyroiditis, and pseudotumor of the orbit has also been reported.[375]

Fibrosing mediastinitis is characterized by progressive proliferation of fibrous tissue within the mediastinum that encases and eventually obstructs vital structures such as the vena cava, the pulmonary arteries and veins, and the airways. Fibrosis due to histoplasmosis is usually focal in nature, whereas idiopathic cases more often result in diffuse mediastinal fibrosis.[376]

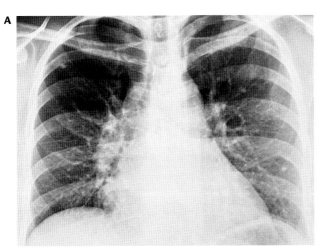
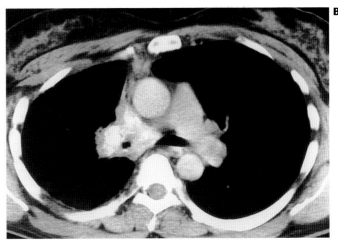

Fig. 14.75 Fibrosing mediastinitis due to histoplasmosis. **A**, Frontal chest radiograph shows right hilar, paratracheal, and subcarinal lymph node enlargement. Note the small calcified nodules in the lungs. **B**, Contrast-enhanced CT shows a calcified infiltrative mediastinal mass that surrounds and narrows the bronchus intermedius and right pulmonary artery.

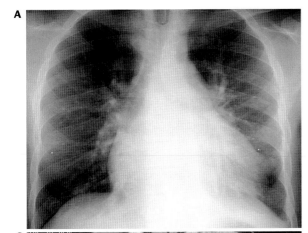
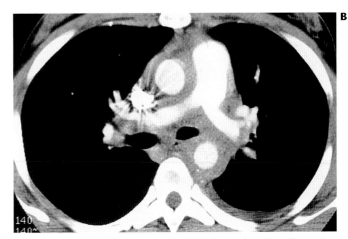
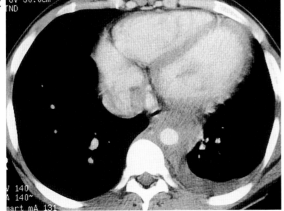

Fig. 14.76 Fibrosing mediastinitis in a patient with sickle cell anemia. **A**, Frontal chest radiograph shows diffuse mediastinal widening. **B** and **C**, Contrast-enhanced CT shows diffuse encasement of the mediastinum by an infiltrating, noncalcified soft tissue mass. Note the narrowing of the proximal right and left pulmonary arteries and encasement of the descending thoracic aorta (**C**).

In areas where histoplasmosis is endemic, affected patients usually present in the second through fifth decades of life with signs and symptoms of cough, recurrent pulmonary infection, hemoptysis, or chest pain.[371] Pulmonary venous obstruction may result in symptoms that mimic mitral stenosis. Patients with superior vena cava obstruction may present with swelling of the face and distension of the neck veins.[377] In other parts of the world where histoplasmosis is unusual, the age range at presentation is much broader.[373]

Chest radiographs frequently underestimate the extent of mediastinal disease (Fig. 14.74) and can be normal.[378–386] When abnormal, chest radiographic findings vary depending on the

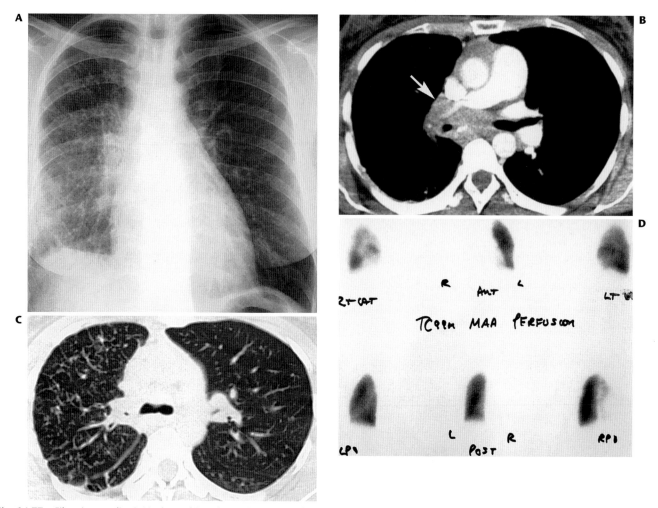

Fig. 14.77 Fibrosing mediastinitis due to histoplasmosis. **A**, Frontal chest radiograph shows volume loss in the right hemithorax and diffuse septal thickening in the right lung. **B**, Contrast-enhanced CT shows an infiltrative, partially calcified mass that narrows the right pulmonary artery and bronchus intermedius. Note the complete obstruction of the superior pulmonary vein (arrow). **C**, CT shows diffuse septal thickening in the right lung due to pulmonary venous obstruction. **D**, Perfusion scintigraphy shows complete absence of perfusion to the right lung. The ventilation scan (not shown) was normal. (With permission from Rossi SE, McAdams HP, Rosado-de-Christenson ML, Franks TJ, Galvin JR. Fibrosing mediastinitis. RadioGraphics 2001;21:737–757.)

etiology of fibrosis and the site and nature of the mediastinal abnormality. Disease due to infection, usually histoplasmosis, typically results in focal calcified mediastinal masses that may be evident radiographically (Fig. 14.75). Idiopathic or noninfectious fibrosis more commonly results in a diffuse mediastinal abnormality without evident calcification (Fig. 14.76).[387] In either setting, the effects of mediastinal fibrosis may also be evident on chest radiographs. These include findings of airway narrowing, parenchymal consolidation or atelectasis due to airway obstruction, oligemia due to pulmonary artery obstruction, or septal thickening and pleural effusion due to pulmonary venous obstruction (Fig. 14.77).

CT or MRI are most useful for evaluation of fibrosing mediastinitis.[205,371,373,384,388–390] When disease is due to histoplasmosis or tuberculosis, CT usually shows a focal, infiltrative mediastinal or hilar mass that may be extensively calcified (Figs 14.74, 14.75 and 14.77). When disease occurs idiopathically, CT generally shows more diffuse encasement of mediastinal structures by soft tissue attenuation masses that obliterate normal fat planes (Fig. 14.76). In either setting, CT is also useful for demonstrating airway, pulmonary arterial and venous involvement.

On MRI, the process is typically of heterogeneous signal intensity on T1- and T2-weighted images.[369] Markedly decreased signal intensity on T2-weighted images is occasionally seen and is suggestive of the fibrotic or calcific nature of the process.[391,392] MRI can demonstrate the infiltrative nature of the fibrosis and the narrowing of the major vessels and bronchi as well as, if not better than, CT.[379,389,391,393,394] However, CT is better for demonstrating calcification within the lesion, a finding that is critical for differentiating fibrosing mediastinitis from other infiltrative disorders of the mediastinum such as metastatic carcinoma or lymphoma.

Radionuclide ventilation–perfusion scanning can be used to diagnose pulmonary arterial or airway obstruction (Fig. 14.77).[392,395] Venography and pulmonary arteriography (Fig. 14.74) show smooth, tapered narrowing of the superior vena cava and brachiocephalic veins, together with numerous dilated collateral veins, and may also show narrowing of the central pulmonary arteries.[371,386] Barium swallow may show narrowing of the esophagus and, in rare instances, may show varices resulting from esophageal venous collaterals, so-called downhill varices.

The prognosis for affected patients is often unpredictable; disease may progress, remain stable for many years, or even spontaneously regress.[369] Mortality rates up to 30% are reported.[371] Patients with subcarinal or bilateral fibrosis may have a slightly higher mortality than patients with more localized disease.[371] Causes of death include recurrent pneumonia, hemoptysis or cor pulmonale.[369] Because many cases in the United States are caused by an inflammatory reaction to *H. capsulatum* infection, some patients have been treated with systemic antifungal agents or corticosteroids, with variable success.[369] If disease is localized, surgical resection can be curative or result in symptomatic improvement. Bilateral mediastinal involvement may preclude surgery, however. Symptomatic patients may also be treated by percutaneous therapies directed at occluded or severely stenosed airways, pulmonary arteries or vena cava. Laser therapy, balloon dilation, and intravascular or endobronchial stent placement have all been used with success to treat affected patients (Fig. 14.78).[369]

Mediastinal panniculitis

Panniculitis is an inflammatory process of fat leading to focal fat necrosis. It is most commonly encountered in subcutaneous mesenteric fat. Mediastinal panniculitis is a very rare condition that is usually seen in patients with Weber–Christian disease. It may cause focal mediastinal widening, and may therefore be mistaken for neoplasm (Fig. 14.79). CT in the case reported by Ashizawa et al[396] showed masslike accumulations of soft tissue (shown to be fibrosis and inflammation on histopathologic examination) interspersed with fat in the mediastinum. On MRI the mass was very heterogeneous.[396]

Neurogenic tumors of the mediastinum (Box 14.14)

For purposes of discussion, the neurogenic tumors can be classified as those tumors of nerve sheath origin, those of ganglion cell origin, and tumors of the paraganglionic cells.[397–399]

The *nerve sheath tumors* include schwannomas, neurofibromas, and malignant tumors of nerve sheath origin. Schwannomas are the most common intrathoracic nerve sheath tumors.[400] All these tumors are more common in patients with neurofibromatosis. Although histologically distinct, both schwannomas and neurofibromas are derived from Schwann cells. In their classic form, schwannomas are eccentric and encapsulated and have no nerve fibers passing through them, whereas neurofibromas are unencapsulated and have nerve fibers scattered throughout

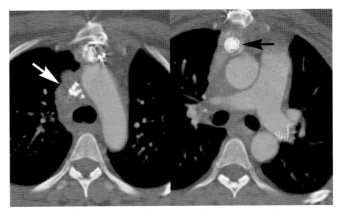

Fig. 14.78 Fibrosing mediastinitis due to histoplasmosis. Contrast-enhanced CT shows a calcified mass (white arrow) obstructing the superior vena cava. A conduit (black arrow) that bypasses the obstructed vena cava is seen anterior to the ascending aorta. Note also the stent in the distal left pulmonary artery.

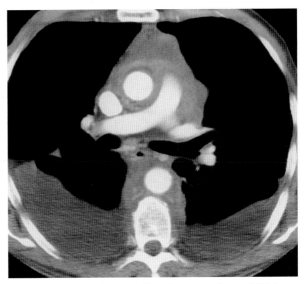

Fig. 14.79 Mediastinal panniculitis. Contrast-enhanced CT shows extensive mediastinal infiltration by soft tissue as well as bilateral pleural effusions.

Box 14.14 Neurogenic tumors of the mediastinum

Nerve sheath tumors
Schwannoma
Neurofibroma
Malignant tumor of nerve sheath origin

Ganglion cell tumors
Ganglioneuroma
Ganglioneuroblastoma
Neuroblastoma

Paragangliomas
Chemodectoma
Pheochromocytoma

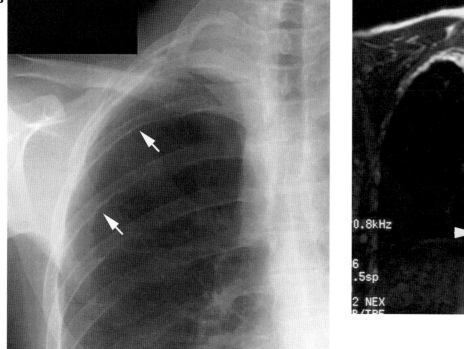

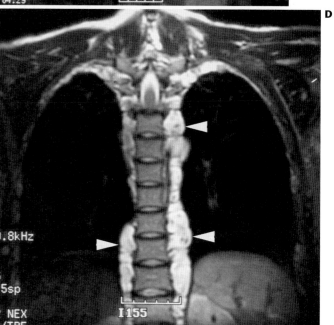

Fig. 14.80   Neurofibromatosis. **A**, Frontal chest radiograph shows lobulated masses in both apices and along both sides of the superior mediastinum. **B**, Coned view shows extensive rib notching (arrows). **C** and **D**, Coronal T1-weighted MRI confirms multiple mediastinal, apical, and axillary plexiform neurofibromas (arrowheads). Note the central regions of low signal intensity ("target sign"). (With permission from Rossi SE, Erasmus JJ, McAdams HP, Donnelly LF. Thoracic manifestations of neurofibromatosis-1. AJR Am J Roentgenol 1999;173:1631–1638.)

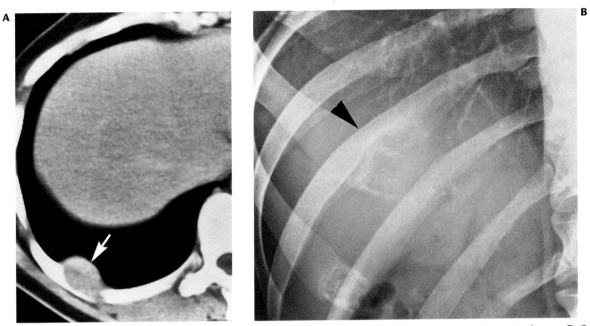

Fig. 14.81 Intercostal nerve schwannoma. **A**, CT shows a well-marginated soft tissue mass (arrow) arising from an intercostal nerve. **B**, Coned view of a frontal chest radiograph shows a smooth, well-corticated pressure erosion of the adjacent rib (arrowhead).

the tumor. Patients with neurofibromatosis may develop large plexiform masses of neurofibromatous tissue in the mediastinum (Fig. 14.80).[401–403] *Granular cell myoblastomas*, which are believed to be of Schwann cell origin, are rarely found in the mediastinum.[404,405]

Almost all intrathoracic nerve sheath tumors arise either from the intercostal (Fig. 14.81) or sympathetic nerves, the rare exceptions being neurofibromas or schwannomas of the phrenic or vagus nerves. Many arise adjacent to the spine and, in about 5% of cases,[14,406] extend through the neural foramina into the spinal canal (the so-called "dumbbell tumor") (Fig. 14.82).

Most nerve sheath tumors of the mediastinum are benign, affected patients are typically asymptomatic, and the tumors are often discovered as incidental findings on chest imaging studies. In contrast to the ganglion cell tumors, nerve sheath tumors are rare in patients below the age of 20 and virtually nonexistent in patients who are under 10 years old, except in patients with neurofibromatosis. Malignant tumors of nerve sheath origin are uncommon and usually occur in patients with neurofibromatosis.[397,399] Affected patients typically present with pain.

Tumors of *Ganglion cell origin* comprise a spectrum from benign ganglioneuroma to malignant neuroblastoma; ganglioneuroblastoma is an intermediate form of low malignant potential.[407] Neuroblastoma and ganglioneuroblastoma may occasionally mature into the more benign form.[408] The mediastinum is the second most common primary site (after the adrenal gland) for tumors of ganglion cell origin.[409] Approx-

imately one-third to one-half of mediastinal neuroblastomas arise primarily in the mediastinum.[410,411] The remainder occur secondary to either lymph node metastases or to intrathoracic spread from a tumor arising primarily in the adrenal gland.

Neuroblastoma and ganglioneuroblastoma are essentially tumors of childhood.[410,412] Less than 10% occur in patients older than 20 years of age.[400,413] In children under 1 year of age, a neurogenic tumor is virtually certain to be one of these two types.[414] Ganglioneuroma has a broader and more even age distribution, ranging from 1 to 50 years.[400,414] Urinary vanillylmandelic acid and homovanillylmandelic acid levels may be elevated in patients with neuroblastoma and ganglioneuroblastoma and are useful diagnostic markers.[415]

Imaging (Box 14.15)

Most neurogenic tumors manifest as well-defined masses with smooth or lobulated contours (Figs 14.83 and 14.84).[400,413,416] When localized, it is not possible to distinguish benign from malignant lesions. The tumors may be almost any size and some are very large, occupying most of a hemithorax. Except for vagal and phrenic nerve tumors, and the occasional neuroblastoma, neurogenic tumors are typically situated in the posterior mediastinum[414] or grow along intercostal nerves. Those that arise adjacent to the upper thoracic spine may occupy the lung apex and appear as a well-marginated apical mass (Fig. 14.85).

Most neurogenic tumors are spherical in nature, but some ganglion cell tumors are elongated along the spine, paralleling the vertical orientation of the sympathetic chain (Fig. 14.86). It

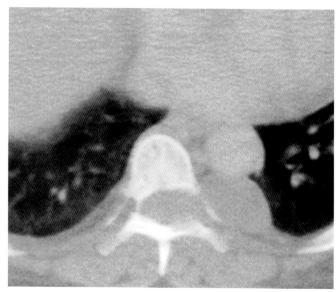

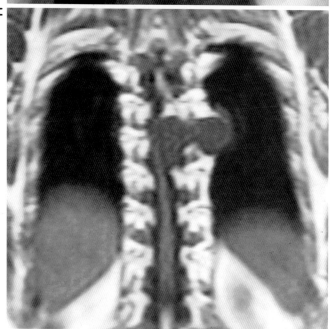

Fig. 14.82 "Dumbbell" neurofibroma. **A**, Coned view of a lateral chest radiograph shows a well-marginated paraspinal mass (arrows). Note the pressure erosion along the posterior surface of the vertebral body (arrowheads). **B**, CT shows marked widening of the neural foramen by a soft tissue mass. **C**, Coronal T1-weighted MRI shows extension of the mass through the foramen into the spinal canal.

Box 14.15 Imaging of neurogenic tumors

Tumors of nerve sheath origin
Chest radiography
- Round or oval
- Enlarged neural foramina
- Pressure erosion on bone
- Rarely calcify

CT
- Neurofibroma – homogeneous soft tissue mass, can be near water attenuation and mimic a cyst
- Schwannoma – usually more heterogeneous
- Both enhance heterogeneously
- Malignant nerve sheath tumor—heterogeneous, bone destruction, metastases

MRI
- Intraspinal extension ("dumbbell" lesion) in 5%
- Neurofibroma – target lesion on T1, T2

Tumors of ganglion cell origin
Chest radiography
- Elongated along axis of spine
- May also cause bone changes
- May calcify

CT
- Ganglioneuroma – homogeneous soft tissue mass
- Neuroblastoma – heterogeneous, invasive
- Calcification is common

MRI
- Intraspinal extension

Paraganglioma
Soft tissue mass on CT/MRI
Intense enhancement with contrast

---

may be possible to distinguish between a ganglion cell tumor and a nerve sheath tumor by observing: (1) the shape of the tumor mass, since the ganglion cell tumors are frequently elongated along the mediastinum with tapered superior and inferior margins, whereas nerve sheath tumors are more spherical in shape with more acute angles at their margins; and (2) that ganglion cell tumors arise slightly more anteriorly with their center alongside the vertebral body, whereas nerve sheath tumors are centered on the neural foramen, or are closely adherent to the chest wall.

Calcification can be seen in all types of neurogenic tumors (Figs 14.86 and 14.87). Approximately 10% of primary mediastinal neuroblastomas are visibly calcified on chest radiographs,[400,410] a figure considerably lower than that reported for with neuroblastomas arising in the abdomen. The incidence of calcification detectable at CT is substantially higher. In neuroblastoma, the calcification is usually finely stippled, whereas in ganglioneuroblastoma and ganglioneuroma (Fig. 14.86), it is

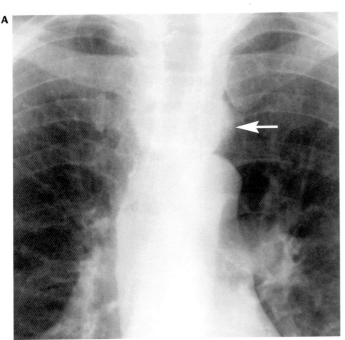

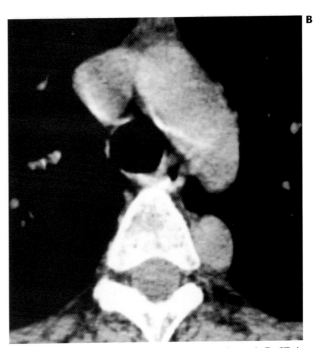

Fig. 14.83 Mediastinal schwannoma. **A**, Coned view of a frontal chest radiograph shows a well-marginated supraaortic mass (arrow). **B**, CT shows that the mass is homogeneous and of soft tissue attenuation.

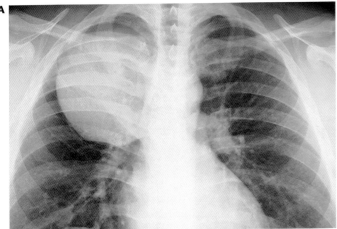

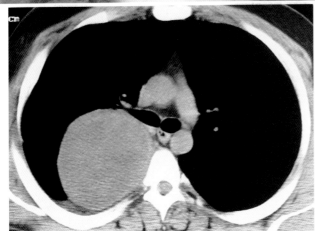

Fig. 14.84 Mediastinal schwannoma. **A**, Frontal chest radiograph shows a large well-marginated mass in the right upper thorax. Note minimal pressure erosion of the posterior ribs. **B**, Noncontrast CT shows a homogeneous, low-attenuation (20 HU) mass with no evidence of extension into the spinal canal.

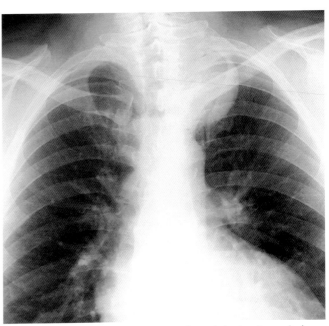

Fig. 14.85 Apical nerve sheath tumor. Frontal chest radiograph shows a well-marginated left apical mass without rib or bone erosion.

denser and coarser, occurring most frequently in the larger, more benign lesions. Nerve sheath tumors calcify only occasionally. Reed et al[400] reported that only two of 65 nerve sheath tumors had visible calcifications on chest radiographs; both lesions were neurofibromas. Carey et al[401] reported that only seven of 67 nerve sheath tumors had visible calcifications on chest radiographs; all seven lesions were schwannomas. In these seven cases, the calcification was curvilinear and peripheral in nature and occurred only in the largest masses.

Because neurogenic tumors tend to arise adjacent to bone and grow slowly, they can cause pressure erosions of adjacent

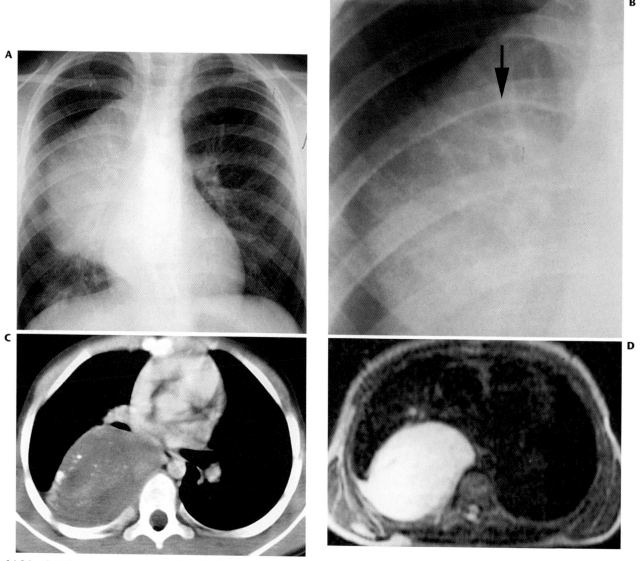

Fig. 14.86 Ganglioneuroma in a 7-year-old girl with cough. **A**, Frontal chest radiograph shows an oblong mass in the right paraspinal region. The lateral margins of the mass are indistinct and there is right lower lobe pneumonia. **B**, Coned view shows minimal pressure erosion (arrow) of the posterior ribs. **C**, Contrast-enhanced CT shows that the mass is heterogeneous and contains punctuate and chunklike calcification. **D**, Axial T2-weighted MRI shows that the mass is of high signal intensity.

ribs and vertebrae (Figs 14.81, 14.84 and 14.86) – an important diagnostic feature. The bone in immediate contact with the tumor shows a scalloped edge; usually the bony cortex is preserved, and frequently it is thickened. The ribs may be thinned and splayed apart, and the intervertebral foramina may appear enlarged. With larger lesions, the absence of changes in the adjacent bones argues against the diagnosis of a neurogenic tumor. Bone changes are most frequently seen with the tumors of ganglion cell origin, perhaps because these tumors are frequently large at presentation and occur in pediatric patients with a rapidly growing skeleton. Large tumors may be associated with scoliosis.[401] Frank destruction of bone appears to be a sign of malignancy,[400,401,417] as is associated pleural effusion.[414]

On noncontrast CT, schwannomas are often of mixed attenuation, and may have regions that are close to water attenuation[399,413,417,418] due either to hypocellularity or cystic degeneration (Fig. 14.84).[419,420] Neurofibromas tend to be more homogeneous on noncontrast CT.[399] Nerve sheath tumors are typically vascular and enhance after administration of intravascular contrast. A variety of enhancement patterns have been described including homogeneous, diffuse heterogeneous (with cystlike regions of nonenhancement), rim enhancement, and central enhancement with a hypoattenuating rim.[399,417] Malignant nerve sheath tumors are typically heterogeneous on both contrast-enhanced and noncontrast CT; the presence of local invasion and bone destruction as well as metastatic foci to the pleura or lungs suggests the diagnosis (Fig. 14.88).[399,420] Ganglioneuromas usually manifest as homogeneous or heterogeneous masses of low-attenuation lesions on both contrast-enhanced and noncontrast CT (Fig. 14.86).[399] Neuroblastomas manifest as heterogeneous soft tissue masses that show extensive local invasion (Fig. 14.89).[399]

CT can show spinal and intraspinal involvement

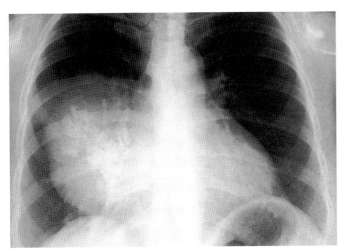

Fig. 14.87   Calcified nerve sheath tumor. Frontal chest radiograph shows a large calcified paraspinal mass.

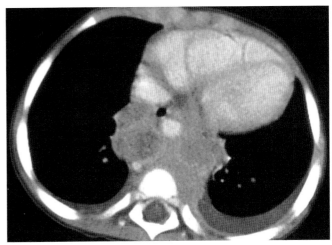

Fig. 14.89   Neuroblastoma. Contrast-enhanced CT shows an infiltrative posterior mediastinal mass that encases the descending thoracic aorta. (Courtesy of Donald Frush, Durham, NC)

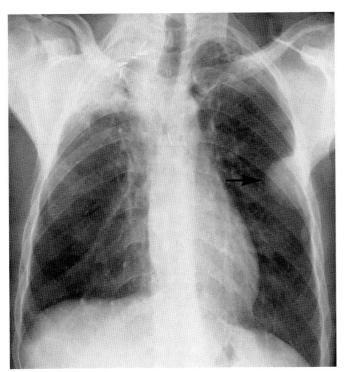

Fig. 14.88   Malignant nerve sheath tumor in a patient with neurofibromatosis. Frontal chest radiograph obtained 1 year after resection of a right sided malignant nerve sheath tumor (note the surgical clips) shows a new mass (arrow) in the left hemithorax. Biopsy confirmed metastatic disease.

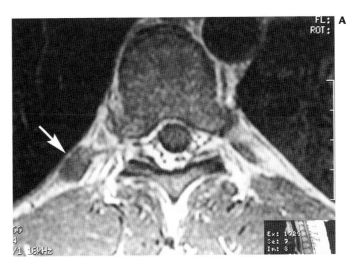

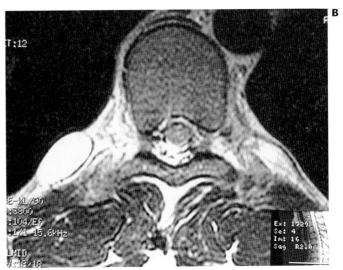

Fig. 14.90   Neurofibroma. **A,** Axial T1-weighted MRI shows a small well-circumscribed mass (arrow) of intermediate signal intensity in the right paraspinal region. **B,** The mass enhances intensely after administration of gadolinium based contrast material.

(Fig. 14.82),[421,422] particularly if intrathecal contrast has been administered. However, MRI is considered the standard for imaging neurogenic tumors because it better demonstrates spinal and intraspinal involvement (Fig. 14.82).[335,423] Predictably, CT is superior to MRI for detecting calcification in neurogenic tumors.[421] The signal pattern at MRI is variable (Figs 14.80, 14.82, 14.86 and 14.90 to 14.92). Neurogenic tumors may show uniform signal intensity similar to muscle on T1-weighted sequences and signal intensity considerably higher than muscle on T2-weighted sequences. Neurofibromas and schwannomas, on

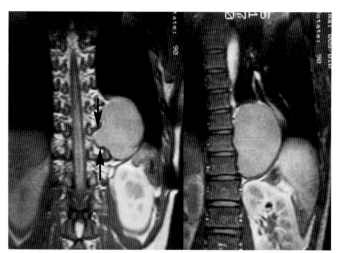

Fig. 14.91 Ganglioneuroma in a young woman. Coronal MRI shows a well-circumscribed oblong mass of intermediate signal intensity in the left paraspinal region. Note the limited extension into the neural foramen (arrow).

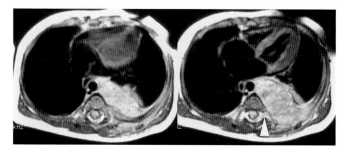

Fig. 14.92 Neuroblastoma. Axial gadolinium-enhanced MRI shows invasion of the chest wall and extension into the neural foramen (arrowhead).

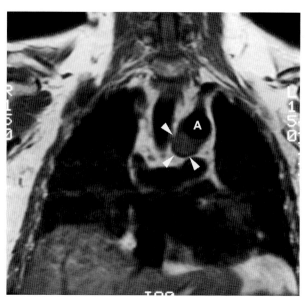

Fig. 14.93 Mediastinal paraganglioma. Coronal T1-weighted MRI shows a mass (arrowheads) of intermediate signal intensity in the aortopulmonary window. Note the relationship of the mass to the under surface of the aortic arch (A).

occasion, show the so-called "target pattern" with different signal in the central portion of the lesion compared with the periphery (see Fig. 14.80).[424–426] On T1-weighted images, the central portion is of higher signal, whereas on T2-weighted spin-echo images, the periphery is of higher intensity than the center, corresponding to the histopathologic finding of central nerve tissue and peripheral myxoid degeneration.[427] Schwannomas and ganglioneuromas may show heterogeneous high signal intensity throughout the lesion on T2-weighted images, and low to intermediate signal intensity on T1-weighted images.[31] In these cases, the high signal intensity on T2-weighted images is probably due to cystic degeneration.[427] Ganglioneuromas may have a whorled appearance on MRI, corresponding to whorls of collagenous fibrous tissue and neural tissue.

Because most neurogenic tumors in adults are benign, the role of imaging is to facilitate differential diagnosis and to evaluate local extent prior to resection. MRI is probably the imaging test of choice for imaging neurogenic tumors because it best shows intraspinal extension. For malignant tumors, notably neuroblastoma, chest radiography and MRI appear to be the best imaging modalities for staging (Fig. 14.92).[415,428] Radionuclide imaging with agents such as meta-iodobenzylguanidine (MIBG) or ^{18}F-FDG PET scanning can also be used to assess the extent of tumor and for staging.[429,430]

Mediastinal paragangliomas

Paragangliomas are tumors of paraganglionic cells that may be benign or malignant.[431,432] In the chest, paragangliomas may be chemodectomas or pheochromocytomas (functioning paragangliomas).[432] Mediastinal paragangliomas are rare, comprising only 2% of thoracic neurogenic tumors in one large series.[400] In a review of 51 nonfunctioning mediastinal paragangliomas, two-thirds arose in the region of the aortic arch (aortic body tumors) and one-third arose in the paravertebral region (Figs 14.93 and 14.94).[433] Aortic body tumors may occur in one of four locations: lateral to the brachiocephalic artery; anterolateral to the aortic arch; at the angle of the ductus arteriosus; or above and to the right of the right pulmonary artery.[433] Multifocal lesions are also reported.[434]

Fewer than 2% of pheochromocytomas occur in the chest.[435] Most are in the posterior mediastinum[436] or adjacent to the heart and pericardium, particularly in the wall of the left atrium or the interatrial septum (Fig. 14.95).[437–439] The left atrial lesions may indent the left atrium from the pericardial surface, rather than growing into the lumen of the atrium.[438] Approximately one-third of mediastinal pheochromocytomas are nonfunctioning and asymptomatic; the remainder present with symptoms, signs, and laboratory findings of overproduction of catecholamines.[436]

The various types of paragangliomas are indistinguishable by chest radiography, CT, or MRI (see Box 14.15). They manifest as round soft tissue masses on CT that, because they are highly vascular, can enhance intensely after administration of intravenous contrast.[29] Arteriography demonstrates enlarged feeding vessels, pathologic vessels within the tumor, and an intense tumor blush.[440] Radioiodine MIBG (Fig. 14.94) and somatostatin receptor scintigraphy all show increased activity in paragangliomas, and are useful methods for identifying extraadrenal pheochromocytomas.[437,441–444]

The MRI findings of thoracic paragangliomas are the subject of case reports only.[445–447] Based on these reports, it seems that

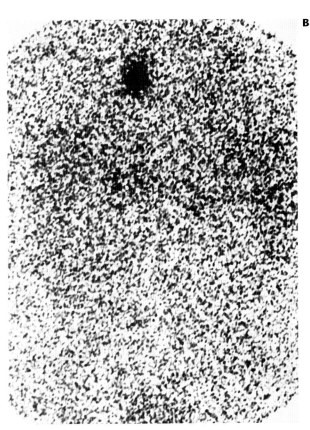

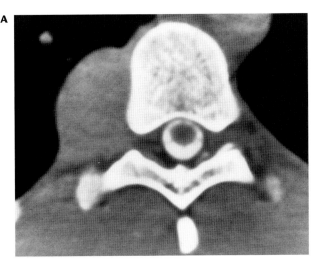

Fig. 14.94 Mediastinal pheochromocytoma. **A**, CT performed after myelography shows a well-marginated right paravertebral mass. **B**, MIBG scan shows increased activity in the mass, but no other sites of tumor.

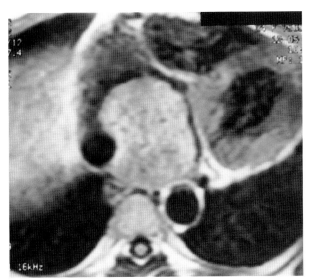

Fig. 14.95 Intracardiac pheochromocytoma arising from the wall of the left atrium. Axial MRI shows a mass of intermediate signal intensity that occupies most of the lumen of the left atrium. Note that the mass contains foci of decreased signal, typical of paraganglionic tumors.

the MRI appearance of thoracic lesions is similar to that of lesions more commonly encountered in the head and neck: the masses are isointense to muscle on T1-weighted images and are of substantially higher signal than muscle on T2-weighted images (Fig. 14.96).[448] Numerous serpiginous vascular channels

may also be seen coursing through the larger lesions. MRI is particularly advantageous for showing intracardiac pheochromocytoma (Fig. 14.95).

Parathyroid lesions of the mediastinum

Primary hyperparathyroidism is usually caused by a parathyroid adenoma in the neck. Surgeons frequently do not obtain preoperative imaging studies to localize the parathyroid glands because neck exploration is curative in over 90% of affected patients.[449] However, about 10% of adenomas arise in ectopic parathyroid glands in the mediastinum, usually in or around the thymus gland.[450,451] In one large series, the two most common ectopic locations were intrathymic and paraesophageal.[452] Affected patients may have four parathyroid glands in the normal position in addition to the ectopic mediastinal adenoma. Although the ectopic adenoma is usually solitary, at least one patient with multiple mediastinal adenomas has been reported.[453]

Because ectopic adenomas can be missed at surgical exploration, preoperative localization with imaging studies can reduce operative time, postoperative morbidity and requirement for repeat surgery.[335] Imaging techniques for localizing ectopic mediastinal parathyroid glands include radionuclide imaging (99mTc-MIBI, 99mTc-Tetrofosmin),[454,455] CT, and MRI.[456-458] Mediastinal parathyroid glands are probably best demonstrated using 99mTc-sestamibi radionuclide imaging.[454-457,459,460] CT or MRI are usually reserved for anatomic localization of an abnormality detected on the 99mTc-sestamibi scan.[335]

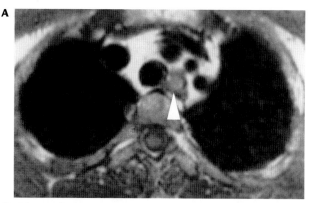

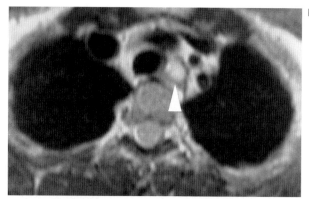

Fig. 14.96 Mediastinal paraganglioma. MRI shows a small mediastinal mass of **A**, intermediate signal intensity on the T1-weighted image, and **B**, of very high signal intensity on the T2-weighted image.

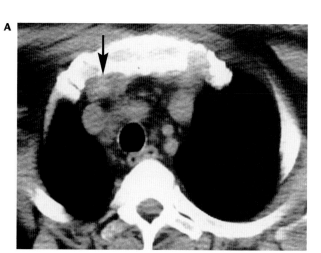

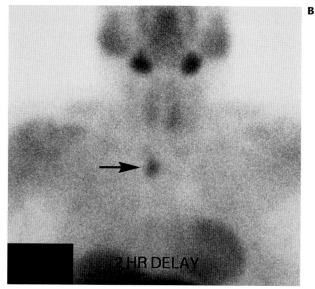

Fig. 14.97 Mediastinal parathyroid adenoma in a patient with persistent hyperparathyroidism after parathyroidectomy. **A**, Noncontrast CT shows a small soft tissue mass in the prevascular space (arrow). **B**, ^{99m}Tc-sestamibi scan shows uptake within the mass (arrow).

On noncontrast CT, mediastinal parathyroid adenomas manifest as small (usually <2 cm diameter) homogeneous masses of soft tissue attenuation (Fig. 14.97). Diagnosis on noncontrast CT can be difficult as they are easily confused with normal mediastinal lymph nodes, thymic remnants or blood vessels. Diagnosis on contrast-enhanced CT is usually more straightforward, although the lesions may sometimes enhance intensely. It is important to realize that a mediastinal parathyroid adenoma may be found as low as the aortopulmonary window and, therefore, the search for such lesions must extend at least to the level of the tracheal carina.[461]

Parathyroid adenomas are usually of intermediate signal intensity on T1-weighted MRI and of markedly increased signal intensity on T2-weighted images (Fig. 14.98).[462] However, up to 13% of abnormal glands do not have high signal intensity on T2-weighted images, possibly due to fibrosis or hemorrhage.[335,462] MRI has comparable sensitivity (78%) and specificity (90%) with other imaging modalities for detecting parathyroid pathology, but its most appropriate use is as an adjunct to ^{99m}Tc-MIBI radionuclide imaging.[462] MRI provides accurate anatomic localization of the adenoma and can predict the need for mediastinotomy or lateral cervical incision. MRI is also useful in "second look operations" and in high risk patients. In such patients, the success rate for surgery is reduced and the combined use of ^{99m}Tc-MIBI and MRI is 89% sensitive and 95% specific for preoperative localization.[459]

Mediastinal parathyroid cysts are quite rare.[463] Most are discovered incidentally, although they can compress the trachea or recurrent laryngeal nerve, causing symptoms.[464,465] About one-third of patients present with hyperparathyroidism.[463] Adenomas are occasionally cystic as well.[466] The radiographic, CT and MRI findings are those of a superior mediastinal cystic mass with a thin, enhancing rim (Fig. 14.99). Adjacent structures may be displaced and deformed.

Pneumomediastinum

The presence of gas in the mediastinum (pneumomediastinum) indicates perforation of a portion of either the respiratory or alimentary tracts. Perforation need not be within the mediastinum; indeed, it often lies beyond the confines of the mediastinum itself. Gas-forming mediastinal infection is a very

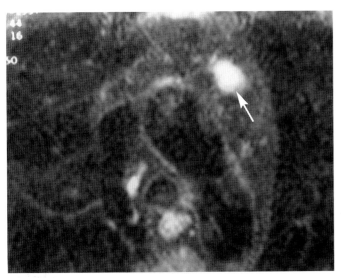

Fig. 14.98 Mediastinal parathyroid adenoma. T2-weighted MRI shows a small mass (arrow) of high signal intensity in the prevascular region.

rare cause of air within the mediastinum. The causes of pneumomediastinum are shown in Box 14.16.[481]

Patients with pneumomediastinum due to *spontaneous alveolar rupture* are usually young and have a history of asthma or severe coughing or vomiting.[467,482] Conditions reported in association with spontaneous pneumomediastinum[85,481–483] include asthma, croup,[468] strenuous exercise, marijuana or crack cocaine smoking,[470] nitrous oxide inhalation,[471] pneumonia, diabetic ketoacidosis,[473,474] diffuse interstitial pulmonary fibrosis,[475] and childbirth. When *spontaneous alveolar rupture* occurs, air dissects through the pulmonary interstitium into the mediastinum.[484] Air may also rupture into the pleural space producing pneumothorax. The patient may complain of chest pain aggravated by deep breathing and dyspnea. Fever and

leukocytosis without apparent infection are also frequently noted,[482] and may cause diagnostic confusion with acute mediastinitis. Spontaneous pneumomediastinum due to alveolar rupture, though it may cause symptoms, does not usually adversely affect patient outcome, and is therefore not treated[473,481] unless accompanied by pneumothorax. However, on rare occasions, air may collect in the mediastinum under pressure (tension pneumomediastinum) and cause impairment of venous return.[485,486] In these rare cases, percutaneous catheter drainage can be life saving.[485,486]

A

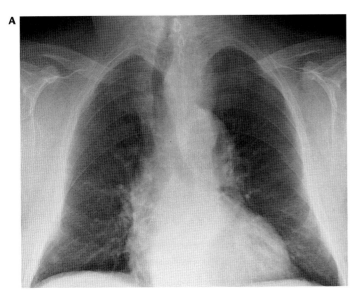

B

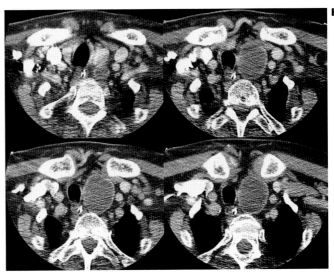

Fig. 14.99 Mediastinal parathyroid cyst. **A**, Frontal chest radiograph shows a left superior mediastinal mass that deviates the trachea to the right. **B**, Contrast-enhanced CT shows that the mass is homogeneous, of water attenuation, and has a thin enhancing rim. Note that the origin of the mass is just posterior to the left thyroid lobe.

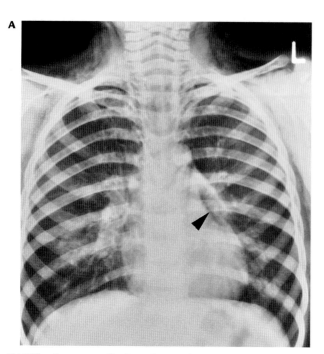

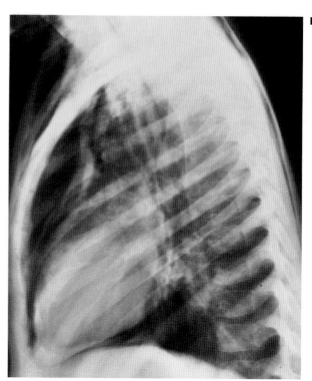

Fig. 14.100 Pneumomediastinum in an asthmatic child. **A**, Frontal and **B**, lateral chest radiographs show extensive mediastinal and subcutaneous air. Note air below the thymus (arrowhead).

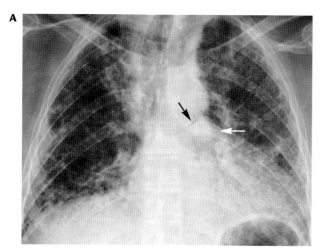

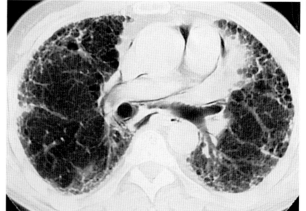

Fig. 14.101 Pneumomediastinum in a patient with pulmonary fibrosis. **A**, Frontal chest radiograph shows findings of end-stage pulmonary fibrosis and air surrounding the left and main pulmonary arteries (arrows). **B**, CT shows extensive mediastinal air to greater advantage.

Alveolar rupture is also common in patients who are on mechanical ventilation, particularly those with small airway obstruction or noncompliant lungs[487] due to hyaline membrane disease, meconium aspiration, neonatal pneumonia or acute respiratory distress syndrome. In these patients, pneumomediastinum itself rarely affects patient outcome and is not treated, but may be a harbinger of more serious problems such as pneumothorax. In such cases, reduction of ventilatory pressures to the minimum needed is advisable.

Air in the chest wall following rib fracture or placement of a chest tube may dissect into the mediastinum, usually by way of the neck. This is particularly common in patients on mechanical ventilation. Usually the chest wall emphysema is severe, and the

cause of the pneumomediastinum is not in doubt. Bubbles of air within the mediastinum are often seen on the first day following mediastinoscopy. In one series of 10 patients examined serially following uncomplicated mediastinoscopy, these bubbles had all cleared by the third day and fluid levels were never seen.[488] Air is also common in the mediastinum after cardiac surgery and may persist for days.

Radiographic findings

Pneumomediastinum manifests on chest radiographs as streaks, bubbles, or larger collections of gas outlining mediastinal blood vessels, major airways, esophagus, or diaphragm (Figs 14.100 to 14.103).[85,357,483] Dissection of air along tissue planes

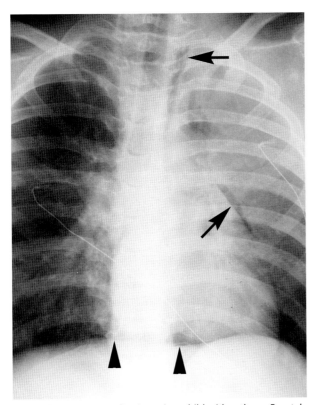

Fig. 14.102 Pneumomediastinum in a child with asthma. Frontal chest radiograph shows mediastinal air along the left heart border and in the left lower neck (arrows). Note that the superior surface of the diaphragm (arrowheads) is continuously visible across the mediastinum – "the continuous diaphragm sign". Note also the findings of left upper lobe atelectasis.

may be more obvious on the lateral projection than on the frontal view. The air may dissect under the parietal layer of the mediastinal pleura so that a thick linear opacity representing the combined parietal and visceral pleura can be seen along the heart and great vessels. Air may also dissect extrapleurally over the apices, simulating the appearance of pneumothorax. The air is usually greatest in amount anteriorly. When limited in quantity, the only sign of pneumomediastinum on chest radiography may be a lucent line or bands seen in the retrosternal area.

An important radiographic finding of pneumomediastinum is air dissecting under, and medial to, the thymus. The outlining of the thymus by air is quite specific for pneumomediastinum and may be the most striking sign of the condition (Fig. 14.100). Air may also track extrapleurally along the upper surface of the diaphragm. Air between the heart and diaphragm gives rise to the "continuous diaphragm sign" (Fig. 14.102)[489] – so-called because air beneath the heart may form a visible lucent line that permits the entire upper surface of the diaphragm to be seen, even within the mediastinum.

It may, on occasion, be difficult to distinguish pneumomediastinum from pneumothorax or pneumopericardium on chest radiographs (Fig. 14.103). The distinction depends on the anatomic extent of the air.[85] Pneumothorax is rarely confined solely to the mediastinal border. It can usually be traced out over the lung apex to the lateral portion of the thoracic cavity. A lateral decubitus view will confirm the pleural location of the air, though it is rarely needed. Pneumopericardium may extend from the diaphragm to just below the aortic arch, but will not extend around the aortic arch or into the superior mediastinum. Pneumopericardium can mimic the continuous diaphragm sign and can lift the thymus away from the great vessels, but the bilateral nature of the air and anatomic conformity to the

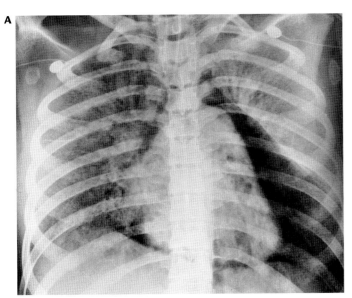

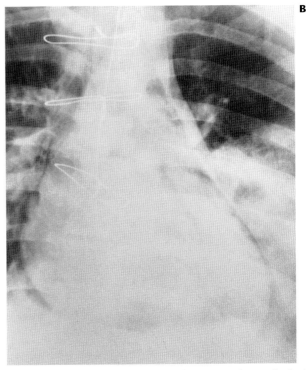

Fig. 14.103 Pneumomediastinum in a patient with acute respiratory distress syndrome. **A,** Frontal chest radiograph shows extensive mediastinal air and the "continuous diaphragm" sign. Contrast this appearance to that of pneumopericardium **B,** after pericardiocentesis.

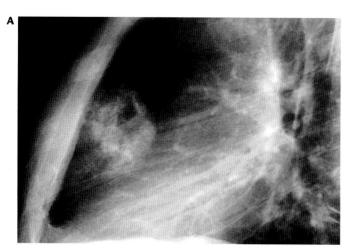

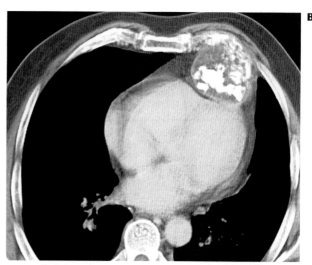

Fig. 14.104 Chest wall chondrosarcoma. **A**, Lateral chest radiograph shows an anteriorly situated, well-circumscribed mass within internal calcification. **B**, CT shows that the mass originates from the anterior rib and contains chondroid calcification. Note the mass effect on the heart.

pericardium is usually evident. A thin line of apparent radiolucency is frequently seen along the heart borders and aorta in healthy individuals due to the "Mach band" phenomenon. The Mach band may have an identical degree of radiolucency to a small pneumomediastinum. The distinction from pneumomediastinum[490] depends on analyzing both the anatomic extent and the border of the radiolucent line. A Mach band will be adjacent to a normally visualized contour, and its lateral boundary will either be unrecognizable or will be formed by a pulmonary blood vessel. The outer margin of a pneumomediastinum, on the other hand, will be the displaced mediastinal pleura.

The diagnosis of mediastinal emphysema is made readily at CT (Fig. 14.101), as the anatomic location of the air is self evident on cross-sectional images.[470] CT is both more sensitive and specific than chest radiographs for the diagnosis of pneumomediastinum and can be used to confirm the diagnosis in patients with the clinical suspicion of pneumomediastinum when the chest radiograph is normal or equivocal. This is usually only necessary in patients with suspected rupture of the trachea or central bronchi, or in cases of suspected esophageal perforation.

Sarcomas of the mediastinum

Primary mediastinal sarcomas are uncommon[491] and include fibrosarcoma, osteosarcoma,[492] rhabdomyosarcoma[493] and liposarcoma (see p. 919). Chest wall tumors, such as chondrosarcoma or giant cell tumor, may project into the mediastinum and simulate the appearance of a mediastinal mass on chest radiographs or CT (Fig. 14.104).[494] Chordomas are usually tumors of the spinal canal but are occasionally found in the posterior mediastinum.[495,496]

Patients with mediastinal sarcomas may be asymptomatic at presentation, or may present with complaints due to compression or invasion of mediastinal structures such as the superior vena cava or trachea. On chest radiographs, they manifest as smooth or lobulated masses that may have either well- or poorly-defined margins. On CT, they are usually heterogeneous soft tissue attenuation masses and may show extensive local invasion. As such, these lesions are generally indistinguishable from other

> ### Box 14.17 Causes of superior vena cava syndrome[497]
>
> *Malignant (78%)*
> Lung cancer
> Lymphoma
> Germ cell malignancy
> Metastatic disease
>
> *Benign (22%)*
> Fibrosing mediastinitis
> Venous catheters
> External compression by
> • Aneurysms
> • Mediastinal cysts

soft tissue attenuation mediastinal masses. The diagnosis of osteosarcoma or liposarcoma may be suggested by the presence of extensive ossification or fat, respectively, within the lesions.[492]

Superior vena cava syndrome

The most common cause of superior vena cava obstruction is compression and invasion by bronchogenic carcinoma (see Box 14.17).[497,498] Other causes include mediastinal tumors, notably metastatic breast and testicular neoplasms and lymphoma, mediastinal fibrosis (see above), and thrombosis due to venous catheters.[497] In one large review, 78% of cases were due to malignant neoplasms (two-thirds of which were lung carcinomas) and 22% were due to benign causes.[497]

Clinically, the features of superior vena cava obstruction are edema and visible distension of the veins of the face, neck, arms, and anterior chest wall. Dyspnea, choking, dysphagia, and a feeling of congestion are common symptoms. Cerebral edema may rarely develop. The severity of the symptoms and signs depends on the degree of venous collateral formation.[499] There may be no symptoms at all, even with complete superior vena cava obstruction, if the obstruction develops slowly and numerous collaterals form.

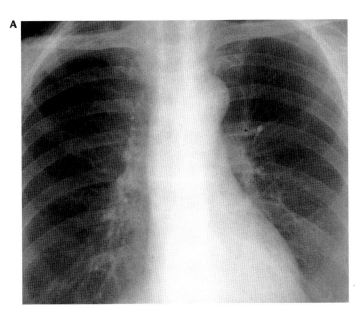

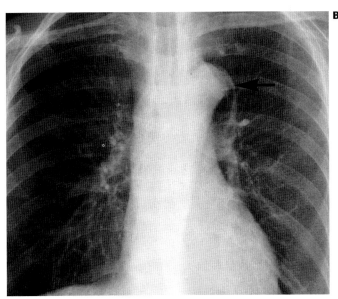

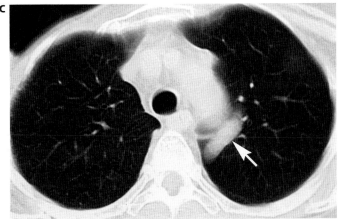

Fig. 14.105   Superior vena cava obstruction in a patient with breast cancer. **A**, Baseline frontal chest radiograph shows a normal mediastinum. **B**, Radiograph obtained 2 weeks later shows dilation of the left superior intercostal vein ("aortic nipple", arrow) and **C**, confirmed at CT (arrow).

Many imaging techniques can be used to diagnose superior vena cava obstruction.[498] On occasion, the presence of obstruction can be inferred from the radiograph appearance of dilation of collateral venous structures, such as the azygos or left superior intercostal vein (aortic nipple) which drains the hemiazygos system (Fig. 14.105).[500] In cases of superior vena cava thrombosis around an indwelling catheter, the superior mediastinum may become visibly widened on chest radiography.[501] This observation may allow a diagnosis of thrombosis even when it is not suspected clinically.[501] Venography shows the obstruction, demonstrates collateral pathways, and is an excellent technique for demonstrating intraluminal thrombus. In general, however, it provides relatively little information about the cause of the obstruction. CT with intravenous contrast enhancement is an excellent test that can show narrowing or filling defects in the superior vena cava (Fig. 14.106), optimally show collateral vessels[502] and demonstrate the responsible pathologic process (Fig. 14.107).[503–505] MRI can show the same features (Fig. 14.108)[506,507] and has the advantages of direct multiplanar imaging and the ability to distinguish rapidly flowing blood from slowly flowing blood and thrombus.[506] The disadvantage of MRI is that it will not demonstrate calcification – an important feature in the diagnosis of mediastinal fibrosis (see above). Contrast-enhanced MR venography using 3D gradient

echo sequences can also be useful for diagnosis of mediastinal venous obstruction; dilute solutions of gadolinium chelate can be injected into the veins of both arms to produce excellent images (Fig. 14.109).[508]

Thymic lesions (Box 14.18)

Thymic masses are usually caused by tumors, occasionally by cysts and, rarely by hyperplasia or infection.[510,511] The most common thymic tumor in adults is thymoma. Other tumors that may occur in the thymus include thymolipoma, lymphoma (notably Hodgkin disease), thymic carcinoid, and thymic carcinoma.

Normal thymus

The thymus is a bilobed, triangular shaped gland that occupies the thyropericardiac space of the anterior mediastinum and extends inferiorly to the heart. The normal morphology and size of the thymus changes markedly with age.[512] There is wide variation in normal size of the thymus, particularly in children and young adults (Figs 14.110 and 14.111). In the newborn, the thymus gland is often larger than the heart. Thymic size decreases with age as the gland undergoes fatty infiltration. The atrophied thymus is often visualized on CT in patients in their fourth

A

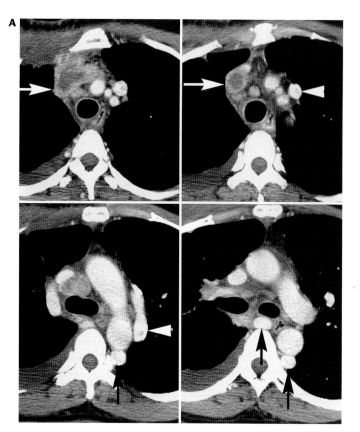

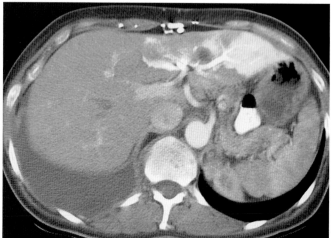

Fig. 14.106 Superior vena cava obstruction in a patient with breast cancer. **A**, Contrast-enhanced CT shows thrombosis of the brachiocephalic vein and proximal superior vena cava (arrows). Note dilation of numerous collateral venous pathways, including the left superior intercostal vein (arrowheads) and the azygos and accessory hemiazygos veins. **B**, CT through the upper abdomen shows recanalization of the umbilical vein and preferential enhancement of the left hepatic lobe.

B

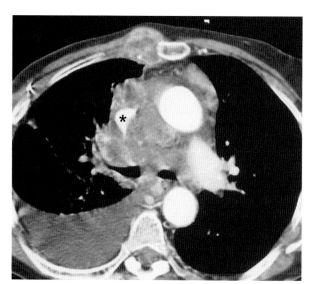

Fig. 14.107 Superior vena cava obstruction in a patient with metastatic breast cancer. Contrast-enhanced CT shows a heterogeneous enhancing mediastinal mass that encases and compresses the superior vena cava (*). Note also the anterior chest wall metastases.

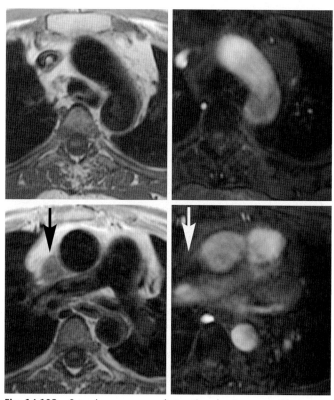

Fig. 14.108 Superior vena cava obstruction due to a central venous catheter. Paired axial T1-weighted and gradient recalled echo sequence MRI shows occlusion of the distal superior vena cava (arrow). Note that it can be difficult to distinguish slowly flowing blood from thrombosis on T1-weighted images (left panels) and that the issue can be resolved by using bright blood GRE images (right panels).

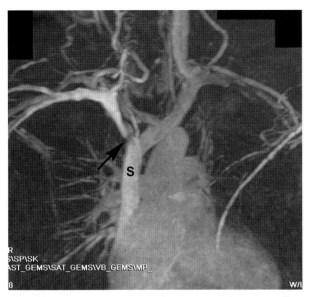

Fig. 14.109 Venous stenosis secondary to a central venous catheter. Coronal maximum intensity projection image from a contrast-enhanced MR venogram shows focal stenosis of the proximal right brachiocephalic vein (arrow). Note the numerous collateral veins in the right neck. S = superior vena cava.

Box 14.18 Causes of thymic masses

Thymic neoplasms
Thymoma, benign or invasive
Carcinoma
Lymphoma, notably Hodgkin disease
Carcinoid (may secrete ACTH)
Thymolipoma
Germ cell tumors

Thymic cysts
Simple cysts
Multilocular cysts
Cystic neoplasms
- Thymoma
- Lymphoma
- Germ cell tumor

Thymic hyperplasia
- Myasthenia gravis
Rebound hyperplasia following
- Severe stress
- Corticosteroid therapy
- Treatment for Cushing disease
- Chemotherapy
- Radiotherapy
- Bone marrow transplant[509]

---

decade of life, but is seen in <50% of patients over 40 years of age.[512] The most useful CT measurement is the thickness of the lobes measured perpendicular to the long axis of the gland. The normal maximal thickness before age 20 years is 18 mm and 13 mm in older patients.[513] Although these measurements are useful indicators of thymic abnormality, thymic shape is also important; focal contour abnormality of the normal thymus gland is a finding suggestive of an underlying mass.[513,514]

On CT, the normal thymus manifests as a homogeneous, bilobed structure of soft tissue attenuation in the anterior mediastinum (Figs 14.110 and 14.111).[3] It is usually seen at the level of the aortic arch and the origin of the great vessels. The left lobe is usually slightly larger than the right. Rarely, a lobe is congenitally absent. The normal thymus is easily demonstrated on MRI.[335] Characteristically, the thymus is homogeneous with intermediate signal intensity (less than that of fat) on T1-weighted images (Fig. 14.112).[514] Because the thymus begins to involute at puberty, and is replaced by fat in older patients, the

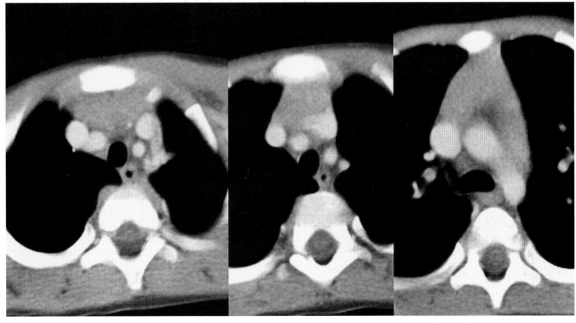

Fig. 14.110 Normal thymus in a 5-year-old child. Contrast-enhanced CT images show that the normal thymus is homogeneous, of soft tissue attenuation, and, in a child of this age, may have laterally convex margins.

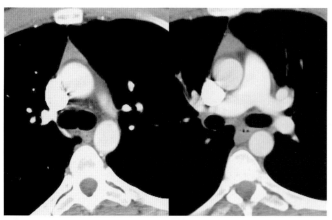

Fig. 14.111 Normal thymus in a 30-year-old adult. Contrast-enhanced CT images show that the thymus in a young adult is usually more heterogeneous due to fatty involution and should have lateral margins that are either straight or concave.

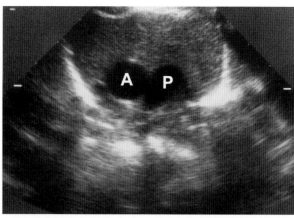

Fig. 14.113 Normal thymus in an infant. Transthoracic ultrasound shows that the gland is homogeneous with low level echoes throughout. A = aorta; P = pulmonary artery. (Courtesy of Helen Carty, Liverpool, UK)

T1-weighted signal intensity of the thyroid increases with age.[515–517] On T2-weighted images the thymus has high signal intensity similar to fat in all age groups and this can make identification of the thymus difficult in patients with abundant mediastinal fat.

Ultrasonography can be used to evaluate a prominent thymus in infants. The suprasternal approach shows a homogeneous low echo pattern without compression of the major vessels (Fig. 14.113).[518–520] Tumors or lymph nodes show mixed echodensity or higher reflectivity than normal thymus.[519]

Thymic masses, on occasion, can be difficult to distinguish from normal thymus. A few important rules should be remembered: (1) The normal thymus conforms to the shape of the adjacent great vessels on CT and MRI, whereas a thymic mass tends to displace these structures; (2) thymic masses usually manifest on CT or MRI as round masses and do not conform to the shape of the normal thymus; (3) on CT, thymic masses are usually heterogeneous with areas of decreased attenuation and possibly calcification; (4) on MRI, thymic masses are also heterogeneous with areas of abnormal signal intensity compared to normal thymus; and (5) thymic masses may show invasion with obliteration of adjacent fat planes.

Thymic hyperplasia
Lymphofollicular thymic hyperplasia
Germinal centers (focal collections of mostly B lymphocytes) are occasionally found in the medulla of the normal thymus but are characteristic of myasthenia gravis; >50% of patients with myasthenia gravis have some degree of lymphofollicular thymic hyperplasia.[155] Lymphofollicular thymic hyperplasia is also seen in other conditions, including thyrotoxicosis (Fig. 14.114),[155,521–523] systemic lupus erythematosus, polyarteritis nodosa, Hashimoto thyroiditis, Addison disease, autoimmune hemolytic anemia, and Behçet disease.[524]

Lymphofollicular thymic hyperplasia in adults and older children is usually detected only by cross-sectional imaging. It very rarely manifests as a mediastinal mass on chest radiographs (Fig. 14.114). On CT or MRI, thymic hyperplasia manifests as enlargement of both lobes of an otherwise normally shaped gland (Fig. 14.114). CT attenuation or MR signal characteristics are those of normal thymic tissue,[516] sometimes interspersed with fat.[525] The size and shape of the thymus is often within the normal range.[526,527] In one report, the size of the hyperplastic thymus increased as symptoms of myasthenia worsened.[528] Lymphofollicular thymic hyperplasia very rarely causes a focal mass that mimics thymic neoplasm on CT.[521,526,529,530]

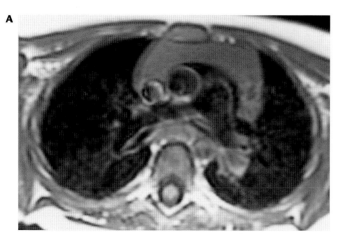

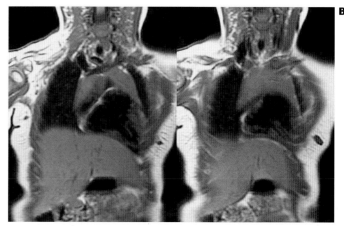

Fig. 14.112 Normal thymus in a 2-year-old child. **A**, Axial and **B**, coronal T1-weighted MRI shows that the normal thymus is homogeneous and of intermediate signal intensity.

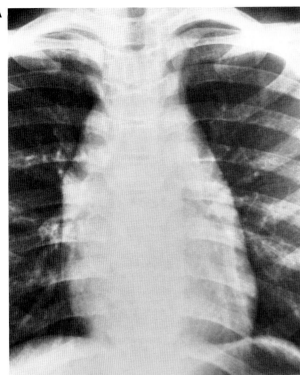

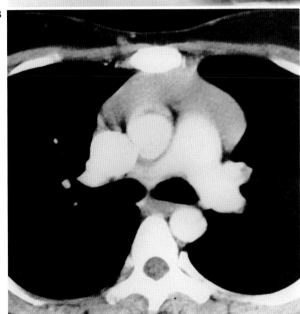

Fig. 14.114 Thymic hyperplasia due to thyrotoxicosis. **A**, Frontal chest radiograph shows a well-marginated mediastinal mass. **B**, Contrast-enhanced CT shows an enlarged, but homogeneous thymus gland.

Rebound thymic hyperplasia

The thymus gland may atrophy rapidly in response to stress or corticosteroid therapy, antineoplastic drugs, or radiotherapy. Atrophy is seen in up to 90% of patients receiving chemotherapy for extrathoracic malignancies.[531,532] The gland usually returns to its original size upon recovery or cessation of treatment. Occasionally, the gland grows back to an even larger size than normal – a phenomenon known as rebound thymic hyperplasia (Fig. 14.115).[531–534] In patients younger than 35 years of age, and

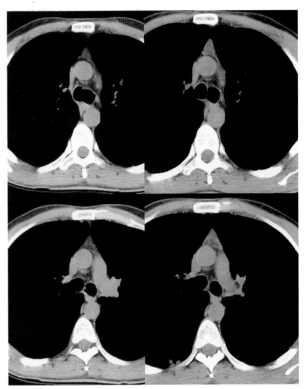

Fig. 14.115 Thymic rebound after treatment of metastatic malignancy. Paired CT images obtained before (left panel) and after (right panel) treatment shows that the "rebounding" thymus retains its normal triangular shape and contains interspersed fat.

particularly in children, the rebounding thymus may exceed its original volume by >50%.[531,533] Histologically, the gland shows hyperplasia of the cortex and medulla.[535] In one review, the average interval between the termination of chemotherapy and the discovery of rebound thymic hyperplasia was 6 months for children and 9 months for adults,[536] though it may be seen as early as 2 months and as late as 5 years after treatment.[532,534,536,537] Rebound hyperplasia after steroid therapy can be more rapid and may be seen in children 2 or 3 weeks after cessation of therapy and in adults after a slightly longer interval.[536]

Rebound thymic hyperplasia has been reported after treatment of Cushing syndrome and after recovery from a wide variety of stresses, including burns, surgery, and tuberculosis.[538–542] When rebound thymic hyperplasia is seen in patients previously treated for a malignant neoplasm that could involve the thymus, there may be difficulty in distinguishing recurrent neoplasm from thymic rebound. The diagnosis depends on the absence of clinical or other features, indicating recurrence of tumor in a patient with a reason for thymic rebound.[543] In one series of children treated for mediastinal Hodgkin disease, thymic enlargement was more likely to be due to hyperplasia than recurrent lymphoma.[544] Helpful features on CT (see Fig. 14.122) are that the gland, though enlarged, may retain a normal shape with a smooth nonlobular outline, that it conforms to the shape of adjacent structures, and that the enlargement is symmetrical rather than asymmetrical (as is the case with most tumors). The attenuation of the hyperplastic gland is the same as that of the normal gland at CT and the signal at MRI is also similar to normal thymic tissue.[517] One case of transient calcification in a child has been reported.[545] Gallium uptake in thymic hyperplasia following treatment for Hodgkin disease has been reported, leading to difficulty in distinguishing between thymic hyperplasia and recurrent Hodgkin disease.[546,547] A normal thymus will shrink on steroid therapy and, in those instances where the diagnosis is uncertain, a trial of steroids can be used to confirm thymic hyperplasia.[548] Lymphomas and leukemias may, however, also be responsive to steroid administration.[543] ^{18}F-FDG PET imaging has also been investigated for distinguishing thymic tumor from thymic hyperplasia with mixed results.[12,549] In difficult cases, biopsy may be required.

Thymoma

Thymomas are the most common primary tumor of the anterior mediastinum in adults and account for about 20% of all mediastinal tumors.[150,550,551] The great majority (90%) occurs in the anterior mediastinum; a few occur in ectopic locations such as the posterior mediastinum.[552,553] About 75% of affected patients present in the fifth and sixth decades of life,[150,550,551] and most are older than 40 years of age at presentation. Thymomas rarely occur in children. There is an equal incidence in men and women. Many thymomas are detected on routine chest radiographs in asymptomatic patients. About a third of lesions are detected because of symptoms of chest pain or cough due to compression of adjacent structures.[150,550,551]

As noted above, thymomas can be clinically silent or they may be associated with a paraneoplastic syndrome such as myasthenia gravis (50%), hypogammaglobulinemia (10%) or pure red cell aplasia (5%) (Box 14.19).[150,550,554,570–572] Up to 50% of patients with thymoma have myasthenia gravis; 10–20% of patients with myasthenia gravis have a thymoma. Sixty-five percent of patients with myasthenia gravis, however, have lymphoid hyperplasia of the thymus (see above). CT may justifiably be performed in patients with myasthenia gravis to exclude thymoma, even if the chest radiograph is normal.

Thymomas typically manifest on chest radiographs as well marginated, smooth or lobulated anterior mediastinal masses (Box 14.20, Figs 14.116 and 14.117). They are typically unilateral

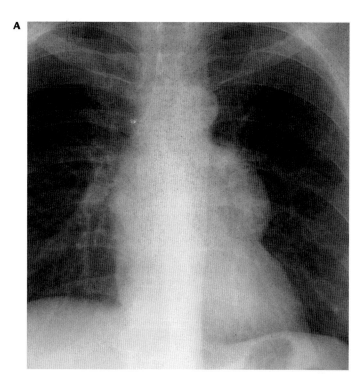

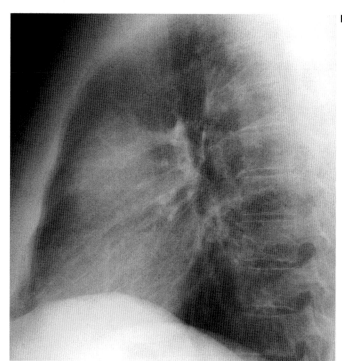

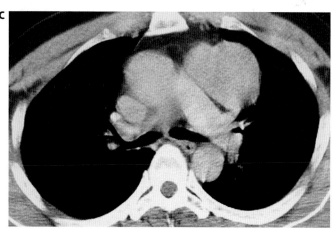

Fig. 14.116 Thymoma. **A**, Frontal and **B**, lateral chest radiographs show a well-marginated left sided mediastinal mass. **C**, CT shows that the mass is lobulated, homogeneous, and of soft tissue attenuation. There is no evidence of invasion beyond the capsule. At surgery, the mass was completely resectable.

Box 14.19 Paraneoplastic syndromes associated with thymoma (adapted from references[524,554–556])

Syndromes with a well-established relationship to thymoma
Myasthenia gravis
Pure red cell aplasia
Acquired hypogammaglobulinemia
Nonthymic cancers

Other reported conditions in patients with thymoma (usually also with myasthenia gravis)
Hematologic
- Pancytopenia[557]
- Autoimmune hemolytic anemia[558]
Neurologic
- Lambert–Eaton myasthenic syndrome[559]
- Peripheral neuropathy[560]
- Limbic encephalitis[561]
- Myeloradiculopathy[561]
Endocrinologic
- Hashimoto thyroiditis[562]
- Addison disease[563]
Rheumatologic[564]
- Rheumatoid arthritis
- Dermatomyositis
- Progressive systemic sclerosis
- Systemic lupus erythematosus[565]
- Myocarditis (giant cell)
Intestinal
- Enteropathy and colitis[566,567]
Miscellaneous
- Nephrotic syndrome[568]
- Hypertrophic osteoarthropathy[569]

Box 14.20 Imaging of thymoma

Location
Upper anterior mediastinum (prevascular) – most common
Cardiophrenic angle
Neck – rare

Chest radiography
Smooth or lobular mediastinal mass
Typically unilateral
Calcification uncommon

CT or MRI
Homogeneous or heterogeneous soft tissue mass
May contain cystlike spaces
Calcification in one-third (on CT)
Invasive
- Poorly defined or infiltrative margins
- Vascular or chest wall invasion
- Irregular interface with adjacent lung
- Focal or diffuse pleural mass (unilateral)

Staging of invasive thymoma (adapted[573])
Stage 1: no capsular invasion
Stage 2: capsular or pleural invasion
Stage 3: invasion of adjacent organs such as lung, pericardium, superior vena cava or aorta
Stage 4A: disseminated tumor in thoracic cavity
Stage 4B: widespread metastatic disease

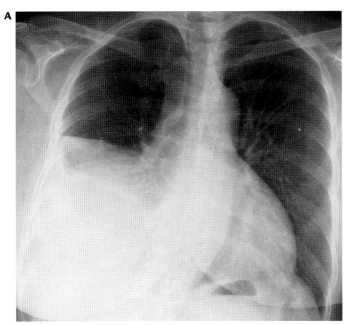

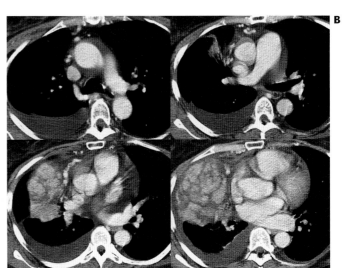

Fig. 14.117 Thymoma in a woman with red cell aplasia and thrombocytopenia. **A**, Frontal chest radiograph shows a large mass in the inferior right thorax. **B**, Contrast-enhanced CT shows a large heterogeneously enhancing mass along the right heart border. Large blood vessels are seen at the superior margin. At surgery, the mass was pedunculated with a vascular pedicle to the prevascular space.

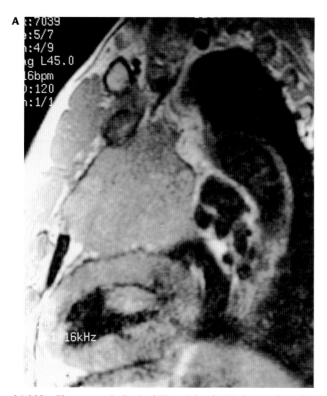

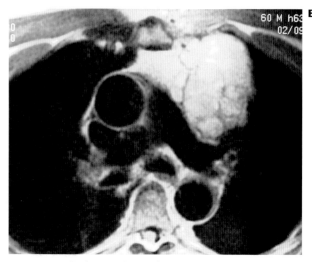

Fig. 14.118 Thymoma. **A,** Sagittal T1-weighted MRI shows a large heterogeneous mass in the anterior mediastinum. **B,** On T2-weighted images, the mass is predominantly of increased signal intensity although low signal intensity septations are seen.

and located anterior to the aortic arch, but can also occur in the cardiophrenic angle.[23,32,150,550,551,555] On cross-sectional imaging, they are smooth or lobulated masses that distort the normal contour of the thymus. They characteristically arise from one lobe of the thymus gland, although bilateral mediastinal involvement can occur. On CT, they manifest as either homogeneous or heterogeneous masses of soft tissue attenuation (Figs 14.116 and 14.117).[3] Intratumoral cysts or areas of necrosis are occasionally seen and the lesions enhance to a variable degree after intravenous contrast administration (Fig. 14.117). Calcification is seen in up to 7% of cases and is usually thin, linear, and located in the capsule. Thymomas usually show low to intermediate signal intensity (similar to skeletal muscle) on T1-weighted MRI and high signal intensity on T2-weighted images (Fig. 14.118).[170,550,574] Because up to 33% of thymomas contain areas of necrosis, hemorrhage or cystic degeneration, thymomas can be fairly heterogeneous in appearance on MRI. Furthermore, MRI will occasionally show fibrous septa within the lesions.

Local invasion is found at surgery in up to 34% of patients with thymoma (Box 14.20).[550] These lesions are best described as invasive, rather than malignant, thymomas. This is because there are no specific histologic features that predict biologic behavior with this particular tumor. Tumor size also does not seem to affect the propensity for invasive behavior.[550,551,555] Furthermore, it can be quite difficult to predict the subsequent biologic behavior of thymomas on the basis of CT or MRI findings (or indeed, histologic features). Surgical exploration is the most reliable means for determining invasion. Findings that suggest invasive thymoma on cross-sectional imaging include poorly defined or infiltrative margins (Fig. 14.119), definite

vascular or chest wall invasion (Fig. 14.119), an irregular interface with adjacent lung, and evidence of spread to ipsilateral pleura (Figs 14.119 and 14.120). Pleural spread manifests either as isolated pleural nodules ("drop metastases") or as a contiguous pleural mass, often mimicking mesothelioma.[575] Because the tumor can spread to the abdomen via normal hiatuses in the diaphragm, staging studies should include the upper abdomen.[335] Pleural effusions are uncommon, despite often extensive pleural metastases.

There is considerable interest in using molecular imaging techniques for evaluating patients with benign and malignant thymic tumors, especially thymoma.[576] Two groups of radiopharmaceuticals have been investigated. The first includes oncotropic tracers that are concentrated in thymic tumors, such as ^{201}Tl chloride, ^{99m}Tc-sestamibi, and ^{18}F-FDG.[577–580] Uptake of these agents within the tumors generally correlates with tumor grade and cellularity,[576] and several agents show promise for more accurate staging of invasive thymoma.[578] Kubota et al[580] reported that the degree of ^{18}F-FDG uptake correlated well with the aggressiveness of the tumor and its propensity for invasion and recurrence. The second group of agents under investigation includes radioligands such as [^{111}In-DTPA-D-Phe1]-octreotide and [^{111}In-DTPA-Arg1]-substance P.[576] [^{111}In-DTPA-D-Phe1]-octreotide binds to the somatostatin receptor and is concentrated in deposits of thymoma.[581] Furthermore, this agent is not concentrated in patients with myasthenia gravis who have only benign lymphofollicular thymic hyperplasia (see above).[581] This differential uptake may be useful for distinguishing between benign hyperplasia and early thymoma, and for selecting patients with advanced thymoma who might benefit from a somatostatin analog based treatment.[581]

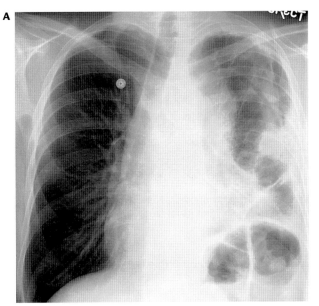

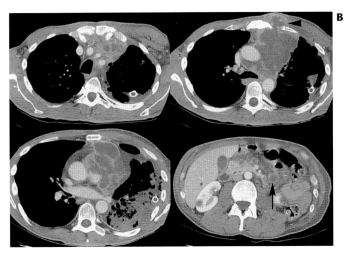

Fig. 14.119 Invasive thymoma. **A**, Frontal chest radiograph shows an ill-defined left mediastinal mass, left pleural thickening, and elevation of the left diaphragm. **B**, Contrast enhanced CT shows that the mass is heterogeneous and shows extensive mediastinal invasion. Note also extension into the left anterior chest wall (arrowhead) and tumor deposits within the upper abdomen (arrow).

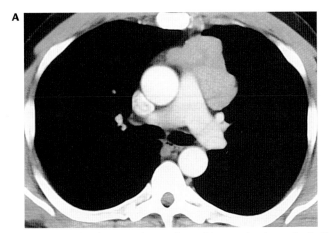

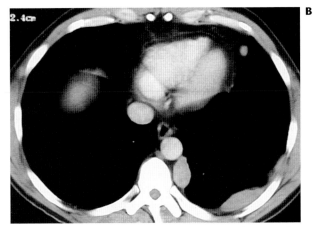

Fig. 14.120 Invasive thymoma in a patient with myasthenia gravis. **A**, Contrast-enhanced CT shows a homogeneous lobulated prevascular mass. **B**, CT at a lower level shows multiple left pleural masses, consistent with so-called "drop metastases".

Thymic carcinoma

Thymic carcinomas account for about 20% of thymic tumors in adults.[150] These are aggressive malignancies that often show marked local invasion and dissemination to regional lymph nodes and distant sites.[582] Distant metastases (lung, liver, brain, and bone) are found in 50–65% of patients at presentation.[150] Prognosis is poor despite therapy.[583] These tumors are histopathologically distinguished from thymoma by the presence of nucleolar prominence, vesicular chromatin, abundant mitotic activity and a markedly increased nucleus:cytoplasm ratio.[556,582,584] Thymic carcinomas are generally not associated with paraneoplastic syndromes, although an association with hypercalcemia has been reported.[585]

Thymic carcinomas on chest radiography are typically large, poorly defined mediastinal masses. Intrathoracic lymphadenopathy, and pleural and pericardial effusions are also common.[582] On CT (Fig. 14.121), the masses are usually heterogeneous, often show necrosis and calcification, have poorly defined infiltrative margins and show invasion along the pleura, pericardium, or mediastinum.[582,585] Focal pleural implants, as are seen in cases of invasive thymoma, are uncommon.[586] Thymic carcinomas typically show intermediate signal intensity (slightly higher than skeletal muscle) on T1-weighted MRI and high signal intensity on T2-weighted images. Signal intensity can be heterogeneous because of hemorrhage and necrosis within the masses.[587] MRI can be helpful for revealing local soft tissue and vascular invasion.

Thymic lymphoma

Lymphomatous involvement of the thymus usually occurs in the setting of more generalized disease. Hodgkin disease accounts for the majority of cases of thymic lymphoma. The overall incidence of thymic involvement by Hodgkin disease is difficult to determine; estimates have varied from 30 to 56%. In

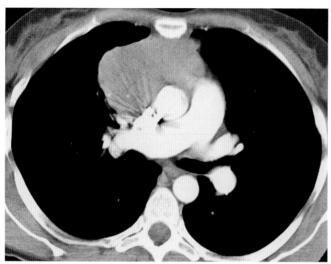

Fig. 14.121 Thymic carcinoma. Contrast-enhanced CT shows a large poorly marginated soft tissue mass within the anterior mediastinum. (Courtesy of Jeremy Erasmus, Houston, TX)

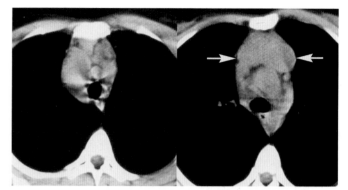

Fig. 14.122 Thymic lymphoma. Noncontrast CT shows diffuse enlargement of the thymus gland (arrows) as well as mediastinal lymphadenopathy.

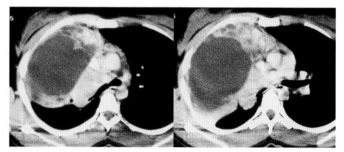

Fig. 14.123 Thymic lymphoma. Contrast-enhanced CT shows a heterogeneous prevascular mass with a significant cystic component.

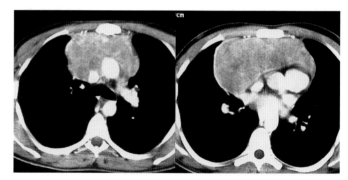

Fig. 14.124 Thymic carcinoid tumor in a patient with multiple endocrine neoplasia, type I. Contrast-enhanced CT shows a large, heterogeneous thymic mass.

most cases, both mediastinal nodes and the thymus are affected; isolated thymic disease is quite rare.[544,588,589]

Thymic lymphoma manifests on chest radiography as a unilateral or bilateral, frequently well-circumscribed, mediastinal mass. On cross-sectional imaging, thymic lymphoma is seen as either diffuse thymic enlargement or as solitary or multiple thymic masses (Fig. 14.122).[589] The lesions may be quite heterogeneous, with an area of focal necrosis appearing as cysts (Fig. 14.123).[590] When the thymus is diffusely enlarged due to lymphoma, it can be difficult to differentiate from a large normal thymus in young patients. Distinguishing rebound thymic hyperplasia in children and young adults from recurrent lymphoma can be even more problematic. Unfortunately, neither CT attenuation or signal intensity at MRI have proved to be very reliable techniques for distinguishing a normal enlarged gland from rebound hyperplasia or tumor. However, pronounced heterogeneity on MR signal may suggest neoplasm.[517,591] ^{18}F-FDG PET imaging is being investigated for evaluation of anterior mediastinal lymphoma after treatment and shows promise in early reports.[592,593] Unfortunately, the normal thymus of children can show uptake on ^{18}F-FDG PET scans.[594] Furthermore, false positive scans have been reported in patients with rebound thymic hyperplasia after treatment of malignancy.[593,594] Thoracic lymphoma is further discussed in Chapter 13.

Neuroendocrine tumors of the thymus

Neuroendocrine tumors are uncommon tumors of variable malignant potential. Histologically, these range from relatively benign (thymic carcinoid) to highly malignant tumors (small cell carcinoma of the thymus).[150,550,595–598] Thymic carcinoid tumor is the most common of this group of tumors.[595] Affected patients are typically in the fourth and fifth decades of life; there is a male predominance. Up to 50% of affected patients have hormonal abnormalities and up to 35% have Cushing syndrome due to tumor production of adrenocorticotrophic hormone.[599–602] Nonfunctioning thymic carcinoid tumors can occur in association with multiple endocrine neoplasia syndrome type 1,[603,604] and thymic and pulmonary carcinoid tumors may coexist.[155,605]

Neuroendocrine tumors of the thymus manifest on chest radiographs as well- or ill-defined anterior mediastinal masses and may contain calcification (Fig. 14.124).[606,607] On CT or MRI, the masses are typically large, of heterogeneous attenuation or signal intensity, and may show local invasion. Radionuclides such as radiolabeled somatostatin, MIBG and ^{201}Tl, may concentrate in the lesions.[581,608–610]

Thymolipoma

Thymolipomas are rare benign tumors that occur in both children and adults and have an equal incidence in men and women. Although there is a wide age range at presentation (2–66 years), most are diagnosed in young adulthood. They are

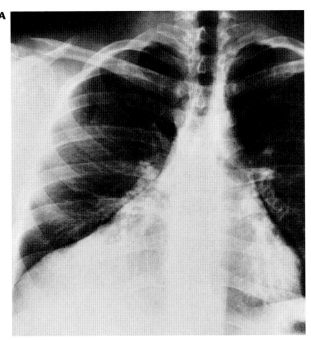

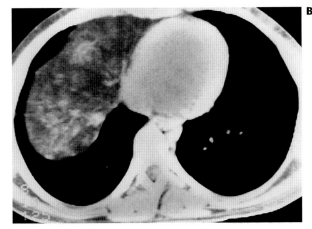

Fig. 14.125 Thymolipoma. **A**, Frontal chest radiograph shows a large right mediastinal mass that drapes the diaphragm. **B**, Contrast-enhanced CT shows that the mass is predominantly of fat attenuation with a few strands of interspersed soft tissue.

composed of a mixture of mature fat and normal or involuted thymic tissue and usually occur low in the anterior mediastinum, often in the cardiophrenic angles.[611,612] Only five of 27 thymolipomas in the largest reported series were located in the upper anterior mediastinum.[612] Individual cases have been reported in association with a variety of conditions, including myasthenia gravis,[613,614] aplastic anemia, Grave disease, and hypogammaglobulinemia.[615]

Thymolipomas frequently grow to a very large size before discovery. Being soft, they mold themselves to the adjacent mediastinum and diaphragm and often mimic cardiomegaly, lobar collapse, or diaphragmatic elevation on chest radiographs (Fig. 14.125).[612,616,617] On CT, thymolipomas manifest as large, well-circumscribed masses of fat attenuation that conform to adjacent structures (Fig. 14.125). Linear bands of soft tissue that histopathologically represent either residual thymic tissue or fibrous septa are frequently identified in the mass.[611,612,615,616,618] On MRI, the masses are of high signal intensity on T1-weighted images; lower signal intensity bands that course through the mass can also be seen, again due to fibrous septa or thymic tissue.[526,611,612,615]

Thymic cysts (Box 14.21)
Thymic cysts account for approximately 3% of all anterior mediastinal masses and are either congenital or acquired in origin.

Congenital thymic cysts
Congenital thymic cysts most likely arise from remnants of the thymopharyngeal duct and are usually thin walled, unilocular lesions <6 cm in diameter.[619] However, cysts up to 30 cm in diameter have been described.[610] Congenital thymic cysts are most frequently encountered in children[621] and affected patients are usually asymptomatic[622]; however, patients can present with

---

Box 14.21 Thymic cysts

Causes
Congenital
Acquired
- Infection
- HIV
- Prior thoracotomy
Neoplasm
- Thymoma
- Germ cell tumor
- Lymphoma (especially Hodgkin disease)

Imaging
Congenital
- Unilocular
- Variable size
- Thin to imperceptible wall
- Water–soft tissue attenuation
Acquired/neoplasm
- Multilocular
- Variable size
- Thick, enhancing septa
- Heterogeneous attenuation

---

cough or dyspnea[623] or with pain if bleeding into the cyst occurs.[624,625] On chest radiographs, congenital thymic cysts are indistinguishable from other nonlobulated thymic masses, notably thymoma. Radiographically visible calcification of the wall of the cyst has been reported,[622] but is uncommon.

On CT, congenital thymic cysts are homogeneous water attenuation masses that have very thin or imperceptible walls

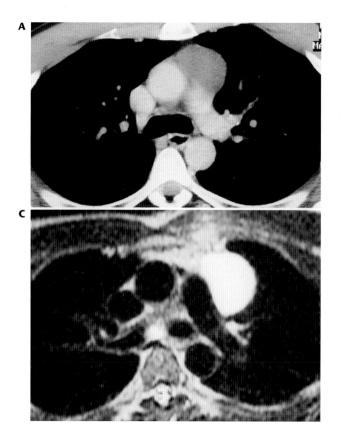

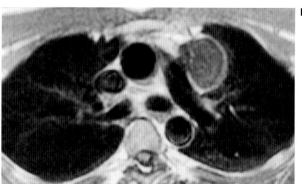

Fig. 14.126 Congenital thymic cyst. **A**, Contrast-enhanced CT shows a homogeneous well-circumscribed mass in the prevascular space. The mass was of slightly higher attenuation than water. **B**, T1- and **C**, T2- weighted MRI shows that the mass is homogeneous and has signal intensity characteristics similar to water. MRI can be useful for demonstrating the cystic nature of masses that appear solid on CT.

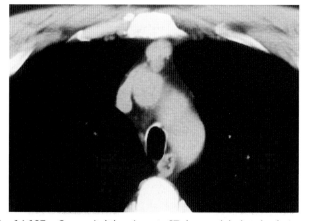

Fig. 14.127 Congenital thymic cyst. CT shows a lobulated soft tissue mass in the prevascular space. Resection showed a congenital thymic cyst that contained proteinaceous debris.

(Fig. 14.126).[626] Occasionally, thymic cysts appear as solid masses on CT because they are filled with proteinaceous fluid (Fig. 14.127).[529] In these cases, MRI can be useful for confirming the cystic nature of the lesion.[335] On MRI, they manifest as well-circumscribed, anterior mediastinal masses of high signal intensity on T2-weighted images (Fig. 14.127).[627,628] Signal intensity usually increases with increasing repetition time (TR). If spontaneous hemorrhage occurs within the cyst, the mass can have high signal intensity on both the T1- and T2-weighted images.[516]

Acquired thymic cysts

Acquired thymic cysts usually occur in the setting of infection, inflammation, or malignancy. Associated malignancies include Hodgkin disease,[589,590,629] seminoma, thymoma,[622,630] and thymic carcinoma. Some acquired cysts result from cystic degeneration within a focus of Hodgkin disease, unrelated to therapy.[589] When radiotherapy eradicates the Hodgkin disease, the cyst may remain unchanged in size[629] or disappear.[589] In some cases, the cysts first develop after irradiation of the mediastinum or following chemotherapy,[631-633] and at least some of these cysts are benign. If a cystic thymic mass develops in a patient with Hodgkin disease following radiotherapy, the possibility of a benign cyst should be considered before further treatment for Hodgkin disease is given.[634]

Suster et al[31] reported that some acquired thymic cysts are the result of inflammatory or infectious processes. Large multilocular thymic cysts are seen in up to 1% of children with human immunodeficiency virus (HIV) infection.[635-639] These multilocular cysts, which can also be seen in adults with HIV infection, may be very large and are easily demonstrated by ultrasonography, CT, or MRI.[635,636] Jaramillo et al[640] reported that some acquired thymic cysts may be associated with prior thoracotomy.

On CT or MRI, acquired thymic cysts are usually multilocular, have walls of variable thickness, and range in size from 3 to 17 cm (Fig. 14.128).[641] The cysts can contain areas of hemorrhage or calcification. The CT and MRI findings of acquired thymic cysts are more variable than those of congenital cysts. Because of their association with thymic neoplasia, care must be taken in the interpretation of cystic lesions of the anterior mediastinum. If an anterior mediastinal cyst is multilocular, heterogeneous in attenuation, thick walled, or associated with a soft tissue

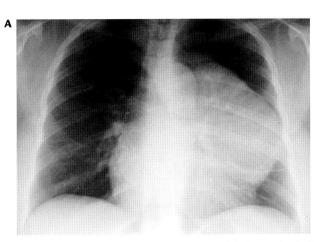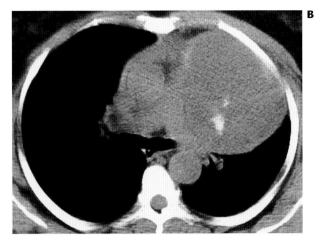

Fig. 14.128 Multilocular thymic cyst in a woman with chest pain. **A**, Frontal chest radiograph shows a lobulated left sided mediastinal mass. **B**, CT shows a cystic mass in the prevascular space. Note the calcified internal septa.

Box 14.22 **Imaging features of intrathoracic thyroid masses**

Well-defined spherical or lobular outline
Displacement or narrowing of the trachea is common
Calcification in benign disease is common, though it can also
  be seen in some malignant thyroid tumors
Multinodular goiter often contains cystic areas
Contiguity with the thyroid gland in the neck is almost
  invariable
Most intrathoracic thyroid masses contain normal thyroid
  tissue which
  • Is of higher attenuation than muscle on noncontrast CT
  • Enhances after administration of intravenous contrast
    material
  • Concentrates radionuclides, notably ^{123}I and [131]I
Intrathoracic goiter can be diagnosed on CT with high
  confidence if
  • Mass is contiguous with the thyroid gland
  • Mass is heterogeneous
  • Portions of the mass are of high attenuation on
    noncontrast CT
  • Portions of the mass enhance intensely after contrast
    administration
  • Mass contains coarse calcifications

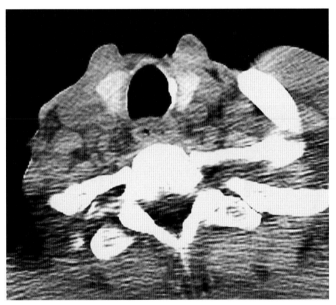

Fig. 14.129 Normal thyroid gland. On noncontrast CT, the gland is normally homogeneous and of high attenuation due to its iodine content.

component, it must be evaluated further (biopsy or resection) to exclude malignancy.

Thyroid lesions (Box 14.22)

The normal thyroid gland consists of two wedge shaped lobes adjacent to the trachea. A narrow isthmus connects the lobes anteriorly. The normal gland is usually seen at or just below the level of the cricoid cartilage on CT.[3] It is typically homogeneous and, due to its iodine content, may be of increased attenuation compared to skeletal muscle on noncontrast CT (Fig. 14.129).[642–644] The normal gland typically enhances homogeneously following administration of intravenous contrast material, and is usually of intermediate signal intensity on T1-weighted MRI and of increased signal intensity on T2-weighted MRI.[645–647]

Benign multinodular goiter is the most common mediastinal mass of thyroid origin. Intrathoracic goiters almost invariably result from downward extension of neck masses into the mediastinum.[14] Consequently, continuity between the mediastinal mass and the thyroid gland in the neck is an important diagnostic feature on chest radiographs and cross-sectional imaging. Goiters typically extend anterior to the recurrent laryngeal nerve and brachiocephalic vessels. Extension posterior to the trachea occurs in up to 25%. Retroesophageal extension is quite rare. Intrathoracic thyroid masses that develop from ectopic thyroid tissue in the mediastinum are also quite rare.[14,648–650]

On chest radiographs, intrathoracic goiters manifest as well-defined spherical or lobular masses (Figs 14.130 and 14.131) that frequently displace and narrow the trachea. Narrowing is occasionally substantial and can result in symptoms of cough, shortness of breath, or even stridor. The direction of tracheal displacement depends on the location of the mass. As noted

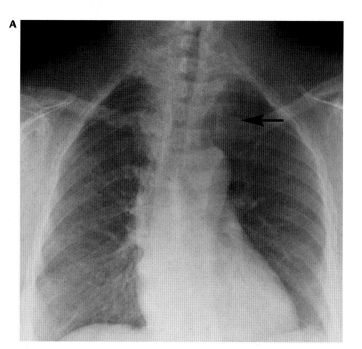

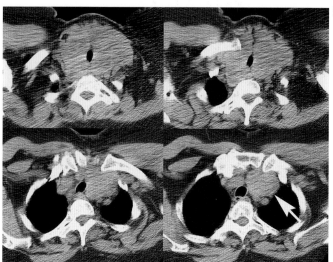

Fig. 14.130 Intrathoracic goiter. **A,** Frontal chest radiograph shows a left superior mediastinal mass (arrow) and bilateral tracheal compression. **B,** Noncontrast CT shows that the thyroid gland is diffusely enlarged, of heterogeneous attenuation, and extends into the left prevascular space (arrow).

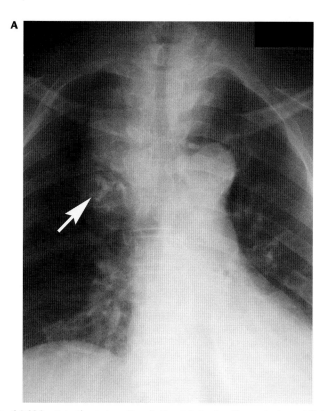

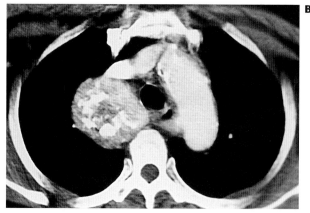

Fig. 14.131 Intrathoracic goiter. **A,** Frontal chest radiograph shows bilateral superior mediastinal masses and tracheal narrowing. Note the extensive calcification within the inferior aspect of the lesion (arrow). **B,** Contrast-enhanced CT shows marked enhancement as well as central chunklike calcification.

above, most masses descend anterior and lateral to the trachea; however, up to 25% may descend posterior to the trachea (Fig. 14.132). Such posteriorly located masses may separate the trachea and esophagus and displace the trachea anteriorly (Fig. 14.133). This finding can also be seen in patients

with bronchogenic cysts or submucosal tumors of the esophagus, but is almost never seen in patients with other mediastinal masses.

Calcification, often in a nodular, curvilinear, or circular configuration (Fig. 14.131), is another characteristic radio-

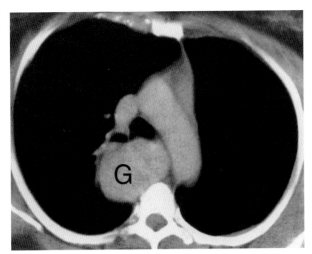

Fig. 14.132 Intrathoracic goiter. CT shows an intrathoracic goiter (G) that extends posterior to the trachea and displaces it anteriorly.

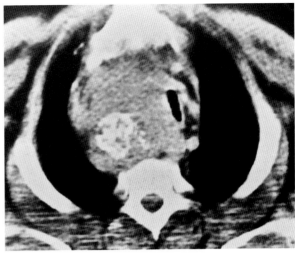

Fig. 14.134 Thyroid carcinoma. CT shows a heterogeneous mediastinal mass with extensive central calcification. Note loss of tissue planes surrounding the mass and marked tracheal displacement.

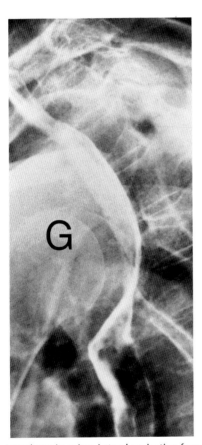

Fig. 14.133 Intrathoracic goiter. Lateral projection from a barium swallow examination shows that the goiter (G) extends between the trachea anteriorly and the esophagus posteriorly.

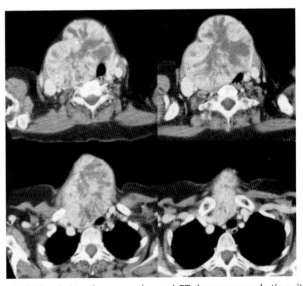

Fig. 14.135 Goiter. Contrast-enhanced CT shows an exophytic goiter that extends into the anterior mediastinum. Note the mass effect upon the trachea and intense contrast enhancement.

graphic feature of intrathoracic goiter. In general, the longer the goiter has been present, the more frequently calcifications are seen.[651] Calcification can also be seen in thyroid carcinomas (Fig. 14.134).[651–654] In general, calcification within a thyroid malignancy is psamommatous in nature (fine, clustered, and punctate), whereas calcification in a goiter is typically larger, less numerous, and more well defined. Unfortunately, calcifications

within a medullary thyroid carcinoma can exactly simulate the appearance of calcification within a goiter.

CT optimally demonstrates the shape, size, and position of the intrathoracic thyroid mass (Figs 14.130 to 14.132).[642–644,655] On CT, thyroid goiters usually manifest as masses of mixed attenuation in a paratracheal or retrotracheal location, often cradled by the brachiocephalic vessels. Compression of the brachiocephalic veins can result in the superior vena cava syndrome.[656] On noncontrast CT, regions of high attenuation due to normal thyroid tissue are often admixed with focal rounded areas of low attenuation. At least some portion of the mass enhances intensely (at least 25 HU) following administration of intravenous contrast material (Fig. 14.135).[644] Regions of low attenuation are typically more conspicuous after contrast administration (Fig. 14.135).[644] Calcification, a common finding, is better seen at CT than on chest radiographs.[644] The

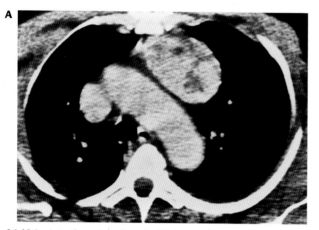

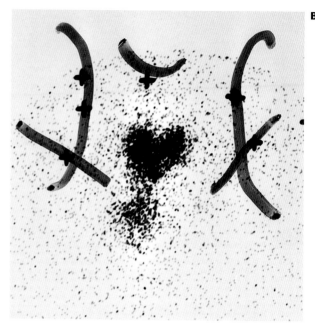

Fig. 14.136 Intrathoracic goiter. **A,** CT shows a heterogeneous mass in the prevascular space. **B,** [131]I radionuclide scan shows uptake within the intrathoracic portion of the goiter. Lines indicate the neck, clavicles, and mandible.

mass is usually continuous with the thyroid gland. Occasionally the only connection is a narrow fibrous or vascular pedicle that is not visible at CT.[644] Distinguishing benign from malignant thyroid masses is not possible with CT unless the tumor has clearly spread beyond the thyroid gland or is invasive.

MRI can be useful for evaluating intrathoracic thyroid masses. MRI well identifies cystic and solid components within the lesions but does not show the characteristic calcifications.[645,647,657] T1-weighted MRI shows signal intensity similar to muscle, but high intensity regions can be seen in areas of hemorrhage or colloid cyst formation.[645,646,658] On T2-weighted MRI, the masses are usually heterogeneous and of increased signal intensity; occasionally, foci of very high signal are seen in what are likely cystic spaces within the goiter. Adenomas cannot be distinguished from carcinomas based on signal intensities; both usually show increased signal on T2-weighted images.

Radionuclide imaging of the thyroid shows some functioning thyroid tissue in almost all intrathoracic goiters (Fig. 14.136).[659] The most appropriate imaging agents are ^{123}I or ^{131}I in older patients partly because they have a higher energy radiation that can penetrate the sternum, and also because they can be seen on delayed images, thus avoiding appreciable background blood pool activity. [99m]Tc images are degraded by the background blood pool activity and ^{125}I energy levels are too low to adequately penetrate the sternum.[659] Radionuclide imaging is a very sensitive and specific method for determining the thyroid nature of an intrathoracic mass. CT, however, is a more useful initial test because it provides better information about the mass should it be something other than thyroid, and is almost as specific for diagnosing a thyroid origin.

DISEASES OF THE THORACIC AORTA (Box 14.23)

Chest radiography is limited in its ability to diagnose diseases of the aorta. Much of the ascending aorta is not border forming

Box 14.23 Diseases of the aorta

Atherosclerotic aneurysm
Traumatic aneurysm
Mycotic aneurysm
Cystic medial necrosis
Acute aortic syndromes
• Aortic dissection
• Intramural hematoma
• Penetrating atherosclerotic ulcer
Congenital aortic aneurysm
Aneurysm resulting from aortitis

on the frontal chest radiograph and, thus, even very large ascending aortic aneurysms may be invisible.[660,661] Lesions of the aortic arch and descending aorta are, however, frequently detectable on chest radiographs and can, in some instances, be confused with soft tissue mediastinal masses (Fig. 14.137). Aortography via an arterially placed catheter was the standard technique for evaluation of the aorta for many years. However, less invasive techniques such as CT, MRI or ultrasonography (transesophageal or endovascular), can show aortic disease as well as or, in some cases, better than conventional catheter angiography.[662–667] Thus, these techniques are now the standard for evaluation of most diseases of the aorta. Depending on the information required, standard axial display CT or MRI may suffice for the diagnosis of most aortic diseases. However, multiplanar reconstruction and 3D display techniques have become very sophisticated with the advent of contrast-enhanced volumetric CT.[668–673] These techniques can generate views and projections that simulate those obtained by catheter angiography (Fig. 14.138). While these views may not be necessary for diagnosis, they may improve confidence of interpretation and may be requested by referring clinicians.

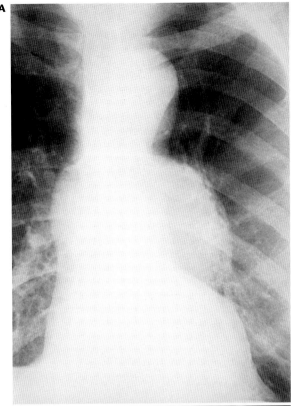

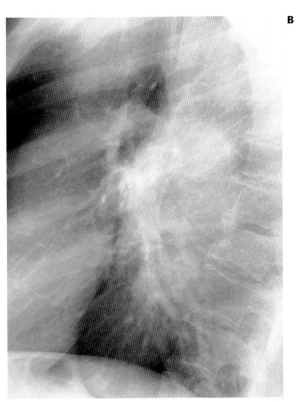

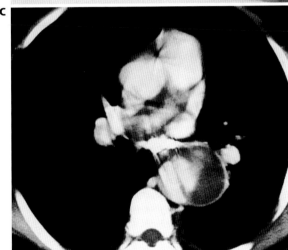

Fig. 14.137 Atherosclerotic aneurysm. **A**, Frontal and **B**, lateral chest radiographs show fusiform dilation of the descending thoracic aorta. **C**, Contrast-enhanced CT shows extensive peripheral thrombus within the aneurysm.

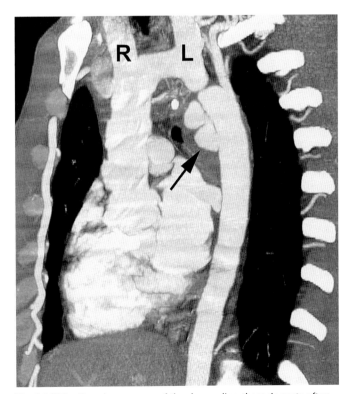

Fig. 14.138 Pseudoaneurysm of the descending thoracic aorta after aortic coarctation repair. Sagittal reformat image from a contrast-enhanced CT clearly shows the relationship of the pseudoaneurysm (arrows) to the aortic arch and branch vessels. R = right brachiocephalic artery; L = left brachiocephalic artery.

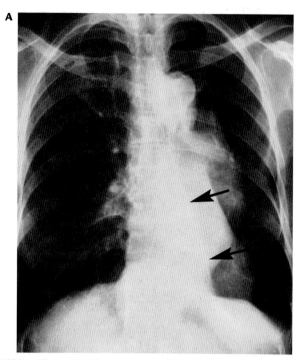

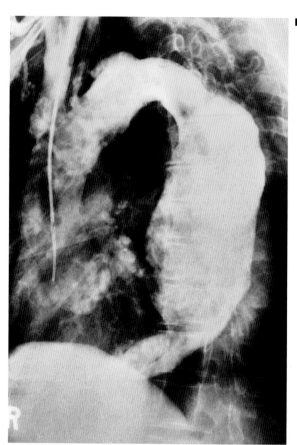

Fig. 14.139 Atherosclerotic aneurysm. **A**, Frontal chest radiograph shows a large fusiform aneurysm of the descending thoracic aorta. Note the findings of left lower lobe collapse (arrows) secondary to compression of the left lower lobe bronchus by the aneurysm. **B**, Aortogram confirms the aneurysm.

Atherosclerotic aortic aneurysm

Atherosclerotic aneurysms, along with generalized ectasia, are extremely common degenerative phenomena and may be fusiform or saccular in shape. Systemic hypertension is a clearly identified risk factor. Atherosclerotic aneurysms are often first discovered on imaging studies when the patient is still asymptomatic. Chest pain and compression effects are the most common symptoms. A hoarse voice may occur because of pressure on the recurrent laryngeal nerve as it passes around and under the aortic arch. Compression of the left main or lower lobe bronchus may result in atelectasis of the left lung or left lower lobe (Fig. 14.139). Compression of the esophagus may cause dysphagia and an extrinsic deformity may be seen on barium swallow examination. Compression of the right and left pulmonary arteries has also been reported.[674,675] Rupture is the most feared complication (Figs 14.140 and 14.141). An ascending aortic aneurysm that is >6 cm in diameter has a 31% lifetime risk of rupture and a descending thoracic aortic aneurysm >7 cm in diameter has a 43% lifetime risk of rupture.[676] A patient with a thoracic aneurysm >6 cm in diameter has a 3.6% yearly risk of rupture, a 3.7% yearly risk of dissection, and a 10.8% yearly risk of death.[676,677] These data suggest that ascending aortic aneurysms >5.5 cm in diameter and descending aortic aneurysms >6.5 cm in diameter should be repaired.[676–678] Saccular aneurysms are at particular risk for rupture.

Most atherosclerotic aneurysms are fusiform but a few are saccular in shape. Fusiform aneurysms usually arise in the aortic arch or descending aorta (Figs 14.137 and 14.139). They do not pose a diagnostic problem because their anatomic relationship to the aorta is obvious. Saccular aneurysms usually arise from the descending aorta (Fig. 14.142) or, infrequently, from the aortic arch (Fig. 14.143). They are extremely unusual in the ascending aorta. Occasionally, they are misdiagnosed on chest radiographs as a neoplastic mediastinal mass (Fig. 14.143).[679] They are usually easily differentiated from the majority of neoplastic or cystic masses by noting their relationship with the aorta and the presence of curvilinear calcification in the wall of the aneurysm (Fig. 14.143). Such calcification is usually present, though it may be difficult to identify on chest radiographs. Peripheral calcification of the wall of the aneurysm is well demonstrated at CT,[680] particularly prior to contrast enhancement. After intravenous contrast administration, the enlarged lumen in the region of the aneurysm is easily demonstrated with CT (Figs 14.137 and 14.141 to 14.143); multiplanar and 3D reconstructions from CT data can show the precise anatomy of atherosclerotic aneurysms to advantage (Fig. 14.142).[681–683] Most atherosclerotic aneurysms have significant amounts of thrombus lining the periphery of the aneurysm; flecks of calcification along the inner margin of the thrombus are common (Fig. 14.143).[684] The thrombus is usually crescent shaped along the wall of the aorta and some luminal dilation at the level of the aneurysm is

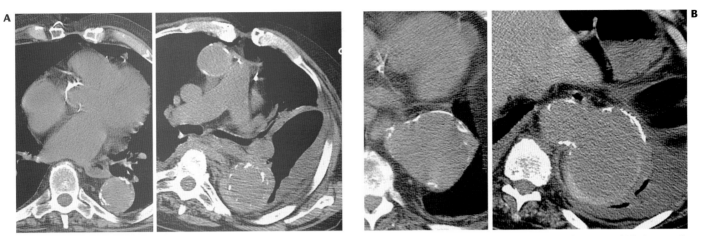

Fig. 14.140   Ruptured thoracic aortic aneurysm. Non-contrast CT images obtained one year prior to admission (left panels on **A** and **B**) shows a 6-cm fusiform aneurysm of the descending thoracic aorta. Non-contrast CT obtained one year later (right panels on **A** and **B**) when the patient presented with severe chest pain shows crescentic high attenuation in the wall of the aneurysm, a new left pleural effusion, and soft tissue stranding in the soft tissues around the aneurysm. These findings are suggestive of aneurysm rupture, confirmed at surgery.

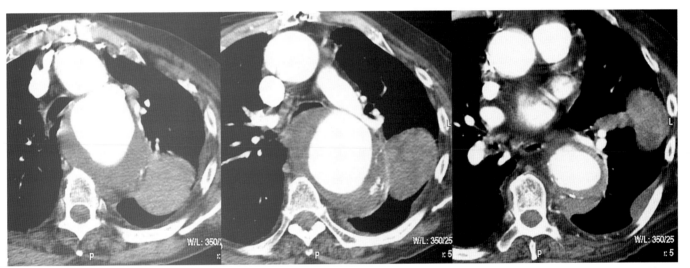

Fig. 14.141   Ruptured thoracic aortic aneurysm. Contrast-enhanced CT shows a large fusiform aneurysm of the descending thoracic aorta with peripheral thrombus. Note the high-attenuation fluid in the soft tissues around the aneurysm and in the major fissure indicative of bleeding. Aneurysm rupture was confirmed at surgery.

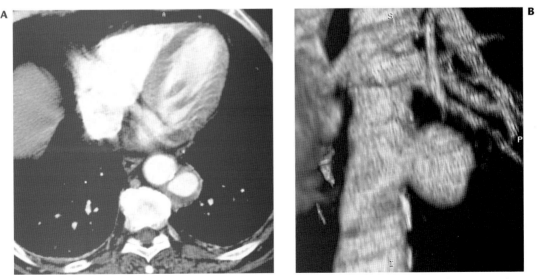

Fig. 14.142   Saccular aneurysm. Contrast-enhanced CT shown in **A**, axial and **B**, 3D shaded surface display shows a saccular aneurysm of the descending thoracic aorta.

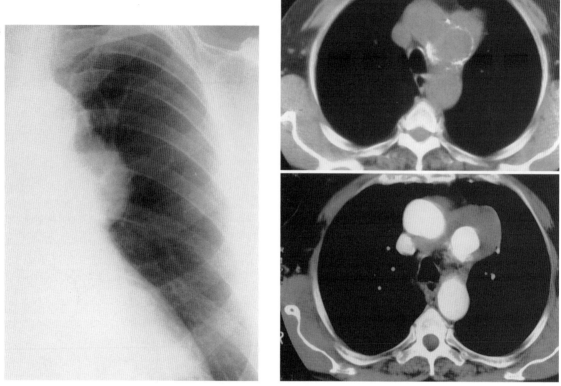

Fig. 14.143 Saccular aneurysm. **A,** Frontal chest radiograph shows a mediastinal mass with peripheral curvilinear calcification. **B,** Noncontrast CT shows peripheral calcification within the mass, suggesting aneurysm. **C,** Contrast-enhanced CT confirms the aneurysm and shows extensive peripheral thrombus.

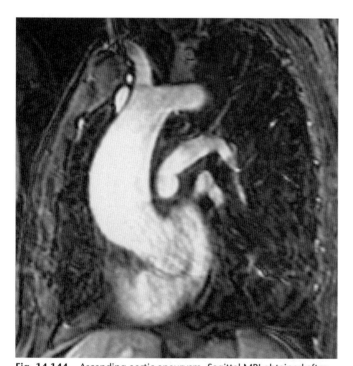

Fig. 14.144 Ascending aortic aneurysm. Sagittal MRI obtained after dynamic injection of gadolinium based contrast material shows a fusiform aneurysm of the ascending aorta. MRI can be a useful technique for reevaluating aortic aneurysms because it does not use ionizing radiation.

almost invariable (Fig. 14.141). Rarely, the lumen of the aneurysm is totally filled with thrombus.[679]

The ability to use multiplanar imaging and to differentiate the wall, lumen, and thrombus makes MRI an excellent method for assessing the size and shape of stable thoracic aortic aneurysms (Fig. 14.144), to show the relationship to branch vessels, and to demonstrate any compressive effects.[685] MRI can also be of value in showing mediastinal hematoma if the aneurysm is leaking.

Traumatic aortic injury and pseudoaneurysm

Traumatic aortic injury is discussed in Chapter 17. In the rare patient that survives aortic injury without surgery, a chronic pseudoaneurysm may develop.[686,687] These pseudoaneurysms characteristically arise at the anteromedial wall of the distal aortic arch or upper descending aorta, near the ligamentum arteriosum.[688] It has been suggested that aortic injury and hematoma at this site is more easily contained in a pseudoaneurysm by surrounding structures than is a posterior

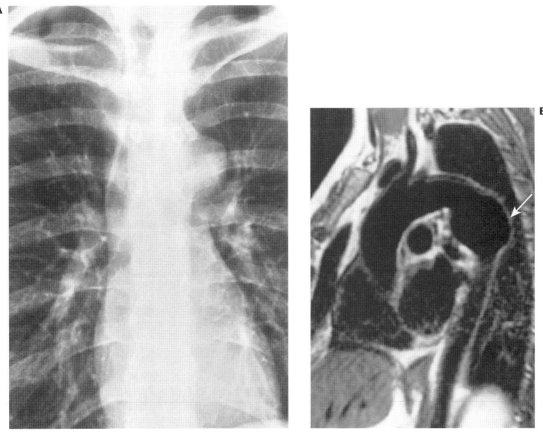

Fig. 14.145 Posttraumatic aortic pseudoaneurysm. **A**, Frontal chest radiograph shows a mass in the aortopulmonary window. **B**, Coronal cardiac gated T1-weighted MRI shows a pseudoaneurysm (arrow) at the ligamentum arteriosum.

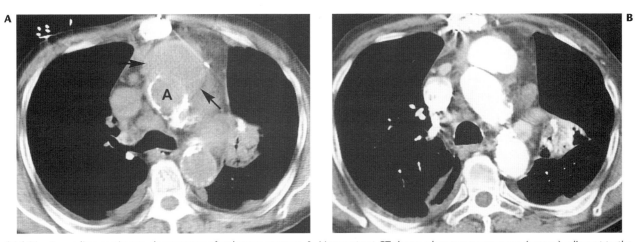

Fig. 14.146 Ascending aortic pseudoaneurysm after bypass surgery. **A**, Noncontrast CT shows a homogeneous mass (arrows) adjacent to the ascending aorta. **B**, Contrast-enhanced CT shows that this mass is a pseudoaneurysm at the aortotomy site.

laceration which tends to hemorrhage uncontrollably.[686] Affected patients may become hoarse because of pressure on the recurrent laryngeal nerve or complain of dysphagia due to compression of the esophagus. Other symptoms include chest pain, dyspnea, and shortness of breath. When small, these aneurysms are often invisible on chest radiographs. As they enlarge, they manifest as aortopulmonary window masses (Fig. 14.145). Chronic post-traumatic pseudoaneurysms are saccular in shape and in time

will develop calcification in their wall or thrombus along the wall.[686,687] At this stage, they are indistinguishable from saccular atherosclerotic aneurysms on chest radiographs, CT, and MRI, except that the patient is often young and there is usually no other evidence of atherosclerotic disease.

Other causes of aortic pseudoaneurysms include prior aortic or cardiac surgery (Figs 14.146 and 14.147), aortic dissection, and penetrating atherosclerotic ulcer (see below).

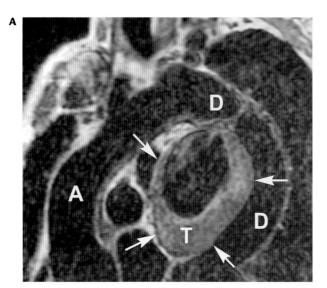
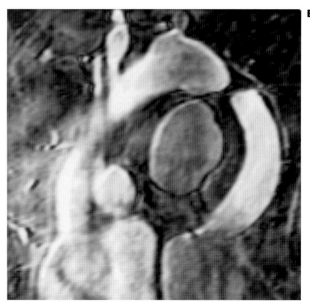

Fig. 14.147 Aortic pseudoaneurysm after repair of a descending thoracic aortic aneurysm. The patient presented with recurrent laryngeal nerve paralysis. **A,** Sagittal T1-weighted MRI shows a large pseudoaneurysm (arrows) with peripheral lining thrombus (T). Note the relationship of the pseudoaneurysm to the descending thoracic aorta (D). A = ascending aorta. **B,** Dynamic MRI obtained after administration of gadolinium based contrast material confirms slow flow within the center of the pseudoaneurysm.

Mycotic aneurysm of the aorta

Mycotic aneurysms of the aorta typically occur in patients with such known predisposing causes as intravenous drug abuse, valvular disease or congenital disorders of the heart or aorta, previous cardiac or aortic surgery, adjacent pyogenic infection[689] or immunocompromise.[690,691] All 20 patients with mycotic aneurysms of the aortic root in the series of Feigl et al[692] had either preexisting aortic valve disease or infected aortic valve prostheses.[692] Mycotic aneurysms may occur in any site in the aorta, depending upon the predisposing factor. Affected patients present with fever and leukocytosis. Mycotic aneurysms are usually saccular in shape. Important differentiating features between mycotic aneurysms and other types of saccular aneurysms are that mycotic aneurysms tend to enlarge rapidly and do not typically have calcium in their walls. Lee et al[693] reviewed CT scans of eight patients with mycotic aneurysms of the aorta. They reported the following CT findings as suggestive of the diagnosis in the appropriate clinical setting: ill-defined aortic wall with evidence of rupture; inflammatory changes around the aneurysm with gas bubble; periaortic fluid collections; and thrombus formation within a false lumen after rupture. Because of their tendency to enlarge and rupture, these aneurysms are frequently fatal unless expeditiously diagnosed and treated.[694]

Cystic medial necrosis

Cystic medial necrosis is characterized by deposition of acellular basophilic material within the aortic media which, when significant in amount, is associated with disruption of the structure of the aortic wall.[695] Severe cystic medial necrosis occurs in patients with Marfan syndrome and in an idiopathic form known as primary dilation of the aorta. Focal aneurysms due to cystic medial necrosis usually involve both the ascending

aorta and the aortic annulus – so-called annuloaortic ectasia – resulting in aortic regurgitation.[660, 696–698] Lesser degrees of this condition are very common in older individuals, possibly as a response to hemodynamic stresses such as hypertension and aortic stenosis.[695] Carlson et al[699] examined the ascending aorta in 250 autopsies. Having excluded cases of Marfan syndrome, idiopathic dilation of the aorta, and aortic dissection, they found that the incidence of cystic medial necrosis increased progressively with age from 10% in the first two decades to 60 and 64% in the 7th and 8th decades of life, respectively. They also found that the incidence of cystic medial necrosis was consistently higher in hypertensive patients than in normotensive subjects of comparable ages.

Acute aortic syndromes

Aortic dissection, intramural hematoma, and penetrating atherosclerotic ulcer are often considered together in discussions of acute nontraumatic aortic syndromes because they share common etiologic associations (atherosclerosis, systemic hypertension), occur in similar patient populations (elderly adults), and are often clinically indistinguishable.[700,701]

Aortic dissection

Aortic dissections are collections of blood within the aortic media that communicate with the lumen through one or more tears in the intima.[695,701] Progressive separation of the intimal layer from the media results in a false channel or lumen within the wall of the aorta. The dissection channel usually spirals so that the false lumen lies anterior and to the right in the ascending aorta, and posterior and to the left in the descending aorta. Degenerative changes in the media and hypertension are the most important predisposing factors.[702] Aortic dissections can be classified as acute (first 14 days) or chronic (after 14 days).[703]

Three-quarters of deaths occur within the acute phase. Patients who survive 2 weeks or more have a better prognosis,[703] although an aneurysm may subsequently develop and rupture, accounting for about 30% of deaths in the late phase.[704]

The classic DeBakey classification characterizes aortic dissections as types I, II, or III.[705] Type I dissections begin in the ascending aorta and extend into the descending aorta. Type II dissections are confined to the ascending aorta, and Type III dissections begin just beyond the left subclavian artery and are confined to the descending aorta. The so-called Stanford classification is simpler, classifying a dissection as type A if any part of the aorta proximal to the left subclavian artery is involved (DeBakey types I or II) or as Type B if the dissection begins at or distal to the left subclavian artery (DeBakey III).[706,707] Type A dissections can cause aortic regurgitation, can rupture into the pericardium and cause tamponade, or can compress the major arteries arising from the aortic arch, including the coronary arteries. The rationale for this classification is that the survival of patients with acute ascending aortic dissections is significantly better when they are treated surgically,[703,708,709] whereas patients with type B aortic dissections fare equally well with medical or surgical therapy. It is therefore recommended that type B dissections be treated initially with medical therapy, holding surgery in reserve for patients with persistent symptoms, progression of dissection, or life-threatening ischemic complications.[710–712]

Clinically, affected patients usually have high blood pressure or other clinical evidence of hypertension and present with the acute onset of severe chest pain, often radiating to the mid back, circulatory shock, pulse deficits, or ischemic symptoms due to the involvement of the coronary arteries or branch vessels.[713] Painless aortic dissection is, however, encountered in up to 15% of patients.[713] Patients with ascending aortic dissections may present with signs and symptoms of left ventricular failure due to acute aortic regurgitation. Pericardial tamponade is a life-threatening complication. Less common manifestations include syncope, cerebrovascular insufficiency, paraplegia, and lower extremity ischemia.

Intramural hematoma

Intramural hematoma without intimal disruption (non-communicating aortic dissection)[714–718] may be caused by intramural ischemia and bleeding from the vasa vasorum, trauma, or a penetrating ulcer (see below).[701] The distribution of intramural hematoma is described using the same terminology as is used for classic aortic dissection (Type A or B). The clinical presentation of intramural hematoma is usually indistinguishable from a classic communicating aortic dissection.[716,717] Some authors, however, have noted an older age at presentation.[719]

Intramural hematoma may regress, stabilize, or progress to form an aneurysm or a classic aortic dissection.[700,719–722] Evangelista et al[721] prospectively followed (mean follow-up period 45 months) 50 patients with intramural hematoma. At the end of the follow-up period, intramural hematoma had regressed completely without sequelae in 17 patients (34%), progressed to classic dissection in six (12%), evolved to fusiform aneurysm in 11 (22%), evolved to saccular aneurysm in four (8%), and evolved to pseudoaneurysm in 12 (24%). They also found a significant correlation between longitudinal extent of intramural hematoma and evolution to dissection.[721] Kaji et al[722] retrospectively compared groups of patients with type B

intramural hematoma and classic dissection. Eleven of 53 patients with intramural hematoma showed progression to either classic dissection or aneurysm on follow-up studies.[722] Further, they found that patients with type B intramural hematoma had better longterm prognosis than patients with classic dissection and less frequently required surgery for complications. Ide et al[723] reported that 40% of patients in their series with aortic intramural hematoma developed a classic communicating aortic dissection or an aortic aneurysm on follow-up examination. Interestingly, in the series of Murray et al,[718] four of five patients with intramural hematoma of the ascending aorta developed classic aortic dissection on follow-up examination, whereas only one of 17 patients with intramural hematoma of the descending aorta did so. Motoyoshi et al[719] studied 36 patients with acute type A intramural hematoma. All 10 patients with intramural hematoma and cardiac tamponade or aortic rupture received surgery; 26 patients without complications were initially treated medically, but seven eventually required surgery due to complications. Motoyoshi et al[719] concluded that patients with Type A intramural hematoma without complications, such as cardiac tamponade or aortic rupture, could be managed medically, but that up to half would eventually require surgical repair of the ascending aorta.

Penetrating atherosclerotic ulcer

Penetrating atherosclerotic ulcers[700, 724–728] result from ulceration of an atheromatous plaque. The ulcer, which is most frequent in the descending aorta, penetrates the internal elastic lamina of the aorta and causes intramural hematoma that may then resolve or progress to aortic rupture or classic dissection.[729] The clinical features of penetrating atherosclerotic ulcer are similar to those of classic aortic dissection, except that affected patients are usually older, there is a marked male predominance, there is a stronger association with severe atherosclerosis, and the ulcerated aorta may be more prone to rupture than is a typical dissection.[730–733] The optimal management of these patients is debated.[727,734]

Ganaha et al[735] reported a retrospective comparison of 34 patients with intramural hematoma associated with penetrating atherosclerotic ulcer (group 1) and 31 patients with intramural hematoma alone (group 2). They noted that the vast majority of ulcers occurred in the descending aorta and that the patients with ulcers were more likely to show progression on follow up. They also noted that persistent or recurrent chest pain, increasing pleural effusion, and both the maximum diameter and depth of the ulcer were significant predictors of disease progression.

Imaging of acute aortic syndromes
(Boxes 14.24–14.26)

The role of imaging in patients with symptoms of an acute nontraumatic aortic syndrome is to: (1) confirm the presence of a dissection, intramural hematoma, or penetrating ulcer; and (2) differentiate between type A and B lesions – information used not only for major management decisions (surgery versus medical therapy), but also for surgical planning. Identification of complications such as associated aortic regurgitation, pericardial, mediastinal or pleural hemorrhage, aortic rupture or coronary artery involvement is also important.[700,739,740]

Box 14.24 Diagnostic information required in patients with acute nontraumatic aortic syndromes (modified from references[736,737])

Confirm presence of aortic dissection, intramural hematoma, or penetrating ulcer

Evaluate extent of disease
- Involvement of the ascending aorta
- Sites of entry and reentry tears
- Branch vessel involvement
- Coronary artery involvement
- Thrombus in the false lumen

Diagnose complications
- Aortic dilation
- Aortic rupture
- Integrity of aortic valve
- Severity of aortic regurgitation
- Pericardial, mediastinal, or pleural hemorrhage

Box 14.25 Chest radiographic findings of acute aortic dissection (none is specific; modified from references[723,736])

Enlarged ascending aorta
Enlarged descending aorta
Enlarged aortic arch
Indistinct aortic arch
Widened paraspinal reflection
Tracheal shift
Displacement of left main bronchus
Displaced intimal calcification
Pleural effusion, notably on left side

Box 14.26 CT of acute aortic syndromes

Aortic dissection
Noncontrast CT
- Displaced intimal calcification
- ± Aortic dilation
- ± Complications
- Mediastinal, pericardial, pleural hemorrhage

Contrast CT
- Opacification of two (or more) lumens separated by thin intimal flap

Pitfalls
- Thrombosed false lumen
- Pulsation artifacts in ascending aorta
- Periaortic atelectasis, tumor

Intramural hematoma
Noncontrast CT
- Crescentic high-attenuation rim
- ± Aortic dilation

Contrast CT
- No intimal flap or false lumen
- No enhancement of rim

Penetrating ulcer
Noncontrast CT
- Extensive, calcified atheromatous plaque
- Associated intramural hematoma
- ± Aortic dilation

Contrast CT
- Focal contrast collection penetrating into media
- No intimal flap or false lumen

Aortic dissection

Chest radiography

The primary role of chest radiography in patients with suspected aortic dissection is to exclude other conditions. Though chest radiographic findings may suggest the diagnosis in up to one-half of affected patients,[741] these findings are not considered reliable for definitive diagnosis.[742] While unusual, the chest radiograph can be completely normal in patients with acute aortic dissection. A major diagnostic problem is that affected patients are often critically ill and that portable radiographs obtained in this situation are frequently suboptimal. Furthermore, dissections confined to the aortic root are often hidden on chest radiographs. The arch and descending aorta are, however, border-forming structures and dissections involving these portions of the aorta usually produce recognizable findings on chest radiographs (Figs 14.148 and 14.149). Enlargement of the aorta, the most frequent finding, tends to involve long segments, although focal dilation is occasionally seen. Sometimes the aorta is distinctly undulating in appearance (Fig. 14.149), and, occasionally, the dissection may manifest as a focal aneurysm of the aorta.[738] It may not be possible to distinguish aortic dissection from atherosclerotic disease on chest radiographs.[743] Progressive enlargement of the aorta over a few hours or days is a fairly specific sign, however, and is therefore a most important observation.

In appropriate clinical circumstances, atheromatous calcification that projects >1.0 cm inside the lateral aortic contour on the frontal chest radiograph is suggestive of aortic dissection (Fig. 14.150). Displacement of intimal calcification to this degree is not a common finding, however, being seen in only 4% of cases in one large series.[742] This sign must, however, be used with caution. The calcification must be unequivocally seen in profile along the lateral aortic contour. This sign is therefore of limited utility in the region of aortic arch where the frontal projection shows a foreshortened view of the obliquely curving aorta (Fig. 14.151). Furthermore, this sign is not specific because the lateral wall of the aorta may be substantially thickened in patients with severe atherosclerosis or aortitis. Additionally, a soft tissue mass that abuts the lateral margin of the aorta may give rise to a false positive finding. Absence of this sign cannot be used to exclude aortic dissection as intimal calcification may not be visibly displaced on chest radiographs of patients with acute aortic dissection.[744]

Hemorrhage from acute aortic dissection may also cause recognizable well- or ill-defined mediastinal widening on chest radiographs (Figs 14.148 to 14.150). Perihilar pulmonary opacities may also be seen due to dissection of mediastinal blood into the lungs. Pleural effusions due to leakage of blood from the mediastinum are common; they are usually left sided or, if bilateral, are often worse on the left than the right. Rupture into the pericardium is an extremely serious, often fatal complication. The presence of pericardial blood can rarely be diagnosed on

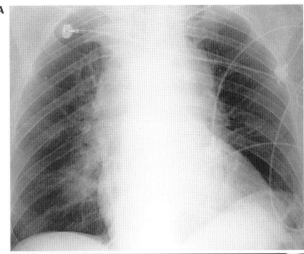

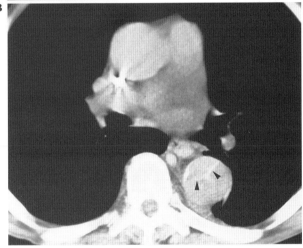

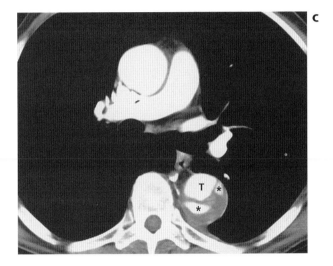

Fig. 14.148   Acute type B aortic dissection. **A**, Frontal chest radiograph shows bilateral mediastinal widening, elevation of the left diaphragm, and perihilar heterogeneous opacity in the right lower lobe. **B**, Noncontrast CT shows displaced intimal calcification (arrowheads) in the lumen of the descending thoracic aorta. **C**, Contrast-enhanced CT shows a complex type B dissection with at least two false lumens (*). T = true lumen.

chest radiographs but is suggested by a rapid increase in the diameter of the cardiopericardial silhouette.

Aortography

For many years, catheter based aortography was the standard for diagnosis of aortic dissection. The reported sensitivity of aortography for diagnosis of aortic dissection varies from 88% in a large multicenter study[745] up to 97%.[746] The principal angiographic finding is a false lumen separated from the true lumen by an intimal flap (Fig. 14.152). False negative results occur when the false lumen is thrombosed,[747] in patients with intramural hematoma, and when the true and false channels opacify equally and the intimal flap is not tangential to the x-ray beam.[748] Conversely, aortic wall thickening may mimic an unopacified false lumen. Aortography can also diagnose aortic regurgitation and, if necessary, the coronary arteries can be evaluated at the same time. The major disadvantages to aortography are that it can delay surgery with possibly deleterious effect and it can have potentially disastrous complications.[749]

Computed tomography

CT, particularly volumetric CT, is a highly sensitive and specific technique for the diagnosis of aortic dissection.[700,739,748,750–754] It is as, if not more, accurate, than aortography for demonstrating the presence and extent of dissection.[748,750–754] Demos et al[746] reported that the average accuracy of CT for aortic dissection

was 95%. Neinaber et al,[755] in a large multicenter study with 110 patients, showed conventional CT to have a sensitivity of 94% and a specificity of 87%. Studies using spiral CT report sensitivities approaching 100% and specificities >95%.[752,753] CT also allows rapid detection of associated mediastinal, pericardial, or pleural hemorrhage. A disadvantage of CT compared to conventional aortography is that it does not allow evaluation of aortic regurgitation or the coronary vessels. Further, CT may not be quite as sensitive as aortography for diagnosis of branch vessel involvement.

CT technique varies from center to center and depends, of course, upon the type of machine available. With modern multislice[756] or ultrafast CT scanners,[757–759] images can be obtained so rapidly that the entire thoracic and upper abdominal aorta can often be imaged in a single breath hold. Most centers use relatively thin sections (2.5 or 1.25 mm collimation) and maximum table speed to image the aorta from the thoracic inlet to the upper abdomen. Contrast material should be power injected at a fairly brisk rate (2–3 ml/s) through a large bore intravenous catheter. If dissection is identified in the descending aorta, the scan should continue into the abdomen to identify the distal extent of the dissection. These parameters will allow high quality multiplanar reconstructions as needed (Fig. 14.153). Many, if not most centers, also obtain at least three noncontrast scans (aortic arch, aortic root, descending aorta) prior to administration of contrast material to facilitate diagnosis of intramural hematoma

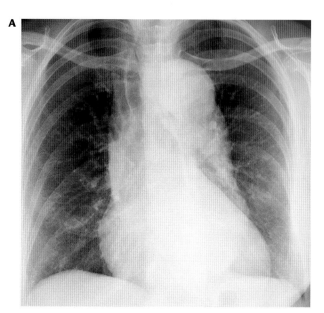

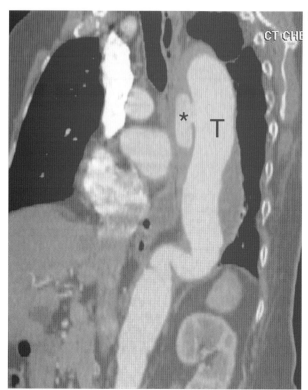

Fig. 14.149 Acute type B aortic dissection. **A,** Frontal chest radiograph shows dilation and tortuosity of the descending thoracic aorta. Note that the lateral contour of the aorta is undulating. **B,** Oblique coronal reformat image from a contrast-enhanced CT shows a limited type B aortic dissection. Note that the reformat image clearly shows the communication between the true (T) and false lumens (*) and that the majority of the false lumen is filled with thrombus.

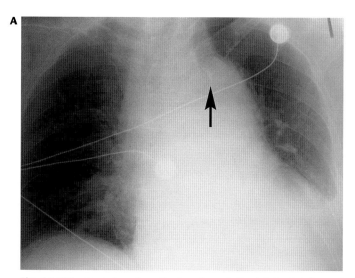

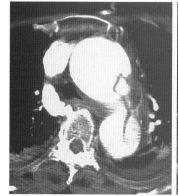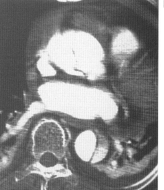

Fig. 14.150 Acute type A aortic dissection. **A,** Frontal chest radiograph shows a widened mediastinum, a left pleural effusion, and displaced intimal calcification (arrow). **B,** Contrast-enhanced CT shows a thin dissection flap in the ascending and descending thoracic aorta consistent with a Type A dissection.

(see below).

The diagnostic features of communicating aortic dissection on contrast-enhanced CT scans are similar to those seen at aortography: namely, the recognition of two lumens separated by an intimal flap (Figs 14.148 to 14.150 and 14.153; see Box 14.26). The intimal flap is seen as a curvilinear lucency within the opacified aorta in some three-quarters of cases. Sometimes, particularly in the aortic arch, the intimal flap may assume a serpiginous course. Plaques of calcification are sometimes seen along the intimal flap (Fig. 14.153). It is sometimes possible to see

the intimal flap on noncontrast scans,[754] particularly when the flap is calcified (Fig. 14.148) or in patients who are anemic.[760] The false lumen may be partially filled with thrombus (Fig. 14.153). It usually fills and empties in a delayed fashion compared with the true lumen. Differential opacification can be a very useful sign in cases where the intimal flap is invisible or uncertain, but often requires dynamic scans at a single level. Equal opacification of both lumina along with failure to see an intimal flap is one of the causes of false negative interpretations using CT. It should be remembered that the false lumen may not

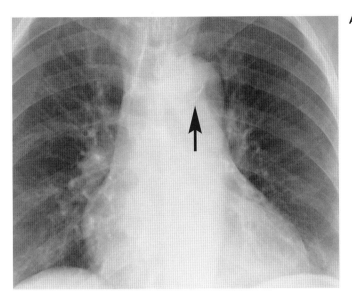

Fig. 14.151 Frontal chest radiograph in an asymptomatic woman with apparently displaced intimal calcification (arrow) due to the normal obliquity of the transverse aortic arch.

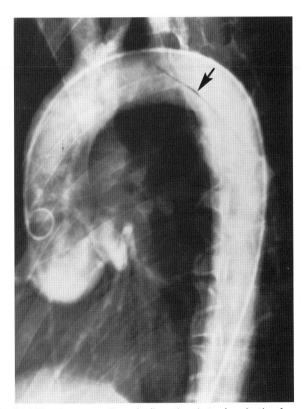

Fig. 14.152 Acute type B aortic dissection. Lateral projection from an aortogram shows an obvious intimal flap (arrow) separating the true from the false lumen.

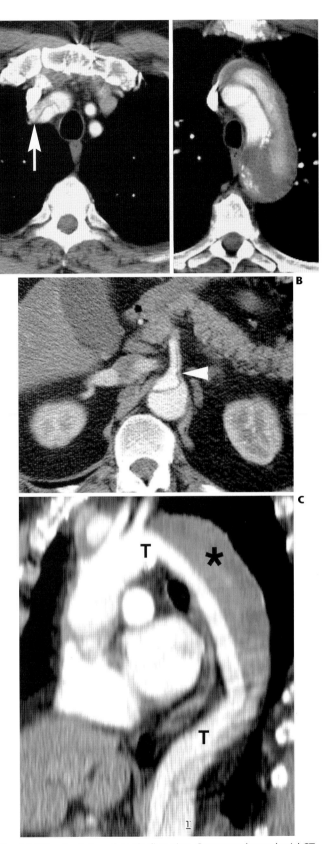

Fig. 14.153 Acute type A aortic dissection. Contrast enhanced axial CT (**A** and **B**) shows an intimal flap within the right brachiocephalic artery (arrow on **A**) and aortic arch. Note extension of the dissection flap into the celiac artery (arrowhead on **B**). Sagittal reformat image (**C**) clearly shows the full extent of the dissection. Furthermore, note that a significant portion of the false lumen (*) is thrombosed. T = true lumen.

enhance, either because it is totally filled by thrombus or because there is an intramural hematoma with no connection to the aortic lumen. The appearance of two lumens separated by an intimal flap is specific for aortic dissection, but care must be taken not to misdiagnose an extraaortic structure as a false lumen. The left innominate vein, the superior vena cava, the left superior intercostal vein, the left superior pulmonary vein, and the superior pericardial recesses can all mimic a false channel,

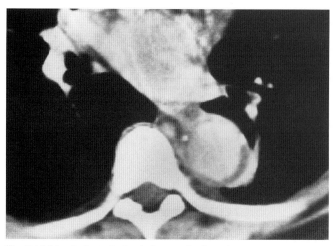

Fig. 14.154 Atelectasis simulating aortic dissection. Contrast-enhanced CT shows enhancing atelectatic lung adjacent to atheromatous plaque in the descending thoracic aorta, simulating the appearance of aortic dissection.

as can adjacent pleural or pericardial thickening and adjacent atelectasis of the lung (Fig. 14.154). Other potential mimics of a false lumen are: apparent asymmetrical thickening of the wall of the aorta caused by motion artifact due to systolic aortic motion,[761–763] and partial volume averaging of densities in the section above or below that may closely resemble a false lumen and give the impression of displaced intimal calcification (Fig. 14.155).[764] These artifacts can be overcome with the use of thinner collimation or by changing the CT reconstruction algorithm (partial reconstruction).[765] Streak artifacts can mimic an intimal flap (Fig. 14.155).[766] Intimal flaps are

gently curved structures of uniform thickness conforming to the configuration of the aorta. Streak artifacts are straight and vary in thickness. Also, their orientation may change markedly from one CT section to the next, and they often extend outside the aorta.

The affected portions of the aorta are often, though by no means always, enlarged. In some reports,[767] aortic dilation was always present, but in the series of Vasile et al,[754] almost 60% of patients with dissection showed no aortic dilation.

Differentiating a thrombosed aortic dissection from severe atherosclerotic disease of the aorta can be difficult. Classically, dissection displaces intimal calcification into the lumen of the aorta, whereas atherosclerotic disease does not. However, calcification may, on occasion, occur along the inner surface of the thrombus in an atherosclerotic aneurysm.[684,768] simulating the appearance of a thrombosed dissection. The shape of the opacified lumen can be a useful differentiating feature. In atherosclerotic aneurysm, the lumen is almost always round (Fig. 14.156), whereas in aortic dissection the true lumen is frequently flattened because of compression by the false lumen (Fig. 14.157).[684,769]

Current CT technique has some limitations.[736] It cannot reliably identify the presence of aortic regurgitation or depict coronary artery involvement. It may be slightly less sensitive than angiography for delineating branch vessel involvement.

Magnetic resonance imaging

MRI is being used with increasing frequency to evaluate known or suspected aortic dissection because it overcomes some of the limitations of CT. The ability to recognize flowing blood without the need for contrast media, together with the multiplanar imaging capability, are significant advantages for MRI, and the sensitivity and specificity of MRI is at least as good as

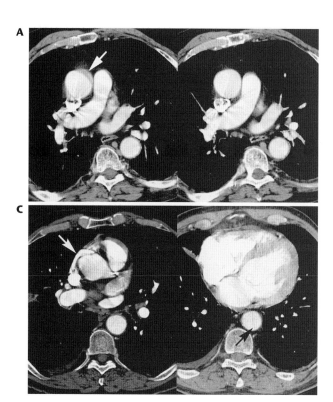

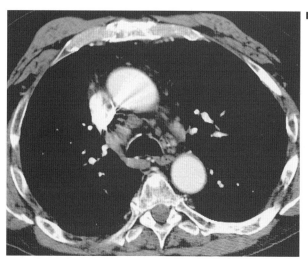

Fig. 14.155 Various artifacts that may simulate aortic dissection on CT. **A**, Pulsation artifact in the ascending aorta (arrow) may simulate aortic dissection. Image obtained 1 mm cephalad (right panel) shows a normal aortic contour. **B**, Streak artifact from the superior vena cava simulates a dissection flap in the ascending aorta. **C**, Enhancement of the closely applied right atrial appendage (white arrow) may also simulate the appearance of a dissection flap in the ascending aorta. Streak artifact in the same patient (black arrow) simulates a dissection flap in the descending aorta.

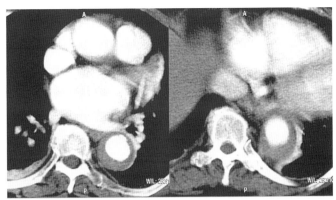

Fig. 14.156   Atherosclerotic aneurysm. Contrast-enhanced CT shows a fusiform saccular aneurysm of the descending thoracic aorta lined by thrombus. Note that the opacified aortic lumen remains round in contour.

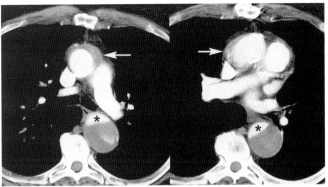

Fig. 14.157   Acute type A aortic dissection. Contrast-enhanced CT shows crescentic soft tissue opacity surrounding the ascending aorta (arrows), dilation of the descending thoracic aorta, and marked compression the true lumen (*). Note that the opacified true lumen in the descending aorta has a flattened contour. These findings suggest acute type A aortic dissection with near complete thrombosis of the true lumen.

CT.[663,739,753,770–774] MRI has been reported to have sensitivities as high as 95–100% for diagnosing aortic dissection.[772] Nienaber et al[775] prospectively studied 53 patients with possible aortic dissection with MRI and reported 100% sensitivity and specificity for the diagnosis. These optimistic numbers dropped slightly to a sensitivity of 98% and a specificity of 97% in a later report.[755]

A variety of MR techniques can be used to study the aorta. ECG gated conventional or fast spin-echo images show fast flowing blood as a signal void. When the blood flow is above a critical rate an intimal flap and the aortic wall are readily demonstrated as separately definable curvilinear structures. For the most part, blood in the true lumen of the aorta flows at a rate above this threshold.[685] Slow flowing blood in the false lumen produces a variety of signal patterns which can be difficult to distinguish from thrombus (Figs 14.158 and 14.159), but gradient echo and MR angiographic sequences can usually help resolve this problem. Gradient echo techniques also allow faster imaging, including breath-hold sequences, and 3D gradient echo sequences with intravenous gadolinium enhancement permit high quality images without flow related loss of signal (Figs 14.158 and 14.159).[665–667,685,773,776–778]

The basic signs of communicating aortic dissection at MRI (Figs 14.158 and 14.159) are the same as those described for CT:

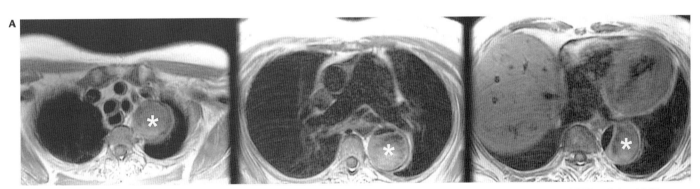

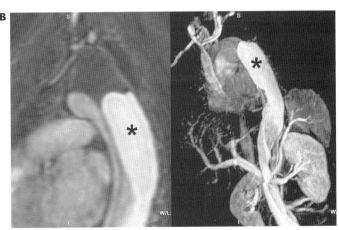

Fig. 14.158   Type B aortic dissection. **A**, Axial T1-weighted MRI shows typical findings of aortic dissection on MRI. Note that it is difficult to distinguish thrombus from slowly flowing blood in the false lumen (*) on this pulse sequence. **B**, Images obtained after dynamic administration of gadolinium based contrast material clearly show flow in the false lumen (*) on both the sagittal image (left panel) and maximum intensity projection (MIP) reconstruction (right panel).

A

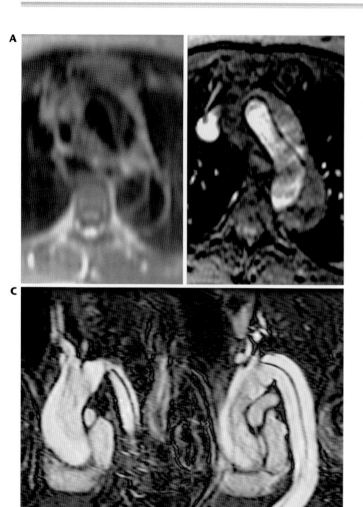

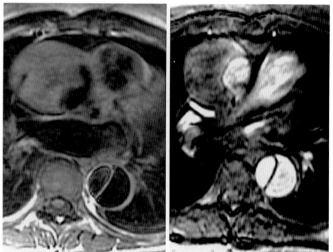

B

Fig. 14.159 Type A aortic dissection. **A** and **B**, Paired axial T1-weighted and bright blood gradient recalled echo sequence images at two different levels clearly show a dissection flap in both the ascending and descending thoracic aorta. Note the differential flow within the true and false lumen in the aortic arch and possible thrombosis of the false lumen at the aortic root (**A**). **C**, Sagittal MRI following dynamic administration of gadolinium based contrast material show flow in the false lumen with no evidence of thrombus.

C

an intimal flap separating true and false lumina. Eccentric or concentric aortic wall thickening may, on occasion, be the only MRI finding.[779] In approximately one-quarter of cases, cords or bands of soft tissue intensity (cobwebs) may be seen traversing the false lumen, a useful marker that the lumen in question is indeed the false lumen.[780] The multiplanar imaging capability of MRI[773] can be an advantage compared with CT; oblique sagittal and coronal planes may be the optimal imaging planes to demonstrate the entry site,[781] extent of dissection, and the relationship of the dissection to the major aortic branches, particularly those arising from the aortic arch.[736,748] MRI can also be used to evaluate the integrity of the aortic valve in patients with Type A dissections and to quantify associated aortic regurgitation. Disadvantages of MRI include lack of access in an emergency setting, the time required to image the patient, and difficulty with monitoring very sick patients in the magnet.[736] Many of these difficulties are not insurmountable, though.[663,773]

As with CT there are a number of diagnostic pitfalls using MRI.[782–784] Adjacent structures, such as the left brachiocephalic vein (Fig. 14.160), the left superior intercostal vein, left superior

pulmonary vein, hemiazygos or azygos vein may mimic a false lumen, as may the origins of the arteries arising from the aortic arch and the superior pericardial recesses. Apparent thickening of the aortic wall due to motion artifact, atherosclerotic plaques, aortitis (Fig. 14.161), or fibrosing mediastinitis may also be confused with a thrombosed false lumen.

Echocardiography

Echocardiography, particularly transesophageal echocardiography (TEE), has proved useful for diagnosis of aortic dissection. Standard transthoracic echocardiography[785,786] can show ascending aortic dissection, the aortic valve, and hemopericardium. Color flow Doppler ultrasonography can diagnose and grade aortic regurgitation. For the diagnosis of aortic dissection, regardless of type, transthoracic cardiac ultrasonography has been shown to be 60% sensitive and 83% specific, the sensitivity for dissections of the descending aorta being particularly poor.[663]

TEE, which allows examination of the aorta at multiple levels, can provide an extensive view of the ascending and descending

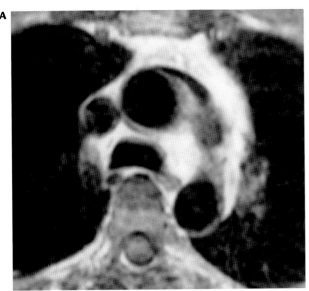

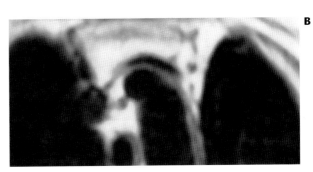

Fig. 14.160 Pitfalls in the diagnosis of aortic dissection on spin-echo MRI. **A,** Shows dissection mimicked by the anterior portion of superior pericardial recess. Pericardial fluid is typically of low signal intensity because it is moving due to cardiac pulsation. **B,** Shows aortic dissection mimicked by the left brachiocephalic vein passing anterior to aortic arch.

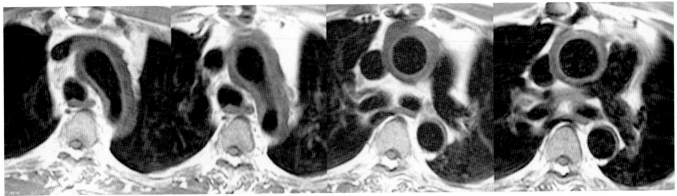

Fig. 14.161 Aortic dissection mimicked by aortitis. Axial T1-weighted MRI shows diffuse aortic wall thickening simulating the appearance of a thrombosed aortic dissection. However, note that the aortic lumen remains round in shape.

aorta, and can also show the aortic arch and proximal coronary arteries. Reports suggest sensitivities >95%, which can be increased to close to 100% for combined transthoracic and transesophageal ultrasonography.[745,747,775,787–789] One problem with ultrasonography is the inability to see through the air in the trachea; thus, if the dissection is confined to the ascending aorta, it may not be visible from the transducer in the esophagus.[663,774] The reported specificities for diagnosis are more variable; one large series showed specificities well above 95%,[790] but another equally large study[663] showed a specificity of 80%, mainly because of false positive findings in the ascending aorta. High frequency ultrasonography probes mounted on the tips of intraarterial catheters have been tested and shown to be accurate in diagnosing aortic dissection.[791] The basic signs of dissection at ultrasonography are the same as those described for CT/MRI and aortography, namely a double lumen separated by an intimal flap. If the false lumen is thrombosed, central displacement of intimal calcification or separation of intimal layers are looked for. The entry tear can be identified at ultrasonography as interruption in the continuity of the intimal flap with associated fluttering of the edges. A major advantage of transthoracic/transesophageal ultrasonography is that it can be performed at the patient's bedside and in operating rooms.

Intramural hematoma

The principal CT finding of intramural hematoma[714,716,717,792,793] is a crescent shaped rim of high attenuation in the wall of the aorta (Fig. 14.162, see Box 14.26). The diameter of the aorta may also be enlarged, but the lumen is not usually compressed. The hyperattenuating rim is best appreciated on noncontrast CT; it can be misdiagnosed as crescentic thrombus on contrast-enhanced CT scans. The attenuation of the hematoma typically declines with time. Unless complicated by classic dissection, the hematoma should not opacify on contrast-enhanced CT scans.

It can be difficult to differentiate intramural hematoma from atherosclerotic disease. Helpful findings include: (1) atherosclerotic wall thickening is rare in the ascending aorta;

A

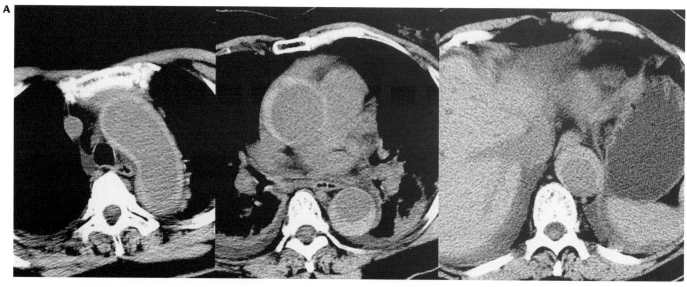

B

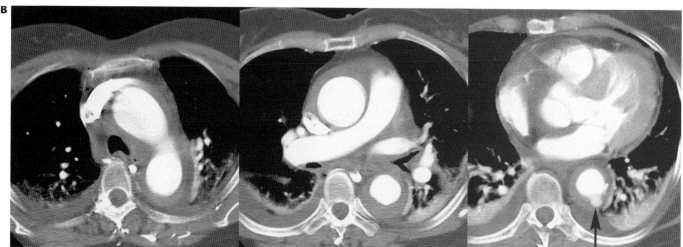

C

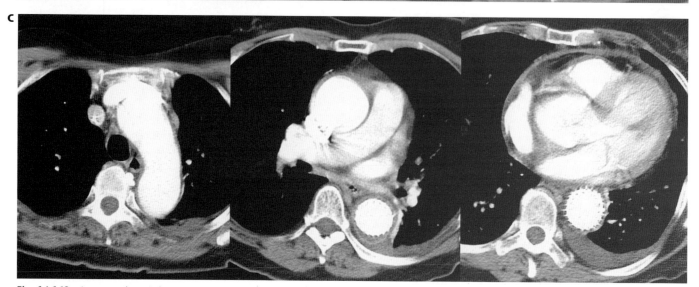

Fig. 14.162 Intramural aortic hematoma. **A,** Noncontrast CT shows crescentic high attenuation in the wall of the aorta, extending from the ascending to the descending aorta. **B,** Contrast-enhanced CT shows no dissection flap. However, a penetrating atherosclerotic ulcer is seen (arrow) in the descending thoracic aorta. **C,** Follow-up contrast-enhanced CT after placement of an aortic stent graft shows near complete resolution of the intramural hematoma. However, the patient eventually required surgical repair of the descending thoracic aorta due to a leak.

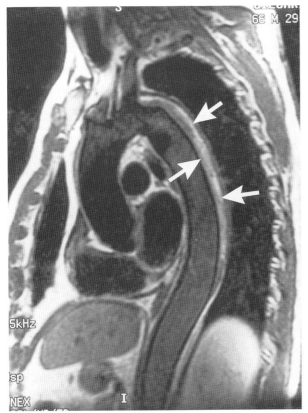

Fig. 14.163 Intramural aortic hematoma. Cardiac gated T1-weighted spin-echo MRI shows fairly uniform high signal in the aortic wall consistent with maturing hematoma (arrows). (Courtesy of TB Oliver, MD, Edinburgh, UK. With permission from Oliver TB, Murchison JT, Reid JH. Spiral CT in acute non-cardiac chest pain. Clin Radiol 1999;54:38–45, Blackwell Publishing Ltd.)

(2) atherosclerosis causes an irregular inner margin whereas the aortic wall is smooth with intramural hematoma; and (3) atherosclerosis is patchy, whereas intramural hematoma extends smoothly up and down the affected part of the aorta (see Fig. 14.162).

Differentiating intramural hematoma from a thrombosed aortic dissection can also be problematic because, in both cases, neither a double contrast-enhanced channel nor an intimal flap is seen on CT. In this circumstance, the spiral shape of the thrombosed false channel and displaced intimal calcification suggests the diagnosis of dissection with a thrombosed lumen. Conversely, crescentic high attenuation in the wall of the aorta on noncontrast CT suggests intramural hematoma (Fig. 14.162).

The features of intramural hematoma on MRI[714–717,792,794] are similar to those seen on CT: a crescent shaped rim with signal characteristics of hematoma (Fig. 14.163). Intramural hematoma is readily diagnosed by TEE as circular or crescentic thickening of the aortic wall showing a partial or complete "thrombus-like echo pattern" with displacement of intimal calcification and some differential movement between the layers of the aortic wall.[716,795]

Penetrating atherosclerotic ulcer

Penetrating ulcers are diagnosed on imaging studies (Figs 14.162, 14.164 and 14.165), such as aortography, CT, or MRI by the presence of a focal contrast-filled outpouching into the aortic wall with associated intramural hematoma (see Box 14.26).[701] Unless

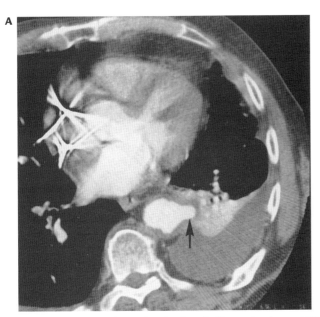

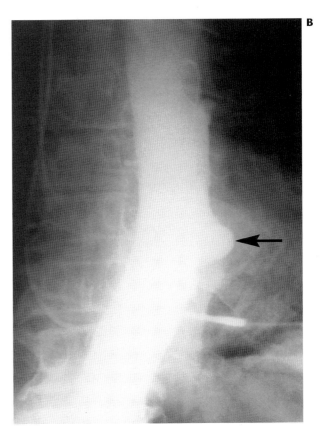

Fig. 14.164 Penetrating atherosclerotic ulcer. **A**, Contrast-enhanced CT and **B**, aortogram shows a focal ulceration (arrow) in the descending thoracic aorta, left lower lobe ateletasis and a left pleural effusion. (Courtesy of TB Oliver, MD, Edinburgh, UK. With permission from Oliver TB, Murchison JT, Reid JH. Spiral CT in acute non-cardiac chest pain. Clin Radiol 1999;54:38–45, Blackwell Publishing Ltd.)

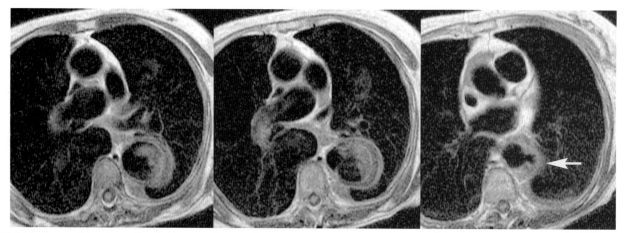

Fig. 14.165 Penetrating atherosclerotic ulcer. Axial T1-weighted MRI shows a focal ulceration in the descending thoracic aorta (arrow), focal dilation of the descending thoracic aorta, and high signal intensity in the aortic wall consistent with intramural hematoma.

the ulcer is complicated by classic dissection, an intimal flap is not seen.[725,727,796–799] Ulcers typically occur in the setting of extensive atheromatous plaque, which may be calcified. Displacement of intimal calcification, similar to that seen with classic aortic dissection, is a common finding on CT, as is the presence of intramural hematoma.

Optimal imaging of an acute nontraumatic aortic syndrome

The four primary imaging methods – CT, MRI, TEE, and aortography – each have important advantages and disadvantages in the evaluation of suspected acute nontraumatic aortic syndrome.[738,753] The ideal examination should confirm or exclude the diagnosis, correctly evaluate the extent of the lesion, and identify all possible complications, including aortic regurgitation and coronary artery involvement (see Box 14.24), all with 100% accuracy. Furthermore, the ideal test should be performed in a rapid and timely fashion, and be applicable to even the most sick and critically ill patients. Unfortunately, no single such test exists![737] Instead, the choice of imaging modality used in a given patient depends upon institutional experience, availability of certain services such as TEE or emergency MRI, and the status of the patient.[736,737] Furthermore, the minimum diagnostic information that a surgeon requires before proceeding to the operating room varies.[737] Some surgeons require detailed knowledge about the status of the aortic valve, coronary arteries and branch vessels before proceeding to surgery, whereas others do not. In many instances, therefore, multiple studies (e.g. CT and TEE) may be required.

Aortography was for many years regarded as the best diagnostic test for patients with suspected acute aortic dissection, but aortography is time consuming, invasive and, very importantly, has lower sensitivity than CT or MRI. Transesophageal ultrasonography has a high sensitivity, but its specificity only becomes as good as CT or MRI when strict criteria are applied to the diagnosis of dissection – criteria which lower its overall sensitivity. MRI is not available on an emergency basis in many hospitals, and the need for patient transport together with the length of the procedure may make it less desirable for patients who are unstable or those requiring particularly close monitoring. TEE is readily available and fast; it can be

performed at the bedside, making it ideal for use in patients who are unstable. It is, however, very operator dependent.

Many authors have opined that TEE, when available, should be considered first in cases of suspected dissection, because of its accuracy, safety, speed, and convenience. As MRI compatible monitoring and life support systems become available, the use of MRI as the primary imaging modality for acute aortic dissection is likely to increase because of its excellent accuracy and high quality images. However, in many, and perhaps most, hospitals, CT scanning, particularly multidetector CT, is the first choice for the rapid screening of patients with suspected acute aortic dissection.

Both echocardiography and MRI are excellent techniques for following up patients with known or treated acute aortic syndromes[800,801] because they are noninvasive and do not involve ionizing radiation.

Congenital aortic aneurysm

Congenital aneurysms of the aorta are rare.[802] Almost all of those encountered in clinical practice are sinus of Valsalva aneurysms.[802] Normally, the media of the wall of the proximal aorta is firmly attached to the fibrous annulus of the aortic valve. In patients with congenital sinus of Valsalva aneurysm, the media avulses from its attachment to the annulus and an aneurysm results.[695] These aneurysms most commonly arise from the posterior noncoronary or right aortic sinus. An aneurysm of the posterior aortic sinus bulges into the right atrium, and if it ruptures the result is an aortic to right atrial shunt. An aneurysm of the right aortic sinus bulges into the right ventricle and rupture, therefore, causes an aortic to right ventricular shunt. The aortic valve lies deep within the mediastinal shadow and congenital sinus of Valsalva aneurysms must, therefore, reach substantial size to be recognizable on chest radiographs. Occasionally, they do reach such a size. Calcification may be visible in the wall of the aneurysm. The signs of left-to-right shunt may be visible if rupture has occurred. CT and MRI can show the aneurysm to advantage.[803–805]

Very occasionally, congenital aneurysms are associated with coarctation of the aorta (Fig. 14.166) or other aortic anomalies, such as right sided aortic arch.[806] Whether the aneurysms in

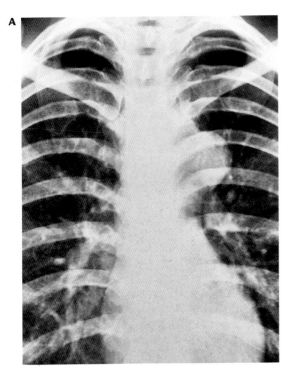

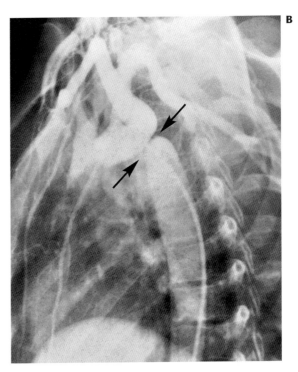

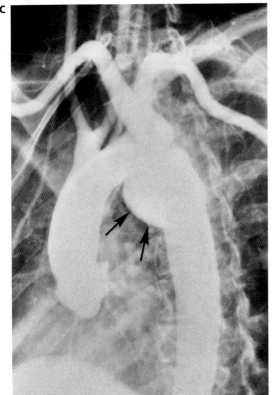

Fig. 14.166 Slowly enlarging aortic aneurysm in a young woman with aortic coarctation. **A**, Frontal chest radiograph shows a saccular aneurysm of the proximal descending thoracic aorta. **B**, Early phase of the aortogram shows the coarctation (arrows). **C**, Later phase of the aortogram shows opacification of the aneurysm (arrows).

encountered in clinical practice are due to giant cell[807] or Takayasu arteritis.[808,809] The latter is a large vessel vasculitis that affects the aorta, branch vessels, and pulmonary arteries. It occurs most commonly in the Orient, but has a worldwide distribution. Though more often a stenosing disease, Takayasu arteritis may, on occasion, cause saccular or fusiform aortic aneurysms (Fig. 14.167).[810–814] Aneurysms in this condition may be single or multiple and may be seen anywhere in the aorta. Aortic wall thickening, which may be calcified, can be seen with CT angiography[815] and aortic dissection may be a complication.

Aortic anomalies that may simulate a mediastinal mass

There are three congenital aortic variants that can simulate a mediastinal mass[816] on chest radiographs or noncontrast CT: right aortic arch, double aortic arch, and pseudocoarctation of the aorta.

Right aortic arch

A right aortic arch is commonly mistaken for a mediastinal mass on chest radiographs and patients may be referred for CT. Most asymptomatic adults with a right sided aortic arch (about one in 200 patients) have an aberrant left subclavian artery. Other anatomic configurations such as mirror image branching of the great vessels are less common and are associated with congenital heart disease. This discussion will be confined to

patients with coarctation are truly congenital or acquired secondary to prolonged hypertension is debatable.

Aortic aneurysm resulting from aortitis

Aortic aneurysm as a result of aortitis is a rare phenomenon now that tertiary syphilis is so uncommon.[374] Most cases

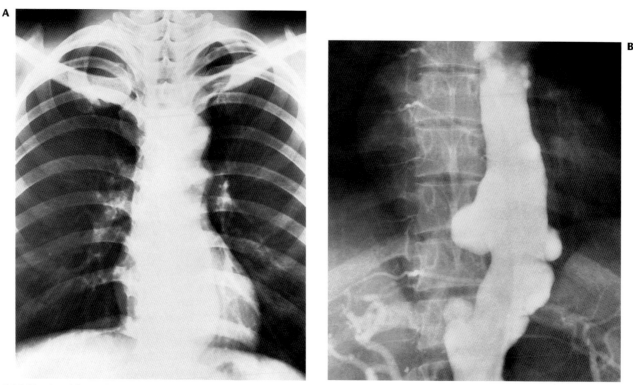

Fig. 14.167 Arteritis causing aortic aneurysms in a young man. **A**, Frontal chest radiograph shows a dilated, irregular descending aorta. **B**, Aortogram shows multiple aneurysms of the descending thoracic aorta.

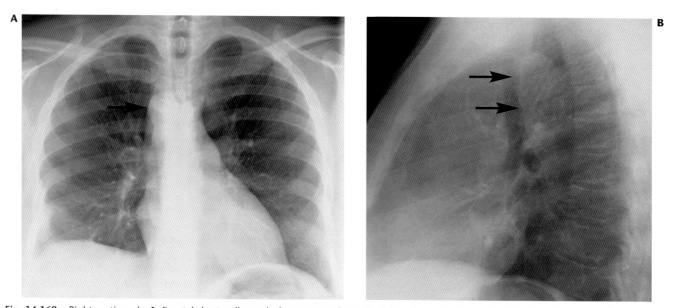

Fig. 14.168 Right aortic arch. **A**, Frontal chest radiograph shows a round opacity that indents the right side of the intrathoracic trachea (arrow). Note the absence of the normal left sided aortic impression. **B**, Lateral radiograph shows a retrotracheal opacity with slight anterior bowing of the trachea (arrows), consistent with an aberrant left subclavian artery.

right aortic arch in patients without cardiac malformation. In these patients, the right arch passes to the right of the trachea and usually descends in the right posterior mediastinum; only rarely is the descending aorta on the left. In the usual branching pattern, the left carotid artery arises first, followed by the right carotid and right subclavian arteries. The left subclavian artery, which arises as the fourth and most distal branch of the aortic arch, is known as an "aberrant subclavian artery". The aberrant left subclavian artery passes behind the esophagus to reach the

root of the neck on the left side. The left subclavian artery may take origin from a diverticulum in the proximal descending aorta, which embryologically represents a remnant of the left arch.

On frontal chest radiographs, the right arch appears as a round mass in the right paratracheal region that indents the right lateral margin of the trachea, and may deviate the trachea to the left (Fig. 14.168). There may, however, be a small round density in the expected location of the left arch, caused either by the diverticulum or by leftward displacement of the aorta. An

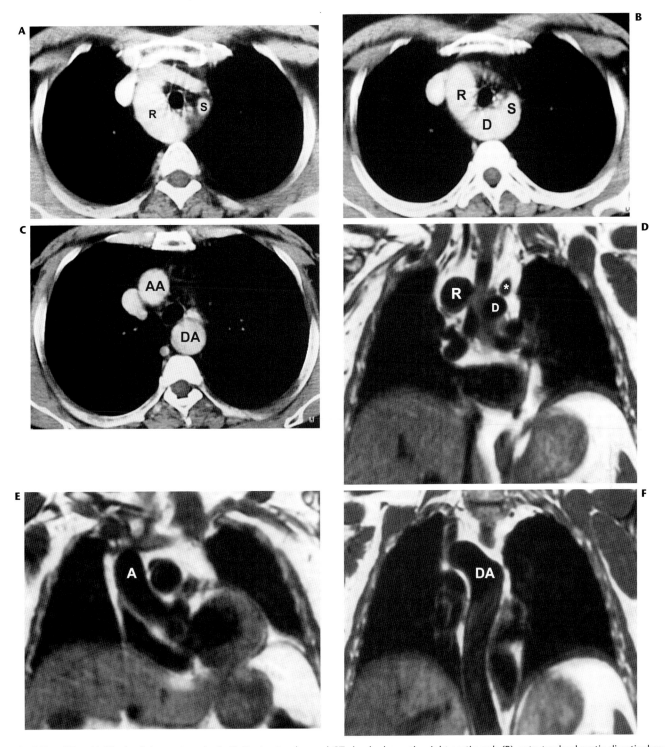

Fig. 14.169   CT and MRI of a right aortic arch. **A–C**, Contrast-enhanced CT clearly shows the right aortic arch (R), retrotracheal aortic diverticulum (D), aberrant left subclavian artery (S), and the midline descending thoracic aorta (DA). AA = ascending aorta. **D–F**, Coronal T1-weighted MRI also clearly shows the right sided ascending aorta (A), high right aortic arch (R), retrotracheal and left sided aortic diverticulum (D), left subclavian artery (*), and midline descending thoracic aorta (DA).

important clue to the correct diagnosis is the absence of the normal left sided tracheal indentation that is seen when the arch is normally situated. The descending aorta is to the right of the midline in almost all cases.

On lateral chest radiographs, a density posterior to the esophagus that is variable in size will be seen (Fig. 14.168).[817] This density is sometimes due to the aortic diverticulum and aberrant left subclavian artery and sometimes to medial displacement of the proximal descending aorta. The posterior impression on the esophagus at barium swallow examination and on the trachea on chest radiography and CT is often striking.

For the most part, the findings of a right arch on chest radiographs are distinctive enough to suggest the correct diagnosis. In difficult cases, or in patients with symptoms of a vascular ring, CT or MRI may be performed (Fig. 14.169). CT or MRI easily identifies the aortic arch to the right of the trachea.

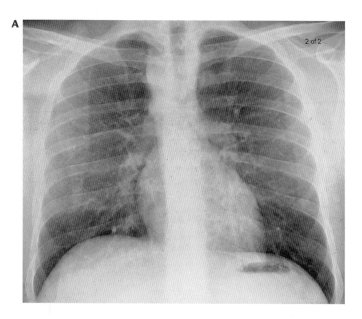

The aberrant right subclavian artery arises as the last and most posterior vessel off the right sided aortic arch, crosses the mediastinum behind the trachea and esophagus, and continues into the neck and axilla along the left side of the trachea. Frequently, a diverticulum is seen at the origin of the aberrant left subclavian artery from the aorta.

Double aortic arch

Most patients with double aortic arch present early in life with tracheal obstruction and swallowing difficulties. Occasionally, the condition remains undetected until later in childhood or adult life. The two aortic arches pass to either side of the trachea and join posteriorly, at which point they often displace the trachea and esophagus forward, thus potentially causing confusion with a middle mediastinal mass. The descending aorta is usually in the midline. On chest radiographs, the features of double aortic arch are similar to those of a right arch with aberrant subclavian artery.

The diagnostic features of double aortic arch on cross-sectional imaging studies (Fig. 14.170)[817] are:

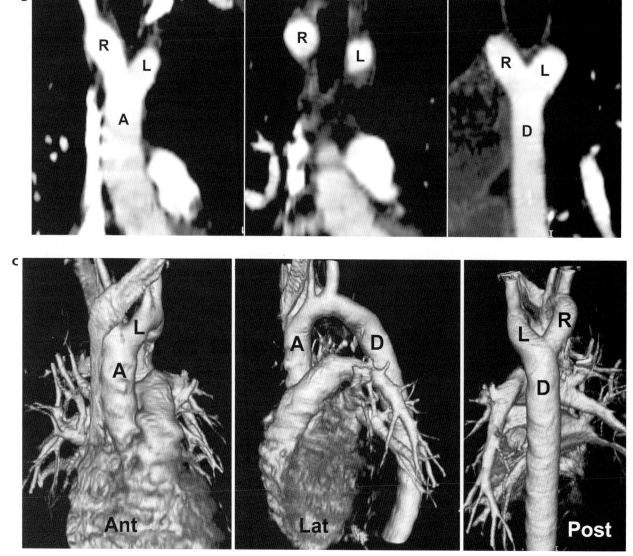

Fig. 14.170 Double aortic arch. **A**, Frontal chest radiograph shows a high right sided aortic arch. **B**, Coronal reformat images from a contrast-enhanced CT shows, from anterior to posterior, the ascending aorta (A), larger right and smaller left aortic arches (R, L), and the midline descending thoracic aorta (D). **C**, These relationships are shown to better advantage by 3D shaded surface display reconstructions.

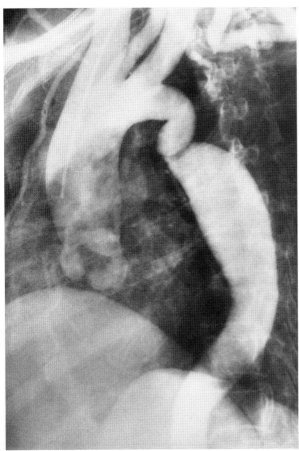

Fig. 14.171 Pseudocoarctation of the aorta. Typical features of pseudocoarctation are shown in this lateral view from an aortogram. Note the high aortic arch, proximal kinking of the aorta, and absence of collateral vessels.

- The right arch is almost always larger and higher than the left arch. This observation is particularly important at barium swallow, where the arches indent the esophagus from either side. Furthermore, the tracheal indentation from the right arch is almost always more pronounced than that of the left arch.
- The branching pattern of the vessels to the head and neck is distinctive. Each arch gives rise to two vessels – a carotid and a subclavian artery – each artery of the pair lying one in front of the other.
- The arches fuse posterior to the esophagus and trachea and may create a masslike density in the middle mediastinum.

Pseudocoarctation of the aorta

Pseudocoarctation of the aorta is a congenital anomaly that many authorities believe to be in the spectrum of true coarctation, but without a gradient producing narrowing of the aorta. The aorta is kinked at the level of the ligamentum arteriosum, the same position as the usual site of coarctation (Fig. 14.171). The ascending aorta is typically more vertical in orientation, the arch higher, and the curve of the arch tighter than normal. This results in a very high aortic arch that may simulate a mass on chest radiographs (Fig. 14.172). Pseudocoarctation, like true coarctation, is associated with an increased tendency to aneurysm formation and aortic dissection. Thus, the aorta above or below the kink may be significantly enlarged, leading to the possibility of even greater confusion with a mass lesion (Fig. 14.173).[818,819] CT or MRI can be diagnostic[697,820,820–822] Absence of significant collateral vessels suggests pseudocoarctation as opposed to true coarctation. However, pressure gradient measurements across the area of kinking or narrowing must be obtained to exclude a hemodynamically significant coarctation.

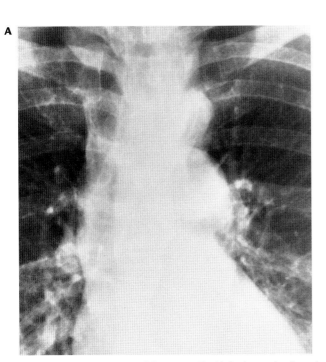

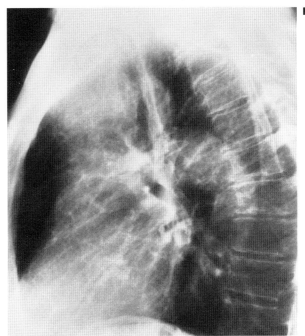

Fig. 14.172 Pseudocoarctation of the aorta. The kinked aorta is aligned such that the portion distal to the kink simulates either an enlarged pulmonary artery or a mediastinal mass on **A**, frontal and **B**, lateral chest radiographs.

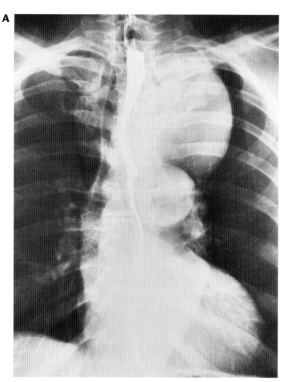 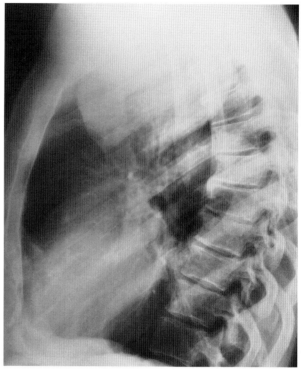

Fig.14.173 Aortic aneurysm proximal to a pseudocoarctation. **A,** Frontal and **B,** lateral chest radiographs with barium in the esophagus show a large well-marginated left mediastinal mass. Aortography (not shown) showed an aneurysm proximal to the pseudocoarctation.

REFERENCES

1. Williams HJ, Alton HM. Imaging of paediatric mediastinal abnormalities. Paediatr Respir Rev 2003;4:55–66.
2. Chieng DC, Jhala D, Jhala N, et al. Endoscopic ultrasound-guided fine-needle aspiration biopsy: a study of 103 cases. Cancer 2002;96:232–239.
3. McAdams HP, Erasmus JJ, Tarver RD, et al. The Mediastinum. In: Haaga JR, Lanzieri CF, Gilkeson RC, eds. CT and MR imaging of the whole body, 4th edn. St Louis: Mosby, 2003: 937–996.
4. Brink JA, Heiken JP, Forman HP, et al. Hepatic spiral CT: reduction of dose of intravenous contrast material. Radiology 1995;197:83–88.
5. Rankin SC. Spiral CT: vascular applications. Eur J Radiol 1998;28:18–29.
6. Boiselle PM, Dippolito G, Copeland J, et al. Multiplanar and 3D imaging of the central airways: comparison of image quality and radiation dose of single-detector row CT and multi-detector row CT at differing tube currents in dogs. Radiology 2003;228:107–111.
7. Brady F, Luthra SK, Brown GD, et al. Radiolabelled tracers and anticancer drugs for assessment of therapeutic efficacy using PET. Curr Pharm Des 2001;7:1863–1892.

8. Jerusalem G, Hustinx R, Beguin Y, et al. PET scan imaging in oncology. Eur J Cancer 2003;39:1525–1534.
9. Patz EF Jr, Lowe VJ, Hoffman JM, et al. Focal pulmonary abnormalities: evaluation with F-18 fluorodeoxyglucose PET scanning. Radiology 1993;188: 487–490.
10. Verboom P, Van Tinteren H, Hoekstra OS, et al. Cost-effectiveness of FDG-PET in staging non-small cell lung cancer: the PLUS study. Eur J Nucl Med Mol Imaging 2003;30:1444–1449.
11. Friedberg JW, Chengazi V. PET scans in the staging of lymphoma: current status. Oncologist 2003;8:438–447.
12. Liu RS, Yeh SH, Huang MH, et al. Use of fluorine-18 fluorodeoxyglucose positron emission tomography in the detection of thymoma: a preliminary report. Eur J Nucl Med 1995;22:1402–1407.
13. von Schulthess GK. Cost considerations regarding an integrated CT-PET system. Eur Radiol 2000;10 Suppl 3:S377–380.
14. Wychulis AR, Payne WS, Clagett OT, et al. Surgical treatment of mediastinal tumors: a 40 year experience. J Thorac Cardiovasc Surg 1971;62:379–392.
15. Azarow KS, Pearl RH, Zurcher R, et al. Primary mediastinal masses. A

comparison of adult and pediatric populations. J Thorac Cardiovasc Surg 1993;106:67–72.
16. Temes R, Allen N, Chavez T, et al. Primary mediastinal malignancies in children: report of 22 patients and comparison to 197 adults. Oncologist 2000;5:179–184.
17. Takeda S, Miyoshi S, Akashi A, et al. Clinical spectrum of primary mediastinal tumors: a comparison of adult and pediatric populations at a single Japanese institution. J Surg Oncol 2003;83:24–30.
18. Benjamin SP, McCormack LJ, Effler DB, et al. Primary tumors of the mediastinum. Chest 1972;62: 297–303.
19. Cohen AJ, Thompson L, Edwards FH, et al. Primary cysts and tumors of the mediastinum. Ann Thorac Surg 1991;51:378–384; discussion 385–386.
20. Whooley BP, Urschel JD, Antkowiak JG, et al. Primary tumors of the mediastinum. J Surg Oncol 1999; 70:95–99.
21. Heitzman ER. The mediastinum: radiologic correlations with anatomy and pathology. Berlin: Springer-Verlag, 1988.

22. Rendina EA, Venuta F, Ceroni L, et al. Computed tomographic staging of anterior mediastinal neoplasms. Thorax 1988;43:441–445.

23. Ahn JM, Lee KS, Goo JM, et al. Predicting the histology of anterior mediastinal masses: comparison of chest radiography and CT. J Thorac Imaging 1996;11:265–271.

24. Woodring JH, Johnson PJ. Computed tomography distinction of central thoracic masses. J Thorac Imaging 1991;6:32–39.

25. Merten DF. Diagnostic imaging of mediastinal masses in children. AJR Am J Roentgenol 1992;158:825–832.

26. Glazer HS, Molina PL, Siegel MJ, et al. High-attenuation mediastinal masses on unenhanced CT. AJR Am J Roentgenol 1991;156:45–50.

27. Glazer HS, Siegel MJ, Sagel SS. Low-attenuation mediastinal masses on CT. AJR Am J Roentgenol 1989;152: 1173–1177.

28. Glazer HS, Wick MR, Anderson DJ, et al. CT of fatty thoracic masses. AJR Am J Roentgenol 1992;159:1181–1187.

29. Spizarny DL, Rebner M, Gross BH. CT evaluation of enhancing mediastinal masses. J Comput Assist Tomogr 1987;11:990–993.

30. Barakos JA, Brown JJ, Brescia RJ, et al. High signal intensity lesions of the chest in MR imaging. J Comput Assist Tomogr 1989;13:797–802.

31. Suster S, Rosai J. Multilocular thymic cyst: an acquired reactive process. Study of 18 cases. Am J Surg Pathol 1991;15: 388–398.

32. Tecce PM, Fishman EK, Kuhlman JE. CT evaluation of the anterior mediastinum: spectrum of disease. RadioGraphics 1994;14:973–990.

33. Wachsberg RH, Yaghmai V, Javors BR, et al. Cardiophrenic varices in portal hypertension: evaluation with CT. Radiology 1995;195:553–556.

34. Takeda S, Miyoshi S, Minami M, et al. Clinical spectrum of mediastinal cysts. Chest 2003;124:125–132.

35. Sasaka K, Kurihara Y, Nakajima Y, et al. Spontaneous rupture: a complication of benign mature teratomas of the mediastinum. AJR Am J Roentgenol 1998;170:323–328.

36. Reed JC, Sobonya RE. Morphologic analysis of foregut cysts in the thorax. Am J Roentgenol Radium Ther Nucl Med 1974;120:851–860.

37. Snyder ME, Luck SR, Hernandez R, et al. Diagnostic dilemmas of mediastinal cysts. J Pediatr Surg 1985;20:810–815.

38. Sirivella S, Ford WB, Zikria EA, et al. Foregut cysts of the mediastinum. Results in 20 consecutive surgically treated cases. J Thorac Cardiovasc Surg 1985;90:776–782.

39. Salo JA, Ala-Kulju KV. Congenital esophageal cysts in adults. Ann Thorac Surg 1987;44:135–138.

40. Jang KM, Lee KS, Lee SJ, et al. The spectrum of benign esophageal lesions: imaging findings. Korean J Radiol 2002;3:199–210.

41. Jeung MY, Gasser B, Gangi A, et al. Imaging of cystic masses of the mediastinum. RadioGraphics 2002; 22 Spec No:S79–93.

42. Kuhlman JE, Fishman EK, Wang KP, et al. Esophageal duplication cyst: CT and transesophageal needle aspiration. AJR Am J Roentgenol 1985;145:531–532.

43. Weiss LM, Fagelman D, Warhit JM. CT demonstration of an esophageal duplication cyst. J Comput Assist Tomogr 1983;7:716–718.

44. Whitaker JA, Deffenbaugh LD, Cooke AR. Esophageal duplication cyst. Case report. Am J Gastroenterol 1980;73:329–332.

45. LeBlanc J, Guttentag AR, Shepard JA, et al. Imaging of mediastinal foregut cysts. Can Assoc Radiol J 1994;45:381–386.

46. Pader E, Kirschner PA. Pericardial diverticulum. Dis Chest 1969;55:344–346.

47. Kittredge RD, Finby N. Pericardial cysts and diverticula. Am J Roentgenol Radium Ther Nucl Med 1967;99:668–673.

48. Feigin DS, Fenoglio JJ, McAllister HA, et al. Pericardial cysts. A radiologic-pathologic correlation and review. Radiology 1977;125:15–20.

49. Wychulis AR, Connolly DC, McGoon DC. Pericardial cysts, tumors, and fat necrosis. J Thorac Cardiovasc Surg 1971;62:294–300.

50. Brunner DR, Whitley NO. A pericardial cyst with high CT numbers. AJR Am J Roentgenol 1984;142:279–280.

51. Demos TC, Budorick NE, Posniak HV. Benign mediastinal cysts: pointed appearance on CT. J Comput Assist Tomogr 1989;13:132–133.

52. Pugatch RD, Braver JH, Robbins AH, et al. CT diagnosis of pericardial cysts. AJR Am J Roentgenol 1978;131:515–516.

53. Klatte EC, Yune HY. Diagnosis and treatment of pericardial cysts. Radiology 1972;104:541–544.

54. Singhal BS, Parekh HN, Ursekar M, et al. Intramedullary neurenteric cyst in mid thoracic spine in an adult: a case report. Neurol India 2001;49:302–304.

55. Boyd DP, Midell AI. Mediastinal cysts and tumors. An analysis of 96 cases. Surg Clin North Am 1968;48:493–505.

56. Madewell JE, Sobonya RE, Reed JC. Clinical conference: RPC from the AFIP. Radiology 1973;109:707–712.

57. Wilson ES Jr. Neurenteric cyst of the mediastinum. Am J Roentgenol Radium Ther Nucl Med 1969;107:641–646.

58. Wittich GR, Karnel F, Schurawitzki H et al. Percutaneous drainage of mediastinal pseudocysts. Radiology 1988;167:51–53.

59. Zeilender S, Turner MA, Glauser FL. Mediastinal pseudocyst associated with chronic pleural effusions. Chest 1990;97:1014–1016.

60. Kirchner SG, Heller RM, Smith CW. Pancreatic pseudocyst of the mediastinum. Radiology 1977;123:37–42.

61. Herrmann F, Reichenberger F, Leupold U, et al. Recurrent pleural effusion and a mediastinal mass. Respiration 2000;67:471–472.

62. Owens GR, Arger PH, Mulhern CB Jr, et al. CT evaluation of mediastinal pseudocyst. J Comput Assist Tomogr 1980;4:256–259.

63. Ito H, Matsubara N, Sakai T, et al. Two cases of thoracopancreatic fistula in alcoholic pancreatitis: clinical and CT findings. Radiat Med 2002;20:207–211.

64. Geier A, Lammert F, Gartung C, et al. Magnetic resonance imaging and magnetic resonance cholangiopancreaticography for diagnosis and pre-interventional evaluation of a fluid thoracic mass. Eur J Gastroenterol Hepatol 2003;15:429–431.

65. Tan MH, Kirk G, Archibold P, et al. Cardiac compromise due to a pancreatic mediastinal pseudocyst. Eur J Gastroenterol Hepatol 2002;14: 1279–1282.

66. Tanaka A, Takeda R, Utsunomiya H, et al. Severe complications of mediastinal pancreatic pseudocyst: report of esophagobronchial fistula and hemothorax. J Hepatobiliary Pancreat Surg 2000;7:86–91.

67. Strollo DC, Rosado-de-Christenson ML, Jett JR. Primary mediastinal tumors: part II. Tumors of the middle and posterior mediastinum. Chest 1997;112: 1344–1357.

68. Miles J, Pennybacker J, Sheldon P. Intrathoracic meningocele. Its development and association with neurofibromatosis. J Neurol Neurosurg Psychiatry 1969;32:99–110.

69. Chen SS, Shao KN, Feng RJ, et al. Multiple bilateral thoracic meningoceles without neurofibromatosis: a case report. Zhonghua Yi Xue Za Zhi (Taipei) 1998;61:736–740.

70. Edeiken J, Lee KF, Libshitz H. Intrathoracic meningocele. Am J Roentgenol Radium Ther Nucl Med 1969;106:381–384.

71. Nakasu Y, Minouchi K, Hatsuda N, et al. Thoracic meningocele in neurofibromatosis: CT and MR findings. J Comput Assist Tomogr 1991;15:1062–1064.

72. Weinreb JC, Arger PH, Grossman R, et al. CT metrizamide myelography in multiple bilateral intrathoracic meningoceles. J Comput Assist Tomogr 1984;8:324–326.

73. Wax MK, Treloar ME. Thoracic duct cyst: an unusual supraclavicular mass. Head Neck 1992;14:502–505.

74. Karajiannis A, Krueger T, Stauffer E, et al. Large thoracic duct cyst – a case report and review of the literature. Eur J Cardiothorac Surg 2000;17:754–756.

75. Mattila PS, Tarkkanen J, Mattila S. Thoracic duct cyst: a case report and review of 29 cases. Ann Otol Rhinol Laryngol 1999;108:505–508.

76. Pramesh CS, Deshpande MS, Pantvaidya GH, Sharma S, Deshpande RK. Thoracic duct cyst of the mediastinum. Ann Thorac Cardiovasc Surg 2003;9:264–265.

77. Kaplan J, Davidson T. Intrathoracic desmoids: report of two cases. Thorax 1986;41:894–895.

78. Black WC, Armstrong P, Daniel TM, et al. Computed tomography of aggressive fibromatosis in the posterior mediastinum. J Comput Assist Tomogr 1987;11:153–155.

79. Casillas J, Sais GJ, Greve JL, et al. Imaging of intra- and extraabdominal desmoid tumors. RadioGraphics 1991;11:959–968.

80. Ko SF, Ng SH, Hsiao CC, et al. Juvenile fibromatosis of the posterior mediastinum with intraspinal extension. AJNR Am J Neuroradiol 1996;17:522–524.

81. Peled N, Babyn PS, Manson D, et al. Aggressive fibromatosis simulating congenital lung malformation. Can Assoc Radiol J 1993;44:221–223.

82. Tam CG, Broome DR, Shannon RL. Desmoid tumor of the anterior mediastinum: CT and radiologic features. J Comput Assist Tomogr 1994;18:499–501.

83. Dosios TJ, Angouras DC, Floros DG. Primary desmoid tumor of the posterior mediastinum. Ann Thorac Surg 1998;66:2098–2099.

84. Shankwiler RA, Athey PA, Lamki N. Aggressive infantile fibromatosis. Pulmonary metastases documented by plain film and computed tomography. Clin Imaging 1989;13:127–129.

85. Cyrlak D, Milne EN, Imray TJ. Pneumomediastinum: a diagnostic problem. Crit Rev Diagn Imaging 1984;23:75–117.

86. Quinn SF, Erickson SJ, Dee PM, et al. MR imaging in fibromatosis: results in 26 patients with pathologic correlation. AJR Am J Roentgenol 1991;156:539–542.

87. Sundaram M, McGuire MH, Schajowicz F. Soft-tissue masses: histologic basis for decreased signal (short T2) on T2-weighted MR images. AJR Am J Roentgenol 1987;148:1247–1250.

88. Cardoso PF, da Silva LC, Bonamigo TP, et al. Intrathoracic desmoid tumor with invasion of the great vessels. Eur J Cardiothorac Surg 2002;22:1017–1019.

89. Kocak Z, Adli M, Erdir O, et al. Intrathoracic desmoid tumor of the posterior mediastinum with transdiaphragmatic extension. Report of a case. Tumori 2000;86:489–491.

90. Hudson TM, Vandergriend RA, Springfield DS, et al. Aggressive fibromatosis: evaluation by computed tomography and angiography. Radiology 1984;150:495–501.

91. Maziak DE, Todd TR, Pearson FG. Massive hiatus hernia: evaluation and surgical management. J Thorac Cardiovasc Surg 1998;115:53–60; discussion 61–62.

92. Hartley WS, Schabel SI, Scruggs MC, et al. Communicating intrathoracic hydrocele. Clin Imaging 1991;15:280–282.

93. Godwin JD, MacGregor JM. Extension of ascites into the chest with hiatal hernia: visualization on CT. AJR Am J Roentgenol 1987;148:31–32.

94. Rabushka LS, Fishman EK, Kuhlman JE. CT evaluation of achalasia. J Comput Assist Tomogr 1991;15:434–439.

95. Donner MW, Saba GP, Martinez CR. Diffuse diseases of the esophagus: a practical approach. Semin Roentgenol 1981;16:198–213.

96. Gonlachanvit S, Fisher RS, Parkman HP. Diagnostic modalities for achalasia. Gastrointest Endosc Clin N Am 2001;11:293–310.

97. Raider L, Landry BA, Brogdon BG. The retrotracheal triangle. RadioGraphics 1990;10:1055–1079.

98. Putman CE, Curtis AM, Westfried M, et al. Thickening of the posterior tracheal stripe: a sign of squamous cell carcinoma of the esophagus. Radiology 1976;121:533–536.

99. Cohen AM, Cunat JS. Giant esophageal leiomyoma as a mediastinal mass. J Can Assoc Radiol 1981;32:129–130.

100. Miettinen M, Sarlomo-Rikala M, Sobin LH, et al. Esophageal stromal tumors: a clinicopathologic, immunohistochemical, and molecular genetic study of 17 cases and comparison with esophageal leiomyomas and leiomyosarcomas. Am J Surg Pathol 2000;24:211–222.

101. Greenson JK. Gastrointestinal stromal tumors and other mesenchymal lesions of the gut. Mod Pathol 2003;16:366–375.

102. Miettinen M, Lasota J. Gastrointestinal stromal tumors (GISTs): definition, occurrence, pathology, differential diagnosis and molecular genetics. Pol J Pathol 2003;54:3–24.

103. Miettinen M, Lasota J. Gastrointestinal stromal tumors – definition, clinical, histological, immunohistochemical, and molecular genetic features and differential diagnosis. Virchows Arch 2001;438:1–12.

104. Ghanem N, Altehoefer C, Furtwangler A, et al. Computed tomography in gastrointestinal stromal tumors. Eur Radiol 2003;13:1669–1678.

105. Gaerte SC, Meyer CA, Winer-Muram HT, et al. Fat-containing lesions of the chest. RadioGraphics 2002;22 Spec No:S61–78.

106. Heitzman ER. Radiological diagnosis of mediastinal lymph node enlargement. J Can Assoc Radiol 1987;39:151–157.

107. Homer MJ, Wechsler RJ, Carter BL. Mediastinal lipomatosis. CT confirmation of a normal variant. Radiology 1978;128:657–661.

108. Koerner HJ, Sun DI. Mediastinal lipomatosis secondary to steroid therapy. Am J Roentgenol Radium Ther Nucl Med 1966;98:461–464.

109. Price JE Jr, Rigler LG. Widening of the mediastinum resulting from fat accumulation. Radiology 1970;96:97–500.

110. Teates CD. Steroid-induced mediastinal lipomatosis. Radiology 1970;96:501–502.

111. Glickstein MF, Miller WT, Dalinka MK, et al. Paraspinal lipomatosis: a benign mass. Radiology 1987;163:79–80.

112. Lee WJ, Fattal G. Mediastinal lipomatosis in simple obesity. Chest 1976;70:308–309.

113. Bein ME, Mancuso AA, Mink JH, et al. Computed tomography in the evaluation of mediastinal lipomatosis. J Comput Assist Tomogr 1978;2:379–383.

114. Streiter ML, Schneider HJ, Proto AV. Steroid-induced thoracic lipomatosis: paraspinal involvement. AJR Am J Roentgenol 1982;139:679–681.

115. Smith PD, Stadelmann WK, Wassermann RJ, et al. Benign symmetric lipomatosis (Madelung's disease). Ann Plast Surg 1998;41:671–673.

116. Ahuja AT, King AD, Chan ES. Ultrasound, CT and MRI in patients with multiple symmetric lipomatosis. Clin Radiol 2000;55:79.

117. Enzi G, Biondetti PR, Fiore D, et al. Computed tomography of deep fat masses in multiple symmetrical lipomatosis. Radiology 1982;144:121–124.

118. Borges A, Torrinha F, Lufkin RB, et al. Laryngeal involvement in multiple symmetric lipomatosis: the role of computed tomography in diagnosis. Am J Otolaryngol 1997;18:127–130.

119. Schweitzer DL, Aguam AS. Primary liposarcoma of the mediastinum. Report of a case and review of the literature. J Thorac Cardiovasc Surg 1977;74:83–97.

120. Quinn SF, Monson M, Paling M. Spinal lipoma presenting as a mediastinal mass: diagnosis by CT. J Comput Assist Tomogr 1983;7:1087–1089.

121. Shub C, Parkin TW, Lie JT. An unusual mediastinal lipoma simulating cardiomegaly. Mayo Clin Proc 1979;54:60–62.

122. Mendez G Jr, Isikoff MB, Isikoff SK, et al. Fatty tumors of the thorax demonstrated by CT. AJR Am J Roentgenol 1979;133:207–212.

123. Federici S, Cuoghi D, Sciutti R. Benign mediastinal lipoblastoma in a 14-months-old infant. Pediatr Radiol 1992;22:150–151.

124. Black WC, Burke JW, Feldman PS, et al, Swanson S. CT appearance of cervical lipoblastoma. J Comput Assist Tomogr 1986;10:696–698.

125. Whyte AM, Powell N. Mediastinal lipoblastoma of infancy. Clin Radiol 1990;42:205–206.

126. Seidel FG, Magill HL, Burton EM, et al. Cases of the day. Pediatric. Lipoblastoma. RadioGraphics 1990;10:728–731.

127. Udwadia ZF, Kumar N, Bhaduri AS. Mediastinal hibernoma. Eur J Cardiothorac Surg 1999;15:533–535.

128. Santambrogio L, Cioffi U, De Simone M, et al. Cervicomediastinal hibernoma. Ann Thorac Surg 1997;64:1160–1162.

129. Kline ME, Patel BU, Agosti SJ. Noninfiltrating angiolipoma of the mediastinum. Radiology 1990;175: 737–738.

130. Kim K, Koo BC, Davis JT, et al. Primary myelolipoma of mediastinum. J Comput Tomogr 1984;8:119–123.

131. Eisenstat R, Bruce D, Williams LE, et al. Primary liposarcoma of the mediastinum with coexistent mediastinal lipomatosis. AJR Am J Roentgenol 2000;174:572–573.

132. Paci M, De Franco S, Cavazza A, et al. Well-differentiated giant "lipoma-like" liposarcoma of the posterior mediastinum: a case report. Chir Ital 2003;55:101–104.

133. Jung JI, Kim H, Kang SW, et al. Radiological findings in myxoid liposarcoma of the anterior mediastinum. Br J Radiol 1998;71:975–976.

134. Yeager BA, Guglielmi GE, Schiebler ML, et al. Magnetic resonance imaging of Morgagni hernia. Gastrointest Radiol 1987;12:296–298.

135. Wyatt SH, Fishman EK. Diffuse pulmonary extramedullary hematopoiesis in a patient with myelofibrosis: CT findings. J Comput Assist Tomogr 1994;18:815–817.

136. Long JA Jr, Doppman JL, Nienhuis AW. Computed tomographic studies of thoracic extramedullary hematopoiesis. J Comput Assist Tomogr 1980;4:67–70.

137. Papavasiliou C, Gouliamos A, Andreou J. The marrow heterotopia in thalassemia. Eur J Radiol 1986;6:92–96.

138. Leong CS, Stark P. Thoracic manifestations of sickle cell disease. J Thorac Imaging 1998;13:128–134.

139. Ross P, Logan W. Roentgen findings in extramedullary hematopoiesis. Am J Roentgenol Radium Ther Nucl Med 1969;106:604–613.

140. Gumbs RV, Higginbotham-Ford EA, Teal JS, et al. Thoracic extramedullary hematopoiesis in sickle-cell disease. AJR Am J Roentgenol 1987;149:889–893.

141. Martin J, Palacio A, Petit J, et al. Fatty transformation of thoracic extramedullary hematopoiesis following splenectomy: CT features. J Comput Assist Tomogr 1990;14:477–478.

142. Savader SJ, Otero RR, Savader BL. MR imaging of intrathoracic extramedullary hematopoiesis. J Comput Assist Tomogr 1988;12:878–880.

143. Yamato M, Fuhrman CR. Computed tomography of fatty replacement in extramedullary hematopoiesis. J Comput Assist Tomogr 1987;11:541–542.

144. Hines GL. Paravertebral extramedullary hematopoiesis (as a posterior mediastinal tumor) associated with congenital dyserythropoietic anemia. J Thorac Cardiovasc Surg 1993;106: 760–761.

145. Stebner FC, Bishop CR. Bone marrow scan and radioiron uptake of an intrathoracic mass. Clin Nucl Med 1982;7:86–87.

146. Adams BK, Jacobs P, Byrne MJ, et al. Fe-52 imaging of intrathoracic extramedullary hematopoiesis in a patient with beta-thalassemia. Clin Nucl Med 1995;20:619–622.

147. Harnsberger HR, Datz FL, Knochel JQ, Taylor AT. Failure to detect extramedullary hematopoiesis during bone-marrow imaging with indium-111 or technetium-99m sulfur colloid. J Nucl Med 1982;23:589–591.

148. Rosado-de-Christenson ML, Templeton PA, Moran CA. From the archives of the AFIP. Mediastinal germ cell tumors: radiologic and pathologic correlation. RadioGraphics 1992;12:1013–1030.

149. Dulmet EM, Macchiarini P, Suc B, Verley JM. Germ cell tumors of the mediastinum. A 30-year experience. Cancer 1993;72:1894–1901.

150. Strollo DC, Rosado de Christenson ML, Jett JR. Primary mediastinal tumors. Part 1: tumors of the anterior mediastinum. Chest 1997;112:511–522.

151. Drevelegas A, Palladas P, Scordalaki A. Mediastinal germ cell tumors: a radiologic-pathologic review. Eur Radiol 2001;11:1925–1932.

152. Sham JS, Chan FL, Lau WH, Choi PH, Choy D. Primary mediastinal endodermal sinus tumors: CT evaluation. Clin Imaging 1989;13:299–304.

153. Strollo DC, Rosado-de-Christenson ML. Primary mediastinal malignant germ cell neoplasms: imaging features. Chest Surg Clin N Am 2002;12:645–658.

154. Nichols CR. Mediastinal germ cell tumors. Clinical features and biologic correlates. Chest 1991;99:472–479.

155. Levine GD, Rosai J. Thymic hyperplasia and neoplasia: a review of current concepts. Hum Pathol 1978;9:495–515.

156. Allen MS. Presentation and management of benign mediastinal teratomas. Chest Surg Clin N Am 2002;12:659–664.

157. Lewis BD, Hurt RD, Payne WS, Farrow GM, Knapp RH, Muhm JR. Benign teratomas of the mediastinum. J Thorac Cardiovasc Surg 1983;86:727–731.

158. Lyons HA, Calvy GL, Sammons BP. The diagnosis and classification of mediastinal masses. A study of 782 cases. Ann Intern Med 1959;51:897–932.

159. Moeller KH, Rosado-de-Christenson ML, Templeton PA. Mediastinal mature teratoma: imaging features. AJR Am J Roentgenol 1997;169:985–990.

160. Dobranowski J, Martin LF, Bennett WF. CT evaluation of posterior mediastinal teratoma. J Comput Assist Tomogr 1987;11:156–157.

161. Sidani AH, Oberson R, Deleze G, Barras MH, Genton N, Laurini R. Infected teratoma of lower posterior mediastinum in a six-year-old boy. Pediatr Radiol 1991;21:438–439.

162. Kurosaki Y, Tanaka YO, Itai Y. Mature teratoma of the posterior mediastinum. Eur Radiol 1998;8:100–102.

163. Ochsner JL, Ochsner SF. Congenital cysts of the mediastinum: 20-year experience with 42 cases. Ann Surg 1966;163: 909–920.

164. Yeoman LJ, Dalton HR, Adam EJ. Fat–fluid level in pleural effusion as a complication of a mediastinal dermoid: CT characteristics. J Comput Assist Tomogr 1990;14:307–309.

165. Brown LR, Muhm JR, Aughenbaugh GL, Lewis BD, Hurt RD. Computed tomography of benign mature teratomas of the mediastinum. J Thorac Imaging 1987;2:66–71.

166. Suzuki M, Takashima T, Itoh H, Choutoh S, Kawamura I, Watanabe Y. Computed tomography of mediastinal teratomas. J Comput Assist Tomogr 1983;7:74–76.

167. Fulcher AS, Proto AV, Jolles H. Cystic teratoma of the mediastinum: demonstration of fat/fluid level. AJR Am J Roentgenol 1990;154:259–260.

168. Seltzer SE, Herman PG, Sagel SS. Differential diagnosis of mediastinal fluid levels visualized on computed tomography. J Comput Assist Tomogr 1984;8:244–246.

169. Choi SJ, Lee JS, Song KS, Lim TH. Mediastinal teratoma: CT differentiation of ruptured and unruptured tumors. AJR Am J Roentgenol 1998;171:591–594.

170. Ikezoe J, Takeuchi N, Johkoh T, et al. MRI of anterior mediastinal tumors. Radiat Med 1992;10:176–183.

171. Ikezoe J, Morimoto S, Arisawa J, et al. Ultrasonography of mediastinal teratoma. J Clin Ultrasound 1986; 14:513–520.

172. Wu TT, Wang HC, Chang YC, Lee YC, Chang YL, Yang PC. Mature mediastinal teratoma: sonographic imaging patterns and pathologic correlation. J Ultrasound Med 2002;21:759–765.

173. Shih JY, Wang HC, Chang YL, Chang YC, Lee YC, Yang PC. Echogenic floating spherules as a sonographic sign of cystic teratoma of mediastinum: correlation with CT and pathologic findings. J Ultrasound Med 1996;15:603–605.

174. Moran CA, Suster S, Koss MN. Primary germ cell tumors of the mediastinum: III. Yolk sac tumor, embryonal carcinoma, choriocarcinoma, and combined nonteratomatous germ cell tumors of the mediastinum – a clinicopathologic and immunohistochemical study of 64 cases. Cancer 1997;80:699–707.

175. Moran CA, Suster S, Przygodzki RM, Koss MN. Primary germ cell tumors of the mediastinum: II. Mediastinal seminomas – a clinicopathologic and immunohistochemical study of 120 cases. Cancer 1997;80:691–698.

176. Polansky SM, Barwick KW, Ravin CE. Primary mediastinal seminoma. AJR Am J Roentgenol 1979;132:17–21.

177. Holbert BL, Libshitz HI. Superior vena caval syndrome in primary mediastinal germ cell tumors. Can Assoc Radiol J 1986;37:182–183.

178. deMent SH. Association between mediastinal germ cell tumors and hematologic malignancies: an update. Hum Pathol 1990;21:699–703.

179. Nichols CR, Roth BJ, Heerema N, et al. Hematologic neoplasia associated with primary mediastinal germ-cell tumors. N Engl J Med 1990;322:1425–1429.

180. Cohen D, Weintrob N. Case 9-2003: mediastinal germ-cell tumor. N Engl J Med 2003;348:2469–2470; author reply 2469–2470.

181. Hainsworth JD, Greco FA. Germ cell neoplasms and other malignancies of the mediastinum. Cancer Treat Res 2001;105:303–325.

182. Blomlie V, Lien HH, Fossa SD, et al. Computed tomography in primary non-seminomatous germ cell tumors of the mediastinum. Acta Radiol 1988;29:289–292.

183. Lee KS, Im JG, Han CH, et al. Malignant primary germ cell tumors of the mediastinum: CT features. AJR Am J Roentgenol 1989;153:947–951.

184. Levitt RG, Husband JE, Glazer HS. CT of primary germ-cell tumors of the mediastinum. AJR Am J Roentgenol 1984;142:73–78.

185. el-Khatib M, Chew FS. Embryonal carcinoma of the anterior mediastinum. AJR Am J Roentgenol 1998;170:722.

186. Mori K, Eguchi K, Moriyama H, et al. Computed tomography of anterior mediastinal tumors. Differentiation between thymoma and germ cell tumor. Acta Radiol 1987;28:395–398.

187. Cox JD. Primary malignant germinal tumors of the mediastinum. A study of 24 cases. Cancer 1975;36:1162–1168.

188. Panicek DM, Toner GC, Heelan RT, et al. Nonseminomatous germ cell tumors: enlarging masses despite chemotherapy. Radiology 1990;175:499–502.

189. Afifi HY, Bosl GJ, Burt ME. Mediastinal growing teratoma syndrome. Ann Thorac Surg 1997;64:359–362.

190. Iyoda A, Hiroshima K, Yusa T, et al. The primary mediastinal growing teratoma syndrome. Anticancer Res 2000;20: 3723–3726.

191. Andre F, Fizazi K, Culine S, et al. The growing teratoma syndrome: results of therapy and long-term follow-up of 33 patients. Eur J Cancer 2000;36:1389–1394.

192. Nimkin K, Gupta P, McCauley R, et al. The growing teratoma syndrome. Pediatr Radiol 2004;34:259–262.

193. Coscojuela P, Llauger J, Perez C, et al. The growing teratoma syndrome: radiologic findings in four cases. Eur J Radiol 1991;12:138–140.

194. Daly BD, Leung SF, Cheung H, et al. Thoracic metastases from carcinoma of the nasopharynx: high frequency of hilar and mediastinal lymphadenopathy. AJR Am J Roentgenol 1993;160:241–244.

195. McLoud TC, Kalisher L, Stark P, et al. Intrathoracic lymph node metastases from extrathoracic neoplasms. AJR Am J Roentgenol 1978;131:403–407.

196. Earls JP, Cerva D Jr, Berman E, et al. Inhalational anthrax after bioterrorism exposure: spectrum of imaging findings in two surviving patients. Radiology 2002;222:305–312.

197. Niimi H, Kang EY, Kwong JS, et al. CT of chronic infiltrative lung disease: prevalence of mediastinal lymphadenopathy. J Comput Assist Tomogr 1996;20:305–308.

198. Slanetz PJ, Truong M, Shepard JA, et al. Mediastinal lymphadenopathy and hazy mediastinal fat: new CT findings of congestive heart failure. AJR Am J Roentgenol 1998;171: 1307–1309.

199. Ngom A, Dumont P, Diot P, et al. Benign mediastinal lymphadenopathy in congestive heart failure. Chest 2001;119:653–656.

200. Erly WK, Borders RJ, Outwater EK, et al. Location, size, and distribution of mediastinal lymph node enlargement in chronic congestive heart failure. J Comput Assist Tomogr 2003;27:485–489.

201. Jung JI, Kim HH, Jung YJ, et al. Mediastinal lymphadenopathy in pulmonary fibrosis: correlation with disease severity. J Comput Assist Tomogr 2000;24:706–710.

202. Bergin C, Castellino RA. Mediastinal lymph node enlargement on CT scans in patients with usual interstitial pneumonitis. AJR Am J Roentgenol 1990;154:251–254.

203. Sampson C, Hansell DM. The prevalence of enlarged mediastinal lymph nodes in asbestos-exposed individuals: a CT study. Clin Radiol 1992;45:340–342.

204. McAdams HP, Erasmus J, Winter JA. Radiologic manifestations of pulmonary tuberculosis. Radiol Clin North Am 1995;33:655–678.

205. McAdams HP, Rosado-de-Christenson ML, Lesar M, et al. Thoracic mycoses from endemic fungi: radiologic-pathologic correlation. RadioGraphics 1995;15:255–270.

206. Archibald N, Dalzell KG, Fernando CC, et al. Infectious mononucleosis complicated by mediastinal lymphadenopathy causing transient pulmonary artery stenosis. Intern Med J 2003;33:324–325.

207. Mayor B, Schnyder P, Giron J, et al. Mediastinal and hilar lymphadenopathy due to Pneumocystis jiroveci infection in AIDS patients: CT features. J Comput Assist Tomogr 1994;18:408–411.

208. Jernigan JA, Stephens DS, Ashford DA, et al. Bioterrorism-related inhalational anthrax: the first 10 cases reported in the United States. Emerg Infect Dis 2001;7:933–944.

209. Bryant KA. Tularemia: lymphadenitis with a twist. Pediatr Ann 2002;31: 187–190.

210. Krishna G, Chitkara RK. Pneumonic plague. Semin Respir Infect 2003;18:159–167.

211. Thomas KW, Hunninghake GW. Sarcoidosis. JAMA 2003;289:3300–3303.

212. Baldwin DR, Lambert L, Pantin CF, et al. Silicosis presenting as bilateral hilar lymphadenopathy. Thorax 1996;51: 1165–1167.

213. Kinoshita T, Itoh H. Coal worker's pneumoconiosis mimicking pulmonary sarcoidosis. Clin Nucl Med 1994;19: 544–545.

214. Zinck SE, Schwartz E, Berry GJ, et al. CT of noninfectious granulomatous lung disease. Radiol Clin North Am 2001;39:1189–1209, vi.

215. Rossman MD, Kreider ME. Is chronic beryllium disease sarcoidosis of known etiology? Sarcoidosis Vasc Diffuse Lung Dis 2003;20:104–109.

216. Fireman E, Haimsky E, Noiderfer M, et al. Misdiagnosis of sarcoidosis in patients with chronic beryllium disease. Sarcoidosis Vasc Diffuse Lung Dis 2003;20:144–148.

217. George TM, Cash JM, Farver C, et al. Mediastinal mass and hilar adenopathy: rare thoracic manifestations of Wegener's granulomatosis. Arthritis Rheum 1997;40:1992–1997.

218. Prakash UB. Respiratory complications in mixed connective tissue disease. Clin Chest Med 1998;19:733–746.

219. Wechsler RJ, Steiner RM, Spirn PW, et al. The relationship of thoracic lymphadenopathy to pulmonary interstitial disease in diffuse and limited

systemic sclerosis: CT findings. AJR Am J Roentgenol 1996;167:101–104.

220. Yoshioka K. Mediastinal lymphadenopathy preceding skin and lung fibrosis in systemic sclerosis. Respiration 1994;61:169–171.

221. Kaplan JO, Morillo G, Weinfeld A, et al. Mediastinal adenopathy in myeloma. J Can Assoc Radiol 1980;31:48–49.

222. Pavlidis N, Briasoulis E, Hainsworth J, et al. Diagnostic and therapeutic management of cancer of an unknown primary. Eur J Cancer 2003;39:1990–2005.

223. McAdams HP, Rosado-de-Christenson M, Fishback NF, et al. Castleman disease of the thorax: radiologic features with clinical and histopathologic correlation. Radiology 1998;209:221–228.

224. Gross BH, Schneider HJ, Proto AV. Eggshell calcification of lymph nodes: an update. AJR Am J Roentgenol 1980;135:1265–1268.

225. Urschel JD, Urschel DM. Mediastinal amyloidosis. Ann Thorac Surg 2000;69:944–946.

226. Takeshita K, Yamada S, Sato N, et al. An unusual case of mediastinal lymphadenopathy caused by amyloidosis. Intern Med 2000;39:839–842.

227. Hiller N, Fisher D, Shmesh O, et al. Primary amyloidosis presenting as an isolated mediastinal mass: diagnosis by fine needle biopsy. Thorax 1995;50:908–909.

228. Kubaska SM, Shepard JA, Chew FS, et al. Whipple's disease involving the mediastinum. AJR Am J Roentgenol 1998;171:364.

229. Wolfert AL, Wright JE. Whipple's disease presenting as sarcoidosis and valvular heart disease. South Med J 1999;92:820–825.

230. Samuels T, Hamilton P, Shaw P. Whipple disease of the mediastinum. AJR Am J Roentgenol 1990;154:1187–1188.

231. Sussman SK, Halvorsen RA Jr, Silverman PM, et al. Paracardiac adenopathy: CT evaluation. AJR Am J Roentgenol 1987;149:29–34.

232. Vock P, Hodler J. Cardiophrenic angle adenopathy: update of causes and significance. Radiology 1986;159:395–399.

233. Thomas RD, Blaquiere RM. Reactive mediastinal lymphadenopathy in bronchiectasis assessed by CT. Acta Radiol 1993;34:489–491.

234. Boiselle PM, Patz EF Jr, Vining DJ, et al. Imaging of mediastinal lymph nodes: CT, MR, and FDG PET. RadioGraphics 1998;18:1061–1069.

235. Garber SJ, Wells AU, duBois RM, et al. Enlarged mediastinal lymph nodes in the fibrosing alveolitis of systemic sclerosis. Br J Radiol 1992;65:983–986.

236. Castleman B, Iverson L, Menendez VP. Localized mediastinal lymph node hyperplasia resembling thymoma. Cancer 1956;9:822–830.

237. Palestro G, Turrini F, Pagano M, et al. Castleman's disease. Adv Clin Path 1999;3:11–22.

238. Kim JH, Jun TG, Sung SW, et al. Giant lymph node hyperplasia (Castleman's disease) in the chest. Ann Thorac Surg 1995;59:1162–1165.

239. Keller AR, Hochholzer L, Castleman B. Hyaline-vascular and plasma-cell types of giant lymph node hyperplasia of the mediastinum and other locations. Cancer 1972;29:670–683.

240. Olscamp G, Weisbrod G, Sanders D, et al. Castleman disease: unusual manifestations of an unusual disorder. Radiology 1980;135:43–48.

241. Kirsch CF, Webb EM, Webb WR. Multicentric Castleman's disease and POEMS syndrome: CT findings. J Thorac Imaging 1997;12:75–77.

242. Gossios K, Nikolaides C, Bai M. Widespread Castleman disease: CT findings. Eur Radiol 1995;6:95–98.

243. Chen KT. Multicentric Castleman's disease and Kaposi's sarcoma. Am J Surg Pathol 1984;8:287–293.

244. Frizzera G, Banks PM, Massarelli G, et al. A systemic lymphoproliferative disorder with morphologic features of Castleman's disease. Pathological findings in 15 patients. Am J Surg Pathol 1983;7:211–231.

245. Phelan MS. Castleman's giant lymph node hyperplasia. Br J Radiol 1982;55:158–160.

246. Samuels TH, Hamilton PA, Ngan B. Mediastinal Castleman's disease: demonstration with computed tomography and angiography. Can Assoc Radiol J 1990;41:380–383.

247. Aalbers R, vd Jagt E, Poppema S, et al. Left paravertebral mass: giant lymph node hyperplasia. Chest 1987;91:889–890.

248. Fiore D, Biondetti PR, Calabro F, et al. CT demonstration of bilateral Castleman tumors in the mediastinum. J Comput Assist Tomogr 1983;7:719–720.

249. Meisel S, Rozenman J, Yellin A, et al. Castleman's disease. An uncommon computed tomographic feature. Chest 1988;93:1306–1307.

250. Onik G, Goodman PC. CT of Castleman disease. AJR Am J Roentgenol 1983;140:691–692.

251. Charig MJ. Mediastinal Castleman's disease: a missed pre-operative diagnosis? Clin Radiol 1990;42:440–442.

252. Walter JF, Rottenberg RW, Cannon WB, et al. Giant mediastinal lymph node hyperplasia (Castleman's disease): angiographic and clinical features. AJR Am J Roentgenol 1978;130:447–450.

253. Moon WK, Im JG, Han MC. Castleman's disease of the mediastinum: MR imaging features. Clin Radiol 1994;49:466–468.

254. Hsieh ML, Quint LE, Faust JM, et al. Enhancing mediastinal mass at MR: Castleman disease. Magn Reson Imaging 1993;11:599–601.

255. Ferrozzi F, Tognini G, Spaggiari E, et al. Focal Castleman disease of the lung: MRI findings. Clin Imaging 2001;25:400–422.

256. Johkoh T, Müller NL, Ichikado K, et al. Intrathoracic multicentric Castleman disease: CT findings in 12 patients. Radiology 1998;209:477–481.

257. Mallens WM, Nijhuis-Heddes JM, Bakker W. Calcified lymph node metastases in bronchioloalveolar carcinoma. Radiology 1986;161:103–104.

258. Oguchi M, Higashi K, Taniguchi M, et al. Calcified mediastinal metastases from ovarian cancer imaged with Tc-99m MDP SPECT. Clin Nucl Med 1998;23:479–481.

259. Lautin EM, Rosenblatt M, Friedman AC, et al. Calcification in non-Hodgkin lymphoma occurring before therapy: identification on plain films and CT. AJR Am J Roentgenol 1990;155:739–740.

260. Panicek DM, Harty MP, Scicutella CJ, et al. Calcification in untreated mediastinal lymphoma. Radiology 1988;166:735–736.

261. Levitt RG, Glazer HS, Roper CL, et al, Murphy WA. Magnetic resonance imaging of mediastinal and hilar masses: comparison with CT. AJR Am J Roentgenol 1985;145:9–14.

262. Groskin SA, Massi AF, Randall PA. Calcified hilar and mediastinal lymph nodes in an AIDS patient with Pneumocystis jiroveci infection. Radiology 1990;175:345–346.

263. Radin DR, Baker EL, Klatt EC, et al. Visceral and nodal calcification in patients with AIDS-related Pneumocystis jiroveci infection. AJR Am J Roentgenol 1990;154:27–31.

264. Israel HL, Lenchner G, Steiner RM. Late development of mediastinal calcification in sarcoidosis. Am Rev Respir Dis 1981;124:302–305.

265. Jacobson G, Fleson B, Pendergrass EP. Eggshell calcifications in coal and metal miners. Semin Roentgenol 1967;2:276–282.

266. Gawne-Cain ML, Hansell DM. The pattern and distribution of calcified mediastinal lymph nodes in sarcoidosis and tuberculosis: a CT study. Clin Radiol 1996;51:263–267.

267. Landay MJ, Rollins NK. Mediastinal histoplasmosis granuloma: evaluation with CT. Radiology 1989;172:657–659.

268. Pombo F, Rodriguez E, Mato J, et al. Patterns of contrast enhancement of tuberculous lymph nodes demonstrated by computed tomography. Clin Radiol 1992;46:13–17.

269. Scatarige JC, Fishman EK, Kuhajda FP, et al. Low attenuation nodal metastases in testicular carcinoma. J Comput Assist Tomogr 1983;7:682–687.

270. Yousem DM, Scatarige JC, Fishman EK, et al. Low-attenuation thoracic metastases in testicular malignancy. AJR Am J Roentgenol 1986;146:291–293.

271. Hopper KD, Diehl LF, Cole BA, et al. The significance of necrotic mediastinal lymph nodes on CT in patients with newly diagnosed Hodgkin disease. AJR Am J Roentgenol 1990;155:267–270.

272. Im JG, Song KS, Kang HS, et al. Mediastinal tuberculous lymphadenitis: CT manifestations. Radiology 1987;164:115–119.

273. Müller NL, Webb WR, Gamsu G. Subcarinal lymph node enlargement: radiographic findings and CT correlation. AJR Am J Roentgenol 1985;145:15–19.

274. Mountain CF, Dresler CM. Regional lymph node classification for lung cancer staging. Chest 1997;111:1718–1723.

275. Müller NL, Webb WR, Gamsu G. Paratracheal lymphadenopathy: radiographic findings and correlation with CT. Radiology 1985;156:761–765.

276. Keats TE, Lipscomb GE, Betts CS 3rd. Mensuration of the arch of the azygos vein and its application to the study of cardiopulmonary disease. Radiology 1968;90:990–994.

277. Blank N, Castellino RA. Patterns of pleural reflections of the left superior mediastinum. Normal anatomy and distortions produced by adenopathy. Radiology 1972;102:585–589.

278. Patz EF Jr, Stark P, Shaffer K, et al. Identification of internal mammary lymph nodes: value of the frontal chest radiograph. J Thorac Imaging 1993;8:81–84.

279. Ravenel JG, Erasmus JJ. Azygoesophageal recess. J Thorac Imaging 2002;17:219–226.

280. Yoon HK, Jung KJ, Han BK, et al. Mediastinal interfaces and lines in children: radiographic-CT correlation. Pediatr Radiol 2001;31:406–412.

281. Miller FH, Fitzgerald SW, Donaldson JS. CT of the azygoesophageal recess in infants and children. Radiographics 1993;13:623–634.

282. Hammersley JR, Grum CM, Green RA. The correlation of subcarinal density visualized on plain chest roentgenograms with computed tomographic scans. Chest 1990;97:869–872.

283. Haramati LB, Cartagena AM, Austin JH. CT evaluation of mediastinal lymphadenopathy: noncontrast 5 mm vs postcontrast 10 mm sections. J Comput Assist Tomogr 1995;19:375–378.

284. Kozuka T, Tomiyama N, Johkoh T, et al. Coronal multiplanar reconstruction view from isotropic voxel data sets obtained with multidetector-row CT: assessment of detection and size of mediastinal and hilar lymph nodes. Radiat Med 2003;21:23–27.

285. Cascade PN, Gross BH, Kazerooni EA, et al. Variability in the detection of enlarged mediastinal lymph nodes in staging lung cancer: a comparison of contrast-enhanced and unenhanced CT. AJR Am J Roentgenol 1998;170:927–931.

286. Patz EF Jr, Erasmus JJ, McAdams HP, et al. Lung cancer staging and management: comparison of contrast-enhanced and nonenhanced helical CT of the thorax. Radiology 1999;212:56–60.

287. Genereux GP, Howie JL. Normal mediastinal lymph node size and number: CT and anatomic study. AJR Am J Roentgenol 1984;142:1095–1100.

288. Glazer GM, Gross BH, Quint LE, et al. Normal mediastinal lymph nodes: number and size according to American Thoracic Society mapping. AJR Am J Roentgenol 1985;144:261–265.

289. Ingram CE, Belli AM, Lewars MD, et al. Normal lymph node size in the mediastinum: a retrospective study in two patient groups. Clin Radiol 1989;40:35–39.

290. Schnyder PA, Gamsu G. CT of the pretracheal retrocaval space. AJR Am J Roentgenol 1981;136:303–308.

291. Quint LE, Glazer GM, Orringer MB, et al. Mediastinal lymph node detection and sizing at CT and autopsy. AJR Am J Roentgenol 1986;147:469–472.

292. Platt JF, Glazer GM, Orringer MB, et al. Radiologic evaluation of the subcarinal lymph nodes: a comparative study. AJR Am J Roentgenol 1988;151:279–282.

293. Kono M, Adachi S, Kusumoto M, et al. Clinical utility of Gd-DTPA-enhanced magnetic resonance imaging in lung cancer. J Thorac Imaging 1993;8:18–26.

294. Crisci R, Di Cesare E, Lupattelli L, et al. MR study of N2 disease in lung cancer: contrast-enhanced method using gadolinium-DTPA. Eur J Cardiothorac Surg 1997;11:214–217.

295. Nguyen BC, Stanford W, Thompson BH, et al. Multicenter clinical trial of ultrasmall superparamagnetic iron oxide in the evaluation of mediastinal lymph nodes in patients with primary lung carcinoma. J Magn Reson Imaging 1999;10:468–473.

296. Pannu HK, Wang KP, Borman TL, et al. MR imaging of mediastinal lymph nodes: evaluation using a superparamagnetic contrast agent. J Magn Reson Imaging 2000;12:899–904.

297. Müller NL, Webb WR. Imaging of the pulmonary hila. Invest Radiol 1985;20:661–671.

298. Park CK, Webb WR, Klein JS. Inferior hilar window. Radiology 1991;178:163–168.

299. Glazer GM, Francis IR, Shirazi KK, et al. Evaluation of the pulmonary hilum: comparison of conventional radiography, 55 degrees posterior oblique tomography, and dynamic computed tomography. J Comput Assist Tomogr 1983;7:983–989.

300. Remy-Jardin M, Duyck P, Remy J, et al. Hilar lymph nodes: identification with spiral CT and histologic correlation. Radiology 1995;196:387–394.

301. Armstrong P. Tomographic evaluation of the questionably enlarged pulmonary hilum. In: Armstrong P, ed. Critical problems in diagnostic radiology. Philadelphia: JB Lippincott, 1983.

302. Naidich DP, Khouri NF, Scott WW Jr, et al. Computed tomography of the pulmonary hila: 1. normal anatomy. J Comput Assist Tomogr 1981;5:459–467.

303. Naidich DP, Khouri NF, Stitik FP, et al. Computed tomography of the pulmonary hila: 2. abnormal anatomy. J Comput Assist Tomogr 1981;5:468–475.

304. Webb WR, Gamsu G, Glazer G. Computed tomography of the abnormal pulmonary hilum. J Comput Assist Tomogr 1981;5:485–490.

305. Webb WR, Hirji M, Gamsu G. Posterior wall of the bronchus intermedius: radiographic-CT correlation. AJR Am J Roentgenol 1984;142:907–911.

306. Webb WR, Gamsu G. Computed tomography of the left retrobronchial stripe. J Comput Assist Tomogr 1983;7:65–69.

307. Gotway MB, Patel RA, Webb WR. Helical CT for the evaluation of suspected acute pulmonary embolism: diagnostic pitfalls. J Comput Assist Tomogr 2000;24:267–273.

308. Webb WR, Gamsu G, Stark DD, et al. Magnetic resonance imaging of the normal and abnormal pulmonary hila. Radiology 1984;152:89–94.

309. Baker HL Jr, Berquist TH, Kispert DB, et al. Magnetic resonance imaging in a routine clinical setting. Mayo Clin Proc 1985;60:75–90.

310. Buirski G, Jordan SC, Joffe HS, et al. Superior vena caval abnormalities: their occurrence rate, associated cardiac abnormalities and angiographic classification in a paediatric population with congenital heart disease. Clin Radiol 1986;37:131–138.

311. Glazer HS, Aronberg DJ, Sagel SS. Pitfalls in CT recognition of mediastinal lymphadenopathy. AJR Am J Roentgenol 1985;144:267–274.

312. Proto AV, Rost RC. CT of the thorax: pitfalls in interpretation. RadioGraphics 1985;5:693–712.

313. Kurihara Y, Nakajima Y, Ishikawa T. Case report: saccular aneurysm of the azygos vein simulating a paratracheal tumour. Clin Radiol 1993;48:427–428.

314. Mehta M, Towers M. Computed tomography appearance of idiopathic aneurysm of the azygos vein. Can Assoc Radiol J 1996;47:288–290.

315. Podbielski FJ, Sam AD 2nd, Halldorsson AO, et al. Giant azygos vein varix. Ann Thorac Surg 1997;63:1167–1169.

316. Burkill GJ, Burn PR, Padley SP. Aneurysm of the left brachiocephalic vein: an unusual cause of mediastinal widening. Br J Radiol 1997;70:837–839.

317. Pasic M, Schopke W, Vogt P, et al. Aneurysm of the superior mediastinal veins. J Vasc Surg 1995;21:505–509.

318. Rappaport DC, Ros PR, Moser RP Jr. Idiopathic dilatation of the thoracic venous system. Can Assoc Radiol J 1992;43:385–387.

319. Choi YW, McAdams HP, Jeon SC, et al. The "High-Riding" superior pericardial recess: CT findings. AJR Am J Roentgenol 2000;175:1025–1028.

320. Kodama F, Fultz PJ, Wandtke JC. Comparing thin-section and thick-section CT of pericardial sinuses and recesses. AJR Am J Roentgenol 2003;181:1101–1108.

321. Davis J, Mark G, Green R. Benign blood vascular tumors of the mediastinum: report of four cases and review of the literature. Radiology 1987;126:581–587.

322. Tarr RW, Page DL, Glick AG, et al. Benign hemangioendothelioma involving posterior mediastinum: CT findings. J Comput Assist Tomogr 1986;10:865–867.

323. Hayashi A, Takamori S, Tayama K, et al. Primary hemangiopericytoma of the superior mediastinum: a case report. Ann Thorac Cardiovasc Surg 1998;4:283–285.

324. Rubinowitz AN, Moreira AL, Naidich DP. Mediastinal hemangioendothelioma: radiologic—pathologic correlation. J Comput Assist Tomogr 2000;24:721–723.

325. Angtuaco EJ, Jimenez JF, Burrows P, et al. Lymphatic-venous malformation (lymphangiohemangioma) of mediastinum. J Comput Assist Tomogr 1983;7:895–897.

326. Riquet M, Briere J, Le Pimpec-Barthes F, et al. Lymphangiohemangioma of the mediastinum. Ann Thorac Surg 1997;64:1476–1478.

327. Toye R, Armstrong P, Dacie JE. Lymphangiohaemangioma of the mediastinum. Br J Radiol 1991;64:62–64.

328. McAdams HP, Rosado-de-Christenson ML, Moran CA. Mediastinal hemangioma: radiographic and CT features in 14 patients. Radiology 1994;193:399–402.

329. Cohen AJ, Sbaschnig RJ, Hochholzer L, et al. Mediastinal hemangiomas. Ann Thorac Surg 1987;43:656–659.

330. Bedros AA, Munson J, Toomey FE. Hemangioendothelioma presenting as posterior mediastinal mass in a child. Cancer 1980;46:801–803.

331. Kronthal AJ, Heitmiller RF, Fishman EK, et al. Mediastinal seroma after esophagogastrectomy. AJR Am J Roentgenol 1991;156:715–716.

332. Buckner S, McAllister J, D'Altorio R. Case of the season. Hemangioma of the middle mediastinum. Semin Roentgenol 1994;29:98–99.

333. Schurawitzki H, Stiglbauer R, Klepetko W, et al. CT and MRI in benign mediastinal haemangioma. Clin Radiol 1991;43:91–94.

334. Seline TH, Gross BH, Francis IR. CT and MR imaging of mediastinal hemangiomas. J Comput Assist Tomogr 1990;14:766–768.

335. Erasmus JJ, McAdams HP, Donnelly LF, et al. MR imaging of mediastinal masses. Magn Reson Imaging Clin N Am 2000;8:59–89.

336. Fishman SJ. Vascular anomalies of the mediastinum. Semin Pediatr Surg 1999;8:92–98.

337. Yoo SY, Hong SH, Chung HW, et al. MRI of Gorham's disease: findings in two cases. Skeletal Radiol 2002;31:301–306.

338. Yoo SY, Goo JM, Im JG. Mediastinal lymphangioma and chylothorax: thoracic involvement of Gorham's disease. Korean J Radiol 2002;3:130–132.

339. Brown LR, Reiman HM, Rosenow EC 3rd, et al. Intrathoracic lymphangioma. Mayo Clin Proc 1986;61:882–892.

340. Halliday DR, Dahlin DC, Pugh DG. Massive osteolysis and angiomatosis. Radiology 1964;82:637–643.

341. Ellison RT 3rd, Corrao WM, Fox MJ, et al. Spontaneous mediastinal hemorrhage in patients on chronic hemodialysis. Ann Intern Med 1981;95:704–706.

342. Aalbers R, Piers B, Eygelaar A, et al. Sudden superior mediastinal enlargement. Chest 1991;99:209–210.

343. Bethancourt B, Pond GD, Jones SE, et al. Mediastinal hematoma simulating recurrent Hodgkin disease during systemic chemotherapy. AJR Am J Roentgenol 1984;142:1119–1120.

344. Pezzulli FA, Aronson D, Goldberg N. Computed tomography of mediastinal hematoma secondary to unusual esophageal laceration: a Boerhaave variant. J Comput Assist Tomogr 1989;13:129–131.

345. Stilwell ME, Weisbrod GL, Ilves R. Spontaneous mediastinal hematoma. J Can Assoc Radiol 1981;32:60–61.

346. Woodring JH, Loh FK, Kryscio RJ. Mediastinal hemorrhage: an evaluation of radiographic manifestations. Radiology 1984;151:15–21.

347. Simeone JF, Minagi H, Putman CE. Traumatic disruption of the thoracic aorta: significance of the left apical extrapleural cap. Radiology 1975;117:265–268.

348. Panicek DM, Ewing DK, Markarian B, et al. Interstitial pulmonary hemorrhage from mediastinal hematoma secondary to aortic rupture. Radiology 1987;162:165–166.

349. Bradley WG Jr. MR appearance of hemorrhage in the brain. Radiology 1993;189:15–26.

350. Burnett CM, Rosemurgy AS, Pfeiffer EA. Life-threatening acute posterior mediastinitis due to esophageal perforation. Ann Thorac Surg 1990;49:979–983.

351. Payne WS, Larson RH. Acute mediastinitis. Surg Clin North Am 1969;49:999–1009.

352. Levine TM, Wurster CF, Krespi YP. Mediastinitis occurring as a complication of odontogenic infections. Laryngoscope 1986;96:747–750.

353. Marty-Ane CH, Alauzen M, Alric P, et al. Descending necrotizing mediastinitis. Advantage of mediastinal drainage with thoracotomy. J Thorac Cardiovasc Surg 1994;107:55–61.

354. Pollack MS. Staphylococcal mediastinitis due to sternoclavicular pyarthrosis: CT appearance. J Comput Assist Tomogr 1990;14:924–927.

355. Ablin DS, Reinhart MA. Esophageal perforation with mediastinal abscess in child abuse. Pediatr Radiol 1990;20:524–525.

356. Breatnach E, Nath PH, Delany DJ. The role of computed tomography in acute and subacute mediastinitis. Clin Radiol 1986;37:139–145.

357. Rogers LF, Puig AW, Dooley BN, et al. Diagnostic considerations in mediastinal emphysema: a pathophysiologic-roentgenologic approach to Boerhaave's syndrome and spontaneous pneumomediastinum. Am J Roentgenol Radium Ther Nucl Med 1972;115:495–511.

358. Carrol CL, Jeffrey RB, Federle MP. CT evaluation of mediastinal infections. J Comput Assist Tomog 1989;11:449–454.

359. Fields JM, Schwartz DS, Gosche J, et al. Idiopathic bilateral anterior mediastinal abscesses. Pediatr Radiol 1997;27:596–597.

360. White CS, Templeton PA, Attar S. Esophageal perforation: CT findings. AJR Am J Roentgenol 1993;160:767–770.

361. Gobien RP, Stanley JH, Gobien BS, et al. Percutaneous catheter aspiration and drainage of suspected mediastinal abscesses. Radiology 1984;151:69–71.

362. Kiernan PD, Hernandez A, Byrne WD, et al. Descending cervical mediastinitis. Ann Thorac Surg 1998;65:1483–1488.

363. Goodman LR, Kay HR, Teplick SK, et al. Complications of median sternotomy: computed tomographic evaluation. AJR Am J Roentgenol 1983;141:225–230.

364. Jolles H, Henry DA, Roberson JP, et al. Mediastinitis following median sternotomy: CT findings. Radiology 1996;201:463–466.

365. Kay HR, Goodman LR, Teplick SK, et al. Use of computed tomography to assess mediastinal complications after median

sternotomy. Ann Thorac Surg 1983;36:706–714.

366. Bitkover CY, Cederlund K, Aberg B, et al. Computed tomography of the sternum and mediastinum after median sternotomy. Ann Thorac Surg 1999;68: 858–863.

367. Robicsek F. Postoperative sterno-mediastinitis. Am Surg 2000;66: 184–192.

368. Carter AR, Sostman HD, Curtis AM, et al. Thoracic alterations after cardiac surgery. AJR Am J Roentgenol 1983;140:475–481.

369. Rossi SE, McAdams HP, Rosado-de-Christenson ML, et al. Fibrosing mediastinitis. RadioGraphics 2001;21:737–757.

370. Goodwin RA, Nickell JA, Des Prez RM. Mediastinal fibrosis complicating healed primary histoplasmosis and tuberculosis. Medicine (Baltimore) 1972;51:227–246.

371. Loyd JE, Tillman BF, Atkinson JB, et al. Mediastinal fibrosis complicating histoplasmosis. Medicine (Baltimore) 1988;67:295–310.

372. Davis AM, Pierson RN, Loyd JE. Mediastinal fibrosis. Semin Respir Infect 2001;16:119–130.

373. Mole TM, Glover J, Sheppard MN. Sclerosing mediastinitis: a report on 18 cases. Thorax 1995;50:280–283.

374. Hofmann-Wellenhof R, Domej W, Schmid C, et al. Mediastinal mass caused by syphilitic aortitis. Thorax 1993;48:568–569.

375. Light AM. Idiopathic fibrosis of mediastinum: a discussion of three cases and review of the literature. J Clin Pathol 1978;31:78–88.

376. Flieder DB, Suster S, Moran CA. Idiopathic fibroinflammatory (fibrosing/sclerosing) lesions of the mediastinum: a study of 30 cases with emphasis on morphologic heterogeneity. Mod Pathol 1999;12:257–264.

377. Ramakantan R, Shah P. Dysphagia due to mediastinal fibrosis in advanced pulmonary tuberculosis. AJR Am J Roentgenol 1990;154:61–63.

378. Goodwin RA, Loyd JE, Des Prez RM. Histoplasmosis in normal hosts. Medicine (Baltimore) 1981;60:231–266.

379. Kirchner SG, Hernanz-Schulman M, Stein SM, et al. Imaging of pediatric mediastinal histoplasmosis. RadioGraphics 1991;11:365–381.

380. Christoforidis AJ. Radiologic manifestations on histoplasmosis. Am J Roentgenol Radium Ther Nucl Med 1970;109:478–490.

381. Conces DJ Jr. Histoplasmosis. Semin Roentgenol 1996;31:14–27.

382. Connell JV, Muhm JR. Radiographic manifestations of pulmonary histoplasmosis: a 10-year review. Radiology 1976;121:281–285.

383. Feigin DS, Eggleston JC, Siegelman SS. The multiple roentgen manifestations of sclerosing mediastinitis. Johns Hopkins Med J 1979;144:1–8.

384. Kountz PD, Molina PL, Sagel SS. Fibrosing mediastinitis in the posterior thorax. AJR Am J Roentgenol 1989; 153:489–490.

385. Wieder S, Rabinowitz JG. Fibrous mediastinitis: a late manifestation of mediastinal histoplasmosis. Radiology 1977;125:305–312.

386. Wieder S, White TJ 3rd, Salazar J, et al. Pulmonary artery occlusion due to histoplasmosis. AJR Am J Roentgenol 1982;138:243–251.

387. Sherrick AD, Brown LR, Harms GF, et al. The radiographic findings of fibrosing mediastinitis. Chest 1994; 106:484–489.

388. Barnett SM. CT findings in tuberculous mediastinitis. J Comput Assist Tomogr 1986;10:165–166.

389. Rodriguez E, Soler R, Pombo F, et al. Fibrosing mediastinitis: CT and MR findings. Clin Radiol 1998;53:907–910.

390. Weinstein JB, Aronberg DJ, Sagel SS. CT of fibrosing mediastinitis: findings and their utility. AJR Am J Roentgenol 1983;141:247–251.

391. Rholl KS, Levitt RG, Glazer HS. Magnetic resonance imaging of fibrosing mediastinitis. AJR Am J Roentgenol 1985;145:255–259.

392. Mallin WH, Silberstein EB, Shipley RT, et al. Fibrosing mediastinitis causing nonvisualization of one lung on pulmonary scintigraphy. Clin Nucl Med 1993;18:594–596.

393. David RA, Weiner MA, Rakow JI. Chronic active mediastinitis in a 7-year-old boy: MRI findings. Pediatr Radiol 1996;26:669–671.

394. Farmer DW, Moore E, Amparo E, et al. Calcific fibrosing mediastinitis: demonstration of pulmonary vascular obstruction by magnetic resonance imaging. AJR Am J Roentgenol 1984;143:1189–1191.

395. Moreno AJ, Weismann I, Billingsley JL, et al. Angiographic and scintigraphic findings in fibrosing mediastinitis. Clin Nucl Med 1983;8:167–169.

396. Ashizawa K, Hayashi K, Minami K, et al. CT and MR findings of posterior mediastinal panniculitis. J Comput Assist Tomogr 1997;21:324–326.

397. Reeder LB. Neurogenic tumors of the mediastinum. Semin Thorac Cardiovasc Surg 2000;12:261–267.

398. Topcu S, Alper A, Gulhan E, et al. Neurogenic tumours of the mediastinum: a report of 60 cases. Can Respir J 2000;7:261–265.

399. Lee JY, Lee KS, Han J, et al. Spectrum of neurogenic tumors in the thorax: CT and pathologic findings. J Comput Assist Tomogr 1999;23:399–406.

400. Reed JC, Hallet KK, Feigin DS. Neural tumors of the thorax: subject review from the AFIP. Radiology 1978;126: 9–17.

401. Carey LS, Ellis FH, Good CA. Neurogenic tumors of the mediastinum: a clinicopathologic study. AJR Am J Roentgenol 1960;84:189–205.

402. Chalmers AH, Armstrong P. Plexiform mediastinal neurofibromas. A report of two cases. Br J Radiol 1977;50:215–217.

403. Gossios KJ, Guy RL. Case report: imaging of widespread plexiform neurofibromatosis. Clin Radiol 1993;47:211–213.

404. Aisner SC, Chakravarthy AK, Joslyn JN, et al. Bilateral granular cell tumors of the posterior mediastinum. Ann Thorac Surg 1988;46:688–689.

405. Machida E, Haniuda M, Eguchi T, et al. Granular cell tumor of the mediastinum. Intern Med 2003;42:178–181.

406. Gale AW, Jelihovsky T, Grant AF, et al. Neurogenic tumors of the mediastinum. Ann Thorac Surg 1974;17:434–443.

407. Lonergan GJ, Schwab CM, Suarez ES, et al. Neuroblastoma, ganglioneuroblastoma, and ganglioneuroma: radiologic-pathologic correlation. RadioGraphics 2002; 22:911–934.

408. Alterman K, Shueller EF. Maturation of neuroblastoma to ganglioneuroma. Am J Dis Child 1970;120:217–222.

409. Alexander F. Neuroblastoma. Urol Clin North Am 2000;27:383–392.

410. Eklof O, Gooding CA. Intrathoracic neuroblastoma. Am J Roentgenol Radium Ther Nucl Med 1967;100: 202–207.

411. Bar-Ziv J, Nogrady MB. Mediastinal neuroblastoma and ganglioneuroma. The differentiation between primary and secondary involvement on the chest roentgenogram. Am J Roentgenol Radium Ther Nucl Med 1975;125:380–390.

412. Filler RM, Traggis DG, Jaffe N, et al. Favorable outlook for children with mediastinal neuroblastoma. J Pediatr Surg 1972;7:136–143.

413. Feinstein RS, Gatewood OM, Fishman EK, et al. Computed tomography of adult neuroblastoma. J Comput Assist Tomogr 1984;8:720–726.

414. Ribet ME, Cardot GR. Neurogenic tumors of the thorax. Ann Thorac Surg 1994;58:1091–1095.

415. Tanabe M, Yoshida H, Ohnuma N, et al. Imaging of neuroblastoma in patients identified by mass screening using urinary catecholamine metabolites. J Pediatr Surg 1993;28: 617–621.

416. Barrett AF, Toye DKM. Sympathicoblastoma: radiological findings in forty-three cases. Clin Radiol 1960;14:33–42.

417. Ko SF, Lee TY, Lin JW, et al. Thoracic neurilemomas: an analysis of computed et al tomography findings in 36 patients. J Thorac Imaging 1998;13:21–26.

418. Coleman BG, Arger PH, Dalinka MK, et al. CT of sarcomatous degeneration in neurofibromatosis. AJR Am J Roentgenol 1983;140:383–387.

419. Cohen LM, Schwartz AM, Rockoff SD. Benign schwannomas: pathologic basis for CT inhomogeneities. AJR Am J Roentgenol 1986;147:141–143.

420. Moon WK, Im JG, Han MC. Malignant schwannomas of the thorax: CT findings. J Comput Assist Tomogr 1993;17: 274–276.

421. Armstrong EA, Harwood-Nash DC, Ritz CR, et al. CT of neuroblastomas and ganglioneuromas in children. AJR Am J Roentgenol 1982;139:571–576.

422. Faerber EN, Carter BL, Sarno RC, et al. Computed tomography of neuroblastic tumors in children. Clin Pediatr (Phila) 1984;23:17–21.

423. Ricci C, Rendina EA, Venuta F, et al. Diagnostic imaging and surgical treatment of dumbbell tumors of the mediastinum. Ann Thorac Surg 1990;50:586–589.

424. Burk DL Jr, Brunberg JA, Kanal E, et al. Spinal and paraspinal neurofibromatosis: surface coil MR imaging at 1.5 T1. Radiology 1987;162:797–801.

425. Freundlich IM, Chasen MH, Varma DG. Magnetic resonance imaging of pulmonary apical tumors. J Thorac Imaging 1996;11:210–222.

426. Suh JS, Abenoza P, Galloway HR, et al. Peripheral (extracranial) nerve tumors: correlation of MR imaging and histologic findings. Radiology 1992;183:341–346.

427. Sakai F, Sone S, Kiyono K, et al. Intrathoracic neurogenic tumors: MR-pathologic correlation. AJR Am J Roentgenol 1992;159:279–283.

428. Slovis TL, Meza MP, Cushing B, et al. Thoracic neuroblastoma: what is the best imaging modality for evaluating extent of disease? Pediatr Radiol 1997;27: 273–275.

429. Shulkin BL, Hutchinson RJ, Castle VP, et al. Neuroblastoma: positron emission tomography with 2-[fluorine-18]-fluoro-2-deoxy-D-glucose compared with metaiodobenzylguanidine scintigraphy. Radiology 1996;199:743–750.

430. Boubaker A, Bischof Delaloye A. Nuclear medicine procedures and neuroblastoma in childhood. Their value in the diagnosis, staging and assessment of response to therapy. Q J Nucl Med 2003;47:31–40.

431. Herrera MF, van Heerden JA, Puga FJ, et al. Mediastinal paraganglioma: a surgical experience. Ann Thorac Surg 1993;56:1096–1100.

432. Suster S, Moran CA. Neuroendocrine neoplasms of the mediastinum. Am J Clin Pathol 2001;115 Suppl:S17–27.

433. Olson JL, Salyer WR. Mediastinal paragangliomas (aortic body tumor): a report of four cases and a review of the literature. Cancer 1978;41:2405–2412.

434. Habe RS. Retroperitoneal and mediastinal chemodectoma: report of a case and review of the literature. AJR Am J Roentgenol 1964;92:1029–1041.

435. van Heerden JA, Sheps SG, Hamberger B, et al. Pheochromocytoma: current status and changing trends. Surgery 1982;91:367–373.

436. McNeill AD, Groden BM, Neville AM. Intrathoracic phaeochromocytoma. Br J Surg 1970;57:457–462.

437. Banzo J, Prats E, Velilla J, et al. Functioning intrapericardial paraganglioma diagnosed by I-123 MIBG imaging. Clin Nucl Med 1991;16:860–861.

438. Shapiro B, Sisson J, Kalff V, et al. The location of middle mediastinal pheochromocytomas. J Thorac Cardiovasc Surg 1984;87:814–820.

439. Shirkhoda A, Wallace S. Computed tomography of juxtacardiac pheochromocytoma. J Comput Tomogr 1984;8:207–209.

440. Castanon J, Gil-Aguado M, de la Llana R, et al. Aortopulmonary paraganglioma, a rare aortic tumor: a case report. J Thorac Cardiovasc Surg 1993;106: 1232–1233.

441. Cornford EJ, Wastie ML, Morgan DA. Malignant paraganglioma of the mediastinum: a further diagnostic and therapeutic use of radiolabelled MIBG. Br J Radiol 1992;65:75–78.

442. Francis IR, Glazer GM, Shapiro B, et al. Complementary roles of CT and ^{131}I-MIBG scintigraphy in diagnosing pheochromocytoma. AJR Am J Roentgenol 1983;141:719–725.

443. Krenning EP, Kwekkeboom DJ, Bakker WH, et al. Somatostatin receptor scintigraphy with [111In-DTPA-D-Phe1]- and [123I-Tyr3]-octreotide: the Rotterdam experience with more than 1000 patients. Eur J Nucl Med 1993;20:716–731.

444. van Gils AP, Falke TH, van Erkel AR, et al. MR imaging and MIBG scintigraphy of pheochromocytomas and extraadrenal functioning paragangliomas. RadioGraphics 1991;11:37–57.

445. Blandino A, Salvi L, Faranda C, et al. Unusual malignant paraganglioma of the anterior mediastinum: CT and MR findings. Eur J Radiol 1992;15:1–3.

446. Andrade CF, Camargo SM, Zanchet M, et al. Nonfunctioning paraganglioma of the aortopulmonary window. Ann Thorac Surg 2003;75:1950–1951.

447. Spector JA, Willis DN, Ginsburg HB. Paraganglioma (pheochromocytoma) of the posterior mediastinum: a case report and review of the literature. J Pediatr Surg 2003;38:1114–1116.

448. Olsen WL, Dillon WP, Kelly WM, et al. MR imaging of paragangliomas. AJR Am J Roentgenol 1987;148:201–204.

449. Satava RM Jr, Beahrs OH, Scholz DA. Success rate of cervical exploration for hyperparathyroidism. Arch Surg 1975;110:625–628.

450. Russell CF, Edis AJ, Scholz DA, et al. Mediastinal parathyroid tumors: experience with 38 tumors requiring mediastinotomy for removal. Ann Surg 1981;193:805–809.

451. Norris EH. The parathyroid adenoma: a study of 322 cases. Int Abst Surg 1947;84:1–41.

452. Kang YS, Rosen K, Clark OH, et al. Localization of abnormal parathyroid glands of the mediastinum with MR imaging. Radiology 1993;189:137–141.

453. Lossef SV, Ziessman HA, Alijani MR, et al. Multiple hyperfunctioning mediastinal parathyroid glands in a patient with tertiary hyperparathyroidism. AJR Am J Roentgenol 1993;161:285–286.

454. Kaczirek K, Prager G, Kienast O, et al. Combined transmission and (99m)Tc-sestamibi emission tomography for localization of mediastinal parathyroid glands. Nuklearmedizin 2003;42:220–223.

455. Itoh K, Ishizuka R. Tc-99m-MIBI scintigraphy for recurrent hyperparathyroidism after total parathyroidectomy with autograft. Ann Nucl Med 2003;17:315–320.

456. Ishibashi M, Nishida H, Hiromatsu Y, et al. Localization of ectopic parathyroid glands using technetium-99m sestamibi imaging: comparison with magnetic resonance and computed tomographic imaging. Eur J Nucl Med 1997;24: 197–201.

457. Ishibashi M, Nishida H, Hiromatsu Y, et al. Comparison of technetium-99m-MIBI, technetium-99m-tetrofosmin, ultrasound and MRI for localization of abnormal parathyroid glands. J Nucl Med 1998;39:320–324.

458. Kelly JD, Forster AM, Higley B, et al. Technetium-99m-tetrofosmin as a new radiopharmaceutical for myocardial perfusion imaging. J Nucl Med 1993;34:222–227.

459. Lee VS, Spritzer CE, Coleman RE, Jr. The complementary roles of fast spin-echo MR imaging and double-phase 99m Tc-sestamibi scintigraphy for localization of hyperfunctioning parathyroid glands. AJR Am J Roentgenol 1996;167: 1555–1562.

460. Mariani G, Gulec SA, Rubello D, et al. Preoperative localization and radioguided parathyroid surgery. J Nucl Med 2003;44:1443–1458.

461. Doppman JL, Skarulis MC, Chen CC, et al. Parathyroid adenomas in the

aortopulmonary window. Radiology 1996;201:456–462.

462. Spritzer CE, Gefter WB, Hamilton R, et al. Abnormal parathyroid glands: high-resolution MR imaging. Radiology 1987;162:487–491.

463. Shields TW, Immerman SC. Mediastinal parathyroid cysts revisited. Ann Thorac Surg 1999;67:581–590.

464. Hauet EJ, Paul MA, Salu MK. Compression of the trachea by a mediastinal parathyroid cyst. Ann Thorac Surg 1997;64:851–852.

465. Landau O, Chamberlain DW, Kennedy RS, et al. Mediastinal parathyroid cysts. Ann Thorac Surg 1997;63:951–953.

466. Soler R, Bargiela A, Cordido F. MRI of mediastinal cystic adenoma causing hyperparathyroidism. J Comput Assist Tomogr 1995;20:166–167.

467. Damore DT, Dayan PS. Medical causes of pneumomediastinum in children. Clin Pediatr (Phila) 2001;40:87–91.

468. Hedlund GL, Wiatrak BJ, Pranikoff T. Pneumomediastinum as an early radiographic sign in membranous croup. AJR Am J Roentgenol 1998;170:55–56.

469. Parker GS, Mosborg DA, Foley RW, et al. Spontaneous cervical and mediastinal emphysema. Laryngoscope 1990;100:938–940.

470. Sullivan TP, Pierson DJ. Pneumomediastinum after freebase cocaine use. AJR Am J Roentgenol 1997;168:84.

471. LiPuma JP, Wellman J, Stern HP. Nitrous oxide abuse: a new cause of pneumomediastinum. Radiology 1982;145:602.

472. Takahashi T, Hoshino Y, Nakamura T, et al. Mediastinal emphysema with Pneumocystis jiroveci pneumonia in AIDS. AJR Am J Roentgenol 1997;169:1465–1466.

473. Girard DE, Carlson V, Natelson EA, et al. Pneumomediastinum in diabetic ketoacidosis: comments on mechanism, incidence, and management. Chest 1971;60:455–459.

474. Ruttley M, Mills RA. Subcutaneous emphysema and pneumomediastinum in diabetic keto-acidosis. Br J Radiol 1971;44:672–674.

475. Fujiwara T. Pneumomediastinum in pulmonary fibrosis: detection by computed tomography. Chest 1993;104:44–46.

476. Sutherland FW, Ho SY, Campanella C. Pneumomediastinum during spontaneous vaginal delivery. Ann Thorac Surg 2002;73:314–315.

477. Sandler CM, Libshitz HI, Marks G. Pneumoperitoneum, pneumomediastinum and pneumopericardium following dental extraction. Radiology 1975;115:539–540.

478. Tomsick TA. Dental surgical subcutaneous and mediastinal emphysema: a case report. J Can Assoc Radiol 1974;25:49–51.

479. Stahl JD, Goldman SM, Minkin SD, et al. Perforated duodenal ulcer and pneumomediastinum. Radiology 1977;124:23–25.

480. Beerman PJ, Gelfand DW, Ott DJ. Pneumomediastinum after double-contrast barium enema examination: a sign of colonic perforation. AJR Am J Roentgenol 1981;136:197–198.

481. Gray JM, Hanson GC. Mediastinal emphysema: aetiology, diagnosis, and treatment. Thorax 1966;21:325–332.

482. Munsell WP. Pneumomediastinum. A report of 28 cases and review of the literature. JAMA 1967;202:689–693.

483. Bejvan SM, Godwin JD. Pneumomediastinum: old signs and new signs. AJR Am J Roentgenol 1996;166:1041–1048.

484. Jamadar DA, Kazerooni EA, Hirschl RB. Pneumomediastinum: elucidation of the anatomic pathway by liquid ventilation. J Comput Assist Tomogr 1996;20: 309–311.

485. Chon KS, vanSonnenberg E, D'Agostino HB, et al. CT-guided catheter drainage of loculated thoracic air collections in mechanically ventilated patients with acute respiratory distress syndrome. AJR Am J Roentgenol 1999;173:1345–1350.

486. Dondelinger RF, Coulon M, Kurdziel JC, et al. Tension mediastinal emphysema: emergency percutaneous drainage with CT guidance. Eur J Radiol 1992;15: 7–10.

487. Rohlfing BM, Webb WR, Schlobohm RM. Ventilator-related extra-alveolar air in adults. Radiology 1976;121:25–31.

488. Astigarraga E, Saez F, Canteli B, et al. Postmediastinoscopy changes in chest CT. J Comput Assist Tomogr 1994;18:566–568.

489. Levin B. The continuous diaphragm sign. A newly-recognized sign of pneumomediastinum. Clin Radiol 1973;24:337–338.

490. Friedman AC, Lautin EM, Rothenberg L. Mach bands and pneumomediastinum. J Can Assoc Radiol 1981;32:232–235.

491. Stark P, Eber CD, Jacobson F. Primary intrathoracic malignant mesenchymal tumors: pictorial essay. J Thorac Imaging 1994;9:148–155.

492. Stark P, Smith DC, Watkins GE, et al. Primary intrathoracic extraosseous osteogenic sarcoma: report of three cases. Radiology 1990;174:725–726.

493. McDermott VG, Mackenzie S, Hendry GM. Case report: primary intrathoracic rhabdomyosarcoma: a rare childhood malignancy. Br J Radiol 1993;66: 937–941.

494. Phillips GW, Choong M. Chondrosarcoma presenting as an anterior mediastinal mass. Clin Radiol 1991;43:63–64.

495. Taki S, Kakuda K, Kakuma K, et al. Posterior mediastinal chordoma: MR imaging findings. AJR Am J Roentgenol 1996;166:26–27.

496. Murphy JM, Wallis F, Toland J, et al. CT and MRI appearances of a thoracic chordoma. Eur Radiol 1998;8: 1677–1679.

497. Parish JM, Marschke RF Jr, Dines DE, et al. Etiologic considerations in superior vena cava syndrome. Mayo Clin Proc 1981;56:407–413.

498. Wudel LJ, Jr., Nesbitt JC. Superior vena cava syndrome. Curr Treat Options Oncol 2001;2:77–91.

499. Mahajan V, Strimlan V, Ordstrand HS, et al. Benign superior vena cava syndrome. Chest 1975;68:32–3.

500. Carter MM, Tarr RW, Mazer MJ, et al. The "aortic nipple" as a sign of impending superior vena caval syndrome. Chest 1985;87:775–777.

501. Brown G, Husband JE. Mediastinal widening – valuable radiographic sign of superior vena cava thrombosis. Clin Radiol 1993;47:415–440.

502. Cihangiroglu M, Lin BH, Dachman AH. Collateral pathways in superior vena caval obstruction as seen on CT. J Comput Assist Tomogr 2001;25:1–8.

503. Barek L, Lautin R, Ledor S, et al. Role of CT in the assessment of superior vena caval obstruction. J Comput Tomogr 1982;6:121–126.

504. Bechtold RE, Wolfman NT, Karstaedt N, et al. Superior vena caval obstruction: detection using CT. Radiology 1985;157:485–487.

505. Moncada R, Cardella R, Demos TC, et al. Evaluation of superior vena cava syndrome by axial CT and CT phlebography. AJR Am J Roentgenol 1984;143:731–736.

506. McMurdo KK, de Geer G, Webb WR, et al. Normal and occluded mediastinal veins: MR imaging. Radiology 1986;159:33–38.

507. Weinreb JC, Mootz A, Cohen JM. MRI evaluation of mediastinal and thoracic inlet venous obstruction. AJR Am J Roentgenol 1986;146:679–684.

508. Li W, David V, Kaplan R, et al. Three-dimensional low dose gadolinium-enhanced peripheral MR venography. J Magn Reson Imaging 1998;8 :630–633.

509. Hara M, McAdams HP, Vredenburgh JJ, et al. Thymic hyperplasia after high-dose chemotherapy and autologous stem cell transplantation: incidence and significance in patients with breast cancer. AJR Am J Roentgenol 1999; 173:1341–1344.

510. FitzGerald JM, Mayo JR, Miller RR, et al. Tuberculosis of the thymus. Chest 1992;102:1604–1605.

511. Freundlich IM, McGavran MH. Abnormalities of the thymus. J Thorac Imaging 1996;11:58–65.

512. Francis IR, Glazer GM, Bookstein FL, et al. The thymus: reexamination of age-related changes in size and shape. AJR Am J Roentgenol 1985;145:249–254.

513. Baron RL, Lee JK, Sagel SS, et al. Computed tomography of the normal thymus. Radiology 1982;142:121–125.

514. de Geer G, Webb WR, Gamsu G. Normal thymus: assessment with MR and CT. Radiology 1986;158:313–317.

515. Boothroyd AE, Hall-Craggs MA, Dicks-Mireaux C, et al. The magnetic resonance appearances of the normal thymus in children. Clin Radiol 1992;45:378–381.

516. Molina PL, Siegel MJ, Glazer HS. Thymic masses on MR imaging. AJR Am J Roentgenol 1990;155:495–500.

517. Siegel MJ, Glazer HS, Wiener JI, et al. Normal and abnormal thymus in childhood: MR imaging. Radiology 1989;172:367–371.

518. Lemaitre L, Marconi V, Avni F, et al. The sonographic evaluation of normal thymus in infants and children. Eur J Radiol 1987;7:130–136.

519. Carty H. Ultrasound of the normal thymus in the infant: a simple method of resolving a clinical dilemma. Br J Radiol 1990;63:737–738.

520. Han BK, Babcock DS, Oestreich AE. Normal thymus in infancy: sonographic characteristics. Radiology 1989;170:471–474.

521. Baron RL, Lee JK, Sagel SS, et al. Computed tomography of the abnormal thymus. Radiology 1982;142:127–134.

522. Franken EA. Radiologic evidence of thymic enlargement in Grave's disease. Radiology 1969;91:20–22.

523. Wortsman J, McConnachie P, Baker JR Jr, et al. Immunoglobulins that cause thymocyte proliferation from a patient with Graves' disease and an enlarged thymus. Am J Med 1988;85:117–121.

524. Rosenow EC 3rd, Hurley BT. Disorders of the thymus. A review. Arch Intern Med 1984;144:763–770.

525. Arliss J, Scholes J, Dickson PR, et al. Massive thymic hyperplasia in an adolescent. Ann Thorac Surg 1988;45:220–222.

526. Nicolaou S, Müller NL, Li DK, et al. Thymus in myasthenia gravis: comparison of CT and pathologic findings and clinical outcome after thymectomy. Radiology 1996;201:471–474.

527. Batra P, Herrmann C Jr, Mulder D. Mediastinal imaging in myasthenia gravis: correlation of chest radiography, CT, MR, and surgical findings. AJR Am J Roentgenol 1987;148:515–519.

528. Goldberg RE, Haaga JR, Yulish BS. Serial CT scans in thymic hyperplasia. J Comput Assist Tomog 1988;11:539–540.

529. Brown LR, Muhm JR, Sheedy PF 2nd, et al. The value of computed tomography in myasthenia gravis. AJR Am J Roentgenol 1983;140:31–35.

530. Fon GT, Bein ME, Mancuso AA, et al. Computed tomography of the anterior mediastinum in myasthenia gravis. A radiologic-pathologic correlative study. Radiology 1982;142:135–141.

531. Choyke PL, Zeman RK, Gootenberg JE, et al. Thymic atrophy and regrowth in response to chemotherapy: CT evaluation. AJR Am J Roentgenol 1987;149:269–272.

532. Hendrickx P, Dohring W. Thymic atrophy and rebound enlargement following chemotherapy for testicular cancer. Acta Radiol 1989;30:263–267.

533. Abildgaard A, Lien HH, Fossa SD, et al. Enlargement of the thymus following chemotherapy for non-seminomatous testicular cancer. Acta Radiol 1989;30:259–262.

534. Kissin CM, Husband JE, Nicholas D, et al. Benign thymic enlargement in adults after chemotherapy: CT demonstration. Radiology 1987;163:67–70.

535. Due W, Dieckmann KP, Stein H. Thymic hyperplasia following chemotherapy of a testicular germ cell tumor. Immunohistological evidence for a simple rebound phenomenon. Cancer 1989;63:446–449.

536. Willich E. Clinical features of thymic hyperplasia. In: Walter E, Willich E, Webb WR, eds. The thymus: diagnostic imaging, functions and pathologic anatomy. Berlin: Springer-Verlag, 1992.

537. Chertoff J, Barth RA, Dickerman JD. Rebound thymic hyperplasia five years after chemotherapy for Wilms' tumor. Pediatr Radiol 1991;21:596–597.

538. Caffey J, Silbey R. Regrowth and overgrowth of the thymus after atrophy induced by the oral administration of adrenocorticosteroids to human infants. Pediatrics 1960;26:762–770.

539. Doppman JL, Oldfield EH, Chrousos GP, et al. Rebound thymic hyperplasia after treatment of Cushing's syndrome. AJR Am J Roentgenol 1986;147:1145–1147.

540. Gelfand DW, Goldman AS, Law EJ, et al. Thymic hyperplasia in children recovering from thermal burns. J Trauma 1972;12:813–817.

541. Rizk G, Cueto L, Amplatz K. Rebound enlargement of the thymus after successful corrective surgery for transposition of the great vessels. Am J Roentgenol Radium Ther Nucl Med 1972;116:528–530.

542. Wenger MC, Cohen AJ, Greensite F. Thymic rebound in a patient with scrotal mesothelioma. J Thorac Imaging 1994;9:145–147.

543. Cohen M, Hill CA, Cangir A, et al. Thymic rebound after treatment of childhood tumors. AJR Am J Roentgenol 1980;135:151–156.

544. Luker GD, Siegel MJ. Mediastinal Hodgkin disease in children: response to therapy. Radiology 1993;189:737–740.

545. Foulner D. Case report: transient thymic calcification – association with rebound enlargement. Clin Radiol 1991;44:428–429.

546. Small EJ, Venook AP, Damon LE. Gallium-avid thymic hyperplasia in an adult after chemotherapy for Hodgkin disease. Cancer 1993;72:905–908.

547. Rettenbacher L, Galvan G. Differentiation between residual cancer and thymic hyperplasia in malignant non-Hodgkin's lymphoma with somatostatin receptor scintigraphy. Clin Nucl Med 1994;19:64–65.

548. Ford EG, Lockhart SK, Sullivan MP, et al. Mediastinal mass following chemotherapeutic treatment of Hodgkin's disease: recurrent tumor or thymic hyperplasia? J Pediatr Surg 1987;22:1155–1159.

549. Wittram C, Fischman AJ, Mark E, et al. Thymic enlargement and FDG uptake in three patients: CT and FDG positron emission tomography correlated with pathology. AJR Am J Roentgenol 2003;180:519–522.

550. Strollo DC, Rosado-de-Christenson ML. Tumors of the thymus. J Thorac Imaging 1999;14:152–171.

551. Rosado-de-Christenson ML, Galobardes J, Moran CA. Thymoma: radiologic-pathologic correlation. RadioGraphics 1992;12:151–168.

552. Tan A, Holdener GP, Hecht A, et al. Malignant thymoma in an ectopic thymus: CT appearance. J Comput Assist Tomogr 1991;15:842–844.

553. Cooper GN Jr, Narodick BG. Posterior mediastinal thymoma: case report. J Thorac Cardiovasc Surg 1972;63:561–563.

554. Souadjian JV, Enriquez P, Silverstein MN, et al. The spectrum of diseases associated with thymoma. Coincidence or syndrome? Arch Intern Med 1974;134:374–379.

555. Morgenthaler TI, Brown LR, Colby TV, et al. Thymoma. Mayo Clin Proc 1993;68:1110–1123.

556. Lewis JE, Wick MR, Scheithauer BW, et al. Thymoma. A clinicopathologic review. Cancer 1987;60:2727–2743.

557. Spedini P, D'Adda M, Blanzuoli L. Thymoma and pancytopenia: a very rare association. Haematologica 2002;87:EIM18.

558. Tuncer Elmaci N, Ratip S, Ince-Gunal D, et al. Myasthenia gravis with thymoma and autoimmune haemolytic anaemia. A case report. Neurol Sci 2003;24:34–36.

559. Newsom-Davis J. Therapy in myasthenia gravis and Lambert-Eaton

myasthenic syndrome. Semin Neurol 2003;23:191–198.

560. Vernino S, Cheshire WP, Lennon VA. Myasthenia gravis with autoimmune autonomic neuropathy. Auton Neurosci 2001;88:187–192.

561. Evoli A, Lo Monaco M, Marra R, et al. Multiple paraneoplastic diseases associated with thymoma. Neuromuscul Disord 1999;9:601–603.

562. Weissel M, Mayr N, Zeitlhofer J. Clinical significance of autoimmune thyroid disease in myasthenia gravis. Exp Clin Endocrinol Diabetes 2000;108: 63–65.

563. Bosch EP, Reith PE, Granner DK. Myasthenia gravis and Schmidt syndrome. Neurology 1977;27: 1179–1180.

564. Christensen PB, Jensen TS, Tsiropoulos I, et al. Associated autoimmune diseases in myasthenia gravis. A population-based study. Acta Neurol Scand 1995;91: 192–195.

565. Barbosa RE, Cordova S, Cajigas JC. Coexistence of systemic lupus erythematosus and myasthenia gravis. Lupus 2000;9:156–157.

566. Mais DD, Mulhall BP, Adolphson KR, et al. Thymoma-associated autoimmune enteropathy. A report of two cases. Am J Clin Pathol 1999;112:810–815.

567. Lowry PW, Myers JD, Geller A, et al. Graft-versus-host-like colitis and malignant thymoma. Dig Dis Sci 2002;47:1998–2001.

568. Lasseur C, Combe C, Deminiere C, et al. Thymoma associated with myasthenia gravis and minimal lesion nephrotic syndrome. Am J Kidney Dis 1999;33:e4.

569. Di Cataldo A, Villari L, Milone P, et al. Thymic carcinoma, systemic lupus erythematosus, and hypertrophic pulmonary osteoarthropathy in an 11-year-old boy: a novel association. Pediatr Hematol Oncol 2000;17:701–706.

570. Papatestas AE, Alpert LI, Osserman KE, et al. Studies in myasthenia gravis: effects of thymectomy. Results on 185 patients with nonthymomatous and thymomatous myasthenia gravis, 1941–1969. Am J Med 1971;50:465–474.

571. Moore AV, Korobkin M, Powers B, et al. Thymoma detection by mediastinal CT: patient with myasthenia gravis. AJR Am J Roentgenol 1982;138:217–222.

572. Monden Y, Nakahara K, Kagotani K, et al. Myasthenia gravis with thymoma: analysis of and postoperative prognosis for 65 patients with thymomatous myasthenia gravis. Ann Thorac Surg 1984;38:46–52.

573. Masaoka A, Monden Y, Nakahara K, et al. Follow-up study of thymomas with special reference to their clinical stages. Cancer 1981;48:2485–2492.

574. Sakai F, Sone S, Kiyono K, et al. MR imaging of thymoma: radiologic-pathologic correlation. AJR Am J Roentgenol 1992;158:751–756.

575. Moran CA, Travis WD, Rosado-de-Christenson M, et al. Thymomas presenting as pleural tumors. Report of eight cases. Am J Surg Pathol 1992;16:138–144.

576. Lastoria S, Palmieri G, Muto P, et al. Functional imaging of thymic disorders. Ann Med 1999;31 Suppl 2:63–69.

577. Ohta H, Taniguchi T, Watanabe H. T1-201 and Tc-99m HMPAO SPECT in a patient with recurrent thymoma. Clin Nucl Med 1996;21:902–903.

578. Hashimoto T, Goto K, Hishinuma Y, et al. Uptake of 99mTc-tetrofosmin, 99mTc-MIBI and 201Tl in malignant thymoma. Ann Nucl Med 2000;14: 293–298.

579. Hashimoto T, Takahashi K, Goto M, et al. Tc-99m tetrofosmin uptake of malignant thymoma in primary tumor and metastatic lesions. Clin Nucl Med 2001;26:562–564.

580. Kubota K, Yamada S, Kondo T, et al. PET imaging of primary mediastinal tumours. Br J Cancer 1996;73:882–886.

581. Lastoria S, Vergara E, Palmieri G, et al. In vivo detection of malignant thymic masses by indium-111-DTPA-D-Phe1-octreotide scintigraphy. J Nucl Med 1998;39:634–639.

582. Lee JD, Choe KO, Kim SJ, et al. CT findings in primary thymic carcinoma. J Comput Assist Tomogr 1991;15:429–433.

583. Hsu CP, Chen CY, Chen CL, et al. Thymic carcinoma. Ten years' experience in twenty patients. J Thorac Cardiovasc Surg 1994;107:615–620.

584. Wick MR, Scheithauer BW, Weiland LH, et al. Primary thymic carcinomas. Am J Surg Pathol 1982;6:613–630.

585. Negron-Soto JM, Cascade PN. Squamous cell carcinoma of the thymus with paraneoplastic hypercalcemia. Clin Imaging 1995;19:122–124.

586. Do YS, Im JG, Lee BH, et al. CT findings in malignant tumors of thymic epithelium. J Comput Assist Tomogr 1995;19:192–197.

587. Kushihashi T, Fujisawa H, Munechika H. Magnetic resonance imaging of thymic epithelial tumors. Crit Rev Diagn Imaging 1996;37:191–259.

588. Heron CW, Husband JE, Williams MP. Hodgkin disease: CT of the thymus. Radiology 1988;167:647–651.

589. Wernecke K, Vassallo P, Rutsch F, et al. Thymic involvement in Hodgkin disease: CT and sonographic findings. Radiology 1991;181:375–383.

590. Federle MP, Callen PW. Cystic Hodgkin's lymphoma of the thymus: computed tomography appearance. J Comput Assist Tomogr 1979;3:542–544.

591. Spiers AS, Husband JE, MacVicar AD. Treated thymic lymphoma: comparison of MR imaging with CT. Radiology 1997;203:369–376.

592. Jerusalem G, Beguin Y, Fassotte MF, et al. Early detection of relapse by whole-body positron emission tomography in the follow-up of patients with Hodgkin's disease. Ann Oncol 2003;14:123–130.

593. Bangerter M, Kotzerke J, Griesshammer M, et al. Positron emission tomography with 18-fluorodeoxyglucose in the staging and follow-up of lymphoma in the chest. Acta Oncol 1999;38:799–804.

594. Brink I, Reinhardt MJ, Hoegerle S, et al. Increased metabolic activity in the thymus gland studied with ^{18}F-FDG PET: age dependency and frequency after chemotherapy. J Nucl Med 2001;42:591–595.

595. Rosado de Christenson ML, Abbott GF, Kirejczyk WM, et al. Thoracic carcinoids: radiologic-pathologic correlation. RadioGraphics 1999;19:707–736.

596. Klemm KM, Moran CA. Primary neuroendocrine carcinomas of the thymus. Semin Diagn Pathol 1999;16:32–41.

597. Klemm KM, Moran CA, Suster S. Pigmented thymic carcinoids: a clinicopathological and immunohistochemical study of two cases. Mod Pathol 1999;12:946–948.

598. Chaer R, Massad MG, Evans A, et al. Primary neuroendocrine tumors of the thymus. Ann Thorac Surg 2002;74:1733–1740.

599. Blunt SB, Sandler LM, Burrin JM, et al. An evaluation of the distinction of ectopic and pituitary ACTH dependent Cushing's syndrome by clinical features, biochemical tests and radiological findings. Q J Med 1990;77:1113–1133.

600. Doppman JL, Nieman L, Miller DL, et al. Ectopic adrenocorticotropic hormone syndrome: localization studies in 28 patients. Radiology 1989;172:115–124.

601. Jex RK, van Heerden JA, Carpenter PC, et al. Ectopic ACTH syndrome. Diagnostic and therapeutic aspects. Am J Surg 1985;149:276–282.

602. Vincent JM, Trainer PJ, Reznek RH, et al. The radiological investigation of occult ectopic ACTH-dependent Cushing's syndrome. Clin Radiol 1993;48:11–17.

603. Gibril F, Chen YJ, Schrump DS, et al. Prospective study of thymic carcinoids in patients with multiple endocrine neoplasia type 1. J Clin Endocrinol Metab 2003;88:1066–1081.

604. Teh BT. Thymic carcinoids in multiple endocrine neoplasia type 1. J Intern Med 1998;243:501–504.

605. de Montpreville VT, Macchiarini P, Dulmet E. Thymic neuroendocrine carcinoma (carcinoid): a clinicopathologic study of fourteen cases. J Thorac Cardiovasc Surg 1996;111:134–141.

606. Wang DY, Chang DB, Kuo SH, et al. Carcinoid tumours of the thymus. Thorax 1994;49:357–360.

607. Brown LR, Aughenbaugh GL, Wick MR, et al. Roentgenologic diagnosis of primary corticotropin-producing carcinoid tumors of the mediastinum. Radiology 1982;142:143–148.

608. Cadigan DG, Hollett PD, Collingwood PW, et al. Imaging of a mediastinal thymic carcinoid tumor with radiolabeled somatostatin analogue. Clin Nucl Med 1996;21:487–488.

609. Hirano T, Otake H, Watanabe N, et al. Presurgical diagnosis of a primary carcinoid tumor of the thymus with MIBG. J Nucl Med 1995;36:2243–2245.

610. Tonami N, Yokoyama K, Nonomura A, et al. Intense accumulation of Tl-201 in carcinoid tumor of the thymus. Clin Nucl Med 1994;19:408–412.

611. Casullo J, Palayew MJ, Lisbona A. General case of the day. Thymolipoma. RadioGraphics 1992;12:1250–1254.

612. Rosado-de-Christenson ML, Pugatch RD, Moran CA, et al. Thymolipoma: analysis of 27 cases. Radiology 1994;193:121–126.

613. Otto HF, Loning T, Lachenmayer L, et al. Thymolipoma in association with myasthenia gravis. Cancer 1982;50:1623–1628.

614. Pan CH, Chiang CY, Chen SS. Thymolipoma in patients with myasthenia gravis: report of two cases and review. Acta Neurol Scand 1988;78:16–21.

615. Shirkhoda A, Chasen MH, Eftekhari F, et al. MR imaging of mediastinal thymolipoma. J Comput Assist Tomogr 1987;11:364–365.

616. Chew FS, Weissleder R. Mediastinal thymolipoma. AJR Am J Roentgenol 1991;157:468.

617. Teplick JG, Nedwich A, Haskin ME. Roentgenographic features of thymolipoma. Am J Roentgenol Radium Ther Nucl Med 1973;117:873–880.

618. Moran CA, Rosado-de-Christenson M, Suster S. Thymolipoma: clinicopathologic review of 33 cases. Mod Pathol 1995;8:741–744.

619. Sltzer RA, Mills DS, Baddock SS, et al. Mediastinal thymic cyst. Dis Chest 1968;53:186–196.

620. Gonullu U, Gungor A, Savas I, et al. Huge thymic cysts. J Thorac Cardiovasc Surg 1996;112:835–836.

621. Barrick B, O'Kell RT. Thymic cysts and remnant cervical thymus. J Pediatr Surg 1969;4:355–358.

622. Graeber GM, Thompson LD, Cohen DJ, et al. Cystic lesion of the thymus. An occasionally malignant cervical and/or anterior mediastinal mass. J Thorac Cardiovasc Surg 1984;87:295–300.

623. Sirivella S, Gielchinsky I, Parsonnet V. Mediastinal thymic cysts: a report of three cases. J Thorac Cardiovasc Surg 1995;110:1771–1772.

624. Chalaoui J, Samson L, Robillard P, et al. Cases of the day. General. Benign thymic cyst complicated by hemorrhage. RadioGraphics 1990;10:957–958.

625. Moskowitz PS, Noon MA, McAlister WH, et al. Thymic cyst hemorrhage: a cause of acute, symptomatic mediastinal widening in children with aplastic anemia. AJR Am J Roentgenol 1980;134:832–836.

626. Gouliamos A, Striggaris K, Lolas C, et al. Thymic cyst. J Comput Assist Tomogr 1982;6:172–174.

627. Merine DS, Fishman EK, Zerhouni EA. Computed tomography and magnetic resonance imaging diagnosis of thymic cyst. J Comput Tomogr 1988;12:220–222.

628. Murayama S, Murakami J, Watanabe H, et al. Signal intensity characteristics of mediastinal cystic masses on T1-weighted MRI. J Comput Assist Tomogr 1995;19:188–191.

629. Lindfors KK, Meyer JE, Dedrick CG, et al. Thymic cysts in mediastinal Hodgkin disease. Radiology 1985;156:37–41.

630. Dyer NH. Cystic thymomas and thymic cysts. A review. Thorax 1967;22:408–421.

631. Baron RL, Sagel SS, Baglan RJ. Thymic cysts following radiation therapy for Hodgkin disease. Radiology 1981;141:593–597.

632. Wong-You-Cheong J, Radford JA. Case report: enlargement of a mediastinal mass during treatment for Hodgkin's disease may be due to accumulation of fluid within thymic cysts. Clin Radiol 1995;50:61–62.

633. Veeze-Kuijpers B, Van Andel JG, Stiegelis WF, et al thymic cyst following mantle radiotherapy for Hodgkin's disease. Clin Radiol 1987;38:289–290.

634. Kim HC, Nosher J, Haas A, et al. Cystic degeneration of thymic Hodgkin's disease following radiation therapy. Cancer 1985;55:354–356.

635. Avila NA, Mueller BU, Carrasquillo JA, et al. Multilocular thymic cysts: imaging features in children with human immunodeficiency virus infection. Radiology 1996;201:130–134.

636. Leonidas JC, Berdon WE, Valderrama E, et al. Human immunodeficiency virus infection and multilocular thymic cysts. Radiology 1996;198:377–379.

637. Mercado-Deane MG, Sabio H, Burton EM, et al. Cystic thymic hyperplasia in a child with HIV infection: imaging findings. AJR Am J Roentgenol 1996;166:171–172.

638. Mishalani SH, Lones MA, Said JW. Multilocular thymic cyst. A novel thymic lesion associated with human immunodeficiency virus infection. Arch Pathol Lab Med 1995;119:467–470.

639. Shalaby-Rana E, Selby D, Ivy P, et al. Multilocular thymic cyst in a child with acquired immunodeficiency syndrome. Pediatr Infect Dis J 1996;15:83–86.

640. Jaramillo D, Perez-Atayde A, Griscom NT. Apparent association between thymic cysts and prior thoracotomy. Radiology 1989;172:207–209.

641. Choi YW, McAdams HP, Jeon SC, et al. Idiopathic multilocular thymic cyst: CT features with clinical and histopathologic correlation. AJR Am J Roentgenol 2001;177:881–885.

642. Glazer GM, Axel L, Moss AA. CT diagnosis of mediastinal thyroid. AJR Am J Roentgenol 1982;138:495–498.

643. Morris UL, Colletti PM, Ralls PW, et al. CT demonstration of intrathoracic thyroid tissue. J Comput Assist Tomogr 1982;6:821–824.

644. Bashist B, Ellis K, Gold RP. Computed tomography of intrathoracic goiters. AJR Am J Roentgenol 1983;140:455–460.

645. Higgins CB, McNamara MT, Fisher MR, et al. MR imaging of the thyroid. AJR Am J Roentgenol 1986;147:1255–1261.

646. Gefter WB, Spritzer CE, Eisenberg B, et al. Thyroid imaging with high-field-strength surface-coil MR. Radiology 1987;164:483–490.

647. Higgins CB, Auffermann W. MR imaging of thyroid and parathyroid glands: a review of current status. AJR Am J Roentgenol 1988;151:1095–1106.

648. Hall TS, Caslowitz P, Popper C, et al. Substernal goiter versus intrathoracic aberrant thyroid: a critical difference. Ann Thorac Surg 1988;46:684–685.

649. Sand J, Pehkonen E, Mattila J, et al. Pulsating mass at the sternum: a primary carcinoma of ectopic mediastinal thyroid. J Thorac Cardiovasc Surg 1996;112:833–835.

650. Sussman SK, Silverman PM, Donnal JF. CT demonstration of isolated mediastinal goiter. J Comput Assist Tomogr 1986;10:863–864.

651. Komolafe F. Radiological patterns and significance of thyroid calcification. Clin Radiol 1981;32:571–575.

652. Holtz S, Powers WE. Calcification in papillary carcinoma of the thyroid. AJR Am J Roentgenol 1958;80:997–1000.

653. Margolin FR, Winfield J, Steinbach HL. Patterns of thyroid calcification. Roentgenologic-histologic study of excised specimens. Invest Radiol 1967;2:208–212.

654. Park CH, Rothermel FJ, Judge DM. Unusual calcification in mixed papillary and follicular carcinoma of the thyroid gland. Radiology 1976;119:554.

655. Binder RE, Pugatch RD, Faling LJ, et al. Diagnosis of posterior mediastinal goiter by computed tomography. J Comput Assist Tomogr 1980;4:550–552.

656. Bryk D. Venous compression and obstruction by intrathoracic goiter. J Can Assoc Radiol 1974;25:300–302.

657. von Schulthess GK, McMurdo K, Tscholakoff D, et al. Mediastinal masses: MR imaging. Radiology 1986;158: 289–296.

658. Noma S, Nishimura K, Togashi K, et al. Thyroid gland: MR imaging. Radiology 1987;164:495–499.

659. Irwin RS, Braman SS, Arvanitidis AN, et al. 131I thyroid scanning in preoperative diagnosis of mediastinal goiter. Ann Intern Med 1978;89:73–74.

660. Keene RJ, Steiner RE, Olsen EJ, et al. Aortic root aneurysm – radiographic and pathologic features. Clin Radiol 1971;22:330–340.

661. Szamosi A. Radiological detection of aneurysms involving the aortic root. Radiology 1981;138:551–555.

662. Krinsky GA, Rofsky NM, DeCorato DR, et al. Thoracic aorta: comparison of gadolinium-enhanced three-dimensional MR angiography with conventional MR imaging. Radiology 1997;202:183–193.

663. Boxerman JL, Mosher TJ, McVeigh ER, et al. Advanced MR imaging techniques for evaluation of the heart and great vessels. RadioGraphics 1998;18:543–564.

664. Prince MR, Narasimham DL, Jacoby WT, et al. Three-dimensional gadolinium-enhanced MR angiography of the thoracic aorta. AJR Am J Roentgenol 1996;166:1387–1397.

665. Ho VB, Prince MR. Thoracic MR aortography: imaging techniques and strategies. RadioGraphics 1998;18:287–309.

666. Krinsky G, Weinreb J. Gadolinium-enhanced three-dimensional MR angiography of the thoracoabdominal aorta. Semin Ultrasound CT MR 1996;17:280–303.

667. Leung DA, Debatin JF. Three-dimensional contrast-enhanced magnetic resonance angiography of the thoracic vasculature. Eur Radiol 1997;7:981–989.

668. Chung JW, Park JH, Im JG, et al. Spiral CT angiography of the thoracic aorta. RadioGraphics 1996;16:811–824.

669. Kimura F, Shen Y, Date S, et al. Thoracic aortic aneurysm and aortic dissection: new endoscopic mode for three-dimensional CT display of aorta. Radiology 1996;198:573–578.

670. Kopecky KK, Gokhale HS, Hawes DR. Spiral CT angiography of the aorta. Semin Ultrasound CT MR 1996;17:304–315.

671. Quint LE, Francis IR, Williams DM, et al. Evaluation of thoracic aortic disease with the use of helical CT and multiplanar reconstructions: comparison with surgical findings. Radiology 1996;201:37–41.

672. Rubin GD. Helical CT angiography of the thoracic aorta. J Thorac Imaging 1997;12:128–149.

673. Zeman RK, Berman PM, Silverman PM, et al. Diagnosis of aortic dissection: value of helical CT with multiplanar reformation and three-dimensional rendering. AJR Am J Roentgenol 1995;164:1375–1380.

674. Cramer M, Foley WD, Palmer TE, et al. Compression of the right pulmonary artery by aortic aneurysms: CT demonstration. J Comput Assist Tomogr 1985;9:310–314.

675. Duke RA, Barrett MR 2nd, Payne SD, et al. Compression of left main bronchus and left pulmonary artery by thoracic aortic aneurysm. AJR Am J Roentgenol 1987;149:261–263.

676. Elefteriades JA. Natural history of thoracic aortic aneurysms: indications for surgery, and surgical versus nonsurgical risks. Ann Thorac Surg 2002;74:S1877–1880; discussion S1892–1898.

677. Davies RR, Goldstein LJ, Coady MA, et al. Yearly rupture or dissection rates for thoracic aortic aneurysms: simple prediction based on size. Ann Thorac Surg 2002;73:17–27; discussion 27–28.

678. Coady MA, Rizzo JA, Hammond GL, et al. What is the appropriate size criterion for resection of thoracic aortic aneurysms? J Thorac Cardiovasc Surg 1997;113:476–491; discussion 489–491.

679. Smith TR, Khoury PT. Aneurysm of the proximal thoracic aorta simulating neoplasm: the role of CT and angiography. AJR Am J Roentgenol 1985;144:909–910.

680. Posniak HV, Olson MC, Demos TC, et al. CT of thoracic aortic aneurysms. RadioGraphics 1990;10:839–855.

681. Rubin GD. MDCT imaging of the aorta and peripheral vessels. Eur J Radiol 2003;45 Suppl 1:S42–49.

682. Rubin GD. CT angiography of the thoracic aorta. Semin Roentgenol 2003;38:115–134.

683. Kalender WA, Prokop M. 3D CT angiography. Crit Rev Diagn Imaging 2001;42:1–28.

684. Heiberg E, Wolverson MK, Sundaram M, et al. CT characteristics of aortic atherosclerotic aneurysm versus aortic dissection. J Comput Assist Tomogr 1985;9:78–83.

685. White RD, Higgins CB. Magnetic resonance imaging of thoracic vascular disease. J Thorac Imaging 1989;4:34–50.

686. Gundry SR, Burney RE, Mackenzie JR, et al. Traumatic pseudoaneurysms of the thoracic aorta. Anatomic and radiologic correlations. Arch Surg 1984;119:1055–1060.

687. Heystraten FM, Rosenbusch G, Kingma LM, et al. Chronic posttraumatic aneurysm of the thoracic aorta: surgically correctable occult threat. AJR Am J Roentgenol 1986;146:303–308.

688. Hirsch JH, Carter SJ, Chikos PM. Traumatic pseudoaneurysms of the thoracic aorta: two unusual cases. AJR Am J Roentgenol 1978;130:157–160.

689. Reed DH. Mycotic pseudoaneurysm of the descending thoracic aorta associated with vertebral osteomyelitis. Clin Radiol 1990;41:427–429.

690. Manzi SV, Fultz PJ, Sickel JZ, et al. Chest mass in a patient with leukemia with hemoptysis. Invest Radiol 1994;29: 940–943.

691. Feltis BA, Lee DA, Beilman GJ. Mycotic aneurysm of the descending thoracic aorta caused by Pseudomonas aeruginosa in a solid organ transplant recipient: case report and review. Surg Infect (Larchmt) 2002;3:29–33.

692. Feigl D, Feigl A, Edwards JE. Mycotic aneurysms of the aortic root. A pathologic study of 20 cases. Chest 1986;90:553–557.

693. Lee MH, Chan P, Chiou HJ, et al. Diagnostic imaging of Salmonella-related mycotic aneurysm of aorta by CT. Clin Imaging 1996;20:26–30.

694. Gufler H, Buitrago-Tellez CH, Nesbitt E, et al. Mycotic aneurysm rupture of the descending aorta. Eur Radiol 1998;8:295–297.

695. Edwards JE. Manifestations of acquired and congenital diseases of the aorta. Curr Probl Cardiol 1979;3:1–62.

696. Gelsomino S, Morocutti G, Frassani R, et al. Long-term results of Bentall composite aortic root replacement for ascending aortic aneurysms and dissections. Chest 2003;124:984–988.

697. Pacini D, Ranocchi F, Angeli E, et al. Aortic root replacement with composite valve graft. Ann Thorac Surg 2003;76: 90–98.

698. Gelsomino S, Masullo G, Morocutti G, et al. Sixteen-year results of composite aortic root replacement for non-dissecting chronic aortic aneurysms. Ital Heart J 2003;4:454–459.

699. Carlson RG, Lillehei CW, Edwards JE. Cystic medial necrosis of the ascending aorta in relation to age and hypertension. Am J Cardiol 1970;25:411–415.

700. Castaner E, Andreu M, Gallardo X, et al. CT in nontraumatic acute thoracic aortic disease: typical and atypical features and complications. RadioGraphics 2003;23 Spec No:S93–110.

701. Macura KJ, Corl FM, Fishman EK, et al. Pathogenesis in acute aortic syndromes: aortic dissection, intramural hematoma, and penetrating atherosclerotic aortic ulcer. AJR Am J Roentgenol 2003;181:309–316.

702. Larson EW, Edwards WD. Risk factors for aortic dissection: a necropsy study of 161 cases. Am J Cardiol 1984;53:849–855.

703. Crawford ES. The diagnosis and management of aortic dissection. JAMA 1990;264:2537–2541.

704. DeBakey ME, McCollum CH, Crawford ES, et al. Dissection and dissecting aneurysms of the aorta: twenty-year follow-up of five hundred twenty-seven

patients treated surgically. Surgery 1982;92:1118–1134.

705. DeBakey ME, Henly WS, Cooley DA. Surgical management of dissecting aneurysms of the aorta. J Thorac Cardiovasc Surg 1965;49:130–149.

706. Appelbaum A, Karp RB, Kirklin JW. Ascending vs descending aortic dissections. Ann Surg 1976;183:296–300.

707. Miller DG, Stinson EB, Oyer PB. Operative treatment of aortic dissection: experience with 125 patients over a sixteen-year period. J Thorac Cardiovasc Surg 1979;78:365–382.

708. Wheat MW, Jr. Acute dissection of the aorta. Cardiovasc Clin 1987;17:241–262.

709. Apaydin AZ, Buket S, Posacioglu H, et al. Perioperative risk factors for mortality in patients with acute type A aortic dissection. Ann Thorac Surg 2002;74:2034–2039; discussion 2039.

710. Umana JP, Lai DT, Mitchell RS, et al. Is medical therapy still the optimal treatment strategy for patients with acute type B aortic dissections? J Thorac Cardiovasc Surg 2002;124:896–910.

711. Umana JP, Miller DC, Mitchell RS. What is the best treatment for patients with acute type B aortic dissections – medical, surgical, or endovascular stent-grafting? Ann Thorac Surg 2002;74:S1840–1843; discussion S1857–1863.

712. Elefteriades JA, Lovoulos CJ, Coady MA, et al. Management of descending aortic dissection. Ann Thorac Surg 1999;67:2002–2005; discussion 2014–2019.

713. Spittell PC, Spittell JA Jr, Joyce JW, et al. Clinical features and differential diagnosis of aortic dissection: experience with 236 cases (1980 through 1990). Mayo Clin Proc 1993;68:642–651.

714. Yamada T, Tada S, Harada J. Aortic dissection without intimal rupture: diagnosis with MR imaging and CT. Radiology 1988;168:347–352.

715. Erbel R, Oelert H, Meyer J, et al. Effect of medical and surgical therapy on aortic dissection evaluated by transesophageal echocardiography. Implications for prognosis and therapy. The European Cooperative Study Group on Echocardiography. Circulation 1993;87:1604–1615.

716. Nienaber CA, von Kodolitsch Y, Petersen B, et al. Intramural hemorrhage of the thoracic aorta. Diagnostic and therapeutic implications. Circulation 1995;92:1465–1472.

717. Robbins RC, McManus RP, Mitchell RS, et al. Management of patients with intramural hematoma of the thoracic aorta. Circulation 1993;88:II1–10.

718. Murray JG, Manisali M, Flamm SD, et al. Intramural hematoma of the thoracic aorta: MR image findings and their prognostic implications. Radiology 1997;204:349–355.

719. Motoyoshi N, Moizumi Y, Komatsu T, et al. Intramural hematoma and dissection involving ascending aorta: the clinical features and prognosis. Eur J Cardiothorac Surg 2003;24:237–242; discussion 242.

720. Sueyoshi E, Matsuoka Y, Sakamoto I, et al. Fate of intramural hematoma of the aorta: CT evaluation. J Comput Assist Tomogr 1997;21:931–938.

721. Evangelista A, Dominguez R, Sebastia C, et al. Long-term follow-up of aortic intramural hematoma: predictors of outcome. Circulation 2003;108:583–589.

722. Kaji S, Akasaka T, Katayama M, et al. Long-term prognosis of patients with type B aortic intramural hematoma. Circulation 2003;108 Suppl 1:II307–11.

723. Ide K, Uchida H, Otsuji H, et al. Acute aortic dissection with intramural hematoma: possibility of transition to classic dissection or aneurysm. J Thorac Imaging 1996;11:46–52.

724. Cooke JP, Kazmier FJ, Orszulak TA. The penetrating aortic ulcer: pathologic manifestations, diagnosis, and management. Mayo Clin Proc 1988; 63:718–725.

725. Harris JA, Bis KG, Glover JL, et al. Penetrating atherosclerotic ulcers of the aorta. J Vasc Surg 1994;19:90–98; discussion 98–99.

726. Hussain S, Glover JL, Bree R, et al. Penetrating atherosclerotic ulcers of the thoracic aorta. J Vasc Surg 1989;9: 710–717.

727. Kazerooni EA, Bree RL, Williams DM. Penetrating atherosclerotic ulcers of the descending thoracic aorta: evaluation with CT and distinction from aortic dissection. Radiology 1992;183:759–765.

728. Stanson AW, Kazmier FJ, Hollier LH, et al. Penetrating atherosclerotic ulcers of the thoracic aorta: natural history and clinicopathologic correlations. Ann Vasc Surg 1986;1:15–23.

729. Primack SL, Mayo JR, Fradet G. Perforated atherosclerotic ulcer of the aorta presenting with upper airway obstruction. Can Assoc Radiol J 1995;46:209–211.

730. Troxler M, Mavor AI, Homer-Vanniasinkam S. Penetrating atherosclerotic ulcers of the aorta. Br J Surg 2001;88:1169–1177.

731. Toda R, Moriyama Y, Iguro Y, et al. Penetrating atherosclerotic ulcer. Surg Today 2001;31:32–35.

732. Hayashi H, Matsuoka Y, Sakamoto I, et al. Penetrating atherosclerotic ulcer of the aorta: imaging features and disease concept. RadioGraphics 2000;20: 995–1005.

733. Coady MA, Rizzo JA, Elefteriades JA. Pathologic variants of thoracic aortic dissections. Penetrating atherosclerotic ulcers and intramural hematomas. Cardiol Clin 1999;17:637–657.

734. Coady MA, Rizzo JA, Hammond GL, et al. Penetrating ulcer of the thoracic aorta: what is it? How do we recognize it? How do we manage it? J Vasc Surg 1998;27:1006–1015; discussion 1015–1016.

735. Ganaha F, Miller DC, Sugimoto K, et al. Prognosis of aortic intramural hematoma with and without penetrating atherosclerotic ulcer: a clinical and radiological analysis. Circulation 2002;106:342–343.

736. Cigarroa JE, Isselbacher EM, DeSanctis RW, et al. Diagnostic imaging in the evaluation of suspected aortic dissection. Old standards and new directions. N Engl J Med 1993;328:35–43.

737. Treasure T. Imaging the dissected aorta. Br Heart J 1993;70:497–498.

738. Dee P, Martin R, Oudkerk M, Overbosch E. The diagnosis of aortic dissection. Curr Probl Diagn Radiol 1983;12:3–56.

739. Macura KJ, Szarf G, Fishman EK, et al. Role of computed tomography and magnetic resonance imaging in assessment of acute aortic syndromes. Semin Ultrasound CT MR 2003;24:232–224.

740. Levy JR, Heiken JP, Gutierrez FR. Imaging of penetrating atherosclerotic ulcers of the aorta. AJR Am J Roentgenol 1999;173:151–154.

741. Luker GD, Glazer HS, Eagar G, et al. Aortic dissection: effect of prospective chest radiographic diagnosis on delay to definitive diagnosis. Radiology 1994;193:813–819.

742. Hartnell GG, Wakeley CJ, Tottle A, et al. Limitations of chest radiography in discriminating between aortic dissection and myocardial infarction: implications for thrombolysis. J Thorac Imaging 1993;8:152–155.

743. Jagannath AS, Sos TA, Lockhart SH, et al. Aortic dissection: a statistical analysis of the usefulness of plain chest radiographic findings. AJR Am J Roentgenol 1986;147:1123–1126.

744. Hachiya J, Nitatori T, Yoshino A, et al. CT of calcified chronic aortic dissection simulating atherosclerotic aneurysm. J Comput Assist Tomogr 1993;17:374–378.

745. Erbel R, Engberding R, Daniel W, et al. Echocardiography in diagnosis of aortic dissection. Lancet 1989;1:457–461.

746. Demos TC, Posniak HV, Marsan RE. CT of aortic dissection. Semin Roentgenol 1989;24:22–37.

747. Bansal RC, Chandrasekaran K, Ayala K, et al. Frequency and explanation of false negative diagnosis of aortic dissection by aortography and transesophageal echocardiography. J Am Coll Cardiol 1995;25:1393–1401.

748. Petasnick JP. Radiologic evaluation of aortic dissection. Radiology 1991;180: 297–305.

749. Rizzo RJ, Aranki SF, Aklog L, et al. Rapid noninvasive diagnosis and surgical repair of acute ascending aortic dissection. Improved survival with less angiography. J Thorac Cardiovasc Surg 1994;108:567–574; discussion 574–575.

750. Oudkerk M, Overbosch E, Dee P. CT recognition of acute aortic dissection. AJR Am J Roentgenol 1983;141:671–676.

751. Singh H, Fitzgerald E, Ruttley MS. Computed tomography: the investigation of choice for aortic dissection? Br Heart J 1986;56:171–175.

752. Small JH, Dixon AK, Coulden RA, et al. Fast CT for aortic dissection. Br J Radiol 1996;69:900–905.

753. Sommer T, Fehske W, Holzknecht N, et al. Aortic dissection: a comparative study of diagnosis with spiral CT, multiplanar transesophageal echocardiography, and MR imaging. Radiology 1996;199:347–352.

754. Vasile N, Mathieu D, Keita K, ett al. Computed tomography of thoracic aortic dissection: accuracy and pitfalls. J Comput Assist Tomogr 1986;10: 211–215.

755. Nienaber CA, von Kodolitsch Y, Nicolas V, et al. The diagnosis of thoracic aortic dissection by noninvasive imaging procedures. N Engl J Med 1993;328:1–9.

756. Costello P, Ecker CP, Tello R, et al. Assessment of the thoracic aorta by spiral CT. AJR Am J Roentgenol 1992;158:1127–1130.

757. Hamada S, Takamiya M, Kimura K, et al. Type A aortic dissection: evaluation with ultrafast CT. Radiology 1992;183:155–158.

758. Stanford W, Rooholamini SA, Galvin JR. Ultrafast computed tomography in the diagnosis of aortic aneurysms and dissections. J Thorac Imaging 1990;5:32–39.

759. Thompson BH, Stanford W. Utility of ultrafast computed tomography in the detection of thoracic aortic aneurysms and dissections. Semin Ultrasound CT MR 1993;14:117–128.

760. Demos TC, Posniak HV, Churchill RJ. Detection of the intimal flap of aortic dissection on unenhanced CT images. AJR Am J Roentgenol 1986;146:601–603.

761. Duvernoy O, Coulden R, Ytterberg C. Aortic motion: a potential pitfall in CT imaging of dissection in the ascending aorta. J Comput Assist Tomogr 1995; 19:569–572.

762. Burns MA, Molina PL, Gutierrez FR, et al. Motion artifact simulating aortic dissection on CT. AJR Am J Roentgenol 1991;157:465–467.

763. Posniak HV, Olson MC, Demos TC. Aortic motion artifact simulating dissection on CT scans: elimination with reconstructive segmented images. AJR Am J Roentgenol 1993;161:557–558.

764. Godwin JD. Conventional CT of the aorta. J Thorac Imaging 1990;5:18–31.

765. Loubeyre P, Angelie E, Grozel F, et al. Spiral CT artifact that simulates aortic dissection: image reconstruction with use of 180 degrees and 360 degrees linear-interpolation algorithms. Radiology 1997;205:153–157.

766. Gallagher S, Dixon AK. Streak artefacts of the thoracic aorta: pseudodissection. J Comput Assist Tomogr 1984;8:688–693.

767. Larde D, Belloir C, Vasile N, et al. Computed tomography of aortic dissection. Radiology 1980;136:147–151.

768. White RD, Lipton MJ, Higgins CB, et al. Noninvasive evaluation of suspected thoracic aortic disease by contrast-enhanced computed tomography. Am J Cardiol 1986;57:282–290.

769. Williams DM, Lee DY, Hamilton BH, et al. The dissected aorta: part III. Anatomy and radiologic diagnosis of branch-vessel compromise. Radiology 1997;203:37–44.

770. Barentz JO, Rujis JH, Heystarten JM. Magnetic resonance imaging of the dissected thoracic aorta. Br J Radiol 1987;60:499–502.

771. Geisinger MA, Risius B, O'Donnell JA, et al. Thoracic aortic dissections: magnetic resonance imaging. Radiology 1985;155:407–412.

772. Kersting-Sommerhoff BA, Higgins CB, White RD, et al. Aortic dissection: sensitivity and specificity of MR imaging. Radiology 1988;166:651–655.

773. Panting JR, Norell MS, Baker C, et al. Feasibility, accuracy and safety of magnetic resonance imaging in acute aortic dissection. Clin Radiol 1995;50:455–458.

774. Laissy JP, Blanc F, Soyer P, et al. Thoracic aortic dissection: diagnosis with transesophageal echocardiography versus MR imaging. Radiology 1995;194:331–336.

775. Nienaber CA, Spielmann RP, von Kodolitsch Y, et al. Diagnosis of thoracic aortic dissection. Magnetic resonance imaging versus transesophageal echocardiography. Circulation 1992;85:434–447.

776. Tomiguchi S, Morishita S, Nakashima R, et al. Usefulness of turbo-FLASH dynamic MR imaging of dissecting aneurysms of the thoracic aorta. Cardiovasc Intervent Radiol 1994;17:17–21.

777. Sakuma H, Bourne MW, O'Sullivan M, et al. Evaluation of thoracic aortic dissection using breath-holding cine MR. J Comput Assist Tomog 1996;20:45–50.

778. Fischer U, Vosshenrich R, Kopka L, et al. Dissection of the thoracic aorta: pre- and postoperative findings on turbo-FLASH MR images obtained in the plane of the aortic arch. AJR Am J Roentgenol 1994;163:1069–1072.

779. Wolff KA, Herold CJ, Tempany CM, et al. Aortic dissection: atypical patterns seen at MR imaging. Radiology 1991;181:489–495.

780. Williams DM, Joshi A, Dake MD, et al. Aortic cobwebs: an anatomic marker identifying the false lumen in aortic dissection – imaging and pathologic correlation. Radiology 1994;190:167–174.

781. Chung JW, Park JH, Kim HC, et al. Entry tears of thoracic aortic dissections: MR appearance on gated SE imaging. J Comput Assist Tomogr 1994;18: 250–255.

782. Lotan CS, Cranney GB, Doyle M, et al. Fat-shift artifact simulating aortic dissection on MR images. AJR Am J Roentgenol 1989;152:385–386.

783. Solomon SL, Brown JJ, Glazer HS, et al. Thoracic aortic dissection: pitfalls and artifacts in MR imaging. Radiology 1990;177:223–228.

784. Savit RM, Panico RA. Case report: simulated thoracic aortic dissection on magnetic resonance in a patient with interruption of the inferior vena cava. Br J Radiol 1995;68:425–427.

785. Granato JE, Dee P, Gibson RS. Utility of two-dimensional echocardiography in suspected ascending aortic dissection. Am J Cardiol 1985;56:123–129.

786. Tottle AJ, Wilde P, Hartnell GG, et al. Diagnosis of acute thoracic aortic dissection using combined echocardiography and computed tomography. Clin Radiol 1992;45: 104–108.

787. Ballal RS, Nanda NC, Gatewood R, et al. Usefulness of transesophageal echocardiography in assessment of aortic dissection. Circulation 1991;84: 1903–1914.

788. Chirillo F, Cavallini C, Longhini C, et al. Comparative diagnostic value of transesophageal echocardiography and retrograde aortography in the evaluation of thoracic aortic dissection. Am J Cardiol 1994;74:590–595.

789. Hashimoto S, Kumada T, Osakada G, et al. Assessment of transesophageal Doppler echography in dissecting aortic aneurysm. J Am Coll Cardiol 1989;14: 1253–1262.

790. Erbel R, Borner N, Steller D, et al. Detection of aortic dissection by transoesophageal echocardiography. Br Heart J 1987;58:45–51.

791. Yamada E, Matsumura M, Kyo S, et al. Usefulness of a prototype intravascular ultrasound imaging in evaluation of aortic dissection and comparison with angiographic study, transesophageal echocardiography, computed tomography, and magnetic resonance imaging. Am J Cardiol 1995;75:161–165.

792. Wambeek ND, Cameron DC, Holden A. Intramural aortic dissection. Australas Radiol 1996;40:442–446.

793. Oliver TB, Murchison JT, Reid JH. Spiral CT in acute non-cardiac chest pain. Clin Radiol 1999;54:38–45.

794. Oliver TB, Murchison JT, Reid JH. Serial MRI in the management of intramural haemorrhage of the thoracic aorta. Br J Radiol 1997;70:1288–1290.

795. Mohr-Kahaly S, Erbel R, Kearney P, et al. Aortic intramural hemorrhage visualized by transesophageal echocardiography: findings and prognostic implications. J Am Coll Cardiol 1994;23:658–664.

796. Yucel EK, Steinberg FL, Egglin TK, et al Athanasoulis CA. Penetrating aortic ulcers: diagnosis with MR imaging. Radiology 1990;177:779–781.

797. Patel NH, Mann FA, Jurkovich GJ. Penetrating ulcer of the descending aorta mimicking a traumatic aortic laceration. AJR Am J Roentgenol 1996;166:20.

798. Welch TJ, Stanson AW, Sheedy PF 2nd, et al. Radiologic evaluation of penetrating aortic atherosclerotic ulcer. RadioGraphics 1990;10:675–685.

799. Williams MP, Farrow R. Atypical patterns in the CT diagnosis of aortic dissection. Clin Radiol 1994;49:686–689.

800. Deutsch HJ, Sechtem U, Meyer H, et al. Chronic aortic dissection: comparison of MR Imaging and transesophageal echocardiography. Radiology 1994;192:645–650.

801. Gaubert JY, Moulin G, Mesana T, et al. Type A dissection of the thoracic aorta: use of MR imaging for long-term follow-up. Radiology 1995;196:363–369.

802. Goldberg N, Krasnow N. Sinus of Valsalva aneurysms. Clin Cardiol 1990;13:831–836.

803. Gomes AS, Lois JF, George B, et al. Congenital abnormalities of the aortic arch: MR imaging. Radiology 1987;165:691–695.

804. Soler R, Rodriguez E, Requejo I, et al. Magnetic resonance imaging of congenital abnormalities of the thoracic aorta. Eur Radiol 1998;8:540–546.

805. Azarine A, Lions C, Koussa M, et al. Rupture of an aneurysm of the coronary sinus of Valsalva: diagnosis by helical CT angiography. Eur Radiol 2001;11:1371–1373.

806. Holland P, Fitzpatrick JD. Case report: magnetic resonance imaging of a right-sided cervical aortic arch with a congenital aneurysm. Clin Radiol 1991;43:352–355.

807. Evans JM, Bowles CA, Bjornsson J, et al. Thoracic aortic aneurysm and rupture in giant cell arteritis: descriptive study of 41 cases. Arthritis Rheum 1994;37:1539–1547.

808. Park JH. Conventional and CT angiographic diagnosis of Takayasu arteritis. Int J Cardiol 1996;54 Suppl:S165–171.

809. Angeli E, Vanzulli A, Venturini M, et al. The role of radiology in the diagnosis and management of Takayasu's arteritis. J Nephrol 2001;14:514–524.

810. Lui YQ. Radiology of aortoarteritis. Radiol Clin North Am 1985;23:671–688.

811. Matsunaga N, Hayashi K, Sakamoto I, et al. Takayasu arteritis: protean radiologic manifestations and diagnosis. RadioGraphics 1997;17:579–594.

812. Peterson IM, Guthaner DF. Aortic pseudoaneurysm complicating Takayasu disease: CT appearance. J Comput Assist Tomogr 1986;10:676–678.

813. Sharma S, Rajani M, Kamalakar T, et al. The association between aneurysm formation and systemic hypertension in Takayasu's arteritis. Clin Radiol 1990;42:182–187.

814. Yamato M, Lecky JW, Hiramatsu et al. Takayasu arteritis: radiographic and angiographic findings in 59 patients. Radiology 1986;161:329–334.

815. Yamada I, Nakagawa T, Himeno Y, et al. Takayasu arteritis: evaluation of the thoracic aorta with CT angiography. Radiology 1998;209:103–109.

816. Cole TJ, Henry DA, Jolles H, et al. Normal and abnormal vascular structures that simulate neoplasms on chest radiographs: clues to the diagnosis. RadioGraphics 1995;15:867–891.

817. VanDyke CW, White RD. Congenital abnormalities of the thoracic aorta presenting in the adult. J Thorac Imaging 1994;9:230–245.

818. Kessler RM, Miller KB, Pett S, et al. Pseudocoarctation of the aorta presenting as a mediastinal mass with dysphagia. Ann Thorac Surg 1993;55:1003–1005.

819. Safir J, Kerr A, Morehouse H, Frost A, et al. Magnetic resonance imaging of dissection in pseudocoarctation of the aorta. Cardiovasc Intervent Radiol 1993;16:180–182.

820. Sebastia C, Quiroga S, Boye R, et al. Aortic stenosis: spectrum of diseases depicted at multisection CT. RadioGraphics 2003;23 Spec No:S79–91.

821. Taneja K, Kawlra S, Sharma S, et al. Pseudocoarctation of the aorta: complementary findings on plain film radiography, CT, DSA, and MRA. Cardiovasc Intervent Radiol 1998;21:439–441.

822. Munjal AK, Rose WS, Williams G. Magnetic resonance imaging of pseudocoarctation of the aorta: a case report. J Thorac Imaging 1994;9:88–91.

823. Rossi SE, Erasmus JJ, McAdams HP, Donnelly LF. Thoracic manifestations of neurofibromatosis-I. AJR Am J Roentgenol 1999;173:1631–1638.

CHAPTER 15

Pleura and pleural disorders

PLEURAL PHYSIOLOGY AND PLEURAL EFFUSIONS (Box 15.1)

The outward pull of the chest wall and the inward recoil of the lung tend to separate the parietal and visceral pleura. These membranes are permeable to both gases and liquid, and are kept in apposition only because of mechanisms that keep the pleural space essentially free of gas and liquid. Gas is removed from the pleural space by systemic venous blood because the total gas pressure in venous blood is about 70 cmH$_2$O subatmospheric, and this provides a steep absorption gradient. The mechanisms governing the formation and absorption of pleural fluid are more complex.

Box 15.1 Pleural effusions

Pleural effusions develop when the rate of formation of fluid and its resorption are mismatched.

Pleural fluid may be transudative or exudative; the pleura is usually normal in the presence of a transudate but generally abnormal in the context of an exudative effusion.

Numerous biochemical markers may be useful in determining the etiology of a pleural effusion, though none is entirely specific.

While a small amount of pleural fluid is necessary to lubricate the pleural surfaces, excessive amounts of fluid will interfere with the efficient mechanical coupling between the chest wall and the lung. It is now considered that pleural fluid originates as extracellular interstitial fluid in parietal pleural tissue, and leaks from there into the pleural space through leaky mesothelial junctions. Under physiologic conditions, the rate of fluid formation by the visceral pleura is low because the bronchial arteries which supply the pleura are relatively deep to the surface, and the pleural capillaries, draining into pulmonary veins, are at relatively low pressure, because they drain into the pulmonary veins.[1] Removal of pleural fluid is accomplished by an absorptive pressure gradient through the visceral pleura, and through parietal pleural stomata which lead directly to lymphatic vessels. Physiologically, the pleural space is best considered as part of the parietal pleural extracellular space.[2,3]

Lymphatic drainage of the pleural space allows removal of proteins, particulates, and cells in addition to water and crystalloids. Protein is also removed by active transport by mesothelial cells.[1] Protein removal is particularly important in pathologic states, but even under normal conditions some protein leaks into the pleural space. Were this not removed, the subsequent rise in oncotic pressure in the pleural fluid would lead to progressive pleural fluid accumulation.

Although the pleural space is gas free, it is normally lubricated by a small amount of pleural fluid. This liquid coupling provides instantaneous transmission of perpendicular forces between pleural surfaces and allows the pleural membranes to slide in response to shear forces of respiratory movement.[4] The thickness of the pleural fluid layer at functional residual capacity is 6–15 μm, decreasing as the volume of the lungs increases.[5]

The volume of pleural fluid in the human pleural space, determined by urea dilution, is 0.26 ml/kg.[6] This means that normal individuals may have 15–20 ml of fluid in each pleural space. Using lateral decubitus chest radiographs to detect pleural fluid, a technique that has a threshold sensitivity of about 5 ml,[7] Hessen[8] found a 10% prevalence of definite or probable pleural fluid in healthy adults. The entry rate of fluid into the pleural space averages 7 ml per day in a 30 kg sheep.[9] In humans, it is estimated that about 10 ml of pleural fluid forms each day.[3,10]

Pleural effusions develop when the rate of entry and exit of pleural fluid is mismatched. Mechanisms for the formation of excessive pleural fluid may include increased microvascular hydrostatic pressure, reduced oncotic pressures, impaired lymphatic drainage, and increased mesothelial or vascular permeability.[1,3] Less common mechanisms include reduced pressure in the pleural space (seen with major atelectasis), and transdiaphragmatic passage of fluid from the peritoneum.

A variety of liquids may accumulate in the pleural space: transudate, exudate, blood, chyle, and occasionally more exotic liquids such as bile, urine, cerebrospinal fluid, peritoneal dialysate, and intravenous infusions. By convention, because the character of pleural fluid is often unknown, liquid in the pleural space is usually called pleural effusion. Alternative and more specific terms such as hemothorax, pyothorax, and chylothorax are used when appropriate.

In clinical practice, the majority of effusions are either transudates or exudates; traditionally, the distinction has been based on estimation of specific gravity, protein, and lactic acid dehydrogenase (LDH). Normal pleural fluid has a protein concentration of 1–2 g/dl, a cell count of 1500–4500/ml (60–70% monocytes) and less than half the serum concentration of large protein macromolecules, such as LDH.[11] Characteristically, transudates have a specific gravity of 1.016 and a protein concentration of 3 g/dl. The standard criteria for distinguishing transudates from exudates were defined by Light et al[12] (Box 15.2). Under these criteria, transudates are defined by the following parameters: a pleural fluid:serum protein ratio <0.5; a pleural fluid:serum LDH ratio <0.6; and an absolute pleural fluid LDH concentration <200 IU/L. There is general consensus about the value of Light's criteria,[13] though it has been suggested that an increase in the threshold for the absolute value of pleural LDH (to >0.45 of the upper limits of normal) may be more discriminatory.[14,15] In a recent multicenter metaanalysis, the overall diagnostic accuracy of the three Light's criteria was 92%.[16] However, the discriminatory value of these criteria decreases as any of the test results approaches the cut-off value. It is not always realistic to rely on dichotomous criteria for distinguishing between transudates and exudates. Discrimination is enhanced by the use of a Bayesian approach, with determination of pretest probability, and use of multiple cut-off points for pleural fluid parameters, each with associated likelihood ratios.[16] However, a Bayesian approach is cumbersome

---

Box 15.2 Features which distinguish transudates from exudates

Underlying condition likely to cause transudate (see Box 15.3)

Pleural fluid:serum protein ratio <0.5

Pleural fluid:serum lactate dehydrogenase (LDH) ratio <0.6

Absolute pleural fluid LDH concentration <200 IU/L

Cholesterol level <60 mg/dl

for routine clinical use. Other tests used to distinguish transudates from exudates have included measurement of pleural fluid to serum albumin gradient, the pleural fluid:serum LDH ratio, the pleural fluid cholesterol, and the pleural fluid:serum cholesterol ratio.[16] Pleural fluid cholesterol measurement may be helpful if the patient has equivocal values on one or more of the other tests.[5] A number of studies have shown that transudative effusions may take on the biochemical characteristics of an exudate if they are long standing,[3] or if the patient has received diuretics.[17,18]

Transudates develop because of a change in the physical factors that affect the rate of pleural fluid formation and resorption: microvascular pressure and plasma oncotic pressure. Because of the systemic nature of these changes, transudates are commonly bilateral. Once the altered factor or factors have been identified, attention can be directed away from the pleura, which is itself normal, to the underlying systemic abnormality. The important causes of transudative pleural effusions are listed in Box 15.3.

Box 15.3   Causes of pleural transudates

Raised microvascular pressure
Heart failure
Constrictive pericarditis
Fluid overload

Reduced plasma oncotic pressure
Hepatic cirrhosis
Nephrotic syndrome
Hypoalbuminemia (other causes)

Reduced pleural surface pressure
Major atelectasis (e.g. total lung collapse)

An exudative effusion indicates that the pleural surface is pathologically altered, with an accompanying increase in permeability or a decrease in lymph flow. The typical and less common[19–27] causes of exudative effusions are shown in Box 15.4.

In practice, >90% of effusions (whether symptomatic or asymptomatic) result from heart failure, cirrhosis, ascites, pleuropulmonary infection, malignancy, or pulmonary embolism.[28,29] Very large effusions are seen especially in malignant disease as a result of metastases, notably from the lung or breast, but large effusions may also occur in heart failure, cirrhosis, tuberculosis, empyema, and hemothorax.[30] Bilateral effusions tend to be transudates, though there are notable exceptions, particularly with metastatic disease, lymphoma, pulmonary embolism, rheumatoid arthritis, and systemic lupus erythematosus.

The differential diagnosis of pleural effusion depends on clinical features and a hierarchy of investigations that, depending on possible diagnoses, include blood and urine tests, thoracentesis with an examination of the pleural fluid, and pleural biopsy. Exudates should be examined for glucose concentration, microorganisms, malignant cells, and in appropriate circumstances amylase and triglycerides.[2] If the effusion is thought to be immunologic in origin, measurement of rheumatoid factor or antinuclear antigens may be helpful. Measurements of adenosine deaminase, lysozyme, and gamma interferon have been used in the diagnosis of tuberculous pleural effusion.[5] If initial evaluation is nondiagnostic, other investigations that may be used included thoracoscopy or open biopsy. Image guided pleural biopsy may have a very high diagnostic yield.[31] Imaging procedures play an early and important part in this work-up and may disclose abnormalities both inside and outside the chest that can establish or suggest a probable cause for the effusion. In addition, imaging techniques are used to direct biopsy or interventional therapy.

A subset of exudative pleural effusions are eosinophilic, where eosinophils make up >10% of the white cell count in the pleural fluid. In one review of 343 eosinophilic effusions, the majority (63%) were either idiopathic (35%) or associated with pneumothorax with or without hemothorax (28%).[32] Other causes

---

Box 15.4   Causes of pleural exudates

Infectious
Bacteria (including *Mycobacterium*)
Viruses, *Chlamydia*
Fungi
Protozoa (including *Pneumocystis carinii*), metazoa, worm
   infestation
Adjacent subphrenic abscess, hepatic abscess (including
   amebic)
Vertebral osteomyelitis

Neoplastic
Bronchial carcinoma
Mesothelioma
Metastasis
Lymphoma
Localized fibrous tumor of pleura
Castleman disease, macroglobulinemia
Chest wall neoplasm

Cardiovascular
Postcardiac injury syndrome
Superior vena cava obstruction
Pulmonary thromboembolism

Hepatic
Cirrhosis
Hepatitis

Pancreatic
Pancreatitis (acute, chronic)

Renal
Uremic pleurisy
Acute nephritic syndrome
Renal tract obstruction
Renal infection

Splenic
Abscess
Infarction
Hematoma

Ascitic
Cirrhosis
Meigs syndrome
Ascites (benign, malignant)
Peritoneal dialysis

included infection (11%), with the majority parapneumonic (5%) or tuberculous (4%), malignancy (8%), pulmonary infarction (4%), benign asbestos related effusion (4%), and rheumatologic disease (4%). Eosinophilic pleural collections have been also described in infections with the roundworm *Toxacara cani*,[33] and following trauma.[34] In general, eosinophilic effusions are self-limiting and commonly associated with air or blood in the pleural space.[3] However, Kuhn et al[35] have emphasized the importance of disease prevalence in making judgments concerning the significance of an eosinophilic effusion.[35] In their study, though only four of 84 effusions in patients with malignancy were eosinophilic, 48% of those with eosinophilic effusion were malignant.[35]

Several large series indicate that about one-fifth of pleural effusions examined by thoracocentesis are of indeterminate cause despite extensive investigation.[29,36–38] In a prospective review of patients with pleural effusions, a diagnosis was not initially established in 53 of 394 (13%) cases.[39] In 32 of 40 (80%) of these patients, no cause was ever determined despite a mean follow up of 62 months. In general, there was complete resolution of pleural fluid in all patients.[39] Relapse of pleural effusion was documented in five of 40 (12%) patients of whom one was diagnosed with mesothelioma.

Imaging of pleural effusion (Box 15.5)

Conventional radiography, CT, and ultrasound are the most frequently used tests for demonstrating pleural fluid. The appearance of an effusion depends on the patient's position at the time of the examination and the mobility of the effusion, which may be free or constrained to a variable extent.

With a moderate sized pleural effusion, fluid collects around and under the lung and takes on a characteristic configuration. This shape is determined by the interplay of the hydrostatic pressure in the effusion, the pleural liquid pressure, and the pleural surface pressure in the various zones from apex to base. In the erect subject, fluid collects mainly in the lower zone. Here the hydrostatic pressure is positive and the lung is compressed, so that it floats away from the chest wall and diaphragm.[4,40] Homeostatic mechanisms, particularly tissue interdependence, prevent the lower lung zones from collapsing as much as might be predicted from the local pleural liquid pressure.[41] In contrast, in the highest zone, normal conditions obtain and pleural liquid pressure is much lower than pleural surface pressure. In this zone the fluid is essentially normal in thickness and radiologically undetectable. In the middle zone the visceral–parietal pleural contact is lost and pleural liquid and surface pressures become identical. Descending in this zone, pleural liquid pressure remains subatmospheric but becomes more positive because of the increasing head of effusion, and thus the recoil of the lung has to become less to allow the pleural surface pressure to rise (become less negative). This is achieved by a decrease in lung volume, since at smaller lung volumes recoil is less. Because lung volume decreases, the thickness of pleural fluid increases progressively. The result of the interactions between these forces is that the lung eventually sits in the pleural fluid rather like an egg in an egg cup, and the upper surface of the effusion takes on a meniscus-like shape (Fig. 15.1).

On plain radiographs the classic appearance of a moderate pleural effusion is a homogeneous lower zone opacity with a curvilinear upper border, quite sharply marginated and concave to the lung (Fig. 15.2). A consideration of Figure 15.1 explains how this type of opacity is produced. The transaxial view shows that the x-ray beam is more attenuated laterally (A) than centrally (C) because the marginal beam passes through a greater thickness of fluid. A pleural effusion is therefore dense laterally, and because it presents a tangential fluid–air interface (B), it has a sharp inner margin with the classic meniscus shape produced by the inner fluid envelope. More centrally the x-ray beam is less attenuated and the effusion produces only a general haziness, the upper edge of which cannot be seen because it has a wedge shaped geometry (Fig. 15.2). The meniscus is often higher laterally than medially because lung attachments (hilum and pulmonary ligament) alter the distribution of forces (Fig. 15.2).

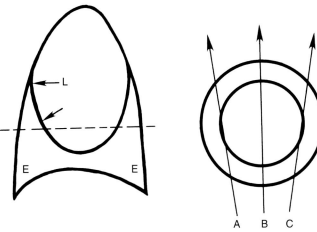

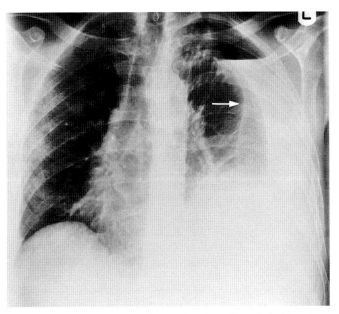

Fig. 15.1 Left, Diagrammatic vertical section through the lungs (L) and a pleural effusion (E) to illustrate the disposition of pleural fluid. Arrows mark lung–pleural fluid interface, which has a meniscus-like shape. Right, Transaxial section at the level indicated in diagram at left. Letters A, B and C represent x-ray beams. See text for explanation. (With permission from Wilson AG. Br J Hosp Med 1987;37:526–534.)

Fig. 15.3 Left hydropneumothorax related to tuberculosis. Note that there are two curvilinear interfaces along the left lateral chest (arrow); the more medial interface is due to invagination of fluid along the left major fissure.

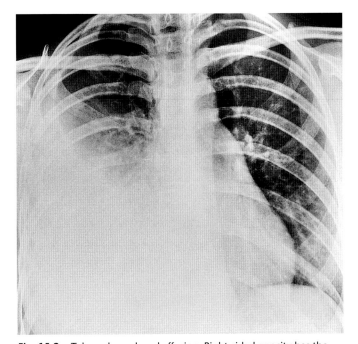

Fig. 15.2 Tuberculous pleural effusion. Right-sided opacity has the classic features of free pleural effusion in an erect patient. The opacity is homogeneous, occupies the inferior part of the chest, and has a concave upper margin that extends higher laterally than medially. The lung–fluid interface is clearly defined where the meniscus is seen in profile along the lateral chest wall, but is poorly defined elsewhere, because the meniscus is seen en face (see Fig. 15.1). Note the left paraspinal widening, which was found to represent a tuberculous paravertebral abscess.

If there is free pleural fluid within fissures, the radiographic appearance depends on the shape and orientation of the fissure, the location of the fluid within it, and the direction of the x-ray beam.[42] A common appearance of fluid in the major fissure is a curvilinear interface on a frontal chest radiograph (Fig. 15.3). Such

an opacity may be faint; typically, it is relatively transradiant medially and more dense laterally and superiorly.[42] The medial curvilinear interface marks the limit of fluid intrusion into the fissure, which may or may not be at the point of fissural fusion.[43] A similar shadow, but higher and more peripheral, may be produced by fluid accumulation between chest wall and the lips of contact of the major fissure.[44] Such tonguelike intrusions of fluid into the margins of fissures are common and may be seen early in the development of a pleural effusion, an observation that has been confirmed in animal studies.[4] Intrusion of fluid into the lateral aspect of the minor fissure gives rise to the thorn sign on a frontal radiograph.[45] A more complex shadow also attributed to fissural intrusion is the middle lobe step (Fig. 15.4). This consists of a steplike accumulation of fluid anteriorly below the minor fissure, thought to result from overlapping fluid intrusion into incomplete major and minor fissures.[42,44]

Moderate or large left pleural effusions may displace the azygoesophageal interface to the left, producing a retrocardiac masslike lesion (Fig. 15.5).[46] Fluid within the azygoesophageal recess may also simulate subcarinal adenopathy.[46]

The radiographic appearance of pleural fluid may be modified when there is associated lung atelectasis.[47] An atelectatic lobe generates increased recoil pressure and perturbs the normally uniform retractile force over the pleural surface; pleural fluid may thus have an atypical distribution. Another unusual appearance with moderate sized effusions is encapsulation of a lobe, particularly the lower lobe, simulating consolidation.[42–44] Sometimes fluid collects preferentially against the mediastinum, particularly on the left, and gives a triangular retrocardiac density simulating lower lobe collapse, from which it can be differentiated by the lack of depression of the lower lobe bronchus. This distribution of fluid has been attributed to the modifying influence of the pulmonary ligament.[48,49]

Early in their development pleural effusions are small and collect in the subpulmonic space, between the lower lobes and

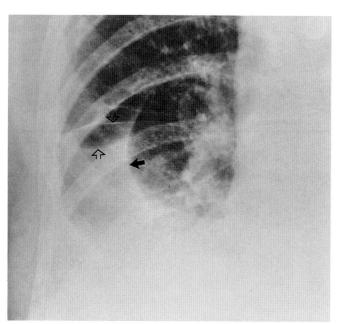

Fig. 15.4 "Middle lobe step". There is a steplike intrusion of pleural fluid into fissures below minor fissure. Features caused by minor fissure (open arrows) and major fissure (closed arrow) are indicated.

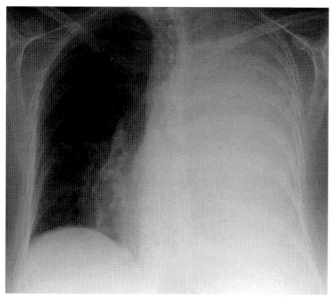

Fig. 15.5 Massive left hepatic hydrothorax with rightward displacement of the azygoesophageal interface. The left hemithorax is completely opacified, with marked displacement of the heart to the right. The curvilinear interface behind the heart is due to the displaced azygoesophageal recess.

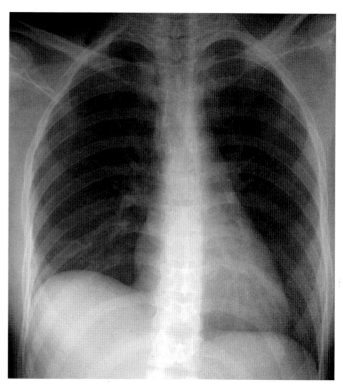

Fig. 15.6 Subpulmonic pleural effusion. Frontal chest radiograph shows apparent elevation of the right hemidiaphragm. However, the peak of the apparently elevated hemidiaphragm is more lateral than would normally be expected, and the lung vessels are not visible through the "hemidiaphragm".

the diaphragm (Fig. 15.6).[40,50] After a variable amount of fluid has accumulated, it spills into the posterior and then into the lateral costophrenic angles and may cause subtle changes in the contour of the inferior aspect of the lower lobe. Because the posterior costophrenic sulcus is deeper than the lateral sulcus, the lateral chest radiograph is more sensitive than the frontal radiograph for detection of pleural effusion. The only study that has assessed the amount of pleural fluid needed to blunt the costophrenic angles on posteroanterior radiographs is an autopsy study in erect cadavers in which it was found that on average the required volume was 175 ml (range 25–525 ml).[51]

When effusions are too small to be detected on conventional posteroanterior and lateral chest radiographs, they may be demonstrated with special radiographic views or by ultrasound or CT. The most widely used special radiographic view is the lateral decubitus (Fig. 15.4)[52] with which it may be possible to detect 3–10 ml of fluid.[7,52] Kocijancic et al,[53] in a study of 36 patients with small pleural effusions, found that expiratory decubitus radiographs were more sensitive than inspiratory decubitus images for detection of fluid. The sensitivity of ultrasound and CT has not been formally assessed, but it is probably similar to that of decubitus radiographs.

Subpulmonic effusion

Occasionally, for reasons that are obscure, large quantities of pleural fluid accumulate in a subpulmonic location rather than escaping into the general pleural cavity. Subpulmonic effusions are often transudates and associated with renal failure, liver cirrhosis, congestive heart failure, and nephrotic syndrome.[52] There are, however, many exceptions. Subpulmonic effusions may be unilateral or bilateral; when unilateral they are more commonly right sided, and when bilateral they can easily be missed on the chest radiograph.[52]

Subpulmonic effusions can be difficult to detect because the upper edge of the fluid mimics the contour of the diaphragm on

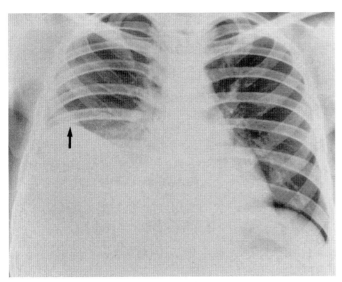

Fig. 15.7 Pleural effusion – subpulmonic. There is apparent elevation of the right hemidiaphragm (arrow). Note that the peak of the "hemidiaphragm" is more lateral than usual, characteristic of a subpulmonic collection.

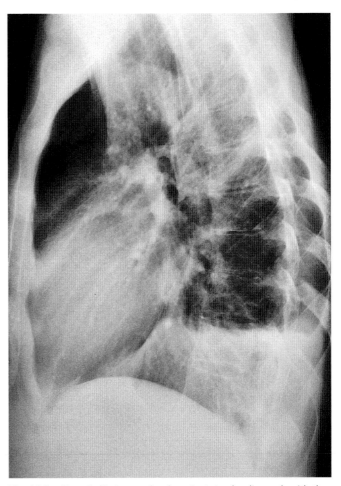

Fig. 15.8 Pleural effusion – subpulmonic. Lateral radiograph with the patient erect demonstrates characteristic horizontal upper border to effusion and abrupt angulation anteriorly against the oblique fissure. The posterior costophrenic sulcus is filled with fluid.

the chest radiograph (Fig. 15.6), so that the principal sign is an apparent elevation of the hemidiaphragm,[52] with the minor fissure appearing closer to the apparent diaphragm than usual. The "elevated hemidiaphragm" may have one or more of the following features, which should suggest the correct diagnosis (Box 15.6):

- The peak of the "hemidiaphragm" is more lateral than usual (Fig. 15.7, see also Fig. 15.24B), and the contour on either side of the peak is straight. The medial slope tends to be gradual, whereas the lateral one is steep.[54–56] These appearances, particularly the lateral peaking, are accentuated on expiration,[56] a phenomenon that has been attributed to the presence of the inferior pulmonary ligament.
- The costophrenic angle is usually ill defined, blunted, or shallow,[52] but exceptionally both the lateral and posterior angles can be clear.
- Because the posterior costophrenic sulcus contains fluid, the aerated lung stops at the level of the "hemidiaphragm", in contrast to the normal situation, where the lung is seen to pass behind the diaphragm on a well-exposed frontal radiograph.[57]
- On the left side, there is increased distance between the lung and the gastric air bubble. However, this distance is variable in healthy patients. Comparison with previous radiographs may help in this assessment. Some authors suggest that a distance of >2 cm is suggestive.[5]

- The frontal radiograph occasionally shows a diaphragmatic spur associated with fluid entering the inferior accessory fissure,[52] or a more substantial triangular retrocardiac shadow. This latter opacity, which effaces the medial "hemidiaphragmatic" contour and the left paravertebral interface, results from paramediastinal extension of the subpulmonic fluid.[58]
- On the lateral radiograph, the posterior aspect of the "hemidiaphragm", beneath the lower lobe, tends to be flat, due to filling of the posterior costophrenic sulcus (Fig. 15.8). At the major fissure the silhouette usually slopes steeply downward (Figs 15.8 and 15.9A and B), and there may be a tail of fluid passing up into the fissure itself.[54,59]

Subpulmonic pleural fluid is rarely loculated, and the diagnosis may therefore be confirmed by taking a decubitus radiograph (Fig. 15.9C).[8] Alternatively, its presence may be confirmed by ultrasound or CT.

Large pleural effusion

Large pleural effusions obscure the border of the heart and displace the mediastinum, airways, and diaphragm. Large

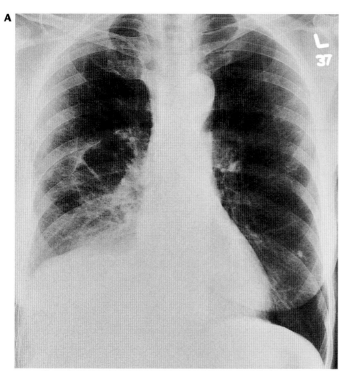

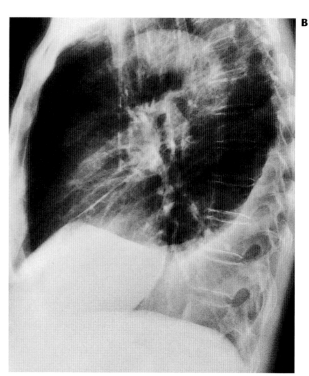

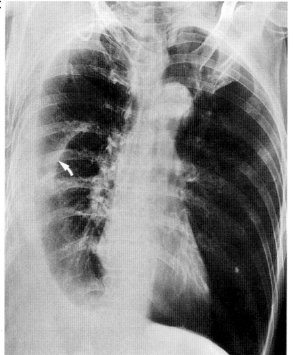

Fig. 15.9 **A**, Pleural effusion – subpulmonic. The right hemidiaphragm is apparently elevated, and though it does not have the classic contour associated with a subpulmonic effusion, there is a longer horizontal medial segment than is usual on the right. The costophrenic angle is clear, but there is haziness in the cardiophrenic angle region. Pulmonary vessels cannot be identified through the "hemidiaphragm", because of filling of the posterior costophrenic sulcus. **B**, Lateral view of the same patient. There is pleural fluid underneath the right lower lobe, but it is not entirely subpulmonic, since the posterior costophrenic angle is obscured and fluid extends up against the posterior chest wall. Rather flat lower margin to the lower lobe and steep downslope at the major fissure are characteristic of subpulmonic fluid. **C**, Right lateral decubitus view. Subdiaphragmatic fluid has extended up along the lateral chest wall, giving a band of soft tissue density. A curvilinear shadow medially (arrow) indicates fluid in the lips of a major fissure.

pleural collections can have significant hemodynamic effects and, depending on the position of the patient, may influence gas exchange.[60–63] Visualization of the pericardial fat as a curvilinear transradiancy sometimes allows assessment of heart size even when the heart border is completely obscured by pleural fluid. Large pleural effusions should lead to contralateral displacement of the mediastinum (Fig. 15.5), and may cause a mediastinally based retrocardiac density as a result of herniation of the fluid filled azygoesophageal recess.[64] A central mediastinum in the presence of a large pleural effusion suggests that either the mediastinum is fixed (most commonly the result of malignant

pleural infiltration by mesothelioma or carcinoma) or obstructive collapse has occurred, usually because of bronchial carcinoma of the underlying lung.[52] In contrast, relaxation collapse of the lung, which normally accompanies a large pleural effusion, is not usually so great that it makes up for the volume of the effusion. On lateral views posterior pleural collections cause anterior displacement of central airways, a helpful differentiating feature from collapse or consolidation.[65]

Inversion of the hemidiaphragm is an occasional but well-recognized finding.[59,66] It is seen with large or moderate effusions, more commonly on the left than on the right,[52] a

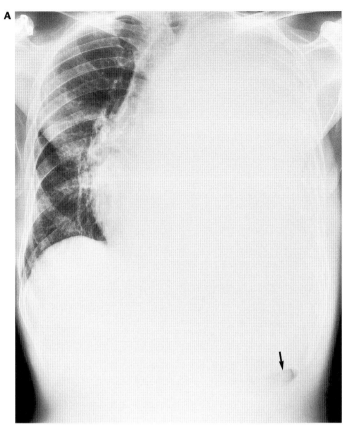

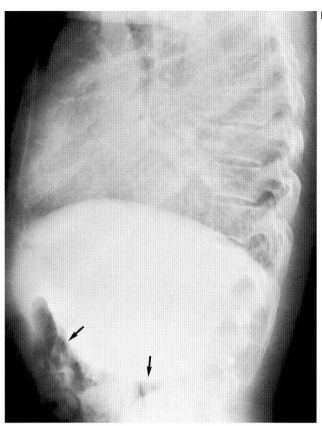

Fig. 15.10 Pleural effusion – hemidiaphragm inversion. **A**, Posteroanterior chest radiograph shows a large left pleural effusion displacing the mediastinum to the right and colonic gas inferiorly (arrow). **B**, Lateral radiograph of the same patient shows more clearly the position of the left hemidiaphragm, indicated by displaced bowel gas (arrows).

difference ascribed to the lack of liver support on the left.[67] On plain chest radiography, diaphragmatic inversion is easier to recognize on the left, where displacement of gastric and colonic gas indicates the shape and position of the left hemidiaphragm (Fig. 15.10). On the right side it may only be evident on ultrasound (Figs 15.11 and 15.12).[67–69] On CT examination, an inverted right hemidiaphragm may mimic a cystlike lesion of the liver (Fig. 15.13), but the inversion is usually readily identifiable on contiguous images.[70–72] Other lesions that may invert the hemidiaphragm include pneumothorax, lobar emphysema, diaphragmatic neoplasm, pericardial cyst, and myocardial aneurysm.[73] Diaphragm inversion generally produces few symptoms. However, the following effects have been described: (1) it may cause or stimulate an upper abdominal mass[74,75]; (2) it can lead to paradoxic diaphragmatic movement[69] that causes dyspnea because of pendulum breathing (expired air from the ipsilateral lung being inspired contralaterally); and (3) should the inversion disappear following thoracocentesis, the apparent size of the pleural effusion on a chest radiograph may not change significantly.

Loculated pleural effusion

Pleural fluid may loculate (encyst) within the fissures, or between parietal and visceral pleura when the pleural layers are partly fused. Loculations occur most typically with exudative pleural effusions, particularly parapneumonic effusions or

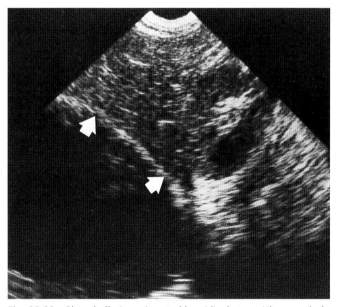

Fig. 15.11 Pleural effusion – inverted hemidiaphragm. Ultrasound of the right upper quadrant of the abdomen. The liver and kidney are separated from the echo free pleural effusion by the hemidiaphragm (arrows), which is convex to liver. (Courtesy of Dr AEA Joseph, London)

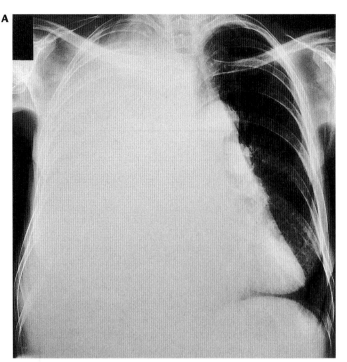

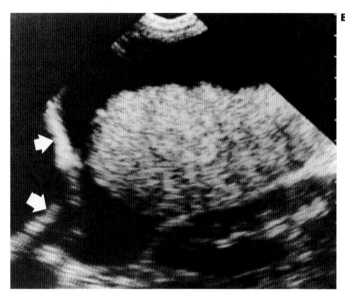

Fig. 15.12 Pleural effusion – hepatic cirrhosis. **A**, Posteroanterior radiograph shows a massive right pleural effusion with mediastinal displacement to the left. The right-sided location of the effusion is characteristic. **B**, Longitudinal ultrasound scan of the right upper quadrant shows an inverted hemidiaphragm (arrows) between the pleural effusion and ascites. The cirrhotic liver is hyperechoic and nodular. (Courtesy of Dr AEA Joseph, London)

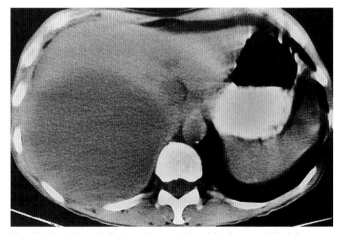

Fig. 15.13 Pleural effusion – inverted hemidiaphragm. CT of the upper abdomen shows large, rounded, low density area apparently lying posteriorly in the liver and caused by a right pleural effusion inverting the right hemidiaphragm.

hemothorax. However, transudative effusions may also loculate, particularly if there has been previous pleural inflammation.

Loculations against the chest wall are the most frequent. They take on a variety of configurations, most commonly a dome shaped projection into the lung (Fig. 15.14). The radiographic appearance depends on the radiographic projection. If the loculation is seen en face or obliquely, it produces a rounded opacity with part of the margin sharp and part ill defined. On a frontal radiograph the sharp margin is usually inferomedial and

the hazy one superolateral (Fig. 15.15). When viewed tangentially a loculation produces a sharply demarcated convex interface with the lung. These lesions tend to have greater length than thickness, and because of the weight of contained fluid the greatest thickness may be towards the inferior part of the mass. The margins of the loculated collection make an obtuse angle with the chest wall, elevating a "tail" of pleura (Fig. 15.14C). Loculated pleural effusions share many radiographic features with chest wall or pleural masses,[76] and they are often indistinguishable. Extrapleural chest wall lesions, however, tend to have thickness more equal to their length, to have their greatest depth opposite the center of attachment, and – most importantly – may show rib involvement (Fig. 15.16).[76] Loculated pleural fluid is typically accompanied by evidence of fluid elsewhere in the pleural cavity.

Pleural fluid may also loculate within fissures, particularly in heart failure.[77,78] Because these collections tend to come and go, they have been called vanishing or phantom tumors and pseudotumors.[77] Such loculations are seen more commonly on the right and in the minor rather than the major fissure despite the greater area of the latter (Fig. 15.17).[77] A fluid collection in the minor fissure on the frontal view may simulate a pulmonary mass because of its sharply demarcated rounded or oval outline. The lateral view is helpful in diagnosis because of the characteristic lenticular shape of intrafissural fluid, often with a pathognomonic tail extending along the fissure for a short distance. Usually the diagnosis is easily made if the distinctive shape and position of the lesion are considered, particularly in the presence of heart failure.

Loculated collections in the major fissure have the expected distinctive lenticular or elliptical configuration on the lateral view

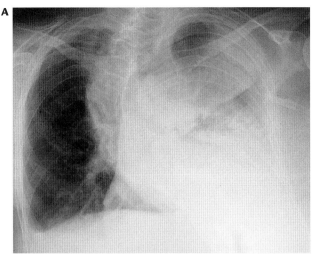

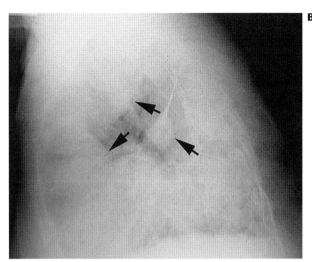

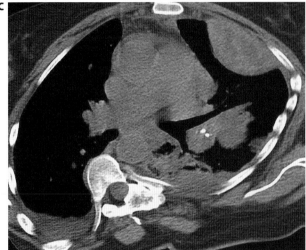

Fig. 15.14 Loculated hemorrhagic empyema. **A**, Frontal chest radiograph shows severe scoliosis and a large left effusion. The sharply delineated opacity in the left upper hemithorax is due to loculated fluid seen en face. **B**, Lateral radiograph shows large anterior loculation, and smaller fissural loculation (arrows). **C**, CT shows the anterior and fissural loculations. Note that the attenuation of the fluid is about the same as that of soft tissue, suggesting the presence of blood. The opacity has the classic shape of a loculated pleural collection; it is sharply marginated and convex to the lung, and it lifts off a tail of pleura, giving its margin an obtuse angle with the chest wall.

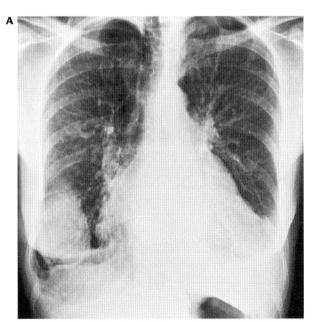

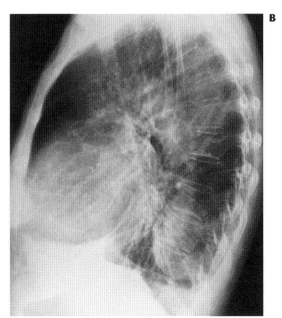

Fig. 15.15 Pleural effusion – loculated. Bilateral pleural effusions in a 68-year-old woman with heart failure secondary to mixed mitral valve disease. Pleural fluid is loculated against the chest wall on the right. **A**, Posteroanterior radiograph shows an oval right lower zone opacity with characteristics of a chest wall or pleural lesion; it is homogeneous, with a sharp inferomedial margin, and an ill-defined superior margin. **B**, Lateral view of the same patient again shows the sharply defined inferior margin of the loculation, and shows blunting of posterior costophrenic angle and fluid entering the major fissure on right.

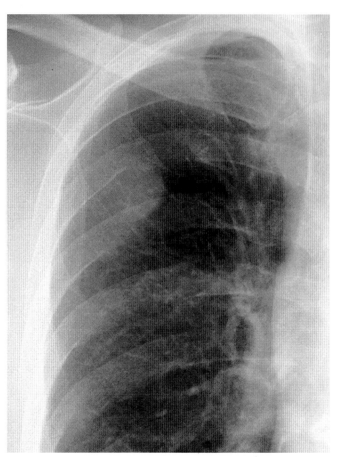

Fig. 15.16 Extrapleural mass due to a neurofibroma. A detailed view of the frontal chest radiograph shows a soft tissue density mass in the right upper chest. Like loculated fluid, the mass has a sharp inferomedial margin, and an indistinct superolateral margin, but the notching of the adjacent right posterior fifth rib indicates that it is extrapleural.

(Fig. 15.18). On the frontal projection, the opacity may be either hazy and veil-like or more discrete and masslike (Fig. 15.19). Loculations in the caudad part of the major fissure (Fig. 15.20) may resemble middle lobe collapse or consolidation (Fig. 15.21). In this situation the following points favor loculated fluid rather than collapse (Fig. 15.22): (1) identification of a separate minor fissure (Fig. 15.18); (2) one or more convex margins in lateral projection (with collapse, usually at least one border is concave or straight); (3) right border of the heart is not effaced on the frontal view; and (4) both ends of the opacity tapering on the lateral view (with collapse the anterior end is usually broad).[59] Two findings that favor collapse are: (1) contact between the anterior end of the shadow and the chest wall; and (2) an air bronchogram (Fig. 15.22).[59]

Loculated pleural fluid along the diaphragm and mediastinum, though less common, may simulate a diaphragmatic or mediastinal mass. The appearances are similar to loculations along the chest wall.

Thickening of the subpleural space due to interstitial lung edema may sometimes cause soft tissue thickening of the lower lateral chest wall mimicking a pleural effusion (Fig. 15.23). This entity was previously called a lamellar pleural effusion, but may be distinguished from pleural effusion by its straight margin parallel to the chest wall, and by the lack of blunting of the costophrenic angle.

Pleural effusion in the supine patient

When a patient is supine, free pleural fluid layers out posteriorly, and though a meniscus effect occurs at the lung–fluid interface, it is not appreciated on a frontal projection because it is oriented at right angles to the x-ray beam. The supine chest radiograph is not particularly sensitive or specific in the diagnosis of pleural effusion,[79] though in one study 90% of effusions between 200

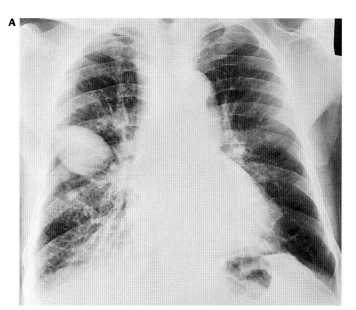

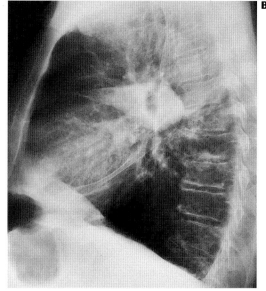

Fig. 15.17 Pleural effusion – loculated. This 77-year-old man is in heart failure. **A**, Posteroanterior chest radiograph shows a 7 × 4 cm well-demarcated oval opacity in the right mid zone projected in the region of minor fissure. **B**, Lateral radiograph shows lenticular opacity occupying the minor fissure, with a characteristic tail anteriorly.

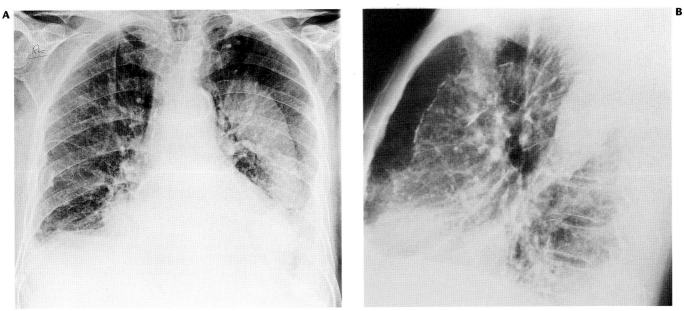

Fig. 15.18   Pleural effusion – loculated. **A**, Anteroposterior and **B**, lateral views of fluid loculated in the major fissure. This effusion is unusual in that most of its margin is sharp in the anteroposterior view. As with many loculated collections, there is also free fluid in the pleural space.

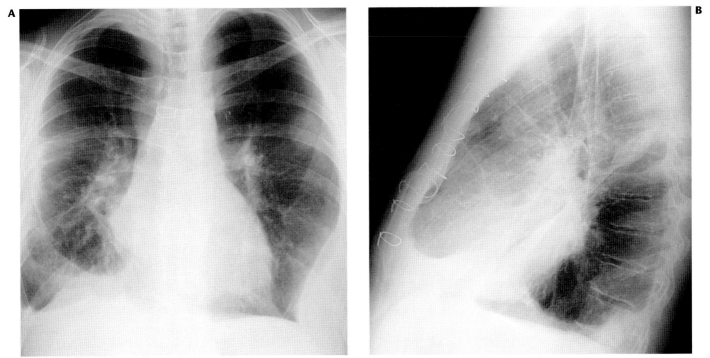

Fig. 15.19   Loculated pleural effusion simulating a mass on frontal radiograph. **A**, Frontal chest radiograph of a lung transplant patient with a large left pleural effusion shows a sharply demarcated masslike lesion in the left upper lung. The inferomedial margin of the mass is better defined than the superolateral margin. **B**, Lateral radiograph shows that the mass is in fact due to fluid loculation within the major fissure.

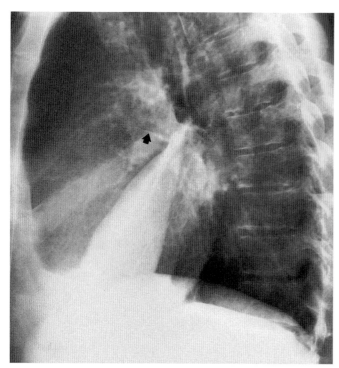

Fig. 15.20   Pleural effusion simulating right middle lobe collapse on lateral view. There is a homogeneous triangular opacity projected over the lower end of the major fissure. Features suggesting that it results from loculated fluid rather than middle lobe collapse are: (1) contact with the diaphragm rather than the sternum anteriorly; and (2) convex borders. Identification of a separate minor fissure (arrow) confirms the diagnosis.

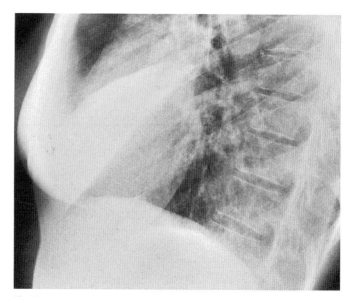

Fig. 15.21   Right middle lobe collapse. In lateral view features that suggest this is a collapsed and consolidated lobe rather than loculated fluid are: (1) anterior contact of the wedge shaped opacity with the sternum; (2) anterior end broader than posterior; (3) one straight border; and (4) absence of a separate minor fissure. The convexity of the upper border is atypical and more commonly a feature of loculated fluid.

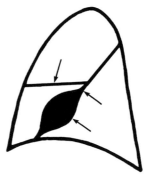 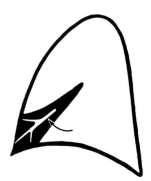

Fig. 15.22   Diagram of collapse versus loculated fluid. Differential diagnosis of loculated fluid in the oblique fissure (left) versus collapse and consolidation (right) of the middle lobe are illustrated. For discussion see text.

and 500 ml were detected.[80] Sensitivity of detection falls when effusions are bilateral. The volume of pleural effusions is generally underestimated in supine patients.[79]

The signs produced by pleural effusions on supine radiographs are as follows:

- Hazy, veil-like opacity of one hemithorax with preserved vascular shadows (Fig. 15.24). When effusions are small, this veiling may occupy only the lower chest, making the lower half of the hemithorax more opaque than the upper, with a gradual transition to more normal lung density.[80]
- Loss of the sharp silhouette of the ipsilateral hemidiaphragm (Fig. 15.24).[80,81]
- Blunting of the costophrenic angle.[82] This sign is less reliable in the supine patient.[79]
- Capping of the lung apex with a pleural shadow.[42] Some regard this as a relatively early sign, explicable because the chest apex has a small capacity and is the most dependent part of the pleural space tangential to a frontal x-ray beam in a supine patient.[42] Others, however, find that effusions have to be at least moderate (>500 ml) before they collect at the apex.[80] With the accumulation of more fluid a bandlike opacity develops and separates the lateral lung margin from the chest wall.
- Thickening of the minor fissure.[42]
- Widening of the paraspinal soft tissues.[83]
- Apparent elevation of the hemidiaphragm and reduced visibility of lower lobe vessels behind the diaphragm.[82]

The modifying effect of additional air in the pleural space on the signs of a supine effusion is discussed by Onik et al.[84] Hydropneumothorax may be recognized by the presence of a pleural line with increased density lateral to it.

CT of pleural fluid

In selected patients CT plays an important role in the assessment of pleural effusion[85] for the following reasons:

- It is a sensitive method for detection and confirmation of the presence of small effusions.[86]
- The configuration of the pleural opacity may allow a distinction between free and loculated fluid. When the

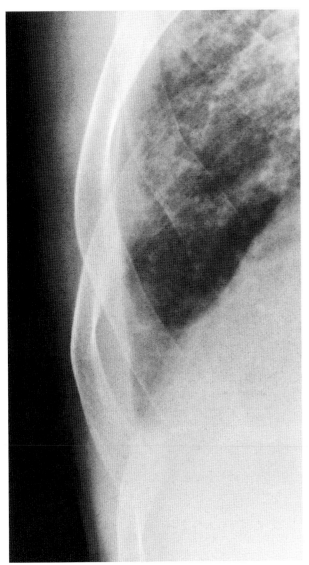

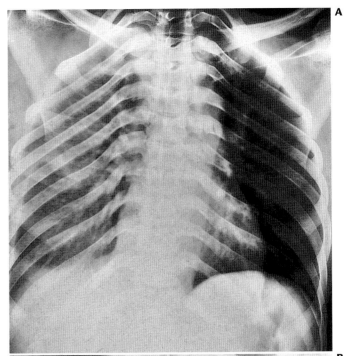

A

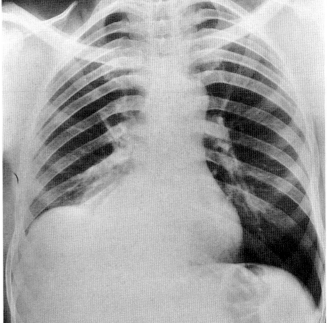

B

Fig. 15.23 Lamellar "effusion" in a patient with heart failure. The localized view of the right costophrenic angle shows a band of soft tissue density parallel to the chest wall. This is due to accumulation of edema in the interstitial space deep to the visceral pleura. Septal lines and a reticular pattern confirm the presence of pulmonary edema. The costophrenic sulcus, though displaced from the chest wall, remains sharp.

Fig. 15.24 Effusion – supine. **A**, Supine view in a patient with right-sided pleural effusion. There is hazy opacification of the right hemithorax with preserved vascular markings. The diaphragm silhouette is hazy. **B**, Radiograph on the same day with patient erect confirms a large, predominantly subpulmonic effusion.

effusion is loculated, CT can assess its extent and localization. If loculation is suspected on the basis of initial supine CT images, it may be confirmed by obtaining a further set of images in decubitus or prone positions.

- CT differentiates between pleural and parenchymal disease and is superior to the chest radiograph in this regard (Fig. 15.25).[87] Such a distinction is greatly helped by the administration of intravenous contrast material, which facilitates identification of lung parenchyma and pleura.[88]
- CT allows assessment of pleural morphology. Some appearances (irregular thickening and focal masses) are highly suggestive of malignancy (Fig. 15.26), and others (mild uniform thickening) of benignity.[89] A normal pleura or one that is thin yet irregular is indeterminate.[89]

- CT may allow identification of underlying lung disease (tumor, pneumonia, abscess).
- It facilitates percutaneous biopsy of abnormal appearing pleura (Fig. 15.26), and drainage of large or loculated fluid collections.

Although comparative studies have not been performed, CT is undoubtedly more sensitive in the detection of pleural fluid than an erect posteroanterior chest radiograph. Pleural effusion

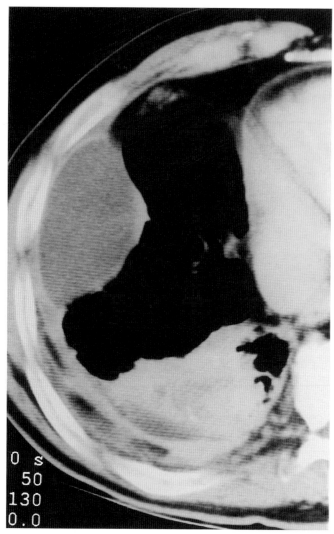

Fig. 15.25 Parapneumonic pleural effusion. CT demonstrates loculated pleural fluid laterally and consolidated lung parenchyma in the right lower lobe.

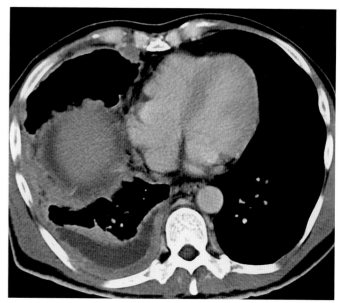

Fig. 15.26 Malignant pleural thickening due to metastatic squamous carcinoma. CT shows a 1 cm rind of parietal pleural thickening along the right chest wall. CT guided percutaneous biopsy confirmed the diagnosis.

gives a homogeneous crescentic opacity in the most dependent part of the pleural cavity. Small effusions are therefore most commonly seen in the mid part of the thorax. The lower CT attenuation of pleural fluid usually allows distinction from pleural thickening and masses (Fig. 15.26).[89] In general, the attenuation coefficient of pleural fluid does not allow reliable differentiation among exudate, transudate, and malignant effusion.[90,91] However, hemothorax is usually recognizable on CT as a nonhomogeneous collection with CT attenuation considerably greater than that of water (Fig. 15.14).[92] The fat content of a chylothorax might be expected to produce low CT numbers, but the associated high protein levels usually result in attenuation values near water density, though occasionally modestly low numbers of –10 to –20 HU may be seen.[93,94] Small amounts of pleural fluid can be difficult to distinguish from pleural thickening, a situation that is clarified by repeat scanning in a changed position.[87]

Analysis of the morphology of the pleura and extrapleural fat may help to differentiate between exudates and transudates.[95] In 36 of 59 exudative effusions, there was CT evidence of parietal

pleural thickening, and of these, 20 patients also had concurrent thickening of the extrapleural fat. By contrast, thickening of the parietal pleura was demonstrated in only a single case with a transudative effusion. In a more recent study of 211 pleural effusions,[96] CT findings of loculation, pleural thickening, pleural nodules, and extrapleural fat of increased density were specific for exudative effusions. Multiple pleural nodules and nodular pleural thickening were seen only in malignant effusions.

Pleural fluid deep in the posterior and lateral costophrenic sulci may be confused with ascites, and a variety of signs have been described to differentiate pleural and ascitic fluid:

- Displaced crus sign. Pleural fluid collects between the crus and the spine and displaces the crus anterolaterally (Fig. 15.27), whereas ascitic fluid collects anterolateral to the crus and causes the opposite displacement.[97,98] This sign is of limited use because it is commonly indeterminate; in one-third of cases in one series.[99]

- Interface sign. The interface between pleural fluid and liver or spleen is hazy (Fig. 15.27),[100] probably because of a partial volume effect from the obliquely sectioned diaphragm. In contrast, the interface between ascitic fluid and intraabdominal organs is sharp. This sign must be assessed away from the dome of the diaphragm, and it becomes less discriminatory when thinner CT sections are obtained (1.5–5 mm).

- Diaphragm sign. If the diaphragm can be identified, fluid inside the dome must be ascites and fluid on the outside must be pleural, provided the diaphragm is not inverted.[98,101] The diaphragm is surprisingly difficult to identify because the diaphragm and liver have similar attenuation values; in a series of 38 patients with peridiaphragmatic fluid the diaphragm could not be identified in one-fifth.[99] Sometimes the curvilinear opacity produced by atelectatic lung mimics the appearance of the

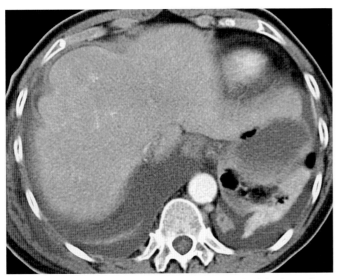

Fig 15.27   Large right pleural effusion on CT. The fluid displaces the diaphragmatic crus anteromedially. The interface with the liver is indistinct. Fluid is present along the posteromedial aspect of the diaphragm, in the region of the bare area of the liver. Note the enhancing curvilinear tongue of atelectatic lung within the fluid, which can sometimes be difficult to distinguish from the diaphragm.

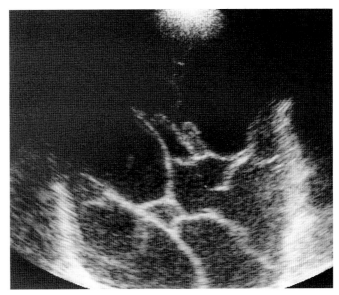

Fig. 15.28   Ultrasound of an empyema demonstrates multiple septa and echo rich spaces in between. Empyema fluid is commonly echogenic because of its content of cells and debris.

diaphragm (Fig. 15.27). In general, atelectatic lung is thicker than the diaphragm, tapers laterally, and is usually interrupted.[102] In addition, contiguous cuts usually show continuity with air containing lung.[102,103] Care must also be taken not to misidentify prominent parietal pleura as diaphragm.[103]

- Bare area sign. Since the posterior portion of the diaphragm is difficult to identify in many individuals, a knowledge of the shape of the various spaces in which peridiaphragmatic fluid may collect is helpful in assessing whether fluid is pleural or ascitic on CT.[98] Pleural fluid is free to collect along the full width of the costophrenic recess behind the liver (Fig. 15.27), whereas ascitic fluid is excluded from the large bare area over the posteromedial surface of the right lobe of the liver. This bare area, which lies between the upper and lower layers of the coronary ligament, is extraperitoneal and not accessible to ascitic fluid.[104] Therefore, fluid posteromedial to liver suggests a pleural location. Some care in interpreting this sign is needed because ascitic fluid can lie above and below the coronary ligament. Therefore assessing multiple scan levels is important.[99]

In a study of 38 patients with peridiaphragmatic fluid the interface and bare area signs proved the most accurate (84 and 92%, respectively).[99] The diaphragm sign (79%) and displaced crus sign (63%) were less accurate. A notable feature of this study was significant intraobserver and interobserver variability.[99] Pitfalls in differentiating pleural effusion from ascites include diaphragmatic inversion and lower lobe atelectasis.[10] Inversion of the hemidiaphragm usually becomes evident on serial CT images as the fluid lying centrally within the hemithorax and progressively decreases in amount on more caudal images. The curving tip of the atelectatic lower lobe adjacent to pleural fluid can be confused with the hemidiaphragm, resulting in erroneous diagnosis of associated ascites. However, review of serial CT

sections will usually demonstrate the contiguity of the atelectatic lung with the remainder of the lower lobe.

On CT a loculated fluid collection usually produces a lenticular opacity with uniform, smooth inner walls. When the pleura of the envelope is thickened, or when it enhances with contrast, a split pleura sign is produced.[105] In addition, loculated fluid produces a mass effect with compression and distortion of adjacent lung. CT of loculated fluid is discussed in more detail in relation to empyema (p. 202), since it is in this condition that CT images play a critical role.

Ultrasonography and pleural fluid

Ultrasound is ideal for imaging pleural fluid, provided there is no intervening air containing lung.[2,10,86] This situation obtains for pleural fluid against the chest wall and for fluid in other situations where there may be ultrasonographic access through a lung free window, such as the liver.

Pleural fluid is commonly anechoic and delineated on its lung aspect by a sharp, highly echogenic line.[86] This echogenic line is due not to posterior echo enhancement but rather to high impedance mismatch resulting in high amplitude reflections at the interface between pleural fluid and air filled lung. Anechoic or hypoechoic effusions may be transudates or exudates.[106,107] Some fluid collections are echogenic and the pattern of echogenicity may be classified as complex, nonseptated, complex septated, or homogeneously echogenic. When pleural lesions are echogenic, a number of signs indicate they are liquid and not solid: (1) change in shape with breathing,[86] which may be relatively subtle because pleural fluid collections often retain their overall shape relatively unchanged despite maneuvers designed to alter their position and outline; (2) presence of septa (Fig. 15.28)[108,109] or fibrinous strands; and (3) dynamic signs elicited during breathing. These include a flapping movement of septa, strands, and atelectatic lung, and a swirling motion of

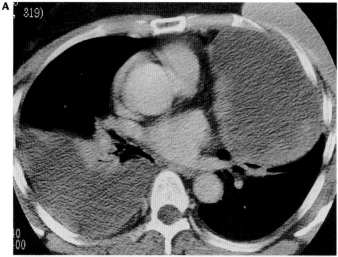

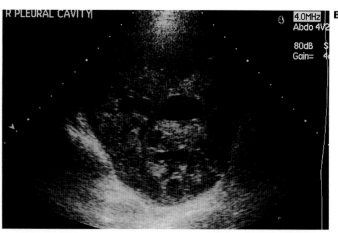

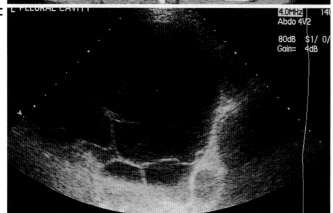

Fig. 15.29 Patient with previous breast carcinoma. **A**, CT suggests bilateral loculated pleural effusions. However, ultrasound revealed **B**, a dominant solid component in the right pleural cavity and **C**, septated pleural fluid on the left. Biopsy of the right-sided lesion confirmed metastatic disease.

finely echogenic material (debris)[110]; and (4) the presence of color Doppler signal during respiratory maneuvers.[111,112] Very occasionally fluid lesions are encountered that are diffusely and homogeneously echogenic and that display no dynamic signs. These structures are indistinguishable from solid pleural lesions. In one series they made up three of 90 cases with pleural fluid collections; one was an empyema and two were parapneumonic exudates.[110]

Ultrasonographic examination is valuable in the evaluation and management of pleural fluid for several reasons:

- It is an excellent method for distinguishing solid from fluid pleural lesions,[113] using the signs described above (Fig. 15.29). However, there are occasional pitfalls in which fluid with abundant cellular or fibrinous content may be misclassified as solid, while hypoechoic solid lesions such as lymphoma or neurogenic tumors can be misinterpreted as fluid.[109]
- It enables differentiation of peripheral lung lesions from pleural fluid,[114] and allows evaluation of their relative extent (Fig. 15.30). Findings that help in this assessment include the angle between the lesion and the chest wall, and in consolidation the presence of vessels on Doppler examination and of airways as evidenced by air or fluid

bronchograms.[86] In general, peripheral lung lesions make an acute angle with the chest wall, whereas with pleural lesions the angle is obtuse. Exceptions to this observation occur when peripheral lung lesions infiltrate the region of the adjacent visceral pleura.

- It may be helpful in evaluation of the opaque hemithorax. In this situation, the absence of air allows ultrasound to identify the relative extent of pleural fluid, and of underlying pulmonary consolidation, mass, or abscess.[115]
- It enables identification of pleural fluid in unusual sites such as in a subpulmonic location.
- It pinpoints localized fluid collections for aspiration, both diagnostic and therapeutic.[116] Indeed, in instances where clinically guided thoracentesis has failed, ultrasound is successful in the majority of cases.[117] Ultrasound guided thoracentesis appears to be associated with a lower risk of pneumothorax than blind thoracentesis, particularly when the effusion is small.[118] It is particularly helpful in intubated patients.[119–122]
- It may identify areas of pleural thickening, raising suspicion of malignancy, and enabling directed biopsy (Fig.15.31).[86,107]
- It can suggest the nature of an effusion. Transudates are typically anechoic and unaccompanied by pleural thickening.[107] Exudates seen with empyema, malignancy,

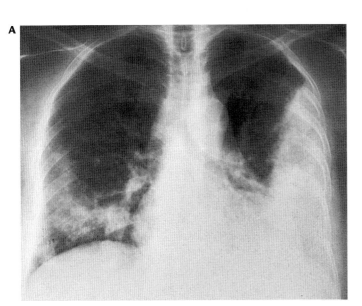

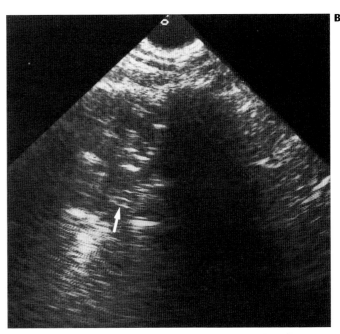

Fig. 15.30 **A**, Posteroanterior chest radiograph of a patient with pneumonia. It was questioned whether or not the opacity against the left chest wall was a loculated pleural effusion. Its overall shape was suggestive, but the irregular inner margin was atypical. **B**, Ultrasound examination shows acoustic shadowing because of ribs. The lesion itself is echogenic and contains parallel linear reflections that could be either fluid filled airways or vessels (arrow). In either case this offers definite evidence that opacity is the result of consolidated lung. Distinction between vessels and airways can be readily made by assessment with color Doppler. (Courtesy of Dr AEA Joseph, London)

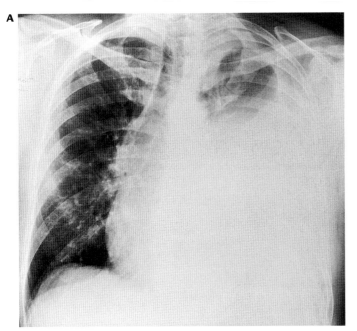

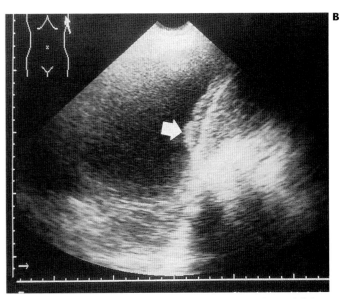

Fig. 15.31 Pleural effusion due to a mesothelioma. **A**, Chest radiograph shows a large left pleural effusion with some rightward mediastinal shift. **B**, Ultrasound demonstrates nodular pleural thickening along the diaphragm (arrow). (Courtesy of Dr MB Rubens, London)

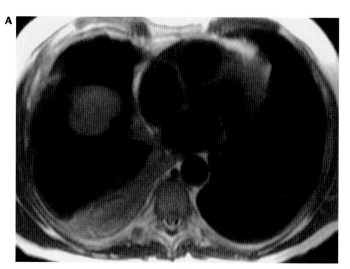

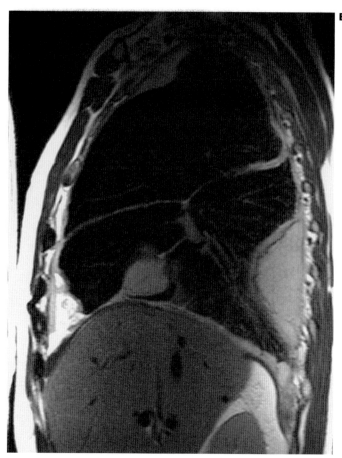

Fig. 15.32 MRI of a malignant pleural effusion in a patient with mesothelioma. **A** Axial T1-weighted image shows posterior fluid of intermediate signal intensity, containing some linear septa. Nodular pleural thickening encircles the entire lung, and involves the major fissure. A mass is present in the major fissure. **B**, Sagittal T2-weighted image shows that the fluid is of high signal intensity. The circumferential nodular pleural thickening is again shown, and the low signal intensity of the diaphragm is focally obliterated due to invasion by tumor.

parapneumonic effusions, and hemothorax typically produce echoes that may be diffuse and homogeneous or structured and complex, e.g. with septation and stranding.[106,107,123] Other features suggesting that an effusion may be an exudate are adjacent pleural thickening and an adjacent parenchymal lung lesion.[107] Effusions that are diffusely and homogeneously echogenic are commonly empyemas or caused by hemorrhage.[107]

• It is helpful in identifying the causes of some effusions, both inside the chest (e.g. pneumonia) and outside, such as those caused by subphrenic or hepatic abscesses.[124]

MRI and pleural fluid

Apart from its established role in the staging of mesothelioma (Fig. 15.32),[125] MRI has no significant role in the investigation of pleural effusions. Pleural fluid has low signal intensity on T1-weighted images and high signal intensity on T2-weighted images (Fig. 15.32) and gradient echo images (Fig. 15.33). The signal is often heterogeneous because motion within the effusion creates flow artifacts. MR signal characteristics can be helpful in identifying hemothorax,[126,127] and pleural thickening or chest wall involvement (Fig. 15.32), but cannot otherwise be used to determine the character of pleural fluid.

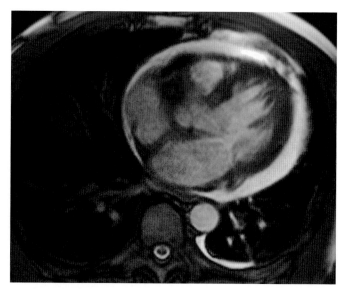

Fig. 15.33 MRI of transudative pleural effusion due to heart failure in a patient with a large malignant pericardial effusion. On this gradient echo image, the left pleural effusion, like the pericardial effusion, shows increased signal intensity.

CAUSES OF PLEURAL EFFUSION

In this section, specific causes of pleural effusion are considered in detail. Effusions caused by pleuropulmonary infection, neoplasm, trauma, asbestos exposure, and collagen vascular diseases[128] are discussed elsewhere. The major causes of pleural effusion are listed in Boxes 15.3 and 15.4.

Pregnancy related pleural effusion

Pleural fluid may be detected both antenatally and in the immediate postnatal period. However, the prevalence of this finding is unclear. In two series which used chest radiographs to detect pleural effusion following normal vaginal delivery, the prevalence was 23[8] and 67%.[129] In 50 nearterm women studied by ultrasound, there was evidence of pleural effusion in six (12%) cases,[20] and fluid persisted into the postpartum period in three of these six patients. However, in another ultrasound study of 50 postpartum women, pleural effusion was found in only one patient who had preeclampsia.

Peripartum pleural effusions, when present, are most commonly small and bilateral. Other causes for pleural effusion associated with pregnancy include infection, pulmonary thromboembolism, fluid overload, cardiomyopathy, preeclampsia, and the HELLP (hemolysis, elevated liver enzymes, low platelet count) syndrome.[130,131]

Adjacent infection

Infectious processes in the upper abdomen commonly cause pleural effusions, which are usually sterile transudates. This happens particularly with subphrenic (and hepatic) abscesses but also occurs with other forms of upper abdominal suppuration, such as perinephric or splenic abscess.[132]

Subphrenic abscess

Subphrenic abscess most commonly follows upper abdominal surgery, particularly involving the stomach and spleen.[133] A significant proportion of cases (10–20%),[133–135] are not directly related to surgery but follow perforation of a hollow viscus, pancreatitis, or trauma, and a small number are cryptogenic. A subphrenic abscess is commonly delayed until 1–3 weeks after surgery but may not develop until many months afterward. With abscesses in contact with the diaphragm there are nearly always changes on the plain chest radiograph.[134] About 80% of patients have a pleural effusion,[133,134,136] which is usually small to moderate in size. Effusions are usually sterile, but occasionally they are empyemas.[137] Additional radiographic findings commonly include an elevated hemidiaphragm, basal collapse and consolidation, and an air–fluid level below the diaphragm. The diagnosis may be established by ultrasound or CT.[138]

Hepatic abscess

In a series of 53 patients with pyogenic liver abscesses the chest radiograph was abnormal in 53%.[139] The most frequent changes were basilar atelectasis (44%), hemidiaphragm elevation (31%),

and pleural effusion (20%). An air–fluid level was present below the hemidiaphragm in 7% of these patients. The possibility of a hepatic abscess (amebic or pyogenic) should be considered in all patients with an obscure right-sided exudative pleural effusion,[140] particularly if fever, anorexia, and abdominal pain are present. Investigation by ultrasound and CT plays a pivotal role in diagnosis and management, but their consideration is beyond the scope of this discussion.

Cardiovascular disease

Heart failure

In clinical practice, heart failure is probably the most common cause of a transudative pleural effusion; the volume of pleural fluid may range from barely detectable to considerable.[30] It is generally thought that pleural effusions in heart failure are more common and larger on the right, and indeed some authors have suggested that isolated left pleural effusion in heart failure indicates an additional disease process such as pulmonary embolism.[141] However, a review of autopsy and clinical series shows that the excess of right-sided effusions in heart failure is not marked: 26% right sided, 16% left sided, 59% bilateral.[142–148] Furthermore, in two autopsy based series, one-fifth of those with right-sided and one-third of those with left-sided effusions had pulmonary infarcts,[147,148] indicating that the side of the pleural effusion is not particularly helpful in determining the likelihood of pulmonary thromboembolism.

Two unusually distributed forms of fluid collection occur particularly in heart failure: fissural loculation forming pseudotumors (see p. 1032), and lamellar "effusion" (see p. 1034).

The mechanism responsible for the development of pleural effusion in heart failure is still debated. Most authors have suggested that a mixture of left and right heart failure is necessary. A much quoted experiment conducted in dogs[149] showed that elevation of right-sided pressures caused a greater accumulation of pleural fluid than elevation of left-sided pressures, but that an increase of right and left-sided pressures together was the most effective. On the other hand, a study of humans in heart failure following myocardial infarction showed that the presence of an effusion correlated much better with elevated left atrial pressure than with elevated right-sided pressures,[150] an observation that fits better with the low prevalence of pleural effusions in cor pulmonale or pulmonary hypertension.[150,151] On balance, it seems most likely that edema fluid in the lung interstitium moves across the nontight mesothelial barrier of the visceral pleura into the pleural space along an interstitial–pleural pressure gradient.[3]

Cardiac surgery

Left-sided pleural effusion occurs in up to 85% of patients undergoing open coronary artery bypass (CABG) surgery.[152] These are usually small, but about 10% of patients have large effusions.[153] Effusions that occur within 1 month of CABG tend to be bloody exudates, and are often associated with eosinophilia, while those occurring later are commonly lymphocytic, and are sometimes associated with visceral pleural thickening and trapped lung or rounded atelectasis.[152,153] The early effusions have been ascribed to left ventricular failure combined with impaired drainage from the left pleural space following internal mammary artery dissection and pleurotomy.[154] The differential diagnosis of pleural effusion occurring after CABG must include heart failure, pulmonary embolism,[155] chylothorax,[156,157] and postcardiac injury syndrome.[158]

Pericardial disease

Pericardial disease, both inflammatory and noninflammatory, may be associated with pleural effusions in a variety of conditions, including congestive heart failure, metastatic malignancy, collagen vascular disease, postcardiac injury syndrome, and infection. Weiss and Spodick[159] assessed a series of 35 patients with pleural effusions and a variety of pericardial diseases and found that effusions were solely left sided in 60% and predominantly left sided in 71% (9% were right predominant and 20% equal bilaterally) (Fig. 15.34).

Postcardiac injury syndrome

Postcardiac injury syndrome follows a variety of myocardial and pericardial injuries and is most commonly seen after myocardial infarction (Dressler syndrome)[160] or cardiac surgery (postpericardiotomy syndrome).[161] Other causes are described, including closed chest trauma,[3] coronary angioplasty and stenting,[162] and implantation of pacemakers or defibrillators.[163–165] The syndrome is characterized by fever, pleuritis, pneumonitis, and pericarditis days or weeks after the precipitating event and often runs an intermittent course. Study of the condition has been hampered by lack of a diagnostic test and by clinical similarities with pneumonia, extension of myocardial infarction, heart failure, and pulmonary embolism, so that this condition remains a diagnosis of exclusion. The prevalence of postcardiac injury

syndrome is probably a few percent following myocardial infarction,[160,166] and somewhat higher after cardiac surgery.[167] An incidence of 31% was reported in 161 patients undergoing surgery for the Wolff–Parkinson–White syndrome.[158] In one series the syndrome developed on average 20 days after cardiac injury (range 2–86 days).[168] The most common clinical features were pleuritic chest pain (91%), fever, pericardial rub, dyspnea, and pleural rub. Nearly all the patients had a high erythrocyte sedimentation rate, and 50% had leukocytosis. None had hemoptysis.

The postcardiac injury syndrome is usually self limiting, though persistence of pleural fluid with consequent fibrosis has been described.[169] Should treatment be required, the usual drugs are aspirin, nonsteroidal antiinflammatory agents, or steroids. Relapse may follow drug withdrawal.[167]

The chest radiograph is abnormal in >90% of patients. The chief findings are pleural effusion, consolidation, and a large heart. Pleural effusions were present in 81% of patients in four combined series,[160,168,170,171] with unilateral and bilateral effusions being equally common. When unilateral, effusions are more common on the left than on the right.[168] About one-half to three-quarters of patients have consolidation, which is usually unilateral (left more than right), and about one-half have a large cardiac silhouette. In the appropriate clinical setting the diagnosis is suspected on radiologic grounds if pleural effusion(s) and consolidation develop with concomitant rapid enlargement of the cardiac silhouette without evidence of heart failure.[172] Echocardiography establishes the pericardial nature of the cardiac enlargement. The pleural fluid is a serosanguineous or bloody exudate.[168] The postcardiac injury syndrome is important to identify if only to avoid iatrogenic complications from unnecessary therapy for incorrect diagnoses such as pulmonary embolism.[3]

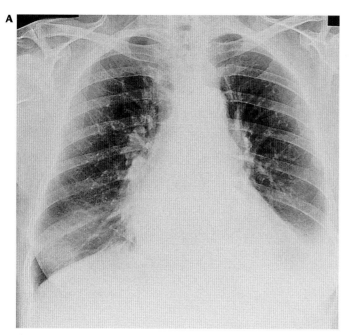
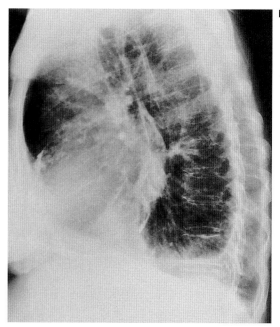

Fig. 15.34 Pleural effusion – pericarditis. **A,** Posteroanterior chest radiograph of a patient with constrictive pericarditis. There is a left pleural effusion. **B,** Lateral chest radiograph of the same patient shows that the pleural fluid is confined to the left side. There is heavy pericardial calcification.

Superior vena cava syndrome

Occlusion of the superior vena cava might be expected to predispose to the formation of pleural effusion[149] because it increases the parietal pleural hydrostatic pressure, thereby increasing fluid filtration from parietal pleural capillaries, and it reduces lymphatic flow from the thoracic duct and right bronchomediastinal trunk.[173] However, pleural effusion secondary to superior vena cava obstruction is uncommon. In a series of 35 patients with superior vena cava syndrome, eight had effusions but in only two did superior vena cava obstruction seem a reasonable explanation for its development.[174] In a larger series of 84 subjects with superior vena cava obstruction all four effusions were the result of malignancy.[175] Apart from these series there are isolated case reports of pleural effusion associated with obstruction of the innominate vein[176] and superior vena cava.[177] In the latter case the effusion followed iatrogenic thrombosis and was a transudate, but in other case reports effusions have been chylous.[178,179] The converse situation in which a large encapsulated pleural effusion causes obstruction of the superior vena cava has also been reported.[61]

Pulmonary embolism

Pleural effusion is common in pulmonary embolism, occurring in one-quarter to one-half of cases.[180–182] Effusions are more likely to occur with pulmonary infarction but can be seen without it.[180,183]

The characteristics of pleural effusions in pulmonary embolism have been well described in a prospective study of 155 patients with pulmonary embolism.[180] Effusion was the only chest radiographic sign in 18% of the patients; more commonly it was associated with other signs of pulmonary embolism. Effusions tended to be small, occupying 15% of a hemithorax on average, and none occupied more than one-third of the hemithorax. The vast majority (98%) were unilateral with no side predilection. Other series have identified a higher prevalence of bilateral effusions.[182,183] The effusions were nearly always associated with pain and tended to be maximal within the first 3 days of clinical illness. Only 3% enlarged after this time, an event that should suggest recurrent embolism, infection, or possibly anticoagulant induced hemorrhage.[184] The effusions tended to disappear within about a week (72% disappearing by 7 days), but effusions accompanied by pulmonary consolidation usually took longer to clear.

Ascitic effusion

Ascitic fluid of any cause may be associated with a pleural effusion. The mechanism of pleural effusion formation in the majority of these patients seems to be the transdiaphragmatic passage of fluid. The association of ascitic and pleural fluid is well recognized with hepatic cirrhosis, peritoneal dialysis, ovarian hyperstimulation syndrome,[185,186] intraperitoneal dextran,[187] and Meigs syndrome (see below).

Hepatic hydrothorax

Pleural effusion is a well-recognized finding in patients with hepatic cirrhosis; the term "hepatic hydrothorax" has been given to the accumulation of a transudative effusion in cirrhotic patients in whom cardiac, pulmonary, and primary pleural causes have been excluded.[188,189] A prevalence varying between 0.4[190] and 12%[191] is recorded in various series, a range that reflects the differing severity of the underlying liver disease. In the context of an intensive care unit, hepatic hydrothorax was an underlying cause in five of 62 (8%) patients with pleural effusion.[192] Effusions may be small to massive, and they show a predilection for the right side (Fig. 15.12). Thus, in 55 cases from six series, 60% were right sided, 22% left sided, and 18% bilateral.[191,193–197] In one series that looked at cirrhosis with isolated left pleural effusion, 18% of effusions were found to be tuberculous.[198] The authors concluded that isolated left-sided effusions in the context of cirrhosis should be fully investigated and not assumed to be the result of liver disease per se.[198]

Although raised lymphatic pressure, azygos vein hypertension, and hypoalbuminemia play a part in generating cirrhotic effusions,[199] evidence indicates that transdiaphragmatic passage of fluid is the most important mechanism.[195] Under these circumstances the development of pleural effusions depends on the presence of ascites, and this is a common, but not universal, finding in hepatic hydrothorax.[191,200] The corollary, that all patients with cirrhotic ascites have pleural effusions, is by no means true. In one series of 330 patients with hepatic ascites only 5.5% had pleural effusions on chest radiography.[194] Transfer of fluid from the peritoneal cavity to the chest has been clearly demonstrated by studies in which blue dye, India ink, and labeled albumin have been introduced into ascitic fluid.[193,194] It is also well recognized that air in the peritoneal cavity can enter the pleural cavity, usually on the right.[194,195,201] Furthermore, defects have been identified in the diaphragm at postmortem examination,[194] at thoracotomy, and thoracoscopy.[194,202] Fluid and air have been seen to pass through these defects.[194] The defects are usually found in the tendinous part of the diaphragm and are probably tears produced by the stretching that occurs in the presence of ascites.[195] Localized muscle thinning where vessels pass through the diaphragm may be another predisposing factor. The pathologic features of these defects were elegantly demonstrated by Lieberman and Peters.[195] Some of the defects were still closed by peritoneum and appeared as fluid filled blebs on the pleural side of the diaphragm, whereas in others the peritoneal membrane had ruptured, leaving a hole. The structure of the blebs, their possible sudden rupture, and their later occlusion by adhesions probably explains why many patients with ascites have no pleural effusion,[194] and why effusions may develop or resolve suddenly.[194,195,197] The right-sided predilection of effusions in ascites may be related to the greater exposure of the tendinous diaphragm on the right, where it is not covered by the heart. Alternatively, it could be due to the action of the liver as a one-way valve, allowing entry of ascitic fluid into the chest on inspiration, but preventing its return to the abdomen on expiration. Drainage of hepatic hydrothorax via chest tube is not usually recommended because the pleural fluid is promptly replenished from the abdomen. Treatment of hepatic hydrothorax is based on management of the underlying ascites, and transjugular portosystemic shunting is usually effective.[189,203,204]

A number of papers have described pleural effusion occurring with hepatitis.[3] Potential etiologies of effusion in this context include hypoproteinemia, sympathetic effusion related to subdiaphragmatic inflammation, and hepatic hydrothorax.

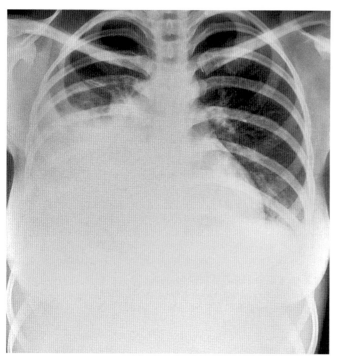

Fig. 15.35 Pleural effusion – Meigs syndrome. This 17 year old had lower abdominal pain and irregular menstrual periods. There was a large pleural effusion, which did not contain malignant cells, and also ascites with an ovarian mass. Removal of the mass (granulosa cell tumor) was followed by resolution of both the ascites and pleural effusion. Three years later the patient remained well.

Meigs syndrome

The earliest descriptions of Meigs syndrome are those of Salmon in 1934 and Meigs and Cass in 1937.[205,206] The syndrome has four components: ascites, pleural effusion, ovarian fibroma, and resolution of ascites and hydrothorax with removal of the tumor. The definition was later extended[207,208] to include other ovarian tumors: theca cell, granulosa cell, and Brenner tumors. More recently there has been a tendency to include all ovarian and uterine neoplasms associated with benign effusions.[209] In particular, there have been numerous case reports of uterine leiomyomata causing a Meigs-like syndrome.[210–214] Some authors call this extended syndrome the atypical (pseudo) Meigs syndrome.[215,216] Majzlin and Stevens[208] reviewed 128 cases of the more limited syndrome and found ovarian fibroma in 82%, theca cell tumor in 9.4%, granulosa cell tumor in 4.7%, and Brenner tumor in 1.6%. The fluid in the chest and abdomen was the same and usually clear, amber colored transudates. However, various appearances of the effusions are described, including hemorrhagic.[217] Pleural effusions are more commonly right sided with a frequency of 65% on the right, 10% on the left, and 22% bilaterally (Fig. 15.35).[208] Meigs syndrome is uncommon; in one series, 51 of 283 patients with ovarian fibromas had ascites but only two had pleural effusions as well.[218] The source of the ascites is not clearly established, but evidence suggests that it is produced by transudation from the surface of the larger tumors, possibly resulting from vascular compromise.[218] Once formed, ascitic fluid almost certainly enters the chest through diaphragmatic defects, as discussed above.

The importance of Meigs syndrome lies in the fact that neither ascites nor pleural effusion necessarily indicates that a pelvic mass is malignant and has metastasized. However, Meigs-type syndromes have been described with malignant tumors.[219]

Pancreatic disease

Pleural effusion occurs in both acute and chronic pancreatitis,[140] and several mechanisms may be pathogenetically important.[3]

The prevalence of pleural effusion in acute pancreatitis is 10–20% but may range from 4[220] to 38%.[221] The presence of an effusion suggests severe or even necrotizing pancreatitis.[222–224] Because of the close relation of the pancreas, particularly the tail, to the left hemidiaphragm, effusions are usually left sided (70%) or bilateral (15%),[221,223,225] and are thought to be lymphatic or sympathetic in origin.[226] There may be additional elevation of the hemidiaphragm together with basal consolidation. The clinical picture is usually dominated by abdominal symptoms, though occasionally the patient has dyspnea or pleuritic chest pain.[140] The effusions usually resolve completely.

The effusions are exudates and often hemorrhagic. The amylase levels of the pleural fluid are high and may exceed those in the serum. Pleural amylase values remain elevated even after serum levels have returned to normal values.[227] An elevated amylase level in pleural fluid is not, however, a specific indicator of pancreatitis and may be seen with esophageal perforation and occasionally with pleural malignancy.[140]

Effusions associated with chronic pancreatitis are often large and recurrent,[226,228–230] and in contrast to acute pancreatitis, chest symptoms usually dominate the clinical picture.[140] The pathogenesis of such effusions is thought to be posterior ductal rupture, allowing pancreatic fluid to move retroperitoneally into the chest via the aortic and esophageal hiatus (Fig. 15.36).[231–233] Ninety-six cases were comprehensively reviewed by Rockey et al.[226] Patients were characteristically young to middle aged men with a history of alcohol abuse (80%). At presentation 94% of patients had chest symptoms (67% without abdominal complaints) and only 52% gave a history of pancreatitis. Plain chest radiographs showed pleural effusions, often large with a left-sided predominance (left 67%, right 19%, bilateral 14%). Since pleural fluid had drained directly from the pancreatic duct, pleural fluid amylase levels were dramatically high.

On CT the majority (79%) of patients demonstrate pancreatic pseudocysts and a fistulous track is shown in about 40%.[233,234] In the remaining patients the CT scan is normal or shows changes of pancreatitis. Endoscopic retrograde pancreatography (ERCP) shows a fistulous track[231,235] in 59% of patients (Fig. 15.36), and when results from ERCP and CT are combined, the track is shown in 70% of patients, and cysts and/or chronic pancreatitis in 25%. MR pancreatography appears to be an effective way of demonstrating pancreatopleural fistulas in these patients.[236–238] Excision of the pancreaticopleural fistula is the treatment of choice if a trial of 2–4 weeks of medical therapy fails.[226] Pleural effusions caused by chronic pancreatitis may cause gross pleural thickening requiring decortication.[140]

Renal disease

Nephrogenic effusions are associated with the following conditions and treatments.[132,239]

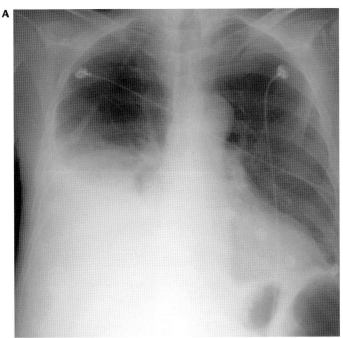

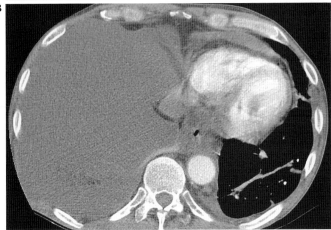

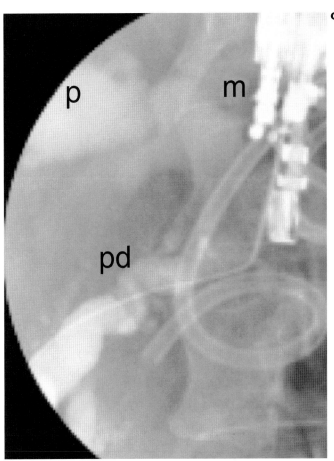

Fig. 15.36   Pleural effusion related to chronic pancreatitis in a 50-year-old man. **A**, Chest radiograph shows a large right effusion. **B**, CT shows fluid extending from the abdomen into the chest around the esophagus. There is a large right effusion and a smaller left effusion, with a small pericardial effusion. Multiple pseudocysts were present in the abdomen. **C**, Endoscopic retrograde pancreatography shows dilated pancreatic duct (pd), with leakage of contrast along the esophageal hiatus into the mediastinum (m) and into the right pleural space (p).

Uremic pleurisy and hemodialysis

A fibrinous pleuritis is common in uremia.[240] It may develop despite hemodialysis[241] and is often accompanied by pericarditis. Patients may be asymptomatic or have chest pain and fever.[241,242] The effusions are exudates[242] and are commonly bloody.[243] In one series 79% were unilateral.[241] The effusions may be small or large. In patients who continue to undergo hemodialysis they often subside over weeks. Sometimes, however, fibrous pleural thickening ensues and decortication is required.[244,245]

Urinothorax

Urinothorax is an unusual condition.[246] It is usually an aftermath of obstruction and rupture of the urinary tract with urinoma formation.[247,248] It may also follow blunt[249] or penetrating trauma, particularly iatrogenic, such as renal biopsy,[246] nephrostomy,[250] or renal transplantation.[251] A few cases are described that are a result of hydronephrosis in which no urinoma is demonstrable.[252–254] It seems likely that a urinothorax develops when retroperitoneal

urine dissects along the posterior pararenal space, which is in contact with the posterior pleural space, allowing urine to escape into the pleural space.[246,248] The effusions are usually unilateral and on the same side as the obstructed or traumatized kidney.[132]

In the appropriate clinical setting a low pH transudate with pleural fluid creatinine levels higher than in the serum establishes the diagnosis.[3] It is important that diagnostic thoracocentesis be performed early before equilibration between pleural and serum levels has had time to develop. The pleural collections subside quite quickly following drainage of the urinomas and relief of the hydronephrosis.

Nephrotic syndrome

Transudative effusions develop in about 20% of patients with nephrotic syndrome because of the associated hypoalbuminemia.[3] The effusions tend to be bilateral and are commonly subpulmonic and recurrent.[255] If the effusion is unilateral[3] or an exudate or bloody, pulmonary embolism should be suspected.[256]

Acute glomerulonephritis

Effusions are common in acute glomerulonephritis, occurring in some 50% of cases.[257] The effusions are often multifactorial in origin, with disturbed fluid balance playing an important role.

Peritoneal dialysis

Acute hydrothorax can develop during peritoneal dialysis.[258,259] The effusions most commonly develop within hours of the initiation of dialysis,[260] though effusions delayed by a year or more are described.[261] Like ascites related pleural effusions, those caused by dialysis are usually on the right,[132] though a few have been left sided.[262] Elevated levels of glucose confirm the presence of dialysate in the pleural effusion.[263] In some and possibly all of the cases the mechanism is believed to be direct transfer of fluid from the peritoneal cavity into the pleural space through diaphragmatic defects. There have, however, been several unsuccessful attempts to demonstrate such communications in patients with pleural effusions who are undergoing peritoneal dialysis.[262,263] It is possible therefore that other mechanisms play a part in the development of dialysis related effusions. Their appearance is a contraindication to peritoneal dialysis, since they usually recur when interrupted dialysis is restarted.[259]

Renal infection and perinephric abscess

Renal[264] and perirenal[132] infections are rare causes of ipsilateral sterile exudative pleural effusion, thought to be sympathetic in origin.

Splenic disease

Splenic disease is an uncommon cause of left-sided pleural effusion. Splenic abscess, most commonly caused by infective endocarditis, is associated with a left pleural effusion in 20–50% of patients and may be accompanied by basal collapse and consolidation and hemidiaphragm elevation.[265–267] Left pleural effusion is also described associated with splenic infarction[268] and splenic hematoma.[269]

Abdominal surgery

Pleural effusions following abdominal surgery are common; one-half of the 200 patients in one series had evidence of pleural fluid on chest radiographs taken within 3 days of surgery.[270] Predisposing factors included upper rather than lower abdominal surgery and postoperative atelectasis. All but one of the effusions settled without complications. The benign nature of early effusions was confirmed in a prospective study of 128 patients having upper abdominal surgery, 70% of whom developed unilateral (37%) or bilateral (63%) effusion.[271]

Small early effusions should be distinguished from larger ones that develop later, since these are more commonly clinically significant, suggesting a complication such as subphrenic abscess (p. 1045).[133]

The development of a unilateral effusion in patients with a chronic traumatic diaphragmatic hernia suggests strangulation and infarction of the contained bowel.[272]

Radiation

Pleural thickening and effusion are recognized complications of radiation therapy.[273,274] Two pathogenetic mechanisms may underlie the development of pleural effusion: radiation pleuritis or lymphatic and venous obstruction caused by mediastinal fibrosis.[3] In one series of 11 patients with carcinoma of the breast, pleural effusions were mostly small, gradually decreasing and sometimes disappearing in an indolent fashion over many months or years.[275] Suggested criteria for the diagnosis of radiation pleuritis are effusion within 6 months of completing radiation therapy, coexisting radiation pneumonitis, and spontaneous resolution.[275] Reaccumulation or rapid increase in the pleural effusion suggests metastasis.

Drugs and the pleura

A number of drugs may cause pleural effusions or pleural thickening. The useful website www.pneumotox.com lists over 50 drugs which may cause pleural effusion, pleural thickening or hemothorax. The main relevant drugs are listed in Box 15.7 and all are considered in this section apart from those associated with systemic lupus erythematosus. Several comprehensive reviews of drug induced pleural disease are available.[276,277]

Antineoplastic drugs

Pleural changes are described with all types of methotrexate regimens: intermittent high dose,[278] intermittent low dose,[279] and maintenance.[280] Urban et al[278] described a 9% prevalence of pleuritis with a high dose regimen that produced thickening of fissures on the radiograph but no free fluid. In another series, a 4% frequency of pleuritic pain and a 1% frequency of pleural effusion were described.[279] An intermittent low dose regimen gave a 4% prevalence of pleuritis, but only about 1% had radiographic evidence of pleural effusion.[278] Maintenance therapy may be associated with pulmonary eosinophilia in which dominant parenchymal shadowing is occasionally accompanied by a small pleural effusion.[280] Treatment with procarbazine has been associated with bilateral interstitial shadowing, blood eosinophilia, and pleural effusions.[281] Pleural effusions have also been described with mitomycin,[282] busulfan,[283] and bleomycin.[284,285]

Interleukin-2, used for its cytotoxic activity in renal cell carcinoma and melanoma, can produce a capillary leak syndrome characterized by pulmonary edema and pleural effusions.[286,287] Uncommonly, pleural effusions are isolated.[288] All-*trans*-retinoic acid (ATRA), used in the treatment of acute promyelocytic leukemia, has also been found to cause effusions, in addition to lung edema.[289]

Antibacterial drugs

Two syndromes are recognized with nitrofurantoin toxicity: an acute syndrome that develops after hours or days and is probably immunologically based, because the patient usually has taken nitrofurantoin in the past and has eosinophilia. The chronic syndrome is less commonly associated with eosinophilia and appears months or years after therapy begins.[167] In one large series, 35% of acute reactions were accompanied by interstitial

Box 15.7 Drugs causing pleural changes

Drugs causing systemic lupus erythematosus
Hydralazine
Isoniazid
Phenytoin
Procainamide
Others (rarely)

Cytotoxic drugs
Bleomycin
Busulfan
Methotrexate
Mitomycin
Procarbazine
Interleukin-2
All-*trans*-retinoic acid

Antibacterial drugs
Nitrofurantoin

Antimigraine drugs
Ergotamine
Methysergide

Antiarrhythmic drugs
Amiodarone

Antithyroid drugs
Propylthiouracil

Skeletal muscle relaxants
Dantrolene

Vasodilator antihypertensives
Minoxidil

Dopaminergic receptor stimulants
Bromocriptine
Pergolide

β-Adrenergic blockers
Acebutolol
Propranolol
Gonadotrophin

lung opacities and pleural effusions, while isolated pleural effusions developed in a further 8%. In the chronic syndrome there was a 7% prevalence of effusions, which were never the sole manifestation.[290]

Antimigraine drugs

Ergot derivatives, such as methysergide and ergotamine, are known to cause pleural and parenchymal disease.[291,292] More than 30 cases of methysergide induced pleuropulmonary disease have been reported in the literature since the first report in 1966.[293] The syndrome may appear between 1 month and 6 years after the beginning therapy.[167] Radiography shows unilateral or bilateral pleural thickening and effusions.[294–296] Pleural effusions sometimes appear to be loculated.[297] Localized pleural and subpleural fibrosis can stimulate a mass lesion.[294] Ergotamine has been implicated in causing unilateral pleural thickening with effusion,[298] and ergonovine may have the same effect.[297]

Pleural thickening with concurrent pericardial fibrosis has also been reported following treatment with ergotamine.[299]

Antiarrhythmic drugs

Amiodarone may produce a variety of changes on the chest radiograph, most commonly parenchymal opacities with either acinar or interstitial characteristics.[300] Pleural thickening and effusions are occasionally present.[301–304] On average the onset is 6 months after the start of treatment, but the delay ranges from 1 month to several years and the changes are rarely seen if the dose is <400 mg/day. The prevalence varies between 1 and 6%.[300] All patients with pleural abnormality have had parenchymal involvement.[302]

Antithyroid drugs

Propylthiouracil has been reported to cause a unilateral, eosinophilic effusion.[305]

Skeletal muscle relaxants

Dantrolene may cause chronic symptomatic pleural effusion, which can be unilateral and rich in eosinophils.[306] Symptomatic improvement occurs within days after the drug is stopped, but radiographic resolution may take months.

Vasodilator antihypertensives

There is one case report of minoxidil administration associated with bilateral pleural and pericardial exudative effusions.[307]

Dopaminergic receptor stimulants

Bromocriptine may cause pleural changes in patients receiving the drug for longterm treatment of Parkinson disease.[308] All patients have been male. Symptoms consist of dyspnea, cough, and pleuritic pain, usually developing 1–2 years after the beginning of treatment. Radiographic findings are pleural thickening and effusion, either unilateral or bilateral.[308] Interstitial lung disease may be present.[309] Although symptoms may abate after withdrawal of bromocriptine, pleural thickening generally persists.[292,308] Pergolide, another dopamine agonist used in Parkinson disease, can cause a similar effect, associated with pericardial and retroperitoneal fibrosis.[310]

β-Adrenergic blockers

Practolol, which was withdrawn from the market in 1976, caused a variety of side effects, including pleural thickening and effusion.[311–314] There is one case report of patchy visceral pleural thickening associated with lung fibrosis caused by acebutolol, which resembles practolol chemically. The radiologic changes were subtle and could be demonstrated only with CT.[315] Propranolol has been implicated in causing a pleural effusion in a patient with sclerosing peritonitis, but the effusion developed after surgery and a clear cause and effect was not established.[316]

Ovarian hyperstimulation syndrome

Occasionally gonadotrophins administered for infertility secondary to ovulation failure cause a syndrome characterized by

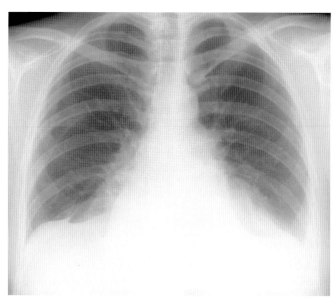

Fig. 15.37 Pleural effusions in a 42-year-old woman treated with gonadotrophins who developed ovarian hyperstimulation syndrome. Chest radiograph shows bilateral effusions. Lung volumes are decreased due to accompanying ascites.

abdominal pain and distension, cystic ovarian enlargement, and ascites with pleural effusion.[185,186] The ovarian hyperstimulation syndrome is associated with high circulating levels of estrogen but the cause of ascites in this condition is unclear. Pleural effusion is usually secondary to the ascites, but patients with isolated pleural effusion and no ascites are recorded.[25,317,318] Although usually bilateral (Fig. 15.37), the effusions may sometimes be unilateral and massive.[319,320] The chest radiograph commonly shows decreased lung volumes due to the accompanying ascites (Fig. 15.37).

Miscellaneous causes

Myxedema

Pleural effusions are described in myxedema,[321] but whether they are more commonly transudates or exudates is not clear,[322] possibly because they have borderline characteristics.[323] In one series of patients with myxedema, about half had a pleural effusion,[324] and these were usually accompanied by pericardial effusions, though isolated pleural effusion is recorded.[325] In another series of 128 patients with hypothyroidism, 28 had a pleural effusion, of which 79% were nonhypothyroid effusions, 4% were associated with pericarditis, and 18% were diagnosed as hypothyroid effusions by exclusion.[323] Effusions were as commonly bilateral as unilateral and occupied less than one-third of the hemithorax. The presence and size of the effusion were not correlated with the degree of hypothyroidism.[323] Effusions disappear with treatment of the myxedema.[325]

Pleural effusion with yellow nails and primary lymphedema

The association between yellow nails and primary lymphedema was first described in 1964,[326] and in the same year the association between pleural effusion and primary lymphedema

was recorded.[327] Two years after these accounts the triad of yellow nails, pleural effusion, and primary lymphedema was reported,[328] and by 1986 nearly 100 cases were on record.[329] The nails are not only yellow but also dystrophic,[330] and subject to both onycholysis and infection. Lymphedema typically affects the lower legs and is mild.[331] The pleural effusions may be unilateral or bilateral, small or large,[330,332] and are characteristically chronic and persistent.[329] The exudates are rich in protein and lymphocytes, but since there is no reflux from the thoracic duct into the lungs, they are not chylous. Other respiratory manifestations are common and include recurrent bronchitis, pneumonia, pleurisy, bronchiectasis,[333] and sinusitis. In an old series, bronchiectasis was present in 25% of patients in two series totaling 32 cases.[330] However, the prevalence of bronchiectasis would probably be higher now that CT is available as a screening technique. Other, less common features are erysipelas and hypogammaglobulinemia.[329]

In a review of 97 patients the male:female ratio was 1:1.6 and the median age at presentation was 40 years.[329] However, the age at presentation and the severity of the manifestations vary widely. At presentation only about half of patients have the classic triad. About one-third of patients have respiratory symptoms at this time, often preceded by a long history of sinopulmonary infections.[3] All elements of the triad are thought to result from impaired lymphatic drainage.[3] In the visceral pleura are dilated lymphatics consistent with downstream obstruction,[334] and lymphatic drainage from the pleural space is reduced.[335] The cause of the changes of the nails is not clear.[331] Neither is the pathogenesis of recurrent sinusitis and bronchiectasis; in some they may be related to hypogammaglobulinemia.

The effusions may require pleurectomy or chemical pleurodesis.[327,329,336,337]

Familial Mediterranean fever

Familial Mediterranean fever is a rare, autosomal recessive disorder characterized by recurrent attacks of abdominal pain, arthralgia, and pleuritic pain accompanied by fever. It has several synonyms, including periodic disease, periodic fever, recurrent polyserositis, and familial paroxysmal polyserositis.[338] It occurs almost exclusively in nonAshkenazic Jews, Armenians, Turks, and Arabs. The disease develops in the first decade in 50% of those affected and before the age of 20 years in 75% (range 1–40 years). Males outnumber females 2:1.[339] The most common presentation is with paroxysmal, recurrent peritonitis and fever lasting 1–4 days, which often lead to unnecessary laparotomy. The peritonitis is commonly accompanied by pleurisy, which is often overlooked. When first examined between 13 and 40% of patients have pleuritis.[339–341] Isolated pleurisy, however, is uncommon at presentation.[339,340,342] Febrile arthropathy, usually of large joints, is the second most common presentation. Colchicine prevents attacks and to some extent suppresses symptoms once an attack has begun.[338] The prognosis is good unless renal amyloidosis develops.

Chest radiographic abnormalities are uncommon and include diaphragmatic elevation, small pleural effusions, diaphragmatic haziness, and discoid atelectasis.[339,341–344]

Atelectasis and trapped lung

If a portion of lung collapses or is reduced in volume and prevented from reexpanding by a postinflammatory pleural peel ("trapped lung"), the pleural pressure is reduced. This fall in pressure may disturb the balance of forces affecting pleural fluid formation and absorption, leading to the accumulation of pleural effusions. Although not well documented, such a mechanism may account for the presence of pleural effusions postoperatively and with neoplastic bronchial obstruction.[3] In such cases, the pleural pressure is likely to be negative rather than positive, as is usually the case with pleural effusions.[345,346] Thoracentesis in patients with trapped lung or atelectasis is highly likely to lead to pneumothorax, as the evacuated fluid is replaced by air, and measurement of pleural pressure during thoracentesis is recommended if the patient is suspected of having trapped lung.[345,346]

CHYLOTHORAX

A chylothorax contains fluid that is largely chyle (lymph of intestinal origin). Because chyle usually contains suspended fat in the form of chylomicrons, chylothorax fluid is milky. A chylothorax should be distinguished from other milky effusions, particularly empyema and pseudochylothorax, which are discussed later. Before the causes of chylothorax are discussed, the anatomy of the thoracic duct and its tributaries and the physiology of chyle need to be considered.

Anatomy of the thoracic duct and its tributaries

The thoracic duct connects the cisterna chyli to the great veins in the root of the neck and transports all of the body lymph except that from most of the lungs and the right upper quadrant of the body (Fig. 15.38).[347–351] The cisterna chyli is formed by the fusion of the two lumbar lymphatic trunks,[349] and lies in front of T12 to L2 vertebral bodies. The thoracic duct arises from the cisterna chyli. It is 2–8 mm in diameter and valved, particularly in its upper half,[349] which effectively prevents retrograde flow.[352] Although the thoracic duct is thought of as a single structure, it is commonly multiple in part of its course,[353] and may consist of up to eight separate channels.[349] Indeed, in one study, entirely single ducts were less common than multiple ones and at the level of the diaphragms, where the duct is commonly ligated therapeutically, about one-third were double.[352] The duct or ducts pass up from the cisterna behind the median arcuate ligament and ascend on the anterior aspect of the vertebral bodies and right intercostal arteries between the azygos vein and aorta. At the level of D6 the thoracic duct crosses to the left of the spine[354] and ascends along the lateral aspect of the esophagus behind the aorta and left subclavian artery. Having reached the neck, it arches forward across the subclavian artery and inserts into a large central vein within 1 cm of the junction of the left internal jugular and subclavian veins. The number of channels and the site of insertion of the terminal thoracic duct vary. Near its termination the thoracic duct receives the left bronchomediastinal trunk, which drains the left lung, left jugular trunk, and left subclavian trunk (Fig. 15.38). Any or all of these vessels may end separately in the great veins.

On the right side is a right lymphatic duct that receives the right jugular, right subclavian, right internal mammary, and right bronchomediastinal trunk. The right bronchomediastinal trunk also receives communications from the left trunk (through which it commonly drains the caudad half of the left

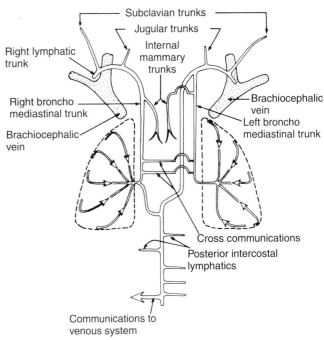

Fig. 15.38 Lymphatics of the thorax. A major feature is extensive lymphatic anastomoses between both lungs, right bronchomediastinal trunk, and thoracic duct. Another important feature is lymphatic-venous connections remote from brachiocephalic vein. The richness of these anastomoses and connections is such that simply obstructing the thoracic duct does not produce chylothorax.

lung) and from the thoracic duct via the right posterior intercostal lymphatics (Fig. 15.38).

Knowledge of thoracic duct anatomy is clinically important for the following reasons:

- Immediately after thoracic duct rupture, chyle commonly collects in the mediastinum and may cause mediastinal swelling.[355] Eventually, however, it bursts through into the pleural space, after a delay that varies from days to months.
- Because the thoracic duct crosses from right to left in the middorsal region, chylothorax tends to be right sided with low chest trauma and left sided with trauma high in the chest.
- The thoracic duct is closely related to the aortic arch and mid esophagus, and surgery to these structures is more likely to cause chylothorax than other cardiothoracic operations.
- Obstruction to the thoracic duct per se does not result in a chylothorax because of the duct's extensive lymphatic and venous communications.[356] This means that it can be tied off therapeutically without adverse consequence,[357] and also implies that obstruction by neoplasm or other process, can cause chylothorax only if it leads to thoracic duct rupture, and not merely obstruction.[352,358]

Mechanisms of chylothorax formation

Four main mechanisms account for chyle collections in the pleural space: leakage from a discrete rupture of the thoracic duct or a large lymphatic vessel; a general oozing from pleural lymphatics; venous obstruction; and passage of chylous ascites through the diaphragm.

Direct leakage from the duct occurs with disruption because of trauma or neoplastic involvement. Chyle will often accumulate within the posterior mediastinum (chyloma), before the mediastinal pleura becomes breached and chyle spills over into the pleural cavity (Fig. 15.39).[359]

Blockage of the thoracic duct can cause extensive collateral formation in the parietal pleura, and these may rupture, allowing seepage of chyle from the parietal pleura (Fig. 15.40). The degree and type of collateral formation with thoracic duct block vary depending on the richness of an individual's lymphatic–lymphatic and lymphatic–venous connections. Another factor that promotes pleural seepage is reflux of chyle into the lungs. With a few exceptions,[360] chyle does not gain access to the lungs or visceral pleura because both the intrapulmonary lymphatics and the thoracic duct are valved.[361] Valvular incompetence, however, allows chyle to reflux into the lungs and to ooze from the visceral pleura over the lung surface (Fig. 15.40). The development of a "lymphangitic" radiologic pattern in the lungs and a chylothorax after obstruction of the thoracic duct and the right bronchomediastinal trunk has been described.[179] The "lymphangitic" pattern in these cases almost certainly represented dilated lung lymphatics distended by chylous reflux (Fig. 15.40). Factors that promote reflux are lymphatic vessel dilatation, increased thoracic duct and lymphatic vessel pressure, and maldevelopment of valves and lymphatic vessel walls.[362] Seepage of chyle from fragile lymphatic vessels and collaterals is possibly the mechanism for chylothorax formation associated with lymphangiomatous malformations.[363]

As might be expected, obstruction of the superior vena cava or of both brachiocephalic veins may produce a chylothorax, since this compromises the drainage of both the thoracic duct and potential anastomotic channels.[178,179,364–366] In an experimental study by Fossum et al,[367] ligation of the superior vena cava below the azygos vein resulted in chylothorax in seven of 10 dogs, but ligation of the thoracic duct did not produce chylothorax.

The fourth mechanism of chylous effusion formation is transdiaphragmatic passage of chylous ascites. This is a recognized but unusual occurrence.[368] The mechanism is the same as that with transdiaphragmatic passage of cirrhotic ascites.

Physiology of chyle

Lymph flowing up the thoracic duct is derived principally from the gut (60%), and to a lesser extent from the liver (35%) and the peripheral lymphatics (5%).[5,350,369] About 1.5–2.5 L/day is produced.[5,370] It flows upward because of contractions of the duct wall, adjacent arterial pulsations, gut contractions, the pressure gradient from the abdomen to the thorax, and vis a tergo (antegrade pressure derived from arterial pressure).[347] Flow is increased by increased fluid intake and particularly by fat ingestion, an effect that may increase flow tenfold for several hours. Between 60 and 70% of the fat absorbed by the gut passes through the thoracic duct. Chyle contains about 0.5–6 g/dl fat, 3 g/dl of protein, and electrolytes as in serum. There are 400–7000 white cells, mostly T lymphocytes, per milliliter of chyle.[5] Loss of chyle from the body, as occurs with drainage of a chylothorax, has serious consequences, including malnutrition, lymphopenia, and immune compromise. Most of the fat in

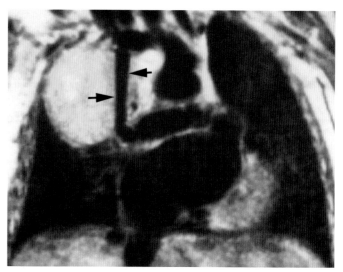

Fig. 15.39 A 3-month-old child who developed a mediastinal chyloma following modified Blalock–Taussig shunt for congenital heart disease. Coronal, T1-weighted MRI shows high-intensity chyle accumulating around the shunt, which extends from the right subclavian artery to the right pulmonary artery (arrows).

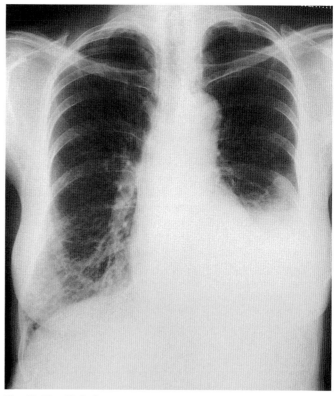

Fig. 15.40 Chylothorax – cryptogenic. Posteroanterior chest radiograph of a 64-year-old woman who presented with dyspnea and was found to have a left chylothorax. At the right lung base there are thick septal lines. The patient had had right chylothorax 7 years previously.

chyle is carried as triglycerides in the form of chylomicrons, which gives chyle its characteristic milky appearance.

Two other types of pleural fluid may appear milky and should be distinguished: (1) empyema, in which the milkiness is due to leukocytes that, unlike chylomicrons, settle out on standing or centrifugation; and (2) pseudochylous effusions, in which the milkiness is due to cholesterol or lecithin–globulin complexes. Pseudochylous effusions may be distinguished from true chylous effusions by their high cholesterol content and by the fact that they usually occur in patients who have long-standing pleural disease with pleural thickening. Not all chylous effusions are milky, and in one series 53% of 38 chylous effusions were initially not diagnosed because they were turbid or bloody.[371] Furthermore, during starvation, as may occur following surgery, flow is reduced and the characteristic milkiness may disappear.[370] The diagnosis of a chylous effusion is made by measuring the triglyceride levels of the effusion.[371] Levels >110 mg/dl are taken as positive, levels <50 mg/dl as negative. In patients with intermediate values, lipoprotein electrophoresis[372] should be performed. With bilateral effusions it should not be assumed that if one is chylous both are.[93] Chyle is bacteriostatic and does not irritate the pleura, so it does not cause pain, pleuritis, or fibrosis.

Causes

The etiology of chylothoraces can be classified (Box 15.8) as neoplastic, traumatic, idiopathic, or of miscellaneous origins.[350,373] In most series, about half are neoplastic,[359,370,374] 25% traumatic, and 15% idiopathic.[350]

Box 15.8 Causes of hemothorax.

Neoplastic
Lymphoma
Metastatic carcinoma

Traumatic
Operative
- Cardiac
- Esophageal
- Thoracic
- Cervical
Penetrating injuries
Closed injuries
- Major
- Minor

Miscellaneous
Systemic venous hypertension
Obstruction of central systemic veins
Scarring process
- Mediastinal
- Nodal (filariasis)
Developmental anomalies
- Thoracic duct atresia
- Lymphangioma
- Lymphangiomatosis
- Lymphangioleiomyomatosis and tuberous sclerosis
Cryptogenic
Hepatic cirrhosis
Gorham syndrome
Myobacterium tuberculosis
Sarcoidosis

Neoplastic causes

Lymphomas account for 75% of the neoplastic causes of chylothoraces.[370,371,374,375] Indeed, a chylothorax may be the first manifestation of lymphoma.[5] When chylothorax is associated with carcinoma, it suggests mediastinal metastasis.[369]

Trauma

Traumatic chylothorax is most commonly related to surgery, particularly cardiac surgery (Fig. 15.39). It usually arises when the thoracic duct is inadvertently stretched, allowing chyle to seep into surrounding tissues. The frequency of chylothorax with cardiothoracic surgery is between 0.2 and 0.56%,[370,376] and the condition is most commonly seen with surgery for Fallot tetralogy, patent ductus arteriosus, and coarctation of the aorta. Mobilization of the left subclavian artery appears to be a risk factor.[5] Chylothorax is also described with coronary artery surgery,[157,377,378] thoracoplasty and pneumonectomy (Fig. 15.41), esophagoscopy,[350] esophageal sclerotherapy,[379] thoracic sympathectomy, and lymph node dissection in the neck or chest.[350,380] Thoracic esophagectomy carries one of the highest risks for chylothorax, with an incidence of 3% of 320 patients in one series.[381]

Closed chest trauma, ranging from major trauma with crush injuries and spinal fractures[365,382] to very minor injuries, is recognized as causing chylothorax. Chylothorax may also follow penetrating injuries such as stab and bullet wounds to the chest and neck.

Chylothorax may occur following straining during childbirth,[130,383] vomiting, weight lifting,[350] coughing,[357] and the hyperextension and stretching that accompany yawning.[384] It has been suggested that for such trivial trauma to cause duct rupture, a duct must be distended by a high postprandial lymphatic flow.[347]

Idiopathic causes

A significant number of cases of chylothorax are cryptogenic. This includes most cases of congenital chylothorax.[5] Congenital chylothorax is increasingly identified on antenatal ultrasound, and is the most common cause of a pleural effusion in the neonatal period.[385] It may be associated with chromosomal anomalies, or with developmental lymphatic anomalies.[359] Neonatal chylothorax may also be related to birth trauma.[359] Most adult cases of cryptogenic chylothorax are thought to be related to minor unnoticed trauma.[5]

Miscellaneous causes

The remaining 10% of chylothoraces have a great variety of causes, many of which fall into one of four subgroups:

- Abnormalities of the lymphatic system. Under this broad heading can be included thoracic duct atresia[375]; tuberous sclerosis, and lymphangioleiomyomatosis[386] (see p. 1074); pulmonary lymphangiectasia, either per se or as part of Noonan syndrome[351,387]; and lymphangiomatosis (Fig. 15.42), which may be either localized to the thorax or systemic, often associated with massive osteolysis.[388–396] In a study by Ryu et al,[386] chylothorax was found in 10% of patients with lymphangiomyomatosis, accounting for 3.5% of cases of chylothorax seen at Mayo Clinic over a 25 year period.

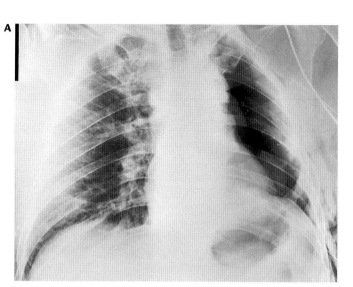

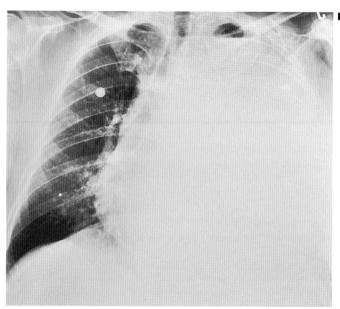

Fig. 15.41 Chylothorax – traumatic (postsurgical). **A**, Anteroposterior chest radiograph immediately following left pneumonectomy for carcinoma of lung. **B**, Just over 1 week later, pleural effusion developed rapidly and proved to be a chylothorax. This complication of cardiothoracic surgery is seen especially following operations for Fallot tetralogy, patent ductus arteriosus, coarctation of the aorta and esophageal carcinoma.

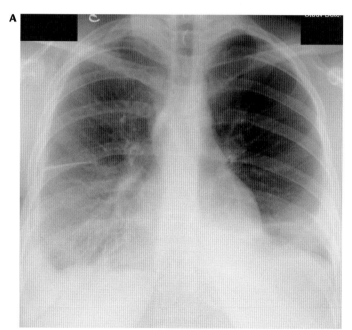

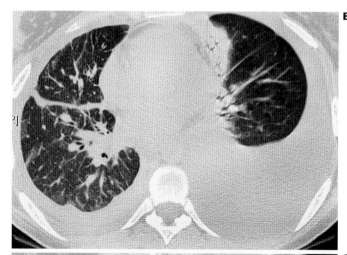

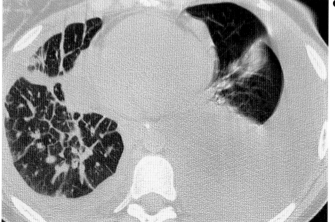

Fig. 15.42 Chylothorax – lymphangiomatosis. A 20-year-old female with chylothorax due to lymphangiomatosis, and prior history of bony involvement. **A**, Chest radiograph shows bilateral effusions. **B** and **C**, High-resolution CT images show thickening of bronchovascular bundles and interlobular septa, mainly on the right.

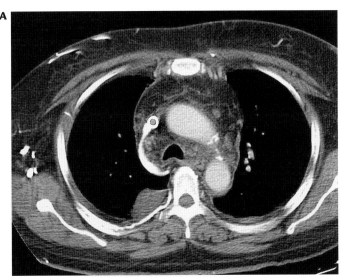
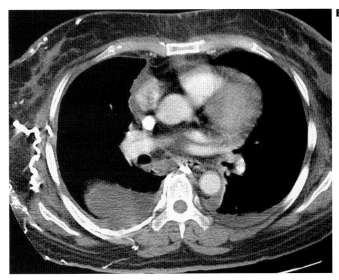

Fig. 15.43   Chylothorax related to superior vena cava obstruction. **A** and **B**, CT shows bilateral effusions due to chylothorax. The right effusion is loculated. Note the dilated enhancing collaterals in the right lateral chest wall, dilated azygos vein, and occluded stent in the superior vena cava.

- Impaired venous drainage. Chylothorax has been recorded with raised venous pressure caused by heart disease,[374,397,398] and with central venous thrombosis that affects subclavian and brachiocephalic veins and the superior vena cava (Fig. 15.43).[178,179,365,399–401] Despite a number of case reports chylothorax remains a rare complication of central venous thrombosis, and in one series of 25 cases no examples were encountered.[402] Compression of the brachiocephalic vessels by a large multinodular goiter has been reported as a rare cause of chylothorax.[403]
- Scarring. This is probably the common mechanism for development of chylothorax in chronic pancreatitis, fibrosing mediastinitis, radiation exposure, tuberculosis,[404] and filariasis.[405,406]
- Transdiaphragmatic passage of chylous ascites.[407–409]

Chylous pleural effusions have been documented as a rare manifestation of sarcoidosis,[410] Gorham syndrome,[411] and infection with *Mycobacterium tuberculosis*.[412]

Radiology

A chylous effusion on plain radiographs cannot be distinguished from other effusions. Chylothoraces vary from small to massive, can be unilateral or bilateral, and are slightly more frequent on the right side.[413] Reference has already been made to the masslike accumulation in the mediastinum that may precede the effusion,[414–416] and the delay, which can vary from days to months, between trauma and the eventual development of chylothorax.[369,374,417]

The CT attenuation of chyle, despite the fat content, is usually close to water attenuation, because the higher attenuation of protein compensates for the lower attenuation of fat (Fig. 15.43), though in one report the CT density was significantly reduced.[93] Because chyle is nonirritant, chylothorax is usually not associated with pleural thickening or loculation.[5] CT may be helpful in identifying an underlying cause for chylothorax, such as

lymphoma, lymphangiomyomatosis, or pulmonary or mediastinal lymphangiomas.

Lymphography has been commonly performed in assessments of chylothorax.[178,351,404,418] Lymphography can show leakage of contrast material into the pleural space,[351] and may also demonstrate the exact site of thoracic duct rupture,[419] which may help in directing surgical repair. It also demonstrates duct blockage with accompanying collaterals,[404,405,419] and lymphatic malformations, including lymphangiectasia.[388] The thoracic duct can be opacified by the use of oral ethiodized oil before CT examination,[420] but this is rarely used in practice. Oral ingestion of fatty compounds labeled with ^{123}I has also been used in a few cases to provide scintigraphic localization of thoracic duct anatomy and site of leak.[421,422]

The exact role of lymphography or lymphoscintigraphy in the investigation of chylothorax is debatable, and these techniques are probably unimportant with current surgical practice and the advent of CT. Once neoplasia is excluded, details about the exact mechanism and point of leakage often play little part in treatment, because if medical management fails, the usual approach is to tie the thoracic duct at the diaphragm[359] or perform a pleurodesis. Chylothorax has also been successfully treated using a pleuroperitoneal shunt.[406] Medical management includes the use of a low fat diet with medium chain triglycerides. Somatostatin may also be helpful.[423]

Pseudochylothorax

Like chylothorax, pseudochylothorax is also a milky effusion, but the milky appearance is the result of cholesterol or lecithin–globulin complexes rather than chylomicrons. Several reviews of the condition have been published.[350,424,425] Pseudochylothorax characteristically occurs in pleural disease of many years' duration, with chronic loculated effusion, pleural thickening, and sometimes calcification. It most commonly follows, or is associated with, tuberculosis[425] and rheumatoid disease.[426]

Unusual causes, including paragonimiasis,[427] are described.[350] The clinical context in which the effusion occurs is so characteristic that pseudochylothorax rarely causes diagnostic confusion with a true chylothorax. Imaging may also help differentiate between these entities, since true chylothorax is rarely associated with pleural thickening, loculation, or calcification.

HEMOTHORAX

Hemothorax usually results from trauma.[428] However, on occasion it occurs in other conditions (Box 15.9). The natural history of hemothorax depends in part on the source of the bleeding. Low pressure bleeding from the lung tends to stop spontaneously because the pleural fluid compresses and collapses the lung. High pressure bleeding from systemic vessels is less susceptible to the tamponade effect of pleural fluid,[448] and the bleeding may be rapid and persistent with the formation of a tension hemothorax.[429] In the context of trauma

---

Box 15.9 Causes of hemothorax

Trauma
Open
Closed (with or without fracture)
Iatrogenic[431]

Infection
Varicella[432]

Coagulopathy
Hemophilia[433]
Anticoagulants[429,434,435]

Vascular abnormality
Arteriovenous malformation[436]
Dissecting aortic aneurysm
Atherosclerotic aneurysm[437]

Rib exostosis[438]

Neurofibromatosis with pregnancy[130]

Pulmonary and pleural neoplasms[437,439]

Extramedullary hemopoiesis[440,441]

Pneumothorax[430,442]

Catamenial hemothorax (endometriosis)[443,444]

Idiopathic[445–447]

---

other causes of rapidly accumulating pleural fluid should be considered, including ruptured esophagus, ruptured thoracic duct, traumatic subarachnoid pleural fistula,[449] and iatrogenic causes, particularly venous perforation from line placement.

In the acute state nothing on the chest radiograph distinguishes hemothorax from other collections of pleural fluid. However, on CT a hemothorax may show areas of hyperdensity (see Fig. 15.14).[450] With clotting of the blood, loculation tends to occur and fibrin bodies may form.[59,430] Hemothorax may eventually organize and cause massive pleural thickening (fibrothorax), necessitating decortication, a

complication that can be avoided by early evacuation of the pleural space.

PLEURAL THICKENING

Pleural thickening can be localized or diffuse, and usually represents the organized end stage of a variety of active processes, particularly infective and noninfective inflammation, hemothorax, and asbestos- and drug-related disease (see Box 15.10). It is virtually always present after thoracotomy and pleurodesis,[451] and may follow irradiation. The most common causes are probably hemothorax, bacterial infection, and tuberculosis.[5] Particularly marked pleural thickening is seen following tuberculosis or irradiation. Identification of diffuse pleural thickening is important because it is commonly associated with significant restrictive physiologic impairment. It can be important to try to distinguish between diffuse pleural thickening, which may be due to a large variety of causes, and localized pleural plaques which are usually related to asbestos exposure (see p. 1043). On the chest radiograph, diffuse postinflammatory pleural thickening almost always involves the costophrenic sulci (Fig. 15.44), while pleural plaques present with localized areas of soft tissue density along the chest wall. The presence of bilateral abnormality favors asbestos related disease.[10]

Box 15.10 Causes of pleural thickening

Infection
Tuberculosis
Empyema

Hemothorax

Asbestos exposure

Surgery or pleurodesis

Radiation

Malignancy
Metastasis
Mesothelioma
Leukemia
Lymphoma

The radiographic changes of diffuse pleural thickening are more commonly unilateral and consist of soft tissue shadowing, characteristically in the more dependent lateral and posterior parts of the chest. There may be radiographic signs of ipsilateral rib enlargement in patients with chronic (particularly tuberculous) pleural disease.[452] Blunting of the costophrenic angle is common and is often angular, distinguishing it from the more smoothly curvilinear pleural fluid. Decubitus radiographs and ultrasonography are particularly helpful in making this distinction. En face, extensive pleural thickening gives a veil-like opacity that has no clear margins and crosses known pulmonary boundaries. Tangentially, it appears as a soft tissue density immediately inside and parallel to the chest wall, sharply marginated on its inner aspect and fading into the soft tissues of the chest wall laterally. Such pleural thickening can extend into and thicken fissures.

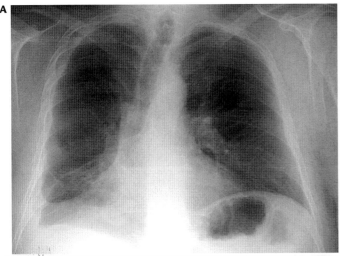

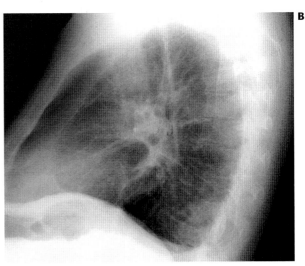

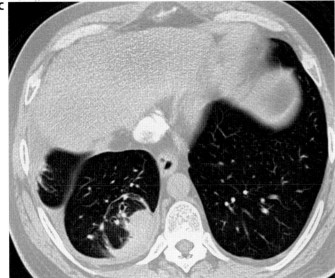

Fig. 15.44 Diffuse pleural thickening related to previous pneumonia. **A**, Frontal chest radiograph shows smooth pleural thickening extending along the right lateral chest wall, with blunting of the costophrenic sulcus, and marked inferior displacement of the right hilum. **B**, Lateral radiograph shows a posterior mass with vessels curving into it. **C**, CT shows dense pleural thickening, with typical features of round atelectasis, with bronchi and vessels curving into the medial and lateral aspects of the mass, and fissural displacement indicating marked right lower lobe volume loss.

On ultrasound, pleural thickening produces a homogeneously echo dense layer subjacent to the chest wall, but it cannot be reliably detected unless it is about 1 cm or more thick.[86] There is no posterior echo enhancement, but this is often difficult to assess because the soft tissue–lung interface is normally so reflective.

On CT, pleural thickening is detected as a layer of soft tissue opacity lying at the chest wall–lung interface. It can be detected almost as well with conventional CT as with HRCT, though the latter is more sensitive in assessing asbestos related plaques.[453] In addition, HRCT may sometimes clarify equivocal findings on conventional CT.[454] On HRCT, pleural thickening is best assessed inside ribs where there should be no discernible soft tissue; exceptions to this "rule" are discussed on page 40.[455] Paravertebrally any thickening of the normally insignificant pleural line is abnormal. HRCT is very sensitive and can detect thickening on the order of 1–2 mm. The extrapleural fat layer, which is normally absent or relatively thin, thickens in chronic pleural disease, particularly with chronic empyema,[455–458] making appreciation of pleural thickening easier. When this fat has higher density than usual, it suggests that there is active inflammation in the pleural space.[459] Both the distribution and

morphology[89] of diffuse pleural thickening are helpful in identifying a cause. In one study the specificity of various CT signs in differentiating a malignant from a benign pleural process was evaluated. The four most useful signs of malignancy (with specificities) were circumferential thickening (100%), nodularity (94%), parietal thickening >1 cm (94%), and mediastinal pleural involvement.[454] Early experience suggests that positron emission tomography (PET) with ^{18}F-fluoro-deoxyglucose (^{18}F-FDG) may have a role in the differentiation between malignant and benign pleural disease.[460] In a study of 23 patients, ^{18}F-FDG PET correctly identified all 16 cases of malignant pleural infiltration; there was intense uptake of ^{18}F-FDG in 14 of 16 cases (Fig. 15.45). Seven of nine benign lesions were characterized by an absence of tracer uptake but there was moderate uptake in two patients, one with a parapneumonic effusion and one with tuberculous pleurisy.[460] Another study found that MRI was more accurate than CT in diagnosis of malignant pleural disease: malignant disease was associated with increased signal intensity on T2-weighted images, and with enhancement following gadolinium administration.[461]

Pleural thickening, particularly when generalized, is often correctly dismissed as an inactive residuum. Care, however, must

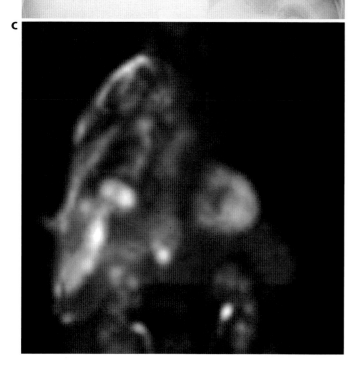

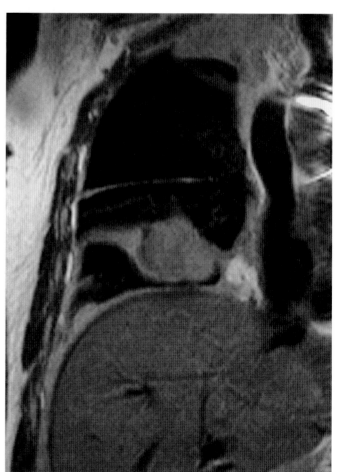

Fig. 15.45 Activity of PET in malignant pleural disease due to mesothelioma (same patient as in Fig. 15.32). **A**, Chest radiograph shows circumferential pleural thickening. **B**, Coronal MRI confirms the presence of circumferential pleural thickening extending into the costophrenic sulci, with a mass in the major fissure. **C**, Coronal PET image obtained with ^{18}F-fluoro-deoxyglucose shows circumferential increase in metabolic activity, extending into the fissures.

be taken to distinguish it from various active processes, some of which are neoplastic. Although a number of these conditions tend to give plaquelike, nodular, or irregular shadowing (Fig. 15.45), they occasionally closely resemble simple inactive pleural thickening. Disorders to consider include mycetoma related pleural thickening,[462] mesothelioma, diffuse pleural metastases (e.g. from thymoma[463]), leukemia,[464] lymphoma, and Wegener granulomatosis. It should also be remembered that a thick pleural peel occurring following empyema will usually decrease progressively over the subsequent 12 weeks.[465]

There are several uncommon syndromes of idiopathic bilateral pleural thickening. In the entity of cryptogenic bilateral fibrosing pleuritis there is widespread thickening of the pleura preceded by effusions (Fig. 15.46).[466,467] Patients may have an elevated erythrocyte sedimentation rate, restrictive lung function, and evidence of rounded atelectasis on CT.[466] Another uncommon idiopathic syndrome is associated with progressive apical pleural and subpleural fibrosis, with restrictive physiology.[468] This syndrome may be familial,[469] and may be associated with renal tubular acidosis.[470]

Mimics

Pleural thickening must be differentiated from apical pleural caps and extrapleural fat. The apical pleural cap, though it looks like pleural thickening, is usually due either to extrapleural fat or to subpleural fibrosis. Older publications refer to serratus

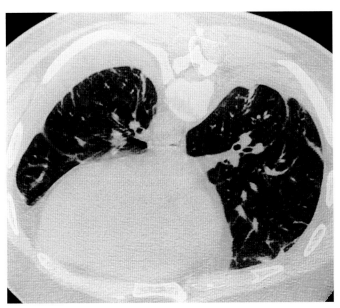

Fig. 15.46 Cryptogenic bilateral fibrosing pleuritis. Prone CT image shows bilateral smooth pleural thickening with bilateral lower lobe volume loss and parenchymal scarring.

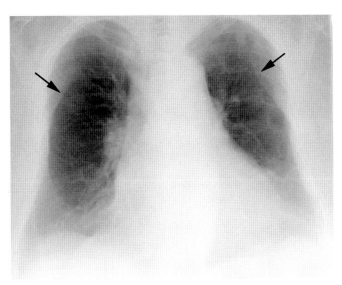

Fig. 15.47 Extrapleural fat in a patient treated with steroids. Chest radiograph shows lobulated smooth thickening along the chest wall bilaterally, extending to the lung apices, and extending. Symmetric curvilinear interfaces in the upper chest (arrows) are due to invagination of fat into the major fissures bilaterally.

anterior shadows and rib companion shadows as mimics of pleural plaques on chest radiographs.[471,472] These are not discussed here because it is very rare for the serratus anterior muscle or ribs to be so sharply outlined by air as to produce a radiographically distinct interface.

Extrapleural fat

Extrapleural fat may generate confusing shadows that can resemble generalized pleural thickening or plaques (Fig. 15.47).[473,474] The distribution varies from patient to patient. Sometimes the fat is widely distributed, mimicking a pleural peel. At other times, it is localized and develops particularly over the fourth to eighth ribs between the anterior axillary line and the rib angles.[473] Excess thoracic fat is more common in obese patients, and associated with mediastinal lipomatosis, but may also be found in thinner individuals. Extrapleural fat may be distinguished from pleural thickening by its symmetry and its undulating outline, often extending to the lung apices but sparing the costophrenic sulci.[473] If doubt remains, CT will readily differentiate thickening from fat, but this distinction is not usually clinically important.[473]

Apical pleural cap

An idiopathic apical pleural cap is an irregular, usually homogeneous, soft tissue density that is found at the extreme lung apex (Fig. 15.48).[475] The lower border is usually sharply marginated and may be smoothly curvilinear, tented, or undulating.[476] Caps are usually <5 mm thick, but the width is variable. In two series caps were about as common unilaterally (11 and 7%) as bilaterally (11 and 12%).[476,477] When bilateral the caps were usually asymmetric. The frequency of occurrence increases with age: 6.2% up to 45 years of age and 15.9% over

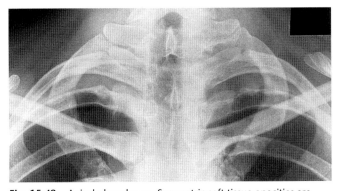

Fig. 15.48 Apical pleural caps. Symmetric soft tissue opacities are projected under both second ribs. They are slightly atypical for pleural caps, being thicker (1 cm) than usual, with some irregularity of their lower margins. The appearance of pleural caps is quite variable.

45 years of age.[475] The opacity is formed by an apical subpleural scar that is nonspecific and unrelated to tuberculosis.[478]

In contrast to the smooth or undulating outline of the apical cap on the chest radiograph, CT usually shows a subpleural irregular linear abnormality, consistent with the pathologic findings of dense subpleural fibrosis, and sometimes difficult to distinguish from a spiculated lung cancer (Fig. 15.49). Indeed, Yousem[479] presented a series of 13 such cases which had been resected because of suspected lung cancer.

The differential diagnosis of an idiopathic apical cap includes nongranulomatous and granulomatous (tuberculous, fungal) infection, radiation pleuritis, lymphoma, pleural and extrapleural neoplasms, extrapleural hematoma, prominent subclavian artery, mediastinal lipomatosis,[480] and apicolateral extrapleural fat.[481] A HRCT study has shown, somewhat surprisingly, that the bulk of the apical "pleural" opacity

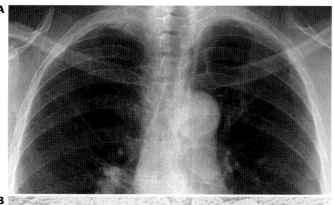

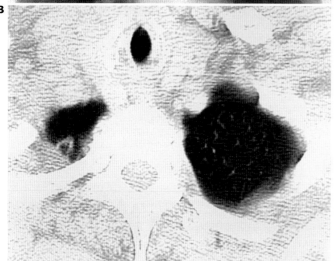

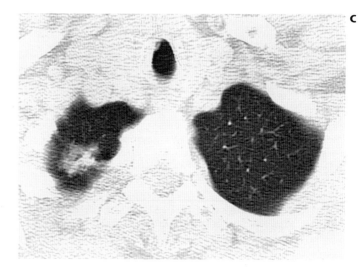

Fig. 15.49 Apical pleural scar. **A**, Chest radiograph shows asymmetric soft tissue thickening at the right apex. **B** and **C**, CT shows irregular subpleural density, with spiculation mimicking lung cancer. The patient was followed for 2 years without evidence of progression.

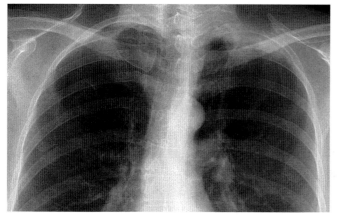

Fig. 15.50 Pancoast tumor. Chest radiograph shows apical pleural thickening associated with destruction of the posterior left second rib.

associated with previous tuberculosis is caused by a thickened (up to 25 mm) layer of fat between visceral pleura and the endothoracic fascia-innermost intercostal muscle stripe.[482] This may be related to contraction of the upper lobe, with filling of the extrapleural space by fat. The most important differential diagnosis is with Pancoast tumor, which should be suspected if there is marked asymmetry or nodularity of apical pleural

thickening, if the patient has local pain, and particularly if there is underlying bone destruction (Fig. 15.50).[480]

RADIOLOGIC APPEARANCE FOLLOWING PLEURODESIS

The most common indications for pleurodesis are recurrent pneumothorax, and malignant pleural effusion. The perfect agent for pleurodesis has not yet been found, but talc is increasingly used in place of chemical agents such as tetracycline or bleomycin, because of its higher success rates and lower rate of local and systemic symptoms.[336,483,484] Talc may be administered either as an aerosolized powder at thoracoscopy,[485,486] or as a slurry via large- or small-bore chest tubes at the bedside.[336,487,488]

After pleurodesis, the pleural space usually undergoes a phase of organization, with pleural thickening and loculations evident on chest radiograph; about 60% of patients have radiographically visible pleural thickening at longterm follow up.[451] On CT obtained after talc pleurodesis, the pleural space usually reveals variable degrees of pleural thickening and nodularity, often with a residual loculated effusion. High-attenuation areas representing talc deposits may mimic pleural calcification (Fig. 15.51).[489] The use of talc as a pleurodesis agent remains controversial, mainly because of recurrent reports of acute respiratory distress syndrome or lung edema occurring after talc pleurodesis.[485,490–492] Although expert opinion favors its use, the search for a better agent continues.

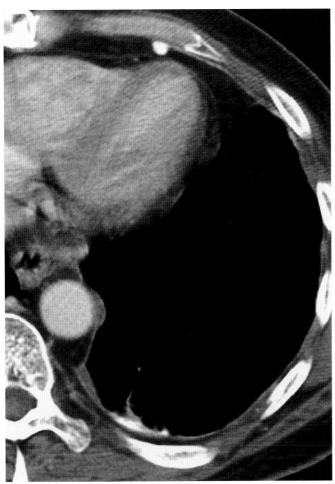

Fig. 15.51 CT appearances following talc pleurodesis. CT in a patient who had aerosolized talc pleurodesis for a left-sided mesothelioma shows a nodular area of hyperattenuation along the left posterior chest wall. A further nodular collection of talc is seen anterior to the heart.

PLEURAL CALCIFICATION

Virtually any process that can cause pleural thickening can be responsible for later pleural calcification,[493] but in practice calcification is usually due to infection, hemorrhage, or asbestos exposure. The recognized causes are listed in Box 15.11.

Calcification in asbestos inhalation and related conditions is morphologically characteristic,[494] and is considered on page 451. Calcification following infection and hemorrhage generally cannot be distinguished from each other. Such calcification is usually unilateral and varies from barely detectable to massive (Fig. 15.52). In the latter circumstance it becomes sheetlike and, reflecting the gravitationally determined distribution of the preceding pleural fluid, is often concentrated posterolaterally.[493] En face it appears as a hazy veil-like opacity, but in profile it is dense and linear, often parallel to the inner chest wall. The calcification in old empyemas occurs in both visceral and parietal pleura.[457,495] Sometimes these calcified layers are separated, an observation that can be made on radiographs or more easily on CT (Fig. 15.53).[457] In a series of 140 calcified fibrothoraces, 15.7% had a persistent effusion that was sandwiched between layers of thickened calcified pleura and was demonstrable on CT by virtue

---

Box 15.11 Causes of pleural calcification

Infection
Tuberculous empyema
Nontuberculous empyema

Hemothorax

Mineral inhalation
Asbestos (including tremolite talc)
Mica
Zeolites

Miscellaneous
Chronic pancreatitis[520]
Chronic hemodialysis[521]
Calcified metastasis
Alveolar microlithiasis[522,523]

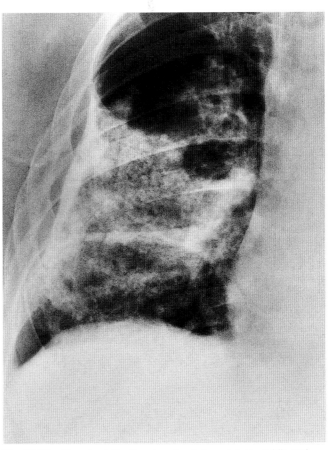

Fig. 15.52 Pleural calcification. Localized view of right middle and lower zone shows sheetlike calcification. Laterally, where calcification is tangential to the x-ray beam, it is dense and homogeneous, but medially – where it is seen en face – it is more broken up and nodular. There is a 1 cm thick band of noncalcified pleural thickening along the lateral chest wall.

of its attenuation, location, homogeneity, and failure to enhance.[457] This can be suspected from the plain radiograph with pleural thickening of >2 cm and a double layer of calcification.[457] Active infection of these loculated collections is manifest by expansion of the pleural opacity and development of an air–fluid level signifying a bronchopleural fistula.[495]

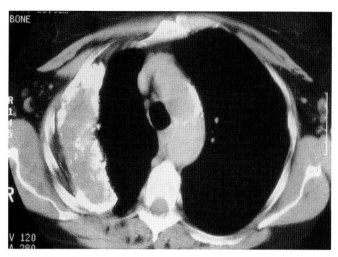

Fig. 15.53 Pleural calcification – old tuberculous empyema. Lenticular pleural opacity shows soft tissue density centrally and is marginated by heavy calcification both in the visceral and parietal pleura.

Occasionally postempyema calcification in the pleural space is manifest as a milk of calcium collection. These are often lenticular in shape and surrounded by mildly thickened pleura. On CT they are high density (200–300 HU) and typically homogeneous.[479]

THORACIC SPLENOSIS

Thoracic splenosis occurs when tissue from a traumatized spleen crosses an injured diaphragm and proliferates within the left hemithorax.[497] It is an uncommon condition[498]; in one prospective review there was evidence of splenic tissue within the thorax in only three of 17 patients who had sustained combined splenic and diaphragmatic injury.[499] Tissue from a traumatized spleen crosses an injured diaphragm and proliferates within the left thorax.[497] The resulting pleural nodules are often multiple and usually <3 cm in diameter, but may be up to 7 cm.[497] The nodules are implanted on parietal or viscera pleura, including fissures.[500]

On radiologic study, lesions of splenosis usually appear as pleural masses of soft tissue attenuation (Fig. 15.54), but they may appear intraparenchymal both on conventional radiographs and CT.[497] It is likely that the majority of apparently intrapulmonary lesions have pleural contact, though possibly some have been implanted in a lung laceration rather than on the pleural surface. On CT, the lesion may be lobulated or smooth and of soft tissue density.[499] On T1- and T2-weighted MRI the masses have been shown to be isointense with paraspinal muscles and subcutaneous fat, respectively.[499] Should the spleen have been removed at the time of trauma, the absence of Howell-Jolly bodies in a blood film would suggest persisting ectopic splenic activity.

The diagnosis may be confirmed with scintiscans using ^{99m}Tc-sulfur colloid, ^{99m}Tc-labeled heat damaged erythrocytes, or ^{111}In-labeled platelets, all of which are taken up by the ectopic splenic tissue.[497,501–503]

PNEUMOTHORAX

Traditionally, pneumothorax is divided into spontaneous and traumatic types. The most common causes in adults are listed in Box 15.12. Only spontaneous pneumothorax is discussed in this chapter, apart from a brief consideration of pneumothorax associated with mechanical ventilation.

Primary spontaneous pneumothorax

A pneumothorax occurring without an obvious precipitating traumatic event is termed *spontaneous*; if, in addition, the individual is apparently healthy, the pneumothorax is termed

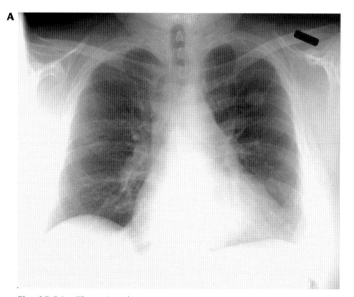
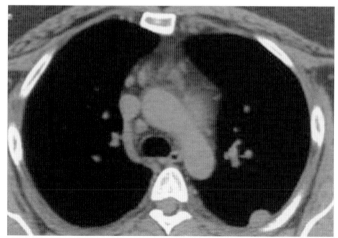

Fig. 15.54 Thoracic splenosis in a patient with a history of previous trauma. **A**, Chest radiograph shows a well-defined soft tissue mass in the left upper chest. **B**, CT confirms a posterior pleural mass. Splenosis was confirmed by sulfur colloid scan.

Box 15.12 Causes and varieties of pneumothorax in adults

Spontaneous
Primary
- Primary spontaneous pneumothorax
- Familial pneumothorax

Secondary
- Airflow obstruction
- Asthma, chronic obstructive pulmonary disorder, cystic fibrosis
- Bronchial atresia
- Spinocerebellar ataxia
- Infection
- Cavitary pneumonias
- Pneumatocele
- Tuberculous, fungal, hydatid disease
- AIDS[547,548]
- Infarction
- Septic, aseptic
- Neoplasm
- Primary, secondary, radiation
- Diffuse lung disease, including Langerhans cell histiocytosis, lymphangiomyomatosis, tuberous sclerosis, idiopathic pulmonary fibrosis, sarcoidosis

Catamenial pneumothorax
Heritable disorders of fibrous connective tissue

Traumatic
Iatrogenic
- Thoracotomy, thoracocentesis
- Percutaneous biopsy (lung, kidney, etc)
- Tracheostomy
- Central venous punctures
- Artificial ventilation
- Feeding tube perforation

Noniatrogenic
Closed
- Ruptured esophagus
- Ruptured trachea
- with or without rib fracture

Penetrating

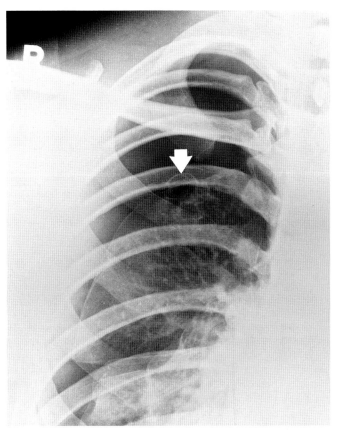

Fig. 15.55 Primary spontaneous pneumothorax. The visceral pleural line is clearly demonstrated together with a lateral avascular space. There is a pleural bleb at the apex of the lung (arrow), a common finding. Such blebs are usually not detectable when the lung reexpands.

primary. Primary spontaneous pneumothorax is strongly associated with smoking.[504,505] Two-thirds of patients are between 20 and 40 years of age.[506] The male:female ratio is approximately 5:1.[506–508] There is a slight predominance of right- over left-sided pneumothorax, which is thought simply to reflect the slightly larger volume of the right lung.[506] Bilateral pneumothoraces occur but are unusual,[509] and are more likely to occur metachronously than simultaneously. Thus, in one series of 242 cases 10% were bilateral but only 2.5% were simultaneous.[510] The incidence is about 10 per 100,000 population per year.[508]

Primary spontaneous pneumothorax is nearly always the result of rupture of an apical pleural bleb. Blebs are said to be detectable on chest radiographs in 15% of cases in the presence of pneumothorax (Fig. 15.55); they are seen in 54% of patients at thoracoscopy and in 92% at thoracotomy.[506] They are rarely seen, however, on chest radiographs obtained after resolution of pneumothorax. CT is much more sensitive than chest radiography in detecting abnormal airspaces in patients with

previous pneumothorax; in one study they were identified by CT in 85% of 20 patients examined 2 months after spontaneous pneumothorax.[511] This compared with a frequency of 30% in control subjects. The most common lesion was paraseptal emphysema (in 80%) with a subpleural and apical predilection, but centrilobular emphysema (in 60%) was almost as common.[511] In another similar study, emphysematous lesions (usually peripheral) were found on chest CT in 22 of 27 young patients with previous spontaneous pneumothorax, and such lesions were seen in 24 of 27 on direct visualization of the lungs.[512] In another CT study the size and number of apical "blebs" (cystic airspaces) was shown to correlate directly with the likelihood of pneumothorax recurrence and need for surgical treatment.[513] The formation or rupture of blebs is probably encouraged by the greater mechanical stresses occurring at the lung apex,[514] where the pleural surface pressure is much more negative than at the base. The transpulmonary pressure, which is the force distending the lungs, is therefore greater at the apex than at the base, causing apical alveoli to be more distended.[515] These stresses are magnified in subjects with long lungs, possibly explaining why pneumothoraces are more common in tall, thin individuals. Interestingly, if the prevalence of spontaneous pneumothorax is compared in male and female groups of the same height, any sex difference in prevalence disappears.[516] There is some difference of opinion regarding the importance of stressful activity in precipitating the actual event.

Some authors suggest that this happens only occasionally,[517] but in other series about one-quarter of patients were engaged in stressful activity, coughing, or sneezing.[506] Unusual atmospheric pressure swings may play a part in precipitating some pneumothoraces.[518]

On presentation patients typically have chest pain (92%) and dyspnea (79%).[506] A few patients are asymptomatic. The pathophysiologic effect is usually mild, but there is a restrictive ventilatory defect,[519] and sometimes transient hypoxemia and widening of the $(A–a)O_2$ gradient.[520] The pneumothorax resorbs once the causal pleural break seals. Absorption is slow, occurring at a rate of about 1.25% of the hemithoracic volume per day.[521] Thus, even a 15% pneumothorax takes 10 days to resolve. In one large series the average time for resorption was 25 days.[506] Breathing 100% oxygen increases the resorption rate.[522] Without definitive treatment the likelihood of having another pneumothorax is about 40%, and this is three times more likely on the ipsilateral side.[506] The chance of recurrence rises with each episode from about 25% with the first to about 50% after several episodes, at which point the risk flattens off.[506] More than 60% of recurrences occur within 2 years,[523] though they are reported up to 12 years after the initial pneumothorax.[506] Risk factors for recurrence include increasing age and height:weight ratio.[523]

Primary spontaneous pneumothorax may be treated conservatively, with chest tube drainage, or with chemical or surgical pleurodesis, the latter usually combined with bullectomy.[506,524]

Familial pneumothorax has been occasionally reported since its first description in 1921.[525] The subject was reviewed in 1960[526] and again in 1979.[527] These last authors found reports of 61 pneumothoraces in 22 families. The male:female ratio was 1.8:1. The reported cases did not allow the mode of inheritance to be determined. Familial pneumothorax does not seem to be definitely related to stature, though in some reports patients have been marfanoid.[528] Other workers have raised the possibility of a relationship to human lymphocyte antigen haplotype (A2, B40) and α_1-antitrypsin phenotype.[525] Concurrent spontaneous pneumothoraces have been reported in 71-year-old identical twins.[529] There is also a report of pneumothoraces associated with large bullae in sisters.[530]

Secondary spontaneous pneumothorax

A pneumothorax developing without a precipitating traumatic event in a patient with predisposing lung disease is said to be a spontaneous secondary pneumothorax. These are generally considered less common than primary spontaneous pneumothoraces. Important causes include the following.

Airflow obstruction

Chronic obstructive pulmonary disease is the most common cause of secondary spontaneous pneumothorax.[531] Patients are predominantly male (3:1 male:female preponderance in one series) and older than patients with primary spontaneous pneumothorax (median age 59 years versus 32 years in the same series).[532] Pneumothorax is a serious complication that can lead to significant morbidity and possibly death.[532–534] The incidence in patients with chronic obstructive pulmonary disease has been estimated to be 0.4% per year, and the mortality is 3% or higher.[506,533]

Pneumothorax is a recognized complication of cystic fibrosis; it occurred in 8% of one large series of patients with cystic fibrosis.[535] It is a late complication (average age 19 years) and usually an ominous one, reflecting advanced disease.[535]

Pneumothorax is an unusual complication of asthma in adults. The frequency in patients with asthma severe enough to warrant hospitalization varies from 0.26[536] to 2.5%.[537] The lower figure is probably the more reliable, since it is based on two very large series. The association is seen more often in children, but even so is uncommon.[538] Recurrent primary spontaneous pneumothorax has been reported as a rare manifestation of bronchial atresia.[539] In this single case, the authors postulated that the hyperinflated lung, within the atretic segment, was predisposed to the development of pneumothorax.[539]

Interstitial lung disease

Pneumothorax may occur with any diffuse lung disease, but is particularly common in patients with cystic lung disease such as Langerhans cell histiocytosis (see p. 432) and lymphangiomyomatosis (see p. 941). Pneumothorax may be the presenting feature in patients with these entities.

Primary and secondary neoplasm

The association of primary bronchial neoplasm and pneumothorax has been reviewed.[540,541] The prevalence of this association is low; well under 1% of pneumothoraces are due to primary carcinoma of the lung.[541,542] Looked at the other way, pneumothorax is the initial manifestation in only 0.5% of lung carcinomas.[541] The suggested mechanisms include coincidental occurrence, possibly associated with chronic obstructive pulmonary disease[509,541]; tumor wall necrosis with direct pleural invasion and rupture (unexpectedly only a few of the carcinomas associated with pneumothorax have been cavitary[540]); rupture of lung that is overexpanded to compensate for adjacent carcinoma induced collapse[541]; and endobronchial obstruction with a check valve effect.[541,543] The suspicion of an underlying bronchial carcinoma is usually raised by the finding of a mass or cavitary lesion in the reexpanded lung. Sometimes, however, the reexpanded lung appears radiographically normal.

Pneumothorax is an unusual presenting feature of pleural mesothelioma; only 11 such cases are reported in the English literature.[544]

In a large series from the Mayo Clinic, about 0.5% of pneumothoraces were associated with lung metastases.[542] Of 45 cases in a literature review, 89% were caused by sarcoma (Fig. 15.56) and only 11% by carcinoma.[545] Osteogenic sarcoma is by far the most common sarcoma.[546,547] Other tumors reported to cause pneumothorax include Wilms tumor,[548] germ cell tumors,[549,550] and lymphoma.[551,552] Many of these patients have been on chemotherapy, and its role is not clear.[553] Pneumothoraces associated with metastases can occur before the deposits are radiographically detectable.[545]

Radiation

The association of radiation and pneumothorax was first reported in 1974.[554] It is unusual, with only 11 cases found in the English literature in a 1985 review.[554] It was reported in 1% of patients receiving mantle irradiation for lymphoma.[554] Usually no malignancy is present in the chest at the time the pneumothorax

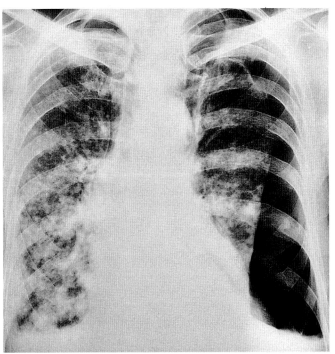

Fig. 15.56 Secondary spontaneous pneumothorax. Left pneumothorax with multiple bilateral nodules, more easily appreciated in the right lung, caused by metastases from a fibrosarcoma of the foot.

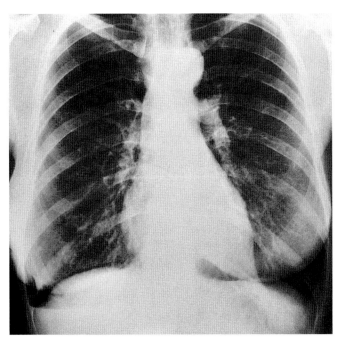

Fig. 15.57 Catamenial pneumothorax in a 34-year-old woman. This was the third episode, and all had been right sided. An air–fluid level in the costophrenic angle draws attention to the pneumothorax, which is otherwise easy to miss.

develops. Typically pneumothoraces occur 4–16 weeks after the end of radiation therapy, and radiographically visible radiation pneumonitis is common. Patients without associated radiation changes in the lung have also been reported.[555] Pneumothoraces tend to be small or moderate in size and heal spontaneously, though some are recurrent and bilateral.[139,556]

Pulmonary infarction

Pulmonary infarcts caused by aseptic emboli are rarely associated with a pneumothorax.[557,558] At the time the pneumothorax develops, the infarct may be sterile,[558,559] or it may have become secondarily infected.[560] Such infarcts are usually large, but only about one-third have had obvious cavities in the consolidation on the chest radiograph.[558] In half of the patients a large or persistent bronchopleural fistula develops.[558] Septic pulmonary emboli may also cause pneumothorax.[561]

Endometriosis and catamenial pneumothorax

Chest involvement in endometriosis is rare. The most common manifestation is catamenial pneumothorax. This disorder together with other aspects of endometriosis is discussed in this section. There are two distinct forms of chest endometriosis: pleurodiaphragmatic and bronchopulmonary.[444] Each has distinct demographic, pathogenetic, and clinical features.

Pleurodiaphragmatic endometriosis

Pleurodiaphragmatic endometriosis manifests clinically as catamenial pneumothorax or less commonly catamenial hemothorax.

Catamenial pneumothorax

Catamenial pneumothorax was first described by Maurer et al in 1958.[562] It is defined as pneumothorax occurring only in relation to the menses, appearing 1 day before or up to 3 days after the periods. It is uncommon; in females with spontaneous pneumothorax, catamenial pneumothorax has been recorded in 1[563] to 5.6%[564] of patients. It usually occurs in parous women who are slightly older than patients with primary spontaneous pneumothorax.[565,566] The pneumothorax is usually small and self resolving.[567] It is nearly always right sided (87% of cases) (Fig. 15.57),[565,568] but about 7% are left sided[566,568] and 6% are bilateral.[568,569] Recurrence is a characteristic feature; indeed, without repeated episodes a clear relationship to the menses cannot be established. Ten or 20 recurrences are not uncommon, and some authors have reported 30 or more.[570] Another characteristic is that recurrence is prevented by pregnancy or drugs that suppress ovulation.[566]

Although 69 cases had been reported by 1987,[568] there is continuing debate regarding pathogenesis. No single concept can explain the occurrence of catamenial pneumothorax in all patients.[567] The most plausible theory is that air enters the peritoneal cavity through the genital tract during menses, the only time the cervix is not occluded by a mucus plug.[571] Having entered the peritoneal cavity, the air passes into the pleural cavity through diaphragmatic holes, which may be either simple defects[562,564,567,572–576] or defects associated with necrotic endometrial implants along the diaphragm or visceral pleura.[562,567,577–579] Some of these latter patients have pelvic endometriosis. In the review by Slasky et al[567] one-third of catamenial pneumothoraces were associated with simple diaphragmatic defects and one-fifth with diaphragmatic endometrial implants. Further support for the genital transdiaphragmatic theory is afforded when cure follows either hormonal suppression of ovulation[481] or tubal ligation.[580]

The above mechanisms cannot account for all cases.[568] In some patients, pulmonary subpleural blebs seem to have been responsible just as in primary spontaneous pneumothorax.[481,568] In other cases endometriosis of the lung itself appears to have caused a direct air leak from the lung.[578,581] Another theory implicating prostaglandin induced bronchiolar constriction in alveolar rupture has been proposed.[566] Finally, the occurrence of recurrent pneumothorax, hemothorax, and hemoptysis in a single patient has also led to the suggestion that microembolization of endometrial tissue may be a pathogenic mechanism.[582] The role played by various mechanisms in catamenial pneumothorax has been critically reviewed.[567,568]

Catamenial hemothorax

A less common manifestation of pleurodiaphragmatic endometriosis in the chest is recurrent hemothorax occurring with the menses. Most patients are nulliparous with an average age of 32 years (range 24–42 years).[443] All patients have had right-sided hemothoraces, pleural endometriosis, and pelvic endometriosis with demonstrated diaphragmatic holes in some,[444] and it seems likely in these patients that pleural implantation has followed transdiaphragmatic spread. Diaphragmatic defects and endometrial tissue in pleural and peritoneal cavities can be demonstrated by both CT and ultrasound.[583,584]

Bronchopulmonary endometriosis

Brochopulmonary endometriosis is a disorder of parous women 30–50 years of age. There is often a clinical history of several spontaneous deliveries or uterine surgery, and the majority of patients do not have pelvic endometriosis.[585] Generally, postmenopausal patients have been symptomless while younger ones have had recurrent hemoptysis at the time of the menses (catamenial hemoptysis). There is usually a single focus of endometrial tissue in the lung parenchyma,[581,586–588] and occasionally in an airway,[589] together with a variable amount of parenchymal hemorrhage.

Radiologic study shows solitary, rounded nodules several centimeters in diameter,[587,588] or thin walled cavitary lesions with septation and focal mural irregularity.[586] Sometimes the dominant radiologic finding is the associated parenchymal bleeding, appearing as consolidation that comes and goes in phase with the menses and hemoptyses (Fig. 15.58).[589,590] Two patients investigated by bronchial and pulmonary arteriography with a view to embolization had normal studies.[591] The chest radiograph can be normal in appearance.[592] In four patients with endobronchial endometriosis, Wang et al[593] found that CT images obtained during hemoptysis were normal in three patients, and demonstrated mild bronchial wall thickening and peribronchial opacity in the right middle lobe in the fourth patient.

Catamenial hemoptysis has been successfully treated with the antigonadotropin danazol.[592] It seems likely that the pulmonary lesions are metastatic, since patients with bronchopulmonary involvement usually give a history of pregnancy or obstetric or gynecologic surgery (cesarean section, dilatation and curettage, abortion, hysterectomy). Experimental evidence in rabbits suggests that this is a realistic possibility, and the finding of decidua in the lungs at postmortem examination is well recognized.[586]

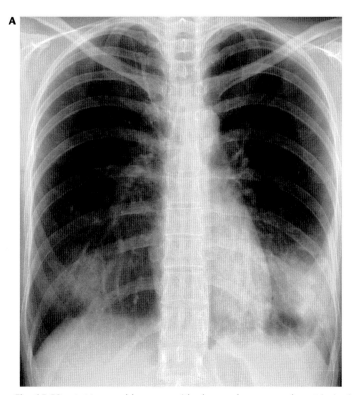
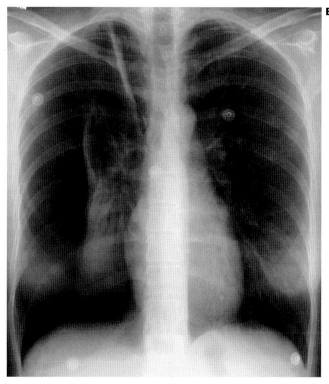

Fig. 15.58   A 44-year-old woman with pleuropulmonary endometriosis. **A**, Chest radiograph shows left lower lobe parenchymal opacity due to bleeding. **B**, Chest radiograph 1 year later shows a right-sided catemenial pneumothorax.

Heritable disorders causing pneumothorax

Five heritable disorders are associated with chest abnormalities; of these, four are disorders of fibrous connective tissue (Table 15.1). Although chest manifestations are uncommon in pseudoxanthoma elasticum, small nodules may be seen.[594]

Marfan syndrome

Marfan syndrome is an autosomal dominant disorder with a variable expression, involving particularly the eyes (myopia, ectopia lentis), aorta and heart (aortic aneurysm, aortic regurgitation, mitral valve disease), and musculoskeletal system (relatively long limbs in relationship to the trunk, arachnodactyly, pectus deformities, kyphoscoliosis, and joint laxity).[595] Marfan syndrome is associated with abnormalities of fibrillin (a glycoprotein component of elastin associated microfibrils) caused by mutations of the fibrillin gene on chromosome 15.[596] New mutations probably account for 15% of cases.[597] Life expectancy is greatly reduced, with most deaths caused by cardiovascular complications.[598]

The chief respiratory abnormalities in Marfan syndrome are pneumothorax, bullae, cysts, and emphysema. These findings are present in some 5–10% of patients. Kyphoscoliosis may be gross and can lead to cor pulmonale and death.[599] Pneumothorax is 30 to several hundred times more likely to occur in patients with Marfan syndrome than in unaffected individuals.[600,601] In such patients the frequency of pneumothorax ranges between 5 and 10%.[600,601] Pneumothoraces are commonly bilateral and recurrent. About two-thirds of affected patients have an underlying chest radiographic abnormality, either bullae or apical fibrosis.[600–602]

A particularly striking manifestation of Marfan syndrome is bullae occurring in young patients.[602,603] The bullae may be apical in position[604] or widely distributed.[601] They can become occupied by an aspergilloma.[601] Other manifestations include emphysema, congenital pulmonary malformations, apical fibrosis, bronchiectasis, and an increased frequency of lower respiratory tract infections.[601] Emphysema (Fig. 15.59) has been recorded at all ages from neonates to adults.[602] It may cause cor pulmonale and death in the pediatric age group.[602] Upper zone fibrosis is rare; only six cases have been reported in the world literature.[605] Associated congenital pulmonary malformations consist mainly of "rudimentary" middle lobes, which do not contribute to mortality or morbidity.[606] Bronchiectasis has been reported in Marfan syndrome,[601,607,608] but it is not clear if this is any more than a chance association.

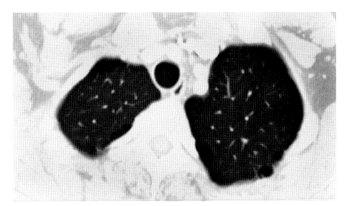

Fig. 15.59 A 43-year-old man with Marfan syndrome. CT shows subpleural emphysema.

Table 15.1 Heritable disorders associated with connective tissue abnormality

Disorder	Major clinical features	Associated chest abnormalities Common	Uncommon
Marfan syndrome	Myopia, ectopia lentis, aortic aneurysm, dissection, mitral valve disease, arachnodactyly, pectus deformity, scoliosis, lax joints	Emphysema, bullae, cysts, pneumothorax, skeletal deformity, aortic abnormality	Cor pulmonale, recurrent infection, bronchiectasis, mycetoma, pulmonary fibrosis, lobar hypoplasia
Ehlers–Danlos syndrome	Hyperextensible but elastic skin, lax joints, tissue fragility, bruising, bleeding	Hemoptysis, bullae, pneumothorax, skeletal deformity	Recurrent infection, bronchiectasis, tracheobronchomegaly, pulmonary fibrosis
Cutis laxa	Loose inelastic skin, doleful facies	Emphysema, cor pulmonale	Recurrent infection, bronchiectasis, tracheobronchomegaly, laryngeal obstruction, tortous or stenotic pulmonary artery, diaphragmatic hernia or eventration
Pseudoxanthoma elasticum		None	Small parenchymal nodules
Spinocerebellar ataxia	Ataxia, dysarthria	Emphysema, bullae, recurrent pneumothorax	

The marfanoid hypermobility syndrome is classed as a separate entity that shares some of the features of both Marfan and Ehlers–Danlos syndromes.[609] Chest abnormalities consist of cysts, pneumothorax, bronchomegaly, and hemoptysis.[610]

Ehlers–Danlos syndromes

The Ehlers–Danlos syndromes are a group of collagen disorders characterized by hyperextensible, doughy skin and joints and abnormal fragility of connective tissue that leads to bleeding, bruising, and atrophic scarring.[611,612] Ten clinical types are recognized.[612] Type IV is the type of Ehlers–Danlos syndrome characterized by vascular fragility and arterial rupture.[613,614] This type of Ehlers–Danlos syndrome is caused by mutation within the COL3AI gene, resulting in the disorder of type III procollagen.[615] The frequency of respiratory abnormality varies among types, but lung involvement is most commonly described in type IV (vascular type).[616–618] Much of the literature has been confined to case reports, indicating a low prevalence, and in one series of 100 patients no respiratory disorder was detected.[619]

The common clinical respiratory findings are hemoptysis, pneumothorax, and bullae. In one series of 20 patients about 50% had respiratory symptoms or abnormal lungs on the chest radiograph,[620] and 25% had hemoptysis, probably related to vascular fragility rather than a bleeding or clotting abnormality. Bullae can occur without pneumothorax[620] and in one patient were both transient and fluid filled.[621] Unlike in cutis laxa, emphysema is not a feature, though exceptional cases are reported.[611]

Pneumothorax is well described, particularly in type IV Ehlers–Danlos syndrome, but appears to be less common in Ehlers–Danlos syndromes than in Marfan syndrome.[620] It may be encountered with[622,623] or without visible bullae on the chest radiograph.[620,624] Cavitation may also be identified.[615–617]

Other findings that have been noted include recurrent sinusitis and pneumonia,[620] and rarely bronchiectasis,[625] tracheobronchomegaly,[620] and upper zone fibrosis.[620] Skeletal abnormalities are commonly seen on the chest radiograph. Of 20 cases in one series, 33% had pectus excavatum, 22% had scoliosis, 17% had straight back, and 17% had thin ribs.[620]

Cutis laxa (generalized elastolysis)

Cutis laxa may be acquired or congenital. Loose, inelastic skin is its characteristic feature. This results in a typical doleful facies with large earlobes, periorbital bagginess, and hook nose. Both forms demonstrate fragile, fragmented elastic tissue that shows normal collagen on histologic study. In the acquired form the abnormality is confined to the skin. Several congenital varieties are recognized. The autosomal recessive form is characterized by neonatal onset of respiratory disease with airflow obstruction, pneumonia, emphysema, and cor pulmonale, resulting in death in childhood.[626,627] The dominant form predominantly involves the skin, though other organ systems are sometimes involved.[628]

The most important respiratory abnormality accompanying this condition is emphysema, which usually develops shortly after birth,[626] but may be delayed until adolescence[629,630] or adulthood.[631,632] Emphysema may be accompanied by bullae or pulmonary arterial hypertension.[630] It commonly leads to death from cor pulmonale or respiratory failure. Other features described in children include repeated pulmonary infections,[626,627]

airflow obstruction caused by large floppy cords, tracheobronchomegaly,[633] and bronchiectasis.[628] The pulmonary arteries may become tortuous and stenotic,[629,634] causing abnormalities that appear on the chest radiograph. Hernias are a feature of cutis laxa and in the chest are manifest as hiatus hernias. In addition, the diaphragm may appear eventrated.[632,634]

Spinocerebellar ataxia

Familial spontaneous pneumothorax has been reported in association with spinocerebellar ataxia (type I).[635] In two siblings with gait ataxia and dysarthria there was a history of recurrent spontaneous pneumothoraces. There were radiographic signs of emphysema in both patients and CT in one demonstrated panacinar emphysema. Thin-section CT in the son of the proband also revealed abnormal parenchymal low density. Serum α_1-antitrypsin was normal in both patients and, though there was a 10 year smoking history in the index case, the sister was a lifelong non-smoker.[635]

Mechanical ventilation

Although pneumothorax was common in patients undergoing ventilation, the prevalence has decreased substantially with modern, low pressure ventilation techniques. Because there are so many modifying factors, a global prevalence rate is meaningless. The likelihood of pneumothorax is increased by high airway pressures, long ventilation times, and abnormal lungs, and is particularly associated with infection,[636] infarction, and chronic obstructive pulmonary disease.[509,637] Many factors cause high airway pressures: stiff lungs, volume cycling, unregulated manual inflation, large tidal volumes, endotracheal tube obstruction, right mainstem bronchus intubation, atelectasis, and positive end-expiratory pressure.[637,638] The development of a pneumothorax may be anticipated by the development of interstitial emphysema. Interstitial emphysema can sometimes be recognized on chest radiograph or chest CT by the presence of perivascular air. Later, this interstitial emphysema may progress to development of parenchymal cysts or pneumatoceles.[637,639] These appear as rounded, thin walled transradiancies, 2–9 cm in diameter; they occur anywhere in the lungs but particularly at the bases, medially, or along the diaphragm. These cysts may presage the development of a tension pneumothorax, unless airway pressure is reduced. Not only are pneumothoraces common with mechanical ventilation, but also they are more likely to be bilateral[509] and under tension (68% in one series).[637] Not surprisingly, pneumothorax occurring with mechanical ventilation may be rapidly fatal.[640] Immediate tube drainage is required.[641,642]

Radiographic signs

As with other pleural processes, the radiologic appearance of a pneumothorax depends critically on the radiographic projection, the patient's position, and the presence or absence of loculation.

Free pneumothorax

In the erect patient, air rises in the pleural space and separates the lung from the chest wall, allowing the visceral pleural line to become visible as a thin curvilinear opacity between vessel containing lung and the avascular pneumothorax space (Fig. 15.56). The pleural line remains approximately parallel to the chest wall. It can be difficult to identify in shallow pneumothoraces, when it may be hidden by ribs and other bony structures. Radiographs taken in expiration may make the line easier to detect as it alters its orientation relative to ribs and also increases the volume of the pneumothorax space relative to the lung volume.[59] However, two studies have shown that expiratory imaging does not improve the detectability of pneumothorax.[643,644] Therefore, only an inspiratory radiograph is obtained for evaluation of pneumothorax in routine practice. However, if clinical suspicion is high, or if findings on inspiratory radiographs are equivocal, an expiratory radiograph may be helpful. Alternatively, a lateral decubitus chest radiograph obtained with the suspect side uppermost may similarly be helpful.[645] In a study on cadavers with controlled pneumothoraces, lateral decubitus radiographs have been shown to be more sensitive than erect radiographs.[646] Somewhat surprisingly, this was not confirmed in an in vivo assessment comparing upright expiratory radiographs and lateral decubitus radiographs.[647] This study did, however, show that both views were equally good at excluding pneumothorax and that in 16% of cases the lateral decubitus view was critical in making the diagnosis of pneumothorax.[647] The difficulty in designing such studies has been discussed.[648]

Curvilinear shadows projected over the lung apex may mimic the visible visceral pleural line of a pneumothorax and cause difficulty in interpretation. Such opacities include those resulting from vascular lines, tubes, clothing, hair, scapulae, skinfolds, and the walls of bullae and cavities. Careful analysis of the structure and shape of these opacities – noting whether or not they extend beyond the inner margin of the chest wall – often allows correct identification. In practice, skinfolds and bullae are the most troublesome. Skinfold artifacts are seen on anteroposterior radiographs of very young or old, seriously ill patients, and are produced when subjects with loose skin slump against a cassette (Fig. 15.60). Sometimes it is clear that the skinfold shadow does not represent a pneumothorax, e.g. when vessels are seen beyond it, when it extends outside the margin of the chest cavity, or when it is located or oriented such that it could not possibly represent the edge of a partially collapsed lung. A helpful feature is that a skinfold generates a broad bandlike opacity with a sharp outer edge that fades off medially and may have a transradiant lateral margin, whereas visceral pleura tends to produce a much thinner linear opacity.[649] The thin marginal transradiancy associated with a skinfold artifact may be a Mach effect,[650,651] or may be due to air trapped beneath the fold of skin. A somewhat similar shadow to that generated by a skinfold may be produced by the scapular companion shadow.[652] Extrapleural dissection of air from a pneumomediastinum may also be mistaken for a pneumothorax on a chest radiograph.[653] The linear abnormality produced by this type of extrapleural air is usually confined to the extreme lung apex, and does not progress over time.

Cysts, bullae, and cavities are probably the most troublesome mimics of pneumothorax because they produce both transradiancy and thin curvilinear opacities (Fig. 15.61). These structures, however, have inner margins that are concave to the chest wall rather than convex.[509] They do not conform to the shape of the costophrenic angle when they are at the lung base,[654] and they may be demonstrably limited to a lobe.[59] Not

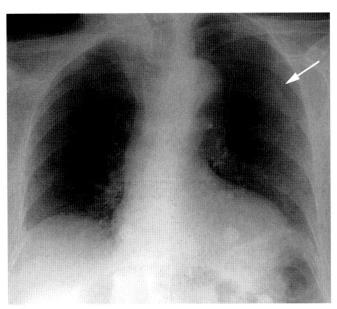

Fig. 15.60 *Skinfold simulating pneumothorax (arrow). The skinfold appears as a bandlike opacity with a sharp outer edge, and a lateral lucency due to air trapped between the skin and the image receptor. The skinfold does not conform to the expected shape of the visceral pleura. Despite these features, the radiograph was erroneously interpreted as showing a pneumothorax, and the patient was admitted with this diagnosis.*

only may a bulla mimic a pneumothorax, but the reverse sometimes occurs when adhesions or fibrous strands traverse the pleural space. These strandlike densities are generally straight, allowing a distinction from the curved linear margins of a cyst or bulla.[509] CT may be used to differentiate bullae from pneumothorax.[655] In patients who have bullae, the "double wall sign" (identification of both sides of the wall of a bulla) may be helpful in the identification of pneumothorax [656]

With a pneumothorax the transradiancy of the ipsilateral hemithorax is variable and is related to the degree of collapse, the presence or absence of disease in the lung itself, and the degree to which perfusion is reduced because of hypoventilation. With a small pneumothorax, transradiancy is unchanged or occasionally slightly increased, but with progressive collapse the lobe's opacity increases until it eventually becomes a fistlike mass of soft tissue density at the hilum. An air bronchogram is often but not invariably present, and its absence does not necessarily indicate obstruction of large airways as has been suggested. As the lung loses volume, the small apical blebs that are almost invariably associated with primary spontaneous pneumothorax frequently become clearly visible (Fig. 15.55). Searching the partially collapsed lung for other predisposing conditions (Fig. 15.62) such as cavities, bullae, interstitial disease, or metastases is also worthwhile. Care should be taken not to misinterpret shadows that simply result from the collapse itself.[59]

Pneumothorax is visible in about 90% of cases on the lateral chest radiograph, commonly as visceral pleural line anteriorly or posteriorly.[657] In the same study 53% of patients had an air–fluid level and in 9% this was the only sign of pneumothorax on the lateral view.[657] In about 15% of cases, the lateral chest radiograph provided information regarding the

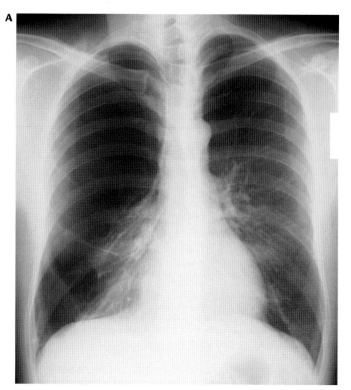

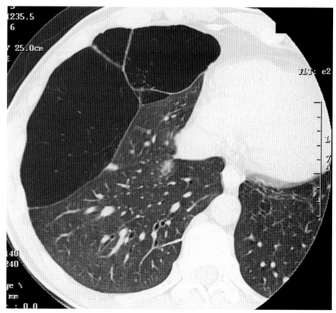

Fig. 15.61 A 36-year-old heavy smoker with very large bulla in right lung, compressing the normal lung parenchyma. **A**, Chest radiograph shows lucency in the right hemithorax simulating pneumothorax, though the hyperlucent space is traversed by some linear strands of parenchyma. **B**, CT confirms the presence of multiple anterior bullae.

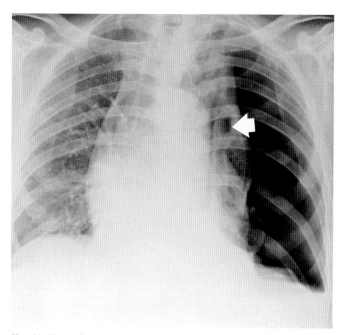

Fig. 15.62 Left pneumothorax secondary to tuberculosis. Anteroposterior chest radiograph of a 58-year-old man with acute dyspnea and pain in the left side of chest. There was a left pneumothorax with a little pleural fluid. The lung, prevented from collapsing completely by apical adhesion, contains a cavity (arrow). The pneumothorax was caused by a tuberculous bronchopleural fistula.

presence, size, or character of the pneumothorax to supplement that obtained from the frontal view.

Numeric estimates of the size of a pneumothorax can be expressed as a percentage of hemithorax volume by making simple measurements[658,659]; the percentage size of a pneumothorax may be accurately computed from measurements of interpleural distances.[660,661] However, such formulae are somewhat cumbersome for routine clinical use. The most commonly used technique, developed by Light, measures the average diameter of the lung and hemithorax, then cubes these diameters and finds their ratio. Thus, with an average 2 cm interpleural distance, if the hemithorax diameter is 10 cm, the percent pneumothorax is $8^3/10^3$, or approximately 50%.[5] The main value of these formulae is that they remind the user that the pneumothorax is usually substantially larger than it seems on a frontal chest radiograph.

Pneumothorax in the supine patient

Many patients, such as those who have sustained trauma and those in intensive care units, undergo radiography while supine. Chest radiographs of a supine patient are not sensitive in the detection of pneumothoraces; a sensitivity of 50–70% has been reported,[662–664] but clearly such figures depend critically on the size of the pneumothorax. Failure to diagnose pneumothorax under these circumstances may have serious consequences because, if untreated, many develop to tension.[637]

In the supine patient the highest part of the chest cavity lies anteriorly or anteromedially at the base and free pleural air rises to this region (Fig. 15.63). If the pneumothorax is small to moderate in size, the lung is not separated from the chest wall

A

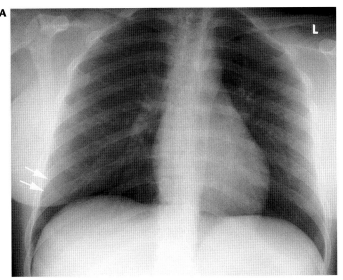

B

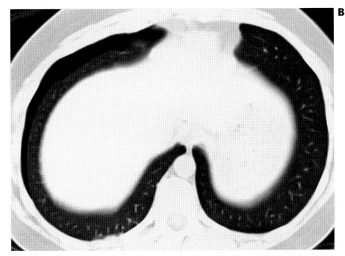

Fig. 15.63 Pneumothorax in a supine patient. **A**, Supine chest radiograph shows a deep lateral costophrenic sulcus on the right with a subtle lateral line indicating a pneumothorax (arrows). **B**, Supine chest CT shows air in the anterior and lateral costophrenic sulci, and air in contact with the anterior mediastinal fat.

laterally (Fig. 15.63) or at the apex. In the absence of a displaced visceral pleural line in these regions the detection of pneumothorax depends on identification of one or more of the following signs:

- Relative transradiancy in the hypochondrial region (Fig. 15.64)[662,665,666] due to air in the anterior costophrenic sulcus. There may also be increased lucency of the whole hemithorax.
- Increased sharpness of the adjacent mediastinal margin (Fig. 15.64) and diaphragm, which may become bordered by a band of relative transradiancy. This effect is particularly well seen in infants and neonates.[667]
- A deep and sometimes rather tonguelike lateral costophrenic sulcus (Fig. 15.63).[668]
- Visualization of the anterior costophrenic sulcus (Fig. 15.64). This recess runs obliquely across the hypochondrium and is sigmoid shaped, with its most cephalad point medially.[669] It may be seen as an interface or, if the undersurface is bordered by gastric or colonic gas, as a line.[665,666] The term "double diaphragm sign" has been applied to the simultaneous visualization of the anterior sulcus and the dome of the true hemidiaphragm.[666]
- Increased sharpness of the cardiac borders (Fig. 15.64), particularly the apex, and a lobulated, rounded, and often masslike appearance to the pericardial fat pads (Fig. 15.65)[666] because they are no longer flattened against the heart.
- Occasionally, anterior pleural air allows the middle lobe to retract medially away from the lateral chest wall while the lower and upper lobes still maintain chest wall contact. Under these circumstances the lateral border of the middle lobe becomes visible as a fine, linear opacity passing caudally from the lateral aspect of the minor fissure, parallel to the chest wall toward the diaphragm.[670]
- Pleural air may also collect in the minor fissure, giving a characteristic transradiancy bounded by two visceral pleural lines.[517,671]

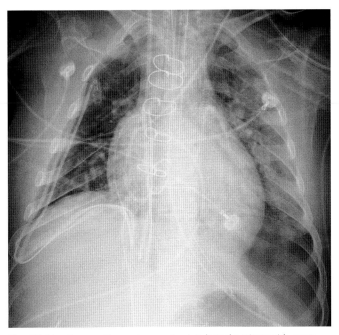

Fig. 15.64 Pneumothorax in a supine intubated patient with acute respiratory distress syndrome. Chest radiograph shows increased lucency over the left upper abdomen, due to air in the anterior costophrenic sulcus. There is increased sharpness of the left heart border.

- Visualization of the inferior edge of the collapsed lung[666] above the diaphragm. This must be distinguished from extrapleural extension of air above the diaphragm, described in pneumomediastinum.[672]
- Depression of the ipsilateral hemidiaphragm.[666]
- In infants the anterior junctional area is occupied by thymus and a junctional line is not normally seen on a frontal radiograph. Its identification on a frontal radiograph of a neonate signifies a bilateral pneumothorax.[673]

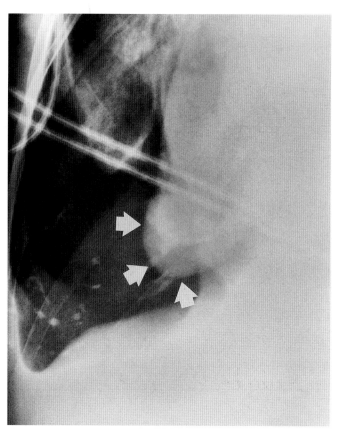

Fig. 15.65 Pneumothorax in a supine patient. Localized view of the right lung base demonstrates a fat pad in the right cardiophrenic angle that has become rounded and masslike (arrows).

If a pneumothorax is suspected on a radiograph of a supine patient, it can be confirmed or excluded by other views, several of which were first described in infants and neonates. The cross-table lateral view[674,675] is probably the least satisfactory because of overlap of the other hemithorax. An alternative is to place a cassette 45° dorsolaterally and angle the x-ray tube so that the central ray is perpendicular to the cassette. However, if the patient can be turned, the best image will result from a lateral decubitus view with the suspect side uppermost.[645]

Clearly CT is more sensitive than conventional radiography in detecting pneumothorax in supine subjects.[662–664] Some authors recommend that a limited CT examination of the lung bases be performed in all patients with severe head trauma at the time of cranial CT[663] to exclude unsuspected pneumothorax. Similarly, in a review of pneumothoraces detected incidentally on abdominal CT scans obtained in trauma victims, Neff et al[676] found that pneumothoraces were present in 230 (74%) of 312 patients, and 126 (55%) of these had not been detected by radiography. Eighty-four (67%) of the 126 patients with radiographically occult pneumothorax underwent chest tube placement.

There is increasing interest in the use of ultrasound to detect pneumothorax, particularly in patients who have had thoracentesis, or in those who have undergone trauma.[677–680] Ultrasonography of the normal pleural interface usually shows an echogenic line beneath which the lung is seen to slide.[679] A "comet tail" artifact may be seen with reverberations extending from the echogenic line to the edge of the image.[681] Diagnosis of pneumothorax by ultrasound depends on the absence of the lung sliding and comet tail signs. For optimal detection, the pleural interfaces should be evaluated at the second to fourth intercostal spaces anteriorly and at the sixth to eighth spaces in the midaxillary line.[682] In a study by Rowan et al,[681] of 27 patients with blunt thoracic trauma, supine chest radiography detected pneumothorax in only four of 11 patients in whom it was present, but ultrasound detected all 11 pneumothoraces, with one false positive due to extensive bullous lung disease. Detection of pneumothorax by ultrasound is operator dependent.

Loculated and localized pneumothorax

Sometimes a pneumothorax is truly loculated because of adhesions.[683] On other occasions a free pneumothorax shows an atypical distribution (Fig. 15.66). Several patterns are recognized.

Subpulmonic pneumothorax

Several papers have described subpulmonic pneumothorax with the visceral pleural line visible just above the diaphragm. This unusual location has been ascribed to preferential collection around diseased basal lobes,[684] or to scarring of the rest of the pleural space, e.g. following tuberculosis.[685] In another series of patients with the adult respiratory distress syndrome, subtle degrees of mediastinal shift and contour changes of the heart and hemidiaphragm suggested that these localized pneumothoraces were under tension.[686] Intrapleural air in this situation must be distinguished from extrapleural air that has dissected outward along the diaphragm from a pneumomediastinum[672,687,688] or from barotraumatic cysts.[637,639]

Loculated pneumothorax

Pneumothorax may loculate in the oblique fissure, giving a cystic opacity in the right mid zone[689,690] or an air–fluid collection with a hemopneumothorax.[691] It may also occur in the inferior accessory fissure.[692]

"Pulmonary ligament pneumatocele"

Following trauma, particularly in children or young adults, a triangular collection of air sometimes develops against the mediastinum with its apex near the hilum. These air collections are more common on the left and may contain an air–fluid level.[693] An obvious ipsilateral pneumothorax may or may not be present, and the air collection generally clears in days or weeks.[694] In the past, these transradiancies have been ascribed to an air collection in the inferior pulmonary ligament.[695–698] CT evaluation, which allows more accurate localization, indicates that such transradiancies are either localized posteromedial pneumothoraces or air collections within the mediastinum.[694,699]

Pneumothorax ex vacuo

Pleural surface pressure would be expected to be more negative over collapsed lung and thus might favor the localization of pneumothorax to that region. Pneumothorax adjacent to collapsed lobes (termed pneumothorax ex vacuo) has been recognized in adults[700,701] and children.[702] The identification of a

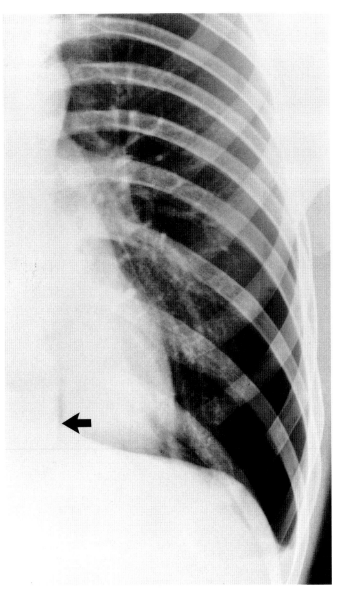

Fig. 15.66   Left pneumothorax in an erect patient. There is an obvious pneumothorax. Pleural air is seen to collect in a linear manner along the left heart border and behind the heart (arrow) and should not be misinterpreted as pneumomediastinum.

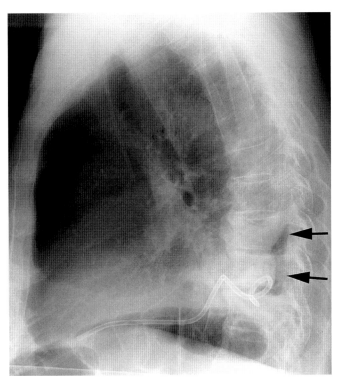

Fig. 15.67   Pneumothorax ex vacuo in a patient with left lower lobe collapse due to lung cancer, who received a chest drain for drainage of a left parapneumonic effusion. Lateral chest radiograph shows a posterior pneumothorax ex vacuo, adjacent to the collapsed left lower lobe (arrows).

pneumothorax confined to the space between collapsed lung and chest wall, the absence of air surrounding noncollapsed lobes, and the acute nature of lobar collapse help to differentiate the entity of pneumothorax ex vacuo from a conventional pneumothorax.[701] Pneumothorax ex vacuo may also occur in patients who undergo thoracentesis for malignant effusions, if thickened visceral pleura or lobar collapse prevents reexpansion of the lung (Fig. 15.67).[703] Pneumothorax ex vacuo is usually asymptomatic, and treatment with chest tube drainage is contraindicated.

Complications

About 20–50% of pneumothoraces are accompanied by *pleural fluid* (Fig. 15.57), which is usually scant and inconsequential.[704,657]

The fluid may be clear, serosanguineous, or sanguineous. On an erect frontal radiograph a small amount of fluid appears as a horizontal air–fluid level or as a C shaped opacity in the costophrenic angle when its horizontal upper border is below the central ray and its anterior and posterior margins are projected separately. Sometimes the air–fluid level generated by a small effusion may be more eye catching than the visceral pleural line and induce the observer to scrutinize the lung apex (Fig. 15.57). Rarely an air–fluid level is the only sign of a pneumothorax on an erect frontal radiograph.[657] If the pneumothorax is very small and pleural separation is present only at the apex, pleural fluid at the base will take on the classic meniscus form. In 3% or fewer of patients a hemothorax develops that is large enough to warrant treatment in its own right.[506,704] *Hemothorax* is much more frequent in primary than in secondary pneumothorax.[704] In keeping with this observation, 93% of patients with hemothorax in one review were men and 92% were under 39 years of age.[705] Torn adhesions between the parietal and visceral pleura are the most common sources of bleeding.[445] Blood can clot in the pleural space and produce a mass – a *fibrin body* or "pleural mouse" – that may mimic a pleural tumor (Fig. 15.68).[430] Pleural thickening is common following hemopneumothorax; in one series 22% of patients needed subsequent decortication.[506]

Uncommonly, purulent fluid accompanies a pneumothorax, giving a *pyopneumothorax*. This is seen with esophageal perforation or necrotizing pneumonia caused most commonly by infection with *Staphylococcus aureus*, *Pseudomonas* spp, *Klebsiella* spp, or anaerobes.[524]

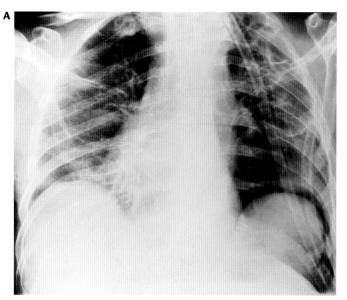
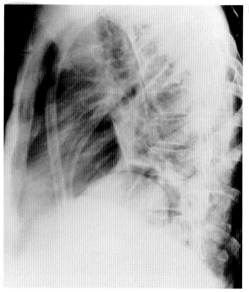

Fig. 15.68 Fibrin body in a patient with previous tuberculous hydropneumothorax (same patient as Figs 15.3 and 15.62). **A**, Frontal and **B**, lateral chest radiographs reveal a 10 cm rounded mobile mass lesion in the pleural space. This is homogeneous and has a smooth, sharp margin. There was no evidence of fungal infection and the mass was assumed to be a fibrin body despite its unusually large size.

Pneumothoraces may be recurrent, and conditions that predispose to recurrence also predispose to bilateral pneumothoraces. *Bilateral pneumothoraces* may be synchronous or, more commonly, metachronous. Conditions particularly associated with bilateral pneumothoraces have been reviewed.[706] They include primary spontaneous pneumothorax and a variety of secondary pneumothoraces, particularly those associated with malignant lung deposits, Langerhans cell histiocytosis, sarcoidosis, lymphangioleiomyomatosis, and exposure to radiation. Catamenial pneumothorax is almost invariably recurrent.

Pneumomediastinum is an unusual association of pneumothorax seen most commonly in neonates. In adults the combination may be seen in patients being mechanically ventilated and with rupture of the esophagus,[707] trachea, or bronchi. It is rare in primary spontaneous pneumothorax.

Pneumoperitoneum is an extremely rare complication of pneumothorax. Diaphragmatic defects may allow pleural air to pass into the peritoneal cavity, resulting in a pneumoperitoneum.[708] Presumably because of the pressure gradient across the diaphragm, the development of pneumothorax after pneumoperitoneum is much more common.

Tension pneumothorax

Tension pneumothorax is a life-threatening complication. It occurs when intrapleural pressure becomes positive for a significant part of the respiratory cycle, compressing the normal lung and causing a restrictive ventilatory defect, an increase in the work of breathing, and a $\dot{V}/\dot{Q}$ imbalance.[509] The cardiovascular effects probably result from respiratory failure rather than directly from the increased pleural pressure.[709,710] The condition must be treated by immediate decompression of the pleural space. It is usually diagnosed clinically, by the presence of tachypnea, tachycardia, cyanosis, sweating, and hypotension. However, it sometimes is first detected on radiographic examination, and the most important signs are mediastinal shift and diaphragmatic depression (Fig. 15.69).

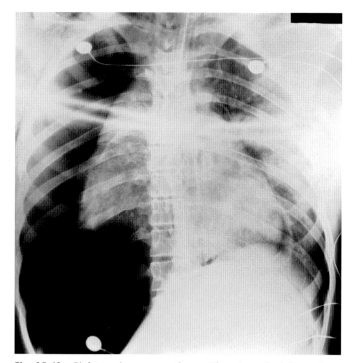

Fig. 15.69 Right tension pneumothorax. There is marked depression of the right hemidiaphragm and shift of the mediastinum to the left, indicated by the position of the heart and endotracheal tube. The patient was being mechanically ventilated, which may account for the relatively slight mediastinal shift compared with the gross diaphragmatic depression. Complete collapse of the right lung is prevented by consolidation. There is also a small left pneumothorax.

Contralateral mediastinal shift must be interpreted with caution because some movement toward the normal side is a frequent finding in a nontension pneumothorax, reflecting the fact that the pressure in the pneumothorax space is usually not as negative as on the normal side. If this shift is any more than mild or mild to moderate, true tension should be considered. Unfortunately, there is no accurate way of relating the amount of mediastinal shift to the degree of tension, because mediastinal compliance varies substantially from person to person. The degree of depression of the ipsilateral hemidiaphragm is a more useful observation than the extent of mediastinal shift, and the hemidiaphragm is invariably depressed with significant tension. In patients receiving mechanical ventilation, diaphragmatic depression is the major sign of tension. In such patients

mediastinal shift is not a marked feature because airway pressure remains positive.[509] It is important to remember that significant tension can occur with little lung collapse if the underlying lung is abnormal (e.g. consolidated).[509] Tension pneumothorax occurs when the leak is through a tear, which behaves like a valve. Tension is unusual in primary pneumothorax and is seen more commonly with trauma or mechanical ventilation,[637] particularly if positive end-expiratory pressure is employed.[641]

Reexpansion pulmonary edema

Reexpansion pulmonary edema (Fig. 15.70) is an uncommon complication of pneumothorax. In one prospective 8 year study the incidence of reexpansion pulmonary edema was 0.9% of

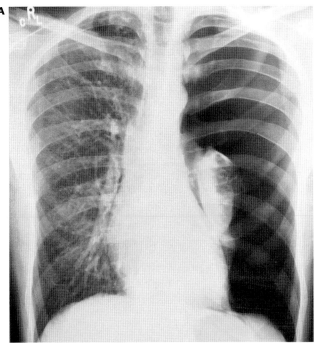

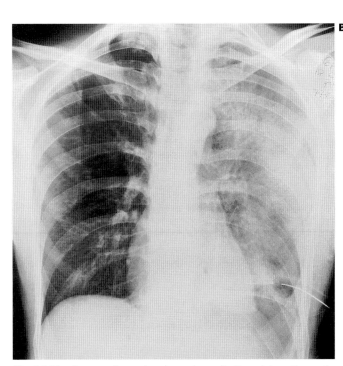

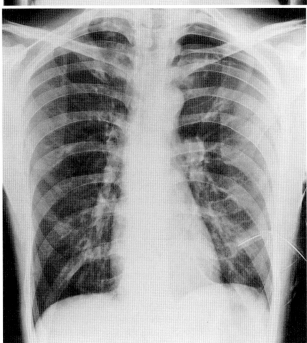

Fig. 15.70 Reexpansion pulmonary edema. **A**, Complete collapse of the left lung following a primary spontaneous pneumothorax that had begun 7 days previously. **B**, Diffuse consolidation of the left lung 2 h after insertion of a left pleural drain attached to an underwater seal drain. **C**, Twenty-four hours after the radiograph in **B**, the airspace opacity has cleared.

320 episodes of spontaneous pneumothorax managed by tube drainage.[711] The mechanism is obscure; some authors suggest it is related to depletion of surfactant,[712–715] and others that it is due to anoxic, mechanical, or mediator induced capillary damage that leads to increased capillary permeability. Considerable evidence supports the latter view.[713,714,716–718] The edema usually develops within 2 h of reexpansion and can progress for 1 or 2 days, resolving within 5–7 days. Reexpansion edema usually causes little morbidity, but patients can become hypotensive and hypoxic,[524,719] and at least one death has been recorded.[720] Predisposing factors are generally considered to be complete pneumothoraces with gross lung collapse, chronicity of the pneumothorax, and high negative aspiration pressures. Most pneumothoraces have been complete and present for at least 3 days,[712,715,721] but shorter durations have been reported.[722] In many patients expansion has been rapid because negative aspiration pressure was used,[720,723,724] but this has not been universal.[715,725,726] The radiograph shows ipsilateral airspace opacity. Exceptional cases are reported with contralateral edema[719,727,728] and recurrent edema with recurrent pneumothorax.[729]

Buffalo chest

Sometimes following major cardiovascular surgery both pleural spaces are in communication, so what would otherwise be a unilateral pneumothorax becomes bilateral[730] and behaves in an atypical shifting fashion.[731] This phenomenon, sometimes called buffalo chest (because the buffalo has a single pleural space)[732] is common in patients who have had double lung transplants or heart–lung transplants. Although buffalo chest can potentially allow drainage of bilateral pneumothorax with a single chest tube,[733] this should be attempted only with great caution.[734] Buffalo chest may occasionally be present in patients without previous surgery.[735]

Following progress and management

Not every pneumothorax requires drainage. Asymptomatic spontaneous pneumothorax with an interpleural distance <2 cm may be successfully managed by observation,[736] with or without oxygen treatment to speed reabsorption. In larger pneumothoraces, or symptomatic pneumothoraces, simple aspiration often suffices.[736] If the pleural surfaces can be completely reapposed by aspiration or drainage, the visceral pleural leak usually resolves quite rapidly.

Changes in the size of a pneumothorax can be followed on serial radiographs by measuring the interpleural distance at the apex or along a specified rib.

The causes to consider for failure of lung expansion include tube malplacement; large airway occlusion by blood, mucus, or foreign body; persistent air leak, airway rupture, pleural adhesions (Fig. 15.62); visceral pleural thickening; and bronchopleural fistula. A number of these conditions may be detected radiographically. Tube malposition may be obvious, but in some cases the radiographic signs are subtle. Malposition in the oblique fissure may be suspected on an anteroposterior radiograph if the chest tube follows a gently curved or straight course upward and medially from its entry point, rather than deviating soon after entry where it is deflected in front of or behind the lung.[737] The outer margin of pleural drainage tubes is seen by virtue of their contrast with surrounding air. Should such a tube become entirely displaced into the soft tissue of the chest wall, the outer margin of the tube will be no longer detectable.[738] However, CT is more accurate than the chest radiograph for the diagnosis of chest tube malposition.

A persistent air leak is relatively common following spontaneous pneumothorax.[739] This complication is of particular importance in patients with preexisting lung disease (emphysema or lung fibrosis), in whom the time to resolution of pneumothorax is greater than in patients with normal lungs and in whom surgical intervention may be necessary.[504,739,740] Provided the degree of collapse is mild, it should be possible to detect any underlying lung diseases that may be responsible for persistent leakage, particularly diffuse interstitial fibrosis, cysts, bullae, or emphysema. Pleural adhesions that may hold open a visceral pleural tear will be seen as band shadows joining visceral to parietal pleura, distorting the lung envelope (Fig. 15.62).

With failure of the lung to reexpand completely, the pneumothorax becomes chronic and persistent. This is an indication for surgery.

BRONCHOPLEURAL FISTULA

While the term bronchopleural fistula has typically been used to refer to a direct communication between a bronchus and the pleural space,[5] others use the term more loosely to indicate a persistent air leak from bronchi or from the lung parenchyma.[741–743] With this broader definition, there is a distinction between central bronchopleural fistula, where there is direct communication between a large bronchus and the pleural space, and peripheral bronchopleural fistula, where the leak is from a peripheral bronchus or from the lung parenchyma.[741–743] Central bronchopleural fistulas are usually large, and usually require surgical treatment. Peripheral fistulas are often smaller, and may respond to nonsurgical management such as bronchial occlusion. Bronchopleural fistula is an important cause of air in the pleural space. Although bronchopleural fistula has a number of causes, the bulk of cases are due to either surgical lung resection or necrotizing infections. The causes of bronchopleural fistulas are listed in Box 15.13.[744,745]

Box 15.13 Causes of bronchopleural fistula

Trauma
Thoracic surgery/lobectomy/pneumonectomy
Other iatrogenic causes (chest tubes, lung biopsy, thoracocentesis, nasogastric tube misplacement, oleothorax)

Infection
Necrotizing pneumonia/empyema (especially anaerobic, tuberculous, pyogenic)
Fungal infection

Pulmonary infarction
Sterile/septic

Miscellaneous
Neoplasms
Radiation
Rheumatoid nodules

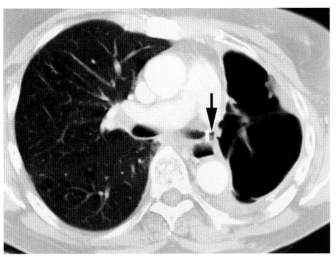

Fig. 15.71 Central bronchopleural fistula in a 70-year-old woman following left pneumonectomy for a bronchial carcinoma. CT shows a large amount of air in the pneumonectomy space. Air leads from the bronchial stump to the pneumonectomy space (arrow).

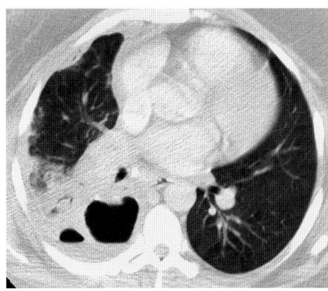

Fig. 15.72 Peripheral bronchopleural fistula in a 37–year-old female following wedge resection of the superior segment of the right lower lobe. There is air in the pleural space, but the fistula is not directly demonstrated.

Bronchopleural fistulas complicating infections (Fig. 15.62) are considered in the discussion of empyema (see p. 203). Postsurgical fistulas are considered here. They occur with a frequency of about 2.5–3%[746,747] and usually develop within 2 weeks of surgery. They should be suspected with the postoperative development of fever, hemoptysis, cough (especially if productive of a large amount of brown sputum), and a persistent large air leak from the pleural drains. Postoperative bronchopleural fistulas are usually associated with infection, and are much more common after surgery performed for pulmonary infections such as tuberculosis.[748]

The chest radiographic signs of bronchopleural fistula following recent pneumonectomy are: (1) a sudden increase in the amount of air in the pneumonectomy space, or in the adjacent chest wall; (2) a decreased amount of fluid; (3) loss of the normal mediastinal shift toward the operated side; and (4) sometimes a contralateral parenchymal opacity due to aspiration of fluid from the pneumonectomy space. Occasionally, unchanged persistence of an airspace following pneumonectomy indicates a fistula. This happens when the residual space is surrounded by pleural fibrosis and scarring so that it cannot change shape.[746] Extensive scarring may also prevent the mediastinal shift sign from being seen.[749] It is not uncommon for radiographic signs (increasing pleural air) of bronchopleural

fistula to appear in otherwise well patients who go on without complication or interference to successful obliteration of the pleural cavity.[750] This is ascribed to a flap valve type of fistula that is self healing. Delayed bronchopleural fistula, occurring after air has been eliminated from the pneumonectomy or lobectomy space, is signaled by the reappearance of air in the pleural space (Fig. 15.71).

A fistula may be detected with ^{133}Xe lung scintigraphy in the washout phase.[751] However, it usually cannot be demonstrated with DTPA aerosol. Injection of water soluble contrast into the relevant bronchus, or into the pleural space may occasionally be helpful. CT can be helpful in depicting the anatomic details of a fistula, particularly in a peripheral bronchopleural fistula which cannot be directly visualized at bronchoscopy.[741,743] Although CT will directly visualize a peripheral bronchopleural fistula in only 30–50% of cases, it will show a probable cause of the bronchopleural fistula (e.g. peripheral cavity, bulla) in most of the others.[742,743] Use of thin sections through areas of suspected fistula may be helpful in directly identifying the site of leakage.[743] Postoperative peripheral bronchopleural fistulas (Fig. 15.72), or those related to bullae, are less likely to be demonstrated than other types of fistulas.[742,743]

REFERENCES

1. Zocchi L. Physiology and pathophysiology of pleural fluid turnover. Eur Respir J 2002;20:1545–1558.
2. Henschke CI, Davis SD, Romano PM, et al. The pathogenesis, radiologic evaluation, and therapy of pleural effusions. Radiol Clin North Am 1989;27:1241–1255.
3. Sahn SA. State of the art. The pleura. Am Rev Respir Dis 1988;138:184–234.
4. Agostoni E. Mechanics of the pleural space. Physiol Rev 1972;52:57–128.
5. Light RW. Pleural diseases, 2nd edn. Philadelphia: Lea and Febiger, 1990.
6. Noppen M, De Waele M, Li R, et al. Volume and cellular content of normal pleural fluid in humans examined by pleural lavage. Am J Respir Crit Care Med 2000;162:1023–1106.
7. Moskowitz H, Platt RT, Schachar R, et al. Roentgen visualization of minute pleural effusion. An experimental study to determine the minimum amount of pleural fluid

visible on a radiograph. Radiology 1973;109:33–35.

8. Hessen J. Roentgen evaluation of pleural fluid: a study of the localization of free effusions, the potentialities of diagnosing minimal quantities of fluid and its existence under physiologic conditions. Acta Radiol 1951;86:7–80.

9. Wiener-Kronish JP, Albertine KH, Licko V, et al. Protein egress and entry rates in pleural fluid and plasma in sheep. J Appl Physiol 1984;56:459–463.

10. Müller NL. Imaging of the pleura. Radiology 1993;186:297–309.

11. Wang NS. Anatomy and physiology of the pleural space. Clin Chest Med 1985;6:3–16.

12. Light RW, Macgregor MI, Luchsinger PC, et al. Pleural effusions: the diagnostic separation of transudates and exudates. Ann Intern Med 1972;77:507–513.

13. Romero S, Martinez A, Hernandez L, et al. Light's criteria revisited: consistency and comparison with new proposed alternative criteria for separating pleural transudates from exudates. Respiration 2000;67:18–23.

14. Heffner JE, Brown LK, Barbieri CA. Diagnostic value of tests that discriminate between exudative and transudative pleural effusions. Primary Study Investigators. Chest 1997;111: 970–980.

15. Gazquez I, Porcel JM, Vives M, et al. Comparative analysis of Light's criteria and other biochemical parameters for distinguishing transudates from exudates. Respir Med 1998;92:762–765.

16. Heffner JE, Highland K, Brown LK. A meta-analysis derivation of continuous likelihood ratios for diagnosing pleural fluid exudates. Am J Respir Crit Care Med 2003;167:1591–1599.

17. Chakko S. Pleural effusion in congestive heart failure. Chest 1990;98:521–522.

18. Romero-Candeira S, Fernandez C, Martin C, et al. Influence of diuretics on the concentration of proteins and other components of pleural transudates in patients with heart failure. Am J Med 2001;110:681–686.

19. Horowitz ML, Schiff M, Samuels J, et al. Pneumocystis carinii pleural effusion. Pathogenesis and pleural fluid analysis. Am Rev Respir Dis 1993;148:232–234.

20. el-Naggar T, Abd-el-Maeboud KH, Abdallah MY, et al. Peripartum pleural effusion. Respir Med 1994;88:541–542.

21. Gourgoulianis KI, Karantanas AH, Diminikou G, et al. Benign postpartum pleural effusion. Eur Respir J 1995;8:1748–1750.

22. Kumagai-Kurata N, Kunitoh H, Nagamine-Nishizawa M, et al. Idiopathic lobular panniculitis with specific pleural involvement. Eur Respir J 1995;8:1613–1615.

23. McNeil KD, Fong KM, Walker QJ, et al. Gorham's syndrome: a usually fatal cause of pleural effusion treated successfully with radiotherapy. Thorax 1996;51:1275–1276.

24. Panchal N, Bhagat R, Pant C, et al. Allergic bronchopulmonary aspergillosis: the spectrum of computed tomography appearances. Respir Med 1997;91:213–219.

25. Man A, Schwarz Y, Greif J. Pleural effusion as a presenting symptom of ovarian hyperstimulation syndrome. Eur Respir J 1997;10:2425–2426.

26. Trudo FJ, Gopez EV, Gupta PK, et al. Pleural effusion due to herpes simplex type II infection in an immunocompromised host. Am J Respir Crit Care Med 1997;155:371–373.

27. Bass SN, Ailani RK, Shekar R, et al. Pyogenic vertebral osteomyelitis presenting as exudative pleural effusion: a series of five cases. Chest 1998;114: 642–647.

28. Jay SJ. Diagnostic procedures for pleural disease. Clin Chest Med 1985;6:33–48.

29. Smyrnios NA, Jederlinic PJ, Irwin RS. Pleural effusion in an asymptomatic patient. Spectrum and frequency of causes and management considerations. Chest 1990;97:192–196.

30. Maher GG, Berger HW. Massive pleural effusion: malignant and nonmalignant causes in 46 patients. Am Rev Respir Dis 1972;105:458–460.

31. Adams RF, Gleeson FV. Percutaneous image-guided cutting-needle biopsy of the pleura in the presence of a suspected malignant effusion. Radiology 2001; 219:510–514.

32. Adelman M, Albelda SM, Gottlieb J, et al. Diagnostic utility of pleural fluid eosinophilia. Am J Med 1984;77:915–920.

33. Jeanfaivre T, Cimon B, Tolstuchow N, et al. Pleural effusion and toxocariasis. Thorax 1996;51:106–107.

34. Ishiura Y, Fujimura M, Nakamura N, et al. Intrapleural corticosteroid injection therapy for post-traumatic eosinophilic pleural effusion. Respir Med 1996;90:501–503.

35. Kuhn M, Fitting JW, Leuenberger P. Probability of malignancy in pleural fluid eosinophilia. Chest 1989;96: 992–994.

36. Hirsch A, Ruffie P, Nebut M, et al. Pleural effusion: laboratory tests in 300 cases. Thorax 1979;34:106–112.

37. Storey DD, Dines DE, Coles DT. Pleural effusion. A diagnostic dilemma. JAMA 1976;236:2183–2186.

38. Ansari T, Idell S. Management of undiagnosed persistent pleural effusions. Clin Chest Med 1998;19:407–417.

39. Ferrer JS, Munoz XG, Orriols RM, et al. Evolution of idiopathic pleural effusion: a prospective, long-term follow-up study. Chest 1996;109:1508–1513.

40. Agostoni E, D'Angelo E. Thickness and pressure of the pleural liquid at various heights and with various hydrothoraces. Respir Physiol 1969;6:330–342.

41. Gillett D, Ford GT, Anthonisen NR. Shape and regional volume in immersed lung lobes. J Appl Physiol 1981;51: 1457–1462.

42. Raasch BN, Carsky EW, Lane EJ, et al. Pleural effusion: explanation of some typical appearances. AJR Am J Roentgenol 1982;139:899–904.

43. Dandy WE Jr. Incomplete pulmonary interlobar fissure sign. Radiology 1978;128:21–25.

44. Heitzman E, editor. Subsegmental anatomy of the lung. In: The lung: Radiographic-pathologic correlations. St Louis: CV Mosby, 1984.

45. Oestreich AE, Haley C. Pleural effusion: the thorn sign. Not a rare finding. Chest 1981;79:365–366.

46. Pecorari A, Weisbrod GL. Computed tomography of pseudotumoral pleural fluid collections in the azygoesophageal recess. J Comput Assist Tomogr 1989;13:803–805.

47. Stark P, Leung A. Effects of lobar atelectasis on the distribution of pleural effusion and pneumothorax. J Thorac Imaging 1996;11:145–149.

48. Mintzer RA, Hendrix RW, Johnson CS, et al. The radiologic significance of the left pulmonary ligament. Experience with 26 patients. Chest 1979;76:401–405.

49. Rabinowitz JG, Wolf BS. Roentgen significance of the pulmonary ligament. Radiology 1966;87:1013–1020.

50. Rigby M, Zylak CJ, Wood LD. The effect of lobar atelectasis on pleural fluid distribution in dogs. Radiology 1980;136:603–607.

51. Colins JD, Burwell D, Furmanski S, et al. Minimal detectable pleural effusions. A roentgen pathology model. Radiology 1972;105:51–53.

52. Vix VA. Roentgenographic recognition of pleural effusion. JAMA 1974;229:695–698.

53. Kocijancic I, Tercelj M, Vidmar K, et al. The value of inspiratory-expiratory lateral decubitus views in the diagnosis of small pleural effusions. Clin Radiol 1999;54:595–597.

54. Petersen J. Recognition of infrapulmonary pleural effusion. Radiology 1960;74:34–41.

55. Fleischner F. Atypical arrangement of free pleural effusion. Radiol Clin North Am 1963;1:347–362.

56. Bryk D. Intrapulmonary effusion. Effect of expiration on the pseudodiaphragmatic contour. Radiology 1976;120:33–36.

57. Schwarz MI, Marmorstein BL. A new radiologic sign of subpulmonic effusion. Chest 1975;67:176–178.

58. Dunbar J, Favreau M. Infrapulmonary pleural effusions with particular

reference to its occurrence in nephrosis. J Can Assoc Radiol 1959;10:24.

59. Felson B. Chest roentgenology. Philadelphia: WB Saunders, 1973.

60. Kaplan LM, Epstein SK, Schwartz SL, et al. Clinical, echocardiographic, and hemodynamic evidence of cardiac tamponade caused by large pleural effusions. Am J Respir Crit Care Med 1995;151:904–908.

61. Lai CL, Tsai TT, Ko SC, et al. Superior vena cava syndrome caused by encapsulated pleural effusion. Eur Respir J 1997;10:1675–1677.

62. Romero S, Martin C, Hernandez L, et al. Effect of body position on gas exchange in patients with unilateral pleural effusion: influence of effusion volume. Respir Med 1995;89:297–301.

63. Agusti AG, Cardus J, Roca J, et al. Ventilation-perfusion mismatch in patients with pleural effusion: effects of thoracentesis. Am J Respir Crit Care Med 1997;156:1205–1209.

64. Pantoja E, Kattan KR, Thomas HA. Some uncommon lower mediastinal densities: a pictorial essay. Radiol Clin North Am 1984;22:633–646.

65. Proto AV, Merhar GL. Central bronchial displacement with large posterior pleural collections. Findings on the lateral chest radiograph and CT scans. J Can Assoc Radiol 1984;35:128–132.

66. Swingle JD, Logan R, Juhl JH. Inversion of the left hemidiaphragm. JAMA 1969;208:863–864.

67. Abu Yousef MM. Case of the fall season. Semin Roentgenol 1980;15:269–271.

68. Lowe SH, Cosgrove DO, Joseph AE. Inversion of the right hemidiaphragm shown on ultrasound examination. Br J Radiol 1981;54:754–757.

69. Subramanyam BR, Raghavendra BN, Lefleur RS. Sonography of the inverted right hemidiaphragm. AJR Am J Roentgenol 1981;136:1004–1006.

70. Katzen BT, Choi WS, Friedman MH, et al. Pseudomass of the liver due to pleural effusion and inversion of the diaphragm. AJR Am J Roentgenol 1978;131:1077–1078.

71. Hertzanu Y, Solomon A. Inversion of the right diaphragm: a thoracoabdominal CT pitfall. Gastrointest Radiol 1986;11: 200–202.

72. Levitt RG, Sagel SS, Stanley RJ, et al. Accuracy of computed tomography of the liver and biliary tract. Radiology 1977;124:123–128.

73. Rogers CI, Meredith HC. Osler revisited: an unusual cause of inversion of the diaphragm. Radiology 1977;125:596.

74. Demos TC, Pieters C. Abdominal pseudotumor due to inverted hemidiaphragm. Radiographic, sonographic, and computed tomographic diagnosis. Chest 1984;86:466–468.

75. Dallemand S, Twersky J, Gordon DH. Pseudomass of the left upper quadrant from inversion of the left hemidiaphragm: CT diagnosis. Gastrointest Radiol 1982;7:57–59.

76. Felson B. The extrapleural space. Semin Roentgenol 1977;12:327–333.

77. Feder B, Wilk S. Localized interlobar effusion in heart failure: phantom lung tumor. Dis Chest 1956;30:289–297.

78. Weiss W, Boucot K, Gefter W. Localized interlobar effusion in congestive heart failure. Ann Intern Med 1953;38: 1177–1186.

79. Ruskin JA, Gurney JW, Thorsen MK, et al. Detection of pleural effusions on supine chest radiographs. AJR Am J Roentgenol 1987;148:681–683.

80. Woodring JH. Recognition of pleural effusion on supine radiographs: how much fluid is required? AJR Am J Roentgenol 1984;142:59–64.

81. Moller A. Pleural effusion. Use of the semi-supine position for radiographic detection. Radiology 1984;150:245–249.

82. Rudikoff JC. Early detection of pleural fluid. Chest 1980;77:109–111.

83. Trackler RT, Brinker RA. Widening of the left paravertebral pleural line on supine chest roentgenograms in free pleural effusions. Am J Roentgenol Radium Ther Nucl Med 1966;96:1027–1034.

84. Onik G, Goodman PC, Webb WR, et al. Hydropneumothorax: detection on supine radiographs. Radiology 1984;152:31–34.

85. Kuhlman JE, Singha NK. Complex disease of the pleural space: radiographic and CT evaluation. Radiographics 1997;17:63–79.

86. McLoud TC, Flower CD. Imaging the pleura: sonography, CT, and MR imaging. AJR Am J Roentgenol 1991;156:1145–1153.

87. Pugatch RD, Faling LJ, Robbins AH, et al. Differentiation of pleural and pulmonary lesions using computed tomography. J Comput Assist Tomogr 1978;2:601–606.

88. Bressler EL, Francis IR, Glazer GM, et al. Bolus contrast medium enhancement for distinguishing pleural from parenchymal lung disease: CT features. J Comput Assist Tomogr 1987;11:436–440.

89. Maffessanti M, Tommasi M, Pellegrini P. Computed tomography of free pleural effusions. Eur J Radiol 1987;7:87–90.

90. Kollins SA. Computed tomography of the pulmonary parenchyma and chest wall. Radiol Clin North Am 1977;15:297–308.

91. Vock P, Effmann EL, Hedlund LW, et al. Analysis of the density of pleural fluid analogs by computed tomography. Invest Radiol 1984;19:10–15.

92. Williford ME, Hidalgo H, Putman CE, et al. Computed tomography of pleural disease. AJR Am J Roentgenol 1983;140: 909–914.

93. Lawton F, Blackledge G, Johnson R. Co-existent chylous and serous pleural effusions associated with ovarian cancer: a case report of Contarini's syndrome. Eur J Surg Oncol 1985;11:177–178.

94. Sullivan KL, Steiner RM, Wechsler RJ. Lymphaticopleural fistula: diagnosis by computed tomography. J Comput Assist Tomogr 1984;8:1005–1006.

95. Aquino SL, Webb WR, Gushiken BJ. Pleural exudates and transudates: diagnosis with contrast-enhanced CT. Radiology 1994;192:803–808.

96. Arenas-Jimenez J, Alonso-Charterina S, Sanchez-Paya J, et al. Evaluation of CT findings for diagnosis of pleural effusions. Eur Radiol 2000;10:681–690.

97. Dwyer A. The displaced crus: a sign for distinguishing between pleural fluid and ascites on computed tomography. J Comput Assist Tomogr 1978;2:598–599.

98. Naidich DP, Megibow AJ, Hilton S, et al. Computed tomography of the diaphragm: peridiaphragmatic fluid localization. J Comput Assist Tomogr 1983;7:641–649.

99. Halvorsen RA, Fedyshin PJ, Korobkin M, et al. CT differentiation of pleural effusion from ascites. An evaluation of four signs using blinded analysis of 52 cases. Invest Radiol 1986;21:391–395.

100. Teplick JG, Teplick SK, Goodman L, et al. The interface sign: a computed tomographic sign for distinguishing pleural and intra-abdominal fluid. Radiology 1982;144:359–362.

101. Alexander ES, Proto AV, Clark RA. CT differentiation of subphrenic abscess and pleural effusion. AJR Am J Roentgenol 1983;140:47–51.

102. Federle MP, Mark AS, Guillaumin ES. CT of subpulmonic pleural effusions and atelectasis: criteria for differentiation from subphrenic fluid. AJR Am J Roentgenol 1986;146:685–689.

103. Silverman PM, Baker ME, Mahony BS. Atelectasis and subpulmonic fluid: a CT pitfall in distinguishing pleural from peritoneal fluid. J Comput Assist Tomogr 1985;9:763–766.

104. Griffin DJ, Gross BH, McCracken S, et al. Observations on CT differentiation of pleural and peritoneal fluid. J Comput Assist Tomogr 1984;8:24–28.

105. Stark DD, Federle MP, Goodman PC, et al. Differentiating lung abscess and empyema: radiography and computed tomography. AJR Am J Roentgenol 1983;141:163–167.

106. Hirsch JH, Rogers JV, Mack LA. Real-time sonography of pleural opacities. AJR Am J Roentgenol 1981;136:297–301.

107. Yang PC, Luh KT, Chang DB, et al. Value of sonography in determining the nature of pleural effusion: analysis of 320 cases. AJR Am J Roentgenol 1992;159:29–33.

108. Marks WM, Filly RA, Callen PW. Real-time evaluation of pleural lesions: new

observations regarding the probability of obtaining free fluid. Radiology 1982;142:163–164.

109. Rosenberg ER. Ultrasound in the assessment of pleural densities. Chest 1983;84:283–285.

110. Lomas DJ, Padley SP, Flower CD. The sonographic appearances of pleural fluid. Br J Radiol 1993;66:619–624.

111. Wu RG, Yuan A, Liaw YS, et al. Image comparison of real-time gray-scale ultrasound and color Doppler ultrasound for use in diagnosis of minimal pleural effusion. Am J Respir Crit Care Med 1994;150:510–514.

112. Wu RG, Yang PC, Kuo SH, et al. "Fluid color" sign: a useful indicator for discrimination between pleural thickening and pleural effusion. J Ultrasound Med 1995;14:767–769.

113. Lipscomb DJ, Flower CD, Hadfield JW. Ultrasound of the pleura: an assessment of its clinical value. Clin Radiol 1981; 32:289–290.

114. Dorne HL. Differentiation of pulmonary parenchymal consolidation from pleural disease using the sonographic fluid bronchogram. Radiology 1986;158:41–42.

115. Yu CJ, Yang PC, Wu HD, et al. Ultrasound study in unilateral hemithorax opacification. Image comparison with computed tomography. Am Rev Respir Dis 1993;147:430–434.

116. O'Moore PV, Mueller PR, Simeone JF, et al. Sonographic guidance in diagnostic and therapeutic interventions in the pleural space. AJR Am J Roentgenol 1987;149:1–5.

117. Weingardt JP, Guico RR, Nemcek AA Jr, et al. Ultrasound findings following failed, clinically directed thoracenteses. J Clin Ultrasound 1994;22:419–426.

118. Grogan DR, Irwin RS, Channick R, et al. Complications associated with thoracentesis. A prospective, randomized study comparing three different methods. Arch Intern Med 1990;150:873–877.

119. Osranek M, Bursi F, O'Leary PW, et al. Hand-carried ultrasound-guided pericardiocentesis and thoracentesis. J Am Soc Echocardiogr 2003;16:480–484.

120. Petersen S, Freitag M, Albert W, et al. Ultrasound-guided thoracentesis in surgical intensive care patients. Intensive Care Med 1999;25:1029.

121. Lichtenstein D, Hulot JS, Rabiller A, et al. Feasibility and safety of ultrasound-aided thoracentesis in mechanically ventilated patients. Intensive Care Med 1999;25:955–958.

122. Keske U. Ultrasound-aided thoracentesis in intensive care patients. Intensive Care Med 1999;25:896–897.

123. Himelman RB, Callen PW. The prognostic value of loculations in parapneumonic pleural effusions. Chest 1986;90: 852–856.

124. Newlin N, Silver TM, Stuck KJ, et al. Ultrasonic features of pyogenic liver abscesses. Radiology 1981;139:155–159.

125. Patz EJ, Shaffer K, Piwnica WD, et al. Malignant pleural mesothelioma: value of CT and MR imaging in predicting resectability. AJR Am J Roentgenol 1992;159:961–966.

126. Imanaka K, Sugimoto K, Aoki M, et al. MRI finding of chronic hemorrhagic empyema: a case report. Radiat Med 1996;14:201–203.

127. Tscholakoff D, Sechtem U, de Geer G, et al. Evaluation of pleural and pericardial effusions by magnetic resonance imaging. Eur J Radiol 1987;7: 169–174.

128. Joseph J, Sahn SA. Connective tissue diseases and the pleura. Chest 1993;104:262–270.

129. Hughson WG, Friedman PJ, Feigin DS, et al. Postpartum pleural effusion: a common radiologic finding. Ann Intern Med 1982;97:856–858.

130. Heffner JE, Sahn SA. Pleural disease in pregnancy. Clin Chest Med 1992;13: 667–678.

131. Haddad B, Barton JR, Livingston JC, et al. HELLP (hemolysis, elevated liver enzymes, and low platelet count) syndrome versus severe preeclampsia: onset at < or = 28.0 weeks' gestation. Am J Obstet Gynecol 2000;183:1475–1479.

132. Sahn SA, Miller KS. Obscure pleural effusion. Look to the kidney. Chest 1986;90:631.

133. Sanders RC. Post-operative pleural effusion and subphrenic abscess. Clin Radiol 1970;21:308–312.

134. DeCrosse JJ, Poulin TL, Fox PS, et al. Subphrenic abscess. Surg Gynecol Obstet 1974;138:841–846.

135. Sherman NJ, Davis JR, Jesseph JE. Subphrenic abscess. A continuing hazard. Am J Surg 1969;117:117–123.

136. Miller WT, Talman EA. Subphrenic abscess. Am J Roentgenol Radium Ther Nucl Med 1967;101:961–969.

137. Ballantyne KC, Sethia B, Reece IJ, et al. Empyema following intra-abdominal sepsis. Br J Surg 1984;71:723–725.

138. Haaga JR, Weinstein AJ. CT-guided percutaneous aspiration and drainage of abscesses. AJR Am J Roentgenol 1980;135:1187–1194.

139. Rubin RH, Swartz MN, Malt R. Hepatic abscess: changes in clinical, bacteriologic and therapeutic aspects. Am J Med 1974;57:601–610.

140. Light RW. Exudative pleural effusions secondary to gastrointestinal diseases. Clin Chest Med 1985;6:103–111.

141. Logue R, Rogers J, Gay B. Subtle radiographic signs of left heart failure. Am Heart J 1963;65:464–473.

142. McPeak E, Levine S. The preponderance of right hydrothorax in congestive heart failure. Ann Intern Med 1946;25:916–927.

143. Leuallen E, Carr D. Pleural effusion: a statistical study of 436 patients. N Engl J Med 1955;252:79–83.

144. Bedford D, Lovibond J. Hydrothorax in heart failure. Br Heart J 1941;3:93–111.

145. Peterman TA, Brothers SK. Pleural effusions in congestive heart failure and in pericardial disease. N Engl J Med 1983;309:313.

146. Weiss JM, Spodick DH. Laterality of pleural effusions in chronic congestive heart failure. Am J Cardiol 1984;53:951.

147. White P, August S, Michie C. Hydrothorax in congestive heart failure. Am J Med Sci 1947;214:243–247.

148. Race G, Scheifley C, Edwards J. Hydrothorax in congestive heart failure. Am J Med 1957;22:83–89.

149. Mellins RB, Levine OR, Fishman AP. Effect of systemic and pulmonary venous hypertension on pleural and pericardial fluid accumulation. J Appl Physiol 1970;29:564–569.

150. Wiener-Kronish JP, Matthay MA, Callen PW, et al. Relationship of pleural effusions to pulmonary hemodynamics in patients with congestive heart failure. Am Rev Respir Dis 1985;132:1253–1256.

151. Wiener-Kronish JP, Goldstein R, Matthay RA, et al. Lack of association of pleural effusion with chronic pulmonary arterial and right atrial hypertension. Chest 1987;92:967–970.

152. Lee YC, Vaz MA, Ely KA, et al. Symptomatic persistent post-coronary artery bypass graft pleural effusions requiring operative treatment : clinical and histologic features. Chest 2001;119:795–800.

153. Light RW. Pleural effusions after coronary artery bypass graft surgery. Curr Opin Pulm Med 2002;8:308–311.

154. Kollef MH. Chronic pleural effusion following coronary artery revascularization with the internal mammary artery. Chest 1990;97:750–751.

155. Parenti C. Pulmonary embolism after coronary artery bypass surgery. Crit Care Nurs Q 1994;17:48–50.

156. Pego-Fernandes PM, Ebaid GX, Nouer GH, et al. Chylothorax after myocardial revascularization with the left internal thoracic artery. Arq Bras Cardiol 1999;73:383–390.

157. Brancaccio G, Prifti E, Cricco AM, et al. Chylothorax: a complication after internal thoracic artery harvesting. Ital Heart J 2001;2:559–562.

158. Kaminsky ME, Rodan BA, Osborne DR, et al. Postpericardiotomy syndrome. AJR Am J Roentgenol 1982;138:503–508.

159. Weiss JM, Spodick DH. Association of left pleural effusion with pericardial disease. N Engl J Med 1983;308: 696–697.

160. Dressler W. The post-myocardial-infarction syndrome: a report on 44 cases. Arch Intern Med 1959;103:28–42.

161. Engle M, Ito T. The postpericardiotomy syndrome. Am J Cardiol 1961;7:73–82.

162. Hearne C, Forjuoh SN. Postcardiac injury syndrome after coronary angioplasty and stenting. J Am Board Fam Pract 2003;16:73–74.

163. Stefanelli CB, Bradley DJ, Leroy S, et al. Implantable cardioverter defibrillator therapy for life-threatening arrhythmias in young patients. J Interv Card Electrophysiol 2002;6:235–244.

164. Spindler M, Burrows G, Kowallik P, et al. Postpericardiotomy syndrome and cardiac tamponade as a late complication after pacemaker implantation. Pacing Clin Electrophysiol 2001;24:1433–1434.

165. Bajaj BP, Evans KE, Thomas P. Postpericardiotomy syndrome following temporary and permanent transvenous pacing. Postgrad Med J 1999;75: 357–358.

166. Liem KL, ten Veen JH, Lie KI, et al. Incidence and significance of heartmuscle antibodies in patients with acute myocardial infarction and unstable angina. Acta Med Scand 1979;206: 473–475.

167. Sahn SA. Immunologic diseases of the pleura. Clin Chest Med 1985;6:83–102.

168. Stelzner TJ, King TE Jr, Antony VB, et al. The pleuropulmonary manifestations of the postcardiac injury syndrome. Chest 1983;84:383–387.

169. Areno JP, McCartney JP, Eggerstedt J, et al. Persistent pleural effusions following coronary bypass surgery. Chest 1998;114:311–474.

170. Levin EJ, Bryk D. Dressler syndrome (postmyocardial infarction syndrome). Radiology 1966;87:731–736.

171. Tabatznik B, Isaacs J. Postpericardiotomy syndrome following traumatic hemopericardium. Am J Cardiol 1961;7:83–96.

172. Soulen RL, Freeman E. Radiologic evaluation of myocardial infarction. Radiol Clin North Am 1971;9:567–582.

173. Szabo G, Magyar Z. Effect of increased systemic venous pressure on lymph pressure and flow. Am J Physiol 1967;212:1469–1474.

174. Hussey H, Katz S, Yater W. The superior vena caval syndrome: report of thirty-five cases. Am Heart J 1946;31:1–26.

175. Perez CA, Presant CA, Van Amburg AL, 3rd. Management of superior vena cava syndrome. Semin Oncol 1978;5:123–134.

176. Javaheri S, Hales CA. Sarcoidosis: a cause of innominate vein obstruction and massive pleural effusion. Lung 1980;157:81–85.

177. Good JT Jr, Moore JB, Fowler AA, et al. Superior vena cava syndrome as a cause of pleural effusion. Am Rev Respir Dis 1982;125:246–247.

178. Diaconis JN, Weiner CI, White DW. Primary subclavian vein thrombosis and bilateral chylothorax documented by lymphography and venography. Radiology 1976;119:557–558.

179. Seibert JJ, Golladay ES, Keller C. Chylothorax secondary to superior vena caval obstruction. Pediatr Radiol 1982;12:252–254.

180. Bynum LJ, Wilson JE 3rd. Radiographic features of pleural effusions in pulmonary embolism. Am Rev Respir Dis 1978;117:829–834.

181. Moses DC, Silver TM, Bookstein JJ. The complementary roles of chest radiography, lung scanning, and selective pulmonary angiography in the diagnosis of pulmonary embolism. Circulation 1974;49:179–188.

182. Talbot S, Worthington BS, Roebuck EJ. Radiographic signs of pulmonary embolism and pulmonary infarction. Thorax 1973;28:198–203.

183. Dalen JE, Haffajee CI, Alpert JS 3rd, et al. Pulmonary embolism, pulmonary hemorrhage and pulmonary infarction. N Engl J Med 1977;296:1431–1435.

184. Simon HB, Daggett WM, DeSanctis RW. Hemothorax as a complication of anticoagulant therapy in the presence of pulmonary infarction. JAMA 1969;208:1830–1834.

185. McArdle CR, Sacks BA. Ovarian hyperstimulation syndrome. AJR Am J Roentgenol 1980;135:835–836.

186. Schenker JG, Weinstein D. Ovarian hyperstimulation syndrome: a current survey. Fertil Steril 1978;30:255–268.

187. Miller WT Jr. Drug-related pleural and mediastinal disorders. J Thorac Imaging 1991;6:36–51.

188. Xiol X, Guardiola J. Hepatic hydrothorax. Curr Opin Pulm Med 1998;4:239–242.

189. Kinasewitz GT, Keddissi JI. Hepatic hydrothorax. Curr Opin Pulm Med 2003;9:261–265.

190. Morrow C, Kantor M, Armen R. Hepatic hydrothorax. Ann Intern Med 1958;49: 193–203.

191. Islam N, Ali S, Kabir H. Hepatic hydrothorax. Br J Dis Chest 1965;59:222–227.

192. Mattison LE, Coppage L, Alderman DF, et al. Pleural effusions in the medical ICU: prevalence, causes, and clinical implications. Chest 1997;111: 1018–1023.

193. Johnston R, Loo R. Hepatic hydrothorax: studies to determine the source of the fluid and report of thirteen cases. Ann Intern Med 1964;61:385–401.

194. Lieberman FL, Hidemura R, Peters RL, et al. Pathogenesis and treatment of hydrothorax complicating cirrhosis with ascites. Ann Intern Med 1966;64:341–351.

195. Lieberman FL, Peters RL. Cirrhotic hydrothorax. Further evidence that an acquired diaphragmatic defect is at fault. Arch Intern Med 1970;125:114–117.

196. McKay D, Sparling H, Robbins S. Cirrhosis of the liver with massive hydrothorax. Arch Intern Med 1947;79:501–509.

197. Williams M. Pleural effusion produced by abdominal-pleural communication in a patient with Laennec's cirrhosis of the liver and ascites. Ann Intern Med 1950;33:216–221.

198. Mirouze D, Juttner HU, Reynolds TB. Left pleural effusion in patients with chronic liver disease and ascites. Prospective study of 22 cases. Dig Dis Sci 1981;26:984–988.

199. Black LF. The pleural space and pleural fluid. Mayo Clin Proc 1972;47:493–506.

200. Frazer IH, Lichtenstein M, Andrews JT. Pleuroperitoneal effusion without ascites. Med J Aust 1983;2:520–521.

201. Bradley JW, Feilding LP. Hydropneumothorax complicating perforated peptic ulcer. Br J Surg 1972;59:72–73.

202. Nakamura A, Kojima Y, Ohmi H, et al. Peritoneal-pleural communications in hepatic hydrothorax demonstrated by thoracoscopy. Chest 1996;109:579–581.

203. Siegerstetter V, Deibert P, Ochs A, et al. Treatment of refractory hepatic hydrothorax with transjugular intrahepatic portosystemic shunt: long-term results in 40 patients. Eur J Gastroenterol Hepatol 2001;13:529–534.

204. Spencer EB, Cohen DT, Darcy MD. Safety and efficacy of transjugular intrahepatic portosystemic shunt creation for the treatment of hepatic hydrothorax. J Vasc Interv Radiol 2002;13:385–390.

205. Salmon V. Benign pelvic tumours associated with ascites and pleural effusion. J Mt Sinai Hosp 1934;1:169–172.

206. Meigs J, Cass J. Fibroma of the ovary with ascites and hydrothorax: with a report of seven cases. Am J Obstet Gynecol 1937;33:249–267.

207. Meigs J. Fibroma of the ovary with ascites and hydrothorax Meigs' syndrome. Am J Obstet Gynecol 1954;67:962–987.

208. Majzlin C, Stevens F. Meigs' syndrome: case report and review of literature. J Int Coll Surg 1964;42:625–630.

209. Solomon S, Farber S, Caruso L. Fibromyomata of the uterus with hemothorax – Meigs' syndrome? Arch Intern Med 1971;127:307–309.

210. Kebapci M, Aslan O, Kaya T, et al. Pedunculated uterine leiomyoma associated with pseudo-Meigs' syndrome and elevated CA-125 level: CT features. Eur Radiol 2002;12 Suppl 3:S127–129.

211. La Fianza A, Alberici E. CT diagnosis of Pseudo-Meigs' syndrome. Clin Radiol 2002;57:315–317.

212. Weise M, Westphalen S, Fayyazi A, et al. Pseudo-Meigs syndrome: uterine

leiomyoma with bladder attachment associated with ascites and hydrothorax – a rare case of a rare syndrome. Onkologie 2002;25:443–446.

213. Amant F, Gabriel C, Timmerman D, et al. Pseudo-Meigs' syndrome caused by a hydropic degenerating uterine leiomyoma with elevated CA 125. Gynecol Oncol 2001;83:153–157.

214. Migishima F, Jobo T, Hata H, et al. Uterine leiomyoma causing massive ascites and left pleural effusion with elevated CA 125: a case report. J Obstet Gynaecol Res 2000;26:283–287.

215. Handler CE, Fray RE, Snashall PD. Atypical Meigs' syndrome. Thorax 1982;37:396–397.

216. O'Flanagan SJ, Tighe BF, Egan TJ, et al. Meigs' syndrome and pseudo-Meigs' syndrome. J R Soc Med 1987;80:252–253.

217. Meigs J. Pelvic tumours other than fibromas of the ovary with ascites and hydrothorax. Obstet Gynecol 1954;3:471–485.

218. Dockerty M, Masson J. Ovarian fibromas: a clinical and pathologic study of 283 cases. Am J Obstet Gynecol 1944;47:741–752.

219. Mokrohisky J. So-called "Meigs' syndrome" associated with benign and malignant ovarian tumors. Radiology 1958;70:578–581.

220. Fishbein R, Murphy G, Wilder R. The pleuropulmonary manifestations of pancreatitis. Dis Chest 1962;41:392–397.

221. Murphy D, Duncan JG, Imrie CW. The "negative chest radiograph" in acute pancreatitis. Br J Radiol 1977;50:264–265.

222. Heller SJ, Noordhoek E, Tenner SM, et al. Pleural effusion as a predictor of severity in acute pancreatitis. Pancreas 1997;15:222–225.

223. Millward SF, Breatnach E, Simpkins KC, et al. Do plain films of the chest and abdomen have a role in the diagnosis of acute pancreatitis? Clin Radiol 1983;34:133–137.

224. Talamini G, Uomo G, Pezzilli R, et al. Serum creatinine and chest radiographs in the early assessment of acute pancreatitis. Am J Surg 1999;177:7–14.

225. Kaye MD. Pleuropulmonary complications of pancreatitis. Thorax 1968;23:297–306.

226. Rockey DC, Cello JP. Pancreaticopleural fistula. Report of 7 patients and review of the literature. Medicine (Baltimore) 1990;69:332–344.

227. McKenna JM, Chandrasekhar AJ, Skorton D, et al. The pleuropulmonary complications of pancreatitis. Clinical conference in pulmonary disease from Northwestern University-McGaw Medical Center and Veterans Administration Lakeside Hospital, Chicago. Chest 1977;71:197–204.

228. Anderson WJ, Skinner DB, Zuidema GD, et al. Chronic pancreatic pleural effusions. Surg Gynecol Obstet 1973;137:827–830.

229. Miridjanian A, Ambruoso VN, Derby BM, et al. Massive bilateral hemorrhagic pleural effusions in chronic relapsing pancreatitis. Arch Surg 1969;98:62–66.

230. Tewari SC, Jayaswal R, Chauhan MS, et al. Bilateral recurrent haemorrhagic pleural effusion in asymptomatic chronic pancreatitis. Thorax 1989;44:824–825.

231. Cameron JL. Chronic pancreatic ascites and pancreatic pleural effusions. Gastroenterology 1978;74:134–140.

232. Kirchner SG, Heller RM, Smith CW. Pancreatic pseudocyst of the mediastinum. Radiology 1977;123:37–42.

233. Louie S, McGahan JP, Frey C, et al. Pancreatic pleuropericardial effusions. Fistulous tracts demonstrated by computed tomography. Arch Intern Med 1985;145:1231–1234.

234. Faling LJ, Gerzof SG, Daly BD, et al. Treatment of chronic pancreatitic pleural effusion by percutaneous catheter drainage of abdominal pseudocyst. Am J Med 1984;76:329–333.

235. Dewan NA, Kinney WW, O'Donohue WJ Jr. Chronic massive pancreatic pleural effusion. Chest 1984;85:497–501.

236. Akahane T, Kuriyama S, Matsumoto M, et al. Pancreatic pleural effusion with a pancreaticopleural fistula diagnosed by magnetic resonance cholangiopancreatography and cured by somatostatin analogue treatment. Abdom Imaging 2003;28:92–95.

237. Mori Y, Iwai A, Inagaki T, et al. Pancreaticopleural fistula imaged with magnetic resonance pancreatography. Pancreatology 2001;1:369–370.

238. Materne R, Vranckx P, Pauls C, et al. Pancreaticopleural fistula: diagnosis with magnetic resonance pancreatography. Chest 2000;117:912–914.

239. Glorioso LW, 3rd, Lang EK. Pulmonary manifestations of renal disease. Radiol Clin North Am 1984;22:647–658.

240. Hopps H, Wissler R. Uremic pneumonitis. Am J Pathol 1955;31:261–274.

241. Berger HW, Rammohan G, Neff MS, et al. Uremic pleural effusion. A study in 14 patients on chronic dialysis. Ann Intern Med 1975;82:362–364.

242. Nidus BD, Matalon R, Cantacuzino D, et al. Uremic pleuritis – a clinicopathological entity. N Engl J Med 1969;281:255–256.

243. Galen MA, Steinberg SM, Lowrie EG, et al. Hemorrhagic pleural effusion in patients undergoing chronic hemodialysis. Ann Intern Med 1975;82:359–361.

244. Gilbert L, Ribot S, Frankel H, et al. Fibrinous uremic pleuritis: a surgical entity. Chest 1975;67:53–56.

245. Rodelas R, Rakowski TA, Argy WP, et al. Fibrosing uremic pleuritis during hemodialysis. JAMA 1980;243:2424–2425.

246. Salcedo JR. Urinothorax: report of 4 cases and review of the literature. J Urol 1986;135:805–808.

247. Barek LB, Cigtay OS. Urinothorax – an unusual pleural effusion. Br J Radiol 1975;48:685–686.

248. Baron RL, Stark DD, McClennan BL, et al. Intrathoracic extension of retroperitoneal urine collections. AJR Am J Roentgenol 1981;137:37–41.

249. Lahiry SK, Alkhafaji AH, Brown AL. Urinothorax following blunt trauma to the kidney. J Trauma 1978;18:608–610.

250. Redman JF, Arnold WC, Smith PL, et al. Hypertension and urino-thorax following an attempted percutaneous nephrostomy. J Urol 1982;128:1307–1308.

251. Carcillo J Jr, Salcedo JR. Urinothorax as a manifestation of nondilated obstructive uropathy following renal transplantation. Am J Kidney Dis 1985;5:211–213.

252. Corriere JN Jr, Miller WT, Murphy JJ. Hydronephrosis as a cause of pleural effusion. Radiology 1968;90:79–84.

253. Laforet EG, Kornitzer GD. Nephrogenic pleural effusion. J Urol 1977;117:118–119.

254. Nusser RA, Culhane RH. Recurrent transudative effusion with an abdominal mass. Urinothorax. Chest 1986;90:263–264.

255. Jenkins PG, Shelp WD. Recurrent pleural transudate in the nephrotic syndrome. A new approach to treatment. JAMA 1974;230:587–588.

256. Llach F, Arieff AI, Massry SG. Renal vein thrombosis and nephrotic syndrome. A prospective study of 36 adult patients. Ann Intern Med 1975;83:8–14.

257. Holzel A, Fawcitt J. Pulmonary changes in acute glomerulonephritis in childhood. J Pediatr 1960;57:695–703.

258. Edwards SR, Unger AM. Acute hydrothorax – a new complication of peritoneal dialysis. JAMA 1967;199:853–855.

259. Rudnick MR, Coyle JF, Beck LH, et al. Acute massive hydrothorax complicating peritoneal dialysis, report of 2 cases and a review of the literature. Clin Nephrol 1979;12:38–44.

260. Finn R, Jowett EW. Acute hydrothorax complicating peritoneal dialysis. Br Med J 1970;2:94.

261. Townsend R, Fragola JA. Hydrothorax in a patient receiving continuous ambulatory peritoneal dialysis: successful treatment with intermittent peritoneal dialysis. Arch Intern Med 1982;142:1571–1572.

262. Nassberger L. Left-sided pleural effusion secondary to continuous ambulatory peritoneal dialysis. Acta Med Scand 1982;211:219–220.

263. Lorentz WB Jr. Acute hydrothorax during peritoneal dialysis. J Pediatr 1979;94:417–419.

264. Polsky MS, Weber CH, Ball TP Jr. Infected pyelocaliceal diverticulum and sympathetic pleural effusion. J Urol 1975;114:301–303.

265. Chun CH, Raff MJ, Contreras L, et al. Splenic abscess. Medicine (Baltimore) 1980;59:50–65.

266. Johnson JD, Raff MJ, Barnwell PA, et al. Splenic abscess complicating infectious endocarditis. Arch Intern Med 1983;143:906–912.

267. Sarr MG, Zuidema GD. Splenic abscess – presentation, diagnosis, and treatment. Surgery 1982;92:480–485.

268. Warren MS, Gibbons RB. Left-sided pleural effusion secondary to splenic vein thrombosis. A previously unrecognized relationship. Chest 1991;100:574–575.

269. Koehler PR, Jones R. Association of left-sided pleural effusions and splenic hematomas. AJR Am J Roentgenol 1980;135:851–853.

270. Light RW, George RB. Incidence and significance of pleural effusion after abdominal surgery. Chest 1976;69:621–625.

271. Nielsen PH, Jepsen SB, Olsen AD. Postoperative pleural effusion following upper abdominal surgery. Chest 1989;96:1133–1135.

272. Aronchick JM, Epstein DM, Gefter WB, et al. Chronic traumatic diaphragmatic hernia: the significance of pleural effusion. Radiology 1988;168:675–678.

273. Libshitz HI, Southard ME. Complications of radiation therapy: the thorax. Semin Roentgenol 1974;9:41–49.

274. Whitcomb ME, Schwarz MI. Pleural effusion complicating intensive mediastinal radiation therapy. Am Rev Respir Dis 1971;103:100–107.

275. Bachman A, Macken K. Pleural effusions following supervoltage radiation for breast carcinoma. Radiology 1959;72:699–709.

276. Antony VB. Drug-induced pleural disease. Clin Chest Med 1998;19:331–340.

277. Miller WT, Jr. Pleural and mediastinal disorders related to drug use. Semin Roentgenol 1995;30:35–48.

278. Urban C, Nirenberg A, Caparros B, et al. Chemical pleuritis as the cause of acute chest pain following high-dose methotrexate treatment. Cancer 1983;51:34–37.

279. Walden PA, Mitchell-Heggs PF, Coppin C, et al. Pleurisy and methotrexate treatment. Br Med J 1977;2:867.

280. Everts CS, Westcott JL, Bragg DG. Methotrexate therapy and pulmonary disease. Radiology 1973;107:539–543.

281. Ecker MD, Jay B, Keohane MF. Procarbazine lung. AJR Am J Roentgenol 1978;131:527–528.

282. Orwoll ES, Kiessling PJ, Patterson JR. Interstitial pneumonia from mitomycin. Ann Intern Med 1978;89:352–355.

283. Smalley RV, Wall RL. Two cases of busulfan toxicity. Ann Intern Med 1966;64:154–164.

284. Holoye PY, Luna MA, MacKay B, et al. Bleomycin hypersensitivity pneumonitis. Ann Intern Med 1978;88:47–49.

285. Pascual RS, Mosher MB, Sikand RS, et al. Effects of bleomycin on pulmonary function in man. Am Rev Respir Dis 1973;108:211–217.

286. Mann H, Ward JH, Samlowski WE. Vascular leak syndrome associated with interleukin-2: chest radiographic manifestations. Radiology 1990; 176:191–194.

287. Saxon RR, Klein JS, Bar MH, et al. Pathogenesis of pulmonary edema during interleukin-2 therapy: correlation of chest radiographic and clinical findings in 54 patients. AJR Am J Roentgenol 1991;156:281–285.

288. Conant EF, Fox KR, Miller WT. Pulmonary edema as a complication of interleukin-2 therapy. AJR Am J Roentgenol 1989;152:749–752.

289. Jung JI, Choi JE, Hahn ST, et al. Radiologic features of all-trans-retinoic acid syndrome. AJR Am J Roentgenol 2002;178:475–480.

290. Holmberg L, Boman G. Pulmonary reactions to nitrofurantoin. 447 cases reported to the Swedish Adverse Drug Reaction Committee 1966–1976. Eur J Respir Dis 1981;62:180–189.

291. Pfitzenmeyer P, Foucher P, Dennewald G, et al. Pleuropulmonary changes induced by ergoline drugs. Eur Respir J 1996;9:1013–1019.

292. Knoop C, Mairesse M, Lenclud C, et al. Pleural effusion during bromocriptine exposure in two patients with pre-existing asbestos pleural plaques: a relationship? Eur Respir J 1997;10:2898–2901.

293. Graham JR, Suby HI, LeCompte PR, et al. Fibrotic disorders associated with methysergide therapy for headache. N Engl J Med 1966;274:359–368.

294. Graham JR. Cardiac and pulmonary fibrosis during methysergide therapy for headache. Am J Med Sci 1967;254:1–12.

295. Hindle W, Posner E, Sweetnam MT, et al. Pleural effusion and fibrosis during treatment with methysergide. Br Med J 1970;1:605–606.

296. Kok-Jensen A, Lindeneg O. Pleurisy and fibrosis of the pleura during methysergide treatment of hemicrania. Scand J Respir Dis 1970;51:218–222.

297. Gefter WB, Epstein DM, Bonavita JA, et al. Pleural thickening caused by Sansert and Ergotrate in the treatment of migraine. AJR Am J Roentgenol 1980;135:375–377.

298. Taal BG, Spierings EL, Hilvering C. Pleuropulmonary fibrosis associated with chronic and excessive intake of ergotamine. Thorax 1983;38:396–398.

299. Allen MB, Tosh G, Walters G, et al. Pleural and pericardial fibrosis after ergotamine therapy. Respir Med 1994;88:67–69.

300. Cooper JA Jr, White DA, Matthay RA. Drug-induced pulmonary disease. Part 2: Noncytotoxic drugs. Am Rev Respir Dis 1986;133:488–505.

301. Kuhlman J, Teigen C, Ren H, Hruban R, et al. Amiodarone pulmonary toxicity: CT findings in symptomatic patients. Radiology 1990;177:121–125.

302. Gonzalez-Rothi RJ, Hannan SE, Hood CI, et al. Amiodarone pulmonary toxicity presenting as bilateral exudative pleural effusions. Chest 1987;92:179–182.

303. Rakita L, Sobol SM, Mostow N, et al. Amiodarone pulmonary toxicity. Am Heart J 1983;106:906–916.

304. Zaher C, Hamer A, Peter T, et al. Low-dose steroid therapy for prophylaxis of amiodarone-induced pulmonary infiltrates. N Engl J Med 1983;308:779.

305. Middleton KL, Santella R, Couser JI Jr. Eosinophilic pleuritis due to propylthiouracil. Chest 1993;103:955–956.

306. Petusevsky ML, Faling LJ, Rocklin RE, et al. Pleuropericardial reaction to treatment with dantrolene. JAMA 1979;242:2772–2774.

307. Webb DB, Whale RJ. Pleuropericardial effusion associated with minoxidil administration. Postgrad Med J 1982;58:319–320.

308. McElvaney NG, Wilcox PG, Churg A, et al. Pleuropulmonary disease during bromocriptine treatment of Parkinson's disease. Arch Intern Med 1988;148:2231–2236.

309. Wiggins J, Skinner C. Bromocriptine induced pleuropulmonary fibrosis. Thorax 1986;41:328–330.

310. Shaunak S, Wilkins A, Pilling JB, et al. Pericardial, retroperitoneal, and pleural fibrosis induced by pergolide. J Neurol Neurosurg Psychiatry 1999;66:79–81.

311. Erwteman TM, Braat MC, van Aken WG. Interstitial pulmonary fibrosis: a new side effect of practolol. Br Med J 1977;2:297–298.

312. Fleming HA, Hickling P. Letter: Pleural effusions after practolol. Lancet 1975;2:1202.

313. Hall DR, Morrison JB, Edwards FR. Pleural fibrosis after practolol therapy. Thorax 1978;33:822–824.

314. Marshall AJ, Eltringham WK, Barritt DW, et al. Respiratory disease associated with practolol therapy. Lancet 1977;2:1254–1257.

315. Wood GM, Bolton RP, Muers MF, et al. Pleurisy and pulmonary granulomas

after treatment with acebutolol. Br Med J (Clin Res Ed) 1982;285:936.

316. Ahmad S. Sclerosing peritonitis and propranolol. Chest 1981;79:361–362.

317. Jewelewicz R, Vande Wiele RL. Acute hydrothorax as the only symptom of ovarian hyperstimulation syndrome. Am J Obstet Gynecol 1975;121:1121.

318. Roden S, Juvin K, Homasson JP, et al. An uncommon etiology of isolated pleural effusion. The ovarian hyperstimulation syndrome. Chest 2000;118:256–258.

319. Tansutthiwong AA, Srisombut C, Rojanasakul A. Unilateral massive pleural effusion as the only principal manifestation of severe ovarian hyperstimulation syndrome. J Assist Reprod Genet 2000;17:454–456.

320. Loret de Mola JR. Pathophysiology of unilateral pleural effusions in the ovarian hyperstimulation syndrome. Hum Reprod 1999;14:272–273.

321. Brown SD, Brashear RE, Schnute RB. Pleural effusion in a young woman with myxedema. Arch Intern Med 1983;143:1458–1460.

322. Chetty KG. Transudative pleural effusions. Clin Chest Med 1985;6:49–54.

323. Gottehrer A, Roa J, Stanford GG, et al. Hypothyroidism and pleural effusions. Chest 1990;98:1130–1132.

324. Marks P, Roof B. Pericardial effusion associated with myxedema. Ann Intern Med 1953;39:230–240.

325. Schneierson S, Katz M. Solitary pleural effusion due to myxedema. JAMA 1958;168:1003–1005.

326. Samman P, White W. The "yellow nail" syndrome. Br J Dermatol 1964;76:153–157.

327. Hurwitz P, Pinals D. Pleural effusion in chronic hereditary lymphedema (Nonne, Milroy, Meige's disease). Radiology 1964;82:246–248.

328. Emerson PA. Yellow nails, lymphoedema, and pleural effusions. Thorax 1966;21:247–253.

329. Nordkild P, Kromann-Andersen H, Struve-Christensen E. Yellow nail syndrome – the triad of yellow nails, lymphedema and pleural effusions. A review of the literature and a case report. Acta Med Scand 1986;219:221–227.

330. Beer DJ, Pereira W Jr, Snider GL. Pleural effusion associated with primary lymphedema: a perspective on the yellow nail syndrome. Am Rev Respir Dis 1978;117:595–599.

331. Anon. Yellow nails and oedema. Br Med J 1972;4:130.

332. Hiller E, Rosenow EC 3rd, Olsen AM. Pulmonary manifestations of the yellow nail syndrome. Chest 1972;61:452–458.

333. Wiggins J, Strickland B, Chung KF. Detection of bronchiectasis by high-resolution computed tomography in the yellow nail syndrome. Clin Radiol 1991;43:377–379.

334. Solal-Celigny P, Cormier Y, Fournier M. The yellow nail syndrome. Light and electron microscopic aspects of the pleura. Arch Pathol Lab Med 1983;107:183–185.

335. Runyon BA, Forker EL, Sopko JA. Pleural-fluid kinetics in a patient with primary lymphedema, pleural effusions, and yellow nails. Am Rev Respir Dis 1979;119:821–825.

336. Glazer M, Berkman N, Lafair JS, et al. Successful talc slurry pleurodesis in patients with nonmalignant pleural effusion. Chest 2000;117:1404–1409.

337. Jiva TM, Poe RH, Kallay MC. Pleural effusion in yellow nail syndrome: chemical pleurodesis and its outcome. Respiration 1994;61:300–302.

338. Cook GC. Periodic disease, recurrent polyserositis, familial Mediterranean fever, or simply 'FMF'. Q J Med 1986;60:819–823.

339. Barakat MH, Karnik AM, Majeed HW, et al. Familial Mediterranean fever (recurrent hereditary polyserositis) in Arabs – a study of 175 patients and review of the literature. Q J Med 1986;60:837–847.

340. Nugent FW, Burns JR. Periodic disease. Med Clin North Am 1966;50:371–378.

341. Sohar E, Gafni J, Pras M, et al. Familial Mediterranean fever. A survey of 470 cases and review of the literature. Am J Med 1967;43:227–253.

342. Mancini JL. Familial paroxysmal polyserositis, phenotype I (familial Mediterranean fever). A rare cause of pleurisy. Case report and review of the literature. Am Rev Respir Dis 1973;107:461–463.

343. el-Kassimi FA. Acute pleuritic chest pain with pleural effusion and plate atelectasis. Familial Mediterranean fever (periodic disease). Chest 1987;91:265–266.

344. Meyerhoff J. Familial Mediterranean fever: report of a large family, review of the literature, and discussion of the frequency of amyloidosis. Medicine (Baltimore) 1980;59:66–77.

345. Villena V, Lopez-Encuentra A, Pozo F, et al. Measurement of pleural pressure during therapeutic thoracentesis. Am J Respir Crit Care Med 2000;162:1534–1538.

346. Light RW, Jenkinson SG, Minh VD, et al. Observations on pleural fluid pressures as fluid is withdrawn during thoracentesis. Am Rev Respir Dis 1980;121:799–804.

347. Bessone LN, Ferguson TB, Burford TH. Chylothorax. Ann Thorac Surg 1971;12:527–550.

348. Dahlgren S. Anatomy of the thoracic duct from the standpoint of surgery for chylothorax. Acta Chir Scand 1963;125:201–206.

349. Rosenberger A, Abrams HL. Radiology of the thoracic duct. Am J Roentgenol Radium Ther Nucl Med 1971;111:807–820.

350. Sassoon CS, Light RW. Chylothorax and pseudochylothorax. Clin Chest Med 1985;6:163–171.

351. Schulman A, Fataar S, Dalrymple R, et al. The lymphographic anatomy of chylothorax. Br J Radiol 1978;51:420–427.

352. Kausel H, Reeve T, Stein A, et al. Anatomic and pathologic studies of the thoracic duct. J Thorac Surg 1957;34:631–641.

353. Van Pernis P. Variations of thoracic duct. Surgery 1949;26:806–809.

354. Meade R, Head J, CW M. The management of chylothorax. J Thorac Surg 1950;19:709–723.

355. Thorne P. Traumatic chylothorax. Tubercle 1958;39:29–34.

356. Neyazaki T, Kupic EA, Marshall WH, et al. Collateral lymphatico-venous communications after experimental obstruction of the thoracic duct. Radiology 1965;85:423–432.

357. Lampson R. Traumatic chylothorax: a review of the literature and report of a case treated by mediastinal ligation of the thoracic duct. J Thorac Surg 1948;17:778–791.

358. Meade R, Head J, Moen C. The management of chylothorax. J Thorac Surg 1950;19:709–723.

359. Valentine VG, Raffin TA. The management of chylothorax. Chest 1992;102:586–591.

360. Grant T, Levin B. Lymphangiographic visualization of pleural and pulmonary lymphatics in a patient without chylothorax. Radiology 1974;113:49–50.

361. Trapnell D. The peripheral lymphatics of the lung. Br J Radiol 1963;36:660–672.

362. Weidner WA, Steiner RM. Roentgenographic demonstration of intrapulmonary and pleural lymphatics during lymphangiography. Radiology 1971;100:533–539.

363. Ducharme JC, Belanger R, Simard P, et al. Chylothorax, chylopericardium with multiple lymphangioma of bone. J Pediatr Surg 1982;17:365–367.

364. Berkenbosch JW, Monteleone PM, Tobias JD. Chylothorax following apparently spontaneous central venous thrombosis in a patient with septic shock. Pediatr Pulmonol 2003;35:230–233.

365. Kramer SS, Taylor GA, Garfinkel DJ, et al. Lethal chylothoraces due to superior vena caval thrombosis in infants. AJR Am J Roentgenol 1981;137:559–563.

366. Thurer RJ. Chylothorax: a complication of subclavian vein catheterization and parenteral hyperalimentation. J Thorac Cardiovasc Surg 1976;71:465–468.

367. Fossum TW, Birchard SJ. Lymphangiographic evaluation of experimentally induced chylothorax

after ligation of the cranial vena cava in dogs. Am J Vet Res 1986;47:967–971.

368. Nix J, Albert M, Dugas J, et al. Chylothorax and chylous ascites; a study of 302 selected cases. Am J Gastroenterol 1957;28:40–53.

369. Ross J. A review of the surgery of the thoracic duct. Thorax 1961;16:12–21.

370. Bower G. Chylothorax: observations in 20 cases. Dis Chest 1964;46:464–468.

371. Staats BA, Ellefson RD, Budahn LL, et al. The lipoprotein profile of chylous and nonchylous pleural effusions. Mayo Clin Proc 1980;55:700–704.

372. Seriff NS, Cohen ML, Samuel P, et al. Chylothorax: diagnosis by lipoprotein electrophoresis of serum and pleural fluid. Thorax 1977;32:98–100.

373. Yeam I, Sassoon C. Hemothorax and chylothorax. Curr Opin Pulm Med 1997;3:310–314.

374. Macfarlane JR, Holman CW. Chylothorax. Am Rev Respir Dis 1972;105:287–291.

375. Roy P, Carr D, Payne W. The problem of chylothorax. Mayo Clin Proc 1967; 42:457–467.

376. Cevese PG, Vecchioni R, D'Amico DF, et al. Postoperative chylothorax. Six cases in 2,500 operations, with a survey of the world literature. J Thorac Cardiovasc Surg 1975;69:966–971.

377. Kshettry VR, Rebello R. Chylothorax after coronary artery bypass grafting. Thorax 1982;37:954.

378. Weber DO, Mastro PD, Yarnoz MD. Chylothorax after myocardial revascularization with internal mammary graft. Ann Thorac Surg 1981;32:499–492.

379. Nygaard SD, Berger HA, Fick RB. Chylothorax as a complication of oesophageal sclerotherapy. Thorax 1992;47:134–135.

380. Shimizu K, Yoshida J, Nishimura M, et al. Treatment strategy for chylothorax after pulmonary resection and lymph node dissection for lung cancer. J Thorac Cardiovasc Surg 2002;124:499–502.

381. Orringer MB, Bluett M, Deeb GM. Aggressive treatment of chylothorax complicating transhiatal esophagectomy without thoracotomy. Surgery 1988;104:720–726.

382. Dulchavsky SA, Ledgerwood AM, Lucas CE. Management of chylothorax after blunt chest trauma. J Trauma 1988;28:1400–1401.

383. Cammarata SK, Brush RE Jr, Hyzy RC. Chylothorax after childbirth. Chest 1991;99:1539–1540.

384. Reilly KM, Tsou E. Bilateral chylothorax. A case report following episodes of stretching. JAMA 1975;233:536–537.

385. van Straaten HL, Gerards LJ, Krediet TG. Chylothorax in the neonatal period. Eur J Pediatr 1993;152:2–5.

386. Ryu JH, Doerr CH, Fisher SD, et al. Chylothorax in lymphangi-

oleiomyomatosis. Chest 2003;123: 623–627.

387. Gardner TW, Domm AC, Brock CE, et al. Congenital pulmonary lymphangiectasis. A case complicated by chylothorax. Clin Pediatr (Phila) 1983;22:75–78.

388. Baltaxe HA, Lee JG, Ehlers KH, et al. Pulmonary lymphangiectasia demonstrated by lymphangiography in 2 patients with Noonan's syndrome. Radiology 1975;115:149–153.

389. Brown LR, Reiman HM, Rosenow EC 3rd, et al. Intrathoracic lymphangioma. Mayo Clin Proc 1986;61:882–892.

390. Duckett JG, Lazarus A, White KM. Cutaneous masses, rib lesions, and chylous pleural effusion in a 20-year-old man. Chest 1990;97:1227–1228.

391. Steiner GM, Farman J, Lawson JP. Lymphangiomatosis of bone. Radiology 1969;93:1093–1098.

392. Aviv R, McHugh K. Mechanisms of chylous effusion in lymphangiomatosis. AJR Am J Roentgenol 2000;175:1191.

393. Swensen SJ, Hartman TE, Mayo JR, et al. Diffuse pulmonary lymphangiomatosis: CT findings. J Comput Assist Tomog 1995;19:348–352.

394. Takahashi K, Takahashi H, Maeda K, et al. An adult case of lymphangiomatosis of the mediastinum, pulmonary interstitium and retroperitoneum complicated by chronic disseminated intravascular coagulation. Eur Respir J 1995;8:1799–1802.

395. Lee WS, Kim SH, Kim I, et al. Chylothorax in Gorham's disease. J Korean Med Sci 2002;17:826–829.

396. Yoo SY, Goo JM, Im JG. Mediastinal lymphangioma and chylothorax: thoracic involvement of Gorham's disease. Korean J Radiol 2002;3:130–132.

397. Brenner WI, Boal BH, Reed GE. Chylothorax as a manifestation of rheumatic mitral stenosis: its postoperative management with a diet of medium-chain triglycerides. Chest 1978;73:672–673.

398. Villena V, de Pablo A, Martin-Escribano P. Chylothorax and chylous ascites due to heart failure. Eur Respir J 1995;8:1235–1236.

399. Effmann EL, Ablow RC, Touloukian RJ, et al. Radiographic aspects of total parenteral nutrition during infancy. Radiology 1978;127:195–201.

400. Hinckley ME. Thoracic-duct thrombosis with fatal chylothorax caused by a long venous catheter. N Engl J Med 1969; 280:95–96.

401. Warren WH, Altman JS, Gregory SA. Chylothorax secondary to obstruction of the superior vena cava: a complication of the LeVeen shunt. Thorax 1990;45: 978–979.

402. Adams J, McEvoy R, DeWeese J. Primary deep venous thrombosis of upper extremity. Arch Surg 1965;91:29–42.

403. Delgado C, Martin M, de la Portilla F. Retrosternal goiter associated with chylothorax. Chest 1994;106:1924–1925.

404. Vennera MC, Moreno R, Cot J, et al. Chylothorax and tuberculosis. Thorax 1983;38:694–695.

405. Freundlich IM. The role of lymphangiography in chylothorax. A report of six nontraumatic cases. Am J Roentgenol Radium Ther Nucl Med 1975;125:617–627.

406. Kitchen ND, Hocken DB, Greenhalgh RM, et al. Use of the Denver pleuroperitoneal shunt in the treatment of chylothorax secondary to filariasis. Thorax 1991;46:144–145.

407. Moss R, Hinds S, Fedullo AJ. Chylothorax: a complication of the nephrotic syndrome. Am Rev Respir Dis 1989;140:1436–1437.

408. Valdes L, Alvarez D, Pose A, et al. Cirrhosis of the liver, an exceptional cause of chylothorax: two cases. Respir Med 1996;90:61–62.

409. Romero S, Martin C, Hernandez L, et al. Chylothorax in cirrhosis of the liver: analysis of its frequency and clinical characteristics. Chest 1998;114:154–159.

410. Jarman PR, Whyte MK, Sabroe I, et al. Sarcoidosis presenting with chylothorax. Thorax 1995;50:1324–1325.

411. Riantawan P, Tansupasawasdikul S, Subhannachart P. Bilateral chylothorax complicating massive osteolysis (Gorham's syndrome). Thorax 1996;51:1277–1278.

412. Anton PA, Rubio J, Casan P, et al. Chylothorax due to Mycobacterium tuberculosis. Thorax 1995;50:1019.

413. Lowell J. Pleural effusions: a comprehensive review. Baltimore: University Park Press, 1977.

414. Fairfax AJ, McNabb WR, Spiro SG. Chylothorax: a review of 18 cases. Thorax 1986;41:880–885.

415. Hom M, Jolles H. Traumatic mediastinal lymphocele mimicking other thoracic injuries: case report. J Thorac Imaging 1992;7:78–80.

416. Suzuki K, Yoshida J, Nishimura M, et al. Postoperative mediastinal chyloma. Ann Thorac Surg 1999;68:1857–1858.

417. Higgins CB, Mulder DG. Mediastinal chyloma, a roentgenographic sign of chylous fistula. JAMA 1970;211:1188.

418. Mine H, Tamura K, Tanegashima K, et al. Non-traumatic chylothorax associated with diffuse lymphatic dysplasia. Lymphology 1984;17:111–112.

419. Ngan H, Fok M, Wong J. The role of lymphography in chylothorax following thoracic surgery. Br J Radiol 1988;61: 1032–1036.

420. Day DL, Warwick WJ. Thoracic duct opacification for CT scanning. AJR Am J Roentgenol 1985;144:403–404.

421. Qureshy A, Kubota K, Ono S, et al. Thoracic duct scintigraphy by orally

administered I-123 BMIPP: normal findings and a case report. Clin Nucl Med 2001;26:847–855.

422. Kettner BI, Aurisch R, Ruckert JC, et al. Scintigraphic localization of lymphatic leakage site after oral administration of iodine-123-IPPA. J Nucl Med 1998;39:2141–2144.

423. Al-Sebeih K, Sadeghi N, Al-Dhahri S. Bilateral chylothorax following neck dissection: a new method of treatment. Ann Otol Rhinol Laryngol 2001;110:381–384.

424. Hillerdal G. Chylothorax and pseudochylothorax. Eur Respir J 1997;10:1157–1162.

425. Hillerdal G. Chyliform (cholesterol) pleural effusion. Chest 1985;88:426–428.

426. Ferguson GC. Cholesterol pleural effusion in rheumatoid lung disease. Thorax 1966;21:577–582.

427. Johnson JR, Falk A, Iber C, et al. Paragonimiasis in the United States. A report of nine cases in Hmong immigrants. Chest 1982;82:168–171.

428. Groskin SA. Selected topics in chest trauma. Radiology 1992;183:605–617.

429. Banks J, Cassidy D, Campbell IA, et al. Unusual clinical signs complicating tension haemothorax. Br J Dis Chest 1984;78:272–274.

430. Willson SA, Sawicka EH, Mitchell IC. Spontaneous pneumothorax: an unusual radiological appearance. Br J Radiol 1985;58:173–175.

431. Milner LB, Ryan K, Gullo J. Fatal intrathoracic hemorrhage after percutaneous aspiration lung biopsy. AJR 1979;132:280–281.

432. Rodriguez E, Martinez J, Javaloyas M, et al. Haemothorax in the course of chickenpox. Thorax 1986;41:491.

433. Rasaretnam R, Chanmugam D, Sivathasan C. Spontaneous haemothorax in a mild haemophiliac. Thorax 1976;31:601–604.

434. Millard CE. Massive hemothorax complicating heparin therapy for pulmonary infarction. Chest 1971;59:235–237.

435. Robinson NMK, Thomas MR, Jewitt DE. Spontaneous haemothorax as a complication of anti-coagulation following coronary angioplasty. Respir Med 1995;89:629–630.

436. Spear BS, Sully L, Lewis CT. Pulmonary arteriovenous fistula presenting as spontaneous haemothorax. Thorax 1975;30:355–356.

437. DeFrance JH, Blewett JH, Ricci JA, et al. Massive hemothorax: two unusual cases. Chest 1974;66:82–84.

438. Castells L, Comas P, Gonzalez A, et al. Case report: haemothorax in herediary multiple exostosis. Br J Radiol 1993;66:269–270.

439. Kravis MMJ, Hutton LC. Solitary plasma cell tumor of the pleura manifested as

massive hemothorax. AJR 1993;161:543–544.

440. Kupferschmid JP, Shahian DM, Villanueva AG. Massive hemothorax associated with intrathoracic extramedullary hematopoiesis involving the pleura. Chest 1993;103:974–975.

441. Sulis E, Floris C. Haemothorax due to thoracic extramedullary erythropoiesis in thalassaemia intermedia. Br Med J 1985;291:1094.

442. Calvert RJ, Smith E. An analytical review of spontaneous haemopneumothorax. Thorax 1955;10:64–72.

443. Shepard MK, Mancini MC, Campbell GD Jr, George R. Right-sided hemothorax and recurrent abdominal pain in a 34-year-old woman. Chest 1993;103:1239–1240.

444. Yeh T. Endometriosis within the thorax: metaplasia, implantation, or metastasis? J Cardiovasc Surg 1967;53:201–205.

445. Deaton W, Johnston F. Spontaneous hemopneumothorax. J Thorac Cardiovasc Surg 1962;43:413–415.

446. Slind RO, Rodarte JR. Spontaneous hemothorax in an otherwise healthy young man. Chest 1974;66:81.

447. Yung CM, Bessen SC, Hingorani V, et al. Idiopathic hemothorax, Chest 1979;103:638–639.

448. Reynolds J, Davis JT. Injuries of the chest wall, pleura, pericardium, lungs, bronchi and esophagus. Radiol Clin North Am 1966;4:383–401.

449. Qureshi MM, Roble DC, Gindin RA, et al. Subarachnoid-pleural fistula. Case report and review of the literature. J Thorac Cardiovasc Surg 1986;91:238–241.

450. Wolverson MK, Crepps LF, Sundaram M, et al. Hyperdensity of recent hemorrhage at body computed tomography: incidence and morphologic variation. Radiology 1983;148:779–784.

451. McLoud TC, Isler R, Head J. The radiologic appearance of chemical pleurodesis. Radiology 1980;135:313–317.

452. Eyler WR, Monsein LH, Beute GH, et al. Rib enlargement in patients with chronic pleural disease. AJR Am J Roentgenol 1996;167:921–926.

453. Aberle DR, Gamsu G, Ray CS. High-resolution CT of benign asbestos-related diseases: clinical and radiographic correlation. AJR Am J Roentgenol 1988;151:883–891.

454. Leung AN, Müller NL, Miller RR. CT in differential diagnosis of diffuse pleural disease. AJR Am J Roentgenol 1990;154:487–492.

455. Im J-G, Webb W, Rosen A, et al. Costal pleura: Appearances at high-resolution CT. Radiology 1989;171:125–131.

456. Hulnick DH, Naidich DP, McCauley DI. Pleural tuberculosis evaluated by computed tomography. Radiology 1983;149:759–765.

457. Schmitt WG, Hubener KH, Rucker HC. Pleural calcification with persistent effusion. Radiology 1983;149:633–638.

458. Waite RJ, Carbonneau RJ, Balikian JP, et al. Parietal pleural changes in empyema: appearances at CT. Radiology 1990;175:145–150.

459. Takasugi JE, Godwin JD, Teefey SA. The extrapleural fat in empyema: CT appearance. Br J Radiol 1991;64:580–583.

460. Bury T, Paulus P, Dowlati A, et al. Evaluation of pleural diseases with FDG-PET imaging: preliminary report. Thorax 1997;52:187–189.

461. Hierholzer J, Luo L, Bittner RC, et al. MRI and CT in the differential diagnosis of pleural disease. Chest 2000;118:604–609.

462. Franquet T, Gimenez A, Cremades R, et al. Spontaneous reversibility of "pleural thickening" in a patient with semi-invasive pulmonary aspergillosis: radiographic and CT findings. Eur Radiol 2000;10:722–724.

463. Chong VF, Fan YF. Invasive thymoma presenting as pleural thickening. AJR Am J Roentgenol 1997;168:568–569.

464. Lee MJ, Breatnach E. Pleural thickening caused by leukemic infiltration: pleural findings. AJR Am J Roentgenol 1994;163:1527–1528.

465. Neff CC, vanSonnenberg E, Lawson DW, et al. CT follow-up of empyemas: pleural peels resolve after percutaneous catheter drainage. Radiology 1990;176:195–197.

466. Buchanan DR, Johnston ID, Kerr IH, et al. Cryptogenic bilateral fibrosing pleuritis. Br J Dis Chest 1988;82:186–193.

467. Lee-Chiong TL Jr, Hilbert J. Extensive idiopathic benign bilateral asynchronous pleural fibrosis. Chest 1996;109:564–565.

468. Oliver RM, Neville E. Progressive apical pleural fibrosis: a 'constrictive' ventilatory defect. Br J Dis Chest 1988;82:439–443.

469. Azoulay E, Paugam B, Heymann MF, et al. Familial extensive idiopathic bilateral pleural fibrosis. Eur Respir J 1999;14:971–973.

470. Hayes JP, Wiggins J, Ward K, et al. Familial cryptogenic fibrosing pleuritis with Fanconi's syndrome (renal tubular acidosis). A new syndrome. Chest 1995;107:576–578.

471. Gilmartin D. The serratus anterior muscle on chest radiographs. Radiology 1979;131:629–635.

472. Collins JD, Brown RK, Batra P. Asbestosis and the serratus anterior muscle. J Natl Med Assoc 1983;75:296–300.

473. Sargent EN, Boswell WD Jr, Ralls PW, et al. Subpleural fat pads in patients exposed to asbestos: distinction from non-calcified pleural plaques. Radiology 1984;152:273–277.

474. Vix VA. Extrapleural costal fat. Radiology 1974;112:563–565.

475. Renner RR, Pernice NJ. The apical cap. Semin Roentgenol 1977;12:299–302.

476. Renner RR, Markarian B, Pernice NJ, et al. The apical cap. Radiology 1974;110:569–573.

471. Jamison H. Anatomic-roentgenographic study of pleural domes and pulmonary apices, with special reference to apical subpleural scars. Radiology 1941;36:302–314.

478. Butler C, 2nd, Kleinerman J. The pulmonary apical cap. Am J Pathol 1970;60:205–216.

479. Yousem SA. Pulmonary apical cap: a distinctive but poorly recognized lesion in pulmonary surgical pathology. Am J Surg Pathol 2001;25:679–683.

480. McLoud TC, Isler RJ, Novelline RA, et al. The apical cap. AJR Am J Roentgenol 1981;137:299–306.

481. Proto AV. Conventional chest radiographs: anatomic understanding of newer observations. Radiology 1992;183:593–603.

482. Im JG, Webb WR, Han MC, et al. Apical opacity associated with pulmonary tuberculosis: high-resolution CT findings. Radiology 1991;178:727–731.

483. Reeder LB. Malignant pleural effusions. Curr Treat Options Oncol 2001;2:93–96.

484. Sahn SA. Management of malignant pleural effusions. Monaldi Arch Chest Dis 2001;56:394–399.

485. de Campos JR, Vargas FS, de Campos Werebe E, et al. Thoracoscopy talc poudrage: a 15-year experience. Chest 2001;119:801–806.

486. Tschopp JM, Frey JG. Treatment of primary spontaneous pneumothorax by simple talcage under medical thoracoscopy. Monaldi Arch Chest Dis 2002;57:88–92.

487. Marom EM, Erasmus JJ, Herndon JE, 2nd, et al. Usefulness of imaging-guided catheter drainage and talc sclerotherapy in patients with metastatic gynecologic malignancies and symptomatic pleural effusions. AJR Am J Roentgenol 2002;179:105–108.

488. Marom EM, Patz EF Jr, Erasmus JJ, et al. Malignant pleural effusions: treatment with small-bore-catheter thoracostomy and talc pleurodesis. Radiology 1999;210:277–281.

489. Murray JG, Patz EF Jr, Erasmus JJ, et al. CT appearance of the pleural space after talc pleurodesis. AJR Am J Roentgenol 1997;169:89–91.

490. Light RW. Talc should not be used for pleurodesis. Am J Respir Crit Care Med 2000;162:2024–2026.

491. Sahn SA. Talc should be used for pleurodesis. Am J Respir Crit Care Med 2000;162:2023–2024; discussion 2026.

492. Brant A, Eaton T. Serious complications with talc slurry pleurodesis. Respirology 2001;6:181–185.

493. Vix VA. Roentgenographic manifestations of pleural disease. Semin Roentgenol 1977;12:277–286.

494. Sargent EN, Jacobson G, Gordonson JS. Pleural plaques: a signpost of asbestos dust inhalation. Semin Roentgenol 1977;12:287–297.

495. Shapir J, Lisbona A, Palayew MJ. Chronic calcified empyema. J Can Assoc Radiol 1981;32:24–27.

496. Im JG, Chung JW, Han MC. Milk of calcium pleural collections: CT findings. J Comput Assist Tomogr 1993;17:613–616.

497. Scales FE, Lee ME. Nonoperative diagnosis of intrathoracic splenosis. AJR Am J Roentgenol 1983;141:1273–1274.

498. Dalton ML Jr, Strange WH, Downs EA. Intrathoracic splenosis. Case report and review of the literature. Am Rev Respir Dis 1971;103:827–830.

499. Normand JP, Rioux M, Dumont M, et al. Thoracic splenosis after blunt trauma: frequency and imaging findings. AJR Am J Roentgenol 1993;161:739–741.

500. Moncada R, Williams V, Fareed J, et al. Thoracic splenosis. AJR Am J Roentgenol 1985;144:705–706.

501. Yammine JN, Yatim A, Barbari A. Radionuclide imaging in thoracic splenosis and a review of the literature. Clin Nucl Med 2003;28:121–123.

502. Naylor MF, Karstaedt N, Finck SJ, et al. Noninvasive methods of diagnosing thoracic splenosis. Ann Thorac Surg 1999;68:243–244.

503. Davis HH, 2nd, Varki A, Heaton WA, et al. Detection of accessory spleens with indium 111-labeled autologous platelets. Am J Hematol 1980;8:81–86.

504. Chee CB, Abisheganaden J, Yeo JK, et al. Persistent air-leak in spontaneous pneumothorax – clinical course and outcome. Respir Med 1998;92:757–761.

505. Abolnik IZ, Lossos IS, Gillis D, et al. Primary spontaneous pneumothorax in men. Am J Med Sci 1993;305:297–303.

506. Killen D, Gobbel W. Spontaneous pneumothorax. Boston: Little, Brown, 1968.

507. Inouye WY, Berggren RB, Johnson J. Spontaneous pneumothorax: treatment and mortality. Dis Chest 1967;51:67–73.

508. Melton LJ, 3rd, Hepper NG, Offord KP. Incidence of spontaneous pneumothorax in Olmsted County, Minnesota: 1950 to 1974. Am Rev Respir Dis 1979;120:1379–1382.

509. Greene R, McLoud TC, Stark P. Pneumothorax. Semin Roentgenol 1977;12:313–325.

510. Ruckley CV, McCormack RJ. The management of spontaneous pneumothorax. Thorax 1966;21:139–144.

511. Lesur O, Delorme N, Fromaget JM, et al. Computed tomography in the etiologic assessment of idiopathic spontaneous pneumothorax. Chest 1990;98:341–347.

512. Bense L, Lewander R, Eklund G, et al. Nonsmoking, non-alpha 1-antitrypsin deficiency-induced emphysema in nonsmokers with healed spontaneous pneumothorax, identified by computed tomography of the lungs [see comments]. Chest 1993;103:433–438.

513. Warner BW, Bailey WW, Shipley RT. Value of computed tomography of the lung in the management of primary spontaneous pneumothorax. Am J Surg 1991;162:39–42.

514. West JB. Distribution of mechanical stress in the lung, a possible factor in localisation of pulmonary disease. Lancet 1971;1:839–841.

515. Glazier JB, Hughes JM, Maloney JE, et al. Vertical gradient of alveolar size in lungs of dogs frozen intact. J Appl Physiol 1967;23:694–705.

516. Melton LJ, 3rd, Hepper NG, Offord KP. Influence of height on the risk of spontaneous pneumothorax. Mayo Clin Proc 1981;56:678–682.

517. Giuffre B. Supine pneumothoraces in adults. Australas Radiol 1984;28:335–338.

518. Scott GC, Berger R, McKean HE. The role of atmospheric pressure variation in the development of spontaneous pneumothoraces. Am Rev Respir Dis 1989;139:659–662.

519. Gilmartin JJ, Wright AJ, Gibson GJ. Effects of pneumothorax or pleural effusion on pulmonary function. Thorax 1985;40:60–65.

520. Norris RM, Jones JG, Bishop JM. Respiratory gas exchange in patients with spontaneous pneumothorax. Thorax 1968;23:427–433.

521. Kircher L, Swartzel R. Spontaneous pneumothorax and its treatment. JAMA 1954;155:24–29.

522. Northfield TC. Oxygen therapy for spontaneous pneumothorax. Br Med J 1971;4:86–88.

523. Lippert HL, Lund O, Blegvad S, et al. Independent risk factors for cumulative recurrence rate after first spontaneous pneumothorax. Eur Respir J 1991;4:324–331.

524. Jenkinson SG. Pneumothorax. Clin Chest Med 1985;6:153–161.

525. Sharpe IK, Ahmad M, Braun W. Familial spontaneous pneumothorax and HLA antigens. Chest 1980;78:264–268.

526. Leites V, Tannenbaum E. Familial spontaneous pneumothorax. Am Rev Respir Dis 1960;82:240–241.

527. Wilson WG, Aylsworth AS. Familial spontaneous pneumothorax. Pediatrics 1979;64:172–175.

528. Sugiyama Y, Maeda H, Yotsumoto H, et al. Familial spontaneous pneumothorax. Thorax 1986;41:969–970.

529. Rashid A, Sendi A, Al-Kadhimi A, et al. Concurrent spontaneous pneumothorax in identical twins. Thorax 1986;41:971.

530. Gibson GJ. Familial pneumothoraces and bullae. Thorax 1977;32:88–90.

531. Light RW, O'Hara VS, Moritz TE, et al. Intrapleural tetracycline for the prevention of recurrent spontaneous pneumothorax. Results of a Department of Veterans Affairs cooperative study [see comments]. JAMA 1990;264: 2224–2230.

532. Videm V, Pillgram-Larsen J, Ellingsen O, et al. Spontaneous pneumothorax in chronic obstructive pulmonary disease: complications, treatment and recurrences. Eur J Respir Dis 1987;71:365–371.

533. Dines DE, Clagett OT, Payne WS. Spontaneous pneumothorax in emphysema. Mayo Clin Proc 1970;45:481–487.

534. George RB, Herbert SJ, Shames JM, et al. Pneumothorax complicating pulmonary emphysema. JAMA 1975;234:389–393.

535. Spector ML, Stern RC. Pneumothorax in cystic fibrosis: a 26-year experience. Ann Thorac Surg 1989;47:204–207.

536. Rebuck AS. Radiological aspects of severe asthma. Australas Radiol 1970;14:264–268.

537. Burke GJ. Pneumothorax complicating acute asthma. S Afr Med J 1979;55: 508–510.

538. Findley LJ, Sahn SA. The value of chest roentgenograms in acute asthma in adults. Chest 1981;80:535–536.

539. Berkman N, Bar-Ziv J, Breuer R. Recurrent spontaneous pneumothorax associated with bronchial atresia. Respir Med 1996;90:307–309.

540. Laurens RG Jr, Pine JR, Honig EG. Spontaneous pneumothorax in primary cavitating lung carcinoma. Radiology 1983;146:295–297.

541. Steinhauslin CA, Cuttat JF. Spontaneous pneumothorax. A complication of lung cancer? Chest 1985;88:709–713.

542. Dines DE, Cortese DA, Brennan MD, et al. Malignant pulmonary neoplasms predisposing to spontaneous pneumothorax. Mayo Clin Proc 1973;48:541–544.

543. Ayres JG, Pitcher DW, Rees PJ. Pneumothorax associated with primary bronchial carcinoma. Br J Dis Chest 1980;74:180–182.

544. Sheard JD, Taylor W, Soorae A, et al. Pneumothorax and malignant mesothelioma in patients over the age of 40. Thorax 1991;46:584–585.

545. Wright FW. Spontaneous pneumothorax and pulmonary malignant disease – a syndrome sometimes associated with cavitating tumours. Report of nine new cases, four with metastases and five with primary bronchial tumours. Clin Radiol 1976;27:211–222.

546. Janetos G, Ochsner S. Bilateral pneumothorax in metastatic osteogenic sarcoma. Am Rev Respir Dis 1963;88: 73–76.

547. Spittle MF, Heal J, Harmer C, et al. The association of spontaneous pneumothorax with pulmonary metastases in bone tumours of children. Clin Radiol 1968;19:400–403.

548. Siegel MJ, McAlister WH. Unusual intrathoracic complications in Wilms tumor. AJR Am J Roentgenol 1980; 134:1231–1234.

549. Singh A, Sethi RS, Singh G. Pneumothorax: an unusual complication of teratoma chest. Chest 1973;63: 1034–1036.

550. Slasky BS, Deutsch M. Germ cell tumors complicated by pneumothorax. Urology 1983;22:39–42.

551. Plowman PN, Stableforth DE, Citron KM. Spontaneous pneumothorax in Hodgkin's disease. Br J Dis Chest 1980;74:411–414.

552. Yellin A, Benfield JR. Pneumothorax associated with lymphoma. Am Rev Respir Dis 1986;134:590–592.

553. Lote K, Dahl O, Vigander T. Pneumothorax during combination chemotherapy. Cancer 1981;47:1743–1745.

554. Libshitz HI, Banner MP. Spontaneous pneumothorax as a complication of radiation therapy to the thorax. Radiology 1974;112:199–201.

555. Blane C, Silberstein R, Sue J. Radiation therapy and spontaneous pneumothorax. J Can Assoc Radiol 1981;32:153–154.

556. Twiford TW Jr, Zornoza J, Libshitz HI. Recurrent spontaneous pneumothorax after radiation therapy to the thorax. Chest 1978;73:387–388.

557. Vaideeswar P. Cavitary pulmonary infarction – a rare cause of spontaneous pneumothorax. J Postgrad Med 1998;44:99–100.

558. Hall FM, Salzman EW, Ellis BI, et al. Pneumothorax complicating aseptic cavitating pulmonary infarction. Chest 1977;72:232–234.

559. Blundell JE. Pneumothorax complicating pulmonary infarction. Br J Radiol 1967;40:226–227.

560. McFadden E, Luparello F. Bronchopleural fistula complication massive pulmonary infarction. Thorax 1969;24:500–505.

561. Jaffe RB, Koschmann EB. Septic pulmonary emboli. Radiology 1970;96:527–532.

562. Maurer E, Schaal J, Mendez F. Chronic recurring spontaneous pneumothorax due to endometriosis of the diaphragm. JAMA 1958;168:2013–2014.

563. Nakamura H, Konishiike J, Sugamura A, et al. Epidemiology of spontaneous pneumothorax in women. Chest 1986;89:378–382.

564. Shearin RP, Hepper NG, Payne WS. Recurrent spontaneous pneumothorax concurrent with menses. Mayo Clin Proc 1974;49:98–101.

565. Carter EJ, Ettensohn DB. Catamenial pneumothorax. Chest 1990;98:713–716.

566. Rossi NP, Goplerud CP. Recurrent catamenial pneumothorax. Arch Surg 1974;109:173–176.

567. Slasky BS, Siewers RD, Lecky JW, et al. Catamenial pneumothorax: the roles of diaphragmatic defects and endometriosis. AJR Am J Roentgenol 1982;138:639–643.

568. Gray R, Cormier M, Yedlicka J, et al. Catamenial pneumothorax: case report and literature review. J Thorac Imaging 1987;2:72–75.

569. Laws HL, Fox LS, Younger JB. Bilateral catamenial pneumothorax. Arch Surg 1977;112:627–628.

570. Davies R. Recurring spontaneous pneumothorax concomitant with menstruation. Thorax 1968;23:370–373.

571. Müller NL, Nelems B. Postcoital catamenial pneumothorax. Report of a case not associated with endometriosis and successfully treated with tubal ligation. Am Rev Respir Dis 1986;134:803–804.

572. Crutcher RR, Waltuch TL, Blue ME. Recurring spontaneous pneumothorax associated with menstruation. J Thorac Cardiovasc Surg 1967;54:599–602.

573. Downey DB, Towers MJ, Poon PY, et al. Pneumoperitoneum with catamenial pneumothorax. AJR Am J Roentgenol 1990;155:29–30.

574. Furman WR, Wang KP, Summer WR, et al. Catamenial pneumothorax: evaluation by fiberoptic pleuroscopy. Am Rev Respir Dis 1980;121:137–140.

575. Stern H, Toole AL, Merino M. Catamenial pneumothorax. Chest 1980;78:480–482.

576. Kirschner PA. Catamenial pneumothorax: an example of porous diaphragm syndromes. Chest 2000;118:1519–1520.

577. Soderberg CH, Dahlquist EH. Catamenial pneumothorax. Surgery 1976;79:236–239.

578. Sakamoto K, Ohmori T, Takei H. Catamenial pneumothorax caused by endometriosis in the visceral pleura. Ann Thorac Surg 2003;76:290–291.

579. Van Schil PE, Vercauteren SR, Vermeire PA, et al. Catamenial pneumothorax caused by thoracic endometriosis. Ann Thorac Surg 1996;62:585–586.

580. Laursen L, Ostergaard AH, Andersen B. Catamenial pneumothorax treated by laparoscopic tubal occlusion using Filshie clips. Acta Obstet Gynecol Scand 2003;82:488–489.

581. Kovarik JL, Toll GD. Thoracic endometriosis with recurrent spontaneous pneumothorax. JAMA 1966;196:595–597.

582. Joseph J, Reed CE, Sahn SA. Thoracic endometriosis. Recurrence following hysterectomy with bilateral salpingo-oophorectomy and successful treatment

with talc pleurodesis. Chest 1994;106:1894–1896.

583. Im JG, Kang HS, Choi BI, et al. Pleural endometriosis: CT and sonographic findings. AJR Am J Roentgenol 1987;148:523–524.

584. Kalapura T, Okadigwe C, Fuchs Y, et al. Spiral computerized tomography and video thoracoscopy in catamenial pneumothorax. Am J Med Sci 2000;319:186–188.

585. Foster DC, Stern JL, Buscema J, et al. Pleural and parenchymal pulmonary endometriosis. Obstet Gynecol 1981;58:552–556.

586. Jelihovsky T, Grant AF. Endometriosis of the lung. Thorax 1968;23:434–437.

587. Lattes R, Shepard F, Tovell H, et al. A clinical and pathologic study of endometriosis of the lung. Surg Gynecol Obstet 1956;103:552–558.

588. Mobbs G, Pfanner D. Endometriosis of the lung. Lancet i 1963:472–474.

589. Rodman M, Jones C. Catamenial hemoptysis due to bronchial endometriosis. N Engl J Med 1962;266:805–808.

590. Hertzanu Y, Heimer D, Hirsch M. Computed tomography of pulmonary endometriosis. Comput Radiol 1987;11:81–84.

591. Katoh O, Yamada H, Aoki Y, et al. Utility of angiograms in patients with catamenial hemoptysis. Chest 1990;98:1296–1297.

592. Rosenberg SM, Riddick DH. Successful treatment of catamenial hemoptysis with danazol. Obstet Gynecol 1981;57:130–132.

593. Wang HC, Kuo PH, Kuo SH, et al. Catamenial hemoptysis from tracheobronchial endometriosis: reappraisal of diagnostic value of bronchoscopy and bronchial brush cytology. Chest 2000;118:1205–1208.

594. Mamtora H, Cope V. Pulmonary opacities in pseudoxanthoma elasticum: report of two cases. Br J Radiol 1981;54:65–67.

595. Magid D, Pyeritz RE, Fishman EK. Musculoskeletal manifestations of the Marfan syndrome: radiologic features. AJR Am J Roentgenol 1990;155:99–104.

596. Tsipouras P, Del Mastro R, Sarfarazi M, et al. Genetic linkage of the Marfan syndrome, ectopia lentis, and congenital contractural arachnodactyly to the fibrillin genes on chromosomes 15 and 5. The International Marfan Syndrome Collaborative Study. N Engl J Med 1992;326:905–909.

597. Pyeritz RE, McKusick VA. The Marfan syndrome: diagnosis and management. N Engl J Med 1979;300:772–777.

598. Murdoch JL, Walker BA, Halpern BL, et al. Life expectancy and causes of death in the Marfan syndrome. N Engl J Med 1972;286:804–808.

599. Wanderman KL, Goldstein MS, Faber J. Letter: cor pulmonale secondary to severe kyphoscoliosis in Marfan's syndrome. Chest 1975;67:250–251.

600. Hall JR, Pyeritz RE, Dudgeon DL, et al. Pneumothorax in the Marfan syndrome: prevalence and therapy. Ann Thorac Surg 1984;37:500–504.

601. Wood JR, Bellamy D, Child AH, et al. Pulmonary disease in patients with Marfan syndrome. Thorax 1984;39:780–784.

602. Dominguez R, Weisgrau RA, Santamaria M. Pulmonary hyperinflation and emphysema in infants with the Marfan syndrome. Pediatr Radiol 1987;17:365–369.

603. Rigante D, Segni G, Bush A. Persistent spontaneous pneumothorax in an adolescent with Marfan's syndrome and pulmonary bullous dysplasia. Respiration 2001;68:621–624.

604. Turner JA, Stanley NN. Fragile lung in the Marfan syndrome. Thorax 1976;31:771–775.

605. Lipton RA, Greenwald RA, Seriff NS. Pneumothorax and bilateral honeycombed lung in Marfan syndrome. Report of a case and review of the pulmonary abnormalities in this disorder. Am Rev Respir Dis 1971;104:924–928.

606. Dwyer E, Troncale F. Spontaneous pneumothorax and pulmonary disease in the Marfan syndrome. Ann Intern Med 1965;62:1285–1292.

607. Foster ME, Foster DR. Bronchiectasis and Marfan's syndrome. Postgrad Med J 1980;56:718–719.

608. Teoh PC. Bronchiectasis and spontaneous pneumothorax in Marfan's syndrome. Chest 1977;72:672–673.

609. Walker BA, Beighton PH, Murdoch JL. The marfanoid hypermobility syndrome. Ann Intern Med 1969;71:349–352.

610. Motoyoshi K, Momoi H, Mikami R, et al. [Pulmonary lesions seen in a family with Marfanoid hypermobility syndrome]. Nihon Kyobu Shikkan Gakkai Zasshi 1973;11:138–144.

611. Cupo LN, Pyeritz RE, Olson JL, et al. Ehlers–Danlos syndrome with abnormal collagen fibrils, sinus of Valsalva aneurysms, myocardial infarction, panacinar emphysema and cerebral heterotopias. Am J Med 1981;71:1051–1058.

612. Pope FM. Ehlers–Danlos syndrome. Baillière's Clin Rheumatol 1991;5:321–349.

613. Francke U. Heritable disorders of connective tissue. In: Humes H, ed. Kelley's textbook of internal medicine. Philadelphia: Lippincott Williams Wilkins 2000:1440–1441.

614. Ehlers–Danlos National Foundation. Types of Ehlers–Danlos syndrome. Online. Available:

http://www.ednf.org/typesofeds.php September 5, 2003.

615. Watanabe A, Kawabata Y, Okada O, et al. Ehlers–Danlos syndrome type IV with few extrathoracic findings: a newly recognized point mutation in the COL3A1 gene. Eur Respir J 2002;19:195–198.

616. Dowton SB, Pincott S, Demmer L. Respiratory complications of Ehlers–Danlos syndrome type IV. Clin Genet 1996;50:510–514.

617. Herman TE, McAlister WH. Cavitary pulmonary lesions in type IV Ehlers–Danlos syndrome. Pediatr Radiol 1994;24:263–265.

618. Yost BA, Vogelsang JP, Lie JT. Fatal hemoptysis in Ehlers–Danlos syndrome. Old malady with a new curse. Chest 1995;107:1465–1467.

619. Beighton P, Thomas ML. The radiology of the Ehlers–Danlos syndrome. Clin Radiol 1969;20:354–361.

620. Ayres JG, Pope FM, Reidy JF, et al. Abnormalities of the lungs and thoracic cage in the Ehlers–Danlos syndrome. Thorax 1985;40:300–305.

621. Baumer JH, Hankey S. Transient pulmonary cysts in an infant with the Ehlers–Danlos syndrome. Br J Radiol 1980;53:598–599.

622. Clark JG, Kuhn C 3rd, Uitto J. Lung collagen in type IV Ehlers–Danlos syndrome: ultrastructural and biochemical studies. Am Rev Respir Dis 1980;122:971–978.

623. Smit J, Alberts C, Balk AG. Pneumothorax in the Ehlers–Danlos syndrome: consequence of coincidence? Scand J Respir Dis 1978;59:239–242.

624. O'Neill S, Sweeney J, Walker F, et al. Pneumothorax in the Ehlers–Danlos syndrome. Ir J Med Sci 1981;150:43–44.

625. Robitaille C. Ehlers–Danlos syndrome and recurrent hemoptysis. Ann Intern Med 1964;61:716–721.

626. Hajjar BA, Joyner EN 3rd. Congenital cutis laxa with advanced cardiopulmonary disease. J Pediatr 1968;73:116–119.

627. Maxwell E, Esterly NB. Cutis laxa. Am J Dis Child 1969;117:479–482.

628. Beighton P. Cutis laxa-a heterogeneous disorder. Birth Defects Orig Artic Ser 1974;10:126–131.

629. Merten DF, Rooney R. Progressive pulmonary emphysema associated with congenital generalized elastolysis (cutis laxa). Radiology 1974;113:691–692.

630. Turner-Stokes L, Turton C, Pope FM, et al. Emphysema and cutis laxa. Thorax 1983;38:790–792.

631. Harris RB, Heaphy MR, Perry HO. Generalized elastolysis (cutis laxa). Am J Med 1978;65:815–822.

632. Lally JF, Gohel VK, Dalinka MK, et al. The roentgenographic

manifestations of cutis laxa (generalized elastolysis). Radiology 1974;113:605–606.

633. Wanderer AA, Ellis EF, Goltz RW, et al. Tracheobronchomegaly and acquired cutis laxa in a child. Physiologic and immunologic studies. Pediatrics 1969;44:709–715.

634. Meine F, Grossman H, Forman W, et al. The radiographic findings in congenital cutis laxa. Radiology 1974;113:687–690.

635. Fukazawa T, Sasaki H, Kikuchi S, et al. Spinocerebellar ataxia type 1 and familial spontaneous pneumothorax. Neurology 1997;49:1460–1462.

636. de Latorre FJ, Tomasa A, Klamburg J, et al. Incidence of pneumothorax and pneumomediastinum in patients with aspiration pneumonia requiring ventilatory support. Chest 1977;72:141–144.

637. Rohlfing BM, Webb WR, Schlobohm RM. Ventilator-related extra-alveolar air in adults. Radiology 1976;121:25–31.

638. McLoud TC, Barash PG, Ravin CE. PEEP: radiographic features and associated complications. AJR Am J Roentgenol 1977;129:209–213.

639. Albelda SM, Gefter WB, Kelley MA, et al. Ventilator-induced subpleural air cysts: clinical, radiographic, and pathologic significance. Am Rev Respir Dis 1983;127:360–365.

640. Kumar A, Pontoppidan H, Falke KJ, et al. Pulmonary barotrauma during mechanical ventilation. Crit Care Med 1973;1:181–186.

641. Steier M, Ching N, Roberts EB, et al. Pneumothorax complicating continuous ventilatory support. J Thorac Cardiovasc Surg 1974;67:17–23.

642. Zwillich CW, Pierson DJ, Creagh CE, et al. Complications of assisted ventilation. A prospective study of 354 consecutive episodes. Am J Med 1974;57:161–170.

643. Seow A, Kazerooni EA, Pernicano PG, et al. Comparison of upright inspiratory and expiratory chest radiographs for detecting pneumothoraces [see comments]. AJR Am J Roentgenol 1996;166:313–316.

644. Schramel FM, Golding RP, Haakman CD, et al. Expiratory chest radiographs do not improve visibility of small apical pneumothoraces by enhanced contrast. Eur Respir J 1996;9:406–409.

645. MacEwan DW, Dunbar JS, Smith RD, et al. Pneumothorax in young infants – recognition and evaluation. J Can Assoc Radiol 1971;22:264–269.

646. Carr JJ, Reed JC, Choplin RH, et al. Plain and computed radiography for detecting experimentally induced pneumothorax in cadavers: implications for detection in patients. Radiology 1992;183:193–199.

647. Beres RA, Goodman LR. Pneumothorax: detection with upright versus decubitus radiography. Radiology 1993;186:19–22.

648. Carr JJ, Reed JC, Choplin RH, et al. Pneumothorax detection: a problem in experimental design. Radiology 1993;186:23–25; discussion 25–26.

649. Fisher JK. Skin fold versus pneumothorax. AJR Am J Roentgenol 1978;130:791–792.

650. Daffner RH. Visual illusions affecting perception of the roentgen image. Crit Rev Diagn Imaging 1983;20:79–119.

651. Lane EJ, Proto AV, Phillips TW. Mach bands and density perception. Radiology 1976;121:9–17.

652. Lams PM, Jolles H. The scapula companion shadow. Radiology 1981;138:19–23.

653. Kurihara Y, Nakajima Y, Niimi H, et al. Extrapleural air collections mimicking pneumothorax: helical CT finding. J Comput Assist Tomogr 1997;21:771–772.

654. Berg RA. Giant congenital bronchogenic cyst, "pseudopneumothorax." Postgrad Med 1970;48:121–126.

655. Bourgouin P, Cousineau G, Lemire P, et al. Computed tomography used to exclude pneumothorax in bullous lung disease. J Can Assoc Radiol 1985;36:341–342.

656. Waitches GM, Stern EJ, Dubinsky TJ. Usefulness of the double-wall sign in detecting pneumothorax in patients with giant bullous emphysema. AJR Am J Roentgenol 2000;174:1765–1768.

657. Glazer HS, Anderson DJ, Wilson BS, et al. Pneumothorax: appearance on lateral chest radiographs. Radiology 1989;173:707–711.

658. Axel L. A simple way to estimate the size of a pneumothorax. Invest Radiol 1981;16:165–166.

659. Rhea JT, DeLuca SA, Greene RE. Determining the size of pneumothorax in the upright patient. Radiology 1982;144:733–736.

660. Collins CD, Lopez A, Mathie A, et al. Quantification of pneumothorax size on chest radiographs using interpleural distances: regression analysis based on volume measurements from helical CT. AJR Am J Roentgenol 1995;165:1127–1130.

661. Noppen M, Alexander P, Driesen P, et al. Quantification of the size of primary spontaneous pneumothorax: accuracy of the Light index. Respiration 2001;68:396–399.

662. Tocino IM, Miller MH, Fairfax WR. Distribution of pneumothorax in the supine and semirecumbent critically ill adult. AJR Am J Roentgenol 1985;144:901–905.

663. Tocino IM, Miller MH, Frederick PR, et al. CT detection of occult pneumothorax in head trauma. AJR Am J Roentgenol 1984;143:987–990.

664. Wall SD, Federle MP, Jeffrey RB, et al. CT diagnosis of unsuspected pneumothorax after blunt abdominal trauma. AJR Am J Roentgenol 1983;141:919–921.

665. Rhea JT, vanSonnenberg E, McLoud TC. Basilar pneumothorax in the supine adult. Radiology 1979;133:593–595.

666. Ziter FM Jr, Westcott JL. Supine subpulmonary pneumothorax. AJR Am J Roentgenol 1981;137:699–701.

667. Moskowitz PS, Griscom NT. The medial pneumothorax. Radiology 1976;120:143–147.

668. Gordon R. The deep sulcus sign. Radiology 1980;136:25–27.

669. Kleinman PK, Raptopoulos V. The anterior diaphragmatic attachments: an anatomic and radiologic study with clinical correlates. Radiology 1985;155:289–293.

670. Lacombe P, Cornud F, Grenier P, et al. A new sign of right anterior pneumothorax in the supine adult. Three case reports. Ann Radiol (Paris) 1982;25:231–236.

671. Spizarny DL, Goodman LR. Air in the minor fissure: a sign of right-sided pneumothorax. Radiology 1986;160:329–331.

672. O'Gorman LD, Cottingham RA, Sargent EN, et al. Mediastinal emphysema in the newborn: a review and description of the new extrapleural gas sign. Dis Chest 1968;53:301–308.

673. Markowitz RI. The anterior junction line: a radiographic sign of bilateral pneumothorax in neonates. Radiology 1988;167:717–719.

674. Hoffer FA, Ablow RC. The cross-table lateral view in neonatal pneumothorax. AJR Am J Roentgenol 1984;142:1283–1286.

675. Morgan RA, Owens CM, Collins CD, et al. Detection of pneumothorax with lateral shoot-through digital radiography. Clin Radiol 1993;48:249–252.

676. Neff MA, Monk JS Jr, Peters K, et al. Detection of occult pneumothoraces on abdominal computed tomographic scans in trauma patients. J Trauma 2000;49:281–285.

677. Wernecke K, Galanski M, Peters PE, et al. Pneumothorax: evaluation by ultrasound – preliminary results. J Thorac Imaging 1987;2:76–78.

678. Goodman TR, Traill ZC, Phillips AJ, et al. Ultrasound detection of pneumothorax. Clin Radiol 1999;54:736–739.

679. Lichtenstein DA, Menu Y. A bedside ultrasound sign ruling out pneumothorax in the critically ill. Lung sliding. Chest 1995;108:1345–1348.

680. Dulchavsky SA, Schwarz KL, Kirkpatrick AW, et al. Prospective evaluation of thoracic ultrasound in the detection of pneumothorax. J Trauma 2001;50:201–205.

681. Lichtenstein D, Meziere G, Biderman P, et al. The comet-tail artifact: an

ultrasound sign ruling out pneumothorax. Intensive Care Med 1999;25:383–388.

682. Rowan KR, Kirkpatrick AW, Liu D, et al. Traumatic pneumothorax detection with thoracic US: correlation with chest radiography and CT – initial experience. Radiology 2002;225:210–214.

683. Nashef SA, Ferguson AD. Occult central pneumothorax. Br J Radiol 1985;58:772–774.

684. Kurlander GJ, Helmen CH. Subpulmonary pneumothorax. Am J Roentgenol Radium Ther Nucl Med 1966;96:1019–1021.

685. Christensen EE, Dietz GW. Subpulmonic pneumothorax in patients with chronic obstructive pulmonary disease. Radiology 1976;121:33–37.

686. Gobien RP, Reines HD, Schabel SI. Localized tension pneumothorax: unrecognized form of barotrauma in adult respiratory distress syndrome. Radiology 1982;142:15–19.

687. Kleinman PK, Brill PW, Whalen JP. Anterior pathway for transdiaphragmatic extension of pneumomediastinum. AJR Am J Roentgenol 1978;131:271–275.

688. Lillard RL, Allen RP. The extrapleural air sign in pneumomediastinum. Radiology 1965;85:1093–1098.

689. Nightingale RC, Flower CD. Encysted pneumothorax, a complication of asthma. Br J Dis Chest 1984;78:98–100.

690. Watanabe A, Shimokata K, Nomura F, et al. Interlobar pneumothorax. AJR Am J Roentgenol 1990;155:1135–1136.

691. Aronberg DJ, Brinkley AB, Jr., Levitt RG, et al. Traumatic fissural hemopneumothorax. Radiology 1980;135:318.

692. Mandell GA, Pizzica AL. Air in the inferior accessory fissure of a neonate. J Can Assoc Radiol 1981;32:249–250.

693. Fagan CJ, Swischuk LE. Traumatic lung and paramediastinal pneumatoceles. Radiology 1976;120:11–18.

694. Godwin JD, Merten DF, Baker ME. Paramediastinal pneumatocele: alternative explanations to gas in the pulmonary ligament. AJR Am J Roentgenol 1985;145:525–530.

695. Felman AH, Rodgers BM, Talbert JL. Traumatic para-mediastinal air cyst. A case report. Pediatr Radiol 1976;4:120–121.

696. Hyde I. Traumatic para-mediastinal air cysts. Br J Radiol 1971;44:380–383.

697. Ravin CE, Smith GW, Lester PD, et al. Post-traumatic pneumatocele in the inferior pulmonary ligament. Radiology 1976;121:39–41.

698. Volberg FM Jr, Everett CJ, Brill PW. Radiologic features of inferior pulmonary ligament air collections in neonates with respiratory distress. Radiology 1979;130:357–360.

699. Friedman PJ. Adult pulmonary ligament pneumatocele: a loculated pneumothorax. Radiology 1985;155:575–576.

700. Lams PM, Jolles H. The effect of lobar collapse on the distribution of free intrapleural air. Radiology 1982;142:309–312.

701. Woodring JH, Baker MD, Stark P. Pneumothorax ex vacuo. Chest 1996;110:1102–1105.

702. Berdon WE, Dee GJ, Abramson SJ, Altman RP, Wung JT. Localized pneumothorax adjacent to a collapsed lobe: a sign of bronchial obstruction. Radiology 1984;150:691–694.

703. Boland GW, Gazelle GS, Girard MJ, et al. Asymptomatic hydropneumothorax after therapeutic thoracentesis for malignant pleural effusions. AJR Am J Roentgenol 1998;170:943–946.

704. Abyholm FE, Storen G. Spontaneous haemopneumothorax. Thorax 1973;28:376–378.

705. Walsh J. Spontaneous pneumohemothorax. Dis Chest 1956;29:329–335.

706. Cohen HL, Cohen SW. Spontaneous bilateral pneumothorax in drug addicts. Chest 1984;86:645–647.

707. Phillips LG Jr, Cunningham J. Esophageal perforation. Radiol Clin North Am 1984;22:607–613.

708. Fataar S, Morton P, Schulman A. Recurrent non-surgical pneumoperitoneum due to spontaneous pneumothorax. Br J Radiol 1981;54:1100–1102.

709. Gustman P, Yerger L, Wanner A. Immediate cardiovascular effects of tension pneumothorax. Am Rev Respir Dis 1983;127:171–174.

710. Rutherford RB, Hurt HH Jr, Brickman RD, et al. The pathophysiology of progressive, tension pneumothorax. J Trauma 1968;8:212–227.

711. Rozenman J, Yellin A, Simansky DA, et al. Re-expansion pulmonary oedema following spontaneous pneumothorax. Respir Med 1996;90:235–238.

712. Miller WC, Toon R, Palat H, et al. Experimental pulmonary edema following re-expansion of pneumothorax. Am Rev Respir Dis 1973;108:654–656.

713. Pavlin J, Cheney FW Jr. Unilateral pulmonary edema in rabbits after reexpansion of collapsed lung. J Appl Physiol 1979;46:31–35.

714. Sewell RW, Fewel JG, Grover FL, et al. Experimental evaluation of reexpansion pulmonary edema. Ann Thorac Surg 1978;26:126–132.

715. Trapnell DH, Thurston JG. Unilateral pulmonary oedema after pleural aspiration. Lancet 1970;1:1367–1369.

716. Buczko GB, Grossman RF, Goldberg M. Re-expansion pulmonary edema:

evidence for increased capillary permeability. Can Med Assoc J 1981;125:460–461.

717. Sprung CL, Loewenherz JW, Baier H, et al. Evidence for increased permeability in reexpansion pulmonary edema. Am J Med 1981;71:497–500.

718. Wilkinson PD, Keegan J, Davies SW, et al. Changes in pulmonary microvascular permeability accompanying re-expansion oedema: evidence from dual isotope scintigraphy. Thorax 1990;45:456–459.

719. Henderson AF, Banham SW, Moran F. Re-expansion pulmonary oedema: a potentially serious complication of delayed diagnosis of pneumothorax. Br Med J (Clin Res Ed) 1985;291:593–594.

720. Sautter RD, Dreher WH, MacIndoe JH, et al. Fatal pulmonary edema and pneumonitis after reexpansion of chronic pneumothorax. Chest 1971;60:399–401.

721. Mahajan VK, Simon M, Huber GL. Reexpansion pulmonary edema. Chest 1979;75:192–194.

722. Sherman S, Ravikrishnan KP. Unilateral pulmonary edema following re-expansion of pneumothorax of brief duration. Chest 1980;77:714.

723. Childress ME, Moy G, Mottram M. Unilateral pulmonary edema resulting from treatment of spontaneous pneumothorax. Am Rev Respir Dis 1971;104:119–121.

724. Ziskind MM, Weill H, George RA. Acute pulmonary edema following the treatment of spontaneous pneumothorax with excessive negative intrapleural pressure. Am Rev Respir Dis 1965;92:632–636.

725. Humphreys RL, Berne AS. Rapid re-expansion of pneumothorax. A cause of unilateral pulmonary edema. Radiology 1970;96:509–512.

726. Waqaruddin M, Bernstein A. Re-expansion pulmonary oedema. Thorax 1975;30:54–60.

727. Steckel RJ. Unilateral pulmonary edema after pneumothorax. N Engl J Med 1973;289:621–622.

728. Heller BJ, Grathwohl MK. Contralateral reexpansion pulmonary edema. South Med J 2000;93:828–831.

729. Shaw TJ, Caterine JM. Recurrent re-expansion pulmonary edema. Chest 1984;86:784–786.

730. Wittich GR, Kusnick CA, Starnes VA, et al. Communication between the two pleural cavities after major cardiothoracic surgery: relevance to percutaneous intervention. Radiology 1992;184:461–462.

731. Engeler CE, Olson PN, Engeler CM, et al. Shifting pneumothorax after heart-lung transplantation. Radiology 1992;185:715–717.

732. Schorlemmer GR, Khouri RK, Murray GF, et al. Bilateral pneumothoraces

secondary to iatrogenic buffalo chest. An unusual complication of median sternotomy and subclavian vein catheterization. Ann Surg 1984;199:372–374.

733. Slebos DJ, Elting-Wartan AN, Bakker M, et al. Managing a bilateral pneumothorax in lung transplantation using single chest-tube drainage. J Heart Lung Transplant 2001;20:796–797.

734. Lee YC, McGrath GB, Chin WS, et al. Contralateral tension pneumothorax following unilateral chest tube drainage of bilateral pneumothoraces in a heart-lung transplant patient. Chest 1999;116:1131–1133.

735. Gruden JF, Stern EJ. Bilateral pneumothorax after percutaneous transthoracic needle biopsy. Evidence for incomplete pleural fusion. Chest 1994;105:627–628.

736. Henry M, Arnold T, Harvey J. BTS guidelines for the management of spontaneous pneumothorax. Thorax 2003;58 Suppl 2:ii39–52.

737. Webb WR, LaBerge JM. Radiographic recognition of chest tube malposition in the major fissure. Chest 1984;85:81–83.

738. Webb WR, Godwin JD. The obscured outer edge: a sign of improperly placed pleural drainage tubes. AJR Am J Roentgenol 1980;134:1062–1064.

739. Mathur R, Cullen J, Kinnear WJ, et al. Time course of resolution of persistent air leak in spontaneous pneumothorax. Respir Med 1995;89:129–132.

740. Miller AC. Management of spontaneous pneumothorax: back to the future. Eur Respir J 1996;9:1773–1774.

741. Stern EJ, Sun H, Haramati LB. Peripheral bronchopleural fistulas: CT imaging features. AJR Am J Roentgenol 1996;167:117–120.

742. Ricci ZJ, Haramati LB, Rosenbaum AT, et al. Role of computed tomography in guiding the management of peripheral bronchopleural fistula. J Thorac Imaging 2002;17:214–218.

743. Westcott JL, Volpe JP. Peripheral bronchopleural fistula: CT evaluation in 20 patients with pneumonia, empyema, or postoperative air leak. Radiology 1995;196:175–181.

744. Friedman PJ, Hellekant CA. Radiologic recognition of bronchopleural fistula. Radiology 1977;124:289–295.

745. Peters ME, Gould HR, McCarthy TM. Identification of a bronchopleural fistula by computerized tomography – a case report. J Comput Tomogr 1983;7:267–270.

746. Malave G, Foster ED, Wilson JA, et al. Bronchopleural fistula – present-day study of an old problem. A review of 52 cases. Ann Thorac Surg 1971;11:1–10.

747. Williams NS, Lewis CT. Bronchopleural fistula: a review of 86 cases. Br J Surg 1976;63:520–522.

748. Kim YT, Kim HK, Sung SW, et al. Long-term outcomes and risk factor analysis after pneumonectomy for active and sequela forms of pulmonary tuberculosis. Eur J Cardiothorac Surg 2003;23:833–839.

749. Lams P. Radiographic signs in post pneumonectomy bronchopleural fistula. J Can Assoc Radiol 1980;31:178–180.

750. O'Meara JB, Slade PR. Disappearance of fluid from the postpneumonectomy space. J Thorac Cardiovasc Surg 1974;67:621–628.

751. Zelefsky MN, Freeman LM, Stern H. A simple approach to the diagnosis of bronchopleural fistula. Radiology 1977;124:843–844.

CHAPTER 16

Congenital anomalies

TRACHEOESOPHAGEAL FISTULAS

BRONCHIAL ATRESIA

CONGENITAL LOBAR OVERINFLATION

ABSENCE OF LUNG OR LOBES OF LUNG

PULMONARY HYPOPLASIA
Primary unilateral pulmonary hypoplasia
Primary bilateral pulmonary hypoplasia
Secondary pulmonary hypoplasia

SCIMITAR SYNDROME

UNILATERAL ABSENCE OF THE PULMONARY ARTERY

PULMONARY ARTERIOVENOUS MALFORMATIONS

CONGENITAL DISORDERS OF LYMPHATIC DEVELOPMENT

BRONCHOGENIC CYSTS

PULMONARY SEQUESTRATION

CONGENITAL CYSTIC ADENOMATOID MALFORMATION OF THE LUNG

CONGENITAL DIAPHRAGMATIC ABNORMALITIES
Congenital diaphragmatic hernia
Bochdalek hernia
Morgagni hernia
Accessory diaphragm

It is apparent from clinical experience that congenital or developmental lesions of the lungs are neither as frequent nor, in general, as significant as their counterparts in the heart. Objective evidence from autopsy series supports this impression. For example, Sotelo-Avila and Skanklin[1] showed that some form of congenital malformation occurred in 46% of >2000 autopsies. Of these, 30% were cardiovascular and 10% were genitourinary – but only 3% were respiratory in nature.

Classification of congenital lesions of the lungs and airways is difficult because the embryogenesis of specific pulmonary malformations is often obscure. Although some of the conditions are not present at birth, they are nevertheless developmental in origin. Because the lungs continue to form for an extended time after birth, deleterious factors operating postnatally can affect their development as, for example, in Swyer–James syndrome (see p. 746). Classification is further complicated by associated congenital heart disease, which can lead to difficulty in deciding whether a particular malformation should be categorized as a lung lesion or as a cardiovascular anomaly.

Box 16.1 shows just one of many arbitrary classifications of developmental lesions of the thorax. Many of the more common (relatively!) conditions are discussed in this or other chapters; the frankly rare conditions are only referenced.

TRACHEOESOPHAGEAL FISTULAS

Most tracheoesophageal fistulas are associated with esophageal atresia and are diagnosed in the neonatal period. However, in rare instances, the so-called H type fistula may not be detected until adult life even though symptoms may have been present from infancy (Fig. 16.1).[22] The H type fistula connects the adjacent trachea and esophagus, with the fistula forming the transverse bar of the "H". This type of fistula constitutes approximately 2–4% of all tracheoesophageal fistulas.[23,24] There is a relatively high association between tracheoesophageal fistula and other congenital abnormalities.[25] These associated anomalies can provide a clue to the presence of an H type fistula. An extensive literature describes the differing patterns of associated anomalies.[7] These patterns have been designated by a series of acronyms: the VATER complex (vertebral, anal, tracheoesophageal, and renal), the VACTEL complex (vertebral, anal, cardiac, tracheoesophageal, and limb), and the ARTICLE ± V complex (anal, renal, tracheal, intestinal, cardiac, limb, and esophageal ± vertebral). Other congenital pulmonary lesions, such as pulmonary hypoplasia, tracheal stenosis, and pulmonary sequestration, occur in approximately 2% of patients with this group of complex malformations.[26]

Symptoms of congenital tracheoesophageal fistula are generally due to recurrent aspiration and include paroxysmal cough, feeding difficulties, and recurrent pneumonia. Pulmonary opacities seen on chest radiographs reflect the extent and severity of aspiration. Excessive air may pass through the fistula into the esophagus and subsequently into the gut. In infants with an H type fistula, an air-filled esophagus may be seen on the chest radiograph and there may be unusual degrees of gaseous distension of the bowel.[27] The condition can be difficult to diagnose with contrast studies of the esophagus because the

Box 16.1 Developmental lesions of the thorax

Abnormalities of development, branching, or separation of the foregut
Absence (agenesis, aplasia) of the lungs or lobes of the lungs
Bridging bronchus
Bronchobiliary fistula[2]
Bronchial atresia
Bronchial stenosis[3]
Bronchomalacia[4]
Bronchiectasis[5]
Bronchopulmonary foregut malformations[6]
Bronchial isomerism syndromes[7]
Congenital lobar overinflation
Ectopia of the lungs[8]
Esophageal bronchus[9,10]
Horseshoe lung
Hypoplasia of the lungs
Potter syndrome (oligohydramnios tetrad)
Tracheal diverticulum[11]
Tracheal agenesis[12]
Tracheal stenosis[13]
Tracheal abnormalities in skeletal dysplasias[14]
Tracheomalacia
Tracheobronchomegaly (Mounier-Kuhn syndrome)
Tracheal bronchus, abnormal bronchial branching patterns
Tracheoesophageal fistula

Abnormalities related to a local or systemic biochemical or cellular defect
Pulmonary microlithiasis (see p. 677)
Immotile cilia syndrome (see p. 734)
α_1-Antiprotease deficiency (see p. 760)
Cystic fibrosis (see p. 729)
Chronic granulomatous disease

Abnormalities of the pulmonary vasculature or lymphatics
Congenital pulmonary lymphangiectasia
Pulmonary arteriovenous fistula
Pulmonary isomerism syndromes[7]
Pulmonary artery aplasia
Peripheral pulmonary stenosis[15]
Scimitar syndrome
Yellow nail syndrome

Abnormalities forming a component of a systemic familial or nonfamilial disease process
Hereditary hemorrhagic telangiectasia
Pulmonary lymphangioleiomyomatosis (see p. 682)

Familial abnormalities of the lungs
Familial primary pulmonary hypertension[16]
Familial spontaneous pneumothorax[17]
Familial fibrocystic pulmonary dysplasia[18]
Familial pulmonary fibrosis[19]

Ectopic or hamartomatous development
Congenital cystic adenomatoid malformation
Intrapulmonary and extrapulmonary sequestration
Hamartomas of the lung (see p. 832)
Interstitial masses, hemangioma, thyroid[20]
Focal muscular hyperplasia of the trachea[21]

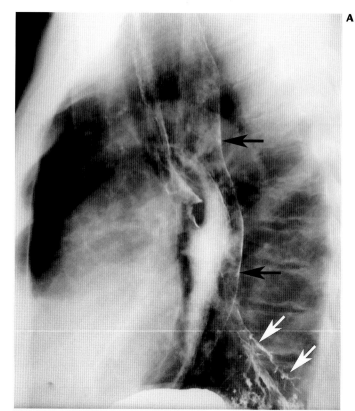

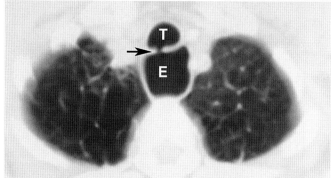

Fig. 16.1 Tracheoesophageal fistula in an elderly man with a history of recurrent pneumonia. **A,** Lateral chest radiograph obtained after a barium swallow examination shows a dilated esophagus (black arrows), barium coating the mid and distal trachea, and barium in the distal airways (white arrows) and airspaces. **B,** CT (lung window) shows an H type fistula (arrow) between the trachea (T) and esophagus (E).

fistula may be relatively small and aspiration through it may be intermittent.[28] The patient should be examined in the prone position, with lateral fluoroscopy and video recording. It is advantageous to inject the contrast medium through a feeding tube while it is withdrawn along the full length of the esophagus. In problematic cases, thin barium suspensions or nonionic water-soluble contrast media are useful. The purpose of these measures is to encourage the contrast medium to enter the fistula.[29] In some cases, repeating the contrast studies on more than one occasion may be necessary to establish the diagnosis.[30] Thus, diagnosis clearly requires a high degree of suspicion.

BRONCHIAL ATRESIA (Box 16.2)

Segmental bronchial atresia is a rare anomaly that results from short segment obliteration of a proximal segmental or subsegmentalal bronchus.[31,32] The distal airways and airspaces develop normally, producing the characteristic triad of findings[33,34]:

1. *Central mucocele*. Proximal bronchial atresia leads to accumulation of mucus within the bronchi distal to the atretic segment. The mucocele manifests on chest radiographs or CT as a central masslike opacity. The opacity is typically round or oval in shape and may not have the branching configuration often associated with acquired mucoceles (Figs 16.2 and 16.3). There may, however, be blunt hornlike protrusions from the main mass.
2. *Hyperlucency* of the affected segment. Aeration of lung beyond the atretic segment occurs through collateral air drift (Figs 16.2 and 16.3).
3. *Hypoperfusion* of the affected segment. Hypoperfusion is presumed to reflect hypoxic vasoconstriction of the segmental vessels and is suggested by a paucity of vessels in that segment (Figs 16.2 and 16.3).

Box 16.2 Segmental bronchial atresia

Etiology
In utero vascular accident (probable)
Proximal short segment atresia of segmental bronchus
Distal airway patent
Distal lung aerates via collateral pathways

Symptoms
Most asymptomatic

Location
Upper lobes most common
Usually apical or posterior segments

Chest radiography
Central masslike opacity (mucocele)
Surrounding hyperlucent lung

Chest CT
Central masslike opacity (mucocele)
Surrounding hyperlucent lung
Used to confirm radiographic findings
Used to exclude endobronchial mass (tumor)
Air-trapping on expiratory images

Differential diagnosis
Allergic bronchopulmonary aspergillosis
Endobronchial mass (tumor, foreign body)

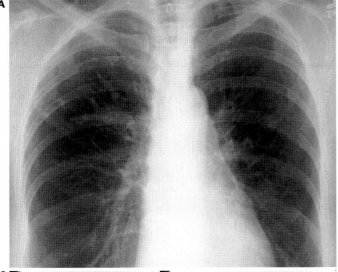

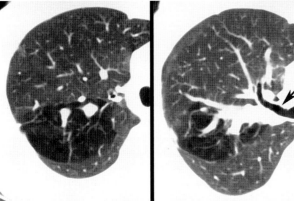

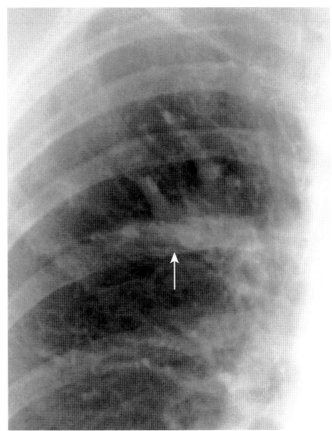

Fig. 16.2   Segmental bronchial atresia in an asymptomatic elderly woman. **A**, Frontal and **B**, coned-down chest radiographs show a branching tubular opacity (arrow on **B**) in the right upper lobe. Note the subtle surrounding lucency. **C**, CT (lung window) shows absence of the posterior segment bronchus, a proximal mucus plug, and hyperlucency of the affected segment. R = right main bronchus, arrow on anterior segment bronchus.

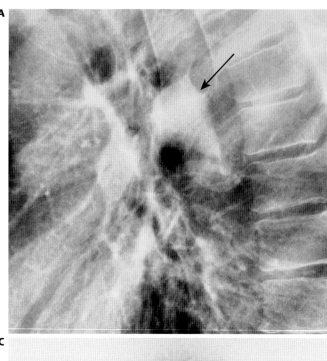

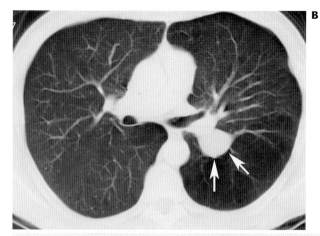

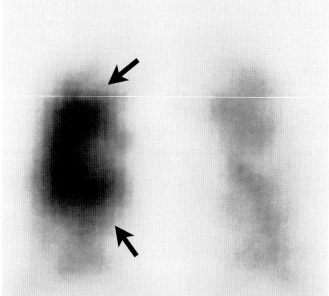

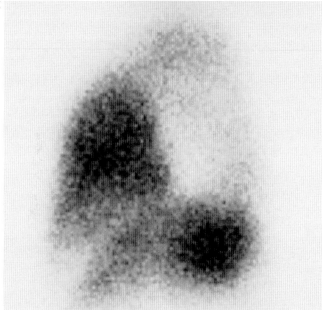

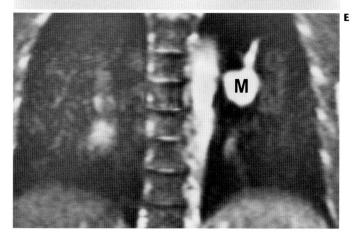

Fig. 16.3   Segmental bronchial atresia in a middle-aged man with a history of cigarette smoking and hemoptysis. **A**, Lateral chest radiograph shows a left hilar mass (arrow). **B**, CT (lung window) shows a hilar mass (arrows) and a hyperlucent superior segment. **C**, Perfusion scintigraphy in the lateral projection shows hypoperfusion of the superior segment. **D**, Ventilation scintigraphy in the frontal projection shows air-trapping in the hyperinflated segment (arrows). **E**, Coronal T2-weighted MRI shows a branching mucocele (M) of high signal intensity distal to the atretic bronchial segment.

Meng et al[35] reviewed 36 cases of bronchial atresia and found that 24 (66%) occurred in the left upper lobe and seven (19%) in the right upper lobe. In the affected upper lobes, it is almost invariably the apical or apicoposterior segments that are involved. Tederlinic et al,[36] however, reported four cases of bronchial atresia in the lower lobes. CT is useful for demonstrating absence of the affected bronchus, the central mucus plug, and the surrounding decreased attenuation and hypoperfused lung.[32,37] Radionuclide $\dot{V}$/Q scanning, now rarely performed for the diagnosis of bronchial atresia, can also demonstrate hypoperfusion and delayed air entry with air-trapping in the affected portion of lung (Fig. 16.3). The central mucus plug is typically of high signal intensity on T2-weighted MRI (Fig. 16.3).[31,38] Bronchial atresia is of little clinical significance. Its importance is that the dilated, mucus-filled bronchus distal to the atresia should not be misdiagnosed as a neoplasm or other important lesion.

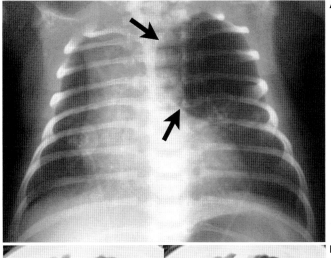

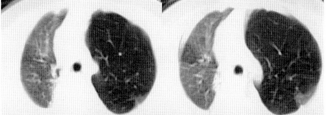

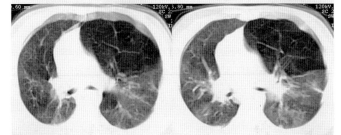

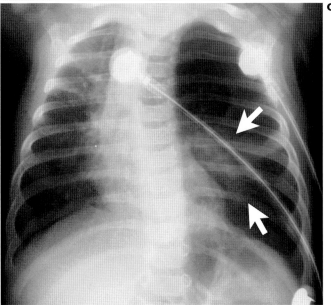

CONGENITAL LOBAR OVERINFLATION
(Box 16.3)

Also known as congenital lobar emphysema, congenital lobar overinflation (CLO) is characterized by progressive hyperexpansion of a lobe of lung. CLO is the preferred term because it best describes the underlying pathophysiology of this disorder – overinflation of normal alveoli, probably due to central obstruction.[39] Although the precise cause of obstruction has been difficult to determine in resected lung specimens, aplasia, hypoplasia, or dysplasia of bronchial support structures is postulated as the primary cause. The congenital nature of the condition has never been unequivocally established even though the circumstantial evidence is strong. There is a definite association with congenital heart disease.[40] A clinically identical but pathologically distinct condition, the polyalveolar lobe, has been described.[41–43] In this condition the airways and the vascular supply to the involved lobe are normal. The lobe contains three to five times the normal number of alveoli for the patient's age. The result is a relatively large lobe that may have all of the compressive effects seen with CLO. This giant lobe is not emphysematous. However, in practical clinical terms the condition is indistinguishable from true lobar overinflation.

In most cases, congenital lobar overinflation manifests in the neonatal period with respiratory distress which may be life threatening. In as many as 25% of cases, however, presentation is delayed until after the first month of life. The classic and by far the most common radiographic appearance is hyperexpansion of a single lobe of lung, usually an upper or middle lobe (Figs 16.4 and 16.5).[44] Remarkably, the lower lobes are

Fig. 16.4 Congenital overinflation of the left upper lobe in a neonate with respiratory distress. **A**, Anteroposterior chest radiograph obtained 1 day after birth shows an overinflated left upper lobe (arrows). **B**, CT (lung window) performed 3 days after birth shows a hyperlucent left upper lobe with no obvious central obstruction. Note the degree of mediastinal shift. **C**, Chest radiograph obtained 4 months later shows progressive overinflation of the left upper lobe with lingular atelectasis (arrows). Resection confirmed overinflation of the left upper lobe. (Courtesy of JR Galvin, Armed Forces Institute of Pathology, Washington, DC)

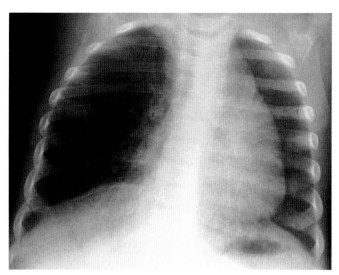

Fig. 16.5 Congenital overinflation of the right upper lobe in a neonate with respiratory distress. Frontal chest radiograph obtained 1 day after birth shows an overinflated right upper lobe.

involved in only about 2% of cases. Involvement of more than one lobe is equally exceptional. The expanded lobe may cause compressive atelectasis of the remainder of the lung, accompanied by displacement of the heart, mediastinum, and diaphragm. The primary differential diagnoses include acquired lobar overinflation due to an endobronchial mass (e.g. foreign body) or extrinsic airway compression, localized pneumothorax, an expanding lung cyst, and, rarely, congenital cystic adenomatoid malformation. Careful study of the chest radiographs should reveal the presence of blood vessels within the hyperexpanded lobe in cases of CLO. Pulmonary interstitial emphysema, an acquired condition most commonly seen in

neonates receiving positive pressure ventilation, may affect a single lobe and closely resemble CLO radiographically. The conditions differ clinically, however, in that interstitial emphysema usually occurs in children who are already receiving mechanical ventilation because of previously known diffuse lung disease. Endobronchial foreign bodies, mucus plugs, or very rarely tumors, can result in obstructive overinflation of a lobe that can appear radiographically identical to CLO. Bronchoscopy to exclude an obstructing lesion should therefore be performed prior to surgical resection of an overexpanded lobe.

Much less commonly, congenital lobar overinflation can manifest as a hyperinflated, fluid-filled lobe.[45] On radiographic examination, the fluid-filled lobe is seen as an expansile mass of soft tissue density (Fig. 16.6). Compression of the remainder of the lung and displacement of the mediastinum may occur exactly as seen with the more common lucent form. In most of these cases, the entrapped fluid drains shortly after birth with resultant conversion to the more conventional appearance of CLO. On rare occasions, a transitional phase between the fluid- and air-filled forms may be encountered.[46] In this transitory phase there are linear interstitial markings resembling septal lines in the hyperexpanded lobe. These opacities disappear, presumably as fluid drains or is absorbed.

The diagnosis of congenital lobar overinflation is usually made on the basis of the clinical and chest radiographic findings.[44] CT may be performed to exclude alternative diagnoses, such as primary pulmonary hypoplasia or scimitar syndrome (Fig. 16.4).[47–50] CT is useful for confirming the presence of lobar overinflation, for better delineating mass effect on adjacent structures, and for excluding endobronchial masses.[44] CT angiography can also be useful for differentiating CLO from various forms of pulmonary hypoplasia.

Resection of the affected lobe is the most common treatment for infants under 2 months old and for patients of any age who have severe respiratory distress related to the overinflated lobe.[44] Patients older than 2 months who have mild to moderate

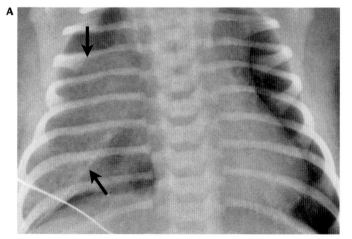
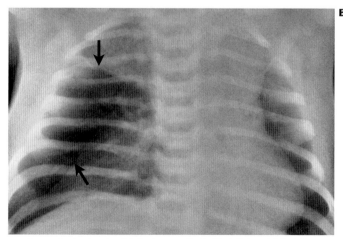

Fig. 16.6 Congenital overinflation of the right middle lobe. **A**, Frontal chest radiograph obtained at birth shows a fluid-filled right middle lobe (arrows). **B**, Chest radiograph obtained several hours later shows an aerated, overinflated lobe (arrows) with mass effect upon the adjacent lung and mediastinum.

symptoms and normal bronchoscopic examination are frequently managed conservatively,[44] with close radiographic follow up.[51] Kennedy et al[47] followed up a group of 12 patients treated conservatively for up to 12 years. They found steady, gradual symptomatic improvement in all cases paralleled by a relative decrease in the lobar hyperexpansion on serial chest radiographs.

ABSENCE OF LUNG OR LOBES OF LUNG
(Table 16.1)

Unilateral absence of a lung or a lobe is a rare congenital abnormality that, in itself, causes surprisingly few clinical problems.[52–54] Indeed, absence of a lung may be encountered de novo in an adult who has had no symptoms referable to the chest. However, the condition is frequently associated with other congenital abnormalities, particularly tracheoesophageal

fistula and the VACTEL syndrome (vertebral, anal, cardiac, tracheoesophageal, and limb).[55–57] When the bronchus to the affected lung is absent, the condition is termed pulmonary agenesis; when there is a rudimentary bronchus, the condition is termed pulmonary aplasia.[58] The ipsilateral pulmonary artery develops but tends to be small or rudimentary.[59] Nearly 10% of patients with tracheobronchial malformations have unilateral pulmonary agenesis. Interestingly, agenesis of the right lung is associated with esophageal atresia,[60–62] whereas agenesis of the left lung is associated with isolated tracheoesophageal fistula without esophageal atresia.[53] Agenesis of the right lung is said to be twice as common as agenesis of the left lung.[63] Absence of one or more lobes of a lung is less common and, when present, is more common on the right. Absence of individual lobes is a form of hypogenetic lung syndrome, which may occur as an isolated entity simulating pulmonary hypoplasia or in association with anomalous pulmonary venous drainage as part of the venolobar syndrome (scimitar syndrome).[59]

Table 16.1 Classification of dysmorphic pulmonary abnormalities

Abnormality	Associated anomalies	Chest radiograph
Aplasia of a pulmonary artery (VB)		• Slight lung volume reduction • Small hilum and diminished vascularity • Contralateral increased vascularity
• Isolated • Associated with hypogenetic lung syndrome • Associated with hypoplastic lung	• Right aortic arch • See below • See below	• See below • See below
Lobar agenesis/aplasia (LB) • Isolated absence of a lobe of lung	• Usually none	• Volume reduction of the affected lung • Mediastinal shift • Retrosternal density
Hypoplasia of lung (LB) • Primary	• Absent pulmonary artery (VB) • Cardiac anomalies	• Volume reduction of the affected lung • Mediastinal shift • Retrosternal density
• Secondary	• See Box 10.4	
Lung agenesis/aplasia (LB) • Agenesis – complete absence of a lung and bronchus • Aplasia – complete absence of a lung but rudimentary bronchus present	Frequent : • Tracheoesophageal • Skeletal • Genitourinary • Cardiac • Gastrointestinal	• No visible aerated lung • Marked mediastinal shift and cardiac rotation • Herniation of the opposite lung • Elevated diaphragm
Scimitar syndrome (VB and LB)	Frequent: • Horseshoe lung • Accessory diaphragm • Diaphragmatic defects • Interrupted inferior vena cava • Sequestration • Cardiac • Systemic arterial supply to lung	Right lung only: • Small volume lung • Dextroposition of the heart • Stunted and deformed vascular pedicle • Scimitar vein(s)

VB = defect of the vascular bud; LB = defect of the lung bud.

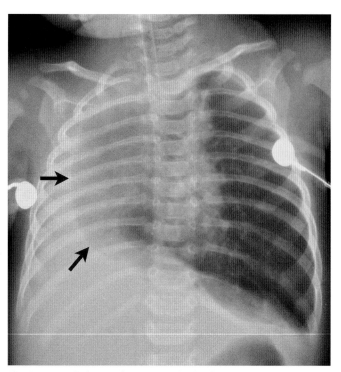

Fig. 16.7 Right lung aplasia in an infant with respiratory distress. Frontal chest radiograph shows marked right sided mediastinal shift, elevation of the right hemidiaphragm, and anterior herniation of the left lung (arrows). Note the characteristic triangular or wedge-shaped opacity in the inferior and lateral aspect of the right hemithorax.

As might be expected, chest radiographs in patients with unilateral absence of a lung show loss of aeration and marked volume loss on the affected side (Figs 16.7 and 16.8). Volume loss is shown as elevation of the ipsilateral hemidiaphragm, shift of the mediastinum toward the abnormal side, and anterior herniation of the contralateral lung. There is usually a characteristic wedge shaped opacity in the inferior and lateral aspect of the affected hemithorax (Fig. 16.8). This opacity is due to herniation of heart and mediastinum into the lower thorax and proliferation of fat to partially compensate for the absence of lung tissue. The obvious differential diagnoses are acquired total lung collapse or prior pneumonectomy. Further investigation with CT or bronchoscopy may be necessary to make the distinction (Fig. 16.8).

In cases of isolated absence of a lobe, there is compensatory hyperexpansion of the remaining lobe or lobes with consequent distortion of the bronchovascular structures. The compensatory expansion is never complete, and lung volume is reduced on the affected side. The chest radiographic findings in congenital absence of a lobe are indistinguishable from those of generalized pulmonary hypoplasia and are discussed below. CT, or now less commonly bronchography, can identify absence of a lobe by demonstrating agenesis or aplasia of the lobar bronchus with an otherwise normal airway.[58] In cases of pulmonary hypoplasia, on the other hand, the number of lobes is normal but the bronchial tree is stunted and deformed.

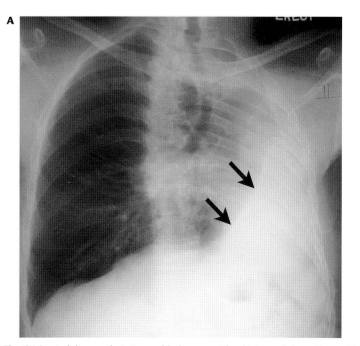

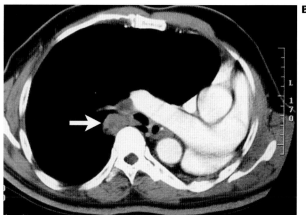

Fig. 16.8 Left lung aplasia in an elderly man with a history of cigarette smoking, despite being told at age 6 that he only had one lung! He now presents with hemoptysis. **A**, Frontal chest radiograph shows left sided volume loss, mediastinal shift, and the characteristic triangular soft tissue opacity (arrows) in the lower lateral hemithorax. **B**, Contrast-enhanced CT shows absence of the left lung and a right hilar mass (arrow). Biopsy confirmed nonsmall cell lung cancer.

Box 16.4 Conditions associated with pulmonary hypoplasia

Pressure effects on developing lung
Pulmonary sequestration
Cystic adenomatoid malformation
Congenital diaphragmatic hernia
Diaphragmatic eventration
Chylothorax
Hydrops fetalis
Ascites or abdominal mass

Conditions associated with reduced or absent fetal respiration
Central nervous system lesions
- Anencephaly
- Arnold–Chiari malformation
Pena–Shokeir syndrome[64]
Phrenic nerve agenesis
Congenital myotonic dystrophy

Restrictive abnormalities of the thoracic cage
Asphyxiating thoracic dystrophy
Achondroplasia
Thanatophoric dwarfism
Ellis–van Creveld syndrome
Osteogenesis imperfecta

Decreased pulmonary vascular perfusion
Bilateral
- Ebstein anomaly
- Hypoplastic right heart syndrome
- Pulmonary stenosis
Unilateral
- Pulmonary artery agenesis
- Scimitar syndrome
Chromosomal abnormalities
- Trisomy 13, 18, and 21

Oligohydramnios
Decreased urine output
- Renal agenesis
- Bladder outlet obstruction
Amniotic fluid leak

PULMONARY HYPOPLASIA (Table 16.1 and Box 16.4)

Pulmonary hypoplasia can be categorized as unilateral or bilateral, and as primary (occurring de novo) or secondary (caused by other fetal developmental anomalies).

Primary unilateral pulmonary hypoplasia

Primary unilateral pulmonary hypoplasia is usually associated with scimitar syndrome or other vascular anomalies (see below).[65] It may be encountered in either a child or an adult. Associated anomalies may be present in other body systems and affect outcome. Affected patients may be asymptomatic or have recurrent episodes of wheezing and pneumonia. The affected lung is small and the mediastinum is displaced into the ipsilateral hemithorax. The pulmonary vasculature is typically deformed and diminutive. The lateral chest film often shows a

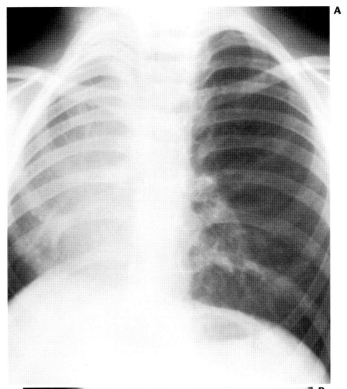

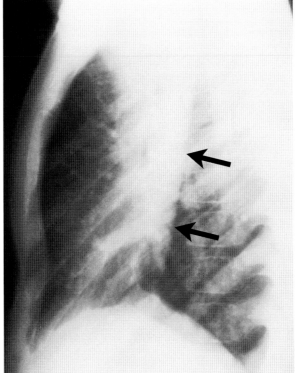

Fig. 16.9 Right pulmonary hypoplasia in an infant. **A**, Frontal and **B**, lateral chest radiographs show right sided volume loss and a characteristic retrosternal soft tissue opacity (arrows).

sharply marginated opacity behind and parallel to the sternum. The appearance is similar to that seen in cases of left upper lobe collapse or combined right upper and middle lobe collapse, but no wedge or fan of tissue extending to the hilum is seen (Figs 16.9 and 16.10). Previously, it was thought that the

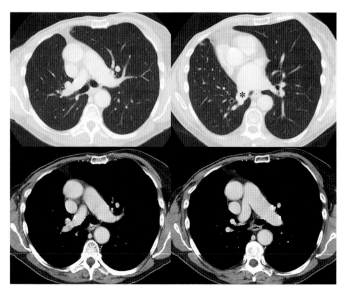

Fig. 16.10 Right pulmonary hypoplasia in an asymptomatic adult. **A**, Frontal chest radiograph shows a small hyperlucent right hemithorax and a diminutive right hilum. **B**, CT shows marked mediastinal shift, a small right lung and pulmonary artery, and normal pulmonary venous drainage (*) into the left atrium.

retrosternal opacity represented extrapleural areolar tissue filling the space that should have been occupied by lung. CT has shown that the density is produced by displacement of heart and mediastinum into the ipsilateral thorax.[66] Cardiac contours may be indistinct on the frontal examination because of rotation of the heart and mediastinum.

Primary bilateral pulmonary hypoplasia

Primary bilateral pulmonary hypoplasia is quite rare and invariably manifests early in the neonatal period. Radiographs reveal small but otherwise aerated lungs with a bell shaped thorax due to marked difference in the size of the thorax and abdomen.[67] Pneumothoraces are frequently present.

Secondary pulmonary hypoplasia

Overall, pulmonary hypoplasia caused by various fetal developmental abnormalities (secondary pulmonary hypoplasia, see Box 16.4) is more common than primary pulmonary hypoplasia. Pulmonary hypoplasia is found in approximately 10% of neonatal autopsies and in 50% of those with congenital anomalies. The mechanisms that cause pulmonary hypoplasia have not been firmly established. The fetal lung communicates freely with the amniotic sac and the fetus is known to exhibit breathing movements in utero. Thus, entry of amniotic fluid into the lungs probably occurs during fetal life. The fetal lung itself produces fluid as evidenced by accumulation of fluid beyond a bronchial obstruction. The presence of lung fluid and respiratory movement appears to play a vital role in normal lung development. Decreased or absent respiratory movement

in utero caused by central nervous system anomalies is associated with pulmonary hypoplasia.[68] Decreased vascular perfusion of the fetal lung in cases of Ebstein anomaly, hypoplastic right heart syndrome, or pulmonary stenosis may impair fetal lung fluid production and be associated with hypoplasia. The most striking example of the influence of fluid on pulmonary development is found in Potter syndrome (oligohydramnios tetrad).[69] Oligohydramnios in these infants is the result of an abnormality in the development of the urinary tract, most commonly renal agenesis (Fig. 16.11). The full tetrad comprises: (1) the underlying renal abnormality that causes oligohydramnios; (2) abnormal facies resulting from pressure effects in utero; (3) abnormal laxity of the skin; and (4) pulmonary hypoplasia.[70] There is debate as to whether pulmonary hypoplasia results from a reduction in the amount of amniotic fluid actually within the developing lung or whether it is secondary to external pressure effects on the developing thorax. Clearly both factors could be operative.

Pulmonary hypoplasia can also occur secondary to in utero conditions that stunt lung growth by virtue of a mass effect. Pulmonary hypoplasia complicating congenital diaphragmatic hernia is a classic example (Fig. 16.12). The ipsilateral lung shows varying degrees of hypoplasia depending on the size of the hernia and the period during which pressure effects on the lung were operative. The contralateral lung may also have a variable degree of hypoplasia depending upon the amount of mediastinal shift. The fundamental problem in such cases is lack of space for growth and development of the lung. The extent of pulmonary hypoplasia is a critical determinant of survival following surgical repair of diaphragmatic hernia or removal of intrathoracic mass lesions.[71] Chest radiographs can be helpful for assessing the degree of hypoplasia and for predicting prognosis in affected infants.[71,72] The radiographic

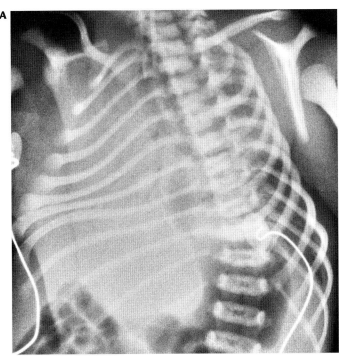

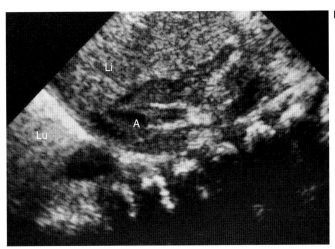

Fig. 16.11   Potter syndrome in a neonate. **A**, Frontal chest radiograph shows largely airless lungs and pressure deformities of the ribs. **B**, Longitudinal ultrasound shows liver (Li), adrenal gland (A), echogenic lung (Lu), and renal agenesis.

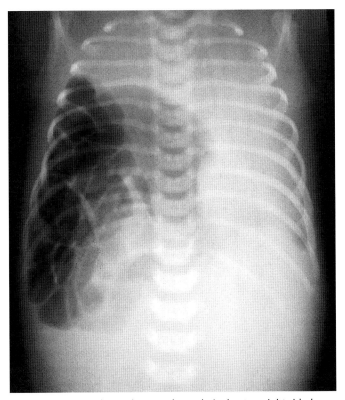

Fig. 16.12   Secondary pulmonary hypoplasia due to a right sided congenital diaphragmatic hernia. Chest radiograph obtained shortly after birth shows air-filled loops of bowel in the right hemithorax with mass effect upon the lung and mediastinum. Both lungs are airless. The patient did not survive despite surgical repair because of severe pulmonary hypoplasia and persistent fetal circulation.

manifestations of secondary pulmonary hypoplasia are the same as those of primary hypoplasia, with the exception that the cause (e.g. congenital diaphragmatic hernia or cystic adenomatoid malformation) may also be identifiable. Rib crowding and deformity may give an indication of intrauterine pressure effects as in cases of Potter syndrome. Respiratory distress is common and the patients are often intubated. Pneumothoraces often complicate the clinical course.

SCIMITAR SYNDROME (Table 16.1 and Box 16.5)

Scimitar syndrome is sometimes termed the "hypogenetic lung syndrome" or the "venolobar syndrome" to emphasize that this anomaly is not simply a variant of pulmonary venous return but is a rather more extensive malformation. Felson[58] coined the term venolobar syndrome and Woodring et al[63] extended the

---

Box 16.5 Scimitar syndrome (also known as venolobar syndrome or hypogenetic lung syndrome)

Associations
Congenital heart disease in 25%
Usually atrial septal defects

Symptoms
Usually asymptomatic
Dyspnea if large left to right shunt

Radiologic findings
Small right lung (pulmonary hypoplasia)
Diminuitive right hilum
Hyparterial right bronchus
Dextroposition of heart
Characteristic "scimitar" veins draining below diaphragm

use of this term to encompass a range of anomalies, including pulmonary hypoplasia and sequestration. However, pulmonary hypoplasia and lobar aplasia can occur in the absence of anomalously draining veins. Therefore, the term "scimitar syndrome" may be the most unambiguous designation of this form of pulmonary dysmorphism, recognizing that cases that deviate from the classical description of the condition do rarely occur.[63,73]

Scimitar syndrome is essentially an anomaly of the right lung. Only very rare cases have been described on the left.[74] The affected lung is hypoplastic, with underdevelopment of both the central airways and vasculature.[75,76] One or more lobes may be absent. The airway on the involved side is stunted and the arterial supply to the right lung may derive in much greater proportion than normal from systemic arteries. The pulmonary artery is correspondingly small and may lie beneath the right bronchus. The syndrome derives its name from the anomalous pulmonary vein that descends vertically in the lung before curving medially to enter the inferior vena cava above or below the diaphragm. The vein broadens as it curves downward and medially, resulting in a configuration resembling a Turkish sword – the scimitar (Figs 16.13 and 16.14). On occasion, two or

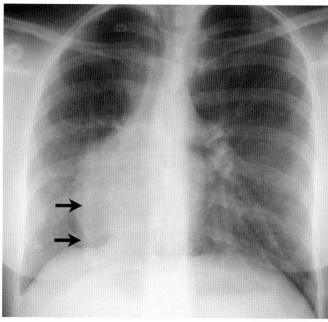

Fig. 16.13 Scimitar syndrome in a young woman with dyspnea. Chest radiograph shows a small right lung, dextroposition of the heart, a diminutive right hilum, and a characteristic scimitar vein (arrows) draining into the inferior vena cava.

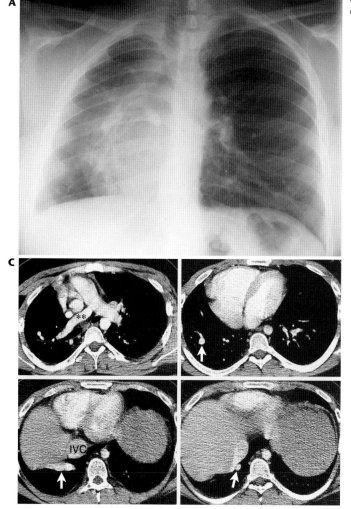

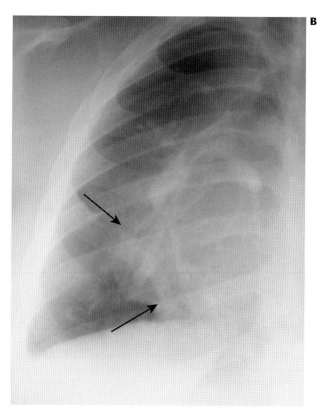

Fig. 16.14 Scimitar syndrome in a young woman with dyspnea. **A**, Chest radiograph and **B**, coned-down view shows a small right lung, dextroposition of the heart, a diminutive right hilum, and characteristic scimitar veins (arrows). **C**, Contrast-enhanced CT shows a small right pulmonary artery (**) and multiple lower lobe pulmonary veins (arrows) that drain into the inferior vena cava (IVC).

more anomalous veins are present. The anomalous vein may drain all or part of the involved lung and empties into the inferior vena cava, the right atrium, coronary sinus, or, rarely, the hepatic veins.

Approximately 25% of patients have associated congenital heart disease, most commonly septal defects.[77] Such cases are more likely to present in infancy or childhood and the outcome depends on the type and severity of the cardiac abnormality.[78] The scimitar syndrome, when isolated, is compatible with a normal life because the consequent left-to-right shunt is typically small.[79] Occasionally, the shunt is large enough to warrant surgical repair.[80] Patients occasionally have symptoms from associated bronchiectasis and tracheal diverticula. Other associated anomalies include eventration or Bochdalek hernia involving the right hemidiaphragm, accessory right hemidiaphragm, and horseshoe lung (see below).

The anomalously draining vein is usually readily visible on chest radiographs in both frontal and lateral projections (Figs 16.13 and 16.14). Associated features include reduced lung volume, shift of trachea and mediastinum to the right, consequent dextroposition of the heart, a diminutive ipsilateral pulmonary artery, and an abnormal bronchovascular pattern in the right hilum. When all of these findings are present, the diagnosis of scimitar syndrome can be made with confidence (Figs 16.13 and 16.14). Partial anomalous pulmonary venous return to the inferior vena cava, right atrium, or coronary sinus may occur without pulmonary hypoplasia, particularly in association with intracardiac lesions such as an atrial septal defect or complex cyanotic lesions. The key distinguishing feature in these cases is the absence of radiographic evidence of pulmonary hypoplasia.

Contrast-enhanced CT provides a noninvasive method for confirming the diagnosis of the scimitar syndrome and identifying the termination of the anomalous veins (Fig. 16.14).[77,81–84] It has the additional advantage that the tracheobronchial anomalies are better delineated and tracheal diverticula and bronchiectasis are readily detected. MRI has been used both to diagnose scimitar syndrome[85–88] and to estimate the degree of left-to-right shunting by means of velocity-encoded cine MRI.[89] CT may also demonstrate the presence of horseshoe lung, a rare associated abnormality.[79] Horseshoe lung is an uncommon malformation where right and left lungs are fused inferiorly by an isthmus of lung tissue crossing the posterior mediastinum.[90–95] Horseshoe lung occurring in the absence of scimitar syndrome is often associated with other lethal malformations. Scimitar syndrome can sometimes be confused radiographically with unilateral agenesis of the pulmonary artery (see below) when systemic collateral vessels simulate scimitar veins.[73] Furthermore, an abnormal "meandering" vein draining a hypoplastic right lung to the left atrium can resemble a scimitar vein.[63]

UNILATERAL ABSENCE OF THE PULMONARY ARTERY

Unilateral absence of the pulmonary artery (UAPA) is a rare anomaly characterized by short segment atresia of the proximal left or right pulmonary artery.[96–102] More distal segments of the arteries in the hila are usually present. The condition is associated with other congenital anomalies, particularly cardiac defects such as tetralogy of Fallot, septal defects, and

pulmonary stenosis.[98] Isolated UAPA also occurs. The atretic segment usually, but not always, occurs on the side opposite the aortic arch.

The majority of patients with isolated UAPA are symptomatic at presentation. In a review of 108 patients with isolated UAPA, Ten Harkel et al[98] found that 87% presented with symptoms that included frequent pulmonary infection (37%), dyspnea or limited exercise tolerance (40%), or hemoptysis (20%). Pulmonary hypertension was present in 44% of the patients. Only 13% were asymptomatic. Hemoptysis is due to systemic collateralization of the lungs.[98,101,102] The etiology of pulmonary hypertension in these individuals is unknown.

Chest radiographs show a reduction in lung volume in the affected hemothorax. The pulmonary hilum is typically diminutive or absent and peripheral perfusion is typically reduced (Figs 16.15 and 16.16). On occasion, increased reticular opacities are noted in the affected lung due to systemic-to-pulmonary collaterals. The vasculature in the normal lung may appear correspondingly plethoric because the entire cardiac output is shunted through that lung. Radioisotope $\dot{V}/Q$ scanning readily demonstrates the total absence of perfusion and the normal ventilation of the lung. CT or MRI clearly show the absence of a pulmonary artery and may also demonstrate evidence of systemic-to-pulmonary arterial collateral vessels.[103,104] CT or MRI should obviate the need for angiography (Fig. 16.16). Acquired conditions, such as Swyer–James syndrome or fibrosing mediastinitis, may, however, closely mimic the findings of UAPA in adults.[105,106] Swyer–James syndrome (see p. 746) should have demonstrably abnormal ventilation of the affected lung, while lung ventilation is normal in cases of UAPA. Fibrosing mediastinitis may sometimes be difficult to distinguish radiologically from UAPA. The presence of calcified

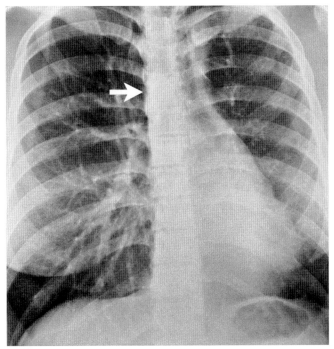

Fig. 16.15 Unilateral absence of the left pulmonary artery in an asymptomatic man. Chest radiograph shows a small left hemithorax, a diminutive left hilum, and a right sided aortic arch (arrow).

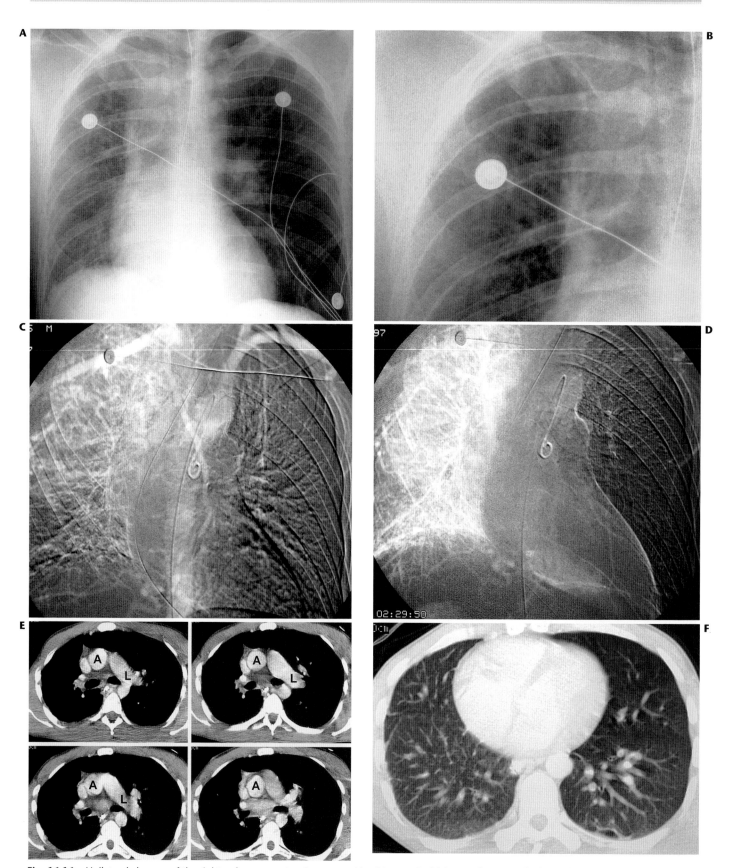

Fig. 16.16 Unilateral absence of the right pulmonary artery in a man with a history of a high speed motor vehicle accident. **A**, Frontal chest radiograph and **B**, coned-down views show a small right hemithorax, a diminutive right hilum, diffuse reticular opacities in the right lung, and unilateral rib notching. **C**, Aortography performed to exclude great vessel injury shows enlarged and tortuous intercostal arteries in the right hemithorax. **D**, A delayed image shows a diffuse vascular blush in the right lung consistent with systemic arterial supply. **E**, CT (mediastinal window) confirms absence of the proximal right pulmonary artery. L = left pulmonary artery; A = ascending aorta. **F**, CT (lung window) also shows thickened interlobular septa due to transpleural collateral vessels.

lymph nodes in the vicinity of the occluded vessel or an associated mediastinal mass suggests fibrosing mediastinitis.[107]

PULMONARY ARTERIOVENOUS MALFORMATIONS (Box 16.6)

Pulmonary arteriovenous malformations (PAVMs) result from abnormal communication between the pulmonary arteries and veins. PAVMs are twice as common in women as in men and the vast majority of lesions are congenital in origin. According to Gossage et al,[108] between 53 and 70% of PAVMs occur in the lower lobes of lung. In a pathologic review of 350 autopsies, Bosher et al[109] found that 75% of affected individuals had unilateral PAVMs, 36% had multiple lesions, and 50% of those with multiple lesions had bilateral PAVMs. Nearly 70% of cases are associated with hereditary hemorrhagic telangiectasia (HHT or Rendu–Osler–Weber disease), and, especially in this disease, the lesions are likely to be multiple.[108] HHT is an autosomal dominant condition characterized by multiple AVMs in the lung, skin, liver and brain.[110,111] Between 15 and 35% of patients with HHT have PAVMs.[108] PAVMs may also be associated with other congenital abnormalities, notably cardiac malformations.

Infants and children with PAVMs may be asymptomatic. However, if the lesions are large enough to cause a significant right-to-left shunt, the patient may present with cyanosis or heart failure (Fig. 16.17). In such cases, a distinct bruit may be heard over the affected hemithorax. Many adult patients with PAVMs are asymptomatic when the lesions are detected on routine chest radiographs. There is evidence, however, that the likelihood of developing symptoms related to PAVMs depends upon the size and number of lesions.[108] Thus, patients with a solitary PAVM >2 cm in diameter or with multiple PAVMs are more likely to have symptoms than those with small, solitary lesions. When present, signs and symptoms include dyspnea, cyanosis, clubbing, hemoptysis, and chest pain. On occasion, the

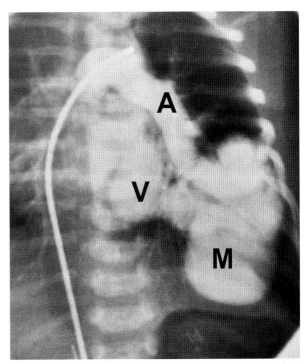

Fig. 16.17 Pulmonary arteriovenous malformation in a cyanotic infant. Angiography shows a large left lower lobe malformation (M). A = feeding artery; V = draining vein.

patient may present with systemic abscesses or infarction, notably of the brain, because right-to-left shunting through the PAVM bypasses the lung (paradoxical embolism, Fig. 16.18).[112–114] One-third of patients in one large series had CT evidence of previous cerebral infarction.[115] On physical examination, patients with HHT and PAVM may have superficial, often perioral, telangiectasias. A bruit is heard over the lesion in up to 46% of patients.[108] Even in asymptomatic adults, right-to-left shunting though the lesion often produces some degree of hypoxia that is often accentuated in the erect position. This finding is known as orthodeoxia, is characterized by detecting a decrease in arterial oxygen saturation when the patient moves from the supine to erect position, and is a typical feature of PAVM. The physiologic explanation for this phenomenon is that the lesions have a predilection for the lower lungs and that shunting is therefore increased in the upright position.[108]

On chest radiographs, arteriovenous malformations manifest as well-circumscribed lung nodules, usually with a lobular contour (Fig. 16.18). The lesions typically range in diameter from 1 to 5 cm.[108] If the lesions are peripheral in location, the feeding arteries and draining veins can usually be seen on the chest radiographs (Figs 16.18 and 16.19) – a diagnostic feature that can be confirmed by CT or MRI. Central lesions are often more difficult to discern among the hilar vessels on chest radiographs (Fig. 16.20), and, even if the lesion itself is detected, the shorter feeding vessels may be difficult or impossible to identify. Multiple lesions can be confused with metastases if the feeding vessels are overlooked.[116] In patients with suspected PAVM, contrast-enhanced echocardiography[108] can be used to confirm the presence of an intrapulmonary right-to-left shunt. Perfusion scintigraphy can also be used to diagnose and, more importantly, quantify the right-to-left shunt.[117–119] Perfusion

---

Box 16.6 Pulmonary arteriovenous malformations: clinical features

Single or multiple lesions: majority associated with hereditary hemorrhagic telangiectasia (HHT) syndrome, an autosomal dominant disorder with incomplete penetrance

Clinical presentation
- Often asymptomatic
- May present with other manifestations of HHT, e.g. epistaxis, gastrointestinal bleeding
- Hypoxia and orthodeoxia with dyspnea and chronic fatigue
- Embolic phenomena: brain abscesses and cerebral ischemia
- Clubbing and polycythemia
- Rarely hemoptysis
- Rarely cyanosis and a chest bruit in infants

Treatment
- Feeding vessel <3 mm: not generally treated
- Feeding vessel >3 mm: occlusion of feeding vessels with detachable balloons or coils. Surgery reserved for very large lesions.

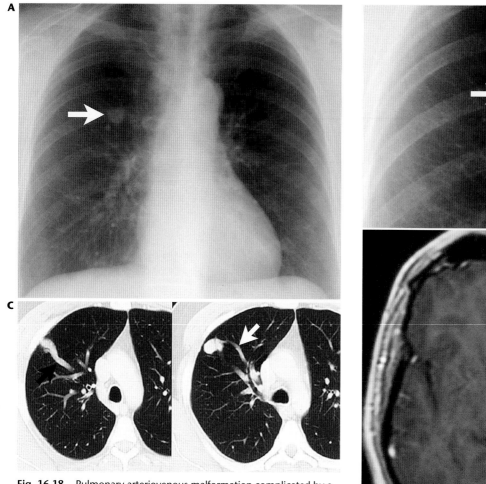

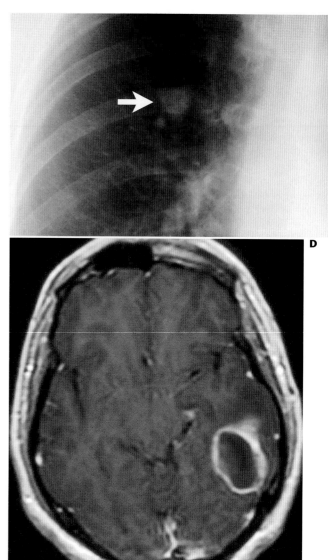

Fig. 16.18 Pulmonary arteriovenous malformation complicated by a brain abscess in a previously healthy man. **A**, Frontal chest radiograph and **B**, coned-down view show a well-circumscribed nodule in the right upper lobe (arrows). Note the associated vessels. **C**, CT (lung window) shows the feeding artery (white arrow) and draining vein (black arrow) to greater advantage. **D**, Gadolinium-enhanced MRI shows a ring-enhancing lesion in the right cerebral hemisphere consistent with an abscess.

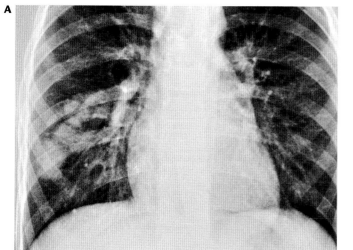

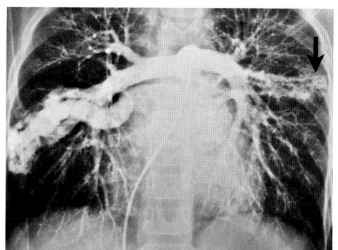

Fig. 16.19 Pulmonary arteriovenous malformations in a patient with hereditary hemorrhagic telangiectasia. **A**, Frontal chest radiograph shows a large arteriovenous malformation in the right lung. No other lesions were seen. **B**, Pulmonary arteriography revealed a second malformation in the left lung (arrow).

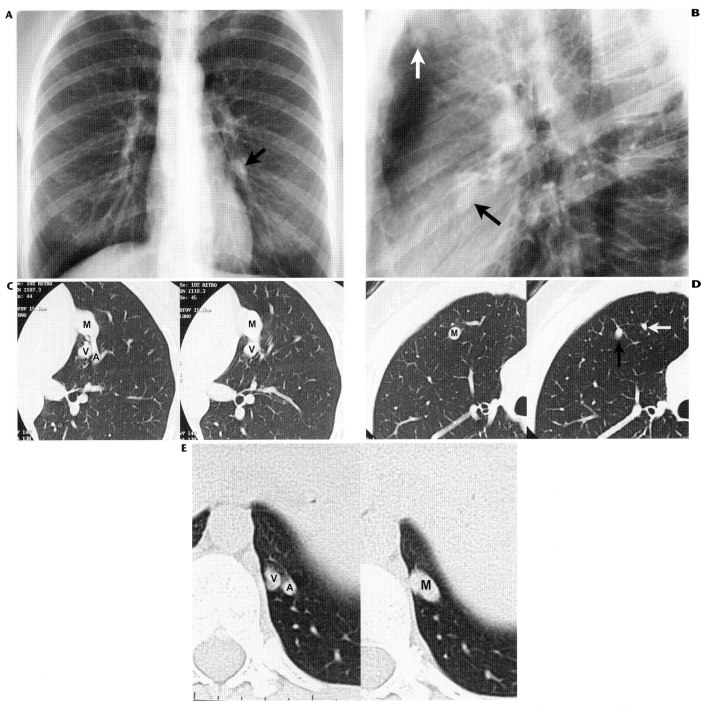

Fig. 16.20 Pulmonary arteriovenous malformations in a patient with hereditary hemorrhagic telangiectasia and dyspnea. **A**, Frontal chest radiograph shows an ovoid nodule (arrow) superimposed upon the left hilum. Associated vessels are not clearly seen. **B**, Lateral radiograph confirms the lingular malformation (black arrow) and shows a second lesion (white arrow) in the retrosternal region. **C–E**, Shows the typical angioarchitecture of the malformations (M) and reveals a third lesion in the left lower lobe (**E**).

scintigraphy cannot, however, distinguish intracardiac from intrapulmonary shunting and thus is used infrequently for diagnosis of PAVM.

Although pulmonary angiography has been considered the "gold standard" for diagnosis of PAVMs (Figs 16.19 and 16.20),[108] CT has recently assumed the dominant role in this regard.[120–125] Contrast-enhanced CT is quite useful for confirming the diagnosis by demonstrating the feeding vessels and

intense contrast enhancement within the lesions (Fig. 16.18). CT is also useful for identifying additional lesions in the lungs (Fig. 16.20). Interestingly, Remy et al[122] found that CT was more sensitive than pulmonary angiography for detecting PAVMs. In their series, CT detected 98% of PAVMs as opposed to 60% detected by pulmonary angiography.

Increasingly, pulmonary arteriovenous malformations are treated by embolotherapy with coils[126–128] or detachable balloons

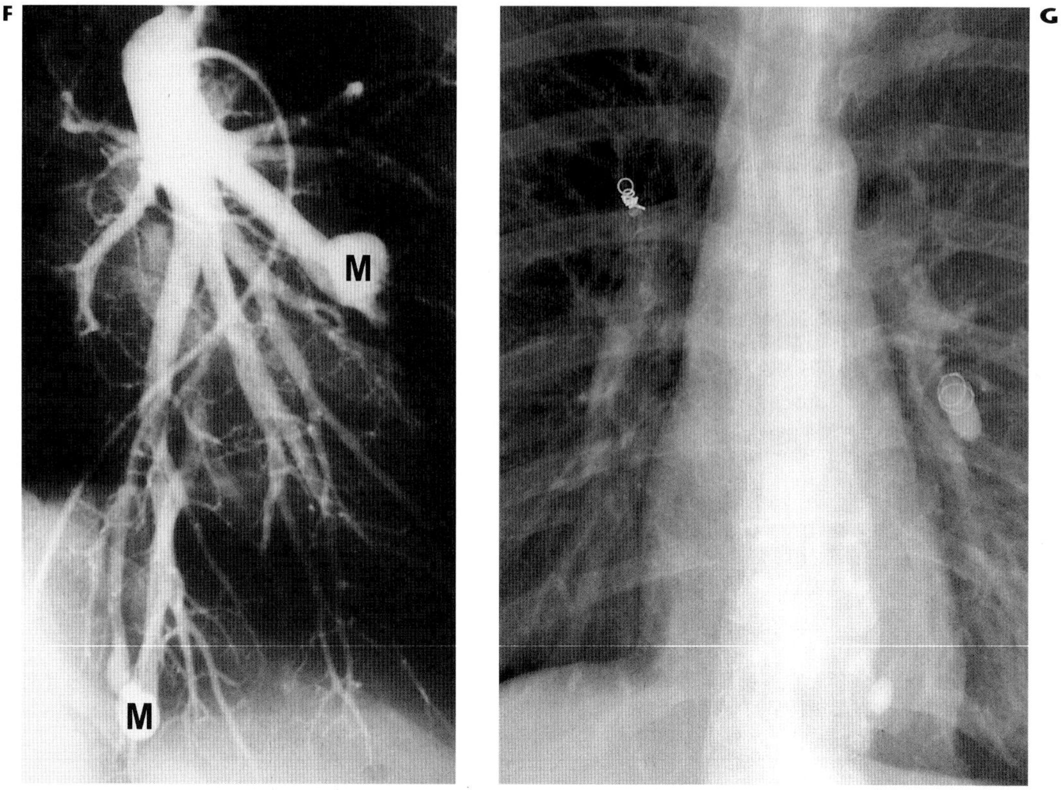

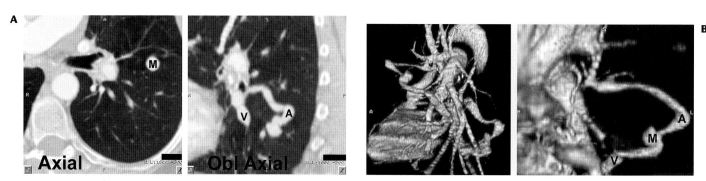

Fig. 16.20 (*cont'd*)   **F**, Angiography confirms that these are simple malformations (one feeding vessel). **G**, Frontal radiograph obtained after embolotherapy shows the coils and detachable balloons used to occlude the lesions. A or white arrow = feeding artery; V or black arrow = draining vein.

Fig. 16.21   Pulmonary arteriovenous malformation. **A**, Axial and oblique axial CT (lung window) shows a malformation in the left lower lobe. **B**, Shaded surface display images clearly delineate the angioarchitecture of the lesion prior to embolotherapy. M = malformation; A = feeding artery; V = draining vein.

(Fig. 16.20).[115,129] The purpose of such intervention is to reduce the risk of systemic embolization and to improve arterial oxygenation by decreasing right-to-left shunting.[130] Treatment of simple PAVMs (single feeding vessel, 80% of lesions)[131] is considered more straightforward than treatment of complex (multiple feeding vessels, 20%) lesions.[108] Furthermore, embolotherapy is usually restricted to malformations with feeding vessels 3 mm or greater in diameter.[115] Thus, information regarding size and number of feeding vessels is considered critical for planning embolotherapy of PAVMs. In past years, pulmonary angiography was performed for this purpose (Fig.

16.20). However, studies have shown that thin-section contrast-enhanced spiral CT with 2D and 3D reconstruction techniques can be quite useful for delineating the often complex angioarchitecture of even small PAVMs (Fig. 16.21).[124,125] Thus, angiography is now performed primarily for the treatment, not diagnosis, of PAVMs.

Large PAVMs can be detected by MRI.[117,132–135] However, MRI remains inferior to CT in terms of spatial resolution, and thus small lesions or feeding vessels may be overlooked. MRI thus does not appear to have a major role in the diagnosis or evaluation of PAVM.

CONGENITAL DISORDERS OF LYMPHATIC DEVELOPMENT (Box 16.7)

Faul et al[136] have proposed the following classification for congenital disorders of lymphatic development: thoracic lymphangioma, lymphangiectasis, lymphangiomatosis, and lymphatic dysplasia syndrome.

Lymphangiomas, or cystic hygromas, are focal masslike proliferations of lymphatic tissue[136] that are classified histopathologically as capillary, cavernous, or cystic. The cystic spaces are typically filled with proteinaceous fluid. They usually present in early infancy, but adult cases are reported.[137] Most occur in the neck and axilla (Fig. 16.22), but 10% extend into the mediastinum and 1% occur only in the mediastinum.[138] On chest radiographs, lymphangiomas manifest as unilateral soft tissue masses in the neck that may demonstrate extension into the mediastinum. Most mediastinal lymphangiomas in adults are found in the anterior or superior mediastinum (Fig. 16.23).[139] Lymphangiomas manifest on ultrasound as uni- or multi-locular cystic masses with walls of variable thickness.[140] They manifest on CT as smoothly marginated multicystic masses (Fig. 16.23)[139,141]; the cyst walls variably enhance follow-

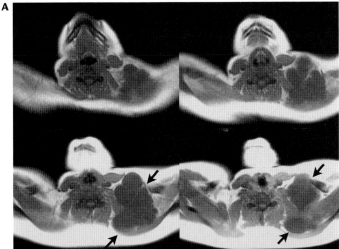

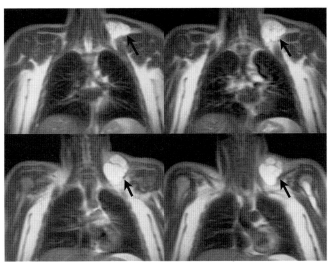

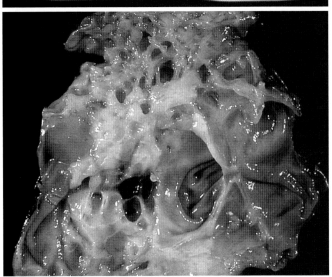

Fig. 16.22 Cervical lymphangioma in a 15-year-old girl. **A**, Axial T1-weighted MRI shows a lobular mass (arrows) in the left supraclavicular fossa with internal septations. The cysts are of low signal intensity. **B**, Coronal T2-weighted MRI shows high signal within the cysts. The mass (arrows) does not extend into the thorax. **C**, Resected specimen. (Courtesy of JR Galvin, Armed Forces Institute of Pathology, Washington, DC)

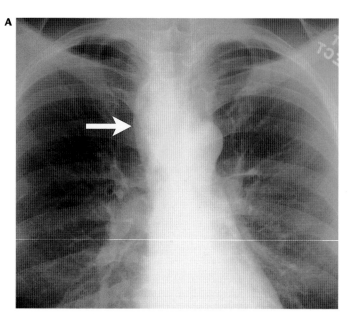

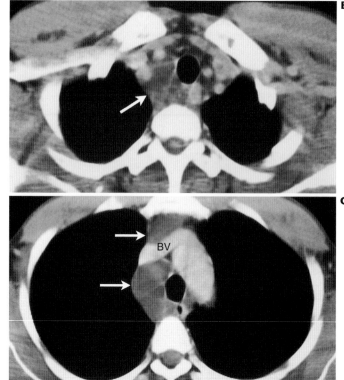

Fig. 16.23 Mediastinal lymphangioma in a middle-aged man. **A,** Frontal chest radiograph shows a right paratracheal soft tissue mass (arrow). Note mass effect on the trachea. **B,** CT (mediastinal window) at the thoracic inlet shows a septated water attenuation mass (arrow). **C,** CT (mediastinal window) at the level of the aortic arch shows that the mass (arrows) extends anterior and posterior to the superior vena cava and brachiocephalic vein (BV). (Courtesy of EF Patz Jr, Durham, NC)

ing administration of intravenous contrast material.[140] In one study, the CT attenuation of the cyst fluid ranged from –4 to 34 HU, likely due to variability in lipid content and intracystic hemorrhage.[140] Unusual CT features include calcification, spiculated margins, and homogeneous soft tissue attenuation.[139] On T1-weighted MRI, the cysts are usually isointense to skeletal muscle. On T2-weighted MRI, they are typically hyperintense to fat (Fig. 16.22).[140] MRI more clearly delineates the extent of the lesion than ultrasound or CT.[139–142]

Generalized dilation of otherwise histopathologically normal lymphatics is known as *lymphangiectasis*.[136] The condition may occur primarily, or be secondary to severe pulmonary venous obstruction in cases of total anomalous pulmonary venous return or hypoplastic left heart syndrome.[143] Primary generalized lymphangiectasis is an extremely rare, lethal abnormality. At least half of affected individuals are stillborn and the remainder die shortly after birth. Lymphangiectasis can be confined to the lung[144,145] and, in such cases, symptoms may be delayed in onset or absent.[146] Pulmonary lymphangiectasis is associated with several genetic diseases, including Noonan, Turner, Ehlers–Danlos and Down syndrome.[136] Chest radiographs in patients with pulmonary lymphangiectasis show diffuse reticulonodular opacities with thickened interlobular septa; the linear opacities may diminish over time if the patient survives (Fig. 16.24).[146,147] Thin-section CT shows thickened interlobular septa and ground-glass opacities (Fig. 16.25); pleural effusions are also common.[148] Echocardiography is useful for excluding a cardiac etiology.

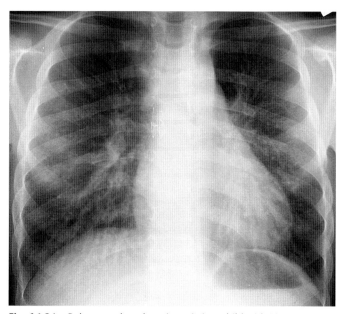

Fig. 16.24 Pulmonary lymphangiectasia in a child with Noonan syndrome. Frontal chest radiograph shows findings of prior median sternotomy and heterogeneous lower lobe opacities due to thickened bronchovascular bundles.

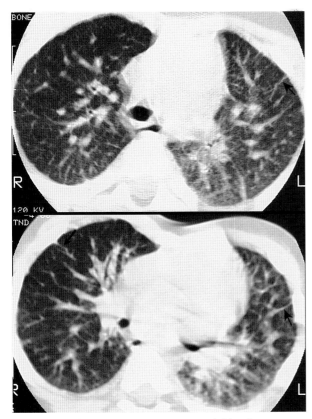

Fig. 16.25 Pulmonary lymphangiectasia in a child with Noonan syndrome. CT (lung window) shows markedly thickened interlobular septa (arrows).

The presence of multiple, often infiltrating lymphangiomas is termed *lymphangiomatosis* (Fig. 16.26). Lymphangiomatosis is often confused with lymphangiectasia, but the conditions are distinct histopathologically.[149] The condition is rare and often fatal.[136] It most often affects lungs and bones, but virtually any organ system can be involved.[150–153] Cystic bone lesions and chylothorax suggest the diagnosis and portend a poor outcome.[136,154] In a review of five patients, Wunderbaldinger et al[154] found that the most common features of generalized lymphangiomatosis were widespread cystic lesions in visceral organs, lytic bone lesions, interstitial lung disease, and diffuse mesenteric thickening on CT or MRI. In a review of eight patients with pulmonary lymphangiomatosis, Swensen et al[155] found that the disease most commonly manifested on thin-section CT scans with smooth thickening of interlobular septa, thickening of bronchovascular bundles, and scattered ground-glass opacities. Diffuse increase in mediastinal fat attenuation was a suggestive finding, seen in all eight patients. Seven of eight also had either bilateral pleural effusions or pleural thickening. The CT appearance of pulmonary lymphangiomatosis is virtually identical to that of pulmonary lymphangiectasia.[148]

The term *lymphatic dysplasia syndrome* has been proposed to encompass the primary lymphedema syndromes, congenital chylothorax, and the yellow nail syndrome.[136] This is a diverse group of disorders with variable prognosis. The yellow nail syndrome typically presents in adulthood; the median age at presentation is between 40 and 50 years.[136] It is characterized by the triad of yellow nails (89%), lymphedema (80%), and pleural effusions (36%) (Fig. 16.27).[156,157] The complete triad is seen in just 20% of patients, however.[156,157] Thus, the presence of two of the three major findings is considered sufficient for diagnosis.[157–160] The respiratory tract is affected in 63% of cases; manifestations include cough, shortness of breath, sinusitis, and bronchiectasis. Wiggins et al[161] evaluated four patients with thin-section CT and found bronchiectasis and bronchial wall

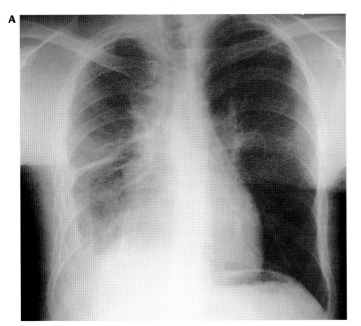

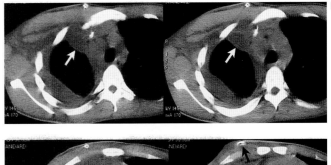

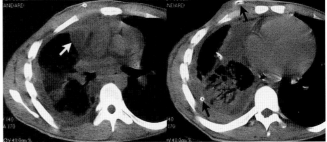

Fig. 16.26 Lymphangiomatosis in a young man. **A**, Frontal chest radiograph shows a possible right sided mediastinal mass, loculated pleural fluid in the right hemithorax, and heterogeneous opacities in the right lung. **B** and **C**, Sequential CT images (mediastinal window) show infiltrating lymphangiomas in the mediastinum (white arrows), right pleural space, and axilla. Note the indwelling pleural catheter (black arrows). (Courtesy of EM Marom, Houston, TX)

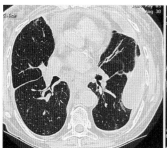 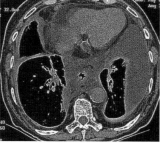

Fig. 16.27 Yellow nail syndrome in a middle-aged man with a history of recurrent pneumonia and pleural effusions. CT shows bilateral loculated pleural effusions and minimal cylindrical bronchiectasis.

thickening in all. Recurrent pericardial effusions and chylous ascites are less common manifestations.[162,163] Chemical pleurodesis has been used to effectively treat symptomatic pleural effusions in affected patients.[164] Cystic lower lobe lesions, not thought to represent bronchiectasis, have also been reported on CT.[165]

BRONCHOGENIC CYSTS (Box 16.8)

Bronchogenic cysts are uncommon, usually isolated, lesions that result from abnormal budding of the ventral foregut between the 26th and 40th days of gestation.[166] This abnormal bud subsequently differentiates into a fluid-filled, blind ending pouch. Bronchogenic cysts typically have a fibrous capsule, contain cartilage, are lined with respiratory epithelium (Fig. 16.28), and contain mucous material that may be remarkably viscid. Most cysts are found in the mediastinum or hila – near the tracheal carina (Fig. 16.29). In the four largest series reported, between 65 and 86% of cysts arose in the mediastinum.[166–169] Less commonly, cysts may occur within the lung parenchyma (Fig. 16.30), pleura, or diaphragm.[166] Paren-

Box 16.8 Bronchogenic cysts

Pathology
Single cyst lined by respiratory epithelium
Contains mucoid material
Associated anomalies (rare)
Location – 85% hilar or mediastinal

Clinical features
May be asymptomatic
Otherwise chest pain, cough, dyspnea, and fever if cyst is infected
Rarely compressive effects, e.g. atelectasis, postobstructive pneumonia
Treatment – usually surgical excision

Chest radiographs
Well-circumscribed hilar or middle mediastinal mass
Air–fluid level if cyst is communicating or infected
Less commonly, a well-circumscribed lung mass – solid or containing an air–fluid level

Chest CT
Well-circumscribed mass usually adjacent to trachea or major bronchi
Molded to adjacent structures without significant compressive effects
Variable CT density of cyst contents – +10 to +120 HU or even higher
About half of water, half of soft tissue attenuation
Cyst wall thin and smooth
Cyst may contain milk of calcium or wall calcification
Gas content indicates communication or infection

MRI
Well-circumscribed mass
Variable signal intensity depending upon cyst content

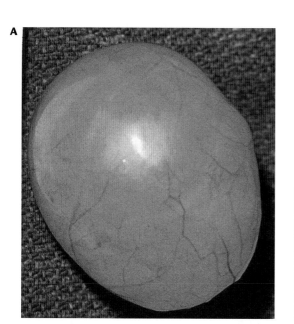 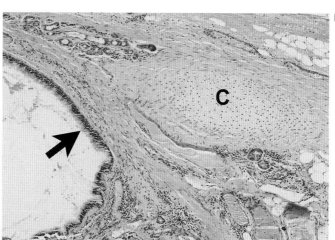

Fig. 16.28 Bronchogenic cyst. **A**, Specimen shows the glistening surface of a water-filled bronchogenic cyst. **B**, Photomicrograph (hematoxylin and eosin stain, ×100) shows the typical features of a bronchogenic cyst, including respiratory epithelium (arrow) and cartilage plates (C). (With permission from McAdams HP, Kirejczyk WM, Rosado-de-Christenson ML, Matsumoto S. Bronchogenic cyst: imaging features with clinical and histopathologic correlation. Radiology 2000;217:441-446.)

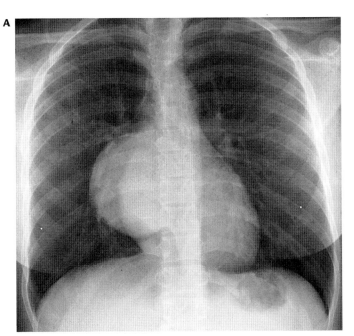
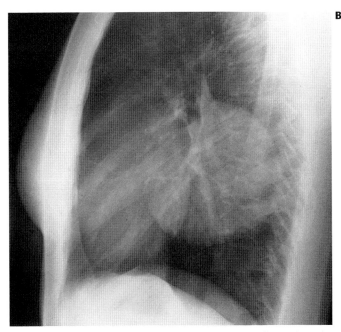

Fig. 16.29   Bronchogenic cyst in a young woman with cough. **A**, Frontal and **B**, lateral chest radiographs show a large, smooth, well-marginated mass in the middle mediastinum – the most common location for a bronchogenic cyst.

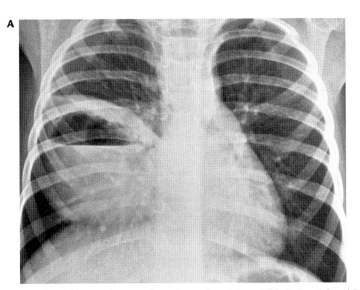
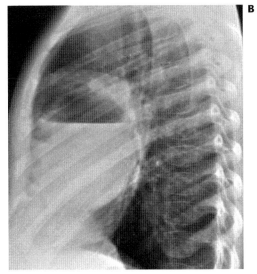

Fig. 16.30   Infected intrapulmonary bronchogenic cyst in a child. **A**, Frontal and **B**, lateral chest radiographs show a large right sided intrapulmonary mass with an air–fluid level. The cyst wall is thickened by inflammation.

chymal cysts are usually perihilar in location (66%). In rare instances, bronchogenic cysts develop in ectopic locations, such as the cervical, infradiaphragmatic, pericardial, and paravertebral regions.[170] Bronchogenic cysts are sometimes found in association with other congenital pulmonary malformations such as sequestration and lobar overinflation.[166] Some pulmonary bronchogenic cysts have a systemic arterial supply and therefore may represent a form of pulmonary sequestration.[171,172] Surgeons must consider the possibility of systemic arterial supply in cases requiring resection.[173]

Most patients with bronchogenic cyst present in the first few decades of life.[166,174] Presentation beyond 50 years of age is distinctly unusual.[175] The clinical features of bronchogenic cyst are variable. Infants may present with respiratory distress due to compression of the central airways.[174,176] In such cases, the chest radiograph may show hyperexpansion of an entire lung as

a result of a ball valve mechanism or collapse of a lobe or entire lung.[177] A mediastinal mass may be visible but may be masked by the thymus. Feeding difficulties caused by pressure effects on the esophagus or edema caused by impaired venous return are less common manifestations.[178,179] Some older children and adults with bronchogenic cyst are asymptomatic at presentation; such lesions are detected on routine chest radiographs.[180] However, most older children and adults are symptomatic at presentation.[166,168,174] St-Georges et al[168] found that 70% of 86 patients had symptoms of chest pain (55%), cough (50%), dyspnea (40%), fever (30%), and purulent sputum (20%). Ribet et al[174] found that 80% of adult patients with bronchogenic cyst had a similar pattern of symptoms. Occasionally, patients complain of dysphagia due to esophageal compression, and there are a few reports of pulmonary artery obstruction by the cyst.[181–183] Rarely, a bronchogenic cyst may undergo a rapid increase in size due to hemorrhage, infection, or distension with air. In such cases, the compressive effects of the enlarging cyst may cause a surgical emergency.[176,177] There is a report of a peripheral bronchogenic cyst presenting with a spontaneous pneumothorax.[184]

On chest radiographs, bronchogenic cysts manifest as well-defined, solitary mediastinal or hilar masses (Fig. 16.29); approximately 10% have a lobular contour.[167] They are usually found in close proximity to the major airways, and therefore one of the surfaces of the cyst usually contacts the trachea or central bronchi. Most cysts occur in the middle mediastinum immediately adjacent to the lower trachea or proximal main bronchi. Anterior and posterior mediastinal cysts are unusual.[185,186] As the cysts enlarge, they displace adjacent lung and esophagus, but the central airways, except in very young children, are usually displaced little, if at all. Calcification, either along the rim or "milk of calcium" within the cyst, is unusual.[167,187,188] The cysts are usually stable in size except when complicated by infection or hemorrhage.[189] When infected, the cyst may become air filled (Fig. 16.30).[167,187] If the cyst contains air or an air–fluid level, the smooth thin wall and the central location of the cavity should indicate its nature and permit distinction from media-

stinal abscess. Barium swallow examination is not usually performed for evaluation of mediastinal masses. If performed, however, perhaps for symptoms of dysphagia, barium swallow shows smooth extrinsic displacement of the esophagus by the cyst in at least half of cases. Typically, the cyst is seen between the airways and the esophagus on the lateral projection.

CT is now the standard technique for diagnosing bronchogenic cysts (Figs 16.31 to 16.34). CT usually reveals a thin walled cystic mass in the middle mediastinum, molded to the adjacent bronchovascular structures.[166] The molding of the cyst may cause one margin of the cyst to have a pointed configuration.[173] The cyst wall is smooth on both its inner and its outer margins and, in uncomplicated masses, is only a few millimeters thick. Most bronchogenic cysts are of water attenuation (–10 to +10 HU) on CT (Figs 16.30 and 16.31).[166] Although the majority are unilocular, multilocular bronchogenic cysts are rarely reported.[188] The CT diagnosis of bronchogenic cyst can be accepted with confidence if the following criteria are met: a well-defined mass with a smooth or lobular outline, a uniformly thin wall, and contents of uniform CT attenuation within a range of –10 to +10 HU. However, a substantial minority of bronchogenic cysts are of soft tissue attenuation on CT

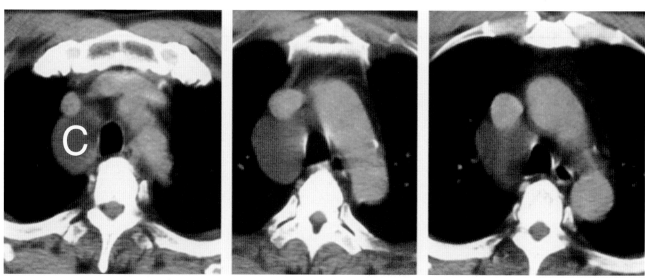

Fig. 16.31 Bronchogenic cyst in a young man. CT shows a well-marginated, homogeneous paratracheal mass (C) of water attenuation.

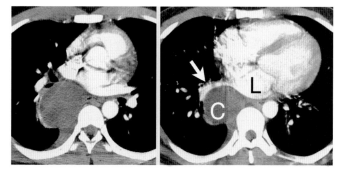

Fig. 16.32 Bronchogenic cyst in a young man. Contrast-enhanced CT shows a well-marginated, homogeneous subcarinal mass (C) of water attenuation. Note mass effect on the left atrium (L) and pulmonary veins (arrow), and a small right pleural effusion.

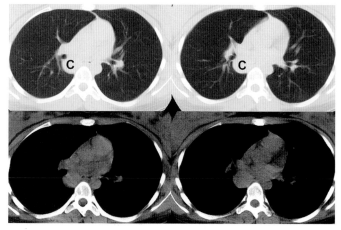

Fig. 16.33 Bronchogenic cyst in a young woman. CT shows a well-marginated homogeneous subcarinal mass (C) of soft tissue attenuation.

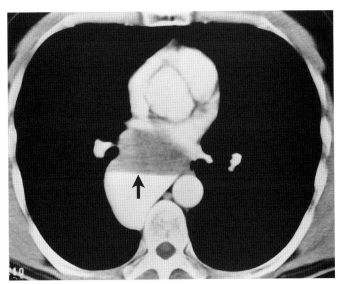

Fig. 16.34 Bronchogenic cyst. CT shows a lobulated well-marginated subcarinal mass with a fluid–fluid level (arrow) due to milk of calcium. (Courtesy of Dr Aksel Ongre, Arendal, Norway)

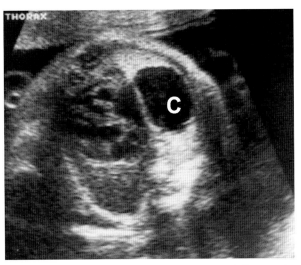

Fig. 16.35 Bronchogenic cyst diagnosed by prenatal ultrasound. Transverse image through the thorax shows a large anechoic mass (C) with distal acoustic enhancement. (With permission from McAdams HP, Kirejczyk WM, Rosado-de-Christenson ML, Matsumoto S. Bronchogenic cyst: imaging features with clinical and histopathologic correlation. Radiology 2000;217:441-446.)

(Fig. 16.33)[166]; cysts with CT numbers as high as 120 HU have been reported. This finding on CT presumably reflects the fact that many cysts contain proteinaceous debris or hemorrhage.[190,191] On rare occasion, a bronchogenic cyst contains milk of calcium, resulting in extremely high CT density (Fig. 16.34).[192]

Ultrasound has been used to diagnose mediastinal bronchogenic cysts in children when there is an appropriate acoustic window (see Boxes 16.6 and 16.7). In two cases described by Ries et al,[193] one lesion was clearly cystic whereas the second was an echogenic solid-appearing mass. Ultrasound can also detect bronchogenic cysts antenatally (Fig. 16.35),[174,194–196] though they appear to be less common than other masses such as pulmonary sequestration or congenital cystic adenomatoid malformation during this period of development.

MRI is often helpful for diagnosis of bronchogenic cyst (Fig. 16.36).[189,197–201] The signal characteristics of bronchogenic cysts generally fall into one of three patterns. First, predominantly water-filled cysts are typically of low signal intensity on T1-weighted images and of high signal intensity on T2-weighted images (Fig. 16.36).[166] Second, cysts that contain proteinaceous debris, blood, or cholesterol may be of high

signal intensity on both T1- and T2-weighted images.[197,200–202] This pattern can also be seen with certain intrathoracic neoplasms that have a relatively high nuclear:cytoplasmic ratio, such as ganglioneuroma, pheochromocytoma, carcinoid tumors, and germ cell tumors as well as in hematomas and lesions with extensive hemorrhage. Third, cysts complicated by hemorrhage or infection may have nonuniform or variable signal intensities.[200] Lyon et al[189] reported one bronchogenic cyst with a fluid–fluid level demonstrable on all pulse sequences, presumably a result of layering of proteinaceous debris.

The diagnosis of bronchogenic cyst is usually established by correlating clinical and characteristic radiologic features. If necessary, the diagnosis can be confirmed nonoperatively by needle aspiration of the cyst contents[203] under either CT guidance[204] or by fiberoptic bronchoscope. The cyst fluid can be examined to exclude malignant cells, and a confirmed diagnosis of bronchogenic cyst may, in appropriate clinical circumstances, obviate the need for operative removal.[205] Many, perhaps most, cysts are surgically removed to either alleviate symptoms or to prevent future problems.

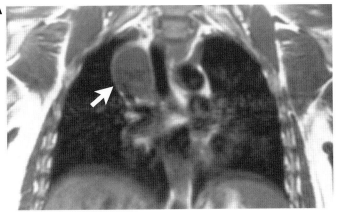

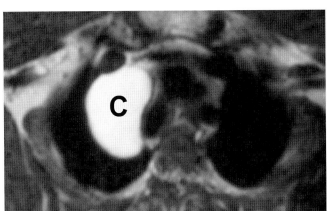

Fig. 16.36 Bronchogenic cyst. **A**, T1-weighted coronal MRI shows a homogeneous well-marginated paratracheal mass (arrow) that is isointense to skeletal muscle. **B**, T2-weighted axial MRI shows that the mass (C) is markedly hyperintense, consistent with fluid.

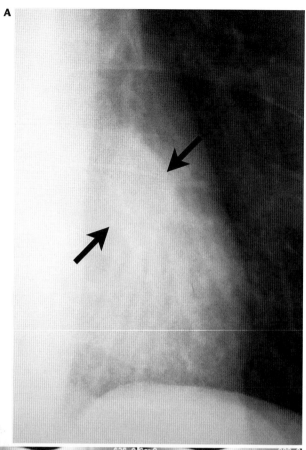

Fig. 16.37 Systemic vascular supply to the left lower lobe in a young woman with hemoptysis. **A**, Coned-down view from a frontal chest radiograph shows tubular opacities (arrows) in the left lower lobe. **B**, CT (lung window) shows increased attenuation in the left lower lobe and enlarged lower lobe vessels. The bronchi (not shown) appeared normal. **C**, Coronal T1-weighted MRI shows a vessel (arrow) arising from aorta to supply left lower lobe. **D**, Gradient recalled echo MRI sequence shows normal pulmonary venous drainage (*) into the left atrium (La). At surgery, the left lower lobe was normal except for systemic arterial supply. (Courtesy of LE Heyneman, Durham, NC)

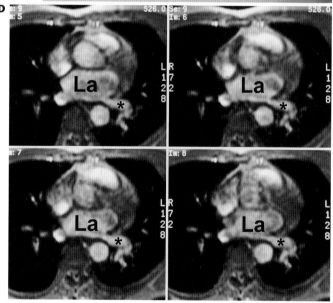

PULMONARY SEQUESTRATION

Pulmonary sequestration is a mass of pulmonary tissue that does not communicate with the central airway through a normal bronchial connection and that receives its blood supply via an anomalous systemic artery. The arterial supply may arise from the descending thoracic aorta or from the abdominal aorta or one of its branches. Pulmonary sequestrations are divided

Table 16.2 Intralobar versus extralobar sequestration

Parameter	Intralobar sequestration	Extralobar sequestration
Etiology	Chronic infection, congenital	Congenital
Relation to normal lung	Within normal lung	Separate with own pleural covering
Venous drainage	Pulmonary	Systemic
Side affected	Left 60–70%	Left 90%
Associated congenital anomalies	Uncommon	Frequent
Age at diagnosis	50% by age 20	60% in first year
Sex ratio	M = F	M:F = 4:1
Infection or communication with normal lung	Common	Rare

into the intralobar and the much less common extralobar types.[206] Key differentiating features are summarized in Table 16.2.[207] However, variants that do not fit neatly into these two categories are sometimes encountered.[208,209] For example, intralobar sequestrations may drain into the systemic venous system and extralobar sequestrations may drain to the left atrium. Furthermore, a portion of normal lung may be supplied by an aberrant systemic artery or be drained by a systemic vein (Fig. 16.37).[210–213]

Extralobar sequestrations are unquestionably congenital abnormalities.[67,214–217] Most are detected in infancy (Fig. 16.38) and there is a high association with other congenital abnormalities such as congenital diaphragmatic hernia, congenital heart disease, and cystic adenomatoid malformation.[218–221] Furthermore, extralobar sequestrations may be detected antenatally by ultrasound.[222,223] On the other hand, most intralobar sequestrations are arguably acquired lesions, possibly due to chronic bronchial obstruction and postobstructive pneumonia.[216,224] The chronic inflammatory process presumably results in parasitization of blood flow from systemic arteries, including the arteries of the inferior pulmonary ligament which may arise from branches off the infradiaphragmatic abdominal aorta.[225] Thus, 98% of intralobar sequestrations occur in the lower lobes (Figs 16.39 and 16.40). The peak incidence of intralobar sequestration is in young adults; the lesions are rarely seen in infants. In some cases, a definite bronchial obstructive lesion has been identified, e.g. a foreign body[226] or a carcinoid tumor.[227] In most cases, no such obstruction is identified and it is not possible to completely discount the possibility of a congenital abnormality that might predispose to chronic infection. For example, in the case illustrated in Figure 16.41, a large branch from the descending thoracic aorta supplied a well-circumscribed portion of the right lower lobe. The portion of lung thus supplied appeared hyperlucent. The patient, a young woman, had at least one episode of lower lobe pneumonia without visible sequela at the time of CT examina-

tion. However, it is conceivable that further episodes of pneumonia might lead to a chronic inflammatory mass. This would necessarily be supplied by a systemic vessel and could have a surrounding hyperlucent margin as has been described in cases of intralobar sequestration.[228,229]

Intralobar sequestrations usually produce symptoms as a result of infection, most commonly in adolescence or in early adult life (Figs 16.39 and 16.40). In very rare instances a considerable shunt through a sequestration may result in high output cardiac failure.[230] This is most likely to occur with the extralobar variety and may compound associated congenital cardiac problems. Extralobar sequestrations are usually asymptomatic and are often discovered incidentally on a chest radiograph or CT (Fig. 16.42), by ultrasound, during angiocardiography, or during surgical repair of a congenital diaphragmatic hernia with which they are frequently associated. Because extralobar sequestrations have a complete serosal covering and may have a narrow vascular pedicle, torsion may occur. The result may be a tension hydrothorax identified either by ultrasound in utero (see Boxes 16.9 and 16.10)[231,232] or on chest radiographs postnatally. An intrauterine tension hydrothorax may obstruct venous return to the heart, producing fetal hydrops.[233–236] Such cases have been successfully treated by intrauterine tube drainage.[237]

Sequestrations typically manifest on chest radiographs as focal opacities in the posterior, inferior, and medial aspect of either hemithorax (Figs 16.39 and 16.40). They are found in the upper half of the thorax in <2% of cases.[238] They are more common on the left than the right. Extralobar sequestrations manifest as masses of uniform density. Their lateral margin is usually well defined because of the pleural envelope. Because the lesions tend to abut the mediastinum, their medial margin is often not appreciated on chest radiographs and they may be confused with a mediastinal mass (Figs 16.38 and 16.42). Extralobar sequestrations can also occur in other locations, including the pericardium, mediastinum, diaphragm, and

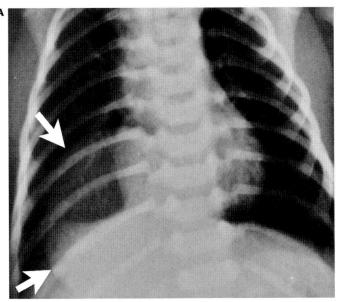
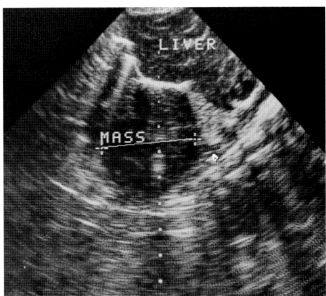

Fig. 16.38 Extralobar sequestration in an infant. **A,** Frontal chest radiograph shows a well-circumscribed right posterior basal soft tissue mass (arrows). **B,** Longitudinal ultrasound shows a mass of mixed echogenicity. Doppler ultrasound (not shown) confirmed systemic vascular supply to the mass.

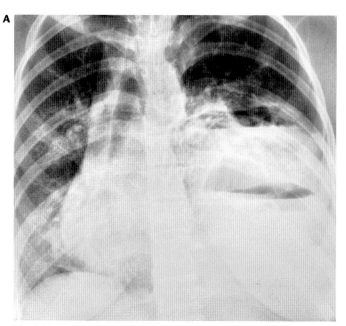 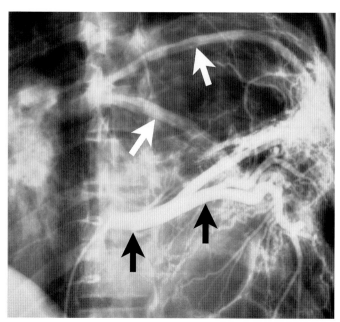

Fig. 16.39 Infected intralobar sequestration in a young woman with cough and fever. **A**, Frontal chest radiograph shows a complex left lower lobe mass with multiple air–fluid levels. Note mass effect on the mediastinum. **B**, Angiography shows a large feeding vessel (black arrows) arising from the descending thoracic aorta and pulmonary venous return (white arrows) to the left atrium.

Box 16.9 Ultrasound of common fetal chest masses

Pulmonary sequestration
Solid hyperechoic mass in lower chest or upper abdomen
Associated anomalies common – cardiac, diaphragmatic hernia
Usually an incidental finding – fetal hydrops and polyhydramnios unusual
May decrease in size during pregnancy
Doppler ultrasound may show systemic arterial supply

Congenital cystic adenomatoid malformation
Most common – cystic with solid components (Types 1 and 2)
Less common – solid hyperechoic mass (Type 3)
Unilateral lesions often with mass effect
May cause fetal hydrops and polyhydramnios
Associated anomalies common
May show an actual or relative decrease in size during pregnancy

Congenital diaphragmatic hernia
Frequently left sided
Diaphragmatic defect may be detected
Abnormal position of gastric bubble
Mediastinal shift and pulmonary hypoplasia frequent
Associated malformations common
May be associated with extralobar sequestration

Box 16.10 Ultrasound of uncommon fetal chest masses

Bronchogenic cyst/esophageal duplication cyst
Rarely seen in utero
Simple centrally located cyst
Mediastinal shift, hydrops fetalis, and polyhydramnios unusual
Associated anomalies rare

Neurenteric cyst
Simple posterior mediastinal cyst
Vertebral anomalies frequent
May cause mediastinal shift

Bronchial obstruction with fluid retention
Fluid retention in a lung or a lobe can result in an echogenic "mass"
Causes – congenital lobar overinflation, pulmonary sling, or bronchial atresia

Intrathoracic neoplasm
Rare causes of solid echogenic masses
Congenital neuroblastoma, pulmonary blastoma

---

retroperitoneum.[215] Communication with the esophagus or the stomach may be demonstrated by barium studies.

Intralobar sequestrations are invariably located above the diaphragm. On chest radiographs they can be homogeneously opaque, round, or lobulated in contour, and resemble an intrapulmonary mass. They can also contain air, have more ill-

defined margins, and resemble an area of pneumonia or lung abscess (Figs 16.39 and 16.40). On occasion, one or more air–fluid levels are seen within sequestered segments. Such air–fluid levels are a consequence of infection with fistula formation to the adjacent bronchi. Although sequestrations may appear solid on plain radiographs, CT usually shows an irregular cystic

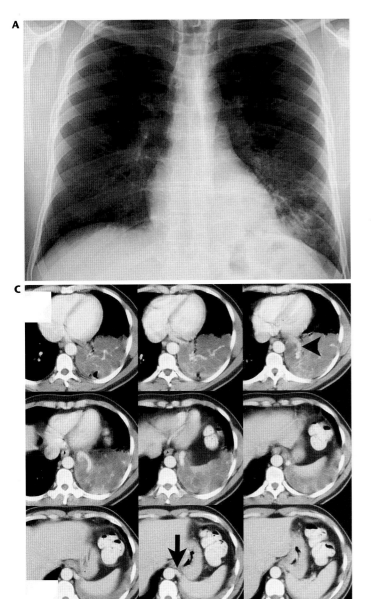

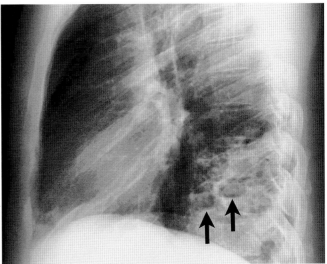

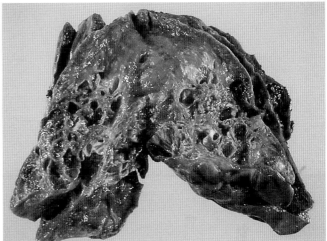

Fig. 16.40 Intralobar sequestration in a young man with recurrent left lower lobe pneumonia. **A**, Frontal and **B**, lateral chest radiographs show poorly defined opacities with multiple air–fluid levels (arrows) in the left lower lobe. **C**, Contrast-enhanced CT shows a heterogeneous mass in the left lower lobe. Note the systemic arterial supply (arrow) and pulmonary venous drainage (arrowhead). **D**, Cut surface of the resected specimen shows multiple cysts of varying size. (Courtesy of JR Galvin, Armed Forces Institute of Pathology, Washington, DC)

component to the lesion (Fig. 16.43).[224,239] Ikezoe et al[239] found a surprisingly high incidence of "emphysema" in the lung adjacent to both intralobar and extralobar sequestrations (Fig. 16.44). Emphysema adjacent to intralobar sequestrations has been explained on the basis of collateral air drift and air-trapping caused by impaired ventilation.[240] Emphysema adjacent to extralobar sequestrations is more difficult to explain because the emphysematous portions of adjacent lung are distinctly separated from the actual sequestration by the pleural envelope. Nevertheless, emphysema appears to be a more constant finding in extralobar sequestration than in the intralobar variety. On rare occasions, calcifications occur in pulmonary sequestration and are readily detected by CT.[239,241] Occasionally, air-trapping and bulla formation are the dominant features,

even on chest radiographs. Thus, a cystic form of pulmonary sequestration may be encountered. This may be caused by infection of a previously solid mass with subsequent communication to the adjacent lung. However, a possible overlap between sequestrations, bronchogenic cysts, and even congenital cystic adenomatoid malformation has been proposed (Fig. 16.45).[242] Demonstration of systemic arterial supply, usually by contrast-enhanced spiral CT or MRI, is the critical diagnostic feature for differentiation from bronchogenic cyst, lobar atelectasis, or other parenchymal abnormality.

Complete delineation of the arterial supply is particularly important if surgical treatment is being considered because inadvertent damage to the artery during surgery can cause significant hemorrhage.[243] The systemic artery is usually well-

A

B

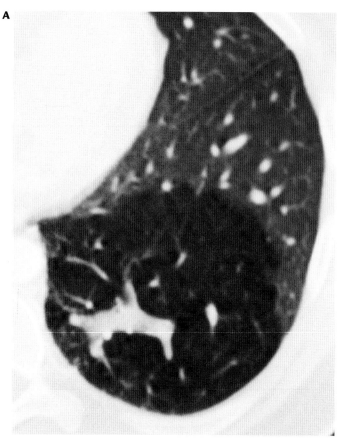

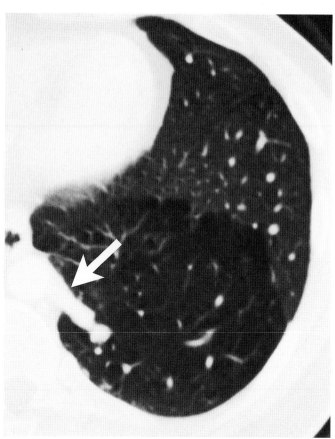

Fig. 16.41 Intralobar sequestration in a 27-year-old woman with one prior episode of left lower lobe pneumonia. **A** and **B**, CT (lung window) shows a well-circumscribed hyperlucent portion of lung supplied by a large vessel from the aorta (arrow). No solid components or bronchi were seen on adjacent sections.

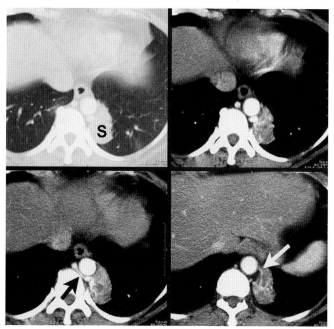

Fig. 16.42 Extralobar sequestration in an asymptomatic middle-aged woman. Sequential images from a contrast-enhanced CT shows a well-marginated soft tissue mass (S) in the left posterior hemithorax. Note the systemic arterial supply from the thoracic aorta (white arrow) and venous drainage (black arrow) into the azygos vein.

demonstrated by thin-section contrast-enhanced spiral CT (Fig. 16.40),[209,239,244–246] color flow Doppler ultrasound,[233,247,248] or MRI (Fig. 16.46).[244,249–256]

The differential diagnosis of pulmonary sequestration includes necrotizing pneumonia, recurrent atelectasis, bronchiectasis and consolidation, lung abscess, neurogenic tumors and meningoceles. The infected pulmonary sequestration may contain air–fluid levels and have ill-defined margins because of inflammatory changes in adjacent lung. The appearance, therefore, may mimic necrotizing pneumonia or simple lung abscess. The correct diagnosis is suggested by the characteristic location of the lesion and a clinical history of recurrent infection in the same location, especially in a young adult. It should be noted, however, that many sequestrations with air–fluid levels are sterile at the time of diagnosis or surgical removal. Some sequestrations, particularly the extralobar variety, can mimic the diagnosis of neurogenic tumor or lateral meningocele. In these lesions, pressure erosions of the vertebrae and the proximal ribs may be observed, a finding not seen with pulmonary sequestration. Other paravertebral masses, such as extramedullary hematopoiesis or pleural tumors, may be indistinguishable from pulmonary sequestration. In essence, the diagnosis of pulmonary sequestration depends as much on the position of the lesion and the clinical features as on the radiologic appearance.

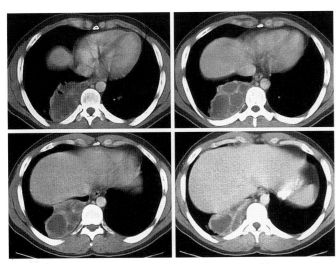

Fig. 16.43 Intralobar sequestration in a young man with recurrent pneumonia. Sequential CT images show a heterogeneous right lower lobe mass containing multiple cysts. Note that most of the cysts are fluid filled.

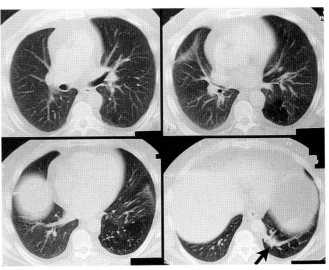

Fig. 16.44 Intralobar sequestration in an asymptomatic elderly woman. Sequential CT images show a hyperlucent region in the left lower lobe with systemic vascular supply (arrow) from the descending aorta. (Courtesy of DP Sponaugle, Elmira, NY)

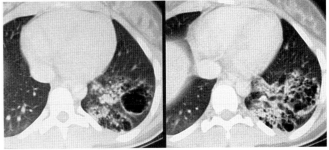

Fig. 16.45 Intralobar sequestration in a young woman with a history of recurrent pneumonia. Sequential CT images show a complex left lower lobe mass with multiple air-filled cysts. Angiography (not shown) confirmed a systemic arterial supply. Elements of congenital cystic adenomatoid malformation were noted at histopathologic examination.

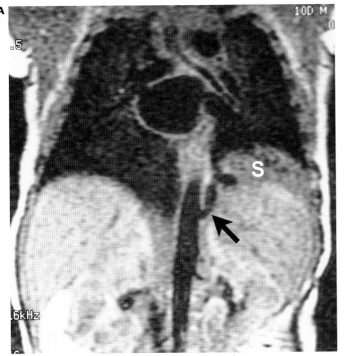

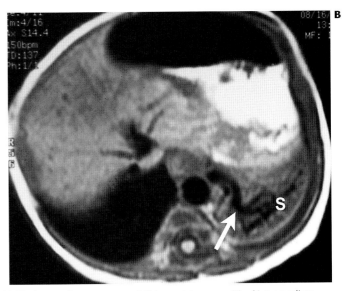

Fig. 16.46 Extralobar sequestration in a neonate. **A**, Coronal T1-weighted MRI shows a heterogeneous left lower lobe mass (S) of intermediate signal intensity. Note flow voids (arrow) in the systemic arteries supplying the lesion. **B**, Axial T2-weighted MRI clearly shows the feeding vessels (arrow). (Case courtesy of Charles White, MD, Baltimore, MD, USA)

A

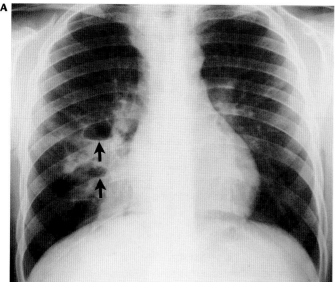

C

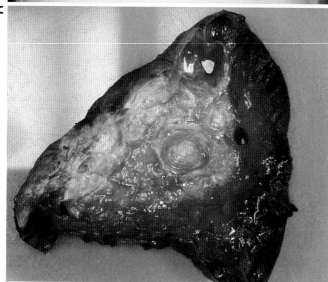

B

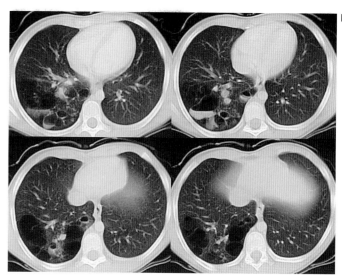

Fig. 16.47 Congenital cystic adenomatoid malformation of the right lung in a 7-year-old boy with a history of recurrent pneumonia. **A,** Frontal chest radiograph shows a heterogeneous right lung mass with multiple air–fluid levels (arrows). **B,** CT (lung window) shows a multicystic mass in the right lower lobe. **C,** Resected specimen shows a complex mass composed of cysts of varying size, consistent with congenital cystic adenomatoid malformation Type 1. (Courtesy of JR Galvin, Armed Forces Institute of Pathology, Washington, DC)

Box 16.11 Congenital cystic adenomatoid malformation

Most important histopathologic types
Type 1: single or multiple cysts 2–10 cm in diameter lined by
  ciliated respiratory epithelium
Type 2: multiple cysts <2 cm in diameter lined by cuboidal
  to columnar epithelium
Type 3: essentially solid lesion with microcysts and
  glandlike (adenomatoid) structures

Effects in utero
Frequently innocuous
Mass effect: fetal hydrops, pleural effusions, and
  polyhydramnios
May decrease in size during pregnancy

Postnatal effects
Small lesions: frequently asymptomatic, may go undetected
  until infancy, childhood or even adult life
Large lesions: secondary pulmonary hypoplasia, respiratory
  distress in neonatal period

Imaging in utero (ultrasound)
See Box 16.9

Postnatal imaging
Unilateral solid or partially cystic lesion with mass effect
Single or multiple air-containing cysts in the mass
Pulmonary hypoplasia or effects of fetal hydrops may be
  evident
CT and ultrasound will usually demonstrate cystic spaces
  even in solid appearing masses on chest radiographs
Differential diagnosis in the neonate – congenital
  diaphragmatic hernia
In the child and adult, CCAMs are predominantly air-
  containing cystic lesions with little solid content by chest
  radiograph or CT

CONGENITAL CYSTIC ADENOMATOID MALFORMATION OF THE LUNG (Box 16.11)

Congenital cystic adenomatoid malformation (CCAM) of the lung is an uncommon, sometimes life-threatening condition that usually manifests in the neonatal period. Adult cases have been reported, but are uncommon.[257] CCAM represents 25% of all congenital lung lesions.[258] The lesion is a hamartomatous mass of fibrous tissue and smooth muscle containing cystic spaces lined by columnar or cuboidal respiratory epithelium.[206,258,259] Unlike pulmonary hamartoma, however, cartilage is notably absent.[260] CCAM is thought to result from failure of pulmonary mesenchyme to induce normal bronchoalveolar differentiation in a portion of the lung bud at about the fifth to seventh weeks of gestation.[220,261] Five pathologic types (CCAM Types 0–4) are now recognized,[259,262] but the imaging features are best characterized for Types 1–3.[263] CCAM Type 1 (cystic CCAM) is the most common (40%) and is characterized by one or more cysts >2 cm in diameter lined by ciliated columnar epithelium (Fig. 16.47).[39,258,259,262] CCAM Type 2 (intermediate type CCAM, 40%) contains cysts <2 cm in

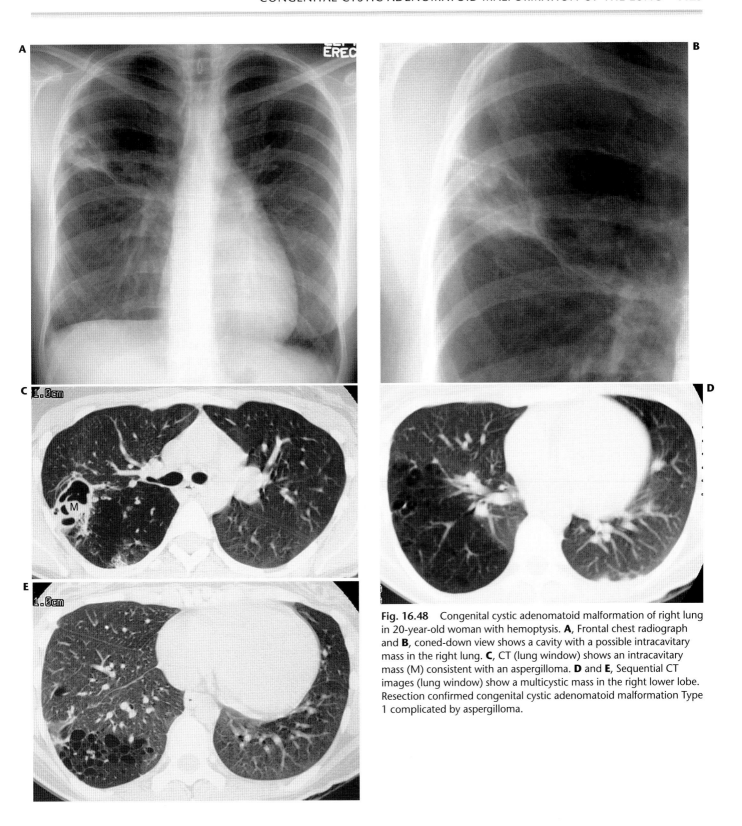

Fig. 16.48   Congenital cystic adenomatoid malformation of right lung in 20-year-old woman with hemoptysis. **A**, Frontal chest radiograph and **B**, coned-down view shows a cavity with a possible intracavitary mass in the right lung. **C**, CT (lung window) shows an intracavitary mass (M) consistent with an aspergilloma. **D** and **E**, Sequential CT images (lung window) show a multicystic mass in the right lower lobe. Resection confirmed congenital cystic adenomatoid malformation Type 1 complicated by aspergilloma.

diameter lined by bronchiolar type epithelium.[39,258,259,262] CCAM Type 3 (solid type CCAM, 10%) is macroscopically solid but microscopically contains glandlike elements, as well as structures resembling bronchioles.[39,258,259,262] Some extralobar pulmonary sequestrations contain elements of CCAM, usually Type 2,[214,261] perhaps reflecting the effect of abnormal mesenchyme on an aberrant lung bud.[156,157] The Stocker

classification has important prognostic significance. Patients with CCAM Type 1 have the best prognosis and these lesions may present in adulthood (Figs 16.48 and 16.49).[257] Patients with CCAM Type 2 may have associated severe or lethal cardiac or renal anomalies such as renal agenesis. Perhaps because CCAM Type 3 lesions tend to be quite large, affected neonates are often stillborn or die in the neonatal period.

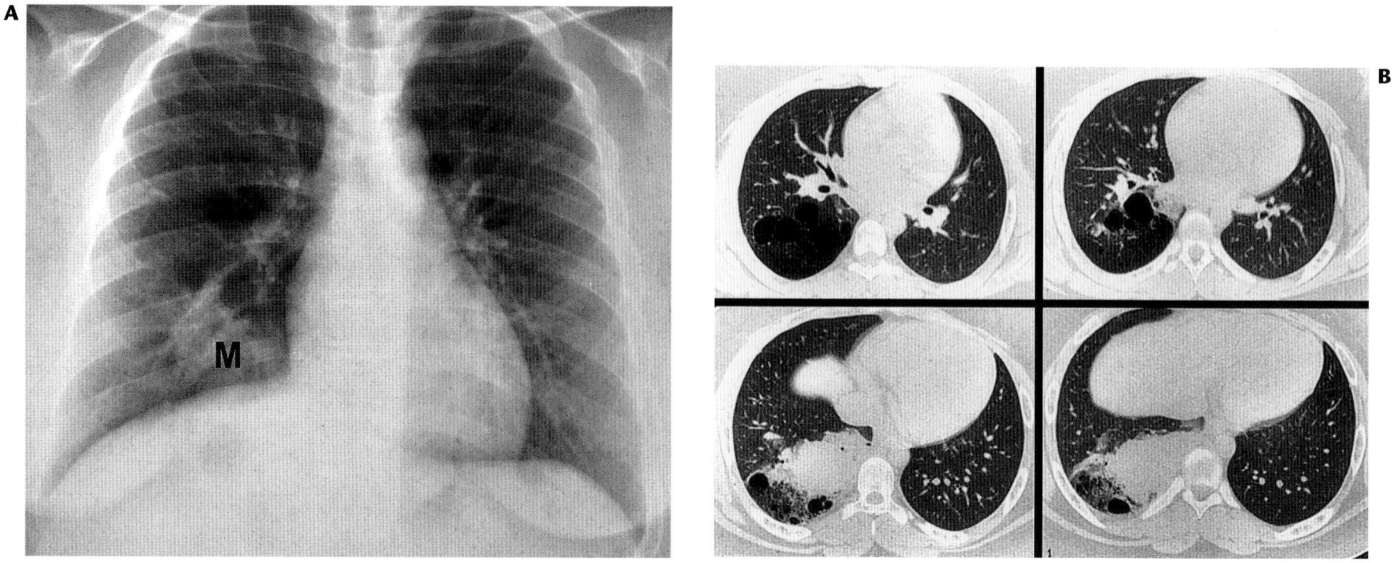

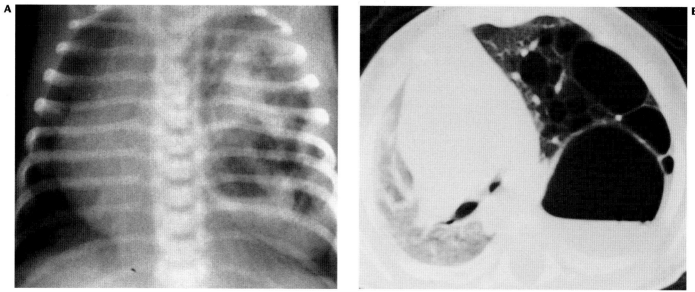

Fig. 16.49 Congenital cystic adenomatoid malformation of the right lung in a young woman. **A,** Frontal chest radiograph shows a masslike opacity (M) in the right lower lobe. **B,** CT (lung window) shows a complex mass with cystic and solid components.

Fig. 16.50 Congenital cystic adenomatoid malformation of the left lung in a neonate. **A,** Frontal chest radiograph shows a complex mass with multiple air–fluid levels in the left hemithorax. Note mass effect on the mediastinum. **B,** CT (lung window) shows a complex mass composed of thin walled cysts. Note compression of the right lung.

CCAM usually manifests in the neonatal period with progressive respiratory distress and cyanosis as a result of mass effect on adjacent lung, diaphragm, and mediastinum (Fig. 16.50). Compression of adjacent lung may result in secondary pulmonary hypoplasia. In utero, the expansile nature of the lesion may result in polyhydramnios and nonimmune hydrops fetalis because of vena cava and, possibly, esophageal obstruction. Approximately 10% of lesions manifest after the first year of life, usually due to chronic respiratory infection.[264–267] Isolated cases have been observed in adults who presented with recurrent pneumonia, pneumothoraces, or hemoptysis, as well as in asymptomatic adults who presented with a pulmonary

mass (Figs 16.48 and 16.49).[257,268–270] The lesion usually involves just one lobe of lung. Involvement of more than one lobe, an entire lung or both lungs is exceedingly rare.[267,268,271,272]

CCAM can be diagnosed antenatally by ultrasound.[222,263,273–277] The cardinal feature on ultrasound is the presence of a solid or cystic intrathoracic mass (Fig. 16.51), sometimes associated with polyhydramnios or nonimmune hydrops fetalis. The finding of hydrops fetalis and polyhydramnios is indicative of a poorer prognosis.[273,276] Antenatally detected CCAMs may decrease in size on serial in utero examinations,[273,276,277] and some may appear to resolve.[263] A similar phenomenon has been noted with pulmonary sequestrations.[222] Decrease in the apparent size

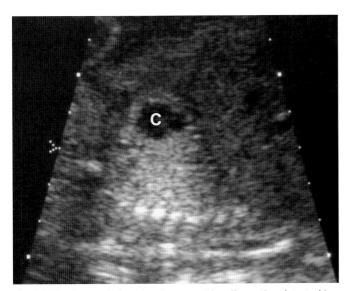

Fig. 16.51 Congenital cystic adenomatoid malformation detected in utero. Longitudinal ultrasound image shows a thick walled cyst (C) with distal acoustic enhancement.

of the lesion in utero, lack of mediastinal shift, and absence of polyhydramnios are favorable prognostic signs.[273,276] Ultrasound examinations identifying CCAM may lead to antenatal intervention in critical cases, either cyst drainage or even fetal lobectomy.[276,278,279]

The radiologic features of CCAM reflect the histopathologic heterogeneity of the condition. Chest radiography is the mainstay for diagnosis in the neonatal period; CT and ultrasound may play a supporting role (Figs 16.47 to 16.50). The chest radiograph typically shows a unilateral mass with evidence of pressure effects on adjacent structures, most notably the mediastinum. Depending upon the type of CCAM, the lesion may appear solid (Fig. 16.49) or contain air-filled cystic spaces of varying size, possibly with air–fluid levels (Figs 16.47 and 16.52). Occasionally, a single large air-filled cyst is the predominant radiographic abnormality.[280] Type 1 or 2 lesions may initially appear solid if the radiograph is obtained before the fetal lung fluid has drained. When the CCAM occurs adjacent to the diaphragm, it may be confused with congenital diaphragmatic hernia.[281] In cases of diaphragmatic hernia, the abdomen tends to be scaphoid with a paucity of gas, whereas the abdominal gas pattern is normal in cases of CCAM. The presence of a nasogastric tube in the thorax confirms diaphragmatic hernia. Immediate diagnosis is essential in both conditions and the treatment for both is surgical. The extent of associated pulmonary hypoplasia is an important determinant of outcome in both conditions.

Ultrasound examinations are more likely to be rewarding for evaluation of radiographically solid intrathoracic masses in the neonatal period (see Box 16.10). On ultrasound, CCAM Types 1 or 2 manifest as masses with one or more fluid-filled cavities of varying size. CCAM Type 3, however, manifests as a solid, diffusely echogenic mass and may be difficult to distinguish from other congenital solid masses, such as neuroblastoma.

When the chest radiograph or ultrasound examination is considered diagnostic for CCAM, CT may not be required.

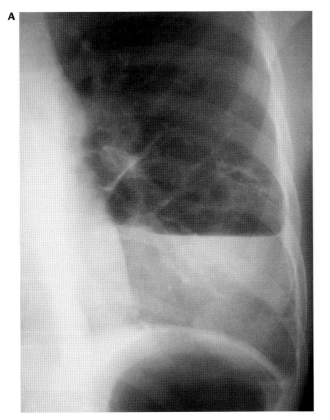

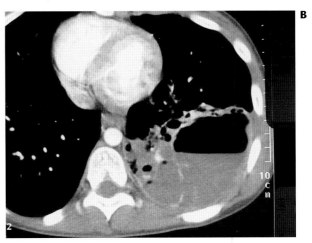

Fig. 16.52 Congenital cystic adenomatoid malformation of the left lung in a child with recurrent pneumonia. **A**, Coned-down view of the left lung shows multiple thin walled cysts of varying size. Note the dominant air–fluid level. **B**, CT (mediastinal window) confirms a complex cystic mass in the left lower lobe. No systemic arterial supply was identified. (Courtesy of DP Frush, MD, Durham, NC)

However, the chest radiographic findings of CCAM can be quite subtle and CT is often required for diagnosis. This may be especially true of the so-called "disappearing" intrathoracic mass on prenatal ultrasound.[277] CT is often applied to confusing cases encountered in childhood or adult life (Figs 16.47 to 16.50 and 16.52).[257,265,282] The CT findings of CCAM depend upon the histopathologic subtype.[258,282,283] As expected, Types 1 and 2 CCAM typically manifest on CT as a mixture of solid and cystic elements; air may or may not be present within the cysts.[283] Solid components are usually not a dominant feature. Occasionally, there is a single dominant air cyst and others are entirely fluid filled. Kim et al[282] reported CT findings of 21 cases of CCAM. Small cystic lesions (<2 cm in diameter) were seen in 90% of cases and large cysts (>2 cm in diameter) were seen in 86%. The diameter of the largest cyst ranged from 1 to 8 cm (median 4.5 cm). Areas of consolidation with heterogeneous attenuation on enhanced scans were seen in 43% of cases. Patz et al[257] reported the CT appearance of seven lesions diagnosed in adult patients. In their series, all of the lesions were in the lower lobes and appeared as complex masses with multiple thin walled cysts ranging from 4 to 12 cm in diameter.

CONGENITAL DIAPHRAGMATIC ABNORMALITIES

The diaphragm develops from four embryologic elements: the septum transversum; the mesentery of the esophagus; the pleuroperitoneal membranes; and ingrowing muscular tissue from the body wall.[284] The septum transversum, a horizontal condensation of mesenchyme, develops into the central tendon of the diaphragm. The mesentery of the esophagus forms the crura of the diaphragm, fusing laterally with the pleuroperitoneal membranes that develop by ingrowth of the pleuroperitoneal folds. The pleuroperitoneal folds grow in from the dorsal and lateral aspects of the embryo to seal the pleuroperitoneal canals, fusing anteriorly with the septum transversum and medially with the esophageal mesentery. Ingrowth of muscular tissue from the body wall completes the diaphragm.[285]

There are many different types of diaphragmatic hernias. The classic congenital diaphragmatic hernia of infancy results from failure of closure of the pleuroperitoneal canal. This usually results in a central diaphragmatic defect of variable size with herniation of abdominal contents into the chest cavity. Bochdalek hernias usually manifest later in life and result from congenital weakness or defects in the posterior aspects of one or both hemidiaphragms. Morgagni hernias also tend to manifest later in life and are the result of a defect or weakness between the sternal and costal attachments of the diaphragm. Defects in the central tendon of the diaphragm that result from failure of development of the septum transversum are extremely rare. In these cases, the abdominal viscera herniate into the pericardial sac and mortality is high.[286,287] The incidence of diaphragmatic defects, typically through the posterior foramina (Bochdalek hernia), increases with age and the presence of emphysema.[288]

Congenital diaphragmatic hernia (Box 16.12)

The incidence of congenital diaphragmatic hernia in the neonatal period is approximately 1 in 2400 births.[289] Hernias are usually unilateral, but may be bilateral in 1% of cases.[290] They

---

Box 16.12 Congenital diaphragmatic hernia

Incidence
1 in 2400 births

Side affected
Almost always unilateral
90% left sided

Clinical presentation
Neonatal respiratory distress

Prenatal diagnosis (ultrasound)
See Box 16.9

Postnatal diagnosis (chest radiograph)
Air-filled loops of bowel in thorax
Orogastric tube terminates in thorax
Contralateral mediastinal shift
Loss of ipsilateral diaphragmatic silhouette
Variable degree of pulmonary hypoplasia

Prognosis
Depends upon degree of pulmonary hypoplasia
Failure of ipsilateral lung to expand or aerate after surgical correction is ominous
Right sided defects have a worse prognosis

---

are more common on the left. Guibaud et al[291] found that 90% of 40 hernias in their series were on the left. There is a high incidence of associated anomalies, both morphologic and chromosomal (particularly trisomy 18).[291]

Classic congenital diaphragmatic hernias are first seen as an emergency in the neonatal period. A major portion of the abdominal viscera may be in one hemithorax with compressive effects on the lungs and mediastinum. Swallowed air enters the stomach and the bowel quickly, and the diagnosis is not usually difficult radiographically (Figs 16.53 and 16.54). The chest radiograph typically shows a mass of soft tissue or mixed soft tissue and air density in the left hemithorax. The lesion is located in the lower chest and ipsilateral aerated lung is displaced into the upper thorax. The silhouette of the left hemidiaphragm is obscured. Mass effect may be considerable, with obvious shift of the mediastinum to the contralateral side and with evidence of compression of the contralateral lung. Air in the lesion may be obviously located in the stomach or may appear loculated due to air in multiple loops of bowel. If a nasogastric tube is inserted, it may either be impeded in the region of the esophagogastric junction or curve up into the thorax if the stomach is included in the herniated viscera (Figs 16.53 and 16.54). The abdomen is likely to be scaphoid instead of showing the protuberance normal in the infant. When the lesion occurs on the right (1–10%), the hernia sac may contain only liver and omentum. Chest radiographs then show a mass of soft tissue density in the lower right hemithorax. Aeration of the lungs may be severely impaired and there is underlying pulmonary hypoplasia, the extent of which cannot always be determined with certainty on the initial radiographs. However, findings on initial chest radiographs can be helpful for predicting survival after repair of congenital diaphragmatic hernia. Saifuddin et al[72] examined a series of preoperative radiographs and correlated radiographic findings with outcome. All patients who had either absent aeration of the contralateral lung or contralateral

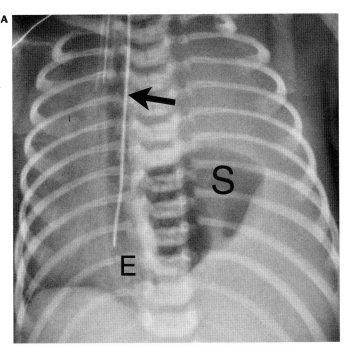 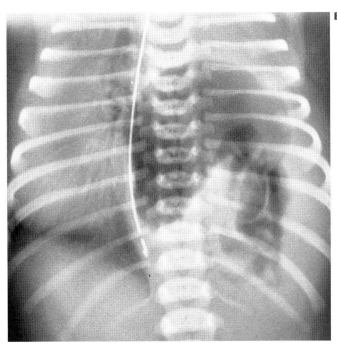

Fig. 16.53 Congenital diaphragmatic hernia in a neonate with respiratory distress. The nasogastric tube could not be advanced into the stomach. **A**, Initial postnatal chest radiograph shows opaque lungs, a nasogastric tube (arrow) in the distal esophagus (E) and gas in the stomach bubble (S). **B**, Repeat chest radiograph now shows gas in the intrathoracic bowel. The patient did not survive despite surgical repair because of severe pulmonary hypoplasia and persistent fetal circulation.

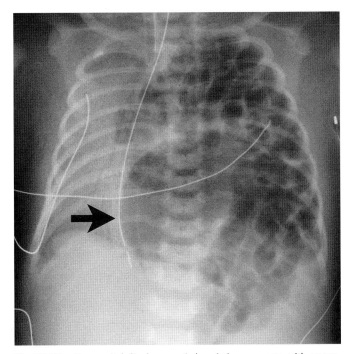

Fig. 16.54 Congenital diaphragmatic hernia in a neonate with severe respiratory distress. Frontal chest radiograph shows the gastric air bubble and multiple loops of bowel in the left hemithorax. The right lung is not aerated and the nasogastric tube (arrow) would not pass beyond the distal esophagus. The patient did not survive despite surgical repair because of severe pulmonary hypoplasia and persistent fetal circulation.

pneumothorax died (Figs 16.53 and 16.54), whereas all patients with visibly aerated ipsilateral lung survived (Fig. 16.55). Donnelly et al[71] found a statistically significant correlation between survival after repair and percentage of both ipsilateral and contralateral lung aeration and degree of mediastinal shift. Other findings associated with a poorer prognosis include right sided defects, fetal hydrops, associated congenital heart disease and intrathoracic position of the stomach.[292–295] It may take several weeks for the lung to expand to fill the thorax where the hernia occurred and full expansion may not occur. However, complete failure of the lung to expand following relief of the pressure effects is ominous.

There are pitfalls in the diagnosis of diaphragmatic hernia, particularly in cases of right sided hernias.[296] The liver or omentum may occlude the defect in the diaphragm and herniation of abdominal contents into the chest may be delayed.[297] Indeed, in a number of cases, the hernia does not manifest until later in life.[298,299] Previous chest radiographs in such patients may be normal (Fig. 16.56).[300,301] Alternatively, the chest radiograph may be intermittently abnormal. Delayed appearance of right sided hernias has been associated with group B streptococcal pneumonia in neonates.[302] Right sided hernias have been noted in association with right pleural effusion, thought to be the result of obstructed hepatic venous outflow.[303] Such an effusion may not only obscure the hernia but also falsely raise the question of primary pulmonary disease such as infection.[299] Solid right sided CCAMs may be difficult or impossible to differentiate from right sided hernias. Left sided cystic CCAMs may radiographically resemble a left sided hernia on chest radiographs. However, in such cases, careful observation will show gas in normally located intraabdominal bowel, a normally protuberant abdomen, and a normal course of the nasogastric tube.

A

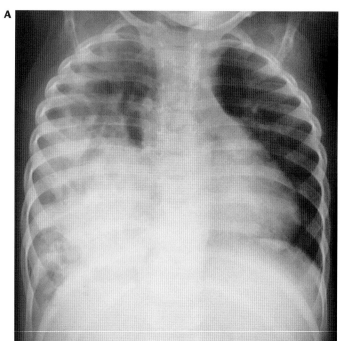

B

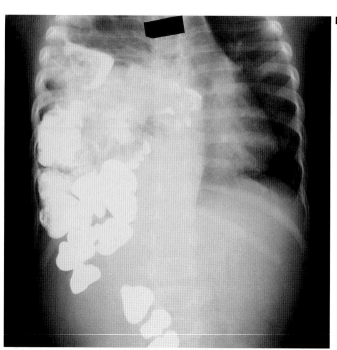

C

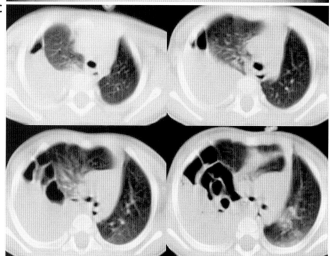

Fig. 16.55 Congenital diaphragmatic hernia in an infant with respiratory distress. **A**, frontal chest radiograph shows multiple loops of bowel in the right hemithorax. The left lung is well aerated. **B**, Frontal radiograph obtained following administration of barium shows colon and small bowel in the right hemithorax. **C**, CT (lung window) shows that the right upper lobe and left lung are well aerated. The patient recovered uneventfully after surgical repair. (Courtesy of JR Galvin, Armed Forces Institute of Pathology, Washington, DC)

Ultrasound is quite useful for both antenatal and postnatal diagnosis of congenital diaphragmatic hernia (see Box 16.9).[284,290,304–307] Peristalsis of bowel within the thorax is observed and the normal, uninterrupted contours of the diaphragm are not seen. Ultrasound is of great use for differentiating other neonatal mass lesions such as pulmonary sequestration and CCAM from hernias. The feeding artery of a pulmonary sequestration may be identified, particularly if Doppler ultrasound is used. Ultrasound examination of a cystic adenomatoid malformation should indicate the presence of an intact diaphragm and the cystic nature of the lesion. Hubbard et al[308] have used MRI in the prenatal period for planning corrective surgery on the fetus. Antenatal MRI may also be useful for evaluating pulmonary hypoplasia and associated defects.[309–311]

Bochdalek hernia

Bochdalek hernias result from herniation through a posterior diaphragmatic defect close to the crura. The defect is a relic of the pleuroperitoneal canal of the embryo.[312] Although the congenital diaphragmatic hernia of infancy is technically also a Bochdalek hernia, the term is customarily reserved for more localized hernias that manifest later in life. Bochdalek hernias may be bilateral and symmetric. Minor degrees of herniation are fairly common and inconsequential, particularly in older individuals.[288] In these instances symmetric hemispherical bulges may be observed on the diaphragmatic contours posteriorly, slightly medial to the midline of each hemithorax. These small herniations contain only perinephric fat. Rarely,

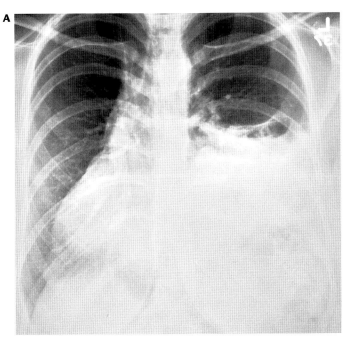

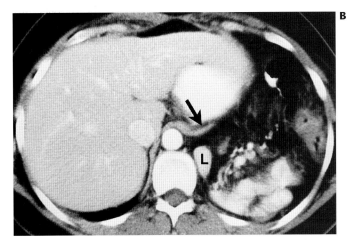

Fig. 16.56   Congenital diaphragmatic hernia in a young woman with numerous congenital anomalies, including cleft lip and palate and limb deformities. **A**, Chest radiograph shows apparent elevation of the left diaphragm and a pleural effusion. **B**, CT (mediastinal window) shows herniated bowel and omentum into the left hemithorax. Note the discontinuity of the left crus of the diaphragm (arrow) and a left sided inferior vena cava (L).

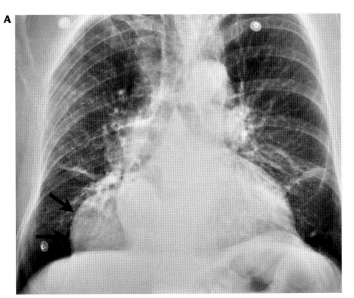

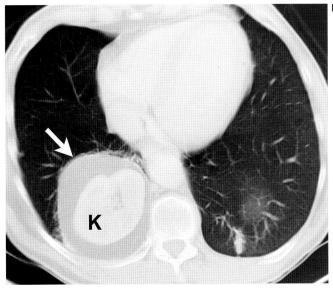

Fig. 16.57   Bochdalek hernia in an asymptomatic middle-aged man. **A**, Frontal chest radiograph shows a well-marginated mass (arrows) in the posterior right hemithorax. **B**, CT (lung window) shows fat and kidney (K) within the hernia sac (arrow).

Bochdalek hernias are larger and contain portions of the kidney, and even the stomach or small bowel (Figs 16.57 and 16.58). Ordinarily the liver prevents visceral herniation on the right side. CT will very clearly determine the presence of a Bochdalek hernia both by determining the nature of the contents of the hernia and by visualization of the actual defect in the diaphragm.[313–316] Small posterior hernias are a common incidental finding on CT, particularly in older adults and patients with emphysema.[288]

Morgagni hernia

Hernias through the foramen of Morgagni can be encountered at any age. They are due to herniation of abdominal contents through the diaphragm between its costal and sternal attachments. The hernia normally develops in the right anterior cardiophrenic sulcus (Figs 16.59 and 16.60), presumably because the heart hinders herniation on the left.[317] Morgagni hernias are normally small and often contain only liver or omentum, in

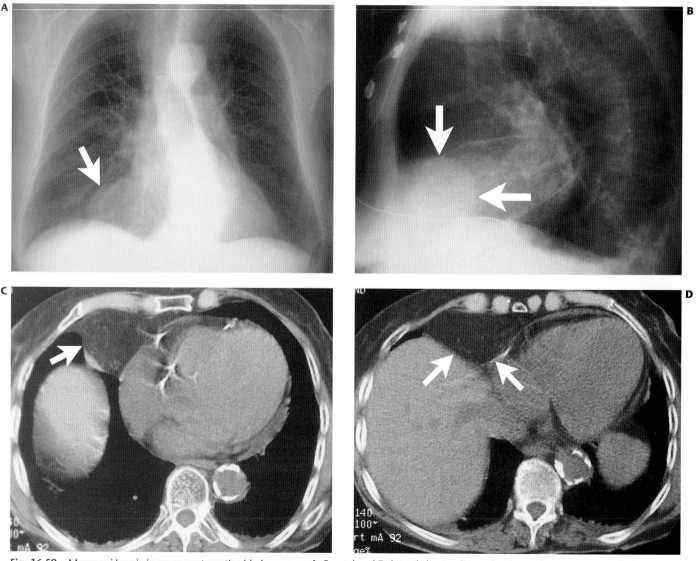

Fig. 16.58 Bochdalek hernia in an asymptomatic elderly man. Sequential CT images show a small left posterior diaphragmatic defect (arrows) with focal herniation of retroperitoneal fat (H).

which case they are of homogeneous soft tissue density on chest radiographs. The margins are smooth and rounded, and the primary differential diagnoses include pericardial cysts, prominent cardiac fat pads, and focal pleural or pulmonary parenchymal masses (Fig. 16.59). CT may be diagnostic by showing omental fat and vessels or liver within the hernia. MRI readily demonstrates a Morgagni hernia with the advantage that scanning may be performed in multiple planes.[316–319] Ultrasound and radionuclide imaging may also be useful in showing herniation of liver into the chest. Radionuclide imaging is limited to determining that a cardiophrenic angle mass contains liver tissue. When the hernia contains bowel, usually transverse colon, the diagnosis is readily made based on chest radiographs (Fig. 16.60). Morgagni hernias are more often a differential diagnostic problem on chest radiography than a clinical problem.

Fig. 16.59 Morgagni hernia in an asymptomatic elderly woman. **A**, Frontal and **B**, lateral chest radiographs show a homogeneous soft tissue mass (arrows) in the right cardiophrenic angle. **C** and **D**, Sequential CT images (mediastinal window) show omental fat (arrows) in the hernia sac. Note the contained mesenteric vessels.

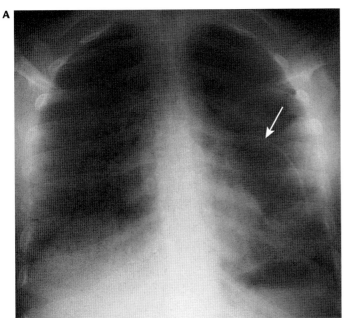

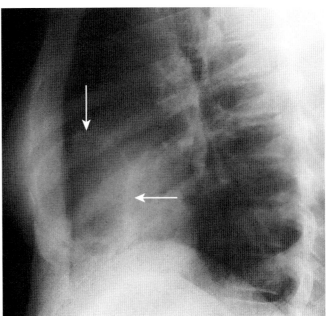

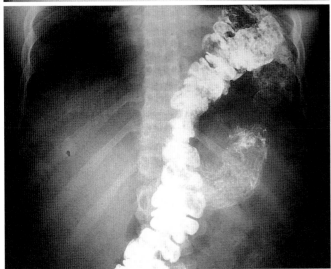

Fig. 16.60 Morgagni hernia. **A**, Frontal and **B**, lateral chest radiographs show an air-filled mass (arrows) in the left cardiophrenic angle. **C**, Frontal view from a barium enema shows colon in the left sided Morgagni hernia.

Accessory diaphragm

An accessory diaphragm is a rare anomaly consisting of an accessory fibromuscular diaphragmatic sheet aligned with the oblique fissure.[320] The hemithorax is thereby separated into two compartments. In an uncomplicated case, the only suggestion of the presence of an accessory diaphragm is the visualization of an unusually thick oblique fissure on that side. An accessory diaphragm may be associated with more significant pulmonary anomalies such as pulmonary hypoplasia[321,322] or the scimitar syndrome.[64]

REFERENCES

1. Sotelo-Avila C, Shanklin DR. Congenital malformations in an autopsy population. Arch Pathol 1967;84:272–279.
2. Sane SM, Sieber WK, Girdany BR. Congenital bronchobiliary fistula. Surgery 1971;69:599–608.
3. Chang N, Hertzler JH, Gregg RH, et al. Congenital stenosis of the right mainstem bronchus. A case report. Pediatrics 1968;41:739–742.
4. MacMahon HE, Ruggieri J. Congenital segmental bronchomalacia. Am J Dis Child 1969;118:923–926.
5. McAdams HP, Erasmus J. Chest case of the day. Williams-Campbell syndrome. AJR Am J Roentgenol 1995;165:190–191.
6. Heithoff KB, Sane SM, Williams HJ, et al. Bronchopulmonary foregut malformations. A unifying etiological concept. Am J Roentgenol 1976;126:46–55.
7. Landing BH. Syndromes of congenital heart disease with tracheobronchial anomalies. Edward BD Neuhauser

Lecture, 1974. Am J Roentgenol Radium Ther Nucl Med 1975;123:679–686.

8. Cunningham MD, Peter ER. Cervical hernia of the lung associated with cri du chat syndrome. Am J Dis Child 1969;118:769–771.

9. Kohne RE, McLeary MS, Kirk GA, Young LW. Esophageal bronchus in an infant diagnosed by fortuitous intubation of the esophagus during ventilation imaging. Clin Nucl Med 1996;21:990–993.

10. Lallemand D, Quignodon JF, Courtel JV. The anomalous origin of bronchus from the esophagus: report of three cases. Pediatr Radiol 1996;26:179–182.

11. Holinger PH, Johnstone KC, Schild JA. Congenital anomalies of the tracheobronchial tree and of the esophagus. Pediatr Clin North Am 1962;9:1113–1124.

12. Warfel KA, Schulz DM. Agenesis of the trachea: report of a case and review of the literature. Arch Pathol Lab Med 1976;100:357–359.

13. Cantrell J, Guild HG. Congenital stenosis of the trachea. Am J Surg 1964;108:297–305.

14. Landing BH, Wells TR. Tracheobronchial anomalies in children. Perspect Pediatr Pathol 1973;1:1–32.

15. Freedom RM, Culham JAG, Moes CAF. Anomalies of pulmonary arteries. In: Angiocardiography of congenital heart disease. New York: Macmillan, 1984:254–273.

16. Rogge JD, Mishkin ME, Genovese PD. The familial occurrence of primary pulmonary hypertension. Ann Intern Med 1966;65:672–684.

17. Leites V, Tannerbaum E. Familial spontaneous pneumothorax. Am Rev Respir Dis 1960;82:240–241.

18. Koch B. Familial fibrocystic pulmonary dysplasia: observations in one family. Can Med Assoc J 1965;92:801–808.

19. Hughes EW. Familial interstitial pulmonary fibrosis. Thorax 1964;19:515–525.

20. Hudson HL, McAlister WH. Obstructing tracheal hemangioma in infancy. AJR Am J Roentgenol 1965;93:428–431.

21. Benisch BM, Wood WG, Kroeger GB Jr, et al. Focal muscular hyperplasia of the trachea. Arch Otolaryngol 1974;99:226–227.

22. Stephens RW, Lingeman RE, Lawson LJ. Congenital tracheoesophageal fistulas in adults. Ann Otol Rhinol Laryngol 1976;85:613–617.

23. Holder TM, Cloud DT, Lewis JE, et al. Esophageal atresia and tracheoesophageal fistula. Pediatrics 1964;34:542–549.

24. Waterston DJ, Carter REB, Aberdeen E. Oesophageal atresia, tracheoesophageal fistula: a study of survival in 218 infants. Lancet 1961:819–822.

25. Barnes JC, Smith WL. The VATER Association. Radiology 1978;126:445–449.

26. Toyama WM. Esophageal atresia and tracheoesophageal fistula in association with bronchial and pulmonary anomalies. J Pediatr Surg 1972;7:302–307.

27. Thomas PS, Chrispin AR. Congenital tracheo-oesophageal fistula without oesophageal atresia. Clin Radiol 1969;20:371–374.

28. Bedard P, Girvan DP, Shandling B. Congenital H-type tracheoesophageal fistula. J Pediatr Surg 1974;9:663–668.

29. Stringer DA, Ein SH. Recurrent tracheo-esophageal fistula: a protocol for investigation. Radiology 1984;151:637–641.

30. Cumming WA. Neonatal radiology. Esophageal atresia and tracheoesophageal fistula. Radiol Clin North Am 1975;13:277–295.

31. Finck S, Milne EN. A case report of segmental bronchial atresia: radiologic evaluation including computed tomography and magnetic resonance imaging. J Thorac Imaging 1988;3:53–57.

32. Ward S, Morcos SK. Congenital bronchial atresia—presentation of three cases and a pictorial review. Clin Radiol 1999;54:144–148.

33. Bighi S, Lupi L, Cardona P, et al. Asymptomatic mucoid impaction in bronchial atresia: roentgenographic and CT patterns. Rays 1987;12:23–26.

34. Kinsella D, Sissons G, Williams MP. The radiological imaging of bronchial atresia. Br J Radiol 1992;65:681–685.

35. Meng RL, Jensik RJ, Faber LP, et al. Bronchial atresia. Ann Thorac Surg 1978;25:184–192.

36. Tederlinic PJ. Congenital bronchial atresia: a report of 4 cases and a review of the literature. Medicine 1986;65:73–83.

37. Kawamoto S, Yuasa M, Tsukuda S, et al. Bronchial atresia: three-dimensional CT bronchography using volume rendering technique. Radiat Med 2001;19:107–110.

38. Matsushima H, Takayanagi N, Satoh M, et al. Congenital bronchial atresia: radiologic findings in nine patients. J Comput Assist Tomogr 2002;26:860–864.

39. Winters WD, Effmann EL. Congenital masses of the lung: prenatal and postnatal imaging evaluation. J Thorac Imaging 2001;16:196–206.

40. Hendren W, McKee DM. Lobar emphysema of infancy. J Pediatr Surg 1966;1:24–39.

41. Case records of the Massachusetts General Hospital (Case 32-1990). N Engl J Med 1990;323:398–406.

42. Hislop A, Reid L. New pathological findings in emphysema of childhood. 1. Polyalveolar lobe with emphysema. Thorax 1970;25:682–690.

43. Tapper D, Schuster S, McBride J, et al. Polyalveolar lobe: anatomic and physiologic parameters and their relationship to congenital lobar emphysema. J Pediatr Surg 1980;15:931–937.

44. Karnak I, Senocak ME, Ciftci AO, et al. Congenital lobar emphysema: diagnostic and therapeutic considerations. J Pediatr Surg 1999;34:1347–1351.

45. Fagan CJ, Swischuk LE. The opaque lung in lobar emphysema. Am J Roentgenol Radium Ther Nucl Med 1972;114:300–304.

46. Allen RP, Taylor RL, Reiquam CW. Congenital lobar emphysema with dilated septal lymphatics. Radiology 1966;86:929–931.

47. Kennedy CD, Habibi P, Matthew DJ, et al. Lobar emphysema: long-term imaging follow-up. Radiology 1991;180:189–193.

48. Markowitz RI, Mercurio MR, Vahjen GA, et al. Congenital lobar emphysema. The roles of CT and V/Q scan. Clin Pediatr (Phila) 1989;28:19–23.

49. Padilla L, Orzel JA, Kreins CM, et al. Congenital lobar emphysema: segmental lobar involvement demonstrated on ventilation and perfusion imaging. J Nucl Med 1985;26:1343–1344.

50. Pardes JG, Auh YH, Blomquist K, et al. CT diagnosis of congenital lobar emphysema. J Comput Assist Tomogr 1983;7:1095–1097.

51. Roghair GD. Nonoperative management of lobar emphysema. Long-term follow-up. Radiology 1972;102:125–127.

52. Jones HE, Howells CHL. Pulmonary agenesis. Br Med J 1961;2:1187–1189.

53. Maltz DL, Nadas AS. Agenesis of the lung. Presentation of eight new cases and review of the literature. Pediatrics 1968;42:175–188.

54. Della Pona C, Rocco G, Rizzi A, et al. Lobar hypoplasia. Eur Respir J 1991;4:1140–1142.

55. Osborne J, Masel J, McCredie J. A spectrum of skeletal anomalies associated with pulmonary agenesis: possible neural crest injuries. Pediatr Radiol 1989;19:425–432.

56. Cunningham ML, Mann N. Pulmonary agenesis: a predictor of ipsilateral malformations. Am J Med Genet 1997;70:391–398.

57. Knowles S, Thomas RM, Lindenbaum RH, et al. Pulmonary agenesis as part of the VACTERL sequence. Arch Dis Child 1988;63:723–726.

58. Felson B. Pulmonary agenesis and related anomalies. Semin Roentgenol 1972;7:17–30.

59. Mata JM, Caceres J. The dysmorphic lung: imaging findings. Eur Radiol 1996;6:403–414.

60. Benson JE, Olsen MM, Fletcher BD. A spectrum of bronchopulmonary

anomalies associated with tracheoesophageal malformations. Pediatr Radiol 1985;15:377–380.

61. Brereton RJ, Rickwood AM. Esophageal atresia with pulmonary agenesis. J Pediatr Surg 1983;18:618–620.

62. Lokare RV, Manvi RS. Esophageal atresia with right pulmonary agenesis. Indian Pediatr 1998;35:555–557.

63. Woodring JH, Howard TA, Kanga JF. Congenital pulmonary venolobar syndrome revisited. RadioGraphics 1994;14:349–369.

64. Pena SD, Shokeir MH. Syndrome of camptodactyly, multiple ankyloses, facial anomalies, and pulmonary hypoplasia: a lethal condition. J Pediatr 1974;85:373–375.

65. Currarino G, Williams B. Causes of congenital unilateral pulmonary hypoplasia: a study of 33 cases. Pediatr Radiol 1985;15:15–24.

66. Mata JM, Caceres J, Lucaya J, et al. CT of congenital malformations of the lung. RadioGraphics 1990;10:651–674.

67. Swischuk LE, Richardson CJ, Nichols MM, et al. Bilateral pulmonary hypoplasia in the neonate. AJR Am J Roentgenol 1979;133:1057–1063.

68. Page DV, Stocker JT. Anomalies associated with pulmonary hypoplasia. Am Rev Respir Dis 1982;125:216–221.

69. Potter EL. Bilateral renal agenesis. J Pediatr 1946;29:68–76.

70. Fraga JR, Mirza AM, Reichelderfer TE. Association of pulmonary hypoplasia, renal anomalies, and Potter's facies. Clin Pediatr (Phila) 1973;12:150–153.

71. Donnelly LF, Sakurai M, Klosterman LA, et al. Correlation between findings on chest radiography and survival in neonates with congenital diaphragmatic hernia. AJR Am J Roentgenol 1999;173:1589–1593.

72. Saifuddin A, Arthur RJ. Congenital diaphragmatic hernia—a review of pre- and postoperative chest radiology. Clin Radiol 1993;47:104–110.

73. Partridge JB, Osborne JM, Slaughter RE. Scimitar etcetera—the dysmorphic right lung. Clin Radiol 1988;39:11–19.

74. Mardini MK, Sakati NA, Lewall DB, et al. Scimitar syndrome. Clin Pediatr (Phila) 1982;21:350–354.

75. Farnsworth AE, Ankeney JL. The spectrum of the scimitar syndrome. J Thorac Cardiovasc Surg 1974;68: 37–42.

76. Neill CA, Ferencz C, Sabiston DC. The familial occurrence of hypoplastic right lung with systemic arterial supply and venous drainage: scimitar syndrome. Bull Johns Hopkins Hosp 1960;107: 1–21.

77. Godwin JD, Tarver RD. Scimitar syndrome: four new cases examined with CT. Radiology 1986;159:15–20.

78. Canter CE, Martin TC, Spray TL, et al.

Scimitar syndrome in childhood. Am J Cardiol 1986;58:652–654.

79. Dupuis C, Charaf LA, Breviere GM, Abou P, Remy-Jardin M, Helmius G. The "adult" form of the scimitar syndrome. Am J Cardiol 1992;70:502–507.

80. Brown JW, Ruzmetov M, Minnich DJ, et al, et al. Surgical management of scimitar syndrome: an alternative approach. J Thorac Cardiovasc Surg 2003;125:238–245.

81. Ang JG, Proto AV. CT demonstration of congenital pulmonary venolobar syndrome. J Comput Assist Tomogr 1984;8:753–757.

82. Olson MA, Becker GJ. The Scimitar syndrome: CT findings in partial anomalous pulmonary venous return. Radiology 1986;159:25–26.

83. Sener RN, Tugran C, Savas R, et al. CT findings in scimitar syndrome. AJR Am J Roentgenol 1993;160:1361.

84. Inoue T, Ichihara M, Uchida T, et al. Three-dimensional computed tomography showing partial anomalous pulmonary venous connection complicated by the scimitar syndrome. Circulation 2002;105:663.

85. Baran R, Kir A, Tor MM, et al. Scimitar syndrome: confirmation of diagnosis by a noninvasive technique (MRI). Eur Radiol 1996;6:92–94.

86. Baxter R, McFadden PM, Gradman M, et al. Scimitar syndrome: cine magnetic resonance imaging demonstration of anomalous pulmonary venous drainage. Ann Thorac Surg 1990;50:121–123.

87. Vrachliotis TG, Bis KG, Shetty AN, et al. Hypogenetic lung syndrome: functional and anatomic evaluation with magnetic resonance imaging and magnetic resonance angiography. J Magn Reson Imaging 1996;6:798–800.

88. Gilkeson RC, Lee JH, Sachs PB, et al. Gadolinium-enhanced magnetic resonance angiography in scimitar syndrome: diagnosis and postoperative evaluation. Tex Heart Inst J 2000;27: 309–311.

89. Henk CB, Prokesch R, Grampp S, et al. Scimitar syndrome: MR assessment of hemodynamic significance. J Comput Assist Tomogr 1997;21:628–630.

90. Ersoz A, Soncul H, Gokgoz L, et al. Horseshoe lung with left lung hypoplasia. Thorax 1992;47:205–206.

91. Frank JL, Poole CA, Rosas G. Horseshoe lung: clinical, pathologic, and radiologic features and a new plain film finding. AJR Am J Roentgenol 1986;146:217–226.

92. Freedom RM, Burrows PE, Moes CA. "Horseshoe" lung: report of five new cases. AJR Am J Roentgenol 1986;146: 211–215.

93. Hawass ND, Badawi MG, al-Muzrakchi AM, et al. Horseshoe lung: differential diagnosis. Pediatr Radiol 1990;20: 580–584.

94. Takeda K, Kato N, Nakagawa T. Horseshoe lung without respiratory distress. Pediatr Radial 1990;20:604.

95. Kamijoh M, Itoh M, Kijimoto C, et al. Horseshoe lung with bilateral vascular anomalies: a rare variant of hypogenetic lung syndrome (scimitar syndrome). Pediatr Int 2002;44:443–445.

96. Kucera V, Fiser B, Tuma S, et al. Unilateral absence of pulmonary artery: a report on 19 selected clinical cases. Thorac Cardiovasc Surg 1982;30:152–158.

97. Finney JO Jr, Finchum RN. Congenital unilateral absence of the left pulmonary artery with right aortic arch and a normal conus. South Med J 1972;65:1079–1082.

98. Ten Harkel AD, Blom NA, Ottenkamp J. Isolated unilateral absence of a pulmonary artery: a case report and review of the literature. Chest 2002; 122:1471–1477.

99. Bouros D, Pare P, Panagou P, et al. The varied manifestation of pulmonary artery agenesis in adulthood. Chest 1995;108:670–676.

100. Mehta AC, Livingston DR, Kawalek W, et al. Pulmonary artery agenesis presenting as massive hemoptysis—a case report. Angiology 1987;38:67–71.

101. Lip GY, Dunn FG. Unilateral pulmonary artery agenesis: a rare cause of haemoptysis and pleuritic chest pain. Int J Cardiol 1993;40:121–125.

102. Rene M, Sans J, Dominguez J, et al. Unilateral pulmonary artery agenesis presenting with hemoptysis: treatment by embolization of systemic collaterals. Cardiovasc Intervent Radiol 1995;18: 251–254.

103. Harris KM, Lloyd DC, Morrissey B, et al. The computed tomographic appearances in pulmonary artery atresia. Clin Radiol 1992;45:382–386.

104. Lynch DA, Higgins CB. MR imaging of unilateral pulmonary artery anomalies. J Comput Assist Tomogr 1990;14:187–191.

105. Kiratli PO, Caglar M, Bozkurt MF. Unilateral absence of pulmonary perfusion in Swyer–James syndrome. Clin Nucl Med 1999;24:706–707.

106. Wieder S, White TJ 3rd, Salazar J, et al. Pulmonary artery occlusion due to histoplasmosis. AJR Am J Roentgenol 1982;138:243–251.

107. Rossi SE, McAdams HP, Rosado-de-Christenson ML, et al. Fibrosing mediastinitis. RadioGraphics 2001;21:737–757.

108. Gossage JR, Kanj G. Pulmonary arteriovenous malformations. A state of the art review. Am J Respir Crit Care Med 1998;158:643–661.

109. Bosher LHJ, Blake DA, Byrd BR. An analysis of the pathologic anatomy of pulmonary arteriovenous aneurysms with particualar reference to the applicability of local excision. Surgery 1959;45:91–104.

110. Haitjema T, Westermann CJ, Overtoom TT, et al. Hereditary hemorrhagic telangiectasia (Osler-Weber-Rendu disease): new insights in pathogenesis, complications, and treatment. Arch Intern Med 1996;156:714–719.

111. Shovlin CL, Letarte M. Hereditary haemorrhagic telangiectasia and pulmonary arteriovenous malformations: issues in clinical management and review of pathogenic mechanisms. Thorax 1999;54:714–729.

112. Case records of the Massachusetts General Hospital (Case 16-1990). N Engl J Med 1990;322:1139–1148.

113. Gibbons JR, McIlrath TE, Bailey IC. Pulmonary arteriovenous fistula in association with recurrent cerebral abscess. Thorac Cardiovasc Surg 1985;33:319–321.

114. Hewes RC, Auster M, White RI, Jr. Cerebral embolism—first manifestation of pulmonary arteriovenous malformation in patients with hereditary hemorrhagic telangiectasia. Cardiovasc Intervent Radiol 1985;8:151–155.

115. White RI Jr, Lynch-Nyhan A, Terry P, et al. Pulmonary arteriovenous malformations: techniques and long-term outcome of embolotherapy. Radiology 1988;169:663–669.

116. Dines DE, Seward JB, Bernatz PE. Pulmonary arteriovenous fistulas. Mayo Clin Proc 1983;58:176–181.

117. Dinsmore BJ, Gefter WB, Hatabu H, et al. Pulmonary arteriovenous malformations: diagnosis by gradient-refocused MR imaging. J Comput Assist Tomogr 1990;14:918–923.

118. Chilvers ER, Peters AM, George P, et al. Quantification of right to left shunt through pulmonary arteriovenous malformations using 99Tcm albumin microspheres. Clin Radiol 1988;39:611–614.

119. Whyte MK, Peters AM, Hughes JM, et al. Quantification of right to left shunt at rest and during exercise in patients with pulmonary arteriovenous malformations. Thorax 1992;47:790–796.

120. Langer R, Langer M. Value of computed tomography in the diagnosis of intrapulmonary arteriovenous shunts. Cardiovasc Intervent Radiol 1984;7:277–279.

121. Rankin S, Faling LJ, Pugatch RD. CT diagnosis of pulmonary arteriovenous malformations. J Comput Assist Tomogr 1982;6:746–749.

122. Remy J, Remy-Jardin M, Wattinne L, Deffontaines C. Pulmonary arteriovenous malformations: evaluation with CT of the chest before and after treatment. Radiology 1992;182:809–816.

123. Remy J, Remy-Jardin M, Artaud D, et al. Multiplanar and three-dimensional reconstruction techniques in CT: impact on chest diseases. Eur Radiol 1998;8:335–351.

124. Hofmann LV, Kuszyk BS, Mitchell SE, et al. Angioarchitecture of pulmonary arteriovenous malformations: characterization using volume-rendered 3-D CT angiography. Cardiovasc Intervent Radiol 2000;23:165–170.

125. Remy J, Remy-Jardin M, Giraud F, et al. Angioarchitecture of pulmonary arteriovenous malformations: clinical utility of three-dimensional helical CT. Radiology 1994;191:657–664.

126. Dutton JA, Jackson JE, Hughes JM, et al. Pulmonary arteriovenous malformations: results of treatment with coil embolization in 53 patients. AJR Am J Roentgenol 1995;165:1119–1125.

127. Hartnell GG, Allison DJ. Coil embolization in the treatment of pulmonary arteriovenous malformations. J Thorac Imaging 1989;4:81–85.

128. Remy-Jardin M, Wattinne L, Remy J. Transcatheter occlusion of pulmonary arterial circulation and collateral supply: failures, incidents, and complications. Radiology 1991;180:699–705.

129. Pollak JS, Egglin TK, Rosenblatt MM, et al. Clinical results of transvenous systemic embolotherapy with a neuroradiologic detachable balloon. Radiology 1994;191:477–482.

130. Chilvers ER, Whyte MK, Jackson JE, et al. Effect of percutaneous transcatheter embolization on pulmonary function, right-to-left shunt, and arterial oxygenation in patients with pulmonary arteriovenous malformations. Am Rev Respir Dis 1990;142:420–425.

131. White RI Jr, Mitchell SE, Barth KH, et al. Angioarchitecture of pulmonary arteriovenous malformations: an important consideration before embolotherapy. AJR Am J Roentgenol 1983;140:681–686.

132. Silverman JM, Julien PJ, Herfkens RJ, et al. Magnetic resonance imaging evaluation of pulmonary vascular malformations. Chest 1994;106:1333–1338.

133. Vrachliotis TG, Bis KG, Kirsch MJ, et al. Contrast-enhanced MRA in pre-embolization assessment of a pulmonary arteriovenous malformation. J Magn Reson Imaging 1997;7:434–436.

134. Ohno Y, Hatabu H, Takenaka D, et al. Contrast-enhanced MR perfusion imaging and MR angiography: utility for management of pulmonary arteriovenous malformations for embolotherapy. Eur J Radiol 2002;41:136–146.

135. Khalil A, Farres MT, Mangiapan G, et al. Pulmonary arteriovenous malformations. Chest 2000;117:1399–1403.

136. Faul JL, Berry GJ, Colby TV, et al. Thoracic lymphangiomas, lymphangiectasis, lymphangiomatosis, and lymphatic dysplasia syndrome. Am J Respir Crit Care Med 2000;161:1037–1046.

137. Kransdorf MJ. Benign soft-tissue tumors in a large referral population: distribution of specific diagnoses by age, sex, and location. AJR Am J Roentgenol 1995;164:395–402.

138. Brown LR, Reiman HM, Rosenow EC 3rd, et al. Intrathoracic lymphangioma. Mayo Clin Proc 1986;61:882–892.

139. Shaffer K, Rosado-de-Christenson ML, Patz EF Jr, et al. Thoracic lymphangioma in adults: CT and MR imaging features. AJR Am J Roentgenol 1994;162:283–289.

140. Pui MH, Li ZP, Chen W, et al. Lymphangioma: imaging diagnosis. Australas Radiol 1997;41:324–328.

141. Charruau L, Parrens M, Jougon J, et al. Mediastinal lymphangioma in adults: CT and MR imaging features. Eur Radiol 2000;10:1310–1314.

142. Fung K, Poenaru D, Soboleski DA, et al. Impact of magnetic resonance imaging on the surgical management of cystic hygromas. J Pediatr Surg 1998;33:839–841.

143. France NE, Brown RJ. Congenital pulmonary lymphangiectasis. Report of 11 examples with special reference to cardiovascular findings. Arch Dis Child 1971;46:528–532.

144. Bouchard S, Di Lorenzo M, Youssef S, et al. Pulmonary lymphangiectasia revisited. J Pediatr Surg 2000;35:796–800.

145. MacLean JE, Cohen E, Weinstein M. Primary intestinal and thoracic lymphangiectasia: a response to antiplasmin therapy. Pediatrics 2002;109:1177–1180.

146. White JE, Veale D, Fishwick D, et al. Generalised lymphangiectasia: pulmonary presentation in an adult. Thorax 1996;51:767–768.

147. Chung CJ, Fordham LA, Barker P, et al. Children with congenital pulmonary lymphangiectasia: after infancy. AJR Am J Roentgenol 1999;173:1583–1588.

148. Copley SJ, Coren M, Nicholson AG, et al. Diagnostic accuracy of thin-section CT and chest radiography of pediatric interstitial lung disease. AJR Am J Roentgenol 2000;174:549–554.

149. Tazelaar HD, Kerr D, Yousem SA, et al. Diffuse pulmonary lymphangiomatosis. Hum Pathol 1993;24:1313–1322.

150. Takahashi K, Takahashi H, Maeda K, et al. An adult case of lymphangiomatosis of the mediastinum, pulmonary interstitium and retroperitoneum complicated by chronic disseminated intravascular coagulation. Eur Respir J 1995;8:1799–1802.

151. Varela JR, Bargiela A, Requejo I, et al. Bilateral renal lymphangiomatosis: US and CT findings. Eur Radiol 1998;8:230–231.

152. Lee BI, Kim BW, Kim KM, et al. Esophageal lymphangiomatosis: a case report. Gastrointest Endosc 2002;56:589–591.

153. Watkins RGt, Reynolds RA, McComb JG, et al. Lymphangiomatosis of the spine: two cases requiring surgical intervention. Spine 2003;28:E45–50.

154. Wunderbaldinger P, Paya K, Partik B, et al. CT and MR imaging of generalized cystic lymphangiomatosis in pediatric patients. AJR Am J Roentgenol 2000;174:827–832.

155. Swensen SJ, Hartman TE, Mayo JR, et al. Diffuse pulmonary lymphangiomatosis: CT findings. J Comput Assist Tomogr 1995;19:348–352.

156. Cordasco EM Jr, Beder S, Coltro A, et al. Clinical features of the yellow nail syndrome. Cleve Clin J Med 1990;57:472–476.

157. Nordkild P, Kromann-Andersen H, Struve-Christensen E. Yellow nail syndrome—the triad of yellow nails, lymphedema and pleural effusions. A review of the literature and a case report. Acta Med Scand 1986;219:221–227.

158. Hershko A, Hirshberg B, Nahir M, et al. Yellow nail syndrome. Postgrad Med J 1997;73:466–468.

159. Fields CL, Roy TM, Ossorio MA, et al. Yellow nail syndrome: a perspective. J Ky Med Assoc 1991;89:563–565.

160. Hiller E, Rosenow EC 3rd, Olsen AM. Pulmonary manifestations of the yellow nail syndrome. Chest 1972;61:452–458.

161. Wiggins J, Strickland B, Chung KF. Detection of bronchiectasis by high-resolution computed tomography in the yellow nail syndrome. Clin Radiol 1991;43:377–379.

162. Malek NP, Ocran K, Tietge UJ, et al. A case of the yellow nail syndrome associated with massive chylous ascites, pleural and pericardial effusions. Z Gastroenterol 1996;34:763–766.

163. Morandi U, Golinelli M, Brandi L, et al. "Yellow nail syndrome" associated with chronic recurrent pericardial and pleural effusions. Eur J Cardiothorac Surg 1995;9:42–44.

164. Jiva TM, Poe RH, Kallay MC. Pleural effusion in yellow nail syndrome: chemical pleurodesis and its outcome. Respiration 1994;61:300–302.

165. Sacco O, Fregonese B, Marino CE, et al. Yellow nail syndrome and bilateral cystic lung disease. Pediatr Pulmonol 1998;26:429–433.

166. McAdams HP, Kirejczyk WM, Rosado-de-Christenson ML, et al. Bronchogenic cyst: imaging features with clinical and histopathologic correlation. Radiology 2000;217:441–446.

167. Reed JC, Sobonya RE. Morphologic analysis of foregut cysts in the thorax. Am J Roentgenol Radium Ther Nucl Med 1974;120:851–860.

168. St-Georges R, Deslauriers J, Duranceau A, et al. Clinical spectrum of bronchogenic cysts of the mediastinum and lung in the adult. Ann Thorac Surg 1991;52:6–13.

169. Di Lorenzo M, Collin PP, Vaillancourt R, et al. Bronchogenic cysts. J Pediatr Surg 1989;24:988–991.

170. Ramenofsky ML, Leape LL, McCauley RG. Bronchogenic cyst. J Pediatr Surg 1979;14:219–224.

171. Bressler S WD. Bronchogenic cyst associated with an anomalous pulmonary artery arising from the thoracic aorta. Surgery 1954;35:815–819.

172. Brower A, Clagett OT, McDonald JR. Anomalous arteries to the lung associated with congenital pulmonary abnormality. J Thorac Surg 1950;19:957–972.

173. Demos TC, Budorick NE, Posniak HV. Benign mediastinal cysts: pointed appearance on CT. J Comput Assist Tomogr 1989;13:132–133.

174. Ribet ME, Copin MC, Gosselin BH. Bronchogenic cysts of the lung. Ann Thorac Surg 1996;61:1636–1640.

175. Rogers LF, Osmer JC. Bronchogenic cyst: a review of 46 cases. AJR Am J Roentgenol 1964;1991:273–283.

176. Eraklis AJ, Griscom NT, McGovern JB. Bronchogenic cysts of the mediastinum in infancy. N Engl J Med 1969;281:1150–1155.

177. Weichert RF 3rd, Lindsey ES, Pearce CW, et al. Bronchogenic cyst with unilateral obstructive emphysema. J Thorac Cardiovasc Surg 1970;59:287–291.

178. Bankoff MS, Daly BD, Johnson HA, et al. Bronchogenic cyst causing superior vena cava obstruction: CT appearance. J Comput Assist Tomogr 1985;9:951–952.

179. Miller DC, Walter JP, Guthaner DF, et al. Recurrent mediastinal bronchogenic cyst. Cause of bronchial obstruction and compression of superior vena cava and pulmonary artery. Chest 1978;74:218–220.

180. Kirwan WO, Walbaum PR, McCormack RJ. Cystic intrathoracic derivatives of the foregut and their complications. Thorax 1973;28:424–428.

181. Watts WJ, Rotman HH, Patten GA. Pulmonary artery compression by a bronchogenic cyst simulating congenital pulmonary artery stenosis. Am J Cardiol 1984;53:347–348.

182. Worsley DF, Johnson RD, Kwong JS. Bronchogenic cyst causing unilateral ventilation-perfusion mismatch. Clin Nucl Med 1996;21:249–250.

183. Worsnop CJ, Teichtahl H, Clarke CP. Bronchogenic cyst: a cause of pulmonary artery obstruction and breathlessness. Ann Thorac Surg 1993;55:1254–1255.

184. Matzinger MA, Matzinger FR, Sachs HJ. Intrapulmonary bronchogenic cyst: spontaneous pneumothorax as the presenting symptom. AJR Am J Roentgenol 1992;158:987–988.

185. Boyd DP, Midell AI. Mediastinal cysts and tumors. An analysis of 96 cases. Surg Clin North Am 1968;48:493–505.

186. Ochsner JL, Ochsner SF. Congenital cysts of the mediastinum: 20-year experience with 42 cases. Ann Surg 1966;163:909–920.

187. Bergstrom JF, Yost RV, Ford KT, et al. Unusual roentgen manifestations of bronchogenic cysts. Radiology 1973;107:49–54.

188. Woodring JH, Vandiviere HM, Dillon ML. Air-filled, multilocular, bronchopulmonary foregut duplication cyst of the mediastinum. Unusual computed tomography appearance. Clin Imaging 1989;13:44–47.

189. Lyon RD, McAdams HP. Mediastinal bronchogenic cyst: demonstration of a fluid-fluid level at MR imaging. Radiology 1993;186:427–428.

190. Mendelson DS, Rose JS, Efremidis SC, et al. Bronchogenic cysts with high CT numbers. AJR Am J Roentgenol 1983;140:463–465.

191. Nakata H, Nakayama C, Kimoto T, et al. Computed tomography of mediastinal bronchogenic cysts. J Comput Assist Tomogr 1982;6:733–738.

192. Yernault JC, Kuhn G, Dumortier P, et al. "Solid" mediastinal bronchogenic cyst: mineralogic analysis. AJR Am J Roentgenol 1986;146:73–74.

193. Ries T, Currarino G, Nikaidoh H, et al. Real-time ultrasonography of subcarinal bronchogenic cysts in two children. Radiology 1982;145:121–122.

194. Albright EB, Crane JP, Shackelford GD. Prenatal diagnosis of a bronchogenic cyst. J Ultrasound Med 1988;7:90–95.

195. Rahmani MR, Filler RM, Shuckett B. Bronchogenic cyst occurring in the antenatal period. J Ultrasound Med 1995;14:971–973.

196. Young G, L'Heureux PR, Krueckeberg ST, et al. Mediastinal bronchogenic cyst: prenatal sonographic diagnosis. AJR Am J Roentgenol 1989;152:125–127.

197. Barakos JA, Brown JJ, Brescia RJ, et al. High signal intensity lesions of the chest in MR imaging. J Comput Assist Tomogr 1989;13:797–802.

198. Brasch RC, Gooding CA, Lallemand DP, et al. Magnetic resonance imaging of the thorax in childhood. Work in progress. Radiology 1984;150:463–467.

199. Marin ML, Romney BM, Franco K, et al. Bronchogenic cyst: a case report emphasizing the role of magnetic resonance imaging. J Thorac Imaging 1991;6:43–46.

200. Naidich DP, Rumancik WM, Ettenger NA, et al. Congenital anomalies of the lungs in adults: MR diagnosis. AJR Am J Roentgenol 1988;151:13–19.

201. Palmer WE, Rivitz SM, Chew FS. Bilateral bronchogenic cysts. AJR Am J Roentgenol 1991;157:950.

202. Suen HC, Mathisen DJ, Grillo HC, et al. Surgical management and radiological characteristics of bronchogenic cysts. Ann Thorac Surg 1993;55:476–481.

203. Schwartz DB, Beals TF, Wimbish KJ, et al. Transbronchial fine needle aspiration of bronchogenic cysts. Chest 1985;88:573–575.

204. Fitch SJ, Tonkin IL, Tonkin AK. Imaging of foregut duplication cysts. Radiographics 1986;6:189–201.

205. Whyte MK, Dollery CT, Adam A, Ind PW. Central bronchogenic cyst: treatment by extrapleural percutaneous aspiration. Br Med J 1989;299:1457–1458.

206. Stocker JT, Drake RM, Madewell JE. Cystic and congenital lung disease in the newborn. In: Rosenberg H, Bolande R, editors. Perspectives in pediatric pathology. Chicago, 1978: 93–154.

207. DeParedes CG, Pierce WS, Johnson DG, et al. Pulmonary sequestration in infants and children: a 20-year experience and review of the literature. J Pediatr Surg 1970;5:136–147.

208. Blesovsky A. Pulmonary sequestration. A report of an unusual case and a review of the literature. Thorax 1967;22:351–357.

209. Felker RE, Tonkin IL. Imaging of pulmonary sequestration. AJR Am J Roentgenol 1990;154:241–249.

210. Kirks DR, Kane PE, Free EA, et al. Systemic arterial supply to normal basilar segments of the left lower lobe. Am J Roentgenol 1976;126:817–821.

211. Chabbert V, Doussau-Thuron S, Otal P, et al. Endovascular treatment of aberrant systemic arterial supply to normal basilar segments of the right lower lobe: case report and review of the literature. Cardiovasc Intervent Radiol 2002;25: 212–215.

212. Kim TS, Lee KS, Im JG, et al. Systemic arterial supply to the normal basal segments of the left lower lobe: radiographic and CT findings in 11 patients. J Thorac Imaging 2002;17:34–39.

213. Ashizawa K, Ishida Y, Matsunaga N, et al. Anomalous systemic arterial supply to normal basal segments of left lower lobe: characteristic imaging findings. J Comput Assist Tomogr 2001;25:764–769.

214. Conran RM, Stocker JT. Extralobar sequestration with frequently associated congenital cystic adenomatoid malformation, type 2: report of 50 cases. Pediatr Dev Pathol 1999;2:454–463.

215. Rosado-de-Christenson ML, Frazier AA, et al. From the archives of the AFIP. Extralobar sequestration: radiologic-pathologic correlation. RadioGraphics 1993;13:425–441.

216. Stocker JT. Sequestrations of the lung. Semin Diagn Pathol 1986;3:106–121.

217. Stocker JT, Kagan-Hallet K. Extralobar pulmonary sequestration: analysis of 15 cases. Am J Clin Pathol 1979;72:917–925.

218. Benya EC, Bulas DI, Selby DM, et al. Cystic sonographic appearance of extralobar pulmonary sequestration. Pediatr Radiol 1993;23:605–607.

219. Hernanz-Schulman M, Johnson JE, Holcomb GW 3rd, et al. Retroperitoneal pulmonary sequestration: imaging findings, histopathologic correlation, and relationship to cystic adenomatoid malformation. AJR Am J Roentgenol 1997;168:1277–1281.

220. Morin C, Filiatrault D, Russo P. Pulmonary sequestration with histologic changes of cystic adenomatoid malformation. Pediatr Radiol 1989;19:130–132.

221. Zangwill BC, Stocker JT. Congenital cystic adenomatoid malformation within an extralobar pulmonary sequestration. Pediatr Pathol 1993;13:309–315.

222. King SJ, Pilling DW, Walkinshaw S. Fetal echogenic lung lesions: prenatal ultrasound diagnosis and outcome. Pediatr Radiol 1995;25:208–210.

223. Luetic T, Crombleholme TM, Semple JP, et al. Early prenatal diagnosis of bronchopulmonary sequestration with associated diaphragmatic hernia. J Ultrasound Med 1995;14:533–535.

224. Frazier AA, Rosado de Christenson ML, Stocker JT, et al. Intralobar sequestration: radiologic-pathologic correlation. RadioGraphics 1997;17:725–745.

225. Stocker JT, Malczak HT. A study of pulmonary ligament arteries. Relationship to intralobar pulmonary sequestration. Chest 1984;86:611–615.

226. Anon. Case records of the Massachusetts General Hospital (Case 48–1983). N Engl J Med 1983;309:1374–1381.

227. Eustace S, Valentine S, Murray J. Acquired intralobar bronchopulmonary sequestration secondary to occluding endobronchial carcinoid tumor. Clin Imaging 1996;20:178–180.

228. Hang JD, Guo QY, Chen CX, et al. Imaging approach to the diagnosis of pulmonary sequestration. Acta Radiol 1996;37:883–888.

229. Orme RI, Pugash RA. Intralobar pulmonary sequestration in the right lower lobe. J Canad Assoc Radiol 1997;48:51–53.

230. Levine MM, Nudel DB, Gootman N, et al. Pulmonary sequestration causing congestive heart failure in infancy: a report of two cases and review of the literature. Ann Thorac Surg 1982;34:581–585.

231. Reece EA, Lockwood CJ, Rizzo N, et al. Intrinsic intrathoracic malformations of the fetus: sonographic detection and clinical presentation. Obstet Gynecol 1987;70:627–632.

232. Stern E, Brill PW, Winchester P, Kosovsky P. Imaging of prenatally detected intra-abdominal extralobar pulmonary sequestration. Clin Imaging 1990;14:152–156.

233. Hernanz-Schulman M, Stein SM, Neblett WW, et al. Pulmonary sequestration: diagnosis with color Doppler sonography and a new theory of associated hydrothorax. Radiology 1991;180:817–821.

234. Kristoffersen SE, Ipsen L. Ultrasonic real time diagnosis of hydrothorax before delivery in an infant with extralobar lung sequestration. Acta Obstet Gynecol Scand 1984;63:723–725.

235. Lucaya J, Garcia-Conesa JA, Bernado L. Pulmonary sequestration associated with unilateral pulmonary hypoplasia and massive pleural effusion. A case report and review of the literature. Pediatr Radiol 1984;14:228–229.

236. Thomas CS, Leopold GR, Hilton S, et al. Fetal hydrops associated with extralobar pulmonary sequestration. J Ultrasound Med 1986;5:668–671.

237. Weiner C, Varner M, Pringle K, Hein H, Williamson R, Smith WL. Antenatal diagnosis and palliative treatment of nonimmune hydrops fetalis secondary to pulmonary extralobar sequestration. Obstet Gynecol 1986;68:275–280.

238. Hoeffel JC, Bernard C. Pulmonary sequestration of the upper lobe in children. Radiology 1986;160:513–514.

239. Ikezoe J, Murayama S, Godwin JD, et al. Bronchopulmonary sequestration: CT assessment. Radiology 1990;176:375–379.

240. Stern EJ, Webb WR, Warnock ML, et al. Bronchopulmonary sequestration: dynamic, ultrafast, high-resolution CT evidence of air trapping. AJR Am J Roentgenol 1991;157:947–949.

241. Van Dyke JA, Sagel SS. Calcified pulmonary sequestration: CT demonstration. J Comput Assist Tomogr 1985;9:372–374.

242. Demos NJ, Teresi A. Congenital lung malformations: a unified concept and a case report. J Thorac Cardiovasc Surg 1975;70:260–264.

243. Carter R. Pulmonary sequestration. Ann Thorac Surg 1969;7:68–88.

244. Cho SY, Kim HC, Bae SH, et al. Case report. Demonstration of blood supply to pulmonary sequestration by MR and CT angiography. J Comput Assist Tomogr 1996;20:993–995.

245. Frush DP, Donnelly LF. Pulmonary sequestration spectrum: a new spin with helical CT. AJR Am J Roentgenol 1997;169:679–682.

246. Miller PA, Williamson BR, Minor GR, et al. Pulmonary sequestration: visualization of the feeding artery by CT. J Comput Assist Tomogr 1982;6:828–830.

247. Smart LM, Hendry GM. Imaging of neonatal pulmonary sequestration including Doppler ultrasound. Br J Radiol 1991;64:324–329.

248. Yuan A, Yang PC, Chang DB, et al. Lung sequestration. Diagnosis with ultrasound and triplex Doppler technique in an adult. Chest 1992;102:1880–1882.

249. Zhang M, Zhu J, Wang Q, et al. Contrast enhanced MR angiography in pulmonary sequestration. Chin Med J (Engl) 2001;114:1326–1328.

250. Lehnhardt S, Winterer JT, Uhrmeister P, et al. Pulmonary sequestration: demonstration of blood supply with 2D and 3D MR angiography. Eur J Radiol 2002;44:28–32.

251. Xu H, Jiang D, Kong X, et al. Pulmonary sequestration: three dimensional dynamic contrast-enhanced MR angiography and MRI. J Tongji Med Univ 2001;21:345–348.

252. Dhingsa R, Coakley FV, Albanese CT, et al. Prenatal sonography and MR imaging of pulmonary sequestration. AJR Am J Roentgenol 2003;180:433–437.

253. Donovan CB, Edelman RR, Vrachliotis TG, et al. Bronchopulmonary sequestration with MR angiographic evaluation. A case report. Angiology 1994;45:239–244.

254. Doyle AJ. Demonstration of blood supply to pulmonary sequestration by MR angiography. AJR Am J Roentgenol 1992;158:989–990.

255. Pessar ML, Soulen RL, Kan JS, et al. MRI demonstration of pulmonary sequestration. Pediatr Radiol 1988;18:229–231.

256. Stannard PA, Sivananthan MU, Robertson RJ. Case report: the use of turbo-FLASH MRI for delineating vascular anatomy in bronchopulmonary sequestration. Clin Radiol 1994;49:286–287.

257. Patz EF, Jr., Müller NL, Swensen SJ, et al. Congenital cystic adenomatoid malformation in adults: CT findings. J Comput Assist Tomogr 1995;19:361–364.

258. Rosado-de-Christenson ML, Stocker JT. Congenital cystic adenomatoid malformation. Radiographics 1991;11:865–886.

259. Stocker JT, Madewell JE, Drake RM. Congenital cystic adenomatoid malformation of the lung. Classification and morphologic spectrum. Hum Pathol 1977;8:155–171.

260. Izzo C, Rickham PP. Neonatal pulmonary hamartoma. J Pediatr Surg 1968;3:77–83.

261. Cass DL, Crombleholme TM, Howell LJ, et al. Cystic lung lesions with systemic arterial blood supply: a hybrid of congenital cystic adenomatoid malformation and bronchopulmonary sequestration. J Pediatr Surg 1997;32:986–990.

262. Bush A. Congenital lung disease: a plea for clear thinking and clear nomenclature. Pediatr Pulmonol 2001;32:328–337.

263. Winters WD, Effmann EL, Nghiem HV, et al. Congenital masses of the lung: changes in cross-sectional area during gestation. J Clin Ultrasound 1997;25:372–377.

264. Pinson CW, Harrison MW, Thornburg et al. Importance of fetal fluid imbalance in congenital cystic adenomatoid malformation of the lung. Am J Surg 1992;163:510–514.

265. Spence LD, Ahmed S, Keohane C, et al. Acute presentation of cystic adenomatoid malformation of the lung in a 9-year-old child. Pediatr Radiol 1995;25:572–573.

266. Walker J, Andmore RE. Respiratory problems and cystic adenomatoid malformations of the lung. Arch Dis Child 1990;65:649–650.

267. Wexler HA, Dapena MV. Congenital cystic adenomatoid malformation. A report of three unusual cases. Radiology 1978;126:737–741.

268. Lackner RP, Thompson AB 3rd, Rikkers LF, et al. Cystic adenomatoid malformation involving an entire lung in a 22–year-old woman. Ann Thorac Surg 1996;61:1827–1829.

269. Merenstein GB. Congenital cystic adenomatoid malformation: report of a case and review of the literature. Am J Dis Child 1979;118:772–776.

270. Torre W, Miguez E, Lorenzo MJ, et al. Type II cystic adenomatoid malformation: late diagnosis in a patient with a pulmonary mass. J Cardiovasc Surg (Torino) 1996;37:647–648.

271. Cloutier MM, Schaeffer DA, Hight D. Congenital cystic adenomatoid malformation. Chest 1993;103:761–764.

272. Plit ML, Blott JA, Lakis N, Murray J, Plit M. Clinical, radiographic and lung function features of diffuse congenital cystic adenomatoid malformation of the lung in an adult. Eur Respir J 1997;10:1680–1682.

273. Bromley B, Parad R, Estroff JA, Benacerraf BR. Fetal lung masses: prenatal course and outcome. J Ultrasound Med 1995;14:927–936.

274. Deacon CS, Smart PJ, Rimmer S. The antenatal diagnosis of congenital cystic adenomatoid malformation of the lung. Br J Radiol 1990;63:968–970.

275. Johnson JA, Rumack CM, Johnson ML, et al. Cystic adenomatoid malformation: antenatal demonstration. AJR Am J Roentgenol 1984;142:483–484.

276. Miller JA, Corteville JE, Langer JC. Congenital cystic adenomatoid malformation in the fetus: natural history and predictors of outcome. J Pediatr Surg 1996;31:805–808.

277. Winters WD, Effmann EL, Nghiem HV, et al. Disappearing fetal lung masses: importance of postnatal imaging studies. Pediatr Radiol 1997;27:535–539.

278. Kuller JA, Yankowitz J, Goldberg JD, et al. Outcome of antenatally diagnosed cystic adenomatoid malformations. Am J Obstet Gynecol 1992;167:1038–1041.

279. Harrison MR, Adzick NS, Jennings RW, et al. Antenatal intervention for congenital cystic adenomatoid malformation. Lancet 1990;336:965–967.

280. Madewell JE, Stocker JT, Korsower JM. Cystic adenomatoid malformation of the lung. Morphologic analysis. Am J Roentgenol Radium Ther Nucl Med 1975;124:436–448.

281. Heij HA, Ekkelkamp S, Vos A. Diagnosis of congenital cystic adenomatoid malformation of the lung in newborn infants and children. Thorax 1990;45:122–125.

282. Kim WS, Lee KS, Kim IO, et al. Congenital cystic adenomatoid malformation of the lung: CT-pathologic correlation. AJR Am J Roentgenol 1997;168:47–53.

283. Shackelford GD, Siegel MJ. CT appearance of cystic adenomatoid malformations. J Comput Assist Tomogr 1989;13:612–616.

284. Langman J. Medical embryology. Baltimore: Williams & Wilkins, 1981.

285. Panicek DM, Benson CB, Gottlieb RH, et al. The diaphragm: anatomic, pathologic, and radiologic considerations. RadioGraphics 1988;8:385–425.

286. Gross BR, D'Agostino C, Coren CV, et al. Prenatal and neonatal sonographic imaging of a central diaphragmatic hernia. Pediatr Radiol 1996;26:395–397.

287. Stevens RL, Mathers A, Hollman AS, et al. An unusual hernia: congenital pericardial effusion associated with liver herniation into the pericardial sac. Pediatr Radiol 1996;26:791–793.

288. Caskey CI, Zerhouni EA, Fishman EK, et al. Aging of the diaphragm: a CT study. Radiology 1989;171:385–389.

289. Harrison MR, Adzick NS, Estes JM, et al. A prospective study of the outcome for fetuses with diaphragmatic hernia. JAMA 1994;271:382–384.

290. Skidmore MD, Morrison SC, Gauderer MW, et al. Imaging case of the month: II. Central diaphragmatic hernia with herniation of the liver into the pericardial sac. Am J Perinatol 1991;8:356–358.

291. Guibaud L, Filiatrault D, Garel L, et al. Fetal congenital diaphragmatic hernia: accuracy of sonography in the diagnosis and prediction of the outcome after birth. AJR Am J Roentgenol 1996;166:1195–1202.

292. Sydorak RM, Goldstein R, Hirose S, et al. Congenital diaphragmatic hernia and hydrops: a lethal association? J Pediatr Surg 2002;37:1678–1680.

293. Cohen MS, Rychik J, Bush DM, et al. Influence of congenital heart disease on

survival in children with congenital diaphragmatic hernia. J Pediatr 2002;141:25–30.

294. Skari H, Bjornland K, Frenckner B, et al. Congenital diaphragmatic hernia in Scandinavia from 1995 to 1998: Predictors of mortality. J Pediatr Surg 2002;37:1269–1275.

295. Garne E, Haeusler M, Barisic I, et al. Congenital diaphragmatic hernia: evaluation of prenatal diagnosis in 20 European regions. Ultrasound Obstet Gynecol 2002;19:329–333.

296. Fu RH, Hsieh WS, Yang PH, et al. Diagnostic pitfalls in congenital right diaphragmatic hernia. Acta Paediatr Taiwan 2000;41:251–254.

297. Young LW, McClead RE, Graham M, et al. Radiological case of the month. Postnatal appearance of diaphragmatic hernia. Am J Dis Child 1978;132:1137–1138.

298. Fisichella PM, Perretta S, Di Stefano A, et al. Chronic liver herniation through a right Bochdalek hernia with acute onset in adulthood. Ann Ital Chir 2001;72:703–705.

299. Gayer G, Bilik R, Vardi A. CT diagnosis of delayed presentation of congenital diaphragmatic hernia simulating massive pleuropneumonia. Eur Radiol 1999;9:1672–1674.

300. Berman L, Stringer DA, Ein S, et al. Childhood diaphragmatic hernias presenting after the neonatal period. Clin Radiol 1988;39:237–244.

301. Malone PS, Brain AJ, Kiely EM, et al. Congenital diaphragmatic defects that present late. Arch Dis Child 1989;64:1542–1544.

302. McCarten KM, Rosenberg HK, Borden St, et al. Delayed appearance of right diaphragmatic hernia associated with group B streptococcal infection in newborns. Radiology 1981;139:385–389.

303. Chilton HW, Chang JH, Jones MD Jr, et al. Right-sided congenital diaphragmatic herniae presenting as pleural effusions in the newborn: dangers and pitfalls. Arch Dis Child 1978;53:600–603.

304. Benacerraf BR, Greene MF. Congenital diaphragmatic hernia: US diagnosis prior to 22 weeks gestation. Radiology 1986;158:809–810.

305. Stiller RJ, Roberts NS, Weiner S, et al. Congenital diaphragmatic hernia: antenatal diagnosis and obstetrical management. J Clin Ultrasound 1985;13:212–215.

306. Fuke S, Kanzaki T, Mu J, et al. Antenatal prediction of pulmonary hypoplasia by acceleration time/ejection time ratio of fetal pulmonary arteries by Doppler blood flow velocimetry. Am J Obstet Gynecol 2003;188:228–233.

307. Sokol J, Bohn D, Lacro RV, et al. Fetal pulmonary artery diameters and their association with lung hypoplasia and postnatal outcome in congenital diaphragmatic hernia. Am J Obstet Gynecol 2002;186:1085–1090.

308. Hubbard AM, Adzick NS, Crombleholme TM, et al. Left-sided congenital diaphragmatic hernia: value of prenatal MR imaging in preparation for fetal surgery. Radiology 1997;203:636–640.

309. Paek BW, Coakley FV, Lu Y, et al. Congenital diaphragmatic hernia: prenatal evaluation with MR lung volumetry—preliminary experience. Radiology 2001;220:63–67.

310. Liu X, Ashtari M, Leonidas JC, et al. Magnetic resonance imaging of the fetus in congenital intrathoracic disorders: preliminary observations. Pediatr Radiol 2001;31:435–439.

311. Williams HJ, Johnson KJ. Imaging of congenital cystic lung lesions. Paediatr Respir Rev 2002;3:120–127.

312. White JJ, Suzuki H. Hernia through the foramen of Bochdalek: a misnomer. J Pediatr Surg 1972;7:60–61.

313. Gale ME. Bochdalek hernia: prevalence and CT characteristics. Radiology 1985;156:449–452.

314. Kumcuoglu Z, Sener RN. Bochdalek's hernia: CT findings. AJR Am J Roentgenol 1992;158:1168–1169.

315. Sener RN, Tugran C, Yorulmaz I, et al. Orguc S. Bilateral large Bochdalek hernias in an adult. CT demonstration. Clin Imaging 1995;19:40–42.

316. Gierada DS, Slone RM, Fleishman MJ. Imaging evaluation of the diaphragm. Chest Surg Clin N Am 1998;8:237–280.

317. Collie DA, Turnbull CM, Shaw TR, et al. Case report: MRI appearances of left sided Morgagni hernia containing liver. Br J Radiol 1996;69:278–280.

318. de Lange EE, Urbanski SR, Mugler JP 3rd, et al. Magnetization-prepared rapid gradient echo (MP-RAGE) magnetic resonance imaging of Morgagni's hernia. Eur J Radiol 1990;11:196–199.

319. Yeager BA, Guglielmi GE, Schiebler ML, et al. Magnetic resonance imaging of Morgagni hernia. Gastrointest Radiol 1987;12:296–298.

320. Wille L, Holthusen W, Willich E. Accessory diaphragm. Report of 6 cases and a review of the literature. Pediatr Radiol 1975;4:14–20.

321. Becmeur F, Horta P, Donato L, et al. Accessory diaphragm—review of 31 cases in the literature. Eur J Pediatr Surg 1995;5:43–47.

322. Smrek M, Vidiscak M. Accessory diaphragm—review of 31 cases in the literature. Eur J Pediatr Surg 1995;5:253.

CHAPTER 17

Chest trauma

Over the past 10–20 years, accidental trauma has been the fourth leading cause of death in men in the United States and the eighth leading cause of death in women.[1] During the same period, accidental trauma was the leading cause of death in young adults between the ages of 10 and 35. Similar figures are reported in Europe.[2] The thorax is a frequent site of significant injury in traumatized patients.[2] The overall mortality rate for chest trauma is approximately 15%, but it approaches 80% when associated with shock and head injury.[3] Survival frequently depends upon rapid diagnosis and treatment of life-threatening thoracic injuries. Some of the more important thoracic injuries include aortic or great vessel injury, rupture of the trachea, esophagus and diaphragm, pulmonary laceration and contusion, and fractures of the ribs or spine.

The supine anteroposterior portable chest radiograph remains one of the first tests ordered for acutely traumatized patients. The chest radiograph provides a wealth of information about potential thoracic injuries and should be carefully scrutinized for signs of pneumothorax or pneumomediastinum, pleural fluid, pulmonary opacities suggesting contusion, rib and spine fractures, or diaphragm rupture. Identification of correct positioning of endotracheal or orogastric tubes or other cardio-vascular support equipment is of equal importance. However, assessment of the mediastinum is perhaps the most critical aspect of interpretation of the chest radiograph in patients with blunt thoracic trauma. Widening of the mediastinum or abnormal mediastinal contours on the chest radiograph are important indicators of mediastinal hemorrhage and, when present, suggest the possibility of aortic or great vessel injury.

The advent of CT scanning, and, in particular, fast helical CT scanning has revolutionized the noninvasive evaluation of the acutely traumatized patient. CT can demonstrate with far greater clarity than the chest radiograph many of the indirect or direct signs of injury. Tracheobronchial tears can be visualized; aortic injury can either be diagnosed conclusively or excluded with confidence; and most diaphragm injuries are well demonstrated on CT. Fractures, contusions, and pneumothoraces are also shown with greater clarity. For these reasons, some authors have advocated the very liberal use of CT in patients with severe blunt thoracic trauma.[3–6] While CT is unlikely to supplant chest radiography as the initial screen in patients with suspected chest trauma, its role in the evaluation of these patients will continue to become more important.

In this chapter, many of the most important manifestations of thoracic injuries are reviewed, emphasizing in particular those due to blunt trauma.

INJURY TO THE AORTA OR GREAT VESSELS

Severe blunt aortic injury (BAI) is often lethal. It is estimated that 85% of affected patients die at the scene of the accident; only 10–20% survive the initial injury.[7] Rapid diagnosis of severe BAI in survivors is critical; undiagnosed, 30% of affected patients die in the first 6 h and 40–50% die in the first 24 h.[4,7] A small percentage of affected patients survive undiagnosed and may develop a chronic pseudoaneurysm (Figs 17.1 and 17.2).[8] The most common causes of BAI are high-speed motor vehicle

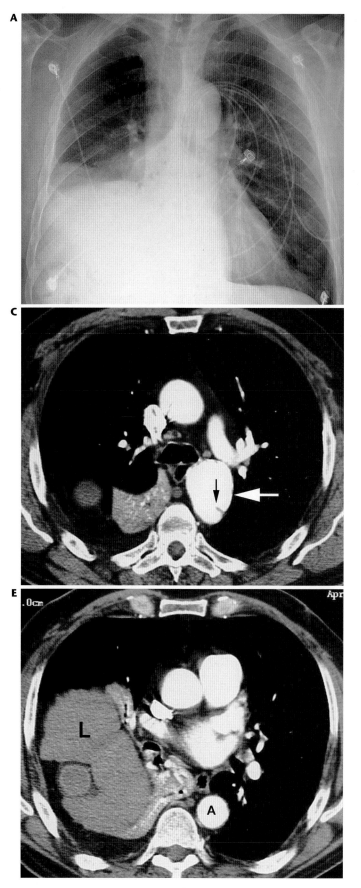

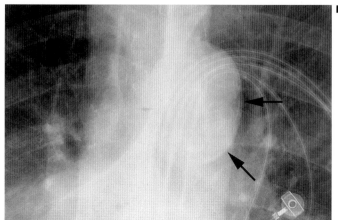

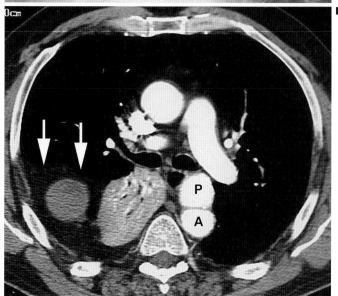

Fig. 17.1 Posttraumatic aortic pseudoaneurysm in a 65-year-old man who presented for evaluation of an abdominal aortic aneurysm 25 years after a severe motor vehicle accident. **A**, Frontal and **B**, coned-down chest radiographs show marked elevation of the right diaphragm and a contour abnormality along the proximal descending thoracic aorta. Note the curvilinear calcification (arrows on **B**). **C–E**, Contrast-enhanced CT scans show a pseudoaneurysm (white arrow on **C**, P on **D**) at the aortic isthmus and an intimal flap (black arrow on **C**). Note also the evidence of prior right diaphragm rupture with herniation of omental fat (white arrows on **D**) and liver (L on **E**) into the right hemithorax. A = descending thoracic aorta.

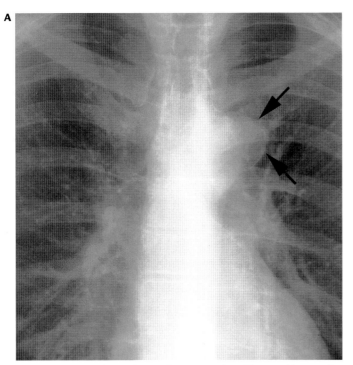 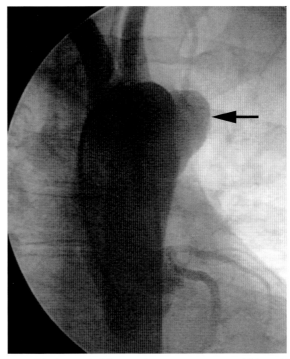

Fig. 17.2 Posttraumatic aortic pseudoaneurysm in a 35-year-old man who presents with chest pain 10 years after a severe motor vehicle accident. **A**, Frontal chest radiograph shows a focal contour abnormality (arrows) of the aortic arch. **B**, Aortogram confirms a focal pseudoaneurysm (arrow) of the proximal descending thoracic aorta.

accidents, falls from significant heights, and airplane crashes. However, BAI has been reported after a wide variety of less severe traumas.

The severity of BAI varies from a minimal intimal tear to complete transection of the aorta. However, the latter injury is rarely encountered in living patients, for obvious reasons. In autopsy series, the three most common sites of BAI are the aortic root, the aortic isthmus (site of the ligamentum arteriosum), and at the diaphragmatic hiatus. Avulsion of a great vessel is another potential, but uncommon, site of injury. The reported distribution of injuries between these sites varies. In autopsy series, BAI is about equally distributed between the aortic root and the isthmus; injuries at the diaphragm are rare.[9] In surviving patients, however, 95% of BAI are found at the isthmus (Figs 17.1 and 17.2).[10] Five percent are found in the ascending aorta (Fig. 17.3) and <1% are found in the descending thoracic aorta (Fig. 17.4).[11]

BAI is generally believed to be due to shearing and twisting stresses that result from rapid deceleration (Box 17.1). These forces are concentrated at sites of aortic attachment: the aortic root, isthmus, and diaphragmatic hiatus. Crass and Cohen[12,13] proposed an alternate mechanism for BAI at the aortic isthmus. They suggested that compression of the anterior chest causes the manubrium to arc posteriorly and inferiorly, the axis of rotation being the spinal attachments of the first ribs. The aortic isthmus is then "pinched" and injured between the manubrium and the spine.[14]

Chest radiography

As noted above, the chest radiograph is frequently the first (along with a lateral view of the cervical spine) imaging test requested on patients with suspected BAI. Fundamentally, the chest radiograph

Box 17.1 Blunt aortic injury

Mechanism of injury
Rapid deceleration in motor vehicle accidents, airplane crashes, and falls

Mechanics of injury
Shearing and twisting forces, particularly at points of transition between relatively mobile and relatively fixed vascular structures
The "osseous pinch" mechanism

Site of injury in surviving patients
95% in the aortic isthmus region
1% in the distal descending aorta
<5% in the ascending aorta

Survival statistics
85% die at the accident site
Of the survivors:
• 30% die within 6 h
• 50% die within 24 h
• 98% die within 4 months
• 2% longterm survivors

is used to screen for mediastinal hemorrhage, an indirect marker for BAI. However, because there are many causes for mediastinal hematoma in seriously injured patients other than BAI (e.g. sternal fracture, venous bleeding, spinal fractures), this finding is quite nonspecific. The great majority of patients with mediastinal hematoma evident on chest radiography (or CT) will prove *not* to have BAI by CT angiography or aortography.

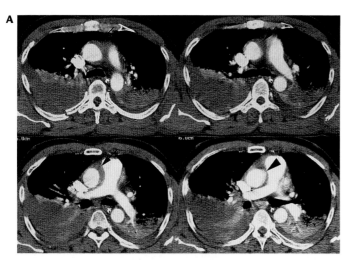

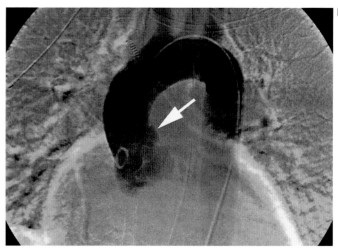

Fig. 17.3 Blunt aortic injury in a 20-year-old man after a high-speed motor vehicle accident. The chest radiograph (not shown) showed a wide mediastinum. **A,** CT shows focal periaortic hematoma (arrows) adjacent to the ascending aorta. The small focal pseudoaneurysm (arrowhead) was not initially appreciated. **B,** Aortogram performed on the basis of periaortic hematoma shows the focal pseudoaneurysm (arrow) in the ascending aorta to better advantage.

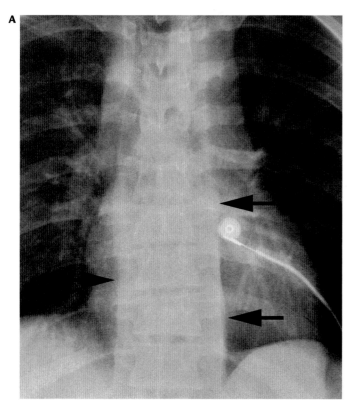

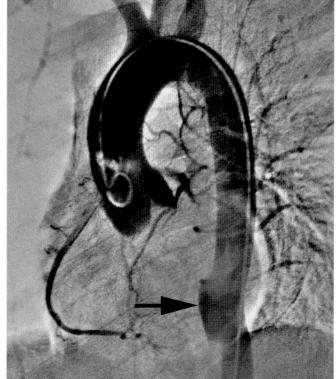

Fig. 17.4 Blunt aortic injury in a young man after a high-speed motor vehicle accident. **A,** Frontal chest radiograph shows widening of both the left and right paraspinal reflections (arrows). No spine fracture is seen. **B,** Aortogram shows a focal pseudoaneurysm (arrow) just above the diaphragm.

Box 17.2 Chest radiographic findings of blunt aortic injury (adapted from reference⁴)

Mediastinal widening
- Width >8 cm above the aortic arch on a supine examination with a film focus distance of 40 inches
- Mediastinal width/thoracic width >0.25 at this level

Obscuration of the aortic arch
Shift of trachea to the right
Shift of orogastric tube (esophagus) to the right
Left apical pleural cap
Widened left paraspinal reflection
Widened right paraspinal reflection
Opacification of the aortopulmonary window
Widened right paratracheal stripe
Displaced superior vena cava
Depressed left main bronchus
Evidence of significant chest trauma
- Multiple rib fractures (especially first rib)
- Lung contusion
- Hemothorax
- Pneumothorax

There is extensive literature documenting the various radiographic findings of mediastinal hematoma, as summarized below and in Box 17.2. (Figs 17.4 to 17.6).[15–17]

Widening of the mediastinum is clearly an important finding of mediastinal hemorrhage after BAI (Figs 17.5 and 17.6). Williams et al[18] found that mediastinal widening was the single most reliable radiographic sign of BAI. However, reliable criteria for diagnosis of mediastinal widening are difficult to establish due to variations in radiographic technique (focal film distance), patient positioning, patient size, obesity, and age. Proposed criteria have included a mediastinal width exceeding 8 cm just above the aortic arch,[19] or a ratio of the width of the mediastinum

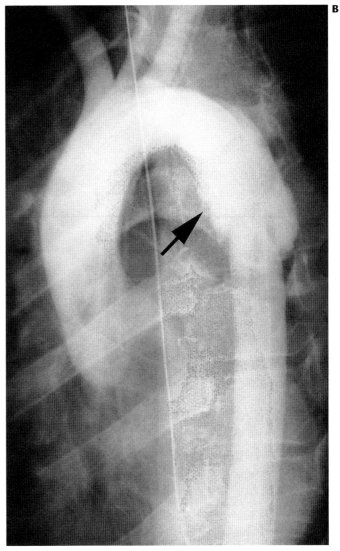

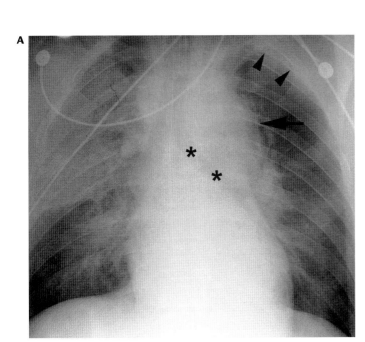

Fig. 17.5 Blunt aortic injury in a middle-aged adult after a high-speed motor vehicle accident. **A**, Frontal chest radiograph shows a wide mediastinum. Note that the aortic arch (arrow) is obscured, the left main bronchus (*) is inferiorly displaced, and there is a left apical cap (arrowheads). The endotracheal and orogastric tubes are not displaced, however. **B**, Aortogram shows a complete aortic disruption with a large pseudoaneurysm (arrow) at the isthmus.

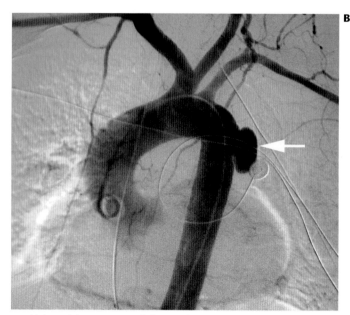

Fig. 17.6   Blunt aortic injury in a middle-aged man after a high-speed motor vehicle accident. **A,** Frontal chest radiograph shows a wide mediastinum and left lung contusion. Note that the aortic arch and descending thoracic aorta are obscured, there is a left apical cap, and both the endotracheal and orogastric tubes (arrowheads) are displaced to the right. **B,** Aortogram shows a focal pseudoaneurysm (arrow) at the isthmus.

to the width of the chest exceeding 0.25 at the same level.[20] However, Williams et al[18] concluded that use of absolute figures for diagnosis of mediastinal hemorrhage was impractical. Furthermore, BAI is occasionally found in patients with normal mediastinal measurements.[21]

Mirvis et al[22] found that an erect anteroposterior view of the chest obtained at full inspiration was more valuable for detecting a true negative mediastinum than a supine view. While such a radiograph performed with pristine technique is clearly most desirable and useful, such views are often difficult to obtain in severely traumatized patients. Thus, many radiographs are obtained with suboptimal technique, so that confident exclusion of mediastinal hematoma, particularly if the patient is thickset or obese, may be impossible.

Obscuration of the normal contours of the aortic arch and descending aorta and opacification of the anteroposterior window are important findings that suggest perivascular mediastinal hematoma (Figs 17.5 and 17.6). Mirvis et al[22] found these signs to be among the best radiographic discriminators for BAI. Furthermore, these signs may be more specifically applied to interpretation of trauma chest radiographs.

Displacement of normal structures such as the trachea, left main bronchus, and esophagus are also important radiographic findings of perivascular hematoma. Hematoma at the aortic isthmus can displace the left main bronchus downward (Fig. 17.5), and the trachea and esophagus to the right (Fig. 17.6). Marnocha et al[23] found that depression of the left main bronchus to below 40° off horizontal was a specific finding of BAI. Tracheal deviation may be more difficult to diagnose because the trachea normally deviates to the right at the level of the aortic arch, and minor degrees of patient rotation can either artificially accentuate or minimize the finding. Because the esophagus descends adjacent to the right lateral wall of the aorta at the isthmus, lateral

deviation of the esophagus (as indicated by the position of an orogastric tube) is also a good indicator of perivascular hematoma (Fig. 17.6).[24,25]

Hemorrhage into anatomically contiguous regions such as the pleural space, paravertebral soft tissues or apex of the thorax can result in further important radiographic findings that suggest BAI. Hemothorax, particularly on the left, should immediately suggest the possibility of BAI. Widening of the paravertebral reflections (Figs 17.4 and 17.7)[26] also suggests mediastinal hemorrhage. Care must be taken not to confuse paraspinal hematoma due to vertebral fractures with mediastinal hematoma due to BAI (Fig. 17.8).[27] Mirvis et al[22] found that widening of the left paraspinal reflection (Fig. 17.4) without associated spine fracture was one of the most discriminating radiographic findings for BAI. Mediastinal hematomas may dissect over the lung apices, forming so-called apical "caps" which are more common on the left (Fig. 17.5).[28] This finding is particularly important when there are no associated fractures of the upper ribs.

Other radiographic findings such as upper rib or scapular fractures, pulmonary contusion, or pneumothorax indicate that a significant transfer of force to the thorax has occurred.[4] The importance of such findings in isolation, particularly upper rib and scapular fractures, and in the context of suspected BAI, is controversial. Most authors have concluded that isolated first rib fractures with an otherwise normal chest radiograph are not sufficient indication for angiography.[29–33]

There is an extensive literature discussing the sensitivity, specificity, and pitfalls of chest radiography for diagnosis of BAI. In summary, the chest radiograph is widely considered a sensitive, but very nonspecific, test for BAI. Mirvis et al[22] reported that a normal chest radiograph had a 98% negative predictive value for BAI. However, there are dissenting opinions.

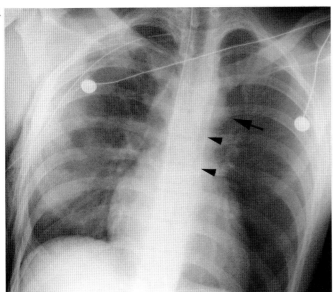

Fig. 17.7 Blunt aortic injury in a 19-year-old man after a high-speed motor vehicle accident. **A**, Frontal chest radiograph shows subtle obscuration of the contour of the descending thoracic aorta (arrow) and mild widening of the left paraspinal reflection (arrowheads). The mediastinum is otherwise normal in appearance. The orogastric tube appears displaced, but this finding is due to rotation. Note the subtle right pneumothorax and right lung contusion. **B**, CT shows perivascular and paraspinal hematoma (arrows). Note the small anterior pseudoaneurysm (*) at the isthmus.

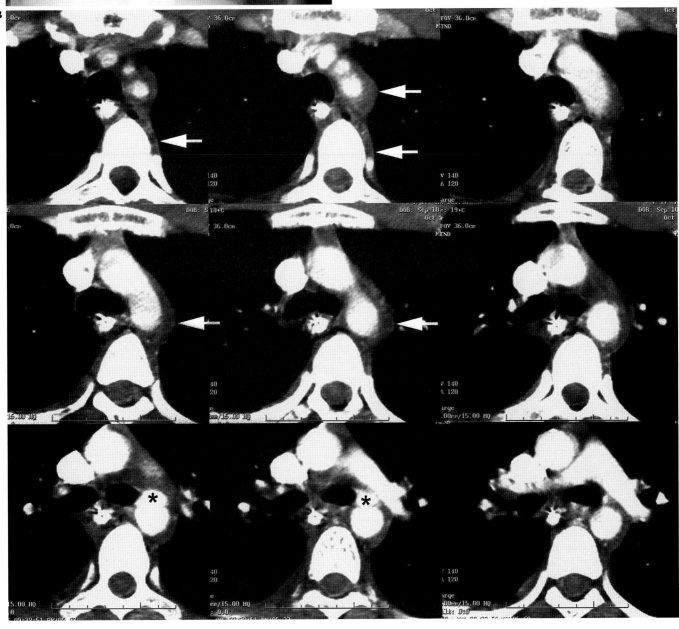

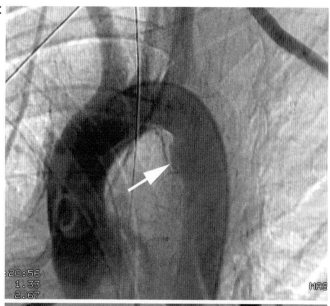

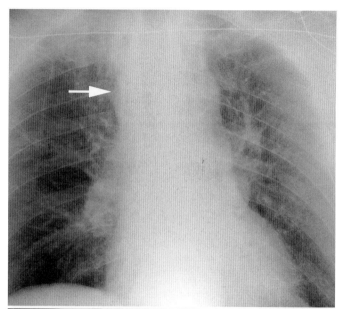

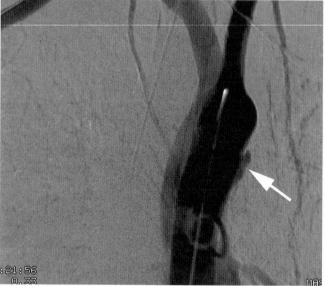

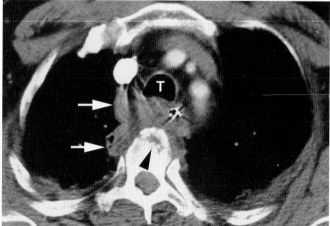

Fig. 17.7 (*cont'd*) **C**, Aortogram confirms the presence of a small pseudoaneurysm (arrows) at the isthmus.

Fig. 17.8 Blunt aortic injury in a middle-aged man after a high-speed motor vehicle accident. **A**, Frontal chest radiograph shows widening of the right paratracheal stripe (arrow). Note that the contours of the aortic arch and descending thoracic aorta are preserved and that the orogastric tube is in the normal position. **B**, CT shows an anterior vertebral body fracture (arrowhead). Note that the paravertebral hematoma displaces the trachea (T) anteriorly and dissects (arrows) along the right side of the mediastinum. The aorta was normal (not shown).

Woodring[17] reviewed 52 published studies of patients with BAI and found that 7% of patients with proved BAI had normal chest radiographs, concluding that a normal chest radiograph does not confidently exclude BAI. However, many of the studies reviewed were quite old, radiographic technique was inconsistent, and the criteria used to diagnose mediastinal hematoma varied. Fabian et al[34] reported that 2% of patients with BAI had a normal chest radiograph. Dyer et al[4] prospectively evaluated over 1500 patients with suspected BAI and found that four of 30 (13%) patients with traumatic aortic injuries had normal chest radiographs. However, they also noted that all four patients had only isolated intimal aortic injuries ("minimal" BAI, see below) and that none of the patients with "significant" aortic injuries had normal radiographs. Their study also confirmed the low specificity and positive predictive value of an abnormal chest radiograph in the setting of chest trauma. Almost two-thirds of their patients had an abnormal chest radiograph, but <3% of these had BAI. Although the value of the chest radiograph for excluding BAI continues to be debated, particularly given the advent of high-speed readily available helical CT scanning, many authors believe that the chest radiograph continues to be a useful examination in this setting.

Computed tomography

There is no doubt that high-speed helical CT scanning has revolutionized the noninvasive evaluation of seriously injured patients. In particular, CT has had a tremendous impact upon the investigation of suspected BAI (Box 17.3). Not only can CT confidently exclude significant BAI,[4,7,35-43] it can diagnose angiographically occult aortic intimal injuries and evaluate the thorax for other injuries.

Historically, CT was first used to select patients for further evaluation with aortography.[44-54] Using this approach, patients with abnormal chest radiographs underwent noncontrast CT (Fig. 17.9). If CT showed mediastinal hematoma, the patient was then referred for aortography. If the mediastinum was normal, aortography was not performed. While such an approach clearly reduces the number of aortograms performed on the basis of abnormal chest radiographs, it is not optimal. Dyer et al,[7] for example, showed that while such an approach detected all cases of BAI (100% sensitivity), the positive predictive value of an abnormal CT was only 7%.

Current generation multidetector CT scanners allow very rapid acquisition of very thin-slice axial images through the thorax. Furthermore, these data sets can be reconstructed in multiple planes.[55,56] In a very real sense, high quality angiography of the thoracic aorta can be performed using CT. A high quality CT angiogram requires rapid bolus administration of intravenous contrast (typically between 2.5 and 4 ml per s), thin-slice collimation (2.5 mm or less), and overlapping reconstruction intervals.

With the advent of helical CT angiography, the focus has shifted from identification of indirect findings, such as mediastinal hematoma, to identification of direct signs of BAI: intimal flaps, aortic contour irregularities and caliber changes, and pseudoaneurysm formation (Figs 17.7, 17.10, and 17.11). A number of large series have now been reported emphasizing the very high sensitivity of this approach for diagnosis of BAI and the very high negative predictive value of a normal study (Figs 17.12 and 17.13). Dyer et al[4,7] reported a sensitivity of 95% for BAI and a 99.9% negative predictive value using only direct signs for diagnosis on CT. When they included periaortic hematoma as an additional positive finding, both their sensitivity and negative predictive value improved to 100%. Fabian et al[35] prospectively evaluated 494 patients with suspected BAI and reported that the sensitivity and negative predictive value of CT was 100 and 100%, respectively. In the same group of patients, the sensitivity and negative predictive value of angiography was 92 and 97%, respectively. Parker et al[38] prospectively evaluated 142 patients with both CT and angiography and reported 100% sensitivity and 100% negative predictive value for both modalities. Other recent studies have also confirmed the high sensitivity for diagnosis of BAI and high negative predictive value for exclusion of BAI by CT angiography.[40,41]

A number of recent articles have debated the merits of using direct versus indirect signs for diagnosis or exclusion of BAI.[36,39,41] Fishman et al[36] found that, when they used direct signs for diagnosis alone, not only did their accuracy of diagnosis improve (with no loss of sensitivity), but the intraobserver variability for

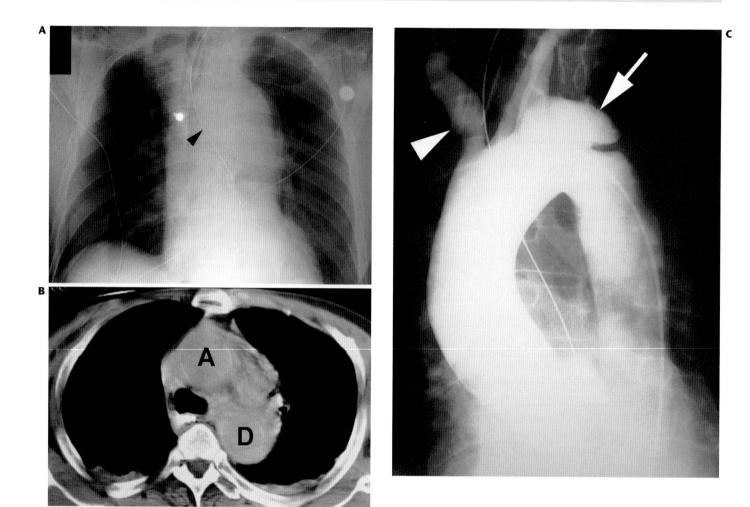

Fig. 17.9 Blunt aortic injury in a middle-aged woman after a high-speed motor vehicle accident. **A**, Frontal chest radiograph shows marked widening of the mediastinum and deviation of the orogastric tube (arrowhead) to the right. **B**, Noncontrast CT shows extensive mediastinal hematoma. A = ascending aorta; D = descending aorta. **C**, Aortogram shows a large pseudoaneurysm (arrow) at the isthmus. Note also the focal dilation of the proximal right brachiocephalic artery (arrowhead), suggesting concomitant branch vessel injury.

diagnosis improved as well. Cleverly et al[39] found that using direct signs enabled diagnosis of all surgically proved cases of BAI. Interestingly, 9% of patients with BAI in their series had no periaortic hematoma.

In summary, there is a growing body of evidence that suggests that helical CT angiography has both a very high sensitivity (close to 100%) and a high negative predictive value (also close to 100%) for diagnosis or exclusion of BAI (Table 17.1).

Furthermore, evidence suggests that if the criteria for diagnosis of BAI are restricted to the direct signs of aortic injury (intimal flaps, aortic contour irregularities and caliber changes, and pseudoaneurysm formation) or periaortic hematoma, specificity can be substantially improved without an adverse effect on either sensitivity or negative predictive value. It almost goes without saying, however, that to achieve these results requires careful attention to CT acquisition technique. Using such an approach,

Table 17.1 Guidelines for aortic imaging (adapted from reference[4])

Clinical suspicion (based on severity of trauma and mechanism of injury)	Findings on chest radiography	Recommended imaging To detect significant aortic injury	To detect all (including intimal) aortic injuries
Medium–high	Suspect mediastinal hematoma	CT	CT
Medium–high	Normal	None	CT
Low	Suspect mediastinal hematoma	CT	CT
Low	Normal	None	None

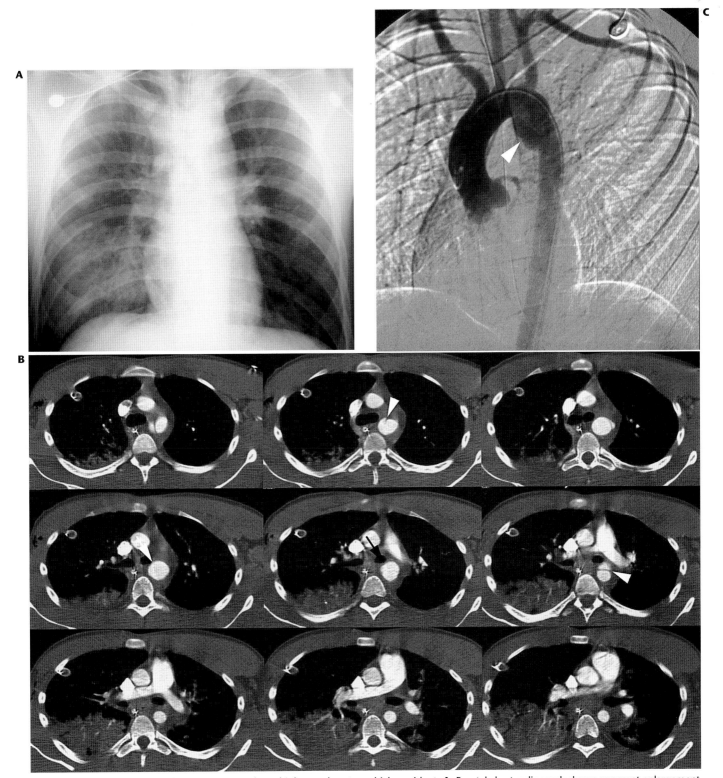

Fig. 17.10   Blunt aortic injury in a young man after a high-speed motor vehicle accident. **A**, Frontal chest radiograph shows apparent enlargement of the proximal descending thoracic aorta and subtle lateral displacement of the orogastric tube. Note the right pneumothorax and right lower lobe contusion. **B**, CT shows a perivascular hematoma, a complex intimal flap (arrowheads), focal dilation of the proximal descending aorta (pseudoaneurysm, arrows), and apparent narrowing of the distal descending aorta (pseudocoarctation). These features are diagnostic of blunt aortic injury. **C**, An aortogram was performed which confirmed the aortic injury (arrowhead), but wasted potentially valuable time.

Fig. 17.11 Blunt aortic injury in a young man who presented after a high-speed motor vehicle accident. The chest radiograph (not shown) suggested mediastinal hematoma. CT shows perivascular hematoma (arrowhead) in the left superior mediastinum, focal dilation of the proximal descending aorta (pseudoaneurysm, arrows), and an intimal flap at the isthmus. These CT features are diagnostic of blunt aortic injury. Angiography was not performed and the injury was promptly repaired.

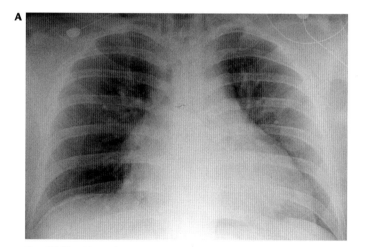

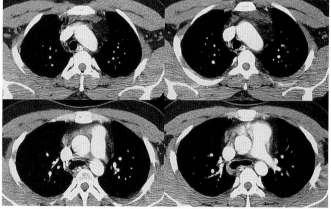

Fig. 17.12 Normal aorta in a 28-year-old man after a high-speed motor vehicle accident. **A,** Frontal chest radiograph shows a wide mediastinum. **B,** CT shows soft tissue in the anterior mediastinum that likely represents residual thymus. The periaortic fat planes are preserved and there are no specific indirect (perivascular hematoma) or direct signs of aortic injury.

patients with a normal appearing aorta and no periaortic hematoma on CT need not undergo further evaluation. Additionally, patients with a normal appearing aorta and isolated anterior mediastinal hematoma need not undergo further evaluation (Figs 17.2 and 17.13). Dyer et al,[4,7] for example, found that no patient with an isolated anterior mediastinal hematoma had BAI. Many authors[4,7,35] recommend that patients with a normal appearing aorta but who have periaortic hematoma should, in the appropriate clinical setting, undergo aortography.

The further management of patients with evidence of BAI on CT angiography is probably the most controversial issue at the present time. There are two important questions that await definitive answers. The first has to do with the management of patients with clearly significant BAI (long intimal tears, pseudoaneurysms) on CT. In many centers, such patients are still referred for angiography to confirm the CT diagnosis and to evaluate the relationship of the injury to the great vessels (Fig. 17.10). The latter information is important for determining

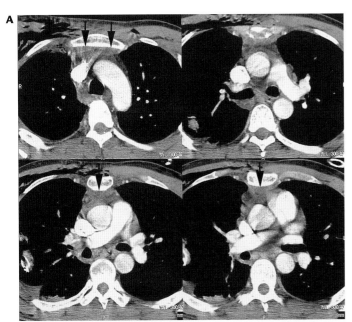

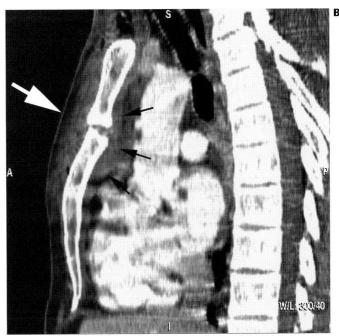

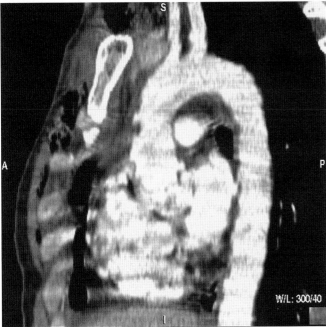

Fig. 17.13   Normal aorta in a 35-year-old man after a high-speed motor vehicle accident. **A**, CT shows an isolated anterior mediastinal hematoma. There are no direct signs of aortic injury. **B**, Sagittal reconstruction shows a fracture dislocation at the sternomanubrial joint (white arrow) and associated hematoma (black arrows). **C**, Sagittal reconstruction confirms a normal aortic isthmus and descending thoracic aorta.

operative approach and need for cardiopulmonary bypass. While this decision ultimately rests on the experience of the operating surgeon, a number of recent studies support the primary use of CT in this regard.[4,7,35,38,40,57] Multiplanar reconstruction techniques can yield images that are quite similar to those obtained at conventional angiography; in particular, sagittal reconstructions are usually adequate for surgical planning (Fig. 17.14).[4] Downing et al[57] reviewed their experience with the treatment of 54 patients with BAI and found that operating on the basis of the CT alone was both safe and expeditious. However, angiography may still be required to exclude great vessel injury in certain cases.[58] Suffice it to say that this issue has not been definitively resolved at the present time.

Perhaps a more interesting open question is the concept of minimal aortic injury (MAI). With the increasing use of high quality CT angiography (or endoscopic ultrasound), more and more subtle aortic intimal injuries are being diagnosed. Frequently, these injuries are detected in the absence of significant periaortic hematoma (Figs 17.15 and 17.16).[4,7,39,59–61] Malhotra et al[61] defined MAI as a small (<1 cm) intimal flap with no other aortic abnormality and no or minimal periaortic hematoma. In their series of 189 patients with BAI, 10% were found to have MAI by CT. Aortography was normal in half the patients with MAI; in these, the diagnosis was confirmed either by surgery or endovascular US. Follow-up studies in six of the nine patients with MAI showed that the lesion resolved in half and that a small

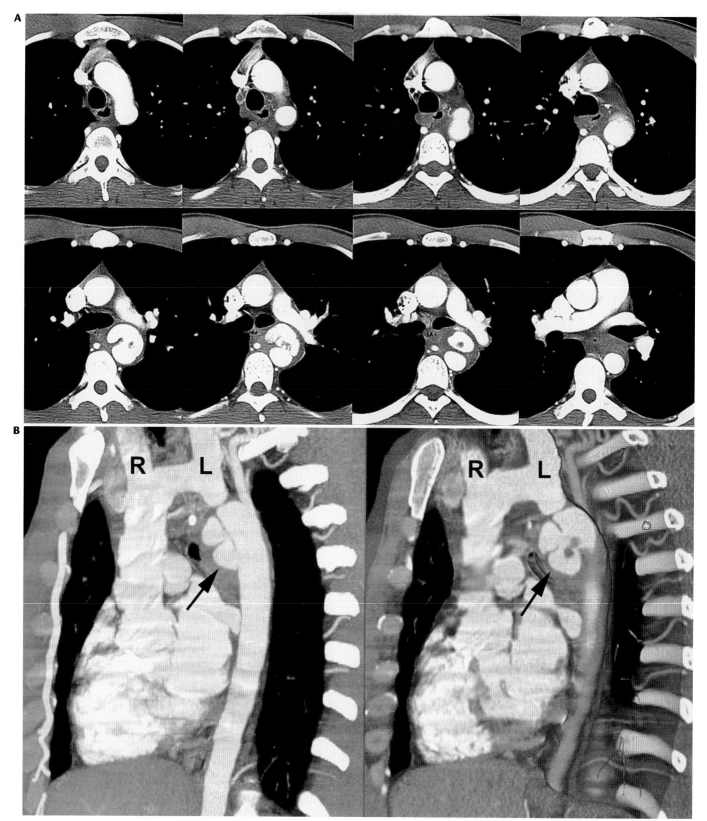

Fig. 17.14 Aortic coarctation and pseudoaneurysm in a 35-year-old man. **A**, CT shows a complex pseudoaneurysm at the aortic isthmus. **B**, Sagittal reconstructed images clearly demonstrate the relationship of the branch vessels to the pseudoaneurysm (arrows). R = right brachiocephalic artery; L = left subclavian artery.

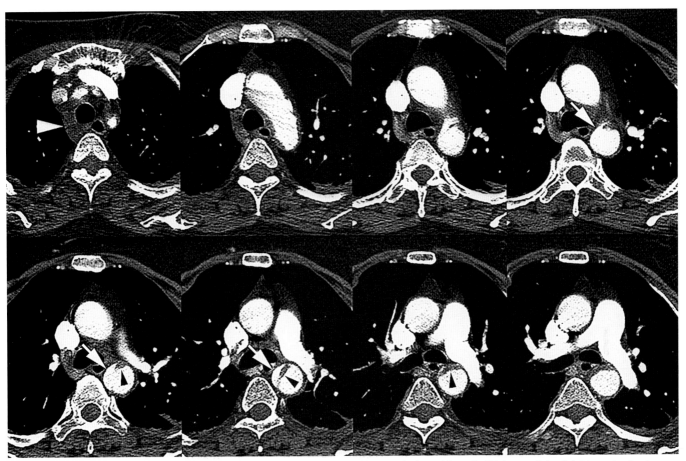

Fig. 17.15 Minimal aortic injury in a 57-year-old woman after a high-speed motor vehicle accident. **A**, CT shows minimal right paratracheal hematoma (white arrowhead) and an intimal flap (black arrowheads). There is also evidence of atheromatous plaque in the arch and questionable irregularity of the aortic contour (arrows) at the isthmus. There is no perivascular hematoma. Aortography (not shown) suggested blunt aortic injury. At surgery, however, the external surface of the aorta was intact and the contour abnormality was reported to be a "ductus bump". Follow-up imaging showed resolution of the intimal flap.

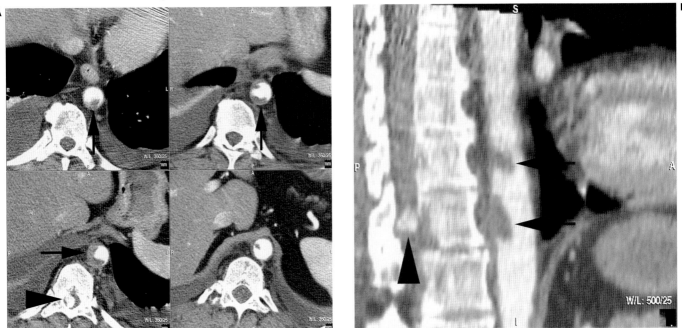

Fig. 17.16 Minimal aortic injury in a 30-year-old man who presented after a high-speed motor vehicle accident with paraplegia. **A**, Axial and **B**, reconstructed sagittal CT shows a complex intimal flap in the descending thoracic aorta at the diaphragm (arrows). The aortic contours are normal and there is only minimal periaortic hematoma. Note the retropulsed vertebral body fragment in the spinal canal (arrowheads) at the same level. The aortic injury was managed conservatively and resolved on follow-up imaging (not shown).

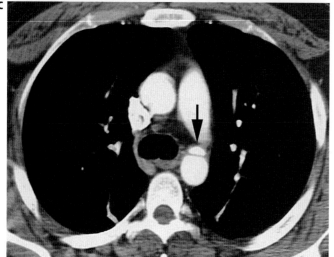

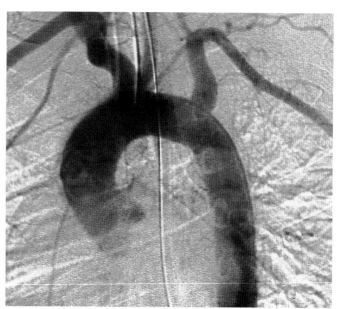

Fig. 17.17 False negative aortogram in an 18-year-old man with blunt aortic injury. **A**, Initial CT shows an intimal flap and small anterior pseudoaneurysm (arrow). **B**, Aortogram was interpreted as normal. **C**, Repeat CT performed 8 days later shows a persistent pseudoaneurysm (arrow).

pseudoaneurysm developed in the other half. Malhotra et al,[61] and others,[59] have suggested that MAI in hemodynamically stable patients can be managed conservatively, but followed carefully until resolution of the lesion is documented. Furthermore, Malhotra et al[61] found that intravascular ultrasound was useful for confirming such limited injuries. The proper management of so-called MAI remains a subject of investigation.

It should be noted that several groups have disparaged the use of CT for evaluation of suspected BAI.[21,62–65] However, the studies from these groups relied upon older generation CT scanners (many nonhelical) with variable technique and inconsistent criteria for diagnosis. Without exception, the experience with later generation helical CT scanners is much more positive, as noted above. Furthermore, the use of CT to screen the mediastinum for signs of hemorrhage,[44,66,67] or to assess the aorta itself for injury,[4,7,60] has been shown to be cost-effective by decreasing the number of negative aortograms performed.

Aortography

Aortography has long been considered the "gold standard" for diagnosis of BAI (Box 17.4, Figs 17.2–17.6, 17.7, 17.9, and 17.10). Prior to the widespread application of helical CT, aortography

---

Box 17.4 Aortographic findings of blunt aortic injury

Pseudoaneurysm
Frank rupture with extravasation of contrast
Intimal tear with intravasation of contrast into the wall
Posttraumatic coarctation
Concomitant great vessel injury
Pitfalls in diagnosis
- Ductus bump or diverticulum
- Ulcerated atheromatous plaque
- Preexistent aortic dissection
- Congenital abnormalities of the arch and the great vessels

---

was performed liberally for evaluation of patients with suspected BAI. Consequently, a large number of negative angiograms were performed; up to 90% of aortograms performed on the basis of an abnormal chest radiograph are negative.[18,22,44,65,68,69] One of the great advantages of CT is to reduce the number of negative angiograms performed. In centers where high quality helical CT is available, aortography is more often reserved for patients

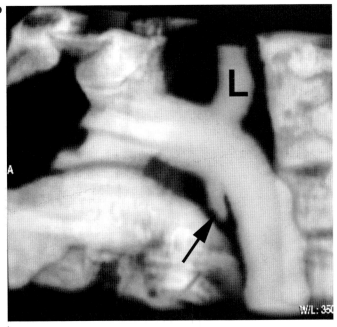

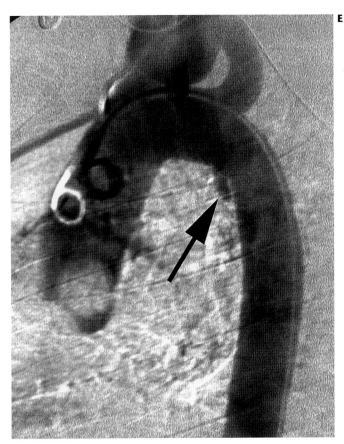

Fig. 17.17 (cont'd) **D**, Oblique sagittal reconstruction clearly shows the relationship of injury (arrow) to the left subclavian artery (L). **E**, Repeat aortogram also shows the lesion (arrow), which was surgically repaired.

with either nondiagnostic scans or minimal periaortic hematoma without aortic contour abnormalities. As discussed above, some centers may also perform aortography in patients with clearly abnormal CT scans. With experience, this practice should occur less and less frequently.

The angiographic diagnosis of BAI is occasionally difficult and both false positive and false negative examinations (Fig. 17.17) are reported.[70,71] Angiographic diagnosis depends upon identifying a disruption of the aortic contour that ranges from a subtle contour irregularity to a focal pseudoaneurysm, and even to evidence of extravasation (Fig. 17.18). The two main pitfalls are ulcerated atheromatous plaque and the ductus diverticulum (ductus bump). Ulcerated plaque can simulate an intimal flap whereas the ductus diverticulum resembles a pseudoaneurysm. Particular care, therefore, needs to be observed in the older individual with other evidence of atheromatous disease. However, this is not a problem with the younger patient and it should be noted that in one large series the mean age of the patients with BAI was 40 years.[46] The ductus diverticulum (bump) can be especially problematic. This outpouching of the aorta occurs at the attachment of the ligamentum arteriosum at the isthmus, and may closely resemble a pseudoaneurysm. Other diagnostic difficulties include BAI in unusual locations, preexistent nontraumatic aortic dissection, and congenital abnormalities of the aorta or great vessels. A detailed review of the problems in the angiographic diagnosis of BAI is beyond the scope of this

text, but the subject is well reviewed with copious illustrations by Mirvis et al[70] and Fisher et al.[72] One potential advantage of aortography over CT and transesophageal echocardiography is that it clearly demonstrates injury to the great vessels (Boxes 17.4 and 17.5).

Box 17.5 Transesophageal echocardiography in blunt aortic injury

Advantages
Bedside examination
Rapidly performed
Highly sensitive and specific with a skilled, experienced operator
Accurate in assessing myocardial and valve function and detecting pericardial effusions

Disadvantages
Cannot be performed on all patients
Operator dependent
Difficult to provide the necessary continuous emergency department coverage
Does not adequately assess the great vessels and the descending aorta

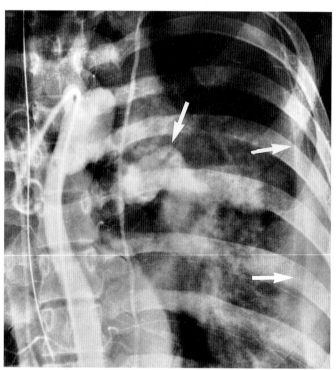

Fig. 17.18 Blunt aortic injury in a young man after a high-speed motor vehicle accident. **A** and **B**, Serial images from an aortogram shows a large pseudoaneurysm with active extravasation into the mediastinum (arrows) and left pleural cavity. The patient expired prior to surgery.

Ultrasonography

Transesophageal echocardiography (TEE) has shown promise in the diagnosis of BAI (Box 17.5).[73–83] Smith et al[84] reported a sensitivity of 100% and a specificity of 98% for TEE in the examination of >90 patients with suspected aortic injury. Buckmaster et al[85] reported comparable results. In their series of 160 patients, TEE was 100% sensitive and specific, whereas aortography had a sensitivity of 73% and a specificity of 99%. On the other hand, Saletta et al[86] and Minard et al[87] reported more modest results with sensitivities of 63 and 57% and specificities of 84 and 91%, respectively. Vignon et al[82] reviewed the literature to 1999 and concluded that the sensitivity and specificity of TEE for BAI was 88% (range 57–100%) and 96% (range 84–100%), respectively. In a more recent study, Goarin et al[79] reported that TEE was more sensitive than either angiography or CT for diagnosis of BAI, primarily because it detected more limited (MAI) intimal injuries. When they compared diagnostic sensitivity for "significant" injuries (those requiring surgical repair), all three modalities were equivalent.

There are certain disadvantages with TEE. It may not be possible to perform the examination because of lack of patient cooperation or maxillofacial trauma.[84] TEE is not suited to diagnosing injury to the arch vessels or distal descending aorta.[82,88] TEE performance is quite dependent on the skill and experience of the operator and it can be difficult to provide continuous TEE coverage with immediate availability by skilled operators. Nevertheless, in experienced hands, TEE seems to be an excellent modality for diagnosing BAI. Although it is not commonly used as a first-line modality, it may be quite useful for assessment of patients with indeterminate or inconclusive CT scans or aortograms.[80,81]

While TEE is clearly an examination of great utility, the role of intravascular ultrasound is less clear. Some authors have reported success in diagnosing BAI with this modality.[61,80,89] This technique is probably too invasive and time consuming to be of value as a primary investigative modality. However, like TEE, its greatest value may be in the assessment of patients with indeterminate or inconclusive CT scans or aortograms.

Magnetic resonance imaging

MRI has not, up to now, played a great role in the acute evaluation of suspected BAI.[3,90,91] There have been, however, considerable recent advances in the quality and speed of high-resolution MRI of the aorta.[92,93] It is now possible to image the aorta with the same clarity and nearly the same speed as helical CT. However, MRI of the acutely traumatized patient remains a daunting task. MRI is now used, and will likely continue to be used, primarily as a problem solving tool for the diagnosis of BAI, after the patient has been stabilized.

Injury to the aortic branch vessels

As has already been noted, injuries to the aortic branch vessels (subclavian, brachiocephalic and intrathoracic carotid arteries) are less common than injuries to the aorta itself in the setting of blunt thoracic trauma.[94] Branch vessel injury due to penetrating

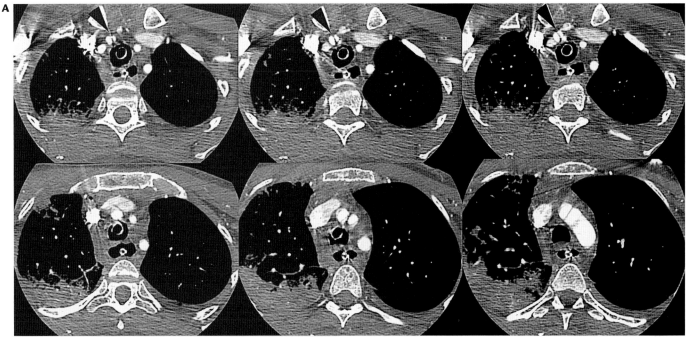

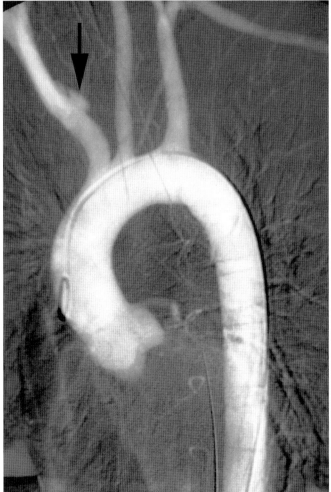

Fig. 17.19   Aortic branch vessel injury in a 62-year-old woman after a high-speed motor vehicle accident. **A**, CT shows extensive perivascular hematoma in the superior mediastinum. There is a subtle intimal flap (arrowheads) in the right carotid artery. The aorta was normal.
B, Aortogram shows a pseudoaneurysm (arrow) of the proximal right carotid artery.

trauma is, for example, far more common. Chen et al[58] retrospectively reviewed 166 arteriograms performed in the setting of blunt trauma to exclude aortic or branch vessel injury. They saw 24 vascular injuries overall; 15 had isolated aortic injury, seven had isolated branch vessel injury, and two had both aortic and branch vessel injuries. They further emphasized that the arteriographic features of the injuries were often quite subtle. The spectrum of branch vessel injuries reported ranges from limited intimal flaps to significant arterial dissection to complete transection with pseudoaneurysm formation.[58,94–102]

Numerous authors have emphasized the difficulties in diagnosing aortic branch vessel injury.[94–102] Chest radiographs in affected patients are usually abnormal, though the sensitivity of the chest radiograph for branch vessel injury has not been studied in detail, perhaps due to the infrequency of these injuries. The role of CT in this regard is even less studied and concerns have been raised regarding the use of CT for diagnosis of branch vessel injury. Certainly, CT can diagnose such injuries (Figs 17.19 and 17.20), but its sensitivity and specificity in the absence of direct signs of vascular injury is unknown. In the practice, patients with significant mediastinal hematoma on CT, but who have no direct signs of arterial injury, frequently undergo arteriography in order to exclude great vessel injury. Furthermore, arteriography is performed if there are suggestive physical examination findings, such as diminished arm blood pressures or pulses or evidence of neurovascular compromise.

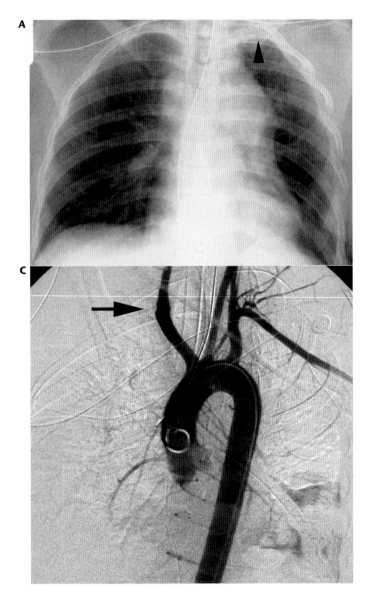

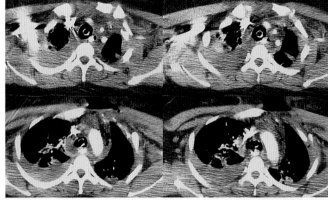

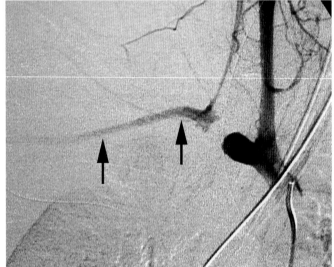

Fig. 17.20 Aortic branch vessel injury in a middle-aged man after a high-speed motor vehicle accident. **A**, Frontal chest radiograph shows a wide mediastinum, multiple left rib fractures, and a left apical cap (arrowhead). **B**, CT shows extensive perivascular hematoma in the superior mediastinum. No direct signs of aortic or great vessel injury are seen. **C**, Aortogram shows nonfilling of the right subclavian artery (arrow). **D**, Selective injection confirms avulsion of the right subclavian artery with distal reconstitution of the vessel (arrows) via collaterals.

Injury to the pulmonary arteries

Injuries to the pulmonary arteries in the setting of blunt trauma are quite rare.[103–107] Penetrating trauma to the pulmonary arteries is much more common. Blunt injury to the pulmonary arteries is often fatal, as intrapericardial rupture may lead to cardiac tamponade. Chest radiographs in all reported cases have been abnormal. CT has been used successfully to diagnose pulmonary artery laceration in the setting of blunt trauma.[103,104,106,107] However, given the rarity of the injury, the sensitivity of CT for pulmonary arterial injury in this setting is unknown.

INJURY TO THE PULMONARY PARENCHYMA
(Box 17.6)

Contusion of the lung parenchyma is quite common in patients with major blunt thoracic trauma and can occur at the site of

injury (coup) or in other parts of the lung (contrecoup injury).[108] Contusion results from laceration of the pulmonary parenchyma by sudden compression and shear forces.[109] Lung injury may be further compounded by fractured ribs or tearing of pleural adhesions. Alveolar hemorrhage and parenchymal destruction are usually greatest during the first 24 h after injury.[108] Nevertheless, radiographs obtained within the first few hours of injury may not show findings of contusion. Radiographs obtained shortly thereafter, however, will show either focal or diffuse homogeneous opacities (Figs 17.21 and 17.22). Because the interlobar fissures do not impede the shock wave, lung contusion does not usually localize in a lobar or segmental pattern. Although the opacities may appear to progress on chest radiographs for a day or two, they tend to stabilize and then clear fairly rapidly, usually within 7 days (Fig. 17.21).[108] Lung contusion can result in significant respiratory distress leading to mechanical ventilation, acute respiratory distress syndrome (ARDS), and, in some cases, longterm respiratory disability.[108]

Box 17.6 Pulmonary parenchymal injuries due to blunt chest trauma

Contusion
Appear rapidly (within a few hours)
Resolve within a few days
Opacities do not respect anatomic boundaries (e.g. fissures)
Peripheral clearing may be noted on CT

Hematoma
May result from focal laceration
Solitary or multiple nodules or masses
Margins initially ill defined but become well defined with time
May cavitate

Posttraumatic lung cysts
Due to parenchymal laceration
Solitary or multiple
May be quite large
Resolve slowly
Residual pneumatocele may occur

Secondary injuries
Pneumothorax
Hemothorax

CT is clearly more sensitive for lung contusion than chest radiography (Figs 17.22 and 17.23).[108,110–113] Schild et al[114] imaged experimentally induced pulmonary contusions with CT and chest radiographs. CT detected 100% of contusions immediately after the trauma, whereas the plain films failed to detect 20% of contusions even on sequential examinations. Miller et al[113] used CT to quantify the volume of contusion and found a correlation between contusion volume and risk for ARDS. Donnelly et al[111] studied 29 children with blunt thoracic trauma and reported a new CT finding for lung contusion: subpleural sparing. They found this sign, seen in 95% of cases of lung contusion, useful for differentiating contusion from other forms of lung injury after trauma, including infection and aspiration.

Pulmonary laceration can also result in formation of post-traumatic lung cysts (pneumatoceles, Figs 17.23 and 17.24) or focal hematomas (Fig. 17.25).[115] Such lesions may be solitary or multiple. Most range from 2 to 5 cm in diameter, but extremely large hematomas, up to 14 cm in diameter, are reported. Pneumatoceles or hematomas may be radiographically apparent within a few hours of injury. However, the lesions may not be apparent on initial chest radiographs because of associated parenchymal contusion. In such instances, the lesions will become more visible as the surrounding pulmonary parenchymal contusion clears. As is the case with lung contusion, CT is more sensitive than chest radiography for detection of posttraumatic lung cysts and parenchymal hematomas. Both lesions tend to resolve with time; pneumatoceles tend to resolve faster than hematomas. Hematomas may take many months to resolve completely and for a considerable period of time may be the only visible sequela of previous injury. Since by this stage a hematoma is a circumscribed lung mass, the lesion may be mistaken for a neoplasm (Fig. 17.25). In such a case, Takahashi et al[116] were able to identify the lesion as a hematoma by its signal characteristics on MRI. During resolution, a hematoma may communicate with the airway and manifest as a cavitary mass (Fig. 17.26). Awareness of these features is important to avoid confusion with more serious pulmonary processes such as lung cancer. Cavitating hematomas resolve without treatment.

Pneumothoraces (Fig. 17.27) and pleural effusions (Fig. 17.28) commonly accompany lung parenchymal injury and may require prompt chest tube drainage. Severely injured patients are usually radiographed in the supine position, which can make detecting air and fluid in the pleural space difficult, unless the fluid or air is localized to the minor fissure, the subpulmonic spaces, or the mediastinal pleural space. In the supine position air tends to collect anteriorly and fluid tends to layer posteriorly. Anterior pneumothoraces can be detected on frontal projections taken with the patient supine, but the findings are subtle and

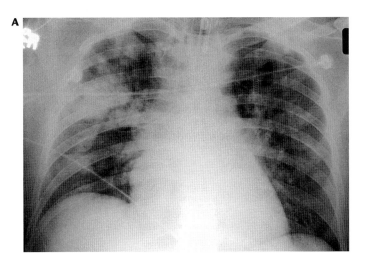
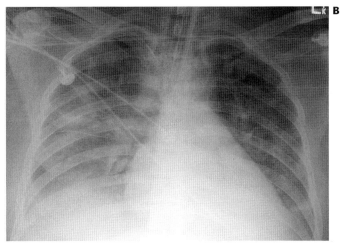

Fig. 17.21 Pulmonary contusion in a young man after a 20 foot fall. **A**, Initial chest radiograph shows homogeneous right upper lobe opacity consistent with contusion. **B**, Radiograph obtained 72 h later shows partial resolution of the right upper lobe opacity and an increasing right pleural effusion.

A

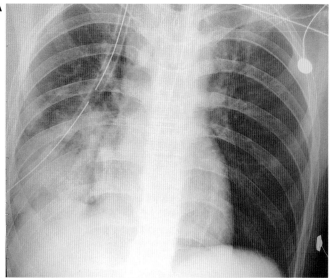

Fig. 17.22 Pulmonary contusion in a 34-year-old man after a motor cycle accident and trauma to the right chest wall. **A**, Frontal chest radiograph shows a wide mediastinum, multiple right rib fractures, a right pleural chest tube, and a right lower lobe opacity consistent with contusion. **B**, CT performed to exclude blunt aortic injury shows homogeneous opacity consistent with contusion in the right lower lobe and possible contrecoup injuries in the left lung (arrows).

B

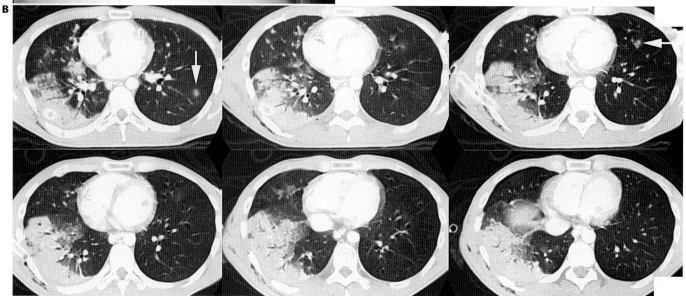

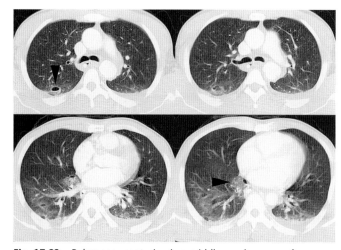

Fig. 17.23 Pulmonary contusion in a middle-aged woman after a motor vehicle accident. CT performed to exclude aortic injury shows subtle, scattered ground-glass opacities and parenchymal cysts (arrowheads) consistent with contusion and laceration. These findings were not seen on the chest radiograph (not shown).

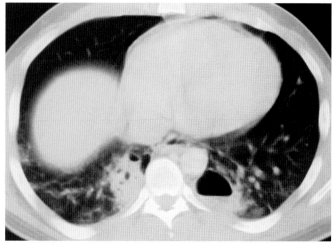

Fig. 17.24 Pulmonary contusion and traumatic lung cysts in a middle-aged man after a motor vehicle accident. CT shows bilateral lower lobe contusions and traumatic lung cysts. (Courtesy of Dr P Goodman, Durham, NC)

A

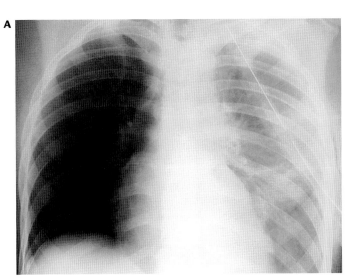

B

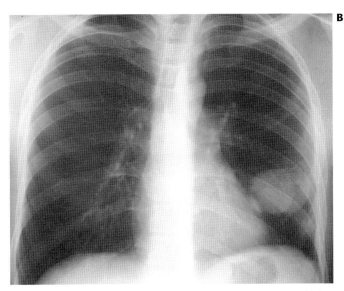

Fig. 17.25 Pulmonary hematomas in a young man after a motor vehicle accident. **A**, Initial chest radiograph shows a wide mediastinum and left lung contusion. **B**, Follow-up radiograph obtained 2 weeks later shows well-defined masses in the left lower lobe consistent with hematomas. (Courtesy of Dr P Goodman, Durham, NC)

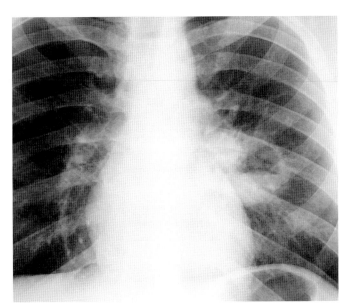

Fig. 17.26 Pulmonary hematomas in an asymptomatic young man with a history of recent chest trauma. Frontal chest radiograph shows a cavitary mass in the left lung. The lesion resolved on follow up, consistent with cavitary hematoma. (Courtesy of Dr P Goodman, Durham, NC)

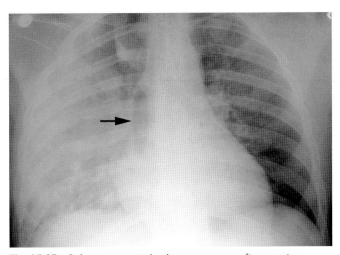

Fig. 17.27 Pulmonary contusion in a young man after a motor vehicle accident. Frontal chest radiograph shows homogeneous opacity in the right lung consistent with contusion and a subtle anteromedial lucency (arrow) indicative of a small anterior pneumothorax.

easily overlooked.[117,118] The mediastinal contours on the affected side may be seen with unusual clarity, and the anterior portion of the diaphragm may be depressed, revealing more of the base of the heart on that side.[117,119] The lateral costophrenic sulcus may also be seen with unusual clarity and appear asymmetrically deep – the co-called "deep sulcus sign".[119] Pleural effusions may cause a diffuse haze over the lungs resulting from the filtering effect of the posteriorly positioned fluid layer. If the effusion is large enough, it may extend around the lung and produce a

band of density along the lateral chest wall and over the apex. Cross-table lateral views can be helpful for detecting both pneumothoraces and pleural effusions. CT is highly accurate for both, and the lung bases should always be covered during the abdominal CT examination for visceral injury.[120] McGonigal et al[121] showed that CT detected 100% of pneumothoraces, whereas supine frontal chest radiographs detected only 40%. Tocino et al[122] and Holmes et al[123] found that supine chest radiographs detected only about 50% of pneumothoraces in trauma

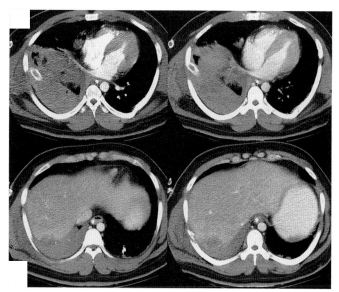

Fig. 17.28 Hemothorax in a young man after a gunshot wound to the right chest. CT shows a large right pleural effusion, parenchymal lung injury, and hepatic laceration. Note that the fluid is of soft tissue attenuation, indicating hemothorax. A small rent in the right diaphragm was repaired at laparoscopy.

patients. However, Holmes et al[123] also found that many of the pneumothoraces detected only by abdominal CT did not require tube thoracostomy. Wolfman et al[124] used CT to grade the size of such incidental pneumothoraces and found that very small ones did not require tube thoracostomy.

INJURY TO THE CENTRAL AIRWAYS (Box 17.7)

Tracheal or bronchial rupture most frequently results from penetrating thoracic injuries or instrumentation.[125] Injury due to blunt trauma is rare and, because of the significant force required, is frequently associated with injuries to other structures such as the aorta and great vessels, thoracic cage, and lungs.[126] Indeed, tracheobronchial rupture due to blunt thoracic trauma is associated with a 30% overall mortality rate, chiefly from associated injuries.[127] Diagnosis can be quite difficult and a significant proportion of cases go undiagnosed until complications develop, either at the site of rupture, such as bronchial stenosis, or in the lung distal to the rupture, such as septic

---

Box 17.7 Central airway injury due to blunt chest trauma

Location
80% occur in main bronchi
Right bronchus > left bronchus
15% occur in trachea
Most occur within 2.5 cm of the carina

Radiographic findings
Persistent pneumothorax despite adequate chest tube drainage
Pneumomediastinum
"Fallen lung" sign (rare)

---

complications or persistent atelectasis.[128–130] The radiologic findings of airway rupture are often subtle and may be overshadowed by other injuries. Definitive diagnosis may require fiberoptic bronchoscopy.

There are two major indirect radiologic manifestations of tracheal or bronchial rupture: evidence of air leakage at the site of rupture and abnormal ventilation of the lung distal to the injury. Evidence of air leak is the more crucial finding and is seen in up to 90% of cases of tracheobronchial fracture.[131] However, if the adventitial sleeve of the bronchus remains intact, an air leak may not occur – the situation in approximately 10% of cases.[131] Absence of air leakage makes the diagnosis of an airway injury difficult, if not impossible. The most common radiologic finding of airway injury is pneumothorax, seen in between 60 and 100% of cases.[132,133] Pneumothoraces due to major airway injury are frequently large and persistent despite insertion of multiple pleural tubes (Fig. 17.29); they may also be under tension. Pneumomediastinum is another important indicator of airway injury (Fig. 17.30),[133,134] and is a more specific sign of a breach of airway integrity. Pneumomediastinum may be the only visible sign of an air leak in patients with rupture of the trachea or intramediastinal bronchi, particularly the left main bronchus.[135] Pneumomediastinum due to airway injury typically manifests on chest radiographs with streaky lucencies around the carina that extend superiorly as the air dissects in the tissue planes around the trachea, aorta, and great vessels. At the margins of the mediastinum, air dissects and elevates the mediastinal parietal pleura from the aorta and heart. On lateral films, pneumomediastinum is best appreciated in the retrosternal space. The presence of both pneumothorax and pneumomediastinum on chest radiographs obtained in patients after severe blunt thoracic trauma is highly suggestive of airway injury.

A rare but characteristic radiographic feature of bronchial rupture is the so-called "fallen lung" sign (Fig. 17.29). This finding occurs in the setting of a complete bronchial transection and a large pneumothorax that allows the lung to sag away from the hilum inferiorly and laterally. The vascular pedicle remains intact and the lung remains perfused though underventilated.[136] The consequent ventilation–perfusion mismatch can result in hypoxia and cyanosis.

The second major indirect manifestation of major airway injury is abnormal ventilation of the affected lung.[137] As noted above, this can result in ventilation–perfusion mismatch with hypoxia and cyanosis. Loss of bronchial continuity combined with intraairway hemorrhage and edema can also result in significant atelectasis. The diagnostic problems in these cases are numerous. In severely traumatized patients, atelectasis may develop for reasons other than bronchial rupture. Furthermore, significant associated pulmonary abnormalities such as lung contusion or aspiration may also be present. Collapse of a lung is expected in the presence of a pneumothorax, particularly if the pneumothorax is large and under tension. Atelectasis in patients with bronchial rupture is usually persistent and unresponsive to normal therapeutic maneuvers. Bronchial stenosis or occlusion at the site of rupture can occur if the injury is not promptly diagnosed and repaired. Septic complications including pneumonia and abscess can also be encountered in the affected lung.

Further important, but infrequently observed, indirect findings of major airway injury include abnormally positioned endotracheal tubes or overdistended endotracheal tube balloons.[138,139] Chen et al[140] reported that balloon overinflation occurred in 71% and balloon herniation through the defect in 29%

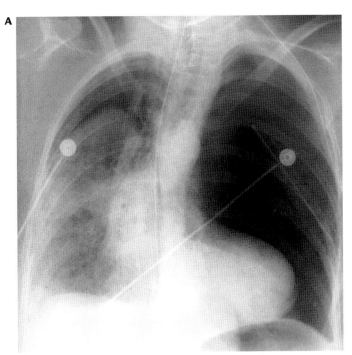

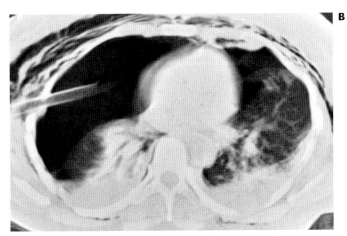

Fig. 17.29 Bronchial injuries in two young men after severe motor vehicle accidents. **A**, Frontal chest radiograph in one man shows a large persistent left pneumothorax despite adequate chest tube drainage. Note that the left lung has collapsed inferiorly away from the hilum – the "fallen lung" sign. Fiberoptic bronchoscopy showed complete transection of the left main bronchus. (Courtesy of Dr Jud Gurney, Omaha, NE) **B**, CT in a second man shows a large right pneumothorax and considerable chest wall emphysema that persisted despite a well placed chest tube. Fiberoptic bronchoscopy confirmed right bronchial transection. (Courtesy of Dr Mark Shogry, Greensboro, NC)

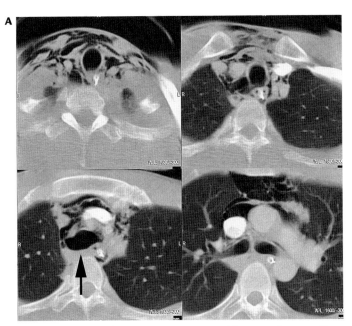

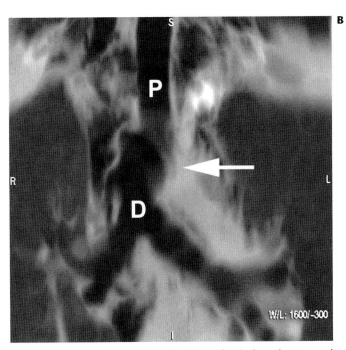

Fig. 17.30 Tracheal injury in a young man with severe dyspnea after a motor vehicle accident. **A**, CT shows extensive mediastinal emphysema and marked focal enlargement and irregularity of the apparent tracheal lumen (arrow). **B**, Coronal reconstruction shows complete transection of the trachea (arrow) with marked separation of the proximal (P) and distal (D) portions.

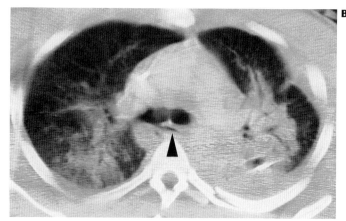

Fig. 17.31 Bronchial injury in a middle-aged man with persistent pneumonia after a motor vehicle accident. **A** and **B**, CT shows an anterior right bronchial wall defect (arrow on **A**) and a posterior sinus tract (arrowhead on **B**). Bronchoscopy confirmed right bronchial injury.

of cases of tracheal rupture. The overinflated balloon may also assume a more rounded configuration than is normally seen. Tracheal perforation due to traumatic intubation can result in the tip of the endotracheal tube projecting too far to the right of the tracheal air column on supine chest radiographs.[125]

CT has been applied with some success to diagnosis of airway injuries (Figs 17.30 and 17.31).[126,140–147] CT is clearly more sensitive than chest radiography for detecting small air leaks in the mediastinum that suggest the presence of airway injury. The sensitivity of CT for direct visualization of the site of injury is less established, however. Chen et al[140] studied a group of patients with tracheal rupture and reported that CT identified the direct site of injury in 71%. However, Kunisch-Hoppe et al[144] saw direct CT evidence of tracheal rupture in only one of 10 patients (10%). The primary role of CT in diagnosis of airway injuries is probably to suggest the possibility of injury when extraluminal air is identified adjacent to major airways. Ultimately, the diagnosis depends on awareness of the possibility of airway injury in cases of severe thoracic trauma. In a significant number of instances the diagnosis is missed in the acute phase and is detected only because of persistent lung or lobar atelectasis. Bronchoscopy should be performed in any case in which the radiographic or CT findings suggest airway rupture.

INJURY TO THE ESOPHAGUS OR THORACIC DUCT (Box 17.8)

Instrumentation is the most common cause of traumatic esophageal rupture. Most noniatrogenic traumatic esophageal ruptures are due to gunshot wounds.[148] Esophageal rupture caused by blunt external thoracic trauma is quite rare, accounting for only 10% of all noniatrogenic cases.[149,150] The radiographic features of esophageal rupture are more fully discussed elsewhere (see p. 943) and include pneumomediastinum, pneumothorax or pleural effusion, most commonly on the left side, and evidence of mediastinitis, including abscess formation. Diagnosis of esophageal rupture in the trauma patient can be quite difficult because these findings may be attributed to other injuries, and a significant delay in diagnosis is common.[149] Unfortunately, this delay in diagnosis results in a higher incidence of infectious complications. The majority of esophageal ruptures due to blunt

Box 17.8 Thoracic duct injuries

Mechanism
 • Penetrating >> blunt trauma
Radiologic findings
 • Chylothorax
 • Lymphocele
Location
 • Left – injuries above T6
 • Right – injuries below T6
Diagnosis
 • Lymphography
 • Lymphoscintigraphy
 • Percutaneous aspiration

trauma occur in the cervical and upper thoracic region (Fig. 17.32), but distal esophageal rupture following blunt external trauma has been described.[151,152] In many cases, particularly with gunshot wounds, the diagnosis is made by surgical exploration. Otherwise, an esophagram using water soluble contrast will readily confirm the injury.

Injuries to the thoracic duct are usually due either to penetrating trauma or to surgical injury during thoracic exploration (Figure 17.27).[153,154] Thoracic duct injury from blunt external trauma is exceedingly rare.[155] Rupture of the thoracic duct can result in chylothorax (Fig. 17.33) or, occasionally, a localized lymphocele (Fig. 17.34).[156] Fluid accumulation is characteristically slow and many days may pass before significant quantities of fluid accumulate. Definitive diagnosis rests on determining that the fluid collection is chylous or that it communicates with the thoracic duct.[156–158] The site of injury to the thoracic duct determines the side on which the fluid accumulates. The duct enters the thorax through the aortic hiatus in the diaphragm and ascends along the right anterolateral aspect of the spine. In the midthoracic region (about the level of the sixth thoracic vertebral body), the duct crosses the midline and ascends along the left anterolateral aspect of the spine. Finally, it arches forward to enter the venous system in the region of the left jugular and subclavian vein junction. As the duct arches into the left cervical

A

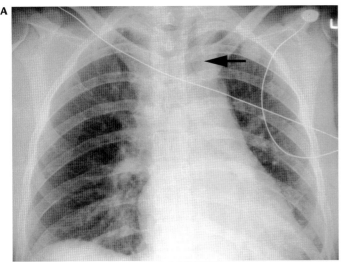

B

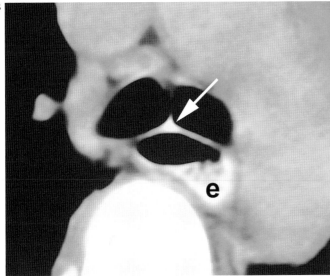

C

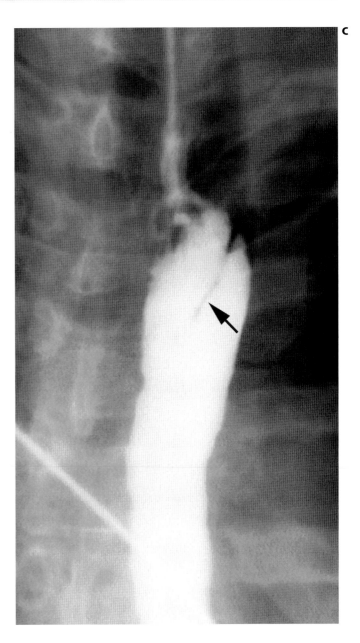

Fig. 17.32   Esophageal injury in a middle-aged man with dysphagia after a recent motor vehicle accident. **A**, Frontal chest radiograph shows air in the proximal esophagus (arrow). **B**, CT performed after administration of a thick barium paste shows a dilated esophagus (e) and extraluminal barium (arrow). **C**, Esophagram shows an intimal flap (arrow) in the proximal esophagus.

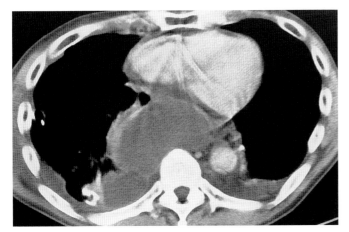

Fig. 17.33   Chylothorax in an elderly man with chest pain after a recent esophagectomy with gastric bypass for esophageal carcinoma. CT shows a large fluid collection in the mediastinum and right pleural space. Aspiration confirmed chylothorax.

region, it is particularly vulnerable to penetrating injury. Worthington et al[159] described eight cases of rupture involving the upper portion of the thoracic duct above the level of the aortic arch, seven of which were caused by knife wounds. All seven were associated with left chylothorax. On the other hand, injuries to the duct below the level of the sixth thoracic vertebral body usually result in right-sided chylothorax or lymphocele formation. Because the duct lies in close proximity to the spine, there is a significant association between thoracic duct injury and fracture dislocation injuries of the thoracic spine.[160] Large persistent pleural effusions in patients with such fractures suggests the possibility of thoracic duct injury.

Lymphography has been used successfully to determine the site of leakage prior to surgical intervention. Sachs et al[161] studied 12 patients with chylous ascites or chylothorax following surgery and found abnormal lymphangiograms in seven. Of five patients

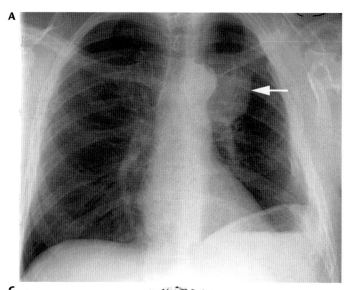

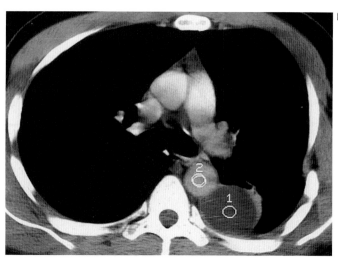

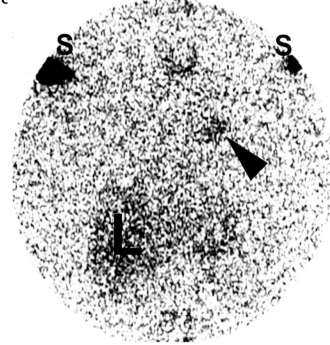

Fig. 17.34 Thoracic lymphocele in a 25-year-old man after a severe motor vehicle accident complicated by aortic transection, and left diaphragm and spleen rupture. **A,** Frontal chest radiograph shows a well-circumscribed left periaortic mass (arrow). Note findings of prior left rib, scapular, and clavicular trauma. **B,** CT shows that the mass is of fluid attenuation. **C,** Frontal view of chest from a ^{99m}Tc-antimony sulfur colloid lymphoscintigram shows activity within the mass (arrowhead), confirming the diagnosis of thoracic lymphocele. S = markers on shoulders; L = liver activity. (With permission from Perusse KR, McAdams HP, Earls JP, Peller PJ. General case of the day. Posttraumatic thoracic lymphocele. Radiographics 1994;14:192–195.)

with normal lymphangiograms, four were successfully treated conservatively and one was found at surgery to have a leak from a gastroplasty anastomosis. These authors did not find that CT gave useful additional information. Lymphoscintigraphy (Fig. 17.34)[156] and CT-guided needle aspiration[158] have also been used to successfully diagnose lymphoceles due to thoracic duct trauma.

INJURY TO THE DIAPHRAGM (Boxes 17.9 and 17.10)

Acute rupture of the diaphragm can result from either penetrating injury or blunt thoracoabdominal trauma (Box 17.9). Rupture may result in herniation of abdominal contents into the chest, either in the acute setting or in a delayed fashion. Herniated

---

Box 17.9 Clinical features of diaphragmatic rupture

Mechanism of injury
Penetrating injury
Blunt trauma, usually high-speed motor vehicle accidents or fall from a height

Incidence
Seen in 3–5% of patients admitted to major trauma centers

Mortality
Approximately 20–25%, mainly due to associated injuries

Associated injuries
>90% have solid abdominal organ injury
10% have associated blunt aortic injury
Pelvic fractures, spinal fractures, and closed head injuries common

Diagnostic peritoneal lavage
Left-sided ruptures – a small number (15–30%) may have a negative lavage (lesser sac sequestration of blood)
Right-sided ruptures – almost invariably positive

viscera can cause respiratory distress because of compression of heart or lung. Herniated bowel may also strangulate with dire consequences, sometimes years after the initial injury.[162]

Penetrating injuries to the diaphragm are usually caused by knife or bullet wounds. These injuries usually cause shorter diaphragmatic tears (typically <3 cm in length) than those seen after blunt trauma.[163] Because the tear is so small in cases of penetrating trauma, herniation of abdominal contents is uncommon (see Fig. 17.28). Furthermore, because the adjacent lung is frequently injured, the contours of the diaphragm may be obscured on the frontal chest radiograph, making detection of small hernias (if present) quite difficult. Thus, the tear is usually not diagnosed radiologically and definitive diagnosis may be delayed. For example, Demetriades et al[164] found herniation of abdominal contents in only 15% of 150 patients with penetrating injuries of the diaphragm. Diagnosis was delayed in almost half of the affected patients. Because associated abdominal injuries that require exploratory laparotomy (e.g. liver, spleen or bowel laceration) occur in at least 75% of affected patients, diaphragmatic injuries due to penetrating trauma are usually detected by direct inspection.

Diaphragmatic rupture due to blunt thoracoabdominal trauma is usually the result of a high-speed motor vehicle accident or a fall from a considerable height. The high incidence of associated injury is reflected in reported mortality rates of up to 25%.[165–167] Over 80% of patients with traumatic rupture of the diaphragm have concomitant intraabdominal injuries, typically liver and splenic lacerations.[168] Pelvic and spinal fractures are frequent, as is closed head injury. There is also an association with thoracic aortic injury. In one series, 10% of patients with diaphragmatic rupture due to blunt trauma also had thoracic aortic injury.[169]

Rupture due to blunt trauma is more commonly seen on the left side, presumably because the liver acts as a buffer on the right. In several large series, between 67 and 88% of ruptures were diagnosed on the left.[163,166,170] Between 12 and 28% were found on the right and 5% were either bilateral or central in location.[163] While the reported left-sided predominance may be due to the protective effects of the liver, it may also reflect the difficulties in diagnosis of right-sided tears. Furthermore, there is also evidence that right diaphragmatic rupture is a more severe injury than is left diaphragmatic rupture. Autopsy studies of trauma victims who died at the accident site or before hospitalization report an equal frequency of right- and left-sided ruptures.[168] This finding is in contrast to the marked left-sided predominance noted in surgical series,[163,166,170] and suggests that patients with right-sided ruptures have more severe associated injuries and are thus more likely to die acutely. This may also account for the findings of Boulanger et al[168] that diagnostic peritoneal lavage is more likely to be positive in patients with right-sided ruptures than in those with left-sided ruptures. In that series, 100% of patients with right-sided ruptures had associated intraabdominal injuries, whereas only 77% of patients with left-sided rupture had associated intraabdominal injuries.

Preoperative diagnosis of diaphragmatic rupture after blunt thoracoabdominal trauma can be difficult. Diagnosis by chest radiography is dependent upon demonstration of herniated abdominal contents within the thorax (see below). However, herniation of abdominal contents does not always occur in cases of traumatic rupture, particularly if positive pressure ventilation is used (Fig. 17.35).[171,172] Thus, a significant number of diaphragmatic injuries are discovered at exploratory laparotomy.[165,166,171] Shah et al[173] reviewed 980 reported cases of traumatic rupture and found that only 44% were diagnosed prior to exploratory surgery. Over 40% of the ruptures were diagnosed during surgery or at autopsy and in 15% of cases the injury was not diagnosed during the initial hospitalization. Beal et al,[174] also using chest radiography, suggested the correct preoperative diagnosis in only 12 of 37 patients. These authors emphasized the diagnostic problems caused by associated lung contusion or laceration, hemothoraces, pneumothoraces, and rib fractures.

Left-sided ruptures appear to be more easily diagnosed radiologically than right-sided ruptures. In cases of left-sided rupture, there are often distinct radiologic findings of herniation, such as identifiable gastrointestinal gas patterns within the thorax or an abnormally positioned orogastric tube. On the other hand, right diaphragmatic ruptures with liver herniation often lack such distinctive radiologic features. Right diaphragmatic rupture may manifest as an "elevated" diaphragm,[175] and associated right basal pulmonary opacities or pleural fluid may not elicit particular concern in a severely injured patient. In the series of Boulanger et al,[168] 37% of the left-sided ruptures were diagnosed by chest radiography whereas none of the right-sided ruptures was so diagnosed. Thus, delayed diagnosis is particularly likely when the right diaphragm is ruptured.[170,176] What is clear from review of the literature is that diagnosis of diaphragmatic rupture by chest radiography first and foremost requires a high index of suspicion for the possibility of such an injury.[163] This is particularly true in regard to the difficult to diagnose right-sided ruptures.

As noted above, confident radiographic diagnosis of diaphragmatic rupture depends upon identifying herniated abdominal contents in the thorax (Box 17.10). Herniation of hollow viscera

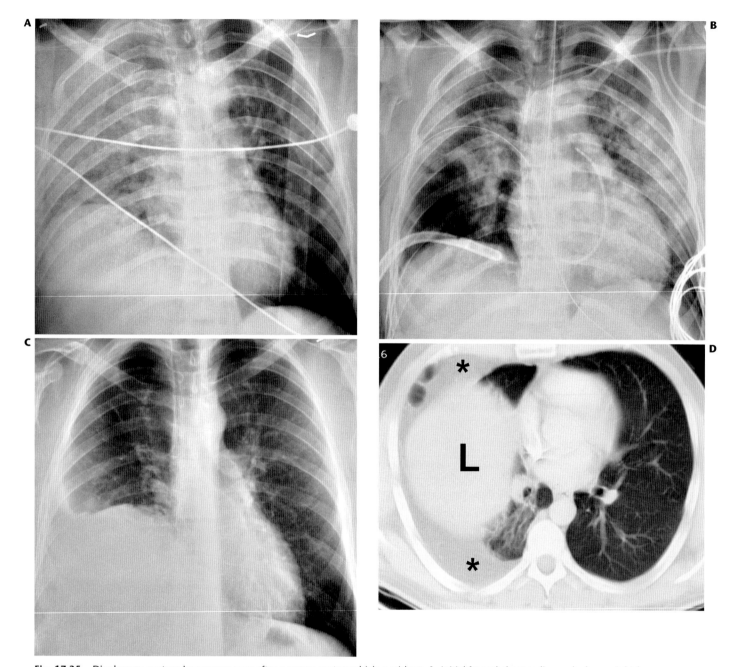

Fig. 17.35 Diaphragm rupture in a young man after a severe motor vehicle accident. **A**, Initial frontal chest radiograph shows right lung contusion and an elevated right diaphragm. **B**, Repeat radiograph obtained after intubation and institution of positive pressure ventilation shows that the previously noted diaphragmatic elevation is no longer apparent. A right hemothorax has been drained. **C**, Chest radiograph obtained at discharge again shows an elevated right diaphragm and an apparent right pleural effusion. **D**, CT shows that the apparent pleural fluid is actually a herniated omentum (*) and bowel, and that the apparently elevated diaphragm is due to the herniated liver (L).

is recognized by the characteristic gas patterns of herniated stomach or bowel (Figs 17.36 and 17.37). Continuity of these loops of bowel with infradiaphragmatic bowel may be apparent, possibly with some constriction or gathering of loops at the site of the rupture. Normal diaphragmatic contours are usually obscured

on the chest radiograph and there may be associated pleural fluid or basal atelectasis. Diagnosis can be difficult if the herniated stomach forms an arclike contour simulating a paralyzed or eventrated diaphragm (Fig. 17.36). Furthermore, if only a small amount of bowel herniates, it may be obscured by pleural fluid

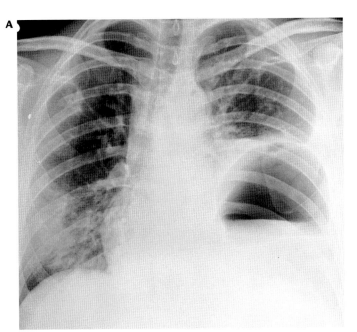

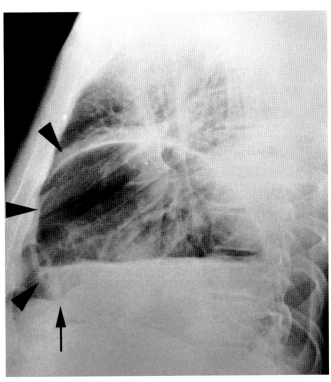

Fig. 17.36 Diaphragm rupture in a young patient after severe blunt abdominal trauma. **A**, Frontal and **B**, lateral chest radiographs show herniated stomach in the left lower hemithorax. The upper margin of the gastric wall simulates the normal appearance of the diaphragm. However, the anterior margin of the stomach (arrowheads) curves down to the actual level of the diaphragm (arrow).

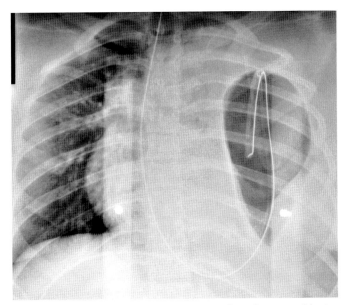

Fig. 17.37 Diaphragm rupture in a young patient after severe blunt abdominal trauma. Frontal chest radiograph shows herniated stomach in the left hemithorax. Note that the orogastric tube turns upwards into the intrathoracic stomach.

and contused or collapsed lung (Fig. 17.38). Placement of an orogastric tube can be helpful with gastric herniation into the left chest; the gastric tube either is held up at the esophageal hiatus or curves upward beyond the hiatus into the left chest (Figs 17.37 and 17.38).[177] Contrast studies of the gastrointestinal tract are rarely necessary or even appropriate in the acute setting. However, such examinations can be useful for evaluation of patients presenting in a delayed fashion.[178–180] Radiographic diagnosis of herniation of solid viscera or omentum is more difficult and accounts in large part for the delays in diagnosis of right diaphragm rupture (Figs 17.35, and 17.39, see also Fig. 17.1).[181] Diaphragmatic herniation can be confused with posttraumatic diaphragmatic paralysis or posttraumatic pneumatoceles.[182]

Because the rent in the diaphragm allows free passage of fluid or air between the abdominal and pleural cavities, the diagnosis is sometimes suggested by seemingly inappropriate passage of air or fluid across this barrier. For example, peritoneal lavage fluid may be detected in the pleural cavity at a subsequent CT examination. An otherwise inexplicable association between pneumothorax and pneumoperitoneum suggests the diagnosis.

CT is now widely performed in patients with blunt thoracoabdominal trauma and is the most appropriate first step beyond the chest radiograph (Figs 17.38 and 17.39). This is particularly true since the advent of high-speed spiral CT. Current

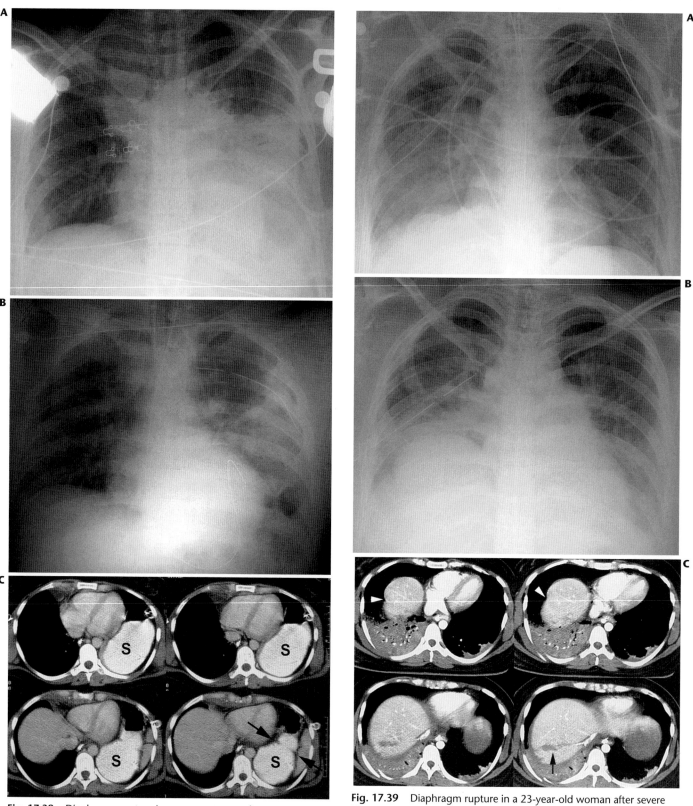

Fig. 17.38 Diaphragm rupture in a young woman after a severe motor vehicle accident. **A**, Initial frontal chest radiograph shows homogeneous left lower lobe opacity that obscures the left diaphragm. The mediastinum is also wide and there is partial right upper lobe collapse. **B**, Repeat radiograph obtained after placement of an orogastric tube now suggests left diaphragm rupture. **C**, CT shows the contrast-filled stomach (S) in the left hemithorax. Note the "waist sign" (arrows) as the stomach herniates through the rent in the diaphragm.

Fig. 17.39 Diaphragm rupture in a 23-year-old woman after severe blunt abdominal trauma. **A**, Initial frontal chest radiograph shows a lobulated contour to the right diaphragm, right lower lobe contusion and hemothorax, and a right chest tube. **B**, Repeat radiograph obtained 5 days later shows apparent elevation of the right diaphragm. **C**, CT shows focal herniation of the medial portion of the right hepatic lobe into the thorax. Note the indentation of the hepatic contour at the site of herniation (arrowheads) and the associated liver laceration (arrow).

generation multidetector scanners allow very rapid acquisition of axial images with thin slice collimation through the entire chest, abdomen, and pelvis. Such data sets can also be rendered in real time into a variety of nonaxial planes for optimal visualization of many structures, including the diaphragm.[183–186] For this reason, CT has assumed an increasingly important role in preoperative diagnosis of diaphragmatic injuries.[187,188] Although CT is clearly useful for demonstrating rupture in the presence of herniation, it can also show ruptures in the absence of herniation.[189] The CT findings of diaphragmatic rupture are well described (Figs 17.38 to 17.42).[172,189–196] Typical findings include direct visualization of the diaphragmatic defect, retraction and thickening of the ruptured diaphragm, and herniation of peritoneal fat or abdominal viscera into the chest. Herniated gut may show a

focal constriction at the site of the rupture; this is known as the "collar" or "waist sign". Bergin et al[197] described the "dependent viscera" sign when the upper third of the liver abuts the posterior right ribs or the bowel or stomach lies in contact with the posterior left ribs on CT. In their experience,[197] this sign was seen in 100% of left-sided ruptures and 83% of right-sided ruptures. Common associated findings on CT include rib fractures, pleural effusions, basal atelectasis or contusion, pneumothorax or pneumomediastinum.

There continues to be debate concerning the reliability of CT for diagnosis of diaphragmatic rupture. Shapiro et al[172] reported that only five of 12 CT scans were diagnostic of rupture in a series of proven diaphragmatic ruptures. These authors further emphasized the difficulty of diagnosing rupture of the right

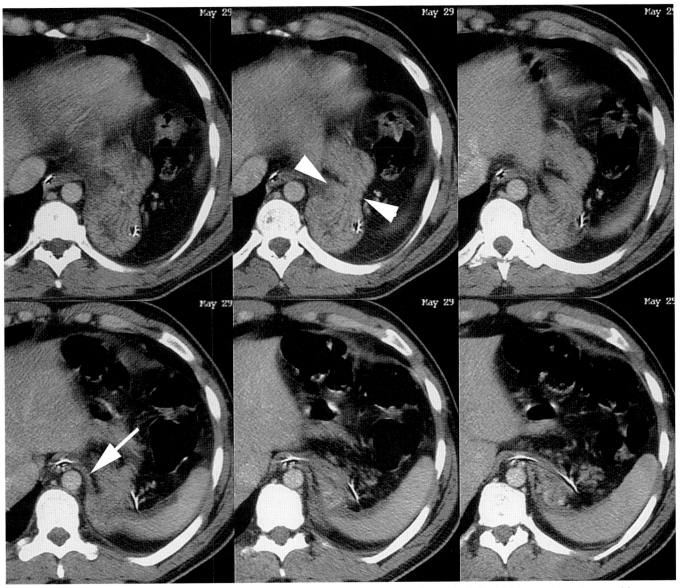

Fig. 17.40   Diaphragm rupture in a young man after severe blunt abdominal trauma. CT shows herniation of the stomach and omental fat through a small diaphragmatic defect (arrow). Note again the classic "waist" or "collar" sign (arrowheads).

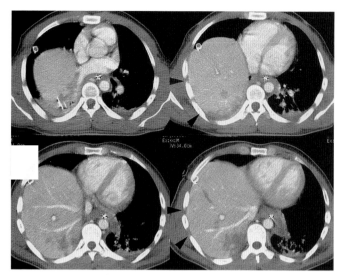

Fig. 17.41 Diaphragm rupture in a young man after severe blunt abdominal trauma. CT shows herniation of the liver into the right hemithorax. Note the dependent viscera sign (arrowheads) and associated hepatic lacerations.

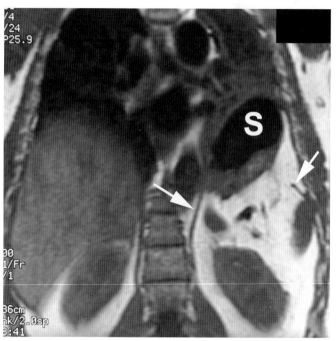

Fig. 17.43 Diaphragm rupture in a young woman after severe blunt abdominal trauma. Coronal T1-weighted MRI clearly demonstrates herniation of the stomach (S) and omental fat into the left chest. Note that the ends of the torn diaphragm (arrows) are well visualized by MRI.

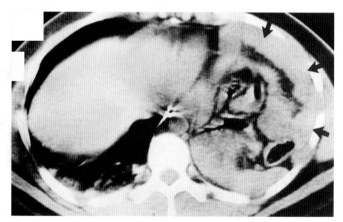

Fig. 17.42 Diaphragm rupture in a young man after severe blunt abdominal trauma. CT shows marked thickening and retraction of the ruptured left diaphragm (arrows) encircling the herniated bowel.

diaphragm and of diagnosing rupture in patients on positive pressure ventilation. Nau et al[198] reported their experience with diaphragmatic injuries (20 blunt, 11 penetrating) over a 10 year period and found that chest radiography and CT diagnosed only a minority of tears. Surprisingly, they reported no significant difference between the diagnostic sensitivity of chest radiographs and CT. However, it should be noted that neither group used the most up to date CT scanners with multiplanar reformat capabilities.[172,198] Other authors have reached different conclusions regarding the accuracy of CT. Worthy et al[196] reported findings diagnostic of rupture in nine of 11 patients. Murray et al[194] reported sensitivity of 61% and specificity 87% for diagnosis of rupture in a series of 32 patients with suspected diaphragmatic

injury. Thus, while CT is clearly not 100% sensitive, it is widely used for the evaluation of seriously injured patients and should detect the majority of diaphragmatic ruptures.[187,188] This should be particularly true with the latest generation multidetector scanners. CT has also been used in cases where the diagnosis has been delayed.[199]

MRI can be a useful adjunct to CT scanning for diagnosis of traumatic diaphragmatic injuries (Figs 17.43 and 17.44).[170,186–188,200–206] Because MRI can directly image multiple planes and identify the entire diaphragm as a distinct and separate structure, it has some advantages compared to conventional CT. Shanmuganathan et al[201] found that MRI was often more definitively positive than CT in diagnosing rupture in seven patients and also correctly excluded rupture in nine others by clearly showing total continuity of the diaphragm. However, the latest generation multidetector CT scanners with multiplanar reformatted images obviate many of the putative advantages of MRI.[185] Furthermore, it remains quite difficult to image acutely injured patients with MRI. Thus, CT remains the mainstay for diagnosis of traumatic diaphragm rupture; MRI is reserved for the more difficult cases (particularly suspected right-sided ruptures) in more stable patients.

There has been little interest in using ultrasound to diagnose traumatic rupture of the diaphragm in humans. However, animal data suggests that ultrasound can be quite sensitive for detecting ruptures.[167] Because both bowel and diaphragm are readily identifiable on ultrasound, diagnosis of visceral herniation in this setting is relatively straightforward.[181,207,208] The edges of the torn diaphragm and actual site of disruption are also frequently detected by ultrasound.[167,208]

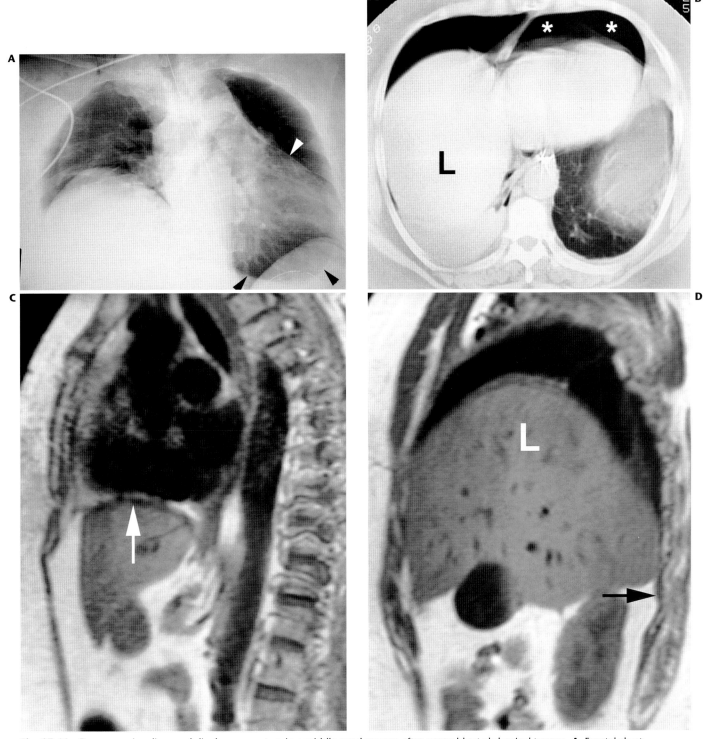

Fig. 17.44   Pneumopericardium and diaphragm rupture in a middle-aged woman after severe blunt abdominal trauma. **A**, Frontal chest radiograph shows an elevated right diaphragm, a right pneumothorax, and air in the pericardial sac (arrowheads). **B**, CT shows a large right pneumothorax and pneumopericardium (*) and suggests a ruptured right diaphragm. Liver **C** and **D**, Sagittal T1-weighted MRI shows lateral herniation of the liver (L) into the right hemithorax. Note that the diaphragm is well visualized medially (arrow on **C**) and posteriorly (arrow on **D**), but is absent over the lateral dome of the liver.

INJURY TO THE HEART OR PERICARDIUM

The heart and pericardium appear to be fairly well protected from the effects of blunt thoracic trauma injury. Cardiac and pericardial injuries due to blunt trauma, other than cardiac contusion, are uncommon. Penetrating trauma, on the other hand, is usually the result of a felonious assault, and the mortality is high (Fig. 17.45). The following injuries may be encountered following blunt chest trauma:

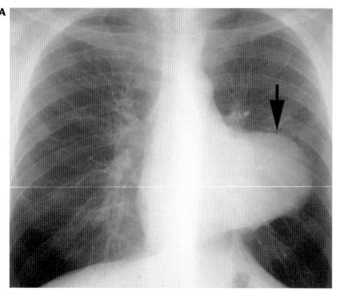
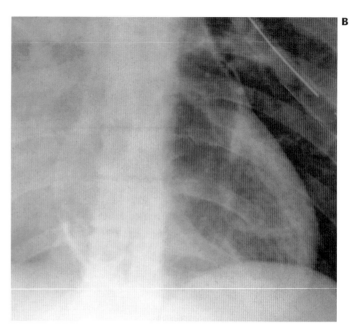

Fig. 17.45 Intracardiac air in a young man who died shortly after arrival because of a stab wound to the right chest. **A**, Frontal and **B**, coned-down chest radiographs show a large right pneumothorax, right pleural effusion, and air in the heart due to a bronchus-to-pulmonary vein fistula. Note that the intracardiac air outlines the intraventricular trabeculations, distinguishing it from pneumopericardium. L = liver. (Courtesy of Dr. P. Goodman, Durham, NC)

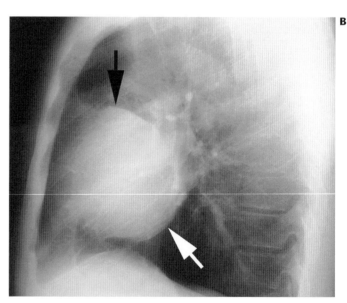

Fig. 17.46 Cardiac herniation in an asymptomatic middle-aged man after pericardial window placement for uremic pericarditis. **A**, Frontal and **B**, lateral chest radiographs show marked lateral displacement of the cardiac apex (arrows) due to herniation of the heart through the pericardial window.

- Myocardial contusion or infarction[209]
- Myocardial rupture, resulting in hemopericardium and tamponade[210,211]
- Septal rupture[212]
- True and false myocardial aneurysms[213,214]
- Coronary artery rupture, resulting in hemopericardium, false aneurysm formation, and infarction[215,216]
- Rupture of chordi tendinii, resulting in valve insufficiency (most commonly the tricuspid valve)[217,218]
- Pneumopericardium (Fig. 17.45)[219,220]

- Postpericardiectomy syndrome and constrictive pericarditis as late sequelae[221,222]
- Herniation of the heart through a pericardial tear (Fig. 17.46).[223,224]

Most of these conditions have clinical and radiologic features that are similar to their nontraumatic counterparts and are beyond the scope of this discussion. Myocardial contusion is probably the most common cardiac injury caused by blunt trauma,[213] and can cause life-threatening arrhythmias and heart failure.[209] Diagnosis is difficult, however, because symptoms are nonspecific and there are few specific tests for myocardial injury. Traditional diagnosis has rested upon the finding of electrocardiographic changes in the setting of blunt thoracic trauma. Recent studies have shown that elevated levels of cardiac troponin I and T are highly sensitive for myocardial injury.[209] Collins et al,[225] however, found that elevated troponin levels did not necessarily correlate with the clinical significance of the contusion. Radiologically, severe cardiac contusions manifest with pulmonary edema that may be misattributed to overvigorous fluid resuscitation.

Cardiac herniation through a pericardial tear is a rare but dramatic form of injury.[223,224,226–230] In the acute setting, this injury is associated with high mortality because torsion of the great vessels results in severely compromised venous return and cardiogenic shock. In the majority of described cases, the diagnosis has been made on the chest radiograph by noting the displaced and distorted cardiac contour (Fig. 17.46). Traumatic pericardial rupture with cardiac herniation has also been diagnosed using CT.[231,232] CT has also been used to diagnose traumatic ruptures of the heart itself.[210,211]

INJURY TO THE THORACIC CAGE

Some of the more important aspects of this topic as they apply to chest imaging are summarized below.

Rib fractures

Rib fractures are very common in clinical practice and most are of limited clinical significance. Occasionally, however, the fractured rib ends lacerate the pleura or lung causing bleeding or pneumothorax. Thus, the primary indication for radiography in patients with suspected rib fractures is to exclude such complications. The diligence with which the clinician works to determine the presence or absence of rib fractures depends on the particular circumstances of the case and, unfortunately, is often driven by medicolegal considerations; inevitably, significant amounts of time, money, and resources are expended with little practical result. A thorough examination of the chest with supplementary rib detail films probably requires a minimum of five films and at least 10 min of room time, when in practice a single frontal upright chest radiograph should suffice to exclude important complications. Danher et al[233] studied radiographs from over 1100 cases of chest trauma and found that only 17 patients were admitted to the hospital for reasons related exclusively to rib trauma. In only two of these cases did oblique views give additional information, and even this information was clinically inconsequential. Other authors have reached similar conclusions.[234–236]

In the absence of significant associated pain, pneumothorax or hemothorax, fractures of single ribs are usually not of major importance. However, fractures of multiple contiguous ribs can result in a flail chest deformity which has significant morbidity and mortality (Figs 17.47 and 17.48).[237–240] This injury causes

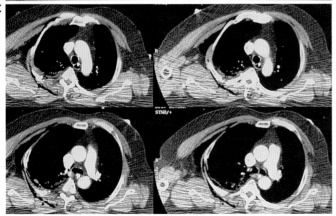

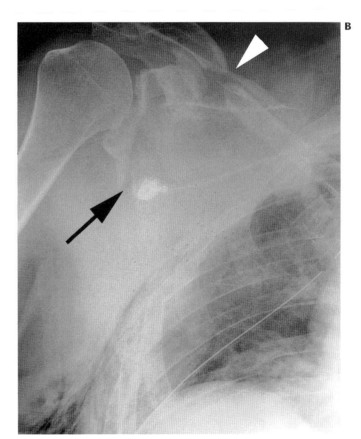

Fig. 17.47 Flail chest deformity in a middle-aged man with severe dyspnea after a motor cycle accident. **A**, Frontal and **B**, coned chest radiographs show multiple contiguous right rib fractures (arrowheads on **A**), as well as fractures of the scapula (arrow on **B**) and clavicle (arrowhead on **B**). The mediastinum is also wide. **C**, CT showed only fat in the anterior mediastinum; the aorta was normal.

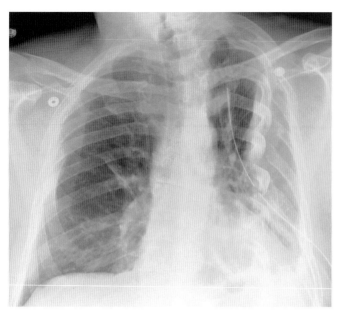

Fig. 17.48 Flail chest deformity and empyema in an elderly man after a crush injury to the left chest. Frontal chest radiograph obtained on discharge shows marked chest wall deformity with multiple contiguous rib fractures.

paradoxical retraction of the affected hemithorax during inspiration, limiting mechanical ventilation.[241] Affected patients often require ventilation and may require surgical stabilization.[238] Although the definition of flail chest varies, contiguous fractures of four or more ribs makes it a distinct clinical possibility. Thin-section CT with three-dimensional reconstructions has been used to assess the flail segment prior to surgical stabilization.[237,242]

Although rib fractures are, of themselves, often of little clinical import (except in the setting of a flail segment), the number or location of fractures can be a marker for the severity of thoracic injury.[243] This is particularly true in the setting of motor vehicle accidents. Generally speaking, the greater the number of rib fractures, the greater the likelihood of severe intrathoracic injury, morbidity, and mortality.[240] Furthermore, fractures of certain ribs indicate severe trauma and may suggest increased likelihood of injury to specific organs. For example, considerable force is required to fracture the first, second, and third ribs because they are well protected by the shoulder girdle and associated muscu-lature.[33] Patients with fractures of these ribs may be at greater risk for injury to important structures such as the aorta and great vessels.[244] Lee et al,[29] in a review of 548 patients with suspected BAI, found a higher incidence of rib fractures in patients with aortic injury than in those without. However, the positive predictive value of fractures for BAI was only 14%, a rate similar to the incidence of aortic injury at major trauma centers. They,[29] and others,[30–33] have concluded that first rib fractures seen in isolation, without other evidence for aortic or great vessel injury (e.g. mediastinal hematoma), are not a sufficient indication for angiography. Fractures of the tenth, eleventh, or twelfth ribs raise the possibility of injury to the liver, kidneys, or spleen. It should be remembered, however, that major internal thoracic injuries can occur in the absence of rib fractures, particularly in younger individuals.[245]

Rib fractures are commonly seen in children subject to physical abuse.[246,247] Indeed, the finding of occult rib fractures may be a critical clue to the fact that the child has been abused. Rib fractures are uncommon in infants and young children and, when present, should be attributable to a known episode of significant trauma.[248] Underlying conditions that may predispose to rib fractures, such as rickets or osteogenesis imperfecta, must be excluded. Rib fractures in abused children are often bilateral and at varying stages of healing. Callus formation may be prominent, a feature that makes the fractures more readily visible.

Certain rib fractures may have distinct or noteworthy features:

- *Stress fractures*. Fractures of the first or second ribs may be stress fractures as a result of activities such as backpacking. The bony reaction and callus formation may give a spurious appearance of an apical pulmonary parenchymal process. Apical lordotic and rib detail views plus the clinical circumstances should clarify the diagnosis.
- *Cough fractures*. These may also be stress fractures but occur in older patients, usually in the posterolateral aspects of the lower ribs. The patient may experience localized rib pain. Callus formation around the fractures may be conspicuous.
- *Excessive callus formation in cushingoid patients*. Patients with Cushing syndrome or who are receiving intensive steroid therapy are frequently osteoporotic and have an increased tendency to develop fractures. An interesting and characteristic feature of fractures in these patients is the exuberant callus formation that occurs in relation to the fractures.[249] This exuberant callus may simulate a pulmonary parenchymal process.
- *Multiple rib fractures in alcoholics*. Hardcore alcoholic patients frequently have multiple bilateral rib fractures in varying stages of healing.[250] Such fractures may be an indicator of other medical consequences of alcohol abuse.
- *Pseudoarthroses of ribs*. On occasion, rib fractures evolve into pseudoarthroses, since ribs are difficult to immobilize. As with stress fractures or excessive callus formation, an unwary or unobservant physician may diagnose a parenchymal lesion on chest radiographs.
- *Pathologic fractures* are clearly of the utmost clinical significance. The diagnosis hinges on identifying a fracture through a destructive process. Obtaining detailed views or tomography may be necessary to confirm the suspicion of focal bone destruction. The majority of such fractures relate to metastatic neoplasm or myeloma, but on occasion they are due to a benign process such eosinophilic granuloma.

Sternal fractures

Up to 8% of patients admitted with blunt chest trauma have sternal fractures.[251,252] These fractures cannot be seen on frontal chest radiographs and may be difficult to diagnose on lateral chest radiographs. In appropriate circumstances, careful attention should be paid to the sternal contours on the lateral view (Figs 17.49, see also Fig. 17.13). Sternal fractures as such do not generally cause problems either in healing or by direct damage to adjacent structures. Costochondral separation may occur in younger individuals and this usually also indicates significant trauma. The diagnosis of costochondral separation, however, is essentially based on clinical findings. The presence of a sternal fracture usually indicates significant chest trauma, and the radiologist should be alert to the possibility of a deceleration injury to the aorta, the great vessels, or the myocardium.[244,251–254]

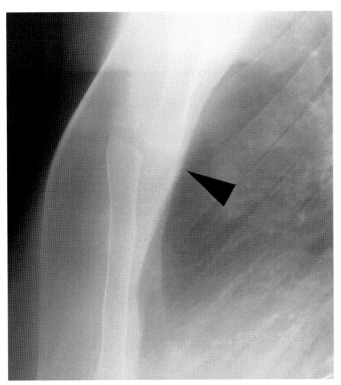

Fig. 17.49 Sternal fracture in a 47-year-old woman with chest pain. Coned view from a lateral chest radiograph shows a fracture dislocation at the sternomanubrial junction.

Sternoclavicular joint and scapula

Dislocation of the sternoclavicular joint with posterior displacement of the inner end of the clavicle may cause compression of the trachea and the adjacent great vessels with significant clinical consequences.[33,256,257] Dislocation of a sternoclavicular joint may be difficult or impossible to detect on chest radiographs, particularly in a patient with major trauma in whom the radiographic examination is restricted. However, tracheal deviation may be noted and paratracheal soft tissue thickening may be apparent. The diagnosis of dislocation of the sternoclavicular joint is readily made with CT.[258–260] Clinical awareness of the possibility of such an injury is the key factor in its recognition, with radiographs often helping to confirm the diagnosis.

Traumatic scapulothoracic dissociation occurs when the attachments of the scapula to the axial skeleton are completely disrupted by a severe rotational force placed on the shoulder.[261] It most commonly occurs in the setting of a motorcycle crash. Scapulothoracic dissociation typically results in injury to the subclavian or axillary vessels, lateral displacement of the scapula, disruption of the clavicular articulations with or without a clavicular fracture, and cervical nerve root avulsion or brachial plexus injury.[261–266] On chest radiographs, the finding of either a clavicular fracture or disruption of either the sternomanubrial or acromioclavicular joints in combination with lateral displacement of the scapula suggests scapulothoracic dissociation (Fig. 17.50).

Vertebral fractures

Fractures of the thoracic spine are not usually of much direct consequence to the respiratory system. Paravertebral hematoma adjacent to these fractures, however, may be conspicuous on the chest radiographs (Fig. 17.51, see also Fig. 17.8), and due allowance should be made when diagnosing lower lobe collapse

On the other hand, Chiu et al[255] could not find any evidence of myocardial injury in over 30 patients with sternal fracture, nor could Sturm et al[68] detect any increase in the incidence of aortic rupture in patients with sternal fracture as opposed to those without.

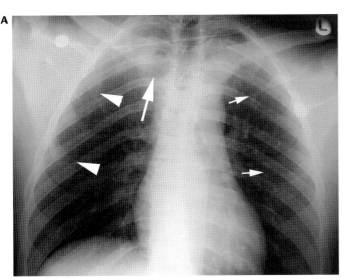

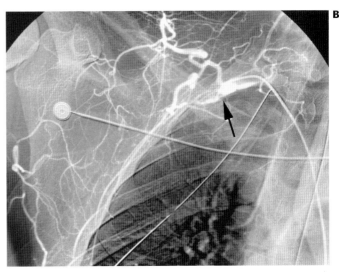

Fig. 17.50 Scapulothoracic dissociation in a 35-year-old man who presented after a motorcycle accident with a diminished right radial pulse. **A**, Frontal chest radiograph shows lateral dislocation of the right clavicle with widening of the sternoclavicular joint (large arrow). Note also that the medial scapular border (arrowheads) is laterally displaced when compared to the left (small arrows). These findings suggest scapulothoracic dissociation. **B**, Selective right subclavian arteriogram shows complete transection of the right subclavian artery (arrow) with abundant collateral vessels. The patient also sustained a significant right brachial plexus injury.

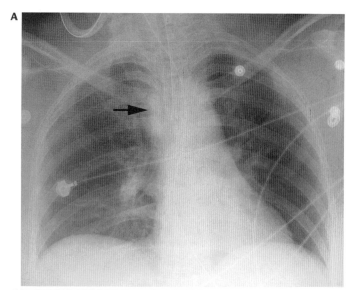

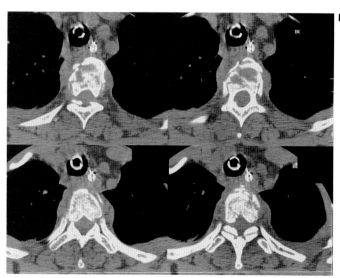

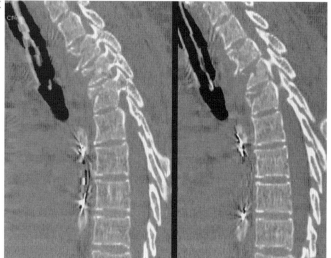

Fig. 17.51 Vertebral fractures in a 37-year-old man after a motor vehicle accident. **A**, Frontal chest radiograph shows widening of the right paratracheal stripe (arrow). **B**, CT shows comminuted vertebral body fractures and bilateral paraspinal hematomas. The aorta was normal. **C**, Sagittal reconstructions show the vertebral body fractures to better advantage.

or aortic injury.[27,267] Nevertheless, when studying the initial chest radiographs on trauma victims, it is important to study the thoracic spine with care. The signs of thoracic spine fracture may not be obvious. Lawrason et al[268] in a study of 34 patients with thoracic spine injury, found that only 18 patients (53%) were initially reported as having fractures, whereas on review fractures were seen in 27 patients (79%). The signs they reported included widening of the paraspinal reflections and apical pleural caps, decreased vertebral body height, lateral offset of vertebral bodies, increased interpediculate and interspinous distances, and rib disarticulation.

MISCELLANEOUS INJURIES

Injury due to gunshot, blast, or stab wounds

Most gunshot wounds to the lungs in civilian practice are the result of low velocity missiles. Although the missiles may fragment, the devastating fragmentation of a high velocity missile is not seen. In addition, the shock waves of low velocity missiles are not nearly so severe or extensive in their effects. The lung is a low density structure of high elasticity, and the degree of damage is much less than in high density, low elasticity structures such as liver or brain.[269] A low velocity missile traversing the lung forms a distinct track that may be air filled or occupied by hematoma (Figs 17.52 to 17.55).[270] Surrounding this track is a variable zone of lung contusion. On occasion the track itself is visible, and gauging the thickness and extent of the surrounding contusion may be possible. This observation applies particularly to cases with an air-filled track radiographed in the axis of the track. Shotgun injuries are generally severe because of the intermediate muzzle velocity of these weapons and the large mass of the shot. Shotgun injuries to the chest are said to be nearly tenfold more lethal than wounds from other weapons.[271] The pleura is inevitably involved in pulmonary damage from gunshots and thus hemothorax or pneumothorax is common. The chest radiographic appearance is a critical factor in determining whether or not the pleural space should be drained. In damage confined to the lungs and pleura, drainage may be the only direct intervention required.

Stab wounds do not generate shock waves, and the resultant contusion of lung parenchyma is less. As with gunshot wounds the significance of stab wounds relates to the extent and severity of damage to major vascular structures and the pleura or pericardium.

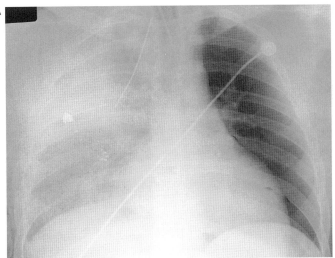

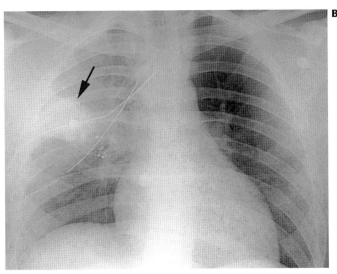

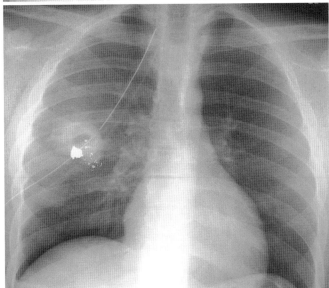

Fig. 17.52 Gunshot wound to the chest in a 19-year-old man. **A**, Initial frontal chest radiograph shows a severe right lung contusion, hemothorax, and metallic bullet fragments overlying the right chest. **B**, Radiograph obtained 4 days later shows resolution of the contusion into a focal hematoma (arrow). **C**, Radiograph obtained 3 days later shows apparent cavitation in the hematoma. This appearance is typical of a "bullet track" in the lung.

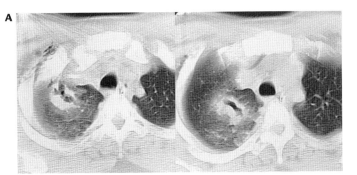

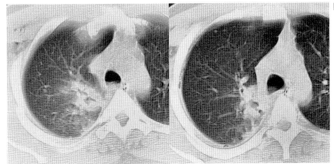

Fig. 17.53 Gunshot wound to the chest in a 21-year-old man. **A** and **B**, CT shows the typical CT appearance of a bullet track in the lung. The linear nature of the abnormality helps distinguish this lesion from other cavitary lung lesions such as abscess.

Blast injuries are relatively uncommon in civilian practice, though clearly of major significance in wartime. Cohn[108] comprehensively reviewed the subject of pulmonary contusion in blast injuries and found that pulmonary hemorrhage was the dominant pathologic finding in such cases. In described cases, the radiographic changes are typically bilateral and centered on the major airways with perihilar edema and contusion.[108,272,273]

Lung torsion

Torsion of a lung or a lobe of lung is an extremely rare but serious condition that can result from compressive trauma to the chest.[274,275] In such cases, the victim is almost invariably a child and has usually been run over by a car. In adults, torsion of the lung is usually associated with thoracic surgery, spontaneous pneumothorax or pneumothorax induced by needle biopsy, pleural effusion, or a neoplasm.[276–284] Predisposing mechanical factors include transection or underdevelopment of the inferior pulmonary ligament, the presence of complete fissures or accessory lobes, the freedom of movement allowed by pneumothoraces or pleural effusions, and the presence of a heavy mass. The condition may be more common than is realized following thoracic surgery: Wong and Goldstraw,[285] in a survey of thoracic surgeons in the United Kingdom, found that 30% of them had encountered at least one case.

Diagnosis of lung torsion is extraordinarily difficult. A key factor is awareness of the existence of this condition and the circumstances under which it occurs. The radiographic findings may be subdivided:

1. *Twisting of the airways and lung vessels.* Airway twisting may result in abrupt cut-off in the bronchus at the hilum with development of distal atelectasis. Twisting of the hilar vessels may result in hemorrhagic infarction of lung. Thus, a spectrum of lung parenchymal findings ranging from normal aeration to varying degrees of lobar or whole lung atelectasis to expansile consolidation of lung is possible. In the immediate period after thoracic surgery (when torsion is most likely to occur), the development of dense consolidation of all or part of the lung or lung remnant should raise the possibility of torsion (Fig. 17.56).
2. *Anatomic malpositioning.* By identifying malpositioning of normal anatomic structures, the radiologist can suggest the diagnosis of lung torsion prior to surgical exploration. Hilar

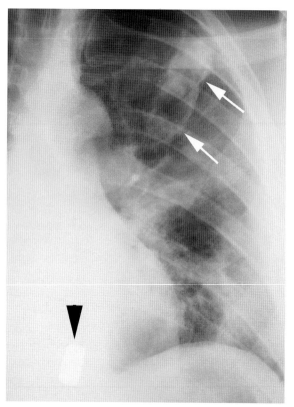

Fig. 17.54 Gunshot wound to the chest in a 28-year-old man. Frontal chest radiograph shows an oblong cavitary mass (arrows) in the left upper lobe, an appearance typical of a "bullet track". Note the position of the bullet (arrowhead).

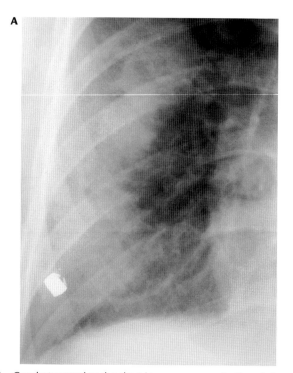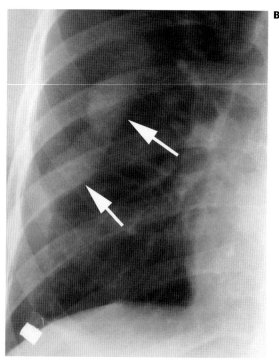

Fig. 17.55 Gunshot wound to the chest in a young man. **A,** Coned-down view from the initial frontal chest radiograph shows a heterogeneous right lung opacity consistent with contusion and a bullet fragment overlying the right lower lobe. **B,** Radiograph obtained several days later shows a residual tubular opacity (arrows) consistent with hematoma along the bullet track.

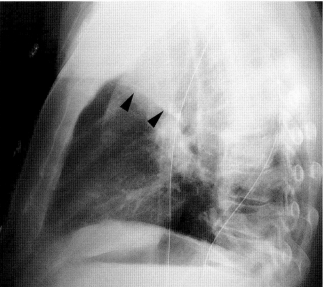

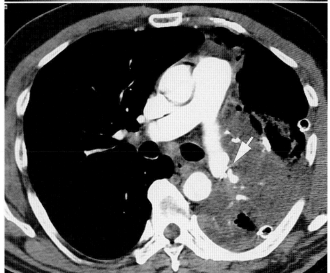

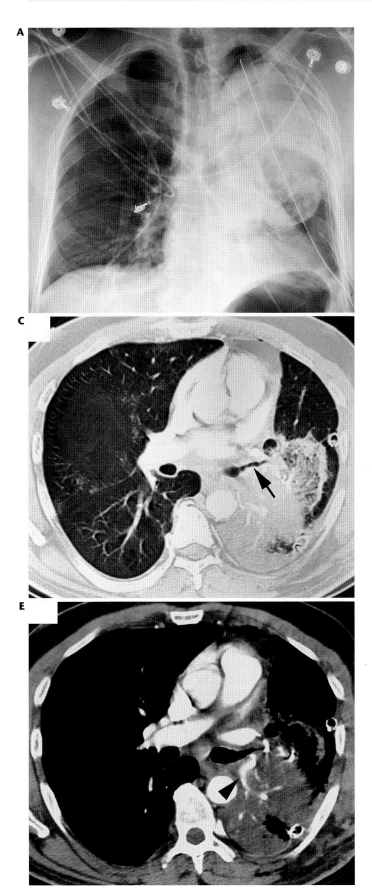

Fig. 17.56 Lung torsion in a middle-aged man with chest pain and hemoptysis 3 days after a lingular sparing left upper lobectomy for lung cancer. **A**, Frontal and **B**, lateral chest radiographs show a large homogeneous opacity in the left upper hemithorax. The fissure between the lower lobe and the lingula (arrowheads) is rotated in a clockwise fashion. **C**, CT (lung window) shows homogeneous opacification of the posteriorly displaced lingula. Note the narrowing of the bronchi (arrow). **D** and **E**, Contrast-enhanced CT (mediastinal window) shows partial vascular occlusion at the arterial stump (arrow on **D**) and unusual curvature of the lingular vessels (arrowhead on **E**). Torsion of the lingula was found at surgical exploration.

vessels or interlobar fissures may be rotated away from their normal position (Fig. 17.56). If previous films are available, an identifiable structure such as a lung nodule or surgical sutures may be shifted in position in an otherwise inexplicable fashion. CT with intravenous contrast material can be particularly useful for diagnosing torsion by demonstrating alterations in vascular orientation (Fig. 17.56).[282–284]

In summary, lung torsion should be suspected when chest radiographs show persistent atelectasis or consolidation of a lobe or lung after prior partial pulmonary resection, or in the setting of trauma or a large pneumothorax. CT can help confirm

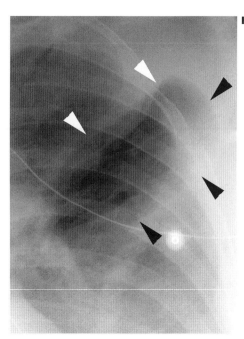

Fig. 17.57 Lung hernia in a middle-aged woman with a crepitant mass over the left upper chest after a motor vehicle accident. **A,** Frontal and **B,** coned-down chest radiographs show a well-circumscribed lucency (arrowheads on **B**) consistent with a posttraumatic lung hernia.

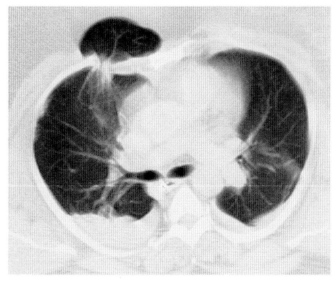

Fig. 17.58 Lung hernia in a middle-aged woman with a crepitant mass over the right upper chest after a motor vehicle accident. CT shows focal anterior lung herniation at the point of costochondral separation.

the diagnosis by demonstrating airway occlusion and alteration of normal vascular anatomy.

Lung herniation

Most lung hernias occur in the cervical region and are not associated with trauma.[286] However, intercostal lung herniation is usually the result of direct trauma or previous surgical intervention such as the placement of chest tubes or thoracotomy.[287–289] Clinically, a chest wall deformity or palpable crepitant mass may be encountered, often varying in size with respirations, coughing, or the Valsalva maneuver. Surprisingly, there are few clinical problems associated with such hernias. They are easily diagnosed by chest radiographs if they can be shown in profile. Alternatively, CT very readily shows the hernias (Figs 17.57 and 17.58).

INDIRECT EFFECTS OF TRAUMA ON THE LUNGS

Severe trauma can have indirect effects on the lungs that may severely complicate the patient's clinical course and affect outcome. Three main processes require consideration: fat embolism, ARDS, and neurogenic pulmonary edema. Only fat embolism is discussed here; the other two conditions are discussed in Chapter 7.

Fat embolism (Box 17.11)

Skeletal trauma, particularly trauma involving the pelvis and major long bones, can cause neutral fat droplets to enter the bloodstream. Presumably, these droplets enter via lacerated veins in the area of trauma, possibly aided by a rise in intraosseous pressure or by movement of bone fragments. Fat embolization is said to be less common in cases of compound or open fractures in which a rise in intraosseous pressure is less likely. Rapid immobilization of fractures, particularly by early operative fixation, decreases the incidence of fat embolization.[290] The fat droplets are typically 20–40 μm in diameter and cause occlusions in the vascular bed of the lungs and other organs. Autopsy and

Box 17.11 Fat embolism syndrome

Clinical setting
Long bone fractures
Orthopedic fixation with intramedullary rod placement
Acute decompression sickness
Pancreatitis
Alcoholism
Burns
Severe infection
Sickle cell anemia (crisis)

Clinical features (usually appear 24–72 h after trauma)
Severe dyspnea
Hypoxemia
CNS symptoms (delirium, obtundation)
Petechial skin and retinal hemorrhages

Chest radiography
Scattered or diffuse pulmonary opacities
Initially may be peripheral in nature

CT
Scattered or diffuse ground-glass opacities
May progress to consolidation
Septal thickening
Centrilobular nodules

Outcome
Usually resolves within 7–14 days (good prognosis)
May progress to acute respiratory distress syndrome (poor prognosis)

clinical studies indicate that subclinical fat embolization is much more common than is generally realized.[291–293] The term "fat embolism syndrome" is usually reserved for patients who have overt clinical findings attributable to the effects of fat embolization on the lungs and other organs such as the brain, kidneys, and skin. Fat embolization may be detected by examination of the blood and urine in as many as 90% of patients following major trauma, whereas the incidence of fat embolism syndrome in this patient group is approximately 3%.[294] The incidence of fat embolism syndrome increases with the number of long bone fractures.[295]

Trauma is the major cause of fat embolism syndrome. However, fat embolization can occur in the absence of trauma in a diverse group of conditions, including diabetes mellitus, acute decompression sickness, chronic pancreatitis, alcoholism, burns, severe infections, sickle cell disease, inhalational anesthesia, and renal infarction.[296] The origin of fat emboli in such nontraumatic cases is debated.[295,297] One theory suggests that the embolic fat is derived from circulating blood lipids and from fat mobilized from fat depots. Neutral fat in the blood is normally emulsified in the form of chylomicrons that are <1 μm in diameter. During periods of stress, chylomicrons may coalesce to form fat globules up to 40 μm in diameter and these globules may cause capillary occlusion.[296] Fat embolism due to bone marrow infarction is believed to be a major cause of acute chest syndrome in patients with sickle cell anemia.[298–301]

However, the deleterious effects of fat embolization are not simply the result of vascular occlusion by neutral fat droplets.[296,302] Hydrolysis of neutral fat by tissue lipase forms free fatty acids that have a toxic effect on the vascular endothelium and lung parenchyma. The result is endothelial damage leading to increased capillary permeability, damage to the alveolar lining cells, loss of surfactant activity, and formation of hyaline membranes. Furthermore, platelets adhere to neutral fat and intravascular coagulation may supervene. Excessive breakdown of platelets releases vasoactive amines such as serotonin and 5-hydroxytryptamine that, together with histamine released from damaged lung parenchyma and vasoactive amines released from the injury site, cause vasospasm and pulmonary capillary congestion. The biochemical and hematologic interactions, therefore, are complex but are certainly crucial to the development of the fat embolism syndrome. In rare cases acute cor pulmonale occurs within hours of an injury, attributable to a major degree of occlusion of the pulmonary vascular bed by neutral fat.[303] A latent period of 12–48 h before fat embolism syndrome occurs is much more common.[304] This latent period is explained by the time required to hydrolyze neutral fat and for the secondary vasculitis and pneumonitis to develop.

The chief clinical manifestations of fat embolism syndrome involve the lungs, central nervous system, and skin. The pulmonary manifestations are generally the first to appear and include dyspnea, tachypnea, and cyanosis that develop within 72 h of the trauma. The arterial oxygen tension decreases to 50 mmHg or less. At the same time, generalized cerebral symptoms may develop, ranging from headache and irritability to delirium, stupor, seizures, and coma. Focal neurologic signs are generally absent. Fundoscopic examination may reveal petechial retinal hemorrhages. A petechial skin rash appears in many, but not all, cases after 2–3 days. The rash is distributed over the neck and trunk.

Chest radiographic findings broadly reflect the severity of fat embolization syndrome. The chest radiograph may remain normal in mild cases. In more severe cases, radiographic findings develop after a 12–72 h latent period. The classic appearance is either that of multifocal homogeneous opacities or more diffuse heterogeneous or homogeneous opacities (pulmonary edema pattern). Pleural effusions are not a typical feature of fat embolization syndrome. On occasion, the degree of opacification becomes remarkably severe, yet clearing generally occurs in 7–14 days. On the other hand, ARDS may develop with prolongation of the clinical course and a significantly increased mortality (Fig. 17.59). Curtis et al[305] studied 30 patients with fat embolization syndrome and found that one-third developed ARDS as a consequence, and that mortality in this group was substantially higher than in the group without ARDS. Two other patients died of the effects of acute paradoxical fat embolization. The radiographic features of ARDS are discussed further on page 407.

The CT findings of fat embolism syndrome have been reported.[306–308] Arakawa et al[308] used CT to evaluate six patients with pulmonary fat embolism syndrome. They saw focal consolidation or ground-glass opacity and nodules in the upper lobes in all six patients. They also saw more diffuse ground-glass opacities in five of six patients (Fig. 17.60). They found that the extent of CT abnormalities correlated with respiratory impairment as assessed by partial pressure of oxygen (PaO_2) measurements and that follow-up CT scans showed rapid improvement in three of six patients. Malagari et al[306] reviewed thin-section CT scans in nine patients with mild fat embolism syndrome. They reported ground-glass opacities in seven

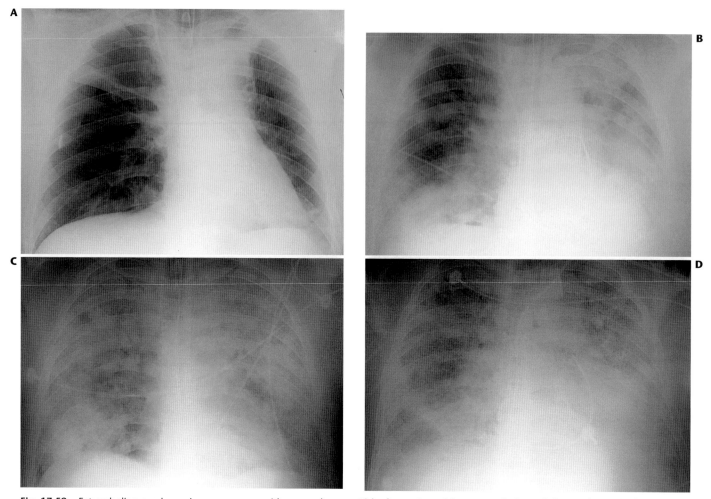

Fig. 17.59 Fat embolism syndrome in a young man with severe dyspnea 48 h after major pelvic trauma. **A,** Frontal chest radiograph obtained on admission shows minimal right upper lobe atelectasis and a wide mediastinum. The lungs are otherwise normal. CT (not shown) showed no evidence of a vascular injury. **B,** Radiograph obtained at the time of symptoms shows bilateral scattered pulmonary opacities. **C,** Radiograph obtained 2 days later shows progression to diffuse pulmonary opacities. By this time, characteristic retinal hemorrhages and a petechial skin rash were evident. **D,** Radiograph obtained 1 week later shows typical findings of acute respiratory distress syndrome. The patient eventually died of respiratory failure.

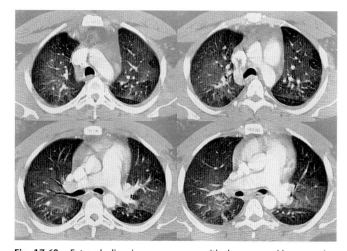

Fig. 17.60 Fat embolism in a young man with dyspnea and hypoxemia after repair of a femur fracture with an intramedullary nail. CT shows scattered nondependent ground-glass opacities, likely due to fat embolism. The patient did not develop further stigmata of fat embolism syndrome and his symptoms improved gradually over the next few days.

patients, thickened interlobular septa in five, and centrilobular nodules in two. In four, the distribution of opacities was quite patchy and geographic in nature. Follow-up CT showed resolution of opacities from 7 to 25 days posttrauma (mean 16 days). Ravenel et al[307] reported a patient with macroscopic fat emboli due to placement of an intramedullary rod. In that case, thromboemboli of fat attenuation were seen in the pulmonary arteries at CT pulmonary angiography.

Posttrauma patients who develop severe hypoxemia despite a normal or near normal chest radiograph may be referred for ventilation–perfusion scintigraphy to exclude pulmonary embolism. Ventilation is normal in patients with fat embolism syndrome. Perfusion scans, however, may show multiple peripheral subsegmental defects that give the scan a diffusely mottled appearance (Fig. 17.61).[304,309] This is quite unlike the larger and more focal defects commonly associated with bland thromboemboli.

The diagnosis of fat embolism syndrome depends on correlation of clinical features, findings on chest radiographs or CT, and laboratory results, especially the results of blood gas

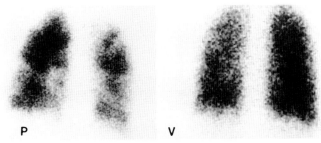

Fig. 17.61 Fat embolism in a patient with dyspnea and hypoxemia after a recent orthopedic procedure. Perfusion (P) and ventilation (V) radionuclide scans show multiple peripheral subsegmental perfusion defects suggestive of fat embolism.

analysis. The radiologic findings are not specific and can be seen in other conditions that affect traumatized patients, including pulmonary contusion, massive aspiration of gastric contents, thermal damage, toxic gas inhalation, transfusion reactions, neurogenic and other causes of pulmonary edema, and gram-negative rod bacterial sepsis. The characteristic latent period before the radiologic and clinical findings of fat embolism syndrome develop has great diagnostic importance. In many of these other conditions, clinical symptoms and radiologic abnormalities are more acute in onset. ARDS may develop in any severely traumatized patients and fat embolization as the precipitating cause may go unrecognized. Although a number of strategies to minimize the severity of fat embolism syndrome have been proposed, treatment is usually supportive.[297]

REFERENCES

1. Anderson RN. Deaths: Leading causes for 2000. National Vital Stat Rep 2000;50:1–86.
2. Wicky S, Wintermark M, Schnyder P, et al. Imaging of blunt chest trauma. Eur Radiol 2000;10:1524–1538.
3. Gavelli G, Canini R, Bertaccini P, et al. Traumatic injuries: imaging of thoracic injuries. Eur Radiol 2002;12:1273–1294.
4. Dyer DS, Moore EE, Ilke DN, et al. Thoracic aortic injury: how predictive is mechanism and is chest computed tomography a reliable screening tool? A prospective study of 1,561 patients. J Trauma 2000;48:673–682; discussion 682–683.
5. Rivas LA, Fishman JE, Munera F, et al. Multislice CT in thoracic trauma. Radiol Clin North Am 2003;41:599–616.
6. Wintermark M, Schnyder P. Imaging of patients post blunt trauma to the chest. Eur J Radiol 2002;83:123–132.
7. Dyer DS, Moore EE, Mestek MF, et al. Can chest CT be used to exclude aortic injury? Radiology 1999;213:195–202.
8. Gundry SR, Burney RE, Mackenzie JR, et al. Traumatic pseudoaneurysms of the thoracic aorta. Anatomic and radiologic correlations. Arch Surg 1984;119:1055–1060.
9. Feczko JD, Lynch L, Pless JE, et al. An autopsy case review of 142 nonpenetrating (blunt) injuries of the aorta. J Trauma 1992;33:846–849.
10. Lundell CJ, Quinn MF, Finck EJ. Traumatic laceration of the ascending aorta: angiographic assessment. AJR Am J Roentgenol 1985;145:715–719.
11. Rabinsky I, Sidhu GS, Wagner RB. Mid-descending aortic traumatic aneurysms. Ann Thorac Surg 1990;50:155–160.
12. Cohen AM, Crass JR, Thomas HA, et al. CT evidence for the "osseous pinch" mechanism of traumatic aortic injury. AJR Am J Roentgenol 1992;159:271–274.
13. Crass JR, Cohen AM, Motta AO, et al. A proposed new mechanism of traumatic aortic rupture: the osseous pinch. Radiology 1990;176:645–649.
14. Javadpour H, O'Toole JJ, McEniff JN, et al. Traumatic aortic transection: evidence for the osseous pinch mechanism. Ann Thorac Surg 2002;73:951–953.
15. Mirvis SE, Bidwell JK, Buddemeyer EU, et al. Imaging diagnosis of traumatic aortic rupture. A review and experience at a major trauma center. Invest Radiol 1987;22:187–196.
16. Sefczek DM, Sefczek RJ, Deeb ZL. Radiographic signs of acute traumatic rupture of the thoracic aorta. AJR Am J Roentgenol 1983;141:1259–1262.
17. Woodring JH. The normal mediastinum in blunt traumatic rupture of the thoracic aorta and brachiocephalic arteries. J Emerg Med 1990;8:467–476.
18. Williams S, Burney RE, MacKenzie JR, et al. Indications for aortography. Radiography after blunt chest trauma: a reassessment of the radiographic findings associated with traumatic rupture of the aorta. Invest Radiol 1983;18:230–237.
19. Marsh DG, Sturm JT. Traumatic aortic rupture: roentgenographic indications for angiography. Ann Thorac Surg 1976;21:337–340.
20. Seltzer SE, D'Orsi C, Kirshner R, et al. Traumatic aortic rupture: plain radiographic findings. AJR Am J Roentgenol 1981;137:1011–1014.
21. Fisher RG, Chasen MH, Lamki N. Diagnosis of injuries of the aorta and brachiocephalic arteries caused by blunt chest trauma: CT vs aortography. AJR Am J Roentgenol 1994;162:1047–1052.
22. Mirvis SE, Bidwell JK, Buddemeyer EU, et al. Value of chest radiography in excluding traumatic aortic rupture. Radiology 1987;163:487–493.
23. Marnocha KE, Maglinte DD. Plain-film criteria for excluding aortic rupture in blunt chest trauma. AJR Am J Roentgenol 1985;144:19–21.
24. Gerlock AJ Jr, Muhletaler CA, Coulam CM, et al. Traumatic aortic aneurysm: validity of esophageal tube displacement sign. AJR Am J Roentgenol 1980;135:713–718.
25. Tisnado J, Tsai FY, Als A, et al. A new radiographic sign of acute traumatic rupture of the thoracic aorta: displacement of the nasogastric tube to the right. Radiology 1977;125:603–608.
26. Peters DR, Gamsu G. Displacement of the right paraspinous interface: a radiographic sign of acute traumatic rupture of the thoracic aorta. Radiology 1980;134:599–603.
27. Dennis LN, Rogers LF. Superior mediastinal widening from spine fractures mimicking aortic rupture on chest radiographs. AJR Am J Roentgenol 1989;152:27–30.
28. Simeone JF, Deren MM, Cagle F. The value of the left apical cap in the diagnosis of aortic rupture: a prospective and retrospective study. Radiology 1981;139:35–37.
29. Lee J, Harris JH Jr, Duke JH Jr, et al. Noncorrelation between thoracic skeletal injuries and acute traumatic aortic tear. J Trauma 1997;43:400–404.
30. Fisher RG, Ward RE, Ben-Menachem Y, et al. Arteriography and the fractured first rib: too much for too little? AJR Am J Roentgenol 1982;138:1059–1062.
31. Poole GV. Fracture of the upper ribs and injury to the great vessels. Surg Gynecol Obstet 1989;169:275–282.
32. Woodring JH, Fried AM, Hatfield DR, et al. Fractures of first and second ribs: predictive value for arterial and bronchial injury. AJR Am J Roentgenol 1982;138:211–215.
33. Gupta A, Jamshidi M, Rubin JR. Traumatic first rib fracture: is angiography necessary? A review of 730 cases. Cardiovasc Surg 1997;5:48–53.

34. Fabian TC, Richardson JD, Croce MA, et al. Prospective study of blunt aortic injury: Multicenter Trial of the American Association for the Surgery of Trauma. J Trauma 1997;42:374–380; discussion 380–383.

35. Fabian TC, Davis KA, Gavant ML, et al. Prospective study of blunt aortic injury: helical CT is diagnostic and antihypertensive therapy reduces rupture. Ann Surg 1998;227:666–676; discussion 676–677.

36. Fishman JE, Nunez D Jr, Kane A, et al. Direct versus indirect signs of traumatic aortic injury revealed by helical CT: performance characteristics and interobserver agreement. AJR Am J Roentgenol 1999;172:1027–1031.

37. Fishman JE. Imaging of blunt aortic and great vessel trauma. J Thorac Imaging 2000;15:97–103.

38. Parker MS, Matheson TL, Rao AV, et al. Making the transition: the role of helical CT in the evaluation of potentially acute thoracic aortic injuries. AJR Am J Roentgenol 2001;176:1267–1272.

39. Cleverley JR, Barrie JR, Raymond GS, et al. Direct findings of aortic injury on contrast-enhanced CT in surgically proven traumatic aortic injury: a multi-centre review. Clin Radiol 2002;57:281–286.

40. Wicky S, Capasso P, Meuli R, et al. Spiral CT aortography: an efficient technique for the diagnosis of traumatic aortic injury. Eur Radiol 1998;8:828–833.

41. Scaglione M, Pinto A, Pinto F, et al. Role of contrast-enhanced helical CT in the evaluation of acute thoracic aortic injuries after blunt chest trauma. Eur Radiol 2001;11:2444–2448.

42. Wintermark M, Wicky S, Schnyder P. Imaging of acute traumatic injuries of the thoracic aorta. Eur Radiol 2002;12:431–442.

43. Gavant ML, Flick P, Menke P, et al. CT aortography of thoracic aortic rupture. AJR Am J Roentgenol 1996;166:955–961.

44. Madayag MA, Kirshenbaum KJ, Nadimpalli SR, et al. Thoracic aortic trauma: role of dynamic CT. Radiology 1991;179:853–855.

45. Agee CK, Metzler MH, Churchill RJ, et al. Computed tomographic evaluation to exclude traumatic aortic disruption. J Trauma 1992;33:876–881.

46. Gavant ML, Menke PG, Fabian T, et al. Blunt traumatic aortic rupture: detection with helical CT of the chest. Radiology 1995;197:125–133.

47. Harris JH, Horowitz DR, Zelitt DL. Unenhanced dynamic mediastinal computed tomography in the selection of patients requiring thoracic aortography for the detection of acute traumatic aortic injury. Emerg Radiol 1995;2:67–76.

48. Hollerman JJ. A rational approach for imaging of blunt thoracic trauma to exclude aortic injury. Emerg Radiol 1994;4:206–208.

49. Mirvis SE, Kostrubiak I, Whitley NO, et al. Role of CT in excluding major arterial injury after blunt thoracic trauma. AJR Am J Roentgenol 1987;149:601–605.

50. Morgan PW, Goodman LR, Aprahamian C, et al. Evaluation of traumatic aortic injury: does dynamic contrast-enhanced CT play a role? Radiology 1992;182:661–666.

51. Raptopoulos V, Sheiman RG, Phillips DA, et al. Traumatic aortic tear: screening with chest CT. Radiology 1992;182:667–673.

52. Richardson P, Mirvis SE, Scorpio R, et al. Value of CT in determining the need for angiography when findings of mediastinal hemorrhage on chest radiographs are equivocal. AJR Am J Roentgenol 1991;156:273–279.

53. Schnyder P, Chapuis L, Mayor B, et al. Helical CT angiography for traumatic aortic rupture: correlation with aortography and surgery in five cases. J Thorac Imaging 1996;11:39–45.

54. Trerotola SO. Can helical CT replace aortography in thoracic trauma. Radiology 1995;197:13–15.

55. Chung JW, Park JH, Im JG, et al. Spiral CT angiography of the thoracic aorta. RadioGraphics 1996;16:811–824.

56. Quint LE, Francis IR, Williams DM, et al. Evaluation of thoracic aortic disease with the use of helical CT and multiplanar reconstructions: comparison with surgical findings. Radiology 1996;201:37–41.

57. Downing SW, Sperling JS, Mirvis SE, et al. Experience with spiral computed tomography as the sole diagnostic method for traumatic aortic rupture. Ann Thorac Surg 2001;72:495–501; discussion 501–502.

58. Chen MY, Regan JD, D'Amore MJ, et al. Role of angiography in the detection of aortic branch vessel injury after blunt thoracic trauma. J Trauma 2001;51:1166–1171; discussion 1172.

59. Pate JW, Gavant ML, Weiman DS, et al. Traumatic rupture of the aortic isthmus: program of selective management. World J Surg 1999;23:59–63.

60. Gavant ML. Helical CT grading of traumatic aortic injuries. Impact on clinical guidelines for medical and surgical management. Radiol Clin North Am 1999;37:553–574.

61. Malhotra AK, Fabian TC, Croce MA, et al. Minimal aortic injury: a lesion associated with advancing diagnostic techniques. J Trauma 2001;51:1042–1048.

62. Durham RM, Zuckerman D, Wolverson M, et al. Computed tomography as a screening exam in patients with suspected blunt aortic injury. Ann Surg 1994;220:699–704.

63. Wills JS, Lally JF. Use of CT for evaluation of possible traumatic aortic injury. AJR Am J Roentgenol 1991;157:1123–1125.

64. McLean TR, Olinger GN, Thorsen MK. Computed tomography in the evaluation of the aorta in patients sustaining blunt chest trauma. J Trauma 1991;31:254–256.

65. Miller FB, Richardson JD, Thomas HA, et al. Role of CT in diagnosis of major arterial injury after blunt thoracic trauma. Surgery 1989;106:596–602; discussion 602–603.

66. Hunink MG, Bos JJ. Triage of patients to angiography for detection of aortic rupture after blunt chest trauma: cost-effectiveness analysis of using CT. AJR Am J Roentgenol 1995;165:27–36.

67. Mirvis SE, Shanmuganathan K, Miller BH, et al. Traumatic aortic injury: diagnosis with contrast-enhanced thoracic CT – five-year experience at a major trauma center. Radiology 1996;200:413–422.

68. Sturm JT, Luxenberg MG, Moudry BM, et al. Does sternal fracture increase the risk for aortic rupture? Ann Thorac Surg 1989;48:697–698.

69. Raptopoulos V. Chest CT for aortic injury: maybe not for everyone. AJR Am J Roentgenol 1994;162:1053–1055.

70. Mirvis SE, Pais SO, Shanmuganathan K. Atypical results of thoracic aortography performed to exclude aortic injury. Emerg Radiol 1994;1:24–31.

71. Morse SS, Glickman MG, Greenwood LH, et al. Traumatic aortic rupture: false-positive aortographic diagnosis due to atypical ductus diverticulum. AJR Am J Roentgenol 1988;150:793–796.

72. Fisher RG, Sanchez-Torres M, Thomas JW, et al. Subtle or atypical injuries of the thoracic aorta and brachiocephalic vessels in blunt thoracic trauma. RadioGraphics 1997;17:835–849.

73. Brooks SW, Cmolik BL, Young JC, et al. Transesophageal echocardiographic examination of a patient with traumatic aortic transection from blunt chest trauma: a case report. J Trauma 1991;31:841–845.

74. Davis GA, Sauerisen S, Chandrasekaran K, et al. Subclinical traumatic aortic injury diagnosed by transesophageal echocardiography. Am Heart J 1992;123:534–536.

75. Goarin JP, Le Bret F, Riou B, Jacquens Y, et al. Early diagnosis of traumatic thoracic aortic rupture by transesophageal echocardiography. Chest 1993;103:618–620.

76. Shapiro MJ, Yanofsky SD, Trapp J, et al. Cardiovascular evaluation in blunt thoracic trauma using transesophageal echocardiography (TEE). J Trauma 1991;31:835–839; discussion 839–840.

77. Sparks MB, Burchard KW, Marrin CA, et al. Transesophageal echocardiography. Preliminary results in patients with

traumatic aortic rupture. Arch Surg 1991;126:711–713; discussion 713–714.

78. Vignon P, Lagrange P, Boncoeur MP, et al. Routine transesophageal echocardiography for the diagnosis of aortic disruption in trauma patients without enlarged mediastinum. J Trauma 1996;40:422–427.

79. Goarin JP, Cluzel P, Gosgnach M, et al. Evaluation of transesophageal echocardiography for diagnosis of traumatic aortic injury. Anesthesiology 2000;93:1373–1377.

80. Patel NH, Hahn D, Comess KA. Blunt chest trauma victims: role of intravascular ultrasound and transesophageal echocardiography in cases of abnormal thoracic aortogram. J Trauma 2003;55:330–337.

81. Lee DE, Arslan B, Queiroz R, et al. Assessment of inter- and intraobserver agreement between intravascular US and aortic angiography of thoracic aortic injury. Radiology 2003;227:434–439.

82. Vignon P, Lang RM. Use of Transesophageal Echocardiography for the Assessment of Traumatic Aortic Injuries. Echocardiography 1999;16: 207–219.

83. Goarin JP, Catoire P, Jacquens Y, et al. Use of transesophageal echocardiography for diagnosis of traumatic aortic injury. Chest 1997;112:71–80.

84. Smith MD, Cassidy JM, Souther S, et al. Transesophageal echocardiography in the diagnosis of traumatic rupture of the aorta. N Engl J Med 1995;332:356–362.

85. Buckmaster MJ, Kearney PA, Johnson SB, et al. Further experience with transesophageal echocardiography in the evaluation of thoracic aortic injury. J Trauma 1994;37:989–995.

86. Saletta S, Lederman E, Fein S, et al. Transesophageal echocardiography for the initial evaluation of the widened mediastinum in trauma patients. J Trauma 1995;39:137–141; discussion 141–142.

87. Minard G, Schurr MJ, Croce MA, et al. A prospective analysis of transesophageal echocardiography in the diagnosis of traumatic disruption of the aorta. J Trauma 1996;40:225–230.

88. Ahrar K, Smith DC, Bansal RC, et al. Angiography in blunt thoracic aortic injury. J Trauma 1997;42:665–669.

89. Williams DM, Simon HJ, Marx MV, et al. Acute traumatic aortic rupture: intravascular US findings. Radiology 1992;182:247–249.

90. Hughes JP, Ruttley MS, Musumeci F. Case report: traumatic aortic rupture: demonstration by magnetic resonance imaging. Br J Radiol 1994;67:1264–1267.

91. Cohn SM, Pollak JS, McCarthy S, et al. Detection of aortic tear in the acute trauma patient using MRI. Magn Reson Imaging 1994;12:963–967.

92. Nakanishi T, Hata R, Tamura A, et al. Breath-hold gadolinium-enhanced three-dimensional MR thoracic aortography: higher spatial resolution imaging with phased-array coil and three-dimensional surface display. Hiroshima J Med Sci 2000;49:129–133.

93. Nienaber CA, Fattori R. Aortic diseases – do we need MR techniques? Herz 2000;25:331–341.

94. Pretre R, Chilcott M, Murith N, et al. Blunt injury to the supra-aortic arteries. Br J Surg 1997;84:603–609.

95. Nunnink L. Blunt carotid artery injury. Emerg Med (Fremantle) 2002;14:412–421.

96. Chomel A, Vernet M, Lile A, et al. Traumatic bilateral dissections of the internal carotid artery: an infrequent diagnosis not to be missed. J Neurosurg Anesthesiol 2002;14:309–312.

97. Stover S, Holtzman RB, Lottenberg L, et al. Blunt innominate artery injury. Am Surg 2001;67:757–759.

98. Klein S, Munshi IA, Engelman D, et al. Innominate artery transection secondary to blunt trauma. J Trauma 2003;54:202.

99. Karkos CD, Thomson GJ. Combined subclavian artery and brachial plexus injury following blunt trauma to the shoulder. Injury 1998;29:395–396.

100. Cox CS Jr, Allen GS, Fischer RP, et al. Blunt versus penetrating subclavian artery injury: presentation, injury pattern, and outcome. J Trauma 1999;46:445–449.

101. Katras T, Baltazar U, Rush DS, et al. Subclavian arterial injury associated with blunt trauma. Vasc Surg 2001;35:43–50.

102. Anastasiadis K, Channon KM, Ratnatunga C. Traumatic innominate artery transection. J Cardiovasc Surg (Torino) 2002;43:697–700.

103. Donaldson B, Ngo-Nonga B. Traumatic pseudoaneurysm of the pulmonary artery: case report and review of the literature. Am Surg 2002;68:414–416.

104. Kanani N, Ting P, Weber B, et al. Blunt trauma resulting in systemic arterial and pulmonary artery injury: case report. Can Assoc Radiol J 2002;53:141–143.

105. Hawkins ML, Carraway RP, Ross SE, et al. Pulmonary artery disruption from blunt thoracic trauma. Am Surg 1988;54:148–152.

106. Weltman DI, Baykal A, Zhang D. CT diagnosis of laceration of the main pulmonary artery after blunt trauma. AJR Am J Roentgenol 1999;173: 1361–1362.

107. Ambrose G, Barrett LO, Angus GL, et al. Main pulmonary artery laceration after blunt trauma: accurate preoperative diagnosis. Ann Thorac Surg 2000;70:955–957.

108. Cohn SM. Pulmonary contusion: review of the clinical entity. J Trauma 1997;42: 973–979.

109. Wagner RB, Crawford WO Jr, Schimpf PP. Classification of parenchymal injuries of the lung. Radiology 1988;167:77–82.

110. Blostein PA, Hodgman CG. Computed tomography of the chest in blunt thoracic trauma: results of a prospective study. J Trauma 1997;43:13–18.

111. Donnelly LF, Klosterman LA. Subpleural sparing: a CT finding of lung contusion in children. Radiology 1997;204:385–387.

112. Guerrero-Lopez F, Vazquez-Mata G, Alcazar-Romero PP, et al. Evaluation of the utility of computed tomography in the initial assessment of the critical care patient with chest trauma. Crit Care Med 2000;28:1370–1375.

113. Miller PR, Croce MA, Bee TK, et al. ARDS after pulmonary contusion: accurate measurement of contusion volume identifies high-risk patients. J Trauma 2001;51:223–228; discussion 229–230.

114. Schild HH, Strunk H, Weber W, et al. Pulmonary contusion: CT vs plain radiograms. J Comput Assist Tomogr 1989;13:417–420.

115. Athanassiadi K, Gerazounis M, Kalantzi N, et al. Primary traumatic pulmonary pseudocysts: a rare entity. Eur J Cardiothorac Surg 2003;23:43–45.

116. Takahashi N, Murakami J, Murayama S, et al. MR evaluation of intrapulmonary hematoma. J Comput Assist Tomogr 1995;19:125–127.

117. Chiles C, Ravin CE. Radiographic recognition of pneumothorax in the intensive care unit. Crit Care Med 1986;14:677–680.

118. Ziter FM Jr, Westcott JL. Supine subpulmonary pneumothorax. AJR Am J Roentgenol 1981;137:699–701.

119. Gordon R. The deep sulcus sign. Radiology 1980;136:25–27.

120. Wall SD, Federle MP, Jeffrey RB, et al. CT diagnosis of unsuspected pneumothorax after blunt abdominal trauma. AJR Am J Roentgenol 1983;141:919–921.

121. McGonigal MD, Schwab CW, Kauder DR, et al. Supplemental emergent chest computed tomography in the management of blunt torso trauma. J Trauma 1990;30:1431–1434; discussion 1434–1435.

122. Tocino IM, Miller MH, Frederick PR, et al. CT detection of occult pneumothorax in head trauma. AJR Am J Roentgenol 1984;143:987–990.

123. Holmes JF, Brant WE, Bogren HG, et al. Prevalence and importance of pneumothoraces visualized on abdominal computed tomographic scan in children with blunt trauma. J Trauma 2001;50:516–520.

124. Wolfman NT, Myers WS, Glauser SJ, et al. Validity of CT classification on management of occult pneumothorax: a

prospective study. AJR Am J Roentgenol 1998;171:1317–1320.

125. Rollins RJ, Tocino I. Early radiographic signs of tracheal rupture. AJR Am J Roentgenol 1987;148:695–698.

126. Wintermark M, Schnyder P, Wicky S. Blunt traumatic rupture of a mainstem bronchus: spiral CT demonstration of the "fallen lung" sign. Eur Radiol 2001;11:409–411.

127. Guest JLJr, Anderson JN. Major airway injury in closed chest trauma. Chest 1977;72:63–66.

128. Harvey-Smith W, Bush W, Northrop C. Traumatic bronchial rupture. AJR Am J Roentgenol 1980;134:1189–1193.

129. Lotz PR, Martel W, Rohwedder JJ, et al. Significance of pneumomediastinum in blunt trauma to the thorax. AJR Am J Roentgenol 1979;132:817–819.

130. Mahboubi S, O'Hara AE. Bronchial rupture in children following blunt chest trauma. Report of five cases with emphasis on radiologic findings. Pediatr Radiol 1981;10:133–138.

131. Chesterman JT, Satsangi PN. Rupture of the trachea and bronchi by closed injury. Thorax 1966;21:21–27.

132. Hood RM, Sloan HE. Injuries of the trachea and major bronchi. J Thorac Cardiovasc Surg 1959;38:458–480.

133. Taskinen SO, Salo JA, Halttunen PE, et al. Tracheobronchial rupture due to blunt chest trauma: a follow-up study. Ann Thorac Surg 1989;48:846–849.

134. Unger JM, Schuchmann GG, Grossman JE, et al. Tears of the trachea and main bronchi caused by blunt trauma: radiologic findings. AJR Am J Roentgenol 1989;153:1175–1180.

135. Stark P. Imaging of tracheobronchial injuries. J Thorac Imaging 1995;10:206–219.

136. Oh KS, Fleischner FG, Wyman SM. Characteristic pulmonary finding in traumatic complete transection of a main-stem bronchus. Radiology 1969;92:371–372 passim.

137. Hartley C, Morritt GN. Bronchial rupture secondary to blunt chest trauma. Thorax 1993;48:183–184.

138. Millham FH, Rajii-Khorasani A, Birkett DF, et al. Carinal injury: diagnosis and treatment – case report. J Trauma 1991;31:1420–1422.

139. Rao PM, Novelline RA, Dobbins JM. The spherical endotracheal tube cuff: a plain radiographic sign of tracheal injury. Emerg Radiol 1996;3:87–90.

140. Chen JD, Shanmuganathan K, Mirvis SE, et al. Using CT to diagnose tracheal rupture. AJR Am J Roentgenol 2001;176:1273–1280.

141. Wan YL, Tsai KT, Yeow KM, et al. CT findings of bronchial transection. Am J Emerg Med 1997;15:176–177.

142. Tack D, Defrance P, Delcour C, et al. The CT fallen-lung sign. Eur Radiol 2000;10:719–721.

143. Epelman M, Ofer A, Klein Y, et al. CT diagnosis of traumatic bronchial rupture in children. Pediatr Radiol 2002;32:888–891.

144. Kunisch-Hoppe M, Hoppe M, Rauber K, et al. Tracheal rupture caused by blunt chest trauma: radiological and clinical features. Eur Radiol 2000;10:480–483.

145. Karmy-Jones R, Avansino J, Stern EJ. CT of blunt tracheal rupture. AJR Am J Roentgenol 2003;180:1670.

146. Nakamori Y, Hayakata T, Fujimi S, et al. Tracheal rupture diagnosed with virtual bronchoscopy and managed nonoperatively: a case report. J Trauma 2002;53:369–371.

147. Marom EM, Goodman PC, McAdams HP. Focal abnormalities of the trachea and main bronchi. AJR Am J Roentgenol 2001;176:707–711.

148. Weiman DS, Walker WA, Brosnan KM, et al. Noniatrogenic esophageal trauma. Ann Thorac Surg 1995;59:845–849; discussion 849–850.

149. Beal SL, Pottmeyer EW, Spisso JM. Esophageal perforation following external blunt trauma. J Trauma 1988;28:1425–1432.

150. Bladergroen MR, Lowe JE, Postlethwait RW. Diagnosis and recommended management of esophageal perforation and rupture. Ann Thorac Surg 1986;42:235–239.

151. Cordero JA, Kuehler DH, Fortune JB. Distal esophageal rupture after external blunt trauma: report of two cases. J Trauma 1997;42:321–322.

152. Micon L, Geis L, Siderys H, et al. Rupture of the distal thoracic esophagus following blunt trauma: case report. J Trauma 1990;30:214–217.

153. Vallieres E, Shamji FM, Todd TR. Postpneumonectomy chylothorax. Ann Thorac Surg 1993;55:1006–1008.

154. Guzman AE, Rossi L, Witte CL, et al. Traumatic injury of the thoracic duct. Lymphology 2002;35:4–14.

155. Dulchavsky SA, Ledgerwood AM, Lucas CE. Management of chylothorax after blunt chest trauma. J Trauma 1988;28:1400–1401.

156. Perusse KR, McAdams HP, Earls JP, et al. General case of the day. Posttraumatic thoracic lymphocele. RadioGraphics 1994;14:192–195.

157. Allen SJ, Koch SM, Tonnesen AS, et al. Tracheal compression caused by traumatic thoracic duct leak. Chest 1994;106:296–297.

158. Hom M, Jolles H. Traumatic mediastinal lymphocele mimicking other thoracic injuries: case report. J Thorac Imaging 1992;7:78–80.

159. Worthington MG, de Groot M, Gunning AJ, et al. Isolated thoracic duct injury after penetrating chest trauma. Ann Thorac Surg 1995;60:272–274.

160. Silen ML, Weber TR. Management of thoracic duct injury associated with fracture-dislocation of the spine following blunt trauma. J Trauma 1995;39:1185–1187.

161. Sachs PB, Zelch MG, Rice TW, et al. Diagnosis and localization of laceration of the thoracic duct: usefulness of lymphangiography and CT. AJR Am J Roentgenol 1991;157:703–705.

162. Aronchick JM, Epstein DM, Gefter WB, et al. Chronic traumatic diaphragmatic hernia: the significance of pleural effusion. Radiology 1988;168:675–678.

163. Mueller CF, Pendarvis RW. Traumatic injury of the diaphragm: report of seven cases and extensive literature review. Emerg Radiol 1994;1:118–132.

164. Demetriades D, Kakoyiannis S, Parekh D, et al. Penetrating injuries of the diaphragm. Br J Surg 1988;75:824–826.

165. Morgan AS, Flancbaum L, Esposito T, et al. Blunt injury to the diaphragm: an analysis of 44 patients. J Trauma 1986;26:565–568.

166. Rodriguez-Morales G, Rodriguez A, Shatney CH. Acute rupture of the diaphragm in blunt trauma: analysis of 60 patients. J Trauma 1986;26:438–444.

167. Simpson J, Lobo DN, Shah AB, et al. Traumatic diaphragmatic rupture: associated injuries and outcome. Ann R Coll Surg Engl 2000;82:97–100.

168. Boulanger BR, Milzman DP, Rosati C, et al. A comparison of right and left blunt traumatic diaphragmatic rupture. J Trauma 1993;35:255–260.

169. Rizoli SB, Brenneman FD, Boulanger BR, et al. Blunt diaphragmatic and thoracic aortic rupture: an emerging injury complex. Ann Thorac Surg 1994;58:1404–1408.

170. Gelman R, Mirvis SE, Gens D. Diaphragmatic rupture due to blunt trauma: sensitivity of plain chest radiographs. AJR Am J Roentgenol 1991;156:51–57.

171. Arendrup HC, Jensen BS. Traumatic rupture of the diaphragm. Surg Gynecol Obstet 1982;154:526–530.

172. Shapiro MJ, Heiberg E, Durham RM, et al. The unreliability of CT scans and initial chest radiographs in evaluating blunt trauma induced diaphragmatic rupture. Clin Radiol 1996;51:27–30.

173. Shah R, Sabanathan S, Mearns AJ, et al. Traumatic rupture of diaphragm. Ann Thorac Surg 1995;60:1444–1449.

174. Beal SL, McKennan M. Blunt diaphragm rupture. A morbid injury. Arch Surg 1988;123:828–832.

175. Baron B, Daffner RH. Traumatic rupture of the right hemidiaphragm: diagnosis by chest radiography. Emerg Radiol 1994;1:231–235.

176. Ball T, McCrory R, Smith JO, et al. Traumatic diaphragmatic hernia: errors in diagnosis. AJR Am J Roentgenol 1982;138:633–637.

177. Perlman SJ, Rogers LF, Mintzer RA. Abnormal course of nasogastric tube in traumatic rupture of left diaphragm. AJR Am J Roentgenol 1985;142:85–88.

178. McHugh K, Ogilvie BC, Brunton FJ. Delayed presentation of traumatic diaphragmatic hernia. Clin Radiol 1991;43:246–250.

179. Schulman A, van Gelderen F. Bowel herniation through the torn diaphragm: I. Gastric herniation. Abdom Imaging 1996;21:395–399.

180. Schulman A, van Gelderen F. Bowel herniation through the torn diaphragm: II. Intestinal herniation. Abdom Imaging 1996;21:400–403.

181. Somers JM, Gleeson FV, Flower CD. Rupture of the right hemidiaphragm following blunt trauma: the use of ultrasound in diagnosis. Clin Radiol 1990;42:97–101.

182. Allbery SM, Swischuk LE, John SD. Post traumatic pneumatoceles mimicking disphragmatic hernia. Emerg Radiol 1997:94–96.

183. Hoy JF, Shortsleeve MJ. Diagnosis of diaphragmatic rupture utilizing spiral computed tomographic reconstruction. Emerg Radiol 1997;4:127–128.

184. Israel RS, Mayberry JC, Primack SL. Diaphragmatic rupture: use of helical CT scanning with multiplanar reformations. AJR Am J Roentgenol 1996;167:1201–1203.

185. Israel RS, McDaniel PA, Primack SL, et al. Diagnosis of diaphragmatic trauma with helical CT in a swine model. AJR Am J Roentgenol 1996;167:637–641.

186. Pomerantz SM, Shanmuganathan K, Siegel EL. Liver herniation through an occult diaphragmatic injury presenting as a solitary pulmonary nodule: value of helical computed tomography and magnetic resonance imaging. Emerg Radiol 1996;3:205–208.

187. Shanmuganathan K, Killeen K, Mirvis SE, et al. Imaging of diaphragmatic injuries. J Thorac Imaging 2000;15:104–111.

188. Iochum S, Ludig T, Walter F, et al. Imaging of diaphragmatic injury: a diagnostic challenge? RadioGraphics 2002;22 Spec No:S103–116; discussion S116–118.

189. Holland DG, Quint LE. Traumatic rupture of the diaphragm without visceral herniation: CT diagnosis. AJR Am J Roentgenol 1991;157:17–18.

190. Demos TC, Solomon C, Posniak HV, et al. Computed tomography in traumatic defects of the diaphragm. Clin Imaging 1989;13:62–67.

191. Catasca JV, Siegel MJ. Posttraumatic diaphragmatic herniation: CT findings in two children. Pediatr Radiol 1995; 25:262–264.

192. Heiberg E, Wolverson MK, Hurd RN, et al. CT recognition of traumatic rupture of the diaphragm. AJR Am J Roentgenol 1980;135:369–372.

193. McCarroll KA, Weintraub J. Traumatic intrapericardial diaphragmatic hernia. Emerg Radiol 1995;2:376–379.

194. Murray JG, Caoili E, Gruden JF, et al, Mackersie RC. Acute rupture of the diaphragm due to blunt trauma: diagnostic sensitivity and specificity of CT. AJR Am J Roentgenol 1996;166:1035–1039.

195. Toombs BD, Sandler CM, Lester RG. Computed tomography of chest trauma. Radiology 1981;140:733–738.

196. Worthy SA, Kang EY, Hartman TE, et al. Diaphragmatic rupture: CT findings in 11 patients. Radiology 1995;194:885–888.

197. Bergin D, Ennis R, Keogh C, et al. The "dependent viscera" sign in CT diagnosis of blunt traumatic diaphragmatic rupture. AJR Am J Roentgenol 2001;177:1137–1140.

198. Nau T, Seitz H, Mousavi M, et al. The diagnostic dilemma of traumatic rupture of the diaphragm. Surg Endosc 2001;15:992–996.

199. Gurney J, Harrison WL, Anderson JC. Omental fat simulating pleural fluid in traumatic diaphragmatic hernia: CT characteristics. J Comput Assist Tomogr 1985;9:1112–1114.

200. Mirvis SE, Shanmuganathan K. MR imaging of thoracic trauma. Magn Reson Imaging Clin N Am 2000;8:91–104.

201. Shanmuganathan K, Mirvis SE, White CS, et al. MR imaging evaluation of hemidiaphragms in acute blunt trauma: experience with 16 patients. AJR Am J Roentgenol 1996;167:397–402.

202. Boulanger BR, Mirvis SE, Rodriguez A. Magnetic resonance imaging in traumatic diaphragmatic rupture: case reports. J Trauma 1992;32:89–93.

203. Carter EA, Cleverley JR, Delany DJ, et al. Case report: cine MRI in the diagnosis of a ruptured right hemidiaphragm. Clin Radiol 1996;51:137–140.

204. Daum-Kowalski R, Shanley DJ, Murphy T. MRI diagnosis of delayed presentation of traumatic diaphragmatic hernia. Gastrointest Radiol 1991;16:298–300.

205. Lawrason JN, Novelline RA, Rhea JT. The magnetic resonance diagnosis of diaphragmatic rupture: a report of two cases. Emerg Radiol 1996;3:137–141.

206. Mirvis SE, Keramati B, Buckman R, et al. MR imaging of traumatic diaphragmatic rupture. J Comput Assist Tomogr 1988;12:147–149.

207. Ammann AM, Brewer WH, Maull KI, et al. Traumatic rupture of the diaphragm: real-time sonographic diagnosis. AJR Am J Roentgenol 1983;140:915–916.

208. Kim HH, Shin YR, Kim KJ, et al. Blunt traumatic rupture of the diaphragm: sonographic diagnosis. J Ultrasound Med 1997;16:593–598.

209. Sybrandy KC, Cramer MJ, Burgersdijk C. Diagnosing cardiac contusion: old wisdom and new insights. Heart 2003;89:485–489.

210. Sliker CW, Mirvis SE, Shanmuganathan K, et al. Blunt cardiac rupture: value of contrast-enhanced spiral CT. Clin Radiol 2000;55:805–808.

211. Wintermark M, Delabays A, Bettex D, et al. Blunt trauma of the heart: CT pattern of atrial appendage ruptures. Eur Radiol 2001;11:113–116.

212. Amorim MJ, Almeida J, Santos A, et al. Atrioventricular septal defect following blunt chest trauma. Eur J Cardiothorac Surg 1999;16:679–682.

213. RuDusky BM. Myocardial contusion culminating in a ruptured pseudoaneurysm of the left ventricle – a case report. Angiology 2003;54:359–362.

214. Moen J, Hansen W, Chandrasekaran K, et al. Traumatic aneurysm and pseudoaneurysm of the right ventricle: a diagnosis by echocardiography. J Am Soc Echocardiogr 2002;15:1025–1026.

215. Sugimoto S, Yamauchi A, Kudoh K, et al. A successfully treated case of blunt traumatic right coronary ostium rupture. Ann Thorac Surg 2003;75:1001–1003.

216. Straub A, Beierlein W, Kuttner A, et al. Isolated coronary artery rupture after blunt chest trauma. Thorac Cardiovasc Surg 2003;51:97–98.

217. Dounis G, Matsakas E, Poularas J, et al. Traumatic tricuspid insufficiency: a case report with a review of the literature. Eur J Emerg Med 2002;9:258–261.

218. van Son JA, Danielson GK, Schaff HV, et al. Traumatic tricuspid valve insufficiency. Experience in thirteen patients. J Thorac Cardiovasc Surg 1994;108:893–898.

219. Roth TC, Schmid RA. Pneumopericardium after blunt chest trauma: a sign of severe injury? J Thorac Cardiovasc Surg 2002;124:630–631.

220. Gould JC, Schurr MA. Tension pneumopericardium after blunt chest trauma. Ann Thorac Surg 2001;72:1728–1730.

221. Loughlin V, Murphy A, Russell C. The post-pericardiotomy syndrome and penetrating injury of the chest. Injury 1987;18:412–414.

222. Rashid MA, Wikstrom T, Ortenwall P. Cardiac injuries: a ten-year experience. Eur J Surg 2000;166:18–21.

223. Janson JT, Harris DG, Pretorius J, et al. Pericardial rupture and cardiac herniation after blunt chest trauma. Ann Thorac Surg 2003;75:581–582.

224. Sharma OP. Pericardio-diaphragmatic rupture: five new cases and literature review. J Emerg Med 1999;17:963–968.

225. Collins JN, Cole FJ, Weireter LJ, et al. The usefulness of serum troponin levels in evaluating cardiac injury. Am Surg 2001;67:821–825; discussion 825–826.

226. Carrillo EH, Heniford BT, Dykes JR, et al. Cardiac herniation producing tamponade: the critical role of early diagnosis. J Trauma 1997;43:19–23.

227. Fulda G, Brathwaite CE, Rodriguez A, et al. Blunt traumatic rupture of the heart and pericardium: a ten-year experience (1979–1989). J Trauma 1991;31:167–172; discussion 172–173.

228. Kermond AJ. The dislocated heart: an unusual complication of major chest injury. Radiology 1976;119:59–60.

229. Furusawa T, Fukaya Y, Amano J. Herniation of the heart due to traumatic rupture of the pericardium. Eur J Cardiothorac Surg 2000;17:752–753.

230. De Amicis V, Rossi M, Monaco M, et al. Right luxation of the heart after pericardial rupture caused by blunt trauma. Tex Heart Inst J 2003;30:140–142.

231. Kirsch JD, Escarous A. CT diagnosis of traumatic pericardium rupture. J Comput Assist Tomogr 1989;13:523–524.

232. Place RJ, Cavanaugh DG. Computed tomography to diagnose pericardial rupture. J Trauma 1995;38:822–823.

233. Danher J, Eyes BE, Kumar K. Oblique rib views after blunt chest trauma: an unnecessary routine? Br Med J (Clin Res Ed) 1984;289:1271.

234. DeLuca SA, Rhea JT, O'Malley TO. Radiographic evaluation of rib fractures. AJR Am J Roentgenol 1982;138: 91–92.

235. Thompson BM, Finger W, Tonsfeldt D, et al. Rib radiographs for trauma: useful or wasteful? Ann Emerg Med 1986;15: 261–265.

236. Verma SM, Hawkins HH, Colglazier S. The clinical utility of rib detail films in the evaluation of trauma. Emerg Radiol 1995;2:264–266.

237. Liman ST, Kuzucu A, Tastepe AI, Ulasan GN, Topcu S. Chest injury due to blunt trauma. Eur J Cardiothorac Surg 2003;23:374–378.

238. Tanaka H, Yukioka T, Yamaguti Y, et al. Surgical stabilization of internal pneumatic stabilization? A prospective randomized study of management of severe flail chest patients. J Trauma 2002;52:727–732.

239. Velmahos GC, Vassiliu P, Chan LS, et al. Influence of flail chest on outcome among patients with severe thoracic cage trauma. Int Surg 2002;87:240–244.

240. Sirmali M, Turut H, Topcu S, et al. A comprehensive analysis of traumatic rib fractures: morbidity, mortality and management. Eur J Cardiothorac Surg 2003;24:133–138.

241. Laghi F, Tobin MJ. Disorders of the respiratory muscles. Am J Respir Crit Care Med 2003;168:10–48.

242. Weyant MJ, Bleier JI, Naama H, et al. Severe crushed chest injury with large flail segment: computed tomographic three-dimensional reconstruction. J Trauma 2002;52:605.

243. Ziegler DW, Agarwal NN. The morbidity and mortality of rib fractures. J Trauma 1994;37:975–979.

244. Ben-Menachem Y. Avulsion of the innominate artery associated with fracture of the sternum. AJR Am J Roentgenol 1988;150:621–622.

245. Vyas PK, Sivit CJ. Imaging of blunt pediatric thoracic trauma. Emerg Radiol 1997;4:16–25.

246. Kleinman PK. Bony thoracic trauma. In: Kleinman PK, ed. Diagnostic imaging of child abuse, 2nd edn. New York: Mosby, 1998.

247. Lonergan GJ, Baker AM, Morey MK, et al. From the archives of the AFIP. Child abuse: radiologic-pathologic correlation. RadioGraphics 2003;23:811–845.

248. Garcia VF, Gotschall CS, Eichelberger MR, et al. Rib fractures in children: a marker of severe trauma. J Trauma 1990;30:695–700.

249. Resnick D. Disorders of other endocrine glands and of pregnancy. In: Resnick D, Niwayama G, eds. Diagnosis of bone and joint disorders. Philadelphia: WB Saunders, 1988.

250. Lindsell DR, Wilson AG, Maxwell JD. Fractures on the chest radiograph in detection of alcoholic liver disease. Br Med J (Clin Res Ed) 1982;285: 597–599.

251. Harley DP, Mena I. Cardiac and vascular sequelae of sternal fractures. J Trauma 1986;26:553–555.

252. Potaris K, Gakidis J, Mihos P, et al. Management of sternal fractures: 239 cases. Asian Cardiovasc Thorac Ann 2002;10:145–149.

253. Athanassiadi K, Gerazounis M, Moustardas M, et al. Sternal fractures: retrospective analysis of 100 cases. World J Surg 2002;26:1243–1246.

254. Rashid MA, Ortenwall P, Wikstrom T. Cardiovascular injuries associated with sternal fractures. Eur J Surg 2001;167: 243–248.

255. Chiu WC, D'Amelio LF, Hammond JS. Sternal fractures in blunt chest trauma: a practical algorithm for management. Am J Emerg Med 1997;15:252–255.

256. Gazak S, Davidson SJ. Posterior sternoclavicular dislocations: two case reports. J Trauma 1984;24:80–82.

257. Hidalgo Ovejero AM, Garcia Mata S, Sanchez Villares JJ, et al. Posterior sternoclavicular dislocation. Report of two cases. Acta Orthop Belg 2003;69:188–192.

258. Brooks AP, Olson LK. Computed tomography of the chest in the trauma patient. Clin Radiol 1989;40:127–132.

259. Ernberg LA, Potter HG. Radiographic evaluation of the acromioclavicular and sternoclavicular joints. Clin Sports Med 2003;22:255–275.

260. Burnstein MI, Pozniak MA. Computed tomography with stress maneuver to demonstrate sternoclavicular joint dislocation. J Comput Assist Tomogr 1990;14:159–160.

261. Clements RH, Reisser JR. Scapulothoracic dissociation: a devastating injury. J Trauma 1996;40:146–149.

262. Oreck SL, Burgess A, Levine AM. Traumatic lateral displacement of the scapula: a radiographic sign of neurovascular disruption. J Bone Joint Surg Am 1984;66:758–763.

263. Lange RH, Noel SH. Traumatic lateral scapular displacement: an expanded spectrum of associated neurovascular injury. J Orthop Trauma 1993;7:361–366.

264. Tsai DW, Swiontkowski MF, Kottra CL. A case of sternoclavicular dislocation with scapulothoracic dissociation. AJR Am J Roentgenol 1996;167:332.

265. Katsamouris AN, Kafetzakis A, Kostas T, et al. The initial management of scapulothoracic dissociation: a challenging task for the vascular surgeon. Eur J Vasc Endovasc Surg 2002;24:547–549.

266. Damschen DD, Cogbill TH, Siegel MJ. Scapulothoracic dissociation caused by blunt trauma. J Trauma 1997;42:537–540.

267. Woodring JH, Lee C, Jenkins K. Spinal fractures in blunt chest trauma. J Trauma 1988;28:789–793.

268. Lawrason JN, Novelline RA, Rhea JT. Early detection of thoracic spine fracture in multiple trauma patient: role of the initial portable chest radiograph. Emerg Radiol 1997;4:309–319.

269. Hollerman JJ, Fackler ML, Coldwell DM, et al. Gunshot wounds: 1. Bullets, ballistics, and mechanisms of injury. AJR Am J Roentgenol 1990;155:685–690.

270. George PY, Goodman P. Radiographic appearance of bullet tracks in the lung. AJR Am J Roentgenol 1992;159:967–970.

271. Shafer N, Wilkenfeld M, Shafer R. Gunshot wounds. Leg Med 1982:1–19.

272. Martin N, Bollaert PE, Bauer P, et al. 2 case reports of pulmonary blast injuries. Cah Anesthesiol 1987;35:133–137.

273. Williams JR, Stembridge VA. Pulmonary contusion secondary to nonpenetrating chest trauma. AJR Am J Roentgenol 1964;91:284–290.

274. Felson B. Lung torsion: radiographic findings in nine cases. Radiology 1987;162:631–638.

275. Selmonosky CA, Flege JB Jr, Ehrenhaft JL. Torsion of a lobe of the lung due to blunt thoracic trauma. Ann Thorac Surg 1967;4:166–170.

276. Graham RJ, Heyd RL, Raval VA, et al. Lung torsion after percutaneous needle biopsy of lung. AJR Am J Roentgenol 1992;159:35–37.

277. Moser ES Jr, Proto AV. Lung torsion: case report and literature review. Radiology 1987;162:639–643.

278. Munk PL, Vellet AD, Zwirewich C. Torsion of the upper lobe of the lung after surgery: findings on pulmonary angiography. AJR Am J Roentgenol 1991;157:471–472.

279. Andresen R, Meyer DR, Kniffert T, et al. Lung torsion – a rare postoperative complication. A case report. Acta Radiol 1997;38:243–245.

280. Chan MC, Scott JM, Mercer CD, et al. Intraoperative whole-lung torsion producing pulmonary venous infarction. Ann Thorac Surg 1994;57:1330–1331.

281. Fogarty JP, Dudek G. An unusual case of lung torsion. Chest 1995;108:575–578.

282. Gilkeson RC, Lange P, Kirby TJ. Lung torsion after lung transplantation: evaluation with helical CT. AJR Am J Roentgenol 2000;174:1341–1343.

283. Spizarny DL, Shetty PC, Lewis JW Jr. Lung torsion: preoperative diagnosis with angiography and computed tomography. J Thorac Imaging 1998;13:42–44.

284. Trotter MC, McFadden PM, Ochsner JL. Spontaneous torsion of the right lung: a case report. Am Surg 1995;61:306–309.

285. Wong PS, Goldstraw P. Pulmonary torsion: a questionnaire survey and a survey of the literature. Ann Thorac Surg 1992;54:286–288.

286. McAdams HP, Gordon DS, White CS. Apical lung hernia: radiologic findings in six cases. AJR Am J Roentgenol 1996;167:927–930.

287. Bhalla M, Leitman BS, Forcade C, et al. Lung hernia: radiographic features. AJR Am J Roentgenol 1990;154:51–53.

288. Sadler MA, Shapiro RS, Wagreich J, et al. CT diagnosis of acquired intercostal lung herniation. Clin Imaging 1997;21:104–106.

289. Seibel DG, Hopper KD, Ghaed N. Mammographic and CT detection of extrathoracic lung herniation. J Comput Assist Tomogr 1987;11:537–538.

290. Riska EB, Myllynen P. Fat embolism in patients with multiple injuries. J Trauma 1982;22:891–894.

291. Chan KM, Tham KT, Chiu HS, et al. Post-traumatic fat embolism – its clinical and subclinical presentations. J Trauma 1984;24:45–49.

292. McCarthy B, Mammen E, Leblanc LP, et al. Subclinical fat embolism: a prospective study of 50 patients with extremity fractures. J Trauma 1973;13:9–16.

293. Palmovic V, McCarroll JR. Fat embolism in trauma. Arch Pathol 1965;80:630–635.

294. Feldman F, Ellis K, Green WM. The fat embolism syndrome. Radiology 1975;114:535–542.

295. Parisi DM, Koval K, Egol K. Fat embolism syndrome. Am J Orthop 2002;31:507–512.

296. Batra P. The fat embolism syndrome. J Thorac Imaging 1987;2:12–17.

297. Mellor A, Soni N. Fat embolism. Anaesthesia 2001;56:145–154.

298. Vichinsky EP, Neumayr LD, Earles AN, et al. Causes and outcomes of the acute chest syndrome in sickle cell disease. National Acute Chest Syndrome Study Group. N Engl J Med 2000;342:1855–1865.

299. Maitre B, Habibi A, Roudot-Thoraval F, et al. Acute chest syndrome in adults with sickle cell disease. Chest 2000;117:1386–1392.

300. Platt OS. The acute chest syndrome of sickle cell disease. N Engl J Med 2000;342:1904–1907.

301. Rucknagel DL. The role of rib infarcts in the acute chest syndrome of sickle cell diseases. Pediatr Pathol Mol Med 2001;20:137–154.

302. Alho A. Fat embolism syndrome: etiology, pathogenesis and treatment. Acta Chir Scand Suppl 1980;499:75–85.

303. Mayron R, Ruiz E, Mestitz ST, et al. Tissue-fat pulmonary embolism occurring in a patient with a severe pelvic fracture. J Emerg Med 1985;2:251–256.

304. Williams AG Jr, Mettler FA Jr, Christie JH, et al. Fat embolism syndrome. Clin Nucl Med 1986;11:495–497.

305. Curtis AM, Knowles GD, Putman CE, et al. The three syndromes of fat embolism: pulmonary manifestations. Yale J Biol Med 1979;52:149–157.

306. Malagari K, Economopoulos N, Stoupis C, et al. High-resolution CT findings in mild pulmonary fat embolism. Chest 2003;123:1196–1201.

307. Ravenel JG, Heyneman LE, McAdams HP. Computed tomography diagnosis of macroscopic pulmonary fat embolism. J Thorac Imaging 2002;17:154–156.

308. Arakawa H, Kurihara Y, Nakajima Y. Pulmonary fat embolism syndrome: CT findings in six patients. J Comput Assist Tomogr 2000;24:24–29.

309. Park HM, Ducret RP, Brindley DC. Pulmonary imaging in fat embolism syndrome. Clin Nucl Med 1986;11:521–522.

Index

Note: Figures, Tables and Boxes are indicated by *italic page numbers*; acronyms: "CT" = "computed tomography"; "HRCT" = "high-resolution computed tomography"; "MRI" = " magnetic resonance imaging"